P9-CEY-344

Exercise Physiology

Energy, Nutrition, and Human Performance

FIFTH EDITION

Exercise Physiology

Energy, Nutrition, and Human Performance

FIFTH EDITION

LIPPINCOTT WILLIAMS & WILKINS
A **Wolters Kluwer** Company
Philadelphia • Baltimore • New York • London
Buenos Aires • Hong Kong • Sydney • Tokyo

William D. McArdle
Professor Emeritus, Department of Family, Nutrition,
and Exercise Science
Queens College of the City of New York
Flushing, New York

Frank I. Katch
Professor, Department of Exercise Science
University of Massachusetts
Amherst, Massachusetts

Victor L. Katch
Professor, Division of Kinesiology
Department of Movement Science
Associate Professor, Pediatrics
University of Michigan
Ann Arbor, Michigan

Editor: Pete Darcy
Managing Editor: Karen Gulliver
Marketing Manager: Christen DeMarco
Production Editor: Lisa JC Franko
Compositor: Graphic World
Printer: RR Donnelley & Sons

351 West Camden Street
Baltimore, Maryland 21201-2436 USA

530 Walnut Street
Philadelphia, Pennsylvania 19106 USA

Printed in the United States of America.

First Edition, 1981; Second Edition, 1986; Third Edition, 1991; Fourth Edition, 1996

Library of Congress Cataloging-in-Publication Data

McArdle, William D.
Exercise physiology : energy, nutrition, and human performance / William D. McArdle, Frank I. Katch, Victor L. Katch.—5th ed.
p. ; cm.
Includes bibliographical references and index.
ISBN 0-7817-2544-5
1. Exercise—Physiological aspects. I. Katch, Frank I. II. Katch, Victor L. III. Title.
[DNLM: 1. Exercise—physiology. 2. Nutrition. 3. Sports Medicine. QT 260 M478e 2001]
QP301 .M375 2001
612′.044—dc21

2001029473

To purchase additional copies of this book, call our customer service department at **(800) 638-3030** or fax orders to **(301) 824-7390.** International customers should call **(301) 714-2324.**

Visit Lippincott Williams & Wilkins on the Internet: http://www.LWW.com. Lippincott Williams & Wilkins customer service representatives are available from 8:30 am to 6:00 pm, EST. Also visit the ancillary website for this text on the internet at http://connection.LWW.com/go/mcardle

02 03 04 05
2 3 4 5 6 7 8 9 10

Dedicated to our wonderful families with Love.

To the many dedicated pioneer physicians and scientists worldwide who nurtured the development of exercise physiology, and to the cadre of past and current students and researchers whose contributions have elevated the field to the respectable status it so richly deserves.

We also dedicate this edition to that special group of former students who earned doctoral degrees in physical education and exercise science, and who have gone on to distinguish themselves as teachers and researchers in the related areas of exercise physiology. These include Denise Agin, Doug Ballor, Dan Becque, George Brooks, Barbara Campaigne, Ed Chaloupka, Ken Cohen, Edward Coyle, Dan Delio, Julia Chase Delio, Chris Dunbar, Patti Freedson, Roger Glaser, Ellen Glickman, Kati Haltiwinger, Everett Harmon, Jay Hoffman, Tibor Hortobagyi, Mitch Kanter, Betsy Keller, Jie Kang, Marliese Kimmerly, George Lesmes, Steve Lichtman, Charles Marks, Karen Nau-White, Laurel Traeger-Mackinnon, Robert Mofatt, Steve Ostrove, James Rimmer, Deborah Rinaldi, Stan Sady, Lapros Sidossis, Bob Spina, John Spring, Bill Thorland, Mike Toner, Lorraine Turcotte, John Villanacci, Jonnis Vrabis, Nancy Wessinger, Stephen Westing, Art Weltman, Anthony Wilcox, and Linda Zwiren.

Finally, a sincere "thank you" to our former professors and cherished colleagues who had a profound influence on our personal and professional development: the late Albert Behnke and Franklin Henry, Jerry Ball, David Benson, John Faulkner, Don Fleming, Guido Foglia, Ernest Michael, Jr., Henry Montoye, George Q. Rich III, Bob Salmons, and Earl Wallis. Without the encouragement, stimulation, and example of these mentors, none of this would have been possible.

Preface

We revised the fourth edition of *Exercise Physiology: Energy, Nutrition, and Human Performance* by incorporating into each topic area considerable new information from the expanding literature in exercise physiology, and adding two new chapters that deal with spaceflight physiology and molecular biology, content areas that we believe will become significant within exercise physiology early in the 21st century. This fifth edition maintains the same seven-section structure as previous editions.

SHAPING THE REVISION

In preparing the fifth edition of this text, we incorporated feedback gathered by the publisher and comments from instructors and students. This feedback guided us to specific areas that needed to be reworked, repositioned, updated, or streamlined.

Significant revisions to the fifth edition include more than 60 new topic headings within the different chapters including:

1. Women scientists and their contributions to exercise physiology (Introduction)
2. Metabolic syndrome X (Chapter 1)
3. Female athlete triad; hyponatremia and exercise (Chapter 2)
4. Extreme ultraendurance sports; glycemic index and exercise nutrition; oral rehydration solutions; high-fat versus low-fat diets for endurance training and performance (Chapter 3)
5. Doubly labeled water to assess energy expenditure (Chapter 8)
6. Delta efficiency in exercise (Chapter 10)
7. Prediction of $\dot{V}O_{2max}$ from non-exercise data (Chapter 11)
8. Exercise implications of gender differences in static and dynamic lung function (Chapter 12)
9. Racial differences in blood lactate threshold (Chapter 14)
10. Venous system as an active vasculature (Chapter 15)
11. Autoregulation of tissue blood flow by nitric oxide (Chapter 16)
12. Muscular force and power comparisons within the animal kingdom (Chapter 18)
13. Expanded information on diabetes mellitus including: insulin-like growth factors; cellular glucose transporters; tests and classifications for diabetes; physical activity and type 2 diabetes risk (Chapter 20)
14. Current fitness guidelines and recommendations for improving cardiovascular fitness, muscular strength, and joint flexibility; tapering for peak performance; expanded discussion of the overtraining syndrome (Chapter 21)
15. Therapeutic benefits of resistance training in HIV; resistance training guidelines for sedentary adults, the elderly, and cardiac patients; expanded information about plyometric training; current thinking on muscle cell remodeling with training (Chapter 22)
16. Supplementation with DHEA, HMB, androstenedione, creatine, chromium, and amino acids and carbohydrate-protein-lipid combinations to enhance performance or augment training responsiveness (Chapter 23)
17. Clothing insulation (clo) and factors affecting a clothing's clo value; exogenous glycerol and thermoregulation (Chapter 25)
18. Sport diving that includes diving history; diving reflex in humans; clothing ensembles; mixed-gas diving (saturation diving, helium-oxygen and trimix diving); technical diving; energy cost of underwater swimming (Chapter 26)
19. New standards for overweight and obese for children and adults; racial and physique adjustments to predict body composition; applicability of BIA in sports and exercise training; BOD POD assessment of body composition (Chapter 28)
20. BMI trends among less-skilled younger athletes; body dimensions of National Basketball Association professional players (Chapter 29)
21. The obesity epidemic; racial factors and body weight; obesity and health risks in childhood and adolescence; aging, exercise, and body composition; National Weight Control Registry; weight loss and improved health risks; exercise training effects on body weight and composition; appropriate weight gain for athletes (Chapter 30)
22. Population age trends; the new gerontology; healthy life expectancy; resistance training for the elderly; endocrine changes with aging; changes in physical activity and improved health outlook; vulnerable plaque and myocardial infarction; homocysteine and CHD; dietary fiber, insulin, and CHD (Chapter 31)
23. Clinical aspects of exercise physiology—regular exercise and hypertension, exercise-induced bronchospasm, the heart transplant patient's responses and adaptations to regular exercise, and exercise stress testing for CHD screening and exercise prescription; training and certification programs for exercise physiologists; blood pressure classification and risk stratification; treatment and rehabilitation in congestive heart failure; worksite health/fitness promotion (Chapter 32)

NEW TO THE FIFTH EDITION

Chapter 27. Microgravity: Exercise Physiology at the Final Frontier

This new chapter begins with an historical overview of early and recent accomplishments in space exploration, including a timeline from Project Mercury to the International Space Station. It explores the nature of the physiologic and anatomic challenges imposed by acute and chronic exposure to a near–zero-g environment and upon return to Earth's gravitational field. An important consideration focuses on the most effective countermeasures to obliterate the negative impact on humans of future, extended-duration missions.

On the Horizon: Molecular Biology—A New Vista for Exercise Physiology

The decision to add the molecular biology content area posed a unique dilemma. Most professors in the exercise physiology field have limited background and formal research experience in genetics and molecular biology. During their graduate preparation, these fields were literally in their infancy with little opportunity for coursework and laboratory training. We empathize with instructors who may feel uncomfortable including this new material as a "must read," perhaps from trepidation about a domain requiring mastery of a new vocabulary. To some extent, this was our reason for placing the material at the end of the textbook. Also, this area does not currently comprise a "standard" component in preparing students in exercise physiology, but rather represents an emerging component of our field that hopefully will soon become commonplace as other traditional content areas. A review of the current literature makes clear that exercise physiology and molecular biology have become undeniably linked by studies concerning the molecular basis of exercise, training responses, body weight and size regulation, injury prevention and rehabilitation, and health-related consequences of physical *inactivity*. Clearly, the topic of molecular biology and human sports performance has already become mainstream for dicussion in exercise physiology, including the lay press (front page *New York Times*, "Someday Soon, Athletic Edge May Be From Altered Genes," May 11, 2001; see listing, Molecular Biology Internet Sites)

In the September, 2000 issue of *Scientific American*, Dr. Bengt Saltin, a premier scientist in our field and featured in an *Up-Close and Personal* interview, coauthored a cover story about gene therapy's significant potential to impact athletic performance. The researchers' poignant concluding statement focused on a fictitious runner in the 2012 Olympic Games who allowed gene therapy to "boost" his muscle cells' force-generating capacity a year before the Games were to begin. The doctor assured the athlete there would be no side effects of the genetic treatment to "express" fast contracting myosin IIb isoform fibers. In the semi-finals, the athlete had lowered the world record to an unbelievable 8.94 seconds, finishing 10 meters ahead of the next competitor. Then, in the finals, . . .

> . . . at 65 meters, far out in front of the field, he feels a sudden twinge in his hamstring. At 80 meters the twinge explodes into overwhelming pain as he pulls his hamstring muscle. A tenth of a second later his patella tendon pulls out part of the tibia bone, which then snaps, and the entire quadriceps shoots up along the femur bone. The runner crumples to the ground his running career over. That is not the scenario that generally springs to mind in connection with the words "genetically engineered superathlete." And some athletes will probably manage to exploit engineered genes while avoiding catastrophe. But it is clear that as genetic technologies begin trickling into the mainstreams of medicine they will change sports profoundly—and not for the better. As a society, we will have to ask ourselves whether new records and other athletic triumphs really are a simple continuation of the age-old quest to show what our species can do."

For non-human athletes, as for example the racing thoroughbred horse, breeders have been carefully mating "select" stallions and mares for hundreds of years to develop blood lines they believe produce genetically superior animals (bigger, stronger, and faster). The same techniques used to study the human genome are now being applied to unravel the complexities of the horse genome (www.uky.edu/Ag/Horsemap/). Teams of equine molecular geneticists worldwide are attempting to unravel the horse's genetic markers on their 32 pairs of chromosomes that code for "athletic potential." The aim, similar to that for human athletes described in the *Scientific American* article, seeks to eventually improve racing performance, while at the same time develop strategies to eliminate debilitating equine diseases that can trigger career-ending injuries (e.g., hyperkalemic periodic paralysis [HYPP], severe combined immunodeficiency [SCID], exercise-induced pulmonary hemorrhage or "bleeding"). As in champion human sprinters (Olympic caliber), champion throroughbreds (Triple Crown caliber) have a high percentage of fast twitch muscle fibers. Thus, any small advantage gained by genetically engineering fibers that increases force output (larger size fibers with improved contractile capacities), or promotes hyperplasia in existing muscles (thereby increasing total force-production capacity), can make the difference between winning and coming in second. In the world of sport, where the economics of winning becomes all-important, the rapidly expanding field of molecular biology applied to human and equine athletes will surely exert an impact in the coming decade.

Up-Close and Personal Interviews

The text's introduction, Exercise Physiology: Roots and Historical Perspectives, reflects our interest and respect for the earliest underpinnings of the field, and the direct and indirect contributions of the men and women physicians/scientists who preceded us. The giants of past generations, scientists and innovators we chronicle from Galen (A.D. 131-201) through the next two thousand years to the current cadre of distinguished scientists/researchers, set the cornerstone for the high standards attained by the current generation of exercise physiologists. In this revision, we feature nine contemporary scientists whose important research contributions and visionary leadership continue the tradition of the scientists of prior generations—Steven Blair, Frank Booth, Claude Bouchard, David Costill, Barbara Drinkwater, John Holloszy, Loring Rowell, Bengt Saltin, and Charles Tipton. These individuals clearly merit recognition, not only for expanding knowledge through their scientific contributions, but also for elucidating mechanisms underlying responses and adaptations to exercise and health enhancement. Each person has been placed within a section linked to their main scholarship interests, yet all of them span one or more sections in terms of scientific contributions. Appendix E lists individual honors and awards for each of these distinguished scientists.

We also consulted the Institute of Scientific Information database, Web of Science (www.webofscience.com/), from January, 1996 through April, 2001 to quantify the frequency that other scientists cite the published work of our featured scholars. The average citation record for the last six years confirmed our initial expectations about the impact that others cite their research. Peers throughout the scientific community consistently refer to their research in their own publications, often citing their numerous publications more than 15,000 times yearly!

Most of us know of these individuals only from journal articles, presentations, and international reputations. But unlike movie icons or top athletes where media scrutiny provides a closer look, those who excel in our field usually remain unknown except to a handful of colleagues who have the privilege of their close association. That's why we are so pleased they agreed to share their thoughts and insights about exercise physiology. Note the similarity in the responses to many of the questions. Despite their diverse educational backgrounds, they make use of their free time in different and often extraordinary ways, and show a great interest and concern for their students. We hope the intimate insights from our "superstars" inspire current exercise physiology students to actualize their potential, whether through accomplishments in graduate school, teaching, research, or numerous other exciting opportunities to achieve excellence.

New Art Program

This fifth edition features an all-new art program.

In a Practical Sense

This new element in every chapter highlights practical applications such as:

- Predict pulmonary function variables and lactate threshold
- Predict $\dot{V}O_{2max}$ from running and swimming performance
- Provide exercise guidelines for diabetic patients and pregnant women
- Provide exercises to protect against lower-back strain
- Identify and treat altitude-related medical problems
- Assess the heat quality of the environment
- Predict body fat in different athletic groups
- Recognize warning signs of disordered eating
- Assess flexibility
- Determine physical activity readiness

Integrative Questions

Another new element in each chapter, "Integrative Questions," poses open-ended questions to encourage students to consider complex concepts without a single "correct" answer.

Ancillaries: The Total Teaching Package

The carefully developed supplementary material for this text will help instructors and students maximize the benefits of the core contents.

Two powerful CDs are available to instructors:

- The *Image Collection for Exercise Physiology, 5th Edition* contains digitized full-color images from the text for easy importing into PowerPoint presentations or printed materials.
- The *Exercise Physiology, 5th Edition Test Generator* contains over 1200 questions faculty can draw from to create tests.

By visiting http://connection.lww.com/go/mcardle instructors and students can access support materials including the following:

Instructor Resources:

Create-Your-Own Website
PowerPoint Presentation Slides for Each Chapter

Student Resources:

Multiple Choice and True/False Quizzes for Each Chapter
Key Words and Concepts for Each Chapter
Study Questions for Each Chapter
Self-Assessment Tests
Search the References of the Book for Reports and Papers
Web Links to Related Sites
Additional Appendices

Acknowledgments

We wish to thank many individuals. First, to Dr. Loring Rowell for his constructive comments on the chapters related to pulmonary and cardiovascular dynamics during rest and exercise, particularly the sections related to the possible role of the venous system as an active vasculature. We thank Drs. Victor Convertino and Charles Tipton for insightful comments and suggestions on the mircogravity chapter.

Stephen Lee (Exercise Physiology Laboratory, Johnson Space Center, Houston) kindly supplied original NASA photos and documents, and Mission Specialist Astronaut Dr. Martin Fettman (Colorado State University, Ft. Collins, CO) provided original slides he took during his Skylab 2 Mission, and Dr. Helen Lane (Chief Nutritionist, Johnson space center, houston), provided pre-publication documents and resource materials. Dr. Ron White, National Space Biomedical Research Institute allowed us to use charts from *Human Physiology In Space Teacher's Manual*. We sincerely appreciate the expertise of Drs. Frank Booth, University of Missouri, Kristin Steumple, Department of Health and Exercise Science at Gettysburg College, and Marvin Balouyt, Division of Kinesiology, University of Michigan, for their expert opinions and suggestions for improving the chapter on molecular biology. Shaun Wallace, Hypoxico Inc., provided photos of the Wallace altitude tent (altitudetent.com). Mr. John Selby (www.hyperlite.co.uk) kindly provided timely information and photos of the portable, collapsible decompression chamber. Gerald J. Nolan, Glenn Research Center and Jim Eckles, White Sands Missile Range, provided original photographs. Many competent staff associates, web curators, and research scientists at various NASA facilities helped to direct us to original documents and photographs. Dr. Alex Knight, York University, UK, graciously provided information about molecular biology techniques he has pioneered (*in vitro* motility assay) and other information and a photograph about myosin, muscle, and single molecules. Yakl Freedman (www.dna2z.com) was supportive in supplying recent information about DNA and molecular biology. Sue Hilt of the American College of Sports Medicine staff headquarters did a superb job of securing the text of the Citation and Honor Awards reproduced in Appendix E. Dr. Martine Thomis, Leuven University, kindly sent original information from his research group's studies about muscular strength in twins. Dr. Sam Case, Western Maryland College, generously supplied original photos of the Iditarod competition. Dr. James A. Freeman, professor of English, University of Massachusetts, unselfishly lent his expertise to make words sing. Dr. Barry Franklin, Beaumont Hospital, Detroit, MI, supplied original information about cardiac rehabilitation. Paul Petrich, Goleta, CA, provided photos of scuba expeditions. The Trustees of Amherst College and Archival Library gave permission to reproduce the photographs and materials of Dr. Hitchcock. Magnus Mueller, the University of Geisen, kindly provided the photo of Liebig's Geisen lab on page xxxii.

We are collectively indebted to the nine researchers/scholars who took time from their busy schedules to answer our interview questions and provide personal photos. Each of those individuals, in their own unique ways, inspired the three of us in our careers by their work ethic, scientific excellence, and generosity of time and advice with colleagues and students. Over the years, we have had the good fortune to come to know these individuals both socially and in the academic arena. We must admit, however, that the interviews provided insights previously unknown to us. We hope you too are as impressed as we are by all they have accomplished and given back to the profession. Frank Katch also wishes to thank Dr. Drinkwater, who served on his MS thesis at UC Santa Barbara. He now fesses up after 33 years that she provided much needed statistical and grammatical assistance beyond the call of duty with that project!

We also acknowledge the following Master's and senior honors students who contributed so much to our research and personal experiences: Pedro Alexander, Christos Balabinis, Margaret Ballantyne, Brandee Black, Michael Carpenter, Steven Christos, Roman Czula, Gwyn Danielson, Toni Denahan, Marty Dicker, Peter Frykman, Scott Glickman, Marion Gurry, Carrie Hauser, Margie King, Peter laChance, Jean Lett, Maria Likomitrou, Robert Martin, Cathi Moorehead, Susan Novitsky, Joan Perry, Sharon Purdy, Michelle Segar, Debra Spiak, Lori Waiter, Stephen Westing, Howard Zelaznik

We also thank the dedicated team of professionals at LWW and their freelancers for their hard work. Editor Pete Darcy was tenacious and garnered needed resources for this project, and his assistant Lisa Manhart provided superb organization skills. Thanks to Nancy Peterson who provided insights, to Karen Gulliver who oversaw the editorial process, and to Lisa Franko for unfailing efforts and dedication to excellence in so many ways and for keeping the project rolling on schedule. Thanks to Christine Cantera whose design enlivens these pages. Kudos to art director Jonathan Dimes for careful scrutiny and polishing of the art program, his assistant Jennifer Clements, and to artists Caitlin Duckwall, Rob Duckwall, and Nancy Held. The efforts of Christine Kushner and Christen DeMarco of the marketing group are much appreciated.

William D. McArdle
GTGAAGGCTGCTAAGACCGATATGATAATGGATAGCACCGGCATAGCTACA
Sound Beach, NY

Frank I. Katch
AAAGGCACCGGTGTTATGAAGATGGTTACCGCAAGACG
Amherst, MA

Victor L. Katch
GGAAAGAGCGCAGTCGGCATGGCTATGGTTACCGCAAGCACG
Ann Arbor, MI

Contents

Introduction: A View of the Past

Exercise Physiology: Roots and Historical Perspectives

Since the first edition of our textbook in 1981, knowledge concerning the physiologic effects of exercise in general, and the body's unique and specific responses to training in particular has exploded. Tipton's search of the 1946 English literature for the terms *exercise* and *exertion* yielded 12 citations in 5 journals.[59] Tipton also cited a 1984 analysis by Booth who reported that in 1962, the number of yearly citations of the term exertion increased to 128 in 51 journals, and by 1981, there were 655 citations to the word exertion in 224 journals. The accompanying figure displays the number of entries for the words exercise or exertion referred to above from a computer search of Index Medicus (Medline) for the years 1966 through 2000. In the almost 6-year period since publication of the fourth edition of this text, the number of listings has increased more than 10-fold to 43,625! In 1994, we stated that the greatest increases occurred between 1976 and 1986, and that citation frequency appeared to level off from 1986 and 1994. Obviously, we were incorrect.

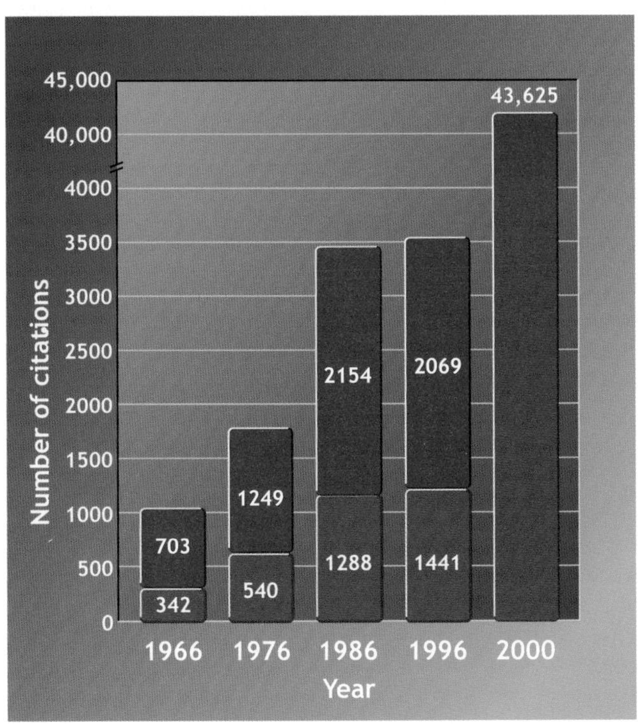

Exercise or *exertion* as a topic (*top bars*) and frequency of the word *exercise* appearing in a scientific journal title (*bottom bars*). 2000. Number of occurrences of the word *exercise*.

As graduate students in the late 1960s, we never dreamed that interest in exercise physiology would increase so dramatically. A new generation of scholars committed to studying the scientific basis of exercise set to work. Some studied the physiologic mechanisms involved in adaptations to regular exercise; others evaluated individual differences in exercise and sports performance. Collectively, both approaches contributed knowledge to the growing field of exercise physiology. At our first scientific conference (American College of Sports Medicine [ACSM] in Las Vegas, 1967), we rubbed elbows with the "giants" of the field, many of whom were themselves students of the leaders of their era. Sitting under an open tent in the Nevada desert with one of the world's leading physiologists, Dr. David Bruce Dill (then age 74), we listened to his researcher—a high school student—lecture about temperature regulation in the desert burro. Later, one of us (FK) sat next to a white-haired gentleman and chatted about a Master's thesis project. Only later did an embarrassed FK learn that this gentleman was Captain Albert R. Behnke, MD (1898–1993; ACSM Honor Award, 1976), the modern-day "father" of human body composition assessment, and whose crucial experiment in the physiology of underwater diving established standards for decompression and use of mixed gases. His pioneering studies of hydrostatic weighing in 1942, the development of a reference man and reference woman model, and the creation of the somatogram based on anthropometric measurements underlie much current work in body composition evaluation (refer to Chapter 28 and its "Focus on Research"). That meeting began a lasting personal and fulfilling professional friendship until Dr. Behnke's death in 1993. Several hundred ACSM members listened attentively as the superstars of exercise physiology and physical fitness (e.g., Per-Olof Åstrand, Erling Asmussen, Bruno Balke, Elsworth Buskirk, Thomas Cureton, Lars Hermansen, Steven Horvath, Henry Montoye, Bengt Saltin, Charles Tipton) presented their research and fielded penetrating questions from an audience of young graduate students eager to savor the latest scientific information.

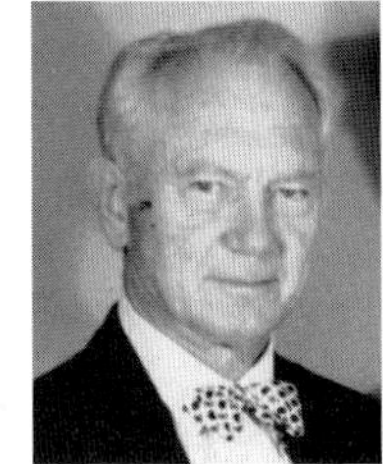

Albert R. Behnke

Over the years, the three of us were fortunate to work with the very best in our field. William McArdle studied for his PhD at the University of Michigan with Dr. Henry Montoye (charter member of ACSM, President of ACSM 1962–1963, Citation

Award, 1973) and Dr. John Faulkner (President of ACSM, 1971–1972, Citation Award, 1973, and ACSM Honor Award, 1992). At the University of California, Berkeley, Victor Katch completed his MS thesis in physical education under the supervision of Dr. Jack Wilmore (ACSM President, 1978–1979, Citation Award 1984, and first editor of *Exercise and Sport Science Reviews*, 1973–1974) and was a doctoral student of Dr. Franklin Henry (ACSM Honor Award, 1975, originator of the "Memory-Drum Concept" about the specificity of exercise, and author of the seminal paper Physical Education—an Academic Discipline, *JOHPER*, 35:32, 1964). Frank Katch completed his MS degree at the University of California, Santa Barbara under the supervision of Dr. Ernest Michael, Jr., (former PhD student of pioneer exercise physiologist–physical fitness scientist Dr. Thomas Kirk Cureton, ACSM Honor Award, 1969), and Dr. Barbara Drinkwater (President of ACSM, 1988–1989; ACSM Honor Award, 1996), and then also completed doctoral studies at the University of California, Berkeley with Professor Henry.

As the three of us examine those earlier times, we realize, like many of our colleagues, that our academic good fortunes prospered because our professors and mentors shared an unwavering commitment to study sport and exercise from a strong scientific and physiologic perspective. These scholars demonstrated why it was crucial for physical educators to be well grounded in both the scientific basics and underlying concepts and principles of exercise physiology.

We would be remiss if we failed to acknowledge the pioneers who created exercise physiology. It is, of course, impossible in an introduction to adequately chronicle the history of exercise physiology from its origins in ancient Asia to the present. Instead, our review presents historical information regarding topics not normally covered in prior exercise physiology textbooks or history texts. Our discussion begins with a brief acknowledgment of the ancient but tremendously influential Greek physicians; along the way, we highlight some milestones (and ingenious experiments), including the many contributions from Sweden, Denmark, Norway, and Finland that fostered the study of sport and exercise as a respectable field of scientific inquiry.

A treasure of information about the early beginnings of exercise physiology in America was uncovered in the archives of Amherst College, Massachusetts, in an anatomy and physiology textbook (incorporating a student study guide) written by the first American father-and-son writing team. The father, Edward Hitchcock, was President of Amherst College; the son, Edward Hitchcock Jr, an Amherst graduate and Harvard-trained physician, made detailed anthropometric and strength measurements of almost every student enrolled at Amherst College from 1861 to 1889. A few years later in 1891, much of what currently forms the college curriculum in exercise physiology, including evaluation of body composition by anthropometry and muscular strength by dynamic measurements, began in the first physical education scientific laboratory at Harvard University's Lawrence Scientific School. Even before the creation of this laboratory, another less formal but still tremendously influential factor impacted the development of exercise physiology: the publication during the 19th century of American textbooks on anatomy and physiology, physiology, physiology and hygiene, and anthropometry. Table 1 lists a sampling of 45 textbooks published between 1801 and 1899 containing information about the muscular, circulatory, respiratory, nervous, and digestive systems—including the influence of exercise and its effects—that eventually shaped the content area of exercise physiology during the next century. Additional textbooks from 1900 to 1947 deal with exercise, training, and exercise physiology.[a]

IN THE BEGINNING: ORIGINS OF EXERCISE PHYSIOLOGY FROM ANCIENT GREECE TO AMERICA IN THE EARLY 1800s.

Exercise physiology arose mainly in early Greece and Asia Minor although the topics of exercise, sports, games, and health concerned even earlier civilizations. These included the Minoan and Mycenaean cultures, the great biblical empires of David and Solomon, Assyria, Babylonia, Media, and Persia, as well as the Empires of Alexander. Other early references to sports, games, and health practices (personal hygiene, exercise, and training) were recorded in the ancient civilizations of Syria, Egypt, Macedonia, Arabia, Mesopotamia and Persia, India, and China. The greatest influence on Western Civilization, however, came from the Greek physicians of antiquity—Herodicus (5th century BC); Hippocrates (460–377 BC), and Claudius Galenus or Galen (131–201 AD[b]).

Herodicus, a physician and athlete, strongly advocated proper diet in physical training. His early writings and devoted followers influenced the famous physician Hippocrates ("father of preventive medicine"), who is credited with producing 87 treatises on medicine—several on health and hygiene—during the Golden Age of Greece.[7] Hippocrates espoused a profound understanding of human suffering, emphasizing a doctor's place at the patient's bedside. Today, physicians take the Hippocratic Oath based on Hippocrates' "Corpus Hippocratum."

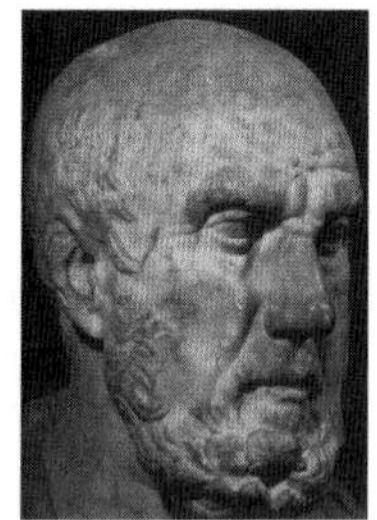
Hippocrates

Five centuries after Hippocrates, during the early decline of the Roman Empire, Galen emerged as perhaps the most well-known and influential physician that ever lived. The son of a wealthy architect, Galen was born in the city of Pergamos[c] and

[a]Buskirk[11] provides a bibliography of books and review articles on exercise, fitness, and exercise physiology from 1920 to 1979. Berryman[7] lists many textbooks and essays from the time of Hippocrates through the Civil War period in the United States.

[b]According to Green, the dates for Galen's birth are estimates based on a notation Galen made when at age 38 he served as personal physician to the Roman emperors Marcus Aurelius and Lucius Verus.[24] Siegel's bibliography contains an excellent source for references to Galen.[57]

[c]An important city on the Mediterranean coast of Asia Minor, Pergamos influenced trade and commerce. From 152–156 AD, Galen studied in Pergamos, renowned at the time for its library of 50,000 books (approximately one-fourth as many as in Alexandria, the greatest city for learning and education) and its famous medical center in the Temple of Asclepios.

TABLE 1 ➤ **SAMPLING OF TEXTBOOKS ON ANATOMY AND PHYSIOLOGY, ANTHROPOMETRY, EXERCISE AND TRAINING, AND EXERCISE PHYSIOLOGY (1801-1947)**

YEAR	AUTHOR AND TEXT
1801	Willich AFM. *Lectures on Diet and Regimen: Being a Systematic Inquiry into the Most Rational Means of Preserving Health and Prolonging Life: Together with Physiological and Chemical Explanations, Calculated Chiefly for the Use of Families, in Order to Banish the Prevailing Abuses and Prejudices in Medicine.* New York: T and J Swords, 1801.
1831	Hitchcock E. *Dyspepsy Forestalled and Resisted, or, Lectures on Diet, Regimen, and Employment.* 2nd ed. Northampton: J.S. & C. Adams, 1831.
1833	Beaumont W. *Experiments and Observations on the Gastric Juice and the Physiology of Digestion.* Plattsburgh: F.P. Allen, 1833.
1839	Carpenter WB. *Principles of Physiology, General and Comparative.* London: John Churchill, 1839. 4th ed., 1854.
1842	Carpenter WB. *Principles of Human Physiology.* London: Churchill, 1842.
1843	Carpenter WB. *Principles of Human Physiology, with Their Chief Applications to Pathology, Hygiene, and Forensic Medicine. Especially Designed for the Use of Students.* Philadelphia: Lea & Blanchard, 1843. Numerous reprints and editions; 9th ed, 1881 (London); 4th American ed., 1890.
1843	Combe A. *The Principles of Physiology Applied to the Preservation of Health, and to the Improvement of Physical and Mental Education.* New York: Harper & Brothers, 1843.
1844	Dunglison R. *Human Health: The Influence of Atmosphere and Locality; Change of Air and Climate; Seasons; Food; Clothing: Bathing and Mineral Springs; Exercise; Sleep; Corporeal and Intellectual Pursuits, on Healthy Man; Constituting Elements of Hygiene.* Philadelphia: Lea & Blanchard, 1844.
1846	Warren JC. *Physical Education and the Preservation of Health.* Boston: William D. Ticknor, 1846.
1848	Cutter C. *Anatomy and Physiology Designed for Academies and Families.* Boston: Benjamin B. Mussey and Co., 1848.
1852	Blackwell E. *The Laws of Life, with Special Reference to the Physical Education of Girls.* New York: George P. Putnam, 1852.
1854	Stokes W. *Diseases of the Heart and Aorta.* Philadelphia: Lindsay, 1854.
1855	Combe A. *The Physiology of Digestion, Considered with the Relation to the Principles of Dietetics.* Philadelphia: Harper and Brothers, 1855.
1856	Beecher C. *Physiology and Calisthenics for Schools and Families.* New York: Harper and Brothers, 1856.
1859	Flint A. *The Clinical Study of the Heart Sounds in Health and Disease.* Philadelphia: Collins, 1859.
1860	Hitchcock E, Hitchcock E Jr. *Elementary Anatomy and Physiology for Colleges, Academies, and Other Schools.* New York: Ivison, Phinney & Co., 1860.
1863	Ordronaux J. *Manual of Instruction for Military Surgeons, on the Examination of Recruits and Discharge of Soldiers.* New York: D. Van Nostrand, 1863.
1866	Flint A. *A Treatise on the Principles and Practice of Medicine; Designed for the Use of Practitioners and Students of Medicine.* Philadelphia: H.C. Les, 1866; 5th edition, 1884.
1866	Flint A. *The Physiology of Man; Designed to Represent the Existing State of Physiological Science as Applied to the Functions of the Human Body. Vol. I. Introduction; The Blood; Circulation; Respiration.* 1866. *Vol. II. Digestion; Absorption;* Lymph and Chyle (1867). *Vol. III. Secretion; Excretion; Ductless Glands; Nutrition; Animal Heat; Movement; Voice and Speech* (1870). Vol. IV. *Nervous System* (1873). *Vol V. Special Senses; Generation* (1874). New York: D. Appleton and Company.
1866	Huxley TH. *Lessons in Elementary Physiology.* London: Macmillan and Co., 1866.
1866	Lewis D. *Weak Lungs and How to Make them Strong.* Boston: Ticknor and Fields, 1866.
1869	Dalton JC. *A Treatise on Physiology and Hygiene; for Schools, Families, and Colleges.* New York: Harper & Brothers, 1869.
1869	Gould BA. *Investigations in the Military and Anthropological Statistics of American Soldiers. Published for the U.S. Sanitary Commission.* New York: Hurd and Houghton, 1869.
1871	Flint A. *On the Physiological Effects of Severe and Protracted Muscular Exercise; with Special Reference to its Influence Upon the Excretion of Nitrogen.* New York: D. Appleton & Co., 1871.
1873	Huxley TH, Youmans WJ. *The Elements of Physiology and Hygiene for Educational Institutions.* New York: D. Appleton & Co., 1873.
1873	Morgan JE. *University Oars.* London: MacMillan, 1873.
1875	Baxter JH. *Statistics, Medical and Anthropological, of the Provost-Marshal-General's Bureau, Derived from Records of the Examination for Military Service in the Armies of the United States During the Late War of the Rebellion, of Over a Million Recruits, Drafted Men, Substitutes, and Enrolled Men. Vol. 1.* Washington, DC: U.S. Government Printing Office, 1875.
1876	Hitchcock E. A part of the course of instruction given in the Department of Physical Education and Hygiene in Amherst College. First issued by the class of 1877 while juniors. Amherst, MA, 1876.
1877	Flint A. *A Text-Book of Human Physiology; Designed for the Use of Practitioners and Students of Medicine.* New York: D. Appleton, 1877. (2nd ed., rev. and cor. 1879; 3rd ed., rev. and cor. 1881, 1882, 1884, 1888; 4th ed., entirely rewritten 1888 and published 1889, 1891, 1892, 1893, 1895, 1896, 1897, 1901.)
1877	Flint A. *The Source of Muscular Power, as Deduced from Observations Upon the Human Subject Under Conditions of Rest, and of Muscular Exercise.* London: 1877.
1878	Flint A. *On the Sources of Muscular Power. Arguments and Conclusions Drawn from Observations Upon the Human Subject, Under Conditions of Rest and of Muscular Exercise.* New York: D. Appleton and Company, 1878.
1878	Foster M. *A Text-Book of Physiology.* London: Macmillan and Co, 1878.
1881	Huxley TH, Youmans WJ. *The Elements of Physiology and Hygiene: A Text-Book for Educational Institutions.* New York: Appleton and Co., 1881.
1884	Martin HN, Martin HC. *The Human Body. A Beginner's Text-book of Anatomy, Physiology and Hygiene.* New York: H. Holt and Company, 1884 (261 p); revised, 1885.
1885	Martin HN, Martin HC. *The Human Body. A Beginner's Text-book of Anatomy, Physiology and Hygiene, with Directions for Illustrating Important Facts of Man's Anatomy from That of the Lower Animals, and with Special References to the Effects of Alcoholic and Other Stimulants, and of Narcotics.* New York: Henry Holt and Son, 1885.
1888	Huxley TH, Martin HN. *A Course of Elementary Instruction in Practical Biology.* Rev. ed. London: Macmillan and Co., 1888.
1888	Lagrange F. *Physiology of Bodily Exercise.* New York: D. Appleton and Company, 1890.
1889	Hitchcock E, Seelye HH. *An Anthropometric Manual, Giving the Average and Mean Physical Measurements and Tests of Male College Students and Method of Securing Them.* 2nd ed. Amherst, MA: Williams, 1889.
1893	Kolb G. *Physiology of Sport.* London: Krohne and Sesemann, 1893.
1895	Galbraith AM. *Hygiene and Physical Culture for Women.* New York: Dodd, Mead and Company, 1895.
1896	Atkinson E. *The Science of Nutrition.* 7th edition. Boston: Damrell & Upham, 1896.
1896	Martin H.N. *The Human Body. An Account of Its Structure and Activities and the Conditions of Its Healthy Working.* New York: Holt & Co., 1881; 3rd ed. rev., 1884; 4th ed. rev. 1885; 5th ed. rev., 1888, 1889 (621 p); 6th ed. rev., 1890, 1894 (621 p); 7th ed., 1896 (685 p); 8th ed. rev., 1896 (685 p).
1896	Seaver JW. *Anthropometry and Physical Examination. A Book for Practical Use in Connection with Gymnastic Work and Physical Education.* New Haven, CN: Press of the O.A. Dorman Co., 1896.
1898	Martin H.N. *The Human Body. A Text-book of Anatomy, Physiology and Hygiene; with practical exercises.* 5th ed., rev. by George Wells Fitz. New York: H. Holt and Company. 1898 (408 p), 1899 (408 p); 5 editions 1900, 1902, 1911, 1912, 1930.
1900	Atwater WO, Bryant AP. Dietary Studies of University Boat Crews. U.S. Department of Agriculture, Office of Experiment Stations, Bulletin no. 25. Washington, DC: U.S. Government Printing Office, 1900.
1900	Howell WH, ed. *An American Text-Book of Physiology. Vol. 1. Blood, Lymph, and Circulation; Secretion, Digestion, and Nutrition; Respiration and Animal Heat; Chemistry of the Body.* 2nd. rev. Philadelphia: W.B. Saunders & Company, 1900.
1901	Howell WH, ed. *An American Text-Book of Physiology. Vol. 2. Muscle and Nerve; Central Nervous System; The Special Senses; Special Muscular Mechanisms; Reproduction.* 2nd. rev. Philadelphia: W.B. Saunders & Company, 1901.
1902	Hastings WW. *A Manual for Physical Measurements for Use in Normal Schools, Public and Preparatory Schools, Boys Clubs, Girls Clubs, and Young Men's Christian Associations.* Springfield: Young Men's Christian Association Training School, 1902.

Year	Author and Text
1903	Demeny G *Les Bases Scientifiques de l'Education Physique.* Paris: Felix Alcan, Editeur, 1903.
1903	Flint A. *Collected Essays and Articles on Physiology and Medicine,* 2 volumes. New York: D. Appleton and Company, 1903.
1904	Butts EL. *Manual of Physical Drill. United States Army.* New York: D. Appleton and Company, 1904.
1904	Mosso A. *Fatigue.* New York: G.P. Putnam's Sons, 1904.
1905	Atwater WO, Benedict FG. *A Respiration Calorimeter with Appliances for the Direct Determination of Oxygen.* Washington, DC: Carnegie Institution of Washington, 1905.
1905	Flint A. *Handbook of Physiology, for Students and Practitioners of Medicine.* New York: The Macmillan Company, 1905.
1906	Hough T, Sedgewick WT. *The Human Mechanism, Its Physiology and Hygiene and the Sanitation of Its Surroundings.* New York: Ginn and Company, 1906.
1906	Sargent DA. *Physical Education.* Boston: Ginn and Company, 1906.
1906	Sherrington SC. *The Integrative Action of the Nervous System.* New Haven, CT: Yale University Press, 1906.
1906	Stevens AW, Darling ED. *Practical Rowing and the Effects of Training.* Boston: Little, Brown and Company, 1906.
1908	Fisher I. *The Effect of Diet on Endurance: Based on an Experiment with Nine Healthy Students at Yale University, January-June, 1906.* New Haven, CT: Tuttle, Morehouse and Taylor Press, 1908.
1908	Fitz GW. *Principles of Physiology and Hygiene.* 2nd ed. rev. New York: H. Holt and Company, 1908; 2nd ed. rev., 1909.
1909	McKenzie RT. *Exercise in Education and Medicine.* Philadelphia: W.B. Saunders Company, 1909.
1911	Cannon WB. *The Mechanical Factors of Digestion.* New York: Longmans, Green and Company, 1911.
1914	Barcroft J. *The Respiratory Function of the Blood.* Cambridge: Cambridge University Press, 1914.
1914	Goodman EH. *Blood Pressure in Medicine and Surgery.* Philadelphia: Lea & Febiger, 1914.
1915	Benedict F, Murchhauser J. *Energy Transformation During Horizontal Walking. Carnegie Institute Publication. No. 231.* Washington, DC: Carnegie Institute of Washington, 1915.
1915	Cannon WB. *Bodily Changes in Pain, Hunger, Fear and Rage.* New York: D. Appleton and Company, 1915.
1917	Haldane JS. *Organism and Environment as Illustrated by the Physiology of Breathing.* New Haven: Yale University Press, 1917.
1918	Fisher I. *The Effect of Diet on Endurance.* New Haven: Yale University Press, 1918.
1918	Lewis T. *The Soldier's Heart and the Effort Syndrome.* New York: P.B. Hoeber, 1918.
1918	Starling EH. *Linacare Lecture; The Law of the Heart.* London: Longmans, Green and Company, 1918.
1918	Wilbur WC. *The Koehler Method of Physical Drill.* Philadelphia: J.B. Lippincott Company, 1918.
1919	Bainbridge FA. *Physiology of Muscular Exercises.* New York: Longmans, Green and Company, 1919.
1919	Love AG, Davenport CB. *Physical Examination of the First Million Draft Recruits: Methods and Results.* Washington, DC: U.S. Government Printing Office, 1919.
1920	Amar J. *The Human Motor.* New York: E.P. Dutton and Company, 1920.
1920	Burton-Ovitz R. *A Textbook of Physiology.* Philadelphia: W.B. Saunders Company, 1920.
1920	Dreyer G. *The Assessment of Physical Fitness.* New York: P.B. Hoeber, 1920.
1920	Gaskell WH. *The Involuntary Nervous System.* New York: Longmans, Green and Company, 1920.
1920	Jansen M. *On Bone Formation: Its Relation to Tension and Pressure.* New York: Longmans, Green and Company, 1920.
1921	Martin EG. *Tests of Muscular Efficiency.* Physiological Reviews 1921;1:454.
1922	Haldane JS. *Respiration.* New Haven, CT: Yale University Press, 1922.
1922	Krogh A. *The Anatomy and Physiology of Capillaries.* New Haven, CT: Yale University Press, 1922.
1923	MacKenzie RT. *Exercise in Education and Medicine.* Philadelphia: W.B. Saunders Company, 1923.
1924	Douglas CG, Priestley JG. *Human Physiology.* Oxford: The Clarendon Press, 1924.
1926	Fulton JF. *Muscular Contraction and Reflex Control of Movement.* Baltimore: Williams & Wilkins Company, 1926.
1926	Hill AV. *Muscular activity.* Lectures on the Herter Foundation, 16th course. "Muscles," 1924. Baltimore: Williams & Wilkins (for the Johns Hopkins University), 1926.
1927	Deutsch F, Kauf E. *Heart and Athletics.* Translation by L.M. Warfield. St. Louis: C.V. Mosby Company, 1927.
1927	DuBois EF. *Basal Metabolism in Health and Disease.* Philadelphia: Lea and Febiger, 1927.
1927	Hill AV. *Living Machinery.* New York: Harcourt, Brace and Company, 1927.
1927	Hill AV. *Muscular Movement in Man.* New York: McGraw-Hill Book Company, 1927.
1928	Henderson LJ. *Blood. A Study in General Physiology.* New Haven, CT: Yale University Press, 1928.
1928	McCurdy HG, McKenzie RT. *The Physiology of Exercise.* Philadelphia: Lea & Febiger, 1928.
1928	Schwartz L, et al. *The Effect of Exercise on the Physical Condition and Development of Adolescent Boys.* U.S. Public Health Service Bulletin 179. Washington, DC: U.S. Government Printing Office, 1928.
1929	Krogh A. *The Anatomy and Physiology of Capillaries.* 2nd ed. New Haven, CT: Yale University Press, 1929.
1929	Macklin CC. The Musculature of the Bronchi and Lungs. *Physiological Reviews* 1929;9:1 (492 references).
1930	Starling EH. *Human Physiology.* Philadelphia: Lea and Febiger, 1930.
1931	Bainbridge FA. *The Physiology of Muscular Exercise.* 3rd edition. Rewritten by AV Bock, DB Dill. London: Longmans Green and Company, 1931.
1931	Hill, A. V. *Adventures in Biophysics.* London: Oxford University Press, 1931.
1931	Schmidt FA, Kohlrasch W. *Physiology of Exercise.* (Translated by C.B. Sputh). Philadelphia: F.A. Davis and Company, 1931.
1932	Boas EP, Goldschmidt EF. *The Heart Rate.* Springfield, IL: Charles C. Thomas, 1932.
1932	Creed R.S., et al. *Reflex Activity of the Spinal Cord.* Oxford, Oxford University Press, 1932.
1932	Gould AG, Dye JA. *Exercise and Its Physiology.* New York: A.S. Barnes and Company, 1932.
1932	Grollman A. *The Cardiac Output of Man in Health and Disease.* Springfield, IL: Charles C Thomas, 1932.
1932	McCloy CH. *The Measurement of Athletic Power.* New York: A.S. Barnes and Company, 1932.
1933	Haggard HW, Greenberg LA. *Diet and Physical Efficiency.* New Haven, CT: Yale University Press, 1933.
1933	Schneider EC. *Physiology of Muscular Activity.* Philadelphia: W.B. Saunders Company, 1933.
1934	Konradi, Slonim D, Farfel VS. *Work Physiology.* Moscow: Medgiz Publishing, 1934.
1935	Boorstein SW. *Orthopedics for the Teacher of Crippled Children.* New York: Aiden, 1935.
1935	Dawson PM. *The Physiology of Physical Education.* Baltimore: Williams & Wilkins, 1935.
1935	Haggard HW, Greenberg LA. *Diet and Physical Efficiency.* New Haven, CT: Yale University Press, 1935.
1935	Haldane JS, Priestley JG. *Respiration.* New York: Oxford University Press, 1935.
1937	Griffin FWW. *The Scientific Basis of Physical Education.* London: Oxford University Press, 1937.
1938	Benedict FG. *Vital Energetics. A Study in Comparative Basal Metabolism.* Washington, DC: Carnegie Institute of Washington, 1938.
1938	Dill DB. *Life, Heat, and Altitude. Physiological Effects of Hot Climates and Great Heights.* Cambridge: Harvard University Press, 1938.
1939	Hrdlicka A. *Practical Anthropometry.* Philadelphia: Wistar Institute of Anatomy and Biology, 1939.
1939	Krestovnikoff A. *Fiziologia Sporta.* Moscow: Fizkultura and Sport, 1939.
1939	McCurdy JH, Larson LA. *The Physiology of Exercise.* Philadelphia: Lea and Febiger, 1939.
1939	Schneider EC. *Physiology of Muscular Activity.* 2nd ed. Philadelphia: W.B. Saunders Company, 1939.
1942	Cureton TK. *Physical Fitness Workbook.* Champaign, IL: Stipes Publishing Company, 1942.
1945	Cureton TK, et al. *Endurance of Young Men.* Washington, DC: National Research Council, National Society for Research in Child Development, 1945.
1947	Adolph EF, et al. *Physiology of Man in the Desert.* New York: Wiley, 1947.
1947	Cureton TK, et al. *Physical Fitness Appraisal and Guidance.* St. Louis: The C.V. Mosby Company, 1947.

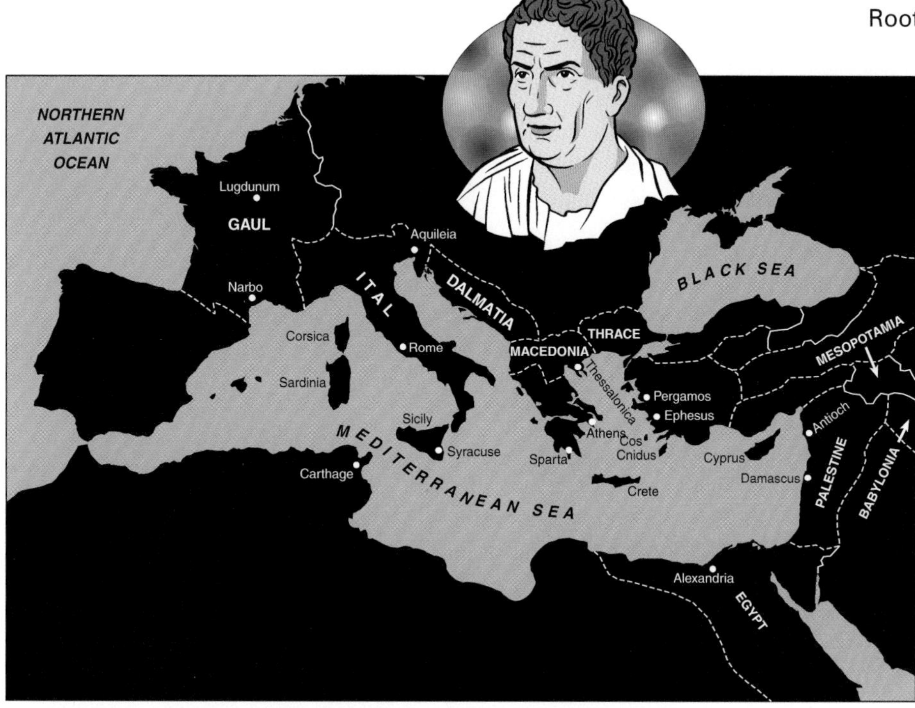

The World According to Galen. The white dots refer to the 14 major cities of that time period.

educated by scholars of the time. He began studying medicine at approximately age 16, and during the next 50 years, he implemented and enhanced the current thinking about health and scientific hygiene, an area that some might consider "applied" exercise physiology. Throughout his life, Galen taught and practiced the "laws of health": breathe fresh air, eat proper foods, drink the right beverages, exercise, get adequate sleep, have a daily bowel movement, and control one's emotions.[7] A prolific writer, Galen produced at least 80 sophisticated treatises (and perhaps 500 essays) on numerous topics, many of which addressed human anatomy and physiology, nutrition, growth and development, the beneficial effects of exercise, the deleterious consequences of sedentary living, and a variety of diseases and their treatment. One of the first "bench physiologists," Galen conducted original experiments in physiology, comparative anatomy, and medicine, including dissections on humans and a variety of animals (e.g., goats, pigs, cows, horses, elephants). Also, as physician to the gladiators of Pergamos, Galen treated torn tendons and muscles by using various surgical procedures he invented, including the procedure depicted in the 1544 woodcut of shoulder surgery shown at the left with commentaries from his Greek text *De fascius*. He also formulated rehabilitation therapies and exercise regimens, including treatment for a dislocated shoulder. Galen followed the Hippocratic school of medicine that believed in logical science grounded in experimentation and observation.

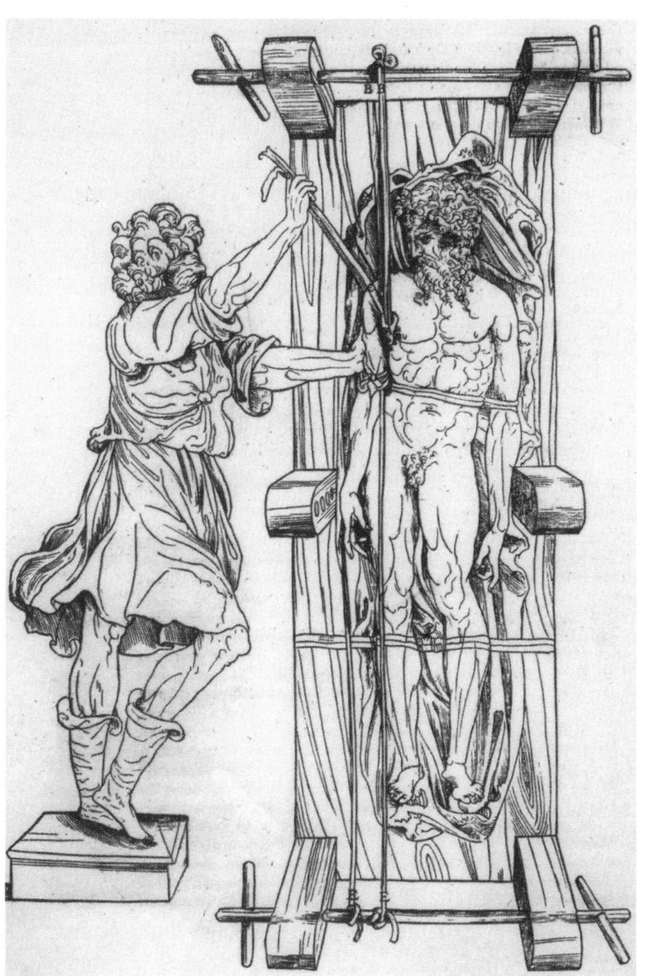

Woodcut by Renaissance artist Francesco Salviati (1544) based on Galen's *De fascius* from the first century B.C. The woodcut showing shoulder surgery provides a direct link with Hippocratic surgical practice that continued through the Byzantine period.

Galen wrote detailed descriptions about the forms, kinds, and varieties of "swift" and vigorous exercises, including their proper quantity and duration. The following definition of exercise is from the first complete English translation by Green[24] of Hygiene (*De Sanitate Tuenda*, pages 53–54) (see Table 2), Galen's insightful and detailed treatise on healthful living:

> To me it does not seem that all movement is exercise, but only when it is vigorous. But since vigor is relative, the same movement might be exercise for one and not for another. The criterion of vigorousness is change of respiration; those movements which do not alter the respiration are not called exercise. But if anyone is compelled by any movement to breathe more or less or faster, that movement becomes exercise from him. This therefore is what is commonly called exercise or gymnastics, from the gymnasium or public-place to which the inhabitants of a city come to anoint and rub themselves, to wrestle, throw the discus, or engage in some other sport. . . . The uses of exercise, I think are twofold, one for the evacuation of the excrements, the other for the production of good condition of the firm parts of the body. For since vigorous motion is exercise, it

must needs be that only these three things result from it in the exercising body—hardness of the organs from mutual attrition, increase of the intrinsic warmth, and accelerated movement of respiration. These are followed by all the other individual benefits which accrue to the body from exercise; from hardness of the organs, both insensitivity and strength for function; from warmth, both strong attraction for things to be eliminated, readier metabolism, and better nutrition and diffusion of all substances, whereby it results that solids are softened, liquids diluted, and ducts dilated. And from the vigorous movement of respiration the ducts must be purged and the excrements evacuated.

During the early Greek period, the Hippocratic school of physicians devised ingenious methods to treat common maladies, including a procedure to reduce pain from dislocated lower lumbar vertebrae. The illustration at the right from the 11th-century Commentaires of Apollonius of Chitiron on the Periarthron of Hippocrates provided details about early Greek surgical "sports medicine" interventions to treat athletes and the common citizen.

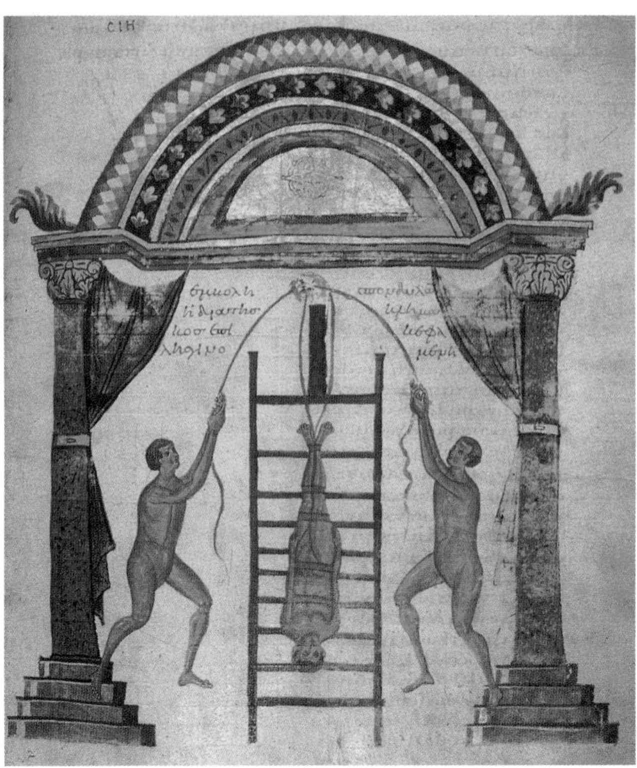

Ancient treatment for low-back pain

TABLE 2 ➤ TABLE OF CONTENTS FOR BOOK 1 AND BOOK 2[a] OF GALEN'S *DE SANITATE TUENDA (HYGIENE)*

Chapter	
	BOOK 1 **THE ART OF PRESERVING HEALTH**
I	Introduction
II	The Nature and Sources of Growth and of Disease
III	Production and Elimination of Excrements
IV	Objectives and Hypothesis of Hygiene
V	Conditions and Constitutions
VI	Good Constitution: A Mean Between Extremes
VII	Hygiene of the Newborn
VIII	The Use and Value of Exercise
IX	Hygiene of Breast-Feeding
X	Hygiene of Bathing and Massage
XI	Hygiene of Beverages and of Fresh Air
XII	Hygiene of the Second Seven Years
XIII	Causes and Prevention of Excrementary Retardation
XIV	Evacuation of Retained Excrements
XV	Summary of Book I
	BOOK 2 **EXERCISE AND MASSAGE**
I	Standards of Hygiene Under Individual Conditions
II	Purposes, Time, and Methods of Exercise and Massage
III	Techniques and Varieties of Massage
IV	Theories of Theon and Hippocrates
V	Definitions of Various Terms
VI	Further Definitions About Massage
VII	Amount of Massage and Exercise
VIII	Forms, Kinds, and Varieties of Exercise
IX	Varieties of Vigorous Exercises
X	Varieties of Swift Exercises
XI	Effects, Exercises, Functions, and Movements
XII	Determination of Diet, Exercise, and Regime

[a]Book III. Apotherapy, Bathing, and Fatigue. Book IV. Forms and Treatment of Fatigue. Book V. Diagnosis, Treatment, and Prevention of Various Diseases. Book VI. Prophylaxis of Pathological Conditions.

The era of more "modern-day" exercise physiology includes the periods of Renaissance, Enlightenment, and Scientific Discovery in Europe. It was then that Galen's ideas impacted the writings of the early physiologists, anatomists, doctors, and teachers of hygiene and health.[45,49] For example, in Venice in 1539, the Italian physician Hieronymus Mercurialis (1530–1606) published *De arte Gymnastica Apud Ancientes* (The Art of Gymnastics Among the Ancients). This text, heavily influenced by Galen and other early Greek and Latin authors, profoundly affected subsequent writings about gymnastics (physical training and exercise) and health (hygiene), not only in Europe (influencing the Swedish and Danish gymnastic systems), but also in early America (the 19th-century gymnastic-hygiene movement). The panel in Figure 1, redrawn from *De Arte Gymnastica*, acknowledges the early Greek influence of one of Galen's famous essays, *Exercise with the Small Ball*, as well as his regimen of specific strengthening exercises (throwing the discus and rope climbing).

RENAISSANCE PERIOD TO NINETEENTH CENTURY

New ideas formulated during the Renaissance exploded almost every idea inherited from antiquity. Johannes Gutenberg's (ca. 1400–1468 AD) printing press disseminated both classic and newly acquired knowledge. The commoner could learn about local and world events. Education became more available because universities sprang up in such centers as Oxford, Cambridge, Cologne, Heidelberg, Prague, Paris, Angiers, Orleans, Vienna, Padua, Bologna, Siena, Naples, Pisa, Montpellier, Toulouse, Valencia, Lisbon, and Salamanca.

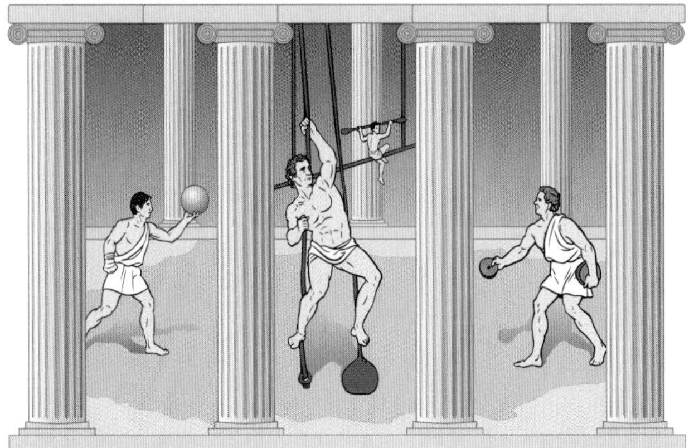

FIGURE 1 • The early Greek influence of Galen's famous essay, *Exercise with the Small Ball* and specific strengthening exercises (throwing the discus and rope climbing), appeared in Mercurialis *De Arte Gumnastica*, a treatise about the many uses of exercise for preventive and therapeutic medical and health benefits. Mercurialis favored discus throwing to aid patients suffering from arthritis and to improve the strength of the trunk and arm muscles. He advocated rope climbing because it did not pose health problems, and he was a firm believer in walking (a mild pace was good for stimulating conversation, and a faster pace would stimulate appetite and help with digestion). He also believed that climbing mountains was good for those with leg problems, long jumping was desirable (but not for pregnant women), but tumbling and handsprings were not recommended because they would produce adverse effects from the intestines pushing against the diaphragm! The three panels above represent the exercises as they might have been performed during the time of Galen.

Art broke with past forms, emphasizing spatial perspective and realistic depictions of the human body.

Although the supernatural still influenced discussions of physical phenomena, many people turned from dogma to experimentation as a source of knowledge. For example, medicine had to confront the new diseases spread by commerce with distant lands. Plagues and epidemics decimated at least 25 million people throughout Europe in just 2 years (1348–1350). New towns and expanding populations in confined cities led to environmental pollution and pestilence, forcing authorities to cope with new problems of community sanitation and care for the sick and dying. Science had not yet solved the medical problems from disease carriers such as insects and rats.

As populations expanded throughout Europe and elsewhere, medical care became more important for all levels of society. But medical knowledge failed to keep pace with need. For roughly 12 centuries, few advances had been made since Greek and Roman medicine. The writings of the early physicians such as Celsus had either been lost or preserved only in the Arab world. Thanks to the prestige of classical authors, Hippocrates and Galen still dominated medical education until the end of the 15th century. Renaissance discoveries greatly modified their theories, however. New anatomists went beyond simplistic notions of four humors when they discovered the complexities of circulatory, respiratory, and excretory mechanisms.

Once rediscovered, these new ideas caused turmoil. The Vatican seemed to ban human dissections, but a number of

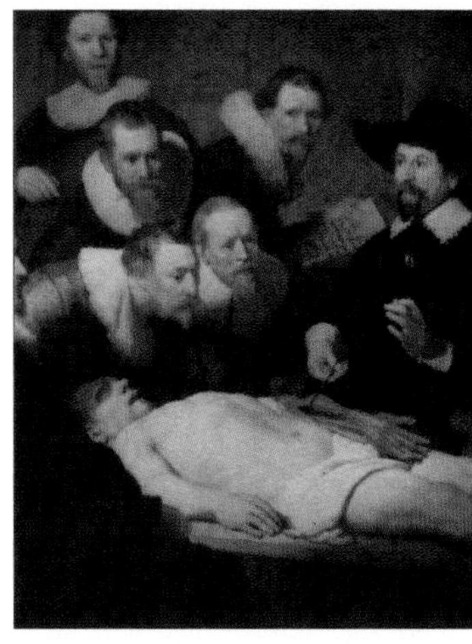

Rembrandt's 1632 *The Anatomy Lesson of Dr. Nicholas Tulp*

medical schools continued to conduct them, usually sanctioning one or two cadavers a year, or with official permission to perform an "anatomy" (the old name for a dissection) every 3 years. Performing autopsies helped physicians to solve legal questions about a person's death, or determine the cause of a disease. In the mid-1200s at the University of Bologna (founded in 1088 as a law school), every medical student had to attend one dissection each year, with 20 students assigned to a male cadaver and 30 students to a female cadaver. The first sanctioned dissection in Paris took place in 1407. In Rembrandt's first major portrait commission shown above, the 1632 *The Anatomy Lesson of Dr. Nicholas Tulp*, medical students listen intensely to the renowned Dr. Tulp as he dissects the arm of a recently executed criminal. The pioneering efforts of Vesalius (p. xxv) and Harvey (p. xxvi) made anatomical study a central focus of medical education, yet conflicted with the Church's strictures against violation of the individual rights of the dead because of the doctrine in resurrection of the body. In fact, the Church considered anatomical dissections a disfiguring violation of bodily integrity, despite the dismemberment of criminals as an extension of punishment. Nevertheless, the art of the period reflected close collaboration between artists and medical school physicians to portray anatomic dissections, essential for medical education, and to satisfy a public thirsty for new information in the emerging fields of physiology and medicine.

In 1316, Mondino de Luzzio (ca. 1275–1326), professor of anatomy at Bologna, published *Anathomia,* the first book of human anatomy. He based his teaching on human cadavers, not Greek and Latin authorities or studies of animals. The 1513 edition of *Anathomia* presented the same drawing as the original edition of the heart with three ventricles, a tribute to his accuracy in translation of the original inaccuracies. Certainly by the turn of the 15th century, anatomic dissections for postmortems were common in the medical schools of France and Italy; they paved the way for the Golden Age of the Renaissance anatomists whose careful observations accelerated understanding of human form and function. Two women from the University of Bologna achieved distinction in the field of anatomy. Laura Bassi (1711–1778), the first woman to earn a doctor of philosophy degree, and the university's first

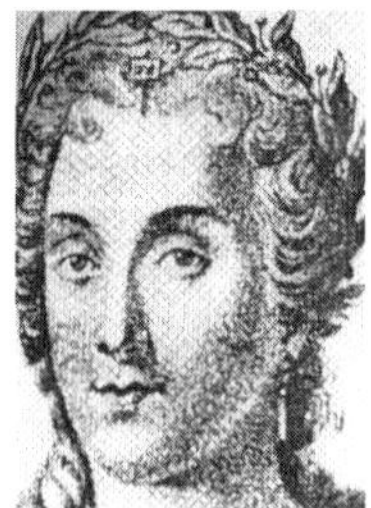
Professor Laura Bassi

female professor, specialized in experimental physics and basic sciences, but had to conduct her experiments at home. Soon after, female scholars were allowed to teach in university classrooms. At the time, Bassi gave her yearly public lectures on topics related to physics (including electricity and hydraulics, correction distortion in telescopes, hydrometry, and the relation between a flame and "stable air"). Anna Morandi Manzolini (1717–1774), also a professor at the University of Bologna, became an expert at creating wax models of internal organs and became the anatomy department's chief model maker. She produced an ear model that students took apart and reassembled to gain a better understanding of the ear's internal structures. Her wax and wood models of the abdomen and uterus were used didactically in the medical school for several hundred years. The wax self-portrait (below) in the Anatomical Museum of the University of Bologna shows Manzolini performing an anatomical dissection, clad in the traditional white lab coat, but also dressed in silks with diamonds and pearl jewelry—the manner expected of a woman of her social and economic status.

Progress in understanding human anatomical form paved the way for specialists in physical culture and hygiene to design specific exercises to improve overall body strength, and training regimens to prepare for rowing, boxing, wrestling, competitive walking, and track and field activities.

Notable Achievements by European Scientists

An explosion of new knowledge in the physical and biological sciences helped prepare the way for future discoveries about human physiology during rest and exercise.

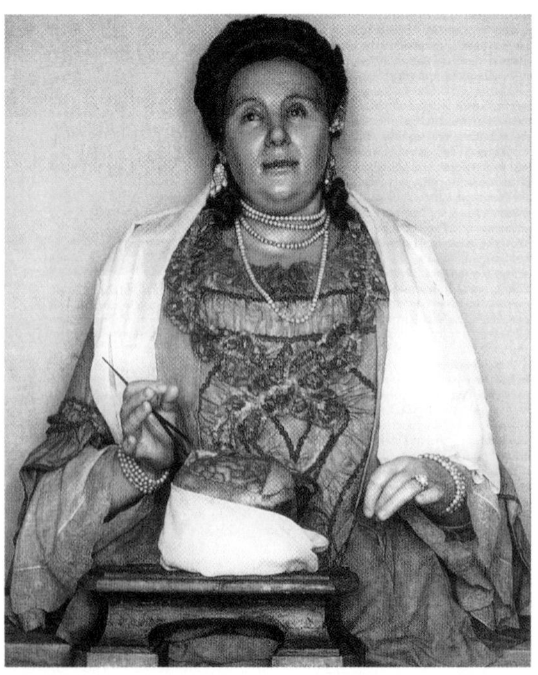
Professor Anna Manzolini

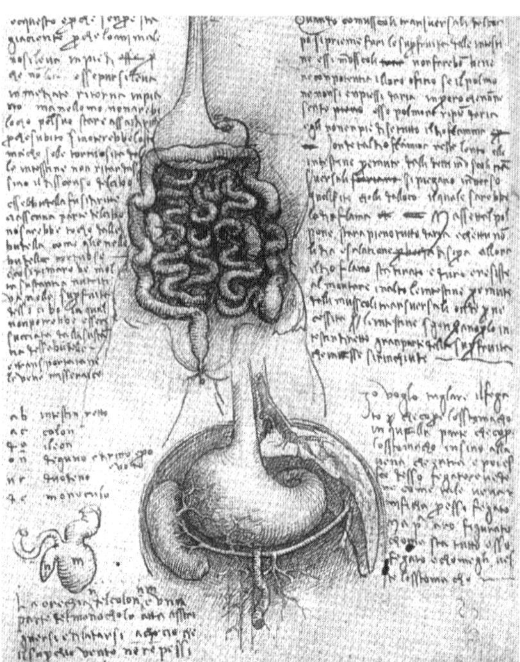
Anatomical sketch by da Vinci

Leonardo da Vinci (1452–1519)

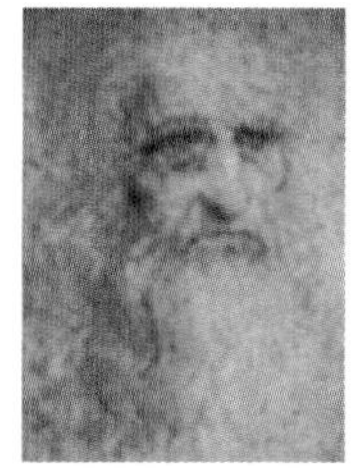

Da Vinci dissected cadavers at the hospital of Santa Maria Nuova in Florence and made detailed anatomical drawings. Accurate as the sketches were, they still preserved Galenic ideas. Although he never saw the pores in the septum of the heart, he included them, believing they existed because Galen had "seen" them. Da Vinci first accurately drew the heart's inner structures and constructed models of valvular function that showed how the blood flowed in only one direction. This observation contradicted Galen's notion about the ebb and flow of blood between the heart's chambers. Because many of da Vinci's drawings were lost for nearly two centuries, they did not influence later anatomical research.

Da Vinci's work built on and led to discoveries by two fellow artists. Leon Battista Alberti (1404-1472), an architect, perfected three-dimensional perspectives, which influenced da Vinci's concepts of internal relationships. Da Vinci's drawings no doubt inspired the incomparable Flemish anatomist Andreas Vesalius (1514–1564). These three exemplary Renaissance anatomists empowered physiologists to understand the systems of the body with technical accuracy, not theoretical bias.

Albrecht Dürer (1471–1528)

Dürer, a German contemporary of da Vinci, extended the Italian's concern for ideal dimensions as depicted on the next page in his famous "Quadrate Man" (see next page) by illustrating age-related differences in body segment ratios. Dürer created a canon of proportion, considering total height as unity. For example, in his schema, the length of the foot was

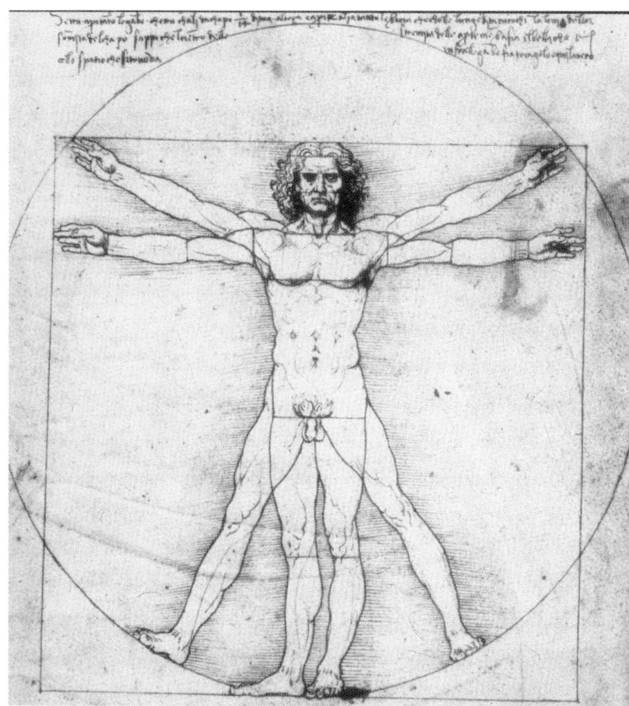

Dürer's *Quadrate Man*

one-sixth of this total, the head one-seventh, and the hand one-tenth. Relying on his artistic skills rather than objective comparison, Dürer made the ratio of height between men and women as 17 to 18 (soon thereafter proved incorrect). Nonetheless, Dürer's work inspired Behnke[23] in the 1950s to quantify body proportions into reference standards to evaluate body composition in men and women (refer to Chapter 28).

Michelangelo Buonarroti (1475–1564)

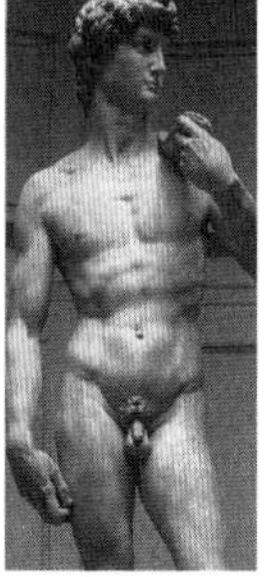

Michelangelo, just as da Vinci, was a superb anatomist. Body segments appear in proper proportion in his accurate drawings. The famous "David" (right) clearly shows the veins, tendons, and muscles enclosing a realistic skeleton. Although his frescos on the Sistine ceiling often exaggerate musculature, they still convey a scientist's vision of the human body.

Andreas Vesalius (1514-1564)

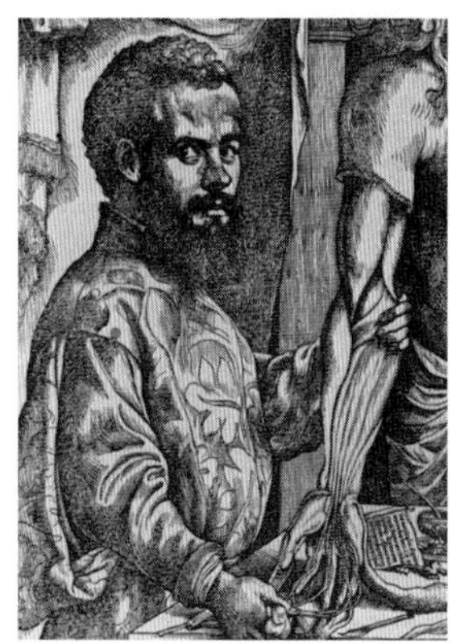

Belgian anatomist and physician Vesalius learned Galenic medicine in Paris, but after making careful human dissections, he rejected the Greek's ideas about bodily functions. At the start of his career, Vesalius authored books on anatomy, originally relying on Arabic texts, but then incorporating observations from his own dissections, including a self-portrait (lower left) from *Fabrica* published at age 29 showing the anatomical details of an upper and lower right arm. His research culminated in the exquisitely illustrated text first published in Basel, Switzerland in 1543, *De Humani Corporis Fabrica* (On the Fabric of the Human Body). Many consider these Vesalius drawings the best anatomical renderings ever made, ushering in the age of modern medicine. The same year, he published *Epitome*, a popular version of *De Fabrica* without Latin text.

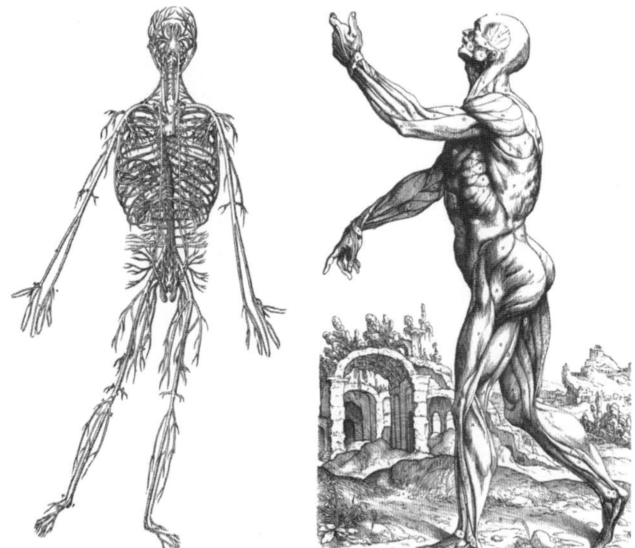

Vesalius' anatomical drawings. Left. Major nerves. Right. Muscular system in action. Note graveyard crypts.

Some physicians and clergymen became outraged, fearful that the new science was overturning Galen's time-honored speculations. Vesalius' treatise accurately rendered bones, muscles, nerves, internal organs, blood vessels (including veins for blood-letting), and the brain, but he differed from Galenic tradition by ignoring what he could not see. His remarkably detailed record of the muscular and skeletal architecture of the human body pared away one muscle layer at a time to reveal the hidden structures underneath.

Despite his attempt at accuracy, some of Vesalius' drawings contain curious inaccuracies. For example, he drew the inferior vena cava as a continuous vessel; he inserted an extra muscle to move the eyeball; and added an extra neck muscle, present only in apes. Despite these minor discrepancies, Vesalius attempted to connect form with function. He showed that a muscle contracted when a longitudinal slice was made along the muscle's belly, but a transverse cut prevented contraction. Vesalius substantiated that nerves controlled muscles and stimulated movement. His two texts profoundly influenced medical education. They demolished traditional theories about human anatomy and emboldened later researchers to explore circulation and metabolism unburdened by past misconceptions. The illuminating work of Vesalius hastened the subsequent important discoveries in physiology and the beginning of modern science.

Santorio Santorio (1561–1636)

A friend of Galileo and professor of medicine at Padua, Italy, Santorio used innovative tools for his research. He recorded changes in daily body temperature with the first air thermometer. He also measured pulse rates with Galileo's pulsilogium (pulsiometer). Ever inventive, Santorio studied digestion by constructing a wooden frame that supported a chair, bed, and worktable (see illustration below). Suspended from the ceiling with scales, the frame recorded changes in body weight.

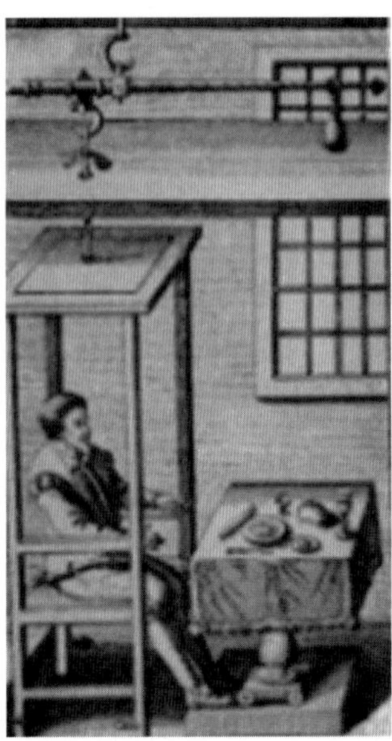

For 30 years, Santorio slept, ate, worked, and made love in the weighing contraption to record how much his weight changed as he ate, fasted, or excreted. He invented the term "insensible perspiration" to account for differences in body weight because he believed that weight was gained or lost through the pores during respiration. Often depriving himself of food and drink, Santorio determined that the daily change in body mass approached 1.25 kg. Santorio's book of medical aphorisms, *De Medicina Statica Aphorismi* (1614), drew worldwide attention. Although he did not explain the role of nutrition in weight gain or loss, Santorio nevertheless inspired later researchers in metabolism, especially during the 18th century.

William Harvey (1578–1657)

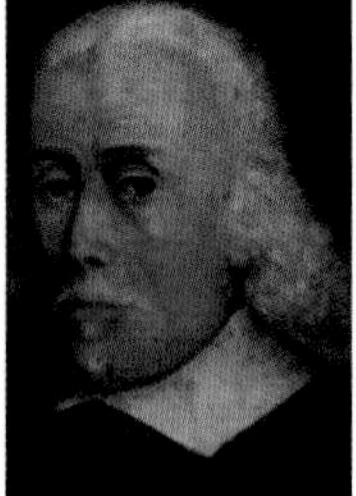

Harvey discovered that blood circulates continuously in one direction and, just as Vesalius had done, he overthrew 2000 years of medical dogma. Animal vivisection disproved the ancient supposition that blood moved from the right to left side of the heart through pores in the septum—pores that even da Vinci and Vesalius acknowledged. Harvey announced his discovery during a 3-day dissection–lecture at the Royal College of Physicians in London on April 16, 1616. Twelve years later, he published the details in a 72-page monograph, *Exercitatio Anatomica de Motu Cordis et Sanguinis in Animalibus* (An Anatomical Treatise on the Movement of the Heart and Blood in Animals).

By combining the new technique of experimentation on living creatures with mathematical logic, Harvey deduced that contrary to conventional wisdom, blood flowed in only one direction—from the heart to the arteries and from the veins back to the heart. It then traversed to the lungs before

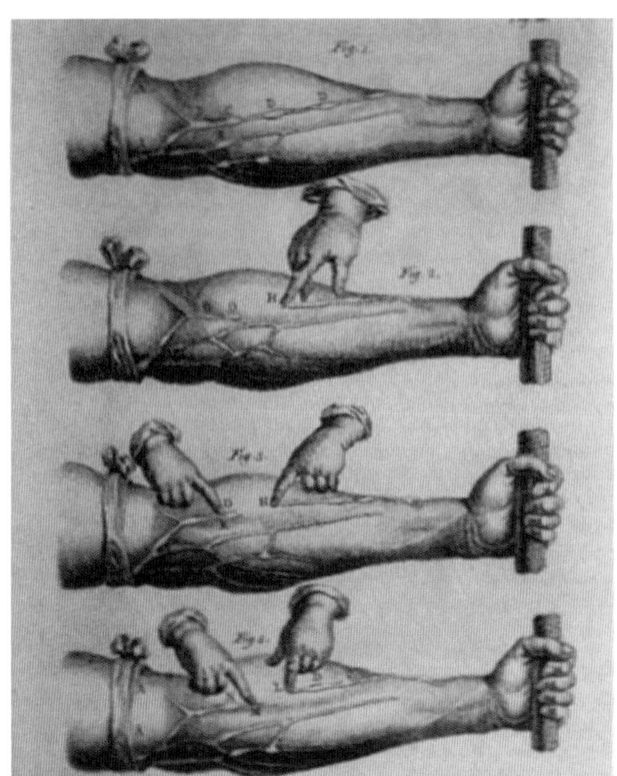

Harvey's famous illustration demonstrating the one-way flow of the circulation.

completing a circuit and re-entering the heart. Harvey publicly demonstrated the one-way flow of blood by placing a tourniquet around a man's upper arm that constricted arterial blood flow to the forearm and stopped the pulse (see illustration above). By loosening the tourniquet, Harvey allowed some blood into the veins. Applying pressure to specific veins forced blood from a peripheral segment where there was little pressure into the previously empty veins. Thus, Harvey proved that the heart pumped blood through a closed, unidirectional (circular) system, from arteries to veins and back to the heart. As he put it:

> It is proved by the structure of the heart that the blood is continuously transferred through the lungs into the aorta as by two clacks of a water bellows to raise water. It is proved by a ligature that there is a passage of blood from the arteries to the veins. It is therefore demonstrated that the continuous movement of the blood in a circle is brought about by the beat of the heart.[21]

Harvey's experiments with sheep proved mathematically that the mass of blood passing through the sheep's heart in a fixed time was greater than the body could produce—a conclusion identical to that concerning the human heart. Harvey reasoned that if a constant mass of blood exists, then the large circulation volumes would require a one-way, closed circulatory system. Harvey did not explain why the blood circulated, only that it did. However, he correctly postulated that circulation might distribute heat and nourishment throughout the body. Despite the validity of Harvey's observations, distinguished scientists criticized them. Jean Riolan, an ardent Galenist who chaired the anatomy and botany departments at the University of Paris in the 1640s, maintained that if anatomical findings differed from Galen's, then the body in question must be abnormal and the results faulty. Nevertheless, Harvey's epic discovery governed subsequent research on circulation.

Giovanni Alfonso Borelli (1608–1679)

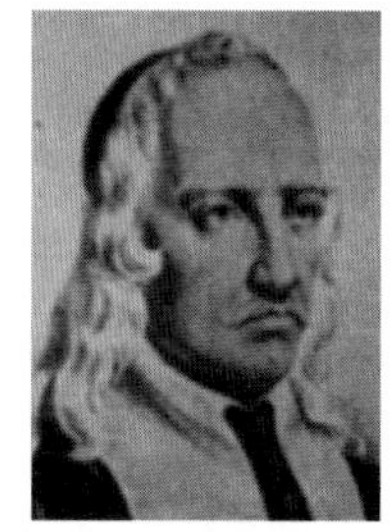

Borelli, a protégé of Galileo and mathematician at the University of Pisa, Italy, used mathematical models to explain how muscles enabled animals to walk, fish to swim, and birds to fly. His ideas explaining how air entered and exited the lungs, though equally important, were less well known. Borelli's accomplished student, Marcello Malpighi (1628–1694), described how he had observed blood flowing through microscopic structures (capillaries) around the lung's terminal air sacs (alveoli). Borelli observed that lungs filled with air because chest volume increased as the diaphragm moved downward. He concluded that air passed through the alveoli and into the blood, a sharp contrast to Galen's notion that air in the lungs cooled the heart, and an advance on Harvey's general observation concerning blood flow.

Robert Boyle (1627–1691)

Working at Gresham College, London with his student Robert Hooke (1635–1703), Boyle devised experiments with a vacuum pump and bell jar (see illustration below) to show that combustion and respiration required air. Boyle partially evacuated air from the jar containing a lit candle. The flame soon died. When he removed air from a jar containing a rodent or bird, it became unconscious; recirculating air back into the jar often revived the animal. Compressing the air produced the same results: animals and flames survived longer.

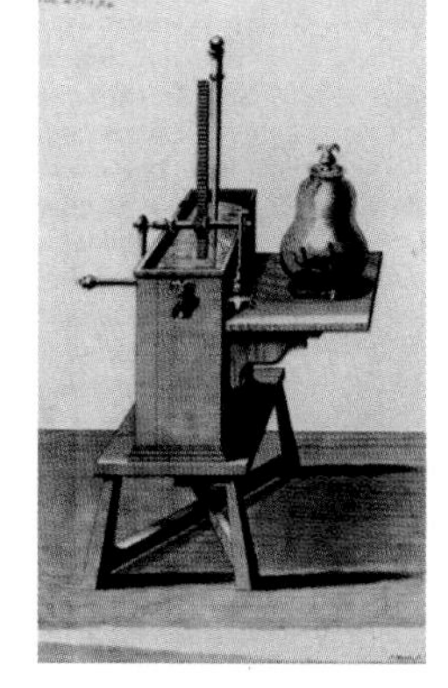

Boyle removed the diaphragm and ribs from a living dog and forced air into its lungs with a bellows. Although the experiment did not prove that air was essential for life, it demonstrated that air pressure alternately contracted and expanded the lungs. He repeated the experiment, this time pricking the lungs so air could escape. Boyle kept the animal alive by forcing air into its lungs, proving that chest movement maintained airflow and disproving the earlier assertion that lungs effected circulation.

Scientific societies and journals broadcasted these discoveries. Boyle belonged to the Royal Society of London, chartered in 1662 by Charles II. Four years later in France, Louis XIV sponsored the Académie Royale des Sciences so its salaried members could conduct a variety of studies. Both societies established journals *(Philosophical Transactions of the Royal Society* and *Journal des Scavans* respectively) to disseminate information in chemistry, physics, medicine, nutrition, and metabolism to scientists and an increasingly educated lay public.

Stephen Hales (1677–1761)

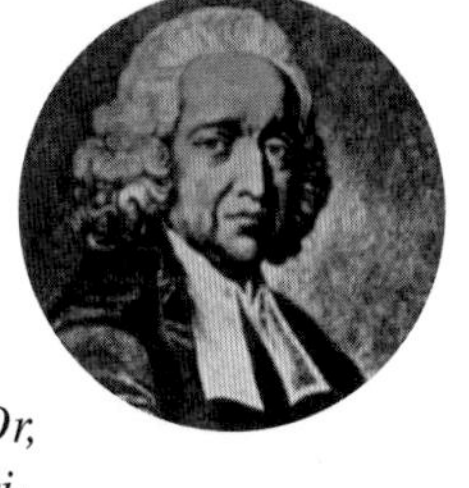

A renowned English plant physiologist and Fellow of the Royal Society, Hales amassed facts from his experiments with animals about blood pressure, the heart's capacity, and velocity of blood flow in *Vegetable Statics: Or, an Account of Some Statical Experiments on the Sap in Vegetables* (1727). In this text, Hales tells how water absorbed air when phosphorus and melted brimstone (sulfur) burned in a closed glass vessel (see illustration [right] that shows the transfer of "air" released from substances burned in a closed vessel). Hales measured the volume of air either released or absorbed, and he demonstrated that air was a constituent of many common substances. His experiments proved that chemical changes occurred in solids and liquids during calcination (oxidation during combustion). Hales developed an idea suggested by Newton in 1713 that provided the first experimental evidence that the nervous system played a role in muscular contraction.

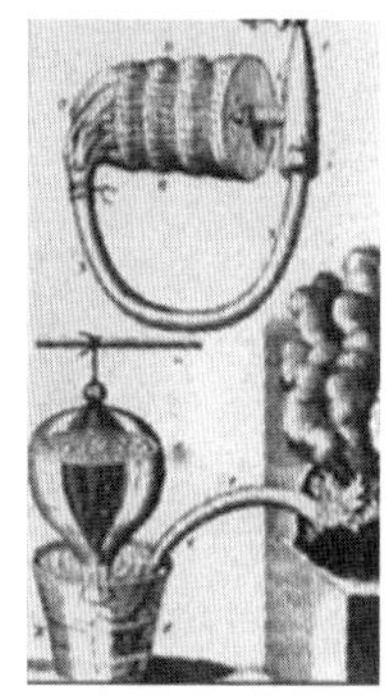

James Lind (1716–1794)

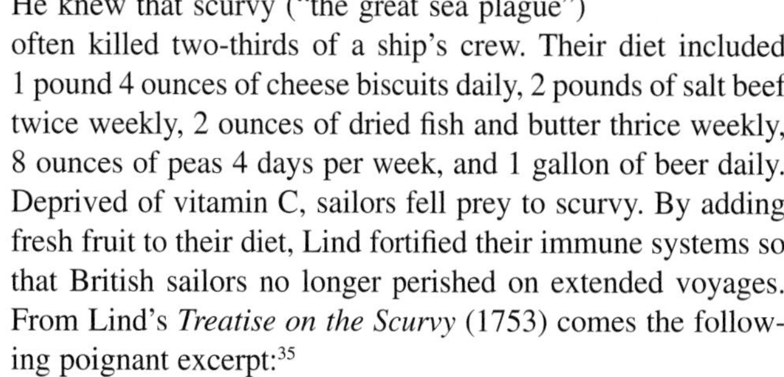

Trained in Edinburgh, Lind entered the British Navy as a Surgeon's Mate in 1739. During an extended trip in the English Channel in 1747 on the 50-gun, 960-ton H.M.S. Salisbury, Lind carried out a decisive experiment (the first planned, controlled clinical trial) that changed the course of naval medicine. He knew that scurvy ("the great sea plague") often killed two-thirds of a ship's crew. Their diet included 1 pound 4 ounces of cheese biscuits daily, 2 pounds of salt beef twice weekly, 2 ounces of dried fish and butter thrice weekly, 8 ounces of peas 4 days per week, and 1 gallon of beer daily. Deprived of vitamin C, sailors fell prey to scurvy. By adding fresh fruit to their diet, Lind fortified their immune systems so that British sailors no longer perished on extended voyages. From Lind's *Treatise on the Scurvy* (1753) comes the following poignant excerpt:[35]

> On the 20th of May, 1747, I selected 12 patients in the scurvy, on board the Salisbury at sea. Their cases were as similar as I could have them. They all in general had putrid gums, the spots and lassitude, with weakness of their knees. . . . The conse-

> quence was, that the most sudden and visible good effects were perceived from the use of oranges and lemons; one of those who had taken them, being at the end of 6 days fit for duty. The spots were not indeed at that time quite off his body, nor his gums sound; but without any other medicine than a gargle for his mouth he became quite healthy before we came into Plymouth which was on the 16th of June. The other was the best recovered in his condition; and being now pretty well, was appointed nurse to the rest of the sick. . . Next to oranges, I thought the cyder had the best effects. It was indeed not very sound. However, those who had taken it, were in a fairer way of recovery than the others at the end of the fortnight, which was the length of time all these different courses were continued, except the oranges. The putrification of their gums, but especially their lassitude and weakness, were somewhat abated, and their appetite increased by it.

Lind published two books:[58] *An Essay on Preserving the Health of Seamen in the Royal Navy* (1757) and *Essay on Diseases Incidental to Europeans in Hot Climates* (1768). Easily available, his books were translated into German, French, and Dutch. Lind's landmark emphasis on the crucial importance of dietary supplements antedates modern practices. His treatment regimen defeated scurvy, but 50 years had to pass with many more lives lost before the British Admiralty required fresh citrus fruit on all ships.

Joseph Black (1728–1799)

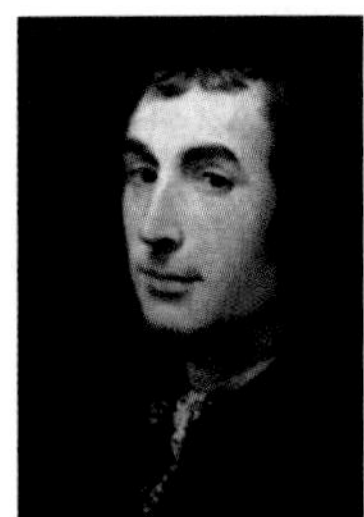

After graduating from the medical school in Edinburgh, Black became professor of chemistry at Glasgow. *Experiments Upon Magnesia Alba, Quicklime, and Some Other Alcaline Substances* (1756) determined that air contained carbon dioxide gas. He observed that carbonate (lime) lost half its weight after burning. Black reasoned that removing air from lime treated with acids produced a new substance he named "fixed air," or carbon dioxide ($CaCO_3 = CaO + CO_2$). Black's discovery that gas existed either freely or combined with other substances encouraged later experiments on the chemical composition of gases.

Joseph Priestley (1733–1804)

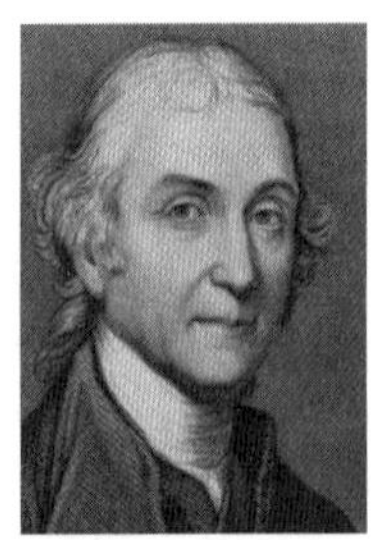

Although Priestley discovered oxygen by heating red oxide of mercury in a closed vessel, he stubbornly clung to the phlogiston theory that had misled other scientists. Dismissing Lavoisier's (1743–1794) proof that respiration produced carbon dioxide and water, Priestley continued to believe in an immaterial constituent (phlogiston) that supposedly escaped from burning substances. He told the Royal Society about oxygen in 1772, and published *Observations on Different Kinds of Air* in 1773. Elated by his discovery, Priestley failed to grasp two facts that later research confirmed: (1) the body needs oxygen, and (2) cellular respiration produces carbon dioxide.

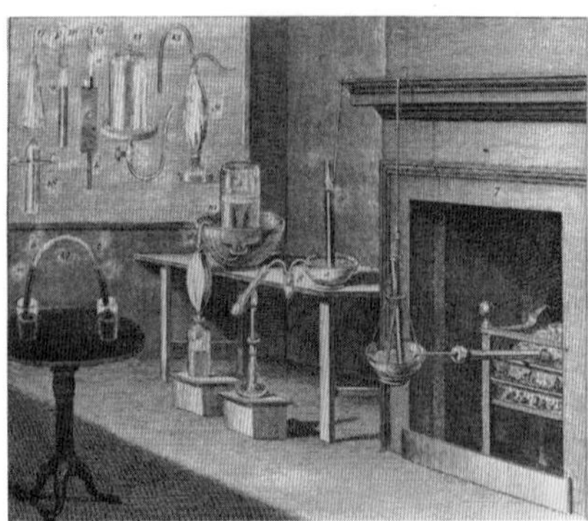

Priestley's laboratory

Carl Wilhelm Scheele (1742–1786)

In one of history's great coincidences, Scheele, a Swedish pharmacist, discovered oxygen independently of Priestley. Scheele noted that heating mercuric oxide released "fire-air" (oxygen); burning other substances in fire-air produced violent reactions. When different mixtures contacted air inside a sealed container, the air volume decreased by 25% and could not support combustion. Scheele named the gas that extinguished fire "foul air." In a memorable experiment, he added two bees to a glass jar immersed in lime water containing fire-air (illustration at left). After a few days, the bees remained alive but the level of lime water had risen in the bottle and became cloudy. Scheele concluded that fixed air replaced the fire-air to sustain the bees. At the end of 8 days, however, the bees died despite ample honey inside the container. Scheele blamed their demise on phlogiston, which he felt was hostile to life. What Scheele called foul-air (phlogisticated air in Priestley's day) was later identified as nitrogen.

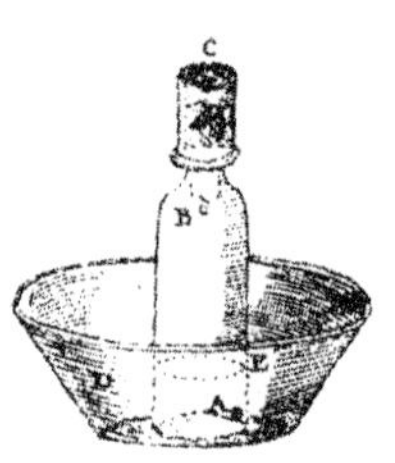

Just as Priestley, Scheele refused to accept Lavoisier's explanations concerning respiration. Although Scheele adhered to the phlogiston theory, he discovered, in addition to oxygen, chlorine, manganese, silicon, glycerol, silicon tetrafluoride, hydrofluoric acid, and copper arsenite (named Scheele's green in his honor).

Henry Cavendish (1731–1810)

Cavendish and his contemporaries Black and Priestley began to identify the constituents of carbohydrates, lipids, and proteins. *On Factitious Air* (1766) describes a highly flammable substance, later identified as hydrogen, which was liberated when acids combined with metals. *Experiments in Air* (1784) showed that "inflammable air" (hydrogen) combined with "deflogisticated air" (oxygen) produced water.

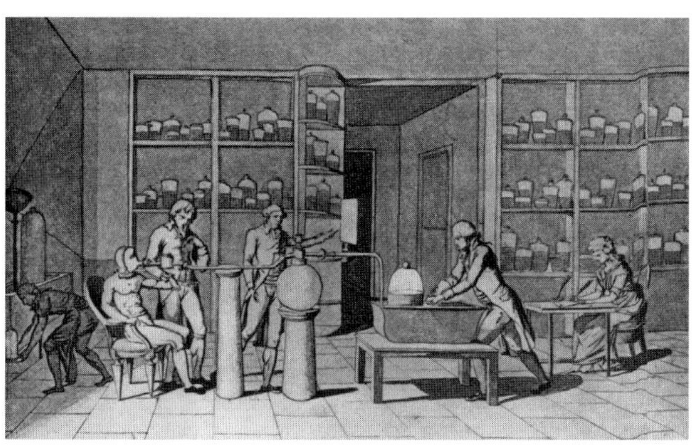

Lavosier supervises the first "true" exercise physiology experiment (heart rate and oxygen consumption measured as the seated subject at the left who breathes through a copper pipe presses a foot pedal to increase external work). Sketched by Madame Lavosier (sitting at the right taking notes).

Antoine Laurent Lavoisier (1743–1794)

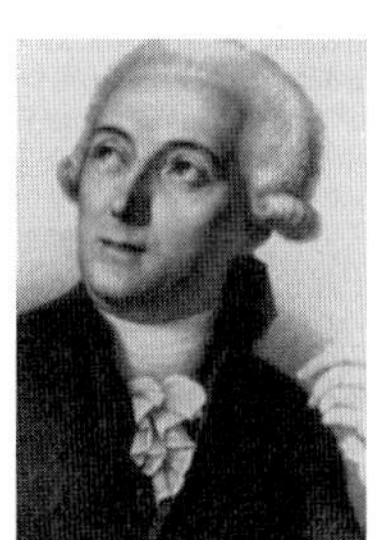

Lavoisier ushered in modern concepts of metabolism, nutrition, and exercise physiology. His discoveries in respiration chemistry and human nutrition were as essential to these fields as Harvey's discoveries were to circulatory physiology and medicine. Lavoisier paved the way for studies of energy balance by recognizing for the first time that the elements involved in metabolism (carbon, hydrogen, nitrogen, and oxygen) appeared neither suddenly nor disappeared mysteriously. He supplied basic truths: only oxygen participates in animal respiration, and the "caloric" liberated during respiration is itself the source of the combustion. In the early 1770s, Lavoisier was the first person to conduct experiments on human respiration. According to Lusk,[43] Lavoisier told of his experiments in a letter written to a friend dated November 19, 1790, as follows:

> The quantity of oxygen absorbed by a resting man at a temperature of 26°C is 1200 pouces de France (1 cubic pouce = 0.0198 L) hourly. (2) The quantity of oxygen required at a temperature of 12° C rises to 1400 pouces. (3) During the digestion of food the quantity of oxygen amounts to from 1800 to 1900 pouces. (4) During exercise 4000 pouces and over may be the quantity of oxygen absorbed.

These discoveries, fundamental to modern concepts of energy balance, could not protect Lavoisier from the intolerance of his revolutionary countrymen. The Jacobean tribunal beheaded him in 1794. Yet once more, thoughtless resistance to innovative science temporarily delayed the triumph of truth.

Lazzaro Spallanzani (1729–1799)

An accomplished Italian physiologist, Spallanzani debunked spontaneous generation as he studied fertilization and contraception in animals. In a famous study of digestion, he refined regurgitation experiments similar to those of the French scientist, René-Antoine Fercault de Réaumur (1683–1757). Réaumur's *Digestion in Birds* (1752) told how he recovered partially digested food from the gizzard of a kite. Spallanzani swallowed a sponge tied to the end of a string and then regurgitated it. He found that the sponge had absorbed a substance that dissolved bread and various animal tissues, thus indirectly observing how gastric juices function. His experiments with animals showed that the tissues of the heart, stomach, and liver consume oxygen and liberate carbon dioxide, even in creatures without lungs.

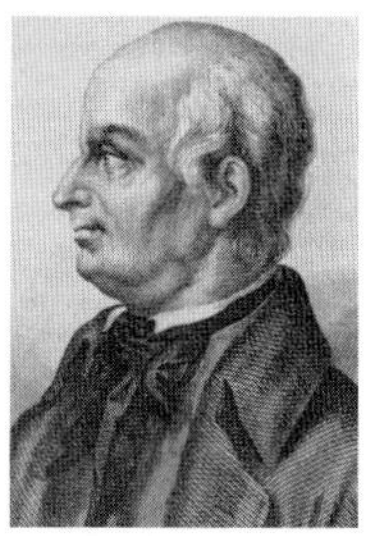

Spallanzani's idea that respiration and combustion took place within the tissues was novel, and appeared posthumously in 1804. A century later, this phenomenon would be called *internal respiration*.

Nineteenth Century Metabolism and Physiology

The untimely death of Lavoisier did not terminate fruitful research in nutrition and medicine. During the next half century, scientists discovered the chemical composition of carbohydrates, lipids, and proteins, and further clarified the energy balance equation.

Claude Louis Berthollet (1748–1822)

A French chemist and contemporary of Lavoisier, Berthollet (in white lab coat in illustration below) identified the "volatile substances" associated with animal tissues. One of these "substances," nitrogen, was produced when ammonia gas burned in oxygen. Berthollet showed that normal tissues did not contain ammonia. He believed that hydrogen united with nitrogen during fermentation to produce ammonia. In 1865, Berthollet took exception to Lavoisier's ideas concerning the amount of heat liberated when the body oxidized an equal weight of carbohydrate or fat. According to Berthollet, "the quantity of heat liberated in the incomplete oxidation of a substance equaled the difference between the total caloric value of the substance and that of the products formed."

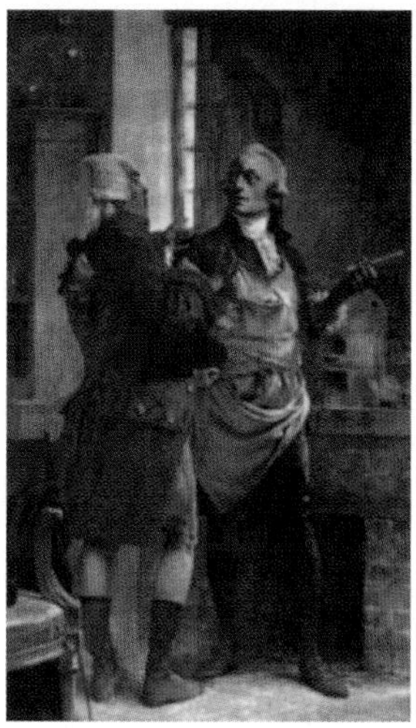

Joseph Louis Proust (1755–1826)

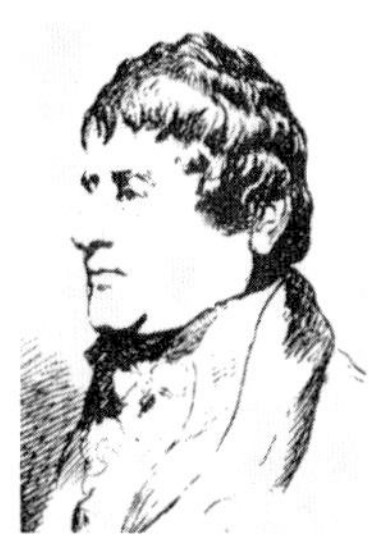

Proust proved that a pure substance isolated in the laboratory or found in nature would always contain the same elements in the same proportions. Known as the "Law of Definite Proportions," Proust's ideas about the chemical constancy of substances provided an important milestone for future nutritional explorers, helping them analyze the major nutrients and calculate energy metabolism as measured by oxygen consumption.

Louis-Joseph Gay-Lussac (1778–1850)

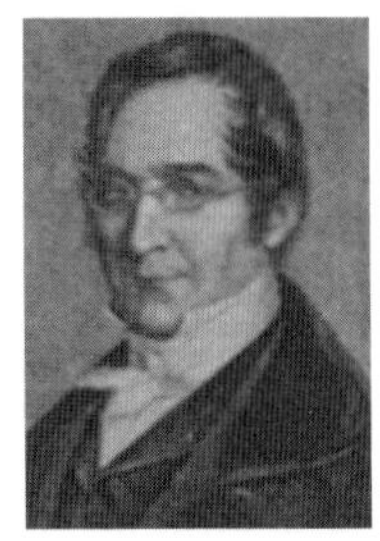

In 1810, Gay-Lussac, a pupil of Berthollet, analyzed the chemical composition of 20 animal and vegetable substances. He placed the vegetable substances into one of three categories, depending on their proportion of hydrogen-to-oxygen atoms. One class of compounds he called saccharine (later identified as carbohydrate) was accepted by William Prout (1785–1850) in his classification of the three basic macronutrients.

William Prout (1785–1850)

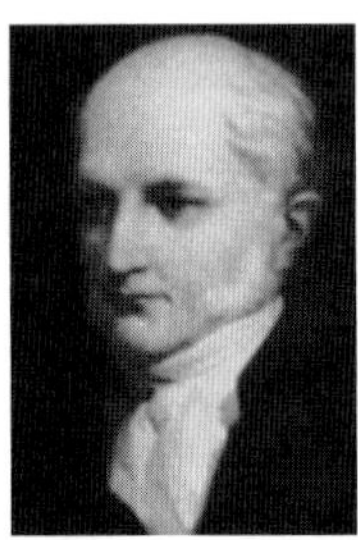

Following up the studies of Lavoisier and Séguin on muscular activity and respiration, Prout, an Englishman, measured the carbon dioxide exhaled by men exercising to fatigue (*Annals of Philosophy* 1813;2:328). Moderate exercise such as walking raised carbon dioxide production to an eventual plateau. This observation heralded the modern concept of steady-state gas exchange kinetics in exercise. Although Prout could not determine the exact amount of carbon dioxide respired because there were no instruments to measure respiration rate, he nevertheless observed that carbon dioxide concentration in expired air decreased dramatically in fatiguing exercise.

François Magendie (1783–1855)

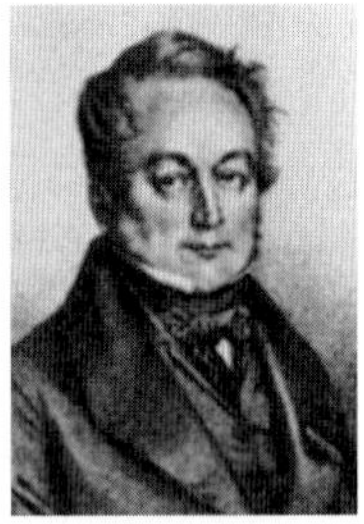

In 1821, Magendie founded the first journal for the study of experimental physiology (*Journal de Physiologie Expérimentale*), a field he literally created. The next year, he showed that anterior spinal nerve roots control motor activities, and posterior roots control sensory functions.

Magendie's accomplishments, however, were not limited to neural physiology. Unlike others who claimed that the tissues derived their nitrogen from the air, Magendie argued that the food they consumed provided the nitrogen. To prove his point, he studied animals subsisting on nitrogen-free diets. Magendie described his 1836 experiment as follows:

> . . . I took a dog of three years old, fat, and in good health, and put it to feed upon sugar alone, and gave it distilled water to drink: it had as much as it chose of both. . . It appeared to thrive very well in this way of living the first 7 or 8 days; it was brisk, active, ate eagerly, and drank in its usual manner. It began to get meagre upon the second week, though it had always a good appetite, and took about 6 or 8 ounces of sugar in 24 hours. . . In the third week its leanness increased, its strength diminished, the animal lost its liveliness, and its appetite was much lessened. At this period there was developed, first upon one eye, and then upon the other, a small ulceration in the center of the transparent cornea; it increased very quickly, and in a few days it was more than a line in diameter; its depth increased in the same proportion; the cornea was very soon entirely perforated, and the humours of the eye ran out. This singular phenomenon was accompanied with an abundant secretion of the glands of the eyelids.
>
> It, however, became weaker and weaker, and lost its strength; and though the animal took from 3 to 4 ounces of sugar every day, it became at length so weak that it could neither chew nor swallow; for the same reason every other motion was impossible. It expired the 32nd day of the experiment. I opened it with every suitable precaution; I found a total want of fat; the muscles were reduced by more than five-sixths of their ordinary size; the stomach and the intestines were also much diminished in volume, and strongly contracted.
>
> The excrements, that were also examined by M. Chevreul, contained very little azote (nitrogen), whilst they generally present a great deal. . . A third experiment produced similar results, and thence I considered sugar incapable of supporting dogs of itself.

William Beaumont (1785–1853)

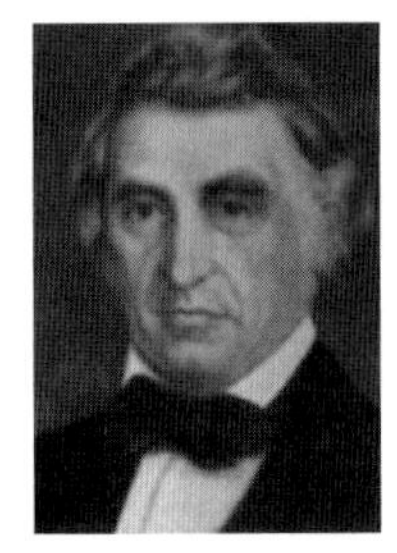

One of the most fortuitous experiments in medicine began on June 6, 1822, at Fort Mackinac, on the upper Michigan peninsula. As fort surgeon, Beaumont tended the accidental shotgun wound that perforated the abdominal wall and stomach of a young French Canadian, Samata St. Martin, a voyageur for the American Fur Company.

The wound healed after 10 months, but continued to provide new insights concerning digestion. Part of the wound formed a small natural "valve" that led directly into the stomach. Beaumont turned St. Martin on his left side, depressing the valve, and then inserted a tube the size of a large quill 5 or 6 inches into the stomach. He began two kinds of experiments on the digestive processes from 1825 to 1833. First, he observed the fluids discharged by the stomach when different foods were eaten (*in vivo*); second, he extracted samples of the stomach's content and put them into glass tubes to determine the time required for "external" digestion (*in vitro*).

Beaumont revolutionized concepts about digestion. For centuries, the stomach was thought to produce heat that somehow "cooked" foods. Alternatively, the stomach was portrayed as a mill, a fermenting vat, or a stew pan.[d]

---

[d]Jean Baptise van Helmont (1577–1644), a Flemish doctor, is credited with being first to prescribe an alkaline cure for indigestion.[24] Observing the innards of birds, he reasoned that acid in the digestive tract could not alone decompose meats, and that other substances ("ferments," now known as digestive enzymes) must break down food.

Beaumont published the first results of his experiments on St. Martin in the *Philadelphia Medical Recorder* in January 1825 and full details in his "Experiments and Observations on the Gastric Juice and the Physiology of Digestion" (1833).[21] Beaumont ends his treatise with a list of 51 inferences based on his 238 separate experiments. Although working away from the centers of medicine, Beaumont used findings from Spallanzini, Carminiti, Viridet, Vauquelin, Tiedemann and Gmelin, Leuret and Lassaigne, Montegre, and Prout. Even with their information, he still obeyed the scientific method, basing all his inferences on direct experimentation. Beaumont concluded:

> Pure gastric juice, when taken directly out of the stomach of a healthy adult, unmixed with any other fluid, save a portion of the mucus of the stomach with which it is most commonly, and perhaps always combined, is a clear, transparent fluid; inodorous; a little saltish; and very perceptibly acid. Its taste, when applied to the tongue, is similar to thin mucilaginous water, slightly acidulated with muriatic acid. It is readily diffusible in water, wine or spirits; slightly effervesces with alkalis; and is an effectual solvent of the materia alimentaria. It possess the property of coagulating albumen, in an eminent degree; is powerfully antiseptic, checking the putrefaction of meat; and effectually restorative of healthy action, when applied to old, fetid sores, and foul, ulcerating surfaces.

Beaumont's accomplishment is even more remarkable because the United States, unlike England, France, and Germany, provided no research facilities for experimental medicine. Little was known about the physiology of digestion. Yet Beaumont, a "backwoods physiologist,"[12] inspired future studies of gastric emptying, intestinal absorption, electrolyte balance, rehydration, and nutritional supplementation with "sports drinks."

Michel Eugene Chevreul (1786–1889)

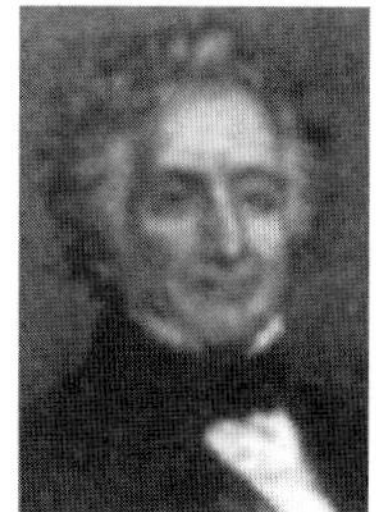

During his long life, Chevreul carried on a 200-year family tradition of studying chemistry and biology. His *Chemical Investigations of Fat* (1823) described different fatty acids. In addition, he separated cholesterol from billiary fats, coined the term *margarine*, and was the first to show that lard consisted of two main fats (a solid he called stearine and the other a liquid called elaine). Chevreul also showed that sugar from a diabetic's urine resembled cane sugar.

Jean Baptiste Boussingault (1802–1884)

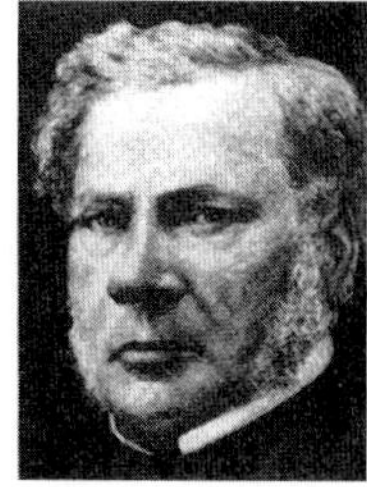

Boussingault's studies of animal nutrition paralleled later studies of human nutrition. He calculated the effect of calcium, iron, and other nutrient intake (particularly nitrogen) on energy balance. His pioneering work among Columbians formed the basis for his recommendations that they receive iodine to counteract goiter. Boussingault also turned his attention to plants. He showed that the carbon within a plant came from atmospheric carbon dioxide. He also determined that a plant derived most of its nitrogen from the nitrates in the soil, not from the atmosphere, as previously believed.

Gerardus Johannis Mulder (1802–1880)

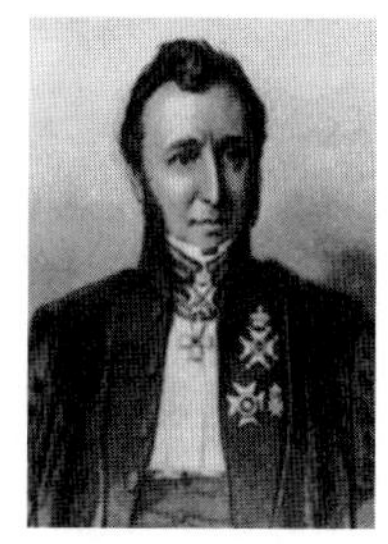

Professor of chemistry at Utrecht, Netherlands, Mulder analyzed albuminous substances that he called "proteine." He postulated a general protein radical identical in chemical composition to plant albumen, casein, animal fibrin, and albumen. This protein would contain substances other than nitrogen available only from plants. Because animals consume plants, substances from the plant kingdom, later called amino acids, served to build their tissues. Unfortunately, an influential German chemist, Justus von Liebig (1803–1873), attacked Mulder's theories about protein so vigorously that they fell out of favor.

Despite the academic controversy, Mulder strongly advocated society's role in promoting quality nutrition. He asked, "Is there a more important question for discussion than the nutrition of the human race?" Mulder urged people to observe the "golden mean" by eating neither too little nor too much food. He established minimum standards for his nation's food supply that he believed should be compatible with optimum health. In 1847, he gave these specific recommendations: laborers should consume 100 g of protein daily; those doing routine work about 60 g. He prescribed 500 g of carbohydrate as starch, and included "some" fat without specifying an amount.

Justus von Liebig (1803–1873)

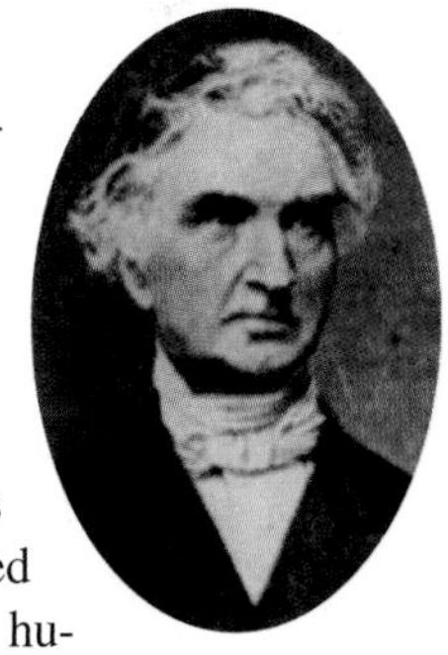

Although embroiled in professional controversies, Liebig established a large, modern chemistry laboratory that attracted numerous students. He developed unique equipment to analyze inorganic and organic substances. Liebig restudied protein compounds (alkaloids discovered by Mulder), and concluded that muscular exertion (by horses or humans) required mainly proteins, not just carbohydrates and fats. Liebig's influential *Animal Chemistry* (1842) communicated his ideas about energy metabolism.

Because Liebig dominated chemistry, his theoretical pronouncements about the relation of dietary protein to muscular activity were usually accepted without critique by other scientists until the 1850s. Despite his pronouncements, Liebig never carried out a physiological experiment or performed nitrogen balance studies on animals or humans. Liebig demeaned physiologists, believing them incapable of commenting on his theoretic calculations unless they themselves achieved his level of expertise.

By midcentury, physiologist Adolf Fick (1829–1901) and chemist Johannes Wislicenus (1835–1903) challenged

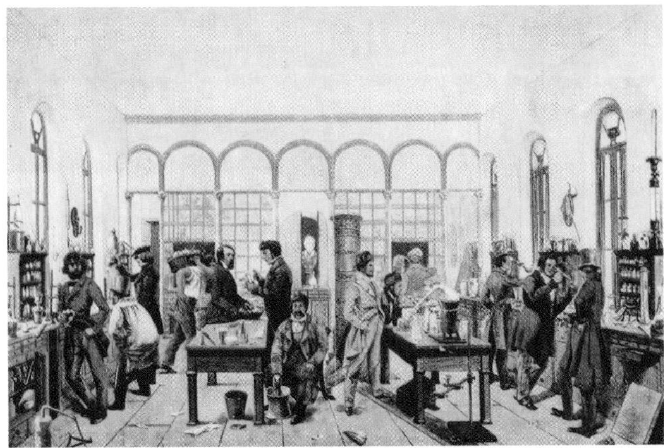

Hundreds of chemists were trained at Liebig's Geisen laboratory, many achieving international reputations for pioneering discoveries in chemistry. (Photo courtesy of Magnus Mueller, Liebig Museum, Giessen, Germany).

Liebig's dogma concerning protein's role in exercise. Their simple experiment measured changes in urinary nitrogen during a mountain climb. The protein that broke down could not have supplied all the energy for the hike. The result discredited Liebig's principle assertion regarding the importance of protein metabolism in supplying energy for exercise.

Although erroneous, Liebig's notions about protein as a primary exercise fuel worked their way into popular writings. By the turn of the 20th century, an idea that survives today seemed unassailable: athletic prowess requires a large protein intake. He lent his name to two commercial products; *Liebig's Infant Food*, advertised as a replacement for breast milk, and *Liebig's Fleisch Extract* (meat extract) that supposedly conferred special benefits to the body. Liebig argued that consuming his extract and meat would help the body perform extra "work" to convert plant material into useful substances. Even today, fitness magazines tout protein supplements for peak performance with little except anecdotal confirmation. Whatever the merit of Liebig's claims, debate continues, building on the metabolic studies of W. O. Atwater (1844–1907), F. G. Benedict (1870–1957), and R. H. Chittenden (1856–1943) in the United States, and M. Rubner (1854–1932) in Germany.

Henri Victor Regnault (1810–1878)

With his colleague Jules Reiset, Henri Regnault, professor of chemistry and physics at the University of Paris, used closed-circuit spirometry to determine the respiratory quotient (RQ; carbon dioxide ÷ oxygen) in dogs, insects, silkworms, earthworms, and frogs (1849). Animals were placed in a sealed, 45-L bell jar surrounded by a water jacket (see illustration below left). A potash solution filtered the carbon dioxide gas produced during respiration. Water rising in a glass receptacle forced oxygen into the bell jar to replace the quantity consumed during energy metabolism. A thermometer recorded temperature, and a manometer measured variations in chamber pressure. For dogs, fowl, and rabbits deprived of food, the RQ was less than when the same animals consumed meat. Regnault and Reiset reasoned that starving animals subsist on their own tissues. Foods were never completely destroyed during their metabolism because urea and uric acid were recovered in the urine.

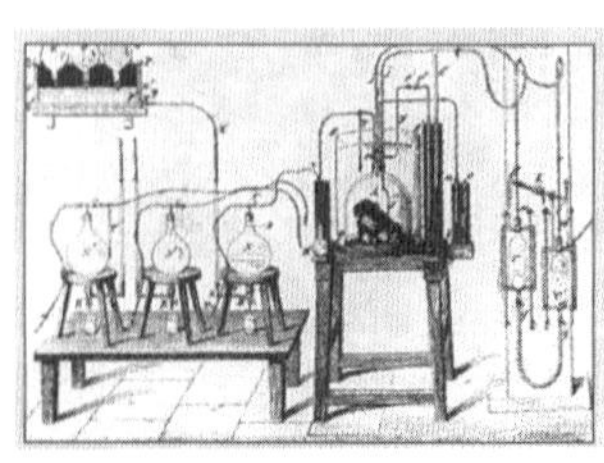

Regnault established relationships between different body sizes and metabolic rates. These ratios preceded the Law of Surface Area and allometric scaling procedures now used in exercise science. Regnault and Reiset related oxygen consumption to heat production and body size in animals:

> The consumption of oxygen absorbed varies greatly in different animals per unit of body weight. It is ten times greater in sparrows than in chickens. Since the different species have the same body temperature, and the smaller animals present a relatively larger area to the environmental air, they experience a substantial cooling effect, and it becomes necessary that the sources of heat production operate more energetically and that respiration increase.

Claude Bernard (1813–1878)

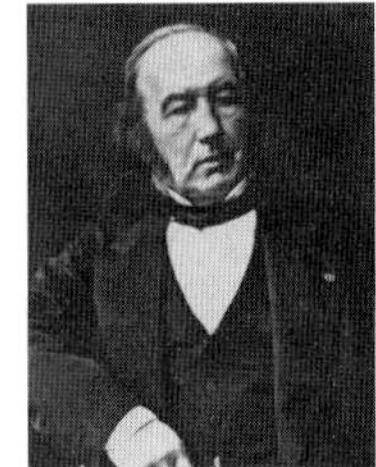

Claude Bernard, typically acclaimed as the greatest physiologist of all time, succeeded Magendie as Professor of Medicine at the Collège de France. Bernard interned in medicine and surgery before serving as laboratory assistant (préparateur) to Magendie in 1839. Three years later, he followed Magendie to the Hôtel-Dieu (hospital) in Paris. For the next 35 years, Bernard discovered fundamental properties concerning physiology. He participated in the explosion of scientific knowledge in the midcentury. Bernard indicated his single-minded devotion to research by producing a doctorate thesis on gastric juice and its role in nutrition (*Du sac gastrique et de son rôle dans la nutrition*; 1843). Ten years later, he received the Doctorate in Natural Sciences for his study entitled *Recherches sur une nouvelle fonction du foie, consideré comme organe producteur de matière sucrée*

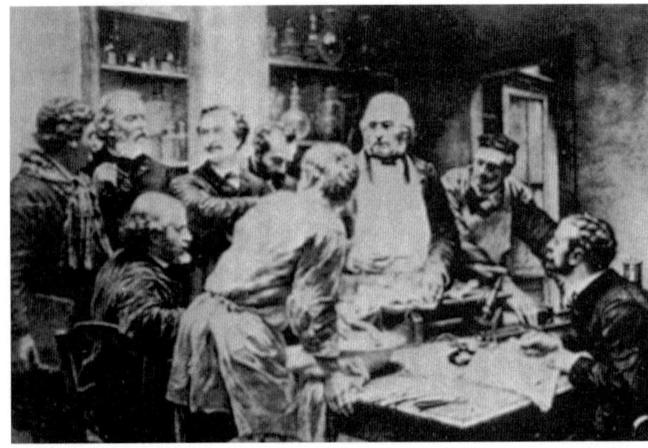

Students observing Bernard perform a dissection as part of their medical training.

chez l'homme et les animaux (Research on a new function of the liver as a producer of sugar in man and animals). Prior to this seminal research, scientists assumed that only plants could synthesize sugar, and that sugar within animals must derive from ingested plant matter. Bernard disproved this notion by documenting the presence of sugar in the hepatic vein of a dog whose diet lacked carbohydrate.

The following lists some of Bernard's experiments that profoundly affected medicine:

1. Discovery of the role of the pancreatic secretion in the digestion of lipids (1848)
2. Discovery of a new function of the liver—the "internal secretion" of glucose into the blood (1848)
3. Induction of diabetes by puncture of the floor of the fourth ventricle (1849)
4. Discovery of the elevation of local skin temperature upon section of the cervical sympathetic nerve (1851)
5. Production of sugar by washed excised liver (1855) and the isolation of glycogen (1857)
6. Demonstration that curare specifically blocks motor nerve endings (1856)
7. Demonstration that carbon monoxide blocks the respiration of erythrocytes (1857)

Bernard's work also influenced other sciences. His discoveries in chemical physiology spawned physiological chemistry and biochemistry, which in turn created molecular biology. His contributions to regulatory physiology helped the next generation of scientists understand how metabolism and nutrition affected exercise. Bernard's influential *Introduction à l'étude de la médecine expérimentale* (The Introduction to the Study of Experimental Medicine, 1865) illustrates the self-control that enabled him to succeed despite external disturbances. Bernard urges researchers to vigorously observe, hypothesize, and then test their hypothesis. In the last third of the book, Bernard shares his strategies for verifying results. His disciplined approach remains valid, and exercise physiologists would profit from reading this book.

Edward Smith (1819-1874)

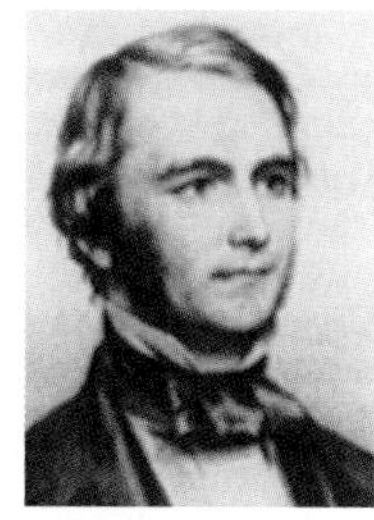

Edward Smith, physician, public health advocate, and social reformer, promoted better living conditions for Britain's lower class, including prisoners. He believed those in prison were maltreated because they received no additional food while toiling on the exhausting "punitive treadmill." Smith had observed prisoners climbing up a treadwheel, whose steps resembled the side paddle wheels of a Victorian steamship. Prisoners climbed for 15 minutes, after which they were allowed a 15-minute rest, for a total of four hours of work three times a week. To overcome resistance from a sail on the prison roof attached to the treadwheel, each man traveled the equivalent of 1.43 miles up a steep hill.

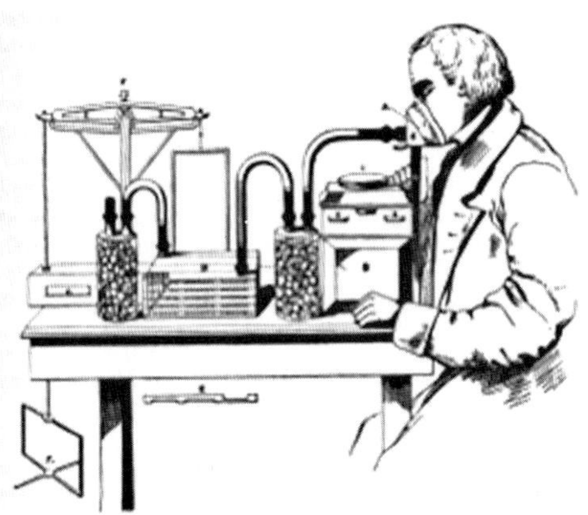

Curious about this strenuous exercise, Smith conducted studies on himself. He constructed a closed-circuit apparatus (facemask with inspiratory and expiratory valves; see above) to measure carbon dioxide production while climbing at Brixton prison.[21] He expired 19.6 more grams of carbon while climbing for 15 minutes and resting for 15 minutes than he expired while resting. Smith estimated that if he climbed and rested for 7.5 hours, his daily total carbon output would increase 66%. Smith analyzed the urine of four prisoners over a 3-week period to show that urea output was related to the nitrogen content of the ingested foods, while carbon dioxide related more closely to exercise intensity.

Smith inspired two German researchers to validate the prevailing idea that protein alone powered muscular contraction. Adolf Eugen Fick (1829–1901), a physiologist at the University of Zurich, and Johannes Wislicenus (1835–1903), professor of chemistry at Zurich, questioned whether protein oxidation or oxidation of carbohydrates and fats supplied energy for muscular work. In 1864, they climbed Mt. Faulhorn in the Swiss Alps. Prior to the climb, they eliminated protein from their diet, reasoning that nonprotein nutrients would have to supply them energy. They collected their urine before and immediately after the ascent and the following morning. They calculated the external energy equivalent of the 1956-m climb by multiplying their body mass by the vertical distance. This external energy requirement exceeded protein catabolism reflected by nitrogen in the urine. Therefore, they concluded that the energy from protein breakdown hardly contributed to exercise energy requirement. Again, these findings posed serious challenge to Liebig's claim that protein served as the primary source of muscular power.

Health and Hygiene Influence in the United States

By the early 1800s in the United States, ideas about health and hygiene were strongly promoted by European science-oriented physicians and experimental anatomists and physiologists. Prior to 1800, only 39 first edition American-authored medical books had been published, a few medical schools had been started (Harvard Medical School was founded in 1782), seven medical societies existed (the New Jersey State Medical Society being the first in 1766[8]), and only one medical journal was available

(*Medical Repository* published in 1797). Outside of the United States, 176 medical journals were being published, but by 1850, the number in the United States had increased to 117.

Medical journal publications in the United States had increased tremendously during the first half of the 19th century, concurrent with a steady growth in the number of scientific contributions, yet the European influence still affected the thinking and practice of U.S. medicine. This influence was particularly apparent in the "information explosion" that reached the public through books, magazines, newspapers, and traveling "health salesmen" who peddled an endless array of tonics, elixirs, and other products for purposes of optimizing health and curing disease. The "hot topics" of the early 19th century (also true today) included nutrition and dieting (slimming), general information concerning exercise, how to best develop overall fitness, training (or gymnastic) exercises for recreation and sport preparation, and all matters relating to personal health and hygiene.

By the middle of the 19th century, fledgling medical schools in the United States began to graduate their own students, many of whom soon assumed positions of leadership in the academic world and allied medical sciences. Interestingly, physicians had the opportunity either to teach in medical school and conduct research (and write textbooks) or become associated with departments of physical education and hygiene. There, they would oversee programs of physical training for students and athletes.

Within this framework, we begin our discussion of the early physiology and exercise physiology pioneers with Austin Flint Jr, MD, a respected physician, physiologist, and successful textbook author (Table 1 lists his texts). His writings provided information for those wishing to place their beliefs about exercise on a scientific footing.

Austin Flint Jr, MD: American Physician–Physiologist

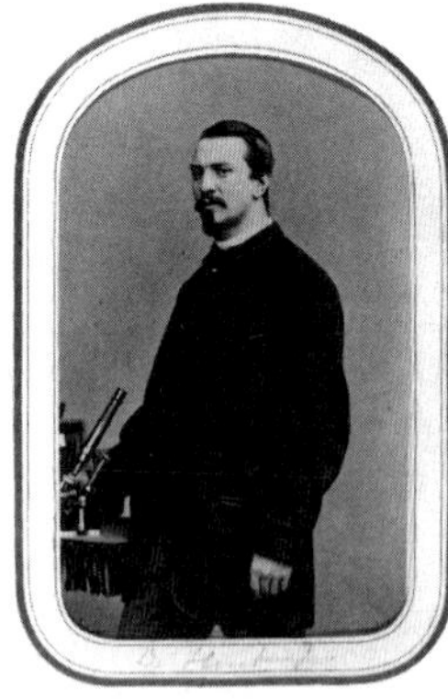

One of the first American pioneer physician–scientists whose writings contributed significantly to the burgeoning literature in physiology was Austin Flint Jr, MD, (1836–1915). He was professor of physiology and physiological anatomy in the Bellevue Hospital Medical College of New York, and chair of the Department of Physiology and Microbiology from 1861 to 1897. In 1866, he published a series of five classic textbooks, the first titled *The Physiology of Man; Designed to Represent the Existing State of Physiological Science as Applied to the Functions of the Human Body. Vol. 1; Introduction; The Blood; Circulation; Respiration*. Eleven years later, Flint published *The Principles and Practice of Medicine*, a synthesis of his first five textbooks, which consisted of 987 pages of meticulously organized sections with supporting documentation. The text included 4 lithograph plates and 313 woodcuts of detailed anatomical illustrations of the body's major systems, along with important principles of physiology. In addition, there were illustrations of equipment used to record physiological phenomena, such as Marey's early cardiograph for registering the wave form and frequency of the pulse, and a refinement of one of Marey's instruments, the sphygomograph, for making pulse measurements—the forerunner of modern cardiovascular instrumentation (Fig. 2).

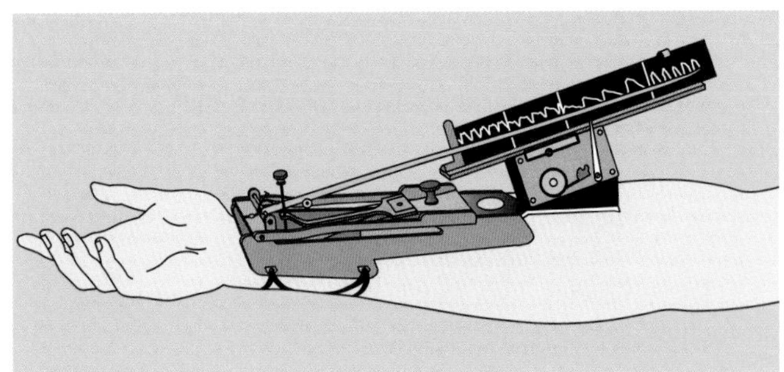

FIGURE 2 • Marey's advanced sphygmograph, including actual portions of four tracings of the pulse under different conditions. It was not until the next century (in 1928) that Boas and Goldschmidt (cited in the 1932 Boas and Goldschmidt text; see Table 1) reported on their human experiments with the first electronic cardiotachometer (Goldschmidt had invented the pulse resonator for recording pulse rate in 1927). The authors present a historical overview of pulse measuring devices, including the clepsydra (water clock) used by the Alexandrian physician Herophilus in the third century.

Dr. Flint, one of six generations of physicians spanning the years 1733–1955, was well trained in the scientific method. In 1858, he received the American Medical Association's prize for basic research on the heart, and his medical school thesis titled, "The Phenomena of Capillary Circulation," was published in 1878 in the *American Journal of the Medical Sciences*. A characteristic of Flint's textbooks was his admiration for the work of other scholars. These included the noted French physician Claude Bernard (1813–1878); the celebrated observations of Dr. William Beaumont; and William Harvey's momentous discoveries.

Dr. Flint was a careful writer. This was a refreshing approach, particularly because so many "authorities" in physical training, exercise, and hygiene in the United States and abroad were uninformed and unscientific about exercise. In his 1877 textbook, Flint wrote about many topics related to exercise. The following sample passages are quoted from Flint's 1877 book to present the flavor of the emerging science of exercise physiology in the late 19th century:

1. Influence of posture and exercise on pulse rate (pp. 52–53)

> It has been observed that the position of the body has a very marked influence upon the rapidity of the pulse. Experiments of a very interesting character have been made by Dr. Guy and others, with a view to determine the difference in the pulse in

different postures. In the male, there is a difference of about ten beats between standing and sitting, and fifteen beats between standing and the recumbent posture. In the female, the variations with position are not so great. The average given by Dr. Guy is, for the male standing, 81; sitting, 71; lying, 66;-for the female: standing, 91; sitting, 84; lying, 80. This is given as the average of a large number of observations.

Influence of age and sex. In both the male and female, observers have constantly found a great difference in the rapidity of the heat's action at different periods of life.

During early life, there is no marked and constant difference in the rapidity of the pulse in the sexes; but, toward the age of puberty, the development of the sexual peculiarities is accompanied with an acceleration of the heart's action in the female, which continues even into old age. The differences at different ages are shown in the following table, compiled from the observations of Dr. Guy:

Ages	Males Average pulsations	Females Average pulsations
From 2 to 7 y	97	98
From 8 to 14 y	84	94
From 14 to 21 y	76	82
From 21 to 28 y	73	80
From 28 to 35 y	70	78
From 35 to 42 y	68	78
From 42 to 49 y	70	77
From 49 to 56 y	67	76
From 56 to 63 y	68	77
From 63 to 70 y	70	78
From 70 to 77 y	67	81
From 77 to 84 y	71	82

Influence of Exercise, etc.—It is a fact generally admitted that muscular exertion increases the frequency of the pulsations of the heart; and the experiments just cited show that the difference in rapidity, which is by some attributed to change in posture (some positions, it is fancied, offering fewer obstacles to the current of blood than others), is mainly due to muscular exertion. Everyone knows, indeed, that the action of the heart is much more rapid after violent exertion, such as running, lifting, etc. Experiments on this point date from quite a remote period. Bryan Robinson, who published a treatise on the *"Animal Economy"* in 1734, states, as the result of observation, that a man in the recumbent position has 64 pulsations per minute; sitting, 68; after a slow walk, 78; after walking four miles in one hour, 100; and 140 to 150 after running as fast as he could. This general statement, which has been repeatedly verified, shows the powerful influence of the muscular system on the heart. The fact is so familiar that it need not be farther dwelt upon.

2. Influence of muscular activity on respiration (pp. 150–151)

Nearly all observers are agreed that there is a considerable increase in the exhalation of carbonic acid during and immediately following muscular exercise. In insects, Mr. Newport has found that a greater quantity is sometimes exhaled in an hour of violent agitation than in twenty-four hours of repose. In a drone, the exhalation in twenty-four hours was 0.30 of a cubic inch, and during violent muscular exertion the exhalation in one hour was 0.34. Lavoisier recognized the great influence of muscular activity upon the respiratory changes. In treating of the consumption of oxygen, we have quoted his observations on the relative quantities of air vitiated in repose and activity.

The following results of the experiments of Dr. Edward Smith on the influence of exercise are very definite and satisfactory:

In walking at the rate of two miles an hour, the exhalation of carbonic acid during one hour was equal to the quantity produced during 1⅘ hour of repose with food, and 2½ hours with, and 3½ hours without food.

One hour's labor at the tread-wheel, while actually working the wheel, was equal to 4½ of rest with food, and 6 hours without food.

The various observers we have cited have remarked that, when muscular exertion is carried so far as to produce great fatigue and exhaustion, the exhalation of carbonic acid is notably diminished.

3. Influence of muscular exercise on nitrogen elimination (pp. 429-430)

We have had an opportunity of settling definitely the vexed question of the influence of muscular exercise upon elimination of nitrogen.[e] In 1871, we made an exceedingly elaborate series of observations upon Mr. Weston, the pedestrian. Of these we can only give here a brief summary. Mr. Weston walked for five consecutive days as follows: First day, 92 miles; second day, 80 miles; third day, 57 miles; fourth day, 48 miles; fifth day, 40.5 miles. The nitrogen of the food was compared with the nitrogen excreted for three periods; viz, five days before the walk, five days walking, and five days after the walk. A trusty assistant was with Mr. Weston day and night for the fifteen days; the food was weighted and analyzed; the excreta were collected; and other observations were made during the entire period. The analyses were made independently, under the direction of Prof. R.O. Doremus, who had no idea of the results until we had classified and tabulated them. The conclusions were most decided, and, as far as possible, all the physiological conditions were fulfilled. As regards the proportion of nitrogen eliminated to the nitrogen of the food, the general results were as follows:

For the 5 days before the walk, with an average exercise of about 8 miles daily, the nitrogen eliminated was 92:82 parts for 100 parts of nitrogen ingested. For the five days of the walk, for every hundred parts of nitrogen ingested, there were discharged 153:99 parts. For the five days after the walk, when there was hardly any exercise, for every hundred parts of nitrogen ingested, there were discharged 84:63 parts. During the walk, the nitrogen excreted was in direct ratio to the amount of exercise; and, what

[e]Flint A, Jr. On the physiological effects of severe and protracted muscular exercise, with special reference to its influence upon the excretion of nitrogen. New York Medical Journal, 1871;xiii:609, et seq.

was still more striking, the excess of nitrogen eliminated over the nitrogen of food almost exactly corresponded with a calculation of the nitrogen of the muscular tissue wasted, as estimated from the loss of weight of the body. Full details of the method of investigation, the processes employed, etc., are given in our original paper.

Through his textbooks, Austin Flint Jr influenced the first medically trained and scientifically oriented professor of physical education, Edward Hitchcock Jr, MD. Hitchcock quoted Flint about the muscular system in his syllabus of Health Lectures, which was required reading for all students enrolled at Amherst College between 1861 and 1905.

The Amherst College Connection

Two physicians, father and son, pioneered the American sports science movement. Edward Hitchcock, DD, LLD (1793–1864), was a professor of chemistry and natural history at Amherst College and also served as President of the College from 1845–1854. He convinced the college President in 1861 to allow his son Edward [(1828–1911); Amherst undergraduate (1849); Harvard medical degree (1853)] to assume the duties of his anatomy course. Subsequently, Edward Hitchcock Jr was officially appointed on August 15, 1861, as Professor of Hygiene and Physical Education with full academic rank in the Department of Physical Culture at an annual salary of $1000, a position he held almost continuously until 1911. This was the second such appointment in physical education to an American college in the United States.[f]

The Hitchcocks geared their textbook to college physical education (Hitchcock E, Hitchcock E Jr. *Elementary Anatomy and Physiology for Colleges, Academies, and Other Schools.* New York: Ivison, Phinney & Co., 1860; Edward Hitchcock Sr had previously published a textbook on hygiene in 1831). The Hitchcock and Hitchcock anatomy and physiology book predated Flint's anatomy and physiology text by 6 years. Topics covered were listed in numerical order by subject, and considerable attention was given to the physiology of species other than humans. The text included questions at the bottom of each page concerning the topics under consideration, making the textbook a "study guide" or "workbook," not an uncommon pedagogical feature (Cutter, 1848; see Table 1). Figure 3 shows sample pages on muscle structure and function from the Hitchcock and Hitchcock text.

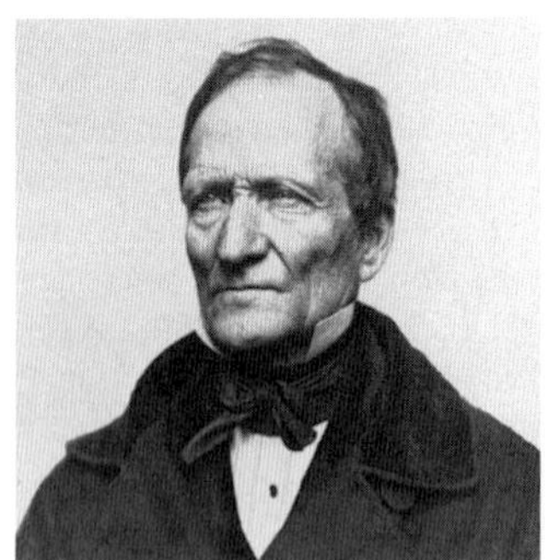

Dr. Edward Hitchcock (1793–1864)

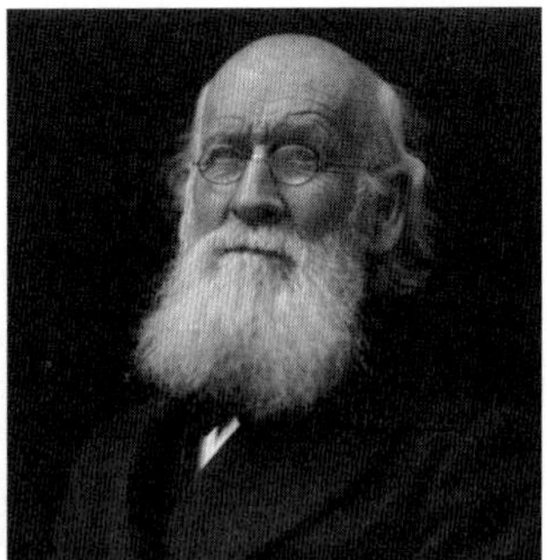

Dr. Edward Hitchcock Jr., M.D. (1828–1911)

From 1865 to approximately 1905, Professor Edward Hitchcock Jr's syllabus of Health Lectures (a 38-page pamphlet titled *"The Subjects and Statement of Facts Upon Personal Health Used for the Lectures Given to the Freshman Classes of Amherst College"*) was part of the required curriculum. The topics included hygiene and physical education, with brief quotations about the topic, including a citation for the quote. In addition to quoting Austin Flint Jr regarding care of the muscles, "The condition of the muscular system is an almost unfailing evidence of the general state of the body," other quotations peppered each section of the pamphlet, some from well-known physiologists such as Thomas Huxley and Henry Pickering Bowditch. For example, with regard to physical education and hygiene, Huxley posited "The successful men in life are those who have stored up such physical health in youth that they can in an emergency work sixteen hours in a day without suffering from it." Concerning food and digestion, Bowditch stated: "A scientific or physiological diet for an adult, per day, is two pounds of bread, and three-quarters of a pound of lean meat," and in regard to tobacco use, "Tobacco is nearly as dangerous and deadly as alcohol, and a man with tobacco heart is as badly off as a drunkard." Other quotations were used for such tissues as skin. Dr. Dudley A. Sargent told readers "Wear dark clothes in winter and light in summer. Have three changes of underclothing—heavy flannels for winter, light flannels for spring and fall, lisle thread, silk or open cotton for summer."

Anthropometric assessment of body build. During the years 1861 to 1888, Dr. Hitchcock Jr obtained 6 measures of segmental height, 23 girths, 6 breadths, 8 lengths, 8 measures of muscular strength, lung capacity, and pilosity (amount of hair on the body) from almost every student who attended Amherst College. From 1882 to 1888, according to Hitchcock, his standardization for measurement was improved

[f]Edward Hitchcock Jr often is accorded the distinction of being the first professor of physical education in the United States, whereas, in fact, John D. Hooker was first appointed to this position at Amherst College in 1860. Because of poor health, Hooker resigned in 1861, and Hitchcock was appointed in his place. The original idea of a Department of Physical Education with a professorship had been proposed in 1854 by William Agustus Stearns, DD, the fourth President of Amherst College, who considered physical education instruction essential for the health of the students and useful to prepare them physically, spiritually, and intellectually. Other institutions were slow to adopt this innovative concept; the next department of physical education in America was not created until 1879. In 1860, the Barrett Gymnasium at Amherst College was completed and served as the training facility where all students were required to perform systematic exercises 30 minutes, four days a week. The gymnasium included a laboratory with scientific instruments (e.g., spirometer, strength and anthropometric equipment), and also a piano to provide rhythm during the exercises. Hitchcock reported to the Trustees that in his first year, he recorded the student's "vital statistics—including age, weight, height, size of chest and forearm, capacity of lungs, and some measure of muscular strength."

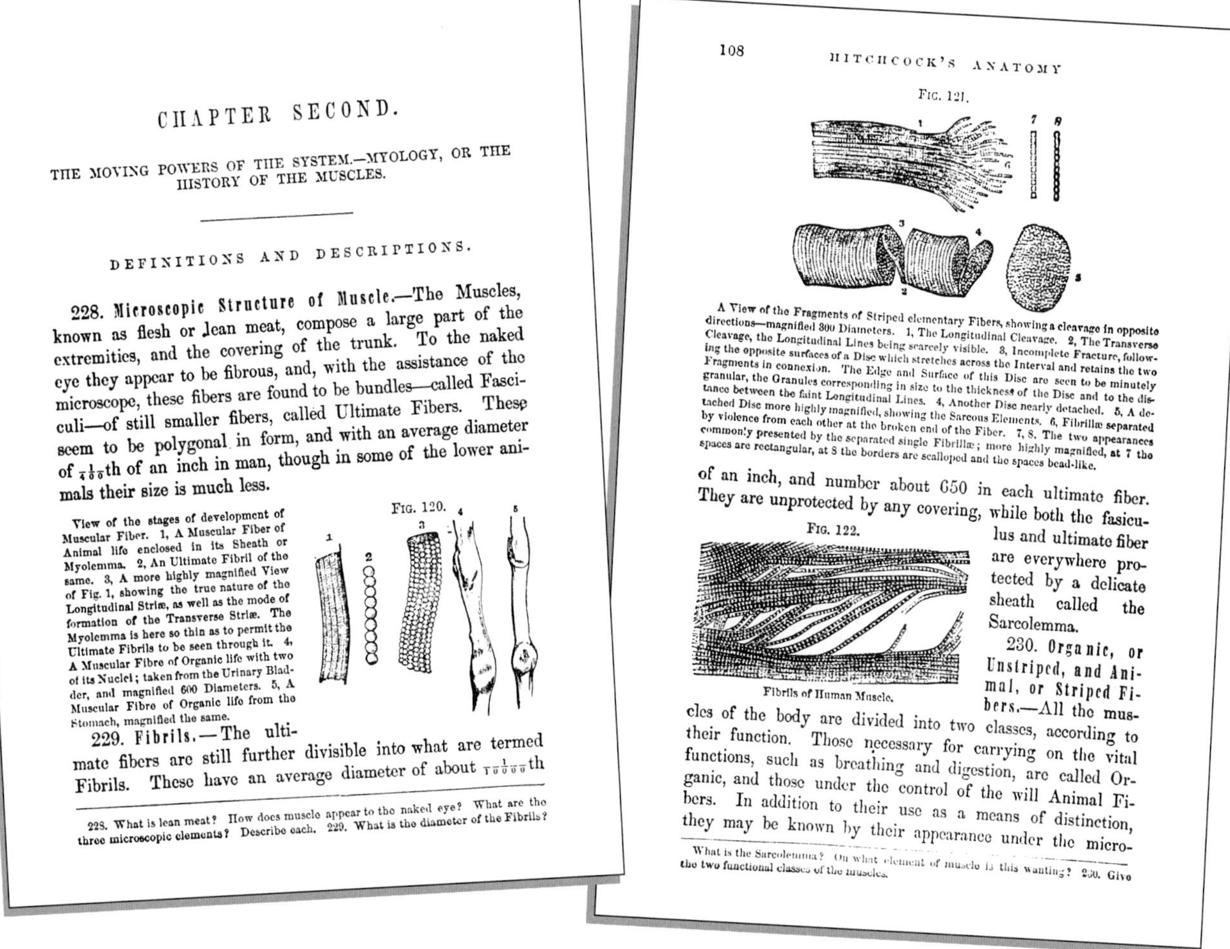

CHAPTER SECOND.

THE MOVING POWERS OF THE SYSTEM.—MYOLOGY, OR THE HISTORY OF THE MUSCLES.

DEFINITIONS AND DESCRIPTIONS.

228. **Microscopic Structure of Muscle.**—The Muscles, known as flesh or lean meat, compose a large part of the extremities, and the covering of the trunk. To the naked eye they appear to be fibrous, and, with the assistance of the microscope, these fibers are found to be bundles—called Fasciculi—of still smaller fibers, called Ultimate Fibers. These seem to be polygonal in form, and with an average diameter of $\frac{1}{400}$th of an inch in man, though in some of the lower animals their size is much less.

FIG. 120.

View of the stages of development of Muscular Fiber. 1, A Muscular Fiber of Animal life enclosed in its Sheath or Myolemma. 2, An Ultimate Fibril of the same. 3, A more highly magnified View of Fig. 1, showing the true nature of the Longitudinal Striæ, as well as the mode of formation of the Transverse Striæ. The Myolemma is here so thin as to permit the Ultimate Fibrils to be seen through it. 4, A Muscular Fibre of Organic life with two of its Nuclei; taken from the Urinary Bladder, and magnified 600 Diameters. 5, A Muscular Fibre of Organic life from the Stomach, magnified the same.

229. **Fibrils.**—The ultimate fibers are still further divisible into what are termed Fibrils. These have an average diameter of about $\frac{1}{10000}$th

228. What is lean meat? How does muscle appear to the naked eye? What are the three microscopic elements? Describe each. 229. What is the diameter of the Fibrils?

108 HITCHCOCK'S ANATOMY

FIG. 121.

A View of the Fragments of Striped elementary Fibers, showing a cleavage in opposite directions—magnified 300 Diameters. 1, The Longitudinal Cleavage. 2, The Transverse Cleavage, the Longitudinal Lines being scarcely visible. 3, Incomplete Fracture, following the opposite surfaces of a Disc which stretches across the Interval and retains the two Fragments in connexion. The Edge and Surface of this Disc are seen to be minutely granular, the Granules corresponding in size to the thickness of the Disc and to the distance between the faint Longitudinal Lines. 4, Another Disc nearly detached. 5, A detached Disc more highly magnified, showing the Sarcous Elements. 6, Fibrillæ separated by violence from each other at the broken end of the Fiber. 7, 8, The two appearances commonly presented by the separated single Fibrillæ; more highly magnified, at 7 the spaces are rectangular, at 8 the borders are scalloped and the spaces bead-like.

of an inch, and number about 650 in each ultimate fiber. They are unprotected by any covering, while both the fasiculus and ultimate fiber are everywhere protected by a delicate sheath called the Sarcolemma.

FIG. 122.

Fibrils of Human Muscle.

230. **Organic, or Unstriped, and Animal, or Striped Fibers.**—All the muscles of the body are divided into two classes, according to their function. Those necessary for carrying on the vital functions, such as breathing and digestion, are called Organic, and those under the control of the will Animal Fibers. In addition to their use as a means of distinction, they may be known by their appearance under the micro-

What is the Sarcolemma? On what element of muscle is this wanting? 230. Give the two functional classes of the muscles.

FIGURE 3 • Examples from the Hitchcock's text on structure and function of muscles. (Reproduced from Hitchcock E, Hitchcock E, Jr. Elementary anatomy and physiology for colleges, academies, and other schools. New York: Ivison, Phinney & Co., 1860: 132, 137. Materials courtesy of Amherst College Archives, and permission of the Trustees of Amherst College, 1995.)

based on suggestions of Dr. W.T. Brigham of Boston and Dr. Dudley A. Sargent (Yale medical degree, 1878; assistant professor of physical training and director of Harvard's Hemenway Gymnasium).

In 1889, Dr. Hitchcock and his colleague in the Department of Physical Education and Hygiene, Hiram H. Seelye, MD (who also served as college physician from 1884–1896), published a 37-page anthropometric manual that included 5 tables of anthropometric statistics of students from 1861 to 1891. This resource compendium provided detailed descriptions for taking measurements that also included eye testing, and an examination of the lungs and heart before testing subjects for muscular strength. In the last section of the manual, Dr. Seelye wrote detailed instructions for using the various pieces of gymnasium apparatus for "enlarging and strengthening the neck, to remedy round or stooping shoulders, to increase the size of the chest and the capacity of the lungs, to strengthen and enlarge the arm, abdominal muscles, and weak back, and to enlarge and strengthen the thighs, calves, legs and ankles." The Hitchcock and Seelye manual, the first of its kind devoted to an analysis of anthropometric and strength data based on detailed measurements, influenced other departments of physical education in the United States (e.g., Yale, Harvard, Wellesley, Mt. Holyoke) to include anthropometric measurements as part of the physical education and hygiene curriculum.

Hitchcock's keen awareness of the history of anthropometry was succinctly stated in a speech titled, "The Need for Anthropometry," delivered as President of the American Association for the Advancement of Physical Education at the second annual meeting held in Brooklyn, New York, November 26, 1886. Hitchcock's claim of the importance of anthropometry in the college curriculum was not universally accepted; in fact, at the same conference, there was heated debate about the need for anthropometric assessment as part of training and exercise programs. Hitchcock was convinced that an important value of anthropometric assessment was its intrinsic relationship to human performance.[g] In fact, in his talk, he laid the groundwork for his rationale based on a historical perspective:

> The study of Anthropometry, or the proportions of the human body, is not modern, but reaches back to the remote civilization of India, when we find a treatise called Silpi Sastri, which investigated the outline of the body by dividing it into 480 parts. In later times, the Greeks proposed a "Canon" or model in the shape of a statue called Doryphoros, which was claimed to be the pattern for the human figure. Still later the mathematical law was applied to the human body, an entirely artificial system; hence, we obtain the terms cubit, hand-breadth, ell, and so on. An Italian sculptor, Alberti, proposed a module of 1 foot in height, which was divided into 10 degrees and minutes, as a standard for the proportions of the human body. In 1854 a German, Carus, proposed an anatomical basis for determining human bodily proportions, assuming the hand length for the unit, and the adult vertebral column of 24 free vertebrae, to be the key to these proportions. But the father of anthropometry is Baron Quetelet of Belgium, who, in the middle part of the present century, offered the actual measurements of the body and the means and averages deduced from them as the true and scientific way of ascertaining human proportions; adopting the Baconian method of reasoning from the effect to the cause, from the concrete to the abstract.

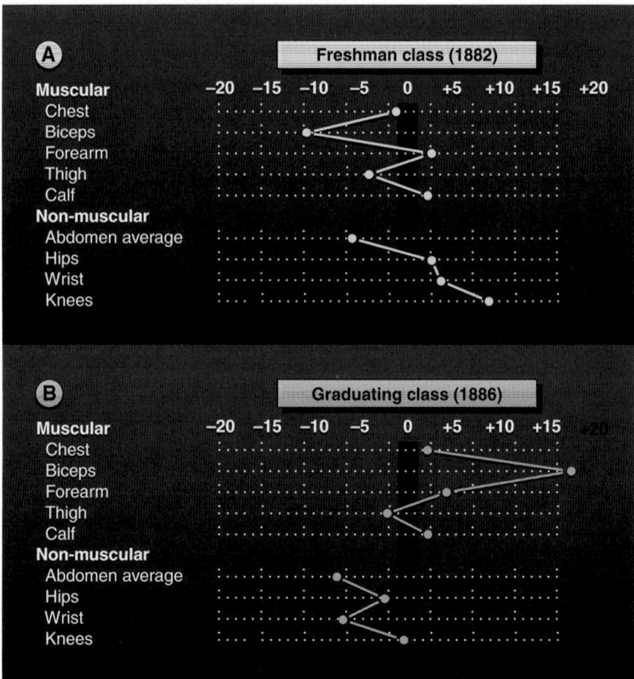

FIGURE 4 • Changes in selected girth measurements of Amherst College men over 4 years of college using Behnke's reference man standards (presented in Chapter 28). **A**. The average body mass of the freshman class in 1882 was 59.1 kg (stature, 171.0 cm). **B**. Four years later, average body mass increased 5.5 kg (11.3 lb) and stature increased by 7.4 cm (2.9 in).

One of the reasons for the early interest in anthropometric measurement was to demonstrate that engaging in daily, vigorous exercise produced desirable results, particularly for muscular development. Although none of the early physical education scientists used statistics to evaluate the outcomes of their exercise programs, it is instructive to apply modern methods of anthropometric analysis to the original data of Hitchcock on entering students at Amherst College in 1882 and on their graduation in 1886. Figure 4 shows how the average student changed in anthropometric dimensions throughout 4 years of college in relation to Behnke's reference standards presented in Chapter 28. Note the dramatic increase in biceps girth and decreases in the nonmuscular abdomen and hip regions. Although data for a nonexercising "control" group of students were not available, these changes coincided with daily resistance training prescribed in the Hitchcock and Seelye *Anthropometric Manual*. This training used Indian club or barbell swinging exercises (Fig. 5) and other strengthening modalities (horizontal bar, rope and ring exercises, parallel bar exercises, dipping machine, inclined presses with weights, pulley weights, and rowing machine workouts). "Old Doc" Hitchcock (as he was affectionately called) would have rejoiced to learn that his required physical education training program produced desirable results, something he fervently believed would occur. The Hitchcock data presentation, a first of its kind initially reported in the *Anthropometric Manual* in March, 1892, used "bodily stature" as the basis of comparison "from measurements of 1322 students between 17 and 26 years of age. The strength tests are derived from 20,761 items." The Hitchcock anthropometric and strength studies were acknowledged in the first formal American textbook on anthropometry published in 1896 by Jay W. Seaver, MD (1855–1915), physician and lecturer on

[g]Probably unknown to Hitchcock was the 1628 manuscript of the Flemish fencing instructor at the French Royal Court, Gerard Thibault, who studied optimal body proportions and success in fencing.[53] This early text, *"L'Académie de l'Espée,"* appeared at a time when important discoveries were being made by European scientists, particularly anatomists and physiologists, whose contributions played such an important role in laboratory experimentation and scientific inquiry. Had Hitchcock known about this early attempt to link anthropometric assessment with success in sport, the acceptance of anthropometry in the college curriculum might have been easier. Nevertheless, just 67 years after Hitchcock began taking anthropometric measurements at Amherst, and 37 years following the creation of Harvard's physical education scientific laboratory in 1891, anthropometric measurements were made of athletes at the 1928 Amsterdam Olympic Games. One of the athletes measured in Amsterdam, Ernst Jokl from South Africa, became a physician and then professor of physical education at the University of Kentucky. Jokl was a charter member and founder of the American College of Sports Medicine. Thus, Hitchcock's visionary ideas about the importance of anthropometry finally caught on, and such assessment techniques are now used routinely in exercise physiology to assess physique status and the dynamics between physiology and performance. The more modern application of anthropometry is now known as *kinanthropometry*. This term, first defined at the International Congress of Physical Activity Sciences in conjunction with the 1976 Montreal Olympic Games,[52] was refined in 1980[53] as follows: "Kinanthropometry is the application of measurement to the study of human size, shape, proportion, composition, maturation, and gross function. Its purpose is to help us to understand human movement in the context of growth, exercise, performance, and nutrition. We see its essentially human-enobling purpose being achieved through applications in medicine, education, and government."

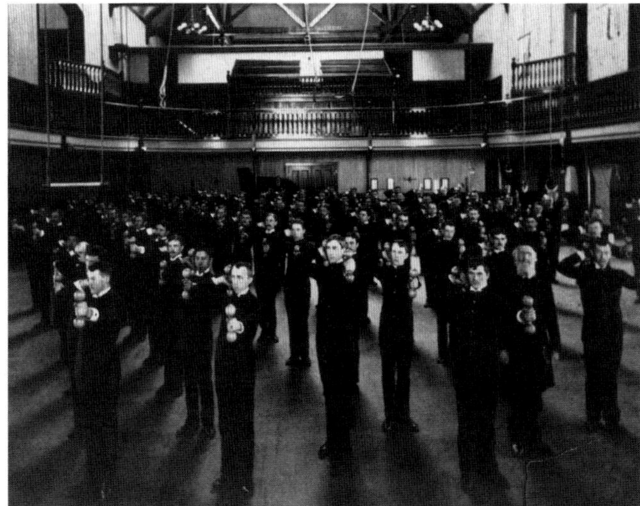

FIGURE 5 • Dr. Edward Hitchcock, Jr. (second from right, with beard) observing the entire class of students perform barbell exercises in the Pratt Gymnasium of Amherst College. (Photo courtesy of Amherst College Archives, and by permission of the Trustees of Amherst College, 1995.)

personal hygiene at Yale University. Table 3 presents a sample of the average and "best" anthropometric values at Amherst College from 1861 to 1900.

While Hitchcock was performing pioneering anthropometric studies at the college level, the military was making the first detailed anthropometric, spirometric, and muscular strength measurements on Civil War soldiers in the early 1860s and published in 1869 by Gould (cited in Table 1). The specially trained military anthropometrists used a unique device, the andrometer (Fig. 6), to secure the physical dimensions to the nearest 1/10th of an inch of soldiers for purposes of fitting uniforms. The andrometer originally was devised in 1855 by a tailor in Edinburgh, Scotland, who was commissioned by the British government to determine the proper size for British soldiers' clothing. This device was set by special gauges to adjust "sliders" for measurement of total height; breadth of the neck, shoulders, and pelvis; and the length of the legs and height to the knees and crotch. Each examiner re-

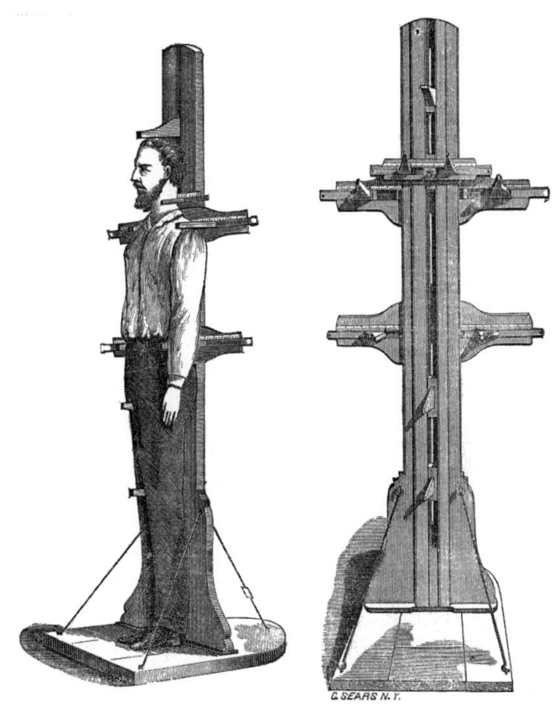

FIGURE 6 • The andrometer was first used by the United States Sanitary Commission at numerous military installations along the Atlantic seaboard during the early 1860s to size soldiers for clothing.

TABLE 3 ➤ **THE AVERAGE AND THE BEST ANTHROPOMETRIC RECORDS OF AMHERST COLLEGE FROM 1861 TO 1900 INCLUSIVE**

	Average		Maxima			
Items	Metric	English	Metric	English	Held By	Date of Record
Weight	61.2	134.9	113.7	250.6	K. R. Otis, '03	Oct. 2, '99
Height	1725	67.9	1947	76.6	B. Matthews '99	Oct. 28, '95
Girth, Head	572	22.5	630	24.8	W. H. Lewis '92	Feb. '92
Girth, Neck	349	13.7	420	16.5	D. R. Knight '91	Feb. '91
Girth, Chest, repose	880	34.6	1140	44.9	K. R. Otis '03	Oct. 2 '99
Girth, Belly	724	28.5	1017	40.1	G. H. Colman '99	May '97
Girth, Hips	893	35.1	1165	45.9	K. R. Otis '03	Oct. 2, '99
Girth, Right Thigh	517	20.3	745	29.3	K. R. Otis '03	Oct. 2, '99
Girth, Right Knee	361	14.2	460	18.1	K. R. Otis '03	Oct. 2, '99
Girth, Right Calf	359	14.1	452	17.8	K. R. Otis '03	Oct. 2, '99
Girth, Upper Right Arm	257	10.1	396	15.6	K. R. Otis '03	Oct. 2, '99
Girth, Right Forearm	267	10.5	327	12.8	K. R. Otis '03	Oct. 2, '99
Girth, Right Wrist	166	6.5	191	7.5	H. B. Haskell '94	April '92
Strength, Chest, Dip	6	—	45	—	H. W. Lane '95	March '95
Strength, Chest, Pull Up	9	—	65	—	H. W. Seelye '79	Oct. '75
Strength, Right Forearm	41	90	86	189.6	A. J. Wyman '98	April '96
Strength, Left Forearm	38	84	73	160.9	A. J. Wyman '98	April '96
Capacity of Lungs	377	230	6.66	406	E. D. Blodgett '87	June '87

From Hitchcock E, et al.: An anthropometric manual, 4th ed. Amherst, MA: Carpenter and Morehouse, 1900.

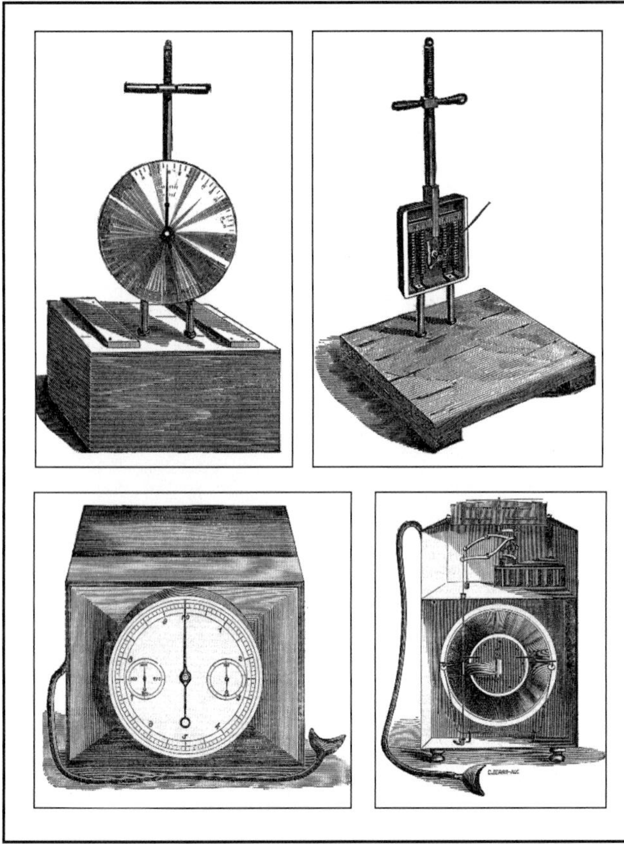

Figure 7 • *Top.* Instrument used to evaluate muscular strength in the military studies of Gould in 1869. The illustration on the left shows the general look of the device, while the right side shows the internal arrangement without face-plate. Gould described the procedure for measuring muscular strength as follows: "The man stands upon the movable lid of the wooden packing box, to which the apparatus is firmly attached, and grasps with both hands the rounded extremities of a wooden bar, of convenient shape and adjustable in height...The handle is conveniently shaped for firm and easy grasp, its height well suited for application and the full muscular power, and the mechanism such as to afford results which are to all appearance very trustworthy." This was not the first dynamometer; Gould cites Regnier (no date given), who published a description of a dynamometer to measure the strength of Parisians; and Péron, who carried a dynamometer on an expedition to Australia. Other researchers in Europe had also used dynamometers to compare the muscular strength of men of different races. Figure 22.1C shows the modern back-leg lift dynamometer still used for assessing muscular strength as part of physical fitness test procedures. *Bottom.* Spirometers, or dry gas meters, were used to measure vital capacity. These instruments were manufactured by the American Meter Company of Philadelphia. According to Gould, the spirometers needed to be rugged "... to undergo the rough usage inseparable from transportation by army trains or on military railroads, which are in danger of being handled roughly at some unguarded moment by rude men..." The spirometers were graduated in cubic centimeters, and were "furnished with a mouth-piece of convenient form, connected with the instrument by flexible tubing."

ceived 2 days of practice to perfect measurement technique before assignment to different military installations (e.g., Fort McHeny in Baltimore, Naval Rendezvous in New York City, Marine Barracks at the Brooklyn Navy Yard, and bases in South Carolina, Washington DC, Detroit, and New Orleans). Data were compiled on the actual and relative proportions of 15,781 men ("Whites, Blacks, Indians") between the ages of 16 and 45 years. One purpose of these military studies was to determine relationships among the anthropometric and other physical measurements, as well as to gather demographic and anthropological statistics on enlisted and commissioned soldiers in the infantry, cavalry, and artillery. These early investigations about muscular strength and body dimensions served as prototypical studies whose measurement techniques led the way to many later studies conducted in the military about muscular strength and human performance per se. Most laboratories in exercise physiology today include assessment procedures to evaluate aspects of muscular strength and body composition.

The top of Figure 7 shows two views of the instrument used to evaluate muscular strength in the military studies; the bottom of the figure shows the early spirometers used to evaluate pulmonary dimensions. The strength device predates the various strength-measuring instruments shown in Figure 8 used by Hitchcock (Amherst), Sargent (Harvard), and Seaver (Yale), as well as anthropometric measuring instruments used in their batteries of physical measurements. The inset shows the price list of some of the equipment from the 1889 and 1890 Hitchcock manuals on anthropometry. Note the progression in complexity of the early spirometers and strength devices used in the 1860 military studies (Fig. 7), and the more "modern" equipment of the 1889–1905 period displayed in Figure 8. Figure 9 includes three recently uncovered photographs (circa 1897–1901) of the strength testing equipment (Kellogg's Universal Dynamometer) acquired by Dr. Hitchcock in 1897 to assess the strength of arms (panel A), anterior trunk and forearm supinators (panel B), and leg extensors, flexors, and adductors (panel C).[h]

The First Exercise Physiology Laboratory and Associated Degree Program in the United States

The first formal exercise physiology laboratory in the United States was established in 1891 at Harvard University and housed in a newly created Department of Anatomy, Physiology, and Physical Training at the Lawrence Scientific School.[22,41] Several instructors in the initial undergraduate BS degree program in Anatomy, Physiology, and Physical Training started at the same time were Harvard-trained physicians; others—including Henry Pickering Bowditch, professor of

[h]According to Hitchcock and Selye's *Anthropometric Manual*, the device consisted "of a lever acting by means of a piston and cylinder on a column of mercury in a closed glass tube. Water keeps the oil in the cylinder from contact with the mercury and various attachments enable the different groups of muscles to be brought to bear on the lever. By means of this apparatus, the strength of most of the large muscles may be tested fairly objectively"(p. 25). In the photographs, note the attachment of the tube to each device. Interestingly, Hitchcock determined an individual's total strength as a composite of body weight multiplied by dip and pull tests, strength of the back, legs, and average of the forearms, and the lung strength. Hitchcock stated, "The TOTAL STRENGTH is purely an arbitrary, and relative, rather than an actual test of strength as its name would indicate. And while confessedly imperfect, it seems decidedly desirable that there should be some method of comparison which does not depend entirely on lifting a dead weight against gravity, or steel springs."

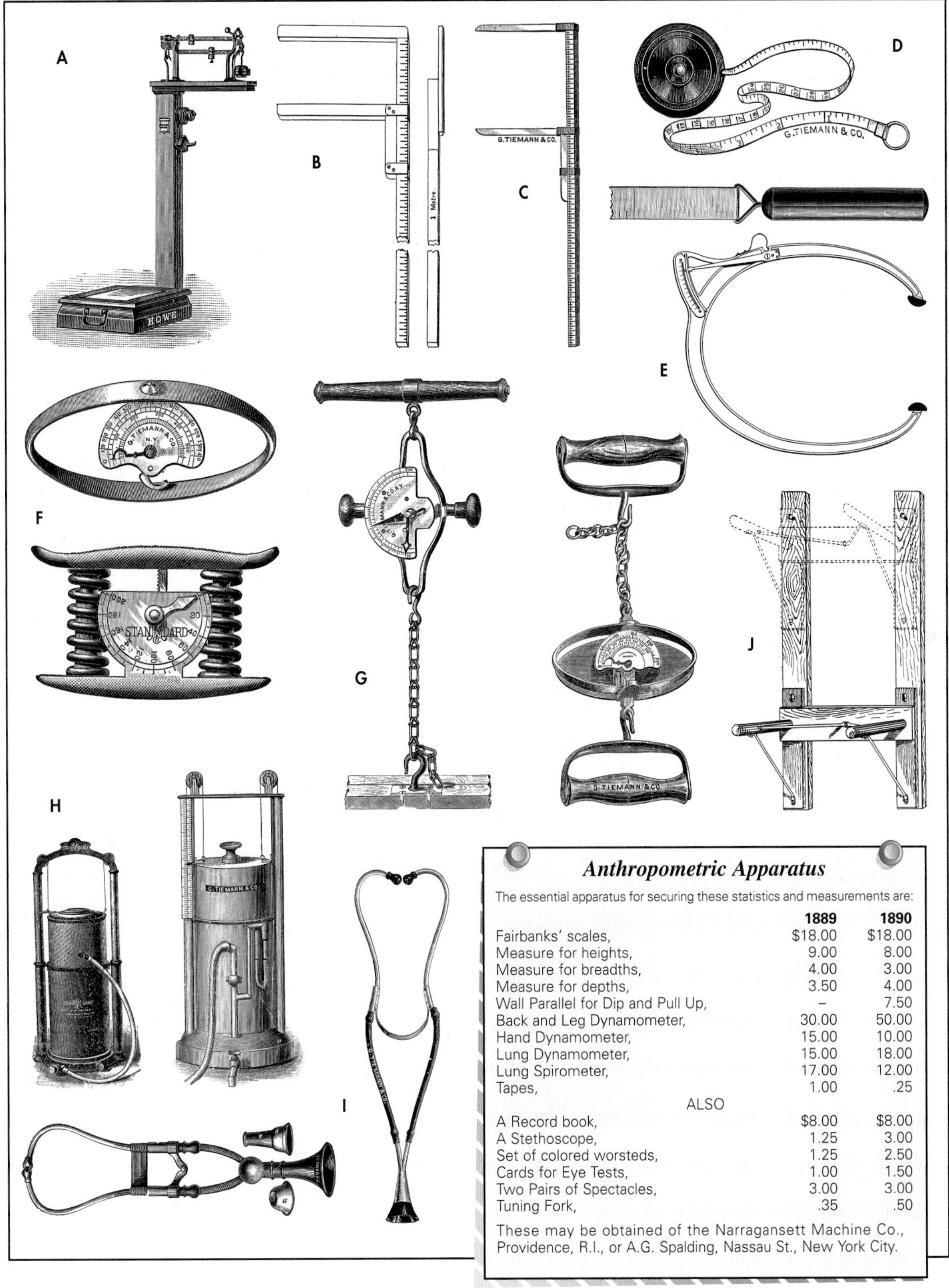

Anthropometric Apparatus

The essential apparatus for securing these statistics and measurements are:

	1889	1890
Fairbanks' scales,	$18.00	$18.00
Measure for heights,	9.00	8.00
Measure for breadths,	4.00	3.00
Measure for depths,	3.50	4.00
Wall Parallel for Dip and Pull Up,	–	7.50
Back and Leg Dynamometer,	30.00	50.00
Hand Dynamometer,	15.00	10.00
Lung Dynamometer,	15.00	18.00
Lung Spirometer,	17.00	12.00
Tapes,	1.00	.25
ALSO		
A Record book,	$8.00	$8.00
A Stethoscope,	1.25	3.00
Set of colored worsteds,	1.25	2.50
Cards for Eye Tests,	1.00	1.50
Two Pairs of Spectacles,	3.00	3.00
Tuning Fork,	.35	.50

These may be obtained of the Narragansett Machine Co., Providence, R.I., or A.G. Spalding, Nassau St., New York City.

Figure 8 • Anthropometric instruments used by Hitchcock, Seaver, and Sargent. Sargent, also an entrepreneur, constructed and sold specialized strength equipment used in his studies. **A**, Metric graduated scale. **B**, Height meter. **C**, Sliding anthropometer. **D**, Cloth tape measure, with an instrument made by the Narragansett Machine Co., at the suggestion of Dr. Gulick (head of the Department of Physical Training of the YMCA Training School, Springfield, MA) in 1887. The modern version of this tape, now sold as the "Gulick tape," was "for attachment to the end of a tape to indicate the proper tension, so that the pressure may be always alike." **E**, Calipers for taking body depths. **F**, Several types of hand dynamometers, including push holder and pull holder instruments. **G**, Back and leg dynamometer, also used to measure the strength of the pectoral and "retractor" muscles of the shoulders. **H**, Vital capacity spirometer and Hutchinson's wet spirometer. **I**, Two stethoscopes. The soft rubber bell was used to "secure perfect coaptation to the surface of the chest." The Albion Stethoscope was preferred because it could be conveniently carried in the pocket. **J**, Parallel bars for testing arm extensors during push-ups, and testing of flexors in pull-ups. In special situations, physiological laboratories used Marey's cardiograph to record pulse, but the preferred instrument was a pneumatic kymograph (or sphygmograph; see Fig.2). The inset shows a price comparison for the testing equipment from the 1889 and 1890 Hitchcock manuals. Note the yearly variation in prices. (Inset courtesy of Amherst College Archives, reproduced by permission of the Trustees of Amherst College, 1995.)

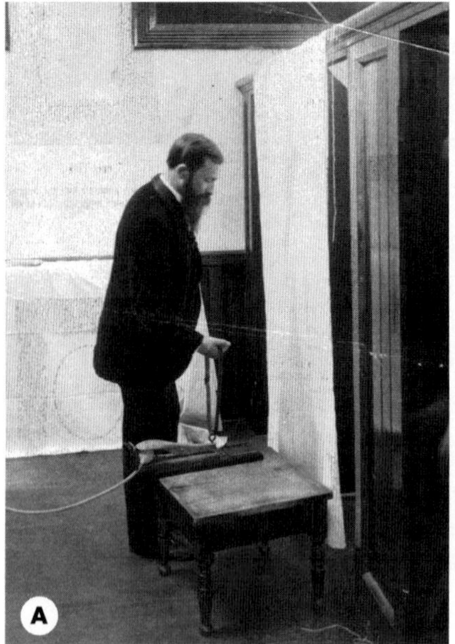

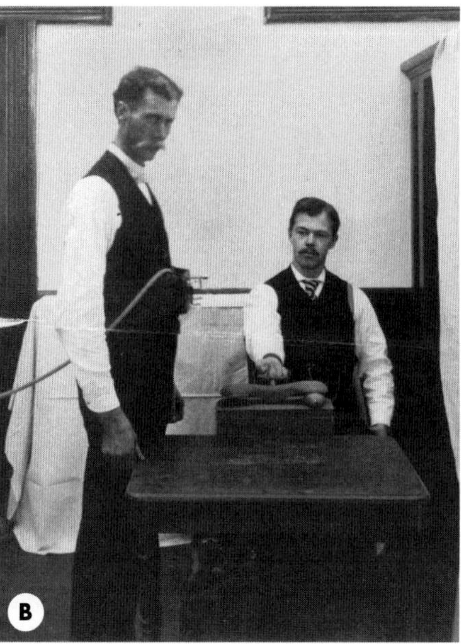

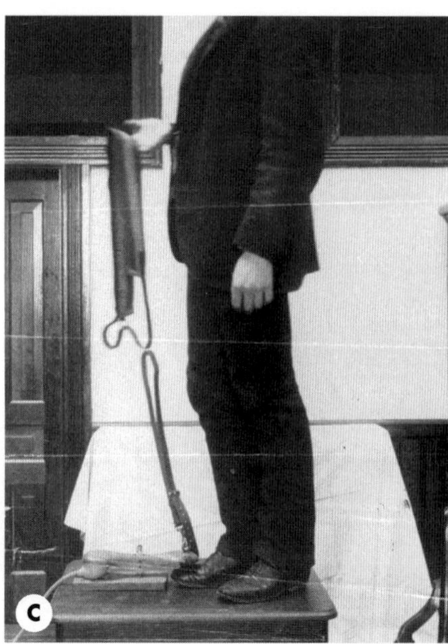

FIGURE 9 • Kellogg's Universal Dynamometer acquired by Dr. Hitchcock to test the muscular strength of Amherst College students. From 1897 to 1900, strength measurements were taken on 328 freshmen, 111 sophomores, and 88 seniors, including re-tests of 58 individuals. Arm strength was measured bilaterally for the forearms and for the latissimus dorsi, deltoid, pectoral, and shoulder "retractor" muscles. Trunk measurements included the anterior trunk, and anterior and posterior neck. The leg measurements included the leg extensors and flexors and thigh adductors. **A**, "Arm pull." **B**, Anterior trunk (standing) and forearm supinators (sitting). **C**, Legs. (Photos courtesy of Amherst College Archives, and by permission of the trustees of Amherst College, 1995.)

physiology who discovered the all-or-none principle of cardiac contraction and treppe, the staircase phenomenon of muscular contraction, and William T. Porter, also a physiologist in the Harvard Medical School—were well respected for their rigorous scientific and laboratory training.

George Wells Fitz, MD: A Major Influence

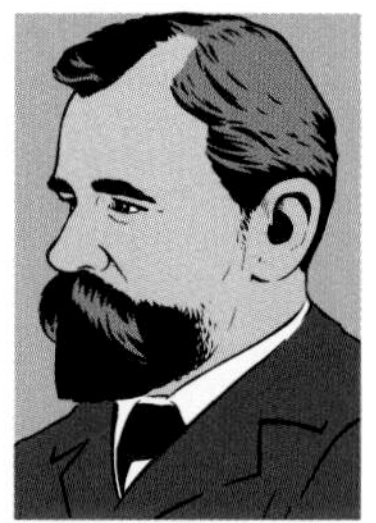

An important influence in creating the new departmental major and recruiting top scientists as faculty in the Harvard program was George Wells Fitz, MD (1860–1934). Fitz vociferously supported a strong, science-based curriculum in preparing the new breed of physical educators. The archival records show that the newly formed major was grounded in the basic sciences, including formal coursework in exercise physiology, zoology, morphology (animal and human), anthropometry, applied anatomy and animal mechanics, medical chemistry, comparative anatomy, remedial exercises, physics, gymnastics and athletics, history of physical education, and English. Physical education students took general anatomy and physiology courses in the medical school; after 4 years of study, graduates could enroll as second-year medical students and graduate in 3 years with an MD degree. Dr. Fitz taught the physiology of exercise course; thus, we believe he was the first person to formally teach such a course. It included experimental investigation and original work and thesis, including 6 hours a week of laboratory study. The course prerequisites included general physiology at the medical school or its equivalent. The purpose of the course was to introduce the student to the fundamentals of physical education and provide training in experimental methods related to exercise physiology. Fitz also taught a more general course titled, "The Elementary Physiology of The Hygiene of Common Life, Personal Hygiene, Emergencies." The course included one lecture and one laboratory section a week for a year (or three times a week for one-half year). The official course description stated: "This is a general introductory course intended to give the knowledge of human anatomy, physiology and hygiene which should be possessed by every student; it is suitable also for those not intending to study medicine or physical training." Fitz also taught a course on "Remedial Exercises. The Correction of Abnormal Conditions and Positions." Course content included observations of deformities such as spinal curvature (and the corrective effects of specialized exercises), and the "selection and application of proper exercises, and in the diagnosis of cases when exercise is unsuitable." Several of Fitz's scientific publications dealt with spinal deformities. In addition to the remedial exercise course, students took a required course in "Applied Anatomy and Animal Mechanics. Action of Muscles in Different Exercises." This thrice-weekly course taught by Dr. Dudley Sargeant was the forerunner of modern biomechanics courses. Its prerequisite was general anatomy at the medical school or its equivalent.

Nine men graduated with BS degrees from the Department of Anatomy, Physiology, and Physical Training up to 1900. The aim of the major was to prepare students to become directors of gymnasia or instructors in physical training, to provide students with the necessary knowledge about the science of exercise, and to offer suitable training for entrance to the medical school. The stated purpose of the new exercise physiology research laboratory was as follows:

> A large and well-equipped laboratory has been organized for the experimental study of the physiology of exercise. The object of this work is to exemplify the hygiene of the muscles, the conditions under which they act, the relation of their action to the body as a whole affecting blood supply and general hygienic conditions, and the effects of various exercises upon muscular growth and general health.

With the activities of the department in full operation, its outspoken and critical director Dr. Fitz was not afraid to speak his mind about academic topics. For example, Fitz reviewed a new physiology text (*American Text-Book of Physiology*, edited by William H. Howell, PhD, MD) in the March 1897 issue of the *American Physical Education Review* (Vol II, No. 1, p. 56). The review praised Dr. Howell's collection of contributions from outstanding physiologists (such as Bowditch, Lee, Lusk, and Sewall), and attacked an 1888 French book by Lagrange that some historians consider the first important text in exercise physiology.[i] The following is Fitz's review:

> No one who is interested in the deeper problems of the physiology of exercise can afford to be without this book [referring to Howell's Physiology test], and it is to be hoped it may be used as a text-book in the normal schools of physical training. These schools have been forced to depend largely on Lagrange's "physiology of exercise" for the discussion of specific problems, or at least for the basis of such discussions. The only value Lagrange has, to my mind, is that he seldom gives any hint of the truth, and the student is forced to work out his own problems. This does very well in well-taught classes, but, Alas! for those schools and readers who take his statements as final in matters physiological. We have a conspicuous example of the disastrous consequences in Treve's contribution of the "Cyclopaedia of Hygiene on Physical Education," in which he quotes freely from Lagrange and rivals him in the absurdity of his conclusions.
>
> The time has surely come for a thoroughly scientific investigation of the physiological problems involved in physical exercise and the promulgation of the exact and absolute. It is not too much to hope that the use of the American text-book of Physiology by training schools and teachers, may aid to bring about this much needed consummation.

For unknown reasons, but coinciding with Fitz's untimely departure from Harvard in 1899,[j] the department changed its curricular emphasis (the term physical training was dropped from the department title), thus terminating at least temporarily this unique experiment in higher education.

One of the legacies of the Fitz-directed "Harvard experience" between 1891 and 1899 was the training it provided to the cadre of young scholars who began their careers with a strong scientific basis in exercise and training and its relationship to health. Unfortunately, it would take about another quarter century before the next generation of science-oriented physical educators (led by physiologists like A. V. Hill and D.B. Dill, not physical educators) would once again exert strong influence on the physical education curriculum.

Exercise Studies in Research Journals

Another notable event in the growth of exercise physiology occurred in 1898: the appearance of three articles dealing with physical activity in the first volume of the *American Journal of Physiology*.[k] This was followed in 1921 with the publication of the prestigious journal *Physiological Reviews*. Table 4 lists the articles in this journal (and two from the *Annual Review of Physiology*) from the first review of the mechanisms of muscular contraction by A. V. Hill in 1922, to Hellebrandt's classic review of exercise in 1940. The German applied physiology publication, *Internationale Zeitschrift fur angewandte Physiologie einschliesslich Arbeitsphysiologie* (1929–1973), was a significant journal for research in exercise physiology. The current title of this journal is *European Journal of Applied Physiology and Occupational Physiology*. The *Journal of Applied Physiology* was first published in 1948. Its first volume contained the now-classic paper on ratio expressions of physiological data with reference to body size and function by Tanner, a must-read for exercise physiologists. The journal *Medicine and Science in Sports* was first published in 1969. Its aim was to integrate both medical and physiological aspects of the emerging fields of sports medicine and exercise science. The official name of this journal was changed in 1980 (Volume 12) to *Medicine and Science in Sports and Exercise*.

The First Textbook in Exercise Physiology: The Debate Continues

What was the first textbook in exercise physiology? Several recent exercise physiology texts give the distinction of being "first" to the English translation of Fernand Lagrange's book, *The Physiology of Bodily Exercise*, originally published in

---

[i]We disagree with Berryman's[6] assessment of the relative historical importance of the translation of the original Lagrange text. We give our reasons for this disagreement in a subsequent section titled, "First Textbook in Exercise Physiology: The Debate Continues."

[j]The reasons for Fitz's early departure from Harvard have been discussed in detail in Park's scholarly presentation of this topic.[46a] His leaving was certainly unfortunate for the next generation of students of exercise physiology. In his 1909 textbook *Principles of Physiology and Hygiene*. (New York, Henry Holt and Company), the title page listed the following about Fitz's affiliation: Sometime Assistant Professor Physiology and Hygiene and Medical Visitor, Harvard University.

[k]The originator of *the American Journal of Physiology* was physiologist W.T. Porter of the St. Louis College of Medicine and Harvard Medical School, who remained editor until 1914.[10] Porter's research focused on cardiac physiology. The three articles in volume 1 concerned (1) spontaneous physical activity in rodents and the influence of diet (C.C. Stewart, Department of Physiology, Clark University), (2) neural control of muscular movement in dogs (R.H. Cunningham, College of Physicians and Surgeons, Columbia University), and (3) perception of muscular fatigue and physical activity (J.C. Welch, Hull Physiological Laboratory, University of Chicago). As pointed out by Buskirk,[10] the next four volumes of the *American Journal of Physiology* (1898–1901) contained six additional articles about exercise physiology from experimental research laboratories at Harvard Medical School, Massachusetts Institute of Technology, The University of Michigan, and The Johns Hopkins University.

TABLE 4 ➤ **REVIEW ARTICLES ABOUT EXERCISE, 1922–1940**

YEAR	AUTHOR AND ARTICLE
1922	Hill, A.V. The mechanism of muscular contraction *Physiol. Rev.* 2: 310, 1922.
1925	Cathcart, E.P. The influence of muscle work on protein metabolism. *Physiol. Rev.* 5: 225, 1925
1925	Cobb, S. Review on the tonus of skeletal muscle. *Physiol. Rev.* 5: 518, 1925.
1928	Vernon, H.M. Industrial fatigue in relation to atomospheric conditions. *Physiol. Rev.* 8: 1, 1921928.
1929	Eggleton, P. The position of phosphorus in the chemical mechansism of muscle contraction. *Physiol. Rev.* 9: 432, 1929.
1929	Richardson, H.B. The respiratory quotient (including: The source of energy used for muscular exertion). *Physiol. Rev.* 9: 61, 1929.
1930	Gasset, H.S. Contracture of skeletal muscle. *Physiol. Rev.* 10: 35, 1930
1931	Milroy, T.H. The present status of the chemistry of skeletal muscular contraction. *Physiol. Rev.* 11: 515, 1931.
1932	Baetzer, A.M. The effect of muscular fatigue upon resistance. *Physiol. Rev.* 12: 453, 1932.
1932	Hill, A.V. The revolution in muscle physiology. *Physiol. Rev.* 12: 56, 1932.
1933	Jordan, H.E. The structural changes in striped muscle during contraction. *Physiol. Rev.* 13: 301, 1933.
1933	Steinhaus, A.H. Chronic effects of exercise. *Physiol. Rev.* 13: 103, 1933.
1934	Hinsey, J.C. The innervation of skeletal muscle. *Physiol. Rev.* 14: 514, 1934.
1936	Dill, D.B. The economy of muscular exercise. *Physiol. Rev.* 16: 263, 1936.
1936	Fenn, W.O. Electrolytes in muscle. *Physiol. Rev.* 16: 450, 1936.
1937	Anderson, W.W. and Williams, H.H. Role of fat in diet. *Physiol. Rev.* 17: 335, 1937.
1939	Bozler, E. Muscle. *Annu. Rev. Physiol.* 1: 217, 1939
1939	Dill, D.B. Applied Physiology. *Annu. Rev. Physiol.* 1: 551, 1939
1939	Millikan, G.A. Muscle hemoglobin. *Physiol. Rev.* 19: 503, 1939.
1939	Tower, S.S. The reaction of muscle to denervation. *Physiol. Rev.* 19: 1, 1939.
1940	Hellebrandt, F.A. Exercise. *Annu. Rev. Physiol.* 2: 411, 1940.

French in 1888.[6,51,60] To deserve such historical recognition, we believe the work should meet the following three criteria:

1. Provide sound scientific rationale for major concepts.
2. Provide summary information (based on experimentation) about important prior research in a particular topic area (e.g., contain scientific references to research in the area).
3. Provide sufficient "factual" information about a topic area to give it academic legitimacy.

After reading the Lagrange book in its entirety, we came to the same conclusion as Fitz. Specifically, it was a popular book about health and exercise with a "scientific" title. It is our opinion that the book is *not* a legitimate scientific textbook of exercise physiology based on any reasonable criteria of the time. Despite Lagrange's assertion that the focus of his book assessed physiology applied to exercise and not hygiene and exercise, it is informed by a 19th century hygienic perspective, not science. We believe Fitz would accept our evaluation.

There was much information available to Lagrange from existing European and American physiology textbooks about the digestive, muscular, circulatory, and respiratory systems, as well as some limited information on physical training, hormones, basic nutrition, chemistry, and the biology of muscular contraction. Admittedly, this information was relatively scarce, but well-trained physiologists such as Flint, Howell, Martin, Huxley, Dalton, Carpenter, and Combe had already produced quality textbooks that contained relatively detailed information about physiology in general, with some reference to muscular exercise. We now understand why Fitz was so troubled by the Lagrange book. By comparison, the two-volume text by Howell, titled *An American Text-Book of Physiology*, was impressive; this edited volume contained articles from acknowledged American physiologists at the forefront of physiological research. This textbook was a high-level physiology text even by today's standards. In his quest to provide the best possible science for his physical education students, Fitz could not tolerate a book that did not live up to his expectations for excellence. In fact, the Lagrange book contained fewer than 20 reference citations, and most of these were ascribed to French research reports or were based on observations of friends performing exercise. This plethora of anecdotal reports must have given Fitz "fits."

Lagrange, an accomplished writer, wrote extensively on exercise. Despite the titles of several of his books,[l] Lagrange

[l]The following books (including translations, editions, and pages) were published by Lagrange beginning in 1888: *Physiologie des exercices du corps.* Paris: Alcan, 1888, 372 pp. (6th ed., 1892); *L'hygiene de l'exercice chez les enfants et les jeunes gens.* Paris: Alcan, 1890, 312 pp. (4th ed., 1893; 6th ed, 1896; 7th ed, 1901, 8th ed, 1905); *Physiology of Bodily Exercise.* New York: D. Appleton, 1890, 395 pp.; *De l'exercice chez les adultes.* Paris: Alcan, 1891, 367 pp. (2nd ed., 1892, 367 pp.; 4th ed., 1900, 367 pp.; Italian translation, *Fisiologia degli esercizj del corpo.* Milano: Dumolard, 1889; Hungarian translation, 1913); *La medication par l'exercice.* Paris: Alcan, 1894, 500 pp.

was not a scientist but probably a practicing "physical culturist." Bibliographic information about Lagrange is limited in the French and American archival records of the period—a further indication of his relative obscurity as a thinker of distinction. As far as we know, there have been no citations to his work in any physiology text or scientific article. For these reasons, we contend the Lagrange book does not qualify as the first exercise physiology textbook.[m]

Other Early Exercise Physiology Research Laboratories

The Nutrition Laboratory at the Carnegie Institute in Washington DC, had been created in 1904 to study nutrition and energy metabolism, and the first research laboratories established in physical education in the United States to study exercise physiology were at George Williams College (1923), the University of Illinois (1925), and Springfield College (1927). However, the real impact of laboratory research in exercise physiology (along with many other research specialties) occurred in 1927 with the creation of the 800-square foot Harvard Fatigue Laboratory in the basement of Morgan Hall of Harvard University's Business School.[33] The outstanding work of this laboratory during the next two decades established the legitimacy of exercise physiology on its own merits as an important area of research and study. Another exercise physiology laboratory started prior to World War II was the Laboratory of Physiological Hygiene at the University of California, Berkeley, in 1934. The syllabus for the Physiological Hygiene course (taught by professor Frank Kleeberger), the precursor of contemporary exercise physiology courses, contained 12 laboratory experiments.[47] Several years later, Dr. Franklin M. Henry assumed responsibility for the laboratory. Dr. Henry began publishing the results of different experiments in various physiology-oriented journals including the *Journal of Applied Physiology*, *Annals of Internal Medicine*, *Aviation Medicine*, *War Medicine*, and *Science*. Henry's first research project as a faculty member in the Department of Physical Education (published in 1938) concerned the validity and reliability of the pulse–ratio test of cardiac efficiency;[26] a later paper dealt with predicting aviators' bends. Henry applied his training in experimental psychology to exercise physiology topics, including individual differences in the kinetics of the fast and slow components of the oxygen uptake and recovery curves during light- and moderate-cycle ergometer exercise; muscular strength; cardiorespiratory responses during steady-rate exercise; assessment of heavy-work fatigue; determinants of endurance performance; and neural control factors related to human motor performance (Fig. 10).

Contributions of the Harvard Fatigue Laboratory (1927–1946)

Many of the great scientists of the 20th century with an interest in exercise were associated with the Harvard Fatigue Laboratory. This research facility was established by Lawrence J. Henderson, MD (1878–1942), a renowned chemist and professor of biochemistry at the Harvard Medical School. The first and only scientific director of the Fatigue Laboratory was David Bruce Dill (1891–1986), a Stanford PhD in physical chemistry. Dill was transformed from a biochemist to an experimental physiologist while at the Fatigue Laboratory, and he was an important driving force behind the laboratory's numerous scientific accomplishments. His early academic association with physician Arlie Bock (a student of famous high-altitude physiologist Dr. Barcroft at Cambridge, England,[5] and Dill's closest friend for 59 years) and contact with 1922 Nobel laureate Archibald Vivian Hill (for his discovery related to heat production in muscles) provided Dill with the confidence to successfully coordinate the research efforts of dozens of scholars from 15 different countries. A. V. Hill convinced Bock to write a third edition of Bainbridge's text, *Physiology of Muscular Activity*. Bock, in turn, invited Dill to coauthor the book republished in 1931.[17]

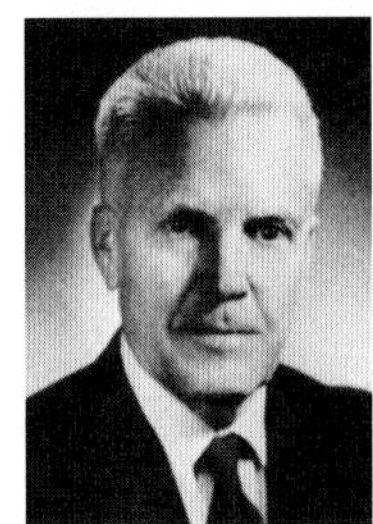

Over a 20-year period, at least 352 research papers, numerous monographs, and a book[18] were published in areas of basic and applied exercise physiology, including methodological refinements concerned with blood chemistry analysis and simplified methods for analyzing the fractional concentrations of expired air. Research at the Fatigue Laboratory included many aspects of acute responses and chronic physiological adaptations to exercise under environmental stresses produced by exposure to altitude, heat, and cold. Most of the key exercise experiments were conducted with humans using treadmill and bicycle ergometer exercise, but several important studies were also conducted with animals. These studies formed the cornerstone for research in modern laboratories of exercise physiology, particularly in areas related to the assessment of physical working capacity and fitness, cardiovascular and hemodynamic responses during maximal exercise, kinetics of oxygen consumption and substrate utilization, metabolism during exercise and recovery, and maximal oxygen consumption. Detailed discussions of each of these topics appear in various chapters of our textbook.

Similar to the legacy of the first exercise physiology laboratory established at Harvard's Lawrence Scientific School in 1892, the Harvard Fatigue Laboratory demanded excellence in research and scholarship. Particularly noteworthy

[m]Possible pre-1900 candidates for "first" exercise physiology textbook listed in Table 1 also include Combe's 1843 text "*The Principles of Physiology Applied to the Preservation of Health, and to the Improvement of Physical and Mental Education*"; Hitchcock and Hitchcock's *Elementary Anatomy and Physiology for Colleges, Academies, and Other Schools* (1860); Kolb's 1887 German monograph, translated into English in 1893 as *Physiology of Sport*; and the 1898 Martin text, *The Human Body. An Account of Its Structure and Activities and the Conditions of Its Healthy Working*.

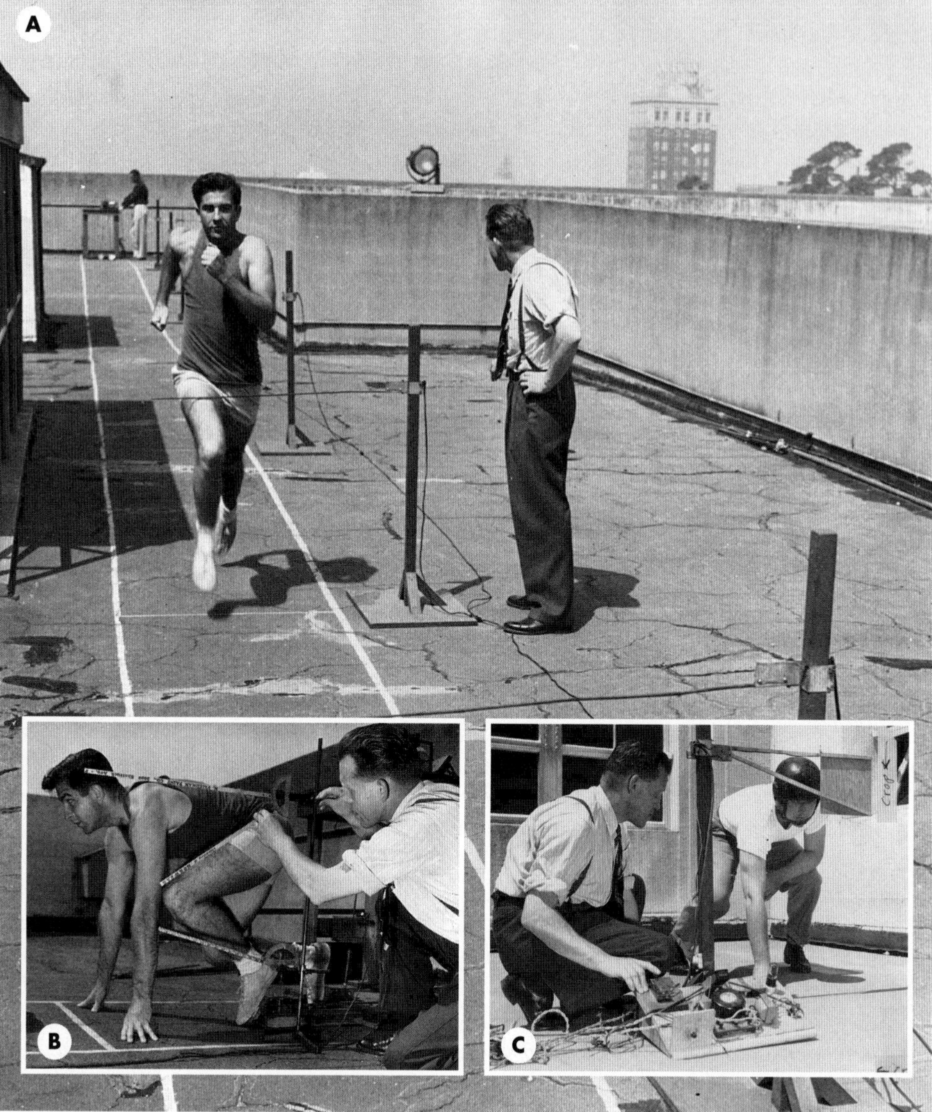

FIGURE 10 • A. Henry supervising 50-yard sprints (at 5-yd intervals) on the roof of Harmon Gymnasium. Henry's study[28] was prompted by A.V. Hill's 1927 observations concerning the "viscosity" factor of muscular contraction that at first helped to explain the large decline in metabolic efficiency at fast rates of movement, and that the oxygen requirement of running increased with the cube of speed. Henry verified that metabolic efficiency was not correlated to a muscle viscosity factor. **B**. Henry making limb and trunk anthropometric measurements on a sprinter during continuous studies of the force-time characteristics of the sprint start[29] to further evaluate A. V. Hill's theoretical equation for the velocity of sprint running. **C**. Henry recording the timing of the initial movements of blocking performance in football players.[44]

was the cooperation among scientists from around the world that fostered lasting collaborations. Furthermore, many of the scientists who had contact with the Fatigue Laboratory profoundly impacted a new generation of exercise physiologists in the United States and abroad. Noteworthy were Ancel Keys, who established the Laboratory of Physiology and Physical Education (later renamed the Laboratory of Physiological Hygiene) at the University of Minnesota; Henry L. Taylor (Keys and Taylor were mentors to exercise physiologist Elsworth R. Buskirk, formerly at the NIH and later the Noll Laboratory at Pennsylvania State University); Robert E. Johnson at the Human Environmental Unit at the University of Illinois; Sid Robinson at Indiana University; Robert C. Darling at the Department of Rehabilitation Medicine at Columbia University; Harwood S. Belding, who started the Environmental Physiology Laboratory at the University of Pittsburgh; C. Frank Consolazio of the U.S. Army Medical Research and Nutrition Laboratory at Denver; Lucien Brouha, who headed the Fitness Research Unit at the University of Montreal, and then went to the Dupont Chemical Company in Delaware; and Steven M. Horvath, who established the Institute of Environmental Stress at the University of California, Santa Barbara, where he worked with visiting scientists and mentored graduate students in the Biology Department and Department of Ergonomics and Physical Education. After the Fatigue Laboratory was unfortunately forced to close in 1946, Dill continued as the deputy director of the U.S. Army Chemical Corps Medical Laboratory in Maryland for 13 years (1948–1961). Thereafter, he worked with Sid Robinson at Indiana University's physiology department. He then started the Desert Research Institute (connected with the University of Nevada at Las Vegas), where he studied the physiological responses of men and animals to hot environments, a topic that culminated in a book on the subject.[20]

The group of scholars associated with the Harvard Fatigue Laboratory mentored the next generation of students who continue to make significant contributions to the field of exercise physiology. The monograph by Horvath and Horvath[33] and the chronology by Dill[19] are the best direct sources of historical information about the Harvard Fatigue Labora-

TABLE 5 ➤ AREAS OF INVESTIGATION AT THE HARVARD FATIGUE LABORATORY THAT HELPED TO ESTABLISH EXERCISE PHYSIOLOGY AS AN ACADEMIC DISCIPLINE

1. Specificity of the exercise prescription
2. Genetic components of an exercise response
3. Selectivity of the adaptive responses by diseased populations
4. Differentiation between central and peripheral adaptations
5. The existence of cellular thresholds
6. Actions of transmitters and the regulation of receptors
7. Feed-forward and feedback mechanisms that influence cardiorespiratory and metabolic control
8. Matching mechanisms between oxygen delivery and oxygen demand
9. The substrate utilization profile with and without dietary manipulations
10. Adaptive responses of cellular and molecular units
11. Mechanisms responsible for signal transduction
12. The behavior of lactate in cells
13. The plasticity of muscle fiber types
14. Motor functions of the spinal cord
15. The ability of hormonally deficient animals to respond to conditions of acute exercise and chronic exercise
16. The hypoxemia of severe exercise

From Tipton CM. Personal communication to F. Katch, June 12, 1995. From a presentation made to the American Physiological Society Meetings, 1995.

tory. Exercise physiology continued to expand after the closing of the Fatigue Laboratory. Subsequent efforts probed the full range of physiologic functions. The depth and breadth of these early investigations, summarized in Table 5, provided much of the current knowledge base for establishing exercise physiology as a respectable academic field of study.

Research Methodology Textbook Focusing on Physiological Research

In 1949, the Research Section of the Research Council of the Research Section of the American Association for Health, Physical Education, and Recreation or AAHPER (an outgrowth of the American Association for the Advancement of Physical Education created in 1885), sponsored publication of the first textbook devoted to research methodology in physical education.[1] Thomas Cureton, PhD, a pioneer researcher in physical fitness evaluation and the director of the exercise physiology research laboratory he established at the University of Illinois in 1944, appointed Dr. Henry to chair the committee to write the chapter on physiological research methods. The other committee members were respected scientists in their own right and included the following: Anna Espenshade (PhD in psychology from Berkeley, specialist in motor development and motor performance during growth); Pauline Hodgson (a Berkeley PhD in physiology who did postdoctoral work at the Harvard Fatigue Laboratory); Peter V. Karpovich, MD (the originator of the Physiological Research Laboratory at Springfield College); Arthur H. Steinhaus, PhD (director of the research laboratory at George Williams College, one of the eleven founders of the American College of Sports Medicine and a research physiologist who authored an important review article [*Physiological Reviews*, 1933] about the chronic effects of exercise); and distinguished Berkeley physiologist Hardin Jones, PhD (from the Donner Research Laboratory of Medical Physics at Berkley).

The resulting book chapter by this distinguished committee stands as a hallmark of research methodology in exercise physiology. The 99 references, many of them key articles in this then-embryonic field, covered such exercise-related topics as the "heart and circulation, blood, urine and kidney function, work, lung ventilation, respiratory metabolism and energy exchange, and alveolar air."

Another masterful compendium of research methodologies published 14 years later, *Physiological Measurements of Metabolic Functions in Man*, by C. F. Consolazio and colleagues provided complete details about specific measurements in exercise physiology.[16] Several sections in this book contained material previously published from the Harvard Fatigue Laboratory one year before its closing in 1946[34] and from another book dealing with metabolic methods[15] published in 1951.

THE NORDIC CONNECTION (DENMARK, SWEDEN, NORWAY, AND FINLAND)

Denmark and Sweden have had a significant historical impact on physical education as an academic field. In 1800, Denmark was the first European country to include physical training (military-style gymnastics) as a requirement in the public school curriculum. Since that time, the Danish and Swedish influences have influenced a large number of scientists who have made outstanding contributions to research in both traditional physiology and exercise physiology.

Danish Influence

In 1909, the University of Copenhagen endowed the equivalent of a Chair in Anatomy, Physiology, and Theory of Gymnastics.[42] The first Docent was Johannes Lindhard, MD (1870–1947). He later teamed with August Krogh (1874–1949), PhD, an eminent scientist specializing in physiological chemistry and research instrument design and construction, to conduct many of the now classic experiments in exercise physiology. For example, Krogh and Lindhard investigated gas exchange in the lungs, pioneered studies of the relative contribution of fat and carbohydrate oxidation during exercise (see "Focus on Research," Chapter 8), measured the redistribution of blood flow during different

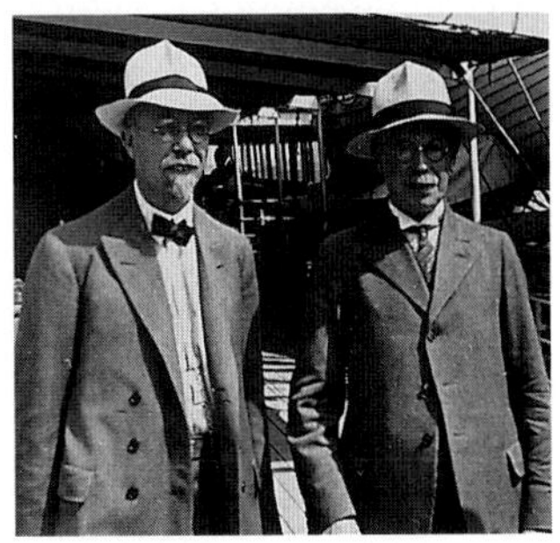

Professors August Krogh and Johannes Lindhard in the early 1930s.

exercise intensities, and measured cardiorespiratory dynamics in exercise (including cardiac output using nitrous oxide gas, a method described by a German researcher in 1770).

By 1910, Krogh and his wife Marie (a physician) had proven through a series of ingenious, decisive experiments[54] that diffusion was how pulmonary gas exchange occurred—not by the secretion of oxygen from lung tissue into the blood during exercise and exposure to altitude, as postulated by British physiologists Sir John Scott Haldane and James Priestley.[25] By 1919, Krogh had published reports of a series of experiments (with three appearing in the *Journal of Physiology*, 1919) concerning the mechanism of oxygen diffusion and transport in skeletal muscles. The details of these early experiments are included in Krogh's 1936 textbook,[37] but he also was prolific in many other areas of science.[36,38–40] In 1920, Krogh received the Nobel Prize in physiology or medicine for discovering the mechanism of capillary control of blood flow in resting and exercising muscle (in frogs). To honor the achievements of this renowned scientist (which included 300 scientific articles), an institute for physiological research in Copenhagen was named for him.

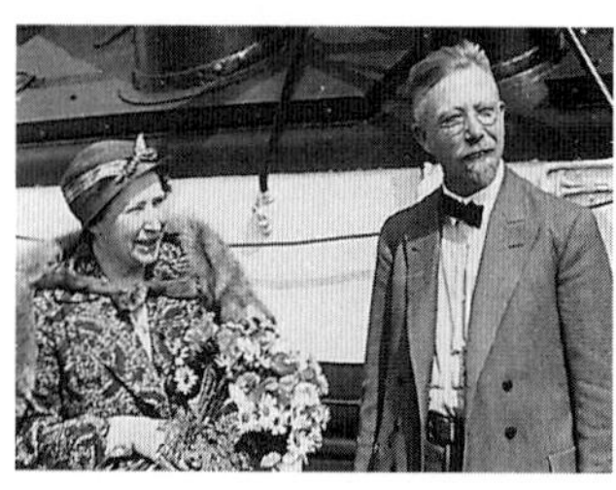

Marie and August Krogh

Three other Danish researcher–physiologists, Erling Asmussen (1907–1991; ACSM Citation Award, 1976 and ACSM Honor Award, 1979), Erik Hohwü-Christensen (b. 1904–; ACSM Honor Award, 1981), and Marius Nielsen (b. 1903–) conducted pioneering studies in exercise physiology. These "three musketeers," as Krogh referred to them, published numerous research papers from the 1930s to the 1970s. Asmussen, initially an assistant in Lindhard's laboratory, became a productive researcher specializing in muscle fiber architecture and mechanics. He also published papers with Nielsen and Christensen as coauthors on many applied topics including muscular strength and performance, ventilatory and cardiovascular response to changes in posture and exercise intensity, maximum working capacity during arm and leg exercise, changes in oxidative response of muscle during exercise, comparisons of positive and negative work, hormonal and core temperature response during different intensities of exercise, and respiratory function in response to decreases in oxygen partial pressure. As evident in his classic review article[2] of muscular exercise that cites many of his own studies (plus 75 references from other Scandinavian researchers), Asmussen's grasp of the importance of the study of biologic functions during exercise is as relevant today as it was more than 35 years ago when the article published. He clearly defines exercise physiology within the context of biological science:

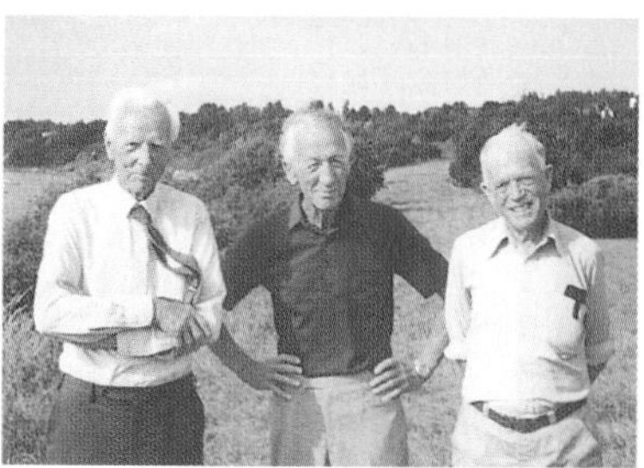

The "three musketeers," Drs. Erling Asmussen (*left*), Erik Hohwü-Christensen (*center*), and Marius Nielsen (*right*) (1988 photo).

> The physiology of muscular exercise can be considered a purely descriptive science: it measures the extent to which the human organism can adapt itself to the stresses and strains of the environment and thus provides useful knowledge for athletes, trainers, industrial human engineers, clinicians, and workers in rehabilitation on the working capacity of humans and its limitations. But the physiology of muscular exercise is also part of the general biological science, physiology, which attempts to explain how the living organism functions, by means of the chemical and physical laws that govern the inanimate world. Its important role in physiology lies in the fact that muscular exercise more than most other conditions, taxes the functions to their uttermost. Respiration, circulation, and heat regulation are only idling in the resting state. By following them through stages of increasing work intensities, a far better understanding of the resting condition is also achieved. Although the physiology of muscular exercise must be studied primarily in healthy subjects, the accumulated knowledge of how the organism responds to the stresses of exercise adds immensely to the understanding of how the organism adapts itself to disease or attempts to eliminate its effects by mobilizing its regulatory mechanisms.

Christensen became Lindhard's student in Copenhagen in 1925. Together with Krogh and Lindhard, Christensen published an important review article in 1936 that described the physiological dynamics during maximal exercise.[14] In his 1931 thesis, Christensen reported on studies of cardiac output with a modified Grollman acetylene method; body temperature and blood sugar concentration during heavy cycling exercise; comparisons of arm versus leg exercise; and the effects of training. Together with Ové Hansen, he used oxygen consumption and the respiratory quotient to describe how diet, state of training, and exercise intensity and duration affected carbohydrate and fat utilization. (In fact, the concept of "carbohydrate loading" was first discovered in 1939!) Other notable studies included core temperature and blood glucose regulation during light-to-heavy fatiguing exercise at various ambient temperatures. A study by Christensen and Nielsen in 1942 used finger plethysmography to study regional blood flow (including skin temperature) during brief periods of constant-load cycle ergometer exercise.[13] Experiments published in 1936 by physician Olé Bang, inspired by his mentor Ejar Lundsgaard, described the fate of blood lactate during exercise of different intensities and durations.[4] The experiments of Christensen, Asmussen, Nielsen, and Hansen were conducted at the Laboratory for the Theory of Gymnastics at the University of Copenhagen. Today, the August Krogh Institute carries on the tradition of basic and applied research in exercise physiology. Since 1973, Swedish-trained scientist Bengt Saltin (the only Nordic researcher besides Erling Asmussen to receive the ACSM Citation Award [1980] and ACSM Honor Award [1990]; former student of Per-Olof Åstrand, discussed

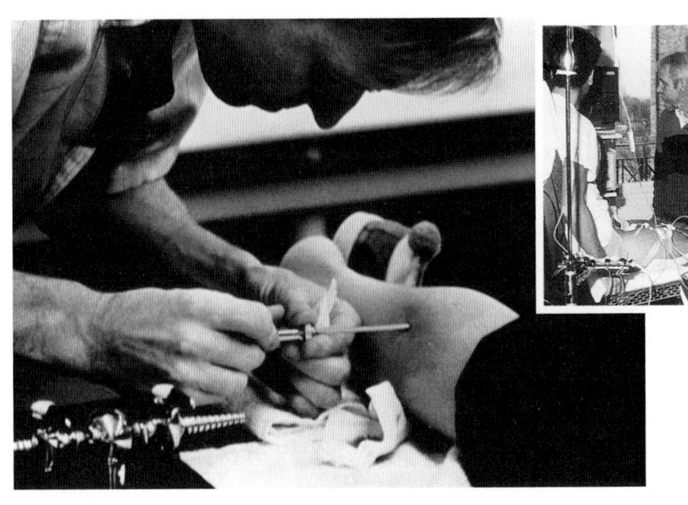

Bengt Saltin taking muscle biopsy of gastrocnemius muscle. (Photo courtesy of Dr. David Costill.) Inset of Saltin (hand on hip) during an experiment at the August Krogh Institute, Copenhagen. (Photo courtesy Per-Olof Åstrand.)

in the next section) has been a professor and continues his significant scientific studies as professor and director of the Copenhagen Muscle Research Centre, University of Copenhagen, Denmark.

Swedish Influence

Modern exercise physiology in Sweden can be traced to Per Henrik Ling (1776–1839), who in 1813 became the first director of Stockholm's Royal Central Institute of Gymnastics.[42] Ling, a specialist in fencing, developed a system of "medical gymnastics." This system, which became part of the school curriculum of Sweden in 1820, was based on his studies of anatomy and physiology.

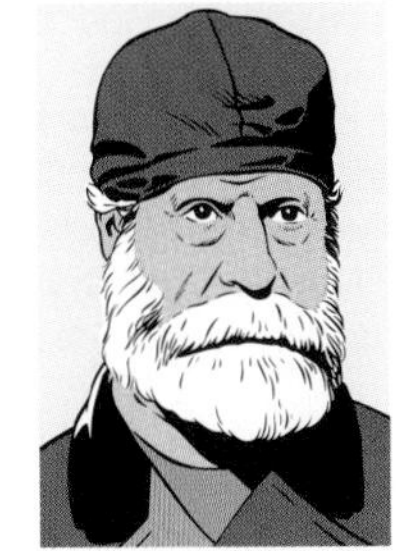

Hjalmar Ling

Ling's son, Hjalmar, also had a strong interest in medical gymnastics and physiology and anatomy, in part owing to his attendance at lectures by physiologist Claude Bernard in Paris, in 1854. Hjalmar Ling published a book on the kinesiology of body movements in 1866. As a result of the Lings' philosophy and influence, the physical educators who graduated from the Stockholm Central Institute were well schooled in the basic biological sciences, in addition to being highly proficient in sports and games. Currently, the College of Physical Education (Gymnastik-Och Idrottshögskolan) and the Department of Physiology in the Karolinska Institute Medical School in Stockholm continue to sponsor studies in exercise physiology.

Per-Olof Åstrand, MD, PhD (1922–) is the most famous graduate of the College of Physical Education (1946); in 1952, he presented his thesis to the Karolinska Institute Medical School. Åstrand taught in the Department of Physiology in the College of Physical Education from 1946 to 1977. When the College of Physical Education became a department of the Karolinska Institute, Åstrand served as professor and department head from 1977 to 1987. Christensen was Åstrand's mentor and supervised his doctoral dissertation, which included data on the physical working capacity of both sexes aged 4 to 33 years. This important study—along with collaborative studies with his wife Irma Ryhming—established a line of research that propelled Åstrand to the forefront of experimental exercise physiology, for which he achieved world-

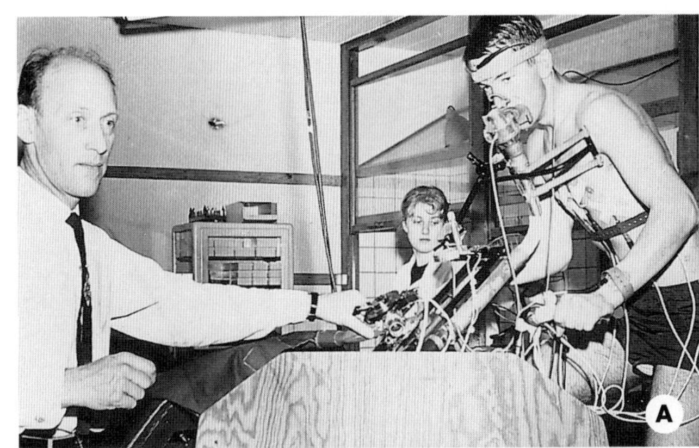

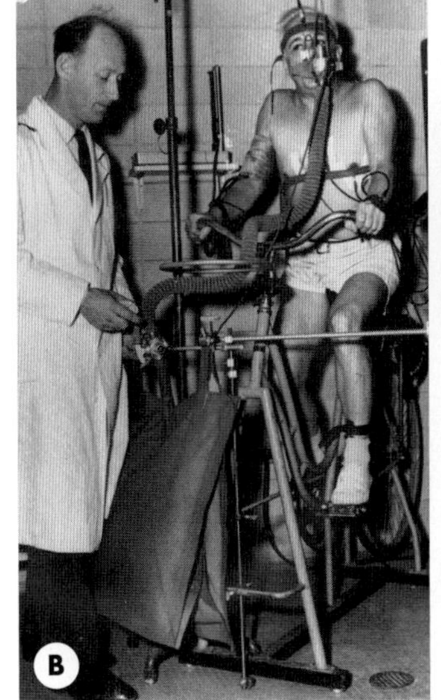

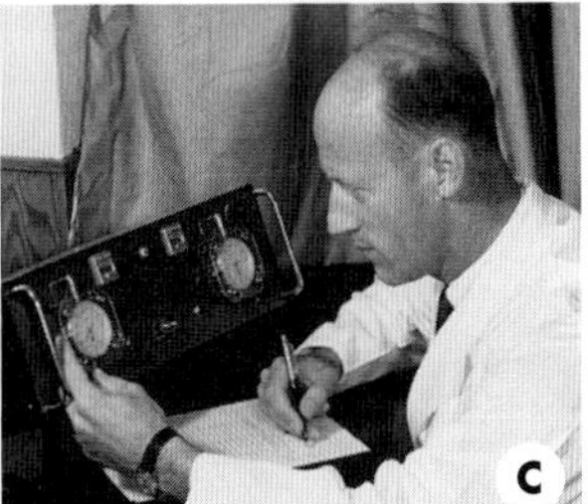

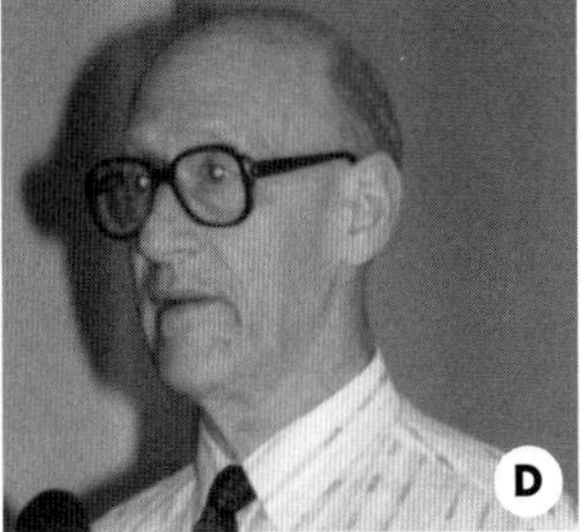

P-O. Åstrand, Department of Physiology. Karolinska Institute, Stockholm. **A**. Measuring maximal performance of Johnny Nilsson, Olympic Gold Medal speed skater, 1964. **B**. Maximal oxygen consumption measured during cycle ergometer exercise, 1958. **C**. Laboratory experiment, 1955. **D**. Invited lecture, 1992 International Conference on Physical Activity, Fitness and Health, Toronto.

wide fame.[n] Four papers published by Åstrand in 1960, with Christensen as one of the authors, stimulated further studies on the physiological responses to intermittent exercise. Åstrand has mentored an impressive group of exercise physiologists, including such "superstars" as Bengt Saltin and Björn Ekblom. Table 6 is a sampling of contributions to the exercise physiology literature by Åstrand and Saltin in books, book chapters, monographs, and research articles. As further evidence of their phenomenal international influence, the bottom part of the table includes the number of times each was cited in the scientific literature from 1996 through April, 2001.

Two Swedish scientists at the Karolinska Institute, Drs. Jonas Bergström and Erik Hultman, performed important experiments with the needle biopsy procedure that have provided a new vista from which to study exercise physiology. With this procedure, it became relatively easy to conduct invasive studies of muscle under various conditions of exercise, training, and nutritional status. Collaborative work with other Scandinavian researchers (Saltin and Hultman from Sweden and Lars Hermanson from Norway) and researchers in the United States (e.g., Phillip Gollnick at Washington State University and David Costill at Ball State University) contributed a whole new dimension to the study of muscular exercise.

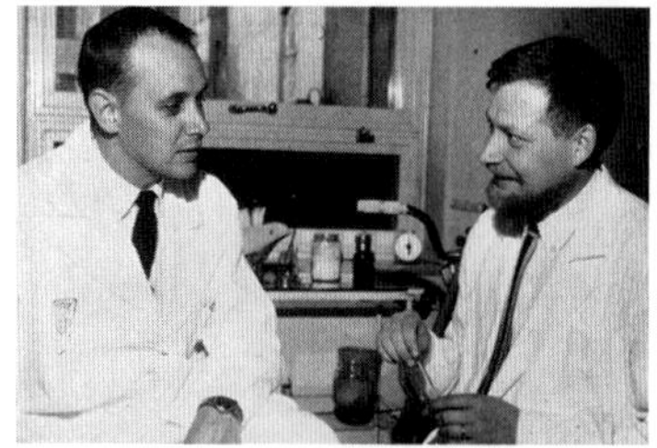

Drs. Jonas Bergström *(left)* and Eric Hultman, Karolinska Institute, mid-1960s.

Norwegian and Finnish Influence

The new generation of exercise physiologists trained in the late 1940s analyzed respiratory gases by means of a highly accurate sampling apparatus that measured relatively small quantities of carbon dioxide and oxygen in expired air. The

TABLE 6 ➤ SELECTED CONTRIBUTIONS TO THE EXERCISE PHYSIOLOGY LITERATURE BY SWEDISH EXERCISE PHYSIOLOGISTS PER-OLOF ÅSTRAND AND BENGT SALTIN

Åstrand P-O. Experimental studies of physical working capacity in relation to sex and age. Copenhagen: Munksgaard, 1952.
Åstrand P-O, and Ryhming I. A nomogram for calculation of aerobic capacity (physical fitness) from pulse rate during submaximal work. J Appl Physiol. 1954;7:218, .
Åstrand P-O, Saltin B. Maximal oxygen uptake and heart rate in various types of muscular activity. J Appl Physiol. 1961;16:977.
Åstrand P-O, et al. Girl swimmers. Acta Paediatr. 1963;(Suppl. 147).
Åstrand P-O, Grimby G. (eds). Physical Activity in Health and Disease: Proceedings of the Second Acta Medica Scandinavica International Symposium. Goteborg, Sweden, June 10-12, 1985.
Åstrand P-O, and Rodahl K. Textbook of Work Physiology, 3rd ed. New York, McGraw-Hill, 1986.
Åstrand P-O, et al. A 33-year followup of peak oxygen uptake and related variables of former physical education students. J Appl Physiol. 1997;82:844.
Ekblom B, Åstrand P-O. Role of physical activity on health in child and adolescents. Acta Paediatr. 2000;89:762.
Saltin B. Aerobic work capacity and circulation of man. Acta Physiol Scand. 1964;(Suppl. 230).
Saltin B and Åstrand P-O. Maximal oxygen uptake in athletes. J Appl Physiol. 1967;23:353.
Saltin B. et al. Physical training in sedentary middle-aged and older men. Scand J Clin Lab Invest. 1967;24:323.
Saltin B, Hermansen L. Glycogen stores and prolonged severe exercise. In Blix, G. (ed.): Nutrition and Physical Activity. Symposia of the Swedish Nutrition Foundation. Stockholm, Almqvist & Wiksell, 1967.
Saltin B. et al. Response to submaximal and maximal exercise after bedrest and training. Circulation. 1968;38:(Suppl. 7).
Saltin B. (ed). International Symposium on Biochemistry of Exercise. Champaign, IL: Human Kinetics, 1986.
Saltin B, et al. Skeletal muscle blood flow in humans and its regulation during exercise. Acta Physiol Scand. 1998;162:421.
Bouvier F, Saltin B, et al. Left ventricular function and perfusion in elderly endurance athletes. Med Sci Sports Exerc. 2001;33:735.

NUMBER OF CITATIONS IN THE SCIENTIFIC LITERATURE

Year	*1996*	*1997*	*1998*	*1999*	*2000*	*2001[a]*
Åstrand	7526	6502	6485	7834	8523	3822
Saltin	20,332	16,780	17,272	21,441	18,060	14,524

Source: Science Citation Index. Numbers refer to the total number of citations ("hits") in the published literature (including books).
[a]Through April 30, 2001.

[n]Personal communication to F. Katch, June 13, 1995, from Dr. Åstrand regarding his professional background. Recipient of five honorary doctorate degrees (Université de Grenoble [1968], University of Jyväskylä [1971], Institut Superieur d'Education Physique, Université Libre de Bruxelles [1987], Loughborough University of Technology [1991], Aristoteles University of Thessaloniki [1992]. Åstrand is an honorary Fellow of nine international societies, a Fellow of the American Association for the Advancement of Science (for "outstanding career contributions to understanding of the physiology of muscular work and applications of this understanding"), and has received many awards and prizes for his outstanding scientific achievements, including the ACSM Honor Award in 1973. Åstrand served on a committee for awarding the Nobel Prize in physiology or medicine from 1977 to 1988 and is coauthor with Kaare Rodahl of *Textbook of Work Physiology,* 3rd edition, 1986 (translated in Chinese, French, Italian, Japanese, Korean, Portuguese, and Spanish). His English publications number about 200 (including book chapters, proceedings, a history of Scandinavian scientists in exercise physiology[3] and monographs), and he has given invited lectures in approximately 50 countries and 150 different cities outside of Sweden. His classic 1974 pamphlet *Health and Fitness* has an estimated distribution of 15 to 20 million copies (about 3 million copies in Sweden)—unfortunately, all without personal royalty!

method of analysis (and also the analyzer) was developed in 1947 by Norwegian scientist Per Scholander (1905–1980). A diagram of Scholander's micrometer gas analyzer[55] is presented in Chapter 8, Figure 8.7, along with its larger counterpart, the Haldane analyzer.

Another prominent Norwegian researcher was Lars A. Hermansen (1933–1984; ACSM Citation Award, 1985) from the Institute of Work Physiology, who died prematurely. Nevertheless, his many contributions include a classic 1969 article entitled "Anaerobic Energy Release" that appeared in the first volume of *Medicine and Science in Sports*.[30] Other papers included work with exercise physiologist K. Lange Andersen.[31]

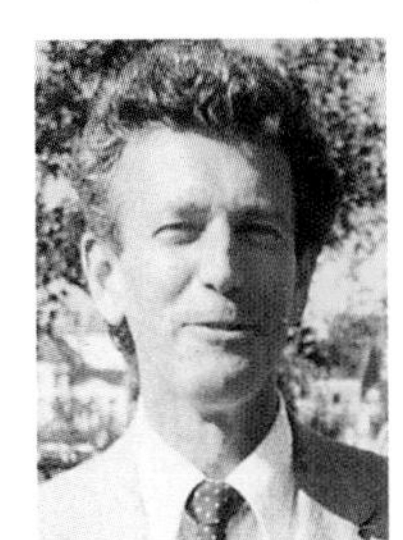

Lars A. Hermansen (1933–1984). Institute of Work Physiology, Oslo.

In Finland, Martti Karvonen, MD, PhD (ACSM Honor Award, 1991) from the Physiology Department of the Institute of Occupational Health, Helsinki, is best known for a method to predict optimal exercise training heart rate, the so-called "Karvonen formula" (see "Focus on Research," Chapter 15). He also conducted studies dealing with exercise performance and the role of exercise in longevity. In 1952, Lauri Pikhala, a physiologist, suggested that obesity was the consequence and not the cause of physical "unfitness." Ilkka Vuori, starting in the early 1970s, reported on hormone responses to exercise. Paavo Komi, from the Department of Biology of Physical Activity, University of Jyväskylä, has been Finland's most prolific researcher, with numerous experiments published in the combined areas of exercise physiology and sport biomechanics. Table 7 lists the Nordic researchers who have received the prestigious ACSM Honor Award or ACSM Citation Award.

TABLE 7 ➤ NORDIC RESEARCHERS[a] AWARDED THE ACSM HONOR AWARD AND ACSM CITATION AWARD

ACSM Honor Award	ACSM Citation Award
Per-Olof Åstrand, 1973	Erling Asmussen, 1976
Erling Asmussen, 1979	Bengt Saltin, 1980
Erik Hohwü-Christensen, 1981	Lars A. Hermansen, 1985
Bengt Saltin, 1990	C. Gunnar Blomqvist, 1987
Martti J. Karvonen, 1991	

[a]Born and educated in a Nordic country.

OTHER CONTRIBUTORS TO THE KNOWLEDGE BASE IN EXERCISE PHYSIOLOGY

In addition to the distinguished American and Nordic applied scientists profiled previously, there have been many other giants" in the field of physiology and experimental science[o] that have made monumental contributions that indirectly added to the knowledge base in exercise physiology. The list includes:

Sir Joseph Barcroft (1872–1947). High-altitude research physiologist who pioneered fundamental work concerning the functions of hemoglobin, later confirmed by Nobel laureate August Krogh. Barcroft also performed experiments to determine how cold affected the central nervous system. For up to 1 hour, he would lie without clothing on a couch in subfreezing temperature and record his subjective reactions.

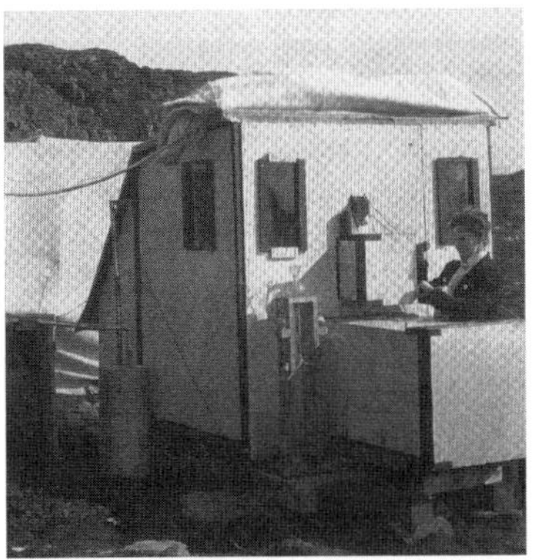

Marie Krogh collects data at Barcroft's high-altitude experimental station to assess oxygen tension of gases.

Christian Bohr (1855–1911). Professor of physiology in the medical school at the University of Copenhagen who mentored August Krogh, and father of nuclear physicist Niels Bohr. Bohr studied with Carl Ludwig in Leipzig in 1881 and 1883, publishing papers on the solubility of gases in various fluids, including oxygen absorption in distilled water and in solutions containing hemoglobin. Krogh's careful experiments using advanced instruments (microtonometer) disproved Bohr's secretion theory that both oxygen and carbon dioxide were secreted across the lung epithelium in opposite directions based on the time required for equalization of gas tension in blood and air.

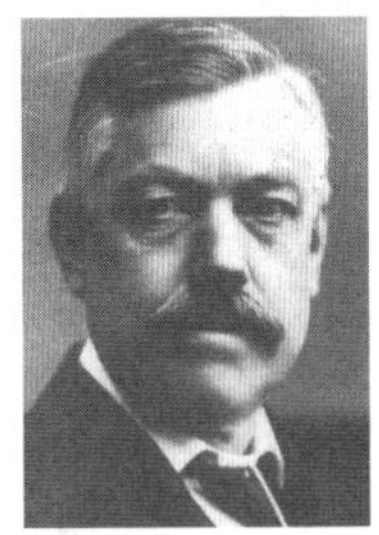

John Scott Haldane (1860–1936). Conducted research in mine safety, investigating principally the action of dangerous gases (carbon monoxide), the use of rescue equipment, and the incidence of pulmonary disease. He devised a decompression apparatus for the safe ascent of deep-sea divers. The British Royal Navy and the United States Navy adopted tables based on this work. In 1905, he discovered that carbon dioxide acted on the brain's respiratory center to regulate

[o]There are many excellent sources of information about the history of science and medicine, including the following: Bettman O. *A Pictorial History of Medicine.* Springfield, IL: Charles C Thomas, 1956; Clendening L. *Source Book of Medical History.* New York: Dover Publications/Henry Schuman, 1960; Coleman W. *Biology in the Nineteenth Century.* New York: Cambridge University Press, 1977; Franklin K. *A Short History of Physiology,* 2nd ed. London: Staples Press, 1949; Fye WB, *The Development of American Physiology. Scientific Medicine in the Nineteenth Century.* Baltimore: Johns Hopkins University Press, 1987; Guthrie D. *A History of Medicine.* London: T. Nelson & Sons, 1945; Haskins T. *Science and Enlightenment.* New York: Cambridge University Press, 1985; Holmes FL. *Lavoisier and the Chemistry of Life.* Madison: University of Wisconsin Press, 1985; Knight B. *Discovering the Human Body.* London: Bloomsbury Books; Lesch JE. *Science and Medicine in France. The Emergence of Experimental Physiology*, 1790–1855. Cambridge, MA: Harvard University Press, 1984; Vertinsky PA. *The Eternally Wounded Woman: Women, Exercise, and Doctors in the Late Nineteenth Century.* Urbana: University of Illinois Press; Walker K. *The Story of Medicine.* London: Arrow Books, 1954.

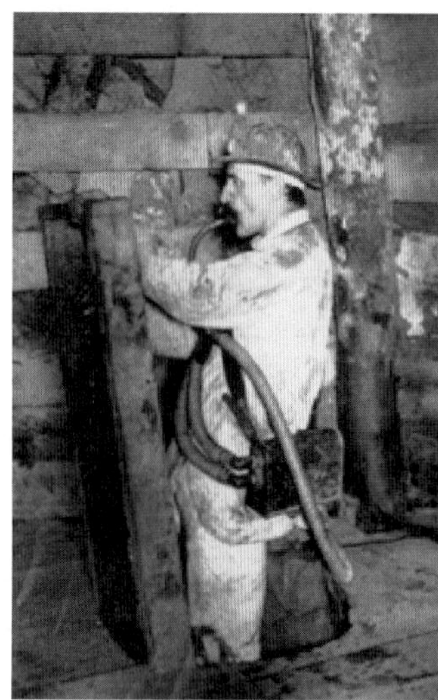
Haldane investigating carbon monoxide gas in an English coal mine at the turn of the 20th century.

breathing. In 1911, he and several other physiologists organized an expedition to Pikes Peak, Colorado, to study the effects of low oxygen pressures at high altitudes. Haldane also showed that the reaction of oxyhemoglobin with ferricyanide rapidly and quantitatively released oxygen and formed methemoglobin. The amount of liberated oxygen could be accurately calculated from the increased gas pressure in the closed reaction system at constant temperature and volume. Haldane devised a microtechnique to fractionate a sample of a mixed gas into its component gases (see Chapter 8, Haldane apparatus). Haldane founded the *Journal of Hygiene*.

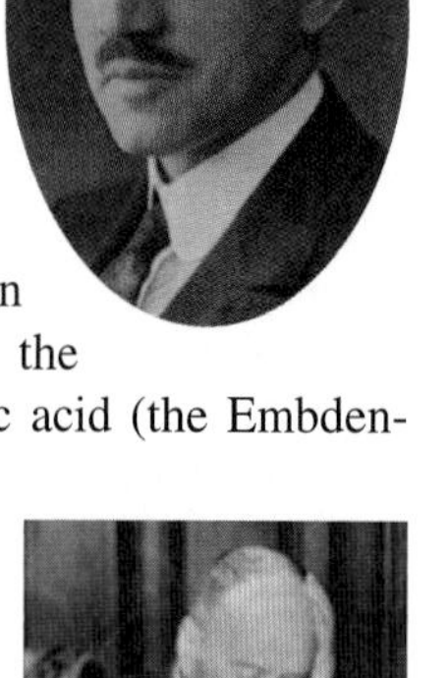

Otto Meyerhof (1884–1951). Meyerhof's experiments on the energy changes during cellular respiration led to discoveries on lactic acid related to muscular activity, research that lead to the Nobel Prize (with A.V. Hill in 1923). In 1925, Meyerhof extracted from muscle the enzymes that convert glycogen to lactic acid. Subsequent research confirmed work done by Gustav Embden in 1933, and together they discovered the pathway that converted glucose to lactic acid (the Embden-Meyerhof pathway).

Nathan Zuntz (1847–1920). Devised the first portable metabolic apparatus to assess respiratory exchange in animals and humans at different altitudes; proved that carbohydrates were precursors for lipid synthesis. He maintained that dietary lipids and carbohydrates should not be consumed equally for proper nutrition. He produced 430 articles concerning blood and blood gases, circulation, mechanics and chemistry of respiration, general metabolism and metabolism of specific foods, energy metabolism and heat production, and digestion.

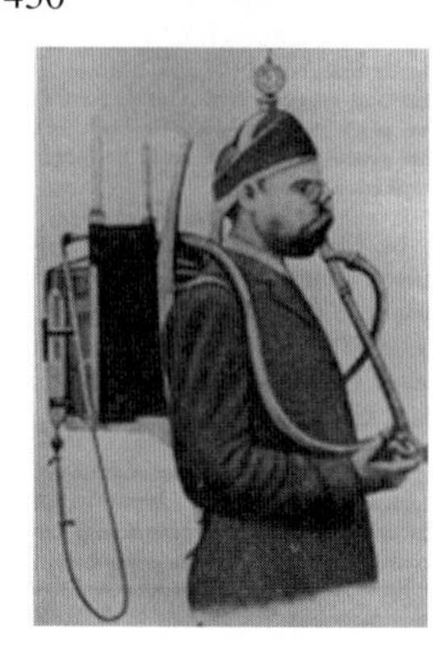
Zuntz tests his portable, closed-circuit spirometer carried on his back. This device made it possible for the first time to measure O_2 consumed and CO_2 produced during ambulation.

Carl von Voit (1831–1908) and his student Max Rubner (1854–1932). Discovered the Isodynamic Law and the calorific heat values of proteins, lipids, and carbohydrates; Rubner's surface area law states that resting heat production is proportional to body surface area, and that consuming food increases heat production. Voit disproved Liebig's assertion that protein was a primary energy fuel by showing that protein breakdown does not increase in proportion to exercise duration or intensity.

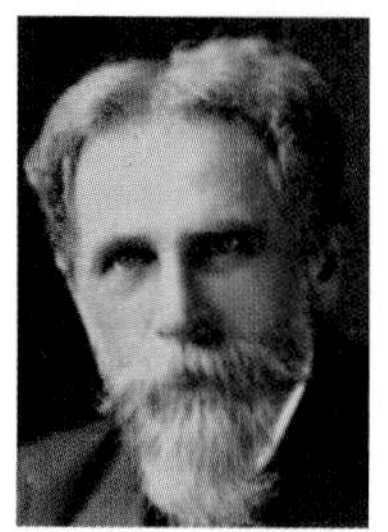

Max Joseph von Pettenkofer (1818–1901). Perfected the respiration calorimeter to study human and animal metabolism; discovered creatinine, an amino acid in urine. The top chamber of the figure below shows the entire calorimeter. The cut-away image shows a human experiment where fresh air was pumped into the sealed chamber and vented air sampled for carbon dioxide.

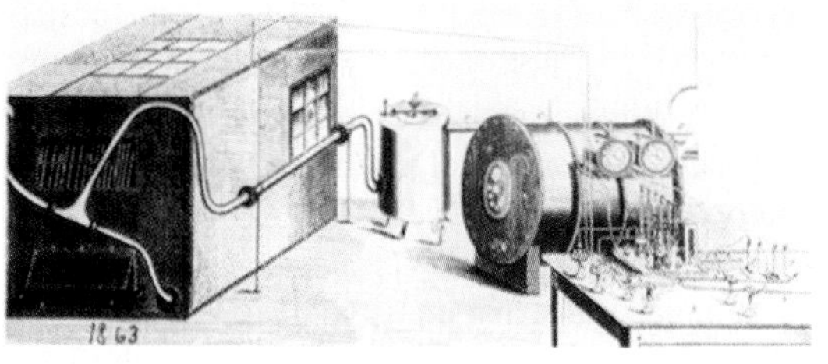

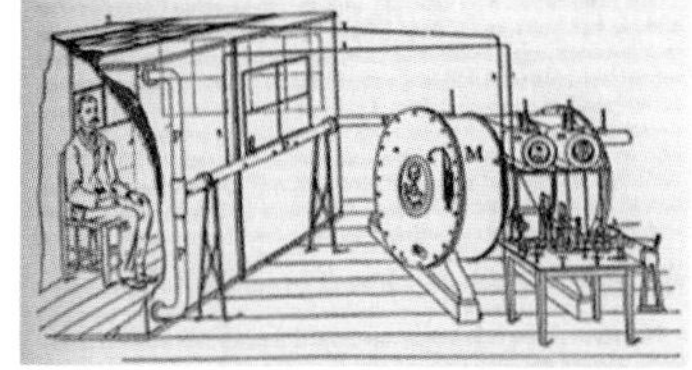
Human respiration calorimeter.

Eduard F.W. Pflüger (1829–1910). First demonstrated that minute changes in the partial pressure of blood gases affect the rate of oxygen release across capillary membranes, thus proving blood flow alone does not govern how tissues receive oxygen.

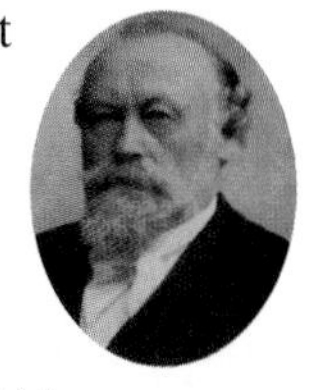

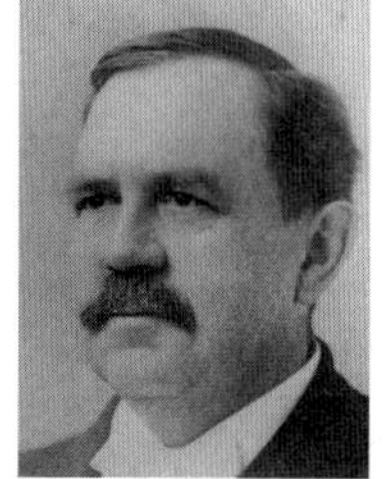

Wilbur Atwater (1844–1907). Published data about the chemical composition of 2600 American foods currently used in databases of food composition. Also performed human calorimetric experiments and confirmed that the Law of Conservation of Energy governs transformation of matter in the human body.

Russel Henry Chittenden (1856–1943). Refocused attention on the minimal protein requirement of humans while resting or exercising; concluded that no debilitation occurred if protein intake equaled 1.0 g · kg

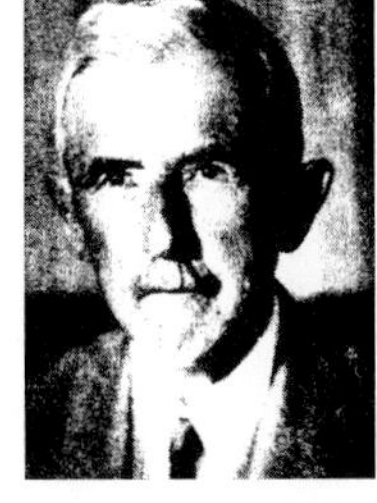

body mass^{-1} in either normal or athletic young men. Chittenden received the first PhD in physiological chemistry given by an American University. Some scholars[10] regard Chittenden as the father of biochemistry in the United States—he believed physiological chemistry would provide basic tools for researchers to study important aspects of physiology and provided the impetus for incorporating biochemical analyses in exercise physiology.

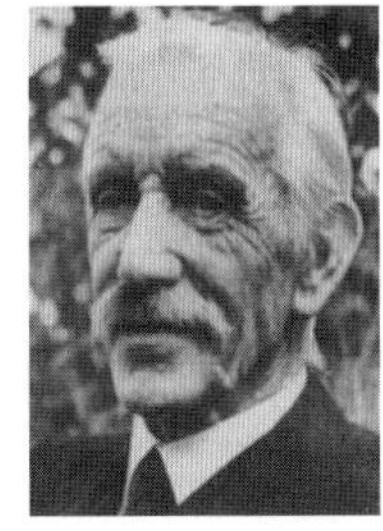

Frederick Gowland Hopkins (1861–1947). Nobel Prize in 1929 for isolating and identifying the structure of the amino acid tryptophan. Hopkins collaborated with W. M. Fletcher (mentor to A. V. Hill) to study muscle chemistry. Their classic 1907 paper in experimental physiology employed new methods to isolate lactic acid in muscle. Fletcher and Hopkins' chemical methods reduced the muscle's enzyme activity prior to analysis to isolate the reactions. They found that a muscle contracting under low oxygen conditions produced lactate at the expense of glycogen. Conversely, oxygen in muscle suppressed lactate formation. The researchers deduced that lactate forms from a nonoxidative (anaerobic) process during contraction; during recovery in a noncontracted state, an oxidative (aerobic) process removes lactate with oxygen present.

Francis Gano Benedict (1870–1957). Conducted exhaustive studies of energy metabolism in newborn infants, growing children and adolescents, starving people, athletes, and vegetarians. Devised "metabolic standard tables" based on sex, age, height, and weight to compare energy metabolism in normals and patients. His last monograph, "Vital Energetics, A Study in Comparative Basal Metabolism" (*Carnegie Institution Monograph* no. 503, 1938) refers to many of his approximately 400 publications.

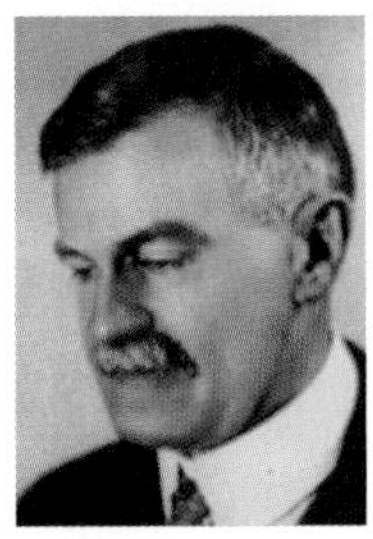

CONTRIBUTIONS OF WOMEN TO SCIENCE AT THE DAWN OF THE 20TH CENTURY

The triumphs and accomplishments during the evolution of exercise physiology reveal a glaring absence of credit to the contributions of women from the 1850s and continuing for the next 100 years. Many reasons can explain this occurrence—but it was not from women's lack of interest in pursuing a career in the sciences. Rather, females who wished to stand with male colleagues found the going difficult. Opposition included hostility, ridicule, and professional discrimination, typically in chemistry, physics, and medicine, but also in related fields such as botany, biology, and mathematics. A few women did break through the almost exclusively male-dominated fields to make significant contributions despite such significant hurdles. The leadership at the "top" of the scientific culture (college presidents, academic deans, curriculum and personnel committees, governing bodies, heads of departments, and review boards for grants and journals) subtly and directly repressed women's attempts to even enter some fields, let alone achieve parity with male scientists. Subtle discrimination included assignment to underequipped, understaffed, and substandard laboratory facilities; having to teach courses without proper university recognition; disallowing membership on graduate thesis or dissertation committees; and having a male colleague's name appear first (or only) on research publications, regardless of his involvement. Male "supervisors" typically presented the results of joint work at conferences and seminars when the woman clearly worked as the lead scientist. Direct suppression included outright refusal to hire women to teach at the university or college level. For those who were hired, many could not directly supervise graduate student research projects. Women also routinely experienced shameful inequity in salary received or were paid no salary as "assistants."

The Nobel Prize in the sciences, the most prestigious award for discoveries in physics, chemistry, and physiology or medicine, has honored 300 men but only 10 women since the award originated in 1901. The Karolinska Institute in Stockholm selects the Nobel laureates in physiology or medicine, and the Swedish Academy of Sciences awards the prizes in chemistry and physics. Considerable controversy has emerged over the years about the role of "in-fighting and politics" in the selection process. The difference in the gender-specific pool of outstanding scientists cannot adequately explain the disparity between male and female Nobel winners. However, reading about the lives and times of the 10 female winners, including others who by all accounts probably deserved the honor, gives a better appreciation for the inequity. Each of the 10 female laureates and the other 3 world-class scientists we chronicle in Table 8 overcame huge "nonscientific" issues before achieving their eventual scientific triumphs.

In a way, some of the same problems faced by women in academia and the private sector over the years help to explain the relatively slow ascendance of women to positions of prominence during the first 100 years of modern exercise physiology. A salient example comes from reviewing the historical record of the ACSM from its inception on January 8, 1955, to the present. Of the 11 founders, one was a woman (Josephine L. Rathbone, PhD, specialist in physical education and rehabilitation). Eighteen months later, three other women joined Dr. Rathbone (Dorothy Ainsworth, PhD, from Smith College, MA; Anna Espenshare, PhD, from UC Berkeley; and Clair Langdon, EdD, from Oregon State College) as part of the 54 original Charter ACSM members.

From ACSM's founding, it would take 33 years before a woman was elected the organization's president. Barbara L. Drinkwater, PhD, from the Institute of Environmental Stress at UC Santa Barbara, became ACSM's first woman president (see "Interview with Barbara L. Drinkwater" in Section 5). Dr. Drinkwater was followed in 1997 to 1998 by Charlotte A. "Toby" Tate, PhD, Dean of the College of Health and Human

TABLE 8 ➤ SCIENTIFIC CONTRIBUTIONS OF THIRTEEN OUTSTANDING FEMALE SCIENTISTS

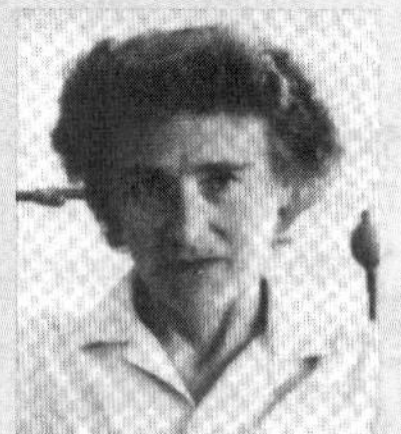

Gerty Radnitz Cori (1896–1954)

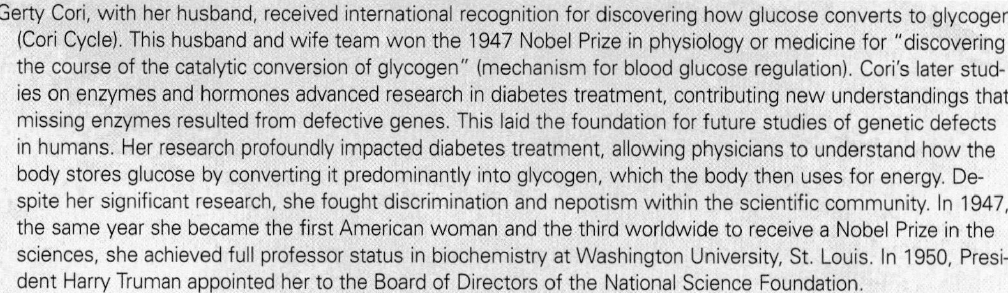

Gerty Cori, with her husband, received international recognition for discovering how glucose converts to glycogen (Cori Cycle). This husband and wife team won the 1947 Nobel Prize in physiology or medicine for "discovering the course of the catalytic conversion of glycogen" (mechanism for blood glucose regulation). Cori's later studies on enzymes and hormones advanced research in diabetes treatment, contributing new understandings that missing enzymes resulted from defective genes. This laid the foundation for future studies of genetic defects in humans. Her research profoundly impacted diabetes treatment, allowing physicians to understand how the body stores glucose by converting it predominantly into glycogen, which the body then uses for energy. Despite her significant research, she fought discrimination and nepotism within the scientific community. In 1947, the same year she became the first American woman and the third worldwide to receive a Nobel Prize in the sciences, she achieved full professor status in biochemistry at Washington University, St. Louis. In 1950, President Harry Truman appointed her to the Board of Directors of the National Science Foundation.

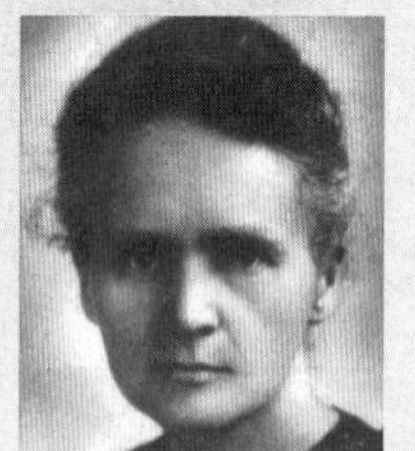

Marie Sklodowska Curie (1867–1934)

Considered the most famous of all women scientists, this Polish researcher "extraordinarie" was the first person (male or female) to win two Nobel Prizes. At age 16, she had already won a gold medal at the Russian lycée in Poland upon completion of her secondary education. In 1891, almost penniless, she began her education at the Sorbonne in Paris and later became the first woman professor to teach there. Marie Curie (with her husband Pierre) discovered that the source of natural radioactivity did not result from a chemical reaction but rather from a property of the element's specific atoms. This led to the discovery in 1898 of two highly radioactive elements, radium and polonium for which they were awarded the 1903 Nobel Prize in physics. Madame Curie continued her work on radioactive elements and again won the Nobel prize in chemistry in 1911 for isolating radium and studying its chemical properties. In 1914, she helped found the Radium Institute in Paris and was the Institute's first director. When World War I broke out, Madame Curie believed that x-rays would help to locate metal fragments and bullets and facilitate surgery. It was also important not to move the wounded, so she invented mobile x-ray vans and trained female attendants. Curie died of leukemia, presumably from extensive exposure to high radiation levels in her research. After her death, the Radium Institute was renamed the Curie Institute in her honor.

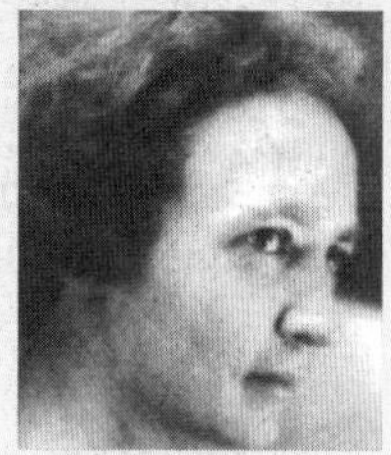

Irene Joliot-Curie (1897–1956)

Daughter of Marie Curie, Irene continued her mother's work in radioactivity with her husband Frédéric (1900–1958). In 1933, they made the important discovery that radioactive elements can be artificially prepared from stable elements. Their experiments bombarded boron with alpha particles, creating an "artificially" radioactive element, an isotope of nitrogen. The Joliot-Curies were awarded the 1935 Nobel Prize in chemistry "for their synthesis of new radioactive elements." In later years, they extended their work to identifying products of nuclear fission. Although Joliot-Curie won many awards for contributions to science, the French Academy of Science never admitted her to membership. In 1911, the Institute de France voted to maintain its all-male status, a policy maintained for the next 40 years, even denying Curie membership after she died in 1956. A social activist who lobbied hard for gender equality, Joliet-Curie planned a fund-raising tour of the United States. Even with a valid visa, she was denied entry and kept in a detention center until the French Embassy in Washington intervened.

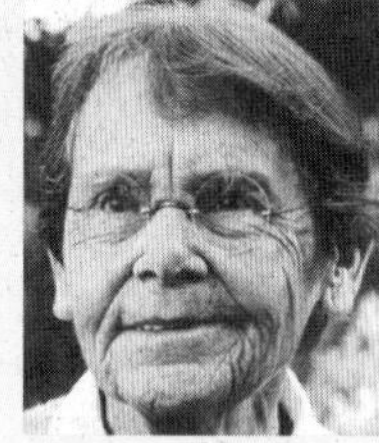

Barbara McClintock (1902–1992)

America's most distinguished cytogeneticist, McClintock studied genetic mutations by examining changes in the color and texture of kernels and leaf pigments of growing plants. In 1951, McClintock first reported that genetic information could transpose from one chromosome to another. Other scientists didn't believe this unorthodox view of genes, assuming instead that genes remained in place in the chromosome like a necklace of beads. By the early 1970's, scientists finally acknowledged McClintock's view of gene transpositions. Her prodigeous research accomplishments clarified our understanding of human disease. The concept of "jumping genes" helped to explain how bacteria develop antibiotic resistance, and provided insight as to how these genes play a role in transforming normal cells to cancerous ones. By the late 1970s, her work with transposable elements (i.e., that mobile genetic elements play important roles in inherited birth defects, resistance to antibiotics, and incidence of cancer) became recognized by the scientific-medical community. During 1980 and 1981, McClintock received eight major awards including the Albert Lasker Basic Medical Research Award, Israel's Wolf Prize in Medicine, and McArthur Foundation Fellowship. In 1983, she was the sole recipient of the Nobel Prize in medicine or physiology. The Nobel Committee called her work "one of the two great discoveries of our times in genetics," the other being the structure of DNA.

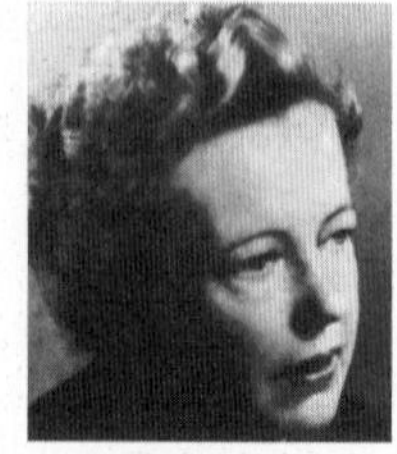

Maria Goeppert Mayer (1906–1972)

The first American woman and the second woman ever to win the Nobel Prize in physics, Maria Mayer made extensive contributions to several different technical fields in physics. Mayer calculated the probability that an electron orbiting an atom's nucleus would emit not one but two photons (quantum units of light) as it jumps to an orbit closer to the nucleus. Because The Johns Hopkins University had strict nepotism rules that forbade her employment (her husband had been hired), she worked without pay or formal academic status. She produced ten papers in nine years applying quantum mechanics to chemistry. She and her husband co-authored *Statistical Mechanics,* a textbook in print for over four decades. At the University of Chicago, Mayer worked part time, supported by a federal grant as senior physicist at the Argonne National Laboratory. There she began her eventual Nobel Prize-winning project elucidating the basic shell model of an atom's nucleus. In 1956, Mayer was elected to the National Academy of Sciences. In 1959, at age 53, after a thirty-year career, she was finally appointed full time professor (with pay), at the University of California, San Diego. In 1963, she received the Nobel Prize in physics for her pioneering research.

TABLE 8 ➤ **SCIENTIFIC CONTRIBUTIONS OF THIRTEEN OUTSTANDING FEMALE SCIENTISTS**

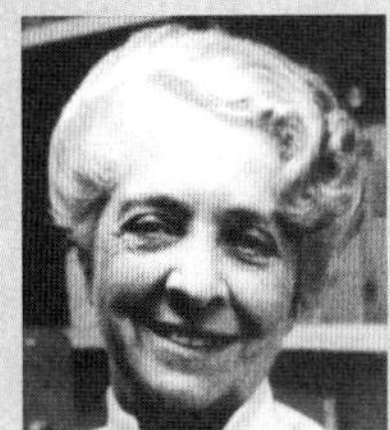

Rita Levi-Montalcini (1909–)

Rita Levi-Montalcini's first studies between 1938 and 1944 investigated the mechanisms controlling vertebrate nervous system development. In 1952, she showed that when tumors from mice were transplanted to chick embryos, they induced potent growth of the embryo's nervous system, specifically the sensory and sympathetic neurons. Since this outgrowth did not require direct contact between tumor and embryo, Levi-Montalcini concluded that the tumor released a nerve growth-promoting factor (NGF) that selectively acted on specific neurons. Following this discovery, Levi-Montalcini focused on a more sensitive cell culture model to measure NGF activity in various extracts. NGF proved to be an extremely potent biological substance in that a sensory or sympathetic nerve cell reacted within 30 seconds to minute quantities of NGF. More specifically, one-billionth of a gram of NGF per mL of culture medium exerted a powerful effect on growth. The biological assay to detect NGF paved the way for the next step of discovery—identification of the active nerve growth-promoting substance. The discovery of NGF opened new fields related to pathology such as developmental malformations, degenerative changes in senile dementia, delayed wound healing, and tumor diseases. Levi-Montalcini received the 1986 Nobel Prize in medicine or physiology (with Stanley Cohen) for their discovery of NGF. From 1993 to 1998, she served as President of the Institute of the Italian Encyclopedia. She is a member of prestigious scientific academics: Accademia Nazionale dei Lincei, Pontifical Academy, Accademia delle Scienze detta dei XL, U.S. National Academy of Sciences, and the Royal Society.

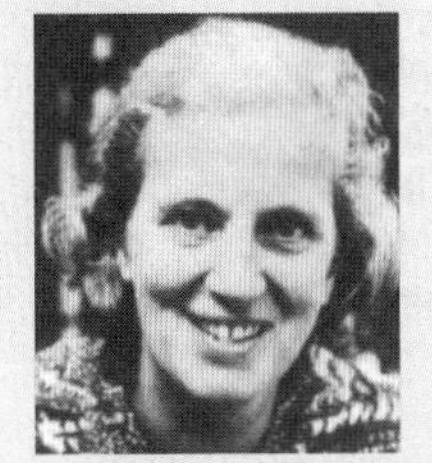

Dorothy Crowfoot Hodgkin (1910–1994)

Applying her expertise as an x-ray crystallographer, Dorothy Hodgkin "developed the analytical methods to identify the structures of penicillin (previously discovered in 1929): cholesteryl iodide (cholesterol), vitamin B_{12} (used to treat pernicious anemia), vitamin B_{12} coenzyme, and the protein hormone insulin. Hodgkin studied more than 100 steroid crystals, reporting on their unit-cell dimensions and refractive indices relative to their crystallographic axes. Her monumental studies of crystalline steroids showed their probable crystal packing and hydrogen-bonding arrangements. Her later studies involved three-dimensional calculations, and established the relative stereochemistry at each carbon atom of the steroids. Hodgkin took the first x-ray diffraction photographs of insulin in 1935 and ultimately resolved this crystal's full structure 34 years later. Hodgkin and colleagues reported the structure of insulin in August 1969. She singly won the 1964 Nobel Prize in chemistry "for her determination by x-ray techniques of the structures of biologically important molecules." In addition to pioneering work in chemistry, she applied computer algorithms to help unravel insulin's complex structure.

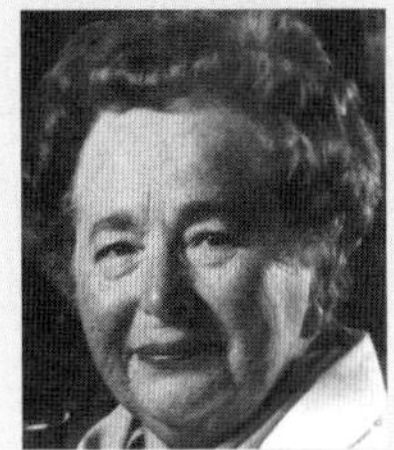

Gertrude B. Elion (1918–1999)

In 1944, with a master's degree in chemistry, Burroughs-Wellcome (now Glaxo-Wellcome) pharmaceutical company hired Gertrude Elion as a $50-a-week research assistant. Prior to that, female scientists had difficulty finding jobs in either academia or the private sector. At Wellcome, however, her strong scientific training paid off. The strategy was to create new medicines by studying the chemical composition of diseased cells. Her research developed acyclovir (Zovirax) for herpes; azathioprine (Imuran) to help prevent rejection of transplanted organs among nonrelated donors and to treat severe rheumatoid arthritis; allopurinol (Zyloprim) for gout; pyriemthamine (Daraprim) for malaria; and trimethoprim (a component of Septra) for bacterial infections. Elion never completed her PhD (she took courses at night, commuting three hours round-trip). Eventually she had to quit because she was told the PhD program at Brooklyn's Polytechnic Institute required full-time attendance, and she could not afford to give up her job. Nonetheless, Gertrude Elion received 25 honorary degrees from prestigious universities, including Duke, Columbia, Brown, Michigan, and Rochester Institute of Technology. In 1988, she shared the Nobel Prize in physiology or medicine with George Hitchings (coworker at Glaxo-Wellcome) for "important principles of drug development." After retirement in 1983, she helped to oversee development of AZT as the first drug against HIV, the AIDS virus. Elion is the only woman inducted into The Inventors Hall of Fame. Her 45 drug patents have provided wide-ranging benefits in many areas, for example a drug that helps the body suppress its immune response to foreign tissue—most important, that of transplanted organs. This drug has thus made relatively routine kidney transplants between non-related donors and patients. In addition to the Nobel Prize, Elion received many top awards: 1991 National Medal of Science presented by President George Bush, who said that her work had "transformed the world;" Garvan Medal from the American Chemical Society; President's Medal from Hunter College; Judd Award from Memorial-Sloan Kettering Institute; Cain Award from the American Association for Cancer Research; Ernst W. Bertner Memorial Award from the M.D. Anderson Cancer Center; City of Medicine Award in Durham, NC; Discoverers Award from the Pharmaceutical Manufacturers Association; Medal of Honor from the American Cancer Society; Ronald H. Brown Innovator Award; and the Lemelson/MIT Lifetime Achievement Award. Elion served as past president of the American Association for Cancer Research, and Presidential appointee on the National Cancer Advisory Board. She belonged to the National Academy of Sciences, the Royal Society, the Institute of Medicine, the American Academy of Arts and Sciences, the National Women's Hall of Fame, and the Engineering and Science Hall of Fame.

TABLE 8 ➤ SCIENTIFIC CONTRIBUTIONS OF THIRTEEN OUTSTANDING FEMALE SCIENTISTS

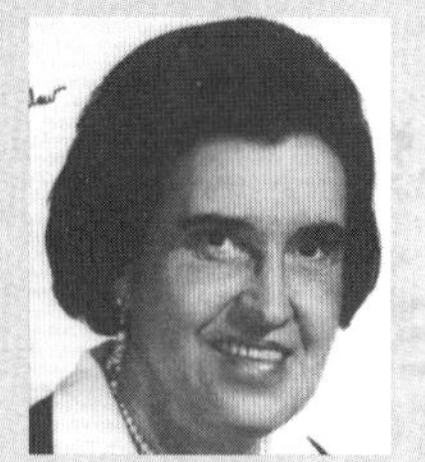
Rosalyn Sussman Yalow (1921–)

Rosalyn Sussman Yalow was the first American woman to win the Albert Lasker Prize for Medicine (1976) and Nobel Prize for physiology or medicine (1977) for developing radioimmunoassay (RIA). This procedure uses radioactive isotopes to "tag" previously undetected concentrations of hormones, viruses, vitamins, enzymes, and drugs to study disease and biochemical reactions. In essence, RIA provided the technique that unlocked the field of endocrinology. On accepting her Nobel Prize, Yalow spoke about women in science careers: "We must believe in ourselves or no one else will believe in us. We must feel a personal responsibility to ease the path for those who come after us. The world cannot afford the loss of the talents of half its people if we are to solve the many problems that beset us." Yalow holds the title of Distinguished Service Professor from The Mount Sinai School of Medicine. She is a member of the National Academy of Sciences. Honors include Albert Lasker Basic Medical Research Award, A. Cressy Morrison Award in Natural Sciences of the New York Academy of Sciences, Scientific Achievement Award of the American Medical Association, Koch Award of the Endocrine Society, Gairdner Foundation International Award, American College of Physicians Award for distinguished contributions in science related to medicine, Eli Lilly Award of the American Diabetes Association, First William S. Middleton Medical Research Award, and 39 honorary degrees.

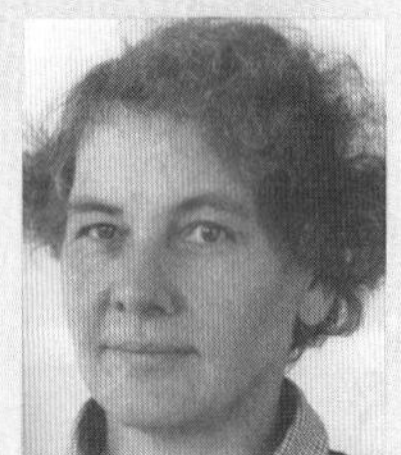
Christiane Nüsslein-Volhard (1942–)

During the 1970s, developmental biologist Christiane Nüsslein-Volhard's research focused on the genetics of mutated fruit-fly embryos. In 1984, she expanded her research by cataloguing 120 well-defined genes that affected the entire embryonic pattern of the fruit fly's development. She received the 1995 Nobel Prize in medicine or physiology (with colleague Eric Wieschaus) for pioneering molecular biology and genetics studies of specific areas of a gene that contributes to mammalian immune system development. Her discoveries had universal application because the same genetic parts that govern gene activity in different cells also similarly operate in plants and many animal organisms, including humans. Defective parts in genes that modulate early growth and development trigger congenital disorders such as spina bifida and cleft palate in humans. Because genes encoding the same protein affect a variety of conditions (e.g., arteriosclerosis, organ rejection, AIDS, and other maladies), the scope of her discoveries had wide-ranging applications. Her awards include membership in the National Academy of Sciences and Royal Society, and honorary degrees from Harvard, Yale, and Princeton.

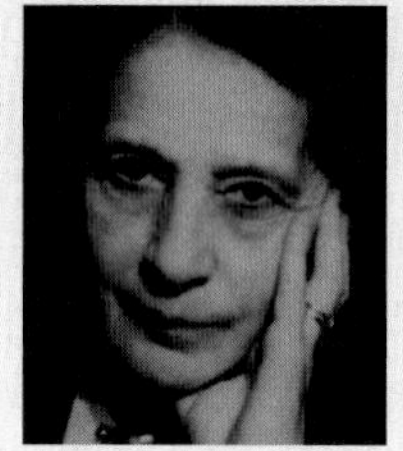
Lise Meitner (1878–1968)

Lise Meitner was the first woman to earn a doctoral degree in physics at the University of Vienna in 1906, which had previously awarded only 14 doctorates to women in the prior 541 years. Meitner worked at the Kaiser-Wilhelm Institute with radiochemist Otto Hahn (eventual Nobel Prize winner). They discovered the 91st element *protactinium* and studied neutron bombardment of uranium. Meitner became joint director of the Institute and head of the Physics Department in 1917. After fleeing Nazi Germany in 1938, she worked at the Nobel Physical Institute in Stockholm, continuing her research with nephew Otto Frisch. Meitner predicted that the atom's nucleus captures neutrons, causing enough instability to pinch it in two, much like a water droplet splitting into two parts. According to Einstein's equation $E = mc^2$, an observed loss of mass must unleash energy. Meitner, combining Bohr's liquid-drop model of the nucleus and Einstein's equation, predicted that a proposed experiment by Hahn should yield barium, krypton, and energy. Within days, she and Frisch worked out a theoretical model for nuclear fission. Frisch, hastily working in Bohr's institute in Copenhagen to test Meitner's expectations, quickly verified the theory. The Meitner-Frisch paper introducing nuclear fission appeared in early 1939. Their momentous discovery (they had split the uranium nucleus) was termed "fission," and predicted the existence of the chain reaction that contributed to the development of the atomic bomb.

During World War II, Meitner refused to work on the atomic bomb. In 1947, the Swedish Atomic Energy Commission established a laboratory where she continued to work on an experimental nuclear reactor. She received the Max Planck Medal, the Leibnitz Medal, and in 1966 she shared the Fermi Award. In 1946, Otto Hahn received the Nobel Prize for his work on fission. Interestingly, he failed to acknowledge that Mietner's ideas had stimulated his research—contributions that many in science believed were considerable. Though denied the Nobel Prize, an international commission in 1994 named element 109, artificially created by slamming bismuth with iron ions, meitnerium.

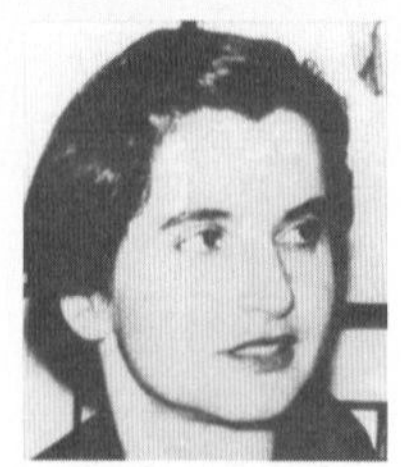
Rosalind Franklin (1920–1958)

A graduate of Cambridge University who specialized in chemistry, Franklin's expertise focused on understanding the chemical (atomic) structure of complex organic compounds. She perfected the technique of x-ray crystallography that locates atoms in any crystal by precisely mapping the image of the crystal under an x-ray beam. Using an extremely fine beam of x-rays, Franklin produced high-resolution photographs of single DNA fibers. These fibers, finer than ever seen before, were then arranged in parallel bundles. Her results showed that DNA's sugar-phosphate backbone lies on its outside; in essence, she elucidated the basic helical structure of the molecule. Unfortunately, Franklin's notes and photographs about the discovery were made available (without her permission) to Watson and Crick at Cambridge University, who were rushing to determine DNA's final structure. Within days, Watson and Crick applied Franklin's data to complete their own detailed and ultimately correct description of DNA's structure. The strained relationship with her immediate supervisor (Maurice Wilkins) and other aspects about King's College where she worked (women scientists were forbidden to eat lunch in the common room with men) led Franklin to seek employment elsewhere. She turned her attention to tobacco mosaic viruses, publishing 17 papers in 5 years—a body of knowledge that formed the basis for structural virology. Franklin began work on the polio virus before succumbing to ovarian cancer in 1958. Ten years after deciphering the double-helix structure (and following Franklin's death), Watson, Crick, and Wilkins received the Nobel Prize in physiology or medicine, thus forever denying Franklin formal credit she richly deserved for her crucial discovery of DNA's helical structure (see •••••• for additional information).

TABLE 8 ➤ SCIENTIFIC CONTRIBUTIONS OF THIRTEEN OUTSTANDING FEMALE SCIENTISTS

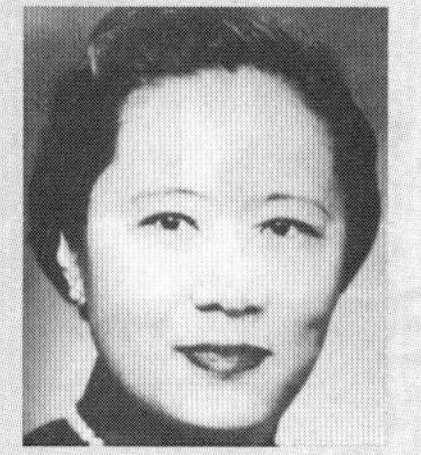
Wu-Chien-Shiung Wu (1912–1997)

A pioneering physicist, Wu radically altered modern physical theory by changing the accepted view of the structure of the universe. Her experiments helped to demolish a proposed "law" of nature concerning the conservation of parity. Wu was the first woman to receive the prestigious Research Corporation Award and the Comstock Prize—given once every 5 years from the National Academy of Sciences—for her contributions to atomic research (understanding of beta decay and the weak interactions) on the Manhattan Project. Wu became the first woman to receive an honorary Doctorate of Science from Princeton University (and 10 other doctorates, including ones from Harvard and Yale), was elected first woman president of the American Physical Society, received the first Wolf Prize from the State of Israel, was awarded a full-professorship and endowed chair (Pupin Professor of Physics) at Columbia University, became the seventh woman elected to the National Academy of Sciences, and was awarded the National Medal of Science prize, the nation's highest science award. And complementing her accomplishments, she was the first living scientist to have an asteroid named after her.

Development Sciences at the University of Illinois at Chicago; in 1999 to 2000 by Priscilla M. Clarkson, PhD, Associate Dean of the School of Public Health and Heath Sciences at the University of Massachusetts at Amherst; and in 2000 to 2001 by Angela D. Smith, MD, Philadelphia's Children's Hospital Sports Medicine & Performance Center. From 1955 to 1980, only Drs. Rathbone and Drinkwater served as officers of the College (as vice presidents); from 1981 to 1992, three additional females achieved elective office (Christine Wells, PhD, Arizona State University; Betty Atwater, PhD, University of Arizona; Mona Shangold, MD, Georgetown Medical Center). Until 1992, no female received the prestigious ACSM Honor Award, delivered the Wolf Memorial Lecture, or won a New Investigator or Scholar Award. Between 1955 to 1992, three women received ACSM's Citation Award (Francis Hellebrandt, 1966; Josephine L. Rathbone, 1974; Barbara L. Drinkwater, 1984).

As the words to a famous song so aptly state: "The times they are a-changin'." In addition to the four female ACSM presidents, many women currently hold key positions as deans, associate deans, chairs of departments of exercise science and kinesiology, principal investigators on major research grants, and directors of exercise physiology laboratories.

We hope the legacy of the 13 women we profile in Table 8 inspires students to strive for excellence in their particular specialty related to exercise physiology. Each scientist trampled many obstacles in her path to achieve success and recognition. However, they all shared common traits—an unyielding passion for science and an uncompromising quest to explore new grounds where others had not ventured. As you progress in your own careers, we hope that you too will experience the pure joy of discovering new truths in exercise physiology. Perhaps the achievements of the 13 women scientists from outside our field will serve as a gentle reminder to support the next generation of scientists based on their accomplishments and passion for the field.

SUMMARY

This introductory section on the historical development of exercise physiology illustrates that interest in exercise and health had its roots with the ancients. During the next 2000 years, the field we now call exercise physiology evolved from a symbiotic (albeit, sometimes rocky) relationship between the classically trained physicians, the academically based anatomists and physiologists, and a small cadre of physical educators who struggled to achieve their identity and academic credibility through research and experimentation in the basic and applied sciences. Although the physiologists used exercise to study the dynamics of human physiology, the early physical educators often used the methodology and knowledge of physiology to study exercise.

Beginning in the mid-1850s in the United States, there was a small but slowly growing effort to raise standards for the scientific training of physical education and hygiene specialists who were primarily involved in teaching at the college and university level. The creation of the first exercise physiology laboratory at Harvard University in 1891 contributed to an already burgeoning knowledge explosion in basic physiology. Originally, medically trained physiologists made the significant scientific advances in most of the subspecialties that are now included in the exercise physiology course curriculum. They studied oxygen metabolism, muscle structure and function, gas transport and exchange, mechanisms of circulatory dynamics, and neural control of voluntary and involuntary muscular activity.

The field of exercise physiology also owes a debt of gratitude to the pioneers of the physical fitness movement in the United States, notably Thomas K. Cureton (1901–1993; ACSM charter member, 1969 ACSM Honor Award) at the University of Illinois, Champaign—a prolific, insightful researcher who trained four generations of physical educators beginning in 1941. Many of these pioneers assumed leadership positions as professors with teaching and research responsibilities in exercise physiology at numerous colleges and universities in the United States and throughout the world.

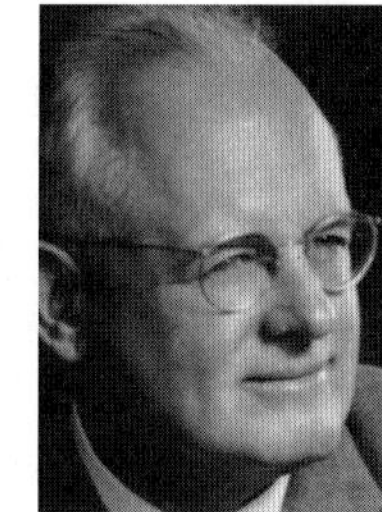
Dr. Thomas Kirk Cureton (1901–1993)

Although we have focused on the contributions of selected early American scientists and physical educators and their counterparts from the Nordic countries to the development of modern-day exercise physiology, we would be ne-

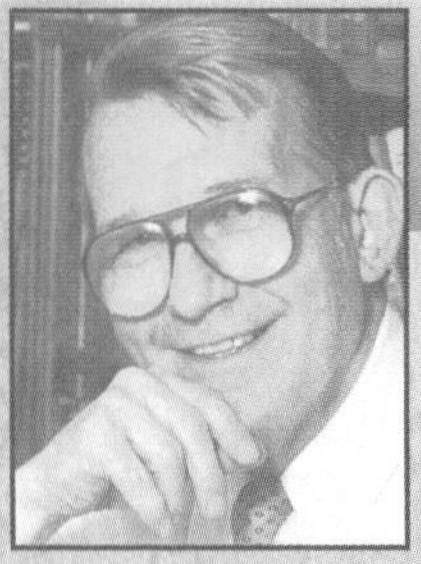

Interview with Dr. Tipton

Education: BA (Springfield College in Springfield, MA); MA, PhD in Physiology, with minors in Biochemistry and Anatomy (University of Illinois, Champaign, IL).

Current Affiliation: Professor Emeritus of Physiology and Surgery at the College of Medicine at the University of Arizona.

Honors and Awards: See Appendix E.

Research Focus: The physiological effects of acute and chronic exercise and their responsible mechanisms.

Memorable Publication: Tipton CM, et al. The influence of exercise, intensity, age, and medication on resting systolic blood pressure of SHR populations. J Appl Physiol 1983:55(4):1305–1310.

Statement of Contributions: ACSM Honor Award
Dr. Tipton is well known for his contributions as an investigator in exercise physiology, his educational vision in establishing the "gold standard" for graduate training in the exercise sciences, and his leadership and driving energy. For almost *25* years, Professor Tipton has excelled as an investigator by using animal models to study the acute and chronic effects of exercise on connective tissue, hormones, metabolism, and the cardiovascular system. This broad scope of knowledge has enabled him to build a graduate training program with an international reputation that has produced researchers and educators who have subsequently achieved prominence in the exercise sciences.

➤ What first inspired you to enter the exercise science field? What made you decide to pursue your degree and/or line of research?

My experiences in athletics and as a Physical Fitness Instructor in an infantry division convinced me that I should secure an education on the G.I. Bill of Rights to be able to teach health and physical education while coaching in a rural high school. Once I realized that I did not enjoy my chosen career, I returned to the University of Illinois for more education in health education. To support a growing family, I secured a summer and part-time position as a 4-H Club Fitness Specialist who conducted fitness tests and clinics through the state of Illinois. When it became apparent that I had to have more physiology and biochemistry to explain what I was testing and advocating, I knew I had to be a physiologist with an expertise in exercise physiology. So I transferred to the Physiology Department, and the rest is history.

➤ What influences did your undergraduate education have on your final career choice?

Very little. Although I had the late Peter V. Karpovich as my exercise physiology instructor at Springfield College, he did not stimulate, motivate, or encourage me to become one. My mind set was to teach and coach in a rural high school, and everything in the undergraduate curriculum or experience was to help me achieve that goal.

➤ Who were the most influential people in your career, and why?

The drive to learn and acquire more education was imprinted by my father, who had to leave school in the eighth grade to help support the family. Early in graduate school at the University of Illinois, I became interested in the physiological and biochemical foundations of physical fitness by the interesting and evangelical lectures of Thomas K.Cureton of the Physical Education Department. However, my interest in physiological research and its scientific foundations was stimulated, developed, and perfected by Darl M. Hall, who was a critical and caring research scientist in the Illinois Extension Service who had the responsibility of testing the fitness levels of 4-H Club members. He made me recognize that functional explanations require in-depth scientific knowledge and encouraged me to transfer into the physiology department to secure such information. Once in physiology, I became exposed to the unique scholarship of Robert E. Johnson and to his example of the scientific attributes necessary to become a productive exercise physiologist. Inherent in this profile of recognition is the fact that without the love and support of my wife, Betty, and our four children, my transition to the various departments — and survival of a poverty state — would have never occurred.

➤ What has been the most interesting/enjoyable aspect of your involvement in science? What was the least interesting/enjoyable aspect

To me, the most interesting and stimulating aspect of exercise physiology was the planning, testing and evaluation of one's hypotheses. The least enjoyable were the administrative aspects of supervising a laboratory and in the conduct of research.

➤ What is your most meaningful contribution to the field of exercise science, and why is it so important?

Exercise science evolved from the discipline of physical education and includes exercise physiology. My most meaning-

ful contribution to the field was the planning and implementation of a rigorous, science-based Ph.D. graduate program in exercise physiology at the University of Iowa, which served as a model for other departments of physical education to follow. It was important to me because it attracted many outstanding individuals to the University of Iowa who became dear friends and help paved the way for exercise science to become an academic entity.

➤ **What advice would you give to students who express an interest in pursuing a career in exercise science research?**

Research requires more than intellectual curiosity and infectious enthusiasm. It is an exciting occupation that demands hard work, while requiring an individual to be disciplined, dedicated, and honest. A future researcher must acquire an education that enables him/her to be well prepared in mathematics, the biological and physical sciences, and the ability to communicate by written and verbal means. Lastly, seek a mentor whose research interests you and one who is concerned about you as a future researcher and not as a contributor to their vitae.

➤ **What interests have you pursued outside of your professional career?**

Becoming a civil war "buff," enjoying the pleasures of dancing and listening to Dixieland jazz, exercising regularly, participating in road races, reading nonfiction, learning about poetry, being a member of a book club, watching televised sports, cheering for the Washington Redskins football team, and observing our grandchildren as they grow up.

➤ **Where do you see the exercise science field (particularly your area of greatest interest) heading in the next 20 years?**

It is my speculation that during the next 20 years exercise physiologists will be emphasizing and investigating molecular mechanisms in all of the known systems. Since the genome will have been characterized during this interval, exercise physiology genomics will have become a well-defined subdiscipline, and countless studies will be underway to determine the interactions between the genome and the exercise response in normal and diseased populations.

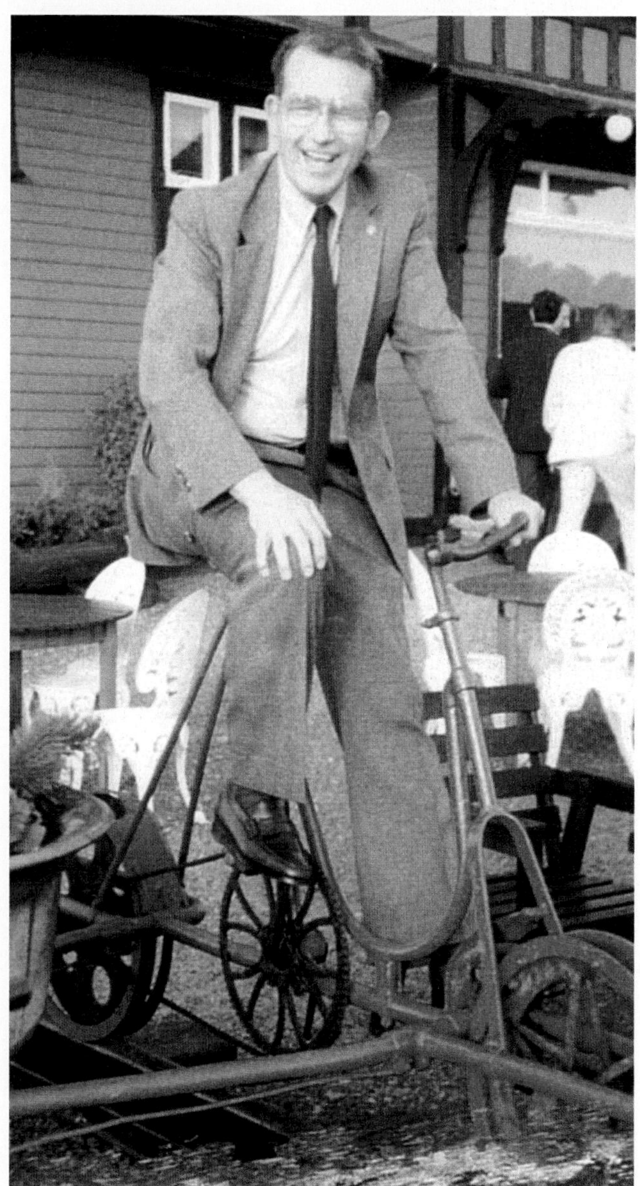

➤ **You have the opportunity to give a "last lecture." Describe its primary focus.**

It would be entitled "Exercise Physiology in the Last Frontier," and would pertain to what is known and unknown about exercising in a microgravity environment.

glectful not to acknowledge the numerous contributions from many scholars in other countries. The group of foreign contributors, many still active, includes but certainly is not limited to the following individuals: Roy Shephard, School of Physical and Health Education, University of Toronto (ACSM Citation Award, 1991); Claude Bouchard, Pennington Biomedical Research Center, Baton Rouge, LA (ACSM Citation Award, 1992); Oded Bar-Or, McMaster University, Hamilton, Ontario, Canada; Rodolfo Margaria and P. Cerretelli, Institute of Human Physiology, Medical School of the Univeristy of Milan; M. Ikai, School of Education, University of Japan; Wildor Holloman, Director of the Institute for Circulation, Research and Sports Medicine, and L. Brauer and H. W. Knipping, Institute of Medicine, University of Cologne, Germany (in 1929, they described the "vita maxima" now called the maximal oxygen consumption); L. G. C. E. Pugh, Medical Research Council Laboratories, London; Z. I. Barbashova, Sechenov Institute of Evolutionary Physiology, Leningrad, U.S.S.R.; Sir Cedric Stanton Hicks, Human Physiology Department, University of Adelaide, Australia; Otto Gustaf Edholm, National Institute for Medical Research, London, England; John Valentine George Andrew Durnin, Department of Physiology, Glasgow University, Scotland; Reginald Passmore, Department of Physiology, University of Edinburgh, Scotland; Ernst F. Jokl (ACSM founder and charter member), Witwatersrand Technical College, Johannesburg, South Africa, and later the University of Kentucky; C. H. Wyndham and N. B. Strydom, University of the Witwatersrand, South Africa. There were also many early German scientific contributions to exercise physiology and sports medicine.[32]

CONCLUDING COMMENT

One theme unites the history of exercise physiology: the value of mentoring by those visionaries who spent an extraordinary amount of their careers "infecting" students with love for hard science. These demanding but inspiring relationships developed researchers who, in turn, nurtured the next generation of productive scholars. This applies not only to the current group of exercise physiologists, but also to scholars of previous generations. Siegel[57] cites Payne,[50] who in 1896 wrote the following about Harvey's 1616 discovery of the mechanism of the circulation, acknowledging the discoveries of the past:

> No kind of knowledge has ever sprung into being without an antecedent, but is inseparably connected with what was known before. . . . We are led back to Aristotle and Galen as the real predecessors of Harvey in his work concerning the heart. It was the labors of the great school of Greek anatomists. . . . that the problem though unsolved, was put in such a shape that the genius of Harvey was enabled to solve it. . . . The moral is, I think, that the influence of the past on the present is even more potent than we commonly suppose. In common and trivial things, we may ignore this connection; in what is of enduring worth we cannot.

We end our overview of the history of exercise physiology with a passage from an American physiology and hygiene textbook written more than 131 years ago by J. C. Dalton, MD, a professor of physiology in the College of Physicians and Surgeons in New York City. It shows how current themes in exercise physiology share a common bond with what was known and advocated at that time (the benefits of moderate physical activity, walking as an excellent exercise, the appropriate exercise intensity, the specificity of training, the importance of mental well-being). Even the "new" thoughts and ideas of Dalton penned in 1869 had their roots in antiquity—reinforcing to us the importance of maintaining a healthy respect for the past.

> Exercise. The natural force of the muscular system requires to be maintained by constant and regular Exercise. If all of the muscles, or those of any particular part, be allowed to remain for a long time unused they diminish in size, grow softer, and finally become sluggish and debilitated. By use and exercise, on the contrary, they maintain their vigor, continue plump and firm to the touch, and retain all the characters of their healthy organization. It is very important, therefore, that the muscles should be trained and exercised by sufficient daily use. Too much confinement by sedentary occupation, in study, or by simple indulgence in indolent habits, will certainly impair the strength of the body and injuriously affect the health. Every one who is in a healthy condition should provide for the free use of the muscles by at least two hours' exercise each day; and this exercise can not be neglected with impunity, any more than the due provision of clothing and food .
>
> The muscular exercise of the body, in order to produce its proper effect, should be regular and moderate in degree. It will not do for any person to remain inactive during the greater part of the week, and then take an excessive amount of exercise on a single day. An unnatural deficiency of this kind cannot be compensated by an occasional excess. It is only a uniform and healthy action of the parts which stimulates the muscles, and provides for their nourishment and growth. Exercise which is so violent and long-continued as to produce exhaustion or unnatural fatigue is an injury instead of an advantage, and creates a waste and expenditure of the muscular force instead of its healthy increase.
>
> Walking is therefore one of the most useful kinds of exercise, since it calls into easy and moderate action nearly all the muscles of the body, and may be continued for a long time without fatigue. Riding on horseback is also exceedingly efficacious, particularly as it is accompanied by a certain amount of excitement and interest which acts as an agreeable and healthy stimulus to the nervous system. Running and leaping, being more violent should be used more sparingly. For children, the rapid and continuous exercise which they spontaneously take in their various games and amusements in the open air is the best. The exact quantity of exercise to be taken is not precisely the same for different persons, but should be measured by its effect. It is always beneficial when it has fully employed the muscular powers without producing any sense of excessive fatigue or exhaustion.
>
> It should be remembered, also, that the object of exercise is not the mere acquisition or increase of muscular strength, but the proper maintenance of the general health. A special increase of strength may be produced to a very great extent by the constant practice or training of particular muscles. Thus the arms of the blacksmith and the legs of the dancer become developed in excessive proportions; and by the continued

practice, in a gymnasium, of raising weights, or carrying loads, the muscular system generally may be greatly increased in force. But this unusual muscular development is not necessary to health, and is not even particularly beneficial about it. The best condition is that in which all the different organs and systems of the body have their full and complete development, no one of them preponderating excessively over the others. The most useful kind of exercise, accordingly, is that which employs equally all the limbs, and cultivates agility and freedom of movement, as well as simple muscular strength.

In all cases, also, the exercise which is taken should be regular and uniform in degree, and should be repeated as nearly as possible for the same time every day.

As a student of Exercise Physiology, you are about to embark on an exciting journey into the world of human physiological response and adaptation to physical activity. We hope our tour of the beginnings of exercise physiology inspires you in your studies to begin your own journey to new discoveries.

References

1. American Association for Health, Physical Education, and Recreation. "Research methods applied to health, physical education, and recreation. Chapter 11. Physiological Laboratory Research (pages 254–274). Washington DC: American Association for Health, Physical Education, and Recreation, 1949.
2. Asmussen E. In: Fenn WO, Rahn H. (eds). Handbook of respiration. Section 3. Respiration. Vol. II. Washington DC: American Physiological Society, 1965:939–978..
3. Åstrand P-O. Influence of Scandinavian scientists in exercise physiology. Scand J Med Sci Sports 1991;1:3–9.
4. Bang O, et al. Contributions to the physiology of severe muscular work. Skand Arch Physiol 1936;74 (suppl):1.
5. Barcroft J. The respiratory function of the blood. Part 1. Lessor from high altitude. Cambridge: University Press, 1925.
6. Berryman JW. Out of many, one. A history of the American College of sports medicine. Champaign, IL: Human Kinetics, 1995.
7. Berryman JW. The tradition of the "six things non-natural": Exercise and medicine from Hippocrates through Ante-Bellum America. Exerc Sport Sci Rev 1989;17:515.
8. Billings JS. Literature and institutions. In: Clarke EH, et al. A century of American medicine. Philadelphia: Henry C. Lea, 1876:294.
9. Breasted JH. The rise of man. Science 1931;74:639.
10. Buskirk ER. Early history of exercise physiology in the United States. Part 1. A contemporary historical perspective. In: History of Exercise and Sport Science. Messengale JD, Swanson RA, (eds). Champaign, IL: Human Kinetics. 1997.
11. Buskirk ER. The emergence of exercise physiology in physical education. In: Brooks GA (ed). Perspectives on the Academic Discipline of Physical Education. Champaign, IL: Human Kinetics Publishers, 1981:55–74.
12. Cathcart EP. The early development of the science of nutrition. In: Bourne GH, Kidder GW (eds). Biochemistry and physiology of nutrition, vol. 1. New York: Academic Press Inc., 1953.
13. Christensen EH, and Nielsen M. Investigations of the circulation in the skin at the beginning of muscular work. Acta Physiol Scand 1942;4:162.
14. Christensen EH, Krogh A, and Lindhard J. Contributions to the physiology of heavy muscular work. Skan Arch Physiol. 1936;Suppl. 10.
15. Consolazio CF. Metabolic methods. St. Louis: The C.V. Mosby Company, 1951.
16. Consolazio CF. Physiological measurements of metabolic functions in man. New York: McGraw-Hill Book Company, 1961.
17. Dill DB. Arlie V. Bock, pioneer in sports medicine. December 30, 1888–August 11, 1984. Med Sci Sports Exerc 1985;17:401.
18. Dill DB. Life, heat, and altitude; physiological effects of hot climates and great heights. Cambridge: Harvard University Press, 1938.
19. Dill DB. The Harvard Fatigue Laboratory: Its development, contributions, and demise. Circ Res 1967;20&21 (supple 1):161.
20. Dill DB. The hot life of man and beast. Springfield, IL: Charles C. Thomas, 1985.
21. Gardner EJ. History of biology, 3rd ed. Minneapolis: Burgess Publishing Co., 1972.
22. Gerber EW. Innovators and institutions in physical education. Philadelphia: Lea & Febiger, 1971.
23. Green H. Fit for America. Health, Fitness, Sport, and American Society. New York: Pantheon Books, 1986.
24. Green RM. A translation of Galen's Hygiene. Illinois: Charles C. Thomas Publisher, 1951.
25. Haldane JS, and Priestly JG. Respiration. New York: Oxford University Press, 1935.
26. Henry FM, and Farmer D. Functional Tests: II. The reliability of the pulse-ratio test. Res Q 1938;4:81.
27. Henry FM, and Kleeberger FL. Functional Tests: I. The validity of the pulse-ratio test of cardiac efficiency. Res Q 1938;4:32.
28. Henry FM, and Trafton IR. The velocity curve of sprint running with some observations on the muscle viscosity factor. Res Q 1951;22:409.
29. Henry FM. Force-time characteristics of the sprint start. Res Q 1952;23:301.
30. Hermansen L. Anaerobic energy release. Med Sci Sports 1969;1:32.
31. Hermansen L, and Anderson KL. Aerobic work capacity in young Norwegian men and women. J Appl Physiol 1965;20:425.
32. Hoberman JM. The early development of sports medicine in Germany. In: Berryman JW, and Park RJ (eds). Sport and Exercise Science. Urbana: University of Illinois Press, 1992: 233–282.
33. Horvath SM, and Horvath EC. The Harvard Fatigue Laboratory: Its history and contributors. Englewood Cliffs: Prentice-Hall, 1973.
34. Johnson RE, et al. Laboratory manual of field methods for the biochemical assessment of metabolic and nutrition conditions. Boston: Harvard Fatigue Laboratory, 1946.
35. Krehl WA. James Lind, MD. J Nutr 1953;50:3.
36. Krogh A. Osmotic regulation in aquatic animals. New York: Dover Publications, 1939.
37. Krogh A. The anatomy and physiology of capillaries. New Haven: Yale University Press, 1936.
38. Krogh A. The comparative physiology of respiratory mechanisms. Philadelphia: University of Pennsylvania Press, 1941.
39. Krogh A. The composition of the atmosphere; An account of preliminary investigations and a programme. Kobehaven: A.F. Host, 1919. (19 p monograph)
40. Krogh A. The respiratory exchange of animals and man. New York: Longmans, Green, 1916. (includes 17 page reference list)
41. Kroll W. Perspectives in physical education. New York: Academic Press, 1971.
42. Leonard FG. A guide to the history of physical education. Philadelphia: Lea & Febiger, 1923.
43. Lusk G. The elements of the science of nutrition. Second edition. Philadelphia: W.B. Saunders Company, 1909.
44. Manolis GG. Relation of charging time to blocking performance in football. Res Q 1955;26:170.
45. Park RJ. Concern for health and exercise as expressed in the writings of 18th century physicians and informed laymen (England, France, and Switzerland). Res Q 1976;47:756.
46. Park RJ. The rise and demise of Harvard's B.S. program in anatomy, physiology, and physical training: a case of conflicts of interest and scarce resources. Res Q Exerc Sport 1992;63:1.
47. Park RJ. Franklin M. Henry—scientist, mentor, pioneer. Res Q Exerc Sports 1994;65:295–307.
48. Park RJ. Physiologists, physicians, and physical educators: nineteenth century biology and exercise, hygienic and educative. J Sport Hist. 1987;14:28.
49. Park RJ. The emergence of the academic discipline of physical education in the United States. In: Brooks GA. (ed). Perspectives on the academic discipline of physical education. Champaign, IL: Human Kinetics Publishers, 1981: 20–45.
50. Payne JF. Harvey and Galen. The Harveyan oration. Oct. 19, 1896. London: Frowde, 1897.
51. Powers SK, and Howley ET. Exercise physiology. Dubuque: Wm. C. Brown Publishers, 1994.
52. Ross WD. Kinanthropometry: an emerging scientific technology. In: Landry F, Orban WAR (eds). Biomechanics of sports and kinanthropometry. Book 6. Miami: Symposia Specialists, Inc., 1978: 269–282.

53. Ross WD, et al. Kinanthropometry: traditions and new perspectives. In: Ostyn M, et al. (ed). Kinanthropometry II. Baltimore: University Park Press, 1980: 3–27.
54. Schmidt-Nielsen B. August and Marie Krogh and respiratory physiology. J Appl Physiol 1984;57:293.
55. Scholander PF. Analyzer for accurate estimation of respiratory gases in one-half cubic centimeter samples. J Biol Chem 1947;167:235.
56. Shaffel N. The evaluation of American medical literature. In: History of American medicine. Marti-Ibanez F. (ed). New York: MD Publications Inc., 1958.
57. Siegel R. Galen's system of physiology and medicine. New York: S. Karger, 1968.
58. Stewart CP, and Guthrie D. Lind's treatise on scurvey. A bicentenary volume containing a reprint of the first edition of A Treatise of the Scurvey by James Lind, MD, with Additional Notes. Edinburgh: University Press, 1953.
59. Tipton CM. A history of exercise physiology in the United States. Part II. A contemporary historical perspective. In: History of exercise and sport science. Messengale JD, Swanson RA (eds). Champaign IL: Human Kinetics, 1997.
60. Wilmore JH, Costill DL. Physiology of sport and exercise. 2nd ed. Champaign IL: Human Kinetics Publishers, 1999.

Additional Resources

Beaumont W. Experiments and observations on the gastric juice and the physiology of digestion. New York: Dover Publications, Inc., 1959.

Bernard C. The introduction to the study of experimental medicine (translated by HC Greene). New York: Henry Schuman, Inc., 1927.

Carpenter KJ. Protein and energy: A study of changing ideas in nutrition. London: Cambridge University Press, 1994.

Carpenter KJ. The history of scurvy and vitamin C. Cambridge: Cambridge University Press, 1986.

Cathcart EP. The early development of the science of nutrition. In: Bourne GH, Kidder GW (eds). Biochemistry and physiology of nutrition, vol. 1. New York: Academic Press Inc., 1953.

Cutter C. Anatomy and physiology designed for academics and families. New York: Benjamin B. Mussey and Co., 1848.

Dunglison R. Human health, or The influence of atmosphere and locality; Change of air and climate; seasons; food; clothing; bathing and mineral springs; exercise; sleep; corporeal and intellectual pursuits, on healthy man; constituting elements of hygiene. A New Edition. Philadelphia: Lea & Blanchard, 1844.

Duveen DI, HS Klickstein. A bibliography of the works of Antoine Laurent Lavosier, 1743–1794. London: W. Dawson & Sons, and E. Weil, 1954.

Foster M. Claude Bernard. New York: Longmans, Green & Co., 1899.

Fruton JS. Claude Bernard the scientist. In: Robin ED (ed). Claude Bernard and the internal environment. A memorial symposium. New York: Marcel Dekker, Inc., 1979.

Grmek MD. Claude Bernard. Dictionary of scientific biography, Volume II. New York: Charles Scribner's Sons, 1971: 87–91.

Guerlac H. "Lavosier." Dictionary of scientific biography. Volume VIII. New York: Charles Scribner's Sons, 1973: 87–91.

Guerlac HG. Essays and papers in the history of modern science. Baltimore: The Johns Hopkins University Press, 1977.

Guggenheim KY. Nutrition and nutritional diseases. Lexington MA: Collamore Press, 1981.

Holmes FL. Claude Bernard and animal chemistry: The emergence of a science. Cambridge, MA: Harvard University Press, 1974.

Holmes FL. Justus von Liebig. Dictionary of scientific biography, Volume VII. New York: Charles Scribner's Sons,

Horsman R. Frontier doctor, William Beaumont, America's first great medical scientist. Columbia: University of Missouri Press, 1996.

Keynes Sir Geoffrey. The life of William Harvey. Oxford: Clarendon, 1966.

Kilgour FG. William Harvey's use of the quantitative method. Yale Journal of Biology and Medicine 1954;26:410–421.

Mayer J. Claude Bernard. J Nutr 1951;45:3.

Myer JS. Life and letters of Dr. William Beaumont. St. Louis: The C.V. Mosby Company, 1939.

Olmsted JMD, Olmsted EH. Claude Bernard and the experimental method in medicine. New York: Schuman, 1952.

Osler W. William Beaumont: A pioneer American physiologist. JAMA Nov. 15, 1902.

Sachflebem R. Nobel prize winners descended from Liebig. J Chem Educ 1958;35:73–75.

Internet Resources

A Treatise of the Scurvy, (www.people.virgina.edu/~rjh9u/scurvy.html)

Claude Bernard (www.santafe.edu/~shalizi/notebooks/bernard.html)

Drawings of Leonardo da Vinci (www.mos.org/sln/Leonardo/)

Four Thousand Years of Women in Science (www.astr.ua.edu/4000ws/4000ws.html)

History Makers: August Krogh (www.sportsci.org/news/history/krogh/krogh.html)

History Makers: Claude Bernard (www.sportsci.org/news/history/bernard/bernard.html)

Life of Dr. William Beaumont (www.james.com/beaumont/dr_life.htm)

Panopticon Lavosier (150.217.52.68/index.htm#5)

Schack August Steenberg Krogh—A Versatile Genius (www.nobel.se/medicine/articles/krogh/index.html)

Vesalius (http://www.mc.vanderbilt.edu/biolib/hc/journeys/book19.html)

Welcome to Exploring Leonardo (www.mos.org/sln/Leonardo/)

William Harvey Medical Research Foundation (www.williamharvey.org/wm_harvey.htm)

Women & Minorities in Science and Engineering. (www.mills.edu/ACAD_INFO/MCS/SPERTUS/Gender/wom_and_min.html).

Woodrow Wilson National Fellowship Foundation. (www.woodrow.org/teachers/ci/1992/Lavosier.html)

PART *One*

EXERCISE PHYSIOLOGY

SECTION

1

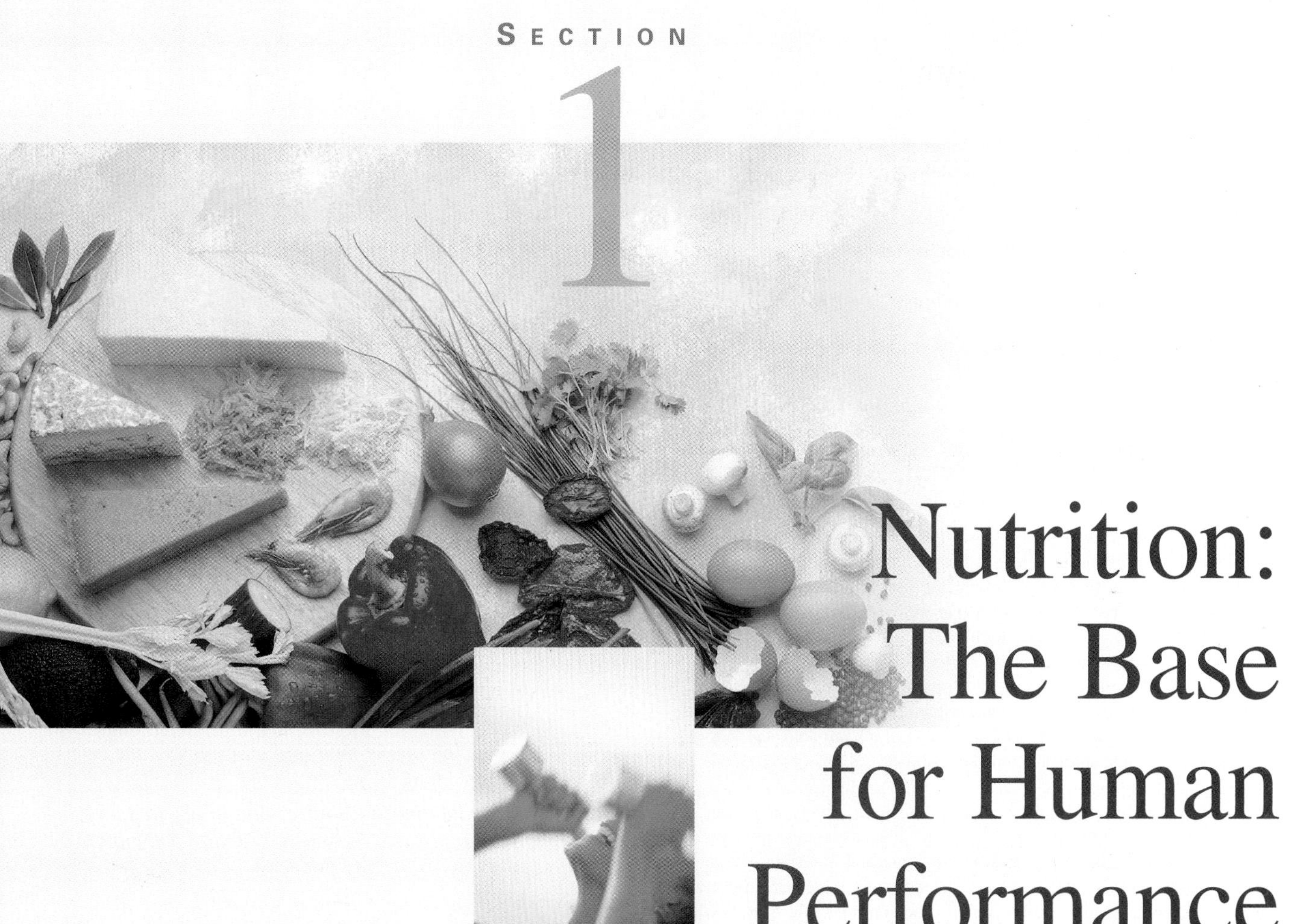

Nutrition: The Base for Human Performance

Overview

Nutrition and exercise physiology share a natural linkage. Proper nutrition forms the foundation for physical performance; it provides fuel for biologic work and chemicals for extracting and using the potential energy within this fuel. Nutrients from food also provide essential elements for repairing existing cells and synthesizing new tissues.

Some may argue that a well-balanced diet readily provides adequate nutrients for exercise, so knowledge of nutrition offers little value to exercise physiologists. We maintain, however, that the study of exercise, viewed within the framework of energy capacities and human performance, must include an understanding of energy sources and the role nutrients play in energy release. With this perspective, the exercise specialist appreciates the importance of "adequate" nutrition and can critically evaluate the validity of claims about special nutritional supplements, including dietary modifications purported to enhance physical performance. Because nutrients provide energy and regulate physiologic processes associated with exercise, many individuals link improved athletic performance with dietary modification. Too often, individuals devote considerable time and effort striving to optimize exercise performance, only to fall short because of inadequate, counterproductive, and sometimes harmful nutritional practices. Finally, nutrition can affect disease conditions for which regular exercise makes important, positive contributions. The three chapters that follow present the six broad categories of nutrients—carbohydrates, lipids, proteins, vitamins, minerals, and water—and explore the following questions: What are they? Where are they found? What are their functions? What is their specific role in physical activity? Also included is a discussion of optimal nutrition for exercise.

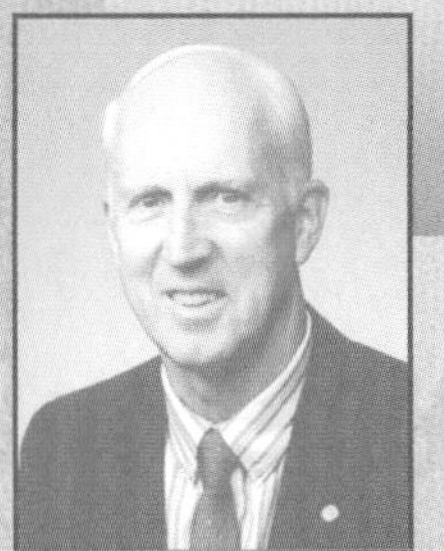

Interview with Dr. David L. Costill

Education: BS (Ohio University, Athens, OH); MEd (Miami University, Oxford, OH); PhD (Physiology, Ohio State University, Columbus, OH)

Current Affiliation: Professor Emeritus, John and Janice Fisher Chair in Exercise Science. Ball State University

Honors and Awards: See Appendix E.

Research Focus: My research interest was aimed at several areas: body fluid balance, carbohydrate metabolism in human muscle, thermal regulation during exercise, physiological characteristics of runners and swimmers, aging distance runners, and changes in muscle fiber function during bed rest and space flight.

Memorable Publication: Costill DL, et al.: Skeletal muscle enzymes and fiber composition in male and female track athletes. J Appl Physiol 1976;40:149.

Statement of Contributions: ACSM Honor Award
In recognition of his lifetime of distinguished scientific achievement in the applied, basic and clinical aspects of exercise physiology, and sports medicine through his research, teaching, lecturing, mentoring of students and colleagues, and professional leadership.

Professor Costill has been one of the pioneers in researching the areas of human performance and sports nutrition. He provided the scientific community with the first complete assessment of the physiological factors which determine distance running performance. His early studies on carbohydrate metabolism and fluid replacement were foundational to understanding the fuel and fluid needs of the endurance athlete, and have provided the stimulus to what has become one of the most active areas in exercise research today. His studies of environmental limitation to endurance performance have contributed greatly to our understanding of how to best prepare individuals to exercise and compete in the heat. His personal interest in and dedication to distance running or swimming led him to conduct an unprecedented series of studies in both sports. The results of these studies have provided the physiologist, coach, and athlete with better understanding of the physiological basis for these sports.

His most recent research in the area of over-training has made major contributions to the training of elite athletes.

Professor Costill has dedicated considerable time and energy to the education of scientists, clinicians, coaches and athletes, through his professional articles, books, and lecturing. No single scientist has impacted the sports community nationally or internationally more than Professor Costill, due largely to his ability to effectively communicate the results of his research and those of others.

Professor Costill has also had a tremendous impact on those who have trained with him as undergraduate students, graduate students, post-doctoral fellows, or visiting colleagues.

Professor Costill's national and international professional leadership is widely acknowledged. He has served the American College of Sports Medicine in many ways, but most importantly as President during a critical time in the growth of the College. He has served as Editor-in-Chief of the *International Journal of Sports Medicine.*

Professor Costill's unceasing search for new insights into the mechanism underlying exercise and sports medicine has received the respect and admiration of the international scientific community. His prolific career has brought honor to his university, his students, his colleagues, and the American College of Sports Medicine.

➤ What first inspired you to enter the exercise science field?

Growing up in Ohio, I was always interested in biology and physiology, although I never thought of it in those terms. Even as an 8-year-old I needed to know why animals differed and what made them work.

In college, I was more interested in anatomy and physiology than in physical education. But I was a poor student who was satisfied with taking all the activities classes and easy grades that I was able to attain. My primary interest was staying eligible for swimming. During my senior year at OSU, I signed up for an independent study and was assigned a research project with 30 rats. The project never amounted to much, but I was left on my own and learned that the research process was challenging.

My first introduction to exercise physiology was as a graduate student at Miami University in Ohio. A faculty member (Fred Zeckman) in the Department of Zoology offered an exercise physiology class to about six students. Again, the class project involved data collection, a process I'd already found interesting. After teaching high school general science and biology for three years, as well as coaching three teams, I decided it was time to see if I could get the credentials to become a coach at a small college. I began working toward a doctorate in higher education. At the same time, I became close friends with Dick Bowers and Ed Fox, fellow graduate students who were majoring in exercise physiology under the direction of Dr. D.K. Mathews. It wasn't long before they persuaded me to switch over to work in the laboratory with them.

➤ What influence did your undergraduate education have on your final career choice?

It enabled me to get a degree and a teaching job. It wasn't until I had been teaching for several years that I identified what I really wanted to do. After one year at OSU, I moved to Cortland (SUNY), where I coached cross-country and swimming for 2 years. Although I enjoyed coaching, I just couldn't take the recruiting and continual exposure to 18-year-olds. So I decided to focus my energy on research. Exercise physiology gave me a chance to do research in an area that held numerous practical questions. My early studies with runners were a natural, considering the experience I'd had in coaching runners at Cortland. Interestingly, a few of those runners (e.g., Bob Fitts and Bob Gregor) have become well known in the exercise science field.

➤ Who were the most influential people in your career, and why?

Dr. Bob Bartels: Bob was my college swimming coach. First, he kept me on the freshman team, even though I was one of the least talented. There were moments during my senior year (as co-captain) when I'm sure he had second thoughts! Bob was also instrumental in getting me admitted to Miami University and OSU. Without his efforts, I'd probably still be teaching junior high science in Ohio.

Dr. David Bruce (D.B.) Dill: I worked with Bruce in the summer of 1968. His words of wisdom and advice headed me in the right direction. Drs. Bengt Saltin and Phil Gollnick: Since I received my PhD after only one year at OSU, I had little research background and no post-doctoral experience. In 1972, I spent 6 months with Bengt and Phil in Bengt's laboratory in Stockholm. I learned a great deal working with them and the "gang" (Jan Karlsson, Björn Ekblom, E.H. Christensen, P.O. Åstrand, etc.), which I consider to be my post-doctoral experience.

➤ What has been the most interesting/enjoyable aspect of your involvement in science?

Most interesting: Meeting people! The professional contact and friendships I had with other scientists (Charles Tipton, Skip Knuttgen, Jack Wilmore, Lars Hermansen, Harm Kuipers, Mark Hargreaves, Reggie Edgerton, Bill Fink, Clyde Williams, Per Blom, George Sheehan, Astronauts from STS-78 flight, and others).

Most enjoyable: Following the success of my ex-students. Since I was a student with little talent but a good work ethic, I tended to recruit those types as graduate students. They were not always the ones with the high GPAs, but they were motivated and knew how to work. A number of them have become well known in our field, including Bill Evans, Ed Coyle, Mike Sherman, Mark Hargreaves, Bob Fitts, Bob Gregor, Paul Thompson, Carl Foster, Joe Houmard, Rick Sharp, Larry Armstrong, Rob Robergs, John Ivy, Hiro Tanaka, Mike Flynn, Scott and Todd Trappe, Abe Katz, Pete Van Handel, Darrell Neufer, Matt Hickey, and others.

One of the most enjoyable aspects of my research has been the opportunity to work with some very interesting subjects, such as Bill Rogers, Steve Prefontaine, Alberto Salazar, Matt Biondi, Derek Clayton, Shella Young, Frank Shorter, Kenny Moore, and Ken Sparks.

➤ What was the least interesting/enjoyable aspect?

I have never liked writing books or chasing after grant money, but I knew that was essential to expand the laboratory and upgrade facilities to continue to do research. Also, seeing students with great talent fail to live up to full potential. Not every student achieved the level of success I expected, but their lives were often altered by events outside the laboratory. I always view my students as a part of my family, so when they had troubles and/or were unsuccessful, it was like watching my own kids' struggle.

➤ What advice would you give to students who express an interest in pursuing a career in exercise science research?

There are six keys to success as a researcher: (1) Identify a worthy question; (2) Design a protocol that will give you the best possible answer; (3) Make sure the question is fundable, i.e., it must be a problem that an outside source is willing to support financially; (4) Be good at and enjoy collecting data. Precision in the laboratory is essential if you want to generate a clear answer to your question; (5) Be capable of reducing the data to an intelligible form and writing a clear/concise paper that is publishable in a creditable journal; and (6) Be capable of presenting your research at scientific forums, as this helps to establish your scientific creditability.

➤ What interests have you pursued outside of your professional career?

Photography (1949-1955): I went to college to study photography (won three national photo contests in HS), but switched to physical education during my sophomore year.

Distance running (1965-1982): I started running for fitness and eventually ran 16 marathons in the late 1970s and early 1980s. Knee injuries forced me back to swimming in 1982. Masters Swimming (1982-present): After training for six months, Doc Counsilman, the famed Indiana University swim coach, talked me into entering a Masters meet, where he promptly beat me in a 500-yard freestyle event. My graduate students Rick Sharp and John Troup convinced me to "shave down" and compete in one more meet. Subsequently, I performed almost as well as I had in college, so I was hooked. At the age of 60, I could still beat my best college times, and set six age-group national records (two that still stand 5 years later).

I have two passions: aviation and auto restoration. I also enjoy fishing, camping, and canoeing. We have a cottage in northern Wisconsin, where we spend as much time in the summer as possible. But I always like to come back to the small town of Muncie, where there is no traffic, a nice house, good airport, and all the activities of the University.

➤ Where do you see the exercise physiology field heading in the next 20 years?

This field has moved from whole body measurements (handgrip and vital capacity) to molecular biology (single muscle fiber physiology). To fully understand the physiology of exercise, the answers lie at the subcellular level. Students need solid training in chemistry and molecular biology in order to contribute to knowledge over the next 20 years.

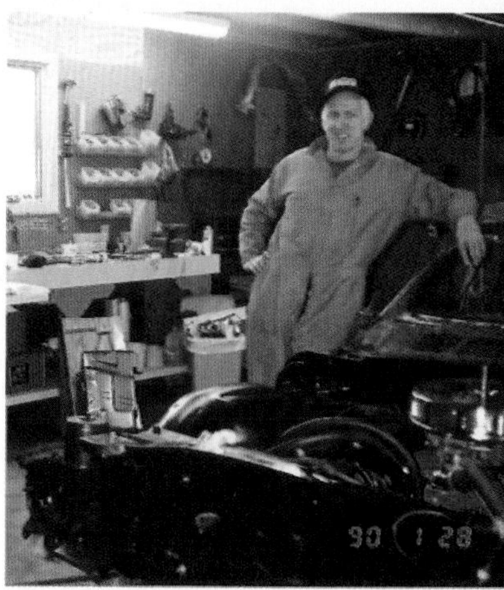

CHAPTER 1

Carbohydrates, Lipids, and Proteins

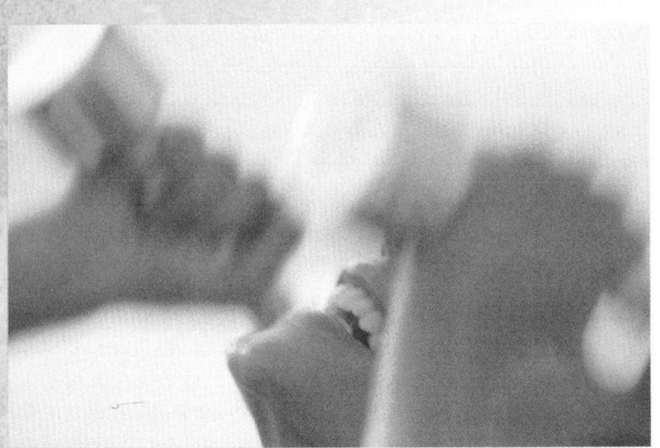

Objectives

- Distinguish among monosaccharides, disaccharides, and polysaccharides
- Identify the two major classifications of dietary fiber and their proposed roles in overall health
- Discuss possible differences in physiologic responses to different forms of dietary carbohydrate in the development of type 2 diabetes and obesity
- Quantify the amount, energy content, and distribution of carbohydrate within an average-sized person
- Summarize carbohydrate's role as an energy source, protein sparer, metabolic primer, and central nervous system fuel
- Outline the dynamics of carbohydrate metabolism during physical activity of various intensities and durations
- Contrast the speed of energy transfer from carbohydrate and fat combustion
- Discuss how diet affects muscle glycogen levels and endurance performance
- Give an example of food sources of diverse fatty acids (including *trans*- and omega-3 fatty acids), their physiologic functions, and their possible role in coronary heart disease risk
- List major characteristics of high- and low-density lipoprotein cholesterol and discuss their role in the development of coronary heart disease
- Make prudent recommendations for dietary lipid intake, including cholesterol and fatty acids
- Quantify the amount, energy content, and distribution of fat within an average-sized person
- Outline the dynamics of fat metabolism during physical activity of various intensities and durations
- List four functions of fat in the body
- Discuss the effects of aerobic exercise training on fat and carbohydrate catabolism during exercise
- Explain how aerobic training affects fat-burning adaptations within skeletal muscle
- Define the terms essential and nonessential amino acids and give food sources for each
- Discuss the advantages and potential limitations of a mainly vegetarian diet in maintaining good health and a physically active lifestyle
- Outline the dynamics of protein metabolism during physical activity of various intensities and durations
- Provide a rationale for increasing protein intake above the recommended dietary allowance (RDA) for individuals who perform heavy endurance or resistance exercise training
- Describe the alanine–glucose cycle and how the body uses amino acids for energy during exercise

The carbohydrate, lipid, and protein nutrients provide the necessary energy to maintain bodily functions during rest and physical activity. Aside from their role as biologic fuel, these nutrients, called **macronutrients**, maintain the structural and functional integrity of the organism. This chapter discusses each macronutrient's general structure, function, and dietary source. We emphasize their importance in sustaining physiologic function during physical activities of differing intensity and duration.

Atoms: Nature's Building Blocks

Of the 103 different atoms or elements identified in nature, the mass of the human organism contains about 3% nitrogen, 10% hydrogen, 18% carbon, and 65% oxygen. These atoms not only make up the structural units for the body's biologically active substances, but they also play the major role in the chemical composition of food nutrients.

The union of two or more atoms produces a molecule. The specific atoms and their arrangement give the molecule its particular properties. Glucose is glucose because of the arrangement (bonding) of three different kinds of 24 atoms within its molecule. An example of chemical bonding occurs when atoms of hydrogen (H) and oxygen (O) join to form the water molecule (H_2O) by sharing electrons in common between the H and O atoms. Forces of attraction between the atoms' positive and negative charges underlie the basis for bonding, serving as "chemical cement" that keeps the atoms and molecules within a substance from readily coming apart. Two or more molecules bound chemically form a larger aggregate of matter termed a substance. A substance can be a gas, a liquid, or a solid, depending on the force of interaction among molecules. Altering these forces by removal, transfer, or exchange of certain electrons releases energy, some of which powers cellular functions.

Carbon: The Versatile Element

All of the nutrients except water and minerals contain carbon. *Carbon-containing compounds compose almost all of the substances within the body.* Carbon atoms easily share their chemical bonds with other carbon atoms, as well as with atoms of other elements, to form large carbon-chain molecules. Atoms of carbon, hydrogen, oxygen, and nitrogen provide the building blocks to construct the diverse nutrients. Lipids and carbohydrates form from linkages of carbon atoms with atoms of hydrogen and oxygen. Protein molecules form when nitrogen combines with carbon, hydrogen, and oxygen atoms and certain minerals. Knowing a protein's nitrogen content makes it possible to chemically analyze any tissue for its protein composition.

➤ PART 1 • Carbohydrates

THE NATURE OF CARBOHYDRATES

Atoms of carbon, hydrogen, and oxygen combine to form a carbohydrate (sugar) molecule in the general formula $(CH_2O)_n$, where *n* ranges from 3 to 7 carbon atoms with hydrogen and oxygen atoms attached by single bonds. Except for lactose and a small amount of glycogen, plants provide the carbohydrate source in the human diet.[130] Figure 1.1 illustrates the most typical sugar, glucose, along with other carbohydrates formed in photosynthesis. Glucose consists of 6 carbon, 12 hydrogen, and 6 oxygen atoms, with the chemical formula $C_6H_{12}O_6$. Each carbon atom has four bonding sites that can link to other atoms, including carbons. Carbon bonds not linked to other carbons are "free" to hold hydrogen (with only one bond site), oxygen (with two bond sites), or an oxygen–hydrogen combination (OH) termed a hydroxyl. Fructose and galactose, two other simple sugars with the same chemical formula as glucose, have a slightly different C-H-O linkage. The alteration in atomic arrangement makes fructose, galactose, and glucose different substances with distinct biochemical characteristics.

KINDS AND SOURCES OF CARBOHYDRATES

Carbohydrates generally classify as monosaccharides, oligosaccharides, and polysaccharides. The number of simple sugars linked within each of these molecules distinguishes each carbohydrate form. Table 1.1 provides specific examples within the general classifications of carbohydrates.

Monosaccharides

The ***monosaccharide*** *represents the basic unit of carbohydrates.* More than 200 monosaccharides exist in nature, categorized by the number of carbon atoms in their ring. The Greek name for this number ending with "ose" identifies them as sugars. For example, trioses are monosaccharides with three carbons; tetroses have four carbons; pentoses, five; hexoses, six; and heptoses, seven. Hexose sugars include the nutritionally important monosaccharides glucose, fructose, and galactose. **Glucose**, also called dextrose or blood sugar, forms naturally in food or in the body through digestion of more complex carbohydrates. **Gluconeogenesis** also synthesizes glucose, primarily in the liver, from the carbon residues of other compounds (generally amino acids, but also glycerol, pyruvate, and lactate).[135] After absorption by the small intestine, glucose either (1) becomes available as an energy source for cellular metabolism, (2) forms glycogen for storage in the liver and muscles, or (3) is converted to triglyceride for later use as energy.

Fructose (fruit sugar or levulose), the sweetest simple sugar, occurs in large amounts in fruits and honey. Some fructose goes directly from the digestive tract into the blood, but all eventually becomes glucose in the liver.[76] **Galactose** does not exist freely in nature; rather, it combines with glucose to form milk sugar in the mammary glands of lactating animals. The body converts galactose to glucose for use in energy metabolism.

Oligosaccharides

Oligosaccharides (*oligo,* Greek, meaning a few) form when 2 to 10 monosaccharides bond chemically. The major oligosaccharides, the **disaccharides** or double sugars,

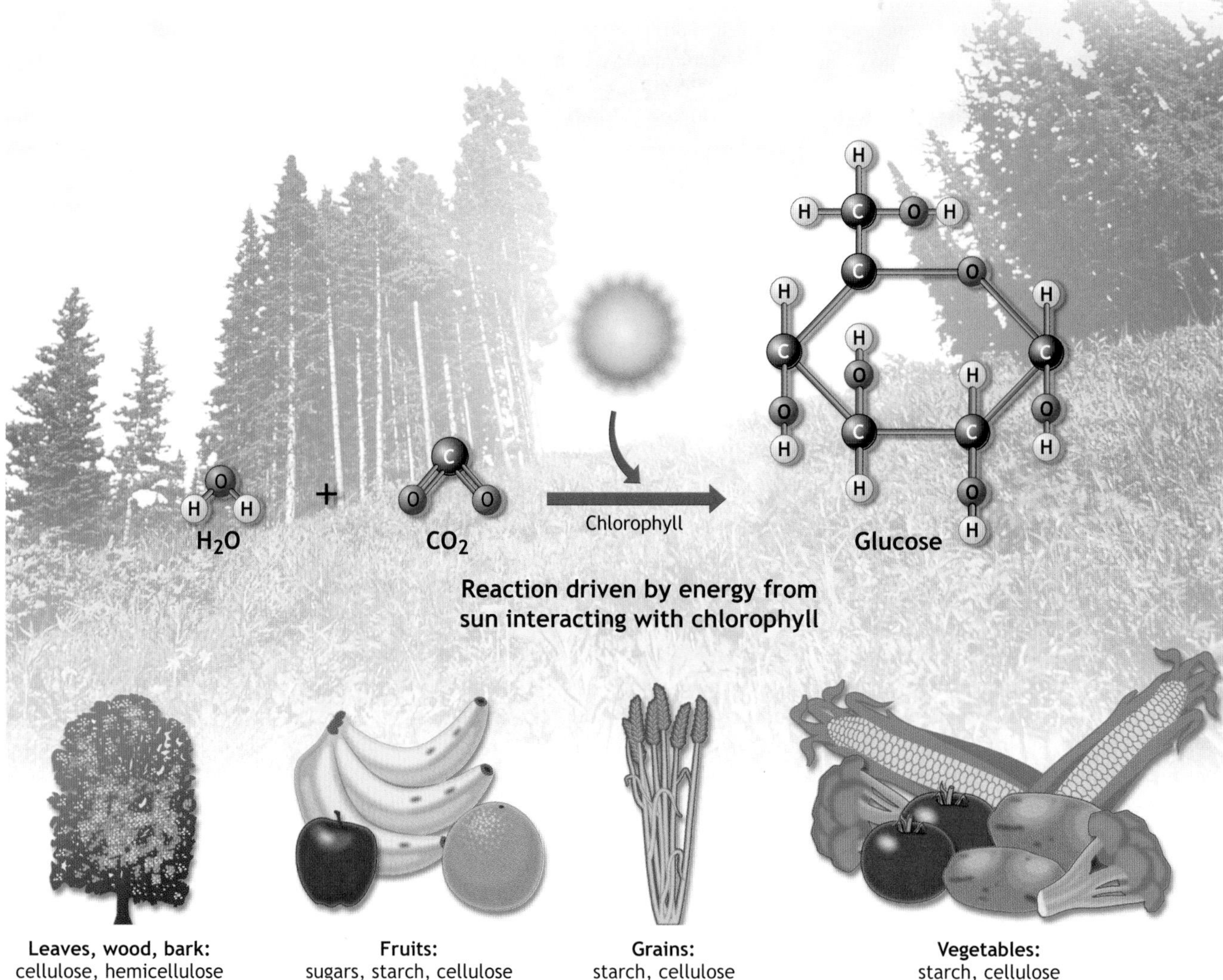

FIGURE 1.1 • Three-dimensional ring structure of the simple sugar glucose molecule formed during photosynthesis when energy from sunlight interacts with water, carbon dioxide, and the green pigment chlorophyll.

form when two monosaccharide molecules combine. Monosaccharides and disaccharides collectively make up the **simple sugars**. These sugars are packaged commercially under a variety of guises—brown sugar, corn syrup, fruit syrup, molasses, barley malt, invert sugar, honey, and "natural sweeteners."

Disaccharides all contain glucose. Three principal disaccharides exist.

- **Sucrose** (glucose plus fructose), the most common dietary disaccharide, contributes up to 25% of the total caloric intake in the United States. It occurs naturally in most foods that contain carbohydrates, especially beet and cane sugar, brown sugar, sorghum, maple syrup, and honey. In many countries, sucrose goes by the common name of table sugar, beet sugar, or cane sugar. Honey, while sweeter than table sugar because of its greater fructose content, is not superior to table sugar either nutritionally or as an energy source.
- **Lactose** (glucose plus galactose), the only sugar *not* found in plants, exists in natural form only in milk as milk sugar. The least sweet of the disaccharides, lactose when artificially processed often becomes an ingredient in carbohydrate-rich, high-calorie liquid meals. A substantial segment of the world's population experiences **lactose intolerance** (9 of every 10 Japanese, Thais, and Filipinos, and nearly 70% of blacks) because they lack adequate quantities of the enzyme lactase that splits lactose to glucose and galactose during digestion. A lactose-intolerant individual who consumes milk or dairy products cannot digest these foods. Consequently, the intestinal lumen draws in a large amount of water because of the osmotic effect caused by the inability to split the lactose molecule for absorption, which then produces cramps and diarrhea.
- **Maltose** (glucose plus glucose) occurs in beer, breakfast cereals, and germinating seeds. Also called malt

TABLE 1.1 ➤ GENERAL CLASSIFICATION OF SOME CARBOHYDRATES

MONOSACCHARIDES		OLIGOSACCHARIDES	POLYSACCHARIDES		
PENTOSES $C_5H_{10}O_5$	HEXOSES $C_6H_{12}O_6$	DISACCHARIDES $C_{12}H_{22}O_{11}$	PENTOSANS $(C_5H_8O_4)n^2$	HEXOSANS $(C_6H_{10}O_5)n^2$	MIXED POLYSACCHARIDES
Arabinose	Fructose	Lactose	Araban	Cellulose	Agar
Ribose	Galactose	Maltose	Xylan	Glycogen	Pectin
Xylose	Glucose	Sucrose		Inulin	Chitin
Deoxyribose	Mannose	Trehalose		Mannan	Hemicelluloses
				Starch (amylose and amylopectin)	Carrageenan
					Vegetable gums

MONOSACCHARIDE DERIVATIVES

Sugar alcohols: glycerol, inositol, mannitol, sorbitol

Amino sugars: galactosamine (formed from galactose—present in cartilage, tendons, and aorta); glucosamine (formed from glucose—present in connective tissues)

Sugar acids: ascorbic acid (vitamin C, not formed in the body); gluconic acid (formed from glucose); glucuronic acid (formed from glucose—aids in detoxification and excretion of other compounds, and is present in connective tissue)

sugar, this sugar easily cleaves into two glucose molecules but makes only a small contribution to the carbohydrate content of the diet.

Polysaccharides

The term **polysaccharide** describes the linkage of three to thousands of sugar molecules. Polysaccharides form during the chemical process of **dehydration synthesis** (water-losing reaction). These large chains of linked monosaccharides come from either plant or animal sources. The designations *plant* and *animal* denote these two polysaccharide subclassifications.

Plant Polysaccharides

Starch and fiber are the common forms of plant polysaccharides.

Starch, the storage form of carbohydrate in plants, is the most familiar form of plant polysaccharide. It occurs in seeds, corn, and various grains of bread, cereal, pasta, and pastries. Large amounts also exist in peas, beans, potatoes, and roots, in which starch serves as an energy store for future use by plants. Starch exists in two forms: (1) **amylose**, a long straight chain of glucose units twisted into a helical coil, and (2) **amylopectin**, a highly branched monosaccharide linkage. The relative proportion of each form of starch in a particular plant species determines the specific characteristics of the starch, including its "digestibility." *Starches with a relatively large amount of amylopectin digest and absorb rapidly, whereas starches with high amylose content have a slower rate of chemical breakdown* (***hydrolysis***).

Plant starch still represents the most important dietary source of carbohydrate in the American diet, accounting for approximately 50% of total carbohydrate intake. Daily starch intake, however, has decreased about 30% since the turn of the twentieth century, while simple-sugar consumption has correspondingly increased from 30% to about 50% of total carbohydrate intake. The term **complex carbohydrate** describes dietary starch.

Fiber, classified as a nonstarch, structural polysaccharide, includes cellulose, the most abundant organic molecule on earth. Fibrous materials resist chemical breakdown by human digestive enzymes, although a portion ferments by action of intestinal bacteria and ultimately participates in metabolic reactions following intestinal absorption. *Fibers occur exclusively in plants;* they make up the structure of leaves, stems, roots, seeds, and fruit coverings. Fibers differ widely in physical and chemical characteristics and physiologic action. Cell walls contain different kinds of fibers (cellulose, hemicellulose, pectin, and the noncarbohydrate lignin); mucilage and gums occur within the plant cell itself.

HEALTH IMPLICATIONS OF FIBER DEFICIENCY. Dietary fiber has received considerable attention from researchers and the lay press. Much of this interest originated from studies that linked high fiber intake, particularly whole-grain cereal fibers, with a lower occurrence of obesity, diabetes, digestive disorders (including cancers of the mouth, pharynx, larynx, esophagus, and stomach), and heart disease.[75,118,123,150] The Western diet contains significant fiber-free animal foods and loses much of its natural plant fiber through processing. Researchers have speculated that a low fiber intake accounts for the higher prevalence of intestinal disorders in Western countries than in countries with diets high in unrefined, complex carbohydrates. For example, the typical American diet contains a daily fiber intake of about 12 g,[92] whereas diets from Africa and India contain between 40 and 150 g per day.[92] (*Note:* Appendix A shows the relationship between metric units and U.S. units, including common expressions of work, energy, and power.) Fibers hold considerable water and thus give "bulk" to the food residues in the small intestine, often increasing stool weight and volume by 40 to 100%.[28] Bulking action may aid gastrointestinal function by (1) exerting a scraping action on the cells of the gut wall, (2) binding or diluting harmful chemicals or inhibiting their activity, and (3) shortening the transit time for food residues (and possibly carcinogenic materials) to pass through the digestive tract. The potential protective effect of fiber on rates and risks of colon cancer remains a hotly debated topic.[18,57]

Fiber intake may *modestly* reduce serum cholesterol in humans, particularly the **water-soluble**, mucilaginous fibers such as psyllium seed husk, β-glucan, pectin, and guar gum present in oats, beans, brown rice, peas, carrots, corn husk, and many fruits.[17,39,52] Adding 100 g of oat bran to the daily diet of men with elevated blood lipids reduced serum cholesterol 13% and favorably affected the ratio of the blood's lipoproteins (see page 24).[84] Also, increasing the daily quar gum fiber intake reduced total cholesterol by lowering the low-density lipoprotein component of the cholesterol profile.[52,136] Dietary fiber exerts no effect on high-density lipoproteins. **Water-insoluble fibers** such as cellulose, hemicellulose, and lignin, and cellulose-rich products such as wheat bran do not lower cholesterol.[17]

Precisely how dietary fibers favorably affect serum cholesterol remains unknown. Possibly, added fiber simply replaces cholesterol-laden items in the diet. Additionally, some fibers may hinder cholesterol absorption while others reduce cholesterol synthesis in the gut. These actions would depress cholesterol synthesis and facilitate excretion of existing cholesterol bound to fiber in the feces. Recent evidence shows fiber consumption to be a better predictor (strong inverse relationship) of insulin levels, weight gain, and diverse coronary artery disease risk factors than is intake of total fat or saturated fatty acids.[99] Heart disease and obesity protection may relate to dietary fiber's regulatory role in reducing insulin secretion by slowing nutrient absorption by the small intestine after a meal. Fiber content of a meal also decreases the total number of calories consumed in subsequent meals. For example, consuming a fiber-rich breakfast decreased the caloric intake during both breakfast and a buffet-type lunch consumed 3.5 hours later. Increased dietary fiber consumption may also confer heart disease protection through beneficial effects on blood pressure, insulin sensitivity, and improved blood clotting characteristics.[95] For nearly 69,000 middle-aged nurses, each 5-g daily increase of cereal fiber (one-half cup of bran-flake cereal contains 4 g of fiber) translated to a 37% decrease in coronary risk.[161] Excessive fiber intake generally blunts the intestinal absorption of calcium, phosphorus, and the trace mineral iron.

Present nutritional wisdom advocates that a well-structured diet contain 20 to 35 g of fiber per day (ratio of 3:1 for water insoluble to soluble fiber) by following the recommendations of the Food Guide Pyramid from the Unites States Department of Agriculture (see Chapter 3, page 85). Table 1.2 lists the fiber content of some common foods, and Table 1.3 presents a sample daily 2,200-kcal menu that includes 31 g of fiber (21 g insoluble fiber). In this particular diet, total lipid calories equal 30% (saturated fat equals 10%); protein, 16%; and carbohydrate, 54% of total calories ingested.

Some Confusion Concerning Dietary Carbohydrates

Controversy exists concerning the potential effects of high-carbohydrate diets on increased risk for obesity and coronary heart disease, particularly among sedentary and obese adults and children.[38,77,122,124,132,140,157] Frequent and excessive intake of some forms of carbohydrate may also increase diabetes risk. The dietary patterns of 65,173 women studied over 6 years showed that women who ate a low-fiber, starchy diet (potatoes and high-glycemic, processed white rice, pasta, and white bread, along with nondiet soft drinks) had 2.5 times the rate of diabetes than women who ate less of those foods and more fiber-containing, whole-grain cereals, fruits, and vegeta-

TABLE 1.2 ➤ FIBER CONTENT OF COMMON FOODS LISTED IN ORDER OF TOTAL FIBER CONTENT

	Serving Size	Total Fiber (g)	Soluble Fiber (g)	Insoluble Fiber (g)
100% bran cereal	½ cup	10.0	0.3	9.7
Peas	½ cup	5.2	2.0	3.2
Kidney beans	½ cup	4.5	0.5	4.0
Apple	1 small	3.9	2.3	1.6
Potato	1 small	3.8	2.2	1.6
Broccoli	½ cup	2.5	1.1	1.4
Strawberries	¾ cup	2.4	0.9	1.5
Oats, whole	½ cup	1.6	0.5	1.1
Banana	1 small	1.3	0.6	0.7
Pasta	½ cup	1.0	0.2	0.8
Lettuce	½ cup	0.5	0.2	0.3
White rice	½ cup	0.5	0	0.5

TABLE 1.3 ➤ SAMPLE DAILY MENU FOR BREAKFAST, LUNCH, AND DINNER (2200 kcal) CONTAINING 31 g OF DIETARY FIBER[a]

BREAKFAST	LUNCH	DINNER
Whole grain cereal (0.75 cup)	Bran muffin (1)	Green salad (3.5 oz)
Whole wheat toast (2 slices)	Milk, 2% (1 cup)	Broccoli, steamed (0.5 cup)
Margarine (2 tsp)	Hamburger on bun, lean beef patty (3 oz) with 2 slices tomato and lettuce, catsup (1 Tbsp) and mustard (1 Tbsp)	Roll, whole wheat (1)
Jelly, strawberry (1 Tbsp)	Whole wheat crackers (4 small)	Margarine (2 tsp)
Milk, 2% (1 cup)	Split-pea soup (1 cup)	Brown rice (0.5 cup)
Raisins (2 Tbsp)	Coffee (or tea)	Chicken breast, skinless, broiled (3 oz)
Orange juice (0.5 cup)		Salad dressing, vinegar and oil (1 Tbsp)
Coffee (or tea)		Pear, medium (1)
		Yogurt, vanilla, lowfat (0.5 cup)

[a]The diet's total cholesterol content is less than 200 mg, and total calcium equals 1242 mg.

bles.[123] Participants who became diabetic developed type 2 diabetes (previously called adult-onset or non-insulin- dependent diabetes; see Chapter 20), the most common form of the disease that afflicts 14 million individuals in the United States. High blood glucose levels in type 2 diabetes can result from (1) inadequate insulin produced by the pancreas to control blood sugar (**relative insulin deficiency**), (2) decreased insulin effects on peripheral tissue (**insulin resistance**), or (3) combined effect of both. Diet-induced insulin resistance/hyperinsulinemia often occurs before manifestations of the **metabolic syndrome** of obesity, insulin resistance, glucose intolerance, dyslipidemia, and hypertension.[9]

NOT ALL CARBOHYDRATES ARE PHYSIOLOGICALLY EQUAL. A possible explanation for a potential carbohydrate intake–diabetes link relates to the digestion and absorption rates of different carbohydrate sources. Low-fiber processed starches (and simple sugars in soft drinks) digest quickly and enter the blood at a relatively rapid rate (these foods have a high glycemic index; see Chapter 3). Dietary fiber slows carbohydrate digestion, minimizing surges in blood glucose. The surge in blood glucose with refined processed starch intake (in contrast to slow-release forms of high-fiber, unrefined complex carbohydrates) increases insulin demand, stimulates overproduction of insulin, and accentuates hyperinsulinemia.[15,53,68,156] Consistently eating such foods may eventually reduce the body's sensitivity to insulin (i.e., peripheral tissues become more resistant to insulin's effects), which would require progressively greater insulin output to control blood sugar levels.

A ROLE IN OBESITY? About 25% of the population produces excessive insulin in response to rapidly absorbed carbohydrates. These insulin-resistant individuals may be at greater risk for obesity if they consistently eat carbohydrates with a rapid absorption rate. This occurs because excessive insulin facilitates glucose oxidation at the expense of fatty acid oxidation; it also stimulates synthesis of very-low-density lipoprotein cholesterol in the liver and fat storage in adipose tissue.[56] If these observations prove correct, obese persons will be most affected because this group shows the greatest insulin resistance and, consequently, the greatest insulin response to a glucose challenge. *For physically active people, however, regular exercise exerts a potent influence to control body weight and improves sensitivity to insulin, thereby reducing the insulin requirement for a given glucose uptake.*

To reduce type 2 diabetes and obesity risks, one should consume more slowly absorbed, unrefined, complex carbohydrate foods with a low glycemic index. These foods provide "slow-release" carbohydrate without triggering rapid fluctuations in blood sugar. If rice, pasta, and bread remain the carbohydrate sources of choice, they should be consumed in unrefined form as brown rice, whole-grain pastas, and multigrain breads. *The same dietary modification would benefit individuals involved in heavy physical training and endurance competition.* In this case, daily dietary carbohydrate intake should approach 800 g (8 to 10 g per kg of body mass).

Animal Polysaccharides

Glycogen is the storage carbohydrate peculiar to mammalian muscle and liver. It forms as a large polysaccharide polymer synthesized from glucose in the glycogen-synthesizing process of **glucogenesis** (catalyzed by the enzyme **glycogen synthase**). Irregularly shaped, glycogen ranges from a few hundred to 30,000 glucose molecules linked together, much like links in a chain of sausages, with branch linkages for joining additional glucose units (see inset stage 4, Fig. 1.2). Figure 1.2 shows that glycogen synthesis involves adding individual glucose units to an existing glycogen polymer. Stage 4 of the figure shows an enlarged view of the chemical configuration of the glycogen molecule. Overall, glycogen synthesis progresses in an irreversible manner. Also, glycogen synthesis requires energy, as one adenosine triphosphate (ATP; stage 1) and one uridine triphosphate (UTP; stage 3) degrade during glucogenesis.

Figure 1.3 shows that a well-nourished 80-kg person stores approximately 500 g of carbohydrate. Of this, muscle glycogen accounts for the largest reserve (approximately 400 g), followed by 90 to 110 g as liver glycogen (highest concentration that represents 3 to 7% of the liver's weight), with only about 2 to 3 g as blood glucose.[50] Because each gram of either glycogen or glucose contains approximately 4 calories of energy, the average

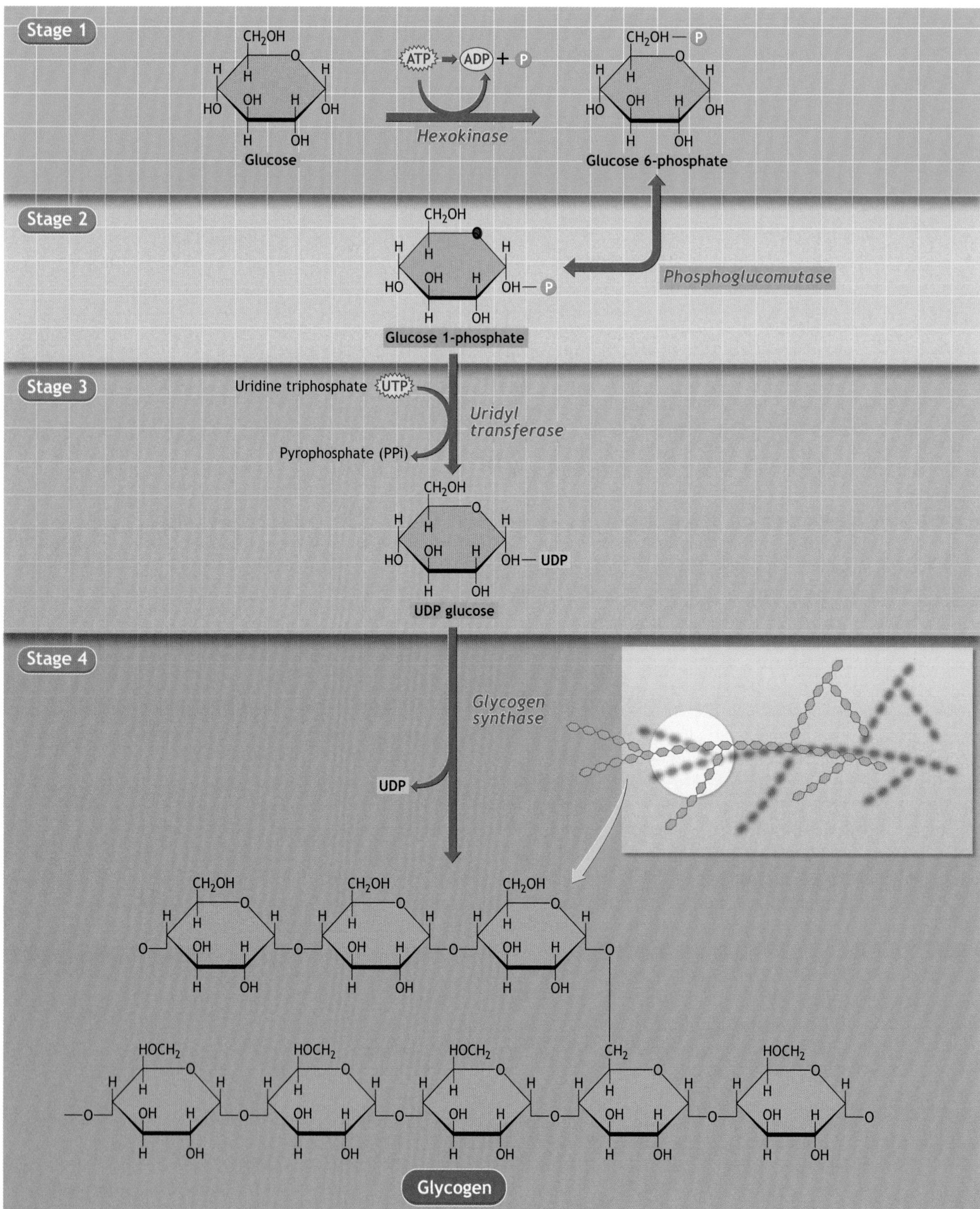

FIGURE 1.2 • Glycogen synthesis consists of a four-stage process. *Stage 1.* ATP donates a phosphate to glucose to form glucose 6-phosphate. This reaction involves the enzyme hexokinase. *Stage 2.* The enzyme phosphoglucomutase catalyzes the isomerization of glucose 6-phosphate to glucose 1-phosphate. *Stage 3.* The enzyme uridyl transferase reacts with glucose 1-phosphate to form UDP-glucose (a pyrophosphate forms in the degradation of uridine triphosphate [UTP]). *Stage 4.* UDP-glucose attaches to one end of an already existing glycogen polymer chain. This forms a new bond (known as a glycoside bond) between the adjacent glucose units, with concomitant release of UDP. For each glucose unit added, two molecules of high-energy phosphate (ATP and UDP) convert to two molecules of ADP and inorganic phosphate. The inset at the upper right of Stage 4 shows a low-resolution view of glycogen; the atomic arrangement of the circled area of the inset appears beneath the inset.

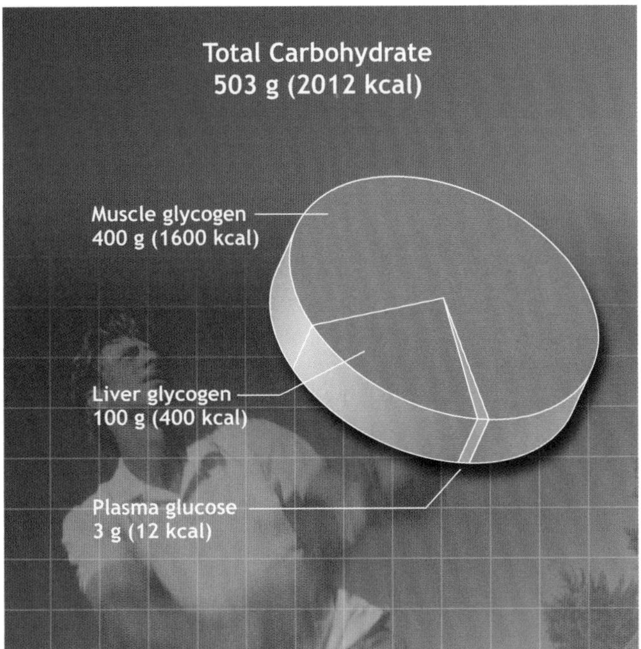

FIGURE 1.3 • Distribution of carbohydrate energy in an average 80-kg person.

person stores 1500 to 2000 calories as carbohydrate—enough total energy to power a 20-mile run at high intensity.

Several factors determine the rate and quantity of glycogen breakdown and resynthesis. During exercise, intramuscular glycogen provides the major carbohydrate energy source for active muscles. In addition, glycogen in the liver rapidly reconverts to glucose (regulated by a specific **phosphatase** enzyme) for release into the blood as an extramuscular glucose supply for exercise. The term **glycogenolysis** describes this reconversion process of glycogen to glucose. In essence, the breakdown of glycogen involves the cleavage of glucose units, one at a time, from the glycogen molecule through the introduction of high-energy phosphates (see Chapter 6). Liver and muscle glycogen depletion by dietary restriction or heavy exercise stimulates glucose synthesis, through gluconeogenic metabolic pathways, from the structural components of other nutrients, especially proteins.

Hormones play a key role in regulating liver and muscle glycogen stores by controlling circulating blood sugar levels. Elevated blood sugar causes the beta (ß) cells of the pancreas to secrete additional insulin, which facilitates cellular glucose uptake and inhibits further insulin secretion. This type of automatic feedback regulation keeps blood glucose at the appropriate physiologic concentration. In contrast, when blood sugar falls below normal, the pancreas's alpha (α) cells secrete **glucagon** (insulin's opposing hormone) to normalize blood sugar concentration. Known as the "insulin antagonist" hormone, glucagon increases blood glucose concentration by stimulating the liver's glycogenolytic and gluconeogenic pathways. Chapter 20 contains further discussion of hormonal regulation in exercise.

Because the body stores comparatively little glycogen, its quantity fluctuates considerably through dietary modifications. For example, a 24-hour fast or low-carbohydrate, normal-calorie diet nearly depletes glycogen reserves.[73] On the other hand, maintaining a carbohydrate-rich diet for several days nearly doubles the body's carbohydrate stores, compared with levels attained with a normal, well-balanced diet.[12] The upper limit for glycogen storage averages about 15 g per kilogram of body mass. This represents a capacity of 1150 g for an average-sized 70-kg man. On page 15, we discuss the effect of enhanced carbohydrate storage on exercise performance.

RECOMMENDED INTAKE OF CARBOHYDRATES

Figure 1.4 lists the carbohydrate content of selected foods. Cereals, cookies, candies, breads, and cakes provide rich carbohydrate sources. The values represent carbohydrate percentage in relation to the food's total weight, including water content. Thus, fruits and vegetables appear as less valuable carbohydrate sources. The dried portion of these foods contains almost pure carbohydrate.

The typical American diet contains between 40 and 50% of total calories as carbohydrate. For a sedentary 70-kg person, this amounts to a daily carbohydrate intake of about 300 g. For more physically active people and those involved in exercise training, carbohydrate should represent about 60% of daily calories (400 to 600 g), predominantly as unrefined, fiber-rich fruits, grains, and vegetables. During heavy training, we recommend an increase in carbohydrate intake to 70% of total calories consumed (8 to 10 g per kg of body mass).

Although nutritious dietary carbohydrate sources consist of fruits, grains, and vegetables, this does not represent the "state of affairs" for all people. The typical American consumes

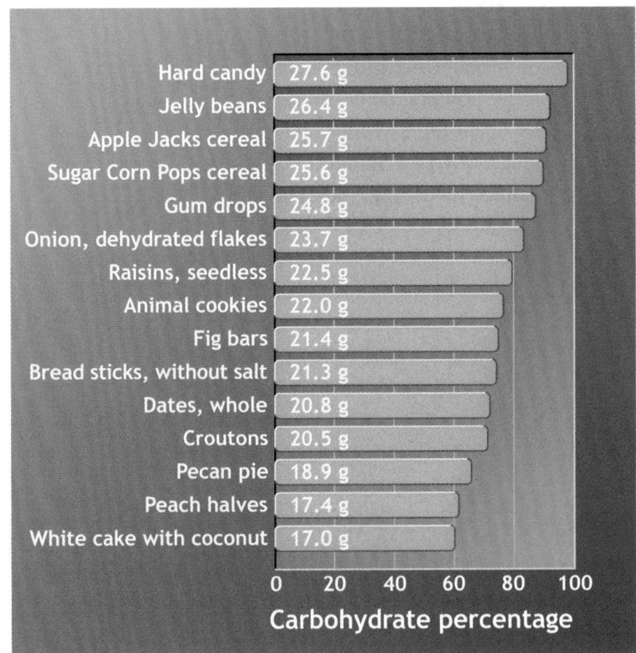

FIGURE 1.4 • Percentage of carbohydrate in common foods arranged by food type. The insert in each bar displays the number of grams of carbohydrate per ounce (28.35 g) of the food.

about 50% of carbohydrate as simple sugars. Intake comes primarily from sugars added in food processing as sucrose and high-fructose corn syrup (formed commercially by enzyme action on cornstarch that emphasizes fructose formation). These added sugars do not come in a nutrient-dense package typical of the simple sugars naturally found in fruits and vegetables. Sodas represent the largest single source of added sugars (33%) in the American diet (e.g., a 12-oz soft drink contains 10 tsp of added sugar). A regular McDonald's shake contains 12 teaspoons, and an 8-oz low-fat, fruit-flavored yogurt contains 7 teaspoons of sugar. On a yearly basis, intake of added sugars per person represents 71 kg (up 25% since 1984), more than the equivalent of 25 to 35 kg of table sugar (20 to 24 tsp of added sugars a day; twice the amount recommended by health experts) and 23 to 36 kg of corn syrup. One-hundred years ago, average yearly simple-sugar intake equaled only 2 kg per person! Excessive fermentable carbohydrate (mainly sucrose) causes tooth decay. Research has not firmly established the precise role that excessive dietary sugar might play in diabetes, obesity, osteoporosis, hypertension, and coronary heart disease.[38] Substituting fructose (a monosaccharide about twice as sweet as table sugar) for sucrose provides equal sweetness with fewer calories. Fructose does not stimulate pancreatic insulin secretion; thus, adding fructose to the diet helps to stabilize blood glucose and insulin levels.[106]

ROLE OF CARBOHYDRATES IN THE BODY

Carbohydrates serve important functions related to energy metabolism and exercise performance.

Energy Source

Carbohydrates primarily serve as an energy fuel, particularly during high-intensity exercise. Energy derived from the catabolism of bloodborne glucose and liver and muscle glycogen ultimately powers the contractile elements of muscle and other forms of biologic work.

Daily carbohydrate intake for physically active individuals must achieve levels that maintain the body's relatively limited glycogen stores. Once cells reach their maximum capacity for glycogen storage, excess sugars readily convert to and store as fat. This biologic "fact of life" should be made crystal clear to individuals who believe that consuming unlimited carbohydrate (in lieu of lipids) confers an advantage for weight control. The interconversion of macronutrients for energy storage explains how body fat can increase when dietary carbohydrate exceeds energy requirements, even if the diet contains little lipid.

Protein Sparer

Adequate carbohydrate intake helps to preserve tissue protein. Depletion of glycogen reserves—readily occurring with starvation, reduced energy and/or carbohydrate intake, and strenuous exercise—dramatically affects the metabolic mixture. Table 1.4 shows the effect of reduced energy intake during a 40-hour fast and 7 days of total food deprivation on plasma glucose and fat breakdown components. After almost 2 days of fasting, blood glucose decreased 35% but did not decrease to a lower level during further prolonged food abstinence. At the same time, circulating fatty acids and **ketone bodies** (acetoacetate and β-hydroxybutyrate, acetone-like byproducts of incomplete fat breakdown) increased rapidly, with plasma ketones rising considerably after 7 days of starvation.

Normally, protein serves a vital role in tissue maintenance, repair, and growth and to a considerably lesser degree as a nutrient energy source. However, in addition to stimulating fat catabolism, glycogen depletion triggers glucose synthesis from protein (amino acids). Gluconeogenic conversion offers a metabolic option for augmenting carbohydrate availability (and maintaining plasma glucose levels) even when glycogen stores deplete. The price paid, however, strains the body's protein levels, particularly muscle protein. In the extreme, this could significantly reduce lean tissue mass and add a solute load on the kidneys, which must excrete the nitrogen-containing byproducts of protein catabolism.

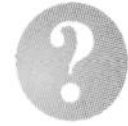

INTEGRATIVE QUESTION

Discuss the rationale for recommending adequate carbohydrate intake rather than an excess of protein to increase muscle mass through heavy resistance training.

Metabolic Primer

Carbohydrates serve as a "primer" for fat catabolism. By-products from carbohydrate breakdown facilitate the body's breakdown of fat. Insufficient carbohydrate breakdown—through either limitations in glucose transport into the cell (e.g., diabetes) or depletion of glycogen through inadequate diet or prolonged exercise—causes fat mobilization to exceed fat oxidation. This produces incomplete fat breakdown and accumulation of ketone bodies. Excessive ketone formation increases body fluid acidity to produce a harmful condition called acidosis, or specifically with regard to fat breakdown, **ketosis**. Chapter 6 continues the discussion of carbohydrate as a primer for fat catabolism.

TABLE 1.4 ➤ **CHANGES IN PLASMA CONCENTRATIONS OF GLUCOSE, FATTY ACIDS, AND KETONES FOLLOWING 40 HOURS OF FASTING AND SUBSEQUENT STARVATION FOR 7 DAYS**

NUTRIENT ($mmol \cdot L^{-1}$)	NORMAL	40 HOURS FASTING	7 DAYS STARVATION
Glucose	5.5	3.6	3.5
Fatty acids	0.3	1.15	1.19
Ketones	0.01	2.9	4.5

Adapted from Bender DA. Introduction to nutrition and metabolism. London: UCL Press, 1993.

Fuel for the Central Nervous System

The central nervous system requires carbohydrate for proper functioning. Under normal conditions and with moderately reduced energy intake, the brain uses blood glucose almost exclusively as its fuel. In poorly regulated diabetes, during starvation, or with a prolonged low carbohydrate intake, the brain adapts after about 8 days and metabolizes relatively large amounts of fat (as ketones) for alternative fuel. Chronic low-carbohydrate, high-fat diets also induce adaptations in skeletal muscle that increase fat use during exercise, thus sparing muscle glycogen.[90,112]

Blood sugar usually remains regulated within narrow limits for two main reasons: (1) glucose serves as a primary fuel for nerve tissue metabolism and (2) glucose represents the sole energy source for red blood cells. At rest and during exercise, liver glycogenolysis primarily maintains normal blood glucose levels, usually at 100 mg · dL^{-1} (5.5 mM). In prolonged, heavy exercise such as marathon running, blood glucose concentration eventually falls below normal levels because liver glycogen depletes, and active muscle continues to use the available blood glucose. Symptoms of significantly reduced blood glucose (**hypoglycemia**) include weakness, hunger, and dizziness, which ultimately impair exercise performance and may partially explain central nervous system fatigue associated with prolonged exercise. Sustained and profound hypoglycemia can trigger unconsciousness and produce irreversible brain damage.

CARBOHYDRATE DYNAMICS IN EXERCISE

Biochemical and biopsy techniques and labeled nutrient tracers assess the energy contribution of intra- and extramuscular nutrients during physical activity. For example, needle biopsies permit serial sampling of specific muscles with little interruption during exercise to assess the kinetics of intramuscular nutrient metabolism. Data obtained from biopsy sample measurements indicate that the intensity and duration of effort and the fitness and nutritional status of the exerciser determine the fuel mixture in exercise.[31,32]

The liver significantly increases glucose release to active muscle as exercise progresses from low to high intensity.[30,85,160] Simultaneously, muscle glycogen supplies the predominant carbohydrate energy source during the early stages of exercise and as intensity increases.[62,120] Compared with fat and protein, carbohydrate remains the preferential fuel in high-intensity aerobic exercise because it rapidly supplies energy (ATP) via oxidative processes. In anaerobic effort (requiring glycolysis reactions; see Chapter 6), carbohydrate becomes the *sole* macronutrient contributor of ATP. Just 3 days of maintaining a diet containing only 5% of its energy as carbohydrate blunts all-out, anaerobic exercise capacity.[91]

Carbohydrate availability in the metabolic mixture controls its use for energy. In turn, carbohydrate intake dramatically affects its availability. It also appears that the concentration of blood glucose provides feedback regulation of the liver's glucose output; an increase in blood glucose inhibits hepatic glucose release during exercise.[71] Carbohydrate availability during exercise also helps to regulate fat mobilization and its use for energy during exercise.[37,41] For example, increasing carbohydrate oxidation by ingesting high-glycemic carbohydrates prior to exercise (with accompanying hyperglycemia and hyperinsulinemia) significantly blunts (1) long-chain fatty acid oxidation by skeletal muscle and (2) free fatty acid (FFA) liberation from adipose tissue. Some speculate that adequate carbohydrate availability (and its resulting increased catabolism) inhibits transport of long-chain fatty acids into the mitochondria, thus controlling the exercise metabolic mixture. This proposition directly opposes the classic notion that fatty acid availability and breakdown inhibit carbohydrate metabolism, as described by the glucose–fatty acid cycle.[58,157]

Intense Exercise

During strenuous exercise, neural–humoral factors increase the output of epinephrine, norepinephrine, and glucagon and decrease insulin release. These hormonal responses activate **glycogen phosphorylase** (indirectly via activation of cyclic AMP; see Chapter 20), the enzyme that facilitates glycogenolysis in the liver and active muscles.[48] Because muscle glycogen provides energy without oxygen, it contributes the most energy in the early minutes of exercise when oxygen use does not meet oxygen demands. As exercise continues, bloodborne glucose increases its contribution as a metabolic fuel. For example, blood glucose may supply 30% of the total energy required by vigorously active muscles, with most of the remaining carbohydrate energy supplied by muscle glycogen.[120]

An hour of high-intensity exercise decreases liver glycogen by about 55%; a 2-hour strenuous workout almost depletes glycogen in the liver and specifically exercised muscles. Figure 1.5 illustrates that the muscles' uptake of circulating

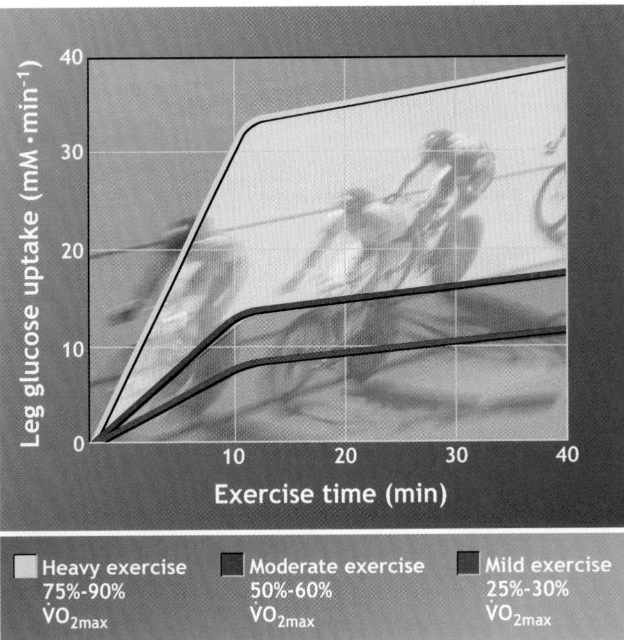

FIGURE 1.5 • Generalized response for blood glucose uptake by the leg muscles during cycling in relation to exercise duration and intensity. Exercise intensity is expressed as a percentage of $\dot{V}O_{2max}$.

blood glucose increases sharply during the initial stage of exercise and continues to increase with further exercise. By the 40th minute, glucose uptake rises to 7 to 20 times the uptake at rest, depending on exercise intensity.[50] *During intense, aerobic exercise, the advantage of a selective dependence on carbohydrate metabolism lies in its rate of energy transfer, which is twice that of fat and protein.* Also, per unit oxygen consumed, carbohydrate generates almost 6% more energy than fat. Chapter 6 presents the specifics of energy release from carbohydrates under anaerobic and aerobic conditions.

Moderate and Prolonged Exercise

Glycogen stored in active muscles supplies almost all of the energy in the transition from rest to submaximal exercise, as is the case in intense exercise. During the next 20 minutes or so, liver and muscle glycogen supply between 40 and 50% of the energy requirement, with the remainder provided by fat catabolism and a small use of protein. This nutrient mixture for energy depends on the relative intensity of exercise. At light intensity, fat remains the main energy substrate throughout exercise (see Fig. 1.20). As exercise continues and glycogen stores decrease, blood glucose becomes the major supplier of carbohydrate energy, while fat catabolism furnishes an increasingly greater percentage of total energy. Eventually, the liver's glucose output fails to keep pace with glucose use by muscle, which lowers the plasma glucose concentration. In such cases, the level of circulating blood glucose may fall to **hypoglycemic levels** (< 45 mg of glucose per 100 mL [dL] blood) during 90 minutes of strenuous exercise.[51]

Figure 1.6 depicts the metabolic profile during prolonged exercise in the glycogen-depleted and glycogen-loaded states.[146] As submaximal exercise progresses in the glycogen-depleted state, blood glucose levels fall and circulating fat increases dramatically compared with levels during exercise under glycogen-loaded conditions. Concurrently, the contribution of protein to energy expenditure increases. As exercise under glycogen depletion continues, work capacity (expressed as percentage of maximum) also progressively decreases. At the end of 2 hours, an exerciser can only maintain about 50% of the initial exercise intensity. Reduced power output results directly from the relatively slow rate of aerobic energy release from fat oxidation, which now becomes the primary energy source.[144]

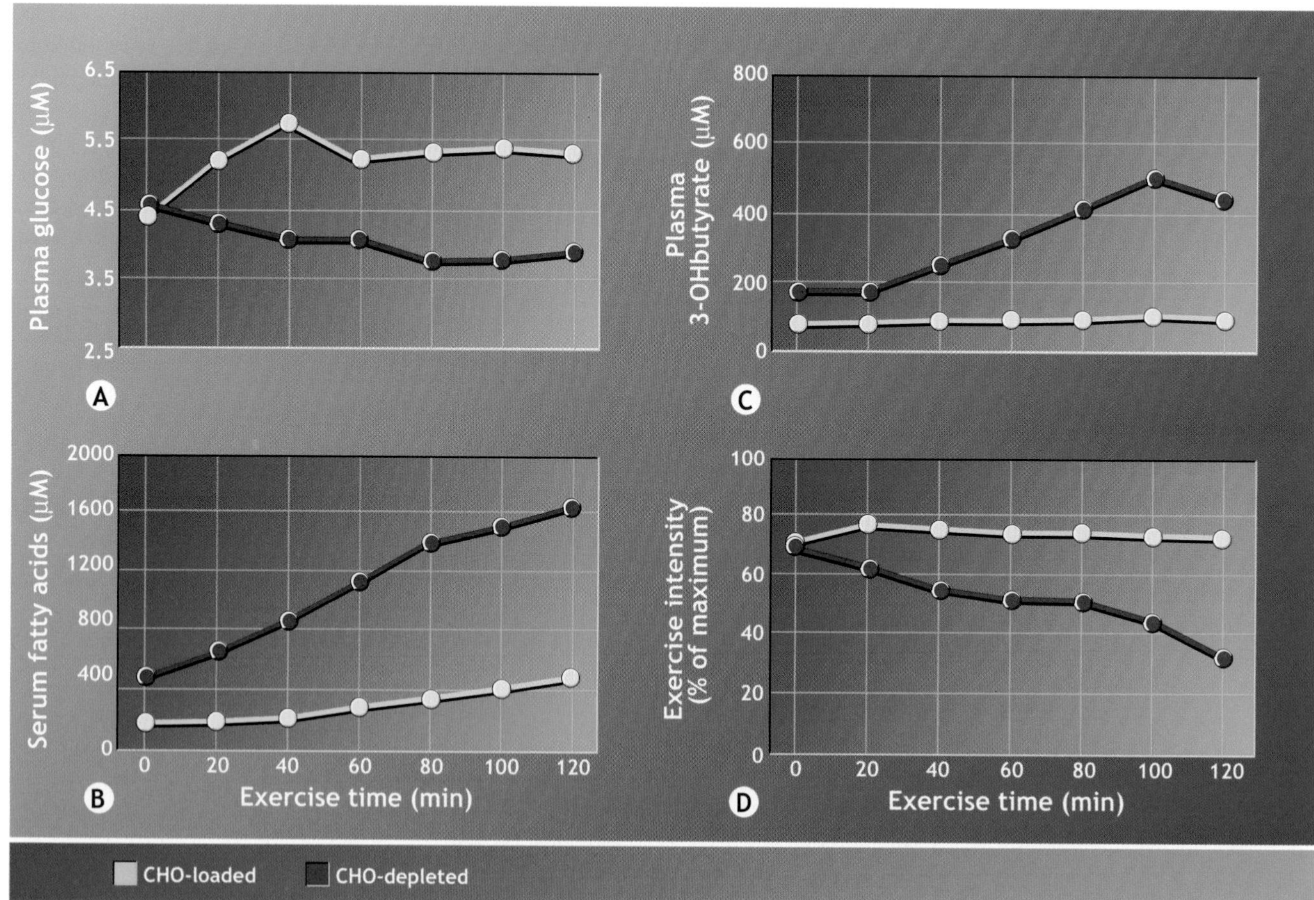

FIGURE 1.6 • Dynamics of nutrient metabolism in the glycogen-loaded and glycogen-depleted states. During exercise with limited carbohydrate availability, blood glucose levels (**A**) progressively decrease, while fat metabolism (**B**) progressively increases compared to similar exercise when glycogen loaded. In addition, protein use for energy (**C**), as indicated by plasma levels of 3-OH butyrate, remains considerably higher with glycogen depletion. After 2 hours, exercise capacity (**D**) decreases to about 50% of maximum in exercise begun in the glycogen-depleted state. (From Wagenmakers AJM, et al. Carbohydrate supplementation, glycogen depletion, and amino acid metabolism. Am J Physiol 1991;260:E883.)

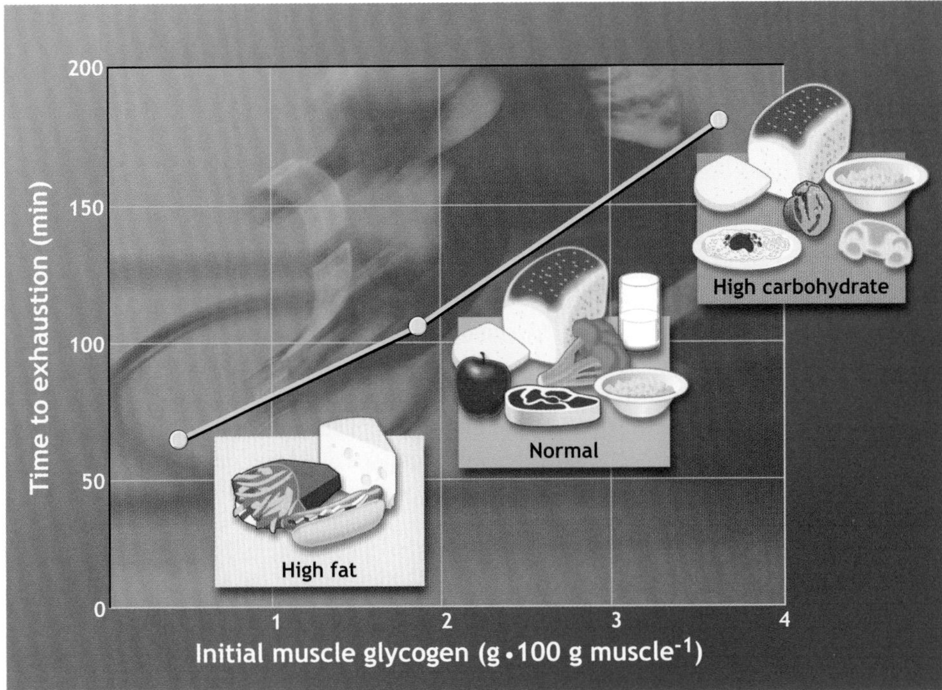

Figure 1.7 • Classic experiment illustrating the effects of a low-carbohydrate diet, a normal diet, and a high-carbohydrate diet on the quadriceps femoris muscle's glycogen content and duration of endurance exercise on a bicycle ergometer. Endurance time with a high-carbohydrate diet is three times that on a low-carbohydrate diet. (Adapted from Bergstrom J, et al. Diet, muscle glycogen and physical performance. Acta Physiol Scand 1967;71:140.)

Carbohydrate and fat breakdown use identical pathways for acetyl-coenzyme A (CoA) oxidation. Consequently, any of a number of the following potential rate-limiting metabolic processes that precede the citric acid cycle could explain the relatively slow rate of fat oxidation compared with that of carbohydrate:

- FFA mobilization from adipose tissue
- FFA transport to skeletal muscle via circulation
- FFA uptake by the muscle cell
- FFA uptake by the muscle from triglycerides in chylomicrons and lipoproteins
- Fatty acid mobilization from intramuscular triglycerides and cytoplasmic transport
- Fatty acid transport into the mitochondria
- Fatty acid oxidation within the mitochondria

Fatigue occurs when exercise continues to the point at which it compromises liver and muscle glycogen supply, despite sufficient oxygen availability to muscle and stored fat's almost unlimited potential energy supply. Endurance athletes commonly refer to this sensation of fatigue as "bonking" or "**hitting the wall**." Without the phosphatase enzyme in muscle, which allows glucose exchange between cells, the relatively inactive muscles maintain their full glycogen content. Why depletion of muscle glycogen coincides with the point of fatigue remains unclear. Part of the answer relates to:

- Use of blood glucose for optimal central nervous system function
- Muscle glycogen's role as a "primer" in fat breakdown
- Significantly slower rate of energy release from fat than from carbohydrate breakdown

Effect of Diet on Muscle Glycogen Stores and Endurance

Diet composition profoundly affects glycogen reserves. Figure 1.7 shows the effects of dietary manipulation on muscle glycogen and endurance performance.[12] In this classic experiment, six subjects maintained normal caloric intake for 3 days but consumed most calories as lipid and 5% or less as carbohydrate (high fat). In the second condition (normal), the 3-day diet contained the recommended daily percentages of carbohydrate, lipid, and protein. The third diet (high carbohydrate) provided 82% of the calories as carbohydrates. The glycogen content of the quadriceps femoris muscle, determined from needle biopsy specimens, averaged 0.63 g of glycogen per 100 g wet muscle with the high-fat diet, 1.75 g for the normal diet, and 3.75 g for the high-carbohydrate diet.

Endurance capacity during cycling exercise varied considerably, depending on what each person consumed 3 days before the exercise test. With the normal diet, exercise lasted an average of 114 minutes, whereas endurance averaged only 57 minutes with the high-fat diet. The high-carbohydrate diet improved endurance performance by more than three times the endurance on the high-fat diet. Interestingly, the point of fatigue coincided with the same low level of muscle glycogen under the three diet conditions. This classic experiment demonstrated conclusively the importance of muscle glycogen for sustaining high-intensity exercise lasting more than an hour. The research emphasized the important role played by nutrition in establishing appropriate energy reserves for long-term exercise and strenuous training.

A carbohydrate-deficient diet rapidly depletes muscle and liver glycogen and negatively affects performance in short-term, anaerobic exercise and prolonged high-intensity aerobic activities. These observations relate particularly to individuals who modify their diets by reducing carbohydrate intake below recommended levels. Reliance on starvation diets or other potentially harmful diets (e.g., high-fat, low-carbohydrate diets, "liquid-protein" diets, or water diets), proves counterproductive for weight control, exercise performance, optimal nutrition, and good health. Low-carbohydrate diets make it difficult from an energy supply standpoint to participate regularly in vigorous, longer-duration physical activities.[36] Chapter 3 discusses optimal provision for carbohydrate needs prior to, during, and in recovery from strenuous exercise.

Summary

1. Atoms provide the basic building blocks of matter and play the major role in the composition of food nutrients and biologically active substances.
2. Carbon, hydrogen, oxygen, and nitrogen represent the primary structural units for most bioactive substances within the body. Specific combinations of carbon with oxygen and hydrogen form carbohydrates and lipids. Proteins form when combinations of carbon, oxygen, and hydrogen bind with nitrogen and minerals.
3. Simple sugars consist of chains of 3 to 7 carbon atoms, with hydrogen and oxygen in the ratio of 2 to 1. Glucose, the most common simple sugar, contains a 6-carbon chain as $C_6H_{12}O_6$.
4. Three major classifications of carbohydrates include monosaccharides (sugars such as glucose and fructose), oligosaccharides (disaccharides such as sucrose, lactose, and maltose), and polysaccharides that contain three or more simple sugars to form starch, fiber, and the large glucose polymer glycogen.
5. Glycogenolysis describes the reconversion of glycogen to glucose; gluconeogenesis refers to glucose synthesis, particularly from protein sources.
6. Americans typically consume 40 to 50% of total caloric intake as carbohydrates, often as simple sugars and refined starches. Excess consumption of simple sugars and other rapidly absorbed carbohydrates may have negative health implications.
7. Carbohydrates, stored in limited quantity in liver and muscle, (1) provide a major source of energy, (2) spare protein breakdown, (3) function as a metabolic primer for fat catabolism, and (4) serve as fuel for the central nervous system.
8. Muscle glycogen provides the primary fuel during intense, anaerobic exercise. The body's glycogen stores (muscle glycogen and glucose from the liver) also contribute substantially to energy metabolism in sustained, high levels of aerobic exercise such as marathon running, distance cycling, and swimming.
9. Fat contributes about 50% of the energy requirement during light and moderate exercise. Stored intramuscular fat and fat derived from adipocytes becomes important during prolonged exercise. In this situation, the fatty acid molecules (mainly as circulating FFAs) supply more than 80% of the exercise energy requirements.
10. A carbohydrate-deficient diet quickly depletes muscle and liver glycogen, and profoundly affects both all-out, maximal exercise capacity as well as the ability to sustain high-intensity, endurance exercise.
11. Individuals who train intensely should consume between 60 and 70% of their daily calories as carbohydrates, predominantly in complex form (400 to 800 g; 8 to 10 g per kg of body mass).
12. With muscles depleted of carbohydrate, exercise intensity decreases to a level determined by the body's ability to mobilize and oxidize fat.

➤ PART 2 • Lipids

THE NATURE OF LIPIDS

A lipid molecule (from the Greek *lipos,* meaning fat) has the same structural elements as carbohydrate, but it differs significantly in its linkage of atoms. Specifically, the lipid's ratio of hydrogen to oxygen considerably exceeds that of carbohydrate. For example, the formula $C_{57}H_{110}O_6$ describes the common lipid stearin with an H:O ratio of 18.3:1; for carbohydrate, the ratio remains constant at 2:1. Lipid, the general term for a heterogeneous group of compounds, includes oils, fats, waxes, and related compounds. Oils become liquid at room temperature, whereas fats remain solid. Approximately 98% of dietary lipid exists as triglycerides (see next section), while about 90% of the body's total fat resides in the adipose tissue depots of the subcutaneous tissues.

KINDS AND SOURCES OF LIPIDS

Plants and animals contain lipids in long hydrocarbon chains. Lipids, generally greasy to the touch, remain insoluble in water but soluble in organic solvents such as ether, chloroform, and benzene. According to common classification, lipids belong to one of three main groups: **simple lipids**, **compound lipids**, and **derived lipids**. Table 1.5 lists the general classification of lipids with specific examples, details about their chemistry, and general comments about each type.

Simple Lipids

The simple lipids or "neutral fats" consist primarily of **triglycerides** (also called triacylglycerols, a preferential term among biochemists because it describes glycerol acylated by three fatty acids). Triglycerides constitute the major storage form of fat in fat cells (**adipocytes**). This molecule contains two different clusters of atoms. One cluster, **glycerol**, consists of a 3-carbon molecule that itself does not qualify as a lipid because of its high solubility in water. Three clusters of carbon-chained atoms, usually in even number, termed **fatty acids**, attach to the glycerol molecule. Fatty acids have straight hydrocarbon chains with as few as 4 carbon atoms or more than 20, although chain lengths of 16 and 18 carbons prevail.

Three molecules of water form when glycerol and fatty acids join in the synthesis (**condensation**) of the triglyceride molecule. Conversely, during hydrolysis, when **lipase** enzymes cleave the fat molecule into its constituents, three molecules of water attach at the point where the fat molecule splits. Figure 1.8 illustrates the basic structure of a **saturated fatty acid** and an **unsaturated fatty acid** molecule. All lipid-containing foods consist of a mixture of different proportions of saturated and unsaturated fatty acids. Fatty acids are so named because the organic acid molecule (COOH) forms part of their chemical structure. Body fat contains both forms of fatty acids.

Saturated Fatty Acids

A saturated fatty acid contains only single bonds between carbon atoms; all of the remaining bonds attach to hydrogen. The fatty acid molecule holds as many hydrogen atoms as chemically possible—thus the term saturated fatty acid.

Saturated fatty acids occur primarily in animal products such as beef (52% saturated fatty acids), lamb, pork, chicken, egg yolk, and dairy fats of cream, milk, butter (62% saturated fatty acids), and cheese. Saturated fatty acids from the plant kingdom include coconut and palm oil, vegetable shortening, and hydrogenated margarine; commercially prepared cakes, pies, and cookies contain plentiful amounts of these fatty acids.

Unsaturated Fatty Acids

Unsaturated fatty acids contain one or more double bonds along the main carbon chain. Each double bond along the chain reduces the number of potential hydrogen-binding sites; the molecule therefore remains unsaturated with respect to hydrogen. A **monounsaturated fatty acid** contains one double bond along the main carbon chain; examples include canola oil, olive oil (77% monounsaturated fatty acids), peanut oil, and the oil in almonds, pecans, and avocados. A **polyunsaturated fatty acid** contains two or more double bonds along the main carbon chain; safflower, sunflower, soybean, and corn oil serve as examples. Figure 1.9 lists the contents of saturated, monounsaturated, and polyunsaturated

TABLE 1.5 ➤ GENERAL CLASSIFICATION OF LIPIDS

TYPE	EXAMPLE	CHEMISTRY	COMMENTS
Simple lipids			
Neutral fats	Triglycerides	3 Fatty acid esters with 1 glycerol	Nature's most abundant lipids Mixed triglycerides with at least two different fatty acids account for 98% of fats in foods and more than 90% of body fat
Waxes	Beeswax	Fatty acid esters with high-molecular-weight alcohols other than glycerol; includes cholesterol esters, vitamins D and A	Most prevalent in cuticle of leaves and fruit
Compound lipids			
Phospholipids	Cephalins Lecithins Lipositols	Water-soluble compounds formed from neutral fat, phosphoric acid, and nitrogenous base	Lecithin, obtained from egg yolks or soybeans, represents largest group of phospholipids
Glycolipids	Cerebrosides Gangliosides	Sugar (glucose or galactose) plus fatty acids plus nitrogen	Component of cell membrane and neural tissues
Lipoproteins	Chylomicrons Very-low-density lipoproteins Low-density lipoproteins High-density lipoproteins	All contain varying amounts of protein, triglycerides, phospholipids, and cholesterol	Synthesized in liver; lipoproteins contain 25 to 35% protein, with the remainder lipids Mode of transporting lipids via blood
Derived lipids			
Fatty acids	Linoleic acid Oleic acid Palmitic acid Stearic acid	Usually contain one acid group (COOH); may be saturated or unsaturated	An even number of carbon atoms usually occurs in the naturally occurring fatty acids
Steroids	Androgens, estrogens, and progesterone Bile acids Cholesterol Cortisol Ergosterol Vitamin D	Chemical structure formed from a series of rings	Collectively referred to as steroid hormones; most researched group of lipids
Hydrocarbons	Terpenes	Compounds containing only hydrogen and carbon	Vitamin A precursor β-carotene an example

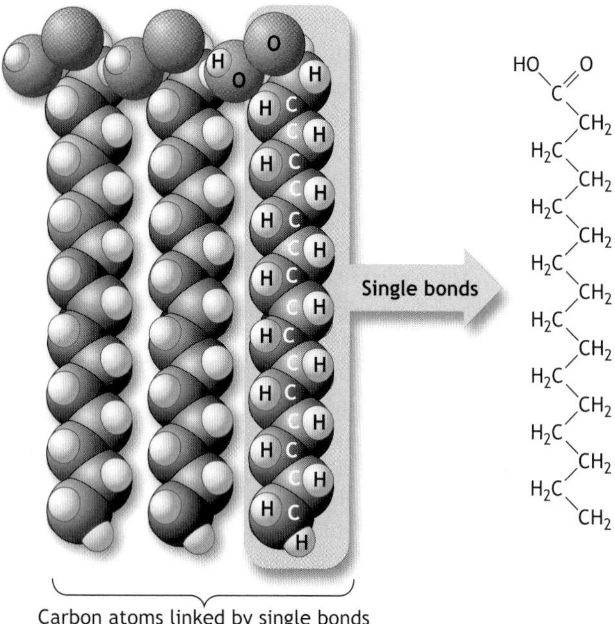

Ⓐ No double bonds; fatty acid chains fit close together

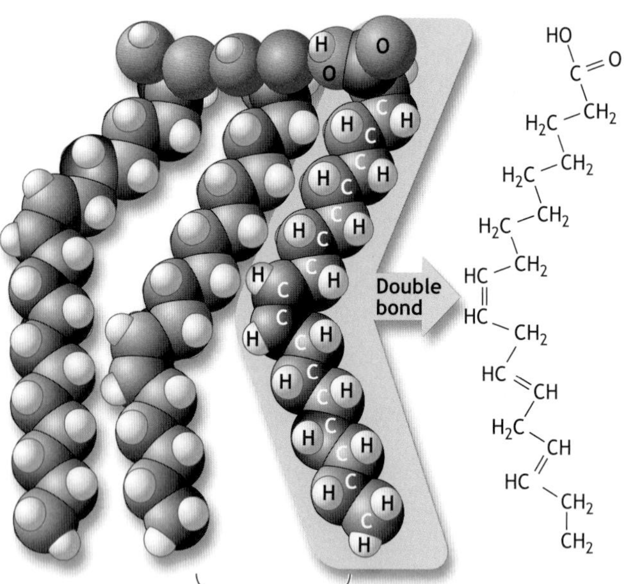

Ⓑ Double bonds present; fatty acid chains do not fit close together

FIGURE 1.8 • The presence or absence of double bonds between the carbon atoms is the major structural difference between saturated and unsaturated fatty acids. **A**. The saturated fatty acid palmitic acid has no double bonds in its carbon chain and thus contains the maximum number of hydrogen atoms. Because they lack double bonds, the three saturated fatty acid chains fit together closely to form a "hard" fat. **B**. The three double bonds in linoleic acid, an unsaturated fatty acid, reduce the number of hydrogen atoms along the carbon chain. Insertion of double bonds into the carbon chain prevents close association of the fatty acids; this produces a "softer" fat, or an oil.

fatty acids in common fats and oils (expressed in g per 100 g of the lipid). The insert table shows the hidden fat percentage in popular food. Several polyunsaturated fatty acids, most notably **linoleic acid** (an 18-carbon fatty acid with two double bonds; present in cooking and salad oils), must originate from dietary sources because they serve as precursors of other fatty acids, which the body cannot synthesize (called **essential fatty acids**). Linoleic acid maintains the integrity of plasma membranes and sustains growth, reproduction, skin maintenance, and general body functioning.

Fatty acids from plant sources generally remain unsaturated and liquefy at room temperature. In contrast, lipids con-

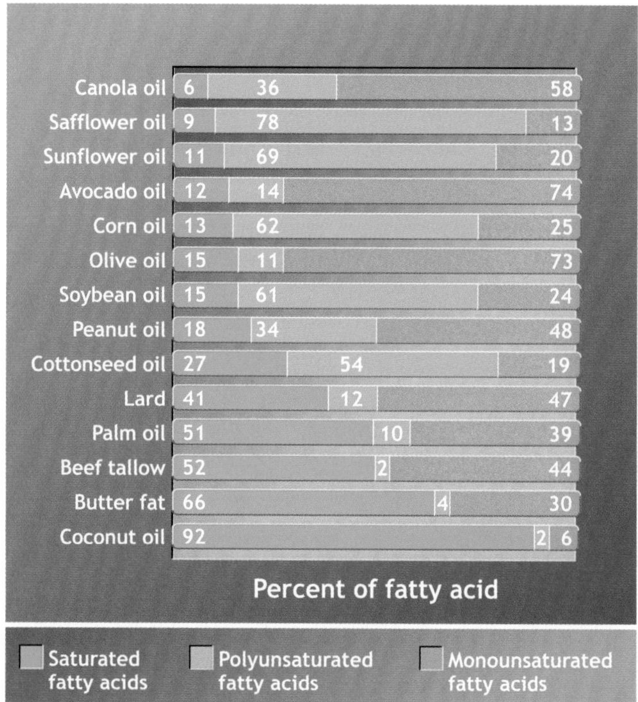

Hidden fat percentage of total calories

Food	Fat %	Food	Fat %
Brazil nuts	67	Lamb roast	19
Walnuts	61	Avocado	16
Almonds	54	Ice cream	13
Peanuts	50	Herring	12
Sunflower seeds	47	Poached eggs	11
Pork sausage	44	Tuna, canned	8
Pork roast	30	Poultry, dark meat	7
Cheese	30	Oatmeal, dry	7
Bologna	28	Salmon	6
Beef roast	25	Whole milk	4
Ham, cured	22	Poultry, light meat	4
Hamburger	20	Shredded wheat cereal	2

FIGURE 1.9 • Composition of diverse fatty acids (g per 100 g) in common lipid sources in the diet. The insert table shows the hidden total fat percentage of total calories in popular foods. (Data from Food Composition Tables, United States Department of Agriculture.)

taining longer (more carbons in the chain) and more saturated fatty acids exist as solids at room temperature; those with shorter and more unsaturated fatty acids remain soft. Oils exist as liquids and contain unsaturated fatty acids. The chemical procedure of **hydrogenation** changes oils to semisolid fats by bubbling liquid hydrogen into vegetable oil (with the addition of the mineral catalyst nickel). This reduces the unsaturated fatty acids' double bonds to single bonds so more hydrogens can attach to carbons along the chain. Firmer fat results because adding hydrogen increases the lipid's melting temperature. Hydrogenated oil thus behaves like a saturated fat; the most common hydrogenated fats include lard substitutes and margarine.

Triglyceride Formation

Figure 1.10 outlines the sequence of reactions in triglyceride synthesis, a process termed **esterification**. Initially, a fatty acid substrate attached to coenzyme A forms fatty acyl-CoA, which then transfers to glycerol (as glycerol 3-phosphate). In subsequent reactions, two additional fatty acyl-CoAs become linked to the single glycerol backbone as the composite triglyceride molecule forms. Triglyceride synthesis increases following a meal because of the (1) increased blood levels of fatty acids and glucose from food absorption and (2) relatively high level of circulating insulin, which facilitates triglyceride synthesis.

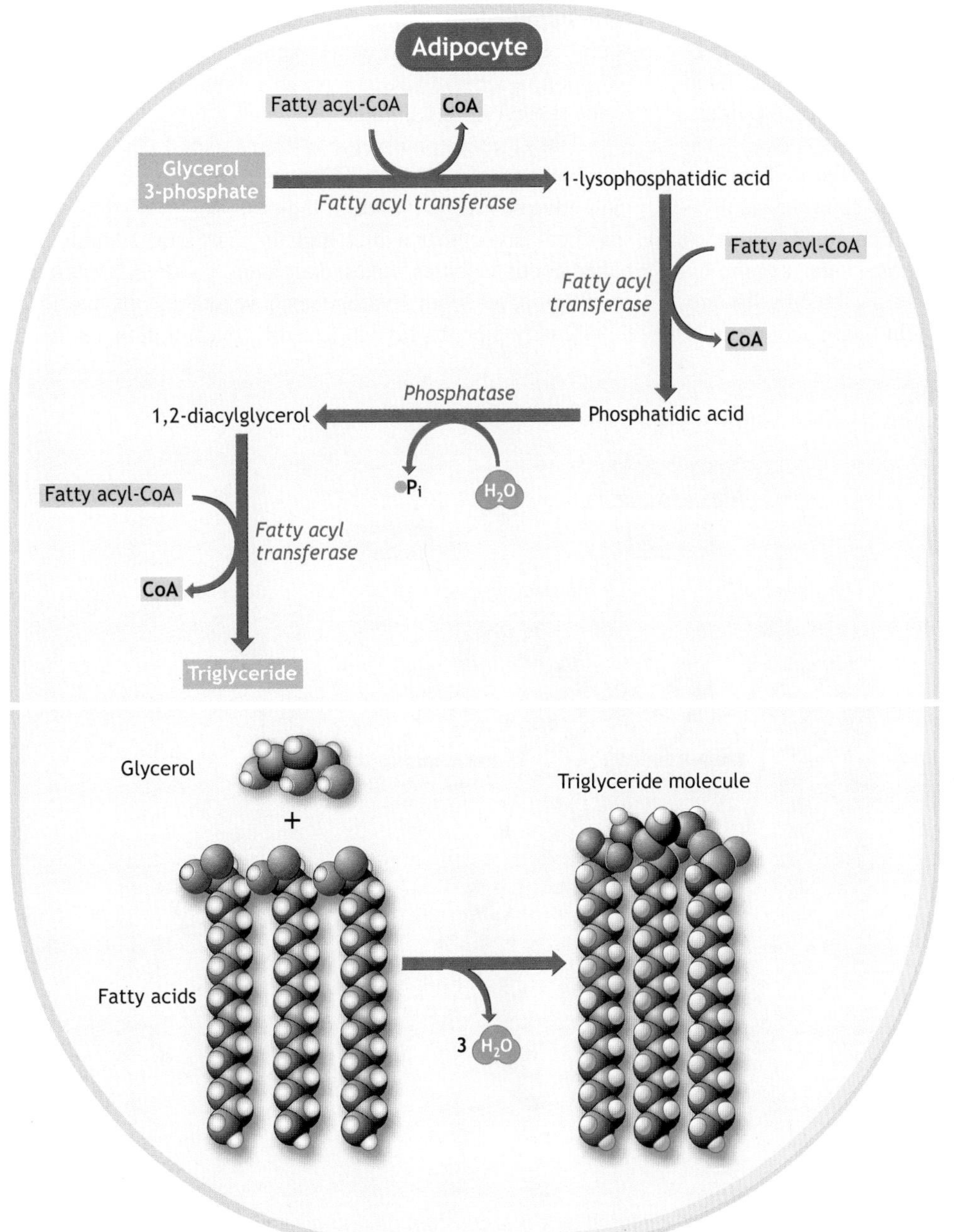

FIGURE 1.10 • Triglyceride formation in adipocytes (and muscle) tissue involves a series of reactions (dehydration synthesis) that link three fatty acid molecules to a single glycerol backbone. The bottom portion of the figure summarizes this linkage.

Triglyceride Breakdown

The term hydrolysis (more specifically **lipolysis**) describes triglyceride catabolism to yield glycerol and the energy-rich fatty acid molecules. Figure 1.11 shows that lipolysis involves the addition of water in three distinct hydrolysis reactions, each catalyzed by hormone-sensitive lipase. The mobilization of fatty acids via lipolysis predominates under conditions of (1) low-to-moderate exercise, (2) low-calorie dieting or fasting, (3) cold stress, and (4) prolonged exercise that depletes the body's glycogen reserves.

Both triglyceride esterification and lipolysis take place in the cytosol of the adipocytes. The fatty acids released during lipolysis can (1) re-esterify to triglyceride following their conversion to a fatty acyl-CoA or (2) exit from the adipocyte, enter the blood, and combine with the blood protein albumin for transport to tissues throughout the body. The term **free fatty acid (FFA)** describes this albumin–fatty acid combination. The glycerol released in lipolysis cannot be reused by adipocytes; instead it exits the cell and circulates in the blood. For this reason, the plasma glycerol concentration provides a convenient index of the degree of lipolysis.

Lipolysis also occurs in tissues other than adipocytes. Hydrolysis of dietary triglyceride takes place in the small intestine, catalyzed by pancreatic lipase; lipoprotein lipase, an enzyme located on the walls of capillaries, catalyzes the hydrolysis of the triglycerides carried by the blood's lipoproteins. Fatty acids released by lipoprotein lipase action can be taken up by adjacent adipose tissue and muscle cells for resynthesis to triglyceride for energy storage.

Butter Versus Margarine: A Health Risk in Trans-Fatty Acids?

Butter and margarine cannot be distinguished by caloric content, only by their fatty acid composition. The manufacture of margarine and some other vegetable shortenings involves the partial hydrogenation of unsaturated corn, soybean, or sunflower oil. A ***trans*-fatty acid** forms in margarine when one of the hydrogen atoms along the restructured carbon chain moves from its naturally occurring position (*cis* position) to the opposite side of the double bond that separates two carbon atoms (*trans* position). From 17 to 25% of margarine's fatty acids exist as *trans*-fatty acids, compared with only 7% in butter. Margarine, consisting of vegetable oil, contains no cholesterol; butter, on the other hand, originates from a dairy source and contains between 11 and 15 mg of cholesterol per teaspoon. *Trans*-fatty acids represent about 5 to 10% of the fat in the typical American diet.

The current controversy over margarine centers on the possible detrimental health effects of *trans*-fatty acids through their adverse effects on serum lipoproteins.[7,8,59,72,113] Some researchers argue that a diet high in margarine, commercial baked goods (cookies, cakes, doughnuts, pies), and deep-fried foods prepared with hydrogenated vegetable oils increases low-density lipoprotein cholesterol concentration by about

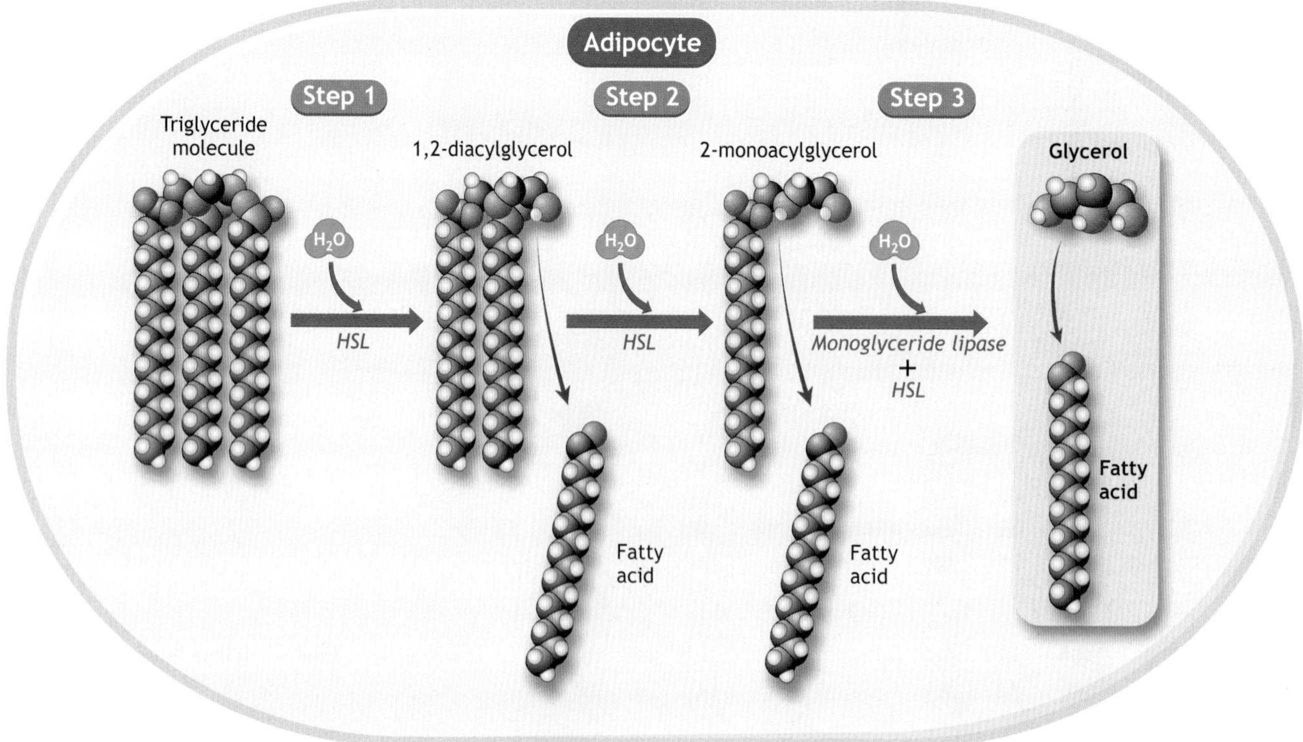

FIGURE 1.11 • Triglyceride catabolism (hydrolysis [lipolysis]) to its glycerol and fatty acid components involves a three-step process regulated by hormone-sensitive lipase (HSL).

the same amount as a diet high in saturated fatty acids (e.g., butter). Unlike saturated fats, however, hydrogenated oils also decrease the concentration of beneficial high-density lipoprotein cholesterol. Dietary *trans*-fatty acids may account for 30,000 deaths annually from heart disease.[151] Figure 1.12 shows heart disease risk associated with the type of fatty acid intake in a 14-year prospective study of 80,082 nurses.[72] Women who consumed the largest amounts of *trans* fats had a 53% higher heart disease risk than those with lower *trans* fat intake. When assessing the combined intake of both polyunsaturated and *trans*-fatty acids, the lowest heart disease risk emerged among women with the lowest intake of *trans*-fat and the highest intake of polyunsaturated fat. In light of the mounting evidence that *trans*-fatty acids do indeed place individuals at increased risk for heart disease, the Food and Drug Administration (FDA) will soon require food companies to include explicit information about *trans* fats on nutrition labels. This represents the first significant change in nutrition-facts labels since the agency began requiring them in 1993.

Lipids in the Diet

Figure 1.13 displays the approximate percentage contribution of some common food groups to the total lipid content of the typical American diet. Plant sources generally contribute about 34% to the daily lipid intake; the remaining 66% comes from animal sources.

The average person in the United States consumes about 15% of total calories as saturated fatty acids (equivalent to over 23 kg of saturated fats per year). This contrasts to the Tarahumara Indians of Mexico, whose diet high in complex, unrefined carbohydrate contains only 2% of total calories as saturated fat.[34] The relationship between saturated fatty acid intake and coronary heart disease risk has prompted health professionals to recommend (1) replacing a portion of the saturated and *trans*-fatty acids with nonhydrogenated monounsaturated and polyunsaturated oils[89] and (2) balancing energy intake with regular physical activity to prevent weight gain and obtain the health benefits of regular exercise.[21,88,150] Estimates indicate that replacement of 5% of energy from saturated fatty acid intake with energy from mono- and polyunsaturated fatty acids reduces coronary heart disease risk in women by 42%.[72] This represents a significantly greater effect on health risk than that

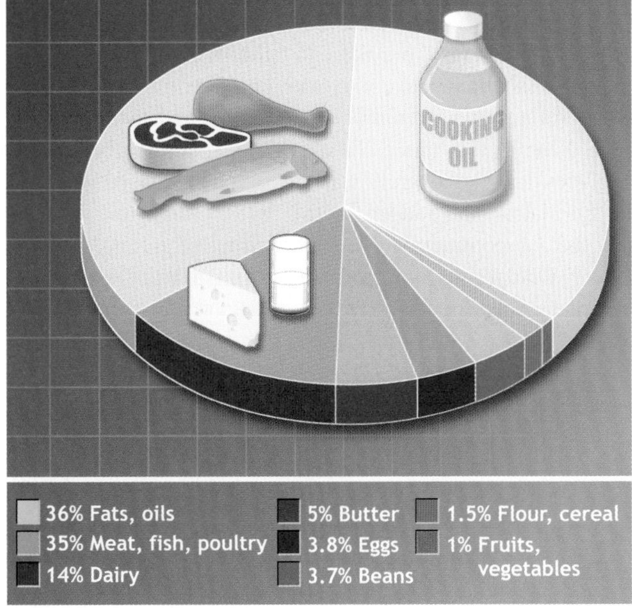

FIGURE 1.13 • Contribution from the major food groups to the lipid content of the typical American diet.

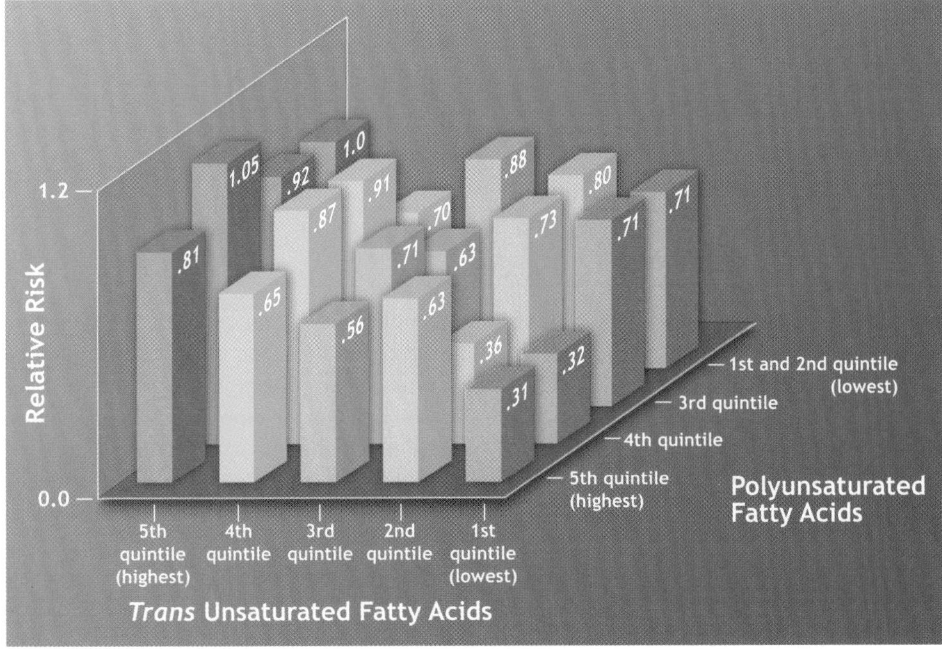

FIGURE 1.12 • Intake of *trans*-unsaturated and polyunsaturated fatty acids and coronary heart disease risk. Each quintile represents 20 percentile units. Relative heart disease risk adjusted for age, time interval, body mass index, cigarette smoking, menopausal status, parental history of premature myocardial infarction, use of multivitamins and vitamin E supplements, alcohol consumption, history of hypertension, aspirin use, physical activity, and dietary lipid and energy intake. (From Hu FB, et al. Dietary fat intake and the risk of coronary heart disease in women. N Engl J Med 1997;337:1491.)

achieved by reducing overall fat intake. Preliminary data also suggest that a high intake of monounsaturates helps to preserve cognitive functions in healthy elderly people. From a health perspective, individuals should consume no more than 10% of total daily energy intake as saturated fatty acids (about 300 kcal or 30 to 35 g for the average young adult male).

FISH OILS ARE HEALTHFUL. Studies of the health profiles of Greenland Eskimos who consumed large quantities of lipids from fish, seal, and whale, yet had low incidence of coronary heart disease, indicated that two long-chain polyunsaturated fatty acids, eicosapentaenoic acid and docosahexaenoic acid, may confer health benefits. These oils belong to the **omega-3 fatty acid** family (also termed *n-3*; the last double bond begins three carbons from the end carbon) found primarily in the oils of shellfish and cold-water tuna, herring, sardines, and mackerel and sea mammals. Regular fish and fish oil intake may benefit the blood lipid profile (particularly plasma triglycerides),[64,148] overall heart disease risk (risk of ventricular fibrillation and sudden death),[2,13,33,40,126] and (for smokers) the risk of contracting chronic obstructive pulmonary disease.[125] One proposed protective mechanism from heart attack asserts that fish oil helps to prevent blood clot formation on arterial walls.

ALL LIPIDS IN MODERATION. The quest for good health through dietary means has touted cooking with and consuming lipids primarily from vegetable sources. This approach may be too simplistic, however, because *total* saturated and unsaturated fatty acid intake may constitute a risk for diabetes and heart disease; if so, then one should reduce the intake of all lipids. Concern also exists over the association of high-fat diets with ovarian, breast, colon, endometrial, and other cancers. Recent research, however, has failed to uncover any relationship between dietary fat intake and breast cancer risk.[69] A beneficial effect of reducing the lipid content of the diet relates to weight control. The energy requirements of various metabolic pathways make the body particularly efficient in converting excess calories from dietary lipid to stored fat.[127] More body fat accumulates when consuming a high-fat diet than with an equivalent caloric excess of carbohydrate.

Compound Lipids

Compound lipids, a triglyceride combined with other chemicals, represent about 10% of the body's total fat. One group of modified triglycerides, the **phospholipids**, contains one or more fatty acid molecules joined with a phosphorus-containing group and a nitrogenous base. These lipids form in all cells, although the liver synthesizes most of them. The phosphorus part of the phospholipids within the plasma membrane bilayer attracts water (hydrophilic), while the lipid portion repels water (hydrophobic). Thus, phospholipids interact with water and lipid to modulate fluid movement across cell membranes. Phospholipids also maintain the structural integrity of the cell, play an important role in blood clotting, and provide structural integrity to the insulating sheath around nerve fibers. **Lecithin**, the most widely distributed phospholipid in food sources (liver, egg yolk, wheat germ, nuts, soybeans), functions in fatty acid and cholesterol transport and use. Lecithin does not qualify as an essential nutrient because the body manufactures the required amount. The FDA has approved lecithin as a food additive; it serves as a stabilizer and emulsifier in baked goods, margarine, chocolate, and some frozen desserts. Other commercial uses of lecithin include its use in cosmetics, paints, soaps, and inks.

Other compound lipids include **glycolipids** (fatty acids bound with carbohydrate and nitrogen) and water-soluble **lipoproteins** (formed primarily in the liver when protein joins with either triglycerides or phospholipids). *Lipoproteins provide the major avenue for transporting lipids in the blood.* If blood lipids did not bind to protein, they literally would float to the top like cream in nonhomogenized, fresh milk.

High-Density and Low-Density Lipoproteins

Figure 1.14 illustrates the general dynamics of cholesterol and lipoproteins, including their transport among the small intestine, liver, and peripheral tissues. Four types of lipoproteins exist on the basis of their gravitational density. **Chylomicrons** form when emulsified lipid droplets (including long-chain triglycerides, phospholipids, and FFAs) leave the intestine and enter the lymphatic vasculature. Under normal conditions, the liver metabolizes chylomicrons and sends them on their way for storage in adipose tissue. Chylomicrons also transport the fat-soluble vitamins A, D, E, and K.

The liver and small intestine produce **high-density lipoproteins (HDLs)**, which contain the highest percentage of protein (about 50%) and the least total lipid (about 20%) and cholesterol (about 20%) of the lipoproteins. Degradation in the liver of a **very-low-density lipoprotein (VLDL)** produces a **low-density lipoprotein (LDL)**. VLDLs, formed in the liver from fats, carbohydrates, alcohol, and cholesterol, contain the highest percentage of lipid (95%), of which about 60% consists of triglyceride. VLDLs transport triglycerides to muscle and adipose tissue. Once the enzyme **lipoprotein lipase** acts on a VLDL, the molecule becomes a denser LDL molecule because then it contains fewer lipids. LDLs and VLDLs have the most lipid and fewest protein components.

"BAD" CHOLESTEROL. Among the lipoproteins, LDL, which normally carries from 60 to 80% of the total serum cholesterol, has the greatest affinity for cells of the arterial wall. LDL delivers cholesterol to arterial tissue where the LDL particles become (1) oxidized to alter their physiochemical properties and (2) taken up by macrophages inside the arterial wall to initiate atherosclerotic plaque development. LDL oxidation ultimately contributes to smooth muscle cell proliferation and other unfavorable cellular changes that damage and narrow arteries.[129,134] A sedentary lifestyle, cigarette smoking, accumulation of excess abdominal body fat, and a diet high in cholesterol and saturated fatty acids (particularly palmitic, which accounts for about two-thirds of the saturated fat in the American diet) raise serum LDL concentration.

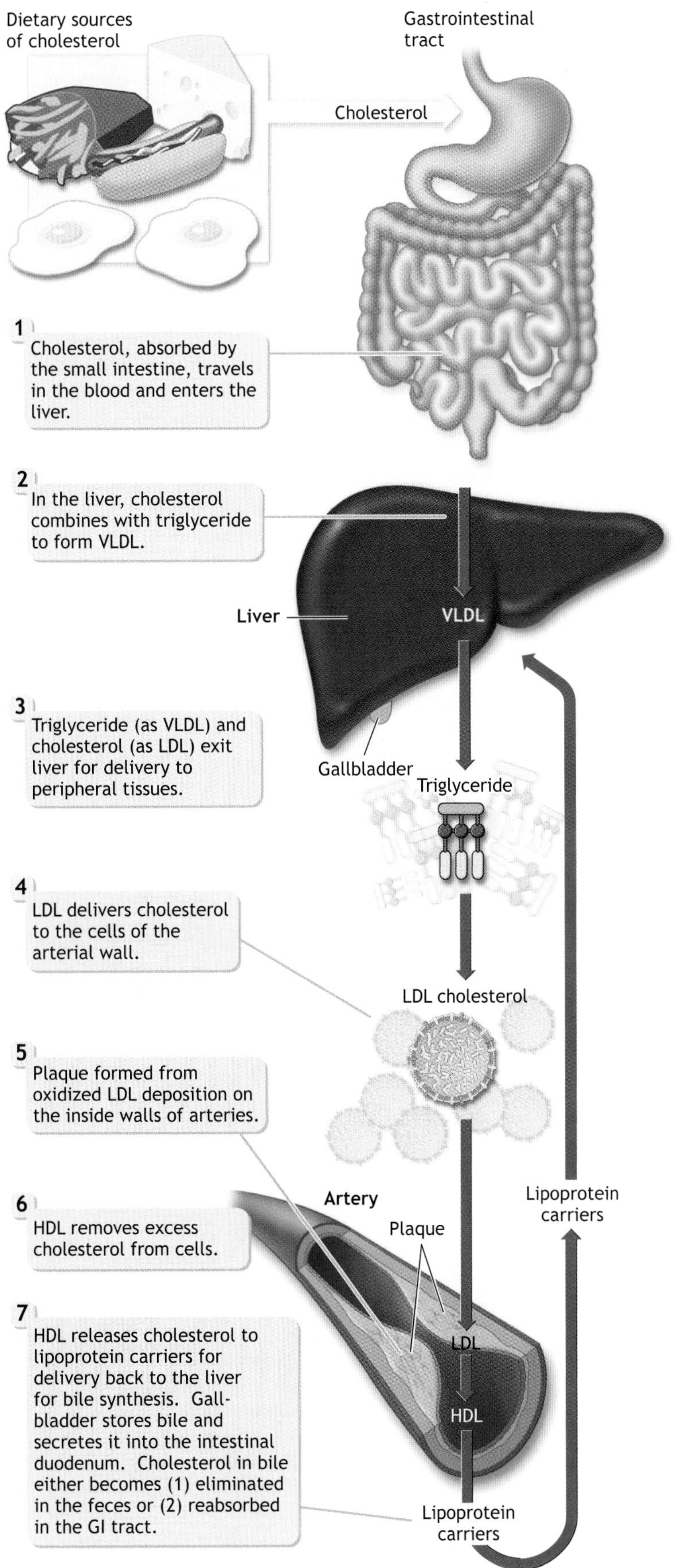

FIGURE 1.14 • General interaction between dietary cholesterol and lipoproteins and their transport among the intestine, liver, and peripheral tissues.

"GOOD" CHOLESTEROL. Unlike LDL, HDL exerts a protective effect against heart disease. HDL acts as a scavenger in the **reverse transport of cholesterol** by removing it from the arterial wall and delivering it to the liver for incorporation into bile and subsequent excretion via the intestinal tract.[42,107]

The amount of LDL and HDL cholesterol and their specific ratios (e.g., HDL ÷ total cholesterol) and subfractions provide more-meaningful indicators of coronary artery disease risk than total cholesterol.[83] Regular aerobic exercise and abstinence from cigarette smoking significantly increase HDL, lower LDL, and favorably alter the LDL:HDL ratio.[47,133,154] We discuss these effects more fully in Chapter 31.

Derived Lipids

Simple and compound lipids form **derived lipids**. Unlike neutral fats and phospholipids with hydrocarbon chains, derived lipids contain hydrocarbon rings. **Cholesterol**, the most widely known derived lipid, exists *only* in animal tissue. Cholesterol does not contain fatty acids, but shares some of a lipid's physical and chemical characteristics. Thus, from a dietary viewpoint, cholesterol classifies as a lipid. Cholesterol, widespread in the plasma membrane of all cells, originates either through the diet (exogenous cholesterol) or through cellular synthesis (endogenous cholesterol). Even if an individual maintains a "cholesterol-free" diet, endogenous daily cholesterol synthesis would vary between 0.5 and 2.0 g. More endogenous cholesterol forms with a diet high in saturated fatty acids, which facilitate LDL-cholesterol synthesis in the liver.[42,45,60] While the liver synthesizes about 70% of the body's cholesterol, other tissues—including the walls of the arteries and intestines—also construct this compound. The rate of endogenous synthesis usually meets the body's needs; hence, severely reducing cholesterol intake, except in pregnant women and infants, would probably have negligible health effects.

Functions of Cholesterol

Cholesterol participates in many bodily functions, including building plasma membranes and serving as a precursor in synthesizing vitamin D, adrenal gland hormones, and the sex hormones estrogen, androgen, and progesterone. Cholesterol furnishes a key component for the synthesis of bile (emulsifies lipids during digestion) and plays a crucial role in forming tissues, organs, and body structures during fetal development.

Egg yolk is a rich source of cholesterol, as are red meats and organ meats (liver, kidney, and brains). Shellfish, particularly shrimp, and dairy products (ice cream, cream cheese, butter, and whole milk) contain relatively large amounts of cholesterol. *Foods of plant origin contain no cholesterol.* Figure 1.15 lists the cholesterol contents of representative foods in the diet.

Cholesterol and Heart Disease Risk

Powerful predictors of increased risk for coronary artery disease include high levels of total serum cholesterol and the cholesterol-rich LDL molecule.[100] These become particularly

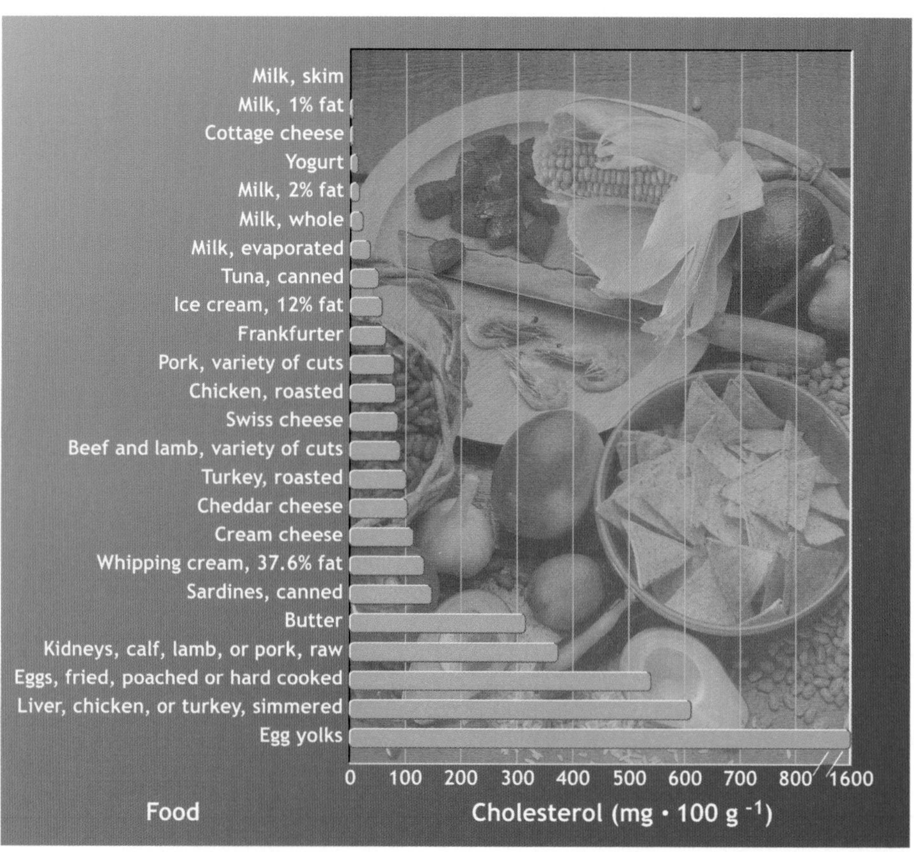

FIGURE 1.15 • Cholesterol content of representative foods in the diet. (Data from Food Composition Tables, United States Department of Agriculture.)

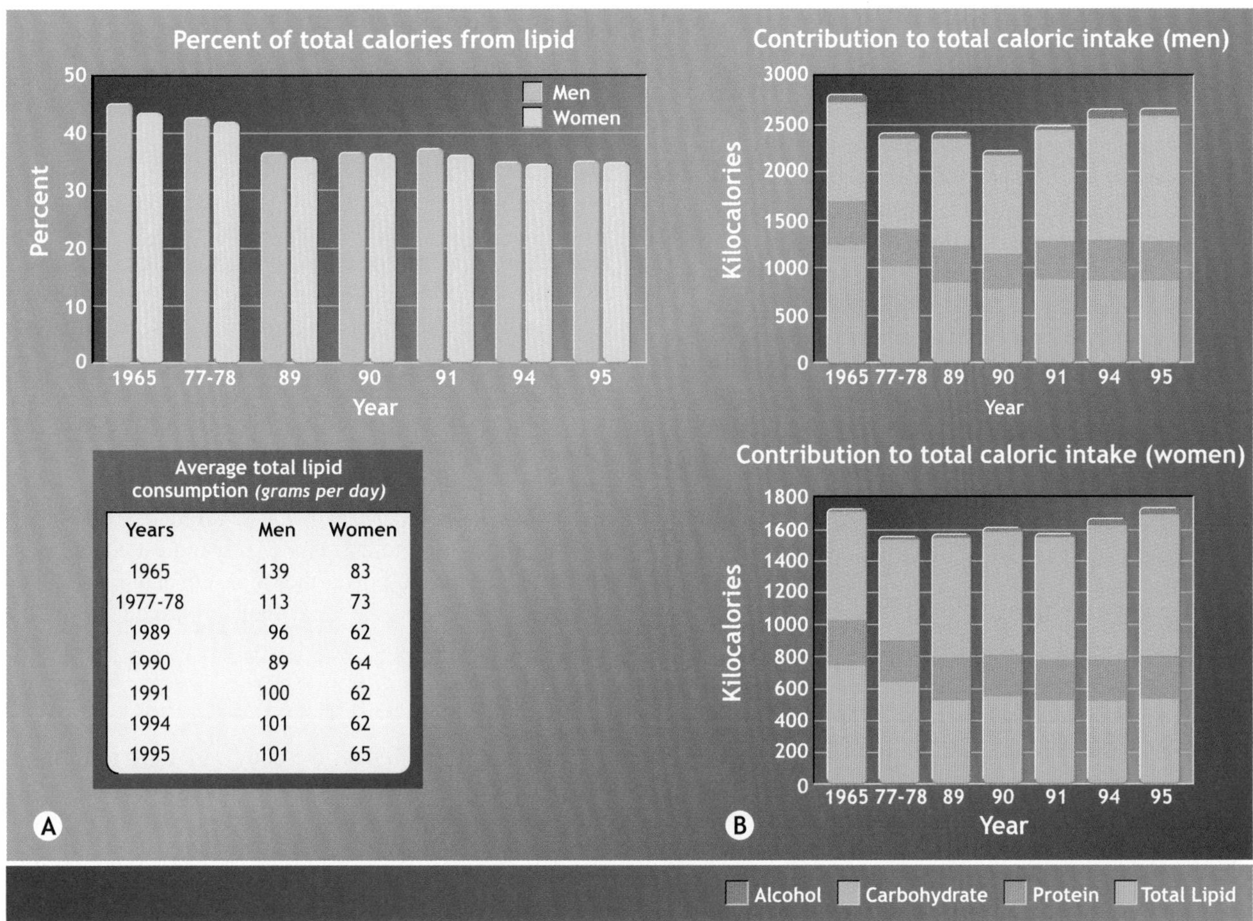

Years	Men	Women
1965	139	83
1977-78	113	73
1989	96	62
1990	89	64
1991	100	62
1994	101	62
1995	101	65

FIGURE 1.16 • Thirty-year trend in lipid consumption of adult U.S. women and men aged 19 to 50 years as (**A**) percentage of total calories (top) and daily average fat intake (bottom) and (**B**) total caloric intake. (From Nutrition insights: is total fat consumption really decreasing? Nutrition Today 1998;33:171.)

potent risks when combined with other risk factors—cigarette smoking, physical inactivity, obesity, and untreated hypertension.[74] A continuous and graded relationship exists between serum cholesterol and death from coronary artery disease.[96,131] Patients with existing heart disease improved coronary blood flow significantly (thus reducing myocardial ischemia during daily life) within 6 months by aggressively using drug and diet therapy that lowered total blood cholesterol and LDL cholesterol (e.g., drugs called statins can reduce cholesterol levels by up to 60 mg · dL^{-1}).[6] Studies with animals show that high cholesterol and saturated fatty acid diets raise serum cholesterol in "susceptible" animals. A dietary excess eventually produces **atherosclerosis**, a degenerative process that forms cholesterol-rich deposits (**plaque**) on the inner lining of the medium and larger arteries, causing them to narrow and eventually close. In humans, reducing saturated fatty acid and cholesterol intake generally lowers serum cholesterol, although for most people the effect remains modest.[22] Similarly, increasing dietary intake of mono- and polyunsaturated fatty acids lowers blood cholesterol.[119]

A controlled 7- to 10-year investigation of nearly 4000 healthy middle-aged men with elevated serum cholesterol levels showed a causal relationship between serum cholesterol and heart disease.[97,98] Lowering cholesterol by 25% significantly reduced heart attack risk and improved survival when a heart attack occurred. Diet and a cholesterol-lowering drug reduced the rate of heart disease by 50%. Improvement in coronary heart disease risk was closely linked to the cholesterol decrease by the factor of 1:2—a 1% reduction in cholesterol caused a 2% reduction in risk! These findings, corroborated in other clinical trials,[23,55] show the wisdom of reducing serum lipids through diet modification, exercise, and control of body weight.

Chapter 31 presents specific recommended values for "desirable," "borderline," and "undesirable" plasma lipid and lipoprotein levels. Research with children and adolescents indicates that maintenance of positive lifestyle habits that include regular exercise and prudent nutrient intake contribute favorably to blood lipid profiles in a manner similar to the effects with adults.[137]

RECOMMENDED DIETARY LIPID

Figure 1.16A shows that lipid consumption declined for men and women from 45% of total calories in 1965 to 34% in 1995. Despite the generally steady decline in percentage of total calories, total daily lipid intake in grams (see insert table) by men declined significantly between 1965 (139 g) and 1990 (89 g) and then increased to 101 g in 1995. For women, daily lipid intake decreased from 83 g in 1965 to 62 g in 1989 and remained relatively stable thereafter. Figure 1.16B shows that between 1990 and 1995 daily total lipid intake increased or remained stable, while total caloric intake increased (largely from increased carbohydrate consumption) at a relatively faster pace than the increased calories from lipids. For example, a 13% increase in total lipid intake by men between 1990 and 1995 accompanied a 21% increase in caloric intake. Consequently, the percentage of total calories from lipids decreased despite little decrease in total fat intake.[4,27]

Recommendations for dietary lipid intake for athletes generally follow prudent health-related recommendations for the general population. Dietary lipid represents between 34 and 38% of total caloric intake in the United States, or about 50 kg of lipid consumed per person each year. No standards for optimal lipid intake have been firmly established. However, the American Heart Association (AHA; www.americanheart.org) and most other major health organizations recommend that, to promote better health, lipid intake should remain below 30% of the diet's energy content. Of this intake, unsaturated fatty acids should equal at least 70% (preferably 80%), equally distributed between poly- and monounsaturates. The American Cancer Society (www.aci.org) advocates a diet that contains only 20% of its calories from lipid to reduce risk of cancers of the colon and rectum, prostate, endometrium, and perhaps breast. Compliance with current dietary recommendations for lipid intake (≤ 30% energy from lipid, 10% from saturated fat, and 300 mg cholesterol daily) should reduce plasma total cholesterol and LDL cholesterol by approximately 5%, compared with serum lipids currently associated with the average American diet.[70] More-drastic lowering of total dietary fat intake toward the 10% level may produce even more pronounced cholesterol-lowering effects, accompanied by clinical improvement for patients with established coronary heart disease.[111]

The AHA recommends a cholesterol intake of no more than 300 mg (0.01 oz) daily, limiting intake to 100 mg per 1000 calories of food consumed. Reducing daily cholesterol intake toward 150 to 200 mg may be even more desirable.[153] The current main sources of dietary cholesterol include the same animal food sources rich in saturated fatty acids. Thus, curtailing these foods in the diet would reduce preformed cholesterol intake and, more importantly, reduce intake of fatty acids known to stimulate endogenous cholesterol synthesis.

ROLE OF LIPID IN THE BODY

Important functions of lipids in the body include:

- Energy source and reserve
- Protection of vital organs
- Thermal insulation
- Vitamin carrier and hunger suppressor

Energy Source and Reserve

Fat constitutes the ideal cellular fuel because each molecule (1) carries large quantities of energy per unit weight, (2) transports and stores easily, and (3) provides a ready source of energy. In well-nourished individuals at rest, fat provides as much as 80 to 90% of the body's energy requirement. One gram of pure lipid contains about 9 calories (38 kJ) of energy, more than *twice* the energy available to the body from equal quantities of carbohydrate or protein, because the lipid molecule has more energy-rich hydrogen atoms. Recall that the synthesis of a triglyceride molecule from glycerol and three fatty acid molecules produces three water molecules. In contrast, when glycogen forms from glucose, each gram of glycogen stores 2.7 g of water. *Whereas fat exists as a relatively water-free, concentrated fuel, glycogen remains hydrated and heavy relative to its energy content.* Migratory birds that fly continuously for up to 2000 miles rely almost exclusively on stored fat reserves to power their nonstop endurance journey. Stored fat represents the ideal fuel for sustaining such prolonged physical effort.

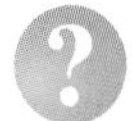

INTEGRATIVE QUESTION

What benefit does the body derive from storing carbohydrate and lipid within muscle cells and specific tissue depots for selective use under diverse exercise conditions?

For young adults, approximately 15% of the body mass of males and 25% of females consists of fat. Figure 1.17 illustrates the total mass (and energy content) of fat from various sources in an 80-kg man. The potential energy stored in the fat molecules of the adipose tissue translates to about 108,000 kcal (12,000 g body fat × 9.0 $kcal \cdot g^{-1}$). A run from

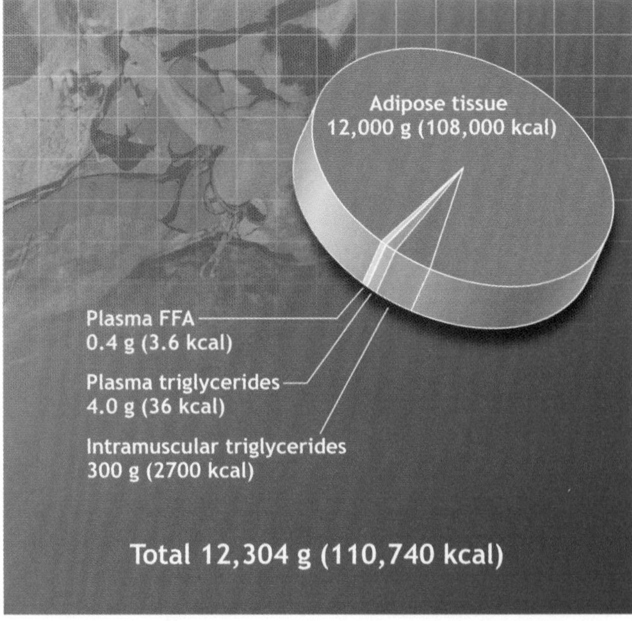

FIGURE 1.17 • Distribution of quantity and energy stored as fat within an average 80-kg man. (FFA, free fatty acids.)

New York City to Madison, Wisconsin (assuming an energy expenditure of about 100 calories per mile) would use up this energy provided from adipose tissue and intramuscular triglycerides and a small amount of plasma FFAs. Contrast this to the limited 2000-calorie reserve of stored carbohydrate that would provide energy for only a 20-mile run. Viewed from a different perspective, the body's energy reserves from carbohydrate could power high-intensity running for about 1.6 hours, while exercise would continue for about 120 hours using the body's fat reserves! Using fat as a fuel "spares" protein to carry out its important functions of tissue synthesis and repair.

Protection of Vital Organs and Thermal Insulation

Up to 4% of the body's fat protects against trauma to vital organs (e.g., heart, liver, kidneys, spleen, brain, spinal cord). Fat stored just below the skin (subcutaneous fat) provides insulation, permitting individuals to tolerate extremes of cold.[141] Swimmers who excelled in swimming the English Channel showed only a slight fall in body temperature while resting in cold water and essentially no lowering effect while swimming.[115] In contrast, the body temperature of leaner, non-Channel swimmers decreased considerably under both conditions. The insulatory layer of fat probably affords little protection except to those regularly engaged in cold-related activities such as deep-sea divers, ocean or channel swimmers, or Arctic inhabitants. Excess body fat hinders temperature regulation during heat stress, most notably during sustained exercise in air, when the body's heat production can increase 20 times above resting levels. In this situation, the shield of insulation from subcutaneous fat retards heat flow from the body.

For large athletes such as football linemen, excess fat storage provides additional cushioning to protect the participant from the sport's normal traumas. Any possible protective benefit, however, must be weighed against the liability imposed by the "dead weight" of excess fat and its impact on exercise energy expenditure, thermal regulation, and subsequent exercise performance.

Vitamin Carrier and Hunger Depressor

Consuming approximately 20 g of dietary fat daily provides the source and transport medium for the fat-soluble vitamins A, D, E, and K. Thus, severely reducing lipid intake depresses the body's level of these vitamins, which ultimately can lead to vitamin deficiency. Dietary lipid also facilitates absorption of vitamin A precursors from nonlipid plant sources such as carrots and apricots. It takes about 3.5 hours after ingesting lipids for the stomach to empty them. Some lipid in the diet, therefore, can delay the onset of "hunger pangs" and contribute to satiety following the meal. This helps to explain why some reducing diets that allow a person to consume a small amount of lipid sometimes prove more successful in blunting the urge to eat than more extreme diet plans advertised as fat free.

FAT DYNAMICS IN EXERCISE

Intracellular and extracellular fat (FFAs, intramuscular triglycerides, and circulating plasma triglycerides bound to lipoproteins as VLDL and chylomicrons) supply between 30 and 80% of the energy for physical activity, depending on nutritional and fitness status and exercise intensity and duration.[11,82,102,120,155,157] Increased blood flow through adipose tissue with exercise increases release of FFAs for delivery and use by muscle. Fat use for energy in light and moderate exercise is three times that in resting conditions. With more-intense exercise (greater percentage of aerobic capacity), adipose tissue release of FFAs fails to increase much above resting levels, which leads to a decrease in plasma FFAs. This in turn stimulates increased muscle glycogen usage[121] and concurrently increases intramuscular triglyceride oxidation (see Fig. 1.20). The energy contribution from intramuscular triglycerides probably ranges between 15 and 35%, with endurance-trained athletes catabolizing the most intramuscular fat.[79,86,103] Chronic consumption of a high-fat diet induces enzymatic adaptations that enhance fat oxidation during submaximal exercise.[90,105] Whether this translates to improved exercise performance remains unproved.

Fatty acids released from triglyceride storage sites and delivered to muscle as FFAs bound to blood albumin and triglycerides within the muscle itself provide the major energy for light to moderate exercise. When exercise begins, a

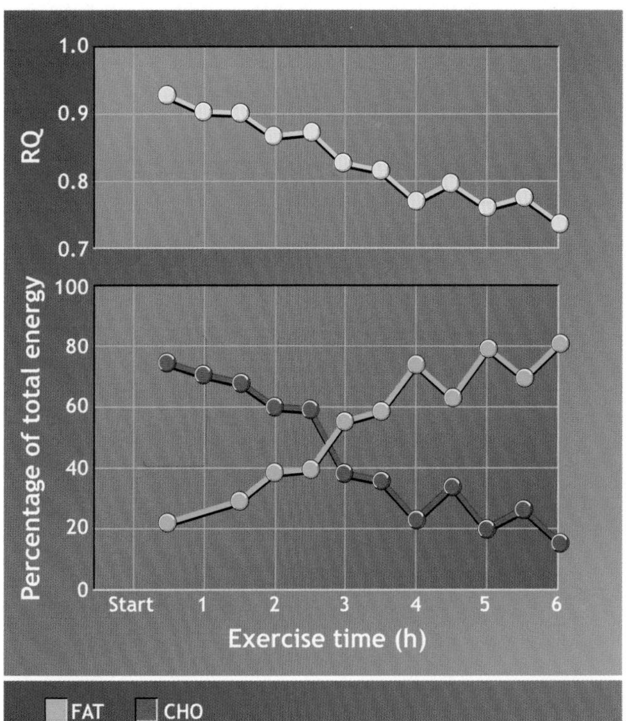

FIGURE 1.18 • Classic 1934 study showing the relationship between respiratory quotient (RQ) and substrate use during long-duration, submaximal exercise. *Top.* Progressive reduction in RQ at an oxygen consumption of 2.36 L · min^{-1} during 6 hours of continuous exercise. *Bottom.* Percentage of energy derived from carbohydrate and fat (1 kcal = 4.2 kJ). (Modified from Edwards HT, et al. Metabolic rate, blood sugar and utilization of carbohydrate. Am J Physiol 1934;108:203.)

transient initial drop in plasma FFA concentration results from increased FFA uptake by active muscles. An increased FFA release from adipose tissue follows (with concomitant suppression of triglyceride formation) owing to (1) hormonal stimulation by the sympathetic nervous system and (2) a decrease in plasma insulin levels. During moderate exercise, approximately equal amounts of carbohydrate and fat supply energy. When exercise continues for an hour or more, fat catabolism gradually supplies a greater percentage of energy, which coincides with the progression of glycogen depletion.

Carbohydrate availability also influences fat use for energy. With adequate reserves, carbohydrate becomes the preferred fuel during high-intensity aerobic exercise, compared with the 30 to 50% slower rate for fat breakdown.[144] Toward the end of prolonged exercise, when glycogen reserves become depleted, fat (mainly as circulating FFAs) supplies nearly 80% of the total energy required. Figure 1.18 shows this phenomenon, observed in the mid-1930s, for a subject who exercised continuously for 6 hours. Carbohydrate combustion (reflected by RQ; see Chapter 8) steadily declined during exercise, with a concomitant increase in fat use. Toward the end of exercise, 84% of the total energy for exercise came from fat breakdown! This experiment, conducted more than 65 years ago, illustrates fat oxidation's important role during extended exercise with glycogen depletion.

Greater fat metabolism during prolonged exercise probably results from a small drop in blood sugar and decreases in insulin (a potent inhibitor of lipolysis), with corresponding increases in the pancreas's glucagon output. These responses ultimately reduce glucose catabolism (and its potential controlling inhibitory effect on long-chain fatty acid breakdown) to further stimulate FFA liberation for energy.[37] The data in Figure 1.19 show that FFA uptake by active muscle rises during hours 1 and 4 of moderate exercise. In the first hour, fat (including intramuscular fat) supplied about 50% of the energy; by the third hour, fat contributed up to 70% of the total energy requirement.[1] *With greater dependence on fat catabolism (e.g., during carbohydrate depletion), high-intensity exercise decreases to a level governed by the body's ability to mobilize and oxidize fat.*

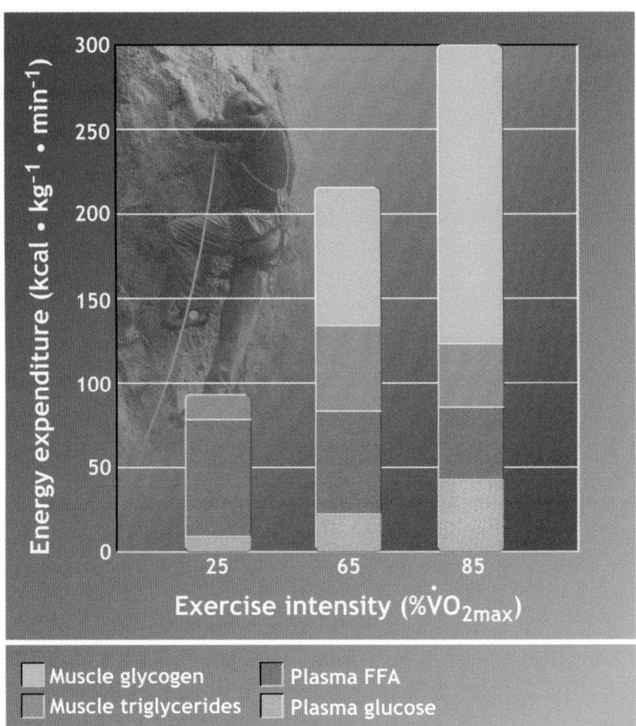

FIGURE 1.20 • Steady-state substrate use calculated using three isotopes and indirect calorimetry in trained men performing cycle ergometer exercise at 25, 65, and 85% of $\dot{V}O_{2max}$. As exercise intensity increases, absolute use of glucose and muscle glycogen increases, while muscle triglyceride and plasma FFA use decreases. (From Romijn JA, et. al. Regulation of endogenous fat and carbohydrate metabolism in relation to exercise intensity and duration. Am J Physiol 1993;265:E380.)

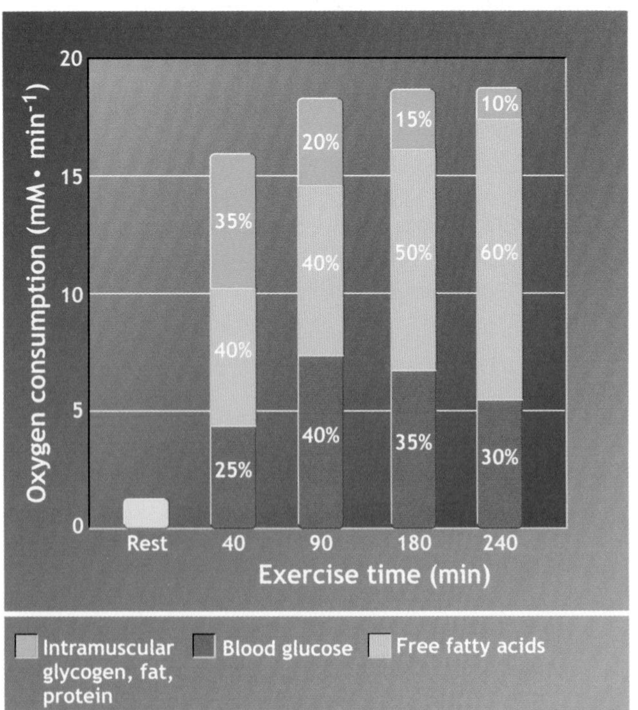

FIGURE 1.19 • Generalized percentage contribution of macronutrient catabolism in relation to oxygen consumption of the leg muscles during prolonged exercise.

Exercise intensity governs fat's contribution to the metabolic mixture in exercise.[120,143] Figure 1.20 illustrates the dynamics of fat use by trained men who exercised between 25 and 85% of their maximum aerobic metabolism. During light to mild exercise (≤40% of maximum), fat provided the main energy source, predominantly as plasma FFAs from adipose tissue depots. Increased exercise intensity produced an eventual *crossover* in the balance of fuel use—total energy from fat breakdown (all sources) remained essentially unchanged, but more-intense exercise required added energy from blood glucose and muscle glycogen. Total energy from fats during exercise at 85% of maximum did not differ from exercise at 25%. *Such data highlight the important role that carbohydrate, particularly muscle glycogen, plays as the major fuel for high-intensity aerobic exercise.*

Exercise Training and Fat Use

Regular aerobic exercise profoundly improves the ability to oxidize long-chain fatty acids, particularly those from triglycerides stored within active muscle, during mild to moderate intensity exercise.[62,78,81,101,108,142] Figure 1.21 illustrates the contribution of various energy substrates during 2 hours of submaximal exercise (8.3 kcal · min^{-1}) in the trained and untrained state.[103] For a total exercise energy expenditure of about 1000 kcal, intramuscular triglyceride combustion supplied about 25% of total energy expenditure before training, which increased to more than 40% following aerobic training. Energy from plasma FFA oxidation decreased from 18% pretraining to about 15% posttraining. Biopsy samples revealed a 41% reduction in muscle glycogen combustion in the trained state, which accounted for the overall decrease in total energy from all carbohydrate fuel sources (58% pretraining to 38% posttraining). The important point concerns the greater uptake of FFAs by the trained limbs and concurrent conservation of glycogen reserves during the same moderate absolute exercise level via the following possible mechanisms:

- Facilitated fatty acid mobilization from adipose tissue through increased rate of lipolysis within adipocytes
- Proliferation of capillaries in trained muscle to increase the total number and density of these microvessels for energy substrate delivery
- Improved transport of FFAs through the muscle fiber's plasma membrane (sarcolemma)
- Increased fatty acid transport within the muscle cell, mediated by carnitine and carnitine acyltransferase

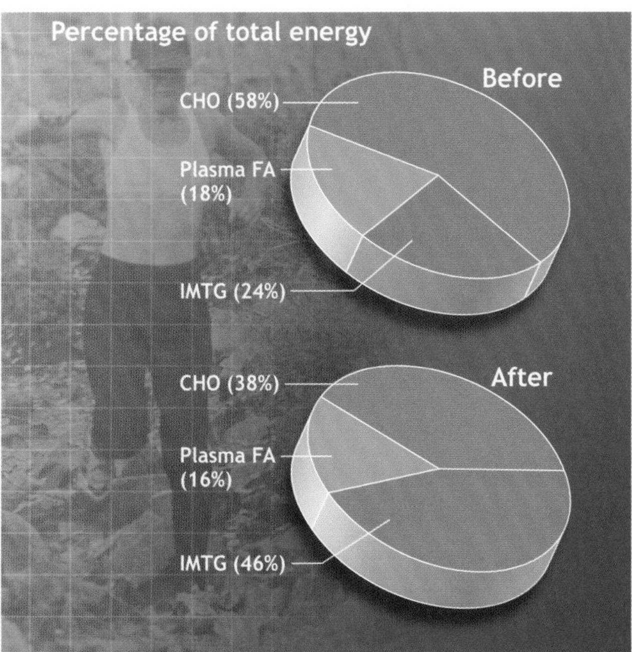

FIGURE 1.21 • Percentage of total energy derived from carbohydrate (CHO), intramuscular triglyceride (IMTG), and plasma fatty acid (FA) fuel sources during prolonged exercise before and after endurance training. (From Martin WH III, et al. Effect of endurance training on plasma free fatty acid turnover and oxidation during exercise. Am J Physiol 1993;265:E708.)

- Increased size and number of mitochondria
- Increased quantity of enzymes involved in ß-oxidation, citric acid cycle metabolism, and the electron-transport chain within specifically trained muscle fibers
- Maintenance of cellular integrity and function (this can enhance endurance performance regardless of the effects of a conservation of glycogen reserves)

Enhanced responsiveness of adipocytes to lipolysis enables endurance athletes to exercise at a higher absolute submaximal exercise level before experiencing the fatiguing effects of glycogen depletion. Improved capacity for fat oxidation, however, does not allow them to sustain the level of aerobic metabolism they can generate when oxidizing glycogen for energy. Consequently, near maximal, sustained aerobic effort in well-nourished endurance athletes still requires almost total reliance on oxidation of stored glycogen.[11]

INTEGRATIVE QUESTION

Explain why a high level of daily physical activity requires regular carbohydrate intake. Additionally, give two "nonexercise" benefits from a diet rich in food sources containing unrefined, complex carbohydrates.

Summary

1. Like carbohydrates, lipids contain carbon, hydrogen, and oxygen atoms, but with a higher ratio of hydrogen to oxygen. The lipid stearin, for example, has the formula $C_{57}H_{110}O_6$. Lipid molecules consist of one glycerol molecule and three fatty acid molecules.
2. Lipids, synthesized by plants and animals, classify into one of three groups: simple lipids (glycerol plus three fatty acids), compound lipids (phospholipids, glycolipids, and lipoproteins) composed of simple lipids combined with other chemicals, and derived lipids such as cholesterol, synthesized from simple and compound lipids.
3. Saturated fatty acids contain as many hydrogen atoms as chemically possible; thus, saturated describes this molecule with respect to hydrogen. Saturated fatty acids exist primarily in animal meat, egg yolk, dairy fats, and cheese. High saturated fatty acid intake elevates blood cholesterol concentration and promotes coronary heart disease.
4. Unsaturated fatty acids contain fewer hydrogen atoms attached to the carbon chain. Unlike saturated fatty acids, double bonds connect carbon atoms; they are either monounsaturated or polyunsaturated with respect to hydrogen. Increasing the diet's proportion of unsaturated fatty acids protects against heart disease.
5. Lowering blood cholesterol, especially that carried by LDL-cholesterol, provides significant protection against coronary artery disease.

6. Dietary lipid currently represents between 34 and 38% of total caloric intake. Prudent recommendations suggest a level of ≤30% for dietary lipid, of which 70 to 80% should consist of unsaturated fatty acids.
7. Lipids provide the largest nutrient store of potential energy for biologic work. They also protect vital organs, provide insulation from the cold, and transport the fat-soluble vitamins A, D, E, and K.
8. Fat contributes 50 to 70% of the energy requirement during light and moderate exercise. Stored fat (intramuscular and derived from adipocytes) plays an increasingly important role during prolonged exercise. In this situation, the fatty acid molecules (mainly circulating FFAs) provide more than 80% of the exercise energy requirements.
9. Carbohydrate depletion reduces exercise intensity to a level determined by the body's ability to mobilize and oxidize fat.
10. Aerobic training increases long-chain fatty acid oxidation, primarily fatty acids from triglycerides within active muscle, during mild- to moderate-intensity exercise.
11. Enhanced fat oxidation spares glycogen, allowing trained individuals to exercise at a higher absolute level of submaximal exercise before experiencing the fatiguing effects of glycogen depletion, compared with untrained counterparts.

➤ PART 3 • Proteins

THE NATURE OF PROTEINS

The body of an average-sized adult contains between 10 and 12 kg of protein, with the largest quantity (6 to 8 kg) located within the skeletal muscle mass. Additionally, approximately 210 g of amino acids exist in free form, largely as glutamine, a key amino acid with functions that include serving as fuel for immune system cells. Humans typically ingest about 10 to 15% of their total calories as protein. During digestion, protein hydrolyzes to its amino acid constituents for absorption by the small intestine. The protein content of most adults remains remarkably stable, and no amino acid "reserves" exist in the body. Amino acids not used for the synthesis of protein or other compounds (e.g., hormones) or for energy metabolism provide substrate for gluconeogenesis or convert to triglyceride for storage in adipocytes.

Structurally, proteins (from the Greek word meaning "of prime importance") resemble carbohydrates and lipids because they contain carbon, oxygen, and hydrogen atoms. Protein molecules also contain about 16% nitrogen, along with sulfur and occasionally phosphorus, cobalt, and iron. Just as glycogen forms from many simple glucose subunits linked together, the protein molecule polymerizes from its **amino acid** "building-block" constituents in endlessly complex arrays. **Peptide bonds** link amino acids in chains that take on diverse forms and chemical combinations; two joined amino acids produce a **dipeptide**, and linking three amino acids produces a **tripeptide**, and so on. Generally, a **polypeptide** chain contains 50 to more than 1000 amino acids. Combination of more than 50 amino acids forms a **protein** of which humans can synthesize about 80,000 different kinds. Single cells contain thousands of different protein molecules; some have a linear configuration, some are folded into complex shapes having three-dimensional properties. In total, approximately 50,000 different protein-containing compounds exist in the body. The biochemical functions and properties of each protein depend on the sequence of specific amino acids as discussed more fully in the final chapter, "On the Horizon."

The 20 different amino acids required by the body each have a positively charged **amine group** at one end and a negatively charged **organic acid group** at the other end. The amine group has two hydrogen atoms attached to nitrogen (NH_2), whereas the organic acid group (technically termed a carboxylic acid group) contains one carbon atom, two oxygen atoms, and one hydrogen atom (COOH). The remainder of the amino acid, referred to as the **R group** or **side chain**, takes on a variety of forms. *The R group's specific structure dictates the amino acid's particular characteristics.* Figure 1.22 shows the four common features that constitute the general structure of all amino acids. The potential for combining the 20 amino acids produces an almost infinite number of possible proteins, depending on their amino acid combinations. For example, linking just three different amino acids could generate 20^3, or 8000, different proteins.

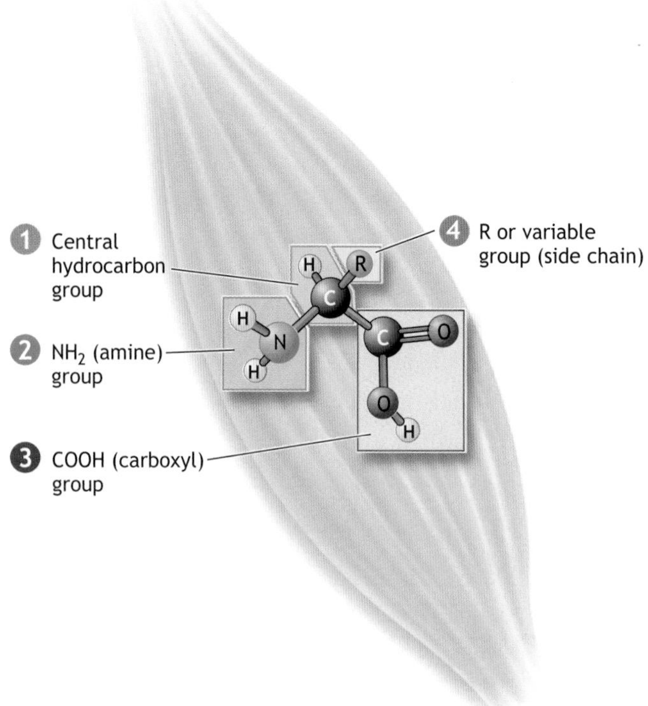

FIGURE 1.22 • Four common features of all amino acids.

KINDS OF PROTEIN

The body cannot synthesize eight amino acids (nine in children and some older adults), so foods containing them must supply the remainder. These make up the **essential amino acids**—isoleucine, leucine, lysine, methionine, phenylalanine, threonine, tryptophan, and valine. In addition, the body synthesizes cystine from methionine and tyrosine from phenylalanine. Infants cannot synthesize histidine, and children have reduced capability for synthesizing arginine. The body manufactures the remaining nine **nonessential** amino acids. The term nonessential does not indicate a lack of importance; rather, other compounds already in the body synthesize these amino acids at a rate that meets demands for normal growth and tissue repair.

Animals and plants manufacture proteins that contain essential amino acids. An amino acid derived from an animal has no health or physiologic advantage over the same amino acid from vegetable origin. Plants synthesize amino acids by incorporating nitrogen from the soil (along with carbon, oxygen, and hydrogen from air and water). In contrast, animals have no broad capability for amino acid synthesis; instead, they consume most of their protein.

Synthesizing a specific protein requires the availability of appropriate amino acids. **Complete proteins**, or higher-quality proteins, come from foods containing all of the essential amino acids in the quantity and correct ratio to maintain nitrogen balance and to allow tissue growth and repair. An **incomplete protein**, or lower-quality protein, lacks one or more essential amino acids. A diet of incomplete protein eventually leads to protein malnutrition, whether or not the food sources contain an adequate amount of energy or protein.

Protein Sources

Sources of complete protein include eggs, milk, meat, fish, and poultry. Eggs provide the optimal mixture of essential amino acids among food sources; hence, eggs receive the highest quality rating (100) for comparison with other foods. Table 1.6 rates some common sources of protein in the diet. Presently, animal sources provide almost two-thirds of dietary protein; 80 years ago plant and animal sources contributed equally to protein consumption. Reliance on animal sources for dietary protein accounts for the current, relatively high cholesterol and saturated fatty acid intake in the world's major industrialized nations.

The **biologic value** of food refers to how well it supplies essential amino acids. High-quality protein foods come from animal sources; vegetables (lentils, dried beans and peas, nuts, and cereals) remain incomplete in one or more essential amino acids, and thus, their proteins have a relatively lower biologic value. *Eating a variety of plant foods (grains, fruits, and vegetables) supplies all of the essential amino acids, each providing a different quality and quantity of amino acids.* See "In a Practical Sense," page 41, for information about reading food labels.

TABLE 1.6 ➤ **COMMON SOURCES OF DIETARY PROTEIN RATED FOR PROTEIN QUALITY**

FOOD	PROTEIN RATING
Eggs	100
Fish	70
Lean beef	69
Cow's milk	60
Brown rice	57
White rice	56
Soybeans	47
Brewer's hash	45
Whole-grain wheat	44
Peanuts	43
Dry beans	34
White potato	34

The Vegetarian Approach

Grains and legumes (a large family of plants with about 13,000 species) provide excellent protein sources, but neither provides the full complement of essential amino acids. An exception may be well-processed, isolated soybean protein, termed soy-protein isolates, whose protein quality matches that of some animal proteins. Grains lack the essential amino acid lysine, while legumes contain lysine but lack the sulfur-containing essential amino acid methionine (found abundantly in grains). Tortillas and beans, rice and beans, rice and lentils, rice and peas, and peanuts and wheat (bread) serve as staples in many cultures because they provide **complementary sources** of all essential amino acids from the plant kingdom.

True vegetarians, or **vegans**, consume nutrients from only two sources—the plant kingdom and dietary supplements. Vegans constitute less than 1% of the U.S. population, although between 5 and 7% of Americans consider themselves "almost" vegetarians. Nutritional diversity remains the key for these individuals. For example, a vegan diet contains all the essential amino acids if the RDA for protein contains 60% of protein from grain products, 35% from legumes, and 5% from green leafy vegetables. A 70-kg person would satisfy the essential amino acid requirement by consuming about 56 g of protein from approximately 1 1/4 cups of beans, 1/4 cup of seeds or nuts, 4 slices of whole-grain bread, 2 cups of vegetables (1 cup leafy green), and 2 1/2 cups from grain sources (brown rice, oatmeal, and cracked wheat). A 100-g serving of cooked lentils (about one-half cup) has a protein value equivalent to that of 1 oz of cooked lean meat.

An increasing number of competitive and champion athletes consume diets consisting predominately of nutrients from varied plant sources, including some dairy and meat products.[109,128] Vegetarian athletes often encounter difficulty in planning, selecting, and preparing nutritious meals from predominantly plant sources without relying on supplementation. The fact remains, however, that two-thirds of the world's population subsist on largely vegetarian diets. In contrast to diets that rely heavily on animal sources for protein, well-balanced vegetarian and vegetarian-type diets provide abundant carbohydrate, crucial in heavy, long-duration training.

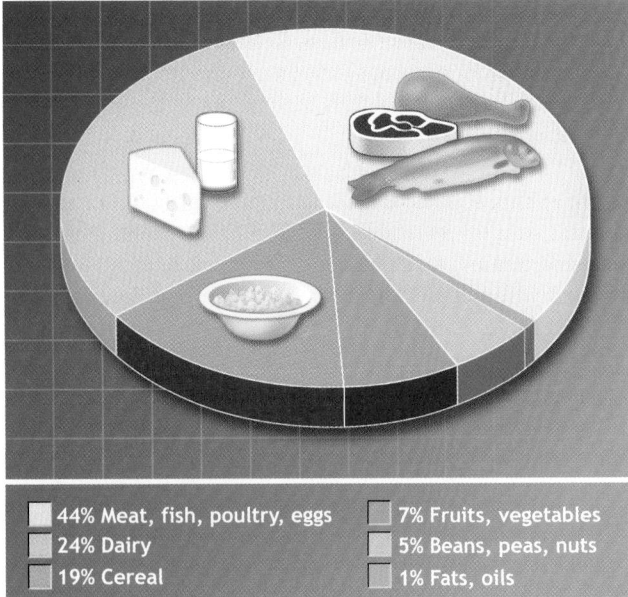

FIGURE 1.23 • Contribution from the major food sources to the protein content of the typical American diet.

Such diets contain little or no cholesterol, contain abundant fiber, and have rich fruit and vegetable sources of antioxidant vitamins. A meta-analysis of 38 controlled clinical trials concluded that substituting soy protein for animal protein significantly decreased plasma triglycerides, total cholesterol, and harmful LDL cholesterol, with no reduction in beneficial HDL cholesterol.[5,10] A **lactovegetarian** diet provides milk and such related products as ice cream, cheese, and yogurt. The lactovegetarian approach minimizes the problem of consuming sufficient high-quality protein and increases the intake of calcium, phosphorus, and vitamin B_{12} (produced by bacteria in the digestive tract of animals). Good meatless sources of iron include fortified ready-to-eat cereals, soybeans, and cooked farina, while cereals, wheat germ, and oysters contain high zinc levels. Adding an egg to the diet (**ovolactovegetarian** diet) ensures intake of high-quality protein.

Figure 1.23 displays the contribution of various food groups to the protein content of the American diet. By far, the greatest protein intake comes from animal sources, with only about 30% from plant sources.

RECOMMENDED DIETARY PROTEIN INTAKE

Despite the beliefs of many coaches, trainers, and athletes, little benefit accrues from eating excessive protein. An intake more than three times the recommended level does not enhance work capacity during intensive training.[35] *For athletes, muscle mass does not increase simply by eating high-protein foods.* If lean tissue synthesis resulted from all of the extra protein consumed by the typical athlete, then muscle mass would increase tremendously. For example, consuming an extra 100 g of protein (400 calories) daily would translate to a daily 500-g (1.1-lb) increase in muscle mass. This obviously does not happen. Excessive dietary protein is catabolized directly for energy (following deamination) or recycled as components of other molecules, including fat stored in subcutaneous depots. Excessive dietary protein intake above recommended values can potentially trigger harmful side effects, particularly strained liver and kidney function from elimination of urea and other compounds.

Many cultures consume more than twice the protein requirement. On a population basis, protein energy intake compared with total energy consumed equals 11% (Germany), 12% (United States), 12% (Sweden), 12.6% (Italy), and 14.4% (Japan). The diets of endurance- and resistance-trained athletes often exceed two to three times the recommended intake, usually as meat.[65,66] This occurs because athletes' diets normally emphasize high-protein foods. Furthermore, an athlete's caloric intake and energy output usually surpass those of the average sedentary counterpart.

The RDA: A Liberal Standard

The **Recommended Dietary Allowance (RDA)** for protein, vitamins, and minerals represents a standard for nutrient intake expressed as a daily average. These guidelines, initially developed in 1943 by the Food and Nutrition Board of the National Research Council/National Academy of Science (www2.nas.edu/iom), have been revised 11 times. RDA levels represent a liberal yet safe excess to prevent nutritional deficiencies in practically all healthy people. In the 11th edition (1999), RDA recommendations included 19 nutrients, energy intake, and the Estimated Safe and Adequate Daily Dietary Intakes (ESADDI) for seven additional vitamins and minerals and three electrolytes.[54] The ESADDI recommendation for certain essential micronutrients (e.g., the vitamins biotin and pantothenic acid and trace elements copper, manganese, fluoride, selenium, chromium, and molybdenum) required sufficient scientific data to formulate a range of intakes considered adequate and safe, yet insufficient for a precise RDA. No RDA or ESADDI exists for sodium, potassium, and chlorine; instead, recommendations refer to a minimum requirement for health. We emphasize that the RDA reflects nutritional needs of a population over a long time; one can only assess a specific individual's requirement by laboratory measurements. Malnutrition occurs from cumulative weeks, months, and even years of inadequate nutrient intake. Also, someone who regularly consumes a diet containing nutrients below the RDA standards may not become malnourished. *The RDA represents a probability statement for adequate nutrition; as nutrient intake falls below the RDA the statistical probability for malnourishment increases for that person, and the probability progressively increases with lower nutrient intake.*

Table 1.7 lists the protein RDAs for adolescent and adult men and women. On average, 0.83 g of protein per kg body mass represents the recommended daily intake. To determine the protein requirement for men and women ages 18 to 65, multiply body mass in kg by 0.83. Thus, for a 90-kg man, total protein requirement equals 75 g (90 x 0.83). The protein RDA holds even for overweight people; it includes a reserve of about 25% to account for individual differences in the protein requirement for about 98% of the population. Generally,

TABLE 1.7 ➤ **PROTEIN RECOMMENDED DIETARY ALLOWANCE (RDA) FOR ADOLESCENT AND ADULT MEN AND WOMEN**

Recommended Amount	Men		Women	
	Adolescent	Adult	Adolescent	Adult
Grams of protein per kg body mass	0.9	0.8	0.9	0.8
Grams per day based on average body mass[a]	59.0	56.0	50.0	44.0

[a]Average body mass based on a "reference" man and woman. For adolescents (ages 14–18), body mass averages 65.8 kg (145 lb) for males and 55.7 kg (123 lb) for females. For adult men, average mass equals 70 kg (154 lb); for adult women, mass averages 56.8 kg (125 lb).

the protein RDA (and the quantity of the required essential amino acids) decreases with age. In contrast, the protein RDA for infants and growing children equals 2.0 to 4.0 g per kg body mass. Pregnant women should increase total daily protein intake by 20 g, and nursing mothers should increase their intake by 10 g. *A 10% increase in the calculated protein requirement, particularly for a vegetarian-type diet, would account for dietary fiber's effect in reducing the digestibility of many plant-based protein sources.* Stress, disease, and injury usually increase the protein requirement.

Current debate focuses on the need for a larger protein requirement for athletes. These include still-growing adolescent athletes, athletes involved in resistance training programs that stimulate muscle growth and endurance training programs that increase protein breakdown, and athletes subjected to recurring tissue microtrauma like wrestlers and football players.[24,67,104,138,139] Inadequate protein intake can induce muscle protein loss, with concomitant performance deterioration. If athletes require additional protein, then more than likely, this need can be met by their generally increased food intake, which compensates for increased energy expenditure in training. However, this may not pertain to athletes with poor nutritional habits or those who reduce energy intake to achieve a desired aesthetic "look" or compete at a lower weight-class category to try and gain a competitive advantage. We present additional information about protein balance in exercise and training in subsequent sections of this chapter and in the "Focus on Research" section, page 40.

Preparations of Simple Amino Acids

Male and female weight lifters, body builders, and other power athletes consume up to four times the RDA for protein.[87] Much of this excess takes the form of liquids, powders, or pills of "purified" protein at a cost exceeding $30 to $50 per pound of actual protein. Such preparations often contain proteins "predigested" to simple amino acids through chemical action in the laboratory. Advocates believe the intestinal tract absorbs the simple amino acid molecule more readily to (1) optimize the expected muscle growth brought on by training or (2) improve strength, power, or "vigor" in the short term for a heavy workout. This, however, does not occur. The healthy small intestine readily absorbs amino acids when they exist in more complex di- and tripeptide forms rather than in simple amino acid form. A concentrated amino acid solution draws water into the intestine. This often precipitates intestinal irritation, cramping, and diarrhea. *Simply stated, adequate research design and methodology has not shown that amino acid supplementation in any form above the RDA significantly increases muscle mass or improves muscular strength, power, or endurance.*

ROLE OF PROTEIN IN THE BODY

Blood plasma, visceral tissue, and muscle represent the three major sources of body protein. No "reservoirs" of this macronutrient exist; all protein contributes to tissue structures or exists as important constituents of metabolic, transport, and hormonal systems. Protein makes up between 12 and 15% of the body mass, but the protein content of different cells varies considerably. A brain cell, for example, consists of only about 10% protein, while red blood cells and muscle cells include up to 20% of their total weight as protein. The protein content of skeletal muscle, which represents about 65% of the body's total protein, can increase to varying degrees with the systematic application of resistance training. Table 1.8 lists examples of different proteins and their functions in the body.

Amino acids provide the major building blocks for synthesizing tissue. They also incorporate nitrogen into the coenzyme electron carriers nicotinamide adenine dinucleotide (NAD^+) and flavin adenine dinucleotide (FAD) (see Chapter 5), the heme components of the oxygen-binding hemoglobin and myoglobin compounds, the catecholamine hormones epinephrine and norepinephrine, and the neurotransmitter serotonin. Amino acids activate vitamins that play a key role in metabolic and physiologic regulation. **Anabolism** refers to tissue-building processes; the amino acid requirement for anabolism can vary considerably. Tissue anabolism accounts for about one third of the protein intake during rapid growth in infancy and childhood. As growth rate declines, so does the percentage of protein retained for anabolic processes. A continual turnover of tissue protein occurs (with no net protein gain or loss) when a person attains a stable body size and growth ceases; normal protein dynamics for adults require adequate protein intake simply to replace the amino acids continually degraded in the turnover process.

Proteins serve as primary constituents for plasma membranes and internal cellular material. As the final chapter, "On the Horizon," discusses in considerable detail, the cell nucleus contains the genetically coded nucleic acid material DNA. DNA replicates itself before the cell divides to ensure that each new cell formed contains identical genetic material. It also provides the instructions, or "master plan," for the cellular manufacture of all the body's proteins via its control over cytoplasmic RNA. Collagenous structural proteins

TABLE 1.8 ➤ DIFFERENT PROTEINS AND THEIR FUNCTIONS

FUNCTION	PROTEIN CLASS	EXAMPLES	USE
Physiologic regulation	Hormones	Thyroxine	Regulates cellular metabolism
		Testosterone	Modulates male secondary sex characteristics
		Oxytocin	Regulates milk production
Mode of transport	Globins	Hemoglobin	Transports O_2 and CO_2 in blood
		Cytochromes	Mitochondrial electron transport
Method of storage	Ion binding	Ferritin	Iron storage
		Calmodulin	Binds calcium ions
Contraction	Muscle	Actin	Contractile protein
		Myosin	Contractile protein
Immune protection	Immunoglobulins	Antibodies	Eliminates foreign proteins (antigens)
Structure	Fibers	Collagen	Connective tissue formation
		Fibrin	Blood clotting
Metabolic regulation	Enzymes	Lysosomes	Hydrolyzes polysaccharides
		Proteases	Catabolizes proteins
		Polymerases	Catalyses nucleic acid synthesis
Membrane transport	Transporters	Sodium-potassium pump	Establishes membrane excitability
		Proton pump	Energy metabolism
Cell recognition	Cell surface antigens	Major histocompatibility complex (MHC) proteins	Encodes proteins for immune recognition
Osmotic regulation	Albumin	Serum albumin	Controls capillary fluid movement
Genetic regulation	Repressors	*lac* repressor	Transcription

compose the hair, skin, nails, bones, tendons, and ligaments. Globular proteins, another class, make up the nearly 2000 different enzymes that speed up chemical reactions and regulate the catabolism of fats, carbohydrates, and proteins for energy release. Blood plasma also contains the specialized proteins thrombin, fibrin, and fibrinogen required for blood clotting. Within red blood cells, the oxygen-carrying compound hemoglobin contains the large globin protein molecule. Proteins help to regulate the acid-base characteristics of the bodily fluids. Buffering neutralizes excess acid metabolites formed during vigorous exercise. The structural proteins actin and myosin slide past each other as muscles shorten and lengthen during movement, thus playing the predominant role in muscle action.

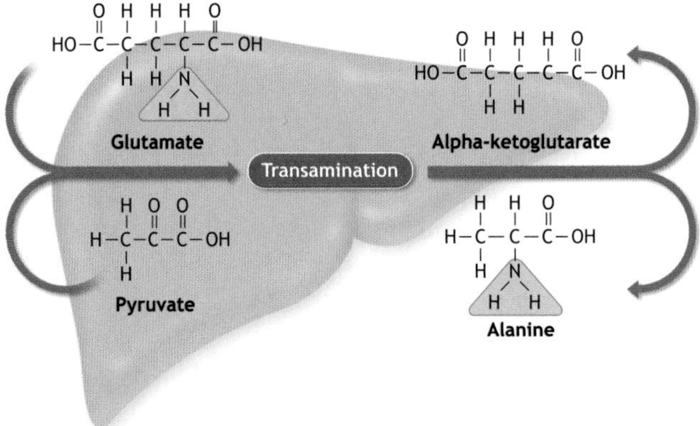

FIGURE 1.24 • Transamination provides for the intramuscular synthesis of amino acids from nonprotein sources. Enzyme action facilitates removal of an amine group from a donor amino acid for transfer to an acceptor, non-nitrogen-containing acid to form a new amino acid.

DYNAMICS OF PROTEIN METABOLISM

Dietary protein's main contribution supplies amino acids to various anabolic processes. In addition, protein is also catabolized for energy. In well-nourished individuals at rest, protein catabolism contributes between 2 and 5% of the body's total energy requirement. Protein undergoes constant degradation because (1) amino acids released during protein's continual turnover that do not immediately participate in protein synthesis are catabolized for energy; (2) dietary protein in excess of recommended values causes more amino acids to convert to fat or catabolize to meet the body's energy needs; and (3) starvation, dieting, prolonged exercise, and uncontrolled diabetes mellitus accelerate amino acid catabolism when carbohydrates are either unavailable or improperly used.

During catabolism, protein first degrades into its component amino acids. The amino acid molecule then loses its nitrogen (amine group) in the liver (**deamination**) to form **urea** (H_2NCONH_2). The remaining deaminated amino acid then is either converted to a new amino acid, converted to carbohydrate or fat, or catabolized directly for energy. Urea formed in deamination (including some ammonia) leaves the body in solution as urine. Excessive protein catabolism promotes fluid loss because urea must be dissolved in water for excretion.

Enzymes in muscle facilitate nitrogen removal from certain amino acids and pass it to other compounds in the reversible biochemical reactions of **transamination** (usually α-keto acid or glutamate; see Fig. 1.24). Transamination occurs when an amine group from a donor amino acid transfers to an acceptor acid to form a new amino acid. A specific transferase enzyme accelerates the transamination reaction. In muscle, transamination uses branched-chain amino acids (BCAAs) that generate branched-chain ketoacids (mediated by BCAA transferase). This allows amino acid formation from non-nitrogen-carrying organic compounds formed in metabolism (e.g., pyruvate). In both deamination and transamination, the resulting carbon skeleton of the nonnitrogenous amino acid residues undergoes further degradation during energy metabolism.

Fate of Amino Acid After Nitrogen Removal

After deamination, the remaining carbon skeletons of α-keto acids such as pyruvate, oxaloacetate, or α-ketoglutarate follow diverse biochemical routes, including the following:

- *Gluconeogenesis*—18 of the 20 amino acids serve as a source for glucose synthesis
- *Energy source*—the carbon skeletons oxidize for energy because they form intermediates in citric acid cycle metabolism or related molecules
- *Fat synthesis*—all amino acids provide a potential source of acetyl-CoA and thus furnish substrate to synthesize fatty acids

Figure 1.25 shows the commonality of the carbon sources from amino acids and the major metabolic paths taken by their deaminated carbon skeletons.

NITROGEN BALANCE

Nitrogen balance exists when nitrogen intake (protein) equals nitrogen excretion as follows:

$$\text{Nitrogen balance} = N_t - N_u - N_f - N_s = 0$$

where N_t = total nitrogen intake from food; N_u = nitrogen in urine; N_f = nitrogen in feces; N_s = nitrogen in sweat.

In **positive nitrogen balance**, nitrogen intake exceeds nitrogen excretion, with the additional protein used to synthesize new tissues. Positive nitrogen balance often occurs in children, during pregnancy, in recovery from illness, and during resistance exercise training, in which muscle cells promote protein synthesis. The body does not develop a protein reserve as it does with fat storage in adipose tissue and to some extent storage of carbohydrate as muscle and liver glycogen. Nevertheless, individuals who consume the recommended protein intake have a higher content of muscle and liver protein than individuals fed a subpar protein diet. Also, research using labeled protein (injecting protein with one or several of its carbon atoms "tagged") indicates that a significant amount of muscle protein becomes recruited for energy metabolism. On

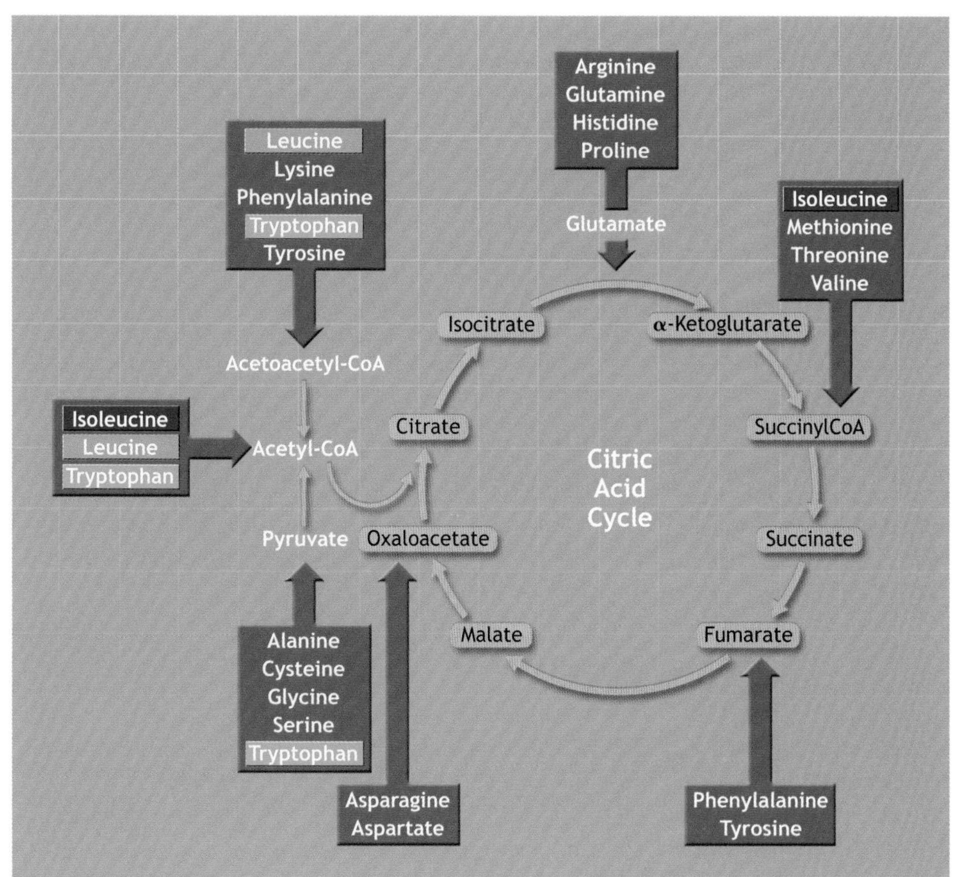

FIGURE 1.25 • Major metabolic pathways for amino acids following removal of nitrogen group by deamination or transamination. Upon removal of their amine group, all amino acids form reactive citric acid cycle intermediates or related compounds. Some of the larger amino acid molecules (e.g., leucine, tryptophan, isoleucine) generate carbon-containing compounds that enter metabolic pathways at different sites.

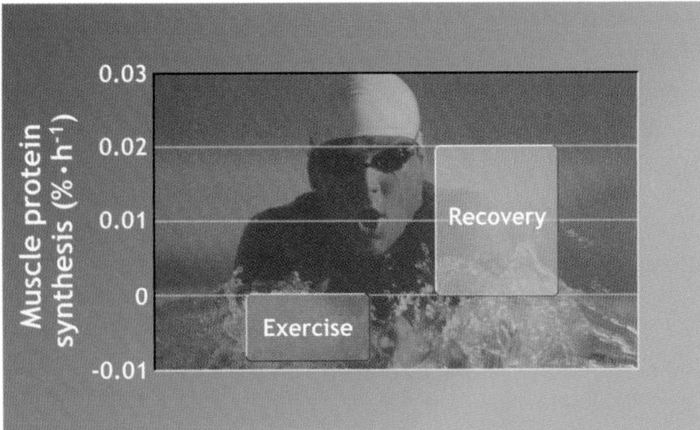

FIGURE 1.26 • Stimulation of human protein synthesis during recovery from aerobic exercise. Values refer to differences between the exercise group and the control group that received the same diet for each time interval. (From Carraro F, et al. Whole body and plasma protein synthesis in exercise and recovery in human subjects. Am J Physiol 1990;258:E821.)

the other hand, proteins in neural and connective tissues remain relatively "fixed" as cellular constituents and cannot be mobilized for energy without harming tissue functions.[49]

Greater nitrogen output than intake, or **negative nitrogen balance**, indicates protein use for energy and possible encroachment on amino acids, primarily from skeletal muscle. Interestingly, a negative nitrogen balance can occur even when protein intake exceeds the recommended standard if the body catabolizes protein because of a lack of other energy nutrients.[20] For example, an individual who participates regularly in heavy training may consume adequate or excess protein but inadequate energy from carbohydrate or lipid. In this scenario, protein becomes a primary energy fuel, which creates a negative protein (nitrogen) balance, resulting in a loss of the body's lean tissue mass. The protein-sparing role of dietary carbohydrate and lipid discussed previously becomes important during tissue growth periods and the high-energy output requirements of intensive exercise training. A negative nitrogen balance can occur during diabetes, fever, burns, dieting, recovery from severe illness, growth, and steroid administration. The greatest negative nitrogen balance occurs during starvation. *Starvation diets, or diets with reduced carbohydrate and/or energy, deplete glycogen reserves and trigger a protein deficiency with accompanying loss of lean tissue.*[147]

While protein breakdown generally increases only modestly with exercise, muscle protein synthesis rises substantially following both endurance and resistance-type exercise. The data for aerobic exercise in Figure 1.26 show that the rate of muscle protein synthesis (determined from labeled leucine incorporation into muscle) increased between 10 and 80% within 4 hours following termination of exercise. It then remained elevated for at least 24 hours.[24] Thus, two factors would justify reexamining protein intake recommendations for those involved in heavy training: (1) increased protein breakdown during long-term exercise and protracted heavy training and (2) somewhat more increased protein synthesis in recovery from exercise.

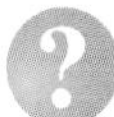

INTEGRATIVE QUESTION

If muscle growth with resistance training results primarily from the deposition of additional protein within the cell, why doesn't extra protein above the RDA facilitate muscle enlargement?

PROTEIN DYNAMICS IN EXERCISE AND TRAINING

The current understanding of protein dynamics and exercise comes from studies that expanded the classic method of determining protein breakdown through urea excretion. For example, release of labeled CO_2 from amino acids injected or ingested increases during exercise in proportion to the metabolic rate.[149] As exercise progresses, the concentration of plasma urea also increases, coupled with a dramatic rise in nitrogen excretion in sweat, often without any change in urinary nitrogen excretion.[63,116] These observations account for prior conclusions concerning minimal protein breakdown during endurance exercise because the early studies only measured nitrogen in urine. Figure 1.27 illustrates that the sweat mechanism serves an important role in excreting the nitrogen from protein breakdown during exercise. Furthermore, urea production may not reflect all aspects of protein breakdown, because the oxidation of both plasma and intracellular leucine (an essential BCAA) increases significantly during moderate exercise independent of changes in urea production.[14,145,159]

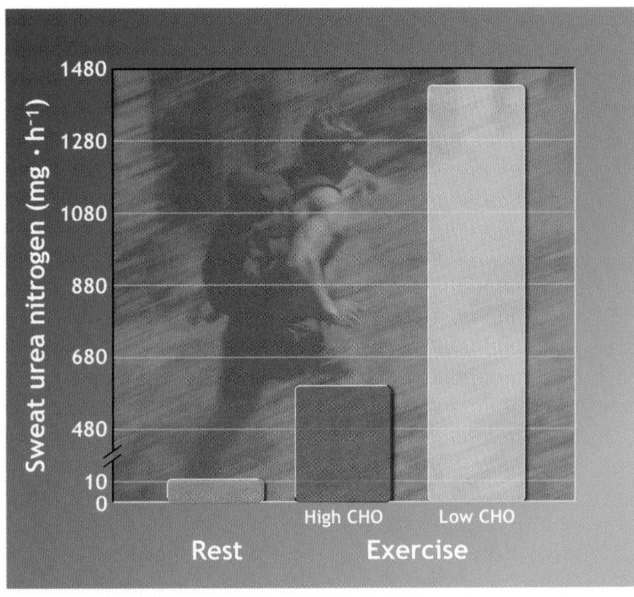

FIGURE 1.27 • Excretion of urea in sweat at rest and during exercise after carbohydrate loading (High CHO) and carbohydrate depletion (Low CHO). The largest use of protein (as reflected by sweat urea) occurs when glycogen reserves are low. (From Lemon PWR, Nagel F. Effects of exercise on protein and amino acid metabolism. Med Sci Sports Exerc 1981;13:141.)

Figure 1.27 also shows that protein use for energy reached its highest level when subjects exercised in the glycogen-depleted state. This emphasizes the important role of carbohydrate as a protein sparer, suggesting that carbohydrate availability affects the demand on protein "reserves" in exercise.[94,146] Protein breakdown and accompanying gluconeogenesis undoubtedly play a role in endurance exercise (or in frequent, high-intensity training) when glycogen reserves diminish.[158]

The increased pattern of protein catabolism during endurance exercise and intense training often mirrors the metabolic mixture during acute starvation. Without glycogen reserves, gluconeogenesis using carbon skeletons from amino acids largely sustains the liver's glucose output. Augmented protein breakdown probably reflects the body's attempt to maintain blood glucose concentration for central nervous system functioning. *These observations support the importance of athletes eating a high-carbohydrate diet with adequate energy intake to conserve muscle protein and to support protracted and hard training.* The potential for increased protein use for energy and depressed protein synthesis during heavy exercise may explain why individuals who undertake resistance training to build muscle size generally refrain from glycogen-depleting, endurance workouts. The beginning phase of an exercise training program also places a transient but increased demand on body protein, perhaps because of both muscle injury and metabolic requirements.[93,114]

Some Modification Required for Recommended Protein Intake

A continuing area of controversy concerns whether the initial, increased protein demand when training commences contributes to a true long-term increase in protein requirement above the RDA.[19,25,46,117] *Although a definitive answer remains elusive, protein breakdown above the resting level does occur during both endurance and resistance training exercise to a greater degree than previously believed.* Protein breakdown occurs mostly when exercising with low carbohydrate reserves and/or low energy intake.[44,93,104] Unfortunately, research has not pinpointed the actual protein requirements for individuals who train 4 to 6 hours daily by resistance exercise. Their requirement for protein may average only slightly greater than that for sedentary individuals (see "Focus on Research," page 40).[138] Despite increased protein use for energy during heavy training, adaptations may augment the body's efficiency in using dietary protein and thus enhance amino acid balance.[3,16] Future research will, one hopes, target protein intake recommendations for different groups of athletes who typically use resistance exercise to increase muscle size, strength, and power and athletes involved in prolonged endurance competitions and heavy training. *We recommend that athletes who train intensely consume between 1.2 and 1.8 g of protein per kg of body mass daily.* This level of protein intake falls within the range of the typical protein intake of the competitive athlete, obviating the need to consume supplementary protein, provided energy intake balances the energy requirements of training.

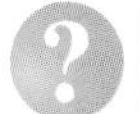

INTEGRATIVE QUESTION

Outline reasons why exercise physiologists debate the adequacy of the current protein RDA for individuals involved in high-intensity exercise training.

The Alanine–Glucose Cycle

Although some body proteins do not readily metabolize for energy, muscle proteins are more changeable. Amino acids participate in energy metabolism when the exercise energy demand increases.[26,29,61] For example, alanine release from active leg muscles is proportional to the severity of exercise.[152] Glutamine, on the other hand, may serve a more important gluconeogenic role than alanine during rest and starvation.[110,145]

Some researchers have proposed that alanine *indirectly* contributes to the exercise energy requirements.[49] Active skeletal muscle synthesizes alanine during transamination from the glucose intermediate pyruvate (with nitrogen derived in part from the amino acid leucine). The residual carbon fragment from the amino acid that formed alanine oxidizes for energy within the muscle cell. The newly formed alanine leaves the muscle and enters the liver for deamination. Alanine's remaining carbon skeleton converts to glucose via gluconeogenesis and enters the blood for delivery to active muscle. Figure 1.28 summarizes the sequence of the **alanine–glucose cycle**. After 4 hours of continuous light exercise, the liver's output of alanine-derived glucose accounts for about 45% of the liver's total glucose release. *The alanine–glucose cycle generates from 10 to 15% of the total exercise energy requirement.* Regular exercise training enhances the liver's synthesis of glucose from the carbon skeletons of noncarbohydrate compounds.[135] This facilitates blood glucose homeostasis during prolonged exercise.

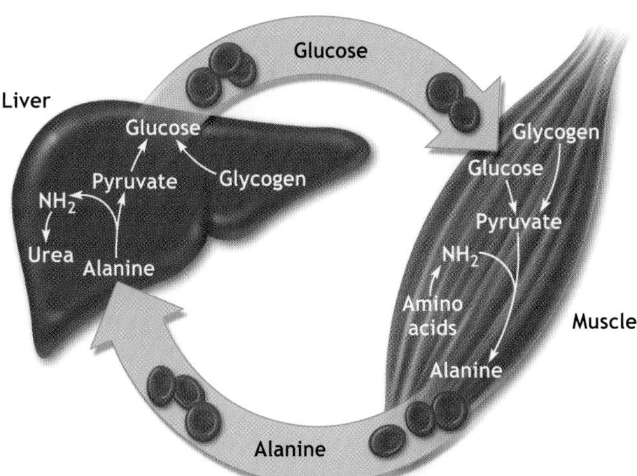

FIGURE 1.28 • The alanine–glucose cycle. Alanine, synthesized in muscle from glucose-derived pyruvate via transamination, enters the blood where the liver converts it to glucose and urea. Glucose release into the blood coincides with its subsequent delivery to the muscle for energy. During exercise, increased production and output of alanine from muscle helps to maintain blood glucose for nervous system and active muscle needs. Exercise training augments hepatic gluconeogenesis.

Focus on Research

Protein and Exercise: How Much Is Enough?

Tarnopolsky MA, et al. Influence of protein intake and training status on nitrogen balance and lean body mass. J Appl Physiol 1988;64:187.

➤ The question of how much dietary protein a physically active person requires to support training and optimize improvements continues to intrigue nutritionists and exercise physiologists. In the mid-1800s, initial studies of human protein needs postulated that muscular contraction destroyed a portion of the muscle's protein content to provide energy for biologic work. Based on this belief, overzealous entrepreneurs and "physical culturists" (the early predecessors of health club fitness trainers) recommended a high-protein diet to carry out heavy physical labor (and exercise training) and support a muscle's structure and its energy needs.

In some ways, many modern-day athletes who devote considerable time and effort training with resistance equipment mimic the older beliefs and practices. They too believe that a significant excess of dietary protein is the most important macronutrient to build bigger muscles and increase strength. For one reason, they believe resistance training in some way damages or "tears down" a muscle's inherent structure. This drain on body protein would require additional dietary protein (above the 0.83 g protein per kg body mass supplied by the RDA) for tissue resynthesis to a new, larger, and more powerful state. Many endurance athletes believe arduous training increases protein catabolism (and consequently its dietary requirement) to sustain the energy requirements of exercise. To some extent, both lines of reasoning have merit. The relevant question, however, concerns whether the protein RDA provides a sufficient reserve should 4 to 6 hours of daily heavy training add demands for protein synthesis and/or catabolism. While the debate continues and sales of protein supplements soar, researchers have attempted to quantify any added protein requirements of intense exercise training.

In one of the earlier attempts to study this problem systematically, Tarnopolsky and colleagues determined the effects of aerobic and resistance training on nitrogen balance in subjects fed a high-protein (HP) or relatively lower-protein (LP) diet. Subject were placed into three groups of six men each: (1) sedentary controls (S), elite endurance athletes (EA), and competitive body builders (BB). Ten-day measurements during training included nitrogen balance evaluation (N-Bal; daily dietary nitrogen intake vs. nitrogen excretion) under HP and LP diets. Quantification of total nitrogen excretion required three sequential 24-hour urine collections, 72-hour fecal collections, and representative samplings of resting and exercise sweat secretion.

The figure shows N-Bal (g of N per day) related to protein intake for each group. The white horizontal line at the zero point on the Y-axis represents the condition when nitrogen intake equals the body's nitrogen requirement. The three lines that intersect the zero point of nitrogen balance theoretically represent a sufficient protein intake: 0.73 $g \cdot kg^{-1} \cdot d^{-1}$ for the S group, 0.82 $g \cdot kg^{-1} \cdot d^{-1}$ for the BB group, and 1.37 $g \cdot kg^{-1} \cdot d^{-1}$ for the EA group. These findings showed that endurance exercise training increased net protein catabolism and protein requirement not evident for the BB group. The researchers recommended that body builders could reduce their typical abnormally high protein intakes, while endurance athletes could possibly benefit from increased protein intake above the RDA level.

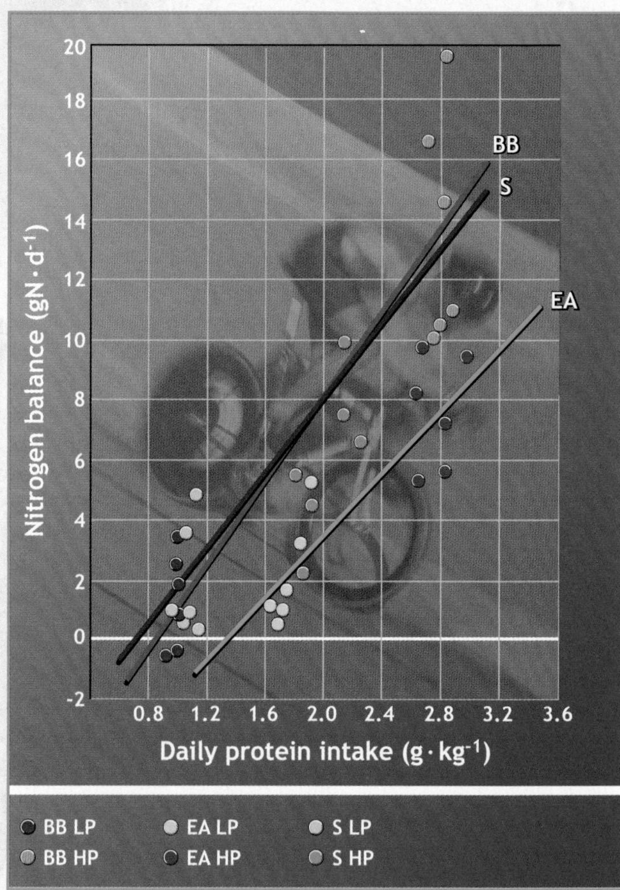

Positive and negative nitrogen balance plotted in relation to daily protein intake of sedentary men *(S)* and groups of elite athletes undergoing either endurance training *(EA)* or resistance training *(BB)*. Subjects consumed either a high-protein *(HP)* diet or a relatively lower-protein *(LP)* diet during the 10-day training period. The *bold horizontal line* at zero nitrogen balance represents the point at which nitrogen intake equals excretion (i.e., nitrogen balance). The point at which each of the three lines crosses the "zero line" indicates the necessary daily protein intake for the group.

IN A PRACTICAL SENSE

➤➤ HOW TO READ FOOD LABELS

In 1990, the United States Congress passed the Nutrition Labeling and Education Act, which brought sweeping changes to regulations for food labeling. The act (including 1993–1998 updates) aimed to (1) help consumers chose more healthful diets and (2) offer an incentive to food companies to improve the nutritional qualities of their products. All foods except those containing only a few nutrients, such as plain coffee, tea, and spices, now provide consistent nutrition information. Leading health and nutrition authorities have petitioned the FDA (www.FDA.gov) to list separately the grams of added sugars in a serving of the food and to indicate how this amount compares with intakes recommended by other organizations (food labels now only list total sugars—sugars naturally in food plus those added by processing). Currently, the food label must display the following information prominently and in words an average person can understand (numbers in insert figure relate to numbered information below).

The figure displays the current food label generated as an outgrowth of regulations from the FDA, the United States Department of Agriculture, and the Nutrition Labeling and Education Act of 1990.

1. Product's common or usual name
2. Name and address of manufacturer, packer, or distributor
3. Net contents for weight, measure, or count
4. All ingredients, listed in descending order of predominance by weight
5. Serving size, number of servings per container, and calorie information
6. Quantities of specified nutrients and food constituents, including total food energy in calories, total fat (g), saturated fat (g), cholesterol (mg), sodium (mg), and total carbohydrate including starch, sugar, fiber (g), and protein (g)
7. Descriptive terms of content
8. Approved health claims stated in terms of the total diet

Terms on Food Labels

COMMON TERMS AND WHAT THEY MEAN:

Free: Nutritionally trivial and unlikely to have physiologic consequences; synonyms include "without," "no," and "zero"

High: 20% or more of the Daily Value (DV) for a given nutrient per serving; synonyms include "rich in," or "excellent in"

Less: At least 25% less of a given nutrient or calories than the comparison food

Low: An amount that allows frequent consumption of the food without exceeding the nutrient's DV

Good source: Product provides between 10 and 19% of a given nutrient's DV per serving

CHOLESTEROL TERMS

Cholesterol-free: Less than 2 mg per serving and 2 g or less saturated fat per serving

Low cholesterol: 20 mg or less of cholesterol per serving and 2 g or less of saturated fat per serving

Less cholesterol: 25% or less cholesterol per serving and 2 g or less saturated fat per serving

FAT TERMS

Extra lean: Less than 5 g of fat, 2 g of saturated fat, and 95 mg of cholesterol per serving and per 100 g of meat, poultry, and seafood

Fat-free: Less than 0.5 g of fat per serving (no added fat or oil)

Lean: Less than 10 g of fat, 4.5 g of saturated fat, and 95 mg of cholesterol per serving and per 100 g of meat, poultry, and seafood

Less fat: 25% or less fat than the comparison food

Low-fat: 3 g or less of fat per serving

Light: 50% or less fat than comparison food (e.g., "50% less fat than our regular cookies")

Less saturated fat: 25% or less saturated fat than the comparison food

ENERGY TERMS

Calorie-free: Fewer than 5 calories per serving

Light: One-third fewer calories than the comparison food

Low-calorie: 40 calories or fewer per serving

Reduced calorie: At least 25% fewer calories per serving than the comparison food

FIBER TERMS

High-fiber: 5 g or more of fiber per serving

SODIUM TERMS

Sodium-free and salt-free: Less than 5 mg of sodium per serving

Low sodium: 140 mg or less of sodium per serving

Light: Low-calorie food with 50% sodium reduction

Light in sodium: No more than 50% of the sodium of the comparison food

Very low sodium: 35 mg or less of sodium per serving.

From the Nutrition Labeling Act of 1990. Federal Register 58(3), 1993. U.S. Government Printing Office, Superintendent of Documents, Washington, DC. (www.fda.gov/opacom/backgrounders/foodlabel/newlabel). (This site provides complete description of the new food label and relevant terms and materials related to the label).

In a Practical Sense

➤➤ How to Read Food Labels—cont'd

7 Descriptive terms if the product meets specified criteria

2 Manufacturer name and address

1 Product name

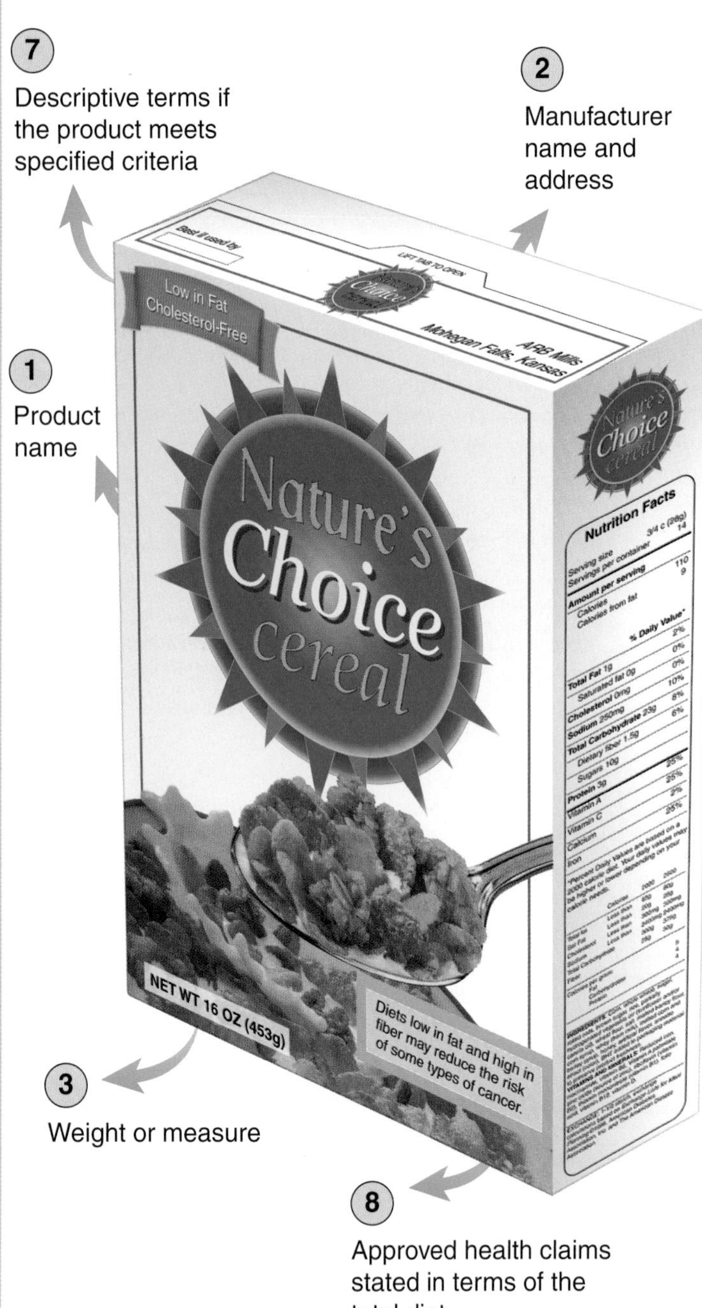

3 Weight or measure

8 Approved health claims stated in terms of the total diet

Nutrition Facts

Serving size	3/4 c (28 g)
Servings per container	14
Amount per serving	
Calories	110
Calories from fat	9
	% Daily Value*
Total Fat 1 g	2%
Saturated fat 0 g	0%
Cholesterol 0 mg	0%
Sodium 250 mg	10%
Total Carbohydrate 23 g	8%
Dietary fiber 1.5 g	6%
Sugars 10 g	
Protein 3 g	
Vitamin A	25%
Vitamin C	25%
Calcium	2%
Iron	25%

*Percent Daily Values are based on a 2000 calorie diet. Your daily values may be higher or lower depending on your calorie needs.

	Calories	2000	2500
Total fat	Less than	65 g	80 g
Sat Fat	Less than	20 g	25 g
Cholesterol	Less than	300 mg	300 mg
Sodium	Less than	2400 mg	2400 mg
Total Carbohydrate		300 g	375 g
Fiber		25 g	30 g

Calories per gram:

Fat	9
Carbohydrates	4
Protein	4

INGREDIENTS: Corn, whole wheat, sugar, rolled oats, brown sugar, rice, partially hydrogenated vegetable oir (sunflower and/or canola oil), wheat flour, salt, malted barley flour, corn syrup, whey (from milk), malted corn and barley syrup, honey, artificial flavor, annatto etract (color), BHT added to packaging material to preserve product freshness.
VITAMINS AND MINERALS: Reduced iron, niacinamide, vitamin B6, Vitamin A palmitate zinc oxide (source of zinc), riboflavin (vitamin B2), thiamin mononitrate (vitamin B1), folic acid, vitamin B12, vitamin D.

EXCHANGE: 1-1/2 starch, exchange calculations based on *Exchange Lists for Meal Planning* ©1995, American Diabetes Association, Inc. and The American Dietetic Association.

5 Serving size, number of servings per container, and calorie information

6 Nutrition information panel provides quantities of nutrients per serving, in both actual amounts and as "% of Daily Values" based on a 2000-calorie energy intake

4 Ingredients in descending order of predominance by weight

Summary

1. Proteins differ chemically from lipids and carbohydrates because they contain nitrogen in addition to sulfur, phosphorus, and iron.
2. Protein forms from subunits called amino acids. The body requires 20 different amino acids, each containing an amine group (NH_2) and an organic acid group (carboxylic acid group; COOH). Amino acids also contain an R group (side chain) that determines the amino acid's particular chemical characteristics.
3. The number of possible protein structures is enormous because of the tremendous number of combinations of 20 different amino acids.
4. Regular exercise training enhances the liver's synthesis of glucose from the carbon skeletons of noncarbohydrate compounds, particularly amino acids.
5. The body cannot synthesize 8 of the required 20 amino acids; these essential amino acids must be consumed in the diet.
6. All animal and plant cells contain protein. Complete (higher-quality) proteins contain all the essential amino acids; incomplete (lower-quality) proteins represent the others. Examples of higher-quality, complete proteins include animal proteins found in eggs, milk, cheese, meat, fish, and poultry.
7. Many physically active people and competitive athletes obtain their nutrients predominantly from plant sources.
8. Proteins provide the building blocks for synthesizing cellular material during anabolic processes. The protein's amino acids also contribute their "carbon skeletons" for energy metabolism.
9. The recommended dietary allowance (RDA) represents a liberal yet safe level of excess to meet the nutritional needs of practically all healthy people. For adults, the protein RDA equals 0.83 g per kg of body mass.
10. Proteins in neural and connective tissues generally do not participate in energy metabolism. The muscle-derived amino acid alanine, however, plays a key role via gluconeogenesis in supporting carbohydrate availability during prolonged exercise. The alanine–glucose cycle accounts for up to 45% of the liver's release of glucose during long-duration exercise.
11. Depleting carbohydrate reserves significantly increases protein catabolism during exercise. Thus, athletes who train vigorously on a regular basis must maintain optimal levels of muscle and liver glycogen to minimize deterioration in athletic performance.
12. Protein serves as an energy fuel to a much greater extent than previously believed. This applies particularly to BCAAs, oxidized in skeletal muscle rather than in the liver.
13. Reexamining the current protein RDA seems justified for athletes who engage in heavy exercise training. This examination must account for increased protein breakdown during exercise and augmented protein synthesis in recovery. Increasing protein intake to 1.2 to 1.8 g per kg body mass daily is reasonable in some situations.

References

1. Ahlborg G, et al. Substrate turnover during prolonged exercise in man. J Clin Invest 1974;53:1080.
2. Albert CM, et al. Fish consumption and risk of sudden cardiac death. JAMA 1998;279:23.
3. Albert JK, et al. Exercise-mediated tissue and whole body amino acid metabolism during intravenous feedings in normal men. Clin Sci 1989;77:113.
4. Anand RS, et al. Rise in amount of total fat and number of calories consumed by Americans. FASEB J 1997;11(3):A183. (Abstract 1064).
5. Anderson JW, et al. Meta-analysis of the effects of soy protein intake on serum lipids. N Engl J Med 1995;333:276.
6. Andrews TC, et al. Effect of cholesterol reduction on myocardial ischemia in patients with coronary disease. Circulation 1997;95:324.
7. Aro A, et al. Stearic acid, *trans* fatty acids, and dairy fat: effects on serum and lipoprotein lipids, apolipoproteins, lipoprotein (a), and lipid transfer proteins in healthy subjects. Am J Clin Nutr 1997;65:1419.
8. ASCN/AIN Task Force on Trans Fatty Acids. Position paper on *trans* fatty acids. 1996;63:663.
9. Barnard RJ, et al. Diet-induced insulin resistance precedes other aspects of the metabolic syndrome. J Appl Physiol 1998;84:1311.
10. Baum JA, et al. Long-term intake of soy protein improves blood lipid profiles and increases mononuclear cell low-density-lipoprotein receptor messenger RNA in hypercholesterolemic, postmenopausal women. Am J Clin Nutr 1998;68:545.
11. Bergman BC, Brooks GA. Respiratory gas-exchange ratios during graded exercise in fed and fasted trained and untrained men. J Appl Physiol 1999;86:479.
12. Bergstrom J, et al. Diet, muscle glycogen and physical performance. Acta Physiol Scand 1967;71:140.
13. Bònaa KH, et al. Effect of eicosapentaenoic and docosahexaenoic acids on blood pressure in hypertension. N Engl J Med 1990;322:795.
14. Bowtell JL, et al. Modulation of whole body protein metabolism, during and after exercise, by variation of dietary protein. J Appl Physiol 1998;85:1744.
15. Brand JC. Importance of glycemic index in diabetes. Am J Clin Nutr 1994;59(suppl):747S.
16. Brooks GA. Amino acid and protein metabolism during exercise and recovery. Med Sci Sports Exerc 1987;19:S150.
17. Brown L, et al. Cholesterol-lowering effects of dietary fiber: a meta-analysis. Am J Clin Nutr 1999;69:30.
18. Burkitt D. Dietary fiber. In: Medical applications of clinical nutrition. New Canaan, CT: Keats, 1983.
19. Butterfield-Hodgen G, Calloway DH. Protein utilization in men under two conditions of energy balance and work. Fed. Proc 1977;39:377.
20. Butterfield GE. Whole body protein utilization in humans. Med Sci Sports Exerc 1987;19:S157.
21. Caggiula AW, Mustak, VA. Effects of dietary fat and fatty acids on coronary artery disease risk and total and lipoprotein cholesterol concentrations: epidemiologic studies. Am J Clin Nutr 1997;65(suppl):1597S.
22. Caggiula AW, et al. The multiple risk factor intervention trial (Mr. Fit): IV. Intervention on blood lipids. Prev Med 1981;10:443.
23. Canner PL, et al. Fifteen year mortality in Coronary Drug Project patients: long-term benefit with niacin. J Am Coll Cardiol 1986;8:1245.
24. Carraro F, et al. Effect of exercise and recovery on muscle protein synthesis in human subjects. Am J Physiol 1990;259:E470.
25. Carraro F, et al. Urea kinetics in humans at two levels of exercise intensity. J Appl Physiol 1993;75:1180.
26. Carraro F, et al. Alanine kinetics in humans during low-intensity exercise. Med Sci Sports Exerc 1994;26:48.
27. Chanmugam P, et al. Reported changes in energy and fat intakes in adults and their food group sources. FASEB J 1998;12(4). (Abstract 4887).

28. Chen H-L, et al. Mechanisms by which wheat bran and oat bran increase stool weight in humans. Am J Clin Nutr 1998;68:711.
29. Christensen HN. Role of amino acid transport and counter transport in nutrition and metabolism. Physiol Rev 1990;70:43.
30. Coggan AR. Plasma glucose metabolism during exercise: effect of endurance training in humans. Med Sci Sports Exerc 1997;29:620.
31. Coggan AR, et al. Plasma glucose kinetics in subjects with high and low lactate thresholds. J Appl Physiol 1992;73:1873.
32. Coggan AR, et al. Glucose kinetics during high-intensity exercise in endurance-trained and untrained humans. J Appl Physiol 1995;78:1203.
33. Connor WE. Do the n-3 fatty acids from fish prevent deaths from cardiovascular disease? Am J Clin Nutr 1997;66:188.
34. Conner WE, et al. The plasma lipids, lipoproteins, and diet of the Tarahumara Indians of Mexico. Am J Clin Nutr 1978;31:1131.
35. Consolazio CF, et al. Protein metabolism during intensive physical training in the young adult. Am J Clin Nutr 1975;28:29.
36. Costill DL, et al. Effects of repeated days of intensified training on muscle glycogen and swimming performance. Med Sci Sports Exerc 1988;20:249.
37. Coyle EF, et al. Fatty acid oxidation is directly regulated by carbohydrate metabolism during exercise. Am J Physiol 1997;273(Endocrinol Metab 36):E268.
38. Daly ME, et al. Dietary carbohydrates and insulin sensitivity: a review of the evidence and clinical implications. Am J Clin Nutr 1997;66:1072.
39. Davidson MH, et al. Long-term effects of consuming foods containing psyllium seed husk on serum lipids in subjects with hypercholesterolemia. Am J Clin Nutr 1998;67:367.
40. Daviglus ML, et al. Fish consumption and the 30-year risk of fatal myocardial infarction. N Engl J Med 1997;336:1046.
41. De Glisezinski I, et al. Effects of carbohydrate ingestion on adipose tissue lipolysis during long-lasting exercise in trained men. J Appl Physiol 1998;84:1627.
42. Dietschy JM. Theoretical considerations of what regulates low-density-lipoprotein and high-density-lipoprotein cholesterol. Am J Clin Nutr 1997;65(suppl):1581S.
43. Djoussé L, et al. Relation between dietary fiber consumption and fibrinogen and plasminogen activator inhibitor type 1: The National Heart, Lung, and Blood Institute Family Heart Study. Am J Clin Nutr 1998;68:568.
44. Dohm GL, et al. Time course of changes in gluconeogenic enzyme activities during exercise and recovery. Am J Physiol 1985;249:E6.
45. Dreon DM, et al. Change in dietary saturated fat intake is correlated with change in mass of large low-density-lipoprotein particles in men. Am J Clin Nutr 1998;67:828.
46. Durnin JVGA. Protein requirements and physical activity. In: Parizkova J, Rogozkin VA, eds. Nutrition, physical fitness and health. Baltimore: University Park Press, 1978.
47. Durstine JL, Haskell WL. Effects of exercise training on plasma lipids and lipoproteins. Exerc Sport Sci Rev 1994;22:477.
48. Febbario MA, et al. Effect of epinephrine on muscle glycogenolysis during exercise in trained men. J Appl Physiol 1998;84:465.
49. Felig P, Wahren J. Amino acid metabolism in exercising man. J Clin Invest 1971;50:2703.
50. Felig P, Wahren J. Fuel homeostasis in exercise. N Engl J Med 1975;293:1078.
51. Felig P, et al. Hypoglycemia during prolonged exercise in normal men. N Engl J Med 1982;306:895.
52. Fernandez ML, et al. Guar gum effects on plasma low-density lipoprotein and hepatic cholesterol metabolism in guinea pigs fed low- and high-cholesterol diets: a dose-response study. Am J Clin Nutr 1995;61:127.
53. Fontvieille AM, et al. The use of low glycemic index foods improves metabolic control of diabetes patients in a 10 week study. Diabet Med 1992;9:444.
54. Food and Nutrition Board. Recommended dietary allowances. 11th ed. Washington, DC: National Academy of Sciences, 1999.
55. Frick MH, et al. Helsinki Heart Study: primary-prevention trial with gemfibrozil in middle-aged men with dyslipidemia. Safety of treatment, changes in risk factors, and incidence of coronary heart disease. N Engl J Med 1987;317:3217.
56. Friedman MI. Fuel partitioning and food intake. Am J Clin Nutr 1998;67(suppl):513S.
57. Fuchs CF, et al. Dietary fiber and risk of colorectal cancer and adenoma in women. N Engl J Med 1999;340:169.
58. Garland PB, Randle PJ. Regulation of glucose uptake by muscle. Effects of alloxan-diabetes, starvation, hypophysectomy and adrenalectomy, and of fatty acids, ketone bodies and pyruvate, on the glycerol output and concentrations of free fatty acids, long-chain fatty acyl-coenzyme A, glycerol phosphate and citrate-cycle intermediates in rat heart and diaphragm muscles. Biochem J 1964;93:678.
59. Gillman MW, et al. Margarine intake and subsequent coronary heart disease in men. Epidemiology 1997;81:144.
60. Grundy SM, Denke MA. Dietary influences of serum lipids and lipoproteins. Am J Clin Nutr 1994;60(suppl):986S.
61. Hall van G, et al. Deamination of amino acids as a source for ammonia production in human skeletal muscle during prolonged exercise. J Physiol 1995;489:251.
62. Hargreaves M. Interactions between muscle glycogen and blood glucose during exercise. Exerc Sport Sci Rev 1997;25:21.
63. Harlambie G, Sensor L. Metabolic changes in man during long-distance swimming. Eur J Appl Physiol 1980;43:115.
64. Harris WS, et al. Fish oils in hypertriglyceridemia: a dose response study. Am J Clin Nutr 1990;51:399.
65. Heyward VH, et al. Anthropometric, body composition and nutritional profiles of bodybuilders during training. J Appl Sports Sci Rev 1989;3:22.
66. Hickson JF, Wolinsky I. Research directions in protein nutrition for athletes. In: Wolinsky I, Hickson JF Jr, eds. Nutrition in exercise and sport. Boca Raton, FL: CRC Press, 1994.
67. Hickson JF, et al. Repeated days of body building exercise do not enhance urinary nitrogen excretions from untrained young males. Nutr Res 1990;10:723.
68. Hill J, Prentice A. Sugar and body weight regulation. Am J Clin Nutr 1995;62(suppl):264S.
69. Holmes MD, et al. Association of dietary intake of fat and fatty acids with risk of breast cancer. JAMA 1999;281:914.
70. Howell WM, et al. Plasma lipid and lipoprotein responses to dietary fat and cholesterol: a meta-analysis. Am J Clin Nutr 1997;65:1747.
71. Howlett K, et al. Effect of increased blood glucose availability on glucose kinetics during exercise. J Appl Physiol 1998;84:1423.
72. Hu FB, et al. Dietary fat intake and the risk of coronary heart disease in women. N Engl J Med 1997;337:1491.
73. Hultman E. Liver as a glucose supplying source during rest and exercise, with special reference to diet. In: Parizkova J, Rogozkin VA, eds. Nutrition, physical fitness, and health. Baltimore: University Park Press, 1978.
74. Iribarren C, et al. Serum total cholesterol and mortality: compound factors and risk modification in Japanese-American men. JAMA 1995;273:1926.
75. Jacobs DR Jr, et al. Is whole grain intake associated in reduced total and cause-specific death rates in older women? The Iowa Women's Health Study. Am J Public Health 1999;89:322.
76. Jandrain BJ, et al. Fructose utilization during exercise in men: rapid conversion of ingested fructose to circulating glucose. J Appl Physiol 1993;74:2146.
77. Jeppesen J, et al. Effects of low-fat, high-carbohydrate diets on risk factors for ischemic heart disease in postmenopausal women. Am J Clin Nutr 1997;65:1027.
78. Jeukendrup AE, et al. Exogenous glucose oxidation during exercise in endurance-trained and untrained subjects. J Appl Physiol 1997;83:835.
79. Jeukendrup AE, et al. Fat metabolism during exercise: a review—part II: Regulation of metabolism and effect of training. Int J Sports Med 1998;19:293.
80. John-Adler HB, et al. Reduced running endurance in gluconeogenesis-inhibited rats. Am J Physiol 1986;251:R137.
81. Kiens B. Effect of endurance training on fatty acid metabolism: local adaptations. Med Sci Sports Exerc 1997;29:640.
82. Kiens B, et al. Skeletal muscle substrate utilization during submaximal exercise in man: effect of endurance training. J Physiol 1993;469:459.
83. Kinosian B, et al. Cholesterol and coronary heart disease: predicting risk by levels and ratios. Ann Intern Med 1994;121:641.
84. Kirby RW, et al. Oat-bran intake selectively lowers serum low-density lipoprotein cholesterol concentrations of hypercholesterolemic men. Am J Clin Nutr 1981;34:824.
85. Kjaer M, et al. Increased epinephrine response and inaccurate glucoregulation in exercising athletes. J Appl Physiol 1986;61:1693.
86. Klein S, et al. Fat metabolism during low intensity exercise in endurance-trained and untrained men. Am J Physiol 1994;267:E934.

87. Kleiner SM, et al. Metabolic profiles, diet and health practices of championship male and female body builders. J Am Diet Assoc 1990;90:962.
88. Kris-Etherton PM, Yu S. Individual fatty acid effects on plasma lipids and lipoproteins. Am J Clin Nutr 1997;65(suppl):1628S.
89. Kris-Etherton PM, et al. Monounsaturated fatty acids and risk of cardiovascular disease. Circulation 1999;100:1253.
90. Lambert EV, et al. Enhanced endurance in trained cyclists during moderate intensity exercise following 2 weeks adaptation to a high fat diet. Eur J Appl Physiol 1994;69:287.
91. Langfort J, et al. The effect of a low-carbohydrate diet on performance, hormonal and metabolic responses to a 30-s bout of supramaximal exercise. Eur J Appl Physiol 1997;76:128.
92. Lanza E, et al. Dietary fiber intake in the U.S. population. Am J Clin Nutr 1987;46:790.
93. Lemon PWR. Protein and exercise: update 1987. Med Sci Sports Exerc 1987; 19:S179.
94. Lemon PWR, Mullin JP. The effect of initial muscle glycogen levels on protein catabolism during exercise. J Appl Physiol 1980;48:624.
95. Levine AS, et al. Effect of breakfast cereals on short-term food intake. Am J Clin Nutr 1989;50:1303.
96. Levy D, et al. Stratifying the patient at risk for coronary disease: new insights from the Framingham Heart Study. Am Heart J 1990;119:712.
97. Lipid Research Clinics Program: The Lipid Research Clinics coronary primary prevention trial results. I. Reduction in incidence of coronary heart disease. JAMA 1984;251:351.
98. Lipid Research Clinics Program: The Lipid Research Clinics coronary primary prevention trial results. II. The relationship of reduction in incidence of coronary heart disease to cholesterol lowering. JAMA 1984;251:365.
99. Ludwig DS, et al. Dietary fiber, weight gain, and cardiovascular disease risk factors in young adults. JAMA 1999;282:1539.
100. Martin MJ, et al. Serum cholesterol, blood pressure, and mortality: implications from a cohort of 361,662 men. Lancet 1986;2:933.
101. Martin WH III. Effect of acute and chronic exercise on fat metabolism. Exerc Sport Sci Rev 1996;24:203.
102. Martin WH III. Effect of endurance training on fatty acid metabolism during whole body exercise. Med Sci Sports Exerc 1997;29:635.
103. Martin WH III, et al. Effect of endurance training on plasma free fatty acid turnover and oxidation during exercise. Am J Physiol 1993;265:E708.
104. Meridith CN, et al. Dietary protein requirements and body protein metabolism in endurance-trained men. J Appl Physiol 1989;66:2850.
105. Mudio DM, et al. Effects of dietary fat on metabolic adjustments to maximal $\dot{V}O_2$ and endurance in runners. Med Sci Sports Exerc 1994;26:81.
106. Murray R, et al. The effects of glucose, fructose, and sucrose ingestion during exercise. Med Sci Sports Exerc 1989;21:275.
107. NIH Consensus Conference. Triglyceride, high-density lipoprotein, and coronary heart disease. JAMA 1993;269:505.
108. Nicklas BJ. Effects of endurance exercise on adipose tissue metabolism. Exerc Sport Sci Rev 1997;25:77–103.
109. Nieman D. Vegetarian dietary practices and endurance performance. Am J Clin Nutr 1998;8:754.
110. Nurjhan N, et al. Glutamine: a major gluconeogenic precursor and vehicle for inter-organ carbon transport in man. J Clin Invest 1995;95:272.
111. Ornish D, et al. Intensive lifestyle changes for reversal of coronary heart disease. JAMA 1998;280:2001.
112. Phinney SD, et al. The human metabolic response to chronic ketosis without caloric restriction: preservation of submaximal exercise capability with reduced carbohydrate oxidation. Metabolism 1993;32:769.
113. Pietinen P, et al. Intake of fatty acids and risk of coronary heart disease in a cohort of Finnish men—The Alpha-Tocopherol, Beta-Carotene Cancer Prevention Study. Am J Epidemiol 1997;145:876.
114. Pivarnik JM, et al. Urinary 3-methylhistidine excretion increases with repeated weight training exercise. Med Sci Sports Exerc 1989;21:283.
115. Pugh LGCE, Edholm OG. The physiology of channel swimmers. Lancet 1955;2:761.
116. Refsum HE, et al. Changes in plasma amino acid distribution and urinary amino acid excretion during prolonged heavy exercise. Scand J Clin Invest 1979;39:407.
117. Rennie MJ, et al. Physical activity and protein metabolism. In: Bouchard C, et al., eds. Physical activity, fitness, and health. Champaign, IL: Human Kinetics, 1994.
118. Rimm EB, et al. Vegetable, fruit, and cereal fiber intake and risk of coronary heart disease among men. JAMA 1996;275:447.
119. Roche HM, et al. Effect of long-term olive oil dietary intervention on postprandial triacylglycerol and factor VII metabolism. Am J Clin Nutr 1998;68:552.
120. Romijn JA, et al. Regulation of endogenous fat and carbohydrate metabolism in relation to exercise intensity and duration. Am J Physiol 1993;265:E380.
121. Romijn JA, et al. Relationship between fatty acid delivery and fatty acid oxidation during strenuous exercise. J Appl Physiol 1995;79:1939.
122. Salmerón JE, et al. Dietary fiber, glycemic load, and risk of NIDDM in men. Diabetes Care 1997;20:545.
123. Salmerón JE, et al. Dietary fiber, glycemic load, and risk of non-insulin-dependent diabetes mellitus in women. JAMA 1997;277:472.
124. Sears B, Lawren W. The zone. New York: Harper Collins, 1995.
125. Shahar E, et al. Dietary n-3 polyunsaturated fatty acids and smoking-related chronic obstructive pulmonary disease. N. Engl J Med 1994;331:228.
126. Simopolous AP. Omega-3 fatty acids in health and disease and in growth and development. Am J Clin Nutr 1991;54:438.
127. Sims EAH, Danforth E Jr. Expenditure and storage of energy in man (perspective). J Clin Invest 1987;79:1019.
128. Slavin JL, et al. Nutritional practices of women cyclists including recreational riders and elite racers. In: Katch FI, ed. Sport, health, and nutrition. Champaign, IL: Human Kinetic Publishers, 1986.
129. Slyper AH, et al. Low-density lipoprotein and atherosclerosis. JAMA 1994;272:305.
130. Southgate DAT. Digestion and metabolism of sugars. Am J Clin Nutr 1995;62:(suppl):203S.
131. Stamler J, et al. Is relationship between serum cholesterol and risk of premature death from coronary heart disease continuous or graded? Findings in 356,222 primary screenees of the Multiple Risk Factor Intervention Trial (Mr Fit). JAMA 1986;256:2823.
132. Starc TJ, et al. Greater dietary intake of simple carbohydrate is associated with lower concentrations of high-density-lipoprotein cholesterol in hypercholesterolemic children. Am J Clin Nutr 1998;67:1147.
133. Stefanick ML, et al. Effects of diet and exercise in men and postmenopausal women with low levels of HDL cholesterol and high levels of LDL cholesterol. N Engl J Med 1998;339:12.
134. Steinberg, D. Low density lipoprotein oxidation and its pathobiological significance. J Biol Chem 1997;272:20963.
135. Sumida KD, Donovan CM. Enhanced hepatic gluconeogenic capacity for selected precursors after endurance training. J Appl Physiol 1995;79:1883.
136. Superko HR, et al. The effect of solid and liquid gum on the reduction of plasma cholesterol in patients with moderate hypercholesterolemia. Am J Cardiol 1988;62:51.
137. Suter E, Hawes MR. Relationship of physical activity, body fat, diet, and blood lipid profile in youths 10–15 yr. Med Sci Sports Exerc 1993;25:748.
138. Tarnopolosky MA, et al. Influence of protein intake and training status on nitrogen balance and lean body mass. J Appl Physiol 1988;64:187.
139. Tarnopolosky MA, et al. Effect of bodybuilding exercise on protein requirements. Can J Sport Sci 1990;15:225.
140. Tiollotson JL, et al. Relation of dietary carbohydrates to blood lipids in the special intervention and usual care groups in the Multiple Risk Factor Intervention Trial. Am J Clin Nutr 1997;65(suppl):3214S.
141. Toner MM, McArdle WD. Human thermoregulatory responses to acute cold stress with special reference to water immersion. In: Fregly MJ, Blatteis CM, eds. Handbook of physiology, section 4: Environmental physiology, vol 1. New York: Oxford University Press, 1996.
142. Turcotte LP, et al. Increased plasma FFA uptake and oxidation during prolonged exercise in trained versus untrained humans. Am J Physiol 1992;262:E791.
143. Turcotte LP. Muscle fatty acid uptake during exercise: possible mechanisms. Exerc Sport Sci Rev 2000;1:4.
144. van der Vusse GJ, Reneman RS. Lipid metabolism in muscle. In: Handbook of physiology, section 12: Exercise: regulation and integration of multiple systems. New York: Oxford University Press, 1996.
145. Wagenmakers AJM. Muscle amino acid metabolism at rest and during exercise: Role in human physiology and metabolism. Exerc Sport Sci Rev 1998;26:287.
146. Wagenmakers AJM, et al. Carbohydrate supplementation, glycogen depletion, and amino acid metabolism. Am J Physiol 1991;260:E883.

147. Walberg JL, et al. Macronutrient content of a hypoenergy diet affects nitrogen retention and muscle function in weight lifters. Int J Sports Med 1988;9:261.
148. Warner JG Jr, et al. Combined effect of aerobic exercise and omega-3 fatty acids in hyperlipidemic persons. Med Sci Sports Exerc 1989;21:498.
149. White TP, Brooks GA. [u-^{14}C]Glucose-alanine and leucine oxidation in rats at rest and two intensities of running. Am J Physiol 1981;240:E155.
150. Willett WC. Nutritional epidemiology. 2nd ed. New York: Oxford University Press, 1998.
151. Willett WC, Ascherio A. Trans fatty acids: are the effects only marginal? Am J Public Health 1994;84:722.
152. Williams BD, et al. Alanine and glutamine kinetics at rest and during exercise in humans. Med Sci Sports Exerc 1998;30:1053.
153. Williams OD, et al. Common methods, different populations: The Lipid Research Clinics program prevalence study. Circulation 1980;62(suppl 4):18.
154. Williams PT. High-density lipoprotein cholesterol and other risk factors for coronary heart disease in female runners. N Engl J Med 1996;334:1298.
155. Winder WW. Malonyl-CoA—Regulator of fatty acid oxidation in muscle during exercise. Exerc Sport Sci Rev 1998;26:117.
156. Wolever TMS, et al. Glycaemic index of 102 complex carbohydrate foods in patients with diabetes. Nutr Res 1994;14:651.
157. Wolfe RR. Metabolic interactions between glucose and fatty acids in humans. Am J Clin Nutr 1998;67(suppl):519S.
158. Wolfe RR, et al. Glucose metabolism in man: response to intravenous glucose infusion. Metabolism 1979;28:210.
159. Wolfe RR, et al. Isotopic analysis of leucine and urea metabolism in exercising humans. J Appl Physiol 1982;52:458.
160. Wolfe RR, et al. Role of changes in insulin and glucagon in glucose homeostasis in exercise. J Clin Invest 1986;77:900.
161. Wolk A, et al. Long-term intake of dietary fiber and decreased risk of coronary heart disease among women. JAMA 1999;281:1998.
162. Yost TJ, et al. Effect of dietary macronutrient composition on tissue-specific lipoprotein lipase activity and insulin action in normal-weight subjects. Am J Clin Nutr 1998;68:296.

CHAPTER 2

Vitamins, Minerals, and Water

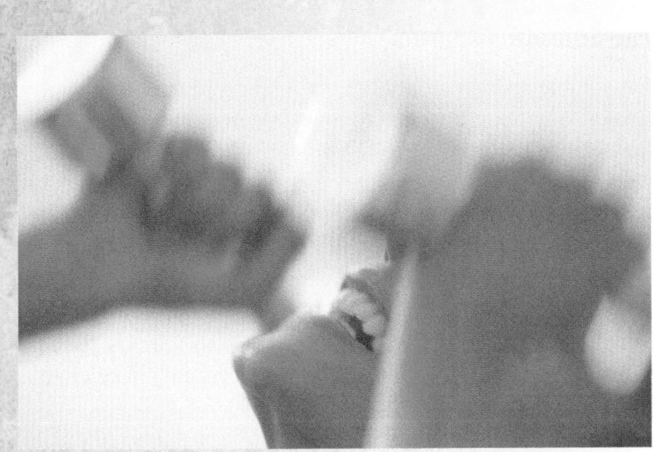

Chapter Objectives

- List one function for each fat- and water-soluble vitamin and potential risks of consuming them in excess
- Outline three broad roles of minerals in the body
- Discuss how free radicals form in the body, particularly during physical activity, and the mechanisms to defend against oxidative stress
- Respond to those who advocate vitamin supplementation above the recommended dietary allowance (RDA) for individuals involved in heavy exercise training
- Define the terms *osteoporosis, exercise-induced anemia,* and *sodium-induced hypertension*
- Describe how regular physical activity affects (1) bone mass and (2) the body's iron stores
- Present a possible explanation for "sports anemia"
- Outline factors related to the "female athlete triad"
- Argue for or against mineral supplementation above the RDA for those involved in heavy exercise training
- List diverse functions of water in the body
- Quantify the volumes of the body's three water compartments
- List five predisposing factors to hyponatremia with prolonged exercise

The effective regulation of all metabolic processes requires a delicate blending of food nutrients in the watery medium of the cell. Of special significance in the metabolic mixture are the **micronutrients**—the small quantities of vitamins and minerals that play highly specific roles in facilitating energy transfer and tissue synthesis. For example, the body requires each year only about 350 g (12 oz) of vitamins from the 862 kg of food consumed by the average adult. We readily obtain these nutrients by consuming well-balanced meals. With proper nutrition from a variety of food sources, the physically active person or competitive athlete need not consume vitamin and mineral supplements; such practices usually prove physiologically and economically wasteful. Furthermore, consuming some micronutrients in excess poses a significant risk to health and safety.

➤ PART 1 • Vitamins

THE NATURE OF VITAMINS

The importance of vitamins was known many centuries before scientists isolated and classified them. For example, the Greek physician Hippocrates advocated eating liver to cure night blindness. While the reason for the cure remained unknown at the time, we now know that vitamin A, which helps to prevent night blindness, is plentiful in this organ meat. In 1897, scientists observed that a regular diet of polished rice caused the disease beriberi, whereas addition of the thiamine-rich rice polishings cured it. In the early 19th century, the disease scurvy was eliminated by adding lemons—then called limes—to the diet of British sailors (nicknamed "limeys"), many of whom would have perished from lack of the then-unknown vitamin C. Not until 1932 did scientists isolate ascorbic acid or vitamin C from lemon juice.

The formal discovery of vitamins revealed they were organic substances needed by the body in minute amounts. Vitamins have no particular chemical structure in common and often are considered accessory nutrients because they neither supply energy nor contribute substantially to the body's mass. With the exception of vitamin D, the body cannot manufacture vitamins; they must be supplied in the diet or through supplementation.

Some foods contain an abundant quantity of vitamins. For example, the green leaves and roots of plants manufacture vitamins during photosynthesis. Animals obtain vitamins from the plants, seeds, grains, and fruits they eat or from the meat of animals that previously consumed these nutrients. Several vitamins, notably vitamins A and D, niacin, and folic acid, are activated from their inactive precursor or **provitamin** form. **Carotenes**, the best-known provitamins, are the yellow and yellow-orange pigmented precursors of vitamin A that give color to vegetables (e.g., carrots, squash, corn, pumpkins) and fruits (e.g., apricots and peaches).

KINDS OF VITAMINS

Thirteen different vitamins have been isolated, analyzed, classified, and synthesized and assigned RDAs. Vitamins are classified as **fat soluble**—vitamins A, D, E, and K—or **water soluble**—vitamin C and the B-complex vitamins: thiamine (B_1), riboflavin (B_2), vitamin B_6 (pyridoxine), niacin (nicotinic acid), pantothenic acid, biotin, folic acid (folacin or folate, its active form in the body), and cobalamin (B_{12}).

Fat-Soluble Vitamins

Fat-soluble vitamins dissolve and remain in the body's fatty tissues, obviating the need to ingest them daily. In fact, years may elapse before symptoms of a fat-soluble vitamin insufficiency emerge. The liver stores vitamins A and D, whereas vitamin E is distributed throughout the body's fatty tissues. Vitamin K is stored only in small amounts, mainly in the liver. Dietary lipid provides the source of fat-soluble vitamins; these vitamins, transported as part of lipoproteins in the lymph, travel to the liver for dispersion to various tissues. Consuming a true "fat-free" diet would certainly accelerate a fat-soluble vitamin insufficiency.

Fat-soluble vitamins should not be consumed in excess without medical supervision. Toxic reactions to excessive fat-soluble vitamin intake occur at a lower multiple of the RDA than water-soluble vitamins. For example, a daily moderate-to-large excess of vitamin A (as retinol but not in carotene form) and vitamin D produces serious toxic effects. Women who consume excess vitamin A early in pregnancy significantly increase the risk of birth defects in utero. In young children, excessive vitamin A accumulation (called hypervitaminosis A) causes irritability, swelling of bones, weight loss, and dry, itchy skin. In adults, symptoms can include nausea, headache, drowsiness, hair loss, diarrhea, and loss of calcium from bones, causing them to become brittle. Discontinuing the high vitamin A intake reverses these symptoms. Regular excessive ingestion of vitamin D can produce kidney damage. Although "overdoses" from vitamins E and K are rare, intakes above the recommended level yield no known health benefits.

Water-Soluble Vitamins

Water-soluble vitamins act largely as **coenzymes**—small molecules combined with a larger, protein compound (apoenzyme) to form an active enzyme that accelerates the interconversion of chemical compounds (see Chapter 5). Figure 2.1 shows examples of the structural relationship of three vitamins to their respective coenzymes. Coenzymes participate directly in chemical reactions; after the reaction runs its course, coenzymes remain intact and participate in additional reactions. Water-soluble vitamins, like their fat-soluble counterparts, consist of carbon, hydrogen, and oxygen atoms. They also contain nitrogen and metal ions including iron, molybdenum, copper, sulfur, and cobalt.

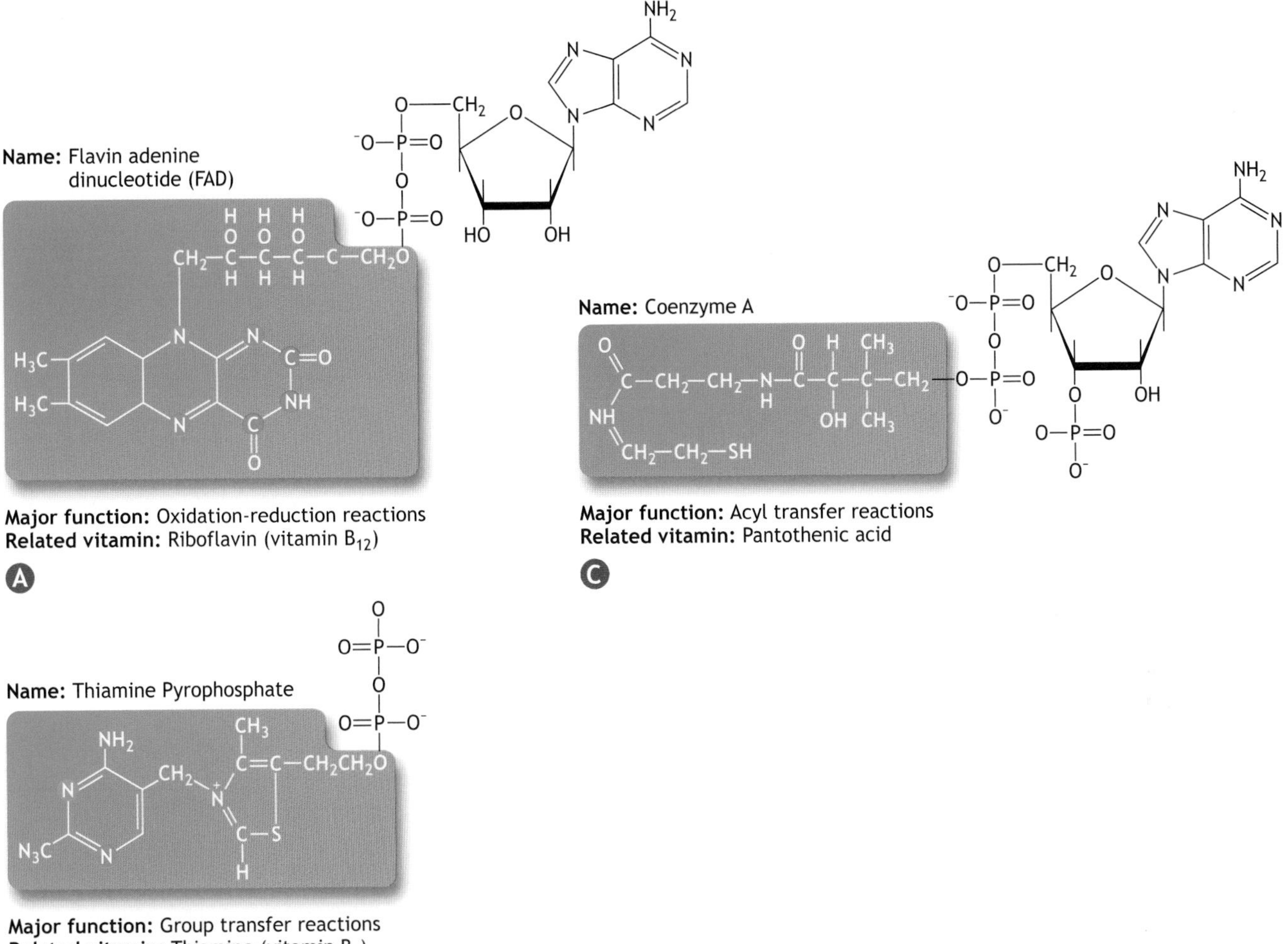

FIGURE 2.1 • Structural relationship of three vitamins to their respective coenzymes. **A**. Riboflavin (vitamin B_{12}). **B**. Thiamine (vitamin B_1). **C**. Pantothenic acid. Vitamins are shown in green.

Because of their solubility in water, water-soluble vitamins disperse in the bodily fluids without being stored to any appreciable extent. If the diet regularly contains less than 50% of the recommended amounts of water-soluble vitamins, marginal deficiencies may develop within 4 weeks. Generally, an excess intake of water-soluble vitamins is voided in the urine. Water-soluble vitamins exert their influence for 8 to 14 hours after ingestion; thereafter, their potency decreases. For maximum benefit, for example, vitamin C supplements should be consumed at least every 12 hours. Some researchers recommend increasing the RDA for vitamin C for healthy people from 60 to 200 mg (not in supplement form but in 2 to 4 daily servings of fruits and 3 to 5 servings of vegetables) to ensure optimal cellular saturation[12,91] The recommended daily 60-mg intake of vitamin C, established in 1980, is currently under revision by the Food and Nutrition Board of the National Academy of Sciences. Figure 2.2 illustrates various food sources for vitamin C and its diverse biologic and biochemical functions. These include serving as an electron donor for eight enzymes and as a chemical reducing agent (antioxidant) in many intracellular and extracellular reactions.

ROLE OF VITAMINS

Figure 2.3 summarizes the major biologic functions of vitamins. Vitamins contain no useful energy for the body; instead they serve as essential links and regulators in metabolic reactions that release energy from food. Vitamins also control tissue synthesis and help to protect the integrity of the cells' plasma membrane. The water-soluble vitamins play important roles in energy metabolism (Tables 2.1 and 2.2). For example,

- Vitamin B_1 facilitates the conversion of pyruvate to acetyl-coenzyme A (CoA) in carbohydrate breakdown
- Niacin and vitamin B_2 regulate mitochondrial energy metabolism
- Vitamins B_6 and B_{12} catalyze protein synthesis
- Pantothenic acid, part of CoA, participates in the aerobic breakdown of the carbohydrate, fat, and protein macronutrients
- Vitamin C acts as a cofactor in enzymatic reactions, as a scavenger of free radicals in antioxidative processes, and as a component in hydroxylation reactions that provide connective tissue stability and wound healing

Food Sources

Source (Portion Size)	Vitamin C (mg)
Fruit	
Cantaloupe (1/4 Medium)	60
Fresh grapefruit (1/2 Fruit)	40
Honeydew melon (1/8 Medium)	40
Kiwi (1 Medium)	75
Mango (1 Cup, sliced)	45
Orange (1 Medium)	70
Papaya (1 Cup, cubes)	85
Strawberries (1 Cup, sliced)	95
Tangerines or tangelos (1 Medium)	25
Watermelon (1 Cup)	15
Juice	
Grapefruit (1/2 Cup)	35
Orange (1/2 Cup)	50
Fortified Juice	
Apple (1/2 Cup)	50
Cranberry juice cocktail (1/2 Cup)	45
Grape (1/2 Cup)	120
Vegetables	
Asparagus, cooked (1/2 Cup)	10
Broccoli, cooked (1/2 Cup)	60
Brussels sprouts, cooked (1/2 Cup)	50
Cabbage	
Red, raw, chopped (1/2 Cup)	20
Red, cooked (1/2 Cup)	25
Raw, chopped (1/2 Cup)	10
Cooked (1/2 Cup)	15
Cauliflower, raw or cooked (1/2 Cup)	25
Kale, cooked (1/2 Cup)	55
Mustard greens, cooked (1 Cup)	35
Pepper, red or green	
Raw (1/2 Cup)	65
Cooked (1/2 Cup)	50
Plantains, sliced, cooked (1 Cup)	15
Potato, baked (1 Medium)	25
Snow peas	
Fresh, cooked (1/2 Cup)	40
Frozen, cooked (1/2 Cup)	20
Sweet potato	
Baked (1 Medium)	30
Vacuum can (1 Cup)	50
Canned, syrup-pack (1 Cup)	20
Tomato	
Raw (1/2 Cup)	15
Canned (1/2 Cup)	35
Juice (6 Fluid oz)	35

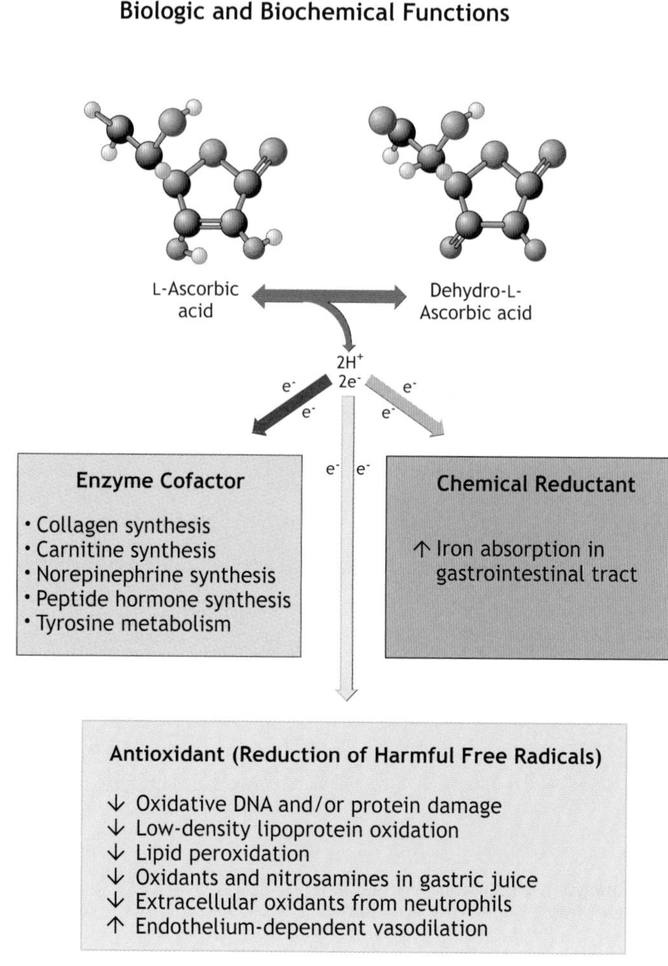

Vitamin C (L-ascorbic acid) oxidation releases donor electrons in pairs for biochemical reactions. The molecular diagrams show carbon atoms in black, oxygen in red, and hydrogen in white. Arrows indicate an increase or decrease in level.

FIGURE 2.2 • Various food sources for vitamin C and diverse biologic and biochemical functions. (Modified from Levine M, et al. Criteria and recommendations for vitamin C intake. JAMA 1999;281:1415.)

Vitamins participate repeatedly in metabolic reactions; thus, the vitamin needs of athletes do not exceed those of sedentary counterparts.

INTEGRATIVE QUESTION

If vitamins play such an important role in energy release, why shouldn't athletes "supercharge" with supplements to enhance exercise performance and training responsiveness?

Table 2.2 lists the bodily functions, dietary requirements, and major dietary sources of the water-soluble and fat-soluble vitamins. Well-balanced meals provide an adequate quantity of all vitamins, regardless of age and physical activity level. Indeed, food intake generally increases to sustain the added energy requirements of exercise. Any additional food intake generally increases the daily vitamin and mineral intake, forgoing the need to consume special foods or supplements that increase the vitamin content above recommended levels.

Several exceptions exist concerning possible need for vitamin supplementation. First, vitamin C and folic acid exist in foods that usually make up only a small part of most Americans' total caloric intake; the availability of these foods also varies by season. Second, different athletic groups

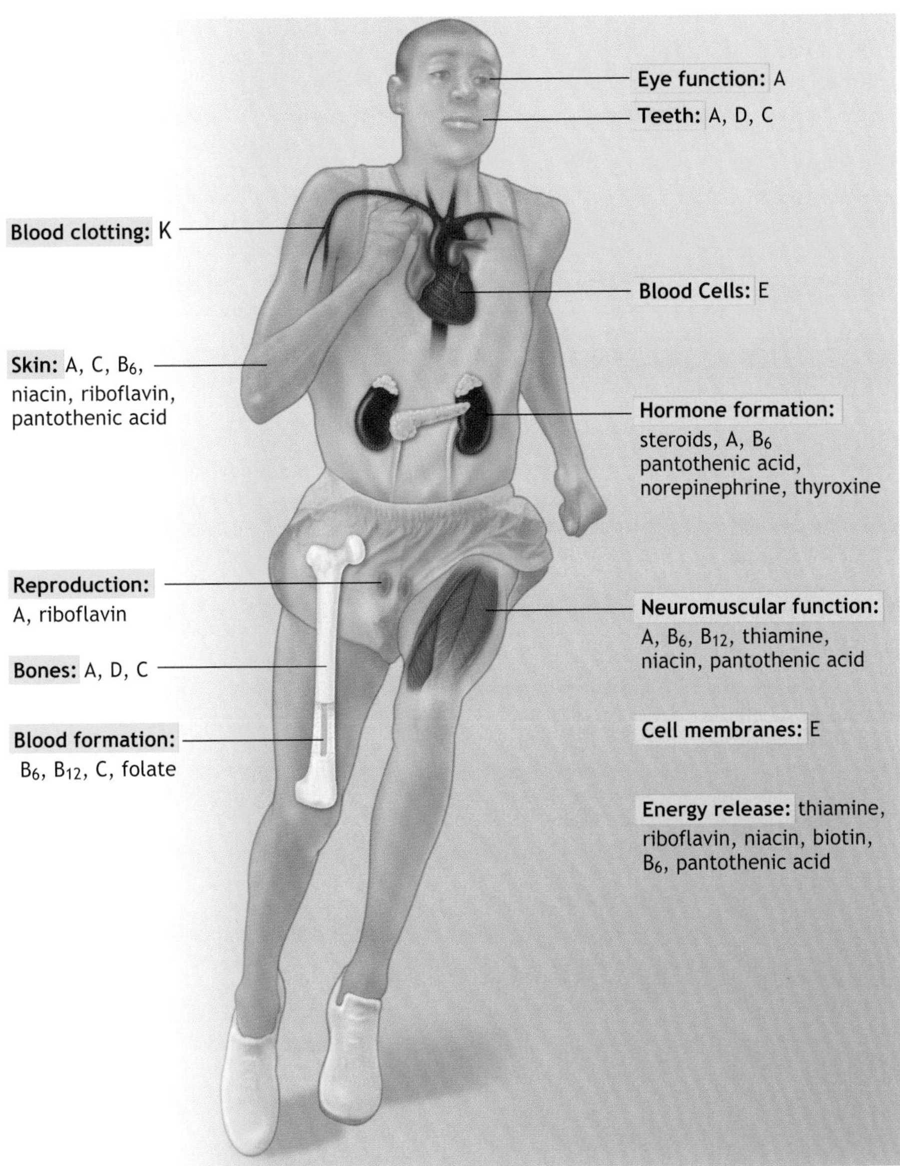

FIGURE 2.3 • Biologic functions of vitamins.

have relatively low intakes of vitamins B_1 and B_6.[43, 139] If the daily diet contains fresh fruit, grains, and uncooked or steamed vegetables, then adequate intake of these two vitamins occurs. Individuals on meatless diets should consume a small amount of milk, milk products, or eggs because vitamin B_{12} exists *only* in foods of animal origin. Recent data indicate that a relatively high intake of the B vitamins folate (400 μg) and B_6 (3 mg) reduces a woman's risk of suffering a heart attack by nearly 50%, in a manner equivalent to quitting smoking, lowering blood cholesterol, or reducing blood pressure.[131] Rich sources of these vitamins include fortified cold cereals, orange juice, spinach and other leafy greens, whole grains, nuts and seeds, bananas, legumes, potatoes, chicken, and fish. The possible protective mechanism of vitamins B_6 and folate may lie in their effects in lowering blood levels of the amino acid homocysteine, which strongly relates to an increased risk of heart attack (see Chapter 31).

Antioxidant Role of Certain Vitamins

Most of the oxygen consumed in the mitochondria during energy metabolism combines with hydrogen to produce water. Normally, 2 to 5% of oxygen forms oxygen-containing **free radicals** such as superoxide (O_2^-), hydrogen peroxide (H_2O_2), and hydroxyl (OH^-) radicals owing to electron "leakage" along the electron transport chain.[151] *A free radical is a highly chemically reactive molecule or molecular fragment that contains at least one unpaired electron in its outer orbital or valence shell.* These are the same free radicals produced by external factors such as heat and ionizing radiation and carried in cigarette smoke, environmental pollutants, and even some medications. Once formed, free radicals interact with other compounds to create new free radical molecules. These new molecules frequently damage electron-dense cellular components such as DNA and lipid-rich cell membranes.

TABLE 2.1 ➤ THE MAJOR COENZYMES, THEIR VITAMIN SOURCE, AND FUNCTION

Name	Abbreviation	Vitamin Source	Function
Biotin		Biotin	CO_2 fixation
Coenzyme A	CoA	Panthothenic acid	Acyl transfer reactions
Flavin adenine dinucleotide	FAD	B_2 (riboflavin)	Oxidation–reduction reactions
Nicotinamide adenine dinucleotide	NAD^+	Niacin	Oxidation–reduction reactions
Pyridoxal phosphate	PLP	B_6 (pyridoxine)	Amino acid metabolism (transamination)
Tetrahydrofolic acid		Folate	Transfer of single-carbon units
Thiamine pyrophosphate	TPP	B_1 (thiamine)	Aldehyde transfer

Many of the vitamins function as coenzymes in metabolic reactions. For example, vitamin B_1 (thiamine) is involved in carbohydrate metabolism and in the citric acid cycle (Krebs cycle). The active coenzyme of thiamine is thiamine diphosphate. Vitamin C is a cofactor in some hydroxylation reactions (e.g., dopamine to noradrenalin), and pantothenic acid is involved in fatty acid synthesis.

TABLE 2.2 ➤ RECOMMENDED DIETARY ALLOWANCE, FOOD SOURCES, MAJOR BODILY FUNCTIONS, AND SYMPTOMS OF DEFICIENCY OR EXCESS OF THE FAT-SOLUBLE AND WATER-SOLUBLE VITAMINS FOR HEALTHY ADULTS (19–50 YEARS)

	RDA (mg)					
Vitamin	Males	Females	Dietary Sources	Major Bodily Functions	Deficiency	Excess
Fat-soluble						
Vitamin A (retinol)	1.0	0.8	Provitamin A (β-carotene) widely distributed in green vegetables; retinol present in milk, butter, cheese, fortified margarine	Constituent of rhodopsin (visual pigment) Maintenance of epithelial tissues; role in mucopolysaccharide synthesis	Xerophthalmia (keratinization of ocular tissue), night blindness, permanent blindness	Headache, vomiting, peeling of skin, anorexia, swelling of long bones
Vitamin D	0.005	0.005	Cod-liver oil, eggs, dairy products, fortified milk, and margarine	Promotes growth and mineralization of bones Increases absorption of calcium	Rickets (bone deformities) in children Osteomalacia in adults	Vomiting, diarrhea, loss of weight, kidney damage
Vitamin E (tocopherol)	10.0	8.0	Seeds, green leafy vegetables, margarines, shortenings	Functions as an antioxidant to prevent cell damage	Possible anemia	Relatively nontoxic
Vitamin K (phylloquinone)	0.08	0.06	Green leafy vegetables, small amounts in cereals, fruits, and meats	Important in blood clotting (involved in formation of active prothrombin)	Conditioned deficiencies associated with severe bleeding; internal hemorrhages	Relatively nontoxic Synthetic forms at high doses may cause jaundice
Water-soluble						
Vitamin B_1 (thiamine)	1.2	1.1	Pork, organ meats, whole grains, nuts, legumes, milk, fruits, and vegetables	Coenzyme (thiamine prophosphate) in reactions involving the removal of carbon dioxide	Beriberi (peripheral nerve changes, edema, heart failure)	None reported
Vitamin B_2 (riboflavin)	1.3	1.1	Widely distributed in foods: meats, eggs, milk products, whole grain and enriched cereal products, wheat germ, green leafy vegetables	Constituent of two flavin nucleotide coenzymes involved in energy metabolism (FAD and FMN)	Reddened lips, cracks at mouth corner (cheilosis), eye lesions	None reported
Niacin (nicotin acid)	16	14	Liver, lean meats, poultry, grains, legumes, peanuts (can be formed from tryptophan)	Constituent of two coenzymes in oxidation-reduction reactions (NAD and NADP)	Pellagra (skin and gastrointestinal lesions, nervous mental disorders)	Flushing, burning and tingling around neck, face, and hands
Vitamin B_6 (pyridoxine)	1.3	1.3	Meats, fish, poultry, vegetables, whole grain, cereals, seeds	Coenzyme (pyridoxal phosphate) involved in amino acid and glycogen metabolism	Irritability, convulsions, muscular twitching, dermatitis, kidney stones	None reported

(continued)

TABLE 2.2 ➤ *continued*

VITAMIN	RDA (MG) MALES	RDA (MG) FEMALES	DIETARY SOURCES	MAJOR BODILY FUNCTIONS	DEFICIENCY	EXCESS
Pantothenic acid	5.0	5.0	Widely distributed in foods: meat, fish, poultry, milk products, legumes, whole grains	Constituent of coenzyme A, which plays a central role in energy metabolism	Fatigue, sleep disturbances, impaired coordination, nausea	None reported
Folate	0.4	0.4	Legumes, green vegetables, whole wheat products, meats, eggs, milk products, liver	Coenzyme (reduced form) involved in transfer of single-carbon units in nucleic acid and amino acid metabolism	Anemia, gastrointestinal disturbances, diarrhea, red tongue	None reported
Vitamin B_{12} (cobalamin)	0.0024	0.0024	Muscle meats, fish, eggs, dairy products, (absent in plant foods)	Coenzyme involved in transfer of single-carbon units in nucleic acid metabolism	Pernicious anemia, neurologic disorders	None reported
Biotin	0.03	0.03	Legumes, vegetables, meats, liver, egg yolk, nuts	Coenzymes required for fat synthesis, amino acid metabolism, and glycogen (animal starch) formation	Fatigue, depression, nausea, dermatitis, muscular pains	None reported
Vitamin C (ascorbic acid)	60	60	Citrus fruits, tomatoes, green peppers, salad greens	Maintains intercellular matrix of cartilage, bone, and dentine; important in collagen synthesis	Scurvy (degeneration of skin, teeth, blood vessels, epithelial hemorrhages)	Relatively nontoxic Possibility of kidney stones

Recommended Dietary Allowances, revised 1989. Food and Nutrition Board, National Academy of Sciences–National Research Council, Washington, DC, and modified from 1998 Dietary Reference Intakes. Food and Nutrition Board Institute of Medicine. National Academy of Sciences. Washington, DC: National Academy Press. (www2.nas.edu/iom)

Fortunately, cells possess mechanisms to immediately counter potential oxidative damage from the challenge of chemical and enzymatic mutagens. Antioxidants scavenge the oxygen radicals or chemically eradicate them by reducing oxidized compounds. When O_2^- forms, the enzyme **superoxide dismutase** rapidly catalyzes its dismutation to form hydrogen peroxide. This enzyme catalyzes the reaction of two identical molecules to produce two molecules in different states of oxidation as follows:

$$O_2^- + O_2^- \xrightarrow[\text{superoxide dismutase}]{2\,H^+} H_2O_2 + O_2$$

The hydrogen peroxide produced in this reaction breaks down further to water and oxygen in a reaction catalyzed by the widely distributed enzyme catalase as follows:

$$2\,H_2O_2 \xrightarrow[\text{catalase}]{} 2\,H_2O + O_2$$

Protection From Disease

An accumulation of free radicals increases the potential for cellular damage (**oxidative stress**) to many biologically important substances through processes that add oxygen to cellular components. These substances include DNA, proteins, and lipid-containing structures, particularly the polyunsaturated fatty acid–rich bilayer membrane that isolates the cell from noxious toxins and carcinogens. During unchecked oxidative stress, the plasma membrane's fatty acids deteriorate through a chain-reaction series of events termed **lipid peroxidation**. These reactions incorporate abnormal amounts of oxygen into lipids and increase the vulnerability of the cell and its constituents.[56] Free radicals also facilitate peroxidation of LDL cholesterol, which accelerates atherosclerosis.[97,158] Oxidative stress ultimately increases the likelihood of cellular deterioration associated with advanced aging, many diseases, and a general decline in central nervous system and immune functions.

Although no way currently exists to stop oxygen reduction and free radical production, the body does provide an elaborate natural defense against their damaging effects. This defense includes the antioxidant scavenger enzymes catalase, glutathione peroxidase, superoxide dismutase, and metal binding (metalloenzyme) proteins.[68,166] In addition, the nutritive-reducing agents vitamins A, C, and E and the vitamin A-precursor, β-carotene (a "carotenoid" in dark green and orange vegetables) serve important protective functions.[86,126,159] Antioxidant vitamins protect the plasma membrane by reacting with and removing free radicals, thus quenching the chain reaction; these vitamins also blunt the damaging effects to cellular constituents of high serum homocysteine levels.[112]

Maintaining a diet with appropriate quantities of antioxidant vitamins and other chemoprotective agents may reduce the risk of several types of cancers.[66,105,132] β-carotene protects against several cancers in humans, yet it paradoxically *increases* lung cancer risk in heavy smokers and workers exposed to asbestos.[119] This contradiction could result from β-carotene's role in increasing the production of enzymes that interact to augment the effects of "procarcinogens" (specific enzymes that convert chemicals into carcinogens) in tobacco smoke.

Reports indicate that a normal to above normal vitamin E intake (in α- and γ-tocopherol forms) and β-carotene and/or high serum levels of carotenoids blunt the progression of coronary artery narrowing and reduce heart attack and possibly diabetes risk in men and women.[57,63,70,80,87] In contrast, a recent large clinical trial of patients at high heart disease risk failed to show any benefit from vitamin E supplements (400 IU daily) in preventing cardiovascular complications and death.[185] Almost 30% of adults in the United States have low blood levels of vitamin E.[45]

A mechanism for heart disease protection proposes that antioxidant vitamins prevent oxidation of LDL cholesterol and its subsequent uptake into foam cells embedded in the arterial wall. In the "**oxidative-modification hypothesis**," the mild oxidation of LDL cholesterol—similar to butter turning rancid—contributes to the plaque-forming, artery-clogging process of atherosclerosis.[34,69,92,160] The reduction in heart disease risk for menopausal women who receive estrogen supplements may also lie in this hormone's antioxidant properties for blunting LDL cholesterol oxidation.[141]

Other Antioxidants

The antioxidant effects of selenium and coenzyme Q_{10} remain unclear. Selenium (and other trace minerals such as copper, manganese, and zinc) may possess antioxidant properties owing to their incorporation within the structure of glutathione peroxidase and other enzymes that protect plasma membranes from free radical damage.[166] Selenium also may offer protection from the development and spread of prostate cancer.[23,184] Coenzyme Q_{10} probably acts as an antioxidant either singularly within the respiratory chain or as a recycler of vitamin E. Little evidence exists to indicate that coenzyme Q_{10} exerts the same direct antioxidant effect as vitamin E. At this time, prudent advice recommends consuming a well-balanced diet with ample fruits, grains, and vegetables to increase the antioxidant capacity of blood. Rich dietary sources of antioxidants include:

- **β-carotene** (best known of the pigmented compounds, or carotenoids, that give color to yellow and green, leafy vegetables): carrots; dark-green leafy vegetables such as spinach, broccoli, turnips, beet and collard greens; sweet potatoes; winter squash; apricots; cantaloupe; mangos; papaya
- **Vitamin C:** citrus fruits and juices, cabbage, broccoli, turnip greens, cantaloupe, tomatoes, strawberries, apples with skin
- **Vitamin E:** vegetable oils, wheat germ, whole-grain bread and cereals, dried beans, green, leafy vegetables

EXERCISE, FREE RADICALS, AND ANTIOXIDANTS

The beneficial effects of physical activity are well known, but consideration of the possibility of negative effects is a recent development.[73] Potentially negative effects may occur because elevated aerobic metabolism in exercise increases production of free radicals.[89] In humans, free-radical production and tissue damage are not directly measured but, rather, inferred from markers of free radical byproducts. Increased free radicals could possibly overwhelm the body's natural defenses and pose a health risk from increased oxidative stress.[68] Free radicals may also play a role in muscle injury and soreness that commonly result from eccentric muscle actions and unaccustomed exercise.

The opposing position maintains that while free radical production increases during exercise, the body's normal antioxidant defenses are either adequate or concomitantly improve. Improvement occurs as natural enzymatic defenses (e.g., superoxide dismutase and glutathione peroxidase) become "upregulated" through both endurance and sprint training adaptations.[48,61,124,125,146,174] *Research supports this latter position; the beneficial effects of regular exercise decrease the incidence of various cancers and heart disease, whose occurrences relate to oxidative stress.* Regular exercise training also protects against myocardial injury from lipid peroxidation induced by short-term tissue ischemia followed by reperfusion.[32]

Increased Metabolism and Free-Radical Production

Exercise produces reactive oxygen in at least two ways. The first occurs via an electron leak in the mitochondria, probably at the cytochrome level, that produces superoxide radicals. The second occurs during alterations in blood flow and oxygen supply—underperfusion during intense exercise followed by substantial reperfusion in recovery—which trigger excessive free-radical generation. The reintroduction of molecular oxygen in recovery produces reactive oxygen species, which magnify oxidative stress. Some argue that the potential for free-radical damage may also increase during trauma, stress, and muscle damage and from environmental pollutants, including smog. The risk of oxidative stress with exercise depends on exercise intensity and the participant's state of training. Also, the type of oxidative stress may vary with the aerobic and anaerobic nature of the exhaustive physical activity (e.g., prolonged running versus isometric exercise).[2] Exhaustive endurance exercise by the untrained generally produces oxidative damage in the active muscles. In addition, high-intensity resistance exercise of the body's major muscle groups increases free-radical production, indirectly measured by the lipid peroxidation byproduct malondialdehyde.[104] For women, variations in estrogen levels during the menstrual cycle do not affect the mild oxidative stress from moderate-intensity exercise.[21]

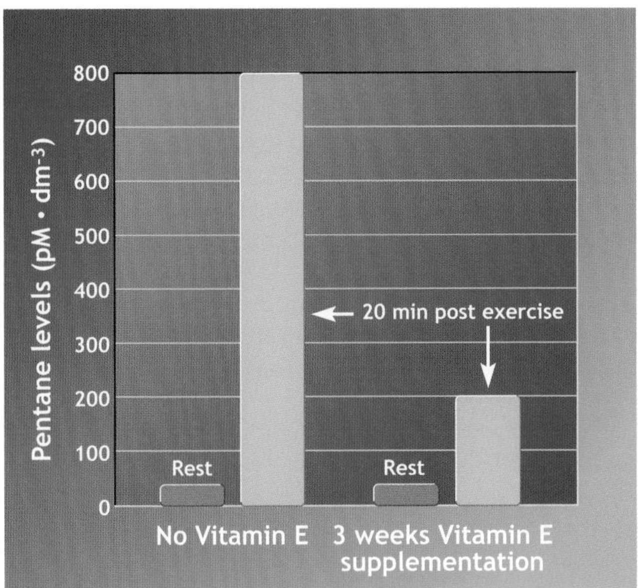

FIGURE 2.4 • Pentane levels before and after 20 minutes of exercise at 100% $\dot{V}O_{2max}$ with and without vitamin E supplementation. (Adapted from Pincemail J, et al. Pentane measurement in man as an index of lipoperoxidation. Bioelectronchem Bioenerg 1987;18:117.)

Important Questions

Two questions arise about the potential for oxidative stress with exercise: (1) are physically active individuals more prone to free-radical damage, and (2) are protective agents with antioxidant properties required in increased quantities in the diets of physically active people?

In answer to the first question, research suggests that in well-nourished humans, the body's natural antioxidant defenses respond adequately to increases in physical activity.[176] Although a single bout of submaximal exercise increased oxidant production, antioxidant defenses coped effectively. Even with repeated multiple bouts of exercise on consecutive days, various indices of oxidative stress indicated no depletion of the body's antioxidant system. The answer to the second question remains equivocal.[173] However, some evidence suggests that exogenous antioxidant compounds either blunt exercise-induced free-radical formation or augment the body's natural defense system.[68] *If supplementation proves beneficial, vitamin E may be the most important antioxidant related to exercise.*[50]

Vitamin E–deficient animals begin an exercise program with plasma membrane function compromised from oxidative damage and thus reach exhaustion earlier than animals with recommended vitamin E levels. In animals fed a normal diet, vitamin E supplements diminished oxidative damage to skeletal muscle fibers and myocardial tissue caused by exercise.[50,51] Figure 2.4 shows the effects of 3 weeks of a daily 200 International Units (IU) vitamin E supplement on pentane elimination (pentane provides a marker of free-radical production) in men after maximal exercise. The vitamin E–supplemented trials dramatically reduced free-radical production. Humans fed a daily antioxidant vitamin mixture of β-carotene, vitamin C, and vitamin E had lower serum and breath markers of lipid peroxidation at rest and following exercise than subjects not receiving supplements.[73] Five months of vitamin E supplementation in racing cyclists reduced markers of oxidative stress induced by extreme endurance exercise. For intense whole-body resistance training, 2 weeks of daily supplementation with 120 IU of vitamin E decreased free-radical interaction with cellular membranes and blunted muscle tissue disruption caused by a bout of heavy exercise.[104]

Recommended vitamin E supplementation ranges between 100 and 400 IU per day. IU is the common unit of measurements on supplement labels. If vitamin E comes from isolated food sources, 1 mg equals 1.5 IU; if taken in supplement form, 1 mg equals 1 IU. This lower conversion reflects a higher concentration of a less active form of vitamin E. Daily supplements of vitamin E containing up to 800 IU probably pose no risk for most people. Higher amounts have produced harmful effects (e.g., internal bleeding) by inhibiting vitamin K metabolism, particularly in people taking anticoagulants.

Antioxidant supplementation with α-lipoic acid (thioctic acid or lipoate), a proglutathione dietary supplement, influenced tissue antioxidant defenses to counteract lipid peroxidation during rest and strenuous exercise.[56] While vitamin C possesses strong antioxidant properties, whether or not it exerts a protective effect in exercise remains unclear.

VITAMIN SUPPLEMENTS: THE COMPETITIVE EDGE?

Figure 2.5 illustrates the progressive increase in money spent on dietary supplements in the United States between 1990 and 1996. Of this total, vitamin–mineral pills and powders represent the most common form of supplement used by the general public, accounting for 70% of the more than \$6.5 billion spent annually. Particularly susceptible marketing targets include the exercise enthusiast, the competitive athlete, and coaches and

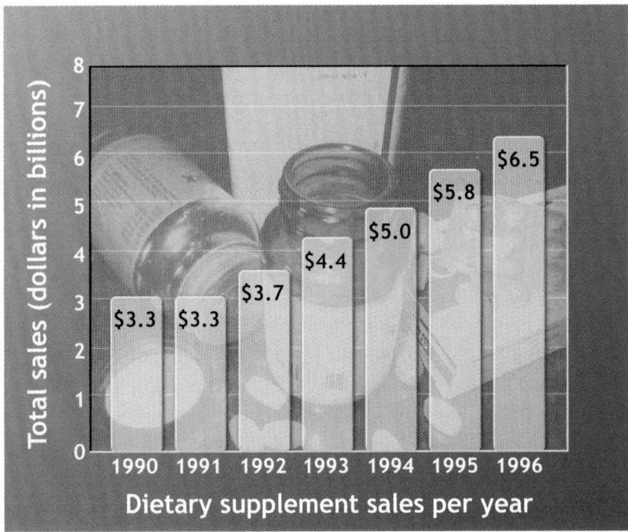

FIGURE 2.5 • Expansion of the dietary supplement industry. (From Packaged Facts Inc., NYC. U.S. Food and Drug Administration. FDA consumer: an FDA guide to dietary supplements. Sep-Oct, 1998.)

personal trainers who assist athletes in achieving peak performance. More than 50% of competitive athletes in some sports consume supplements on a regular basis, either to ensure adequate micronutrient intake or to achieve an excess with the hope of enhancing performance and training responsiveness.[24,25,76]

Vitamins synthesized in the laboratory are no less effective for bodily functions than vitamins from food sources. When deficiencies exist, vitamin supplements can reverse the deficiency symptoms. However, when vitamin intake achieves recommended levels, supplements neither improve exercise performance nor necessarily increase the blood levels of these micronutrients. The facts, however, often become clouded by "testimonials" from coaches and elite athletes who attribute their success to a particular dietary modification (which usually includes specific vitamin supplements). *More than 40 years of research does not support the wisdom of using vitamin (and mineral) supplements to improve exercise performance, the hormonal and metabolic responses to exercise, or the ability to train arduously in healthy people with nutritionally adequate diets.*[13,102,168,178]

Megavitamins

Most nutritionists believe that no harm results from taking a multivitamin capsule containing the recommended quantity of each vitamin. Supplementing daily with vitamin C may actually confer some benefit to individuals engaged in heavy exercise and who have problems with frequent viral upper respiratory tract infections (URTIs).[62] Some athletes take **megavitamins**, or doses at least 10 times and up to 1000 times the RDA, hoping to improve exercise performance by "supercharging" with vitamins. Such a practice warrants concern and may cause harm, except in serious medical illness requiring a pharmacologic dose of vitamins.

INTEGRATIVE QUESTION

Respond to an athlete who asks: "What's wrong with taking megadoses of vitamin and mineral supplements to ensure I'm getting an adequate intake on a daily basis?"

Excess Vitamins Behave as Chemicals

Once the enzyme systems with specific vitamin cofactors become saturated, any excess vitamins taken in megadose function as chemicals (drugs) in the body. For example, a megadose of water-soluble vitamin C can raise serum uric acid levels and precipitate gout in people predisposed to this disease. At intakes above 1,000 mg daily, urinary excretion of oxalate (a breakdown product of vitamin C) increases, accelerating kidney stone formation in susceptible individuals.[91] Also, some American blacks, Asians, and Sephardic Jews have a genetic metabolic deficiency that becomes activated to hemolytic anemia with excessive vitamin C intake. In iron-deficient individuals, taking megadoses of vitamin C may destroy significant amounts of vitamin B_{12}. In healthy people, vitamin C supplements frequently irritate the bowel and cause diarrhea. Further disconcerting news about excesses in vitamin C supplementation comes from British researchers.[123] Thirty healthy men and women who consumed a 500-mg supplement of vitamin C daily for 6 weeks showed undesirable changes in cellular DNA that constitutes an individual's genetic makeup. The favorable antioxidant properties of vitamin C were shown for the guanine base part of the DNA molecule. The unexpected findings came from evaluating a second indicator of DNA oxidation, oxoadenine. With vitamin C supplementation, oxoadenine increased rather than declined, indicating some genetic damage. The potential pro-oxidant effect of excess exogenous vitamin C should serve as a cautionary note to those who significantly exceed the recommended 60-mg daily intake. Importantly, vitamin C in natural form in such foods as orange juice does not appear to exhibit pro-oxidant properties.

Excess vitamin B_6 may induce liver disease and nerve damage. Excessive riboflavin (B_2) can impair vision. A megadose of nicotinic acid (niacin) functions as a potent vasodilator and inhibits fatty acid mobilization during exercise, which could cause more-rapid depletion of glycogen reserves. Folic acid excess in supplement form can trigger an allergic response, producing hives, light-headedness, and breathing difficulties. Possible side effects of vitamin E megadose include headache, fatigue, blurred vision, gastrointestinal disturbances, internal bleeding, muscular weakness, and low blood sugar. The toxicity to the nervous system of a vitamin A megadose and the damaging effects to the kidneys of excess vitamin D are well established.

Data from the U.S. National Health Interview Survey and other surveys provide troubling indications that up to 42% of American adults use vitamin and/or mineral supplements, often at potentially toxic dosages.[170] If vitamin supplementation does offer benefits to physically active individuals, it may only apply to those with marginal vitamin stores. Well-controlled research must fully determine if and under what circumstances such supplementation confers benefits. Perhaps the misuse and abuse of vitamins by individuals hoping to improve athletic performance can be put in proper perspective by the following quotation from nearly 22 years ago: "The sale of vitamins is probably the biggest rip-off in our society today."[120]

VITAMIN C MAY PROTECT AGAINST URTI. A 600-mg daily supplement of vitamin C before and for 3 weeks following a 90-km ultramarathon significantly reduced symptoms of URTI (running nose, sneezing, sore throat, coughing, fever) compared with those in runners who received a placebo.[121] Duration and severity of symptoms also decreased in a nonrunning control group who took vitamin C supplements. For the athletes, risk of infection was inversely related to race performance; those who performed best suffered more URTI symptoms. A greater infection rate also occurred among runners with the most strenuous training regimens.

Vitamins and Exercise Performance

Figure 2.6 illustrates that the B-complex vitamins play key roles as coenzymes to regulate important energy-yielding reactions during carbohydrate, fat, and protein catabolism. They

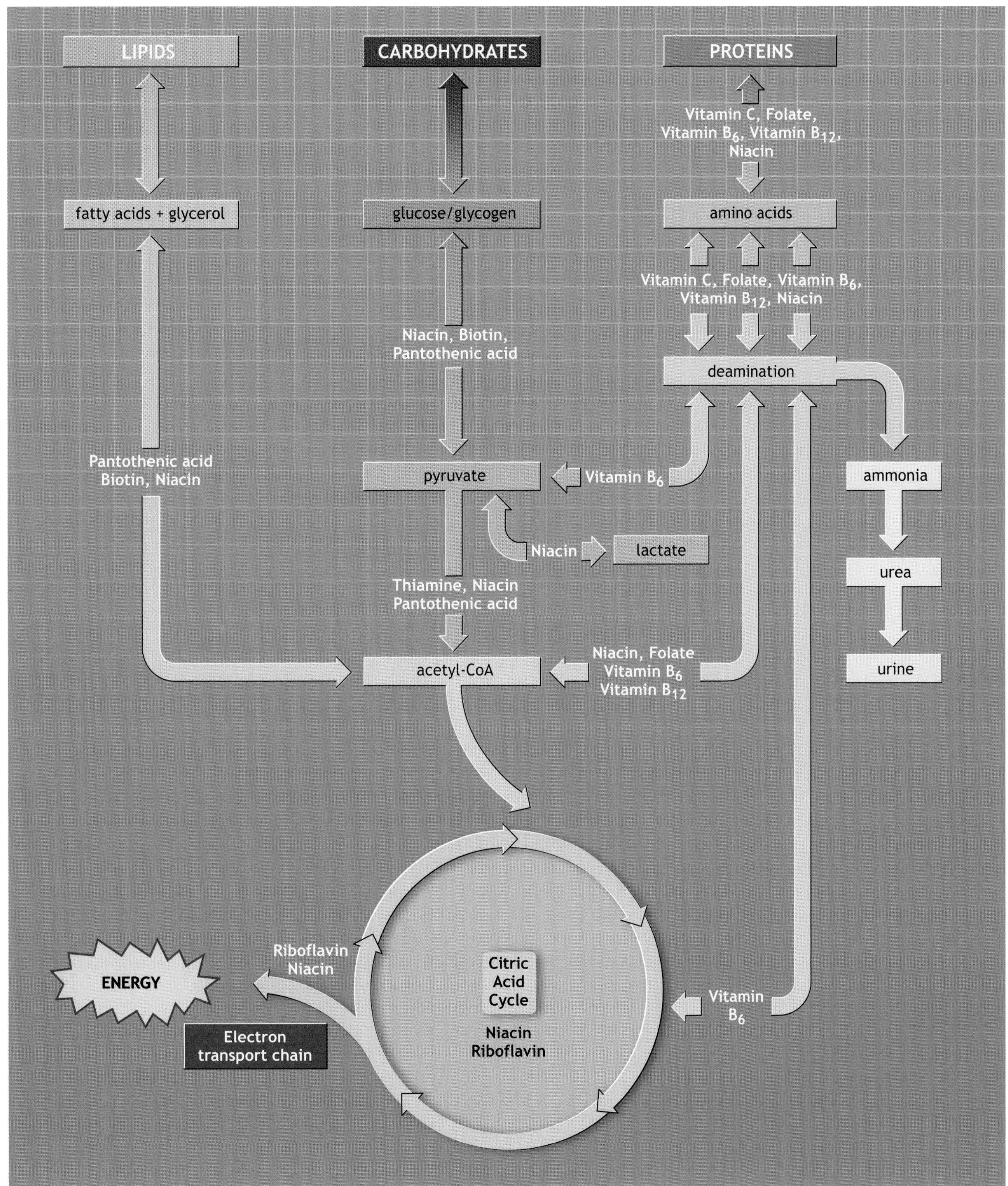

FIGURE 2.6 • General schema for the role of water-soluble vitamins in carbohydrate, fat, and protein metabolism.

also contribute to hemoglobin synthesis and red blood cell production. However, the belief that "if a little is good, more must be better" has led many coaches, athletes, fitness enthusiasts, and even some scientists to advocate using vitamin supplements above recommended levels. Research findings and the overwhelming majority of professional nutritionists simply do not support this approach.

Supplementing with vitamin B_6, an essential cofactor in glycogen and amino acid metabolism, did not benefit the metabolic mixture metabolized by women during high-intensity aerobic exercise. Data indicate that athletes' status for this vitamin equaled reference standards for the population[102] and did not decrease with strenuous exercise to a level warranting supplementation.[138] For endurance-trained men, 9 days of vitamin B_6 supplementation (20 mg per day) provided no ergogenic effect on exercise time to exhaustion while cycling at 71% of aerobic capacity.[175]

Chronic high-potency, multivitamin–mineral supplementation for well-nourished, healthy individuals did not augment aerobic fitness, muscular strength, and athletic performance.[148] In addition to the B-complex group, no exercise benefit exists for excess vitamins C and E on stamina, circulatory function, or energy metabolism. For example, short-term daily supplementation with vitamin E (400 IU) produced no effect on normal neuroendocrine and metabolic responses to strenuous exercise or performance time to exhaustion.[150] Supplementing with vitamin C had negligible effects on endurance performance and did not alter the rate, severity, and duration of injuries from those with a placebo treatment.[47] The energy intake of active people generally increases to match the increased energy requirement of physical activity; thus, a proportionate increase also occurs in micronutrient intake, often in amounts greatly exceeding recommended levels.

Summary

1. Vitamins, organic compounds that neither supply energy nor contribute to body mass, serve crucial functions in almost all bodily processes. They must be obtained from food or dietary supplementation.
2. Plants synthesize vitamins; animals also produce them from precursor substances known as provitamins.
3. Thirteen known vitamins are classified as either water soluble or fat soluble. The fat-soluble vitamins are A, D, E, and K; vitamin C and the B-complex vitamins are the water-soluble vitamins.
4. Excess fat-soluble vitamins accumulate in body tissues and can increase to toxic concentrations. Except in relatively rare instances, excess water-soluble vitamins generally remain nontoxic and are eventually excreted in the urine.
5. Vitamins regulate metabolism, facilitate energy release, and play key functions in bone and tissue synthesis.
6. Vitamins A, C, E, and the provitamin β-carotene serve important protective functions as antioxidants. A diet with appropriate levels of these micronutrients helps to reduce the potential for free-radical damage (oxidative stress) and may protect against heart disease and cancer.
7. Physical activity elevates metabolism and increases the production of potentially harmful free radicals. The daily diet should contain foods rich in antioxidant vitamins and minerals to attenuate the potential for oxidative stress.
8. For well-nourished individuals, the body's natural antioxidant defenses upregulate in response to increased physical activity. Support for this belief comes from research showing the beneficial effects of regular exercise on the incidence of heart disease and various forms of cancer, whose occurrences relate to oxidative stress.
9. Vitamin supplementation above the RDA does not improve exercise performance or the potential to sustain intense physical training. Serious illness can occur from regularly consuming an excess of fat-soluble and, in some instances, water-soluble vitamins.

➤ PART 2 • Minerals

THE NATURE OF MINERALS

In addition to the organic elements carbon, oxygen, hydrogen, and nitrogen, approximately 4% of the body's mass (about 2 kg for a 50-kg woman), consists of 22 mostly metallic elements collectively called **minerals**. Minerals serve as constituents of enzymes, hormones, and vitamins; they combine with other chemicals (e.g., calcium phosphate in bone, iron in the heme of hemoglobin) or exist singularly (e.g., free calcium and sodium in body fluids).

The minerals essential to life include seven **major minerals** (required in amounts $>$100 mg daily) and 14 minor or **trace minerals** (required in amounts $<$100 mg daily). Trace minerals account for less than 15 g (approximately 0.5 oz), or 0.02% of the total body mass. Like consuming excess vitamins, excess mineral intake serves no useful physiologic purpose and can even produce toxic effects. RDAs and recommended ranges of intakes have been established for many minerals; if the diet supplies these mineral requirements, then this ensures an adequate intake of the remaining minerals.

Most minerals, major or trace, occur freely in nature—mainly in the waters of rivers, lakes, and oceans; in topsoil; and beneath the earth's surface. Minerals exist in the root systems of plants and the body structure of animals that consume plants and water containing minerals.

KINDS AND SOURCES OF MINERALS

Table 2.3 lists the important minerals and their functions, food sources, and daily requirements. Mineral supplements, like vitamin supplements, generally confer little benefit because a well-balanced diet readily supplies them. However, some supplementation may be necessary in geographic regions where the soil or water supply lack a particular mineral. For example, relatively poor concentrations of iodine occur in the basin of the Great Lakes and Pacific Northwest of the United States and in central Brazil and the Himalayan mountain region. Iodine is required by the thyroid gland to synthesize the hormones thyroxine and tri-iodothyronine, which accelerate the cells' resting metabolism. Adding iodine

TABLE 2.3 ➤ **THE IMPORTANT MAJOR AND MINOR (TRACE) MINERALS FOR HEALTHY ADULTS (AGE 19–50 YEARS) AND THEIR DIETARY REQUIREMENTS, FOOD SOURCES, FUNCTIONS, AND THE EFFECTS OF DEFICIENCIES AND EXCESSES**

	RDA (MG)			MAJOR BODILY		
MINERAL	MALES	FEMALES	DIETARY SOURCES	FUNCTIONS	DEFICIENCY	EXCESS
Major						
Calcium[a]	1000	1000	Milk, cheese, dark green vegetables, dried legumes	Bone and tooth formation, blood clotting, nerve transmission	Stunted growth, rickets, osteoporosis, convulsions	Not reported in humans
Phosphorus	700	700	Milk, cheese, yogurt, meat, poultry, grains, fish	Bone and tooth formation, acid–base balance of bone, loss of calcium	Weakness, demineralization	Erosion of jaw (phossy jaw)
Potassium	2000	2000	Leafy vegetables, canteloupe, lima beans, potatoes, bananas, milk, meats, coffee, tea	Fluid balance, nerve transmission, acid–base balance	Muscle cramps, irregular cardiac rhythm, mental confusion, loss of appetite; can be life threatening	None if kidneys function normally; poor kidney function causes potassium buildup and cardiac arrythmias
Sulfur	Unknown	Unknown	Obtained as part of dietary protein; present in food preservatives	Acid–base balance, liver function	Unlikely to occur with adequate dietary intake	Unknown
Sodium[b]	1100–3300	1100–3300	Common salt	Acid–base balance, body water balance, nerve function	Muscle cramps, mental apathy, reduced appetite	High blood pressure
Chlorine (chloride)	700	300	Chloride part of salt-containing food; some vegetables and fruits	Important part of extracellular fluids	Unlikely to occur with adequate dietary intake	Along with sodium contributes to high blood pressure
Magnesium[b]	400–420	310–320	Whole grains, green leafy vegetables	Activates enzymes involved in protein synthesis	Growth failure, behavioral disturbances	Diarrhea
Minor						
Iron	10	15	Eggs, lean meats, legumes, whole grains, green leafy vegetables	Constituent of hemoglobin and enzymes involved in energy metabolism	Iron deficiency (weakness, reduced resistance to infection)	Siderosis; cirrhosis of liver
Fluoride	4.0	3.0	Drinking water, tea, seafood	May be important in maintenance of bone structure	Higher frequency of tooth decay	Mottling of teeth, increased bone density
Zinc	15	12	Widely distributed in foods	Constituent of enzymes involved in digestion	Growth failure, small sex glands	Fever, nausea, vomiting, diarrhea
Copper[b]	1.5–3.0	1.5–3.0	Meats, drinking water	Constituent of enzymes associated with iron metabolism	Anemia, bone changes (rare)	Rare metabolic condition (Wilson's disease)
Selenium	0.070	0.055	Seafood, meats, grains	Functions in close association with vitamin E	Anemia (rare)	Gastrointestinal disorders, lung irritations
Iodine (iodide)	150	150	Marine fish and shellfish, dairy products, vegetables, iodized salt	Constituent of thyroid hormones	Goiter (enlarged thyroid)	Very high intakes depress thyroid activity
Chromium[b]	0.075–0.25	0.05–0.25	Legumes, cereals, organ meats	Constituent of some enzymes	Not reported in humans	Inhibition of enzymes
			Fats, vegetable oils, meats, whole grains	Involved in glucose and energy metabolism	Impaired ability to metabolize glucose	Occupational exposures: skin and kidney damage

Recommended Dietary Allowances, revised 1989. Food and Nutrition Board, National Academy of Sciences–National Research Council, Washington, DC, and modified from 1998 Dietary Reference Intakes. Food and Nutrition Board Institute of Medicine. National Academy of Sciences. Washington, DC: National Academy Press. (www2.nas.edu/iom)

[a]800 mg for adults 25 and older.

[b]Because there is less information on which to base allowances, these figures are given in the form of ranges.

to the water supply or to table salt (iodized salt) easily prevents iodine deficiency.

A lack of dietary iron produces a common mineral deficiency in the United States. Between 30 and 50% of American women of childbearing age suffer some form of dietary iron insufficiency (see page 66). Two iron sources exist in the diet: the first is the heme source in meat and animal products (hemoglobin), particularly red meat, liver, kidney, and heart; the second is the inorganic nonheme iron salts in foods of plant origin such as beans, peas, dried uncooked fruits, and leafy green vegetables.

ROLE OF MINERALS

Whereas vitamins catalyze chemical processes without becoming part of the reaction's byproducts, some minerals become part of the structures and existing chemicals in the body. Minerals serve three broad roles in the body:

- Minerals provide *structure* in forming bones and teeth
- In terms of *function*, minerals help maintain normal heart rhythm, muscle contractility, neural conductivity, and acid-base balance
- Minerals *regulate* cellular metabolism by becoming part of enzymes and hormones that modulate cellular activity

Figure 2.7 lists minerals that participate in catabolic and anabolic cellular processes. Minerals activate reactions that release energy during carbohydrate, fat, and protein catabolism. In addition, minerals participate in the synthesis of biologic nutrients—glycogen from glucose, triglycerides from fatty acids and glycerol, and proteins from amino acids. A lack of the essential minerals disrupts the fine balance between catabolism and anabolism. Minerals also form important constituents of hormones. Inadequate thyroxine production from iodine insufficiency, for example, significantly slows the body's resting metabolism. In extreme cases, this could predispose a person to develop obesity. The synthesis of insulin, the hormone that facilitates glucose uptake by the cells, requires zinc (as do approximately 100 enzymes), whereas the mineral chlorine forms the digestive acid hydrochloric acid.

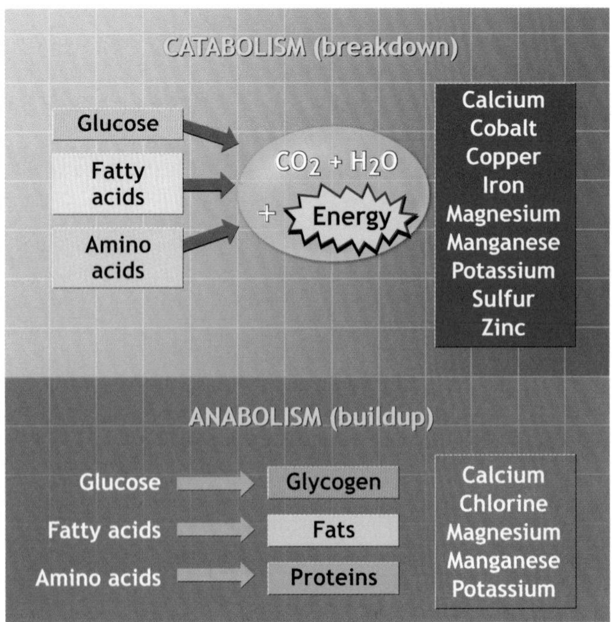

FIGURE 2.7 • Minerals that function in macronutrient catabolism and anabolism.

Mineral Bioavailability

The body varies considerably in its capacity to absorb and use the minerals in food. For example, spinach contains considerable calcium, but only about 5% of it becomes absorbed. The same holds true for dietary iron, which the intestine absorbs with an average efficiency of 5 to 10%. Factors that affect the bioavailability of minerals in the food include

- *Type of food:* The small intestine readily absorbs minerals contained in animal products because plant binders and dietary fibers are not present to hinder digestion and absorption. Also, foods from the animal kingdom generally contain a high mineral concentration (except magnesium, which has a higher concentration in plants).
- *Mineral–mineral interaction:* Many minerals have the same molecular weight and thus compete for intestinal absorption. This makes it unwise to consume an excess of any one mineral, because it can retard another mineral's absorption.
- *Vitamin–mineral interaction:* Various vitamins interact with minerals in a manner that affects mineral bioavailability. From a positive perspective, vitamin D facilitates calcium absorption, while vitamin C improves absorption of iron.
- *Fiber–mineral interaction:* High fiber intake blunts the absorption of some minerals (e.g., calcium, iron, magnesium, phosphorus) by binding to them and causing them to pass unabsorbed through the digestive tract.

In the subsequent sections, we describe specific functions for several of the more important minerals related to physical activity.

CALCIUM

Calcium, the most abundant mineral in the body, combines with phosphorus to form bones and teeth. These two minerals represent about 75% of the body's total mineral content, or about 2.5% of body mass. In its ionized form (about 1% of the body's 1200 mg of calcium), calcium functions in muscle stimulation, blood clotting, transmission of nerve impulses, activation of several enzymes, synthesis of calcitriol (active form of vitamin D), and transport of fluids across cell membranes. It also may contribute to easing premenstrual syndrome, preventing colon cancer, and optimizing blood pressure regulation.[40,103]

Osteoporosis: Calcium, Estrogen, and Exercise

Bone, a dynamic tissue matrix of collagen and minerals, consists of about 50% water. It exists in a continual state of flux, or **remodeling**, in which bone-destroying cells (osteoclasts) cause the breakdown (resorption) of bone under the influence of parathyroid hormone. Bone-forming osteoblast cells induce bone synthesis. Calcium availability significantly affects the dynamics of bone remodeling. Calcium derived from food or calcium derived from the resorption of the bone mass maintains the plasma calcium level. The two broad categories of bone are

- **Cortical bone**: dense, hard outer layer of bone such as the shafts of the long bones of the arms and legs
- **Trabecular bone**: spongy, less dense, and relatively weaker bone most prevalent in the vertebrae and ball of the femur

Growing children require more calcium daily per unit body mass than adults to achieve their full genetic potential for bone mass. As a general guideline, adolescents and young adults require 1200 mg of calcium daily (800 to 1000 mg for adults over age 24), or about as much calcium as in five 8-oz glasses of milk. Unfortunately, calcium remains one of the nutrients frequently lacking in the diet of most individuals including athletes. For an average adult, daily calcium intake ranges between 500 and 700 mg. More than 75% of adults consume less than the RDA, and about 25% of females in the United States consume less than 300 mg of calcium on any given day.[60] *Among athletes, female dancers, gymnasts, and endurance competitors are most prone to calcium dietary insufficiency.*[14,33,109] Inadequate calcium intake or low levels of calcium-regulating hormones cause withdrawal of calcium "reserves" in bone to restore any deficit. Prolonging this restorative imbalance promotes one of two conditions: (1) **osteoporosis**, literally meaning "porous bones," with bone density more than 2.5 standard deviations below normal for age and gender, or (2) **osteopenia**—from the Greek words *osteo,* meaning "bone," and *penia,* meaning poverty—a midway condition in which bones weaken with increased risk of fractures. Osteoporosis develops progressively as bone loses its mineral mass (bone mineral content) and calcium concentration (bone mineral density) and progressively becomes porous and brittle (Fig. 2.8). The stresses of normal living often cause bone to break, with compression fracture of the spine occurring most frequently.

INTEGRATIVE QUESTION

Discuss the interactions among physical activity, calcium intake, and bone health.

A Disease of Growing Prevalence

Osteoporosis currently afflicts 20 to 25 million Americans, of whom 80 to 90% are women; 50% of all women eventually develop osteoporosis. Men are not immune from osteoporosis; 1.5 to 2.0 million men (1 in 8 older than 50 years) suffer from this disease. Osteoporosis has reached near-epidemic proportions, particularly among women above age 60. Osteoporosis accounts for more than 1.5 million fractures (the clinical manifestation of the disease) yearly, including about 500,000 to 600,000 spinal fractures and nearly 300,000 hip fractures. The annual medical cost of hip fractures in the United States may exceed $240 billion by the mid-21st century.

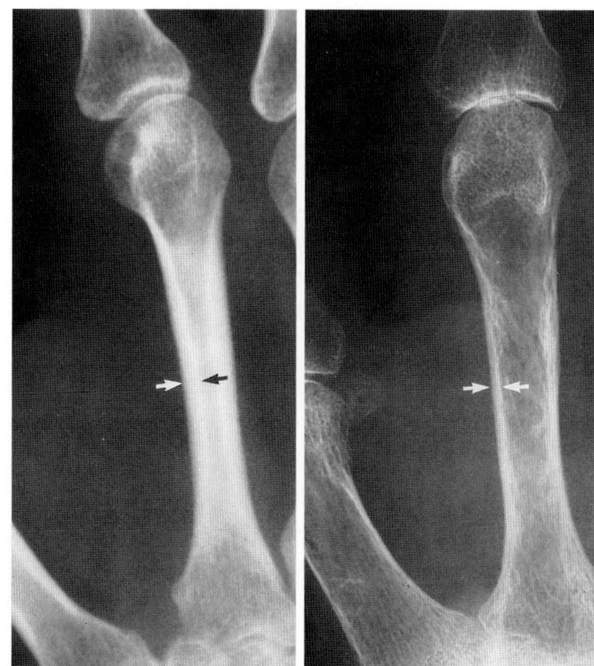

FIGURE 2.8 • Radiograph of mid-second metacarpal of person with normal mineralization (*left*) and of patient with severe osteoporosis (*right*). Under normal conditions, cortical width (arrows) is greater than one-third of the total width of the metacarpal, whereas osteoporosis produces extreme cortical narrowing. Note also the intracortical tunneling that occurs in more aggressive forms of osteoporosis. (From Brant W, Helms C. Fundamentals of diagnostic radiology. 2nd edition. Baltimore: Williams & Wilkins, 1998.)

RISK FACTORS FOR OSTEOPOROSIS

- History of fracture as an adult, regardless of cause
- History of fracture in a parent or sibling
- Cigarette smoking
- Slight build or tendency toward underweight
- White or Asian female
- Sedentary lifestyle
- Early menopause
- Eating disorder
- High protein intake (particularly animal protein)
- Excess sodium intake
- Alcohol abuse
- Calcium-deficient diet in the years before and after menopause
- High caffeine intake (equivocal)
- Vitamin D deficiency, either through inadequate exposure to sunlight or dietary insufficiency (prevalent in about 40% of adults)

Increased susceptibility to osteoporosis among older women coincides with menopause and the marked decrease in estradiol secretion, the most potent naturally occurring human estrogen.[29] Exactly how estrogen exerts its protective effects on bone remains unknown (see page 65 for estrogen's possible actions). Most men normally produce some estrogen into old age—a major reason why they exhibit a relatively lower prevalence of osteoporosis. In addition, a portion of circulating testosterone converts to estradiol, which also promotes positive calcium balance in men. Osteoporosis risk factors for men include low testosterone levels, cigarette smoking, and use of steroid medications.

A Progressive Disease

Between 60 to 80% of an individual's susceptibility to osteoporosis links to genetic factors, while 20 to 40% remains lifestyle related. Proper nutrition (adequate calcium and vitamin D, which maintain normal blood levels of calcium and bone mineralization)[90,167] and regular physical activity enable women to gain bone mass throughout the third decade of life. However, the early teens serve as the prime years to maximize bone mass.[15,164] In reality, osteoporosis for many women begins early in life because the average teenager consumes suboptimal calcium to support growing bones. This often creates an irreversible deficit that cannot be fully eliminated after achieving skeletal maturity. Calcium imbalance worsens into adulthood (particularly among women with genetic predisposition toward the disease).[93,171] By middle age, many adult women consume only one third of the calcium required for optimal bone maintenance.

Beginning at about age 50, the typical man experiences an average bone loss of 0.4% each year, whereas women begin to lose twice this amount at age 35. For men, the rate of bone mineral loss does not usually pose a problem until the eighth decade of life. Menopause, however, makes women highly susceptible to osteoporosis because the ovaries release little or no estrogen. Muscle, adipose tissue, and connective tissues continue to produce estrogen but in limited quantities. The dramatic decrease in estrogen production at menopause coincides with reduced intestinal calcium absorption, reduced calcitonin production (a hormone that blunts bone resorption), and increased bone resorption as bone loss accelerates to 3 to 6% per year in the 5 years after menopause. The rate then drops to approximately 1% yearly. At this rate, the typical woman loses about 15% of bone mass in the first decade after menopause, and some women lose as much as 30% of bone mineral mass by age 70.

Prevention

Adequate calcium intake throughout life remains the prime defense against bone loss with age.[12,71,78,116] For example, increasing the calcium intake of adolescent girls from their normal 80% of the RDA to 110% through supplementation significantly increased total body calcium and spinal bone density. The National Institutes of Health consensus panel recommends that adolescent girls consume 1500 mg of calcium daily. Furthermore, experts recommend increasing daily calcium intake for middle-aged women, particularly estrogen-deprived women after menopause, to 1200 to 1500 mg to improve the body's calcium balance.[59,128] Additional calcium provides beneficial effects in slowing the rate of bone loss, even with inadequate estrogen.[116] Because the typical quantity of calcium present in major meals inhibits iron absorption, adolescents and menstruating and pregnant women with high iron requirements should take calcium supplements (if needed) before going to bed.[55]

Good dietary calcium sources include milk and milk products, sardines and canned salmon, kidney beans, and dark green leafy vegetables. Calcium supplements, best absorbed on an empty stomach, can also correct dietary deficiencies regardless of whether the extra calcium comes from fortified foods or commercial supplements. Calcium citrate causes less stomach upset than other supplement forms and also enhances iron absorption compared to calcium gluconate, calcium carbonate, or commercial products such as Tums. Adequate availability of vitamin D (currently estimated to be 800 IU daily) facilitates calcium uptake, while excessive consumption of meat, salt, coffee, and alcohol inhibits its absorption. A high caffeine intake also relates to a negative bone status in postmenopausal women.[94] Reduced vitamin D levels impair calcium uptake and increase levels of parathyroid hormone, which facilitates bone loss. In postmenopausal women, estrogen supplements, calcitonin, selective estrogen receptor modulators, biophosphonates, or low-dose, slow-release fluoride plus calcium supplements serve as a treatment for severe osteoporosis and substantially reduce risk of bone fracture.[12,29]

Estrogen therapy, usually continued for prolonged periods, increases risk for cancers of the uterus, breast, and other organs. For most women, the beneficial effects of hormone replacement therapy in reducing coronary heart disease risk generally outweigh an increased cancer risk.[26]

EXERCISE PROVIDES BENEFITS. *Regular exercise slows the rate of skeletal aging*. Regardless of age or gender, children and adults who maintain an active lifestyle show significantly greater bone mass than their sedentary counterparts.[4,10,16,20,81,115,148,172] Benefits of regular exercise often accrue into the seventh and even eighth

FIVE PRINCIPLES FOR PROMOTING BONE HEALTH THROUGH EXERCISE

- *Specificity:* exercise provides a local osteogenic effect.
- *Overload:* progressively increasing exercise intensity promotes continued bone deposition.
- *Initial Values:* individuals with the smallest total bone mass show the greatest potential for bone deposition.
- *Diminishing Returns:* as one approaches the biologic ceiling for bone density, further density gains require greater effort.
- *Reversibility:* discontinuing exercise overload reverses the positive osteogenic effects gained through appropriate exercise stress.

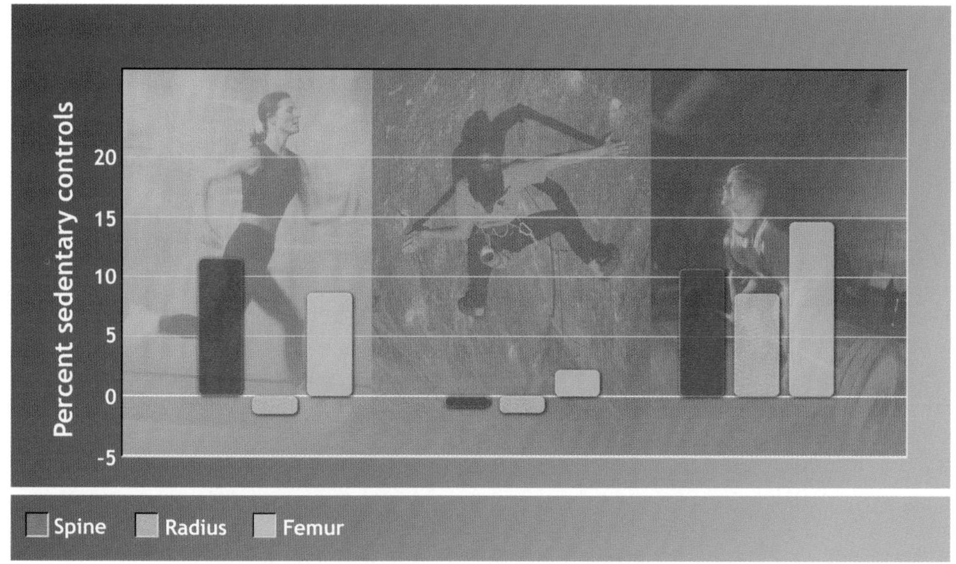

FIGURE 2.9 • Bone mineral density expressed as a percentage of sedentary control values at three skeletal sites for runners, swimmers, and weight lifters. (From Drinkwater BL. Physical activity, fitness, and osteoporosis. In: Bouchard C, et al., eds. Physical activity, fitness, and health. Champaign, IL: Human Kinetics, 1994.)

decades of life.[161] The decline in vigorous exercise with a sedentary lifestyle as a person ages closely parallels the age-related bone mass loss. Regular exercise also counters the accelerated bone loss that accompanies weight reduction in postmenopausal women.[140]

Although not as effective as hormone replacement therapy in preventing bone loss in the early postmenopausal period, mechanical loading of bone through exercise provides a potent stimulus to maintain or increase bone mass in adults.[3] Figure 2.9 illustrates the beneficial effects of heavy resistance exercises and circuit-resistance training or weight-bearing exercise such as walking, running, dancing, rope skipping, or gymnastics. These exercise modes generate significant intermittent force against the body's long bones.[1,38,41,162,180] Walking only 1 mile per day provides beneficial effects during and after menopause. Activities that provide relatively high impact on the skeletal mass (e.g., volleyball, basketball, and gymnastics) induce the greatest increases in bone mass.[35,44] Men and women who participate in strength and power activities have as much or more bone mass than endurance athletes.[136] The exercise effects are site specific to the working muscles and bones to which they attach.[88] In fact, bone mineral density relates directly to measures of muscular strength and regional lean tissue mass;[114] the lumbar spine and proximal femur bone masses of elite teenage weight lifters exceed representative values for fully mature bone of reference adults.[27] Eccentric exercise training may provide a more potent site-specific osteogenic stimulus than concentric muscle training because greater forces usually occur with eccentric muscle loading.[58] Prior exercise and sports experience may provide a residual effect on an adult's bone mineral density. Retrospective cross-sectional studies of ex-athletes and their controls and prospective studies of the same athletes over time indicate that exercise-induced differences in bone mass achieved during teenage and young-adult years do not readily disappear with cessation of active competition.[77,82]

SITE-SPECIFIC EFFECTS. In a normal hormonal milieu for both children and adults, muscle forces acting on specific bones during physical activity (particularly intermittent compression and tension mechanical loading) modify bone metabolism at the point of stress.[9,10,67,74] The lower limb bones of older cross-country runners have greater bone mineral content than the bones of less active counterparts, while the throwing arm of baseball players shows greater bone thickness than their less-used, nondominant arm. Likewise, the bone mineral content of the humeral shaft and proximal humerus of the playing arm of tennis players generally averages 20 to 25% greater than that of the nondominant arm; side-to-side differences in comparisons of the arms of nonplayers generally average only 5%.[82]

Prevailing theory considers that bone reacts as a piezoelectric crystal that converts mechanical stress into electrical energy. The electrical changes stimulate osteoblasts to accumulate calcium. Bone accretion depends on two important factors: (1) magnitude of applied force and (2) frequency of application. Chemicals produced in bone also may contribute to bone formation, while alterations in bone's geometric configuration in response to long-term exercise also enhance its mechanical properties.[9] Figure 2.10 illustrates the anatomic structure and cross-sectional view of a typical long bone and depicts the dynamics of bone growth and remodeling.

The Female Athlete Triad: Unexpected Problem for Women Who Train Intensely

A paradox exists between exercise and bone dynamics for athletic premenopausal women, particularly young athletes who have yet to attain peak bone mass (see "Focus on Research"). Women who train intensely and emphasize weight loss often engage in disordered eating behaviors. This further decreases energy availability, reducing body mass and body fat to a point that (1) creates irregularities in menstrual cycle function (**oligomenorrhea**; 35 to 90 days between periods) or (2) causes cessation of menstruation (**secondary amenorrhea**). Clinicians define secondary amenorrhea as cessation of monthly menstrual cycles for at least 3 consecutive months

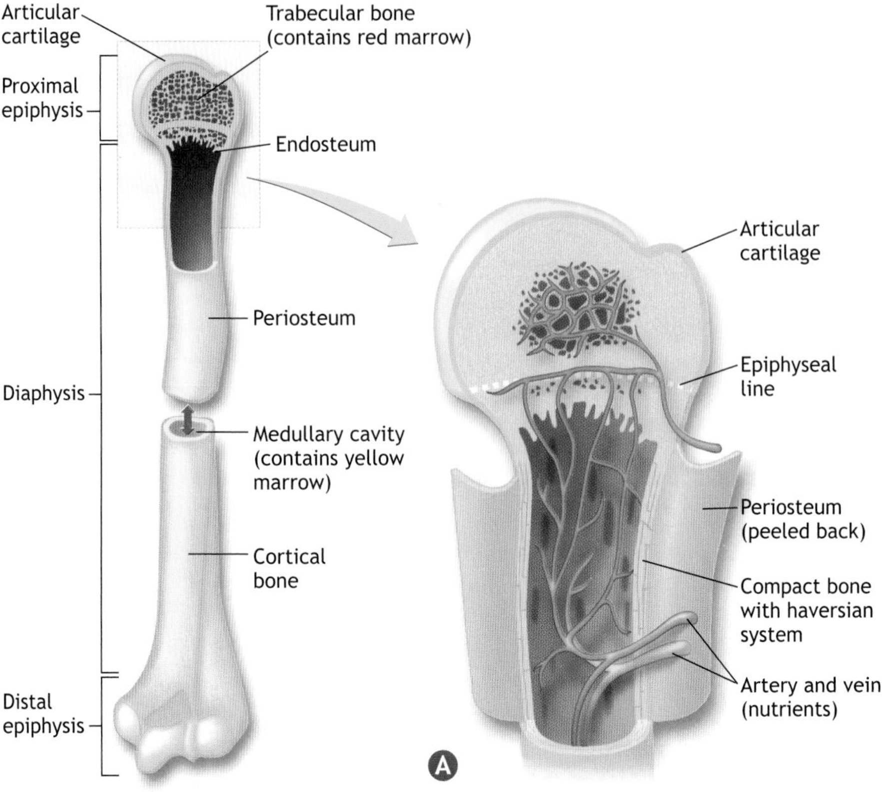

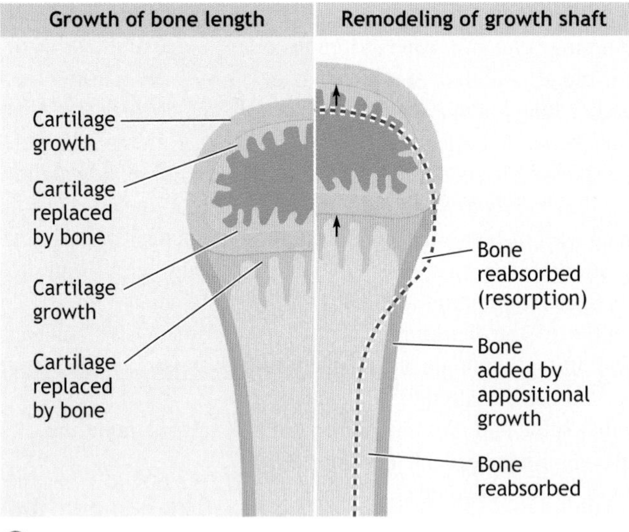

FIGURE 2.10 • Anatomic structure (**A**) and longitudinal view of a typical long bone, and (**B**) bone dynamics during growth and continual remodeling.

after regular cycles have begun. An interacting, tightly bound continuum generally begins with disordered eating—a serious ailment that in the extreme causes life-threatening complications. This leads to a significant energy drain, amenorrhea, and osteoporosis and reflects the clinical entity labeled the **female athlete triad** (Fig. 2.11) at an American College of Sports Medicine conference in 1992.[96,113,152,183] Some researchers and physicians prefer the term female triad because the syndrome of disorders also afflicts physically active women in the general population who do not fit the typical competitive athlete model.

INTEGRATIVE QUESTION

Why do resistance exercises for the body's major muscle groups offer unique benefits to bone mass compared with a typical weight-bearing program of brisk walking?

Limited data exist regarding the prevalence of the triad, mainly from a disagreement about how to define the disorder. However, many young women who play sports likely suffer from at least one of the triad's disorders, particularly disordered eating behaviors, which occur in 15 to 60% of female athletes, based on informal surveys. Figure 2.12 illustrates the contributing factors associated with exercise-related amenorrhea, considered the "red flag," or most recognizable symptom for the triad's presence. Female athletes of the 1970s and 1980s believed the loss of normal menstruation reflected hard training and was the inevitable consequence of athletic success. The prevalence of amenorrhea among female athletes in body weight–related sports (distance running, gymnastics, ballet, cheerleading, figure skating, body building) probably ranges between 25 and 65%; no more than 5% of the general population of women of menstruating age experience this condition. Bone density generally relates closely to (1) menstrual regularity and (2) the total number of menstrual cycles.

INTEGRATIVE QUESTION

Advise a group of high school females about strategies to achieve weight loss to compete successfully and healthfully in competitive gymnastics.

Cessation of menstruation removes estrogen's protective effect on bone, making these young women more vulnerable to calcium loss with concomitant decrease in bone mass.[54,182] The most severe menstrual disorders relate to the greatest negative effect on bone mass.[169] Lowered bone density from extended amenorrhea often occurs at multiple sites, including

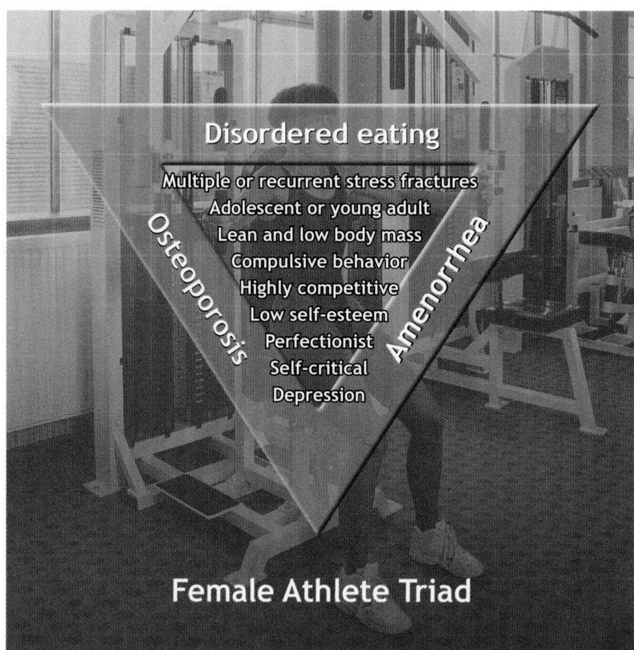

FIGURE 2.11 • The female athlete triad: disordered eating, amenorrhea, and osteoporosis.

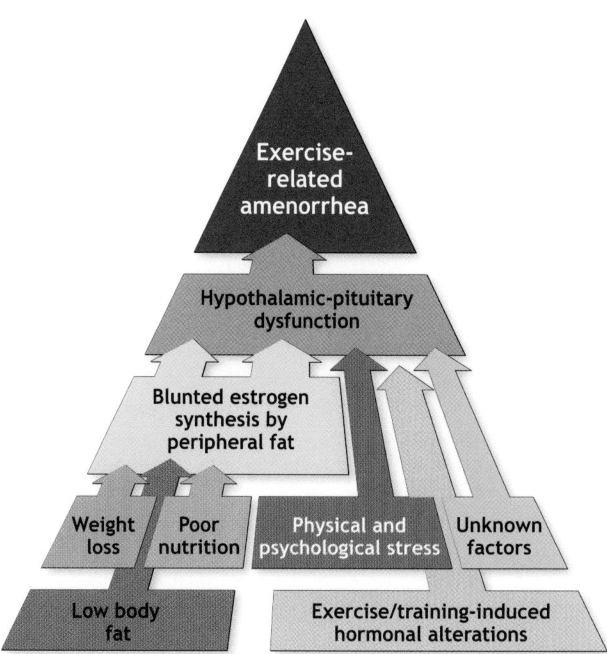

FIGURE 2.12 • Factors contributing to the development of exercise-related amenorrhea.

bone areas subjected to increased force and impact loading during exercise.[129] Concurrently, the problem worsens with low protein, lipid, and energy intakes; in such cases, a poor diet provides inadequate calcium intake. Persistent amenorrhea that begins at an early age blunts the benefits of exercise on bone mass; it also increases the risk of musculoskeletal injuries, particularly repeated stress fractures during exercise.[111] For example, a 5% loss in bone mass increases the risk of stress fracture by nearly 40%. Reestablishing normal menses causes some regain in bone mass but not to levels achieved with normal menstruation. Bone mass may remain *permanently* at suboptimal levels throughout adult life—leaving the woman at increased risk for osteoporosis and stress fractures, even years after competitive athletic participation.[39,106] The American College of Sports Medicine recommends that intervention begin within 3 months of the onset of amenorrhea. Successful treatment of athletic amenorrhea uses a nonpharmacologic, behavioral approach plus diet and training interventions as follows:[36]

- Reduce training level by 10 to 20%
- Gradually increase total energy intake
- Increase body weight by 2 to 3%
- Maintain daily calcium intake at 1500 mg

ESTROGEN'S ROLE IN BONE HEALTH

- Increases intestinal calcium absorption
- Reduces urinary calcium excretion
- Inhibits bone resorption
- Decreases bone turnover

Focus on Research

Female Athletes with Osteoporosis

Drinkwater BL, et al. Menstrual history as a determinant of current bone density in young athletes. JAMA 1990;263:545.

➤ Research on female athletes has focused on their reduced bone mineral density associated with menstrual dysfunctions (oligomenorrhea—irregular menstrual cycle; amenorrhea—menstrual cessation). Persistent amenorrhea often minimizes the benefits of exercise on bone mass, increasing risk of repeated stress fractures during exercise because osteoporosis develops at an early age.

A pioneering 1984 study by Barbara Drinkwater and colleagues linked amenorrhea in 14 female athletes with a statistically significant 13.8% decrease in spinal bone mineral density compared with age-matched eumenorrheic athletes.[1] The researchers hypothesized that early onset and repeated menstrual dysfunction produced permanent suboptimal bone mass throughout life. The condition increased these women's risk for developing early osteoporosis and stress fractures, even after competitive athletics ceased and normal menstruation resumed.

A subsequent study by Drinkwater (6 y later and presented here), demonstrated that women with regular menstrual cycles maintained higher lumbar bone densities (1.27 g · cm^{-2}) than athletic women with oligomenorrhea/amenorrhea interspersed with regular cycles (1.18 g · cm^{-2}) Moreover, the density of the lumbar bone region of both groups exceeded that of athletic women who never had regular cycles (1.05 g · cm^{-2}).

The researchers studied 97 active women aged 18 to 38 years. No woman smoked, and all had exercised regularly at least 4 days per week for 45 minutes or longer per session. None of the women used oral contraceptives, and none experienced medical problems with bone metabolism. The following definitions defined current menstrual status: regular (10 to 13 periods per y), oligomenorrheic (3 to 6 periods per y at intervals longer than 36 days), or amenorrheic (no more than 2 periods per y or no period during the last 6 mo). Assays for estradiol and progesterone levels confirmed menstrual status. Menstrual history included one of three categories: always had regular menses (R), had episodes of oligomenorrhea (O), or amenorrhea (A). Two reproductive endocrinologists ranked subjects on a scale from 1 to 9 about their expectations for bone mass for all combinations of reported present and past menstrual patterns. A pattern of always maintaining regular menses (R/R) ranked first as the most positive affect on bone. Current amenorrheics who also exhibited previous amenorrhea (A/A) received the lowest rank (ninth) for the physician's expectation of identifying women with the most negative bone pattern.

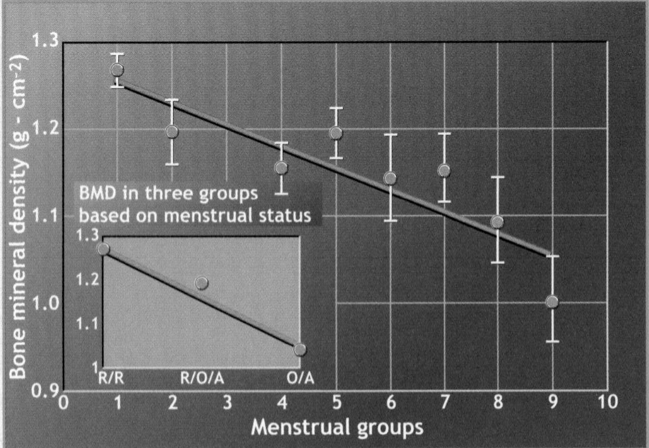

Relationship between vertebral bone mineral density (BMD) and menstrual history for 97 young women. (Inset) Bone mineral densities in three groups based on menstrual status.

The main figure displays actual vertebral bone density versus menstrual history for the 97 women. The plot includes the averages and variability for the menstrual groupings (only $\bar{X}$s with 5 or more subjects plotted) containing the following numbers of subjects per grouping: 1, R/R (n = 21); 2 , R/O (n = 7); 3, O/R (n = 2); 4, O/O (n = 5); 5, R/A (n = 22); 6, A/R (n = 9); 7, O/A (n = 10); 8, A/O (n = 10); 9, A/A (n = 11). Statistical analyses revealed significant bone mineral density differences between group 1 and groups 8 and 9, yet no statistically significant differences among groups 2 through 7. Thus, the researchers merged the nine groups into three subgroups: group 1, women who always maintained regular menses (R/R); group 2, women with bouts of oligomenorrhea or amenorrhea interspersed with regular menses and women with current oligomenorrhea (R/O/A); and group 3, women with current amenorrhea who experienced previous amenorrhea or oligomenorrhea (O/A). The inset figure relates the three subgroups to bone mineral density. Women who always menstruated regularly had the highest bone density values, women with occasional irregularity averaged 6% less bone density, and women who never menstruated regularly averaged 17% less. The third group was younger, weighed less, and experienced menarche at an older age. They also began to train seriously earlier in life, they trained more frequently and for longer durations each day, and traversed more miles than women who always maintained regular menses (group 1).

These studies suggest that prolonged oligomenorrhea/amenorrhea may irreversibly decrease vertebral bone density; the condition becomes exacerbated in women with persistently low body weight.

The work of Drinkwater and colleagues also increased awareness in the research and medical communities about the importance of understanding interactions among bone mineral density and intense physical training, estrogen levels, menstrual dysfunction, low body weight, and suboptimal energy and nutrient intake. The research paved the way for more clinically relevant treatment of female athletes at increased risk of irreversible loss of bone mass.

PHOSPHORUS

Inadequate phosphorus intake may contribute to bone loss in elderly women, because phosphorus combines with calcium to form hydroxyapatite and calcium phosphate compounds that give rigidity to bones and teeth. Phosphorus also serves as an essential component of the intracellular mediator cyclic adenosine monophosphate (AMP) and the intramuscular high-energy compounds adenosine triphosphate (ATP) and phosphocreatine (PCr). ATP supplies the energy for all forms of biologic work. Phosphorus combines with lipids to form phospholipid compounds, integral components of the cells' bilayer plasma membrane. The phosphorous-containing phosphatase enzymes regulate cellular metabolism; phosphorus also participates in buffering acid end products of energy metabolism. For this latter reason, some coaches and trainers recommend consuming special "phosphate drinks" to reduce the effects of acid production in heavy exercise and perhaps enhance oxygen release from red blood cells.[25] In Chapter 23, we discuss the usefulness of buffering agents for augmenting exercise performance. Athletes usually consume adequate phosphorus, with the possible exception of female dancers and gymnasts.[14,109] Rich dietary sources of phosphorus include meat, fish, poultry, milk products, and cereals.

MAGNESIUM

About 300 enzymes that regulate metabolic processes contain magnesium. Magnesium plays a vital role in glucose metabolism by facilitating muscle and liver glycogen formation from blood-borne glucose. The 20 to 30 g of magnesium in the body also participates as a cofactor in glucose, fatty acid, and amino acid breakdown during energy metabolism. Magnesium affects lipid and protein synthesis and contributes to optimal neuromuscular functioning. It acts as an electrolyte, which along with potassium and sodium helps to maintain blood pressure. Sweating generally produces only small losses of magnesium.

IRON

The body normally contains between 2.5 and 4.0 g (about ⅙ oz) of the trace mineral iron. Of this amount, approximately 70% exists in functionally active compounds, predominantly combined with **hemoglobin** in red blood cells (85% of functional iron) and **myoglobin** in muscle fibers (12% of functional iron). The iron-protein compound hemoglobin increases the blood's oxygen-carrying capacity approximately 65 times. Iron serves other important exercise-related functions besides its role in oxygen transport. It is a structural component of myoglobin (about 5% of total iron), a compound similar to hemoglobin, which aids in oxygen storage and transport within the muscle cell. Small amounts of iron also exist in **cytochromes**, the specialized substances that facilitate energy transfer within the cell. About 20% of the body's iron does not combine in functionally active compounds. **Hemosiderin** and **ferritin** constitute the intracellular iron stores in the liver, spleen, and bone marrow. These stores replenish iron lost from the functional compounds; they also provide the iron reserve during periods of insufficient dietary iron intake. An iron-binding plasma protein, **transferrin**, transports iron from ingested food and damaged red blood cells to tissues in need, particularly the liver, spleen, bone marrow, and skeletal muscles. *Plasma levels of transferrin often reflect the adequacy of the current iron intake.*

Athletes should include normal amounts of iron-rich foods in their daily diet. Persons with inadequate iron intake or with limited rates of iron absorption or high rates of iron loss often develop a reduced concentration of hemoglobin in red blood cells. The result of the extreme condition of iron insufficiency, commonly called **iron deficiency anemia**, produces general sluggishness, loss of appetite, and reduced capacity to sustain even mild exercise. "Iron therapy" normalizes the blood's hemoglobin content and exercise capacity. Table 2.4 lists recommendations for iron intake for children and adults.

Females: A Population at Risk

Inadequate iron intake frequently occurs among young children, teenagers, and females of childbearing age, including many physically active women.[25,127] In addition, pregnancy can trigger a moderate iron-deficiency anemia owing to the increased iron demand for both mother and fetus.

Iron loss from the 30 to 60 mL of blood generally lost during a menstrual cycle ranges between 15 and 30 mg. This loss requires an additional 5 mg of dietary iron daily for premenopausal females, which increases the average monthly dietary iron requirement by 150 mg. The healthy small intestine absorbs about 10 to 15% of the total ingested iron, depending on one's iron status, form of iron ingested, and composition of the meal. Thus, an additional 20 to 25 mg of iron becomes available to females each month for synthesizing red blood cells lost during menstruation. Not surprisingly, 30 to 50% of American women experience significant dietary iron insufficiency from menstrual blood loss and limited di-

TABLE 2.4 ➤ **RECOMMENDED DIETARY ALLOWANCES FOR IRON**

	AGE (Y)	IRON (MG)
Children	1–10	10
Males	11–18	12
	19	10
Females	11–50	15
	51	10
	Pregnant	30[a]
	Lactating	15[a]

Recommended Dietary Allowances, revised 1989, Food and Nutrition Board, National Academy of Sciences–National Research Council, Washington, DC.

[a]Generally, this increased requirement cannot be met by ordinary diets; therefore, the use of 30 to 60 mg of supplemental iron is recommended.

etary iron intake, which averages 6 mg of iron per 1000 calories of food consumed, with heme iron providing about 15% of the total iron.

Importance of Iron Source

Intestinal iron absorption varies closely with iron need, yet considerable variation in absorption (bioavailability) occurs in relation to diet composition. For example, the intestine usually absorbs 2 to 5% of iron from plants (trivalent ferric or **nonheme** elemental iron), whereas iron absorption from animal (divalent ferrous or **heme**) sources increases to 10 to 35%. The presence of heme iron, which represents between 35% and 55% of iron in animal sources, also increases iron absorption from nonheme sources. Additional meat consumption maintains iron status in exercising women more effectively than supplementing with commercial iron preparations.[101] Many other factors affect iron absorption, the most important being the body's current iron stores. Increased iron loss or requirement induces increased intestinal iron absorption.

The relatively low bioavailability of nonheme iron places women on vegetarian-type diets at risk for developing iron insufficiency. Female vegetarian runners have a poorer iron status than counterparts who consume the same quantity of iron from predominantly animal sources.[153] Including foods rich in vitamin C in the diet upgrades dietary iron bioavailability (see Fig. 2.2). This occurs because ascorbic acid prevents oxidation of ferrous iron to the ferric form, thus increasing nonheme iron's solubility for absorption at the alkaline pH of the small intestine. The ascorbic acid in one glass of orange juice stimulates a 3-fold increase in nonheme iron absorption from a breakfast.[143] Heme sources of iron include beef, beef liver, pork, tuna, and clams; oatmeal, dried figs, spinach, beans, and lentils are good nonheme sources.

Exercise-Induced Anemia: Fact or Fiction?

Interest in endurance sports, combined with increased participation of women in these activities, has focused research on the influence of hard training on the body's iron status. The term **sports anemia** frequently describes reduced hemoglobin levels approaching clinical anemia (12 g per dL of blood for women and 14 g for men) attributable to intense training. Some researchers maintain that *strenuous* exercise training creates an added demand for iron that often exceeds its intake. This would tax iron reserves and eventually lead to depressed hemoglobin synthesis and/or reduction in iron-containing compounds within the cell's energy transfer system.[31] Individuals susceptible to an "iron drain" could experience reduced exercise capacity because of iron's crucial role in oxygen transport and use.

Heavy training may theoretically create an augmented iron demand (facilitating the development of clinical anemia) from three sources:

1. A small iron loss in sweat (greater in men than women).[17,177]
2. Loss of hemoglobin in urine from red blood cell destruction, with increased temperature, spleen activity, and circulation rates, and from jarring of the kidneys and mechanical trauma from feet pounding on the running surface (foot-strike hemolysis).[72,118]
3. Gastrointestinal bleeding unrelated to age, gender, or performance time also may occur with long-distance running.[18,134]

Such iron loss would certainly stress the body's iron reserves required to synthesize 260 billion new red blood cells daily in the bone marrow of the skull, upper arms and legs, sternum, ribs, spine, and pelvis. Iron losses pose an additional burden to women, who have a greater iron requirement yet lower iron intake than men.

Real Anemia or Pseudoanemia?

Suboptimal hemoglobin concentrations and hematocrits occur more frequently among endurance athletes, thus supporting the possibility of an exercise-induced anemia.[64] On closer scrutiny, however, reductions in hemoglobin concentration are transient, occurring in the early phase of training and then returning toward pretraining values. Figure 2.13 illustrates the general response for hematologic variables for high-school female cross-country runners during a competitive season. The decrease in hemoglobin concentration generally parallels the disproportionately large expansion in plasma volume compared with total hemoglobin with training (see Fig. 13.5).[49,147] Just several days of exercise training increase plasma volume by 20%, while total red blood cell volume remains unchanged. Consequently, *total* hemoglobin (an important factor in endurance performance) remains the same or increases slightly with training, even though hemoglobin concentration decreases in the expanding plasma volume. Despite this hemoglobin dilution, aerobic capacity and exercise performance normally improve with training.

FACTORS AFFECTING IRON ABSORPTION

Increase Iron Absorption

- Acid in the stomach
- Iron in heme form
- High body demand for red blood cells (blood loss, high altitude, physical training, pregnancy)
- Low body iron stores
- Presence of mean protein factor (MPF)
- Presence of vitamin C in small intestine

Decrease Iron Absorption

- Phytic acid (in dietary fiber)
- Oxalic acid
- Polyphenols (in tea and coffee)
- High body iron stores
- Excess of other minerals (Zn, Mn, Ca), particularly when taken as supplements
- Reduction in stomach acid
- Some antacids

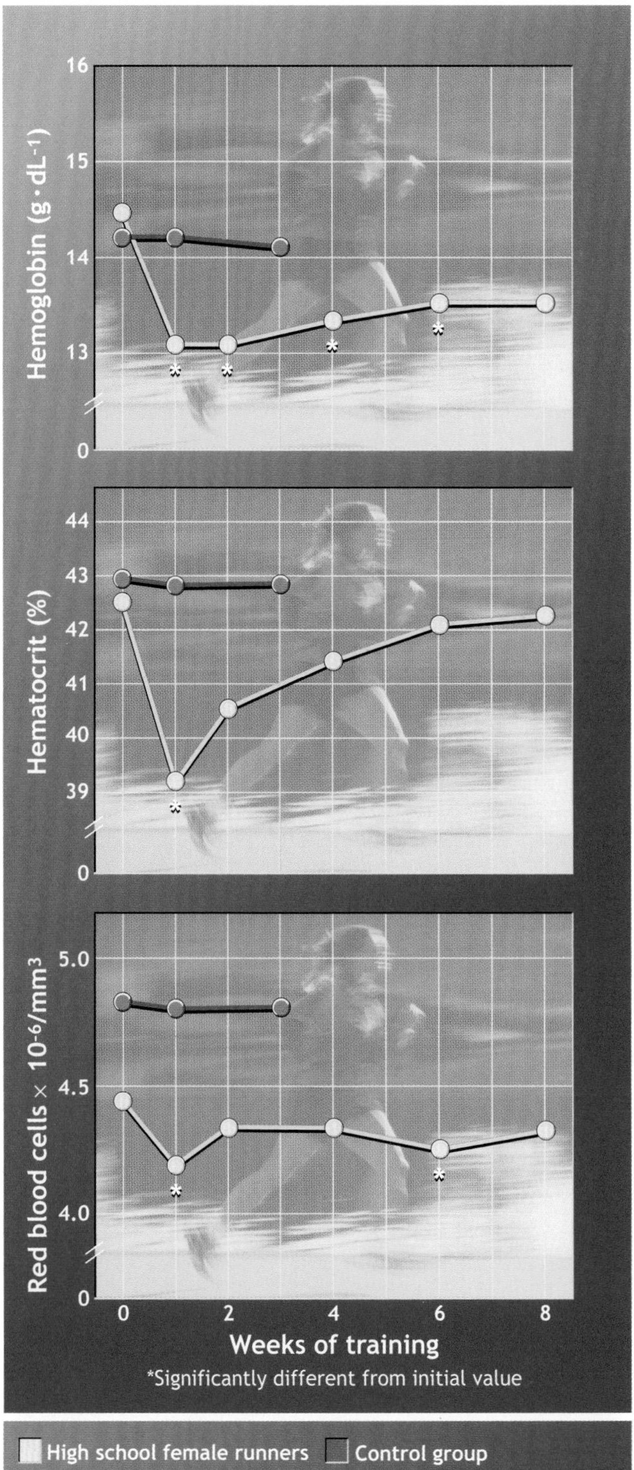

FIGURE 2.13 • Hemoglobin, red blood cell count, and hematocrit in female high school cross-country runners and a comparison group during the competitive season. (Adapted from Puhl JL, et al. Erythrocyte changes during training in high school women cross-country runners. Res Q Exerc Sport 1981;52:484.)

Some mechanical destruction of red blood cells occurs with vigorous exercise, along with some loss of iron in sweat (a potentially important loss for women with low iron absorption).[177] However, no evidence shows that these factors can strain an athlete's iron reserves and precipitate clinical anemia as long as iron intake remains at recommended levels. Applying stringent criteria for both anemia and insufficiency of iron reserves makes sports anemia much less prevalent among highly trained athletes than generally believed.[179] For male collegiate runners and swimmers, no indications of the early stages of anemia were noted despite large changes in training volume and intensity during the competitive season.[122] Data from female athletes further indicate that the prevalence of iron deficiency anemia did *not* differ in comparisons among specific athletic groups or with nonathletic controls.[133]

Should Athletes Take an Iron Supplement?

Any increase in iron loss with exercise training (coupled with poor dietary habits) in adolescent and premenopausal women could strain an already limited iron reserve. This does not mean that all individuals in training should supplement with iron or that all indications of sports anemia result from dietary iron insufficiency or iron loss caused by exercise. Instead, the data suggest that an athlete's iron status should be monitored by twice-yearly evaluation of both hematologic characteristics and iron reserves.[99,100] Measuring serum ferritin concentration provides useful information about iron reserves; values below 20 $\mu g \cdot L^{-1}$ for females and 30 $\mu g \cdot L^{-1}$ for males indicate depleted reserves.

For an individual whose diet contains the recommended iron intake or who shows no clinical signs of iron deficiency, iron supplementation does not increase hemoglobin or hematocrit concentrations or other measures of iron status.[8] Even with mild iron insufficiency without anemia, iron supplementation and an improved iron reserve status may not enhance aerobic capacity or exercise performance.[79]

Potential harm exists from overconsumption or overabsorption of iron (particularly with the widespread use of vitamin C supplements). Iron supplements should not be used indiscriminately because excessive iron can accumulate to toxic levels and contribute significantly to diabetes, liver disease, and heart and joint damage; it may even augment the growth of latent cancers and infectious organisms. Current debate centers on whether men with high levels of body iron stores and/or a high dietary heme iron intake have a higher risk for coronary heart disease than men with iron levels in the low-to-normal range.[30,80,145] If risk exists, one explanation postulates that high serum iron catalyzes free-radical formation, which augments the oxidation of LDL cholesterol to promote atherosclerosis.

SODIUM, POTASSIUM, AND CHLORINE

Sodium, potassium, and chlorine, collectively termed **electrolytes**, remain dissolved in the body fluids as electrically charged particles called **ions**. Sodium and chlorine represent the chief minerals contained in blood plasma and extracellular fluid. Electrolytes modulate fluid exchange within the body's fluid compartments, promoting a constant, well-regulated exchange of nutrients and waste products between the cell and

TABLE 2.5 ➤ ELECTROLYTE CONCENTRATIONS IN BLOOD SERUM AND SWEAT, AND CARBOHYDRATE AND ELECTROLYTE CONCENTRATIONS OF SOME POPULAR BEVERAGES

Substance	Na^+ (mEq · L^{-1})[a]	K^+ (mEq · L^{-1})	Ca^{++} (mEq · L^{-1})	Mg^{++} (mEq · L^{-1})	Cl^- (mEq · L^{-1})	Osmolality (mOsm · L^{-1})[b]	CHO (g · L^{-1})[c]
Blood serum	140	4.5	2.5	1.5–2.1	110	300	—
Sweat	60–80	4.5	1.5	3.3	40–90	170–220	—
Coca Cola	3.0	—	—	—	1.0	650	107
Gatorade	23.0	3.0	—	—	14.0	280	62
Fruit juice	0.5	58.0	—	—	—	690	118
Pepsi Cola	1.7	Trace	—	—	Trace	568	81
Water	Trace	Trace	—	—	Trace	10–20	—

[a]Milliequivalents per liter.
[b]Milliosmoles per liter.
[c]Grams per liter.

its external fluid environment. Potassium is the chief intracellular mineral.

The most important function of sodium and potassium ions concerns their role in establishing the proper electrical gradient across cell membranes. The difference in electrical balance between the cell's interior and exterior facilitates nerve impulse transmission, stimulation and action of muscle, and proper gland functioning. Electrolytes also maintain plasma membrane permeability and regulate the acid and base qualities of bodily fluids, particularly blood. Table 2.5 lists values considered normal for the electrolyte concentrations in serum and sweat and the electrolyte and carbohydrate concentrations of common beverages.

Optimal Sodium Intake

With low-to-moderate dietary sodium intake, the hormone **aldosterone** conserves sodium in the kidneys. In contrast, high dietary sodium blunts aldosterone release, with excess sodium voided in the urine. This maintains sodium balance throughout a wide range of intakes. Some individuals cannot adequately regulate excessive sodium intake. Abnormal sodium accumulation in bodily fluids increases fluid volume and elevates blood pressure to levels that may pose a health risk. **Sodium-induced hypertension** occurs in about one third of individuals with hypertension.

Sodium distributes so widely naturally in foods that one can readily maintain the daily requirement without adding salt. In the United States, sodium intake regularly exceeds the daily recommended range for adults of 1100 to 3300 mg, or the amount of sodium in 0.5 to 1.5 teaspoons of table salt (sodium makes up about 40% of salt [NaCl]). The typical Western diet contains about 4500 mg of sodium (8 to 12 g of salt) each day. This represents 10 times the 500 mg of sodium the body actually needs. The heavy reliance on table salt in processing, curing, cooking, seasoning, and preserving common foods accounts for the large sodium intake. Aside from table salt, common sodium-rich dietary sources include monosodium glutamate (MSG), soy sauce, condiments, canned foods, baking soda, and baking powder.

SALT-SENSITIVE HYPERTENSION. For decades, the first line of defense in treating high blood pressure eliminated excess sodium from the diet. Reducing sodium intake can lower blood pressure via reduced plasma volume. However, considerable variation exists in blood pressure responsiveness to NaCl intake.[83] Sodium restriction does not lower blood pressure in people with normal blood pressure and only minimally affects most people with high blood pressure.[53] However, certain individuals are "**salt sensitive**," perhaps with a genetic variation in the angiotensinogen gene that produces the hormone angiotensinogen.[65] For these individuals, reducing dietary sodium to the low end of the recommended range and upgrading the quality of the diet (see "In a Practical Sense") reduces blood pressure.[157] Debate continues, however, concerning the magnitude of this reduction for most hypertensives.[42,98,107,163] Older adults who lost 4 to 5 kg and limited their daily salt intake to 1800 mg were 53% less likely to have hypertension or require blood pressure medication than individuals making no change in body weight or salt intake.[181] Those who either lost weight or reduced salt intake were 30% less likely to require medication. If dietary constraints prove ineffective in lowering blood pressure, drugs that induce water loss (diuretics) become the next line of defense. Unfortunately, diuretics also produce losses in other minerals, particularly potassium. A potassium-rich diet (e.g., potatoes, bananas, oranges, tomatoes, and meat) becomes a necessity for a patient using diuretics.

MINERALS AND EXERCISE PERFORMANCE

Consuming mineral supplements above recommended levels on a long- or short-term basis does not benefit exercise performance or enhance training responsiveness.

Mineral Loss in Sweat

Excessive water and electrolyte loss impairs heat tolerance and exercise performance and can lead to severe dysfunction culminating in heat cramps, heat exhaustion, or heat stroke. The yearly toll of heat-related deaths during spring and summer football practice provides a tragic illustration of the importance

IN A PRACTICAL SENSE

➤➤ LOWERING HIGH BLOOD PRESSURE WITH DIETARY INTERVENTION: THE DASH DIET

Nearly 50 million Americans have hypertension, a condition that if left untreated increases the risk of stroke, heart attack, and kidney failure. Fifty percent of hypertensives actually seek treatment. Only about one half of these individuals achieve long-term success. One reason for the lack of compliance concerns possible side effects of readily available antihypertensive medication. For example, fatigue and impotence often discourage patients from maintaining a chronic medication schedule required by pharmacologic treatment of hypertension.

The DASH Approach

Research using DASH (Dietary Approaches to Stop Hypertension) to treat hypertension shows that this diet lowers blood pressure in some individuals to the same extent as pharmacologic therapy and often more than other lifestyle changes. Two months of the diet reduced systolic pressure by an average of 11.4 mm Hg; diastolic pressure decreased by 5.5 mm Hg. Every 2 mm Hg reduction in systolic pressure lowers heart disease risk by 5% and stroke risk by 8%. Further good news emerges from the latest research that indicates that the standard DASH diet combined with a daily dietary salt intake of 1500 mg produced even greater blood pressure reductions than achieved with the DASH diet only.

The table below shows the general nature of the DASH diet with its high content of fruits, vegetables, and dairy products and low fat composition.

SAMPLE DASH DIET

The table at the right shows a sample DASH diet consisting of approximately 2,100 calories (kcal). This level of energy intake provides a stable body weight for a typical 70-kg person. More physically active and heavier individuals should boost portion size or the number of individual items to maintain weight. Individuals desiring to lose weight or who are lighter and/or sedentary should eat less, but not less than the minimum number of servings for each food group shown below.

Sacks FM, et al. Rationale and design of the dietary approaches to stop hypertension trial (DASH): a multicenter controlled feeding study of dietary patterns to lower blood pressure. Ann Epidemiol 1995;108:118.

SAMPLE DASH DIET (2100 KCAL)

FOOD	AMOUNT
Breakfast	
Orange juice	6 oz
1% low-fat milk	8 oz (used with corn flakes)
Corn flakes (1 tsp sugar)	1 cup (dry) [equals 2 servings of grains]
Banana	1 medium
Whole-wheat bread	1 slice
Soft margarine	1 tsp
Lunch	
Low-fat chicken salad	3/4 cup
Pita bread	1/2 large
Raw vegetable medley	
Carrot and celery sticks	3–4 sticks each
Radishes	2
Lettuce	2 leaves
Part-skim mozzarella	1 1/2 slices (1.5 oz)
1% low-fat milk	8 oz
Fruit cocktail	1/2 cup
Dinner	
Herbed baked cod	3 oz
Scallion rice	1 cup [equals 2 servings of grain]
Steamed broccoli	1/2 cup
Stewed tomatoes	1/2 cup
Spinach salad (raw spinach)	1/2 cup
Cherry tomatoes	2
Cucumber	2 slices
Light Italian salad dressing	1 Tbsp [equals 1/2 fat serving]
Whole wheat dinner roll	1
Soft margarine	1 tsp
Melon balls	1/2 cup
Snack	
Dried apricots	1 oz (1/4 cup)
Mixed nuts, unsalted	1.5 oz (1/3 cup)
Mini-pretzels, unsalted	1 oz (3/4 cup)
Diet ginger ale	12 oz [does not count as a serving of any food]

Svetkey LP, et al. Effects of dietary patterns on blood pressure: subgroup analysis of the dietary approaches to stop hypertension (DASH) randomized clinical trial. Arch Intern Med 1999;159:285.

DIETARY APPROACHES TO STOP HYPERTENSION (DASH)

FOOD GROUP	EXAMPLE OF ONE SERVING	SERVINGS
Vegetables	1/2 cup of cooked or raw chopped vegetables; 1 cup of raw leafy vegetables; or 6 oz of juice	8 to 12 daily
Fruit	1 medium apple, pear, orange, or banana; 1/2 grapefruit; 1/3 cantaloupe; 1/2 cup of fresh frozen or canned fruit; 1/4 cup of dried fruit; or 6 oz of juice	8 to 12 daily
Grains	1 slice of bread; 1/2 cup of cold, dry cereal; 1/2 cup cooked rice or pasta	6 to 12 daily
Dairy	1 cup of no-fat or low-fat milk or 1 1/2 oz of low-fat or part-skim cheese	2 to 4 daily
Nuts, seeds, and beans	1/3 cup (1 1/2 oz) of nuts; 2 Tbsp of seeds; or 1/2 cup of cooked beans	4 to 7 weekly
Meat, poultry, or fish	3 oz serving (roughly the size of a deck of cards)	1 to 2 daily
Oil or other fats	1 tsp vegetable oil, butter, salad dressings, soft margarine	2 to 4 daily

of fluid and electrolyte replacement. During practice or a game, an athlete may lose up to 5 kg of water from sweating. This corresponds to about 8.0 g of salt depletion, because each kg (1 L) of sweat generally contains about 1.5 g of salt. Despite this potential for mineral loss, replacement of water lost through sweating becomes the crucial and immediate need.

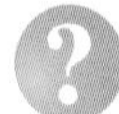

INTEGRATIVE QUESTION

Many young girls and women engaged in sports likely suffer from at least one of the disorders of the female athlete triad. Discuss factors related to this syndrome and how a coach might guard against their occurrence.

Defense Against Mineral Loss

Chronic mineral supplementation does not enhance physical performance in well-nourished active people.[165] Sweat loss during vigorous exercise triggers a rapid, coordinated release of the hormones vasopressin, renin, and aldosterone, which reduces sodium and water loss through the kidneys.[110] An increase in sodium conservation occurs even under extreme conditions like running a marathon in warm, humid weather when sweat output often reaches 2 L per hour. Adding a slight amount of salt to the fluid or food ingested usually replenishes electrolytes lost in sweat. During a 20-day road race in Hawaii, runners maintained plasma minerals at normal levels when they consumed an unrestricted diet without mineral supplements.[37] This and other findings indicate that ingesting "athletic drinks" provides no special benefit in replacing minerals lost through sweating, compared with the same minerals ingested in a well-balanced diet. Salt supplements may be necessary for prolonged exercise in the heat when fluid loss exceeds 4 or 5 kg. This can be achieved by drinking a 0.1 to 0.2% salt solution (adding 0.3 tsp of table salt per L of water).[5] A mild potassium deficiency may occur with intense exercise during heat stress, but a diet containing normal amounts of this mineral usually ensures adequate potassium levels.[28] An 8-oz

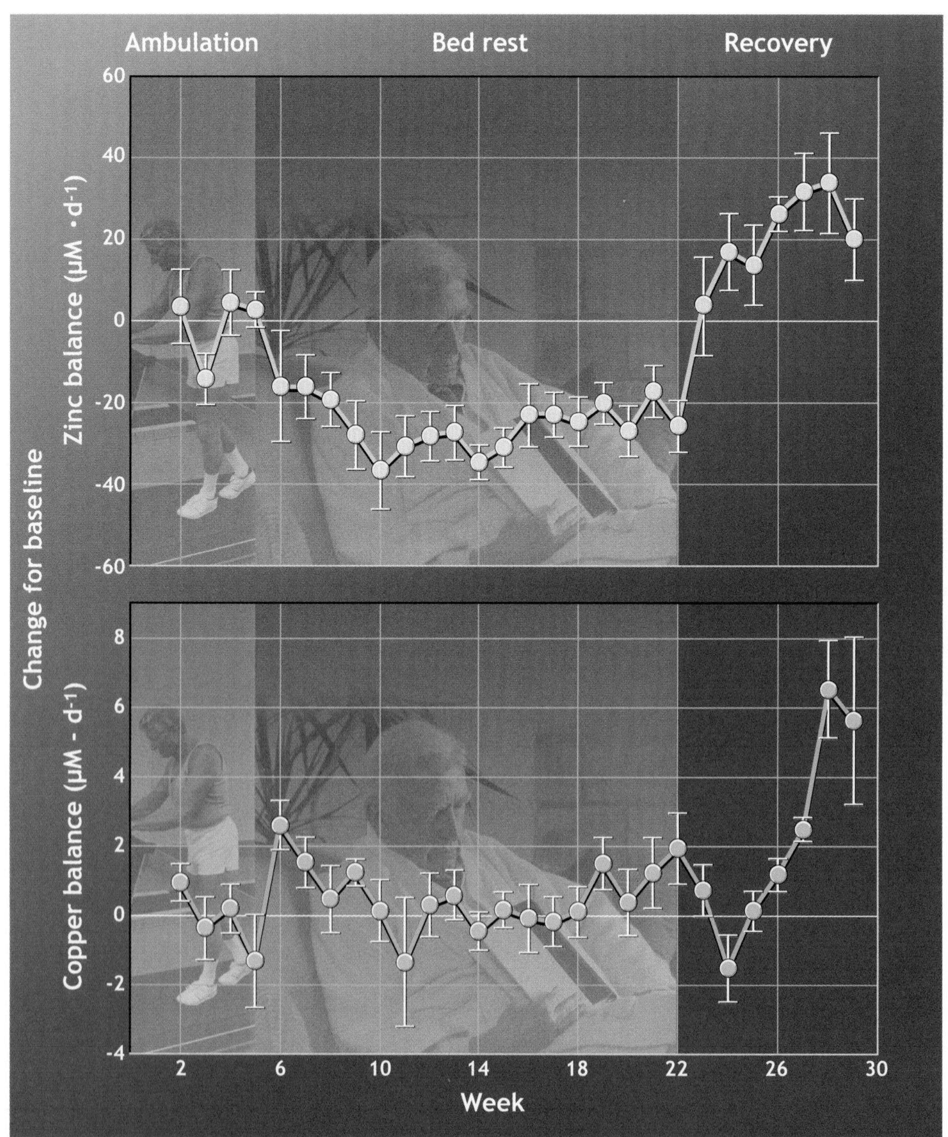

FIGURE 2.14 • Changes in weekly zinc and copper balance during a 5-week control period (ambulation), a 17-week period of bed rest, and a 7-week recovery period. (From Krebs JM, et al. Zinc and copper balances in healthy adult males during and after 17 wk of bed rest. Am J Clin Nutr 1993;58:897.)

glass of orange or tomato juice replaces almost all of the calcium, potassium, and magnesium lost in 3 L (3 kg) of sweat.

Trace Minerals and Exercise

Many individuals believe that supplementing with certain trace minerals enhances exercise performance and counteracts the demands of heavy training. Strenuous exercise may increase excretion of the following trace elements:

- *Chromium:* necessary for carbohydrate and lipid catabolism and proper insulin function and protein synthesis
- *Copper:* required for red blood cell formation; influences gene expression and serves as a cofactor or prosthetic group for several enzymes
- *Manganese:* component of superoxide dismutase in the body's antioxidant defense system
- *Zinc:* component of lactate dehydrogenase, carbonic anhydrase, superoxide dismutase, and enzymes related to energy metabolism, cell growth and differentiation, and tissue repair

Urinary losses of zinc and chromium were 1.5- to 2.0-fold higher after a 6-mile run than on a rest day.[7] In addition, sweat loss of copper and zinc can be relatively high. Documentation of trace mineral losses with exercise does not necessarily mean athletes should supplement with these micronutrients. For example, short-term zinc supplementation (25 mg $\cdot$ d^{-1}) did not benefit metabolic and endocrine responses and endurance performance during strenuous exercise by eumenorrheic women.[150] However, men and women who engage in heavy training (with large sweat production) and have marginal nutrition (e.g., wrestlers, endurance runners, ballet dancers, and female gymnasts) should monitor trace mineral intake to prevent an overt deficiency. *For most athletes, trace mineral deficiency does not appear to pose a problem to exercise performance or overall health.* Collegiate football players who supplemented with 200 μg of chromium (as chromium picolinate) daily for 9 weeks experienced no beneficial changes in body composition and muscular strength during intense weight lifting compared with a control group that received a placebo.[22] Power and endurance athletes also had significantly higher plasma levels of copper and zinc than nontraining controls.[137] Because iron, zinc, and copper interact with each other and compete for the same carrier during intestinal absorption, an excessive intake of one mineral may cause a deficiency in the other.[95]

The muscle and bone masses contain approximately one half of the body's copper and zinc. Thus, prolonged bed rest and perhaps physical inactivity could drain these minerals from the body. Figure 2.14 shows the time course for zinc and copper balance during a 30-week period that included a 5-week control period with ambulation, 17 weeks of continuous bed rest, and a 7-week recovery period when ambulation again occurred.[85] Dietary intake remained constant at approximately 2,688 kcal (11,115 kJ) throughout the observation period. The results were clear; bed rest markedly decreased the body's copper and zinc stores. During recovery with modest physical activity, the trace mineral concentration maintained greater stability than in the bed rest condition. Although this study represented an extreme condition, it indicates that physical *inactivity* can affect trace mineral dynamics in the body. We hope more researchers pursue the fascinating area of trace mineral metabolism in general and the effects of exercise and training on their requirements in particular.[6,24] Chapter 23 discusses the possible ergogenic effects of chromium supplements.

Summary

1. Approximately 4% of body mass consists of 22 elements called minerals that are distributed in all body tissues and fluids.
2. Minerals occur freely in nature, in the waters of rivers, lakes, and oceans and in soil. The root system of plants absorbs minerals; they eventually become incorporated into the tissues of animals that consume plants.
3. Minerals function primarily in metabolism as important parts of enzymes. Minerals provide structure to bones and teeth and serve in synthesizing the biologic macronutrients—glycogen, fat, and protein.
4. A balanced diet generally provides adequate mineral intake, except in some geographic locations that lack minerals such as iodine.
5. Osteoporosis has reached almost epidemic proportions among older individuals, particularly women. Adequate calcium intake and regular weight-bearing exercise and/or resistance training provide an effective defense against bone loss at any age.
6. Women who train intensely often do not match energy intake to energy output. This reduces body weight and body fat to a point that adversely affects menstruation, which contributes to significant bone loss at an early age. Restoration of normal menstruation does not necessarily fully restore bone mass.
7. About 40% of American women of childbearing age suffer from dietary iron insufficiency. This could lead to iron-deficiency anemia, which negatively affects aerobic exercise performance and the ability to perform heavy training.
8. For women on vegetarian-type diets, the relatively low bioavailability of nonheme iron increases risk for developing iron insufficiency. Vitamin C (in food or supplement form) increases intestinal absorption of nonheme iron.
9. Regular physical activity probably does not create a significant drain on the body's iron reserves. If it does, females, with the greatest iron requirement and lowest iron intake, could be at increased risk for anemia. Periodic assessment of the body's iron status should evaluate hematologic characteristics and iron reserves.

10. Excessive sweating during exercise produces significant losses of body water and related minerals; these should be replaced during and following exercise. Sweat loss during exercise usually does not increase the mineral requirement above recommended values.

➤ PART 3 • Water

WATER IN THE BODY

Water makes up from 40 to 70% of body mass, depending on age, gender, and body composition; it constitutes 65 to 75% of the weight of muscle and about 10% of the fat mass. Consequently, differences in total body water between individuals largely result from variations in body composition (i.e., differences in lean versus fat tissue).

Figure 2.15 depicts the fluid compartments of the body, the normal daily body water variation, and specific terminology to describe the various states of human hydration. The body contains two fluid "compartments." The first, **intracellular**, refers to fluid inside the cells. The second, **extracellular**, includes the fluid that flows within the microscopic spaces between cells (**interstitial fluid**) in addition to lymph, saliva, fluid in the eyes, fluid secreted by glands and the digestive tract, fluid that bathes the spinal cord nerves, and fluid excreted from the skin and kidneys. Blood plasma accounts for nearly 20% of the extracellular fluid (3 to 4 L). *Extracellular fluid provides most of the fluid lost through sweating, predominantly from blood plasma.* Of the total body water, an average of 62% (26 L of the body's 42 L of water for an average 80-kg man) represents intracellular water, and 38% comes from extracellular sources. These volumes do not remain static but represent averages from a dynamic exchange of fluid between compartments, particularly in physically active men and women.[142] Exercise training often increases the percentage of water distributed within the intracellular compartment because muscle mass increases, with its accompanying large water content. In contrast, an acute bout of exercise causes a temporary fluid shift from plasma to interstitial and intracellular spaces from the increased hydrostatic (fluid) pressure within the active circulatory system.

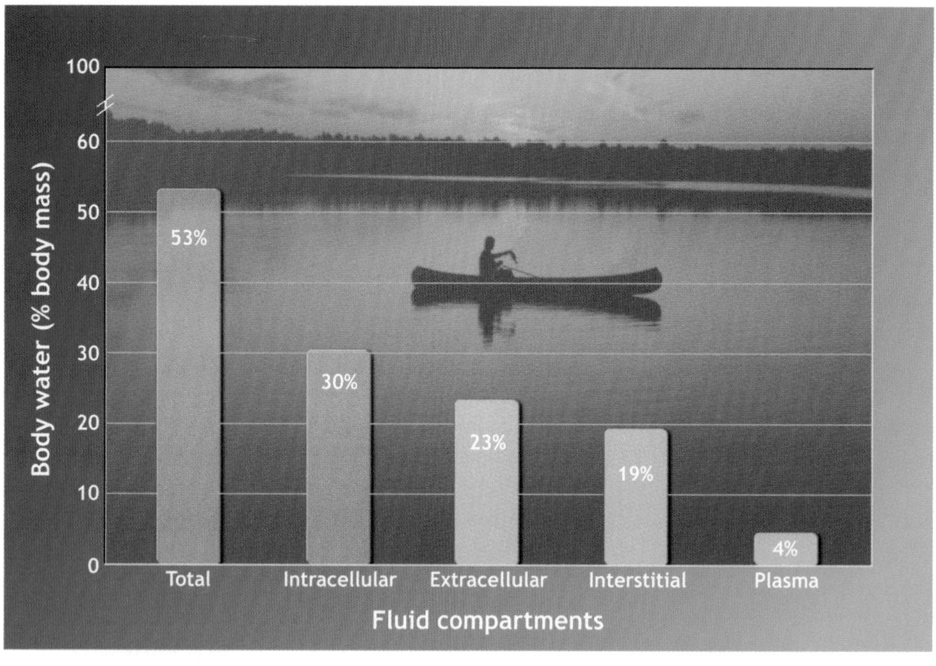

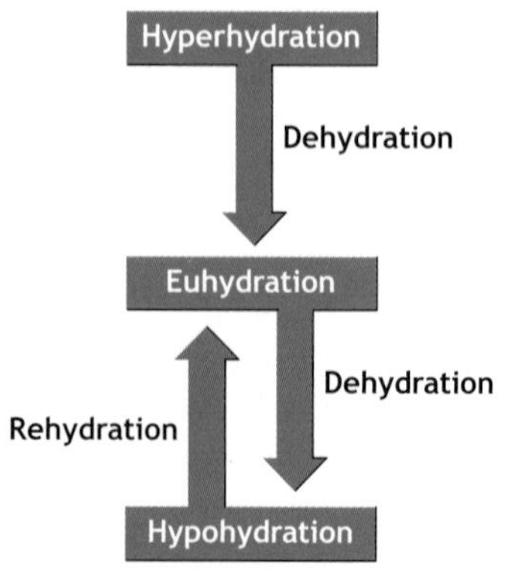

Daily euhydration variability of total body water
Temperate climate: ±0.165 L (±0.2% body mass)
Heat exercise conditions: ±0.382 L (±0.5% body mass)

Daily plasma volume variability
All conditions: ±0.027 L (±0.6% blood volume)

Hydration terminology
Euhydration: normal daily water variation
Hyperhydration: new steady-state of increased water content
Hypohydration: new steady-state of decreased water content
Dehydration: process of losing water either from the hyperhydrated state to euhydration, or from euhydration downward to hypohydration
Rehydration: process of gaining water from a hypohydrated state toward euhydration

FIGURE 2.15 • Fluid compartments, average volumes and variability, and hydration terminology. Volumes represent an 80-kg man. Approximately 55% of the body mass consists of water in striated muscle (80% water), skeleton (32% water), and adipose tissue (50% water). For a man and woman of similar body mass, the woman contains less total water because of her larger ratio of adipose tissue to lean body mass (striated muscle + skeleton). (Adapted from Greenleaf JE. Problem: thirst, drinking behavior, and involuntary dehydration. Med Sci Sports Exerc 1992;24:645.)

FUNCTIONS OF BODY WATER

Water is a ubiquitous, remarkable nutrient. Without water, death occurs within days. It serves as the body's transport and reactive medium; diffusion of gases always takes place across surfaces moistened by water. Nutrients and gases travel in aqueous solution; waste products leave the body through the water in urine and feces. Water, in conjunction with various proteins, lubricates joints and cushions a variety of "moving" organs such as the heart, lungs, intestines, and eyes. Because it is noncompressible, water gives structure and form to the body through the turgor it provides for body tissues. Water has tremendous heat-stabilizing qualities because it absorbs considerable heat with only small changes in temperature. This quality, combined with water's high heat of vaporization, maintains a relatively stable body temperature during (1) environmental heat stress and (2) increased internal heat load generated by exercise. More is said in Chapter 25 on the dynamics of thermoregulation during heat stress and exercise, particularly water's important role.

WATER BALANCE: INTAKE VERSUS OUTPUT

The body's water content remains relatively stable over time. Although considerable water output occurs in physically active individuals, appropriate fluid intake rapidly restores any imbalance in the body's fluid level. Figure 2.16 displays the sources of water intake and output.

Water Intake

A sedentary adult in a thermoneutral environment requires about 2.5 L of water daily. For an active person in a warm, humid environment the water requirement often increases to between 5 and 10 L daily. Three sources provide this water: (1) foods, (2) fluids, and (3) metabolism.

Water from Liquids

The average individual normally consumes 1200 mL of water each day. Exercise and thermal stress can increase the need for fluid intake to five or six times above this amount. At the extreme, an individual lost 13.6 kg of water weight during a 2-day, 17-hour, 55-mile run across Death Valley, California.[135] However, with proper fluid ingestion, including salt supplements, the actual body weight loss amounted to only 1.4 kg. In this example, fluid loss and replenishment represented nearly 4 gallons of liquid!

Water in Foods

Fruits and vegetables contain considerable water (e.g., lettuce, watermelon and cantaloupe, pickles, green beans, and broccoli); in contrast, butter, oils, dried meats, and chocolate, cookies, and cakes have a relatively low water content.

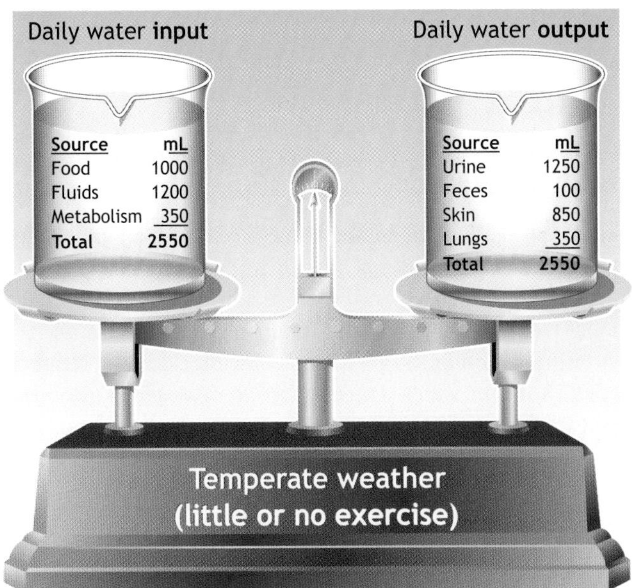

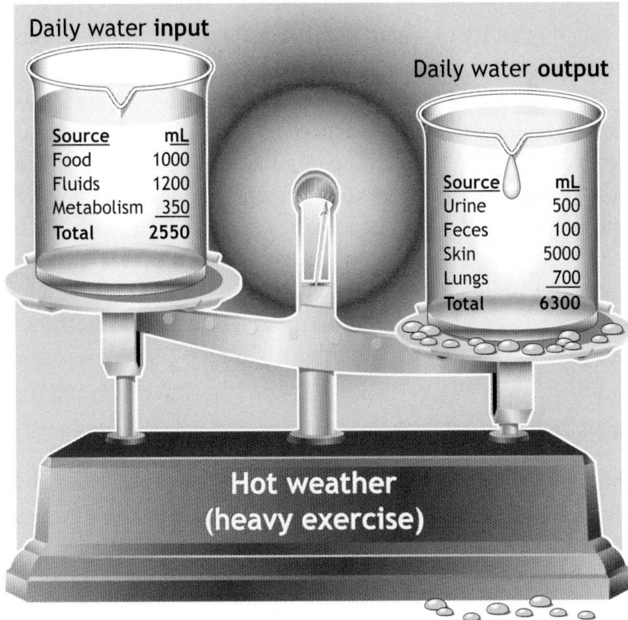

FIGURE 2.16 • Water balance in the body. *Top.* Little or no exercise with thermoneutral ambient temperature and humidity. *Bottom.* Moderate to heavy exercise in a hot, humid environment.

Metabolic Water

The breakdown of macronutrient molecules in energy metabolism forms carbon dioxide and water. Termed **metabolic water**, this fluid provides about 14% of the daily water requirement of a sedentary person. When glucose breaks down, it liberates 55 g of metabolic water. A larger amount of water forms from protein (100 g) and fat (107 g) catabolism. Additionally, each gram of glycogen joins with 2.7 g of water as its glucose units link together; subsequently, glycogen liberates this bound water during its catabolism for energy.

Water Output

Water loss from the body occurs in urine, through the skin, as water vapor in expired air, and in feces.

Water Loss in Urine

Under normal conditions, the kidneys reabsorb about 99% of the 140 to 160 L of renal filtrate formed each day; consequently, the volume of urine excreted daily by the kidneys ranges from 1000 to 1500 mL, or about 1.5 quarts.

Elimination of 1 g of solute by the kidneys requires about 15 mL of water. Thus, a portion of water in urine becomes "obligated" to rid the body of metabolic byproducts such as urea, an end product of protein breakdown. Large quantities of protein used for energy (as occurs with a high-protein diet) actually accelerate dehydration during exercise.

Water Loss Through the Skin

A small quantity of water, perhaps 350 mL, continually seeps from the deeper tissues through the skin to the body's surface as **insensible perspiration**. Water loss also occurs through the skin in the form of sweat produced by specialized sweat glands beneath the skin. Evaporation of sweat provides the refrigeration mechanism to cool the body. Each day under normal thermal and physical activity conditions the body produces 500 to 700 mL of sweat. This by no means reflects sweating capacity, because a well-acclimatized person can produce up to 12 L of sweat (at a rate of 1 L per hour) during prolonged, moderately intense exercise in a hot environment.

Water Loss as Water Vapor

Insensible water loss through small water droplets in exhaled air amounts to between 250 and 350 mL per day from the complete moistening of inspired air as it passes down the pulmonary airways. Exercise affects this source of water loss. For physically active persons, the respiratory passages release 2 to 5 mL of water each minute during strenuous exercise, depending on climatic conditions. Ventilatory water loss is least in hot, humid weather and greatest in cold temperatures (inspired air contains little moisture) and at altitude. The latter occurs because inspired air volumes (which require humidification) are significantly larger than at sea-level conditions.

Water Loss in Feces

Intestinal elimination produces between 100 and 200 mL of water loss because water constitutes approximately 70% of fecal matter. The remainder comprises nondigestible materials including bacteria from the digestive process and the residues of digestive juices from the intestine, stomach, and pancreas. With diarrhea or vomiting, water loss increases to 1500 to 5000 mL, a potentially dangerous situation that can create fluid and electrolyte imbalance.

WATER REQUIREMENT IN EXERCISE

The loss of body water represents the most serious consequence of profuse sweating. The severity of physical activity, environmental temperature, and humidity determine the amount of water lost through sweating. **Relative humidity** (water content of the ambient air) affects the efficiency of the sweating mechanism in temperature regulation. Ambient air becomes completely saturated with water vapor at 100% relative humidity. This blocks any evaporation of fluid from the skin surface to the air, minimizing this important avenue for cooling the body. Under such conditions, sweat beads on the skin and eventually rolls off without providing a cooling effect. On a dry day, the air can hold considerable moisture, and fluid evaporates rapidly from the skin. Thus, the sweat mechanism functions at optimal efficiency and body temperature remains regulated within a narrow range. Chapters 3 and 25 present a more detailed discussion of fluid replacement with exercise. Importantly, a decrease in plasma volume occurs when sweating causes a fluid loss equal to 2 or 3% of body mass. Fluid loss from the vascular compartment places a significant strain on circulatory function, which ultimately impairs exercise capacity and thermoregulation. *Monitoring changes in body weight provides a convenient method to assess fluid loss during exercise and/or heat stress. Each 0.45 kg (1 lb) of body weight loss corresponds to 450 mL (15 oz) of dehydration.*

HYPONATREMIA: SWEATING + PLAIN WATER INTAKE = TOO MUCH OF TWO GOOD THINGS

Major concerns in hot-weather exercise include:

- Dehydration
- Decreased plasma volume and resulting hemoconcentration
- Impaired physical performance and thermoregulatory capacity
- Increased risk of heat injury, particularly heat stroke

The exercise physiology literature contains more than adequate information about the need to consume fluid before, during, and after exercise. In many instances, the recommended beverage remains plain, hypotonic water. However, excessive fluid intake under certain exercise conditions can be counterproductive, producing the potentially serious medical complication of **hyponatremia**, or "water intoxication," first described among athletes in 1985. Symptoms range from mild (headache, confusion, malaise, nausea, cramping) to severe (seizures, coma, pulmonary edema, and death).

Hyponatremia exists when serum sodium concentration falls below 135 $mEq \cdot L^{-1}$; serum sodium below 130 $mEq \cdot L^{-1}$ triggers severe symptoms. The most conducive conditions for hyponatremia include high-intensity, ultramarathon-type, continuous exercise lasting 6 to 8 hours, although it may occur with exercise of only 4 hours. Mild-to-severe hyponatremia from fluid overload has been reported with increasing frequency in ultraendurance athletes competing in hot weather.[156] For example, nearly 30% of the athletes competing in the 1984 Ironman Triathlon had symptoms of hyponatremia, most frequently observed late in the race or in the recovery period. In a large study of more than 18,000 ultraendurance athletes (including triathletes), approximately 9% of collapsed athletes during or following competition had symptoms of hyponatremia.[117] The athletes, on average, drank fluids with low sodium chloride content (< 6.8 $mmol \cdot L^{-1}$). The runner with the most severe hyponatremia (serum Na level = 112 $mEq \cdot L^{-1}$) excreted in excess of 7.5 L dilute urine during the first 17 hours of hospitalization.

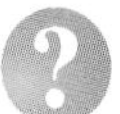

INTEGRATIVE QUESTION

In what way would knowledge about hyponatremia modify your recommendations concerning fluid intake prior to, during, and in recovery from long-duration exercise?

Medical personnel monitored 95 athletes receiving medical care and 169 athletes not requiring care in the 1996 New Zealand Ironman Triathlon (swim 3.8 km, cycle 180 km, run 42 km) for changes in body mass and blood sodium concentration.[155] For athletes with clinical evidence of fluid or electrolyte disturbance, body mass declined 2.5 kg (−2.9 kg in athletes without medical care). Hyponatremia accounted for 9% of medical abnormalities (identical to that reported above[117]). One athlete with hyponatremia (serum Na = 130 $mEq \cdot L^{-1}$) drank 16 L of fluid during the race, and gained 2.5 kg of body mass—consistent with the hypothesis that fluid overload causes hyponatremia. In an ultradistance multisport triathlon (kayak 67 km, cycle 148 km, run 23.8 km), average body mass of the competitors declined 2.5 kg (3% of initial body mass).[154] None of the athletes gained weight, six weighed the same; the one athlete who became hyponatremic (serum Na = 134 $mEq \cdot L^{-1}$) maintained weight and did not seek medical attention. Serum sodium concentration at the end of the race for the 47 athletes averaged 139.3 $mEq \cdot L^{-1}$.

Development of hyponatremia involves extreme sodium loss through prolonged sweating, coupled with dilution of existing extracellular sodium (reduced osmolality) from consuming fluids with low or no sodium. Several hours of exercise in heat can produce significant sodium loss. Exercise in hot, humid weather often produces a sweating rate of more than 1 L per hour, with sweat sodium concentrations ranging from 20 to 100 $mEq \cdot L^{-1}$. Also, frequently ingesting large volumes of plain water draws sodium from the extracellular fluid compartment into the unabsorbed intestinal water, further diluting serum sodium concentration.

Prudent recommendations to reduce the risk of hyponatremia in prolonged exercise include (1) refraining from overhydration by not consuming more than 1000 mL of plain water each hour either before, during, or after exercise and (2) adding a relatively small amount of sodium (approximately 25 $mEq \cdot L^{-1}$) to the ingested fluid. Also, including some glucose in the rehydration drink facilitates intestinal water uptake via the glucose–sodium transport mechanism (see Chapters 3 and 25).

PREDISPOSING FACTORS TO HYPONATREMIA

- Prolonged, high-intensity exercise in hot weather
- Augmented sodium loss associated with sweat production containing high sodium concentration, which often occurs in poorly conditioned individuals
- Beginning physical activity in a sodium-depleted state because of "salt-free" or "low-sodium" diets
- Use of diuretic medication for hypertension
- Frequent intake of large quantities of sodium-free fluid during prolonged exercise

Summary

1. Water makes up 40 to 70% of the total body mass. Muscle contains 70% water by weight, whereas water represents only about 10% of the weight of body fat.
2. Of the total body water, roughly 62% occurs intracellularly (inside the cells) and 38% extracellularly in the plasma, lymph, and other fluids.
3. The typical average daily water intake of 2.5 L comes from (1) liquid (1.2 L), (2) food (1.0 L), and (3) metabolic water produced during energy-yielding reactions (0.35 L).
4. Water loss from the body each day occurs from (1) urine (1 to 1.5 L); (2) skin, as insensible perspiration (0.85 L); (3) water vapor in expired air (0.35 L); and (4) feces (0.10 L).
5. Food and oxygen always are supplied in aqueous solution, and waste products always leave via a watery medium. Water also helps give structure and form to the body and plays a pivotal role in temperature regulation.
6. Exercise in hot weather greatly increases the body's water requirement. Extreme conditions increase fluid needs five or six times above normal requirements.
7. Excessive sweating combined with ingestion of large volumes of plain water during prolonged exercise set the stage for hyponatremia or water intoxication. This potentially dangerous condition relates to a significant decrease in serum sodium concentration.

References

1. Alekel L, et al. Contributions of exercise, body composition, and age to bone mineral density in premenopausal women. Med Sci Sports Exerc 1995;27:1477.
2. Alessio HM, et al. Generation of reactive oxygen species after exhaustive aerobic and isometric exercise. Med Sci Sports Exerc 2000;32:1576.
3. Aloia JF, et al. Calcium supplementation with and without hormone replacement therapy to prevent postmenopausal bone loss. Ann Intern Med 1994;120:97.
4. American College of Sports Medicine. American College of Sports Medicine position stand on osteoporosis and exercise. Med Sci Sports Exerc 1995;27:I.
5. American College of Sports Medicine. Position statement on prevention of heat injuries during distance running. Med Sci Sports Exerc 1984;16:ix.
6. Anderson RA, Guttman HN. Trace minerals and exercise. In: Horton ES, Terjung RL, eds. Exercise, nutrition, and energy metabolism. New York: Macmillan, 1988.
7. Anderson RA, et al. Strenuous running: acute effects on chromium, copper, zinc, and selected variables in urine and serum of male runners. Biol Trace Element Res 1984;6:327.
8. Asheden MJ, et al. The haematological response to an iron injection amongst female athletes. Int J Sports Med 1998;19:474.
9. Ashizawa N, et al. Tomographical description of tennis-loaded radius: reciprocal relation between bone size and volumetric BMD. J Appl Physiol 1999;86:1347.
10. Bailey DA, et al. Growth, physical activity, and bone mineral acquisition. Exerc Sport Sci Rev 1996;24:233.
11. Bailey DA, et al. Altered loading patterns and femoral bone mineral density in children with unilateral Legg-Calvé-Pethees disease. Med Sci Sports Exerc 1997;29:1395.
12. Beck RB, and Shoemaker MR. Osteoporosis: Understanding key risk factors and therapetutic options. Phys Sportsmed 2000;28(2):69.
13. van der Beek EJ. Vitamin supplementation and physical exercise performance. In: Williams C, Devlin LT, eds. Foods, nutrition and sports performance. London: E and FN Spon, 1992.
14. Benson J, et al. Inadequate nutrition and chronic calorie restriction in adolescent ballerinas. Phys Sportsmed 1985;13:79.
15. Bonjour J-P, et al. Critical years and stages of puberty for spinal and femoral bone mass accumulation during adolescence. J Clin Endocrinol Metab 1991;73:555.
16. Boot AM, et al. Bone mineral density in children and adolescents: relation to puberty, calcium intake and physical activity. J Clin Endocrinol Metab 1997;82:57.
17. Brune M, et al. Iron loss in sweat. Am J Clin Nutr 1986;43:438.
18. Buckman MT. Gastrointestinal bleeding in long distance runners. Ann Intern Med 1984;101:127.
19. Cann EC. Decreased spinal mineral content in amenorrheic women. JAMA 1984;251:626.
20. Cassell C, et al. Bone mineral density in elite 7-9-yr-old female gymnasts and swimmers. Med Sci Sports Exerc 1996;28:1243.
21. Chung S-C, et al. Effect of exercise during the follicular and luteal phases on indices of oxidative stress in healthy women. Med Sci Sports Exerc 1999;31:409.
22. Clancy SP, et al. Effects of chromium picolinate supplementation on body composition, strength, and urinary chromium loss in football players. Int J Sport Nutr 1994;4:142.
23. Clark LC, et al. Effects of selenium supplementation for cancer prevention in patients with carcinoma of the skin: a randomized trial. JAMA 1996;276:1957.
24. Clarkson PM. Minerals: exercise performance and supplementation in athletes. J Sports Sci 1991;9:91.
25. Clarkson PM, Haymes EM. Exercise and mineral status of athletes: calcium, magnesium, phosphorus, and iron. Med Sci Sports Exerc 1995;27:831.
26. Col NF, et al. Patient-specific decisions about hormone replacement therapy in postmenopausal women. JAMA 1997;2177:1140.
27. Conroy BP, et al. Bone mineral density in elite junior Olympic weight lifters. Med Sci Sports Exerc 1993;25:1103.
28. Costill DL, et al. Dietary potassium and heavy exercise: effects on muscle water and electrolytes. Am J Clin Nutr 1982;36:266.
29. Cummings SR, et al. Endogenous hormones and the risk of hip and vertebral fractures among older women. N Engl J Med 1998;339:733.
30. Danesh J, Appleby P. Coronary heart disease and iron status: meta-analysis of prospective studies. Circulation 1999;99:852.
31. Davies KJA, et al. Muscle mitochondrial bioenergetics, oxygen supply, and work capacity during dietary iron deficiency and repletion. Am J Physiol 1982;242:E418.
32. Demirel HA, et al. Exercise training reduces myocardial lipid peroxidation following short-term ischemia-reperfusion. Med Sci Sports Exerc 1998;30:1211.
33. Deuster PA, et al. Nutritional survey of highly trained women runners. Am J Clin Nutr 1986;45:954.
34. Diaz MN, et al. Antioxidants and atherosclerotic heart disease. N Engl J Med 1997;337:408.
35. Dook JE, et al. Exercise and bone mineral density in mature female athletes. Med Sci Sports Exerc 1997;29:291.
36. Dueck CA, et al. A diet and training intervention program for the treatment of athletic amenorrhea. Int J Sports Nutr 1996;6:134.
37. Dressendorfer RH, et al. Plasma mineral levels in marathon runners during a 20-day road race. Phys Sportsmed 1982;10:113.
38. Drinkwater BL. C.H. McCloy research lecture: does physical activity play a role in preventing osteoporosis? Res Q Exerc Sport 1994;65:197.
39. Drinkwater BL, et al. Menstrual history as a determinant of current bone density in young athletes. JAMA 1990;263:545.
40. Dwyer JH, et al. Dietary calcium, calcium supplementation, and blood pressure in African American adolescents. Am J Clin Nutr 1998;68:648.
41. Dyson KC, et al. Gymnastics training and bone density in pre-adolescent females. Med Sci Sports Exerc 1997;29:443.
42. Ely DL. Overview of dietary sodium effects on and interactions with cardiovascular and neuroendocrine functions. Am J Clin Nutr 1997;65(suppl):594S.
43. Erp-Bart van AMJ, et al. Nationwide survey on nutritional habits in elite athletes. Part 1: energy, carbohydrate, protein and fat intake. Int J Sports Med 1989;10(Suppl 1):S3.
44. Fehling PC, et al. A comparison of bone mineral densities among female athletes in impact loading and active loading sports. Bone 1995;17:205.
45. Ford ES, Sowell A. Serum α-tocopherol status in United States population: findings from the Third National Health and Nutrition Examination Survey. Am J Epidemiol 1999;150:290.
46. Gardner GW, et al. Cardiorespiratory, hematological and physical performance responses of anemic subjects to iron treatment. Am J Clin Nutr 1975;28:982.
47. Gey GO, et al. Effects of ascorbic acid on endurance performance and athletic injury. JAMA 1970;211:105.
48. Ginsburg GS, et al. Effects of a single bout of ultraendurance exercise on lipid levels and susceptibility of lipids to peroxidation in triathletes. JAMA 1996;276:221.
49. Gledhill N, et al. Haemoglobin, blood volume, cardiac function, and aerobic power. Can J Appl Physiol 1999;24:54.
50. Goldfarb AH, et al. Vitamin E effects on indexes of lipid peroxidation in muscle from DHEA-treated and exercised rats. J Appl Physiol 1994;76:1630.
51. Goldfarb AH, et al. Vitamin E attenuates myocardial oxidative stress induced by DHEA in rested and exercised rats. J Appl Physiol 1996;80:486.
52. Gonzalez ER. Premature bone loss found in some nonmenstruating sports-women. JAMA 1982;248:513.
53. Gradual NA, et al. Effects of sodium restriction on blood pressure, renin, aldosterone, catecholamines, cholesterol, and triglyceride: a meta-analysis. JAMA 1998;279:1383.
54. Gremion G, et al. Oligo-amenorrheic long-distance runners may lose more bone in spine than femur. Med Sci Sports Exerc 2001;33:15.
55. Halberg L. Does calcium interfere with iron absorption (editorial). Am J Clin Nutr 1998;63:3.
56. Halliwell B, Chirico S. Lipid peroxidation: its mechanism, measurement and significance. Am J Clin Nutr (suppl) 1993;57:715S.
57. Harats D, et al. Citrus fruit supplementation reduces lipoprotein oxidation in young men ingesting a diet high in saturated fat: presumptive evidence for an interaction between vitamins C and E in vivo. Am J Clin Nutr 1998;67:240.

58. Hawkins SA, et al. Eccentric muscle action increases site-specific osteogenic response. Med Sci Sports Exerc 1999;31:1287.
59. Heaney R. Bone mass, nutrition and other life style factors. Am J Med 1993;95 (Suppl 5A):29.
60. Heaney RP, et al. Calcium nutrition and bone health in the elderly. Am J Clin Nutr 1982;36:986.
61. Hellsten Y, et al. Effect of sprint cycle training on activities of antioxidant enzymes in human skeletal muscle. J Appl Physiol 1996;81:1484.
62. Hemilä H. Vitamin C and common cold incidence: a review of studies with subjects under heavy physical stress. Int J Sports Med 1996;17:379.
63. Hodis HN, et al. Serial coronary angiographic evidence that antioxidant vitamin intake reduces progression of coronary artery disease. JAMA 1995;273:1849.
64. Hundig A, et al. Runner's anemia and iron deficiency. Acta Med Scand 1981;209:315.
65. Hunt SC, et al. Angiotensinogen genotype, sodium reduction, weight loss, and prevention of hypertension. Trials of Hypertension Prevention, phase II. Hypertension 1998;32:393.
66. Hunter EJ, et al. Dietary carotenoids and vitamins A, C, and E and risk of breast cancer. J Natl Cancer Inst 1999;91:547.
67. Hutchinson TM, et al. Factors in daily physical activity related to calcaneal mineral density in men. Med Sci Sports Exerc 1995;27:745.
68. Ji LL. Exercise and oxidative stress: role of the cellular antioxidant systems. Exerc Sport Sci Rev 1995;23:135.
69. Jialil I, Devaraj S. Low-density lipoprotein oxidation, antioxidants, and atherosclerosis: a clinical biochemistry perspective. Clin Chem 1996;42:498.
70. Jialil I, Grundy SM. Effect of combined supplementation with alpha-tocopherol, ascorbate, and beta carotene on low-density lipoprotein oxidation. Circulation 1993;88:2780.
71. Johnston CC Jr, et al. Calcium supplementation and increases in bone mineral density in children. N Engl J Med 1992;327:82.
72. Jordan J, et al. Red cell membrane skeletal changes in marathon runners. Int J Sports Med 1998;19:16.
73. Kanter MM. Free radicals and exercise: effects of nutritional antioxidant supplementation. Exerc Sport Sci Rev 1995;23:375.
74. Kerr D, et al. Exercise effects on bone mass in postmenopausal women are site-specific and load-dependent. J Bone Miner Res 1996;11:218.
75. Khanna S, et al. α-Lipoic acid supplementation: tissue glutathione homeostasis at rest and after exercise. J Appl Physiol 1999;86:1191.
76. Khoo C-S, et al. Nutrient intake and eating habits of triathletes. Ann Sports Med 1987;3:144.
77. Kirchner EM, et al. Effect of past gymnastic participation on adult bone mass. J Appl Physiol 1996;80:226.
78. Klesges RC, et al. Changes in bone mineral content in male athletes: mechanisms of action and intervention effects. JAMA 1996;276:226.
79. Klingshirn LA, et al. Effect of iron supplementation on endurance capacity in iron-depleted female runners. Med Sci Sports Exerc 1992;24:819.
80. Klipstein-Grobusch K, et al. Dietary antioxidants and risk of myocardial infarction in the elderly: the Rotterdam Study. Am J Clin Nutr 1999;69:261.
81. Kohrt WM, et al. HRT preserves increases in bone mineral density and reductions in body fat after a supervised exercise program. J Appl Physiol 1998;84:1506.
82. Kontulainen S, et al. Changes in bone mineral content with decreased training in competitive young adult tennis players and controls: a prospective 4-yr follow-up. Med Sci Sports Exerc 1999;31:646.
83. Kotchen TA, McCarron DA. Dietary electrolytes and blood pressure. Circulation 1998:68:613.
84. Krebs P, et al. The acute and prolonged effects of marathon running on 20 blood parameters. Phys Sportsmed 1982;10:58.
85. Krebs JM, et al. Zinc and copper balances in healthy adult males during and after 17 wk of bed rest. Am J Clin Nutr 1993;58:897.
86. Kritchevsky SB, et al. Provitamin A carotenoid intake and carotid artery plaques: the Atherosclerosis Risk in Communities Study. Am J Clin Nutr 1998;68:726.
87. Kushi LH, et al. Dietary antioxidant vitamins and death from coronary heart disease in postmenopausal women. N Engl J Med 1996;334:1156.
88. Layne JE, Nelson ME. The effects of progressive resistance training on bone density: a review. Med Sci Sports Exerc 1999;31:25.
89. Leaf DA, et al. The effect of exercise intensity on lipid peroxidation. Med Sci Sports Exerc 1997;29:1036.
90. LeBoff MS, et al. Occult vitamin D deficiency in postmenopausal US women with acute hip fracture. JAMA 1999;281:1505.
91. Levine M, et al. Criteria and recommendations for vitamin C intake. JAMA 1999;281:1415.
92. Lin Y, et al. Estimating the concentration of β-carotene required for maximal protection of low-density lipoproteins in women. Am J Clin Nutr 1998;67:837.
93. Livshits G, et al. Genes play an important role in bone aging. Hum Biol 1998;10:421.
94. Lloyd T, et al. Dietary caffeine intake and bone status of post-menopausal women. Am J Clin Nutr 1997;65:1826.
95. Lönnerdal B. Bioavailability of copper. Am J Clin Nutr 1996;63(suppl):821S.
96. Loucks AB. The reproductive system. In: Bar-Or O, et al., eds. Perspectives in exercise science and sports medicine, vol 9: Exercise and the female—a life span approach. Carmel, IN: Cooper Publishing, 1996.
97. Luc G, et al. Oxidation of lipoproteins and atherosclerosis. Am J Clin Nutr 1991;55:265S.
98. Luft GS, Weinberger MH. Heterogeneous responses to changes in dietary salt intake: the salt-sensitivity paradigm. Am J Clin Nutr 1997;65(suppl):626S.
99. Lukaski HC. Interactions among indices of mineral element nutrition and physical performance of swimmers. In: Kies CV, Driskell JA, eds. Sports nutrition: minerals and electrolytes. Boca Raton, FL: CRC Press, 1995.
100. Lukaski HC, et al. Iron, copper, magnesium and zinc status as predictors of swimming performance. Int J Sports Med 1996;17:535.
101. Lyle RM, et al. Iron status in exercising women: the effect of oral iron therapy vs increased consumption of muscle foods. Am J Clin Nutr 1992;56:1099.
102. Manore, MM. Vitamin B_6 and exercise. Int J Sports Nutr 1994;5:89.
103. Martinez ME, et al. Physical activity, body mass index, and prostaglandin E_2 levels in rectal mucosa. J Natl Cancer Inst 1999;91:950.
104. McBride JM, et al. Effect of resistance exercise on free radical production. Med Sci Sports Exerc 1998;30:67.
105. Michaud DS, et al. Fruit and vegetable intake and incidence of bladder cancer in a male prospective cohort. J Natl Cancer Inst 1999;91:605.
106. Micklesfield LK, et al. Bone mineral density in mature, premenopausal ultramarathon runners. Med Sci Sports Exerc 1995;27:688.
107. Midgley JP, et al. Effect of reduced dietary sodium on blood pressure: a meta-analysis of randomized controlled trials. JAMA 1996;275:1590.
108. Mitchel J, et al. Respiratory weight loss during exercise. J Appl Physiol 1972;32:474.
109. Moffatt RJ. Dietary status of elite female high school gymnasts: inadequacy of vitamin and mineral intake. J Am Diet Assoc 1984;84:1361.
110. Montain SJ, et al. Aldosterone and vasopressin response in the heat: hydration level and exercise intensity effects. Med Sci Sports Exerc 1997;29:661.
111. Myburgh KH, et al. Low bone mineral density at axial and appendicular sites in amenorrheic athletes. Med Sci Sports Exerc 1993;25:1197.
112. Nappo F, et al. Impairment of endothelial functions by acute hyperhomocystinemia and reversal by antioxidant vitamins. JAMA 1999;281:2113.
113. Nattiv A, et al. The female athlete triad. Clin Sports Med 1994;13:405.
114. Nichols DL, et al. Relationship of regional body composition to bone mineral density in college females. Med Sci Sports Exerc 1995;27:178.
115. Nickols-Richardson SM, et al. Premenarcheal gymnasts possess higher bone mineral density than controls. Med Sci Sports Exerc, 2000;32:62.
116. Nieves JN, et al. Calcium potentiates the effect of estrogen and calcitonin on bone mass: review and analysis. Am J Clin Nutr 1998;67:18.
117. Noakes TD, et al. The incidence of hyponatremia during prolonged ultraendurance exercise. Med Sci Sports Exerc 1990;22:165.

118. O'Toole ML, et al. Hemolysis during triathlon races: its relation to race distance. Med Sci Sports Exerc 1988;20:172.
119. Poalini M, et al. Co-carcinogenic effect of β-carotene. Nature 1999;398:760.
120. Percey EC. Ergogenic aids in athletics. Med Sci Sports 1978;10:298.
121. Peters EM, et al. Vitamin C supplementation reduces the incidence of postrace symptoms of upper-respiratory-tract infection in ultramarathon runners. Am J Clin Nutr 1993;57:170.
122. Pizza FX, et al. Serum haptoglobin and ferritin during a competitive running and swimming season. Int J Sports Med 1997;18:233.
123. Podmore I, et al. Vitamin C exhibits pro-oxidant properties. Nature 1998;392:559.
124. Powers SK, et al. Influence of exercise and fiber type on antioxidant enzyme activity in rat skeletal muscle. Am J Physiol (Regulatory Integrative Comp Physiol 35) 1994;266: R375.
125. Powers SK, et al. Exercise training-induced alterations in skeletal muscle antioxidant capacity: a review. Med Sci Sports Exerc 1999;31:987.
126. Praticò D, et al. Vitamin E suppresses isoprostane generation in vivo and reduces atherosclerosis in ApoE-deficient mice. Nature Med 1998;4:1189.
127. Rajaram S, et al. Effects of long-term moderate exercise on iron status in young women. Med Sci Sports Exerc 1995;27:1105.
128. Reid IR, et al. Effect of calcium supplementation on bone loss in postmenopausal women. N Engl J Med 1993;328:460.
129. Rencken ML, et al. Bone density at multiple skeletal sites in amenorrheic athletes. JAMA 1996;276:238.
130. Report of the Council on Scientific Affairs: Diet and cancer: where do matters stand? Arch Intern Med 1993;153:50.
131. Rimm EB, et al. Folate and vitamin B_6 from diet and supplements in relation to risk of coronary heart disease among women. JAMA 1998;279:359.
132. Ripple MO, et al. Effect of antioxidants on androgen-induced AP-1 and NF-kB DNA-binding activity in prostate carcinoma cells. J Natl Cancer Inst 1999;91:1227.
133. Risser WL, et al. Iron deficiency in female athletes: its prevalence and impact on performance. Med Sci Sports Exerc 1988;20:116.
134. Robertson JO, et al. Fecal blood loss in response to exercise. Br Med J 1987;295:303.
135. Robinson S. Cardiovascular and respiratory reactions to heat. In: Yousef MK, et al., eds. Physiological adaptations. New York: Academic Press, 1972.
136. Robinson TL, et al. Gymnasts exhibit higher bone mass than runners despite similar prevalence of amenorrhea and oligomenorrhea. J Bone Miner Res 1995;10:26.
137. Rodriguez Tuya I, et al. Evaluation of the influence of physical activity on plasma concentrations of several trace metals. Eur J Appl Physiol 1996;23:299.
138. Rokitzke L, et al. Acute changes in vitamin B_6 status in endurance athletes before and after a marathon. Int J Sports Nutr 1994;4:154.
139. Rokitzki L, et al. Assessment of vitamin B_6 status of strength and speedpower athletes. J Am Coll Nutr 1994;13:87.
140. Ryan AS, et al. Aerobic exercise maintains regional bone mineral density during weight loss in postmenopausal women. J Appl Physiol 1998;84:1305.
141. Sack MN, et al. Oestrogen and inhibition of oxidation of low-density lipoproteins in postmenopausal women. Lancet 1994;343:269.
142. Sawka MN, Coyle EF. Influence of body water and blood volume on thermoregulation and exercise performance in the heat. Exerc Sport Sci Rev 1999;27:167.
143. Schmid A, et al. Effect of physical exercise and vitamin C on absorption of ferric sodium citrate. Med Sci Sports Exerc 1996;28:1470.
144. Schoene RB, et al. Iron repletion decreases maximal exercise lactate concentrations in female athletes with minimal iron-deficiency anemia. J Lab Clin Med 1983;102:306.
145. Sempos CT, et al. Body iron stores and risk of coronary heart disease. N Engl J Med 1994;330:1119.
146. Shern-Brewer S, et al. Exercise and cardiovascular disease: a new perspective. Atherosclerosis Thromb Vasc Biol 1998;18:11.
147. Shoemaker JD, et al. Relationships between fluid and electrolyte hormones and plasma volume during exercise with training and detraining. Med Sci Sports Exerc 1998;30:497.
148. Sinaki M, et al. A three year controlled, randomized trial of the effect of dose-specified loading and strengthening exercise on bone mineral density of spine and femur in nonathletic, physically active women. Bone 1996;19:233.
149. Singh A, et al. Chronic multivitamin-mineral supplementation does not enhance physical performance. Med Sci Sports Exerc 1992;24:726.
150. Singh A, et al. Neuroendocrine response to running in women after zinc and vitamin E supplementation. Med Sci Sports Exerc 1999;31:536.
151. Sjodin B, et al. Biochemical mechanisms for oxygen free radical formation during exercise. Sports Med 1990;10:233.
152. Smith AD. The female athlete triad: causes, diagnosis, and treatment. Phys Sportsmed 1996;24(7):67.
153. Snyder AC, et al. Importance of dietary iron source on measures of iron status among female runners. Med Sci Sports Exerc 1989;21:7.
154. Speedy DB, et al. Weight changes and serum sodium concentrations after an ultradistance multisport triathlon. Clin J Sport Med 1997;7:100.
155. Speedy DB, et al. Hyponatremia and weight changes in an ultradistance triathlon. Clin J Sport Med 1997;7:180.
156. Speedy DB, et al. Hyponatremia in ultradistance triathletes. Med Sci Sports Exerc 1999;31:809.
157. Stamler J. The INTERSALT study: background, methods, findings, and implications. Am J Clin Nutr 1997;65(suppl):626S.
158. Steinberg D. Low density lipoprotein oxidation and its pathobiological significance. J Biol Chem 1997;272:20963.
159. Steinberg FM, Chait A. Antioxidant vitamin supplementation and lipid peroxidation in smokers. Am J Clin Nutr 1998;68:319.
160. Steinberg DL, et al. Beyond cholesterol modification of low-density lipoprotein that increases its atherogenicity. N Engl J Med 1989;320:915.
161. Suominen H., Rahkila P. Bone mineral density of the calcaneus in 70- to 81-yr-old male athletes and a population sample. Med Sci Sports Exerc 1991;23:1227.
162. Taaffe DR, et al. Differential effects of swimming versus weight bearing activity on bone mineral status of eumenorrheic athletes. J Bone Miner Res 1995;10:586.
163. Taubes G. The (political) science of salt. Science 1998;281:898.
164. Teegarden D, et al. Dietary calcium, protein, and phosphorus are related to bone mineral density and content in young women. Am J Clin Nutr 1998;68:749.
165. Telford R, et al. The effect of 7 to 8 months of vitamin/mineral supplementation on athletic performance. Int J Sports Nutr 1992;2:135.
166. Tessier F, et al. Selenium and training effects on the glutathione system and aerobic performance. Med Sci Sports Exerc 1995;27:390.
167. Thomas MK, et al. Hypovitaminosis D in medical inpatients. N Engl J Med 1998;338:784.
168. Tiidus PM, Houston ME. Vitamin E status and response to exercise training. Sports Med 1995;26:12.
169. Tomten SE, et al. Bone mineral density and menstrual irregularities. A comparative study of cortical and trabecular bone structures in runners with alleged normal eating behavior. Int J Sports Med 1998;19:87.
170. Use of vitamin and mineral supplements in the United States. Nutr Rev 1990;70:43.
171. Uitterlinden AG, et al. Relation of alleles of the collagen type I α I gene to bone density and risk of osteoporotic fractures in postmenopausal women. N Engl J Med 1998;338:1016.
172. Ulrich CM, et al. Bone mineral density in mother-daughter pairs: relations to lifetime exercise, lifetime milk consumption, and calcium supplements. Am J Clin Nutr 1996;63:72.
173. Vasankari TJ, et al. Increased serum and low-density-lipoprotein antioxidant potential after antioxidant supplementation in endurance athletes. Am J Clin Nutr 1997;65:1052.
174. Vincent HK, et al. Exercise training protects against contraction-induced lipid peroxidation in the diaphragm. Eur J Appl Physiol 1999;79:268.
175. Virk RS, et al. Effect of vitamin B-6 supplementation on fuels, catecholamines, and amino acids during exercise in men. Med Sci Sports Exerc 1999;31:400.
176. Viquie CA, et al. Antioxidant status and indexes of oxidative stress during consecutive days of exercise. J Appl Physiol 1993;75:566.

177. Waller MF, Haymes EM. The effects of heat and exercise on sweat iron loss. Med Sci Sports Exerc 1996;28:197.
178. Webster MJ, et al. The effect of a thiamin derivative on exercise performance. Eur J Appl Physiol 1997;75:520.
179. Weight LM, et al. Sports anemia: a real or apparent phenomenon in endurance-trained athletes. Int J Sports Med 1992;13:344.
180. Westerlind KC, et al. Effect of resistance exercise training on cortical and cancellous bone in mature male rats. J Appl Physiol 1998;84:459.
181. Whelton PK, et al. Sodium reduction and weight loss in the treatment of hypertension in older persons: a randomized controlled trial of nonpharmacologic interventions in the elderly (TONE). JAMA 1998;279:839.
182. Winters K, et al. Bone density and cyclic ovarian function in trained runners and active controls. Med Sci Sports Exerc 1996;28:776.
183. Yeager KK, et al. The female athlete triad—disordered eating, amenorrhea and osteoporosis. Med Sci Sports Exerc 1993;25:775.
184. Yoshizawa K, et al. Study of prediagnostic selenium level in toenails and the risk of advanced prostate cancer. J Natl Cancer Inst 1998;90:9219.
185. Yusuf S, et al. Vitamin E supplementation and cardiovascular events in high-risk patients. N Engl J Med 2000;342:154.

CHAPTER 3

Optimal Nutrition for Exercise

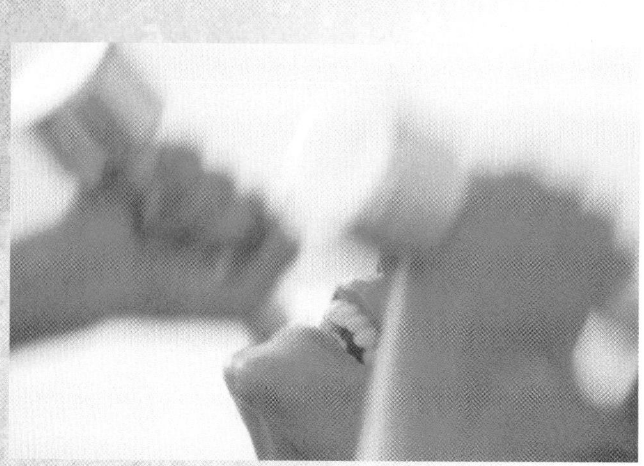

Chapter Objectives

- Compare nutrient and energy intakes of physically active men and women and their sedentary counterparts
- Provide prudent recommendations for carbohydrate, lipid, and protein intake for individuals who (1) maintain a physically active lifestyle and (2) regularly engage in heavy training
- Outline the Food Guide Pyramid recommendations
- Give examples of the energy intakes of men and women involved in training for diverse competitive sport activities
- Advise an athlete concerning timing and composition of the precompetition meal; justify your reasons for limiting lipid and protein intake
- Advise endurance athletes about the (1) potential negative effects of consuming a concentrated sugar drink within 30 minutes of competition and (2) rationale and recommended intake for carbohydrate during intense endurance exercise
- Define the glycemic index; provide examples of high, moderate, and low glycemic index foods; and describe the role of the glycemic index in preexercise and postexercise carbohydrate replenishment
- Outline an optimal glycogen replenishment schedule following a bout of high-intensity endurance exercise that depletes liver and muscle glycogen
- Describe the composition of the ideal sports drink and give the rationale for the drink's composition
- Give recommendations for fluid and carbohydrate replacement during exercise
- Discuss the controversy concerning high-fat versus low-fat diets for exercise training and endurance performance

An optimal diet supplies required nutrients in adequate amounts for tissue maintenance, repair, and growth without excess energy intake. As the understanding of human nutrition evolves, a reasonable estimate of nutritional needs of men and women takes into account normal variation in nutrient digestion, absorption, and assimilation, and daily energy expenditure. Dietary recommendations for men and women at high levels of sports competition should also consider the specific sport's energy requirements and training demands and individual dietary preferences. Reliance on low-calorie "semistarvation" diets or high-fat, low-carbohydrate diets, "liquid-protein" diets, or single-food diets can jeopardize health, exercise performance, and optimum body composition. Excluding sufficient dietary carbohydrate can rapidly lead to a state of relative glycogen depletion, which may eventually produce "staleness" that hinders a person's ability to train and compete.

NUTRIENT REQUIREMENTS

Physically active people do not require additional nutrients beyond those obtained in a balanced diet. Active Americans, including those involved in exceptional endurance activities, consume typical diets remarkably similar in composition to diets of more sedentary counterparts.[7,46] Table 3.1 shows that the main difference in diet entails a larger *quantity* of food consumed; the physically active eat more of the same foods to support the extra energy for their additional exercise. In essence, sound nutrition for athletes equals sound human nutrition. However, individuals involved in heavy training must pay special attention to maintaining adequate, regular carbohydrate intake.

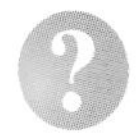

INTEGRATIVE QUESTION

In what ways might the nutritional and energy intake goals for training differ from the requirements for actual competition?

Recommended Nutrient Intake

Figure 3.1 lists the recommended intakes for protein, lipid, and carbohydrate and the food sources for these macronutrients for a resting daily energy requirement of about 1200 kcal. A total daily energy requirement of 2000 kcal for women and 3000 kcal for men represents the average values for typical young adults. *After meeting basic nutrient requirements (as recommended in Fig. 3.1), a variety of food sources based on individual preference can supply the extra energy needs for physical activity.*

Protein

As discussed in Chapter 1, 0.83 g per kg of body mass represents the recommended dietary allowance (RDA) for protein intake. A person weighing 77 kg (170 lb) therefore requires about 64 g, or 2.2 oz, of protein daily. Assuming that even during exercise relatively little protein catabolism occurs through energy metabolism (an assumption not entirely correct), the protein recommendation still remains adequate for most active

TABLE 3.1 ➤ COMPARISON OF CARBOHYDRATE, LIPID, PROTEIN, AND CALORIC INTAKE OF MIDDLE-AGED MALE AND FEMALE RUNNERS AND SEDENTARY CONTROLS[a]

	RUNNERS	SEDENTARY CONTROLS
Males		
Calories (kcal · d^{-1})	2959.0[b]	2361.0
Protein (g · d^{-1})	102.1	93.6
Protein (%)	13.8[b]	15.8
Lipid (g · d^{-1})	134.4[b]	109.0
Lipid (%)	40.8	41.5
Carbohydrate (g · d^{-1})	294.6[b]	225.7
Carbohydrate (%)	39.8	38.6
Cholesterol (mg · 1000 kcal^{-1})	175.0	190.0
Saturated fat (g · 1000 kcal^{-1})	16.2	16.0
Polyunsaturated fat (g · 1000 kcal^{-1})	9.0	9.3
Females		
Calories (kcal · d^{-1})	2386.0[b]	1871.0
Protein (g · d^{-1})	82.2	76.7
Protein (%)	14.2[b]	17.4
Lipid (g · d^{-1})	110.7	83.0
Lipid (%)	41.1	40.3
Carbohydrate (g · d^{-1})	234.3[b]	174.7
Carbohydrate (%)	39.5	39.1
Cholesterol (mg · 1000 kcal^{-1})	190.0	205.0
Saturated fat (g · 1000 kcal^{-1})	16.8	16.5
Polyunsaturated fat (g · 1000 kcal^{-1})	8.5	7.9

From Blair SN et al: Comparisons of nutrient intake in middle-aged men and women runners and controls. Med Sci Sports. Exerc 1981;13:310.
[a]% calories do not total 100% because alcohol calories constitute the difference.
[b]Values for runners are significantly different from controls.

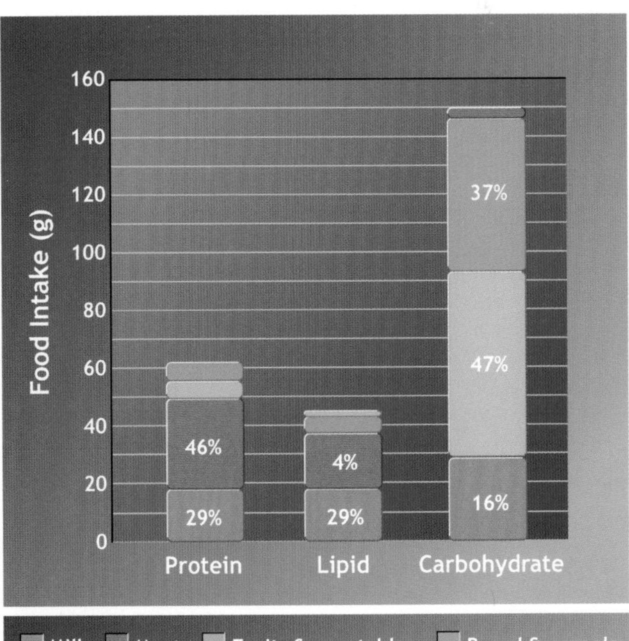

FIGURE 3.1 • Basic recommendations for carbohydrate, lipid, and protein components, and the general categories of food sources in a balanced diet to meet resting daily energy requirement of about 1200 kcal.

individuals. Also, the protein intake in the average American diet significantly exceeds protein's RDA. For athletes in heavy training, a protein intake between 1.2 and 1.8 g per kg body mass should meet any added protein-related nutrient demands. This does not necessarily require protein supplementation as the typical athlete's diet exceeds the protein RDA by two to four times. One nutritional dilemma for the vegetarian athlete concerns obtaining an adequate essential amino acid balance from a diet containing all (or most) protein sources from the plant kingdom. Chapter 1 discussed the use of complementary protein food sources to minimize this concern.

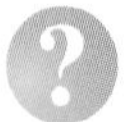

INTEGRATIVE QUESTION

In what situations might a protein intake representing twice the RDA still prove inadequate for an individual involved in heavy exercise training?

Lipid

Standards for optimal lipid intake have not been firmly established. The amount of dietary lipid varies widely depending on personal taste, money spent on food, geographic influences, and availability of lipid-rich foods. For example, lipid furnishes only about 10% of the energy in the average diet of people living in Asia, whereas in many Western countries lipid accounts for 40 to 45% of the total energy intake. *Lipid intake should not exceed 30% of the diet's energy content to promote good health. Of this, at least 70% should be in the form of unsaturated fatty acids.* Significant reductions in dietary lipid, however, may compromise exercise performance. Consuming a low-fat diet during strenuous training makes it difficult to increase carbohydrate and protein intake to furnish sufficient energy to maintain body weight and muscle mass. Also, the essential fatty acids (e.g., linoleic acid) and fat-soluble vitamins become available via dietary lipids; thus, a low-fat or "fat-free" diet could create a relative state of malnutrition.

Carbohydrate

The prominence of dietary carbohydrates varies widely throughout the world, depending on availability and relative cost of lipid-rich and protein-rich foods. Carbohydrate-rich unrefined grains, starchy roots, and dried peas and beans usually cost least relative to their energy value. In the Far East, carbohydrates (rice) contribute 80% of the total energy intake, whereas in the United States only about 40 to 50% of total energy comes from carbohydrates. *Subsisting chiefly on a variety of fiber-rich complex carbohydrates, with adequate intake of essential amino acids, fatty acids, minerals, and vitamins, does not compromise health.* The diet of the Tarahumara Indians of Mexico (see "Focus on Research," page 101) consists of high-fiber and complex-carbohydrate foods and correspondingly low cholesterol, lipid, and saturated fat.[22] The Tarahumaras exhibit little or no hypertension, obesity, or death from cardiac and circulatory complications.

Dietary carbohydrate intake takes on additional importance for individuals involved in a significant amount of physical activity on the job or in exercise training and sports competition. Stored muscle glycogen becomes the prime energy contributor under conditions of inadequate oxygen supply to active muscles. In addition to this anaerobic role of carbohydrates, stored glycogen (and blood glucose) provides substantial energy during intense aerobic exercise.[21] *Considering the body's limited glycogen reserves, the diet of physically active individuals should contain at least 55 to 60% of calories in the form of carbohydrates, predominantly starches from fiber-rich, unprocessed grains, fruits, and vegetables.* For many competitive athletes (e.g., swimmers, rowers, and speed skaters), the importance of maintaining a relatively high daily carbohydrate intake relates more to the considerable energy demands of training than to the short-term demands of competition.

CARBOHYDRATE NEEDS IN INTENSE TRAINING. Athletes training for endurance activities such as distance running, ocean swim-

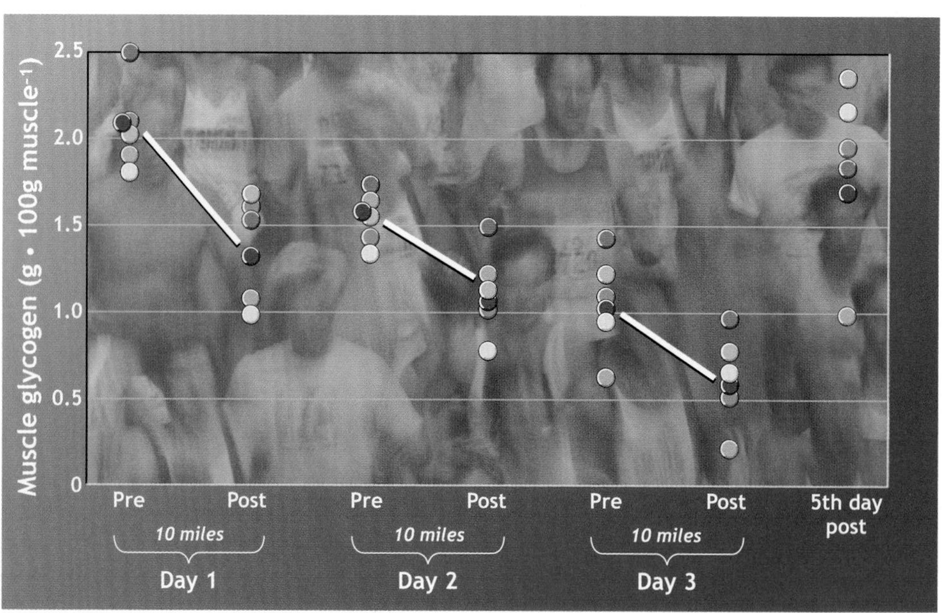

FIGURE 3.2 • Changes in muscle glycogen concentration for six male subjects before and after each 10-mile (16.1-km0 run performed on three successive days. Muscle glycogen measured 5 days after the last run is referred to as "5th day post." (From Costill DL, et al. Muscle glycogen utilization during prolonged exercise on successive days. J Appl Physiol 1971;31:834.)

IN A PRACTICAL SENSE

NUTRITION TO PREVENT CHRONIC ATHLETIC FATIGUE

Endurance runners, swimmers, cross-country skiers, and cyclists frequently experience chronic fatigue as successive days of hard training become progressively more difficult. Normal exercise performance deteriorates because the individual experiences increasing difficulty recovering from each training session. The overtraining syndrome (see Chapter 21) also relates to frequent infections and general malaise and loss of interest in sustaining high-level training. Injuries occur more frequently in the overtrained, stale state.

Depleted Carbohydrate Plays a Role

Gradually depleting carbohydrate reserves with repeated strenuous training most likely contributes to the overtraining syndrome. It requires at least 1 to 2 days of rest or lighter exercise combined with a high carbohydrate intake to reestablish preexercise muscle glycogen levels after exhaustive training or competition. Unduly heavy exercise performed regularly requires an upward adjustment of daily carbohydrate intake to optimize glycogen resynthesis and high-quality training.

The following table provides nutritional recommendations to reduce the likelihood of athletic fatigue or staleness:

PRACTICAL NUTRITIONAL GUIDELINES FOR ATHLETES TO PREVENT CHRONIC FATIGUE

1. Consume easily digested, high-carbohydrate drinks or solid foods 1 to 4 h before training or competition. Consume about 1 g carbohydrate/kg body mass 1 h before exercise and up to 5 g carbohydrate/kg body mass if the feeding occurs 4 h prior to exercise. For example, a 70-kg swimmer could drink 350 mL (12 oz) of a 20% carbohydrate beverage 1 h before exercise or eat 14 "energy bars," each containing 25 g carbohydrate, spread over the 4-h period before exercise.
2. Consume a readily digested, high-carbohydrate liquid or solid food containing 0.35–1.5 g carbohydrate/kg body mass/h immediately after exercise for the first 4 h after exercise. Thus, a 70-kg swimmer could drink 100–450 mL (3.6–16 oz) of a 25% carbohydrate beverage or 1 to 4 energy bars, each containing 25 g of carbohydrate immediately after exercise and every hour thereafter for 4 h.
3. Consume a 15–25% carbohydrate drink or a solid, high-carbohydrate supplement with each meal. For example, reduce consumption of normal foods by 250 kcal and consume a high-carbohydrate beverage or solid food containing 250 kcal of carbohydrate with each meal.
4. Stabilize body weight during all phases of training by matching energy consumption to training's energy demands. This also helps to maintain body carbohydrate reserves.

From Sherman WJ, Maglischo EW. Minimizing chronic athletic fatigue among swimmers: special emphasis on nutrition. Sports Science Exchange. Gatorade Sports Science Institute. 1991;35(4).

ming, cross-country skiing, or cycling frequently experience a state of chronic fatigue in which successive days of hard training become progressively more difficult. This **staleness** often relates to the gradual depletion of the body's glycogen reserves, even though the athlete's diet contains the typical percentage of carbohydrate. Figure 3.2 shows that three successive days of running 16.1 km (10 miles) nearly depleted the glycogen in the thigh muscle. This occurred even though the runners' diet contained 40 to 60% carbohydrates. By the third day, the quantity of glycogen used during the run averaged considerably less than on the first day. Presumably, the body's fat reserves supplied the predominant energy for exercise on day 3. Unmistakably, a person who performs unduly heavy exercise on a regular basis must adjust the daily carbohydrate allowance upward to permit optimal glycogen resynthesis to maintain high-quality training. The need for optimal replenishment of depleted glycogen reserves provides nutritional justification for the recommendation of many coaches to gradually reduce, or taper, the intensity of exercise routines several days prior to competition.[96]

Because glycogen synthesis relates to carbohydrate intake, individuals undergoing heavy training should consume 10 g of carbohydrate per kg of body mass each day to induce protein sparing and ensure adequate glycogen reserves.[11,12,23] Thus, the daily carbohydrate intake for a small 46-kg (100-lb) athlete who expends about 2800 kcal each day should average 450 g, or 1800 kcal. The athlete weighing 68 kg (150 lb) should consume 675 g of carbohydrate (2700 kcal) daily to sustain an energy requirement averaging 4200 kcal. In both examples, carbohydrates exceed the minimum requirement (55 to 60%) to represent 65% of total energy intake. Even with a high-carbohydrate diet, complete glycogen replenishment does not occur rapidly following prolonged effort, particularly in the type I (slow-twitch) muscle fibers. *While liver glycogen replenishes at a faster rate, it takes at least 20 hours to fully restore muscle glycogen after a glycogen-depleting bout of exhaustive exercise.*[27]

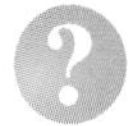

INTEGRATIVE QUESTION

From a nutritional perspective, why might a reduction in the total volume of daily training bring about improved training responsiveness and competitive performance?

The Food Guide Pyramid: The Essentials of Good Nutrition

Two principles of good eating include *variety* and *moderation*. Lobbyists for the beef and dairy industries greatly influenced earlier approaches to formulating recommendations for sound nutrition, such as the Four-Food-Group Plan developed by the U.S. Department of Agriculture (USDA). Research in nutrition, cancer, and heart disease over the past 40 years uncovered the shortcomings of this plan, with an emphasis on meat and milk products, as a guide to healthful eating. To

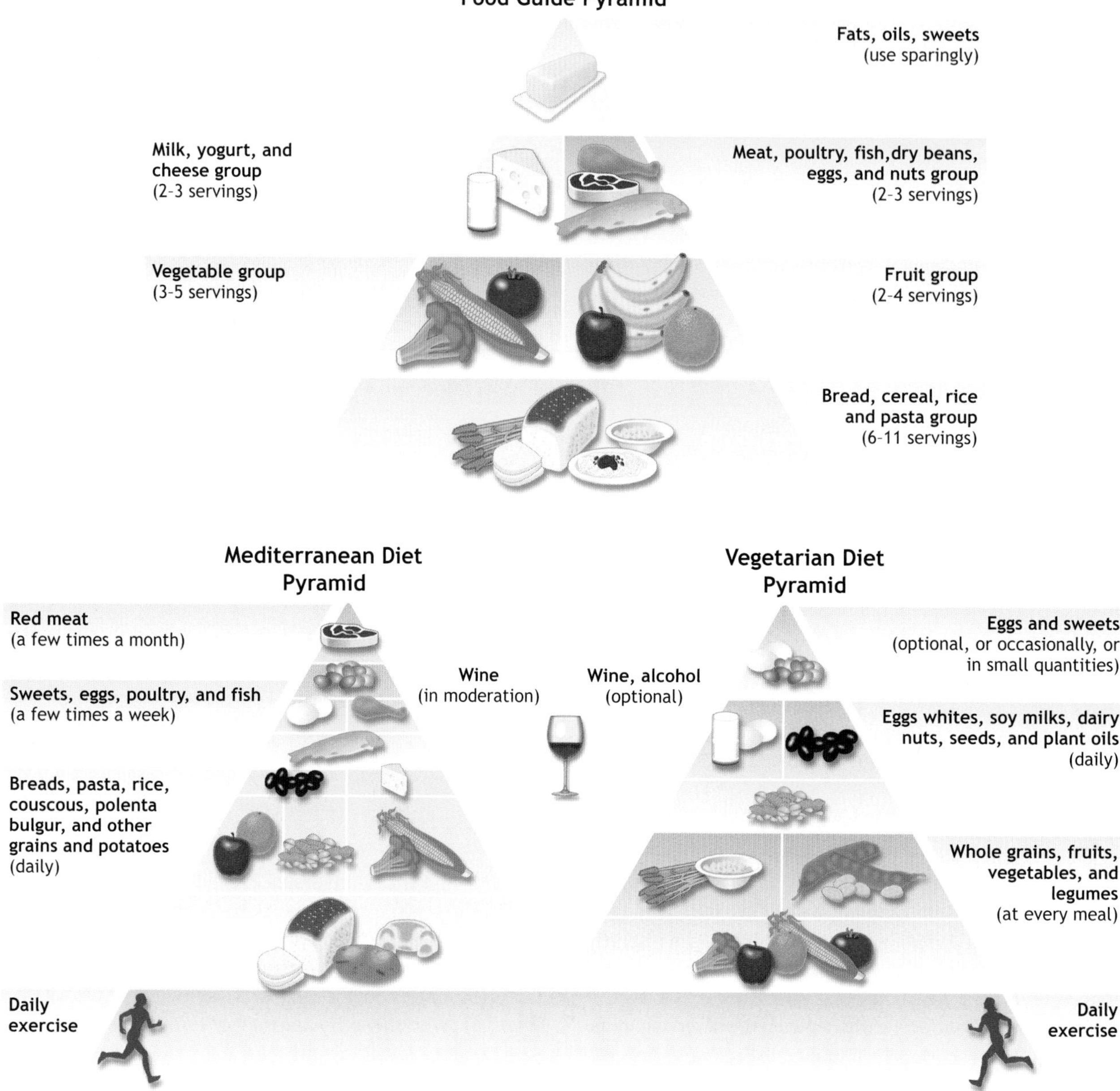

FIGURE 3.3 • The Food Guide Pyramid emphasizes grains, vegetables, and fruits as important sources of nutrients.

reflect the current state of nutritional knowledge more clearly, the USDA developed the **Food Guide Pyramid**, a new model of dietary guidelines for Americans aged 2 years and older (Fig. 3.3).*[97] The two bottom figures present modifications of the basic pyramid for application to individuals whose diet consists largely of (1) foods from the plant kingdom (Vegetarian Diet Pyramid) or (2) fruits, nuts, vegetables, fish, beans, and all manner of grains, with dietary fat composed mostly of mono-unsaturated fatty acids (Mediterranean Diet Pyramid). A Mediterranean-style diet offers protection for individuals at high risk of death from heart disease;[32] its high monounsaturated fatty acid content may also stave off age-related memory loss in healthy, elderly people.[88] Dietary focus of all three pyramids on fruits and vegetables, particularly cruciferous and green leafy vegetables and citrus fruit and juice, also significantly reduces risk for ischemic stroke.[56]

The pyramid's approach to good nutrition and a healthful diet translates the RDAs and *Dietary Guidelines* by categorizing foods that make similar nutrient contributions and recommending the number of servings from each category. Dietary emphasis focuses on whole grains, vegetables, and fruits, all rich in fiber and a myriad of plant chemicals that may exert far stronger effects than the specific antioxidant vi-

*The latest "Dietary Guidelines for Americans" (fifth edition) includes a recommendation to exercise moderately for 30 minutes (e.g. walking, jogging, bicycling, and lawn, garden, and house work) "most, preferably all, days of the week." The Guidelines also advise children to get 60 minutes of moderate physical activity daily. They acknowledge that good nutrition combined with regular exercise provides an important approach to ensure good health, and combat the obesity epidemic in the United States. The Guidelines separate fruits and vegetables from grains and emphasize whole grains.

tamins. The pyramid downplays food sources high in animal protein, lipids, and dairy products. Monounsaturated and polyunsaturated fatty acids constitute the major form of lipids consumed. Because meat, fish, and poultry represent good sources of B vitamins, iron, and zinc, vegetarians must emphasize these nutrients in their nonmeat dietary sources. Although the guidelines for healthful eating focus on the general population, they also provide a sound framework for meal planning for the physically active man and woman.

INTEGRATIVE QUESTION

How would you advise a high school soccer team with individuals from diverse ethnic backgrounds with unique food intake patterns about sound nutrition?

EXERCISE AND FOOD INTAKE

Figure 3.4 illustrates the average energy intakes for males and females in the United States in relation to age for 1988 to 1991.[9] Energy intakes peaked between ages 16 and 29 years and then declined for succeeding age groups. A similar pattern occurred for males and females, although males reported higher daily energy intakes than females at all ages. Between ages 20 and 29 years, the women consumed on average 35% fewer kcal than men on a daily basis (3025 kcal [12,657 kJ] versus 1957 kcal [8188 kJ]). Thereafter, the difference in energy intake between genders was smaller; at age 70 years, women consumed about 25% fewer kcal than their male counterparts.

Individuals who engage regularly in moderate-to-intense physical activity eventually increase daily energy intake to match their higher energy expenditure level. Lumber workers, who expend approximately 4500 kcal daily, unconsciously adjust energy intake to closely balance energy output. Consequently, body mass remains stable despite a seemingly large food intake. The daily food intake of athletes in the 1936 Olympics reportedly averaged more than 7000 calories, or roughly three times the average daily intake.[1] These oft quoted energy values justify what many believe to be an enormous food requirement of athletes in training. However, these figures represent only estimates because objective dietary data do not appear in the original report. They probably depict inflated estimates of energy expended (and required) by the athletes. Distance runners who train upward of 100 miles per week (6-min mile pace at 15 kcal per min) probably do not expend more than 800 to 1300 "extra" kcal each day above their normal energy requirements to balance their increased energy expenditure. Figure 3.5 presents data on energy intake from a large sample of elite male and female

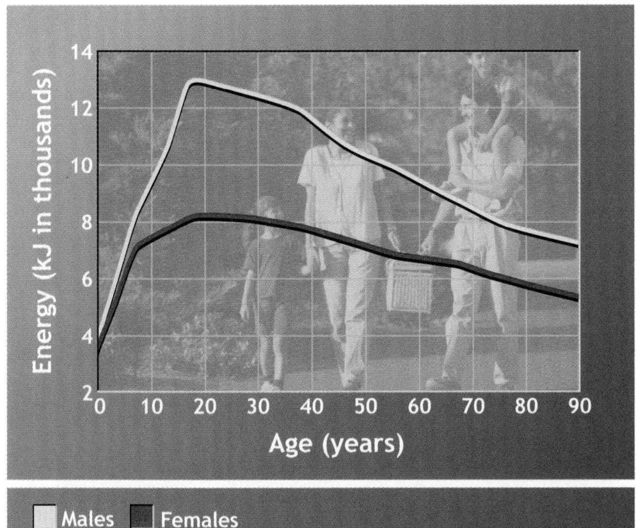

FIGURE 3.4 • Average daily energy intake for males and females by age in the U.S. population during the years 1988 to 1990. Multiply by 0.239 to convert kJ to kcal. (From Briefel RR, et al. Total energy intake of the US population: The third National Health and Nutrition Examination Survey, 1988–1991. Am J Clin Nutr 1995;62(suppl):1072S.)

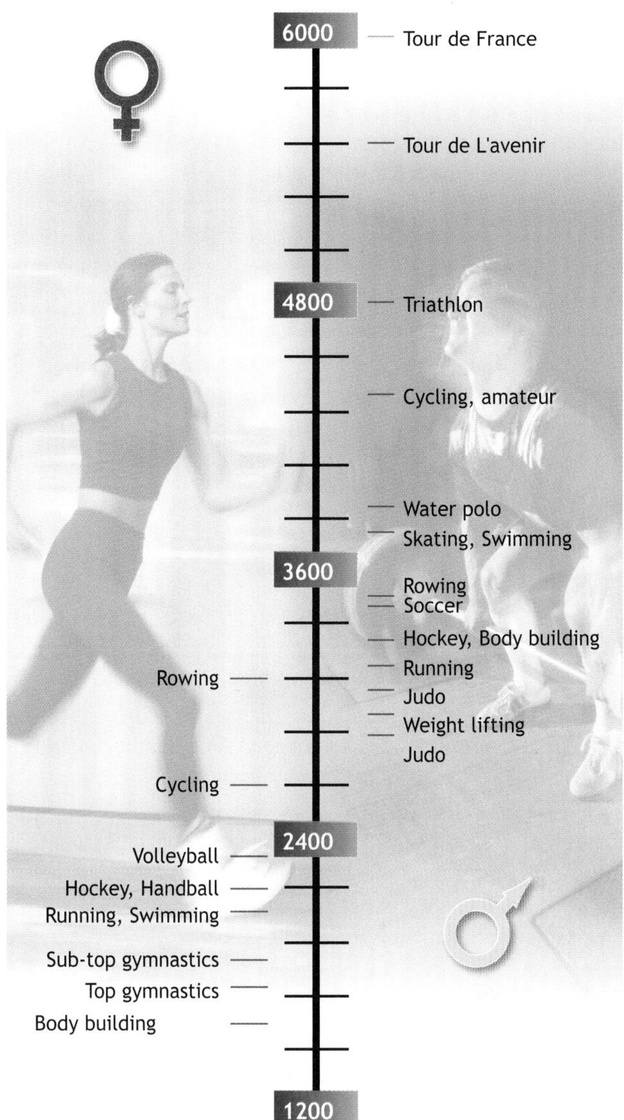

FIGURE 3.5 • Daily energy intake (kcal) of elite male and female endurance, strength, and team sport athletes. (Modified from van Erp-Baart AMJ, et al. Nationwide survey on nutritional habits in elite athletes. Int J Sports Med 1989;10:53.)

endurance, strength, and team sport athletes in the Netherlands.[98] For males, daily energy intake ranged between 2900 and 5900 kcal, whereas female competitors consumed between 1600 and 3200 kcal. With the exception of the large energy intakes of athletes at extremes of performance and training, daily energy intake generally did not exceed 4000 kcal for men and 3000 kcal for women.

To complement these observations, the doubly labeled water technique indicated that daily energy expenditure of elite female swimmers increased to 5593 kcal daily during high-volume training. This value represents the highest level of sustained daily energy expenditure reported for female athletes.[95] However, the swimmers' daily energy intakes did not increase to match training demands. It averaged only 3136 kcal, implying a negative energy balance of 43%. A negative energy balance in the transition from moderate to heavy training may ultimately compromise an athlete's full potential to train and compete.

Tour de France

Figure 3.6 outlines the variation in daily energy expenditure for a male competitor during the Tour de France professional cycling race. In this most grueling of sporting events, energy expenditure averaged 6500 kcal daily for nearly 3 weeks. Large daily variation occurred depending on activity level for a particular day; the daily energy expenditure decreased to about 3000 kcal on a "rest" day and increased to approximately 9000 kcal cycling over a mountain pass. By combining liquid nutrition with normal meals, this cyclist nearly matched daily energy expenditure with energy intake.

Other sport and training activities also require extreme energy output (and correspondingly high energy intake), sometimes in excess of 1000 kcal per hour in elite marathoners. The daily energy requirements of elite cross-country skiers during 1 week of training averaged 3740 to 4860 kcal for women and 6120 to 8570 kcal for men.[86] Another study used the doubly labeled water technique to evaluate the energy balance for two men who pulled sledges with starting weights of 222 kg (10 h · d^{-1} for 95 days) for 2,300 km across Antarctica.[90] During a 10-day period of the expedition, one man averaged a daily energy expenditure of 10,654 kcal, while his counterpart averaged an extraordinary intake of 11,634 kcal. These values approach the 13,975-kcal theoretical daily energy expenditure ceiling attained by ultra–long-distance runners.[17]

Ultraendurance Running Competition

Energy balance was studied during a 1000-km (approximately 600-mile) race from Sidney to Melbourne, Australia.[79] The Greek ultramarathon champion Kouros completed the race in 5 days, 5 hours, and 7 minutes, finishing 24 hours and 40 minutes ahead of the next competitor. Table 3.2 provides relevant features of race conditions, distance covered, average daily speed, and rest and sleep patterns. Kouros did not sleep during the first 2 days of competition. He covered 463 km (287.8 miles) at an average speed of 11.4 km · h^{-1} during day 1 and 8.3 km · h^{-1} on day 2. During the remaining days, he took frequent rest periods, including periodic breaks for short "naps." Weather ranged from spring to winter conditions (30°C to 8°C), and terrain varied. The bottom of Table 3.2 lists the pertinent details of food and water intake.

The near equivalence between Kouros' estimated total energy intake (55,970 kcal) and energy expenditure (59,079 kcal) represents a remarkable aspect of energy balance homeostasis in response to extremes of physical activity. Of

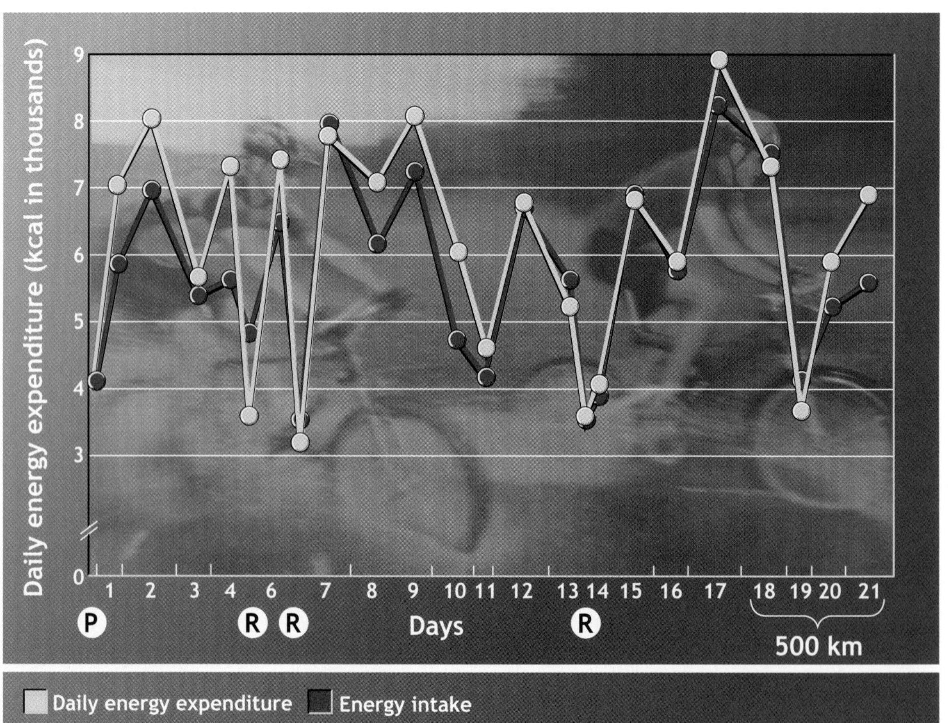

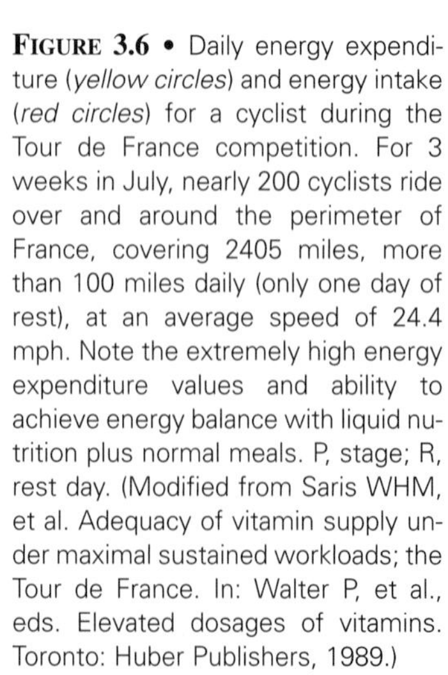
FIGURE 3.6 • Daily energy expenditure (*yellow circles*) and energy intake (*red circles*) for a cyclist during the Tour de France competition. For 3 weeks in July, nearly 200 cyclists ride over and around the perimeter of France, covering 2405 miles, more than 100 miles daily (only one day of rest), at an average speed of 24.4 mph. Note the extremely high energy expenditure values and ability to achieve energy balance with liquid nutrition plus normal meals. P, stage; R, rest day. (Modified from Saris WHM, et al. Adequacy of vitamin supply under maximal sustained workloads; the Tour de France. In: Walter P, et al., eds. Elevated dosages of vitamins. Toronto: Huber Publishers, 1989.)

TABLE 3.2 ➤ *TOP.* **FEATURES ABOUT RACE CONDITIONS, DISTANCE COVERED, AVERAGE DAILY SPEED, REST AND SLEEP PATTERNS, AND NUTRIENT BALANCE DURING AN ELITE ULTRAENDURANCE PERFORMANCE.** *BOTTOM.* **DAILY AND TOTAL ENERGY BALANCE, NUTRIENT DISTRIBUTIONS IN FOOD, AND WATER INTAKE DURING THE RACE.**[a]

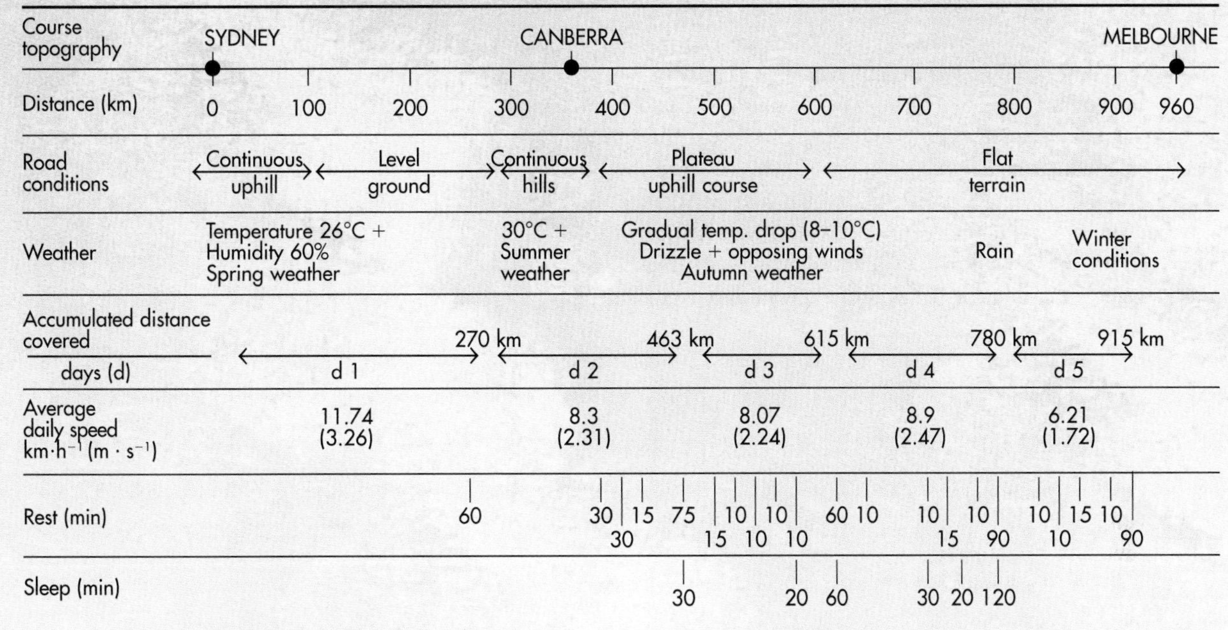

RACE DAY	DISTANCE COVERED (km)	ESTIMATED ENERGY EXPENDITURE (kcal)	ESTIMATED ENERGY INTAKE (kcal)	CARBOHYDRATES (g)	CARBOHYDRATES (%)	CARBOHYDRATES (kcal)	LIPIDS (g)	LIPIDS (%)	LIPIDS (kcal)	PROTEINS (g)	PROTEINS (%)	PROTEINS (kcal)	H_2O (L)
1	270	15367	13770	3375	98.0	13502	20	1.3	180	22	0.7	88	22.0
2	193	10741	8600	1981	92.2	7923	53	5.5	477	50	2.3	200	19.2
3	152	8919	12700	3074	96.8	12297	27	1.9	243	40	1.3	160	22.7
4	165	9780	7800	1758	90.1	7032	56	6.5	504	66	3.4	264	14.3
5	135	7736	12500	3014	96.4	12058	30	2.2	270	43	1.4	172	18.3
5 h	45	2536	550	138	100.0	550	—	—	—	—	—	—	3.2
Total	960	55079	55920	13340		53362	186		1674	221		884	99.7

[a]The runner Kouros weighed 65 kg, stature was 171 cm, percent body fat was 8%, and $\dot{V}O_{2max}$ was 62.5 mL · kg⁻¹ · min⁻¹.
Modified from Rontoyannis GP, et al. Energy balance in ultramarathon running. Am J Clin Nutr 1989;49:976.

the total energy intake, carbohydrates represented 95.3% and lipids 3%, with the remaining 1.7% from proteins. Protein intake from food averaged considerably below recommended levels, but Kouros did take protein supplements in tablet form. The unusually large daily energy intake, which ranged from 8,600 to 13,770 kcal, came from Greek sweets (baklava, cookies, and doughnuts), some chocolate, dried fruit and nuts, various fruit juices, and fresh fruits. Every 30 minutes after the first 6 hours of running, Kouros replaced sweets and fruit with a small biscuit soaked in honey or jam. He consumed a small amount of roasted chicken on day 4, and drank coffee every morning. He took a 500-mg vitamin C supplement every 12 hours and a protein tablet twice daily.

The remarkable achievement by the champion Kouros exemplifies a highly conditioned athlete's exquisite regulatory control for energy balance during strenuous exercise. He performed at a pace that required a continuous energy metabolism averaging 49% of aerobic capacity during the first 2 days of competition and 38% for days 3 through 5. He also finished the competition without compromising overall health (no muscular injuries or thermoregulatory problems, and body mass remained unchanged); reported difficulties included a severe bout of constipation during the run and frequent urination, which persisted for several days post race.

Extreme Ultraendurance Sports

The Iditasport ultramarathon currently consists of a choice of one race event from among the following options: run 120 km, snowshoe 120 km, bicycle 259 km, cross-country ski 250 km, or snowshoe, ski, and bicycle 250 km. Begun in 1983 as a single-event Iditaski, a parallel competition emerged in 1987 consisting of long-distance cycling (Iditabike). In 1991, the two races merged along with foot, snowshoe, and triathlon events. The triathlon was discontinued in 1997, and the lengths of all other races changed to 160 km. The competition begins in late February, and the athletes traverse varied terrain, mostly in the wilderness over frozen rivers and lakes; wooded, rolling hills; and packed snow trails. On any given day, racers can experience extremes in weather conditions, ranging from calm, "balmy" 30°F to harsh −40°F with blizzard conditions. During the 48-hour time limit for the event, racers must carry a minimum of 15 pounds of survival gear; this includes a sleeping bag rated to −20°F, insulated sleeping pad, bivy sack or tent, stove and 8 ounces of fuel with fire starter (matches or lighter), pot to melt snow, insulated water containers to carry 2 quarts of water, headlamp or flashlight, and a minimum of 1 day's supply of emergency food. The supplies are carried in a backpack or pulled by sled (weighing from 15 to 30 lb).

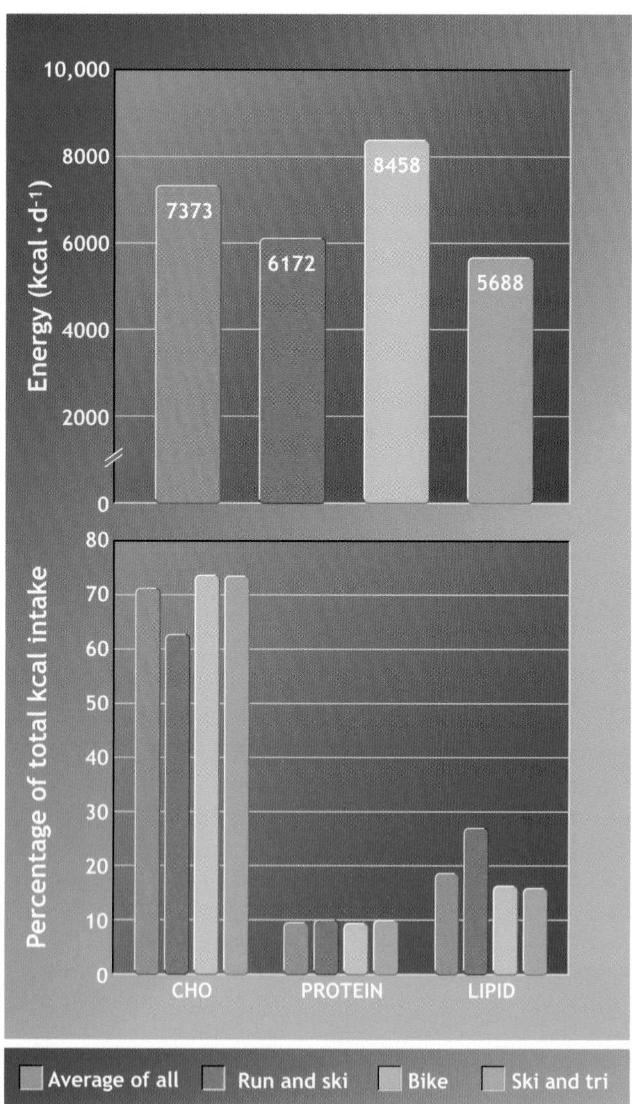

FIGURE 3.7 • Energy and macronutrient content of the diets of Iditasport competitors. Multiply kcal value by 4.182 to convert to kJ. (Data for 1995 from Case D, et al. Dietary intakes of participants in the Iditasport human powered ultra-marathon. Alaska Med 1995;37:20. Data reported in the text for 1997–1998 from Stuempfle K, et al. Dietary factors of participants in the 1994–1998 Iditasport human powered ultra-marathon. Med Sci Sports Exerc 1999;31: S80.)

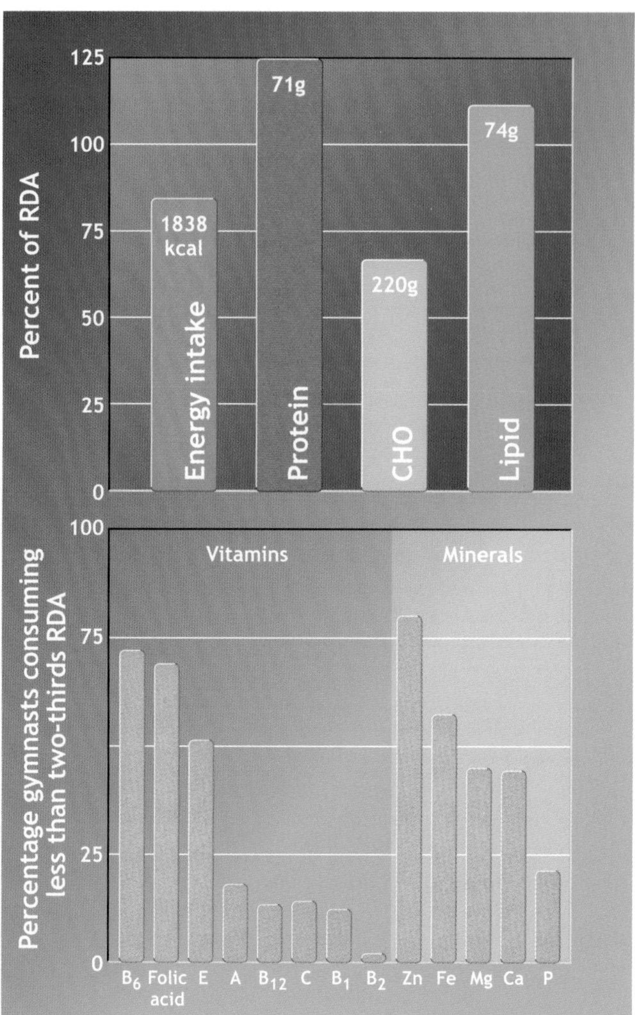

FIGURE 3.8 • Average daily nutrient intake for 97 adolescent female gymnasts (11 to 14 y) related to recommended values (RDA). The RDA on the *y* axis (top) reflects only protein, while energy, CHO, and lipid reflect "recommended" values. Percentage of gymnasts consuming less than two-thirds of the RDA for micronutrients (*bottom*). Mean age, 13.1 y; mean stature, 152.4 cm (60 in); mean body mass, 43.1 kg (94.8 lb). (Modified from Loosli AR, Benson J. Nutritional intake in adolescent athletes. Sports Med 1990;37:1143.)

Researchers estimated the total energy and macronutrient requirements for 14 participants (13 males, 1 female) in the 1995 race with 49 entrants. Figure 3.7 displays the total energy intake and percentage intake of carbohydrate, protein, and fat by runners and snowshoers, bikers, skiers, and triathletes. The bikers consumed the most total calories (8458 kcal), 74.1% as carbohydrate, 9.4% as protein, and 16.5% as fat. A comparison study between 1997–1998 Iditasport athletes and their 1995 counterparts showed only small differences in energy and nutrient contents except for higher intakes of carbohydrate (78.5%) and less fat (14.5%) and protein (7.3%) for skiers. The authors concluded that even though the length of the events differed in 1994–1996 and 1997–1998, few differences existed in the energy content and macronutrient percentages of the diets among the four categories of competitors from the two periods.

Other Athletic Groups

Gymnasts, ballet dancers, ice dancers, and weight-class athletes in boxing, wrestling, and judo engage in arduous training. Owing to the nature of their sport, these men and women continually strive to maintain a lean, relatively light body mass dictated by either esthetic or weight-class considerations. As a result, energy intake often intentionally falls short of energy expenditure, and a relative state of malnutrition develops.[92] Nutritional supplementation for these athletes may prove beneficial, as suggested by the data in Figure 3.8 for daily nutrient intake (% of RDA) of 97 competitive female gymnasts aged 11 to 14 years. Twenty-three percent of the girls consumed less than 1500 kcal daily, and more than 40% consumed less than two-thirds of the RDA for vitamins E and folic acid and the minerals iron, magnesium, calcium, and zinc. Clearly, many of these adolescent gymnasts needed to upgrade the nutritional quality of their diets or consider supplementation. For athletes like these, carbohydrate intake may fail to match the energy requirements of heavy training. As a result, training and competition take place in a carbohydrate-depleted state. Protein supplementation to achieve a daily intake of 1.2 to 1.8 g per kg of body mass may help maintain normal nitrogen balance and optimize training status.

Eat More, Weigh Less

Table 3.1 showed that during endurance training, middle-aged men and women took in 40 to 60% more calories per kg of body mass than their sedentary controls. The extra energy required for running 8 to 10 km daily accounted for the runners' larger caloric intake. Paradoxically, the most active men and women, who ate more on a daily basis, weighed less than those who exercised at a lower total caloric expenditure. Such findings agree with other studies of physically active people. They support the strong argument that regular exercise permits a person to actually "eat more yet weigh less" while maintaining a lower percentage of body fat, despite the age-related tendency toward weight gain in middle age.[14] *Active people maintain a lighter and leaner body and a healthier heart disease risk profile, despite increased intake of the typical, high-fat American diet.* Table 3.3 presents a sample model for food intake for active athletes and an example of a

TABLE 3.3 ➤ SAMPLE TRAINING DIET[a]

BODY WEIGHT	110 LB (50 KG)	132 LB (60 KG)	154 LB (70 KG)	176 LB (80 KG)
Total kcal	**2500[b]**	**3000**	**3500**	**4000**
Milk group (90 kcal) Skim milk, 1 cup Plain, low-fat yogurt, 1 cup	4	4	4	4
Meat group (55–75 kcal) Cooked, lean meat (fish, poultry), 1 oz Egg, 1 Peanut butter, 1 Tbsp Low-fat cheese, 1 oz Cottage cheese, 1/4 cup	5	5	6	6
Fruits	7	9	10	12
Vegetables	3	5	6	7
Grains	16	18	20	24
Lipids	5	6	8	10

Sample high-carbohydrate 2500-kcal menu (350 g)

Breakfast	Lunch	Dinner	Snack 1	Snack 2
1 cup bran cereal 8 oz low-fat milk 1 English muffin 1 tsp margarine 4 oz orange juice	3 oz lean roast beef 1 hard roll 2 tsp mayonnaise or mustard, lettuce and tomato 1/2 cup cole slaw 2 fresh plums 2 oatmeal cookies 8 oz seltzer water with lemon	Chicken stir-fry: 3 oz chicken 1 cup diced vegetables 2 tsp oil 2 cup rice 1 cup orange and grapefruit sections 1 cup vanilla yogurt Iced tea with lemon	3 cups popcorn	8 oz apple cider

[a]An active athlete requires approximately 50 kcal of food per kg (23 kcal per lb) of body mass each day to provide enough calories for optimal athletic performance. A training diet ideally consists of approximately 60% carbohydrates, 15 to 20% proteins, and less than 25% lipids.

[b]Numbers below total kcal values are recommended number of daily servings.

Modified from Carbohydrates and Athletic Performance. Sports Science Exchange, vol. 7. Chicago: Gatorade Sports Science Institute, 1988.

2500-kcal menu containing 350 g of carbohydrates. Chapter 30 discusses the important role of exercise for weight control in more detail.

PRECOMPETITION MEAL

Athletes often compete in the morning following an overnight fast. As Chapter 1 discusses, significant depletion occurs in the body's carbohydrate reserves over an 8- to 12-hour period without eating, even if the athlete has previously followed appropriate dietary recommendations. Consequently, precompetition nutrition takes on considerable importance. *The precompetition meal provides adequate carbohydrate energy and ensures optimal hydration.* Fasting before competition or training makes no sense physiologically because it rapidly depletes liver and muscle glycogen and impairs exercise performance.[34,63,82] Individualizing an athlete's meal plan should consider the following three factors: (1) food preference of the athlete, (2) "psychological set" of competition, and (3) digestibility of foods. As a general rule, competition day should exclude foods high in lipid and protein. Such foods digest slowly and remain in the digestive tract longer than foods containing similar energy content as carbohydrate. Precompetition meal timing also deserves consideration. The increased stress and tension that usually accompany competition significantly reduce blood flow to the digestive tract, causing depressed intestinal absorption. *Three hours usually is a sufficient amount of time to digest and absorb, and benefit from a carbohydrate-rich, precompetition meal.* Extending the time for eating beyond 3 hours may negatively impact subsequent performance in moderate- to high-intensity endurance exercise.[65]

Protein or Carbohydrate?

Many athletes look forward to the classic "steak and eggs" precompetition meal. Such foods may satisfy the athlete, coach, and restaurateur, yet their benefits to exercise performance remain undemonstrated. A meal of this type, with its low carbohydrate content, actually thwarts optimal performance.

The following reasons justify modifying or even abolishing the high-protein precompetition meal in favor of one high in carbohydrates:

- Dietary carbohydrates replenish the significant depletion of liver and muscle glycogen from the overnight fast.
- Carbohydrate digestion and absorption are faster than those of either protein or lipid. Thus, carbohydrate provides energy faster and reduces the feeling of fullness following a meal.
- A high-protein meal elevates resting metabolism more than a high-carbohydrate meal because of protein's greater energy requirements for digestion, absorption, and assimilation. This additional thermic effect could strain the body's heat-dissipating mechanisms and impair exercise performance in hot weather.
- Protein breakdown for energy facilitates dehydration during exercise because the byproducts of amino acid breakdown require water for urinary excretion. About 50 mL of water "accompanies" the excretion of each gram of urea.
- Carbohydrate, not protein, serves as the main energy nutrient for short-term anaerobic activity and high-intensity aerobic exercise.

The ideal precompetition meal maximizes muscle and liver glycogen storage and provides glucose for intestinal absorption during exercise. The meal should:

- Contain 150 to 300 g of carbohydrate (3 to 5 g per kg body mass in either solid or liquid form).
- Be consumed 3 hours before exercising.

The benefits of proper precompetition feeding occur only if the athlete maintains a nutritionally sound diet throughout training. Preexercise feedings cannot correct existing nutritional deficiencies or inadequate nutrient intake during the weeks before competition. Chapter 23 discusses how endurance athletes can augment precompetition glycogen storage in conjunction with specific exercise/diet modifications using "carbohydrate-loading" techniques.

INTEGRATIVE QUESTION

Outline your presentation to a high school class about how to eat well for a physically active and healthy lifestyle.

Liquid and Prepackaged Meals

Commercially prepared liquid meals offer an alternative to precompetition meals. They also effectively enhance the athlete's energy and nutrient intake in training, particularly if daily energy output exceeds food intake because of disinterest or mismanagement of feedings. Liquid meals provide fluid and a high carbohydrate content but also contain enough lipid and protein to contribute to satiety. Liquid meals digest rapidly, leaving essentially no residue in the intestinal tract. They prove particularly effective during day-long swimming and track meets or in tennis, soccer, and basketball tournaments. In these situations, the athlete usually has little time for, or interest in, food. Liquid meals offer a practical approach to supplement energy intake during the high-energy output phases of training. Athletes can also use them if they experience difficulty maintaining a relatively large body mass or as a ready source of calories for weight gain.

CARBOHYDRATE FEEDINGS PRIOR TO, DURING, AND IN RECOVERY FROM EXERCISE

High-intensity aerobic exercise for 1 hour decreases liver glycogen by about 55%, whereas a 2-hour strenuous workout almost depletes the glycogen content of the liver and active muscle fibers. Even supermaximal, repetitive 1- to 5-minute bouts of exercise interspersed with brief rest intervals (e.g., soccer, ice hockey, field hockey, European handball, and tennis) dramatically lower liver and muscle glycogen reserves.

Performance under such conditions improves with carbohydrate supplementation.[71,101,103]

The vulnerability of the body's glycogen stores during strenuous exercise has focused research on the potential benefits of carbohydrate feedings immediately before and during exercise. Scientists also study ways to optimize carbohydrate replenishment in the postexercise recovery period.

During Exercise

Ingested carbohydrate provides a readily available energy nutrient for active muscles during intense exercise.[18,54] *Consuming about 60 g of liquid or solid carbohydrates each hour during exercise benefits high-intensity, long-duration (≥1 h) aerobic exercise and repetitive short bouts of near-maximal effort.*[30,55,66,67] Supplemental carbohydrate during protracted intermittent exercise to fatigue also facilitates skill performance, such as improved stroke quality during the final stages of prolonged tennis play.[101] Little benefit derives from carbohydrate feedings during low-intensity exercise, because fat oxidation fuels exercise, with little demand on carbohydrate breakdown.[2] In contrast, in high-intensity exercise when carbohydrate catabolism predominates, glucose feedings contribute significantly to sustaining exercise. Exogenous carbohydrate either (1) spares muscle glycogen because ingested glucose fuels exercise or (2) maintains a more optimal blood glucose level that prevents headache, lightheadedness, nausea, and other symptoms of central nervous system distress.[15,29,58] Blood glucose maintenance also supplies the needs of muscles when prolonged exercise depletes glycogen reserves.[20,47]

Carbohydrate feeding during exercise at an intensity of 60 to 80% of aerobic capacity postpones fatigue by 15 to 30 minutes.[26] This effect contributes significantly to endurance competition because well-nourished athletes without supplementation usually fatigue within 2 hours when they exercise at 75% of aerobic capacity. A single concentrated carbohydrate feeding about 30 minutes before anticipated fatigue (about 2 hours into exercise) proves as effective as periodic carbohydrate ingestion throughout exercise. This later feeding restores the blood glucose level (Fig. 3.9), which delays fatigue by increasing carbohydrate availability to the active muscles.

The greatest benefits from carbohydrate feedings emerge during prolonged exercise at about 75% of aerobic capacity. When exercise begins above this level, subjects must reduce exercise intensity to about the 75% level to attain the benefits from carbohydrate feedings.[20] Fat provides the primary energy fuel in light-to-moderate exercise below 50% of maximum; at this intensity, glycogen reserves do not decrease to a level that limits endurance in such exercise. Repeated feedings of carbohydrate in solid form (43 g sucrose with 400 mL water) at the beginning and at 1, 2, and 3 hours of exercise maintain blood glucose and slow glycogen depletion during 4 hours of cycling. Glycogen conservation not only extends endurance but also enhances sprint performance to exhaustion at the end of exercise.[5,6,91] *These findings demonstrate that carbohydrate feedings during prolonged, high-intensity aerobic exercise either conserve the muscle's glycogen content for later use or maintain blood glucose for use as exercise progresses and muscle glycogen levels deplete, or both.* The end result is (1) improved endurance at a high steady pace or during intense intermittent exercise and (2) augmented sprint capacity toward the end of prolonged physical effort. In a marathon run, a sustained high-output effort and a final sprint to the finish often determine the winner.

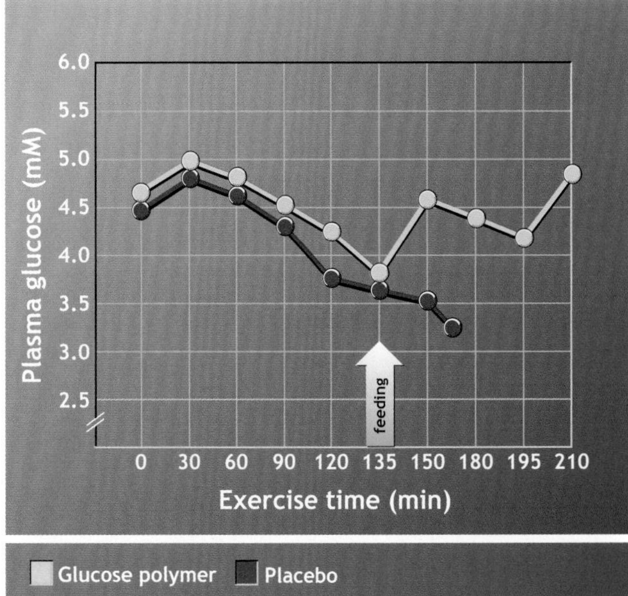

FIGURE 3.9 • Average plasma glucose concentration during prolonged high-intensity aerobic exercise when subjects consumed a placebo or glucose polymer (3 g per kg body mass in a 50% solution). (Modified from Coggan AR, Coyle EF. Metabolism and performance following carbohydrate ingestion late in exercise. Med Sci Sports Exerc 1989;21:59.)

Prior to Exercise

Confusion exists regarding the potential endurance benefits of preexercise ingestion of simple sugars. Some researchers argue that consuming rapidly absorbed, high-glycemic carbohydrates within 1 hour before exercising accelerates glycogen depletion, which negatively affects endurance performance by the following mechanisms:

- It rapidly raises blood sugar, triggering an overshoot in insulin release, which causes a relative hypoglycemia (also called **rebound hypoglycemia**, or reactive hypoglycemia). Significant blood sugar reduction impairs central nervous system function during exercise.
- It facilitates glucose influx into muscle, because of a large insulin release, which disproportionately increases glycogen catabolism in exercise. At the same time, high insulin levels *inhibit* lipolysis, which reduces free fatty acid mobilization from adipose tissue. Augmented carbohydrate breakdown and blunted fat mobilization contribute to premature glycogen depletion and early fatigue.

Research in the late 1970s indicated that drinking a highly concentrated sugar solution within 30 minutes before exercise precipitated early fatigue in endurance activities. For example, when young men and women consumed a 300-mL solution containing 75 g of glucose 30 minutes before cycling exercise, endurance was 19% lower than in similar trials preceded by 300 mL of plain water or a liquid meal of protein, lipid, and carbohydrate.[38] Paradoxically, the concentrated sugar drink depleted muscle glycogen reserves prematurely compared with drinking plain water. The researchers hypothesized that the dramatic rise in blood sugar within 5 to 10 minutes after consuming the concentrated preevent sugar drink caused the pancreas to oversecrete insulin (accentuated hyperinsulinemia). This, in turn, triggered rebound hypoglycemia as glucose moved rapidly into muscle.[48,107] At the same time, insulin inhibited mobilization and use of fat for energy (lipolysis suppression).[89] Consequently, intramuscular glycogen catabolized to a much greater extent, causing early glycogen depletion and fatigue compared with control conditions. Subsequent research has *not* corroborated these negative effects of concentrated preexercise sugar feedings on endurance performance.[3,36,46,89] The discrepancy in research findings has no clear explanation.

One way to eliminate any potential for negative effects of preexercise simple sugars is to ingest them 1 to 3 hours prior to exercising.[44,82] This provides sufficient time to reestablish hormonal balance before exercise begins. When a person consumes significant amounts of carbohydrates *during* endurance exercise, the form of carbohydrate exerts little negative effect on hormonal response, exercise metabolism, or endurance performance.[16] The reason is straightforward: increased levels of sympathetic nervous system hormones (catecholamines) in exercise inhibit insulin release. Concurrently, exercise increases a muscle's absorption of glucose, so any exogenous glucose moves into the cells with a lower insulin requirement.

Debate Concerning Fructose

The small intestine absorbs fructose more slowly than either glucose or sucrose. This causes a minimal insulin response with essentially no decline in blood glucose.[31] This observation has stimulated debate about whether fructose can substitute as an immediate preexercise exogenous carbohydrate fuel source.[69,73] The theoretical rationale for fructose use appears plausible, but its exercise benefits remain inconclusive. From a practical standpoint, gastrointestinal distress (vomiting and diarrhea) often accompanies high-fructose beverage consumption, which in itself negatively affects exercise performance. After absorption, the liver must first convert the fructose to glucose, which further limits the rapidity of fructose availability as an energy source.

In Recovery

Carbohydrates are not all digested and absorbed at the same rate. Researchers devised a physiologically based index to indirectly assess carbohydrate absorption rates. The **glycemic index** provides a relative measure of the increase in blood glucose concentration in the 2 hours after ingestion of a food containing 50 g of carbohydrate, compared with a "standard" for carbohydrate (usually white bread or glucose) with an assigned value of 100.[39,106] Ingesting 50 g of the food with a glycemic index of 45 raises blood glucose concentrations to levels that reach 45% of the value for 50 g of glucose. Figure 3.10 presents a sample of the more than 600 foods classified by their glycemic index, including examples of high– and low–glycemic-index meals of similar calorie and macronutrient composition (see inset table). Interestingly, a food's index rating does not depend simply on its grouping as simple (monosaccharides and disaccharides) or complex (starch and fiber) carbohydrate, since the plant starch in white rice and potatoes has a higher glycemic index than the simple sugars (particularly fructose) in apples and peaches. Because a food's fiber content slows digestion, many vegetables have a low glycemic index such as peas, beans, and other legumes. Clearly, a food with a moderate-to-high glycemic index rating offers more benefit than one rated low for rapid replenishment of carbohydrate following prolonged exercise.[25,104] Dietary lipids and proteins slow food passage into the intestine. This reduces the glycemic index of the meal's accompanying carbohydrate content. Thus, one should limit these foods to optimize carbohydrate replenishment during the recovery period.

Optimal glycogen replenishment benefits individuals involved in (1) regular heavy training, (2) tournament competition with qualifying rounds, or (3) events scheduled with only 1 or 2 days for recuperation. A heavy bout of resistance training also significantly reduces muscle glycogen reserves.[80] Competitive wrestlers who lose considerable glycogen and water attempting to "make weight" (via food and fluid restriction prior to the weigh-in) also benefit from a proper strategy for glycogen replenishment.[53] For collegiate wrestlers, acute weight loss by energy restriction without dehydration impaired anaerobic exercise capacity.[77] When the athletes then consumed a diet containing 75% carbohydrate (21 kcal per kg body mass) over the next 5 hours, anaerobic performance recovered to near-baseline values. No improvement occurred if the refeeding diet contained only 45% carbohydrate. Even without full glycogen replenishment, some replenishment in recovery provides beneficial endurance effects in the next exercise bout. For example, consuming carbohydrate for only 4 hours in recovery from a glycogen-depleting exercise bout significantly improves endurance capacity in subsequent exercise compared with performance when no carbohydrate is eaten in the 4-hour recovery.[53]

INTEGRATIVE QUESTION

Explain why foods with divergent glycemic index values dictate the nutritional recommendations for immediate preexercise versus immediate postexercise feedings.

The glycogen needs of previously exercised muscle significantly affect glycogen resynthesis during recovery.[108] In addition, endurance-trained individuals restore more muscle

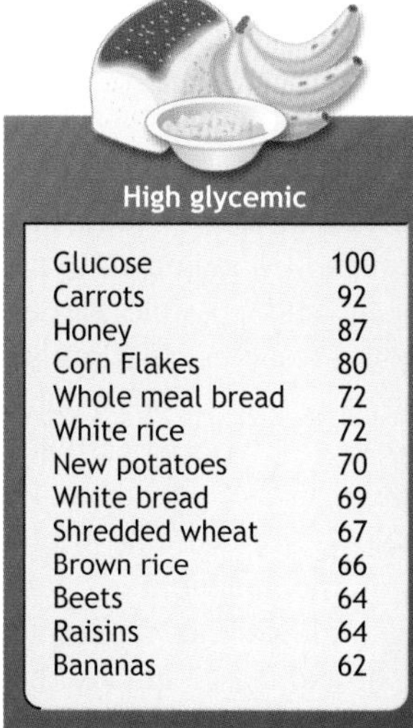

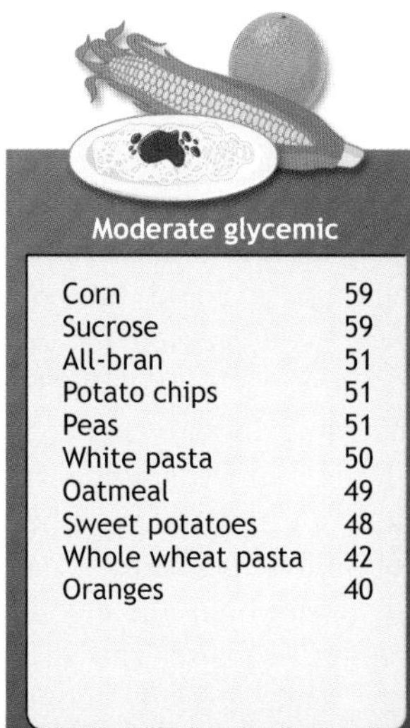

High glycemic	
Glucose	100
Carrots	92
Honey	87
Corn Flakes	80
Whole meal bread	72
White rice	72
New potatoes	70
White bread	69
Shredded wheat	67
Brown rice	66
Beets	64
Raisins	64
Bananas	62

Moderate glycemic	
Corn	59
Sucrose	59
All-bran	51
Potato chips	51
Peas	51
White pasta	50
Oatmeal	49
Sweet potatoes	48
Whole wheat pasta	42
Oranges	40

Low glycemic	
Apples	39
Fish sticks	38
Butter beans	36
Navy beans	31
Kidney beans	29
Lentils	29
Sausage	28
Fructose	20
Peanuts	13

High GI Diet	CHO (g)	Contribution to Total GI	Low GI Diet	CHO (g)	Contribution to Total GI
Breakfast			**Breakfast**		
30 g Corn Flakes	25	9.9	30 g All Bran	24	4.7
1 banana	30	7.8	1 diced peach	8	1.1
1 slice whole meal bread	12	3.8	1 slice grain bread	14	2.2
1 tsp margarine			1 tsp margarine		
			1 tsp jelly		
Snack			**Snack**		
1 crumpet	20	6.4	1 slice grain fruit loaf	20	4.1
1 tsp margarine			1 tsp margarine		
Lunch			**Lunch**		
2 slices wholemeal bread	23.5	7.6	2 slices grain bread	28	4.5
2 tsp margarine			2 tsp margarine		
25 g cheese			25 g cheese		
1 cup diced cantaloupe	8	10.4	1 apple	20	3.6
Snack			**Snack**		
4 plain sweet biscuits	28	10.4	200 g low fat fruit yogurt	26	4.1
Dinner			**Dinner**		
120 g lean steak			120 g lean minced beef		
1 cup of mashed potatoes	32	12.1	1 cup boiled pasta	34	6.4
1/2 cup of carrots	4	1.7	1 cup of tomato and onion sauce	8	2.5
1/2 cup of green beans	2	0.6	Green salad with vinaigrette	1	0.6
50 g broccoli					
Snack			**Snack**		
290 g watermelon	15	5.1	1 orange	10	2.1
1 cup of reduced fat milk throughout day	14	1.9	1 cup of reduced-fat milk throughout day	14	1.9
Total	212	69.8	**Total**	212	39.0

For each diet, the carbohydrate choices are maximized for differences between the two diets.

FIGURE 3.10 • Categorization for glycemic index (GI) of common food sources of carbohydrates. The inset table presents high– and low–glycemic-index diets that contain the same amounts of energy and macronutrients and derive 50% of energy from carbohydrate (CHO) and 30% of energy from lipid. (Diets from Brand-Miller J, Foster-Powell K. Nutr Today 1999;34:64.)

glycogen than untrained counterparts.[52] Consuming food after exercising facilitates glucose transport into muscle cells by:

1. Enhanced hormonal milieu, particularly higher insulin and lower catecholamine levels.
2. Increased tissue sensitivity to insulin and intracellular glucose transporter proteins (e.g., GLUT 1 and GLUT 4; see Chapter 20).
3. Increased activity of a specific form of the glycogen-storing enzyme glycogen synthase.[70]

Practical Recommendations

Consuming high-glycemic, carbohydrate-rich foods as soon as possible after hard training or competition speeds glycogen replenishment. One strategy would be to consume about 50 to 75 g (2 to 3 oz) of high- to moderate-glycemic carbohydrates every 2 hours until reaching 500 g (7 to 10 g per kg of body mass) or until eating a large, high-carbohydrate meal. If this is impractical, an alternative strategy entails eating meals containing 2.5 g of high-glycemic carbohydrate per kg body mass at 2, 4, 6, 8, and 22 hours postexercise. This produces levels of muscle glycogen replenishment similar to those with the same protocol begun immediately postexercise.[74] Legumes, fructose, and milk products have a slow rate of digestion and/or intestinal absorption and should be avoided. Adding protein to an isocaloric postexercise supplement does not facilitate carbohydrate replenishment.[80] Glycogen resynthesis is more rapid if the person remains inactive during the recovery period.[19]

With optimal carbohydrate intake, glycogen stores replenish at about 5 to 7% per hour. Thus, under the best circumstances, it takes at least 20 hours to reestablish glycogen stores after a glycogen-depleting bout of exercise.[27] Postexercise oral glucose also may speed recovery by facilitating removal of free ammonia that forms at an increased rate during strenuous exercise. This results because consuming glucose enhances glutamine and alanine synthesis in skeletal muscle.[43] These compounds provide the primary vehicle to transport ammonia out of muscle tissue.

Cellular Uptake of Glucose

Normal blood glucose concentration (**euglycemia**) approximates 5 mM, equivalent to 90 mg of glucose per dL (100 mL) of blood. Blood glucose can rise above the hyperglycemic level to about 9 mM (162 mg · dL^{-1}) following a meal. A decrease in blood glucose concentration well below normal to 2.5 mM (<45 mg · dL^{-1}) classifies as hypoglycemia; it can occur during starvation or extremes of prolonged exercise.

Entry of glucose into red blood cells, brain cells, and kidney and liver cells depends on the maintenance of a positive concentration gradient of glucose across the cell membrane (termed unregulated glucose transport). In contrast, in large tissue masses such as skeletal and heart muscle and adipose tissue, glucose transport occurs via regulated uptake, with insulin and the predominant intracellular glucose transporter protein GLUT 4 as the regulating compounds.[64] Active skeletal muscle also increases its ability to take up glucose from the blood, independent of the effect of insulin. This effect persists into the early postexercise period and helps to replenish glycogen stores. Thus, maintaining an adequate level of blood glucose during exercise and in recovery decreases possible negative effects from a low blood glucose concentration.

The Glycemic Index and Preexercise Feedings

The ideal meal immediately before exercising should provide a source of carbohydrate to sustain blood glucose and muscle metabolism while minimizing any increase in insulin release. Maintaining a relatively normal plasma insulin level should theoretically preserve blood glucose availability, optimize fat mobilization and catabolism, and at the same time spare liver and muscle glycogen reserves.

Use the glycemic index to formulate the immediate preexercise feeding.[4,33,36] As mentioned on page 93, consuming simple sugars (concentrated high-glycemic carbohydrates) immediately before exercising causes blood sugar to rise rapidly (**glycemic response**), which may trigger excessive insulin release (**insulinemic response**).[8,37] Endurance performance could be compromised by rebound hypoglycemia, depressed fat catabolism, and possible earlier-than-expected depletion of glycogen reserves. In contrast, consuming low-glycemic, carbohydrate-rich foods (starch with high amylose content or moderate-glycemic carbohydrate with high dietary fiber content) in the immediate 45- to 60-minute preexercise period allows a slower rate of glucose absorption, thereby reducing the potential rebound glycemic response. This strategy would eliminate the insulin surge, while a steady supply of "slow-release" glucose becomes available from the digestive tract throughout exercise. This effect should theoretically prove beneficial during prolonged, high-intensity exercise, such as ocean swimming, in which it often becomes impractical to consume carbohydrate during the activity.

Several research studies compared the effects of preexercise, low-glycemic versus high-glycemic carbohydrate ingestion on endurance performance and blood glucose levels during sustained exercise. In one study of trained cyclists who performed high-intensity aerobic exercise, a preexercise low-glycemic meal of lentils significantly extended endurance over that with feedings of glucose or a high-glycemic meal of potatoes of equivalent carbohydrate content.[94] A moderate-glycemic-index breakfast cereal with added dietary fiber eaten 45 minutes before moderately intense exercise increased time to fatigue by 16% compared with control conditions or a high-glycemic meal without fiber.[57] Maintaining relatively high plasma glucose levels during prolonged exercise following a preexercise meal of low-glycemic carbohydrate may also enhance subsequent performance at maximal effort. Ten trained cyclists consumed a low-glycemic or high-glycemic meal 30 minutes before bicycling for 2 hours at 70% $\dot{V}O_{2max}$ followed by bicycling to exhaustion at 100% $\dot{V}O_{2max}$.[31] The low-glycemic meal produced significantly lower plasma insulin levels after 20 minutes of exercise. At the end of 2 hours, carbohydrate oxidation and plasma glucose levels remained significantly higher and ratings of perceived exertion lower than under the high-glycemic conditions. Thereafter, time to exhaustion exercising at $\dot{V}O_{2max}$ averaged 59% longer than high-glycemic maximal effort (Fig. 3.11). All studies, however, do not support the wisdom of preexercise low glycemic feedings for enhancing endurance performance.[104] Further study of the topic certainly seems warranted.

INTEGRATIVE QUESTION

Advise an endurance athlete whose pre-event nutrition consists of a fast-food hamburger and high-protein shake consumed 1 hour before competition.

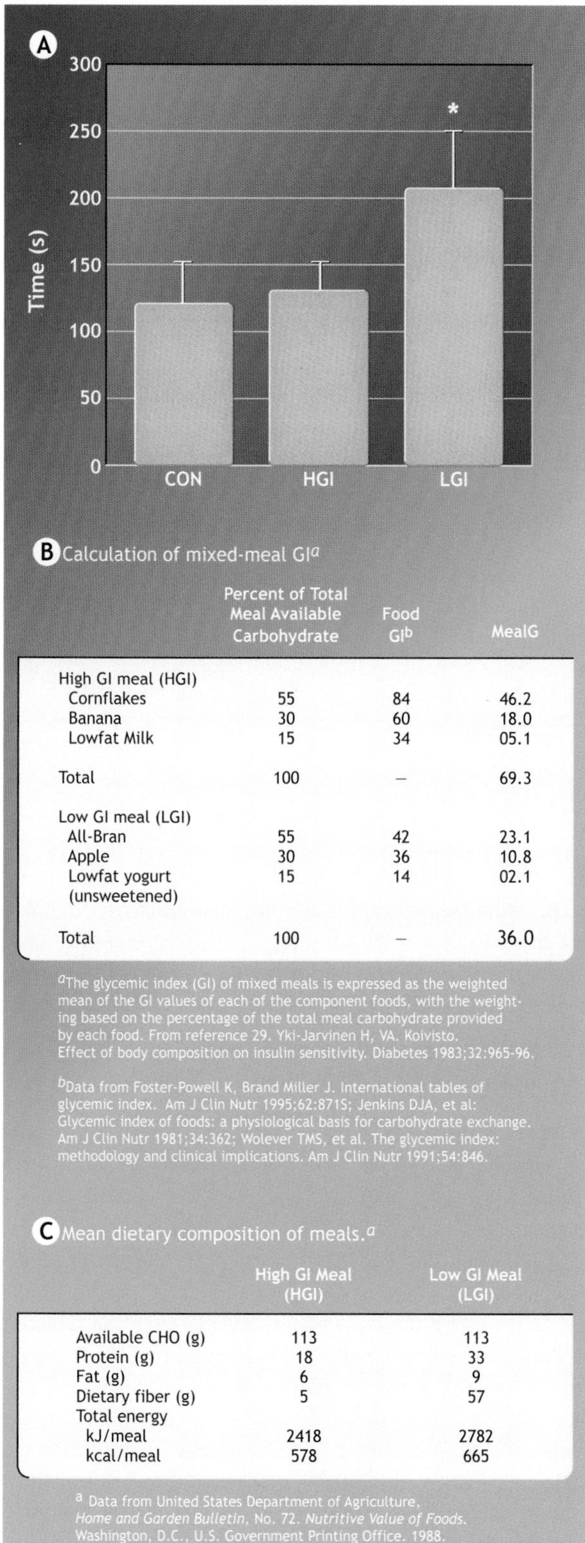

B Calculation of mixed-meal GI[a]

	Percent of Total Meal Available Carbohydrate	Food GI[b]	MealG
High GI meal (HGI)			
Cornflakes	55	84	46.2
Banana	30	60	18.0
Lowfat Milk	15	34	05.1
Total	100	–	69.3
Low GI meal (LGI)			
All-Bran	55	42	23.1
Apple	30	36	10.8
Lowfat yogurt (unsweetened)	15	14	02.1
Total	100	–	36.0

[a]The glycemic index (GI) of mixed meals is expressed as the weighted mean of the GI values of each of the component foods, with the weighting based on the percentage of the total meal carbohydrate provided by each food. From reference 29. Yki-Jarvinen H, VA. Koivisto. Effect of body composition on insulin sensitivity. Diabetes 1983;32:965-96.

[b]Data from Foster-Powell K, Brand Miller J. International tables of glycemic index. Am J Clin Nutr 1995;62:871S; Jenkins DJA, et al: Glycemic index of foods: a physiological basis for carbohydrate exchange. Am J Clin Nutr 1981;34:362; Wolever TMS, et al. The glycemic index: methodology and clinical implications. Am J Clin Nutr 1991;54:846.

C Mean dietary composition of meals.[a]

	High GI Meal (HGI)	Low GI Meal (LGI)
Available CHO (g)	113	113
Protein (g)	18	33
Fat (g)	6	9
Dietary fiber (g)	5	57
Total energy		
kJ/meal	2418	2782
kcal/meal	578	665

[a] Data from United States Department of Agriculture, *Home and Garden Bulletin*, No. 72. *Nutritive Value of Foods.* Washington, D.C., U.S. Government Printing Office. 1988.

FIGURE 3.11 • A. All-out cycling time to exhaustion (after 2h high-intensity exercise) for control (CON), moderately high-glycemic-index meal (HGI), and low-glycemic-index meal (LGI) trials. Values represent the average cycling times for 10 trained cyclists. *Indicates LGI significantly longer than HGI and CON. Inset boxes indicate (**B**) calculation of mixed-meal glycemic index and (**C**) average dietary composition of the meals. (From DeMarco HM, et al. Pre-exercise carbohydrate meals: application of glycemic index. Med Sci Sports Exerc 1999;31:164.)

GLUCOSE FEEDINGS, ELECTROLYTES, AND WATER UPTAKE

As we discuss in Chapter 25, ingesting fluid before and during exercise minimizes the detrimental effects of dehydration on cardiovascular dynamics, temperature regulation, and exercise performance. Adding carbohydrate to an **oral rehydration solution** provides additional glucose energy for exercise. Determining the optimal fluid/carbohydrate mixture and volume becomes important to minimize fatigue and prevent dehydration. Particular concern centers on the dual observations that (1) a large fluid volume intake may impair carbohydrate uptake, while (2) a concentrated sugar solution may impair fluid replenishment.

Important Considerations

The rate the stomach empties greatly affects intestinal absorption of fluid and nutrients. Figure 3.12 shows the important factors that influence gastric emptying. Little negative effect of exercise on gastric emptying occurs up to an intensity of about 75% of maximum, after which emptying rate slows.[83] Gastric volume, however, greatly influences gastric emptying; the emptying rate increases exponentially as fluid volume in the stomach increases. *A major factor to speed gastric emptying (and compensate for any inhibitory effects of the beverage's carbohydrate content) involves keeping a relatively high fluid volume in the stomach.* Consuming 400 to 600 mL of fluid immediately before exercise optimizes the beneficial effect of increased stomach volume on fluid and nutrient passage into the intestine. Then, regularly drinking 150 to 250 mL of fluid at 15-minute intervals throughout exercise continually replenishes fluid passed into the intestine. This protocol maintains a relatively large and constant gastric volume during exercise,[35,60,62] producing a fluid delivery rate to the small intestine of about 1 L per hour, a volume sufficient to meet the fluid needs of most endurance athletes. Moderate hypohydration of up to 4% body mass probably does not negatively affect gastric emptying rate.[81] Although prior research indicated that colder fluid emptied from the stomach at a faster rate than fluid at room temperature, fluid temperature probably does not exert a major effect during exercise. Highly carbonated beverages retard gastric emptying.[75] Beverages containing alcohol or caffeine induce a diuretic effect (alcohol most pronounced) that facilitates water loss from the kidneys, thus making them inappropriate for fluid replacement.

Particles in Solution

Concern exists about the potential negative effect of sugar drinks on water uptake by the digestive tract. Gastric emptying slows when ingested fluids contain a high concentration of particles in solution (**osmolality**), or possess high caloric content.[10,81,102] Whether rehydration beverages hypertonic to plasma ($\geq$280 mOsm $\cdot$ L^{-1}) retard net fluid uptake by the intestine remains unclear. If this does occur, it could negatively

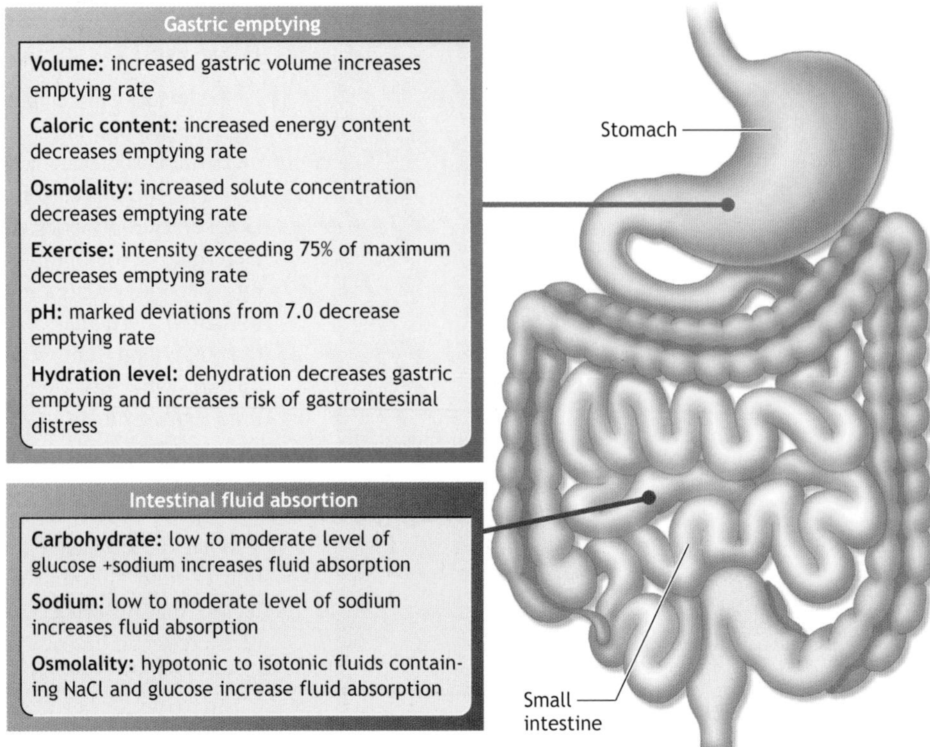

FIGURE 3.12 • Major factors that affect gastric emptying (stomach) and fluid absorption (small intestine).

affect prolonged exercise in hot weather, when adequate fluid intake *and* absorption play prime roles in the participant's health and safety.

Consuming a drink containing glucose polymers (**maltodextrin**) rather than simple sugars minimizes the negative effects of concentrated sugar molecules on gastric emptying and helps to maintain plasma volume.[87] Short-chain polymers (3 to 20 glucose units, derived from cornstarch breakdown) reduce the number of particles in solution, thus aiding water movement from the stomach for absorption by the intestine. Adding small amounts of glucose and sodium (glucose the more important factor) to the oral rehydration solution creates little negative effect on gastric emptying.[40,41] Glucose may actually facilitate fluid uptake by the intestinal lumen because of the rapid, active cotransport of glucose–sodium across the intestinal mucosa. Absorption of these particles stimulates water's passive uptake by osmotic action.[41,62,83] Extra glucose uptake not only effectively replenishes water but also helps to preserve blood glucose. The additional glucose then spares muscle and liver glycogen and/or maintains blood glucose should glycogen reserves decrease as prolonged exercise continues.

Adding sodium, the most abundant ion in the extracellular space, to a fluid probably minimally affects glucose absorption or glucose's contribution to the total energy yield in prolonged exercise.[41,49] Extra sodium, however, can aid in maintaining plasma sodium concentrations. This would benefit the ultraendurance athlete at risk for hyponatremia owing to a large sweat–sodium loss coupled with drinking copious amounts of plain water (see Chapter 2). Maintaining plasma osmolality by adding sodium to the rehydration beverage also reduces urine output, and sustains the sodium-dependent osmotic drive to drink (see Chapter 25).[78] A normal plasma and extracellular fluid osmolality promotes continued fluid intake *and* fluid retention during recovery.

Recommended Oral Rehydration Solution

As a general rule, a 5 to 8% carbohydrate-electrolyte beverage consumed during exercise in the heat contributes to temperature regulation and fluid balance as effectively as plain water. The beverage provides an intestinal energy delivery rate of approximately 5.0 kcal · min^{-1}; this helps to maintain glucose metabolism and glycogen reserves in prolonged exercise.[35,85] To determine a drink's percentage carbohydrate, divide the carbohydrate content (g) by the fluid volume (mL) and multiply by 100. For example, 80 g of carbohydrate in 1 L (1,000 mL) of water represents an 8% solution. Effective fluid absorption during prolonged exercise apparently occurs over a wide range of osmolalities. Total fluid absorption from the intestinal duodenum–jejunum of 6% carbohydrate-electrolyte (17 to 18 mEq Na^+ and 32 mEq K^+) beverages with osmolalities of 197 (hypotonic), 295 (isotonic), and 414 (hypertonic) mOsm per L of H_2O did not differ from the absorption rate of a plain water placebo.[42]

Do not confuse the conventional fluid replacement beverage with more-concentrated carbohydrate beverages designed to provide significant carbohydrate without concern for rapid fluid replenishment. These high-carbohydrate products composed of 20 to 25% carbohydrate, largely as mal-

PRACTICAL RECOMMENDATIONS FOR FLUID AND CARBOHYDRATE REPLENISHMENT DURING EXERCISE

- Monitor dehydration rate from changes in body weight; require urination before postexercise body weight measurement for precise determination of the body's total fluid loss. Each pound of weight loss corresponds to 450 mL (15 oz) of dehydration.
- Drink fluids at the same rate as their estimated depletion (or at least drink at a rate close to 80% of sweating rate) during prolonged exercise that increases cardiovascular stress, metabolic heat load, and dehydration.
- Achieve carbohydrate (30 to 60 g · h^{-1}) and fluid requirements by drinking 4 to 8% carbohydrate beverage each hour (625 to 1250 mL; average 250 mL every 15 min).

todextrins to prevent excessive sweetness, are well suited as carbohydrate sources for use during recovery from heavy training or competition.

Various environmental and exercise conditions interact to influence the rehydration solution's optimal composition. Fluid replenishment becomes crucial to health and safety when intense aerobic effort performed under high thermal stress lasts 30 to 60 minutes. Under these conditions, the individual should consume a more dilute carbohydrate–electrolyte solution (≤5% carbohydrate). In cooler weather, when dehydration does not pose a problem, a more-concentrated 15% carbohydrate beverage would suffice. Little difference exists among liquid glucose, sucrose, or starch as the ingested carbohydrate fuel source during exercise. Fructose is undesirable because of its potential to cause gastrointestinal distress. Furthermore, fructose absorption by the gut does not involve the active cotransport process required for glucose–sodium. This makes fructose absorption relatively slow and promotes less fluid uptake than with an equivalent amount of glucose. *The optimal carbohydrate replacement rate during intense aerobic exercise ranges from 30 to 60 g (about 1 to 2 oz) per hour.*

Figure 3.13 presents a general guideline for fluid intake each hour during exercise for a given amount of carbohydrate replenishment.[28] Acknowledging that a tradeoff exists between how much carbohydrate to consume and gastric emptying, the stomach still empties up to 1700 mL of water per hour, even when drinking an 8% carbohydrate solution. However, 1000 mL (about 1 quart) of fluid consumed each hour probably represents the optimal volume to offset dehydration, because larger fluid volumes often produce gastrointestinal discomfort.

HIGH-FAT VERSUS LOW-FAT DIETS FOR ENDURANCE TRAINING AND PERFORMANCE

Current debate concerns the wisdom of maintaining a high-fat diet (or even fasting) during training or prior to endurance competition.[24,59,68,100] Adaptations to high-fat diets have consistently shown a shift in substrate use toward higher fat oxidation during exercise.[50,51] Based on such findings, proponents of high-fat diets argue that a long-term increased dietary fat intake stimulates fat burning and augments the capacity to mobilize and catabolize this energy nutrient during high-intensity aerobic exercise. Any fat-burning metabolic enhancement should conserve glycogen reserves and/or contribute to improved endurance capacity under conditions of low glycogen reserves.[51] To investigate possible benefits, endurance capacity was compared in two groups of 10 young men matched for aerobic capacity and fed either a high-carbohydrate diet (65% kcal from carbohydrate) or high-fat diet (62% kcal from lipid) for 7 weeks.[50] Each group trained for 60 to 70 minutes at 50 to 85% of aerobic capacity, 3 days a week during weeks 1 to 3 and 4 days a week during weeks 4 to 7. Following 7 weeks of training, the group consuming the high-fat diet switched to the high-carbohydrate diet. Figure 3.14 displays the performance of both groups. The results for endurance were clear—the group consuming the high-carbohydrate diet performed significantly better after 7 weeks of training than the group consuming the high-fat diet (102.4 min versus 65.2 min). When the high-fat diet group switched to the high-carbohydrate diet during week 8 of the experiment, only a small additional improvement in endurance of 11.5 minutes

CHO concentration in drink (g · dL^{-1})	30 g · h^{-1}	40 g · h^{-1}	50 g · h^{-1}	60 g · h^{-1}
2%	1500 mL	2000 mL	2500 mL	3000 mL
4%	750	1000	1250	1500
6%	500	667	833	1000
8%	375	500	625	750
10%	300	400	300	600
15%	200	267	333	400
20%	150	200	250	300
25%	120	160	200	240
50%	60	80	100	120

Volume too large: greater than 1200 mL · h^{-1}

Adequate fluid replacement: 600-1250 mL · h^{-1}

Low fluid replacement: less than 600 mL · h^{-1}

FIGURE 3.13 • Volume of fluid to ingest each hour to obtain the noted amount of carbohydrate. (Modified from Coyle EF, Montain SJ. Benefits of fluid replacement with carbohydrate during exercise. Med Sci Sports Exerc 1992;24:S324.)

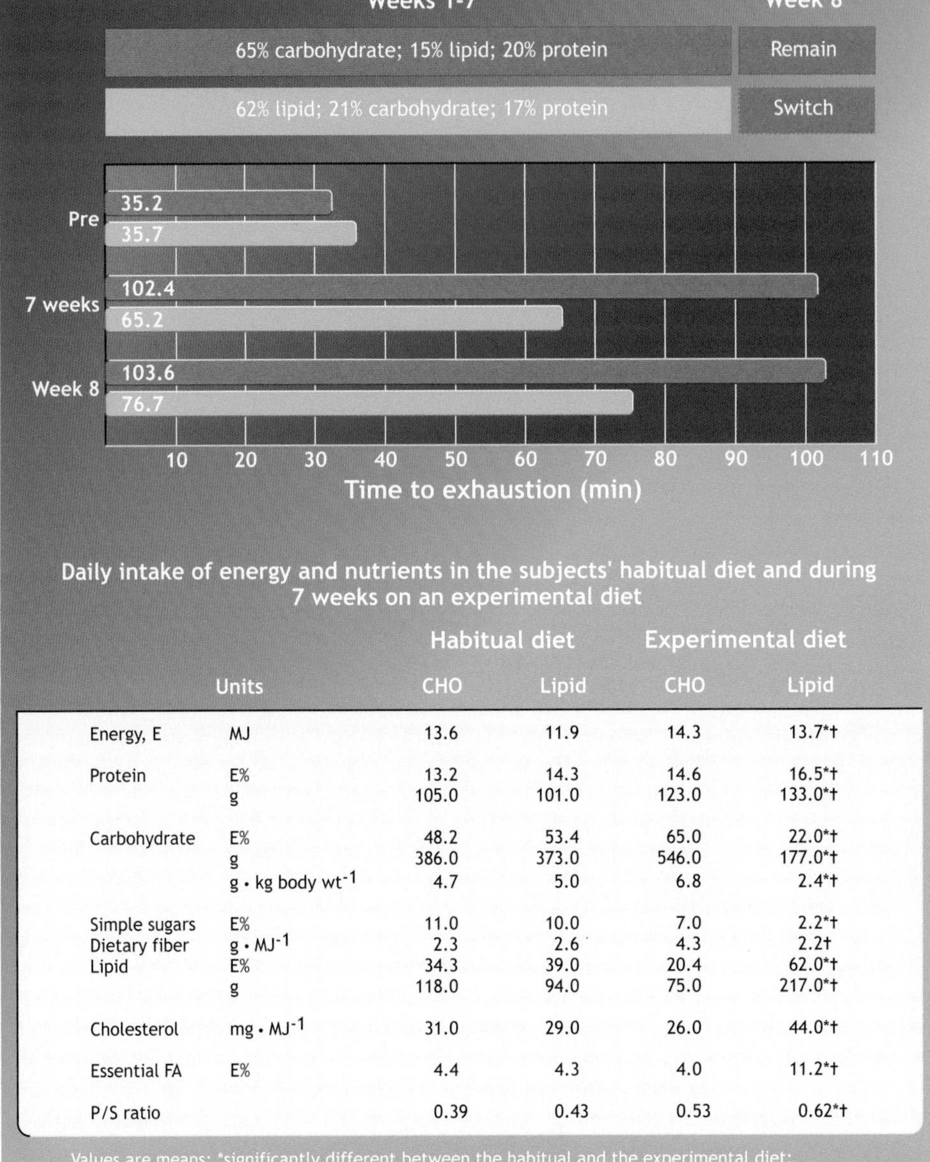

Daily intake of energy and nutrients in the subjects' habitual diet and during 7 weeks on an experimental diet

	Units	Habitual diet CHO	Habitual diet Lipid	Experimental diet CHO	Experimental diet Lipid
Energy, E	MJ	13.6	11.9	14.3	13.7*†
Protein	E%	13.2	14.3	14.6	16.5*†
	g	105.0	101.0	123.0	133.0*†
Carbohydrate	E%	48.2	53.4	65.0	22.0*†
	g	386.0	373.0	546.0	177.0*†
	g • kg body wt^{-1}	4.7	5.0	6.8	2.4*†
Simple sugars	E%	11.0	10.0	7.0	2.2*†
Dietary fiber	g • MJ^{-1}	2.3	2.6	4.3	2.2†
Lipid	E%	34.3	39.0	20.4	62.0*†
	g	118.0	94.0	75.0	217.0*†
Cholesterol	mg • MJ^{-1}	31.0	29.0	26.0	44.0*†
Essential FA	E%	4.4	4.3	4.0	11.2*†
P/S ratio		0.39	0.43	0.53	0.62*†

Values are means; *significantly different between the habitual and the experimental diet; †significantly different between the two experimental diets; MJ, megajoule; E%, percent of total energy

FIGURE 3.14 • Effects of a high-carbohydrate (CHO) versus a high-fat diet on endurance performance. The group consuming the high-fat diet for 7 weeks switched to the high CHO diet during week 8. The endurance test consisted of pedaling a bicycle ergometer at the desired rate. The inset table compares the average daily energy and nutrient intake during the habitual and experimental diets. P/S ratio, polyunsaturated-to-saturated fatty acid ratio. (From Helge JW, et al. Interaction of training and diet on metabolism and endurance during exercise in man. J Physiol 1996;492:293.)

occurred. Consequently, total overall improvement in endurance over the 8-week period reached 115% for the high-fat diet group, and endurance for the group receiving the high-carbohydrate diet while training improved by 194%. The inset table shows daily intakes of energy and nutrients prior to the experimental treatment (habitual diet) and during the 7-week experimental diet. The authors concluded that the high-fat diet produced *suboptimal adaptations* in endurance performance, which did not become fully remedied by switching to a high-carbohydrate diet. Subsequent research from the same laboratory failed to demonstrate any endurance-enhancing effect of a high-fat diet containing only moderate carbohydrate (15% total calories) in rats, regardless of their training status. For sedentary humans, maintaining a low or high dietary fat intake for 4 weeks produced no differences in maximal or submaximal aerobic exercise performance.[76]

While a high-fat diet may stimulate adaptive responses that augment fat use, reliable research has yet to demonstrate consistent exercise or training benefits from this dietary modification. Furthermore, one must carefully consider recommending a diet consisting of 60% of total calories from lipid from the standpoint of potential detrimental health risks. However, this concern may prove unwarranted for athletes with high daily levels of energy expenditure. Increasing the percentage of total lipid calories in the diet to 50% for physically active individuals who maintain a stable body weight and body composition does not appear to adversely affect selected heart disease risk factors, including plasma lipoprotein profiles.[13,61] Overall, available research does not support the popular notion that reducing carbohydrate while increasing fat intake above a 30% level produces a more optimal metabolic "zone" for endurance performance.[84,99] Conversely, sig-

Focus on Research

Potential Effect of Diet on Health Status

Connor WE, et al. The plasma lipids, lipoproteins, and diet of the Tarahumara Indians of Mexico. Am J Clin Nutr 1978;31:1131.

➤ The Tarahumara Indians compose a group of about 50,000 farmers who inhabit the rugged Sierra Madre Occidental Mountains in the north-central state of Chihuahua, Mexico. These individuals, renowned for their endurance capacity, reportedly run distances of up to 200 miles in the competitive sport of "kickball" that lasts 2 days.

Conner and colleagues assessed the diet, blood lipid status, and blood pressure of these 20th-century Spartans. Measurements of 523 Tarahumaras over a 3-year period included plasma cholesterol and triglycerides, lipoprotein fractions, body stature and mass, triceps skinfold, resting blood pressure, and nutrient intake by dietary history and observation of food intake. The most striking findings included extremely low values for total cholesterol, LDL- and VLDL-cholesterol, blood pressure, skinfold thickness, and dietary lipid intake. The average blood cholesterol levels (136 mg · dL^{-1} for men; 117 mg · dL^{-1} for women; and 116 mg · dL^{-1} for children) contrast sharply with typical U.S. values of more than 200 mg · dL^{-1}.

The low plasma cholesterol of the Tarahumaras largely relates to their unique dietary patterns. The diet averaged an extremely low cholesterol intake of 71 mg · d^{-1} (typical U.S. cholesterol intake ranges from 500 to 700 mg · d^{-1}). Additionally, lipid intake averaged only 11% of total energy intake, compared with nearly 40% for the U.S. diet. Corn and beans accounted for 95% of total lipid consumption, mainly from polyunsaturated and monounsaturated fatty acids. Saturated fat constituted only 2% of total calories, compared with 15% in the U.S. Thus, the healthful polyunsaturated:saturated fat ratio exceeded 2.0, compared with only 0.35 for the U.S. diet.

Simple sugars provided only 5% of total energy intake, compared with 25% for the typical North American diet. No obesity or hypertension occurred in the Tarahumara. Vegetable sources provided more than 96% of all dietary protein, while protein intake ranged from 79 to 96 g · d^{-1} and accounted for 236 to 1221% of the total essential amino acid requirements based on the U.S. RDA. The Tarahumaras' high level of physical activity coincided with favorable blood lipid and blood pressure profiles and other low coronary risk factors. Overall, the results illustrated that diet and increased physical activity linked to the group's relatively good health status.

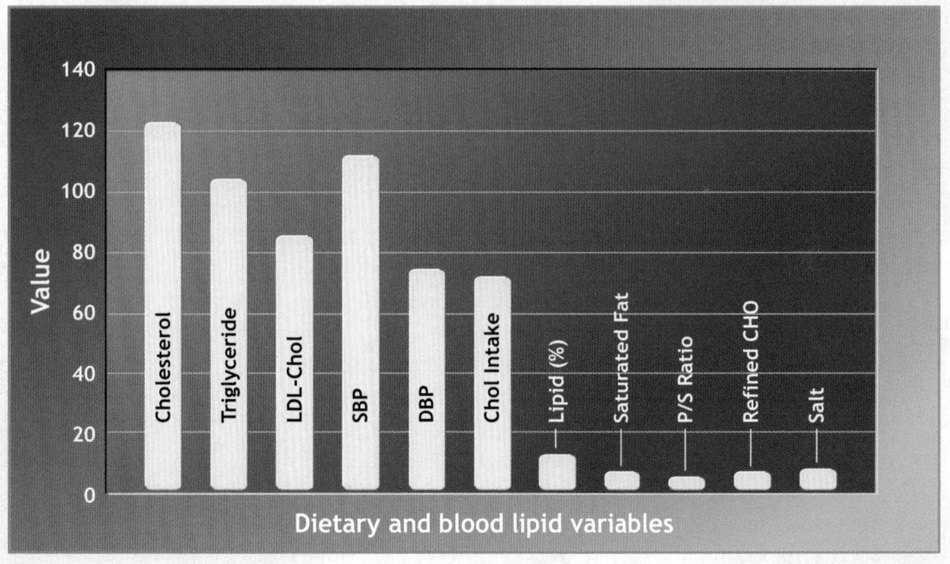

Dietary and blood lipid variables for the Tarahumara Indians of Mexico. Plasma *cholesterol, triglyceride,* and *LDL-chol* in mg per dL. *Chol Intake* is cholesterol intake in mg per day. Lipid intake (*Lipid %*) and saturated fat intake (*Saturated Fat*) expressed as percentage of total caloric intake; *P/S Ratio* represents ratio of polyunsaturated to saturated fatty acid intake; *refined CHO* is the percentage of total calories from refined sugar; *salt* is salt intake in g per day; *SBP* and *DBP* represent systolic and diastolic blood pressure in mm Hg.

nificant restriction of dietary fat intake below recommended levels may impair performance in endurance exercise.[50,99]

Summary

1. Within rather broad limits, a balanced diet provides the nutrient requirements of athletes and other individuals who train regularly. Well-planned daily menus with as few as 1200 kcal can provide the vitamin, mineral, and protein requirements.
2. The recommended protein intake of 0.83 g per kg body mass represents a liberal requirement believed adequate for nearly all people, regardless of physical activity level. A protein intake between 1.2 and 1.8 g per kg of body mass should adequately meet the possibility of added protein need during heavy training. Athletes generally consume two to four times the protein RDA because their greater caloric intake usually provides proportionately more protein.

3. No precise recommendations exist for daily lipid and carbohydrate intake. Prudent advice recommends no more than 30% of daily calories from lipids; of this amount, most should be unsaturated fatty acids. For physically active people, carbohydrates, particularly unrefined polysaccharides, should provide 60% or more of the daily calories (400 to 600 g on a daily basis).
4. Successive days of hard training gradually deplete the body's liver and muscle glycogen reserves and could lead to training staleness, making continued training more difficult.
5. The Food Guide Pyramid provides broad recommendations for healthful nutrition for physically active men and women. It emphasizes fruits, grains, and vegetables, and deemphasizes foods high in animal protein, lipids, and dairy products.
6. Intensity of daily physical activity largely determines energy intake requirements. The daily caloric needs of athletes in strenuous sports probably do not consistently exceed 4000 kcal; the exceptions include individuals with a large body mass or those involved in extreme levels of training or competition.
7. The precompetition meal should include foods high in carbohydrates and relatively low in lipids and proteins so it readily digests and contributes to the energy and fluid requirements of exercise. A low-carbohydrate steak-and-eggs diet does not fulfill the needs for optimal preevent nutrition. Three hours should provide sufficient time to digest and absorb the precompetition meal.
8. Commercially prepared liquid meals offer well-balanced nutritive value, contribute to fluid need, and absorb rapidly, leaving little residue in the digestive tract.
9. Consuming carbohydrate-containing rehydration solutions during exercise enhances high-intensity endurance performance by maintaining blood sugar concentration. Glucose supplied via the blood can (1) spare existing glycogen in active muscles during exercise or (2) serve as reserve blood glucose for later use should muscle glycogen become depleted.
10. The glycemic index provides a relative measure of blood glucose increase after consuming a specific carbohydrate food. For rapid carbohydrate replenishment after exercise, individuals should consume 50 to 75 g of moderate- to high-glycemic index, carbohydrate-containing foods each hour.
11. With optimal carbohydrate intake, glycogen stores replenish at a rate of about 5 to 7% per hour. It takes about 20 hours for full replenishment of liver and muscle glycogen after a glycogen-depleting exercise bout.
12. The glycemic index can formulate the immediate preexercise feeding. Foods with a low glycemic index digest and absorb at a relatively slow rate to provide a steady supply of slow-release glucose from the intestinal tract during prolonged exercise.
13. Consuming 400 to 600 mL of fluid immediately before exercise, followed by regular fluid ingestion during exercise (250 mL every 15 minutes) optimizes gastric emptying by maintaining a relatively large fluid volume in the stomach.
14. The ideal oral rehydration solution to maintain fluid balance during exercise and heat stress contains between 5 and 8% carbohydrates. This beverage formulation permits carbohydrate replenishment without adversely affecting gastric emptying rate, fluid balance, and thermoregulation.
15. Adding a moderate amount of sodium to fluid stabilizes plasma sodium concentrations, which benefits the ultraendurance athlete at risk for hyponatremia. Added sodium in the rehydration beverage also reduces urine production and sustains the sodium-dependent osmotic drive to drink.
16. While a high-fat diet may stimulate adaptive responses that enhance fat use, reliable research has not yet demonstrated consistent exercise or training benefits from this dietary modification.

References

1. Abrahams A. The nutrition of athletes. Br J Nutr 1948;2:266.
2. Ahlborg G, Felig P. Influence of glucose ingestion on the fuel-hormone response during prolonged exercise. J Appl Physiol 1976;41:683.
3. Anantaraman R, et al. Effects of carbohydrate supplementation on performance during 1 hour of high-intensity exercise. Int J Sports Med 1995;16:461.
4. Anderson M, et al. Preexercise meal affects ride time to fatigue in trained cyclists. J Am Diet Assoc 1994;94:1152.
5. Ball TC, et al. Periodic carbohydrate replacement during 50 min of high-intensity cycling improves subsequent sprint performance. Int J Sports Nutr 1995;5:151.
6. Below PR, et al. Fluid and carbohydrate ingestion independently improve performance during 1 h of intense exercise. Med Sci Sports Exerc 1995;27:200.
7. Blair SN, et al. Comparison of nutrient intake in middle-aged men and women runners and controls. Med Sci Sports Exerc 1981;13:310.
8. Brand-Miller J, et al. The G.I. factor: the glycaemic index solution. Sydney, Australia: Hodder and Stoughton, 1996.
9. Briefel RR, et al. Total energy intake of the US population: the third National Health and Nutrition Examination Survey, 1988–1991. Am J Clin Nutr 1995;62(suppl):1072S.
10. Brouns F, Beckers E. Is the gut an athletic organ? Sports Med 1993;15:242.
11. Brouns F, et al. Eating, drinking, and cycling. A controlled Tour de France simulation study, part I. Int J Sports Med 1989;10:532.
12. Brouns F, et al. Eating, drinking, and cycling. A controlled Tour de France simulation study, part II. Effect of diet manipulation. Int J Sports Med 1989;10:541.
13. Brown RC, Cox CM. Effects of high fat versus high carbohydrate diets on plasma lipids and lipoproteins in endurance athletes. Med Sci Sports Exerc 1998;30:1677.
14. Bungard LB, et al. Energy requirements of middle-aged men are modifiable by physical activity. Am J Clin Nutr 1998;68:1136.
15. Burelle Y, et al. Oxidation of an oral [^{13}C]glucose load at rest and prolonged exercise in trained and sedentary subjects. J Appl Physiol 1999;86:52.
16. Burke LM, et al. Carbohydrate intake during prolonged cycling exercise minimizes effect of glycemic index of preexercise meal. J Appl Physiol 1998;85:2228.
17. Cavies CT, Thompson D. Aerobic performance of female marathon and male ultramarathon athletes. Eur J Appl Physiol 1979;41:223.

18. Burke LM, et al. Carbohydrate failed to improve 100-km cycling performance in a placebo-controlled trial. J Appl Physiol 2000;88:1284.
19. Choi D, et al. Effect of passive and active recovery on the resynthesis of muscle glycogen. Med Sci Sports Exerc 1994;26:992.
20. Coggan AR, Coyle EF. Metabolism and performance following carbohydrate ingestion late in exercise. Med Sci Sports Exerc 1989;21:59.
21. Coggan AR, Coyle EF. Carbohydrate ingestion during prolonged exercise: effects on metabolism and performance. Exerc Sport Sci Rev 1991;19:1.
22. Connor WE, et al. The plasma lipids, lipoproteins, and diet of the Tarahumara Indians of Mexico. Am J Clin Nutr 1978;31:1131.
23. Costill DL, Miller J. Nutrition for endurance sports: carbohydrate and fluid balance. Int J Sports Med 1980;1:2.
24. Cox CM, et al. The effects of high-carbohydrate versus high-fat dietary advice on plasma lipids, lipoproteins, apolipoproteins, and performance in endurance trained cyclists. Nutr Metab Cardiovasc Dis 1996;6:227.
25. Coyle EF. Substrate utilization during exercise in active people. Am J Clin Nutr 1995;61:968S.
26. Coyle EF, Coggan AC. Effectiveness of carbohydrate feeding in delaying fatigue during prolonged exercise. Sports Med 1984;1:446.
27. Coyle EF, Coyle E. Carbohydrates that speed recovery from training. Phys Sportsmed 1993;21:111.
28. Coyle EF, Montain SJ. Benefits of fluid replacement with carbohydrate during exercise. Med Sci Sports Exerc 1992;24:S324.
29. Coyle EF, et al. Carbohydrate feeding during prolonged strenuous exercise can delay fatigue. J Appl Physiol 1983;55:230.
30. Coyle EF, et al. Muscle glycogen utilization during prolonged strenuous exercise when fed carbohydrate. J Appl Physiol 1986;61:165.
31. Craig BW. The influence of fructose feeding on physical performance. Am J Clin Nutr 1993;58(suppl):815S.
32. deLorgeril M, et al. Mediterranean diet, traditional risk factors, and the rate of cardiovascular complications after myocardial infarction. Circulation 1999;99:779.
33. DeMarco HM, et al. Pre-exercise carbohydrate meals: application of glycemic index. Med Sci Sports Exerc 1999;31:164.
34. Dohm GL, et al. Metabolic response to exercise after fasting. J Appl Physiol 1986;61:1363.
35. Duchman SM, et al. Upper limit for intestinal absorption of a dilute glucose solution in men at rest. Med Sci Sports Exerc 1997;29:482.
36. Febbraio MA, Stewart KL. CHO feeding before prolonged exercise: effect of glycemic index on muscle glycogenolysis and exercise performance. J Appl Physiol 1996;81:1115.
37. Fontvieille AM, et al. The use of low glycemic index foods improves metabolic control of diabetes patients in a 10 week study. Diabet Med 1992;9:444.
38. Foster C, et al. Effects of pre-exercise feedings on endurance performance. Med Sci Sports 1979;11:1.
39. Foster-Powell K, Brand-Miller J. International tables of glycemic index. Am J Clin Nutr 1995;62(suppl):871S.
40. Gilsolfi CV, et al. Intestinal water absorption from select carbohydrate solutions in humans. J Appl Physiol 1992;7:2142.
41. Gilsolfi CV, et al. Effect of sodium concentration in a carbohydrate-electrolyte solution on intestinal absorption. Med Sci Sports Exerc 1995;27:1414.
42. Gilsolfi CV, et al. Effect of beverage osmolality on intestinal fluid absorption during exercise. J Appl Physiol 1998;85:1941.
43. Glassetti P, et al. Enhanced muscle glucose facilitates nitrogen efflux from exercised muscle. J Appl Physiol 1998;84:1952.
44. Gleeson M, et al. Comparison of the effects of pre-exercise feedings of glucose, glycerol, and placebo on endurance and fuel homeostasis in man. Eur J Appl Physiol 1986;55:645.
45. Goodpaster BH, et al. The effects of pre-exercise starch ingestion on endurance performance. Int J Sports Med 1996;17:366.
46. Grandjean AC. Macronutrient intakes of U.S. athletes compared with the general population and recommendations made for athletes. Am J Clin Nutr 1989;49:1070.
47. Hargreaves M, Briggs CA. Effect of carbohydrate ingestion on exercise metabolism. J Appl Physiol 1988;65:1553.
48. Hargreaves M, et al. Effect of fructose ingestion on muscle glycogen usage during exercise. Med Sci Sports Exerc 1985;17:360.
49. Hargreaves M, et al. Influence of sodium on glucose bioavailability during exercise. Med Sci Sports Exerc 1994;26:365.
50. Helge JW, et al. Interaction of training and diet on metabolism and endurance during exercise in man. J Physiol 1996;492:293.
51. Helge JW, et al. Impact of a fat-rich diet on endurance in man: role of the dietary period. Med Sci Sports Exerc 1998;30:456.
52. Hickson RC, et al. Muscle glycogen accumulation after endurance exercise in trained and untrained individuals. J Appl Physiol 1997;83:897.
53. Ivy JL. Muscle glycogen synthesis before and after exercise. Sports Med 1991;11:6.
54. Jandrain BJ, et al. Metabolic availability of glucose ingested three hours before prolonged exercise in humans. J Appl Physiol 1984;56:1314.
55. Jeukendrup AE, et al. Carbohydrate-electrolyte feedings improve 1 h time trial cycling performance. Int J Sports Med 1997;18:125.
56. Joshipura KJ, et al. Fruit and vegetable intake in relation to risk of ischemic stroke. JAMA 1999;282:1233.
57. Kirwin JP, et al. A moderate glycemic meal before endurance exercise can enhance performance. J Appl Physiol 1998;84:53.
58. Krzentowski B, et al. Availability of glucose given orally during exercise. J Appl Physiol 1984;56:315.
59. Lambert EV, et al. Enhanced endurance in trained cyclists during moderate intensity exercise following 2 weeks adaptation to a high fat diet. Eur J Appl Physiol 1994;69:287.
60. Lambert GP, et al. Simultaneous determination of gastric emptying and intestinal absorption during cycle exercise in humans. Int J Sports Med 1996;17:48.
61. Leddy J, et al. Effect of a high or a low fat diet on cardiovascular risk factors in male and female runners. Med Sci Sports Exerc 1997;29:17.
62. Leiper JB. Intestinal water absorption—implications for the formulation of rehydration solutions. Int J Sports Med 1998;19(Suppl 2):s129.
63. Lukaski HC. Interactions among indices of mineral element nutrition and physical performance of swimmers. In: Kies CV, Driskell JA, eds. Sports nutrition: minerals and electrolytes. Boca Raton, FL: CRC Press, 1995.
64. MacLean PS, et al. Muscle glucose transporters (GLUT4) gene expression during exercise. Exerc Sport Sci Rev 2000;28:148.
65. Mafucci DM, McMurray RG. Toward optimizing the timing of the pre-exercise meal. Int J Sport Nutr Exerc Metab 2000;10:103.
66. McConell G, et al. Effect of timing of carbohydrate ingestion on endurance exercise performance. Med Sci Sports Exerc 1996;28:1300.
67. Mitchell JB, et al. Effects of carbohydrate ingestion on gastric emptying and exercise performance. Med Sci Sports Exerc 1988;20:110.
68. Mudio DM. Effect of dietary fat on metabolic adjustments to maximal $\dot{V}O_2$ and endurance in runners. Med Sci Sports Exerc 1994;26:81.
69. Murray R, et al. The effects of glucose, fructose, and sucrose ingestion during exercise. Med Sci Sports Exerc 1989;21:275.
70. Nakatani A, et al. Effect of endurance exercise training on muscle glycogen supercompensation in rats. J Appl Physiol 1997;82:711.
71. Nicholas CW, et al. Influence of ingesting a carbohydrate-electrolyte solution on endurance capacity during intermittent, high intensity shuttle running. J Sports Sci 1996;13:283.
72. Nicholas CW, et al. Carbohydrate-electrolyte ingestion during intermittent high-intensity running. Med Sci Sports Exerc 1999;31:1280.
73. Okano G, et al. Effect of pre-exercise fructose ingestion on endurance performance in fed man. Med Sci Sports Exerc 1988;20:105.
74. Pabkin JAM, et al. Muscle glycogen storage following prolonged exercise: effect of timing of ingestion of high glycemic index food. Med Sci Sports Exerc 1997;29:220.
75. Ploutz-Snyder L, et al. Gastric gas and fluid emptying assessed by magnetic resonance imaging. Eur J Appl Physiol 1999;79:212.
76. Pogliaghi S, Veicsteinas A. Influence of low and high dietary fat on physical performance in untrained males. Med Sci Sports Exerc 1999;31:149.
77. Rankin JW, et al. Effect of weight loss and refeeding diet composition on anaerobic performance in wrestlers. Med Sci Sports Exerc 1996;28:1292.
78. Ray ML, et al. Effect of sodium in a rehydration beverage when consumed as a fluid or meal. J Appl Physiol 1998;85:1329.
79. Rontoyannis GP, et al. Energy balance in ultramarathon running. Am J Clin Nutr 1989;49:976.
80. Roy BD, Tarnopolsky MA. Influence of differing macronutrient intakes on muscle glycogen resynthesis after resistance exercise. J Appl Physiol 1998;84:890.
81. Ryan AJ, et al. Effect of hypohydration on gastric emptying and intestinal absorption during exercise. J Appl Physiol 1998;84:1581.
82. Schabort EJ, et al. The effect of a preexercise meal on time to fatigue during prolonged cycling exercise. Med Sci Sports Exerc 1999;31:464.
83. Schedl HP, et al. Intestinal absorption during rest and exercise: implications for formulating an oral rehydration solution (ORS). Med Sci Sports Exerc 1994;26:267.

84. Sears B, Lawren W. The zone. New York: Harper Collins, 1995.
85. Shi X, Gisolfi CV. Fluid and carbohydrate replacement during intermittent exercise. Sports Med 1998;25:157.
86. Sjödin AM, et al. Energy balance in cross-country skiers: a study using doubly labeled water. Med Sci Sports Exerc 1994;26:720.
87. Sole CC, Noakes TD. Faster emptying for glucose-polymer and fructose solutions than for glucose in humans. Eur J Appl Physiol 1989;58:605.
88. Solfrizzi V, et al. High monounsaturated fatty acids intake protects against age-related cognitive decline. Neurology 1999;52:1563.
89. Sparks MJ, et al. Pre-exercise carbohydrate ingestion: effect of the glycemic index on endurance exercise performance. Med Sci Sports Exerc 1998;30:844.
90. Stroud MA, et al. Energy expenditure using isotope-labeled water ($^2H^{18}O$), exercise performance, skeletal muscle enzyme activities and plasma biochemical parameters in humans during 95 days of endurance exercise with inadequate energy intake. Eur J Appl Physiol 1997;76:243.
91. Sugiura K, Kibayashi K. Effect of carbohydrate ingestion on sprint performance following continuous and intermittent exercise. Med Sci Sports Exerc 1998;30:1624.
92. Sundgot-Borgen J. Prevalence of eating disorders in elite female athletes. Int J Sports Nutr 1993;3:30.
93. Taub IA. Optimizing the design of combat rations. In: Marriot BM, ed. Food components to enhance performance. Food and Nutrition Board. Institute of Medicine. Washington, DC: National Academy Press, 1994.
94. Thomas DE, et al. Carbohydrate feeding before exercise: effect of glycemic index. Int J Sports Med 1991;12:180.
95. Trappe TA, et al. Energy expenditure of swimmers during high volume training. Med Sci Sports Exerc 1997;29:950.
96. Trappe S, et al. Effect of swim taper on whole muscle and single muscle fiber contractile properties. Med Sci Sports Exerc 2001;32:48.
97. USDA, Center for Nutrition Policy and Promotion. USDA/HHS dietary guidelines for Americans. Washington, DC: CNPP, 1996.
98. van Erp-Baart AMJ, et al. Nationwide survey on nutritional habits in elite athletes. Part I. Energy, carbohydrate, protein, and fat intake. Int J Sports Med 1989;10:53.
99. Venkatraman JT, Pendergast D. Effects of the level of dietary fat intake and endurance exercise on plasma cytokines in runners. Med Sci Sports Exerc 1998;30:1198.
100. Venkatraman JT, et al. Influence of the level of dietary lipid intake and maximal exercise on the immune status in runners. Med Sci Sports Exerc 1997;29:333.
101. Vergauwen L, et al. Carbohydrate supplementation improves stroke performance in tennis. Med Sci Sports Exerc 1998;30:1289.
102. Vist GE, Maughan RJ. Gastric emptying of ingested solutions in man: effect of beverage glucose concentration. Med Sci Sports Exerc 1994;26:1269.
103. Wagenmakers AJM. Carbohydrate feedings improve 1 h time trial cycling performance. Med Sci Sports Exerc 1996;28:S37.
104. Walton P, Rhodes EC. Glycaemic index and optimal performance. Sports Med 1997;33:164.
105. Wee S-L, et al. Influence of high and low glycemic index meals on endurance running capacity. Med Sci Sports Exerc 1999;31:393.
106. Wolever TMS, et al. Glycaemic index of 102 complex carbohydrate foods in patients with diabetes. Nutr Res 1994;14:651.
107. Yannick C, et al. Oxidation of corn starch, glucose, and fructose ingested before exercise. Med Sci Sports Exerc 1989;21:45.
108. Zachwieja JJ, et al. Influence of muscle glycogen depletion on the rate of resynthesis. Med Sci Sports Exerc 1991;23:44.

SECTION 2

Energy for Physical Activity

Biochemical reactions that do not consume oxygen generate considerable energy for short durations. The rapid generation of energy becomes crucial in maintaining a high standard of performance in sprint activities and other bursts of all-out exercise. In comparison, longer-duration aerobic exercise extracts energy more slowly from food through reactions that require oxygen. For greatest effectiveness, training the various physiologic systems requires an understanding of how the body generates energy to sustain exercise, the sources that provide energy, and the energy requirements of diverse physical activities.

This section presents a broad overview of how cells extract the chemical energy bound within the food molecules and use it to power biologic work. We emphasize the importance of the food nutrients and processes of energy transfer to sustain physiologic function during light, moderate, and strenuous exercise.

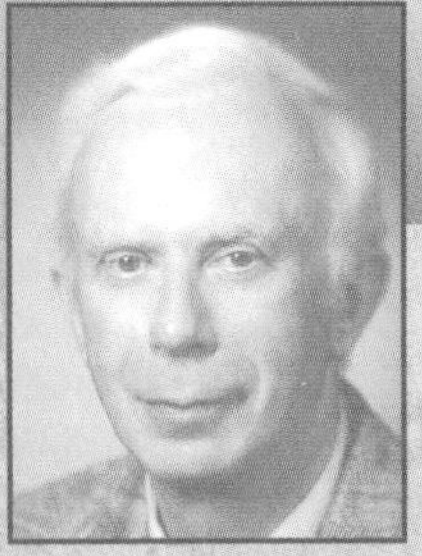

Interview with Dr. John O. Holloszy

Education: BS (Oregon State College, Salem, OR); MD (Washington University School of Medicine, St. Louis, MO); Postgraduate Training (NIH Special Research Fellow, Department of Biological Chemistry, Washington University School of Medicine, St. Louis, MO)

Current Affiliation: Professor of Internal Medicine; Chief, Division of Geriatrics and Gerontology, and Director, Section of Applied Physiology, Washington University School of Medicine, St. Louis, MO

Honors and Awards: See Appendix E.

Research Focus: The biological adaptations to exercise.

Memorable Publication: Holloszy JO. Biochemical adaptations in muscle. J Biol Chem 1967;242:2278–2282.

Statement of Contributions: ACSM Honor Award

Over the past twenty-five years, John O. Holloszy has been the most important individual responsible for the development of cellular exercise research. His contributions have advanced knowledge in glucose transport, substrate provision, skeletal muscle metabolism, biochemical adaptations induced by training, fiber type responses, blood lipids, the aging process, and rehabilitation.

His innovative work, which has been applied to health related aspects of exercise, has spawned a wealth of research inquiries by other investigators. He was the first to introduce postdoctoral training to exercise science. Our valued colleague, whose work has always exemplified quality, has fused exercise science with other disciplines.

➤ What first inspired you to enter the exercise science field? What made you decide to pursue your advanced degree and/or line of research?

After completing medical school and four years of training in Internal Medicine and Endocrinology and Metabolism, I worked for two years as a Lt. Commander in the U.S. Public Health Service. Because of my interest in the prevention of coronary heart disease through diet and exercise, I was stationed at the Physical Fitness Research Laboratory at the University of Illinois.

At the time, Dr. Tom Cureton, Director of the Laboratory and pioneer in the area of endurance exercise training, conducted a year-round, daily exercise program, staffed by his graduate students, for university faculty and other individuals in the community. Most of the participants were middle-aged men, and I was tasked with obtaining information on the physiological and metabolic effects induced by the exercise program. With the help of some of Dr. Cureton's students and junior faculty, particularly James S. Skinner, who used this research for his doctoral dissertation, I conducted a series of studies on the effect of a six-month exercise program on body composition, blood lipids, and cardiovascular function.

This was my first experience with the effects of endurance training. I became fascinated with the remarkable improvements in endurance and exercise capacity that developed rapidly in response to training. I was also impressed by the decrease in body fat, reduction in serum triglycerides, and improvement in cardiovascular function. I had become convinced by the epidemiological evidence that obesity, ischemic heart disease, and type 2 diabetes were largely diseases of exercise deficiency. But, at the time, there was little research being done on the effects of exercise at the time, and research on the biological effects of exercise was a low priority, generally viewed as unimportant and not prestigious. Therefore, because I had become extremely interested in the biological mechanisms responsible for the adaptive responses to exercise at the cellular level, and because I thought that exercise deficiency had become the country's number one health problem, I decided to devote my career to research on the effects of exercise. My goals were to: 1) elucidate the biological mechanisms underlying the improvements in performance and metabolism induced by exercise training; 2) evaluate the roles of exercise in the maintenance of health, treatment of disease, and prevention of loss of independence with advancing age, and, in the process; 3) bring research on the biology of exercise into the scientific mainstream.

➤ Who were the most influential people in your career, and why?

The only person who had a major influence on my career was Dr. Hiro Narahara, my mentor during my two years of postdoctoral research training in biochemistry. Like many physicians who come to basic research relatively late in their careers, I tended to be sloppy in laboratory work. Hiro forced me to become careful and accurate in my technical work, although, because of a lack of natural aptitude, I never did become a skilled bench researcher. My other mentors generally tried to dissuade me from devoting my research career to the biology of exercise, because they thought that I would ruin my academic career by working in what was at the time a low-prestige area of science.

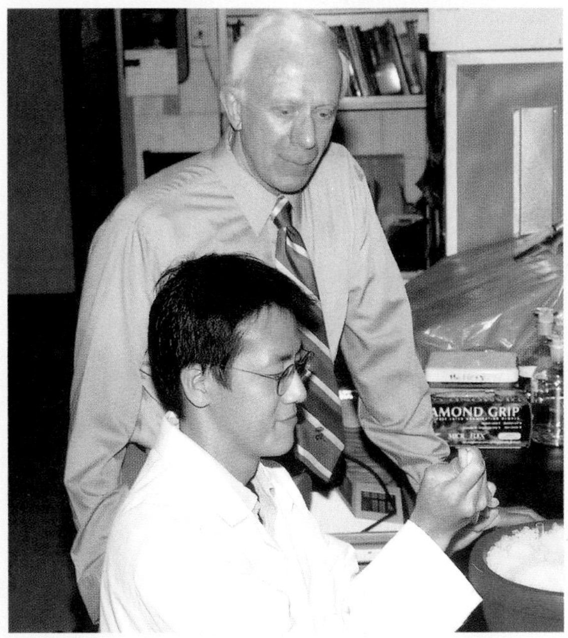

➤ What has been the most interesting/enjoyable aspect of your involvement in science? What was the least interesting/enjoyable aspect?

The most interesting and enjoyable aspects of my involvement in science have been the excitement and intellectual stimulation that comes from making new discoveries.

➤ What is your most meaningful contribution to the field of exercise science, and why is it so important?

Although it is difficult to single out, the most meaningful contribution that I have made to exercise science—the one that has probably had the greatest impact—is the discovery that endurance training induces an increase in muscle mitochondria. The importance of this finding is that it plays a major role in explaining how endurance training improves endurance and alters the metabolic response to exercise.

➤ What advice would you give to students who express an interest in pursuing a career in exercise science research?

A career in research in any area of biology can be extremely exciting and rewarding. This is particularly true of exercise science, a field in which there are still so many interesting, unanswered questions. However, biological research is extremely competitive in terms of coming up with novel, important ideas; obtaining research funding; keeping current with new methodology; and getting papers published. I would, therefore, strongly discourage students from pursuing a research career if they are not: 1) highly intelligent, able to think independently and originally, with the ability to identify important problems and devise approaches for solving them; 2) highly motivated; 3) persevering and not easily discouraged; and 4) able to write well. There is probably nothing more discouraging than having to struggle for support and advancement, yet to be unsuccessful in ones chosen profession; but the chance for both is extremely high in biological research. A sensible approach for individuals who have an interest in exercise science but are not sure that they can succeed in a research career is to get a professional degree (MD, DO, PT, RN, RD, etc.), preferably along with a PhD. This way, one can remain associated with the research area and yet still be assured of making a good living.

➤ What interests have you pursued outside of your professional career?

My interests unrelated to my professional career include literature, particularly historical novels, opera, and gourmet food.

➤ Where do you see the exercise science field (particularly your area of greatest interest) heading in the next 20 years?

The most discouraging aspect of working in the field of exercise science is that, despite the now rather general perception that exercise is necessary for maintenance of health and functional capacity, the majority of people in North America are sedentary. Therefore, it seems likely to me that the major emphasis during the next 20 years will be: 1) from a practical aspect, trying to get people to exercise; and 2) from a basic research perspective, trying to find pharmacological and other approaches that induce some of the same health benefits as exercise.

➤ You have the opportunity to give a "last lecture." Describe its primary focus.

The adaptive response of muscle mitochondria to endurance exercise.

CHAPTER 4

Energy Value of Food

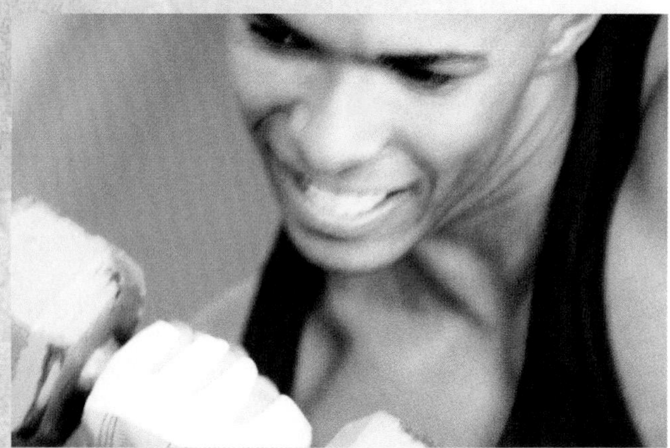

Chapter Objectives

- Describe the method for directly determining the energy content of the macronutrients
- Discuss various factors that influence the difference between a food's gross energy value and its net physiologic energy value
- Define the following: (1) heat of combustion, (2) digestive efficiency, and (3) Atwater factors
- Compute the energy content of a meal from its macronutrient composition

MEASUREMENT OF FOOD ENERGY

The Calorie As a Measurement Unit

In terms of food energy, one calorie expresses the quantity of heat needed to raise the temperature of 1 kg (1 L) of water 1°C (specifically, from 14.5 to 15.5°C). Thus, kilogram calorie or **kilocalorie (kcal)** more accurately defines calorie. For example, if a particular food contains 300 kcal, then releasing the potential energy trapped within this food's chemical structure increases the temperature of 300 L of water 1°C. Different foods contain different amounts of potential energy. One-half cup of peanut butter with a caloric value of 759 kcal contains the equivalent heat energy to increase the temperature of 759 L of water 1°C.

A corresponding unit of heat using Fahrenheit degrees is the British thermal unit, or BTU. One BTU represents the quantity of heat necessary to raise the temperature of 1 lb (weight) of water 1°F from 63 to 64°F. A clear distinction exists between temperature and heat. Temperature reflects a quantitative measure of an object's hotness or coldness. Heat describes energy transfer or exchange from one body or system to another. (The following conversions apply: 1 cal = 4.184 J; 1 kcal = 1,000 cal = 4,184 J or 4.184 kJ; 1 BTU = 778 ft-lb = 252 cal = 1,055 J.)

The joule, **or kilojoule (kJ)**, reflects the standard international unit for expressing food energy. To convert kilocalories to kilojoules, multiply the kilocalorie value by 4.184. The kilojoule value for one-half cup of peanut butter, for example, would equal 759 kcal × 4.184 or 3,176 kJ. The **megajoule (MJ)** equals 1,000 kJ; its use avoids unmanageably large numbers. Appendix A presents a listing of metric system transpositions and conversion constants commonly used in exercise physiology.

Gross Energy Value of Foods

Laboratories use bomb calorimeters similar to the one illustrated in Figure 4.1 to measure the total or **gross energy value** of various food macronutrients. Bomb calorimeters operate on the principle of **direct calorimetry**, measuring the heat liberated as the food burns completely.

Figure 4.1 shows food within a sealed chamber charged with oxygen at high pressure. An electrical current moving through the fuse at the tip ignites the food–oxygen mixture. As the food burns, a water jacket surrounding the bomb absorbs the heat (energy) liberated. Because the calorimeter remains fully insulated from the ambient environment, the increase in water temperature directly reflects the heat released during a food's oxidation (burning).

Heat of combustion refers to the heat liberated by oxidizing a specific food; it represents the food's total energy value. For example, a teaspoon of margarine releases 100 kcal of heat energy when burned completely in a bomb calorimeter. This equals the energy required to raise 1.0 kg (2.2 lb) of ice water to the boiling point. Although the oxidation pathways of the intact organism and the bomb calorimeter differ, the quantity of energy liberated in the complete breakdown of a food remains the same.

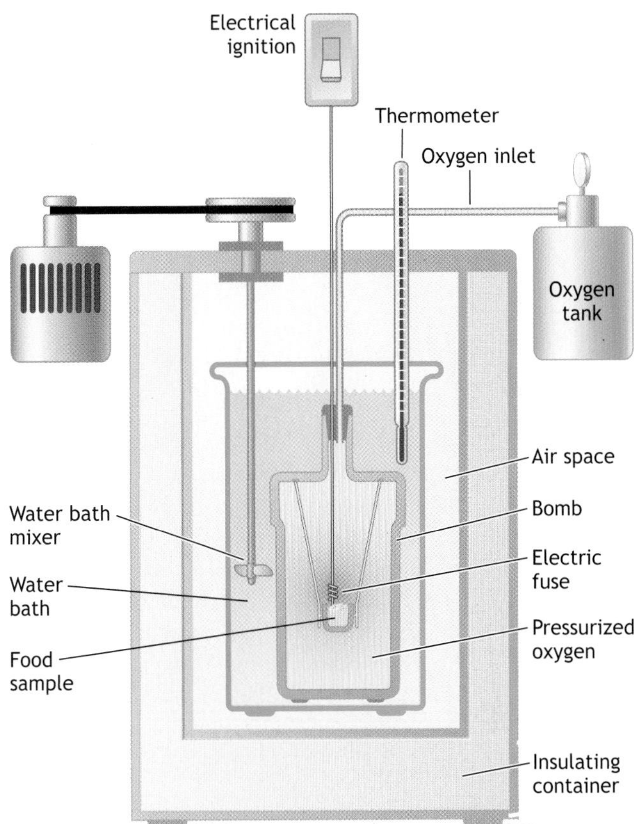

FIGURE 4.1 • A bomb calorimeter directly measures the energy value of food.

Heat of Combustion: Lipid

The heat of combustion for lipid varies with the structural composition of the triglyceride molecule's fatty acids. For example, 1 g of either beef or pork fat yields 9.50 kcal, whereas oxidizing 1 g of butterfat liberates 9.27 kcal. The average caloric value for 1 g of lipid in meat, fish, and eggs equals 9.50 kcal. In dairy products, the calorific equivalent amounts to 9.25 kcal per gram and in vegetables and fruits, 9.30 kcal. *The average heat of combustion for lipid equals 9.4 kcal per gram.*

Heat of Combustion: Carbohydrate

The heat of combustion for carbohydrate also varies, depending upon the arrangement of atoms in the particular carbohydrate molecule. The heat of combustion for glucose equals 3.74 kcal per gram, whereas larger values result for glycogen (4.19 kcal) and starch (4.20 kcal). *A value of 4.2 kcal generally represents the heat of combustion for a gram of carbohydrate.*

Heat of Combustion: Protein

Two factors affect energy release during combustion of a food's protein component: (1) the type of protein in the food and (2) the relative nitrogen content of the protein. Common proteins in eggs, meat, corn (maize), and beans (jack, Lima, navy, soy) contain approximately 16% nitrogen and have corresponding heats of combustion that average 5.75 kcal per gram. Proteins in other foods have a somewhat higher nitrogen content (e.g., most nuts and seeds [18.9%] and whole-kernel wheat, rye, millets, and barley [17.2%]). Other foods contain a slightly lower nitrogen percentage, for example, whole milk (15.7%) and bran (15.8%). *The heat of combustion for protein averages 5.65 kcal per gram.*

Comparing the Energy Value of Nutrients

The average heats of combustion for the three macronutrients (carbohydrate, 4.2 kcal · g^{-1}; lipid, 9.4 kcal · g^{-1}; protein, 5.65 kcal · g^{-1}) demonstrate that the complete oxidation of lipid in the bomb calorimeter liberates about 65% more energy per gram than protein oxidation and 120% more energy than the oxidation of carbohydrate. Recall from Chapter 1 that lipid molecules contains more hydrogen atoms than either carbohydrate or protein molecules. The common fatty acid palmitic acid, for example, has the structural formula $C_{16}H_{32}O_2$. The ratio of hydrogen atoms to oxygen atoms in fatty acids always greatly exceeds the 2:1 ratio in carbohydrates. Simply stated, lipid molecules have more hydrogen atoms available for cleavage and subsequent oxidation for energy than carbohydrates and proteins.

INTEGRATIVE QUESTION

Respond to a student who asks: "How can the oxygen required to burn food indicate the number of calories in the meal I'm going to eat tonight?"

One can conclude from the above discussion that lipid-rich foods have a higher energy content than relatively fat-free foods. One cup of whole milk, for example, contains 160 kcal, whereas the same quantity of skim milk contains only 90 kcal. If a person who normally consumes one quart of whole milk each day switches to skim milk, the total calories ingested each year would decrease by the equivalent of the calories in 25 pounds of body fat. In 3 years, all other things remaining constant, the loss of body fat would approximate 75 pounds! Such a theoretical comparison merits serious consideration because of the almost identical nutrient composition between whole milk and skim milk except for lipid content. Drinking skim rather than whole milk also significantly reduces saturated fatty acid intake (0.4 versus 5.1 g; 863%) and cholesterol (0.3 versus 33 mg; 910%).

Net Energy Value of Foods

Differences exist in the energy value of foods when the heat of combustion (gross energy value) determined by direct calorimetry is compared with the **net energy** actually available to the body. This pertains particularly to protein because the body cannot oxidize the nitrogen component of this nutrient. In the body, nitrogen atoms combine with hydrogen to form urea (NH_2CONH_2), which the kidneys excrete in the urine. Elimination of hydrogen in this manner represents a loss of approximately 19% of the protein molecule's potential energy. This hydrogen loss reduces protein's heat of combustion to approximately 4.6 kcal per gram instead of 5.65 kcal per gram released during oxidation in the bomb calorimeter. In contrast, the physiologic fuel values of carbohydrates and lipids (which contain no nitrogen) are *identical* to their heats of combustion in the bomb calorimeter.

COEFFICIENT OF DIGESTIBILITY. The efficiency of the digestive process influences the ultimate energy yield from the food macronutrients. Numerically defined as the **coefficient of digestibility**, digestive efficiency indicates the percentage of ingested food actually digested and absorbed to meet the body's metabolic needs. The food remaining unabsorbed in the intestinal tract is voided in the feces. Dietary fiber reduces the coefficient of digestibility; a high-fiber meal has less total energy absorbed than does a fiber-free meal of equivalent caloric content. This variance occurs because fiber moves food through the intestine more rapidly, reducing time for absorption. Fiber also may cause mechanical erosion of the intestinal mucosa, which is then resynthesized through energy-requiring processes.

Table 4.1 shows different digestibility coefficients, heats of combustion, and net energy values for nutrients in the various food groups. *The relative percentage of the macronutrients digested and absorbed averages 97% for carbohydrate, 95% for lipid, and 92% for protein.* Little difference exists in digestive efficiency between obese and lean individuals. However, considerable variability exists in efficiency percentages for any food within a particular category. Proteins in particular have digestive efficiencies ranging from a low of about 78% for protein in legumes to a high of 97% for protein from animal sources. Some advocates promote the use of vegetables in weight-loss diets because of plant protein's relatively low coefficient of digestibility. Those who choose vegetarian-type diets should consume adequate, diverse protein food sources to obtain all the essential amino acids.

From the data in Table 4.1, one can round the average net energy values to whole numbers referred to as **Atwater general factors**.

These values, named for Wilbur Olin Atwater (1844–1907), the 19th-century chemist who pioneered human nutrition and energy balance studies at Wesleyan College, indicate the net metabolizable energy available to the body from ingested foods. If precise energy values for experimental or therapeutic diets are not required, the Atwater general factors provide a good estimate of the energy content of the daily diet (see "In a Practical Sense"). For alcohol, 7 kcal (29.4 kJ) represents each g (mL) of

ATWATER GENERAL FACTORS

- 4 kcal per gram for dietary carbohydrate
- 9 kcal per gram for dietary lipid
- 4 kcal per gram for dietary protein

TABLE 4.1 ➤ **FACTORS FOR DIGESTIBILITY, HEATS OF COMBUSTION, AND NET PHYSIOLOGIC ENERGY VALUES[a] OF PROTEIN, LIPID, AND CARBOHYDRATE**

FOOD GROUP	DIGESTIBILITY (%)	HEAT OF COMBUSTION (KCAL · G^{-1})	NET ENERGY (KCAL · G^{-1})
Protein			
Animal food	97	5.65	4.27
Meats, fish	97	5.65	4.27
Eggs	97	5.75	4.37
Dairy products	97	5.65	4.27
Vegetable food	85	5.65	3.74
Cereals	85	5.80	3.87
Legumes	78	5.70	3.47
Vegetables	83	5.00	3.11
Fruits	85	5.20	3.36
Average Protein	92	5.65	4.05
Lipid			
Meat and eggs	95	9.50	9.03
Dairy products	95	9.25	8.79
Animal food	95	9.40	8.93
Vegetable food	90	9.30	8.37
Average Lipid	95	9.40	8.93
Carbohydrate			
Animal food	98	3.90	3.82
Cereals	98	4.20	4.11
Legumes	97	4.20	4.07
Vegetables	95	4.20	3.99
Fruits	90	4.00	3.60
Sugars	98	3.95	3.87
Vegetable food	97	4.15	4.03
Average Carbohydrate	97	4.15	4.03

[a]Net physiologic energy values are computed as the coefficient of digestibility × heat of combustion adjusted for energy loss in urine.
From Merrill AL, Watt BK. Energy values of foods: basis and derivation. Agricultural Handbook no. 74, Washington, DC: USDA, 1973.

pure (200-proof) alcohol ingested. In terms of potential energy available to the body, alcohol's efficiency of use equals that of other carbohydrates.

Use of Tabled Values

Computing the kilocalorie content of foods requires considerable time and labor. Various governmental agencies in the United States and elsewhere have evaluated and compiled nutritive values for thousands of foods. The most comprehensive data bank resources include the United States Nutrient Data Bank (USNDB), maintained by the U. S. Department of Agriculture's Consumer Nutrition Center, and a computerized data bank maintained by the Bureau of Nutritional Sciences of Health and Welfare Canada. Appendix B presents the energy and nutritive values for common foods, including specialty and fast-food items.

A brief review of Appendix B indicates that large differences exist between the energy values of various foods. Consuming an equal number of calories from different foods often requires a tremendous intake of a particular food or relatively little of another. For example, to consume 100 kcal from each of six common foods—carrots, celery, green peppers, grapefruit, medium-sized eggs, and mayonnaise—one must eat 5 carrots, 20 stalks of celery, 6.5 green peppers, 1 large grapefruit, 1 1/4 eggs, but only 1 tablespoon of mayonnaise. Consequently, a typical sedentary adult female who expends 2100 kcal each day must consume about 420 celery stalks, 105 carrots, 136 green peppers, 26 eggs, yet only 1 1/2 cup of mayonnaise or 8 ounces of salad oil to meet daily energy needs. These examples illustrate dramatically that foods high in lipid content contain considerably more calories than food low in lipid and correspondingly high in water content.

IN A PRACTICAL SENSE

➤➤ DETERMINING A FOOD'S MACRONUTRIENT COMPOSITION AND ENERGY CONTRIBUTION

Food labels must indicate a food's macronutrient content (g) and total calories (kcal). Knowing the energy value per gram for carbohydrate, lipid, and protein in a food allows one to readily compute the percentage kcal derived from each macronutrient. The net energy value, referred to as Atwater general factors, equals 4 kcal for carbohydrate, 9 kcal for lipid, and 4 kcal for protein.

Calculations

The table shows the macronutrient composition for one large serving of McDonald's French fries (weight, 122.3 g [4.3 oz]). [*Note:* McDonald's publishes the weight of each of the macronutrients for one serving along with the total kcal value.]

1. Calculate kcal value of each macronutrient (column 4).
   Multiply the weight of each nutrient (column 2) by the appropriate Atwater factor (column 3).
2. Calculate percentage weight of each nutrient (column 5).
   Divide weight of each macronutrient (column 2) by the food's total weight.
3. Calculate percentage kcal for each macronutrient (column 6).
   Divide kcal value of each macronutrient (column 4) by food's total kcal value.

Learn to Read Food Labels

Computing the percentage weight and kcal of each macronutrient in a food fosters wise decisions in choosing foods. Manufacturers must state the absolute and percentage weights for each macronutrient, but computing their absolute and percentage energy contributions completes the more important picture. In the example for French fries, lipid represents only 17% of the food's total weight. However, the percentage of total calories from lipid jumps to 48.3%, or about 195 kcal of this food's 402 kcal energy content. This information becomes crucial for those interested in maintaining a low-fat diet.

Similar computations can estimate the caloric value of any food serving. Of course, increasing or decreasing portion sizes or adding lipid-rich sauces or creams, or using fruits or calorie-free substitutes, affects the caloric content accordingly.

MACRONUTRIENT ENERGY CONTENT AND PERCENTAGE COMPOSITION OF MCDONALD'S FRENCH FRIES, LARGE (TOTAL WEIGHT, 122.3 G [4.3 OZ])

(1) NUTRIENT	(2) WEIGHT	(3) ATWATER (g) FACTOR	(4) KCAL	(5) % OF WEIGHT	(6) % OF KCAL
Protein	6	4 kcal · g^{-1}	24	4.9	6.0
Carbohydrate	45.9	4 kcal · g^{-1}	183.6	37.5	45.7
Lipid	21.6	9 kcal · g^{-1}	194.4	17.7	48.3
Ash	3.2		0	2.6	0
Water	45.6		0	37.3	0
Total	122.3		402	100	100

INTEGRATIVE QUESTION

What factors could account for a discrepancy between computations of the energy value of daily food intake using the Atwater general factors and those from direct measurement via the bomb calorimeter?

Also note that a calorie reflects the food energy *regardless* of the food source. Thus, from an energy standpoint, 100 calories from mayonnaise equals the same 100 calories in 20 celery stalks. The more a person eats of any food, the more calories that person consumes. However, a small amount of fatty food represents a considerable number of calories; thus, the term *fattening* often describes these foods. An individual's caloric intake equals the sum of *all* energy consumed from either small or large quantities of foods. Celery would become a fattening food if consumed in excess! Chapter 3 considered variations in daily energy intake among diverse groups of male and female athletes.

Summary

1. A calorie or kilocalorie (kcal) represents a measure of heat used to express the energy value of food.
2. Burning food in the bomb calorimeter permits direct quantification of the food's energy content.
3. The heat of combustion quantifies the amount of heat liberated in the complete oxidation of a food. Average gross energy values equal 4.2 kcal per gram for carbohydrate, 9.4 kcal per gram for lipid, and 5.65 kcal per gram for protein.
4. The coefficient of digestibility represents the proportion of food consumed that is actually digested and absorbed.
5. Coefficients of digestibility average approximately 97% for carbohydrates, 95% for lipids, and 92% for proteins. Thus, the net energy values equal 4 kcal per gram of carbohydrate, 9 kcal per gram of lipid, and 4 kcal per gram of protein. These values, known as Atwater general factors, provide an accu-

Focus on Research

Obesity-Related Thermogenic Response

Segal KR, Gutin B. Thermic effects of food and exercise in lean and obese women. Metabolism 1983;32:581.

➤ Considerable research has linked obesity and impaired thermogenesis—a diminished capacity to increase metabolism in response to different stimuli. These studies note a lower rise in metabolism for obese individuals than for lean individuals after ingestion of a meal, exposure to cold, infusion of noradrenaline, or the combination of eating and exercising. A diminished thermogenic response probably plays an accessory role in total energy conservation, contributing to the onset and persistence of human obesity.

The research of Segal and Gutin evaluated thermogenic difference between obese and lean women in response to food intake, two levels of exercise, and the possible potentiation of the thermic effect of food with physical activity. Subjects included 10 obese (% fat, 37; body mass, 77.9 kg) and 10 lean (% fat, 18.8; body mass, 53.2 kg) women, measured under six different conditions: (a) resting metabolism ($\dot{V}O_2$) for 4 hours; (b) $\dot{V}O_2$ for 4 hours following consumption of a 910-kcal meal (14% protein, 46% carbohydrate, 40% lipid); (c) $\dot{V}O_2$ during exercise at a constant submaximal intensity of 300 kg-m · min^{-1} (cycling for 5 min every 0.5 h for 4 h); (d) $\dot{V}O_2$ during exercise at an intensity equal to the subject's lactate threshold (cycling for 5 min every 0.5 h for 4 h); (e) and (f) same as protocols c and d, except the subjects consumed the test meal before exercising.

The figure indicates that consumption of the 910-kcal meal increased exercise $\dot{V}O_2$ more for the lean than for the obese women. Stated somewhat differently, a greater difference emerged between the fed and fasting conditions for the lean group at both exercise intensities. The postprandial exercise $\dot{V}O_2$ for the lean group also remained elevated above the corresponding fasting value at the end of the 4 hours, while for the obese group, the postprandial value at 4 hours equaled their fasting exercise metabolism. Thus, using a 4-hour measurement underestimated the total amount that eating augmented energy expenditure during exercise for the lean women. These subjects exhibited a larger thermic effect of food during exercise than during rest. Obese subjects, on the other hand, showed similar thermic effects of food for exercise and rest conditions, with no added thermogenic bonus from exercise after eating.

The researchers concluded that exercise significantly potentiated the thermic effect of food for lean but *not* for obese women. The large differences in response to the combination of food and subsequent exercise emerged despite similar thermogenic responses of the lean and obese women to food alone and exercise alone. Therefore, the cumulative effect of a lower metabolic rate of the obese (compared with lean subjects) during exercise that follows eating favors energy conservation rather than energy dissipation.

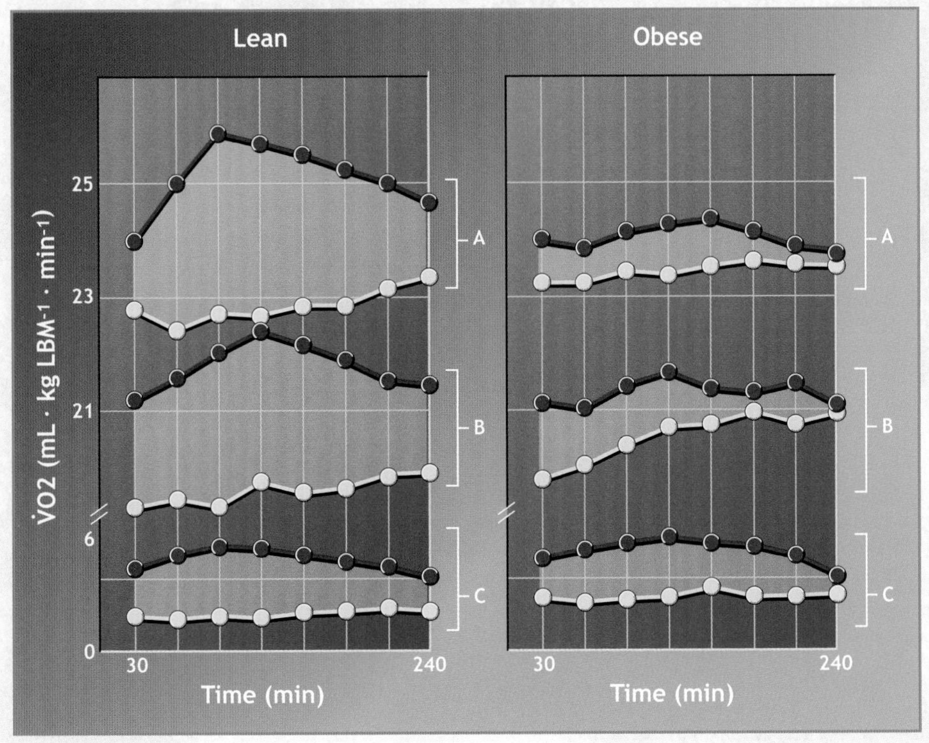

Effects of exercise and a 910-kcal meal on metabolic rates of lean and obese men and women. *A,* Exercise at lactate threshold; *B,* exercise at 300 kg-m · min^{-1}; and *C,* rest. The *red circles* represent postprandial (after the meal) data; *yellow circles* represent postabsorptive (after fasting) data. The *shaded areas* indicate the thermic effect of food under each condition.

rate estimate of the net energy value of typical foods a person consumes.

6. The Atwater calorific values allow one to compute the caloric content of any meal from the carbohydrate, lipid, and protein compositions of the food.
7. Calories represent heat energy regardless of the food source. From an energy standpoint, 500 kcal of peppermint ice cream topped with whipped cream and Brazil nuts is no more fattening than 500 kcal of watermelon, 500 kcal of cheese and pepperoni pizza, or 500 kcal of an egg bagel with salmon, onions, and sour cream.

Suggested Reading

Atwater WO, Woods CD. The chemical composition of American food materials. USDA Bulletin no. 28. Washington, DC: USDA, 1896.

Boyle M. Personal Nutrition. 4th ed. Belmont, CA: Wadsworth Publishing, 2001.

Brody T. Nutritional biochemistry. New York: Academic Press, 1998.

Brown J. Nutrition now. Belmont, CA: Wadsworth Publishing, 1999.

Brooks GA, et al. Exercise physiology: human bioenergetics and its applications. 3rd ed. Mountain View, CA: Mayfield, 2000.

Gibson RS. Principles of nutritional assessment. New York: Oxford University Press, 1990.

Groff JL, Gropper SS. Advanced nutrition and human metabolism. Belmont, CA: Wadsworth Publishing, 1999.

Guyton AC. Textbook of medical physiology. 10th ed. Philadelphia: WB Saunders, 2000.

Health and Welfare Canada. Nutrient value of some common foods. Ottawa, Canada: Health Services and Promotion Branch, Health and Welfare, 1988.

Katch FI. U.S. government raises serious questions about reliability of U.S. Department of Agriculture's food composition tables. Int J Sports Nutr 1995;5:62.

Mahan IK, Escott-Stump S. Krause's food, nutrition, & diet therapy. Philadelphia: WB Saunders, 2000.

McCance RA, Widdowson EM. The composition of foods. 5th ed. London: Royal Society of Chemistry. Ministry of Agriculture, Fisheries and Food, 1991.

Miles CW, et al. Effect of dietary fiber on the metabolizable energy of human diets. J Nutr 1988;118:1075.

Pennington JAT, Church HN. Bowes and Church's food values of portions commonly used. 17th ed. Baltimore: Lippincott Williams & Wilkins, 1989.

Rand WM, et al., eds. Food composition data: a user's perspective. Tokyo: United Nations University, 1987.

Rumpler WV, et al. Energy value of moderate alcohol consumption by humans. Am J Clin Nutr 1996;64:108.

Shils ME, et al. Modern nutrition in health and disease. 9th ed. Baltimore: Lippincott Williams & Wilkins, 1999.

US Department of Agriculture. Composition of foods—raw, processed, and prepared. No. 8. Washington, DC: US Department of Agriculture, 1963–1987.

CHAPTER 5

Introduction to Energy Transfer

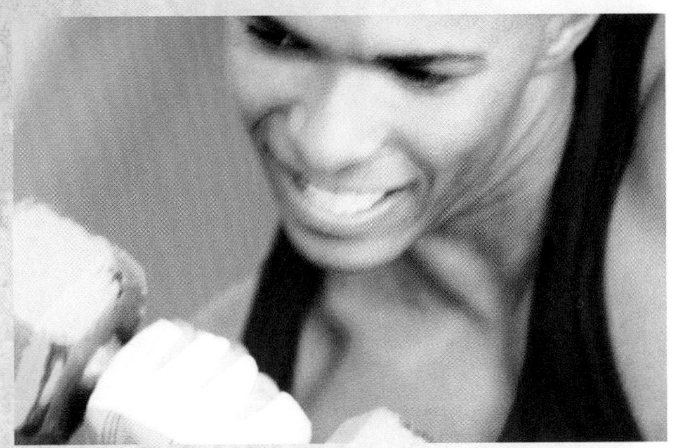

Chapter Objectives

- Describe the first law of thermodynamics as it relates to energy balance and work within biologic systems
- Define the terms potential energy and kinetic energy and give examples of each
- Discuss the role of free energy in biologic work
- Give examples of exergonic and endergonic chemical processes within the body and indicate their importance
- State the second law of thermodynamics and give a practical application of this law
- Discuss the role of coupled reactions in biologic processes within the body
- Differentiate between photosynthesis and respiration and give the biologic significance of each
- Identify and give examples of the three forms of biologic work
- Describe the effects of enzymes and coenzymes on energy metabolism
- Differentiate between hydrolysis and condensation and give their importance in physiologic function
- Discuss the role of redox chemical reactions in energy metabolism

The capacity to extract energy from food macronutrients and continually transfer it at a high rate to the contractile elements of skeletal muscle largely determines one's capacity for swimming, running, or skiing long distances. Likewise, specific energy-transferring capacities that demand all-out, "explosive" power output for brief durations determine success in weight lifting, sprinting, jumping, and football line play. Although muscular activity represents the main frame of reference in this text, *all* forms of biologic work require power generated from the direct transfer of chemical energy.

The sections that follow introduce general concepts about bioenergetics. They provide the basis for understanding energy metabolism during physical activity.

ENERGY—THE CAPACITY FOR WORK

Extracting energy from the stored nutrients and transferring it to the contractile proteins of skeletal muscle greatly influences exercise performance, but unlike the physical properties of matter, one cannot define energy in concrete terms of size, shape, or mass. Rather the term energy suggests a dynamic state related to change; thus, the presence of energy emerges only when a change occurs. Within this context, energy relates to the performance of work—as work increases so does energy transfer, thus producing a change.

The **first law of thermodynamics** describes one of the most important principles related to biologic work. The basic tenet states that energy cannot be created or destroyed but, instead, transforms from one form to another without being depleted. In essence, this law describes the immutable principle of the **conservation of energy** that applies to both living and nonliving systems. In the body, chemical energy stored within the bonds of macronutrients does not immediately dissipate as heat during energy metabolism; instead, a large portion remains as chemical energy, which the musculoskeletal system then changes into mechanical energy (and then ultimately to heat energy). *The first law of thermodynamics dictates that the body does not produce, consume, or use up energy; rather it transforms it from one form into another as physiologic systems undergo continual change.*

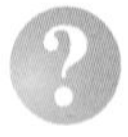

INTEGRATIVE QUESTION

Based on the first law of thermodynamics, why is it imprecise to refer to energy "production" in the body?

Potential and Kinetic Energy

***Potential energy** and **kinetic energy** constitute the total energy of a system.* Figure 5.1 shows potential energy as energy of position, similar to a boulder tottering atop a cliff or water at the top of a hill before it flows downstream. In the example of flowing water, the energy change is proportional to the water's vertical drop—the greater the vertical drop, the greater the potential energy at the top. The waterwheel harnesses a portion of the energy from the falling water to produce useful

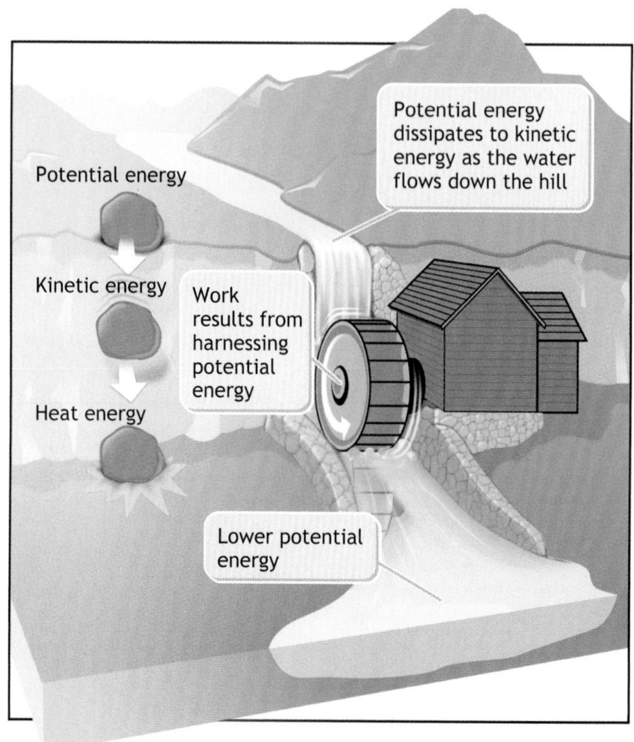

FIGURE 5.1 • High-grade potential energy capable of performing work degrades to a useless form of kinetic energy. In the example of falling water, the water wheel harnesses potential energy to perform useful work. For the falling boulder, all of the potential energy dissipates to kinetic energy (heat) as the boulder crashes to the surface.

work. In the case of the boulder, *all* potential energy transforms to kinetic energy and dissipates as useless heat.

Other examples of potential energy include bound energy within the internal structure of a battery, a stick of dynamite, or a macronutrient before release of its stored energy in metabolism. *Releasing potential energy transforms it into kinetic energy of motion.* In some cases, bound energy in one substance directly transfers to other substances to increase their potential energy. Energy transfers of this type provide the necessary energy for the body's chemical work of **biosynthesis**. In this process, specific building-block atoms of carbon, hydrogen, oxygen, and nitrogen become activated and join other atoms and molecules to synthesize important biologic compounds and tissues. Some newly created compounds provide structure as in bone or the lipid-containing plasma membrane that encloses each cell. Other synthesized compounds such as adenosine triphosphate (ATP) and phosphocreatine (PCr) serve the cell's energy requirements.

Energy-Releasing and Energy-Conserving Processes

The term **exergonic** describes any physical or chemical process that results in the release (freeing) of energy to its surroundings. Such reactions represent "downhill" processes; they result in a decline in free energy—"useful" energy for biologic work that encompasses all of the energy-requiring, life-sustaining processes within cells. Within a cell, where pressure and volume remain relatively stable, free energy (denoted by the symbol G to honor Willard Gibbs [1839–1903] whose research provided the foundation of biochemical thermodynamics) equals the potential energy within a molecule's chemical bonds (called enthalpy, or H), minus the energy unavailable because of randomness (S), times the absolute temperature (°C + 273). The equation $G = H - TS$ describes free energy quantitatively.

Chemical processes that store or absorb energy are termed **endergonic**; these reactions represent "uphill" processes and proceed with an increase in free energy for biologic work. In some instances, exergonic processes link or couple with endergonic reactions to transfer some energy to the endergonic process. In the body, such coupled reactions conserve in a usable form a large portion of the chemical energy stored within the macronutrients.

Figure 5.2 illustrates the flow of energy in exergonic and endergonic chemical reactions. Changes in free energy occur when the bonds in the reactant molecules form new product molecules with different bonding. The equation that expresses these changes, under conditions of constant temperature, pressure, and volume, takes the following form:

$$\Delta G = \Delta H - T\Delta S$$

The symbol Δ designates change. The change in free energy represents a keystone of chemical reactions. In exergonic reactions, ΔG is negative; the products contain *less* free energy than the reactants, with the energy differential released as heat. For example, the union of hydrogen and oxygen to form water releases 68 kcal per mole (molecular weight of substance in g) of free energy in the following reaction:

$$H_2 + O \rightarrow H_2O \; -\Delta G \; 68 \text{ kcal} \cdot \text{mol}^{-1}$$

In the reverse endergonic reaction, ΔG is positive because the product contains *more* free energy than the reactants. The infusion of 68 kcal of energy per mole of water causes the chemical bonds of the water molecule to split apart, freeing the original hydrogen and oxygen atoms. This "uphill" process of energy transfer provides the hydrogen and oxygen atoms with their original energy content to satisfy the principle of the first law of thermodynamics—the conservation of energy.

$$H_2 + O \leftarrow H_2O + \Delta G \; 68 \text{ kcal} \cdot \text{mol}^{-1}$$

Energy transfer in cells follows the same principles in the waterfall–waterwheel example. Carbohydrate, lipid, and protein macronutrients possess considerable potential energy. The formation of product substances progressively reduces the nutrient molecule's original potential energy, with a corresponding increase in kinetic energy. Enzyme-regulated transfer systems harness or conserve a portion of this chemical energy in new compounds for use in biologic work. In essence, living cells serve as transducers with the capacity to extract and use chemical energy stored within a compound's atomic structure. Conversely, and equally important, they also bond atoms and molecules together, raising them to a higher level of potential energy.

The transfer of potential energy in any spontaneous process always proceeds in a direction that decreases the capacity to perform work. The tendency of potential energy to degrade to kinetic energy of motion with a lower capacity for work (i.e., increased **entropy**) reflects the **second law of thermodynamics**. A flashlight battery provides a good illustration. The electrochemical energy stored within its cells slowly dissipates, even if the battery remains unused. The energy from sunlight also continually degrades to heat energy when light strikes and becomes absorbed by a surface. Food and other chemicals represent excellent stores of potential energy, yet this energy continually decreases as the compounds decompose through normal oxidative processes. Energy, like water, always runs downhill, so potential energy decreases. *Ultimately, all of the potential energy in a system degrades to the unusable form of kinetic or heat energy.*

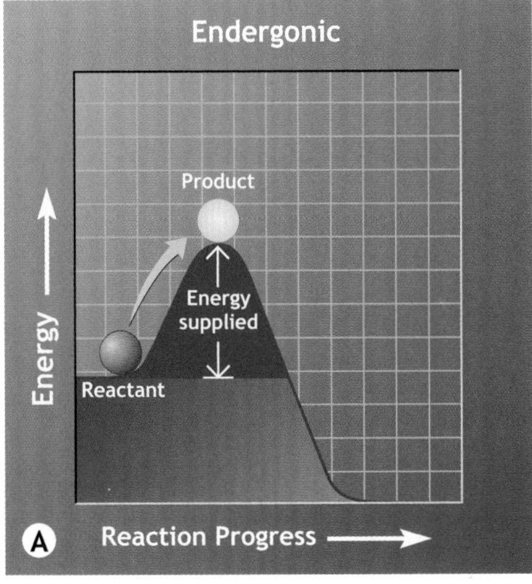

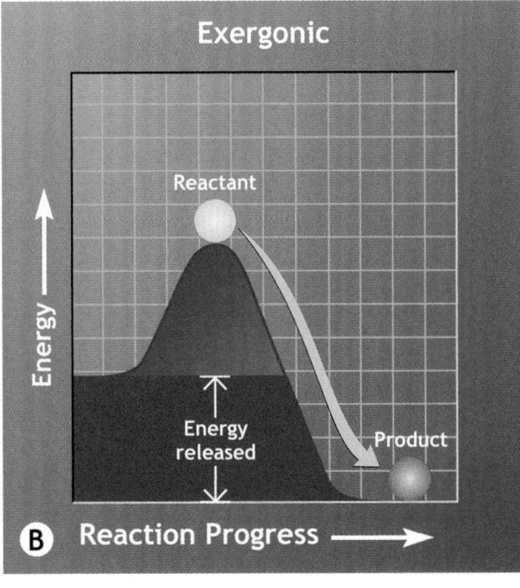

FIGURE 5.2 • Flow of energy in chemical reactions. **A**. Energy supply is required for endergonic reaction to proceed because the reaction's product contains *more* energy than the reactant. **B**. Exergonic reaction releases energy, which results in *less* energy in the product than in the reactant.

INTERCONVERSIONS OF ENERGY

Because the total energy in an isolated system remains constant, a decrease in one form of energy is matched by an equivalent increase in another form. During energy conversions, a loss of potential energy from one source often produces a temporary increase in the potential energy of another source. In this way, nature harnesses vast quantities of potential energy for useful purposes. But even under such favorable conditions, the net flow of energy in the biologic world moves toward entropy, which ultimately results in the loss of potential energy.

Entropy, discovered by the German chemist Ludwig Boltzmann (1844–1906) in the late 1800s, reflects the continual process of energy change. All chemical and physical processes proceed in a direction in which total randomness or disorder *increases* and the energy available for work *decreases.* In coupled reactions during biosynthesis, part of a system may show a decrease in entropy while another part shows an increase. However, no way exists to circumvent the second law—the entire system always shows a net increase in entropy. In a more global sense, the biochemical reactions within the body's trillions of cells (as within the universe as a whole) "tilt" in the direction of spontaneity that favors disorder and randomness (i.e., entropy).

Forms of Energy

Figure 5.3 shows energy categorized into one of six forms: chemical, mechanical, heat, light, electric, and nuclear.

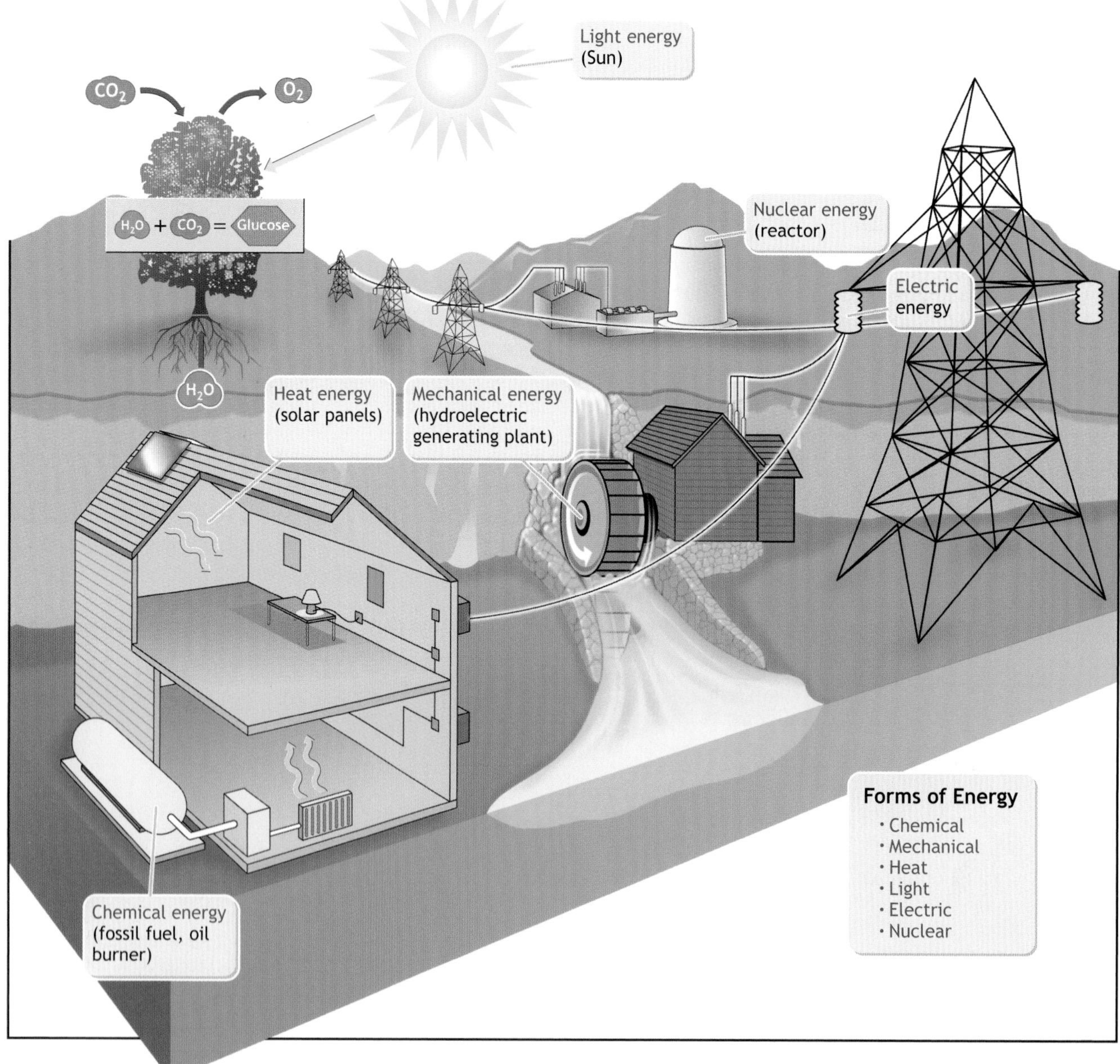

FIGURE 5.3 • Interconversions of six forms of energy.

Examples of Energy Conversions

The conversion of energy from one form to another occurs readily in the inanimate and animate worlds. **Photosynthesis** and **respiration** represent the most fundamental examples of energy conversion in living cells.

PHOTOSYNTHESIS. In the sun, with a temperature of several million degrees Fahrenheit, nuclear fusion releases part of the potential energy stored in the nucleus of the hydrogen atom. This energy, in the form of gamma radiation, then converts to radiant energy.

Figure 5.4 depicts the dynamics of photosynthesis, an endergonic process powered by energy from sunlight. The pigment chlorophyll, contained in large chloroplasts (organelles within the leaf's cells), absorbs radiant (solar) energy to synthesize glucose from carbon dioxide and water, while oxygen flows to the environment. The plant also converts carbohydrates to lipids and proteins for storage as a future reserve for energy and growth. Animals then ingest plant nutrients to serve their own energy needs. *In essence, solar energy coupled with photosynthesis powers the animal world with food and oxygen.*

CELLULAR RESPIRATION. Figure 5.5 shows that the reactions of respiration are the reverse of those of photosynthesis as the plant's stored energy is recovered for use in biologic work. During these exergonic reactions, the cells extract, in the presence of oxygen, the chemical energy stored in the carbohydrate, lipid, and protein molecules. For glucose, this releases 689 kcal per mole (180 g) oxidized. *A portion of the energy released during cellular respiration becomes conserved in other chemical compounds for use in energy-requiring processes; the remaining energy flows to the environment as heat.*

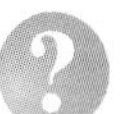

INTEGRATIVE QUESTION

From the perspective of human bioenergetics, discuss the significance of a bumper sticker that reads: "Have you thanked a green plant today?"

BIOLOGIC WORK IN HUMANS

Figure 5.5 also illustrates that biologic work takes one of three forms:

- **Mechanical work** of muscle contraction
- **Chemical work** that synthesizes cellular molecules
- **Transport work** that concentrates various substances in the intracellular and extracellular fluids

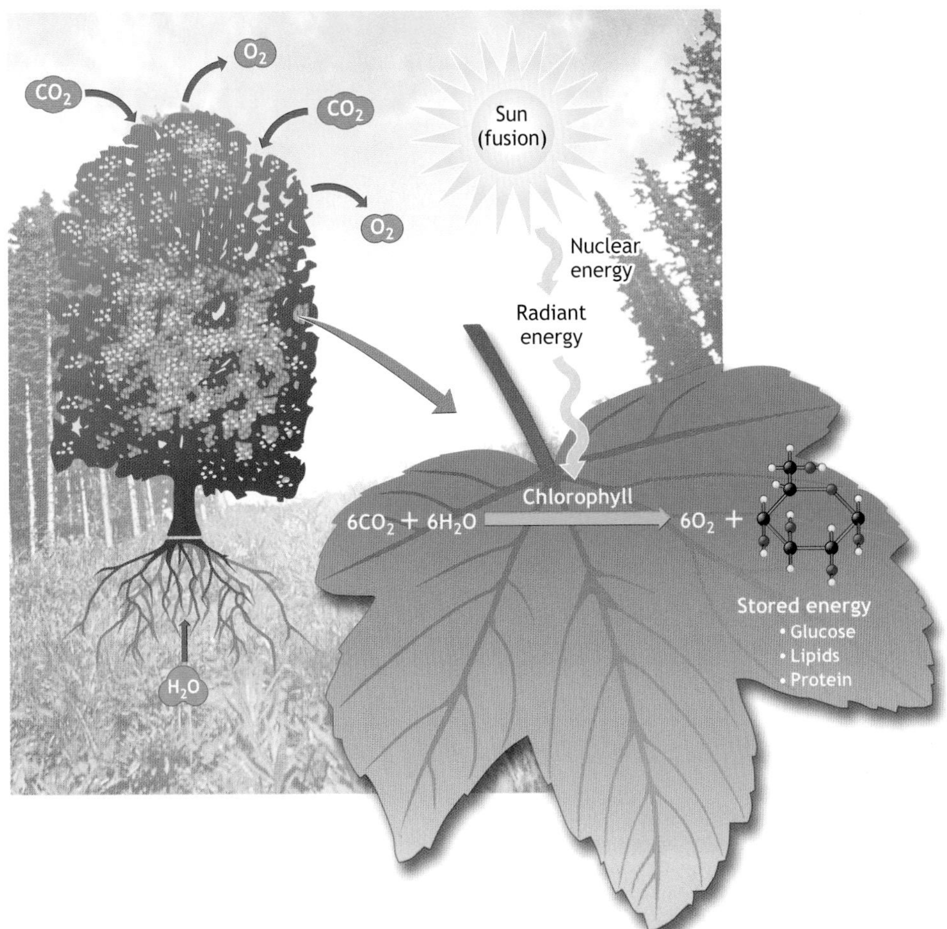

FIGURE 5.4 • The endergonic process of photosynthesis in plants, algea, and some bacteria serves as the mechanism for synthesizing carbohydrates, lipids, and proteins. In this example, a glucose molecule forms from the union of carbon dioxide and water, with a positive free energy (useful energy) change ($+\Delta G$).

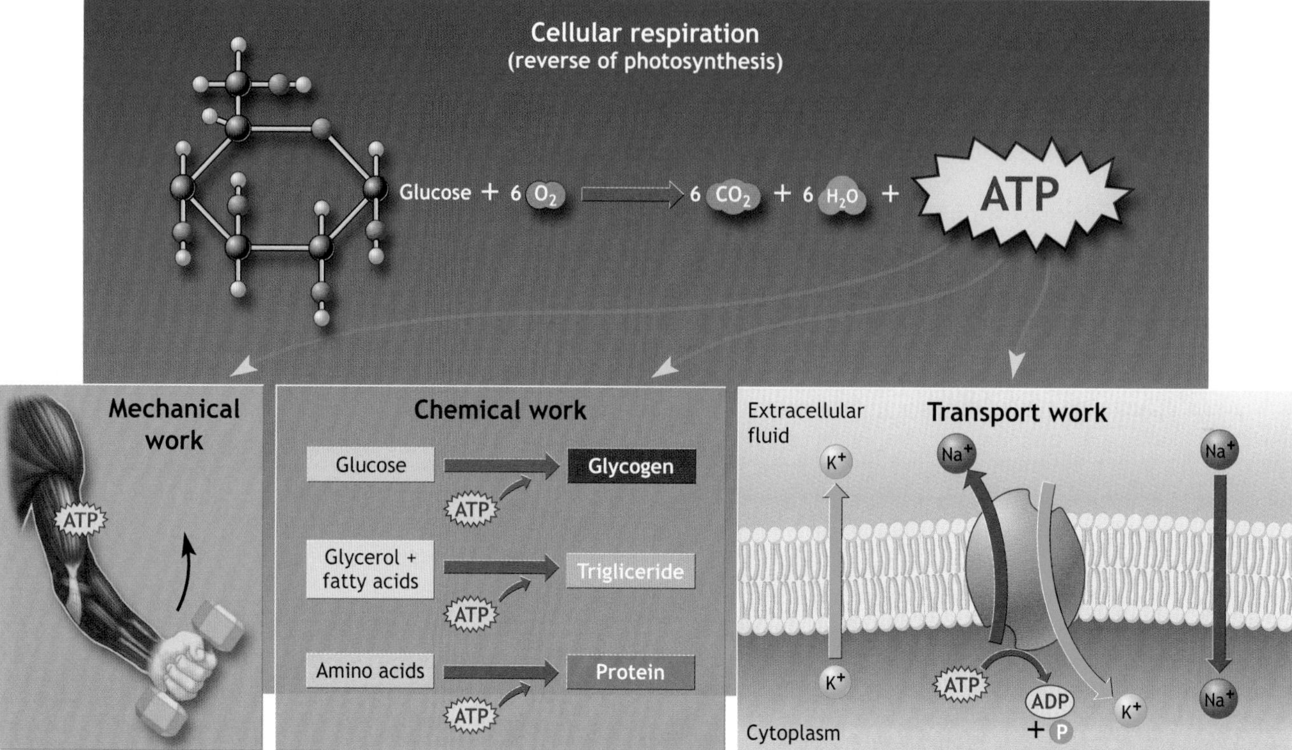

FIGURE 5.5 • The exergonic process of cellular respiration. Exergonic reactions, such as the burning of gasoline or the oxidation of glucose, release potential energy. This results in a negative standard free energy change (i.e., reduction in total energy available for work; $-\Delta G$). In this illustration, cellular respiration harvests the potential energy in food to form ATP. Subsequently, the energy in ATP powers all forms of biologic work.

Mechanical Work

Mechanical work generated by muscle contraction and subsequent movement provides the most obvious example of energy transformation. The molecular motors in a muscle fiber's protein filaments directly convert chemical energy into mechanical energy. However, this does not represent the body's only form of mechanical work. In the cell nucleus, for example, contractile elements literally tug at the chromosomes to facilitate cell division. Specialized structures such as cilia also perform mechanical work in many cells. "In a Practical Sense" shows the methods for quantifying work (and power) on three common exercise modes.

Chemical Work

All cells perform chemical work for maintenance and growth. Continuous synthesis of cellular components takes place as other components break down. The extreme muscle tissue synthesis that occurs in response to chronic overload in resistance training vividly illustrates chemical work.

Transport Work

The biologic work of concentrating substances in the body (transport work) progresses much less conspicuously than mechanical or chemical work. Cellular materials normally flow from an area of high concentration to one of lower concentration. This passive process of **diffusion** requires no energy. For proper physiologic functioning, certain chemicals require transport uphill, against their normal concentration gradients from an area of lower to one of higher concentration. **Active transport** describes this energy-requiring process. Secretion and reabsorption in the kidney tubules use active transport mechanisms, as does neural tissue in establishing the proper electrochemical gradients about its plasma membranes. These "quiet" forms of biologic work require a continual expenditure of stored chemical energy.

FACTORS THAT AFFECT THE RATE OF BIOENERGETICS

The limits of exercise intensity ultimately depend on the rate that cells extract, conserve, and transfer the chemical energy in the food nutrients to the contractile filaments of skeletal muscle. *The sustained pace of the marathon runner at close to 90% of maximum aerobic capacity, or the rapid speed achieved by the sprinter in all-out exercise, directly reflects the body's capacity to transfer chemical energy into mechanical work.* Enzymes and coenzymes significantly affect the rate of energy release during chemical reactions.

Enzymes as Biologic Catalysts

*An **enzyme**, a highly specific and large protein catalyst, accelerates the forward and reverse rates of chemical reactions within the body without being consumed or changed in the reaction.* Enzymes only govern reactions that would normally

IN A PRACTICAL SENSE

➤➤ MEASUREMENT OF WORK ON A TREADMILL, CYCLE ERGOMETER, AND STEP BENCH

An ergometer is an exercise apparatus that quantifies and standardizes physical exercise in terms of work and/or power output. The most common ergometers include treadmills, cycle and arm-crank ergometers, stair steppers, and rowers.

Work (W) represents application or force (F) through a distance (D):

$$W = F \times D$$

For example, for a body mass of 70 kg and vertical jump score of 0.5 m, work accomplished equals 35 kilogram-meters (70 kg × 0.5 m). The most common units of measurement to express work include: kilogram-meters (kg-m), foot-pounds (ft-lb), joules (J), Newton-meters (Nm), and kilocalories (kcal).

Power (P) represents W performed per unit time (T):

$$P = F \times D \div T$$

Calculation of Treadmill Work

Picture the treadmill as a moving conveyor belt with variable angle of incline and speed. Work performed on a treadmill equals the product of the weight (mass) of the person (*F*) and the vertical distance (*vert dist*) the person achieves walking or running up the incline. Vert dist equals the sine of the treadmill angle (theta or θ) multiplied by the distance traveled (*D*) along the incline (treadmill speed × time).

$$W = \text{body mass (force)} \times \text{vertical distance}$$

EXAMPLE

For an angle θ of 8° (measured with an inclinometer or determined by knowing the percent grade of the treadmill), the sine of angle θ equals 0.1392 (see table). The *vert dist* represents treadmill speed multiplied by exercise duration multiplied by sine θ. For example, *vert dist* on the incline while walking at 5000 $m \cdot h^{-1}$ for 1 hour equals 696 m (5000 × 0.1392). If a person with a body mass of 50 kg walked on a treadmill at an incline of 8° (% grade, approximately 14%) to 60 minutes at 5000 $m \cdot h^{-1}$, work accomplished computes as:

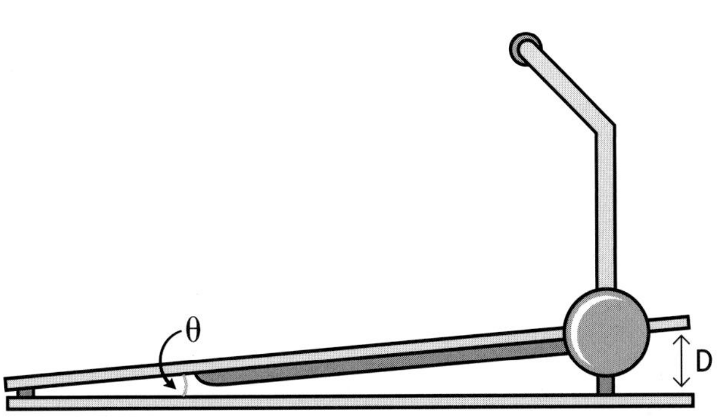

$$W = F \times \textit{vert dist} \ (\text{sine } \theta \times D)$$
$$= 50 \text{ kg} \times (0.1392 \times 5{,}000 \text{ m})$$
$$= 34{,}800 \text{ kg-m}$$

The value for power equals 34,800 kg-m ÷ 60 minutes or 580 kg-m · min^{-1}.

ANGLE (DEG)	SINE θ	PERCENT GRADE
1	0.0175	1.75
2	0.0349	3.49
3	0.0523	5.23
4	0.0698	6.98
5	0.0872	8.72
6	0.1045	10.51
7	0.1219	12.28
8	0.1392	14.05
9	0.1564	15.84
10	0.1736	17.63
15	0.2588	26.80
20	0.3420	36.40

Calculation of Cycle Ergometer Work

The mechanically braked cycle ergometer contains a flywheel with a belt around it connected by a small spring at one end and an adjustable tension lever at the other end. A pendulum balance indicates the resistance against the flywheel as it turns. Increasing the tension on the belt increases flywheel friction, which increases resistance to pedaling. The force (flywheel friction) represents braking load in kg or kilopounds (kp = force acting on 1-kg mass at the normal acceleration of gravity). The distance traveled equals number of pedal revolutions times flywheel circumference.

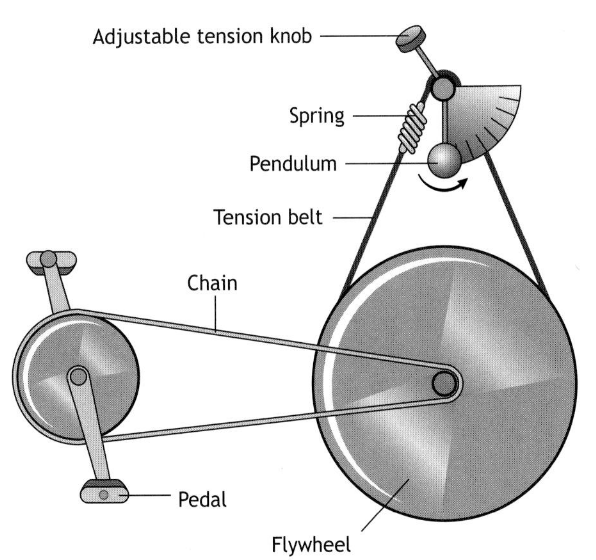

IN A PRACTICAL SENSE

MEASUREMENT OF WORK ON A TREADMILL, CYCLE ERGOMETER, AND STEP BENCH—CONT'D

EXAMPLE

A person pedaling a bicycle ergometer with a 6-m flywheel circumference at 60 rpm for 1 minute covers a distance (*D*) of 360 m each minute (6 m × 60). If the frictional resistance on the flywheel equals 2.5 kg, total work computes as

W = F × D
= frictional resistance × distance traveled
= 2.5 kg × 360 m
= 900 kg-m

Power generated by the effort equals 900 kg-m in 1 minute or 900 kg-m · min^{-1} (900 kg-m ÷ 1 min).

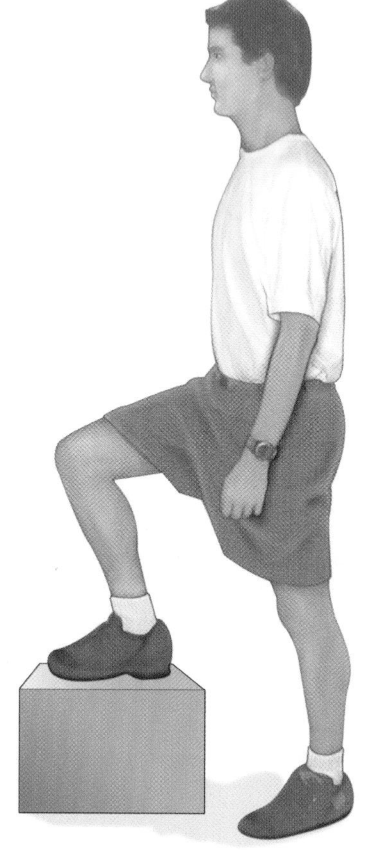

Calculation of Work During Bench Stepping

Only the vertical (positive) work can be calculated in bench stepping. Distance (*D*) computes as bench height times the number of times the person steps; force (*F*) equals the person's body mass (kg).

EXAMPLE

If a 70-kg person steps on a bench 0.375-m high at a rate of 30 steps per minute for 10 minutes, total work computes as

W = F × D
= body mass, kg × (vertical distance [m] × steps per min × 10 min)
= 70 kg × (0.375 m × 30 × 10)
= 7875 kg-m

Power generated during stepping equals 787 kg-m · min^{-1} (7,875 kg-m ÷ 10 min).

take place but at a much slower rate. In a way, enzymes reduce the required **activation energy**—the energy input to initiate a reaction—so its rate changes. Enzyme action takes place without altering the equilibrium constants and total energy released (free energy change or ΔG) in the reaction. Figure 5.6 contrasts the effectiveness of a catalyst in initiating a chemical reaction with initiation in the uncatalyzed state. The vertical axis represents the energy required to activate each reaction; the horizontal axis plots the reaction's progress. Clearly, initiation (activation) of an uncatalyzed reaction requires considerably more energy than a catalyzed one. The rate of a catalyzed reaction can be 10^6 to 10^{20} times faster than the uncatalyzed reaction under similar conditions. Biochemists estimate that without enzyme action, the complete digestion of a breakfast meal might take 50 years!

In its simplest form, an enzyme-catalyzed reaction occurs when a single reactant converts to a single product. The reaction proceeds in one direction so that all substrate (substance acted upon by an enzyme) molecules convert into product molecules. Alternatively, the reaction could reverse so that given enough time, an equilibrium establishes, with the ratio of product concentration to substrate concentration described by the equilibrium constant. Most enzyme-catalyzed reactions proceed in discrete steps. The enzyme first combines with its substrate to form an enzyme–substrate complex. This complex then converts to an enzyme–intermediate complex, which then changes to an enzyme–product complex that quickly dissociates into free product and the enzyme released unchanged.

Enzymes possess the unique property of not being readily altered by the reactions they affect. Consequently, enzyme turnover in the body remains relatively slow, and the specific enzymes are continually reused. A typical mitochondrion may contain up to 10 billion enzyme molecules, each carrying out millions of operations within a brief time. During strenuous exercise, the rate of enzyme activity increases tremendously within the cell, as energy demands increase some 100 times above the resting level. A single cell contains thousands of different enzymes, each with a specific function that catalyzes a distinct cellular reaction. For example, glucose breakdown to carbon dioxide and water requires 19 different chemical re-

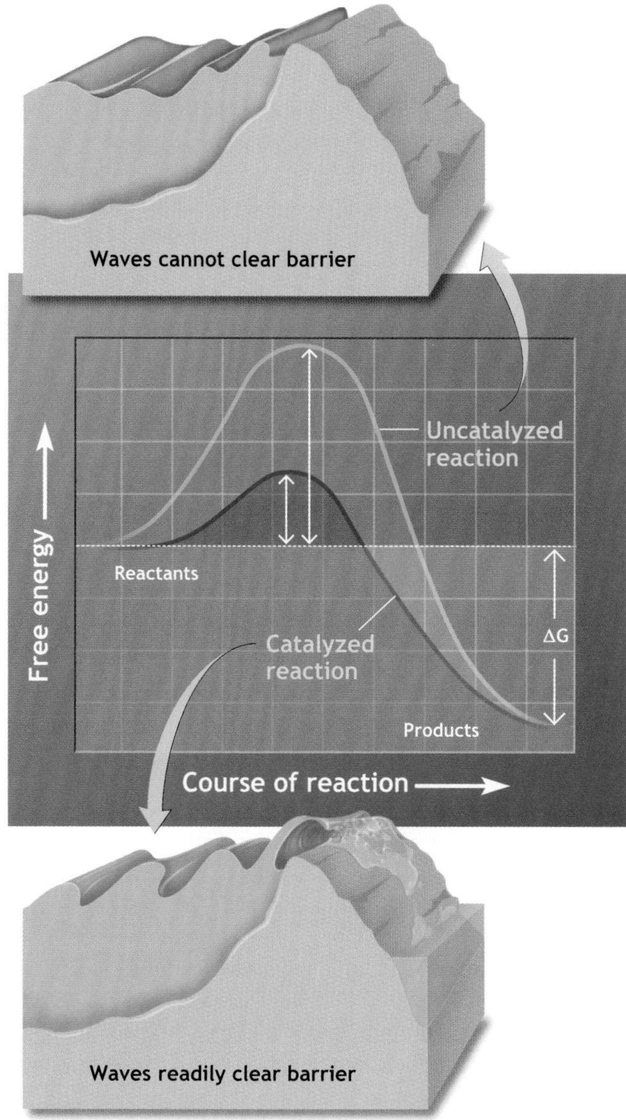

FIGURE 5.6 • The presence of a catalyst greatly reduces the activation energy required to initiate a chemical reaction compared with the energy for an uncatalyzed reaction. For the reaction to proceed, the reactant must have a higher free-energy than the product.

actions, each catalyzed by its own specific enzyme. Enzymes contact precise locations on the surfaces of cell structures; they also operate within the structure itself. Many enzymes operate outside the cell—in the bloodstream, digestive mixture, or intestinal fluids.

Enzymes usually take the names of the functions they perform. The suffix *-ase* appended to the enzyme whose prefix often indicates its mode of operation or the substance with which it interacts. For example, hydrol*ase* adds water during hydrolysis reactions, prote*ase* interacts with protein, oxid*ase* adds oxygen to a substance, and ribonucle*ase* splits ribonucleic acid (RNA).

Reaction Rates

Enzymes do not all operate at the same rate; some operate slowly, others much more rapidly. Consider the enzyme carbonic anhydrase, which catalyzes the hydration of carbon dioxide to form carbonic acid. Its maximum **turnover number**—number of moles of substrate that react to form product per mole of enzyme per unit time—is 800,000. On the other hand, the turnover number for tryptophan synthetase, which catalyzes the final step in tryptophan synthesis, is 2. Enzymes often work cooperatively among their binding sites. While one substance "turns on" at a particular site, its neighbor "turns off" until the process completes. The operation then can reverse, with one enzyme becoming inactive and the other active. Enzymes also can act along small regions of the substrate, each time working at a different rate than previously. Some enzymes delay initiating their work. The precursor digestive enzyme trypsinogen, manufactured by the pancreas in inactive form, serves as a good example. Trypsinogen enters the small intestine, where upon activation (by intestinal enzyme action) it becomes the active enzyme trypsin to digest complex proteins into simple amino acids. Proteolytic action describes this catabolic process. Without the delay in activity, trypsinogen would literally digest the pancreatic tissue that produced it.

Figure 5.7 shows that pH and temperature dramatically affect enzyme activity. For some enzymes, peak activity requires relatively high acidity, while others function opti-

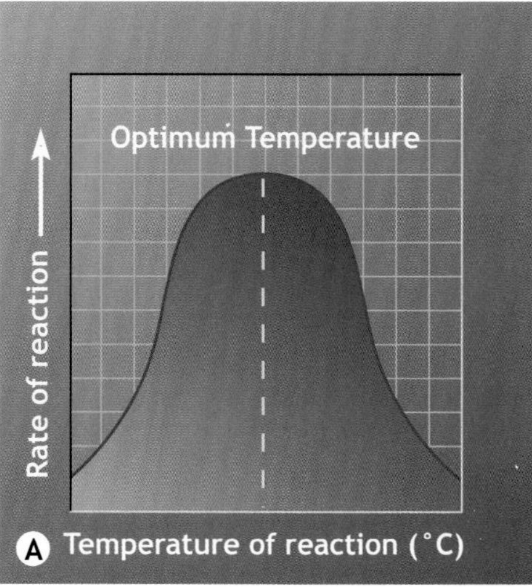

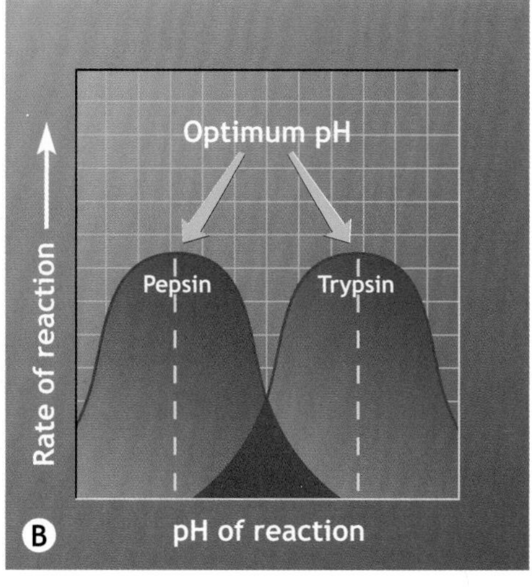

FIGURE 5.7 • Effects of (**A**) temperature and (**B**) pH on the enzyme action turnover rate.

mally on the alkaline side of neutrality. Note that the two enzymes pepsin and trypsin have different pH profiles that modify their activity rates and determine optimal function. Pepsin operates optimally at a pH between 2.4 and 2.6, whereas trypsin's optimum range is close to that of saliva and milk (6.2 to 6.6). This pH effect on enzyme dynamics takes place because changing a fluid's hydrogen ion concentration alters the balance between positively and negatively charged complexes in the enzyme's amino acids. Increases in temperature generally accelerate enzyme reactivity. As temperature rises above 40 to 50°C, however, the protein enzymes become permanently denatured, and their activity ceases.

Mode of Action

Interaction with its specific substrate represents a unique characteristic of an enzyme's three-dimensional globular protein structure. Interaction works like a key fitting a lock as illustrated in Figure 5.8. The enzyme turns on when its **active site** (usually a groove, cleft, or cavity on the protein's surface) joins in a "perfect fit" with the substrate's active site. Upon forming an **enzyme–substrate complex**, the splitting of chemical bonds forms a new product with new bonds, freeing the enzyme to act on additional substrate. The example depicts the interaction sequence of the enzyme maltase as it disassembles maltose into its component two glucose building blocks:

Step 1: The active site of the enzyme and substrate line up to achieve a perfect fit, forming an enzyme–substrate complex.

Step 2: The enzyme catalyzes (greatly speeds up) the chemical reaction with the substrate. Note that the hydrolysis reaction adds a water molecule.

Step 3: An end-product (two glucose molecules) forms releasing the enzyme to act on another substrate.

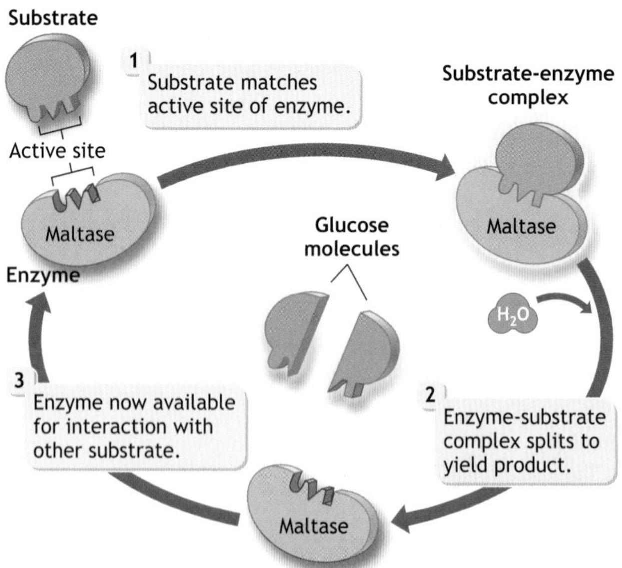

FIGURE 5.8 • Sequence of steps in the "lock and key" mechanism of an enzyme with its substrate. The example shows how two monosaccharide glucose molecules form when maltase interacts with its disaccharide substrate maltose.

A "**lock and key mechanism**," first proposed in the early 1890s by the German chemist and Nobel laureate Emil Fischer (1852–1919), describes the enzyme–substrate interaction. This interactive process ensures that the correct enzyme "mates" with its specific substrate to perform a particular function. Once the enzyme and substrate join, a conformational change in enzyme shape takes place as it molds to the substrate. Even if an enzyme links with a substrate, unless the specific conformational change occurs in the shape of the enzyme, it will not interact chemically with the substrate. A more contemporary hypothesis considers the lock and key more of an "induced fit" because of the required conformational characteristics of enzymes.

The lock-and-key mechanism serves a protective function so only the correct enzyme activates a given substrate. Consider the enzyme hexokinase, which accelerates a chemical reaction by linking with a glucose molecule. When this occurs, a phosphate molecule transfers from ATP to a specific binding site on one of glucose's carbon atoms. Once the two binding sites join to form a glucose–hexokinase complex, the substrate begins its stepwise degradation (controlled by other specific enzymes) to form less complex molecules during energy metabolism.

Coenzymes

Some enzymes remain totally dormant without activation by additional substances termed **coenzymes**. These complex, nonprotein, organic substances facilitate enzyme action by binding the substrate with its specific enzyme. Coenzymes then regenerate to assist in further similar reactions. The metallic ions iron and zinc play coenzyme roles, as do the B vitamins or their derivatives. Oxidation–reduction reactions use the B vitamins riboflavin and niacin, while other vitamins serve as transfer agents for groups of compounds in other metabolic processes (see Table 2.1). Some advertisements for vitamins imply that taking vitamin supplements provides immediate usable energy for exercise. Although vitamins as coenzymes "make the reactions go," they contain *no* chemical energy for biologic work.

A coenzyme requires less specificity in its action than an enzyme because the coenzyme affects a number of different reactions. It either acts as a "cobinder" or serves as a temporary carrier of intermediary products in the reaction. For example, the coenzyme **nicotinamide adenine dinucleotide (NAD^+)** forms NADH in transporting hydrogen atoms and electrons that split from food fragments during energy metabolism. The electrons then pass to other special transporter molecules in another series of chemical reactions that ultimately deliver the electrons to oxygen.

ENZYME INHIBITION. A variety of substances can inhibit enzyme activity to slow the rate of a reaction. **Competitive inhibitors** closely resemble the structure of the normal substrate for an enzyme, so they bind to the enzyme's active site but cannot be changed by the enzyme. The inhibitor repetitively occupies the active site and blunts the enzyme's ability to interact with its substrate. **Noncompetitive inhibitors** do not resemble the enzyme's substrate and do not bind to its active site. Instead, they bind to the enzyme at a site other than the active site, which causes a change in the enzyme's structure and ability to catalyze the reaction because of the presence of the bound inhibitor. Many drugs act as noncompetitive enzyme inhibitors.

HYDROLYSIS AND CONDENSATION: THE BASIS FOR DIGESTION AND SYNTHESIS

Hydrolysis Reactions

***Hydrolysis** catabolizes complex organic molecules—carbohydrates, lipids, and proteins—into simpler forms the body easily absorbs and assimilates.* This basic decomposition process splits chemical bonds by adding H^+ and OH^- (constituents of water) to the reaction byproducts. Examples of hydrolytic reactions include digestion of starches and disaccharides to monosaccharides, proteins to amino acids, and lipids to glycerol and fatty acids. Specific enzymes catalyze each step of these breakdown processes. For disaccharides, the enzymes are lactase (lactose), sucrase (sucrose), and maltase (maltose). The lipid enzymes (lipases) degrade the triglyceride molecule by adding water, which cleaves the fatty acids from their glycerol backbone. During protein digestion, protease enzymes accelerate amino acid release when the addition of water splits the peptide linkages. The following represents the general form for all hydrolysis reactions:

$$AB + HOH \longrightarrow A\text{-}H + B\text{-}OH$$

Water added to the substance AB causes the chemical bond that joins AB to decompose to produce the breakdown products A-H (H refers to a hydrogen atom from water) and

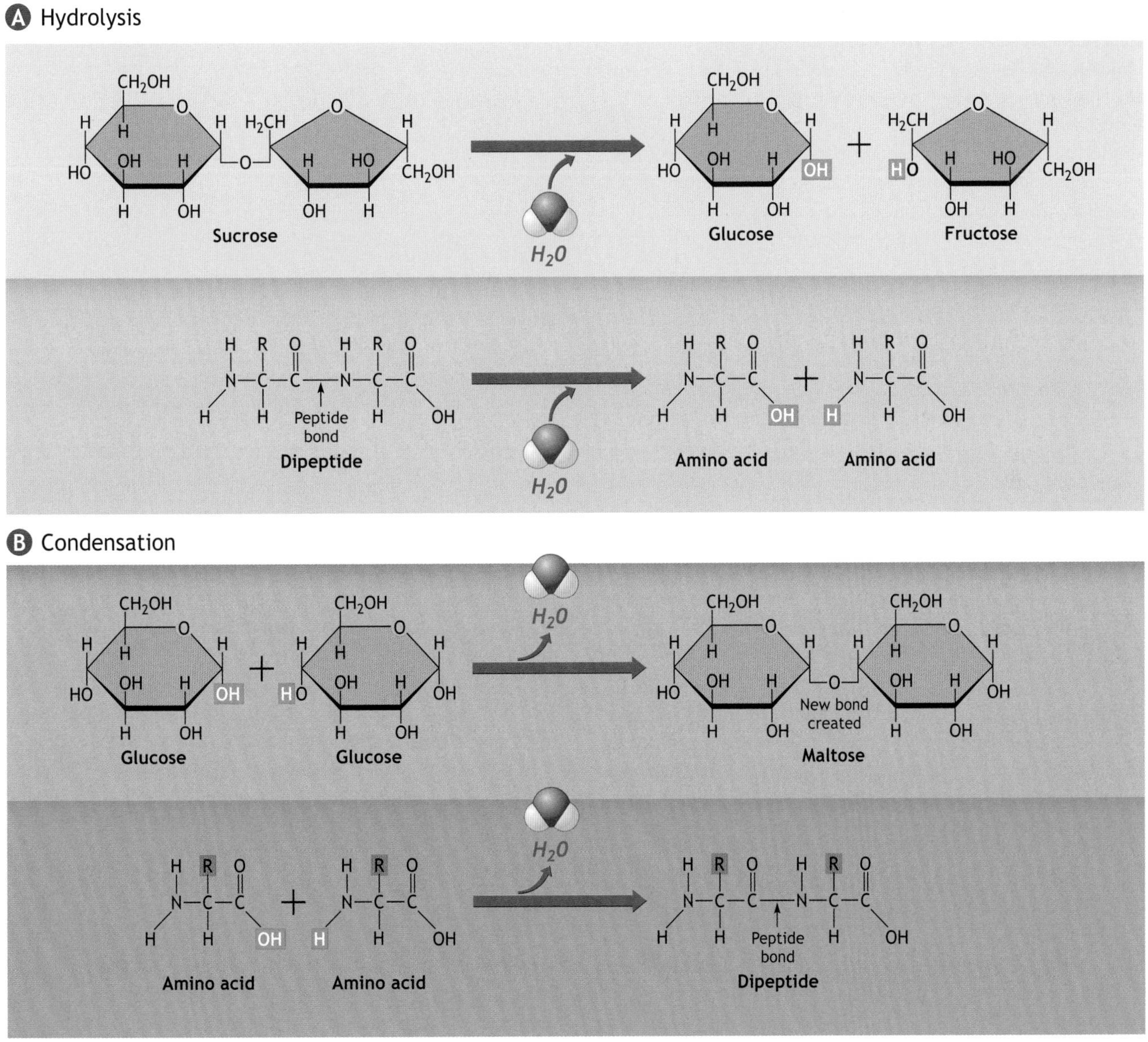

A Hydrolysis

B Condensation

Figure 5.9 • **A**. Hydrolysis of the disaccharide sucrose to the end-product molecules glucose and fructose and the hydrolysis of a dipeptide (protein) into two amino acid constituents. **B**. A condensation chemical reaction for synthesizing maltose from two glucose units and creation of a protein dipeptide from two amino acid subunits. Note that the reactions in (**B**) illustrate the reverse of the hydrolysis reaction for the dipeptide. The symbol *R* represents the remainder of the molecule.

B-OH (OH refers to the remaining hydroxyl group from water). Figure 5.9A illustrates the hydrolysis reaction for the disaccharide sucrose to its end-product molecules glucose and fructose. The figure also shows the hydrolysis of a dipeptide (protein) into its two constituent amino acid units. Intestinal absorption occurs quickly following hydrolysis of the carbohydrate, lipid, and protein macronutrients.

Condensation Reactions

The reactions illustrated for hydrolysis can occur in the opposite direction. In the reverse reaction, the compound AB is synthesized from A-H and B-OH, and a water molecule forms in the building, or anabolic, process of **condensation**. The structural components of the nutrients bind together in condensation reactions to form more-complex molecules and compounds. Figure 5.9B shows the condensation reactions for maltose synthesis from two glucose units and the synthesis of a more-complex protein from two amino acid units. During protein synthesis, a hydroxyl removed from one amino acid and a hydrogen from the other amino acid join to create a water molecule. **Peptide bond** describes the new bond that forms for the protein. Water also forms in the synthesis of more-complex carbohydrates from simple sugars; for lipids, water forms when glycerol and fatty acid components combine.

Oxidation and Reduction Reactions

Literally thousands of simultaneous chemical reactions occur in the body that involve the transfer of electrons from one substance to another. ***Oxidation** reactions transfer either oxygen atoms, hydrogen atoms, or electrons.* A loss of electrons always occurs in oxidation reactions, with a corresponding gain in valence. For example, removing hydrogen from a substance yields a net gain of valence electrons. ***Reduction** involves any process in which the atoms in an element gain electrons, with a corresponding decrease in valence.*

The term **reducing agent** describes the substance that donates or loses electrons as it oxidizes; the substance being reduced or gaining electrons is called the electron acceptor or **oxidizing agent**. Electron transfer requires both an oxidizing agent and a reducing agent. Oxidation and reduction reactions become characteristically **coupled**. Whenever oxidation occurs, the reverse reduction also takes place; when one substance loses electrons, the other substance gains them. The term **redox reaction** commonly describes an oxidation–reduction reaction.

An excellent example of an oxidation reaction involves the transfer of electrons within the mitochondria. Here, special carrier molecules transfer oxidized hydrogen atoms and their removed electrons for delivery to oxygen, which becomes reduced. The carbohydrate, fat, and protein substrates provide the body with a ready source of hydrogen. Dehydrogenase (oxidase) enzymes speed up the redox reactions. Two hydrogen-accepting dehydrogenase coenzymes are the vitamin B–containing NAD^+ and flavin adenine dinucleotide (FAD). Transferring electrons from NADH and $FADH_2$ harnesses energy in the form of ATP.

In glucose oxidation, the energy release occurs as electrons reposition (shift) as they move closer to their final destination—oxygen atoms. The close-up illustration of a mitochondrion in Figure 5.10 shows the various chemical events that take place on the outer and inner membranes and matrix. The inset table summarizes the mitochondrion's diverse molecular reactions related to its structures. Most of the energy-generating "action," including the redox reactions, takes place within the matrix. The inner membrane is rich in protein (70%) and lipid (30%), two key macromolecules whose configurations encourage transfer of substances through membranes.

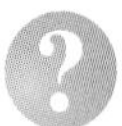

INTEGRATIVE QUESTION

From a biologic perspective, what benefit comes from the characteristic coupling of oxidation and reduction reactions?

*The transport of electrons by specific carrier molecules constitutes the **respiratory chain**.* **Electron transport** represents the final common pathway in aerobic (oxidative) metabolism. For each pair of hydrogen atoms, two electrons flow down the chain and reduce one atom of oxygen. The process ends when oxygen accepts two hydrogens and forms water. This coupled redox process constitutes hydrogen oxidation and subsequent oxygen reduction. Chemical energy trapped (conserved) in cellular oxidation–reduction reactions forms ATP, the energy-rich molecule that powers all biologic work.

Figure 5.11 illustrates a redox reaction during vigorous physical activity. As exercise intensifies, hydrogen atoms are stripped from the carbohydrate substrate faster than they are oxidized in the respiratory chain. To continue energy metabolism, a substance other than oxygen must "accept" the nonoxidized excess hydrogens. A molecule of pyruvate, an intermediate compound formed in the initial phase of carbohydrate catabolism, temporarily accepts a pair of hydrogens (electrons). A new compound, lactate (ionized form of lactic acid, as always exists in body), forms when reduced pyruvate accepts additional hydrogens. As illustrated in Figure 5.11, more-intense exercise produces a greater flow of excess hydrogens to pyruvate, and lactate concentration rises rapidly within the active muscle. During recovery, the excess hydrogens in lactate are oxidized (electrons are removed and passed to NAD^+) to re-form a pyruvate molecule. The enzyme lactate dehydrogenase (LDH) facilitates this reaction. Chapter 6 more fully discusses oxidation–reduction reactions in energy metabolism.

The Mass Action Effect

The effect of the concentration of chemicals in solution on the occurrence of a particular chemical reaction embodies the law of mass action, often referred to as the **mass action effect**. In essence, a chemical reaction progresses to the right with the addition of reactants and to the left with the addition of byproducts. In a simple chemical reaction, the formation of product increases linearly with the concentration of chemicals

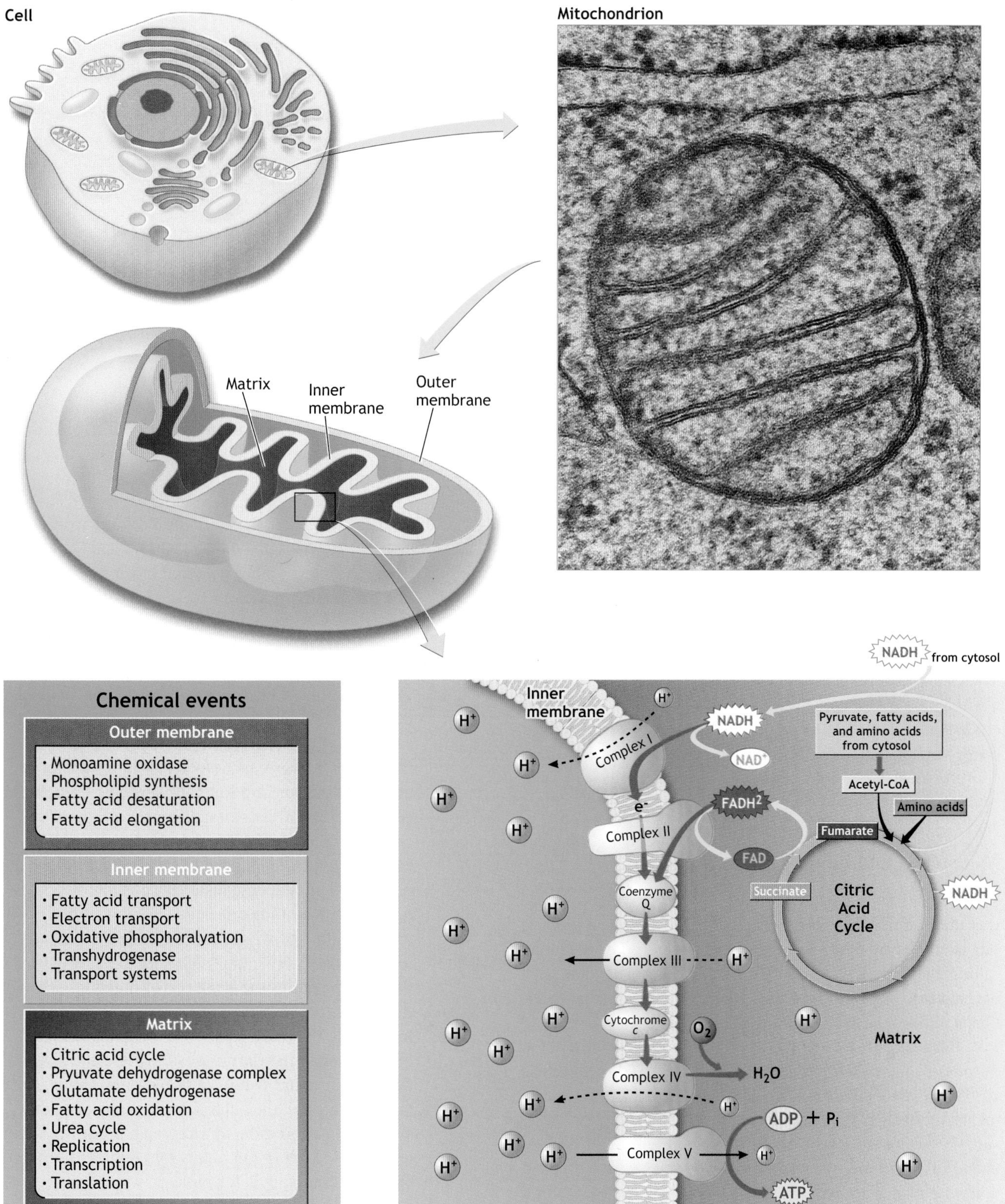

FIGURE 5.10 • The mitochondrion, its intramitochondrial structures, and primary chemical reactions. The inset table summarizes the different chemical events in relation to mitochondrial structures.

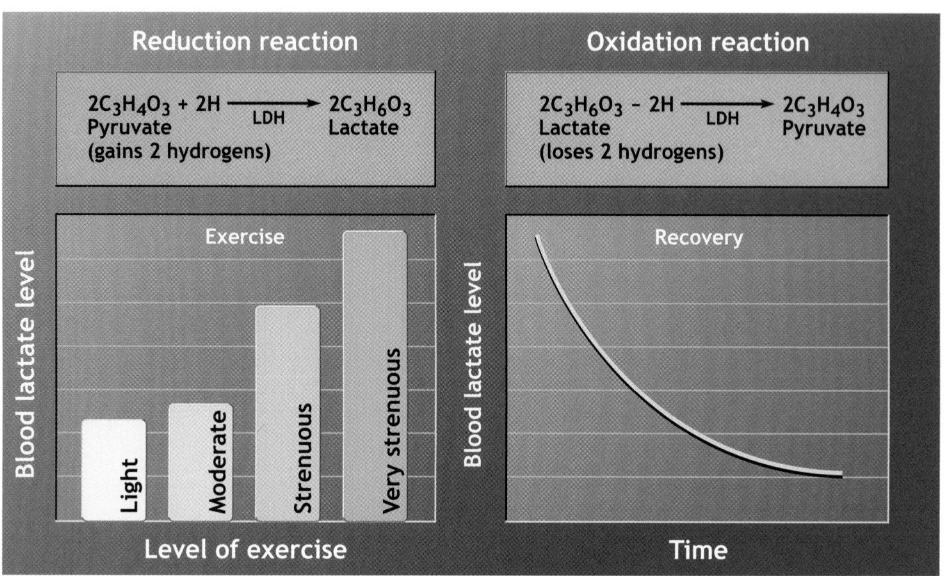

FIGURE 5.11 • Example of a redox (oxidation–reduction) reaction. During progressively more strenuous exercise when oxygen supply (or use) becomes inadequate, some pyruvate formed in energy metabolism gains two hydrogens (two electrons) and becomes *reduced* to a new compound, lactate. In recovery, when oxygen supply becomes adequate, lactate loses two hydrogens (two electrons) and *oxidizes* back to pyruvate. This example shows how a redox reaction enables the continuance of energy metabolism, despite limited oxygen availability (or use) in relation to exercise energy demands.

available to enter the reaction. In an enzyme-mediated reaction, however, the rate of product formation increases dramatically with a small change in substrate concentration, which generally produces a relatively large effect on product formation. Certain substances in the body frequently link to several reactions; thus, the products of one reaction become reactant substances for other reactions. Simply changing the concentration of one substance profoundly affects a number of different reactions. Also, some molecules play key roles in a whole chain of chemical events. Oxygen, for example, exerts a significant mass action effect on reactions required for energy transfer. If oxygen supply to tissues diminishes, several chemical processes cease, and the net energy available for biologic work decreases dramatically.

Measuring Energy Release in Humans

The gain or loss of heat in a biologic system provides a simple way to determine the energy dynamics of any chemical process. For example, in food catabolism, within the body, a human calorimeter (Fig. 8.1), similar to the bomb calorimeter described in Chapter 4, measures the energy change directly as heat (kcal) liberated from the reactions.

Because complete combustion of food takes place at the expense of molecular oxygen, the heat generated in these exergonic reactions can readily be determined from measurements of oxygen consumption. Oxygen consumption measurement forms the basis of indirect calorimetry and enables one to infer the energy metabolism of humans during rest and diverse physical activities (see Focus on Research). Chapter 8 discusses how direct and indirect calorimetry determine heat production (energy metabolism) in humans.

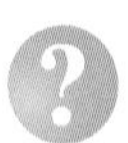

INTEGRATIVE QUESTION

Discuss the implications of the second law of thermodynamics for the measurement of energy expenditure.

Summary

1. Energy, defined as the ability to perform work, emerges only when a change takes place.
2. Energy exists in either potential or kinetic form. Potential energy refers to energy associated with a substance's structure or position; kinetic energy refers to energy of motion. Potential energy can be measured when it transforms into kinetic energy.
3. The six forms of energy are chemical, mechanical, heat, light, electric, and nuclear. Each energy form can convert or transform to another form.
4. Exergonic energy reactions result in a transfer of energy to the surroundings. Endergonic energy reactions result in the storage, conservation, or increase in free energy. All potential energy ultimately degrades into kinetic (heat) energy. Living organisms, however, conserve a portion of potential energy within the structure of new compounds, some of which contributes to power biologic work.
5. Entropy describes the tendency of potential energy to degrade to kinetic energy with a lower capacity for work.
6. Plants transfer the energy of sunlight to the potential energy bound within carbohydrates, lipids, and proteins through the endergonic process of photosynthesis. Respiration, an exergonic process, releases stored energy in plants for coupling to other chemical compounds for biologic work.
7. Energy transfer in humans supports one of three forms of biologic work: chemical (biosynthesis of cellular molecules), mechanical (muscle contraction), or transport (transfer of substances among cells).
8. Enzymes represent highly specific protein catalysts that greatly accelerate chemical reaction rates without being consumed or changed in the reaction.

Focus on Research

Valid Determination of Oxygen Consumption

Wilmore JH., Costill DL. Adequacy of the Haldane transformation in the computation of exercise VO_2 in man. J Appl Physiol 1973;35:85.

➤ Oxygen consumption using open-circuit spirometry represents a fundamental measurement in exercise physiology. This methodology assumes no nitrogen production or retention by the body, so the nitrogen volume remains equal in the inspired and expired air. Because of this intrinsic relationship, no need exists to collect and analyze both inspired and expired air volumes during measurement of oxygen consumption and carbon dioxide production. The following mathematical relationship, known as the Haldane transformation, exists between inspired and expired air volumes:

$$V_I = V_E \times F_{EN_2} \div F_{IN_2}$$

where V_I equals air volume inspired, V_E equals air volume expired, and F_{EN_2} and F_{IN_2} equal the fractional concentrations of nitrogen in the expired and inspired air. Because the fractional concentrations for inspired oxygen, carbon dioxide, and nitrogen are known, only V_E (or V_I) and the concentrations in expired air of CO_2 (F_{ECO_2}) and O_2 (F_{EO_2}) are required to calculate the oxygen consumed each minute ($\dot{V}O_2$):

$$\dot{V}O_2 = \dot{V}_E \times F_{EN_2} / F_{IN_2} \times F_{IO_2} - \dot{V}_E \times F_{EO_2}$$

In this formula, F_{EN_2} usually equals 1.00 − (F_{EO_2} + F_{ECO_2}).

The study by Wilmore and Costill determined any nitrogen retention or production and how it influenced the accuracy of oxygen consumption computations using the traditional Haldane transformation during light-to-heavy exercise. Six subjects completed treadmill exercise by walking on the level at 4 mph; a 5-minute jog followed at 6.0 mph, followed again by a 5-minute run at 7.5 mph. Oxygen consumption, continuously monitored using open-circuit spirometry, included measurement of inspired and expired ventilation volumes. Measurements also included barometric pressure, inspired and expired gas temperatures, relative humidity, and F_{EO_2}, F_{ECO_2}, F_{IO_2}, and F_{ICO_2}.

The figure shows $\dot{V}O_2$ calculated from the inspired and expired air volumes (actual) for all subjects compared with the values estimated from the Haldane transformation. The slope of the regression line deviates only 0.003 units from unity (the intercept equals nearly zero), demonstrating the closeness between the actual oxygen consumption and that predicted by use of the Haldane transformation. The largest difference between the 68 actual and estimated $\dot{V}O_2$ values was 230 mL, an error of 7.3%. The average difference of 0.8% for all subjects fell within the measurement error of the instruments. For the nitrogen data, a difference of 1.6% occurred between the minute volume of nitrogen inspired and expired for any subject at any exercise intensity; 11 of 17 subjects' work rates exhibited less than 1% difference. The largest difference, 1099 mL of $N_2 \cdot min^{-1}$, occurred during heavy exercise (2.1% difference).

The researchers noted that the major sources of variation in assessing $\dot{V}O_2$ included the measurement of ventilation volume, gas meter calibration, and determination of the inspired air's water vapor pressure (P_{H_2O}). Ventilation volume posed a problem because accuracy depended on the subject being "switched in" and "switched out" at the same phase of the tidal volume at the beginning and end of the collection period. Because this remains difficult (if not impossible) to achieve, an inspired-to-expired volume differential nearly always occurs. Also, a 10 percentage point difference in inspired P_{H_2O} (e.g., from 50 to 60% relative humidity) produces more than a 100-mL difference between the inspired and expired N_2 volumes.

This study supported the continued use of the Haldane transformation to calculate exercise $\dot{V}O_2$. While production and/or retention of N_2 can occur during exercise, it exerts little or no effect on the $\dot{V}O_2$ computation.

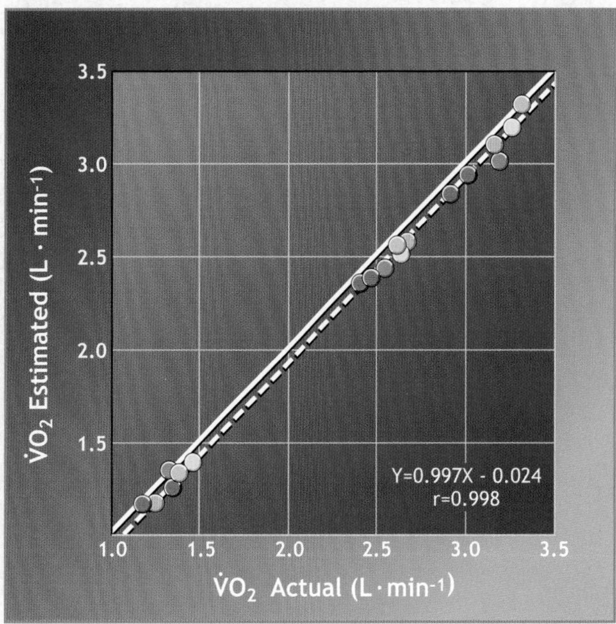

Actual versus estimated exercise oxygen consumption for six subjects. The *solid line* represents the line of identity, and the *dashed line* represents the regression line that predicts oxygen consumption estimated from the Haldane transformation (*y* axis) from the actual oxygen consumption (*x* axis). Note the slope of nearly 1.00 and intercept of 0. Colored data points indicate same subjects measured under each condition.

9. Coenzymes consist of nonprotein organic substances that facilitate enzyme action by binding a substrate to its specific enzyme.
10. Hydrolysis (catabolism) of complex organic molecules performs critical functions in digestion and energy metabolism. Condensation (anabolism) reactions synthesize complex biomolecules for the body's maintenance and growth.
11. The linking (coupling) of oxidation–reduction (redox) reactions enables oxidation (in which a substance loses electrons) to coincide with the reverse reaction of reduction (in which a substance gains electrons). Redox reactions represent the basis for the body's energy-transfer processes.
12. The transport of electrons by specific carrier molecules constitutes the respiratory chain. Electron transport represents the final common pathway in aerobic metabolism.

Suggested Readings

Åstrand PO, Rodahl K. Textbook of work physiology. 3rd ed. New York: McGraw-Hill, 1986.

Atkins PW. The second law. San Francisco: WH Freeman, 1984.

Brooks GA, et al. Exercise physiology: human bioenergetics and its applications. 2nd ed. Mountain View, CA: Mayfield, 2000.

Campbell MK. Biochemistry. New York: WB Saunders, 1991.

Doolittle RF. Proteins. Sci Am 1985;253(4):88.

Kraut J. How do enzymes work? Science 1988;242:533.

Lehninger AL. Bioenergetics: the molecular bases of biological energy transformations. Menlo Park, CA: WA Benjamin, 1971.

Lehninger AL, et al. Principles of biochemistry. 2nd ed. New York: Worth, 1993.

Mathews CK, Van Holde KE. Biochemistry. Menlo Park, NJ: Benjamin/Cummings, 1996.

Raven PH, Hohnson GB. Biology. 4th ed. Dubuque, IA: CW Brown, 1996.

Stryker L. Biochemistry. 4th ed. New York: WH Freeman, 1995.

Szent-Györgyi A. Chemistry of muscular contraction. New York: Academic Press, 1951.

Vander JA, et al. Human physiology: the mechanisms of body function. 6th ed. New York: McGraw-Hill, 1993.

Watson JD, et al. Molecular biology of the cell. 4th ed. Menlo Park, NJ: Benjamin/Cummings, 1995.

CHAPTER 6

Energy Transfer in the Body

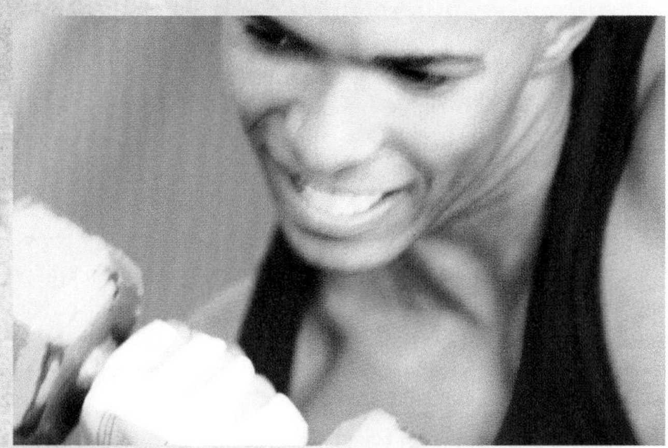

Chapter Objectives

- Identify the high-energy phosphates and discuss their contributions to powering biologic work
- Quantify the body's reserves of adenosine triphosphate (ATP) and phosphocreatine (PCr) and give examples of physical activities in which each of these energy sources predominates
- Outline electron transport–oxidative phosphorylation
- Discuss the role of oxygen in energy metabolism
- List important functions of carbohydrate in energy metabolism
- Describe cellular energy release during anaerobic metabolism
- Contrast the energy-conserving efficiencies of aerobic and anaerobic metabolism
- Discuss the dynamics of lactate formation and its accumulation in blood during increasing exercise intensity
- Indicate the role of the citric acid cycle in energy metabolism
- Outline the general pathways for energy release during macronutrient catabolism
- Contrast ATP yield from carbohydrate, fat, and protein catabolism
- Indicate the role of the Cori cycle in exercise energy metabolism
- Outline diverse interconversions among carbohydrate, fat, and protein
- Discuss the statement: "Fats burn in a carbohydrate flame"

The human body demands a continual supply of chemical energy to perform its many complex functions. Energy derived from the oxidation of food does not release suddenly at some kindling temperature (Fig. 6.1A), because the body, unlike a mechanical engine, cannot use heat energy. If this did happen, the body fluids would actually boil, and tissues would burst into flames. *Instead, human energy dynamics involve transferring energy by chemical bonds.* Potential energy within carbohydrate, fat, and protein bonds releases stepwise in small quantities when bonds split, with energy conserved when new bonds form during enzymatically controlled reactions in the relatively cool, watery medium of the cell (Fig. 6.1B). Some energy lost by one molecule transfers to the chemical structure of other molecules without appearing as heat. This provides greater efficiency in energy transformations. Biologic work occurs when compounds relatively low in potential energy become "juiced up" from energy transfer via high-energy phosphate bonds. In essence, the cells receive energy as needed.

The story of how the body maintains its continuous energy supply begins with ATP, the body's special carrier of free energy.

➤ Part 1 • Phosphate Bond Energy

ADENOSINE TRIPHOSPHATE: THE ENERGY CURRENCY

The energy in food does not transfer directly to the cells for biologic work. Rather, energy from macronutrient oxidation becomes harvested and funneled through the energy-rich nucleotide compound **adenosine triphosphate (ATP)**. The potential energy within the ATP molecule powers *all* of the cell's energy-requiring processes. In essence, this energy donor–energy receiver cycle represents the cells' two major energy-transforming activities:

- Extract potential energy from food and conserve it within the bonds of ATP
- Extract and transfer the chemical energy in ATP to power biologic work

ATP serves as the ideal energy-transfer agent. In one respect, ATP's phosphate bonds "trap" a large portion of the original food molecule's potential energy. ATP also readily transfers this energy to other compounds to raise them to a higher activation level. The cell contains other high-energy compounds, but ATP is by far the most important. Figure 6.2 shows how ATP forms from a molecule of adenine and ribose (called adenosine) linked to three phosphates, each consisting of phosphorus and oxygen atoms. The bonds that link the two outermost phosphates (symbolized ~) represent high-energy bonds because they release considerable useful energy during hydrolysis. A new compound, **adenosine diphosphate (ADP)** forms when ATP joins with water, catalyzed by the enzyme **adenosine triphosphatase (ATPase)**. The reaction cleaves ATP's outermost phosphate bond to release a phosphate ion (inorganic phosphate) and liberates approximately 7.3 kcal of free energy (i.e., energy available for work) per mole of ATP hydrolyzed to ADP. The value 7.3 kcal $\cdot$ mol^{-1} represents the standard free energy change under standard conditions. In the intracellular environment, the value may actually approach 10 kcal $\cdot$ mol^{-1}.

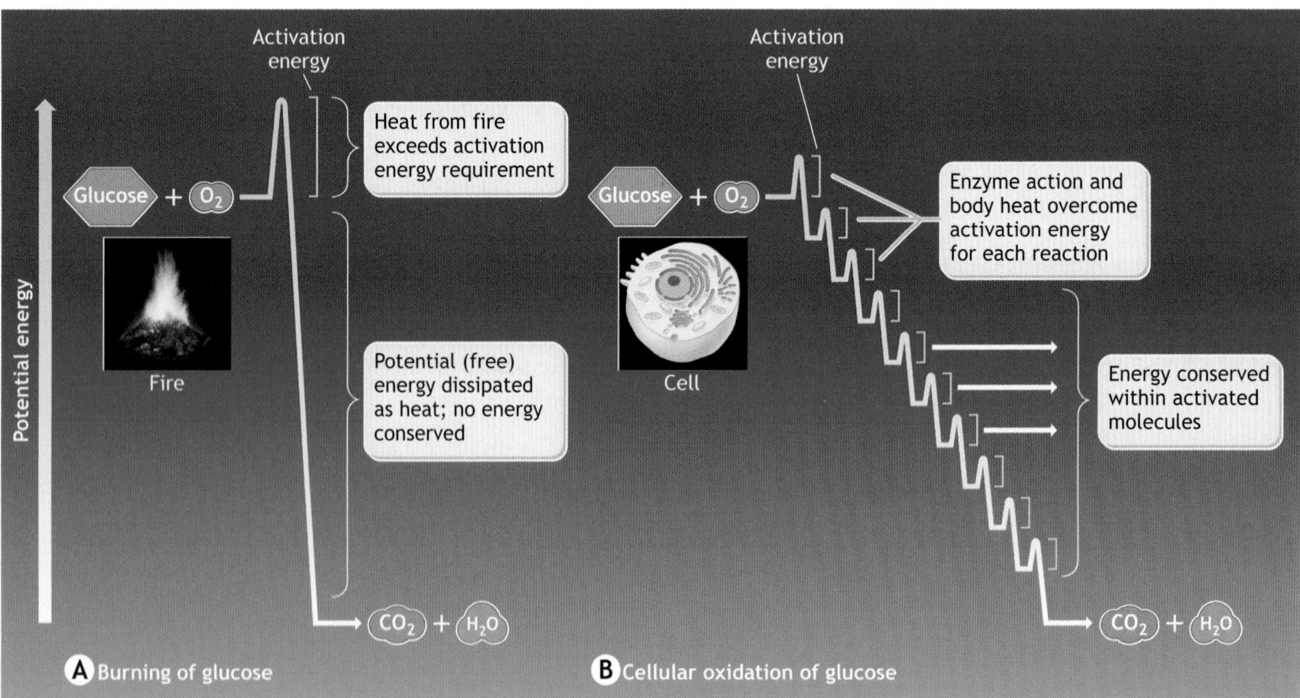

Figure 6.1 • **A**. The heat generated by fire exceeds the activation energy requirement of a macronutrient (e.g., glucose), causing all of the molecule's potential energy to release suddenly at kindling temperature and dissipate as heat. **B**. Human energy dynamics involve release of potential energy from carbohydrate, fat, and protein in small quantities when bonds split during enzymatically controlled reactions. Energy conservation occurs with the formation of new molecules.

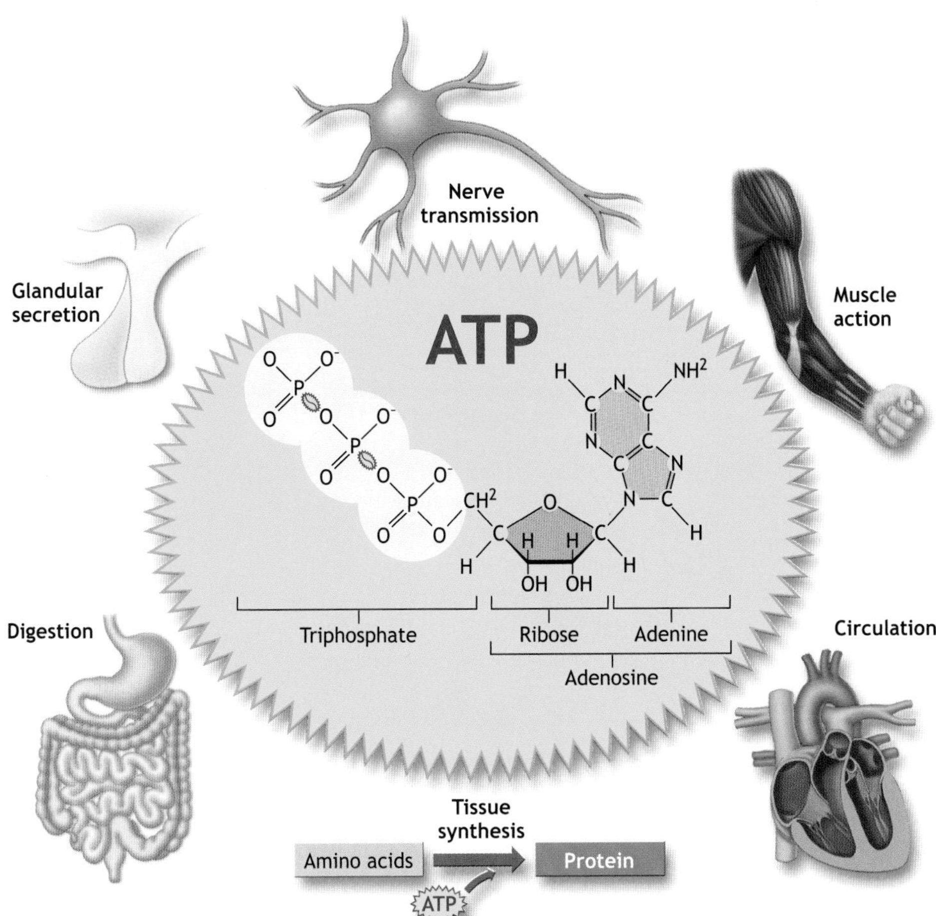

FIGURE 6.2 • Structure of ATP, the energy currency that powers all forms of biologic work. The symbol ~ represents high-energy bonds.

$$ATP + H_2O \xrightarrow{ATPase} ADP + P_i \; -\Delta G \; 7.3 \text{ kcal} \cdot \text{mol}^{-1}$$

The free energy liberated in ATP hydrolysis reflects the energy difference between the reactant and end products. Because this reaction generates considerable free energy, we refer to ATP as a **high-energy phosphate** compound. Infrequently, additional energy releases when another phosphate splits from ADP. In some reactions of biosynthesis, ATP donates its two terminal phosphates simultaneously to construct new cellular material. Adenosine monophosphate (AMP) is the new molecule, with a single phosphate group.

The energy liberated during ATP breakdown directly transfers to other energy-requiring molecules. In muscle, for example, the energy stimulates specific sites on the contractile elements to activate the molecular motors that power the shortening of muscle fibers. *Because energy from ATP hydrolysis powers all forms of biologic work, ATP constitutes the cell's "energy currency."* Figure 6.3 illustrates the role of ATP as energy currency for biologic work and its subsequent recycling from ADP and a phosphate ion (P_i) via the oxidation of stored macronutrients.

An ATP molecule splits almost instantaneously, without the need for oxygen. The cell's capability to hydrolyze ATP

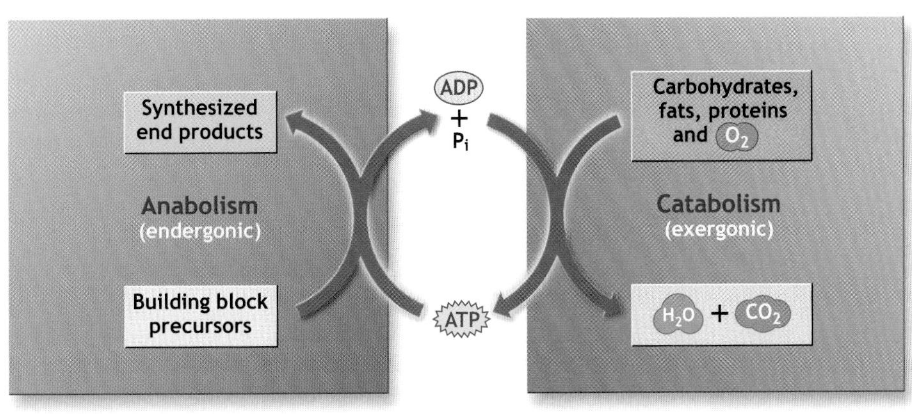

FIGURE 6.3 • Catabolism–anabolism interactions. Continual recycling of ATP for biologic work from intracellular ADP, P_i, and energy released from stored macronutrients.

anaerobically generates energy for rapid use; this would not occur if energy metabolism required oxygen at all times. For this reason, any body movement can happen immediately without consuming oxygen; examples include sprinting for a bus, lifting an object, swinging a golf club, spiking a volleyball, or doing a push-up. The well-known practice of holding one's breath during a sprint swim provides a clear example of ATP splitting (and subsequent resynthesis) without consuming atmospheric oxygen. Withholding air (oxygen) would not preclude a 50-yard sprint on the track, lifting a barbell, or a dash up several flights of stairs. In each case, energy metabolism proceeds uninterrupted because the energy required to perform the activity derives almost exclusively from intramuscular anaerobic sources.

The body maintains a continuous ATP supply through different metabolic pathways; some are located in the cell's cytosol while others operate within the mitochondria (Fig. 6.4). For example, the cytosol contains the pathways for ATP production from the anaerobic breakdown of PCr, glucose, glycerol, and the carbon skeletons of some deaminated amino acids, whereas reactions that harness cellular energy to generate ATP aerobically—the citric acid cycle, β-oxidation, and the respiratory chain—reside within the mitochondria.

A Limited Currency

Cells store a small quantity of ATP and must therefore continually resynthesize it at its rate of use. Only under extreme exercise conditions do skeletal muscle ATP levels decrease. A limited ATP supply provides a biologically useful mechanism for regulating energy metabolism. By maintaining only a small amount of ATP, its relative concentration (and the corresponding concentration of ADP) changes rapidly in response to only a small increase in a cell's energy use. Any increase in energy requirement immediately disrupts the balance between ATP and ADP. This imbalance stimulates the breakdown of other stored energy-containing compounds to resynthesize ATP. In this way, diverse systems for energy transfer increase rapidly when movement begins. As one might expect, increases in energy transfer depend on exercise intensity. Energy transfer increases about fourfold in the transition from sitting in a chair to slow walking. Changing from a walk to an all-out sprint almost immediately accelerates the rate of energy transfer within active muscles about 120 times.

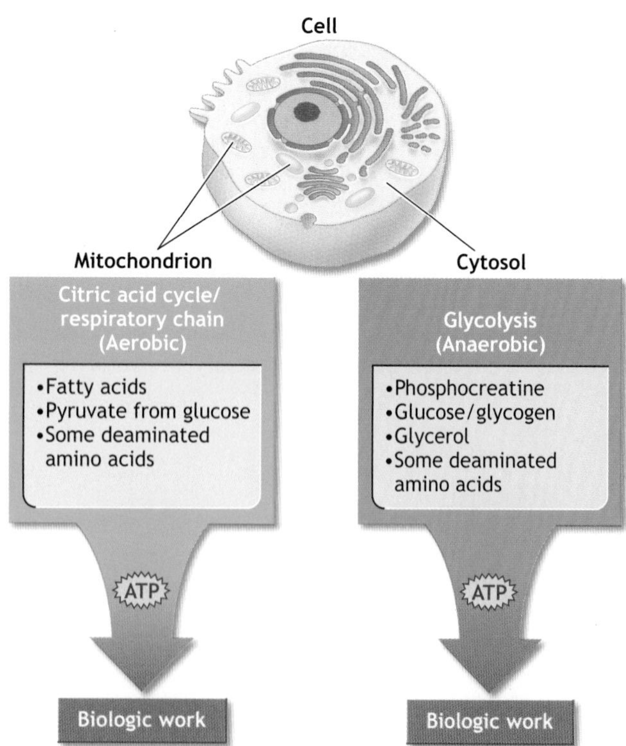

FIGURE 6.4 • Contributors to the anaerobic and aerobic resynthesis of ATP.

The body stores only 80 to 100 g (about 3.0 oz) of ATP at any time. This quantity makes available each second approximately 2.4 mmol of ATP per kg wet muscle weight, or about 1.44×10^{10} molecules of ATP—enough intramuscular stored energy to power several seconds of explosive, all-out exercise. Thus, ATP alone does not represent a significant energy reserve. However, maintaining a limited quantity of ATP fuel provides additional advantages because of the relatively heavy weight of the ATP molecule. Biochemists estimate that a sedentary person resynthesizes an amount of ATP each day equal to about 75% of body mass. For an endurance athlete who generates 20 times the resting energy expenditure throughout a 2.5-hour marathon race, this could amount to 80 kg of ATP resynthesis during the run!

PHOSPHOCREATINE: THE ENERGY RESERVOIR

To overcome its storage limitation, ATP resynthesis proceeds uninterrupted to supply energy for biologic work. Fat and glycogen represent the major energy sources for maintaining continual ATP resynthesis. Some energy for ATP resynthesis also comes directly from the anaerobic splitting of a phosphate from **phosphocreatine (PCr)**, another intracellular high-energy phosphate compound. Figure 6.5 schematically illustrates the release and use of phosphate-bond energy in ATP and PCr. The term **high-energy phosphate** describes these compounds.

The PCr and ATP molecules have a similar characteristic; a large amount of free energy releases when the bond cleaves between the creatine and phosphate molecules in PCr. The arrow in the reaction points in both directions, indicating a reversible reaction. In other words, phosphate (P) and creatine (Cr) can rejoin to form PCr. This also applies to ATP;ADP plus P re-forms ATP. Because PCr has a larger free energy of hydrolysis than ATP, its hydrolysis (catalyzed by the enzyme **creatine kinase**—4 to 6% on the outer mitochondrial membrane, 3 to 5% in the sarcomere, and 90% in the cytosol) drives the phosphorylation of ADP to ATP. Cells store approximately four to six times more PCr than ATP.

Transient increases in ADP within the muscle's contractile unit during muscle action shift the creatine kinase reaction toward PCr hydrolysis and ATP production; the reaction does not require oxygen and reaches a maximum energy yield in about 10 seconds.[35] Thus, PCr serves as a

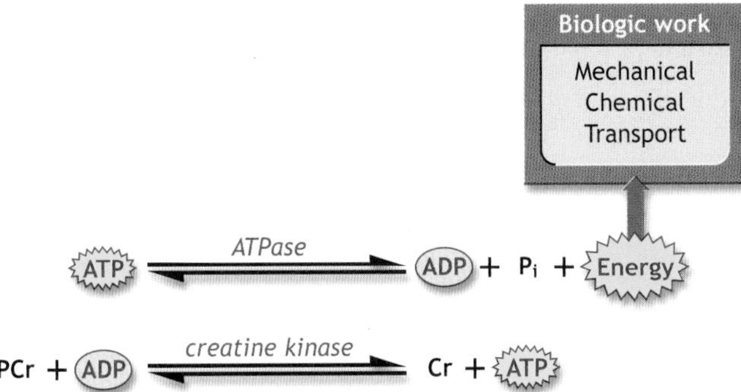

FIGURE 6.5 • ATP and PCr provide anaerobic sources of phosphate-bond energy. The energy liberated from hydrolysis (splitting) of PCr rebonds ADP and P_i to form ATP.

"reservoir" of high-energy phosphate bonds. Its rapidity for ADP phosphorylation considerably exceeds anaerobic energy transfer from stored muscle glycogen because of the high activity rate of creatine kinase.[18] If maximal effort continues beyond 10 seconds, energy for continual ATP resynthesis must originate from less-rapid catabolism of the stored macronutrients.[16] Chapter 23 discusses the potential for exogenous creatine supplementation to enhance short-term, all-out exercise performance.

The **adenylate kinase reaction** represents another single-enzyme–mediated reaction for ATP regeneration. The reaction uses two ADP molecules to produce one molecule of ATP and AMP as follows:

$$2\ ADP \xrightleftharpoons{\text{adenylate kinase}} ATP + AMP$$

The creatine kinase and adenylate kinase reactions not only augment the muscle's ability to rapidly increase energy output (ATP availability), they also produce molecular byproducts (AMP, P_i, ADP) that activate the initial stages of glycogen and glucose catabolism and the respiration pathways of the mitochondrion.

CELLULAR OXIDATION

Most energy for phosphorylation derives from the oxidation ("biologic burning") of dietary carbohydrate, lipid, and protein macronutrients. Recall from Chapter 5 that a molecule becomes reduced when it accepts electrons from an electron donor. In turn, the molecule that gives up the electron becomes oxidized. Oxidation reactions (those that donate electrons) and reduction reactions (those that accept electrons) remain coupled, because every oxidation coincides with a reduction. *In essence, cellular oxidation–reduction constitutes the biochemical mechanism that underlies energy metabolism.* This process continually provides hydrogen atoms from the catabolism of stored carbohydrate, fat, and protein molecules. The mitochondria, the cell's "energy factories," contain carrier molecules that remove electrons from hydrogen (oxidation) and eventually pass them to oxygen (reduction). ATP synthesis occurs during oxidation–reduction reactions.

Electron Transport

Figure 6.6 illustrates the general scheme for hydrogen oxidation and accompanying electron transport to oxygen. During cellular oxidation, hydrogen atoms are not merely turned loose in intracellular fluids. Rather, substrate-specific **dehydrogenase enzymes** catalyze hydrogen's release from the nutrient substrate. The coenzyme component of the dehydrogenase (usually the niacin-containing coenzyme **nicotinamide adenine dinucleotide** [**NAD^+**]) accepts pairs of electrons (energy) from hydrogen. While the substrate oxidizes and gives up hydrogens (electrons), NAD^+ gains hydrogen and two electrons and reduces to NADH; the other hydrogen appears as H^+ in the cell fluid. The riboflavin-containing coenzyme, **flavin adenine dinucleotide** (**FAD**) serves as the other important electron acceptor in oxidizing food fragments. Like NAD^+, FAD catalyzes dehydrogenation and accepts electron pairs. Unlike NAD^+, however, FAD becomes $FADH_2$ by accepting both hydrogens. *The NADH and $FADH_2$ formed in the breakdown of food provide energy-rich molecules because they carry electrons with a high energy-transfer potential.*

The **cytochromes**, a series of iron-protein electron carriers on the inner membranes of the mitochondrion, then pass (in "bucket brigade" fashion) pairs of electrons carried by NADH and $FADH_2$. The iron portion of each cytochrome exists in either its oxidized (ferric, or Fe^{3+}) or reduced (ferrous, or Fe^{2+}) ionic state. By accepting an electron, the ferric portion of a specific cytochrome reduces to its ferrous form. In turn, ferrous iron donates its electron to the next cytochrome, and so on down the line. By shuttling between these two iron forms,

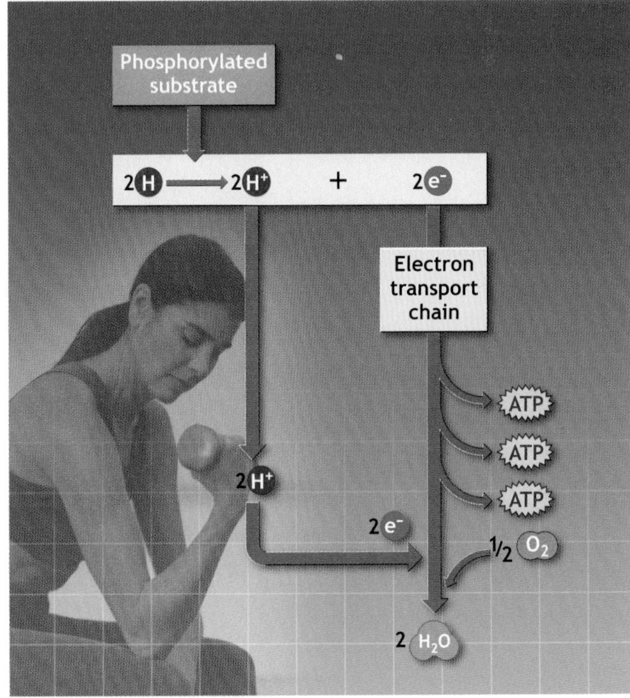

FIGURE 6.6 • A general scheme for oxidizing (removing electrons) hydrogen and the accompanying electron transport. In this process, oxygen is reduced (gain of electrons) and water forms. Energy liberated powers the synthesis of ATP from ADP.

the cytochromes transfer electrons to their ultimate destination, where they reduce oxygen to form water. NAD^+ and FAD then recycle for subsequent use in energy metabolism.

Electron transport by specific carrier molecules constitutes the ***respiratory chain****, the final common pathway where electrons extracted from hydrogen pass to oxygen.* For each pair of hydrogen atoms, two electrons flow down the chain and reduce one atom of oxygen to form one water molecule. Of the five specific cytochromes, only the last, cytochrome oxidase (cytochrome aa_3, with strong affinity for oxygen), discharges its electron directly to oxygen. Figure 6.7A shows the route for hydrogen oxidation, electron transport, and energy transfer in the respiratory chain. The respiratory chain releases free energy in relatively small amounts. In several of the electron transfers, the formation of high-energy phosphate bonds conserves energy. Each electron acceptor in the respiratory chain has a progressively greater affinity for electrons. In biochemical terms, this affinity represents a substance's **re-**

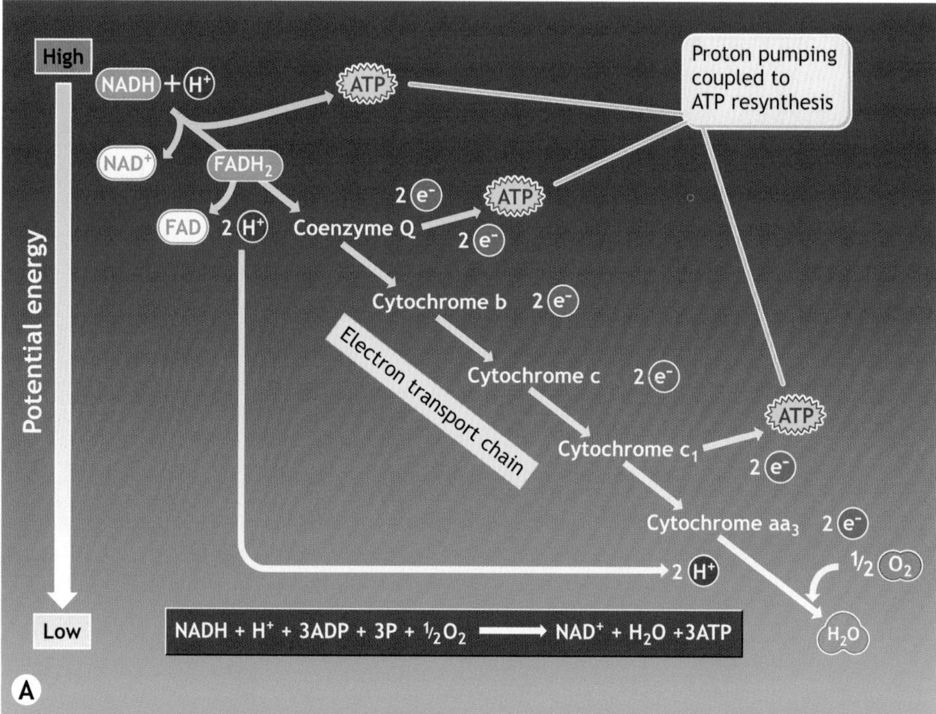

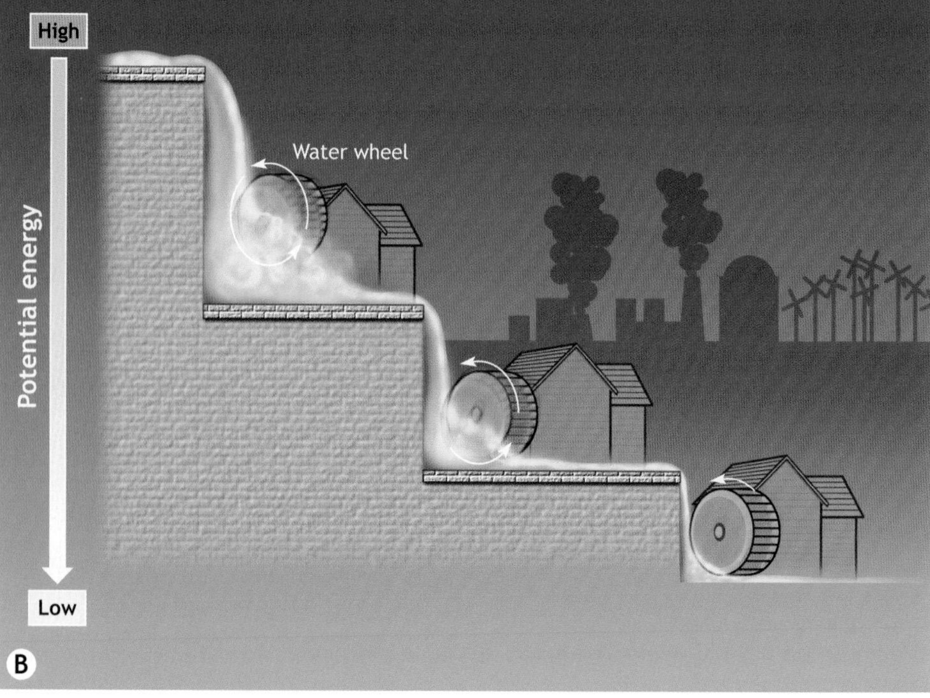

Figure 6.7 • Examples of harnessing potential energy. **A**. *In the body,* the electron transport chain removes electrons from hydrogens for ultimate delivery to oxygen. In oxidation–reduction, much of the chemical energy stored within the hydrogen atom does not dissipate to kinetic energy, but instead becomes conserved within ATP. **B**. *In industry,* energy from falling water becomes harnessed to turn the waterwheel, which in turn performs mechanical work.

duction potential. Oxygen, the last electron receiver in the transport chain, possesses the largest reduction potential. Thus, mitochondrial oxygen ultimately drives the respiratory chain as well as other catabolic reactions that depend on continual availability of NAD^+ and FAD.

Oxidative Phosphorylation

Oxidative phosphorylation synthesizes ATP by transferring electrons from NADH and $FADH_2$ to oxygen. Figure 6.8 shows that the energy generated in the reactions of electron transport pumps protons across the inner mitochondrial membrane into the intermembrane space. The electrochemical gradient generated by this reverse flow of protons represents stored potential energy. It provides the coupling mechanism that binds ADP and a phosphate ion to synthesize ATP. (Because the mitochondrion's inner membrane remains impermeable to ATP, the protein complex ATP/ADP translocase exports the newly synthesized ATP molecule. In turn, ADP and P_i move into the mitochondrion for subsequent synthesis to ATP.) Biochemists refer to this union as **chemiosmotic coupling**, the cell's primary endergonic means of extracting and trapping chemical energy in the high-energy phosphates. *More than 90% of ATP synthesis takes place in the respiratory chain by oxidative reactions coupled with phosphorylation.*

In a way, oxidative phosphorylation can be likened to a waterfall divided into several separate cascades by the intervention of waterwheels at different heights. Figure 6.7B depicts the waterwheels harnessing the energy of the falling water; similarly, electrochemical energy generated in the electron transport chain becomes harnessed and transferred (coupled) to ADP. Energy transfer from NADH to ADP to re-form ATP (Fig. 6.7A) happens at three distinct coupling sites during electron transport. Oxidation of hydrogen and subsequent phosphorylation occurs as follows:

$$NADH + H^+ + 3ADP + 3P_i + 1/2\,O_2 \rightarrow NAD^+ + H_2O + 3ATP$$

The ratio of phosphate bonds formed to oxygen atoms consumed (**P/O ratio**) reflects quantitatively the coupling of ATP production to electron transport. Note in the above reaction that the P/O ratio equals 3 for each NADH plus H^+ oxidized. However, if $FADH_2$ originally donates hydrogen,

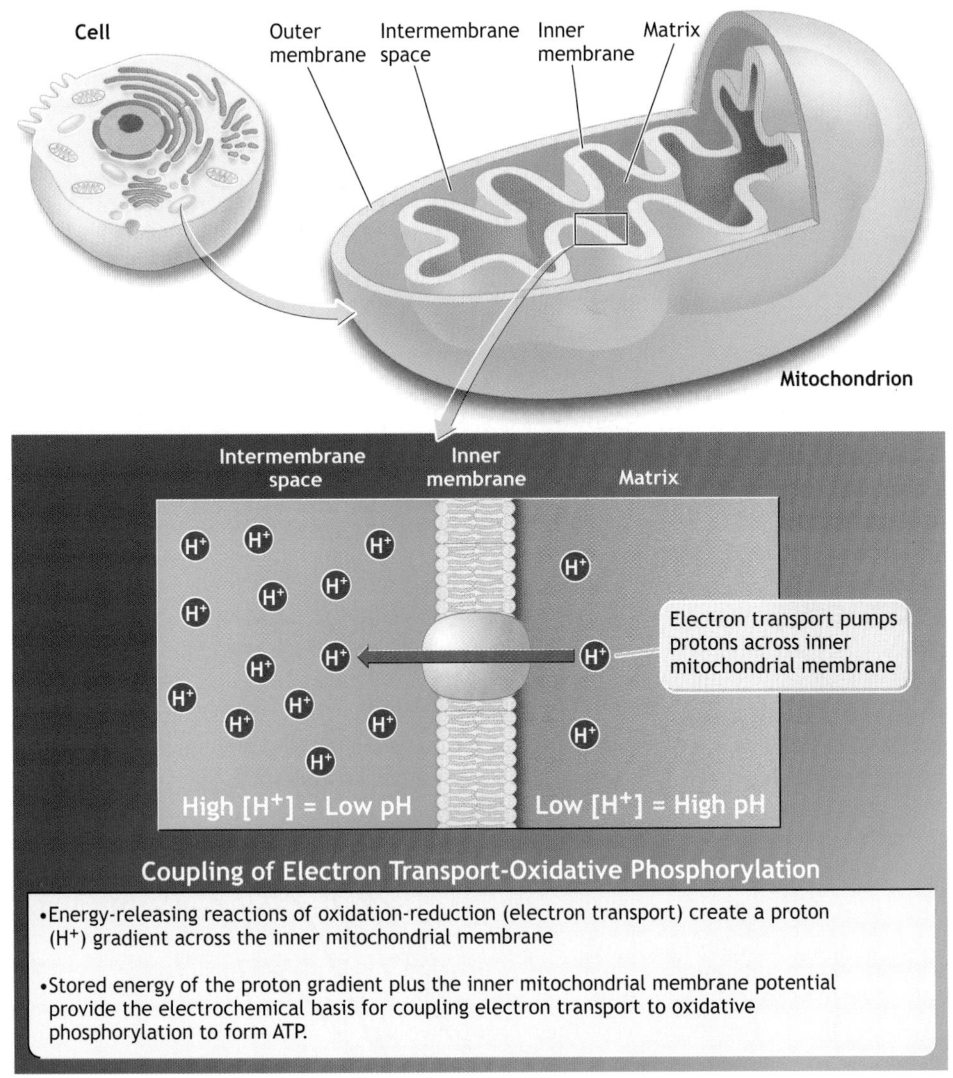

FIGURE 6.8 • The mitochondrion: the site for aerobic energy metabolism. Electron transport creates a proton (H^+) gradient across the inner mitochondrial membrane. This leads to a net flow of protons to provide the coupling mechanism to drive ATP resynthesis.

only two molecules of ATP form (P/O ratio = 2) for each hydrogen pair oxidized. This occurs because $FADH_2$ enters the respiratory chain at a lower energy level at a point beyond the site of the first ATP synthesis.

Efficiency of Electron Transport–Oxidative Phosphorylation

Each mole of ATP formed from ADP conserves approximately 7 kcal of energy. Because 3 moles of ATP regenerate from the total of 52 kcal of energy released to oxidize 1 mole of NADH, about 21 kcal (7 kcal per mol × 3) is conserved as chemical energy. This represents a relative efficiency of 40% for harnessing chemical energy via electron transport–oxidative phosphorylation (21 kcal ÷ 52 kcal × 100). The remaining 60% of the energy dissipates as heat. If the intracellular energy change for ATP hydrolysis (or synthesis) approaches 10 $kcal \cdot mol^{-1}$, then efficiency of energy conservation approximates 60%. Because the number of ATPs synthesized per NADH oxidized is not necessarily an integral number (probably closer to 2.5), some biochemists estimate energy transfer efficiency at nearly 50%. Considering that a steam engine transforms its fuel into useful energy at only about 30% efficiency, the value of 40% or larger for the human body represents a remarkably high efficiency rate.

OXYGEN'S ROLE IN ENERGY METABOLISM

Three prerequisites exist for the continual resynthesis of ATP during coupled oxidative phosphorylation. Satisfying these three conditions causes hydrogen and electrons to shuttle uninterrupted down the respiratory chain to oxygen during energy metabolism.

1. Availability of the reducing agent NADH (or $FADH_2$) in the tissues
2. Presence of the oxidizing agent oxygen in the tissues
3. Sufficient concentration of enzymes and mitochondria to ensure that energy transfer reactions proceed at their appropriate rate

In strenuous exercise, inadequacy in oxygen delivery (condition 2) or its rate of use (condition 3) creates a relative imbalance between hydrogen release and its final acceptance by oxygen. If either of these deficiencies exists, electron flow down the respiratory chain "backs up," and hydrogens accumulate bound to NAD^+ and FAD. On page 143, we describe how the compound pyruvate, a product of carbohydrate breakdown, temporarily binds excess hydrogens (electrons) to form lactate. Lactate formation allows electron transport–oxidative phosphorylation to continue.

Aerobic metabolism *refers to energy-generating catabolic reactions in which oxygen serves as the final electron acceptor in the respiratory chain and combines with hydrogen to form water.* In one sense, the term aerobic seems misleading because oxygen does not participate directly in ATP synthesis. On the other hand, oxygen's presence at the "end of the line" largely determines the capacity for ATP production. This, in turn, largely determines the ability to sustain high-intensity, endurance exercise.

Summary

1. Energy within the chemical structure of carbohydrate, fat, and protein molecules does not suddenly release in the body at some kindling temperature. Rather, it releases slowly in small amounts during complex, enzymatically controlled reactions. This enables more efficient energy transfer and conservation.
2. About 40% of the potential energy in food nutrients transfers to the high-energy compound ATP.
3. Splitting the terminal phosphate bond of ATP liberates free energy to power all forms of biologic work. This makes ATP the body's energy currency, despite its limited quantity of only about 3.0 oz.
4. PCr interacts with ADP to form ATP; this nonaerobic, high-energy reservoir replenishes ATP almost instantaneously.
5. Phosphorylation refers to energy transfer via phosphate bonds as ADP and creatine continually recycle into ATP and PCr.
6. Cellular oxidation occurs on the inner lining of the mitochondrial membranes; it involves transferring electrons from NADH and $FADH_2$ to oxygen. Electron transport–oxidative phosphorylation produces coupled transfer of chemical energy to form ATP from ADP plus phosphate ion.
7. During aerobic ATP resynthesis, oxygen serves as the final electron acceptor in the respiratory chain and combines with hydrogen to form water.

➤ PART 2 • Energy Release From Food

Energy release in macronutrient catabolism serves one crucial purpose—to phosphorylate ADP to re-form the energy-rich compound ATP. Figure 6.9 outlines three broad stages that ultimately lead to the release and conservation of energy for use by the cell for biologic work. *Stage 1* involves the digestion, absorption, and assimilation of relatively large food macromolecules into smaller subunits for use in cellular metabolism. Within the cytosol, *stage 2* degrades amino acid, glucose, and fatty acid and glycerol units into acetyl-coenzyme A (CoA) (formed within the mitochondrion), with limited production of ATP and NADH. In *stage 3* within the mitochondrion, acetyl-CoA degrades to CO_2 and H_2O with considerable ATP production. The specific pathways of degradation differ, depending on the nutrient substrate catabolized. In the sections that follow, we show how ATP resynthesis occurs from extraction of the potential energy in carbohydrate, fat, and protein.

Figure 6.10 outlines the macronutrient fuel sources that supply substrate for oxidation and subsequent formation of ATP. These sources consist primarily of (1) triglyceride and

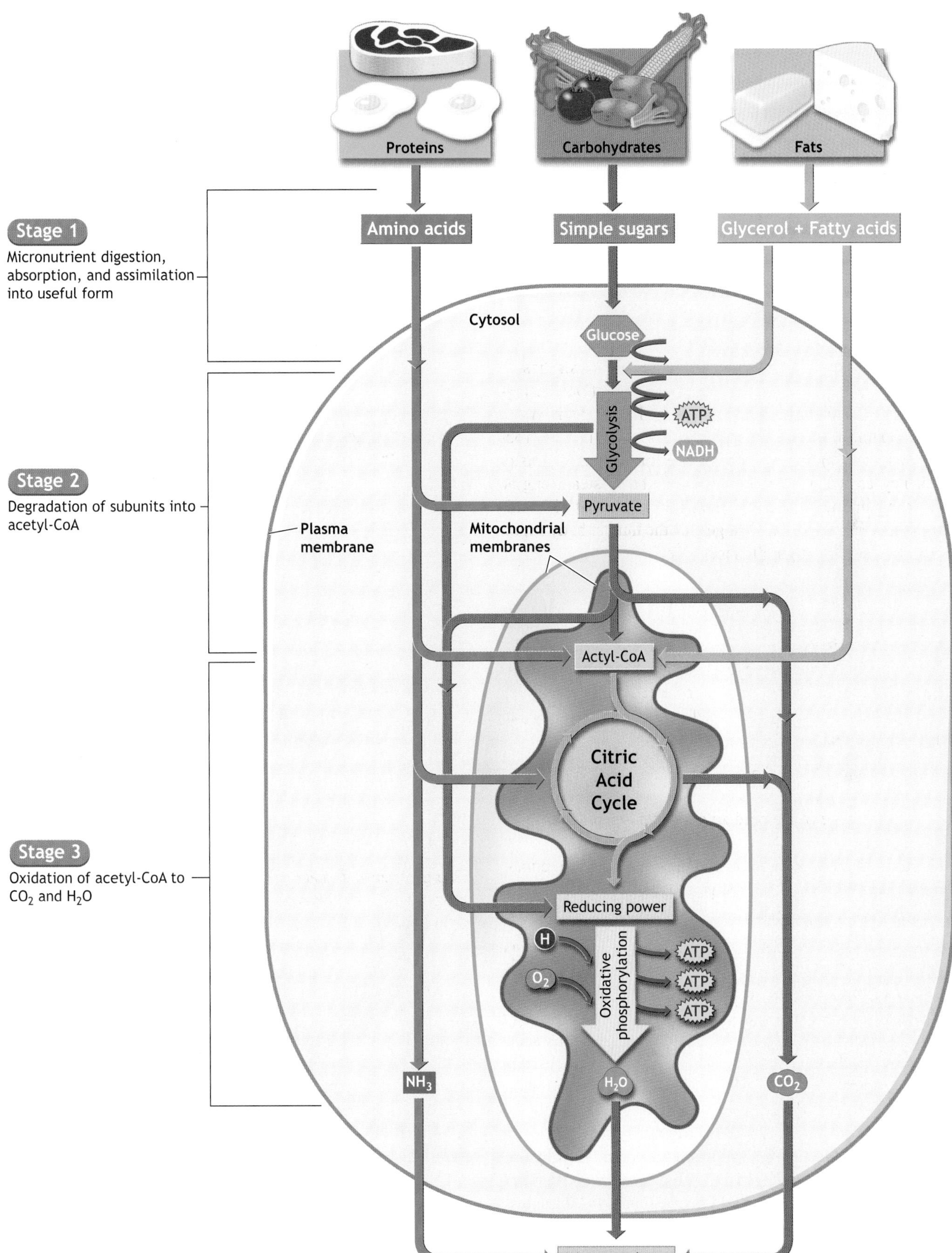

FIGURE 6.9 • Broad stages for the use of macronutrient constituents for energy metabolism.

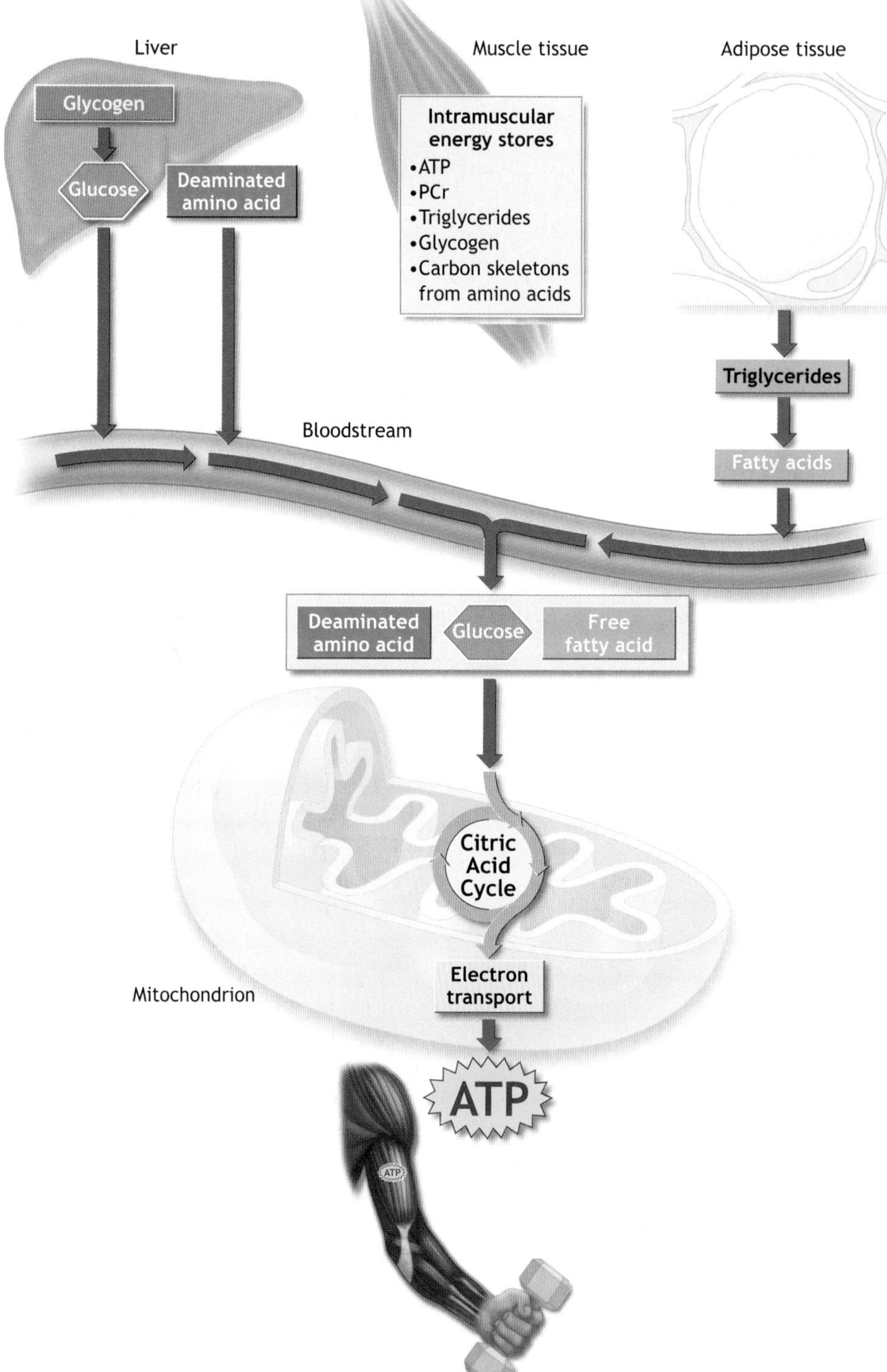

FIGURE 6.10 • Macronutrient fuel sources that supply substrates for regenerating ATP. The liver provides a rich source of amino acids and glucose, while adipocytes generate large quantities of energy-rich fatty acid molecules. After their release, the bloodstream delivers these compounds to the muscle cell. Most of the cells' energy production takes place within the mitochondria. Mitochondrial proteins carry out their roles in oxidative phosphorylation in the inner membranous walls of this architecturally elegant complex. The intramuscular energy sources consist of the high-energy phosphates ATP and PCr and triglycerides, glycogen, and amino acids.

glycogen molecules stored within muscle cells, (2) glucose (derived from liver glycogen), (3) free fatty acids (derived from triglycerides in liver and adipocytes) and, (4) intramuscular- and liver-derived carbon skeletons of amino acids. A small amount of ATP also forms from (5) anaerobic reactions in the cytosol in the initial phase of glucose or glycogen breakdown and (6) phosphorylation of ADP by PCr under enzymatic control by creatine kinase and adenylate kinase.

ENERGY RELEASE FROM CARBOHYDRATE

Carbohydrate's primary function is supplying energy for cellular work. Our discussion of macronutrient energy metabolism begins with carbohydrates for several reasons:

- Carbohydrate provides the only macronutrient substrate whose stored energy generates ATP anaerobically. This becomes important in maximal exercise

that requires rapid energy release above levels supplied by aerobic metabolism. In this case, intramuscular glycogen supplies most of the energy for ATP resynthesis.
- During light and moderate aerobic exercise, carbohydrate supplies about one-third of the body's energy requirements.
- Processing large quantities of fat for energy requires some carbohydrate catabolism.
- Aerobic hydrolysis of carbohydrate for energy occurs more rapidly than energy generation from fatty acid breakdown. Thus, depleting glycogen reserves significantly reduces exercise power output. In prolonged aerobic exercise such as marathon running, athletes often experience nutrient-related fatigue—a state associated with muscle and liver glycogen depletion.

The complete breakdown of one mole (180 g) of glucose to carbon dioxide and water yields a maximum of 686 kcal of chemical free energy available for work.

$$C_6H_{12}O_6 + 6\ O_2 \rightarrow 6\ CO_2 + 6\ H_2O\ \ -\Delta G\ 686\ \text{kcal} \cdot \text{mol}^{-1}$$

Complete glucose breakdown conserves only some of the released energy as ATP. Recall that the synthesis of 1 mole of ATP from ADP and a phosphate ion requires 7.3 kcal of energy. Therefore, coupling all of the energy in glucose oxidation to phosphorylation could theoretically form 94 moles of ATP per mole of glucose (686 kcal $\div$ 7.3 kcal $\cdot$ mol^{-1} = 94 mol). In the muscle, phosphate bond formation conserves only 38%, or 263 kcal of energy, with the remainder dissipated as heat. Consequently, glucose breakdown regenerates 36 moles of ATP (263 kcal $\div$ 7.3 kcal $\cdot$ mol^{-1} = 36 mol) with an accompanying free energy gain of 263 kcal.

Glucose degradation occurs in two stages. In stage one, glucose breaks down relatively rapidly into two molecules of pyruvate. Energy transfer for phosphorylation occurs without oxygen (anaerobic). In stage two, pyruvate degrades further to carbon dioxide and water. Energy transfers from these reactions require electron transport and accompanying oxidative phosphorylation (aerobic).

Glycolysis Generates Anaerobic Energy From Glucose

Figure 6.11 illustrates the first stage of glucose degradation in a series of fermentation reactions collectively termed **glycolysis**, or the Embden-Meyerhof pathway for its discoverers.[3] Glycolysis occurs in the watery medium of the cell, outside the mitochondrion. In a sense, the reactions represent a more primitive form of rapid energy transfer well developed in amphibians, reptiles, fish, and marine mammals. In humans, the cells' capacity for glycolysis becomes crucial during physical activities that require maximal effort for up to 90 seconds.

In reaction 1, ATP acts as a phosphate donor to phosphorylate glucose to glucose 6-phosphate. In most tissues, the glucose molecule becomes "trapped" in the cell. Liver, and to a small extent, kidney cells, contain the enzyme **phosphatase**, which splits the phosphate from glucose 6-phosphate. This frees glucose from the cell for transport throughout the body. In the presence of the enzyme **glycogen synthase**, glucose can now link (become polymerized) with other glucose molecules to form glycogen (see Fig. 1.2). During energy metabolism, glucose 6-phosphate changes to fructose 6-phosphate. At this stage, no energy is extracted, yet energy has been incorporated into the original glucose molecule at the expense of one ATP molecule. In a sense, phosphorylation "primes the pump" for energy metabolism to proceed. The fructose 6-phosphate molecule gains an additional phosphate and changes to fructose 1,6-diphosphate under control of the enzyme **phosphofructokinase (PFK)**. The activity level of PFK probably limits the rate of glycolysis during maximum-effort exercise. Fructose 1,6-diphosphate then splits into two phosphorylated molecules with three carbon chains; these further decompose to pyruvate in five successive reactions. Fast-twitch muscle fibers (see Chapter 7, p 163) contain relatively large quantities of PFK; this makes them ideally suited for generating anaerobic energy via glycolysis.

Metabolism of Glucose to Glycogen and Glycogen to Glucose

The cytoplasm of liver and muscle cells contains glycogen granules and the enzymes for both glycogen synthesis (glycogenesis) and breakdown (glycogenolysis). Under normal conditions glucose does not accumulate in the blood following a meal. Depending on the cells' energy status, surplus glucose stores as either glycogen or fat or enters the pathways of energy metabolism. Under high cellular activity, available glucose oxidizes via the glycolytic pathway, the citric acid cycle, and the respiratory chain to form ATP. On the other hand, low cellular activity levels and/or depleted glycogen reserves inactivate key enzymes in glycolysis, causing surplus glucose to channel into glycogen formation.

Glycogenolysis describes the cleavage of glucose from the glycogen molecule. The glucose residue then reacts with a phosphate ion to produce glucose 6-phosphate, bypassing step 1 of the glycolytic pathway. Thus, when glycogen provides a glucose molecule for glycolysis, a net gain of three ATPs occurs rather than two ATPs during glucose breakdown (see p 148).

REGULATION OF GLYCOGEN METABOLISM. In the liver, **glycogen phosphorylase** enzymes become inactive following a meal, while glycogen synthase activity increases to facilitate storage of the glucose obtained from food. Conversely, between meals when glycogen reserves decrease, liver phosphorylase becomes active (concurrent depression of glycogen synthase activity) to maintain blood glucose for body tissues. Skeletal muscle at rest shows higher synthase activity, while physical activity induces increased phosphorylase activity with concomitant blunting of the synthase enzyme. **Epinephrine**, a sympathetic nervous system hormone, accelerates the rate that phosphorylase cleaves one glucose component at a time from the glycogen molecule.[9,13] Epinephrine's action has been termed the **glycogenolysis cascade** whereby the hormone effects progressively greater

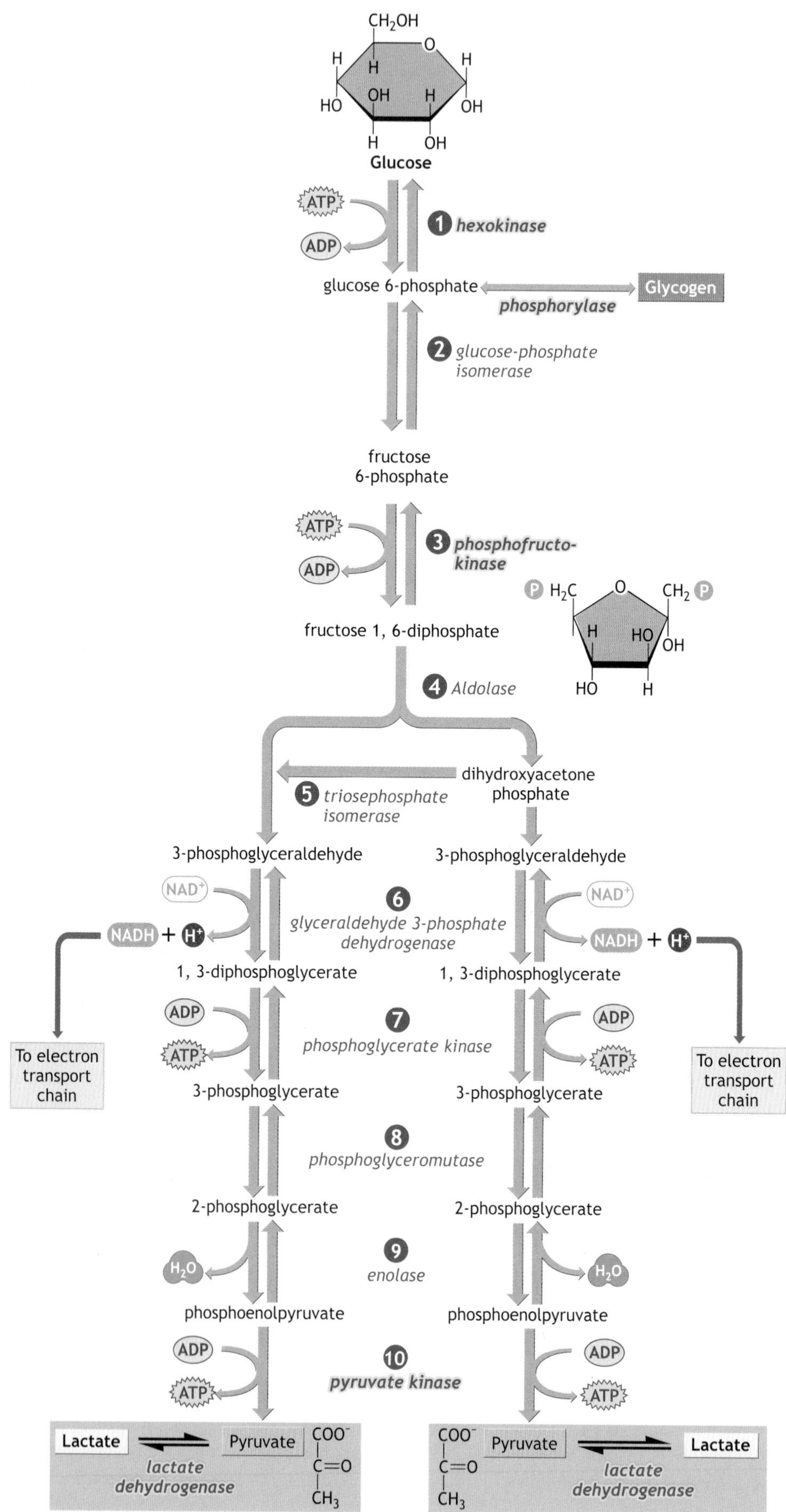

FIGURE 6.11 • Glycolysis: a series of 10 enzymatically controlled chemical reactions create two molecules of pyruvate from the anaerobic breakdown of glucose. Lactate forms when NADH oxidation does not keep pace with its formation in glycolysis. Enzymes colored *yellow-purple* are those that play a key regulatory role in these metabolic reactions.

phosphorylase activation to ensure rapid glycogen mobilization. Thus, phosphorylase activity becomes most active during intense exercise when sympathetic activity increases and carbohydrate provides the optimum fuel. Sympathetic outflow and subsequent glycogen catabolism decrease considerably during low- to moderate-intensity exercise when fatty acid oxidation adequately maintains ATP concentrations in active muscle.

Substrate-Level Phosphorylation in Glycolysis

Most of the energy generated in glycolysis (44 kcal · mol^{-1}) does not result in ATP resynthesis. Instead, it dissipates as heat. In reactions 7 and 10, however, the energy released from the glucose intermediates stimulates the direct transfer of a phosphate group to four ADP molecules, generating four molecules of ATP. *Because two molecules of ATP contribute to the initial phosphorylation of the glucose molecule, glycolysis generates a net gain of two ATP molecules. This represents an endergonic conservation of 14.6 kcal · mol^{-1}*. The specific energy transfers from substrate to ADP by phosphorylation in glycolysis do not require oxygen. Rather, energy directly transfers via phosphate bonds in the anaerobic reactions called **substrate-level phosphorylation**. Energy conservation during glycolysis operates at an efficiency of about 30%.

Glycolysis generates only about 5% of the total ATP during the glucose molecule's complete breakdown. However, owing to the high concentration of glycolytic enzymes and the speed of these reactions, significant energy for muscle action occurs rapidly during glycolysis. The following represent examples of activities that rely heavily on ATP generated by anaerobic glycolytic reactions: sprinting at the end of a mile run, swimming all-out from start to finish in a 50- and 100-m swim, routines on gymnastics apparatus, and sprint running up to 200 m. Note that anaerobic energy transfer from macronutrients occurs *only* from carbohydrate breakdown during glycolytic reactions.

Regulation of Glycolysis

The regulation of glycolysis depends on (1) concentrations of the key glycolytic enzymes hexokinase, phosphofructokinase, and pyruvate kinase, (2) levels of the substrate fructose 1,6-disphosphate, and (3) oxygen, which in abundance inhibits glycolysis. In addition, glucose delivery to cells influences its subsequent use in energy metabolism.

Glucose locates in the surrounding extracellular fluid for transport across the cell's plasma membrane. A family of five proteins collectively termed facilitative glucose transporters mediates this process of **facilitative diffusion**. Muscle fibers and adipocytes contain an insulin-dependent transporter known as Glu T4, or simply **GLUT 4**. In response to insulin and physical activity (independent of insulin), GLUT 4 migrates from vesicles within the cell to the plasma membrane. Its action facilitates glucose transport into the sarcoplasm, where it subsequently is used for ATP formation. Another glucose transporter, GLUT 1, accounts for basal levels of glucose transport into muscle.

Hydrogen Release in Glycolysis

Glycolytic reactions strip two pairs of hydrogen atoms from the glucose substrate during glycolysis and pass their electrons to NAD^+ to form NADH (Fig. 6.11, reaction 6). Normally, if the respiratory chain processed these electrons directly, three ATP molecules would generate for each NADH molecule oxidized (P/O ratio = 3). Within heart, kidney, and liver cells, extramitochondrial hydrogen (NADH) appears as NADH in the mitochondrion (a mechanism termed the **malate-aspartate shuttle**). This produces three ATP molecules from the oxidation of each NADH molecule from glycolysis. The mitochondrion in skeletal muscle and brain cells remains impermeable to NADH formed in the cytoplasm during glycolysis. Consequently, electrons from extramitochondrial NADH shuttle indirectly into the mitochondrion. This route ends with electrons passing to FAD to form $FADH_2$ (a mechanism termed the **glycerol-phosphate shuttle**) at a point below the first formation of ATP (see Fig. 6.7A). *Thus two, rather than three ATP molecules form when the respiratory chain oxidizes cytoplasmic NADH (P/O ratio = 2). Because two molecules of NADH form in glycolysis, four molecules of ATP generate aerobically by subsequent electron transport–oxidative phosphorylation in skeletal muscle.*

Lactate Formation

Sufficient oxygen bathes the cells during light to moderate levels of energy metabolism. Consequently, the hydrogens (electrons) stripped from the substrate and carried by NADH oxidize within the mitochondria to form water when they join with oxygen. In a biochemical sense, a "steady state," or more precisely a "steady rate," exists because hydrogen oxidizes at about the same *rate* that it becomes available. Biochemists frequently refer to this relatively steady dynamic condition as **aerobic glycolysis**, with pyruvate as the end product.

In strenuous exercise, when energy demands exceed either oxygen supply or its rate of use, the respiratory chain cannot process all of the hydrogen joined to NADH. Continued release of anaerobic energy in glycolysis depends on NAD^+ availability to oxidize 3-phosphoglyceraldehyde (see reaction 6, Fig. 6.11); otherwise, the rapid rate of glycolysis "grinds to a halt." During **anaerobic glycolysis**, NAD^+ "frees up" as pairs of "excess" nonoxidized hydrogens combine temporarily with pyruvate to form lactate. Lactate formation requires one additional step, catalyzed by the enzyme **lactate dehydrogenase**, in the reversible reaction shown in Figure 6.12.

Lactate accumulation, not simply its production, signifies the onset of anaerobic energy metabolism. During rest and moderate exercise, some lactate continually forms in two ways: (1) the energy metabolism of red blood cells that contain no mitochondria and (2) limitations posed by enzyme activity in muscle fibers with high glycolytic capacity. However, any lactate that forms in this manner readily oxidizes in neighboring muscle fibers with high oxidative capacity or in more-distant tissues such as the heart. Consequently, lactate does not accumulate because its removal rate equals its rate of production. Endurance athletes show an enhanced ability for lactate clearance (turnover) during exercise.[21]

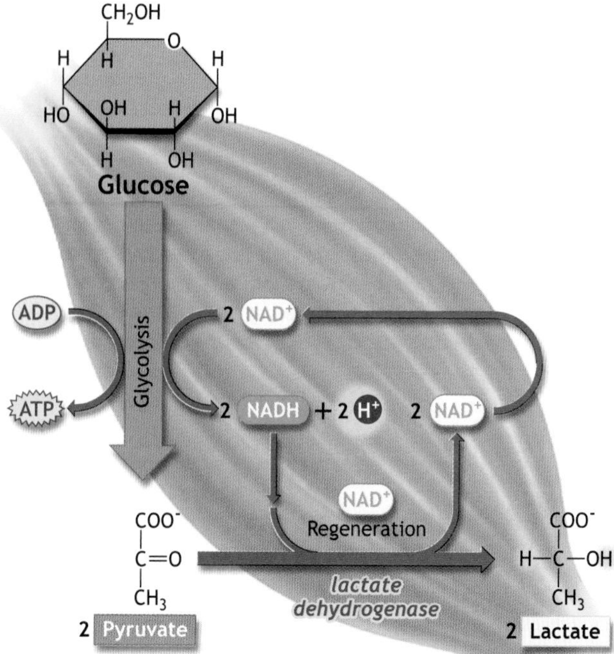

FIGURE 6.12 • Under physiologic conditions in muscle, lactate forms when hydrogens from NADH combine temporarily with pyruvate. This frees up NAD to accept additional hydrogens generated in glycolysis.

The temporary storage of hydrogen with pyruvate represents a unique aspect of energy metabolism because it provides a ready "sump" for temporary storage of the end products of anaerobic glycolysis. Also, once lactate forms in muscle, it diffuses rapidly into the interstitial space and blood for buffering and removal from the site of energy metabolism. In this way, glycolysis continues to supply anaerobic energy for ATP resynthesis. This avenue for extra energy remains temporary because blood and muscle lactate levels increase and ATP regeneration fails to keep pace with its rate of use. Fatigue soon sets in, and exercise performance diminishes. Increased intracellular acidity and other disruptions mediate fatigue by inactivating various enzymes in energy transfer and impairing the muscle's contractile properties.[2,8,17,22] However, increased acidity (decreased pH) does not singularly explain the decrement in exercise capacity during heavy physical effort.[19]

Lactate should not be viewed as a metabolic waste product. To the contrary, it provides a valuable source of chemical energy that accumulates as a result of intense exercise.[15] When sufficient oxygen once again becomes available during recovery, or when exercise pace slows, NAD^+ scavenges hydrogens attached to lactate for subsequent oxidation to form ATP. The carbon skeletons of the pyruvate molecules re-formed from lactate during exercise become either oxidized for energy or synthesized to glucose (gluconeogenesis) in the **Cori cycle** (Fig. 6.13). The Cori cycle not only removes lactate but also uses it to replenish glycogen reserves depleted in heavy exercise.[33]

In strenuous exercise with elevated carbohydrate catabolism, the glycogen within inactive tissues can become available to supply the needs of active muscle. Such active glycogen turnover through the **exchangeable lactate pool** progresses as inactive tissues release lactate into the circulation. The lactate provides a gluconeogenic precursor to synthesize carbohydrate (via the Cori cycle in liver and kidneys) to support blood glucose homeostasis and the energy requirements of exercise.[5,21]

LACTATE SHUTTLE: BLOOD LACTATE AS AN ENERGY SOURCE. Isotope tracer studies of muscle and other tissues show that lactate produced in fast-twitch muscle fibers can circulate to other fast-twitch or slow-twitch fibers for conversion to pyruvate. Pyruvate, in turn, converts to acetyl-CoA for entry into the citric acid cycle for aerobic energy metabolism. Such **lactate shuttling** among cells enables glycogenolysis in one cell to supply other cells with fuel for oxidation. *This makes muscle not only a major site of lactate production, but also a primary tissue for lactate removal via oxidation.*[6]

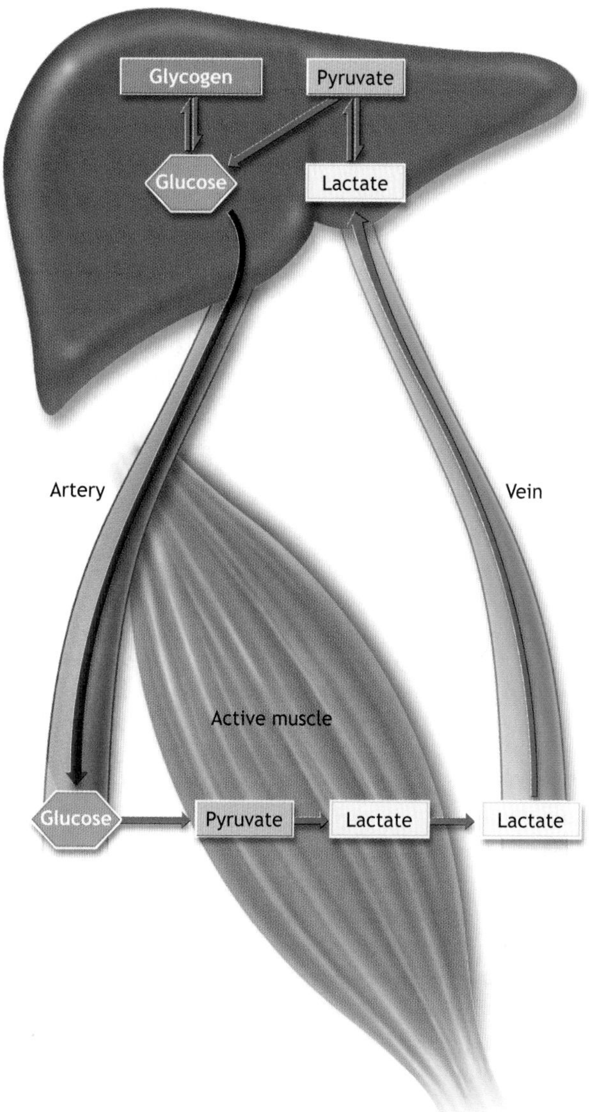

FIGURE 6.13 • The biochemical reactions of the Cori cycle in the liver synthesize glucose from the lactate released from active muscles. This gluconeogenic process helps to maintain carbohydrate reserves.

Citric Acid Cycle

Anaerobic reactions of glycolysis release only about 10% of the energy within the original glucose molecule. Extraction of the remaining energy continues when pyruvate *irreversibly* converts to **acetyl-CoA**, a form of acetic acid. Acetyl-CoA enters the **citric acid cycle** (also termed Krebs cycle or tricarboxylic acid cycle), the second stage of carbohydrate breakdown. This sequence of metabolic events often bears the name of its discoverer, 1953 Nobel chemist Sir Hans Krebs.[4] As shown schematically in Figure 6.14, the citric acid cycle degrades the acetyl-CoA substrate to carbon dioxide and hydrogen atoms within the mitochondria. ATP forms when hydrogen atoms oxidize during electron transport–oxidative phosphorylation.

Figure 6.15 shows pyruvate preparing to enter the citric acid cycle by joining with the vitamin B derivative coenzyme A (*A* for acetic acid) to form the 2-carbon compound acetyl-CoA. The two hydrogens released transfer their electrons to NAD^+, forming one molecule of carbon dioxide as follows:

$$\text{Pyruvate} + NAD^+ + \text{CoA} \rightarrow \text{Acetyl-CoA} + CO_2 + NADH^+ + H^+$$

The acetyl portion of acetyl-CoA joins with **oxaloacetate** to form **citrate**, the same 6-carbon citric acid compound found in citrus fruits, which then proceeds through the citric acid cycle. The citric acid cycle continues its operations because it retains the original oxaloacetate molecule to join with a new acetyl fragment that enters the cycle.

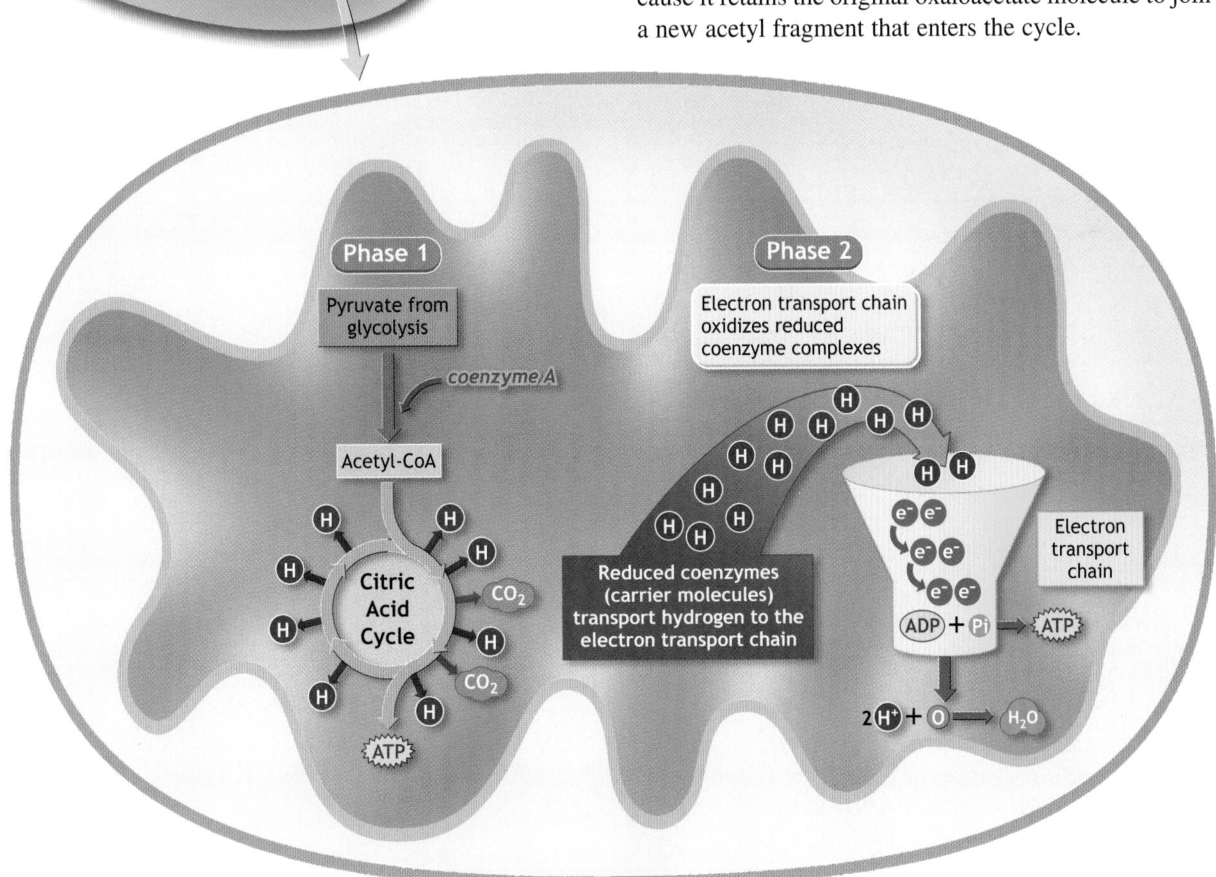

FIGURE 6.14 • Aerobic energy metabolism. *Phase 1.* In the mitochondria, the citric acid cycle generates hydrogen atoms during acetyl-CoA breakdown. *Phase 2.* Significant quantities of ATP regenerate when these hydrogens oxidize via the aerobic process of electron transport–oxidative phosphorylation (electron transport chain).

Each acetyl-CoA molecule entering the citric acid cycle releases two carbon dioxide molecules and four pairs of hydrogen atoms. One molecule of ATP also regenerates directly by substrate-level phosphorylation from citric acid cycle reactions (reaction 7, Fig. 6.15). As summarized at the bottom of Figure 6.15, the formation of two acetyl-CoA molecules from two pyruvate molecules created in glycolysis releases four hydrogens, and the citric acid cycle releases 16 hydrogens. *Generating electrons (H^+) for passage in the respiratory chain to NAD^+ and FAD represents the most important function of the citric acid cycle.*

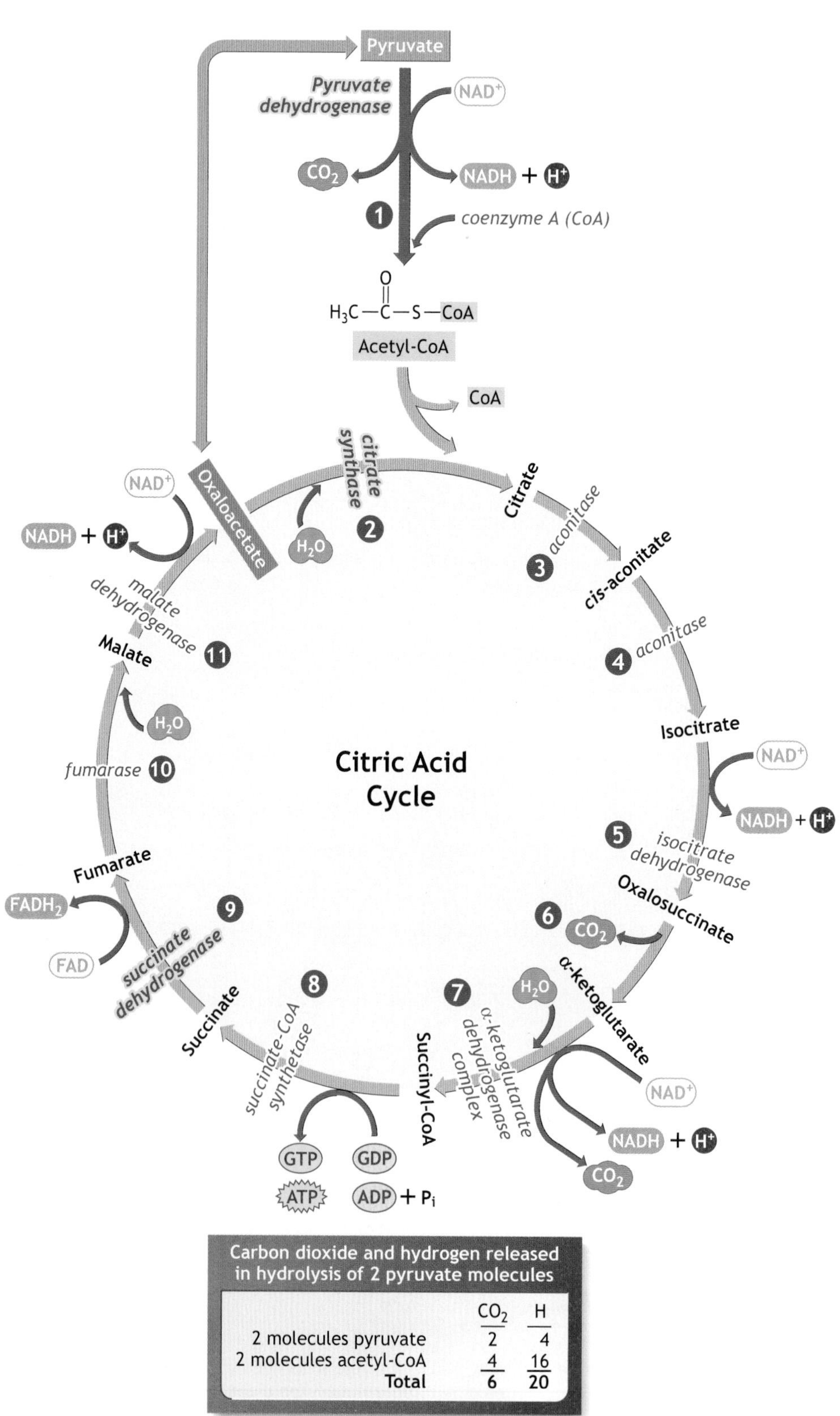

Carbon dioxide and hydrogen released in hydrolysis of 2 pyruvate molecules

	CO_2	H
2 molecules pyruvate	2	4
2 molecules acetyl-CoA	4	16
Total	6	20

FIGURE 6.15 • Flow sheet for the release of hydrogen and carbon dioxide in the mitochondrion during the breakdown of one pyruvate molecule. All values are doubled when computing the net gain of hydrogen and carbon dioxide because two molecules of pyruvate form from one glucose molecule in glycolysis. Enzymes colored yellow-purple are key regulatory enzymes.

Oxygen does not participate directly in citric acid cycle reactions. The major portion of the chemical energy within pyruvate transfers to ADP through the subsequent aerobic process of electron transport–oxidative phosphorylation. With adequate oxygen, including enzymes and substrate, NAD^+ and FAD regeneration takes place, and citric acid cycle metabolism proceeds unimpeded. The citric acid cycle, electron transport, and oxidative phosphorylation represent the three components of aerobic metabolism.

Total Energy Transfer From Glucose Catabolism

Figure 6.16 summarizes the pathways for energy transfer during glucose catabolism in skeletal muscle. Two ATPs (net gain) form from substrate-level phosphorylation in glycolysis; similarly, two ATPs emerge from acetyl-CoA degradation in the citric acid cycle. The 24 released hydrogen atoms can be accounted for as follows:

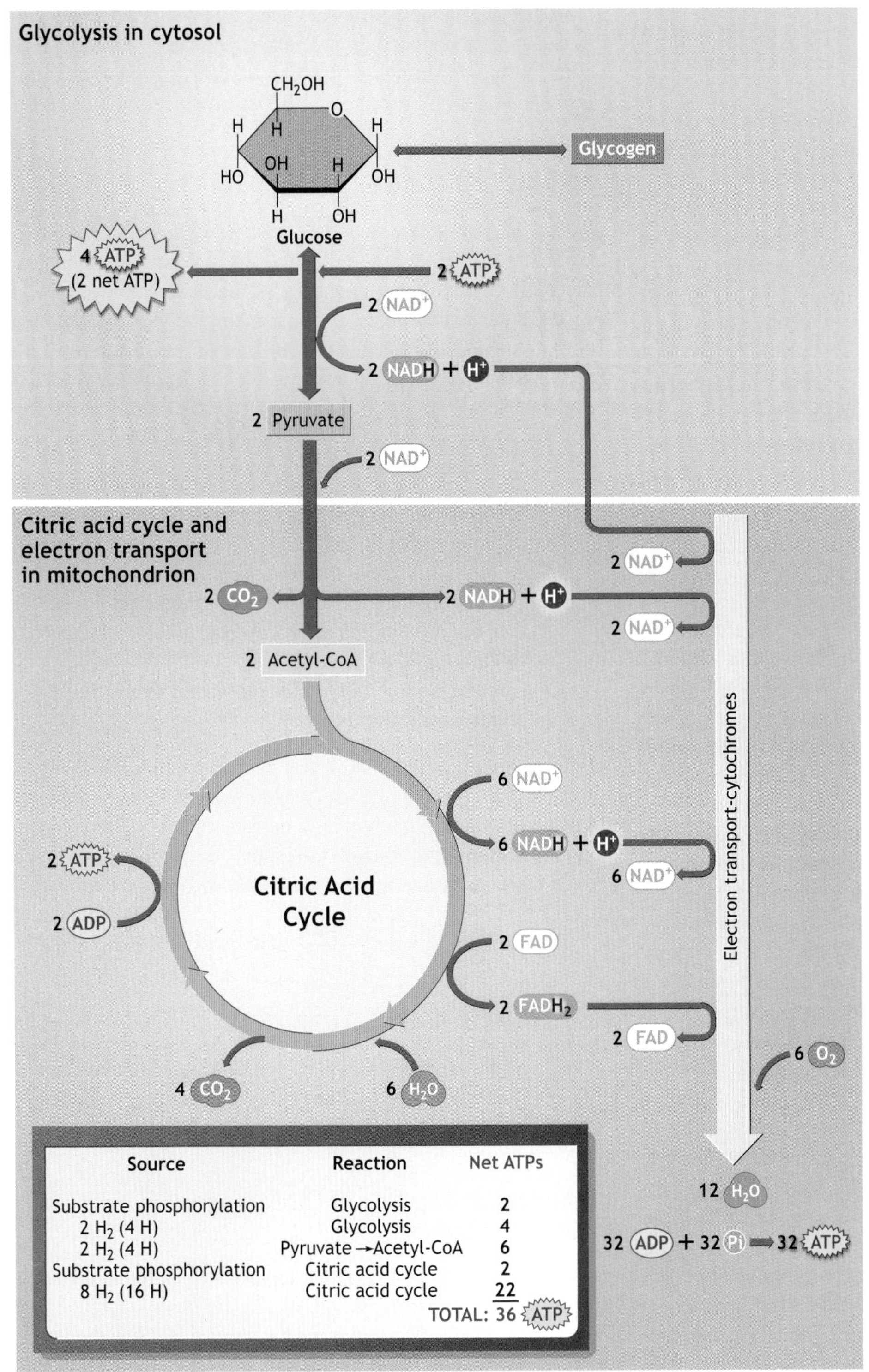

Source	Reaction	Net ATPs
Substrate phosphorylation	Glycolysis	2
$2\ H_2$ (4 H)	Glycolysis	4
$2\ H_2$ (4 H)	Pyruvate→Acetyl-CoA	6
Substrate phosphorylation	Citric acid cycle	2
$8\ H_2$ (16 H)	Citric acid cycle	22
	TOTAL:	36 ATP

FIGURE 6.16 • A net yield of 36 ATPs from energy transfer during the complete oxidation of one glucose molecule in glycolysis, the citric acid cycle, and electron transport.

- Four extramitochondrial hydrogens (2 NADH) generated in glycolysis yield 4 ATPs during oxidative phosphorylation (6 ATPs in heart, kidney, and liver)
- Four hydrogens (2 NADH) released in the mitochondrion as pyruvate degrades to acetyl-CoA yield 6 ATPs
- Twelve of the 16 hydrogens (6 NADH) released in the citric acid cycle yield 18 ATPs
- Four hydrogens joined to FAD (2 $FADH_2$) in the citric acid cycle yield 4 ATPs

Thirty-eight ATPs represent the total ATP yield from the complete breakdown of glucose. Because 2 ATPs initially phosphorylate glucose, 36 ATP molecules equal the net ATP yield from glucose catabolism in skeletal muscle. Four ATP molecules form directly from substrate-level phosphorylation (glycolysis and citric acid cycle), whereas 32 ATP molecules regenerate during oxidative phosphorylation.

Some textbooks quote 38 while others give 36 as the net ATP yield from glucose catabolism. The disparity depends on which shuttle system (the glycerol phosphate or malate/aspartate) transports NADH + H^+ into the mitochondrion. (Many scientists in the ever-evolving field of biochemistry have modified the range from 36 to 38 down to 30 to 32.) As discussed previously, 4 ATPs represent the final yield from the glycerol phosphate shuttle (skeletal muscle and brain) as opposed to 6 ATPs from the malate/aspartate shuttle (myocardium, liver, and kidneys) during the complete breakdown of a single glucose molecule.

What Regulates Energy Metabolism?

Under normal conditions, electron transfer and subsequent energy release tightly couple to ADP phosphorylation. Without ADP availability for phosphorylation to ATP, electrons generally do not shuttle down the respiratory chain to oxygen. *Compounds that either inhibit or activate enzymes at key control points in the oxidative pathways modulate regulatory control of glycolysis and the citric acid cycle.*[16,19,28] Each pathway contains at least one enzyme considered rate limiting, because the enzyme controls the overall speed of that pathway's reactions. *Cellular ADP concentration exerts the greatest effect on the rate-limiting enzymes controlling the energy metabolism of carbohydrates, fats, and proteins.* This mechanism for respiratory control makes sense because any increase in ADP signals a need to supply energy to restore ATP levels. Conversely, high levels of cellular ATP indicate a relatively low energy requirement. From a broader perspective, ADP concentrations function as a cellular feedback mechanism to maintain a relative constancy (homeostasis) in the level of energy currency available for biologic work. Other rate-limiting modulators include cellular levels of phosphate, cyclic AMP, AMP-activated protein kinase (AMPK), calcium, NAD^+, citrate, and pH. More specifically, ATP and NADH act as enzyme inhibitors, while intracellular calcium, ADP, and NAD^+ serve as activators. Such chemical feedback allows rapid metabolic adjustment to the cells' energy needs. Within the resting cell, the ATP concentration considerably exceeds the concentration of ADP by about 500:1. However, a decrease in the ATP/ADP ratio and intramitochondrial NADH/NAD^+ ratio, as occurs in the beginning of exercise, signals a need for increased metabolism of stored nutrients. On the other hand, relatively low levels of energy demand maintain high ratios of ATP/ADP and NADH/NAD^+, which blunts the rate of energy metabolism.[1]

INDEPENDENT EFFECTS. No single chemical regulator dominates in affecting mitochondrial ATP production. In vitro and in vivo experiments show that changes in each of these compounds independently alter the rate of oxidative phosphorylation. Thus, it appears that all exert regulatory effects, each contributing differently depending on energy demands, cellular conditions, and the specific tissue involved.

ENERGY RELEASE FROM FAT

Stored fat represents the body's most plentiful source of potential energy. Relative to carbohydrate and protein, stored fat provides almost unlimited energy. The fuel reserves in a typical young adult male come from two main sources: (1) between 60,000 and 100,000 kcal (23,900 kJ) from triglyceride in fat cells (**adipocytes**) and (2) about 3,000 kcal from intramuscular triglyceride (12 mmol · kg · muscle^{-1}). In contrast, carbohydrate energy reserves generally amount to less than 2,000 kcal (8,400 kJ). Energy sources for fat catabolism include:

- Triglycerides stored directly within the muscle fiber in close proximity to the mitochondria (more in slow-twitch than in fast-twitch muscle fibers)
- Circulating triglycerides in lipoprotein complexes that lipoprotein lipase hydrolyzes on the surface of a tissue's capillary endothelium
- Circulating free fatty acids mobilized from triglycerides in adipose tissue

Prior to energy release from fat, hydrolysis (**lipolysis**) in the cell's cytosol splits the triglyceride molecule into glycerol and three water-insoluble fatty acid molecules. The enzyme **hormone-sensitive lipase** (activated by cyclic AMP; see page 149) catalyzes triglyceride breakdown as follows:

$$\text{Triglyceride} + 3\ H_2O \xrightarrow{\text{lipase}} \text{Glycerol} + 3\ \text{Fatty acids}$$

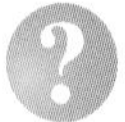

INTEGRATIVE QUESTION

Discuss the claim that regular low-intensity exercise stimulates greater body fat loss than high-intensity exercise of equal total caloric expenditure.

Adipocytes: The Site of Fat Storage and Mobilization

Figure 6.17 outlines the dynamics of fatty acid mobilization (lipolysis) in adipose tissue and delivery for use by skeletal muscle. Although all cells store some fat, adipose tissue serves as an active, major supplier of fatty acid molecules. Adipocytes spe-

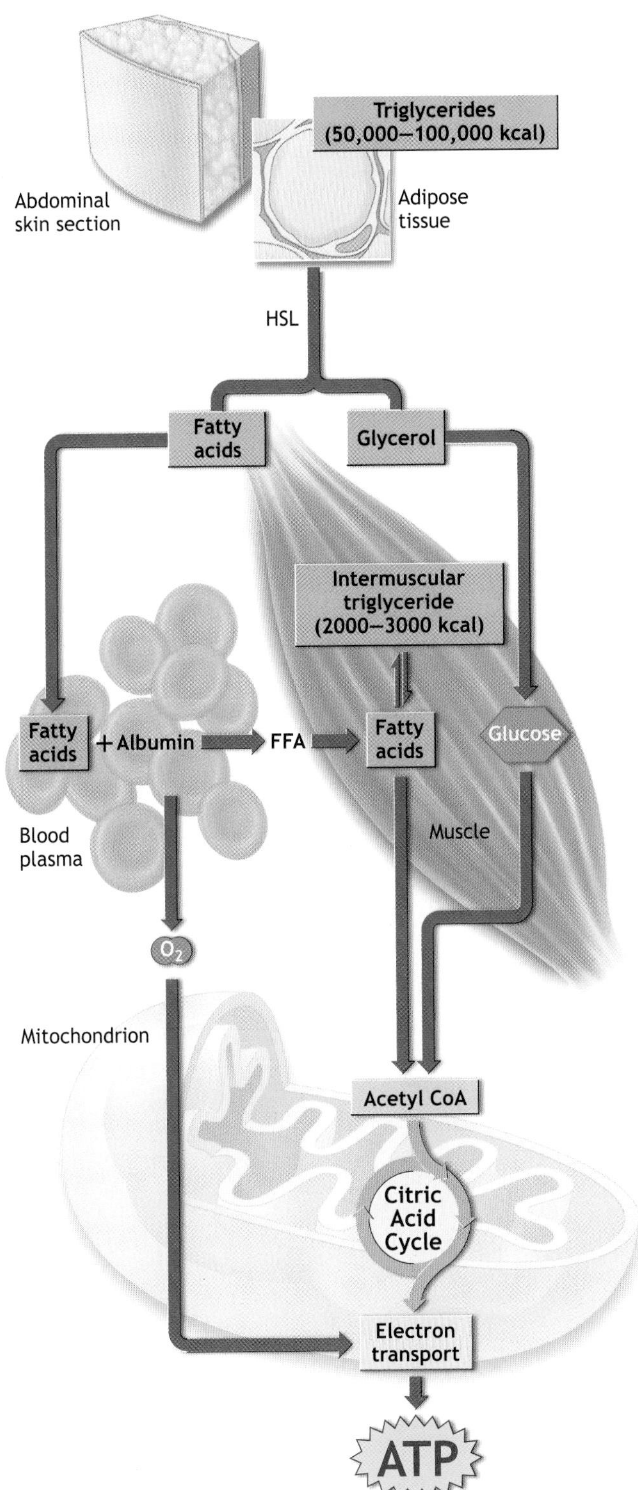

FIGURE 6.17 • Dynamics of fat mobilization and fat use. Hormone-sensitive lipase (HSL) stimulates triglyceride breakdown into its glycerol and fatty acid components. The blood transports free fatty acids (FFAs) released from adipocytes and bound to plasma albumin. Triglycerides stored within the muscle fiber also degrade to glycerol and fatty acids to provide energy.

cialize in synthesizing and storing triglycerides. Triglyceride fat droplets occupy up to 95% of the adipocyte cell's volume. Once hormone-sensitive lipase stimulates fatty acids to diffuse from the adipocyte into the circulation, nearly all bind to plasma albumin for transport to active tissues as **free fatty acids (FFAs)**.[29] Hence, FFAs are not truly "free" entities. At the muscle site, FFAs release from the albumin–FFA complex for transport by diffusion and/or a protein-mediated carrier system across the plasma membrane. Once inside the muscle fiber, FFAs can (1) reesterify to form triglycerides or (2) bind with intramuscular proteins and enter the mitochondria for energy metabolism by enzymatic action of **carnitine acyltransferase**, located on the inner mitochondrial membrane. This enzyme catalyzes the transfer of an acyl group to carnitine to form acyl carnitine, a compound that readily crosses the mitochondrial membrane. Medium- and short-chain fatty acids do not depend on enzyme-mediated transport; most diffuse freely into the mitochondria.

The water-soluble glycerol molecule formed during lipolysis readily diffuses from the adipocyte into the circulation. As a result, plasma glycerol levels often reflect the level of triglyceride catabolism.[27] When delivered to the liver, glycerol serves as a gluconeogenic precursor for glucose synthesis. The relatively slow rate of this process explains why exogenous glycerol supplementation contributes little as an energy substrate (or glucose replenisher) during exercise.[24]

Adipose tissue release of FFAs and their subsequent use for energy in light and moderate exercise increase directly with blood flow through adipose tissue (threefold increase not uncommon) and active muscle. FFA catabolism increases principally in slow-twitch muscle fibers, whose ample blood supply and large, numerous mitochondria make them ideal for fat breakdown.

Circulating triglycerides carried in lipoprotein complexes also provide an energy source. **Lipoprotein lipase (LPL)**, an enzyme synthesized within the cell and then localized on the surface of its surrounding capillaries, catalyzes the hydrolysis of these triglycerides. LPL facilitates a cell's uptake of fatty acids for use either as energy or for resynthesis (reesterfication) of triglycerides stored in muscle and adipose tissues.[29,31]

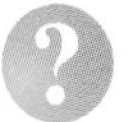

INTEGRATIVE QUESTION

If the average person stores enough energy as body fat to power a 750-mile run, why do athletes often experience impaired performance toward the end of a marathon performed under high-intensity, steady-rate aerobic metabolism?

Hormonal Effects

The hormones epinephrine, norepinephrine, glucagon, and growth hormone augment lipase activation and subsequent lipolysis and FFA mobilization from adipose tissue. Plasma concentrations of these lipogenic hormones increase during exercise to provide active muscles with a continual supply of energy-rich substrate. An intracellular mediator, **adenosine 3′,5′-cyclic monophosphate**, or **cyclic AMP**, activates hormone-sensitive lipase and thus regulates fat breakdown. The

Focus on Research — Aerobic Metabolism and Exercise

Hill AV, Lupton H. Muscular exercise, lactic acid and the supply and utilization of oxygen. Q J Med 1923;16:135.

➤ Perhaps no scientist has contributed more to the field of exercise physiology than Archibald Vivian Hill. Although he won the Nobel Prize in physiology or medicine for studies of energy metabolism using mostly frog muscle, A. V. Hill also pioneered studies of the physiology of running in humans. His careful experiments on oxygen consumption ($\dot{V}O_2$) during exercise and recovery enhanced understanding of the dynamics of exercise energy metabolism and mechanical efficiency. Hill and Lupton's 1923 research investigated interrelationships among exercise intensity, and lactate production and recovery $\dot{V}O_2$. This lengthy article reported the results of many experiments on several individuals (including the researchers) performing different athletic events like running, continuous jumping, and "violent" gymnastics for 10 to 40 minutes. Measurements included $\dot{V}O_2$ and blood lactate during exercise and recovery, using what currently seem crude techniques.

> The subject finished the exercise in front of a stand carrying a wide pipe with nine projecting tubes. To one of these tubes the valves and mouth piece were fixed: to the others were attached rubber bags through single-way stopcocks. The subject on cessation of exercise adopted the standard resting position adjusted the valves, and nose clip, and commenced to expire into the first bag. At the end of about one-half minute (end of nearest expiration) the first bag was turned off, and the second one turned on for a like interval. This process was continued, the intervals of collection being gradually increased.

Topics covered in this article included the following: role of lactate in muscle; heat release in exercise; metabolic efficiency and speed of recovery from different levels of exercise; lactate production in humans; interrelation between lactate formation and oxygen debt; maximal lactate accumulation in exercise; exercise steady state; maximal $\dot{V}O_2$; relation between exercise intensity and $\dot{V}O_2$; and acid–base balance during exercise.

The inclusion of a detailed description of the $\dot{V}O_2$ in recovery from different exercise intensities represents a notable feature of this pioneering article in exercise physiology. The figure shows that the time course of recovery $\dot{V}O_2$ related to the intensity of previous exercise and accompanying lactate accumulation (not shown). Nearly 80 years of subsequent research has confirmed most of Hill and Lupton's astute observations.

The researchers also presented data for near-maximal (peak) oxygen consumption ($\dot{V}O_{2peak}$). Prior to 1923, little information existed on oxygen consumption in individuals "of athletic disposition" during high-intensity exercise. Hill and Lupton reported $\dot{V}O_{2peak}$ for five men during running (last row of values in table inset). We also include other $\dot{V}O_{2peak}$ data for high-intensity exercise, collected between 1913 and 1934. Compare the average value of 3.95 $L \cdot min^{-1}$ for the Hill and Lupton data with the $\dot{V}O_{2max}$ data presented in Figure 11.9 (assume 70-kg body mass to convert data to $mL\ O_2 \cdot kg^{-1} \cdot min^{-1}$). How might you account for the discrepancy in the values?

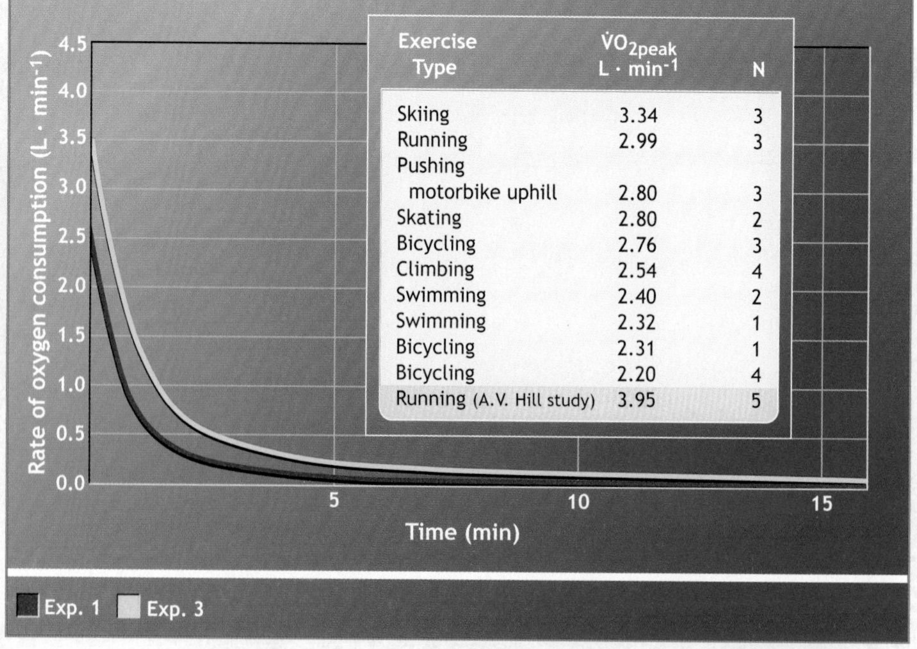

Exercise Type	$\dot{V}O_{2peak}$ $L \cdot min^{-1}$	N
Skiing	3.34	3
Running	2.99	3
Pushing motorbike uphill	2.80	3
Skating	2.80	2
Bicycling	2.76	3
Climbing	2.54	4
Swimming	2.40	2
Swimming	2.32	1
Bicycling	2.31	1
Bicycling	2.20	4
Running (A.V. Hill study)	3.95	5

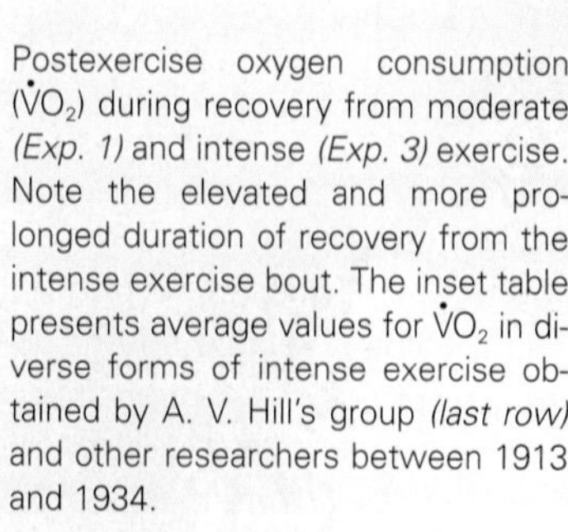

Postexercise oxygen consumption ($\dot{V}O_2$) during recovery from moderate *(Exp. 1)* and intense *(Exp. 3)* exercise. Note the elevated and more prolonged duration of recovery from the intense exercise bout. The inset table presents average values for $\dot{V}O_2$ in diverse forms of intense exercise obtained by A. V. Hill's group *(last row)* and other researchers between 1913 and 1934.

various lipid-mobilizing hormones, which themselves do not enter the cell, activate cyclic AMP.[30] Circulating lactate, ketones, and particularly insulin inhibit cyclic AMP activation.[12] Exercise training-induced increases in the activity level of skeletal muscle and adipose tissue lipases, including biochemical and vascular adaptations in the muscles themselves, contribute to enhanced fat use for energy during moderate exercise.[10,11,20,31] Chapter 20 presents a more detailed evaluation of hormone regulation in exercise and training.

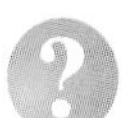

INTEGRATIVE QUESTION

Respond to a person who asks: "If elite marathoners run at an exercise intensity that does not cause appreciable accumulation of blood lactate, why do some of these athletes appear disoriented and fatigued and forced to slow down toward the end of the race?"

Fat breakdown or synthesis depends on availability of the building-block fatty acid molecules. After a meal, when energy metabolism remains relatively low, digestive processes increase FFA and triglyceride delivery to cells; this in turn stimulates triglyceride synthesis. In moderate exercise, on the other hand, the increased fatty acid use for energy reduces their cellular concentration. The decrease in intracellular FFAs stimulates triglyceride breakdown into its glycerol and fatty acid components. Concurrently, hormonal release triggered by exercise stimulates adipose tissue lipolysis to further augment FFA delivery to active muscle.

Catabolism of Glycerol and Fatty Acids

Figure 6.18 summarizes the pathways for degrading the glycerol and fatty acid fragments of the triglyceride molecule.

Glycerol

The anaerobic reactions of glycolysis accept glycerol as 3-phosphoglyceraldehyde, which then degrades to pyruvate to form ATP by substrate-level phosphorylation. Hydrogen atoms pass to NAD^+, and the citric acid cycle oxidizes pyruvate. *The complete breakdown of the single glycerol molecule in a triglyceride synthesizes a total of 19 ATP molecules.* Glycerol also provides carbon skeletons for glucose synthesis (see "In a Practical Sense"). The gluconeogenic role of glycerol becomes important when glycogen reserves significantly deplete from either dietary restriction of carbohydrates or long-term exercise or heavy training.

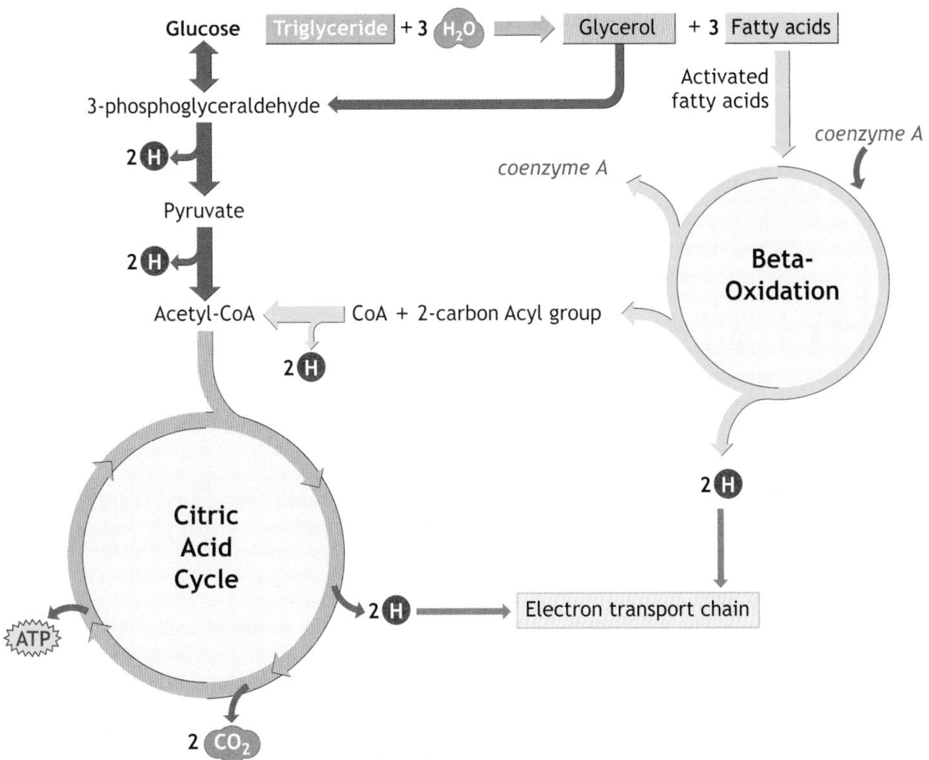

Source	Pathway	ATP yield per molecule neutral fat
1 molecule glycerol	Glycolysis + Citric acid cycle	19
3 molecules of 18-carbon fatty acid	ß-oxidation + Citric acid cycle	441
		TOTAL: 460 ATP

FIGURE 6.18 • General scheme for the breakdown of the glycerol and fatty acid components of a triglyceride molecule. Glycerol enters the energy pathways during glycolysis. Fatty acids prepare to enter the citric acid cycle through β-oxidation. The electron transport chain accepts hydrogens released during glycolysis, β-oxidation, and citric acid cycle metabolism.

Fatty Acids

The fatty acid molecule transforms to acetyl-CoA in the mitochondrion during **beta- (β-) oxidation**, which involves successive splitting of 2-carbon acyl fragments from the long chain of the fatty acid. ATP phosphorylates the reactions, water is added, hydrogens pass to NAD^+ and FAD, and the acyl fragment joins with coenzyme A to form acetyl-CoA. *β-oxidation provides the same acetyl unit as that generated from glucose catabolism.* β-oxidation continues until the entire fatty acid molecule degrades to acetyl-CoA for direct entry into the citric acid cycle. The hydrogens released during fatty acid catabolism oxidize through the respiratory chain. *Note that fatty acid breakdown relates directly to oxygen consumption.* For β-oxidation to proceed, oxygen must join with hydrogen. Under anaerobic conditions, hydrogen remains with NAD^+ and FAD, bringing a halt to fat catabolism.

Total Energy Transfer From Fat Catabolism

The breakdown of a fatty acid molecule progresses as follows:

- β-oxidation produces NADH and $FADH_2$ by cleaving the fatty acid molecule into 2-carbon acyl fragments
- Citric acid cycle degrades acetyl-CoA into carbon dioxide and hydrogen atoms
- Hydrogen atoms oxidize via electron transport–oxidative phosphorylation

For each 18-carbon fatty acid molecule, 147 molecules of ADP phosphorylate to ATP during β-oxidation and citric acid cycle metabolism. Because each triglyceride molecule contains 3 fatty acid molecules, 441 ATP molecules form from the triglyceride's fatty acid components (3 × 147 ATP). Also, 19 ATP molecules form during glycerol breakdown, generating a total of 460 molecules of ATP for each triglyceride molecule catabolized. This represents a considerable energy yield, compared with the 36 ATPs that form during a glucose molecule's catabolism in skeletal muscle. The efficiency of energy conservation for fatty acid oxidation amounts to about 40%, a value similar to that with glucose oxidation.

Depending on a person's state of nutrition and level of training and the intensity and duration of physical activity, intra- and extracellular lipid molecules usually supply between 30 and 80% of the energy for biologic work.[27,34] When high-intensity, long-duration exercise depletes glycogen, fat becomes the *primary* energy fuel for exercise and recovery.[20] Furthermore, prolonged exposure to a high-fat, low-carbohydrate diet brings about enzymatic adaptations that enhance one's capacity for fat oxidation during exercise.[23]

ENERGY RELEASE FROM PROTEIN

Chapter 1 emphasized that protein, primarily the branched-chain amino acids leucine, isoleucine, valine, glutamine, and aspartate, plays a contributory role as an energy substrate during endurance activities and heavy training. The amino acids first convert to a form that readily enters pathways for energy release. This conversion requires nitrogen removal from the amino acid molecule. Whereas the liver serves as the main site for **deamination**, skeletal muscle also contains enzymes that remove nitrogen from an amino acid and pass it to other compounds during **transamination** (see Fig. 1.24). For example, the citric acid cycle intermediate α-ketoglutarate accepts a nitrogen-containing amine group (NH_2) to form a new amino acid, glutamate. In this way, the muscle can use the carbon-skeleton byproducts of donor amino acids for ATP formation. The levels of enzymes for transamination increase with exercise training, which may further facilitate protein's use as an energy substrate.

Some amino acids are **glucogenic**; when deaminated, they yield pyruvate, oxaloacetate, or malate—intermediates for glucose synthesis via gluconeogenesis. For example, pyruvate forms when alanine loses its amino group and gains a double-bonded oxygen. The gluconeogenic role of certain amino acids provides an important component of the Cori cycle for furnishing glucose during prolonged exercise. Regular exercise training enhances the liver's capacity for glucose synthesis from alanine.[33] Other amino acids such as glycine are **ketogenic**; when deaminated, they yield the intermediates acetyl-CoA or acetoacetate. These compounds cannot be used to synthesize glucose, but instead synthesize to triglyceride or catabolize for energy in the citric acid cycle.

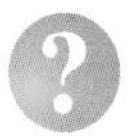

INTEGRATIVE QUESTION

Give examples of where the quantity of ATP produced varies depending on where a deaminated amino acid enters the catabolic pathways.

PROTEIN BREAKDOWN FACILITATES WATER LOSS. When protein provides energy, the body eliminates the nitrogen-containing amine group and other solutes produced from protein breakdown. These waste products must leave the body dissolved in "obligatory" fluid (urine). For this reason, excessive protein catabolism increases the body's water needs.

THE METABOLIC MILL: INTERRELATIONSHIPS AMONG CARBOHYDRATE, FAT, AND PROTEIN METABOLISM

The citric acid cycle plays a much more important role than simply degrading pyruvate produced during glucose catabolism. Fragments from other organic compounds formed from fat and protein breakdown generate useful energy during the citric acid cycle and subsequent electron transport–oxidative phosphorylation. Figure 6.19 illustrates that deaminated residues of excess amino acids enter the citric acid cycle at various intermediate stages, whereas the glycerol fragment of triglyceride catabolism gains entrance via the glycolytic pathway. Fatty acids become oxidized via β-oxidation to acetyl-CoA, which then enters the citric acid cycle directly.

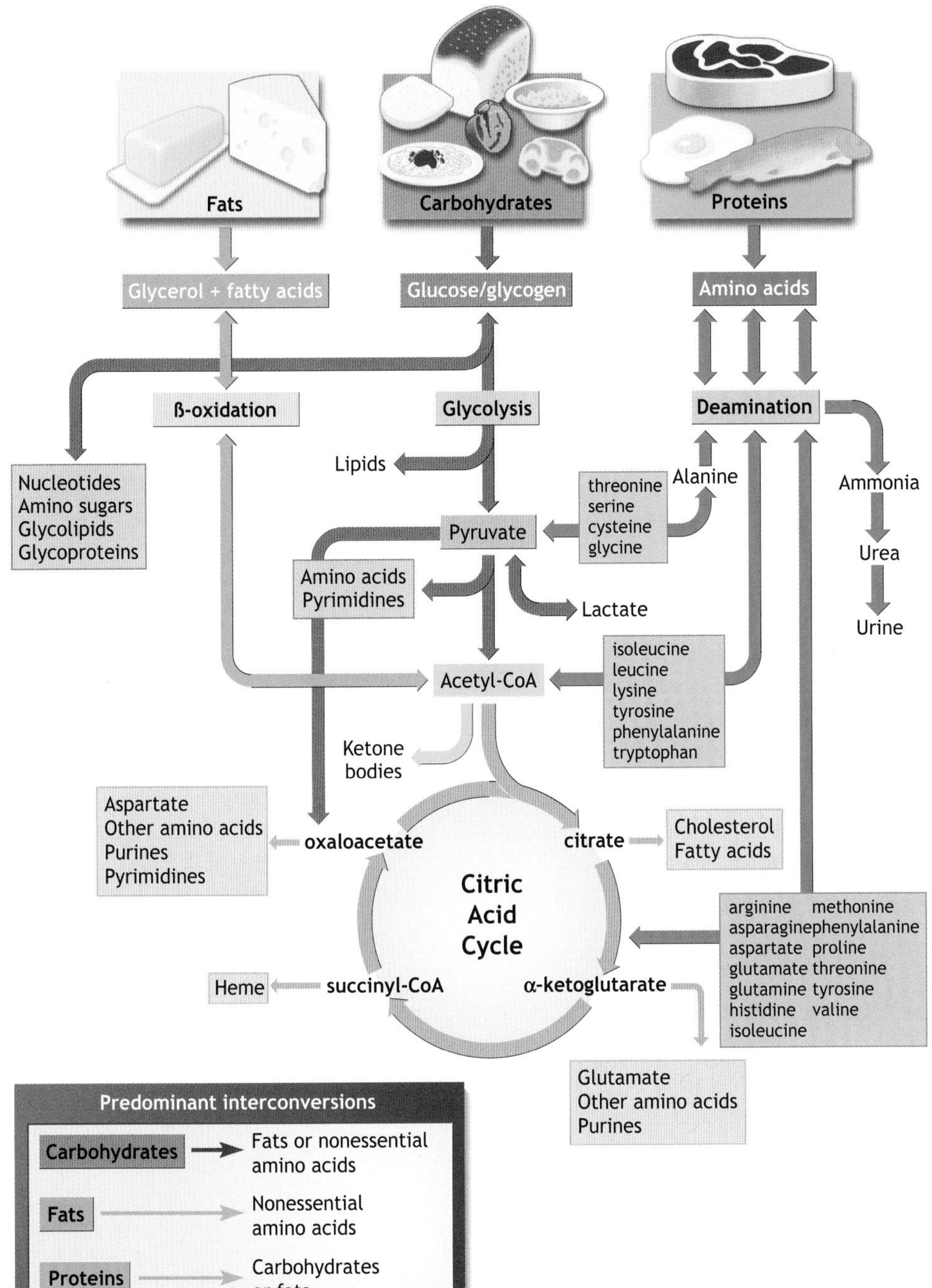

FIGURE 6.19 • The "metabolic mill" allows important interconversions for catabolism and anabolism among carbohydrates, fats, and proteins.

The "metabolic mill" depicts the citric acid cycle as the vital link between food (macronutrient) energy and the chemical energy in ATP. However, the citric acid cycle also serves as a metabolic hub to provide intermediates that cross the mitochondrial membrane into the cytosol for synthesis to bionutrients for maintenance and growth. For example, excess carbohydrates provide the glycerol and acetyl fragments to synthesize triglyceride. Acetyl-CoA functions as the starting point for synthesizing cholesterol and many hormones. Fatty acids *cannot* contribute to glucose synthesis because the conversion of pyruvate to acetyl-CoA does not reverse (notice the one-way arrow in Fig. 6.18). Many of the carbon compounds generated in citric acid cycle reactions also provide the organic starting points for synthesizing nonessential amino acids.

Glucose Conversion to Fat

The filling of muscle and liver glycogen stores causes any excess caloric intake as carbohydrate to convert to fat. Glucose enters the **pentose-phosphate pathway**, whose end products

IN A PRACTICAL SENSE

➤➤ POTENTIAL FOR GLUCOSE SYNTHESIS FROM TRIGLYCERIDE COMPONENTS

Circulating glucose provides vital fuel for brain and red blood cell functions. Maintaining blood glucose homeostasis becomes a challenge during prolonged starvation or high-intensity endurance exercise, when muscle and liver glycogen reserves rapidly deplete. When this occurs, the central nervous system eventually metabolizes ketone bodies as an energy fuel. Concurrently, muscle protein (amino acids) degrades to gluconeogenic constituents to sustain plasma glucose levels. Muscle protein catabolism eventually produces a muscle-wasting effect. Reliance on protein catabolism, coincident with depleted glycogen, continues because fatty acids from triglyceride hydrolysis in muscle and adipose tissue fail to provide gluconeogenic substrates.

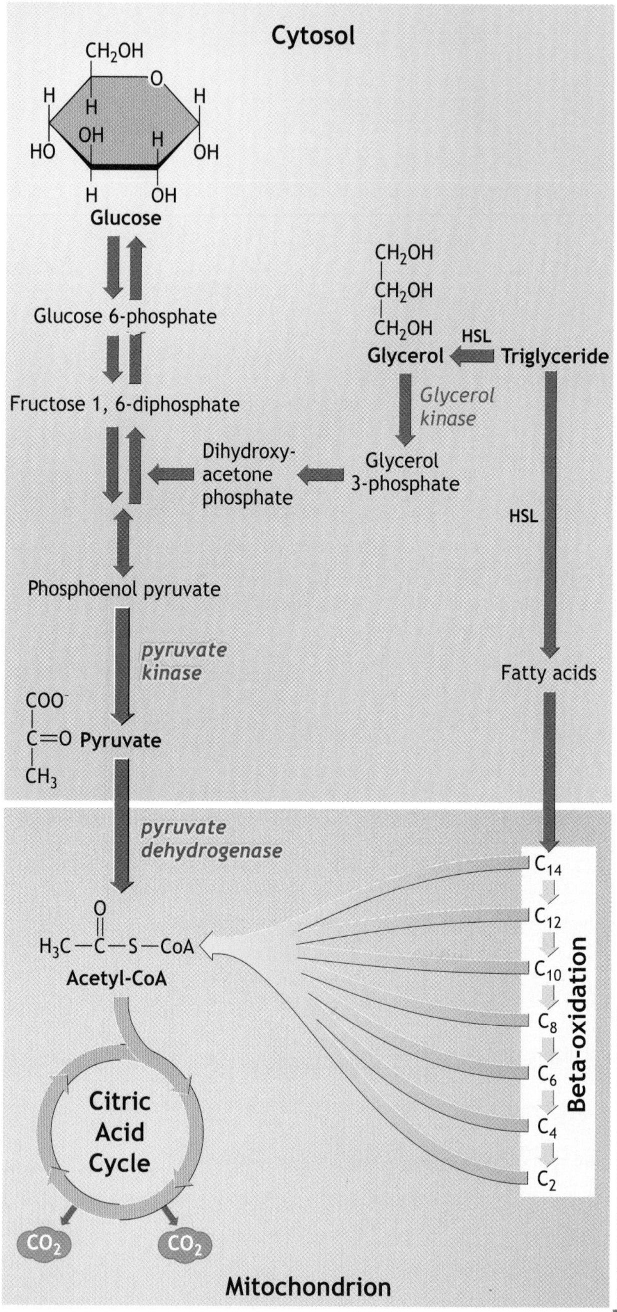

No Glucose Synthesis From Fatty Acids

The figure illustrates why humans cannot convert fatty acids (palmitate in example) from triglyceride breakdown to glucose. Fatty acid oxidation within the mitochondria produces acetyl-CoA. Because the *pyruvate dehydrogenase* and *pyruvate kinase* reactions proceed irreversibly, acetyl-CoA cannot simply form pyruvate by carboxylation and synthesize glucose by reversing glycolysis. Instead, the two-carbon acetyl group formed from acetyl-CoA degrades further when it enters the citric acid cycle. Hence, in humans, fatty acid hydrolysis produces *no* net synthesis of glucose.

Limited Glucose From Triglyceride-Derived Glycerol

The figure also shows that triglyceride hydrolysis via hormone-sensitive lipase (HSL) also produces a single three-carbon glycerol molecule. Unlike fatty acids, the liver can use glycerol for glucose synthesis. After delivery of glycerol in the blood to the liver, *glycerol kinase* phosphorylates it to glycerol 3-phosphate. Further reduction produces dihydroxyacetone phosphate, a substance that provides the carbon skeleton for glucose synthesis.

There is a clear "practical application" to sports and exercise nutrition from an understanding of the limited metabolic pathways available for glucose synthesis from the body's triglyceride energy depots. Because replenishment and maintenance of liver and muscle glycogen reserves so intimately depend on exogeneous carbohydrate intake, the physically active person must make a concerted effort to regularly consume nutritious, low-to moderate-glycemic sources of this macronutrient.

form a temporary diversion from the glycolytic pathway. The metabolites eventually rejoin the main glycolytic route, pass into the mitochondrion, and enter the citric acid cycle for oxidation. In the well-fed state, however, citrate diverts from the mitochondrion into the cytosol for fatty acid synthesis. After a meal, for example, insulin release from the pancreas causes a 30-fold increase in glucose transport into adipocytes. Insulin initiates the translocation of a latent pool of GLUT 4 transporters from the adipocyte cytosol to the plasma membrane. GLUT 4 action facilitates glucose transport into the cytosol for synthesis to triglycerides and subsequent storage within the adipocyte.

Protein Conversion to Fat

As in the case of carbohydrate, surplus dietary protein readily converts to fat. The amino acids absorbed by the small intestine after protein's digestion are transported to the liver. Carbon skeletons derived from these amino acids after deamination convert to pyruvate as shown in Figure 6.19. The pyruvate then enters the mitochondrion for conversion to acetyl-CoA for either (1) catabolism in the citric acid cycle or (2) fatty acid synthesis.

Fats Burn in a Carbohydrate Flame

Interestingly, in metabolically active tissues, fatty acid breakdown depends somewhat on continual background levels of carbohydrate catabolism. Recall that acetyl-CoA enters the citric acid cycle by combining with oxaloacetate to form citrate. Oxaloacetate generates from pyruvate during carbohydrate breakdown under enzymatic control of pyruvate carboxylase, which adds a carboxyl group to the pyruvate molecule. The degradation of fatty acids in the citric acid cycle continues only if sufficient oxaloacetate and other intermediates combine with acetyl-CoA formed during β-oxidation. However, these intermediates are continually lost or removed from the cycle and need to be replenished. Pyruvate formed during glucose metabolism plays an important role in maintaining a proper level of oxaloacetate (Figs. 6.15 and 6.19). Low pyruvate levels bring about reduced levels of citric acid cycle intermediates (oxaloacetate and malate), which slows citric acid cycle activity.[7,14,25,26,32,36] In this sense, "fats burn in a carbohydrate flame."

A Slower Rate of Energy Release From Fat

A rate limit exists for fatty acid use by active muscle.[37] Aerobic training enhances this limit, although the power generated solely by fat breakdown represents only about one-half that achieved with carbohydrate as the chief aerobic energy source. Thus, depleting muscle glycogen must decrease a muscle's maximum aerobic power output. Just as the hypoglycemic condition coincides with a "central" or neural fatigue, muscle glycogen depletion probably causes "peripheral" or local muscle fatigue during exercise.

Gluconeogenesis provides a metabolic option for synthesizing glucose from noncarbohydrate sources, but it cannot replenish or even maintain glycogen stores without regular carbohydrate consumption. Appreciably reducing carbohydrate availability seriously limits energy transfer capacity. Glycogen depletion can occur in prolonged exercise (marathon running), consecutive days of heavy training, inadequate energy intake, dietary elimination of carbohydrates (as advocated with high-fat, low-carbohydrate "ketogenic diets"), or diabetes. Aerobic exercise intensity is depressed even though large amounts of fatty acid substrate circulate to muscle. With extreme carbohydrate depletion, the acetate fragments produced in β-oxidation (acetoacetate and β -hydroxybutyrate) accumulate in extracellular fluids because they cannot enter the citric acid cycle. The liver readily converts these compounds to ketone bodies, some of which pass in the urine. If ketosis persists, the acid quality of the body fluids can increase to potentially toxic levels.

Summary

1. Food macronutrients provide the major sources of potential energy to form ATP from the rejoining of ADP and phosphate ion.
2. The complete breakdown of 1 mole of glucose liberates 689 kcal of energy. Of this, ATP bonds conserve about 263 kcal (38%), with the remainder dissipated as heat.
3. During glycolytic reactions in the cell's cytosol, a net of two ATP molecules forms during anaerobic substrate-level phosphorylation.
4. Pyruvate converts to acetyl-CoA during the second stage of carbohydrate breakdown within the mitochondrion. Acetyl-CoA then progresses through the citric acid cycle.
5. Hydrogen atoms released during glucose breakdown oxidize via the respiratory chain; the released energy couples with ADP phosphorylation.
6. The complete oxidation of a glucose molecule in skeletal muscle yields a total of 36 ATP molecules.
7. Oxidation of hydrogen atoms at their rate of formation establishes a biochemical steady state or "steady rate."
8. During heavy exercise, when hydrogen oxidation does not keep pace with its production, pyruvate temporarily binds hydrogen, and lactate forms. This allows progression of anaerobic glycolysis for an additional time.
9. Compounds that either inhibit or activate enzymes at key control points in the oxidative pathways modulate enzymatic regulatory control of glycolysis and the citric acid cycle.
10. By far, cellular ADP concentration exerts the greatest effect on the rate-limiting enzymes that control energy metabolism.
11. The complete oxidation of a triglyceride molecule yields about 460 ATP molecules. Fatty acid catabolism requires oxygen; the term aerobic describes such reactions.
12. Protein serves as a potentially important energy substrate. After nitrogen removal from the amino acid molecule during deamination, the remaining carbon skeletons enter various metabolic pathways to produce ATP aerobically.
13. Numerous interconversions take place among the food nutrients. Fatty acids represent a noteworthy exception; they cannot yield glucose.
14. Fats require intermediates generated in carbohydrate breakdown for their continual catabolism for energy in the metabolic mill. To this extent, "fats burn in a carbohydrate flame."

References

1. Balban RS. Regulation of oxidative phosphorylation in the mammalian cell. Am J Physiol 1990;258:C377.
2. Bertocci LA, Gollnick PD. pH effect on mitochondria and individual enzyme function. Med Sci Sports Exerc 1985;17:244.
3. Bodner GM. Metabolism: Part I. Glycolysis, or the Embden-Myerhof pathway. J Chem Educ 1986;63:566.
4. Bodner GM. The tricarboxylic acid (TCA), citric acid, Krebs cycle. J Chem Educ 1986;63:673.
5. Brooks GA. Physical activity and carbohydrate metabolism. In: Bouchard C, et al., eds. Physical activity, fitness, and health. Champaign, IL: Human Kinetics, 1994.
6. Brooks GA. Intra- and extra-cellular lactate shuttles. Med Sci Sports Exerc 2000;35:778.
7. Campbell MK. Biochemistry. 2nd ed. Philadelphia: WB Saunders, 1999.
8. Carins SP, et al. Role of extracellular [Ca^{2+}] in fatigue of isolated mammalian skeletal muscle. J Appl Physiol 1998;84:1395.
9. Chasiotis D. Role of cyclic AMP and inorganic phosphate in the regulation of muscle glycogenolysis during exercise. Med Sci Sports Exerc 1988;20:545.
10. Coggan AR, et al. Plasma glucose kinetics during exercise in subjects with high and low lactate thresholds. J Appl Physiol 1992;73:1873.
11. Coggan AR, et al. Isotopic estimation of CO_2 production during exercise before and after endurance training. J Appl Physiol 1993;75:70.
12. Coppack SW, et al. In vivo regulation of lipolysis in humans. J Lipid Res 1994;35:177.
13. Febbario MA, et al. Effect of epinephrine on muscle glycogenolysis during exercise in trained men. J Appl Physiol 1998;84:465.
14. Gibala MJ, et al. Tricarboxylic acid cycle intermediates in human muscle at rest and during prolonged cycling. Am J Physiol 1997;272(Endocrinol Metab 35):E239.
15. Gladden BL. Muscle as a consumer of lactate. Med Sci Sports Exerc 2000;32:764.
16. Greehnaff PL, Timmons JA. Interaction between aerobic and anaerobic metabolism during intense muscle contraction. Exerc Sport Sci Rev 1998;26:1.
17. Hogan MC, et al. Increased [lactate] in working dog muscle reduces tension development independent of pH. Med Sci Sports Exerc 1995;27:371.
18. Hultman E, et al. Energy metabolism and fatigue. In: Taylor AW, et al., eds. Biochemistry of exercise VII. Champaign, IL: Human Kinetics, 1990.
19. Jacobs I, et al. Effects of prior exercise or ammonium chloride ingestion on muscular strength and endurance. Med Sci Sports Exerc 1993;25:809.
20. Kiens B, et al. Skeletal muscle substrate utilization during submaximal exercise in man: effect of endurance training. J Physiol 1993;469:459.
21. MacRae HS-H, et al. Effects of training on lactate production and removal during progressive exercise. J Appl Physiol 1992;72:1649.
22. Mainwood GW, Renaud JM. The effect of acid-base on fatigue of skeletal muscle. Can J Physiol Pharmacol 1985;63:403.
23. Mudio DM, et al. Effects of dietary fat on metabolic adjustments to maximal $\dot{V}O_2$ and endurance in runners. Med Sci Sports Exerc 1994;26:81.
24. Murray R, et al. Physiological responses to glycerol ingestion during exercise. J Appl Physiol 1991;71:144.
25. Owen OE, et al. Protein, fat, and carbohydrate requirements during starvation: anaplerosis and cataplerosis. Am J Clin Nutr 1998;68:12.
26. Richter EA. Interaction of fuels in muscle metabolism during exercise. Integration of medical and sport sciences. Basal: Karger, 1992.
27. Romijn JA, et al. Regulations of endogenous fat and carbohydrate metabolism in relation to exercise intensity and duration. Am J Physiol 1993;265:E380.
28. Rennie, MJ. How to avoid running on empty. J Physiol 2000;528(Pt1):3.
29. Seip RL, Semenkovich CF. Skeletal muscle lipoprotein lipase: molecular regulation and physiological effects in relation to exercise. Exerc Sport Sci Rev 1998;26:191.
30. Shepherd RE, Bah MD. Cyclic AMP regulation of fuel metabolism during exercise: regulation of adipose tissue lipolysis during exercise. Med Sci Sports Exerc 1988;20:531.
31. Stefanick ML, Wood PD. Physical activity, lipid and lipoprotein metabolism, and lipid transport. In: Bouchard C, et al., eds. Physical activity, fitness, and health. Champaign, IL: Human Kinetics, 1994.
32. Stryer L. Biochemistry. 4th ed. San Francisco: WH Freeman, 1995.
33. Sumida KD, et al. Enhanced gluconeogenesis from lactate in perfused livers after endurance training. J Appl Physiol 1993;74:782.
34. Thompson DL, et al. Substrate use during and following moderate- and low-intensity exercise: implications for weight control. Eur J Appl Physiol 1998;78:43.
35. Trump ME, et al. Importance of muscle phosphocreatine during intermittent maximal cycling. J Appl Physiol 1996;80:1574.
36. Turcoatte LP, et al. Impaired plasma FFA oxidation imposed by extreme CHO deficiency in contracting rat skeletal muscle. J Appl Physiol 1994;77:517.
37. van der Vusse GJ, et al. Lipid metabolism in muscle. Handbook of physiology, section 12: Exercise: regulation and integration of multiple systems. New York: Oxford Press, 1996.

Suggested Resources

Bjorntorp P. Importance of fat as a support nutrient for energy: metabolism of athletes. In: Williams C, Devlin JT, eds. Foods, nutrition and sports performance. London: E & FN Spon, 1992.

Brooks GA, et al. Exercise physiology: human bioenergetics and its applications. 3rd ed. Mountain View, CA: Mayfield, 2000.

Cerretelli P. Energy sources for muscular exercise. Int J Sports Med 1992;13(Suppl 1):S106.

Hargreaves M. Interactions between muscle glycogen and blood glucose during exercise. Exerc Sport Sci Rev 1997;25:21.

Horton ES, Terjung RL, eds. Exercise, nutrition, and energy metabolism. 2nd ed. New York: Macmillan, 1994.

Marieb EN. Human anatomy and physiology. 3rd ed. Redwood City, CA: Benjamin Cummings, 1999.

Martin WH III, et al. Effect of endurance training on plasma free fatty acid turnover and oxidation during exercise. Am J Physiol 1993;E708.

Mott-Smith M. The concept of energy simply explained. New York: Dover, 1964.

Nelson DL, Cox MM. Lehninger's principles of biochemistry. 3rd ed. New York: Worth, 2000.

Nicklas BJ. Effects of endurance exercise on adipose tissue metabolism. Exerc Sport Sci Rev 1997;25:77.

Shils ME, et al. Modern nutrition in health and disease. 9th ed. Baltimore: Lippincott Williams & Wilkins, 1999.

Stryer L. Biochemistry. 4th ed. San Francisco: WH Freeman, 1995.

Vander AJ, et al. Human physiology: the mechanisms of body function. 7th ed. New York: McGraw-Hill, 1997.

CHAPTER 7

Energy Transfer in Exercise

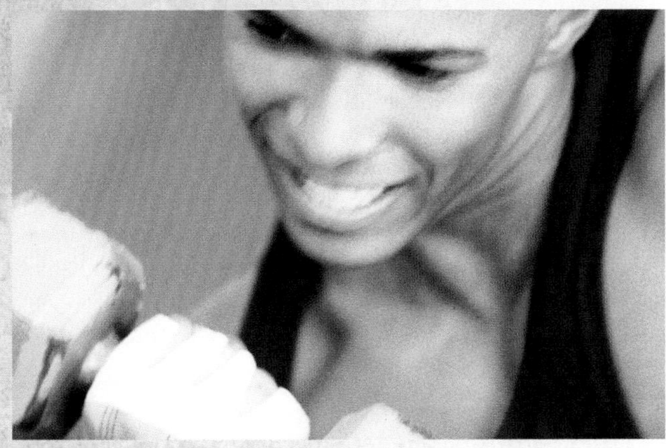

Chapter Objectives

- Identify the body's three energy systems and outline the relative contribution of each in terms of exercise intensity and duration; relate your discussion to specific sport activities
- Discuss blood lactate threshold, indicating differences between sedentary and endurance-trained individuals
- Outline the time course for oxygen consumption during 10 minutes of moderate exercise
- Draw a figure to illustrate oxygen consumption during progressive increments in exercise intensity up to maximum
- Differentiate between type I and type II muscle fibers
- Discuss differences in recovery oxygen consumption patterns from moderate and exhaustive exercise; what factors account for the excess postexercise oxygen consumption (EPOC) from each form of exercise?
- Outline optimal recovery procedures from steady-rate and non–steady-rate exercise
- Discuss the rationale for using intermittent exercise for interval training

Physical activity provides the greatest demand for energy. In sprint running and swimming, for example, energy output from active muscles exceeds their resting value by 120 times or more. During less-intense but sustained exercise such as marathon running, the whole-body energy requirement increases 20 to 30 times above resting levels. The relative contribution of the different energy transfer systems differs markedly depending on intensity and duration of exercise and the specific fitness status of the participant.

IMMEDIATE ENERGY: THE ATP–PCr SYSTEM

Exercise of short duration and high intensity such as a 100-m dash, 25-m swim, or lifting a heavy weight requires an immediate energy supply provided almost exclusively from the intramuscular high-energy phosphates, or phosphagens, adenosine triphosphate (ATP) and phosphocreatine (PCr). Each kilogram of skeletal muscle contains 3 to 8 mmol of ATP and 4 to 5 times more PCr.[43] For a 70-kg person with a muscle mass of 30 kg, this represents between 570 and 690 mmol of high-energy phosphates. Assuming that 20 kg of muscle becomes active during "big-muscle" exercise, sufficient stored phosphagen energy exists to walk briskly for 1 minute, run at marathon pace for 20 to 30 seconds, or sprint run for 5 to 8 seconds. (The maximum rate of energy transfer from the intramuscular high-energy phosphates exceeds by four to eight times the maximal energy transfer from aerobic metabolism.) In a world record 100-m sprint (9.84 s, or 27.1 mph), the runner cannot maintain maximum speed throughout the run. During the last few seconds, the runner actually slows, with the winner often slowing down least. In this situation, the quantity of intramuscular high-energy phosphates significantly affects performance.

All sports use the high-energy phosphates, but many rely almost exclusively on this means of energy transfer. For example, success in football, weight lifting, field events, baseball, and volleyball requires brief but maximal efforts during the performance. Visualize a breakaway for the goal in ice hockey or soccer, driving for a lay-up in basketball, thrusting upward in a pole vault, or an end run in football without the capability for generating energy rapidly from the stored phosphagens. However, the ability to sustain exercise beyond a brief period and recover from a prior all-out effort requires additional energy for ATP replenishment. If this does not occur, the "fuel" supply diminishes, and high-intensity movement ceases. As we discuss subsequently, the carbohydrate, fat, and protein macronutrients within the cellular fluids and tissue depots stand ready to continually recharge the available pool of high-energy phosphates to sustain exercise.

Nuclear Magnetic Resonance Spectroscopy to Study Exercise Muscle Metabolism

Nuclear magnetic resonance (**NMR**) spectroscopy provides a noninvasive means to study intracellular metabolism. NMR applies radio-frequency energy to probe and identify the con-

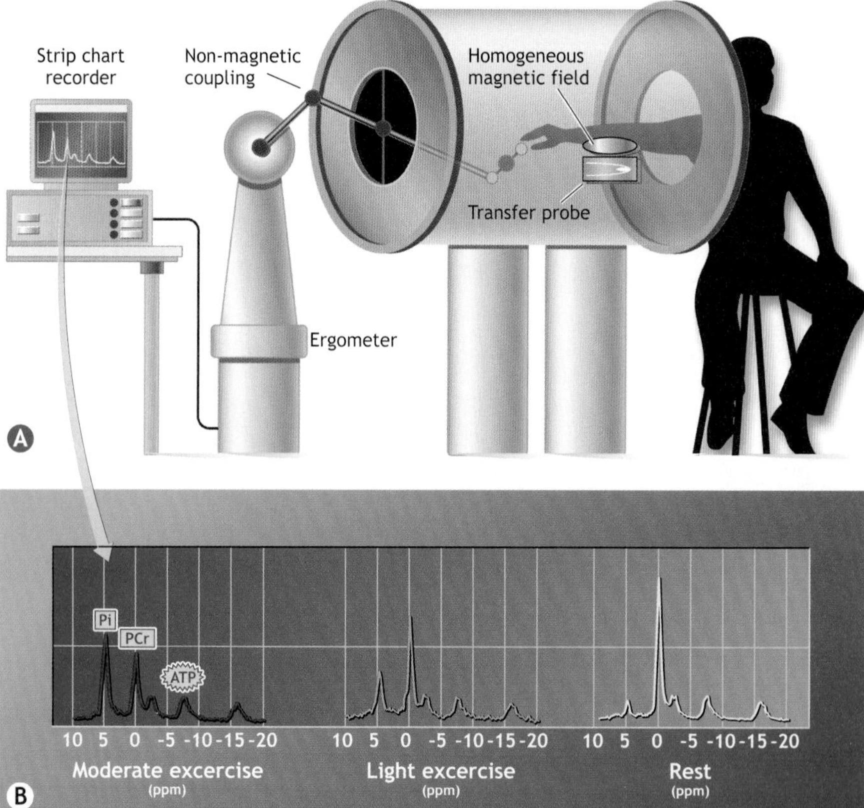

FIGURE 7.1 • NMR spectroscopy. **A**. The wrist flexor muscles are placed on a surface coil in a superconducting magnet. The subject grasps a handle attached to an isokinetic dynamometer (constant velocity, variable force output) while observing a recorder that provides feedback on the level of force production. **B**. Example of NMR spectroscopy spectra for ATP, PCr, and inorganic phosphate (Pi) during rest and two levels of exercise. Ppm, parts per million. (From McCully KK, et al., Application of ^{31}P magnetic resonance spectroscopy to the study of athletic performance. Sports Med 1988;5:312.)

tent of chemical elements and compounds within living tissue. The technique provides the opportunity to continuously monitor relative concentrations and turnover rates of phosphorylated high-energy compounds and other metabolic events within muscle during exercise.[11,54,55] Measurements take place at regular intervals without the disruptive consequences of the muscle biopsy technique. Figure 7.1A illustrates the NMR method during wrist flexion exercise. The active muscles are placed over a superconducting magnet while the subject exercises under conditions that control for power output, contraction speed, and exercise duration. Application of specific radio-frequency pulses within a strong magnetic field determines concentrations of diverse bioactive compounds. Figure 7.1B shows the results for ATP, PCr, and inorganic phosphate during rest and low- and moderate-intensity exercise. The areas under the peaks correspond to relative concentrations of free phosphorus compounds, including the three phosphorus atoms of ATP. Such elegant studies of the ratio of inorganic phosphate (phosphate ion) to PCr provide insight into the rate of mitochondrial respiration. With this methodology, investigators have studied muscle injury, glycolytic metabolism, and the effects of training on the intricacies of muscle metabolism, including the relationships among local muscle substrate catabolism, cardiovascular functional capacity, and exercise performance.[12,50]

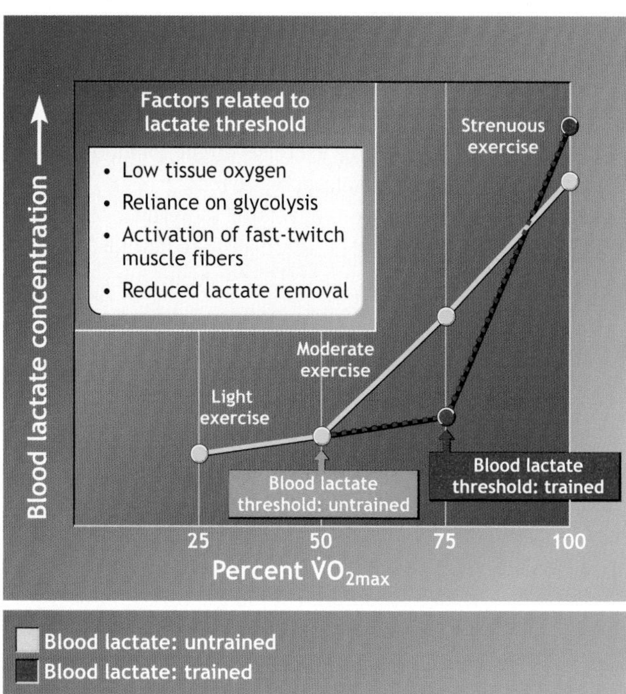

FIGURE 7.2 • Blood lactate concentration for trained and untrained subjects at different levels of exercise expressed as a percentage of maximal oxygen consumption ($\dot{V}O_{2max}$).

SHORT-TERM ENERGY: THE LACTIC ACID SYSTEM

Resynthesis of the high-energy phosphates must proceed at a rapid rate for strenuous exercise to continue. The energy to phosphorylate ADP during intense exercise derives mainly from stored muscle glycogen through anaerobic glycolysis (maximal energy transfer rate 45% that of the high-energy phosphates), with resulting lactate formation. In a way, anaerobic glycolysis with lactate formation buys time. It allows ATP to form rapidly by substrate-level phosphorylation, even though the oxygen supply remains inadequate and/or energy demands outstrip the muscle's capacity to resynthesize ATP aerobically. Anaerobic energy for ATP resynthesis in glycolysis can be viewed as reserve fuel activated when a person accelerates during the last few hundred yards of a mile run or performs all-out during a 440-yard run or 100-yard swim. *Rapid, large accumulations of blood lactate occur during maximal exercise lasting between 60 and 180 seconds.* Decreasing the intensity of such arduous exercise to extend the exercise period correspondingly decreases both the rate of accumulation and the final level of blood lactate.[46]

Lactate Accumulation

Blood lactate does not accumulate at all levels of exercise. Figure 7.2 illustrates the general relationship between oxygen consumption, expressed as a percentage of maximum, and blood lactate during light, moderate, and heavy exercise by endurance athletes and untrained subjects. Oxygen-consuming reactions adequately meet the energy demands of the trained and untrained during relatively light exercise ($<50\%$ aerobic capacity). In biochemical terms, energy generated from the oxidation of hydrogen provides the predominant ATP for muscular activity. Any lactate formed in one part of a working muscle becomes rapidly oxidized by muscle fibers with high oxidative capacity (heart and other fibers in the same muscle or less-active neighboring muscles).[14,45,47] When lactate oxidation equals its production, blood lactate level remains stable, even though exercise intensity and oxygen consumption increase.

For healthy, untrained persons, blood lactate begins to accumulate and rise in an exponential fashion at about 55% of their maximal capacity for aerobic metabolism.[21] The usual explanation for a blood lactate accumulation in exercise assumes a relative tissue hypoxia. When glycolytic metabolism predominates, nicotinamide adenine dinucleotide (NADH) production exceeds the cell's capacity for shuttling its hydrogens (electrons) down the respiratory chain because insufficient oxygen exists at the tissue level. The imbalance in hydrogen release and subsequent oxidation (more precisely, the cytoplasmic $NAD^+/NADH$ ratio) causes pyruvate to accept the excess hydrogens, which results in lactate accumulation.[49]

Research using radioactive tracers to label the carbon in the glucose molecule provides an alternate explanation for lactate buildup in muscle and its subsequent appearance in blood.[13,23] These studies show that lactate continuously forms during rest and moderate exercise. Under aerobic conditions, lactate's rate of removal by other tissues matches its rate of formation, resulting in no *net* lactate accumulation (i.e., blood lactate concentration remains stable). Only when removal does not match production does blood lactate accumulate. Adaptations within muscle from aerobic training allow high rates of lactate turnover; thus lactate accumulates at higher exercise levels than in the untrained state.[63] Another explanation for lactate accumulation during exercise might include the tendency for the enzyme lactate dehydrogenase (LDH) in fast-twitch muscle fibers to favor conversion of pyruvate to lactate. On the other hand, the LDH level in slow-twitch fibers favors conversion of lactate to pyruvate. Therefore, recruitment of the fast-twitch fibers with increasing exercise intensity favors lactate formation, independent of tissue oxygenation.

Lactate production and accumulation accelerate as exercise becomes more intense and the muscle cells can neither meet the additional energy demands aerobically nor oxidize lactate at its rate of production. A similar pattern exists for untrained subjects and endurance athletes, except the threshold for lactate buildup, termed the **blood lactate threshold**, occurs at a higher percentage of the athlete's aerobic capacity.[20,28,67,69,70] Trained endurance athletes, for example, perform steady-rate aerobic exercise at intensities between 80 and 90% of their maximum capacity for aerobic metabolism.[66] This favorable aerobic response can be explained by the athletes' specific genetic endowment (e.g., muscle fiber type, muscle blood flow responsiveness), specific local training adaptations that favor less lactate production,[17,18,27,41] or a more rapid rate of lactate removal (lactate clearance or turnover) at any exercise intensity.[14,52] For example, capillary density and the size and number of mitochondria increase with endurance training, as does the concentration of enzymes and transfer agents in aerobic metabolism.[30,41,64] This training response remains unimpaired with aging.[19] Such adjustments and training adaptations certainly enhance cellular capacity to generate ATP aerobically through glucose and fatty acid catabolism. Maintaining a low lactate level also conserves glycogen reserves, which extends the duration of high-intensity aerobic effort. Chapter 14 further develops the concept of the blood lactate threshold, its measurement, and its relation to endurance performance and in Chapter 2 we discuss adaptations with training.

Lactate-Producing Capacity

The ability to generate high blood lactate levels during maximal exercise increases with specific sprint-power anaerobic training and subsequently decreases with detraining. Sprint-power athletes generally achieve 20 to 30% higher blood lactate levels than untrained counterparts during maximal short-duration exercise. The mechanism for this response likely results from one or more of the following factors: (1) improved motivation accompanying the trained state, (2) increased intramuscular glycogen stores that accompany training, which probably allow a greater contribution of energy via anaerobic glycolysis, and (3) a training-induced approximately 20% increase in enzymes that regulate glycolysis, particularly phosphofructokinase, However, their increases fall well below the two- to threefold increase in aerobic enzymes with endurance training.[41,45] Because tissues continually metabolize lactate during exercise and recovery, blood lactate accumulation measured at a specific time in recovery does not fully account for an individual's capacity for anaerobic metabolism as reflected by lactate accumulation.[28]

LONG-TERM ENERGY: THE AEROBIC SYSTEM

The reactions of glycolysis form relatively little ATP. Consequently, aerobic metabolism provides most of the energy transfer when intense exercise lasts beyond several minutes.

Oxygen Consumption During Exercise

Figure 7.3 illustrates oxygen consumption—also referred to as **pulmonary oxygen uptake** because oxygen measurements occur at the lung and not the active muscles—during each minute of a steady, relatively slow, 10-minute run. Oxygen consumption rises exponentially during the first minutes of exercise (fast component of exercise oxygen consumption) to reach a plateau between the third and fourth minutes.[10] It then remains relatively stable for the duration of the exercise. The terms **steady state** or **steady rate** generally describe the flat portion (plateau) of the oxygen consumption curve. Steady rate reflects a balance between energy required by the working muscles and ATP production in aerobic metabolism. Within this region, oxygen-consuming reactions supply the energy for exercise; any lactate produced either oxidizes or reconverts to glucose via the Cori cycle in the liver and pos-

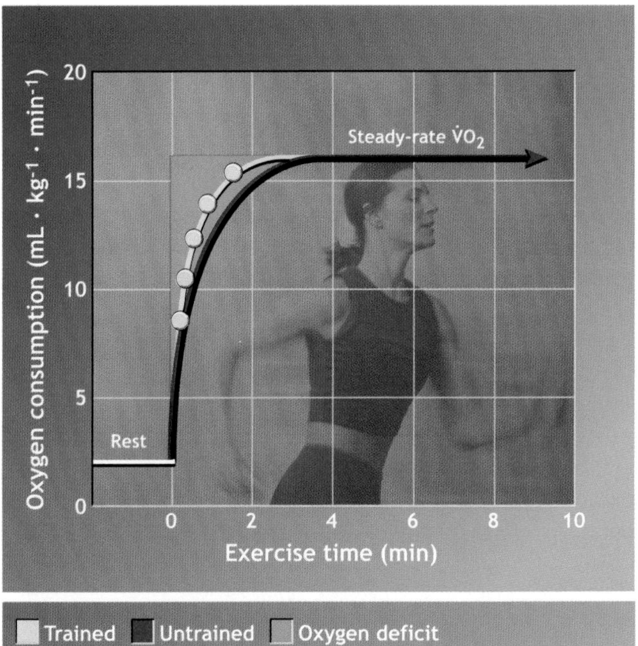

FIGURE 7.3 • Time course for oxygen consumption during a continuous jog at a relatively slow pace by an endurance-trained and an untrained individual. The *shaded area* indicates the oxygen deficit or quantity of oxygen that would have been consumed had oxygen consumption reached the steady-rate immediately.

sibly the kidneys. *Blood lactate does not accumulate under steady-rate metabolic conditions.*

Once a person attains a steady rate of aerobic metabolism, exercise could theoretically progress indefinitely if the individual possessed the will to continue. This, of course, assumes that steady-rate aerobic metabolism singularly determines one's capacity to sustain submaximal exercise. Fluid loss and electrolyte depletion often pose significant limiting factors, especially during exercise in hot weather. In addition, maintaining adequate reserves of both liver glycogen for central nervous system function and muscle glycogen to power exercise takes on added significance at high intensities of prolonged aerobic effort. Glycogen depletion dramatically reduces exercise capacity.

Individuals possess many exercise steady-rate levels. For some, the spectrum might range from sitting and watching TV to pushing a power lawn mower for 20 minutes. An elite endurance runner maintains a steady rate of aerobic metabolism throughout a 26.2-mile marathon, averaging slightly less than 5 minutes per mile, or during a 658-mile ultramarathon, averaging 118 miles a day over 5.6 days! These magnificent endurance accomplishments result from a high capacity of the central circulation to *deliver* oxygen to the working muscles and a high capacity of those muscles to *use* the oxygen available.

Oxygen Deficit

Once exercise begins, the oxygen consumption curve shown in Figure 7.3 does not increase instantaneously to steady rate. In the beginning transitional stage of constant-load exercise, oxygen consumption falls considerably below the steady-rate level, even though the energy requirement remains unchanged throughout the exercise period. A lag in oxygen consumption early in exercise should not be surprising, because the energy for muscle contraction comes directly from the immediate, anaerobic breakdown of ATP. Even with experimentally increased oxygen availability and increased oxygen diffusion gradients at the tissue level, the initial increase in exercise oxygen consumption always lags behind energy expenditure.[33,34] Owing to the interaction of (1) intrinsic inertia in cellular metabolic signals and enzyme activation and (2) the sluggishness of oxygen delivery to the mitochondria, the hydrogens produced in energy metabolism do not immediately oxidize and combine with oxygen.[58,66] Oxygen consumption becomes evident in subsequent energy transfer reactions when oxygen combines with the hydrogens liberated in glycolysis, β-oxidation of fatty acids, or the reactions of the citric acid cycle. In other words, without substrate (hydrogens), oxygen is not consumed. After several minutes of submaximal exercise, hydrogen production and subsequent oxidation becomes proportional to exercise intensity, and oxygen consumption attains a steady rate.

*The **oxygen deficit** quantitatively expresses the difference between the total oxygen actually consumed during exercise and the total that would have been consumed had steady-rate aerobic metabolism been reached from the start.* The energy derived in the early stage of exercise represents immediate energy transfer from the hydrolysis of intramuscular high-energy phosphates and glycolysis until steady-rate oxygen consumption matches energy demands. The kinetics of oxygen consumption at the onset of exercise do not differ in children and adults.[37]

Figure 7.4 depicts the relationship between the size of the oxygen deficit and the contribution of energy from the ATP–PCr and lactate energy systems. The high-energy phosphates are substantially depleted in exercise that generates about a 3- to 4-L oxygen deficit. Consequently, further exercise only progresses on a "pay-as-you-go" basis, with continual ATP resynthesis through either anaerobic glycolysis or the aerobic breakdown of macronutrients. Interestingly, lactate begins to increase in active muscle well before the high-energy phosphates reach their lowest levels. This indicates that glycolysis also contributes anaerobic energy in the early stages of vigorous exercise, even before full use of the high-energy phosphates. *Energy for exercise does not simply result from activation of a series of energy systems that "switch on" and "switch off" but rather from smooth blending, with considerable overlap of one mode of energy transfer to another.*[35,63]

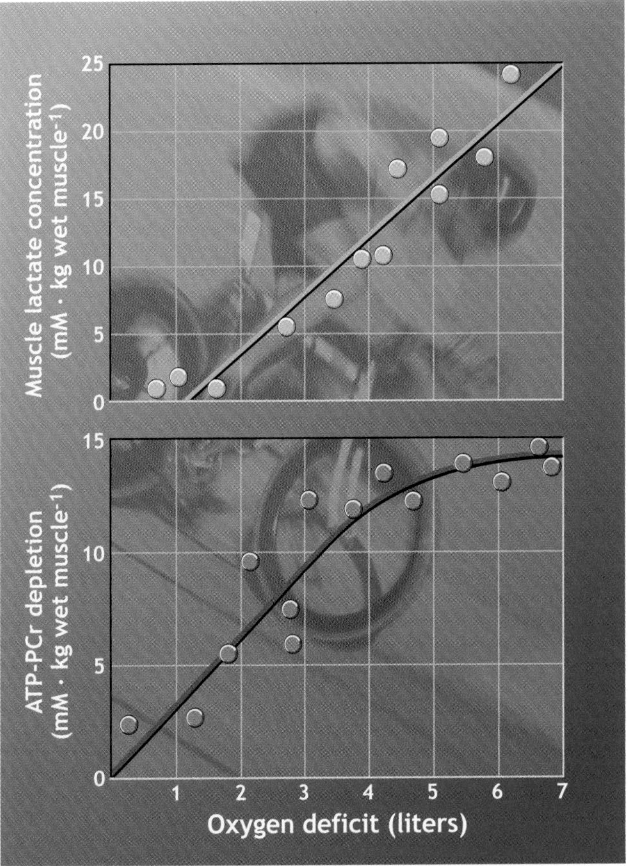

FIGURE 7.4 • Muscle ATP and PCr depletion and muscle lactate concentration in relation to the oxygen deficit. (Adapted from Pernow B, Karlsson J. Muscle ATP, PCr and lactate in submaximal and maximal exercise. In: Pernow B, Saltin B, eds. Muscle metabolism during exercise. New York: Plenum, 1971.)

Oxygen Deficit in the Trained and Untrained

Trained and untrained individuals attain similar steady-rate oxygen consumption values. The endurance-trained person, however, reaches steady rate more rapidly with a smaller oxygen deficit than the untrained (Fig. 7.3), sprint-power athletes, and cardiac patients.[24,36,42,51] Consequently, the aerobically trained person consumes a greater total amount of oxygen during steady-rate exercise and, presumably, the anaerobic component of exercise energy transfer becomes proportionately smaller. *A facilitated rate of aerobic metabolism in the early stages of exercise may result from a more rapid increase in overall blood flow (cardiac output) and/or a disproportionately large regional blood flow to active muscle complemented by training-induced cellular adaptations. Many of these adaptations increase cellular capacity to generate ATP aerobically (see Chapter 21).*

INTEGRATIVE QUESTION

Respond to a student who asks: "At what exercise level does the body switch to anaerobic energy metabolism?"

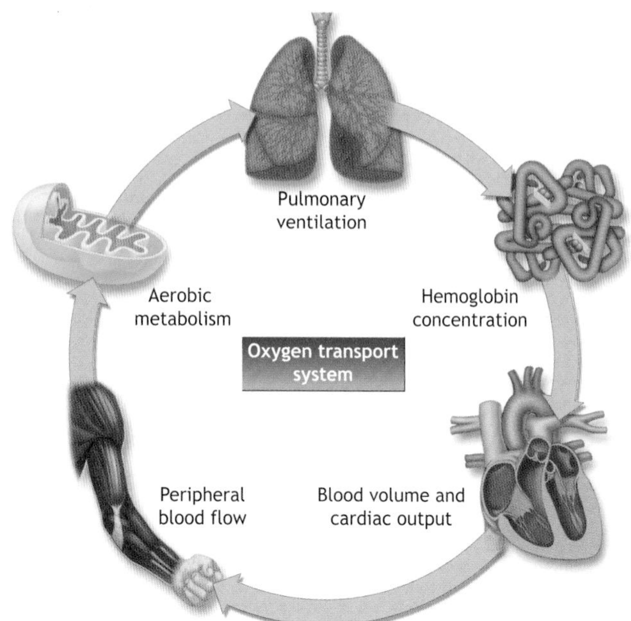

FIGURE 7.6 • The oxygen transport system. The physiologic significance of $\dot{V}O_{2max}$ relates to its dependence upon the functional capacity and integration of systems required for oxygen supply, transport, delivery, and use.

Maximal Oxygen Consumption

Figure 7.5 depicts oxygen consumption during a series of constant-speed runs up six progressively steeper hills. The laboratory simulates these hills by increasing the elevation of a treadmill or step bench or increasing the resistance to pedaling a bicycle ergometer. Each successive hill requires a greater energy output that places an additional demand on the capacity for aerobic ATP resynthesis. During the first several hills, oxygen consumption increases rapidly, with each new steady-rate value in direct proportion to exercise severity. The runner maintains speed up the two last hills, but oxygen consumption does not increase as rapidly or to the same extent as with the previous hills. No increase in oxygen consumption occurs during the run up the last hill. *The region in which oxygen consumption plateaus or increases only slightly with additional increases in exercise intensity represents the* ***maximal oxygen consumption****—also called maximal oxygen uptake, maximal aerobic power, aerobic capacity, or, simply* $\dot{V}O_{2max}$. Performing more-intense exercise results only from energy transfer in glycolysis, with a resulting lactate accumu-

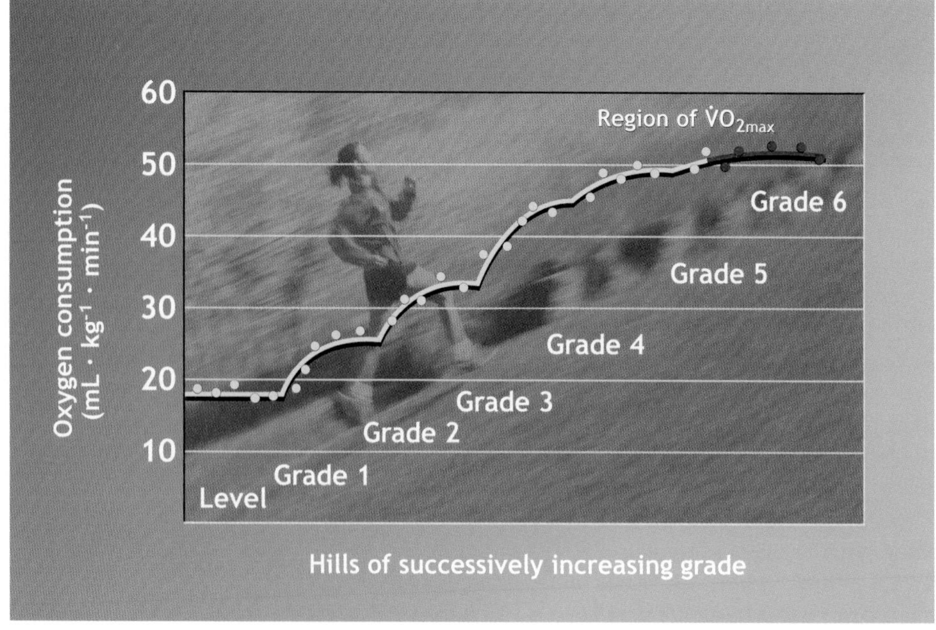

FIGURE 7.5 • Attainment of maximal oxygen consumption ($\dot{V}O_{2max}$) while running up hills of increasing slope. $\dot{V}O_{2max}$ occurs in the region where further increases in exercise intensity produce a less-than-expected increase (or no increase) in oxygen consumption. The *dots* represent measured values of oxygen consumption while running up each of the hills.

lation. Under these conditions, the runner soon becomes exhausted and unable to continue.

The $\dot{V}O_{2max}$ provides a quantitative measure of a person's *capacity* for aerobic ATP resynthesis. This makes the $\dot{V}O_{2max}$ an important determinant of the ability to sustain high-intensity exercise for longer than 4 or 5 minutes. Attainment of a high $\dot{V}O_{2max}$ has important physiologic meaning in addition to its role in sustaining energy metabolism. High aerobic power requires the integrated and high-level response of diverse physiologic support systems illustrated in Figure 7.6. In subsequent chapters, we discuss various aspects of $\dot{V}O_{2max}$, including its physiologic significance, measurement, and role in exercise performance and cardiovascular health.

Fast- and Slow-Twitch Muscle Fibers

Extracting about 20 to 40 mg of tissue (the size of a grain of rice) during surgical biopsy gives exercise physiologists the means to study functional and structural characteristics of human skeletal muscle. Two distinct types of muscle fiber exist in humans. A **fast-twitch (FT)**, or **type II**, fiber has two primary subdivisions, type IIa and type IIb, each possessing rapid contraction speed and high capacity for anaerobic ATP production in glycolysis. The type IIa fiber also possesses somewhat higher aerobic capacity. Type II fibers become active during change-of-pace and stop-and-go activities like basketball, soccer, and ice hockey. They also contribute increased force output when running or cycling up a hill while maintaining a constant speed or during all-out effort requiring rapid, powerful movements that depend almost exclusively on energy from anaerobic metabolism.

The second fiber-type, the **slow-twitch (ST)**, or **type I**, muscle fiber, generates energy primarily through aerobic pathways. This fiber possesses a relatively slow contraction speed compared with its fast-twitch counterpart. Its capacity to generate ATP aerobically intimately relates to numerous large mitochondria and high levels of enzymes required for aerobic metabolism, particularly fatty acid catabolism. Slow-twitch muscle fibers primarily sustain continuous activities requiring a steady rate of aerobic energy transfer. Fatigue in prolonged running is associated with glycogen depletion in the leg muscles' type I and type IIa muscle fibers.[2,31] This selective glycogen depletion pattern also occurs in the arms of wheelchair-dependent athletes during extended periods of exercise.[62] More than likely, the predominance of slow-twitch muscle fibers greatly contributes to high blood lactate thresholds observed among elite endurance athletes.[47,61] Figure 7.7 illustrates the muscle fiber type composition of two athletes in sports that rely on distinctly different energy systems that would be favored by a specific fiber type predominance. For the 50-m sprint swim champion, type II fibers represent nearly 80% of the total muscle fibers, whereas the endurance cyclist possesses 80% type I fibers. From a practical perspective, most sports require relatively slow, sustained muscle actions interspersed with short bursts of powerful effort (e.g.,

IN A PRACTICAL SENSE

➤➤ INTERPRETING $\dot{V}O_{2MAX}$—ESTABLISHING CARDIOVASCULAR FITNESS CATEGORIES

Cardiovascular fitness reflects the maximal amount of oxygen consumed during each minute of near-maximal exercise. These values for maximal oxygen consumption, or $\dot{V}O_{2max}$, generally are expressed in milliliters of oxygen per kg of body mass per minute ($mL \cdot kg^{-1} \cdot min^{-1}$). Individual values can range from about 10 $mL \cdot kg^{-1} \cdot min^{-1}$ in cardiac patients to 80 or 90 $mL \cdot kg^{-1} \cdot min^{-1}$ in world-class runners and cross-country skiers. Men and women distance runners, swimmers, cyclists, and cross-country skiers generally attain $\dot{V}O_{2max}$ values nearly double those of sedentary persons (see Fig. 11.8).

Researchers have measured the $\dot{V}O_{2max}$ of thousands of individuals of different ages. The average values and respective ranges for men and women of different ages establish category values to classify individuals for cardiovascular fitness. The table presents a five-part classification based upon data from the literature.

CARDIOVASCULAR FITNESS CLASSIFICATIONS

GENDER	AGE	POOR	FAIR	AVERAGE	GOOD	EXCELLENT
Men	≤29	≤24.9	25-33.9	34-43.9	44-52.9	≥53
	30-39	≤22.9	23-30.9	31-41.9	42-49.9	≥50
	40-49	≤19.9	20-26.9	27-38.9	39-44.9	≥45
	50-59	≤17.9	18-24.9	25-37.9	38-42.9	≥43
	60-69	≤15.9	16-22.9	23-35.9	36-40.9	≥41
Women	≤29	≤23.9	24-30.9	31-38.9	39-48.9	≥49
	30-39	≤19.9	20-27.9	28-36.9	37-44.9	≥45
	40-49	≤16.9	17-24.9	25-34.9	35-41.9	≥42
	50-59	≤14.9	15-21.9	22-33.9	34-39.9	≥40
	60-69	≤12.9	13-20.9	21-32.9	33-36.9	≥37

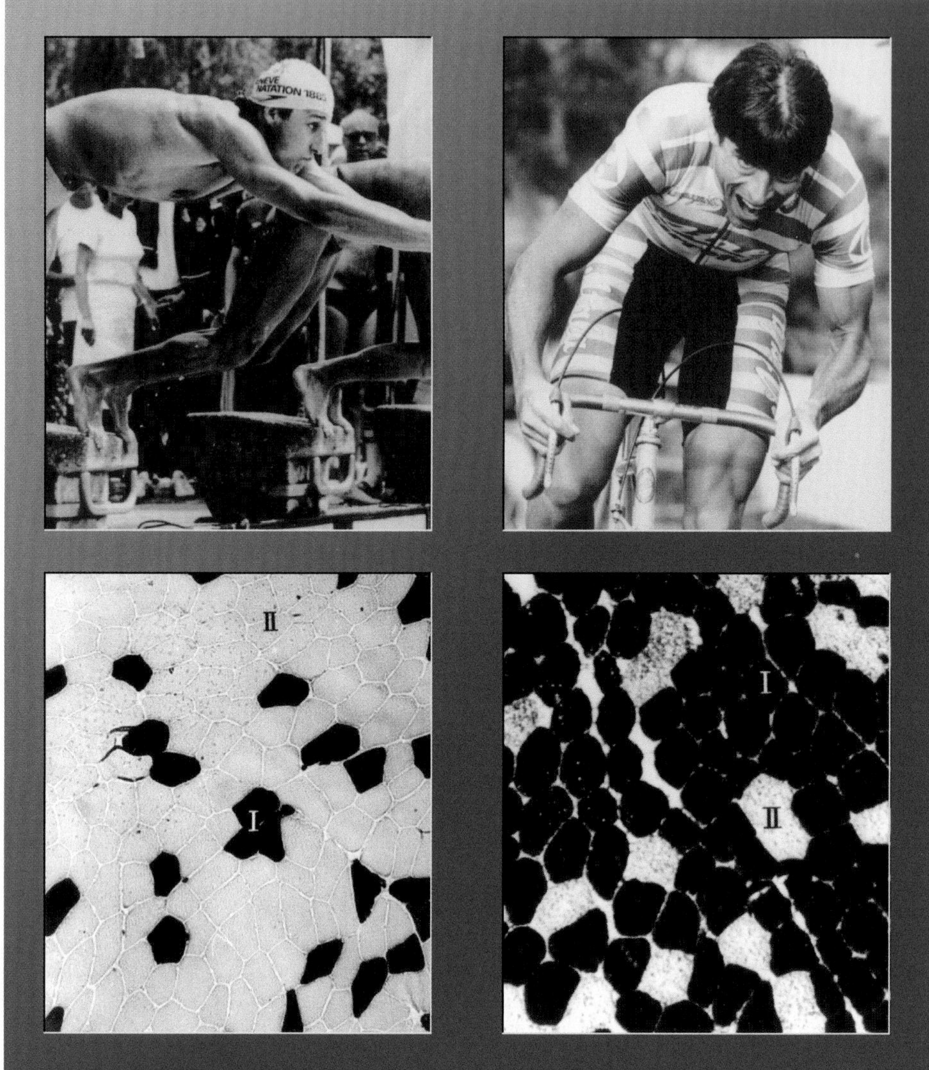

FIGURE 7.7 • Differences in muscle-fiber type composition between a sprint swimmer and endurance cyclist. The type I and type II muscle fibers were sampled from the vastus lateralis muscle and stained for myofibrillar ATPase after incubation at pH 4.3. Type I fibers stain dark, while type II fibers remain unstained. (Photos and photomicrographs courtesy of Dr. R. Billeter, Department of Anatomy, University of Bern, Switzerland.)

basketball, soccer, field hockey). These activities require activation of both muscle fiber types.

The preceding discussion suggests that a muscle's predominant fiber type significantly contributes to success in certain sports or physical activities. Chapter 18 explores this idea more fully, including other considerations concerning metabolic, contractile, and fatigue characteristics of each fiber type, the various subdivisions, proposed classification system, and effects of exercise training.

ENERGY SPECTRUM OF EXERCISE

Figure 7.8 illustrates the relative contribution of anaerobic and aerobic energy sources in relation to maximal exercise duration. Table 7.1 also shows the approximate percentage energy yield from these energy transfer systems, including the relative contributions of the major energy fuels during various running competitions. These data, derived from laboratory experiments involving all-out running, easily transpose to other activities by drawing the appropriate time relationships. For example, a 100-m sprint run corresponds to any all-out exercise lasting 10 seconds, while an 800-m run and 200-m swim last about 2 minutes. All-out 1-minute exercise includes the 400-m run, the 100-m swim, and repeated full-court presses at the end of a basketball game.

One should view the allocation of energy in exercise from each form of energy transfer as progressing on a continuum. At one extreme, the intramuscular high-energy phosphates supply almost all energy for exercise. The ATP–PCr and lactic acid systems supply about one-half the energy for intense exercise lasting 2 minutes; aerobic reactions supply the remainder. To excel under these conditions requires a well-developed capacity for both anaerobic and aerobic metabolism. Intense exercise of intermediate duration, performed for 5 to 10 minutes (e.g., middle-distance running and swimming, or basketball) places greater demand on aerobic energy transfer. Long-duration performances like marathon running, distance swimming, cycling, recreational jogging, and hiking and trekking require a constant supply of aerobic energy and place little reliance on energy from anaerobic sources with subsequent lactate formation.

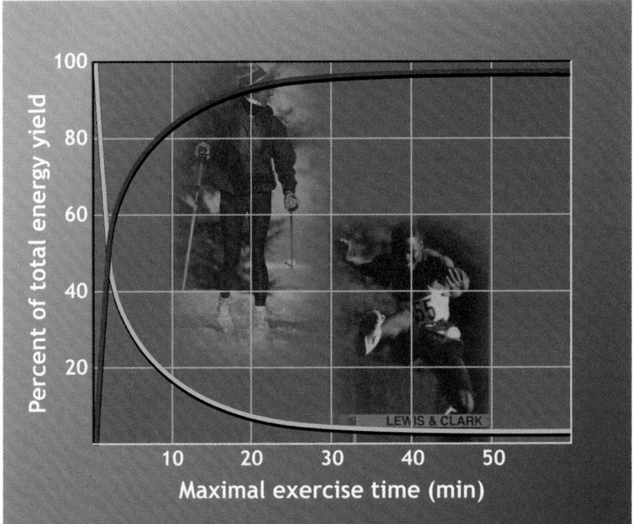

Duration of maximal exercise

	Seconds			Minutes					
	10	30	60	2	4	10	30	60	120
Percent anaerobic	90	80	70	50	35	15	5	2	1
Percent aerobic	10	20	30	50	65	85	95	98	99

FIGURE 7.8 • Relative contribution of aerobic and anaerobic energy metabolism during maximal physical effort of various durations. Note that 2 minutes of maximal effort requires about 50% of the energy from both aerobic and anaerobic processes. A world-class 4-minute-mile pace derives approximately 65% of its energy from aerobic metabolism, with the remainder generated from anaerobic processes. A 2-hour marathon, on the other hand, generates almost all of its energy from aerobic processes. (Adapted from Åstrand PO, Rodahl K. Textbook of work physiology. New York: McGraw-Hill, 1977.)

An understanding of the energy demands of diverse physical activities provides some explanation of why a world-record holder in the 1-mile run does not necessarily excel in distance running. Conversely, premier marathon runners rarely can run 1 mile in less than 4 minutes yet complete 26.2 miles at a 5-minute-per-mile pace. The appropriate approach to exercise training analyzes an activity for its specific energy components and then formulates training strategies to ensure optimal adaptations in physiologic and metabolic function. *Improved capacity for energy transfer usually translates into improved exercise performance.*

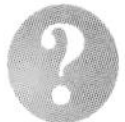

INTEGRATIVE QUESTION

If athletes generally perform marathon running under high-intensity but steady-rate conditions, explain why some experience a reduced capacity to sprint to the finish at the end of the race.

OXYGEN CONSUMPTION DURING RECOVERY

Following exercise, bodily processes do not immediately return to resting levels. After relatively light, short-duration physical effort, recovery proceeds rapidly and unnoticed. On the other hand, stressful exercise, such as running a one-half mile race or swimming 200 yards as fast as possible, requires considerable time for resting metabolism to recover. Variation in recovery from light, moderate, and strenuous exercise results from specific metabolic and physiologic processes during and in recovery from each form of effort.[5]

Figure 7.9 illustrates oxygen consumption during exercise and recovery from different exercise intensities. Light exercise (A), with rapid attainment of steady-rate oxygen consumption, produces a small oxygen deficit. The magnitude of recovery oxygen consumption approximates the size of the oxygen deficit at the beginning of exercise. Recovery proceeds rapidly; oxygen consumption follows a logarithmic

TABLE 7.1 ➤ ESTIMATE OF THE PERCENTAGE CONTRIBUTION OF DIFFERENT FUELS TO ATP GENERATION IN VARIOUS RUNNING EVENTS

	Percentage Contribution to ATP Generation				
		Glycogen			
Event	Phosphocreatine	Anaerobic	Aerobic	Blood Glucose (Liver Glycogen)	Triglyceride (Fatty Acids)
100 m	50	50	—	—	—
200 m	25	65	10	—	—
400 m	12.5	62.5	25	—	—
800 m	6	50	44	—	—
1,500 m	[a]	25	75	—	—
5,000 m	[a]	12.5	87.5	—	—
10,000 m	[a]	3	97	—	—
Marathon	—	—	75	5	20
Ultramarathon (80 km)	—	—	35	5	60
24-h race	—	—	10	2	88
Soccer game	10	70	20	—	—

[a]In such events phosphocreatine will be used for the first few seconds and, if it has been resynthesized during the race, in the sprint to the finish.
From Newsholme EA, et al. Physical and mental fatigue: metabolic mechanisms and importance of plasma amino acids. Brit Med Bull 1992;48:477.

curve, decreasing by about 50% over each subsequent 30-second period until reaching the preexercise level.

Oxygen consumption during steady-rate and non-steady-rate (heavy) exercise and recovery plot as a logarithmic function in relation to time.[10,69] The function increases in exercise or decreases in recovery by some constant fraction for each unit of time as oxygen consumption approaches an asymptote, or level value. Consider the example of recovery from 10 minutes of light, steady-rate exercise at an oxygen consumption of 2000 mL · min^{-1}. If recovery oxygen consumption decreased by one half over 30 seconds, then oxygen consumption would equal 1000 mL · min^{-1} at 30-seconds recovery and 500 mL · min^{-1} at 60 seconds, with the resting value of 250 mL · min^{-1} achieved in about 90 seconds.

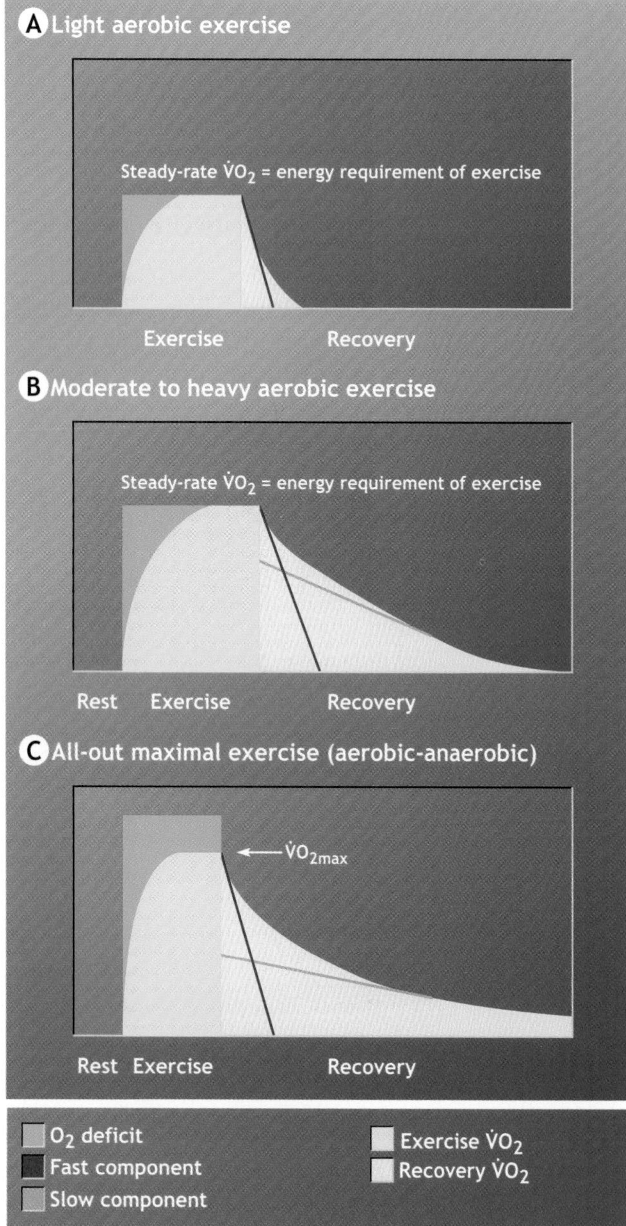

FIGURE 7.9 • Oxygen consumption during exercise and in recovery from (**A**) light steady-rate exercise, (**B**) moderate-to-heavy steady-rate exercise, and (**C**) exhaustive exercise that does not produce a steady-rate of aerobic metabolism. Note that in exhaustive exercise, the exercise oxygen requirement significantly exceeds the actual exercise oxygen consumption.

Moderate-to-heavy aerobic exercise (Fig. 7.9B) requires a longer time to reach steady rate, which creates a larger oxygen deficit than less-intense exercise. Consequently, it takes longer for oxygen consumption to return to the resting level in recovery. The oxygen consumption recovery curve demonstrates an initial rapid decline (similar to recovery from light exercise) followed by a more gradual decline to baseline resting levels. In Figures 7-9A and B, the oxygen deficit and recovery oxygen consumption are computed by using the steady-rate oxygen consumption to represent the oxygen (energy) requirement of exercise. Figure 7.9C shows that maximal exercise does not produce a steady rate of aerobic metabolism. Such exercise demands a larger energy requirement than aerobic processes can supply. Under these conditions anaerobic energy transfer increases and blood lactate accumulates, with considerable time required to achieve complete recovery. Failure to achieve steady-rate oxygen consumption makes it unfeasible to quantify the true oxygen deficit accurately.

Each of the curves in Figure 7.9 shows that oxygen consumption in recovery always exists in excess of the resting value, regardless of exercise intensity. The excess has classically been termed the **oxygen debt** or more appropriately, **recovery oxygen consumption** (indicated by the yellow shaded area under each recovery curve). One computes it as the total oxygen consumed in recovery minus the total oxygen theoretically consumed at rest during the recovery period. For example, if a total of 5.5 L of oxygen was consumed in recovery until attaining the resting value of 0.310 L · min^{-1}, and recovery required 10 minutes, the recovery oxygen consumption would equal 5.5 L minus 3.1 L (0.310 L × 10 min), or 2.4 L. This indicates that the preceding exercise caused physiologic alterations during exercise *and* recovery that required an additional 2.4 L of oxygen before oxygen consumption returned to the preexercise resting level. The inference assumes that resting oxygen consumption remains unchanged during exercise and recovery. As we discuss below, this assumption is not entirely correct, particularly following strenuous exercise.

The curves in Figure 7.9 illustrate two important characteristics of recovery oxygen consumption:

1. With mild aerobic exercise of relatively short duration (little disruption in body temperature and hormonal milieu), about one-half of the total recovery oxygen consumption takes place within 30 seconds, with complete recovery within several minutes. The decline in oxygen consumption follows a single-component exponential curve termed the **fast component** of recovery oxygen consumption.[8]
2. Recovery from strenuous exercise, when blood lactate, body temperature, and thermogenic hormone levels increase substantially, presents a different

picture. In addition to the fast component of the recovery phase, a second phase of recovery exists, termed the **slow component**. Depending on the intensity and duration of the previous exercise, the slow component may take up to 24 hours to reach the preexercise oxygen consumption.[7,32,57,59] Even with shorter, intermittent bouts of "supermaximal" exercise (e.g., three 2-minute bouts at 108% $\dot{V}O_{2max}$ interspersed with a 3-minute rest), recovery oxygen consumption remains elevated for 1 hour or longer.[4]

Aerobic training accelerates the rate of recovery. Trained subjects show a more rapid rate of recovery oxygen consumption to baseline when exercising at either the same absolute or relative exercise intensity as untrained counterparts.[60] More than likely, training adaptations that facilitate the rapid achievement of steady rate also contribute to a facilitated recovery.

Metabolic Dynamics of Recovery Oxygen Consumption

A precise biochemical explanation for the recovery oxygen consumption, particularly the role of lactate, remains elusive, because no comprehensive explanation exists about specific contributory factors.[26]

Traditional Concepts

Nobel laureate Archibald Vivian Hill and colleagues first coined the term oxygen debt in 1922. These scientists discussed energy metabolism during exercise and recovery in financial–accounting terms.[39] Within this framework, the body's carbohydrate stores were likened to energy "credits." Expending stored credits during exercise incurred an energy "debt." The greater the energy "deficit" (use of available stored energy credits), the larger the energy debt. Hill believed that the recovery oxygen consumption represented the cost of repaying this debt—hence the term oxygen debt.

Lactate accumulation from the anaerobic component of exercise represented use of glycogen, the stored energy credit. The ensuing oxygen debt served two purposes: (1) reestablishing the original glycogen stores (credits) by synthesizing approximately 80% of the lactate back to glycogen in the liver (Cori cycle) and (2) catabolizing the remaining lactate through the pyruvate–citric acid cycle pathway. The ATP generated in this process presumably powered glycogen resynthesis from lactate. This early explanation of the dynamics of recovery oxygen consumption was subsequently termed the "lactic acid theory of oxygen debt."

In 1933, after the work of Hill, researchers at the Harvard Fatigue Laboratory attempted to explain their observation that the initial phase of recovery oxygen consumption ended before blood lactate began decreasing.[53] In fact, they showed that one could incur an oxygen debt of almost 3 L without any appreciable blood lactate accumulation. To resolve these findings, they proposed two phases of oxygen debt: (1) **alactic** (or **alactacid) oxygen debt** (without lactate buildup) and (2) **lactic acid** or **(lactacid) oxygen debt** associated with elevated blood lactate levels. They based these two explanations on speculation, because they could not measure ATP and PCr replenishment or the relationship between blood lactate and glucose and glycogen levels. For nearly 65 years, the following model served to explain the energetics of oxygen debt:

- **Alactacid debt:** The alactacid portion of the oxygen debt depicted in the recovery from light, steady-rate exercise in Figure 7.9A or the rapid phase of recovery from more strenuous exercise (Figs. 7.9, B and C), resulted from restoration of the intramuscular high-energy phosphates ATP and PCr depleted during exercise. This restoration came from the aerobic breakdown of the stored macronutrients during recovery. A small portion of the recovery oxygen consumption also reloaded muscle myoglobin and hemoglobin in blood returning from previously active tissues.
- **Lactacid debt:** In keeping with A. V. Hill's explanation, most of the lactacid oxygen debt represented the reconversion of lactate to glycogen in the liver.

Controversy with Traditional Explanation of Oxygen Debt. Several relationships must exist to support the contention that (1) anaerobic energy sources temporarily compensate for an aerobic energy deficit during exercise and (2) the recovery oxygen consumption reflects the magnitude of the anaerobic energy contribution in exercise. For example, only a moderate relationship exists between the oxygen deficit and the excess oxygen consumption in recovery (oxygen debt). To accept the traditional explanation for the lactacid phase of the oxygen debt, one must show that most lactate accumulated in exercise actually contributes to glycogen resynthesis in recovery, as Hill and others had speculated. This has never been shown. In experiments with humans, no substantial replenishment of glycogen occurred 10 minutes following strenuous exercise, even though blood lactate levels decreased significantly. *This suggests that most lactate oxidizes for energy* (see "Focus on Research").[5,9] This takes place because heart, liver, kidney, and skeletal muscle tissues use lactate as an energy substrate during exercise and recovery.

Contemporary Concepts

The elevated aerobic metabolism in recovery restores the body to its preexercise condition. In short-duration, light-to-moderate exercise, recovery oxygen consumption generally replenishes the high-energy phosphates depleted by exercise. Recovery typically proceeds rapidly within several minutes.[5,8] In longer-duration (>60 min), high-intensity aerobic exercise, recovery oxygen consumption remains elevated for a considerably longer period.[6,59] Figure 7.10 clearly illustrates the effect of exercise duration on the magnitude of recovery oxygen consumption. Eight trained women walked at 70% of $\dot{V}O_{2max}$ for 20, 40, or 60 minutes. Recovery oxygen consumption, also termed **excess postexercise oxygen consumption**

Focus on Research

A Challenge to Conventional Wisdom

Brooks GA, et al. Glycogen synthesis and metabolism of lactic acid after exercise. Am. J Physiol 1973;224:1162.

➤ The early research of A. V. Hill and colleagues postulated that the elevated oxygen consumption ($\dot{V}O_2$) in recovery from exercise (so-called oxygen debt) resulted from oxidation of about one-fifth of the lactate produced in exercise. Lactate oxidation provided the necessary energy to resynthesize the remaining lactate to glycogen. Subsequent research by Margaria (see "Focus on Research," Chapter 9) retained this traditional "lactic acid interpretation" of the elevated $\dot{V}O_2$ in recovery from exercise. Until the 1973 publication by Brooks and coworkers, few investigators had directly challenged the conventional wisdom that lactate produced in strenuous exercise caused significant glycogen resynthesis during the postexercise repayment of the oxygen debt.

Female rats served as subjects during two experiments to test the lactic acid–oxygen debt theory. *Experiment 1* placed animals into either a sedentary group or an exercise group that ran at intensities that produced significant lactate buildup and a large postexercise $\dot{V}O_2$. Following exercise, the researchers periodically sacrificed some animals and measured glycogen, glucose, and lactate in muscle, liver, and blood during a 24-hour recovery. The top figure displays liver and muscle glycogen concentrations during recovery from exercise. Compared with sedentary controls (*purple and blue squares*) little glycogen remained in the muscles and liver at the end of exhaustive exercise (0 min). Furthermore, no significant glycogen resynthesis occurred in the postexercise period; liver and muscle glycogen concentrations after 24 hours' recovery did not exceed the immediate postexercise values. These findings did not support the hypothesis set forth by Hill and colleagues that the elevated postexercise $\dot{V}O_2$ largely related to glycogen resynthesis from lactate produced during exhaustive exercise.

In a parallel experiment (*experiment 2,* bottom figure), the researchers infused ^{14}C-labeled lactate into exercise-exhausted and pair-fasted sedentary control rats. Measurements included release of labeled CO_2 in recovery to assess the fate of the infused ^{14}C-labeled lactate. If lactate resynthesized to glycogen in recovery—as proposed by the "lactic acid theory of oxygen debt"—then little of the injected isotope should have appeared in expired CO_2. Conversely, if oxidation explains the primary fate of lactate then most of the labeled carbon in the infused lactate should indeed appear as $^{14}CO_2$ in expired air. The experiment produced unequivocal results: 70 to 90% of the isotope appeared as CO_2.

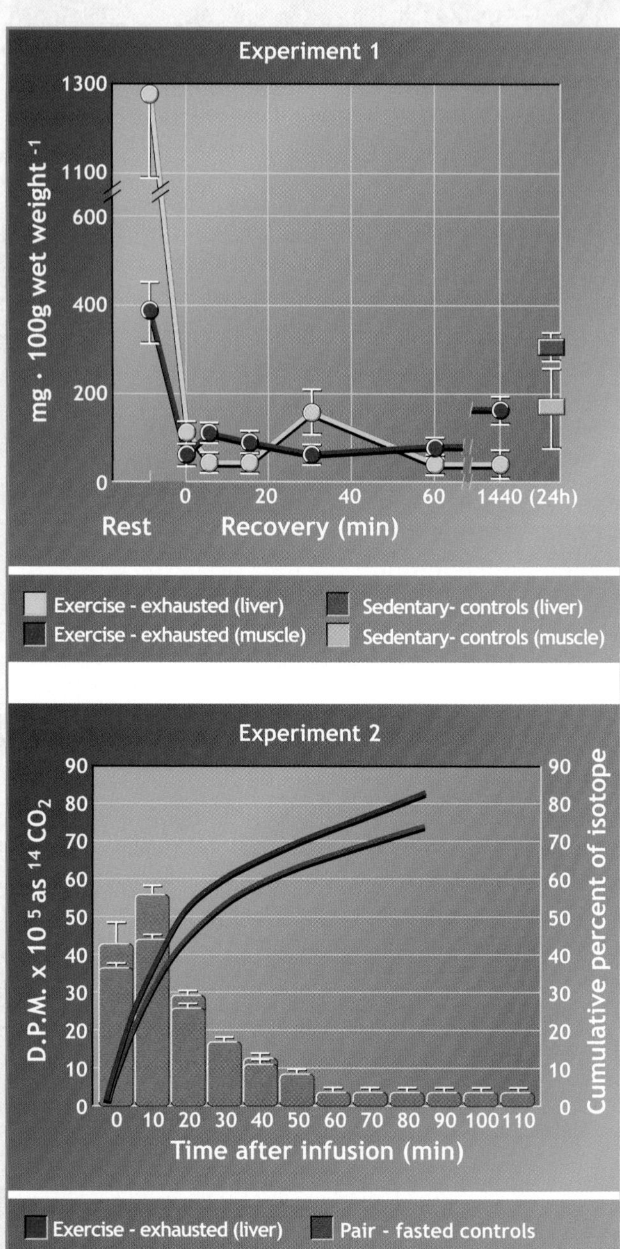

Experiment 1. Liver and muscle glycogen concentrations over time after exhaustive exercise in rats previously fasted for 10 to 12 hours. *Experiment 2.* Production of labeled CO_2 after infusion of ^{14}C-labeled lactate in exercise-exhausted and pair-fasted rats (*bar graph, left ordinate*). Expiration of labeled CO_2 also expressed as a cumulative percentage of ^{14}C-labeled lactate (*line graph, right ordinate*).

Under the conditions of Brooks' experiment, glycogen resynthesis from elevated lactate did not represent a predominant process to explain the oxygen debt proposed by Hill and colleagues in the 1920s. Subsequent research by Brooks and other investigators continues to redefine and expand the biochemical and physiologic factors that affect recovery $\dot{V}O_2$.

(EPOC), totaled 8.6 L for the 20-minute exercise period and 9.8 L for the 40-minute session, while the cost of recovery from the 60-minute workout nearly doubled, to 15.2 L. The increase in EPOC in each bout of steady-rate exercise did not relate to lactate accumulation. Rather, other disequilibriums in physiologic function elevate the recovery metabolism.

In exhaustive exercise with its significant anaerobic component and lactate accumulation, a small portion of EPOC resynthesizes lactate to glycogen. This gluconeogenic mechanism also progresses during exercise, particularly among trained individuals.[23,52] Of course, the main source for replenishing glycogen remains dietary carbohydrate, not resynthesized lactate. A significant component of EPOC relates to physiologic processes that actually take place *during* recovery, in addition to metabolic events during exercise. Such factors probably account for the considerably larger oxygen debt than oxygen deficit in prolonged aerobic exercise and exhaustive anaerobic exercise. Body temperature, for example, rises about 3°C (5.4°F) during a long bout of intense aerobic exercise and can remain elevated for several hours in recovery. Elevated body temperature directly stimulates metabolism to increase recovery oxygen consumption.[5,6,15]

Other factors also affect EPOC. As much as 10% of the recovery oxygen consumption reloads the blood returning to the lungs from the previously active muscles. An additional 2 to 5% restores oxygen dissolved in bodily fluids and bound to myoglobin in the muscle itself. Ventilation volumes in intense exercise increase 8 to 10 times above the resting requirement, a cost that can equal 10% of the EPOC.[48] The heart also works harder and requires a greater oxygen supply during recovery. Tissue

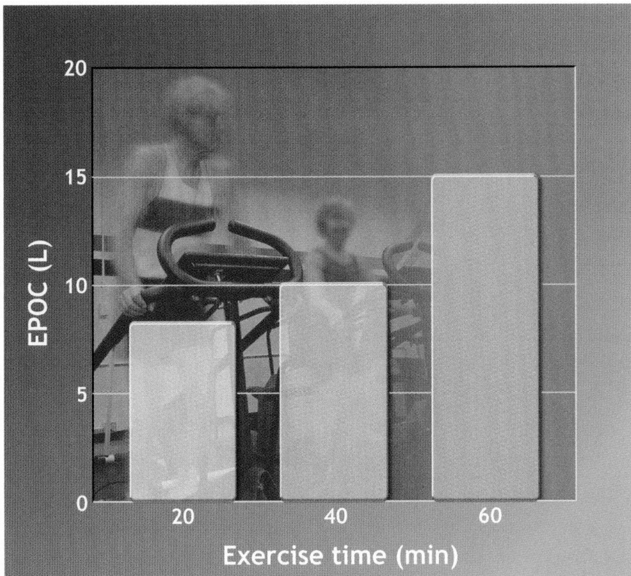

FIGURE 7.10 • Total excess postexercise oxygen consumption (EPOC) during a 3-hour recovery from 20, 40, and 60 minutes of treadmill walking at 70% $\dot{V}O_{2max}$. EPOC for the 60-minute exercise significantly exceeded the 20- or 40-minute workouts. (From Quinn TJ, et al. Postexercise oxygen consumption in trained females: effect of exercise duration. Med Sci Sports Exerc 1994;26:908.)

repair and the redistribution of calcium, potassium, and sodium ions within muscle and other body compartments require additional energy, while the residual effects of the thermogenic hormones epinephrine, norepinephrine, and thyroxine and the glucocorticoids released in exercise keep metabolism elevated for a considerable time in recovery.[29] In essence, all of the physiologic systems activated in exercise increase their own particular need for oxygen during recovery (Fig. 7.11). EPOC does not appear to be affected by different phases of the menstrual cycle.[25] *The recovery oxygen consumption, or EPOC, reflects two factors: (1) the level of anaerobic metabolism in previous exercise and (2) the respiratory, circulatory, hormonal, ionic, and thermal adjustments that exert influence during recovery.*

Implications of EPOC for Exercise and Recovery

Understanding the dynamics of EPOC provides a basis for structuring exercise intervals and optimizing recovery. No appreciable lactate accumulates either with steady-rate aerobic exercise or with brief 5 to 10-second bouts of all-out effort powered by the intramuscular high-energy phosphates. Consequently, recovery progresses rapidly (fast component predominantly), and exercise can begin again with only a short rest period. In contrast, longer periods of anaerobic exercise produce considerable lactate buildup (in active muscles and blood) and significant disruption in physiologic functions. In such cases, EPOC consists of both a fast component and a slower component that often requires considerable time. Prolonged recovery between exercise intervals would impair performance in such sports as basketball, hockey, soccer, tennis, and badminton. An athlete pushed to a high level of anaerobic metabolism may not fully recover during brief time-out periods or intermittent intervals of less-intense exercise.

Procedures for speeding recovery from exercise generally are either active or passive. In **active recovery** (often termed "cooling-down" or "tapering-off"), the individual performs submaximal exercise, believing that continued physical activity in some way prevents muscle cramps and stiffness and facilitates overall recovery. With **passive recovery**, the person usually lies down, presuming that total inactivity reduces the resting energy requirements and thus "frees" oxygen for the recovery process. Modifications of passive recovery have included massage, cold showers, specific body positions, and ingestion of cold liquids.

Optimal Recovery From Steady-Rate Exercise

Most people generally perform exercise in steady rate with little lactate accumulation at oxygen consumptions below 55 to 60% of $\dot{V}O_{2max}$. Recovery entails resynthesis of high-energy phosphates; replenishment of oxygen in the blood, bodily fluids, and muscle myoglobin; and a small energy cost to sustain elevated circulation and ventilation. Under these circumstances, passive procedures facilitate recovery because any additional exercise only serves to elevate total metabolism and delay recovery.

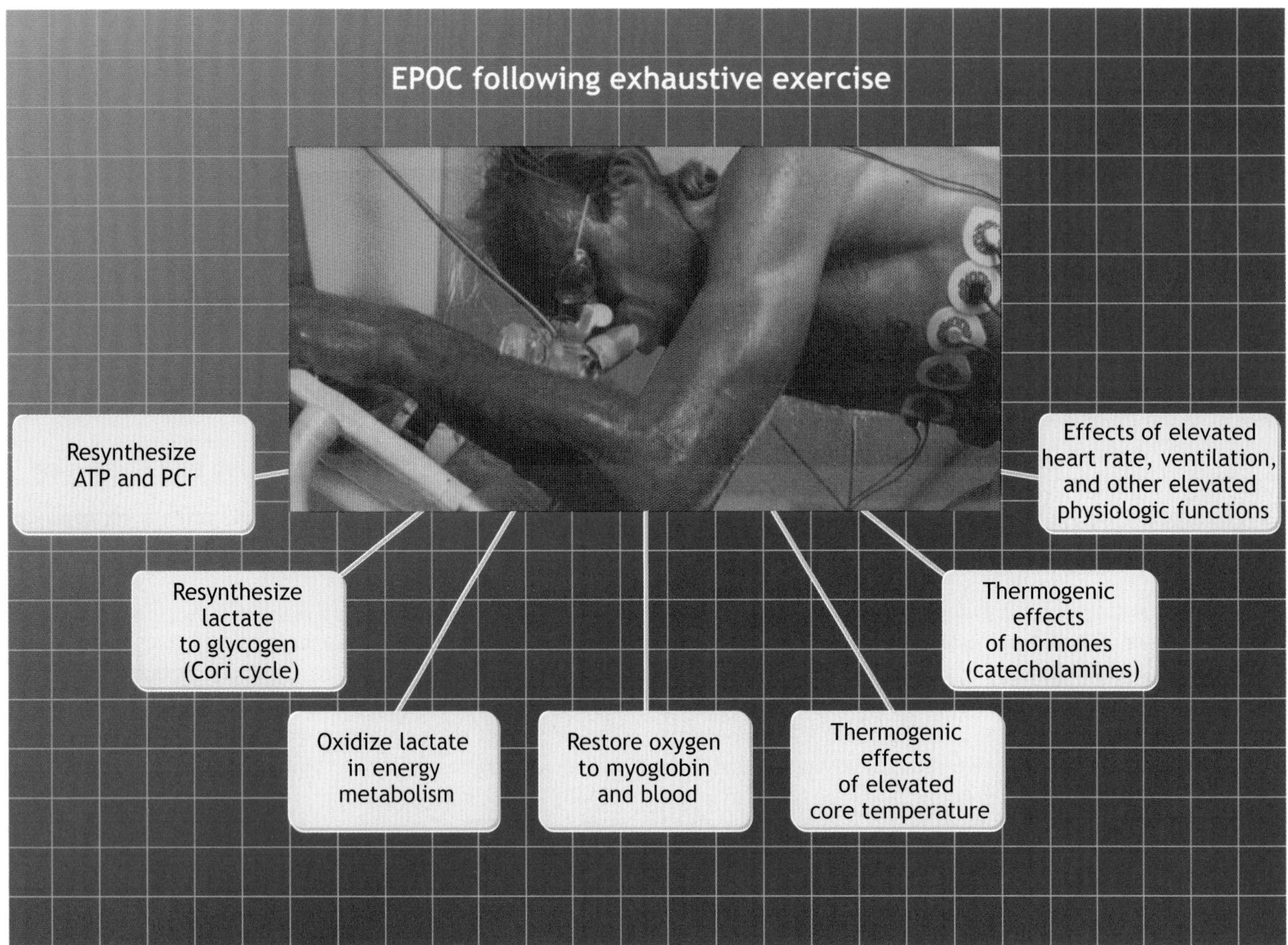

FIGURE 7.11 • Factors that contribute to the EPOC following exhaustive exercise.

Optimal Recovery From Non–Steady-Rate Exercise

When exercise intensity exceeds the maximum steady-rate level, lactate formation in muscle exceeds its removal rate, and blood lactate accumulates. As exercise intensity increases, blood lactate levels rise sharply, and the exerciser soon becomes exhausted. Although the precise mechanisms for exhaustion during anaerobic exercise remain unclear, blood lactate levels can provide an objective indication of the relative strenuousness of exercise; they also reflect the adequacy of recovery.[44] Because the lactate anion produces a fatiguing effect on skeletal muscle, independent of associated reductions in pH,[40] any procedure that accelerates lactate removal probably augments subsequent exercise performance.[1]

Performing aerobic exercise in recovery accelerates blood lactate removal.[1,16,28] The optimal level of recovery exercise ranges between 30 and 45% $\dot{V}O_{2max}$ for bicycle exercise, and 55 to 60% $\dot{V}O_{2max}$ when the recovery involves treadmill running.[56] This difference between exercise modes probably reflects the more-localized muscle involvement in bicycling, which lowers the threshold for blood lactate accumulation.[38]

Figure 7.12 illustrates blood lactate recovery patterns for trained men who performed 6 minutes of supermaximal exercise on a bicycle ergometer. Active recovery involved 40 minutes of continuous exercise at either 35 or 65% $\dot{V}O_{2max}$. A combination of 65% $\dot{V}O_{2max}$ (7 min) followed by 35% $\dot{V}O_{2max}$ (33 min) evaluated whether a higher-intensity exercise interval early in recovery would expedite lactate removal.[22] These data show clearly that moderate aerobic exercise performed in recovery facilitates lactate removal, compared with passive recovery procedures. The combination of higher-intensity followed by lower-intensity exercise provided no greater benefit than a single exercise level at moderate intensity. Performing recovery exercise above the lactate threshold offers no added benefit and may even prolong recovery by initiating lactate formation and accumulation.[22,28] In a practical sense, if left to their own choice, most individuals select an optimal recovery exercise intensity.

The facilitated lactate removal with active recovery likely results from increased perfusion of blood through the "lactate-using" liver and heart.[3] In addition, increased blood flow through the muscles in active recovery certainly enhances lactate removal, because this tissue readily oxidizes lactate via citric acid cycle metabolism.

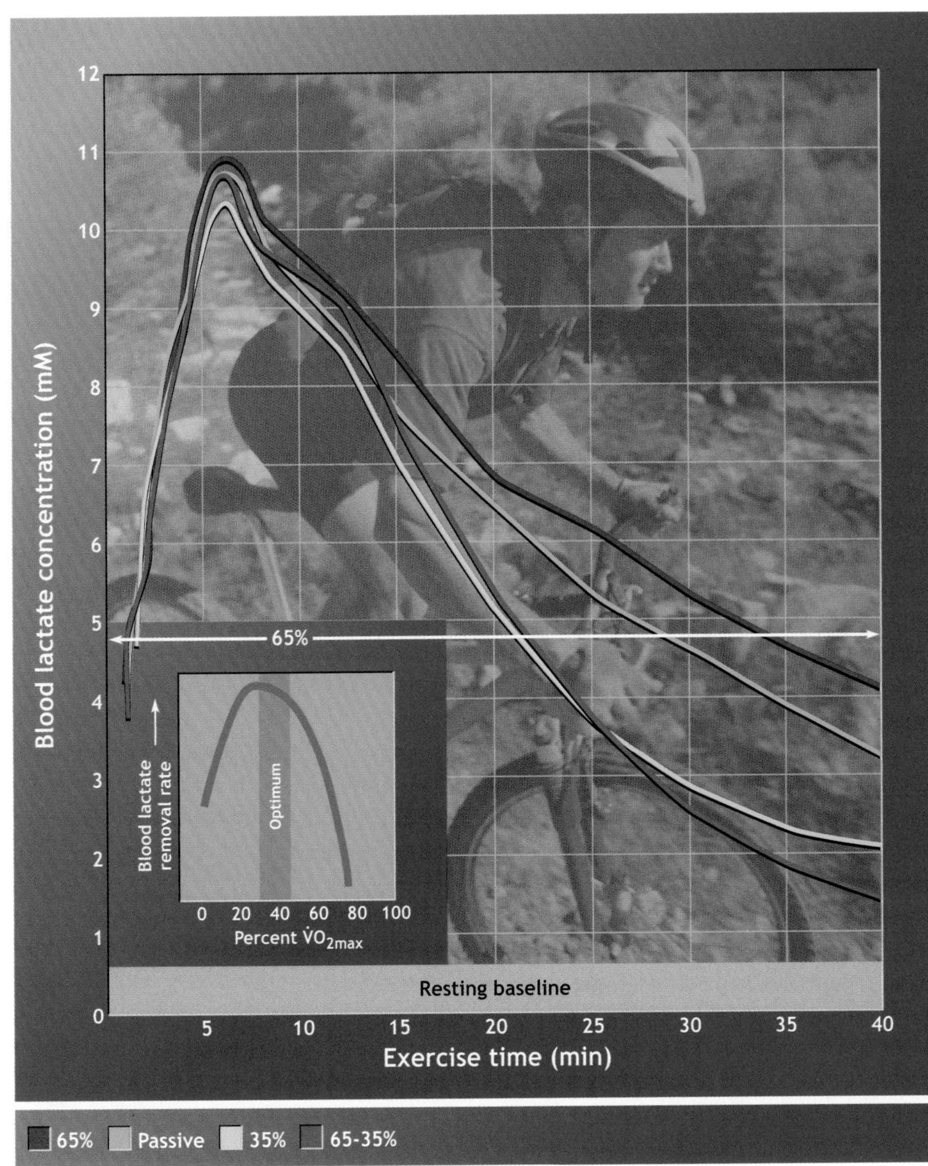

FIGURE 7.12 • Blood lactate concentration following maximal exercise using passive recovery and active recoveries at 35, 65, and a combination 35% and 65% $\dot{V}O_{2max}$. The *horizontal white line* indicates the blood lactate level produced by exercise at 65% $\dot{V}O_{2max}$ without previous exercise. The inset curve depicts the generalized relationship between exercise intensity and rate of lactate removal. (Adapted from Dodd S, et al. Blood lactate disappearance at various intensities of recovery exercise. J Appl Physiol: Respir Environ Exerc Physiol 1984;57:1462.)

Intermittent (Interval) Exercise

An approach to performing exercise that would normally cause exhaustion within several minutes if performed continuously requires exercising *intermittently* using a preestablished spacing of exercise and rest intervals. The physical conditioning program of **interval training** characterizes this approach. This training applies various work-to-rest intervals, using supermaximal exercise to overload the energy transfer systems. For example, with all-out exercise for up to 8 second's duration, the intramuscular high-energy phosphates provide most of the energy, with minimal reliance on the glycolytic pathway. This produces rapid recovery (alactic, fast component), enabling a subsequent bout of heavy exercise to begin, following a brief recovery.

Table 7.2 summarizes the results of a classic series of experiments that combined exercise and rest intervals. On one

TABLE 7.2 ➤ EXPERIMENTAL RESULTS WITH INTERMITTENT EXERCISE

Exercise–Rest Periods	Total Distance Run (yards)	Average Oxygen Consumption ($L \cdot min^{-1}$)	Blood Lactate Level ($mg \cdot dL\ blood^{-1}$)
4 min continuous	1422	5.6	150
10 s exercise 5 s rest	7294	5.1	44
10 s exercise 10 s rest	5468	4.4	20
15 s exercise 30 s rest	3642	3.6	16

From data of Christenson EH, et al. Intermittent and continuous running. Acta Physiol Scand 1960;50:269.

day, the subject ran at a speed that would normally exhaust him within 5 minutes. The continuous run covered about 0.8 mile, and the runner attained a $\dot{V}O_{2max}$ of 5.6 L · min^{-1}. A high blood lactate level (last column of the table), owing to substantial anaerobic metabolism, verified a relative state of exhaustion. On another day, the subject ran at the same fast speed but intermittently, with periods of 10 seconds of exercise and 5 seconds of recovery. During 30 minutes of intermittent exercise, the actual time spent running amounted to 20 minutes, and the distance covered equaled 4 miles, compared with less than 5 minutes and 0.8 miles with a continuous run! The effectiveness of the intermittent exercise protocol becomes even more impressive considering that the blood lactate remained low, even though the oxygen consumption averaged 5.1 L · min^{-1} (91% $\dot{V}O_{2max}$) during the 30-minute period. Thus, a relative balance existed between the energy requirements of exercise and aerobic energy transfer within the muscles throughout the exercise and rest intervals.

Manipulating the duration of exercise and rest intervals can effectively overload a specific energy-transfer system. When the rest interval increased from 5 to 10 seconds, oxygen consumption averaged 4.4 L · min^{-1}; 15-second work and 30-second recovery intervals produced only a 3.6-L oxygen consumption. For each 30-minute bout of intermittent exercise, however, the runner achieved a longer distance and a substantially lower blood lactate level than when exercising continuously at the same intensity. Chapter 21 focuses on the specific application of the principles of intermittent exercise for aerobic and anaerobic training and sports performance.

Summary

1. The relative contribution of the pathways for ATP production differs, depending on exercise intensity and duration. In short-duration, intense exercise (100-m dash, repetitive lifting of heavy weights), the intramuscular stores of ATP and PCr (immediate energy system) provide the energy for exercise. For less-intense exercise of longer duration (1 to 2 min), anaerobic reactions of glycolysis (short-term energy system) generate most of the energy. As exercise progresses beyond several minutes, the aerobic system (long-term energy system) predominates.
2. Humans possess two distinct types of muscle fibers, each with unique metabolic and contractile properties: (1) low glycolytic–high oxidative, slow-twitch fibers (type I) and (2) low oxidative–high glycolytic, fast-twitch (type II) fibers. Intermediate fibers of the fast-twitch type also exist, with overlapping metabolic characteristics.
3. Understanding the energy spectrum of exercise makes it possible to train for specific improvement in each of the body's energy transfer systems.
4. A steady rate of oxygen consumption represents a balance between the energy requirements of the active muscles and the aerobic resynthesis of ATP.
5. The term oxygen deficit defines the difference between the oxygen requirement of exercise and the oxygen actually consumed during exercise.
6. Maximum oxygen consumption ($\dot{V}O_{2max}$) quantitatively defines a person's maximum capacity to resynthesize ATP aerobically. $\dot{V}O_{2max}$ provides an important indicator of overall physiologic functional capacity and ability to sustain high-intensity exercise.
7. Oxygen consumption remains elevated above the resting level following exercise. Recovery oxygen consumption reflects the metabolic demands of exercise in addition to physiologic imbalances caused by exercise that last into recovery.
8. Moderate physical activity performed following intense exercise (active recovery) facilitates recovery, compared with passive procedures. In most cases, active recovery produces faster blood lactate removal and enhanced performance in subsequent exercise.

References

1. Ahmaidi S, et al. Effects of active recovery on plasma lactate and anaerobic power following repeated intensive exercise. Med Sci Sports Exerc 1996;28:450.
2. Asp S, et al. Muscle glycogen accumulation after a marathon: roles of fiber type and pro- and macroglycogen. J Appl Physiol 1999;86:474.
3. Baher SK, et al. Training-intensity dependent and tissue-specific increases in lactate uptake and MCT-1 in heart muscle. J Appl Physiol 1998;84:987.
4. Bahr R. Effects of supramaximal exercise on excess postexercise oxygen consumption. Med Sci Sports Exerc 1992;24:66.
5. Bahr R. Excess postexercise oxygen consumption—magnitude, mechanisms and practical implications. Acta Physiol Scand 1992;(suppl)605:1.
6. Bahr R, Sejersted OM. Effect of intensity of exercise on excess postexercise oxygen consumption. Metabolism 1991;40:836.
7. Bahr R, et al. Triglyceride/fatty acid cycling is increased after exercise. Metabolism 1990;39:993.
8. Bangsbo J, et al. Anaerobic energy production and O_2 deficit-debt relationship during exhaustive exercise in humans. J Physiol 1990;422:539.
9. Bangsbo JP, et al. Substrates for muscle glycogen synthesis in recovery from intense exercise in man. J Physiol 1991;434:423.
10. Barstow TJ. Characterization of $\dot{V}O_2$ kinetics during heavy exercise. Med Sci Sports Exerc 1994;26:1327.
11. Bernús G, et al. ^{31}P-MRS of quadriceps reveals quantitative differences between sprinters and long-distance runners. Med Sci Sports Exerc 1993;25:479.
12. Bertocci LA, et al. Oxidation of lactate and acetate in rat skeletal muscle: analysis by ^{13}C–nuclear magnetic resonance spectroscopy. J Appl Physiol 1997;83:32.
13. Brooks GA. Anaerobic threshold: review of the concept and directions for future research. Med Sci Sports Exerc 1985;17:22.
14. Brooks GA. Physical activity and carbohydrate metabolism. In: Bouchard C, et al., eds. Physical activity, fitness, and health. Champaign, IL: Human Kinetics, 1994.
15. Brooks GA, et al. Temperature, skeletal muscle mitochondrial functions and oxygen debt. Am J Physiol 1971;220:1053.
16. Choi D, et al. Effect of passive and active recovery on the resynthesis of muscle glycogen. Med Sci Sports Exerc 1994;26:992.
17. Coggan AR, et al. Endurance training decreases plasma glucose turnover and oxidation during moderate-intensity exercise in men. J Appl Physiol 1990;68:990.
18. Coggan AR, et al. Plasma glucose kinetics during exercise in subjects with high and low lactate thresholds. J Appl Physiol 1992;73:1873.
19. Coggan AR, et al. Skeletal muscle adaptations to endurance training in 60- to 70 yr-old men and women. J Appl Physiol 1992;72:1780.

20. Coyle EF. Blood lactate threshold in some well trained ischemic heart disease patients. J Appl Physiol 1983;54:18.
21. Davis JA, et al. Anaerobic threshold alterations caused by endurance training in middle-aged men. J Appl Physiol 1979;46:1039.
22. Dodd S, et al. Blood lactate disappearance at various intensities of recovery exercise. J Appl Physiol 1984;57:1462.
23. Donovan CM, Brooks GA. Endurance training affects lactate clearance, not lactate production. Am J Physiol 1983;244(Endocrinol Metab 7):E83.
24. Edwards AM, et al. $\dot{V}O_2$ kinetics determined by PRBS techniques differentiate elite endurance runners from elite athletes. Int J Sports Med 1999;20:1.
25. Fukubay Y, et al. The effect of dietary restriction and menstrual cycle on excess on post-exercise oxygen consumption (EPOC) in young women. Clin Physiol 2000;20:165.
26. Gaesser GA, Brooks GA. Metabolic basis of excess post-exercise oxygen consumption: a review. Med Sci Sports Exerc 1984;16:29.
27. Gayagay G, et al. Elite endurance athletes and the ACE I allele—the role of genes in athletic performance. Hum Genet 1998;103:48.
28. Gladden LB. Lactate uptake by skeletal muscle. Exerc Sport Sci Rev 1989;17:115.
29. Gladden LB, et al. Norepinephrine increases and canine skeletal muscle $\dot{V}O_2$ during recovery. Med Sci Sports Exerc 1982;14:371.
30. Gollnick PD, Saltin B. Significance of skeletal muscle oxidative enzyme enhancement with endurance training. Clin Physiol 1983;2:1.
31. Gollnick PD, et al. Glycogen depletion patterns in human skeletal muscle fibers after varying types and intensities of exercise. In: Howard H, Poortmans J, eds. Metabolic adaptation to prolonged exercise. Basel: Birkhausen Verlag, 1975.
32. Gore CJ, Withers RI. Effects of exercise intensity and duration on postexercise metabolism. J Appl Physiol 1990;68:2362.
33. Grassi B, et al. Faster adjustment of O_2 delivery does not affect $\dot{V}O_2$ kinetics in isolated in situ canine muscle. J Appl Physiol 1998;85:1394.
34. Grassi B, et al. Peripheral oxygen diffusion does not affect $\dot{V}O_2$ on-kinetics in isolated in situ canine muscle. J Appl Physiol 1998;85:1404.
35. Greenhaff PL, Timmons JA. Interaction between aerobic and anaerobic metabolism during intense muscle contraction. Exerc Sport Sci Rev 1998;26:1.
36. Hagberg JM, et al. Faster adjustment to and recovery from submaximal exercise in the trained state. J Appl Physiol 1980;48:218.
37. Hebestreit H, et al. Kinetics of oxygen uptake at the onset of exercise in boys and men. J Appl Physiol 1998;85:1833.
38. Hermansen L, Stensvold I. Production and removal of lactate during exercise in man. Acta Physiol Scand 1972;86:191.
39. Hill AV, et al. Muscular exercise, lactic acid and the supply and utilization of oxygen. Proc R Soc Lond (Biol) 1924;96:438.
40. Hogan MC, et al. Increased [lactate] in working dog muscle reduces tension development independent of pH. Med Sci Sports Exerc 1995;27:371.
41. Holloszy JO, Coyle EF. Adaptations of skeletal muscle to endurance training and their metabolic consequences. J Appl Physiol 1984;56:831.
42. Hughson RL, Tschakovsky ME. Cardiovascular dynamics at the onset of exercise. Med Sci Sports Exerc 1999;31:1005.
43. Hultman E. Studies on muscle metabolism of glycogen and active phosphate in man with special reference to exercise and diet. Scand J Clin Lab Invest Suppl 1967:94.
44. Jacobs I. Blood lactate: implications for training and sports performance. Sports Med 1986;3:10.
45. Jacobs I, et al. Sprint training effects on muscle myoglobin, enzymes, fiber types, and blood lactate. Med Sci Sports Exerc 1987;19:368.
46. Karlsson J. Lactate and phosphagen concentrations in working muscle of man. Acta Physiol Scand Suppl 1971:358.
47. Karlsson J, Jacobs I. Onset of blood lactate accumulation during muscular exercise as a threshold concept. I. Theoretical considerations. Int J Sports Med 1982;3:190.
48. Katch FI, et al. The influence of the estimated oxygen cost of ventilation on oxygen deficit and recovery oxygen intake for moderately heavy bicycle ergometer exercise. Med Sci Sports 1972;4:71.
49. Katz A, Sahlin K. Role of oxygen in regulation of glycolysis and lactate production in human skeletal muscle. Exerc Sport Sci Rev 1990,18:1.
50. Kent-Braun JA, et al. Human skeletal muscle metabolism in health and disease: utility of magnetic resonance spectroscopy. Exerc Sport Sci Rev 1995;23:305.
51. Koike A, et al. Oxygen uptake kinetics are determined by cardiac function at onset of exercise rather than peak exercise in patients with prior myocardial infarction. Circulation 1994;90:2324.
52. MacRae HS-H, et al. Effect of training on lactate production and removal during progressive exercise. J Appl Physiol 1992;72:1649.
53. Margaria R, et al. The possible mechanism of contracting and paying the oxygen debt and the role of lactic acid in muscular contraction. Am J Physiol 1933;106:687.
54. McCann DJ, et al. Phosphocreatine kinetics in humans during exercise and recovery. Med Sci Sports Exerc 1995;27:378.
55. McCully KK, et al. Simultaneous in vivo measurements of HbO_2 saturation and PCr kinetics after exercise in normal humans. J Appl Physiol 1994;77:5.
56. McLellan TM, Skinner JS. Blood lactate removal during active recovery related to aerobic threshold. Int J Sports Med 1982;3:224.
57. Poehlman EA, et al. The impact of exercise and diet restriction on daily energy expenditure. Sports Med 1991;11:78.
58. Poole DC. $\dot{V}O_2$ slow component: physiological and functional significance. Med Sci Sports Exerc 1994;26:1354.
59. Quinn TJ, et al. Postexercise oxygen consumption in trained females: effect of exercise duration. Med Sci Sports Exerc 1994;26:908.
60. Short KR, Sedlock DA. Excess postexercise oxygen consumption and recovery rate in trained and untrained subjects. J Appl Physiol 1997;83:153.
61. Sjödin B, Jacobs I. Onset of blood lactate accumulation and marathon running performance. Int J Sports Med 1981;2:23.
62. Skirnar GS, et al. Glycogen utilization in wheelchair-dependent athletes. Int J Sports Med 1982;3:215.
63. Spencer MR, Gastin PB. Energy system contribution during 200- to 1500-m running in highly trained athletes. Med Sci Sports Exerc 2001;33:157.
64. Stainsby WN, Brooks GA. Control of lactic acid metabolism in contracting muscles and during exercise. Exerc Sport Sci Rev 1990;18:29.
65. Starritt EC, et al. Effect of short-term training on mitochondrial ATP production rate in human skeletal muscle. J Appl Physiol 1999;86:450.
66. Tschakovsky ME, Hughson RL. Interaction of factors determining oxygen uptake at the onset of exercise. J Appl Physiol 1999;86:1101.
67. Wasserman K, et al. Respiratory physiology of exercise: metabolism gas exchange and ventilatory control. Int Rev Respir Physiol 1981;111:149.
68. Weltman A, et al. Reliability and validity of a continuous incremental treadmill protocol for the determination of lactate threshold, fixed blood lactate concentrations and $\dot{V}O_{2max}$. Int J Sports Med 1990;11:26.
69. Whipp BJ. The slow component of O_2 uptake kinetics during heavy exercise. Med Sci Sports Exerc 1994;26:1319.
70. Wilber RL, et al. Physiological profiles of elite off-road and road cyclists. Med Sci Sports Exerc 1997;29:1090.
71. Wyatt FB. Comparison of lactate and ventilatory threshold to maximal oxygen consumption: a meta-analysis. J Strength Cond Res 1999;13:67.

CHAPTER 8

Measurement of Human Energy Expenditure

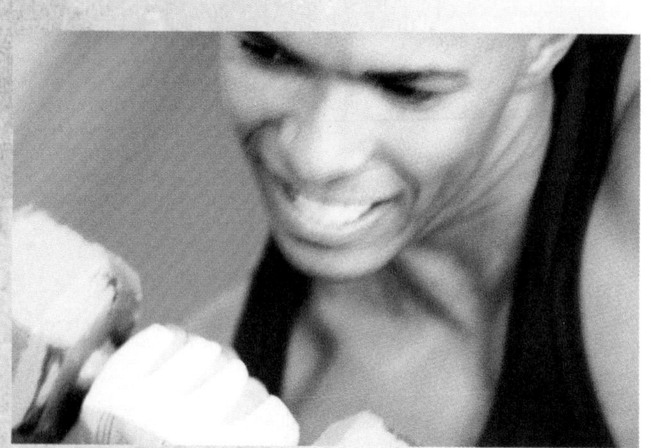

Chapter Objectives

- Define direct calorimetry, indirect calorimetry, closed-circuit spirometry, and open-circuit spirometry
- Diagram the closed-circuit spirometry system for oxygen consumption determinations
- Describe portable spirometry, bag technique, and computerized instrumentation systems of open-circuit spirometry
- Outline the basics of the micro-Scholander and Haldane techniques for chemical analysis of expired air samples
- Discuss the application of the doubly labeled water technique to estimate human daily energy expenditure and give advantages and limitations of the method
- Define respiratory quotient (RQ), and discuss its use to quantify (1) energy release in metabolism and (2) the composition of the food mixture metabolized during rest and steady-rate exercise
- Discuss the difference between RQ and respiratory exchange ratio (R) and factors that affect each

METHODS OF MEASURING THE BODY'S HEAT PRODUCTION

Two different approaches, **direct calorimetry** and **indirect calorimetry**, accurately quantify energy expenditure (energy generated by the body) during rest and physical activity.

Direct Calorimetry

All of the body's metabolic processes ultimately result in heat production. The early experiments of Lavoisier and Seguin and Lavoisier and LaPlace in the 1770s provided the impetus to measure the body's heat production directly during rest and physical activity. The idea, similar to that used in the bomb calorimeter described in Chapter 4 to determine food energy, provides a convenient (though elaborate) methodology to directly measure heat production in humans.

In the 1890s, at Wesleyan University, professors W. O. Atwater (a chemist) and E. B. Rosa (a physicist) used the first human calorimeter of major scientific importance.[1,28] Their elegant calorimetric experiments relating energy input (food consumption) to energy expenditure verified the law of the conservation of energy and established the validity of indirect calorimetry. The calorimeter diagramed schematically in Figure 8.1 consisted of a small chamber where a subject could live, eat, sleep, and exercise on a bicycle ergometer. The experiments lasted from several hours to 13 days, and some experiments involved cycling exercise performed for up to 16 hours, with total energy expenditure exceeding 10,000 kcal! A staff of 16, working in teams of 8 for 12-hour shifts, operated the airtight, thermally insulated calorimeter.[1] A known volume of water at a specified temperature circulated through a series of coils at the top of the chamber. Circulating water absorbed the heat produced and radiated by the subject. Insulation protected the entire chamber so that any change in water temperature (measured in 0.01°C with a microscope mounted alongside a thermometer) related directly to the subject's energy metabolism. For adequate ventilation, exhaled air continually passed from the room through chemicals that removed moisture and absorbed carbon dioxide. Oxygen was added to the air recirculated through the chamber.

In the 100 years since the publication of the seminal papers by Atwater and Rosa, other calorimetric methods have emerged for inferring energy expenditure from metabolic gas exchange (see next section) for extended periods in respiration chambers,[5,9,18,19] and via metabolic and thermal balance with water flow and airflow calorimeters.[17,22] For example, the modern space suit worn by astronauts during extravehicular activities represents a suit calorimeter designed to maintain respiratory gas exchange, thermal balance, and protection from a potentially dangerous ambient environment. These suits have application for performing extended work outside an orbiting space vehicle, on the lunar surface, and, eventually, while constructing space stations.[21]

Over the years, various other heat-measuring devices have been developed, each based on a different principle of operation. In an **airflow calorimeter**, the temperature change in air that flows through an insulated space, multiplied by the air's mass and specific heat (including calculations for evaporative heat loss), determines heat production. A **water flow calorimeter** operates similarly, except that a change in temperature occurs in water flowing through coils that make up part of an

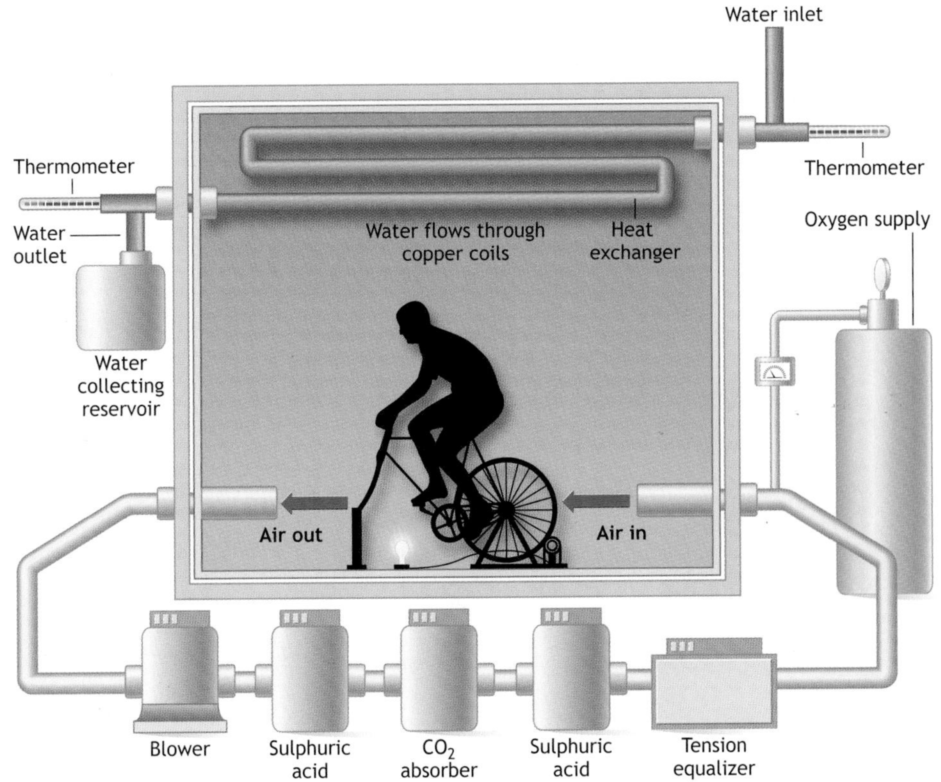

FIGURE 8.1 • A human calorimeter directly measures the body's rate of energy metabolism (heat production). In the Atwater-Rosa calorimeter depicted, a thin sheet of copper lines the interior wall to which heat exchangers attach overhead and through which cold water passes. Water cooled to 2°C moves at a high flow rate, rapidly absorbing the heat radiated from the subject during exercise. As the subject rests, warmer water flows at a slower rate. In the original bicycle ergometer shown in the schematic, the rear wheel contacts the shaft of a generator that powers a light bulb. In later-version ergometers, copper composed part of the rear wheel. The wheel rotated through the field of an electromagnet, producing an electric current for accurately determining power output.

environmentally self-contained body suit like that worn by astronauts. **Gradient layer calorimetry** measures body heat that flows from the subject through a sheet of insulating materials (with appropriate piping and cooler water flowing on the outside of the gradient). In **storage calorimetry**, the subject sits in an insulated tank surrounded by a known mass of water at a constant temperature. The heat given off by the subject changes the temperature of the surrounding water.

Direct measurement of heat production in humans has considerable theoretical implications but limited applications. Accurate measurements of heat production in the calorimeter require considerable time and expense and formidable engineering expertise. Thus, calorimeters remain inapplicable for energy determinations for most sport, occupational, and recreational activities. Their use is highly impractical in large-scale studies in underdeveloped and poor countries. Still, great need exists for total nutritional and energy assessment that includes measures of energy expenditure under deprivation conditions, particularly during undernutrition and starvation.[4]

Indirect Calorimetry

All energy-releasing reactions in the body ultimately depend on oxygen use. Measuring a person's oxygen consumption during physical activities therefore gives researchers an indirect, yet highly accurate, estimate of energy expenditure.[2,23] Compared with direct calorimetry, indirect calorimetry remains simple and less expensive to maintain and staff.

Studies with the bomb calorimeter show the release of approximately 4.82 kcal of energy when a blend of carbohydrate, lipid, and protein burns with 1 L of oxygen. Even with large variations in the metabolic mixture, this **calorific value for oxygen** varies only slightly, generally within 2 to 4%. Assuming the combustion of a mixed diet, a rounded value of 5.0 kcal per liter of oxygen consumed is an appropriate conversion factor for estimating energy expenditure under steady-rate conditions of aerobic metabolism. An energy–oxygen equivalent of 5.0 kcal per liter provides a suitable yardstick for expressing any aerobic physical activity in energy units (see Appendix C).

Indirect calorimetry yields results comparable to those from direct measurement in the human calorimeter.[22] **Closed-circuit spirometry** and **open-circuit spirometry** represent the two applications of indirect calorimetry.

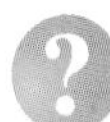

INTEGRATIVE QUESTION

What rationale underlies early experiments that quantified energy metabolism of small animals by measuring the rate that ice melted in a container surrounding the animal?

Closed-Circuit Spirometry

Figure 8.2 illustrates the technique of closed-circuit spirometry, developed in the late 1800s and currently used in hospitals and research laboratories to estimate resting energy expenditure. The subject breathes 100% oxygen from a prefilled

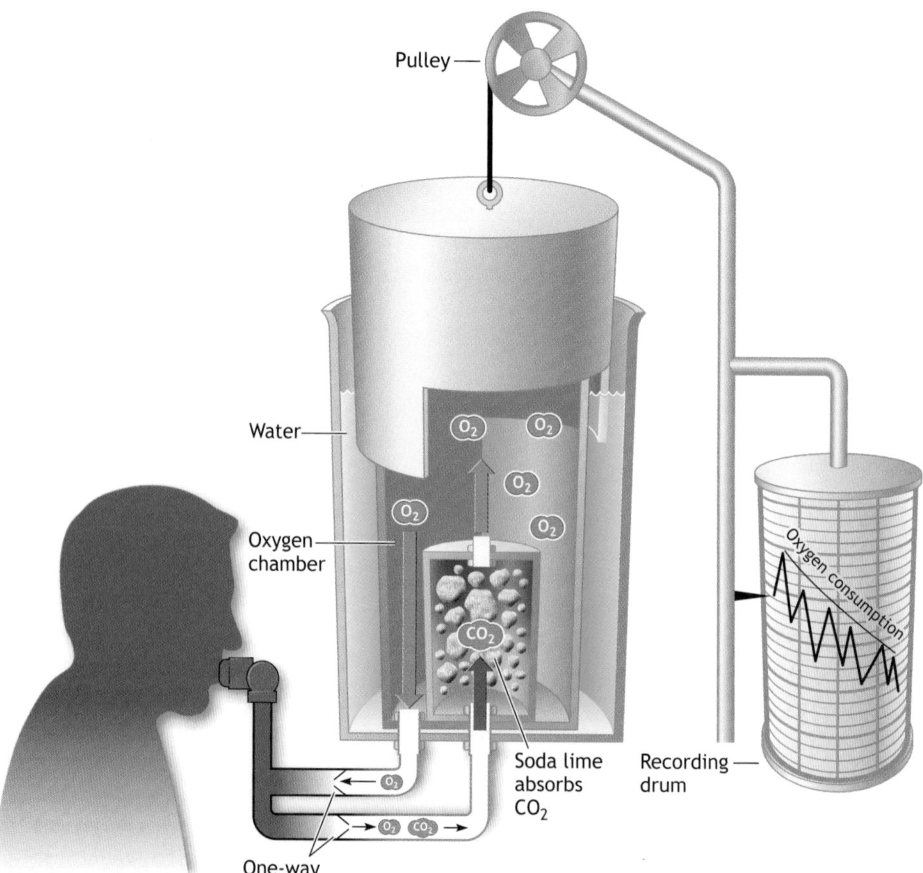

FIGURE 8.2 • The closed-circuit method employs a spirometer prefilled with 100% oxygen. As the subject rebreathes from the spirometer, soda lime removes the expired air's carbon dioxide. The difference between the initial and final volumes of oxygen in the calibrated spirometer indicates oxygen consumption during the measurement interval.

container (spirometer). The equipment is a closed system because the subject rebreathes only the gas in the spirometer. A canister of soda lime (potassium hydroxide) placed in the breathing circuit absorbs the carbon dioxide in the exhaled air. A drum attached to the spirometer revolves at a known speed to record the oxygen removed (oxygen consumption) from changes in the system's total volume.

During exercise, closed-circuit spirometry measurement becomes problematic. The subject must remain close to the bulky equipment, considerable resistance exists from the circuit's resistance to accommodating the large breathing volumes during exercise, and carbon dioxide removal lags behind its production rate during heavy exercise. For these reasons, open-circuit spirometry remains the most widely used procedure to measure exercise oxygen consumption.

Open-Circuit Spirometry

The open-circuit method provides a relatively simple way to measure oxygen consumption. A subject inhales ambient air that has a constant composition of 20.93% oxygen, 0.03% carbon dioxide, and 79.04% nitrogen (includes a small quantity of inert gases). The changes in oxygen and carbon dioxide percentages in expired air, compared with the percentages in inspired ambient air, indirectly reflect the ongoing process of energy metabolism. Thus, analysis of two factors—the volume of air breathed during a specified time period and the composition of exhaled air—provides a useful way to measure oxygen consumption and infer energy expenditure.

Three common indirect calorimetry procedures measure oxygen consumption during various physical activities:

- Portable spirometry
- Bag technique
- Computerized instrumentation

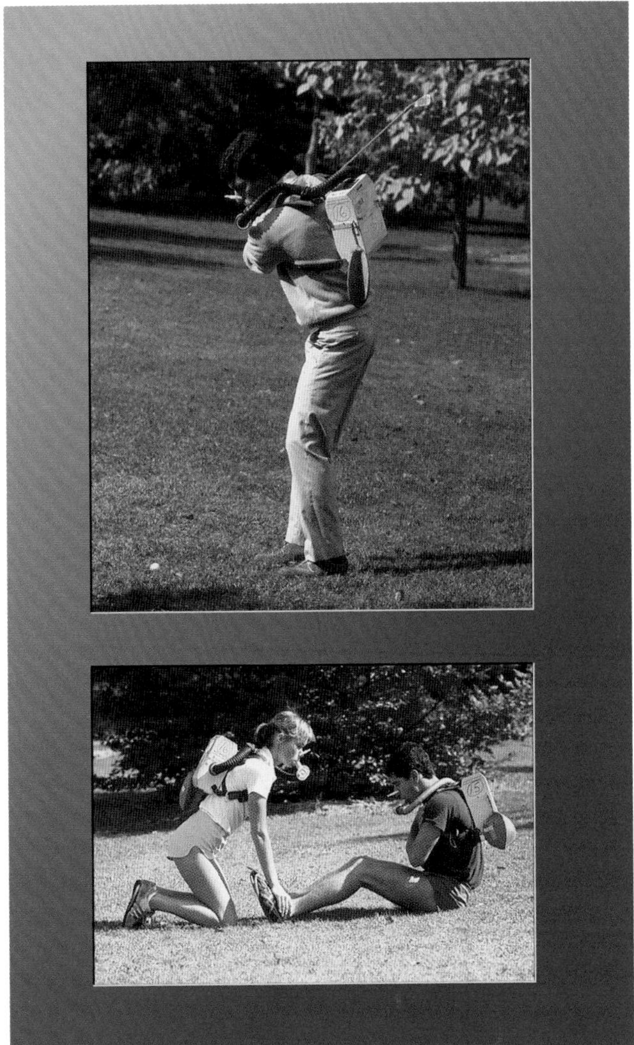

FIGURE 8.3 • Portable spirometer to measure oxygen consumption via the open-circuit method during golf and calisthenics exercise.

Portable Spirometry

Two German scientists in the early 1940s perfected a lightweight, portable system (first devised by German respiratory physiologist Nathan Zuntz [1847–1920] at the turn of the century) to determine energy expenditure indirectly during physical activity.[12] The activities included war-related operations such as traveling over different terrains with full battle gear, operating transportation vehicles including tanks and aircraft, and performing physical tasks that soldiers encounter during combat operations. With this system, the subject carries the 3-kg box-shaped apparatus shown in Figure 8.3 on the back, like a backpack. Through a two-way breathing valve, ambient air is inspired, and expired air exits through a gas meter. The meter measures total expired air volume and collects a small gas sample for later analysis of oxygen and carbon dioxide content and determination of oxygen consumption and energy expenditure for the measurement period.

Carrying the portable spirometer allows considerable freedom of movement in physical activities as diverse as mountain climbing, downhill skiing, sailing, golf, and common household activities (Appendix C). However, the equipment becomes cumbersome during vigorous activity, and the meter begins to underrecord air flow volume during heavy exercise with rapid breathing.[15]

Bag Technique

Figure 8.4 A and B depicts the classic bag technique. The subject in Figure 8.4A rides a stationary bicycle ergometer, wearing headgear attached to a two-way, high-velocity, low-resistance breathing valve. He breathes ambient air through one side of the valve and expels it through the other side. The expired air then passes into either large plastic or canvas Douglas bags (named for the distinguished British respiratory physiologist Claude G. Douglas [1882–1963]) or rubber meteorologic balloons or directly through a gas meter that continually measures expired air volume. The meter draws off a small sample of expired air for subsequent analysis of O_2 and CO_2 composition.

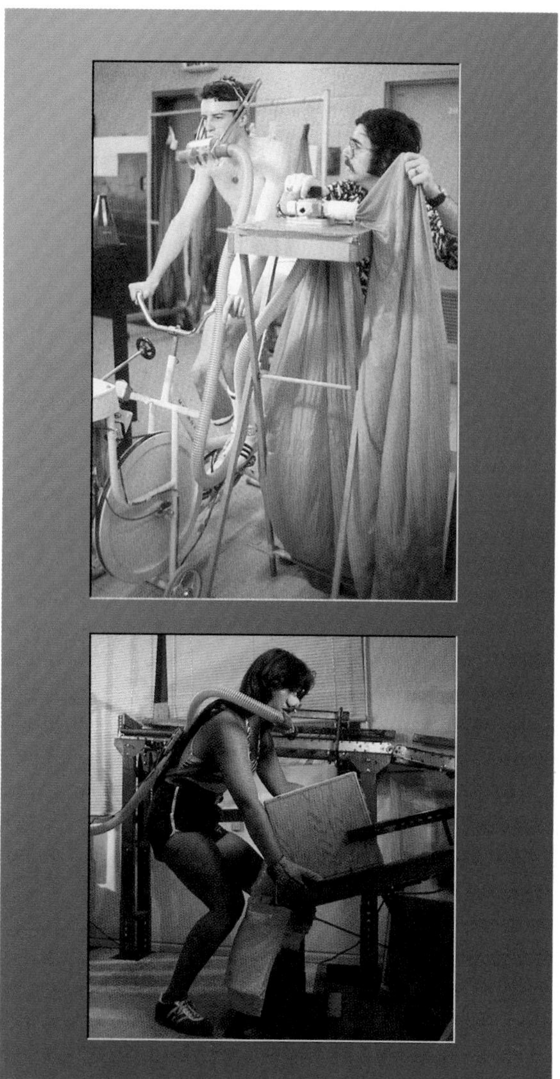

Figure 8.4 • Measurement of oxygen consumption with open-circuit spirometry (classic bag technique) during (**A**) stationary cycle ergometer exercise, and (**B**) box loading and unloading.

Figure 8.4B illustrates oxygen consumption measured by the bag technique while the subject lifts boxes of different weights and sizes, to evaluate the energy requirements of a specific occupational task.

Computerized Instrumentation

With advances in computer and microprocessor technology, the exercise scientist can measure metabolic and physiologic responses to exercise accurately and rapidly.[11,31] A computer interfaces with at least three instruments: a system to continuously sample the subject's expired air, a flow-measuring device to record air volume breathed, and oxygen and carbon dioxide analyzers to measure the expired gas mixture's composition. The computer performs metabolic calculations based on electronic signals it receives from the instruments. A printed or graphic display of the data appears throughout the measurement period. More-advanced systems include automated blood pressure, heart rate, and temperature monitors, as well as preset instructions to regulate speed, duration, and exercise intensity with a treadmill, bicycle ergometer, stepper, rower, swim flume, or other exercise apparatus. Figure 8.5 depicts computerized instrumentation for assessing and monitoring metabolic and physiologic responses during exercise.

The system illustrated in Figure 8.6 provides wireless telemetric transmission of data for metabolic measurement—pulmonary ventilation and oxygen and carbon dioxide analysis—during a broad range of exercise, sport, and occupational activities.[30] The lightweight and miniaturized components (~1 kg) include a voice-sensitive chip that provides feedback on pacing, duration of exercise, energy expenditure, heart rate, and pulmonary ventilation. The unit's microprocessor stores several hours of exercise data for later downloading to a computer. By use of telemetry, data appear in "real time" on a host computer. With proper calibration, commercially available miniaturized equipment provides reasonable accuracy for quantifying the energy cost in vivo of diverse sport and occupational activities.[3] Computerized systems offer tremendous advantages in terms of ease of operation and speed of data analysis, but distinct disadvantages also exist. These include the high cost of equipment and delays owing to system breakdowns. Of course, good results require good data. *Regardless of the apparent sophistication of a particular automated system, the output data still reflect the accuracy of the measuring device. Therefore, accuracy and validity of measurement devices require careful and frequent calibration using established reference standards.*

INTEGRATIVE QUESTION

Discuss the common energy basis for equating food intake and physical activity.

Chemical Gas Analyzers for Calibration Purposes. Figure 8.7 illustrates two common chemical procedures for analyzing gas mixtures for oxygen, carbon dioxide, and nitrogen and for calibrating and/or validating electronic analyzers. The **micro-Scholander** technique measures oxygen and carbon dioxide concentration in expired air to an accuracy of ±0.015 mL per 100 mL of gas.[20] A skilled technician can perform one analysis of a 0.5-mL microsample of the gas in about 10 minutes. The **Haldane** method provides another technique for gas analysis.[7] It uses a 10-mL air sample and requires between 10 and 15 minutes to complete one analysis. The Haldane method has a slightly lower accuracy than the Scholander method because of the larger gas sample.

Before the conversion to computerized instrumentation to measure oxygen and carbon dioxide concentrations in expired air, oxygen consumption determinations used either the Scholander or Haldane gas analysis methods. These methods involved hundreds of time-consuming separate analyses for a single experiment, with frequent duplicate measurements to verify results. This partly explains why energy metabolism studies from the early exercise physiology literature often only relied on one or two subjects and took so long to complete. When performed properly with attention to detail,

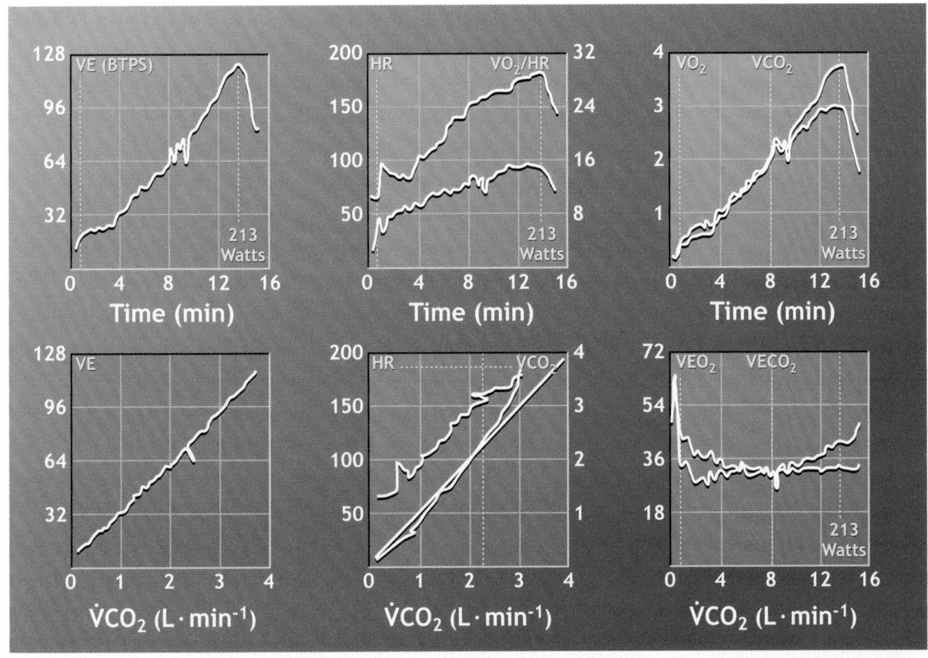

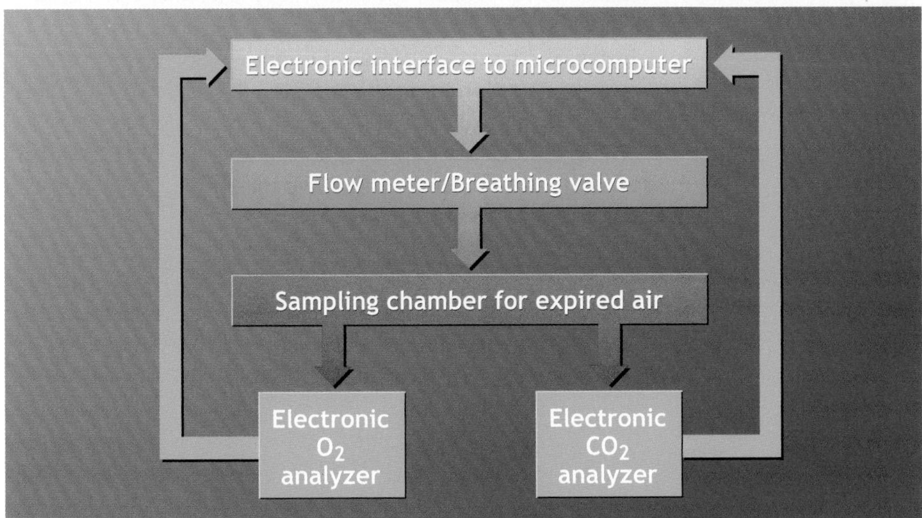

FIGURE 8.5 • Computer systems approach to collecting, analyzing, and monitoring physiologic and metabolic data. (Graphics courtesy of Fitco, a division of PhysioDyne Instrument Corporation, Farmingdale, NY.)

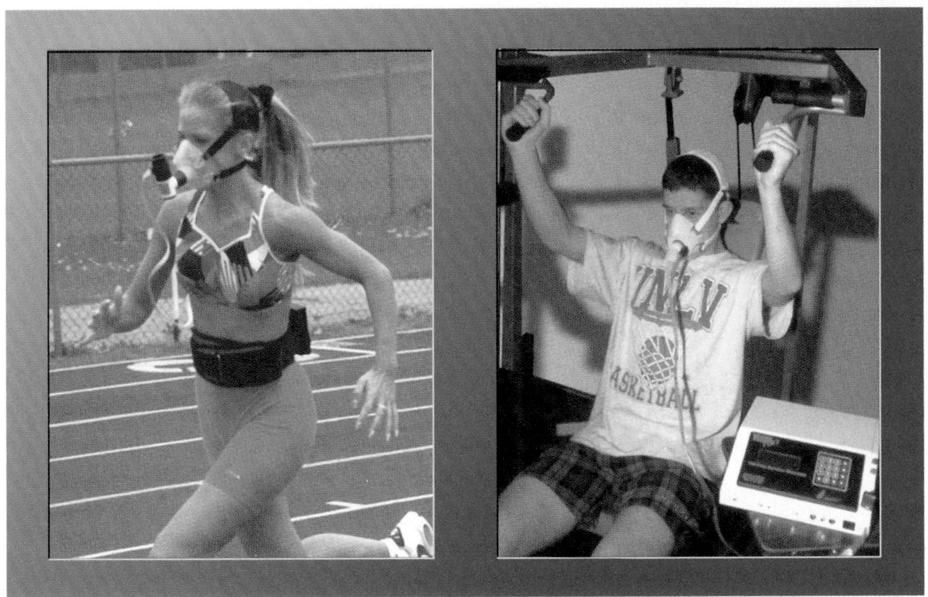

FIGURE 8.6 • Miniaturized metabolic system. The 3 × 6–inch system fits in a chest-vest containing the electronic instrumentation, battery, oxygen and carbon dioxide sensors, and telemetry connections to a microcomputer that permits infrared transmission to a source computer. Easily transported during physical activity, the metabolic system weighs approximately 1.13 kg (2.5 lb). The headpiece contains all of the electronic instrumentation, including the microcomputer. (Photo courtesy of P. Howard, AeroSport Inc., Ann Arbor, MI.)

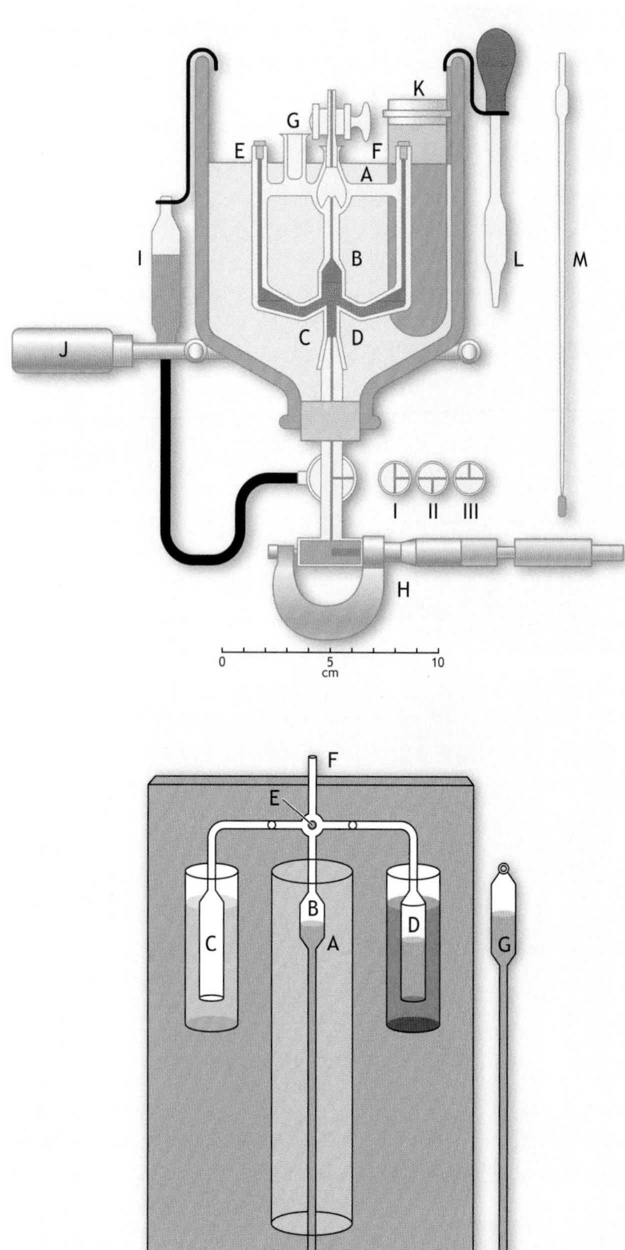

FIGURE 8.7 • General schematic for two common analytical procedures for gas calibration. *Top.* Micro-Scholander gas analyzer. *A,* Compensating chamber; *B,* reaction chamber; *C,* side arm for CO_2 absorber; *D,* side arm for O_2 absorber; *E* and *F,* solid vaccine bottle stoppers; *G,* receptacle for stopcock; *H,* micrometer burette; *I,* leveling bulb containing mercury; *J,* handle for tilting apparatus; *K,* tube for storing the acid rinsing solution; *L,* pipette for the rinsing acid; *M,* transfer pipette. *Bottom.* Haldane gas analyzer. *A,* Water jacket surrounding the measuring burette; *B,* calibrated measuring burette containing a gas sample for measurement; *C,* vessel containing CO_2 absorber (potassium hydroxide); *D,* vessel containing O_2 absorber (pyrogallate); *E,* glass valve; *F,* entry for gas sample; *G,* mercury-leveling bulb. The gas introduced into the burette is exposed to the O_2 and CO_2 absorbers by alternately lowering and raising the mercury-leveling bulb. The O_2 and CO_2 gas volumes are determined by subtracting the initial volume.

these chemical analyzers produced data that were highly accurate and reliable. Chemical gas analyzers are used to check the accuracy of the more modern electronic gas analyzers.

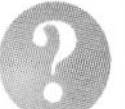

INTEGRATIVE QUESTION

Justify the use of the measurement of only CO_2 production to estimate energy expenditure during steady-rate exercise.

Direct Versus Indirect Calorimetry

Comparisons of energy metabolism with both direct and indirect calorimetry provide convincing evidence for the validity of the indirect method. Research at the turn of the century compared the two calorimetry methods over 40 days on three men who lived in a calorimeter similar to the one shown in Figure 8.1. Daily energy expenditure averaged 2723 kcal when measured directly by heat production and 2717 kcal when computed indirectly by closed-circuit oxygen-consumption measures. Other experiments with animals and humans, using moderate (steady-rate) exercise, also showed close agreement between direct and indirect methods; in most instances, the difference averaged less than 1%. In Atwater and Rosa's calorimetry experiments, the error of the method averaged only 0.2%. This remarkable achievement, using mostly handmade instruments, resulted from these scientists' dedication to precise calibration methods, long before the availability of electronic instrumentation.

DOUBLY LABELED WATER TECHNIQUE

The doubly labeled water technique provides an isotope-based method to estimate total daily energy expenditure of groups of children and adults in free-living conditions without the normal constraints imposed by laboratory procedures.[26,32] The technique does not provide sufficient refinement for accurate estimates of an individual's energy expenditure.[24] Because of the expense in using doubly labeled water and the need for sophisticated measurement equipment, few studies routinely use this method, and subject number remains small. Nevertheless, its measurement does serve as a criterion or standard to validate other methods that estimate total daily energy expenditure over prolonged time periods.[6,15,21]

The subject consumes a quantity of water containing a known concentration of the stable isotopes of hydrogen (^2H, or deuterium) and oxygen (^{18}O or oxygen-18)—hence the term **doubly labeled water**. The isotopes distribute throughout all bodily fluids. Labeled hydrogen leaves the body as water (^2H_2O) in sweat, urine, and pulmonary water vapor, while labeled oxygen leaves as both water ($H_2{}^{18}O$) and carbon dioxide ($C^{18}O_2$) produced during macronutrient oxidation in energy metabolism. Differences between elimination rates of the two isotopes (determined by an isotope ratio mass spectrometer) relative to the body's normal background levels estimate total CO_2 production during the measurement

Focus on Research

Respiratory Gas Exchange Infers Metabolic Mixture

Krogh A, Lindhard J. The relative value of fat and carbohydrate as sources of muscular energy. Biochem J 1920;14:290.

➤ In this 73-page research report, Nobel laureate August Krogh and colleague Johannes Lindhard made 220 determinations of respiratory gas exchange on 6 subjects (including themselves) who consumed varied diets to determine macronutrient combustion during rest and exercise. For 2 days prior to testing, subjects maintained a high-carbohydrate, low-protein diet or a high-fat, low-protein diet. Krogh and Lindhard believed that different respiratory quotients (RQs) for the same exercise undergoing different diets would indicate the preferential use of a particular fuel substrate.

The researchers made careful energy expenditure measurements during rest and 2 hours of cycling, using a closed-circuit, air current flow-through apparatus common to that time period. Subjects rode the stationary bicycle within the chamber, with appropriate tubing placed between the subject and a gas collection system outside the chamber (see figure). Typical of Krogh's research, extreme care in data collection ensured high accuracy and reliability of data. Respiratory gas exchange measurements achieved accuracy to within ±1.0%, a remarkable figure considering the handmade equipment used.

The research's major finding was that the energy expended to perform a standard physical effort varied inversely with the RQ. This meant that different energy values existed for the oxidation of fat and carbohydrate; specifically, fat released less energy than carbohydrate per liter of oxygen consumed during exercise. Although subjects consumed exclusively either lipid or carbohydrate (with protein held constant), RQ values did not indicate combustion of fat only or carbohydrate only. This permitted quantifying the relationship between RQ and the relative amounts of fat and carbohydrate oxidized. The researchers found that the percentage of total energy derived from fat oxidation approximated a straight-line function of the RQ.

In a second series of experiments performed on two trained athletes during rest and exercise, the proportion of carbohydrate to fat catabolized varied with the relative availability of the two substrates. Krogh and Lindhard hypothesized that neither fat nor carbohydrate exclusively supplied energy during exercise, but that a blend of the macronutrients probably served simultaneously as fuel.

Overall, this important 1920 experiment showed the following:

1. Efficiency of constant-load exercise is higher with carbohydrate as the energy fuel than with fat.
2. Performance deteriorates in high-intensity exercise when fat (not carbohydrate) serves as the preferential energy nutrient.
3. Preexercise nutrition influences the metabolic mixture during rest and exercise.
4. The RQ changes in the transition from rest to moderate exercise and increases with higher-intensity exercise, indicating greater reliance on carbohydrate oxidation.
5. Fat oxidation predominates during the latter portion of 1 hour of constant-intensity exercise.

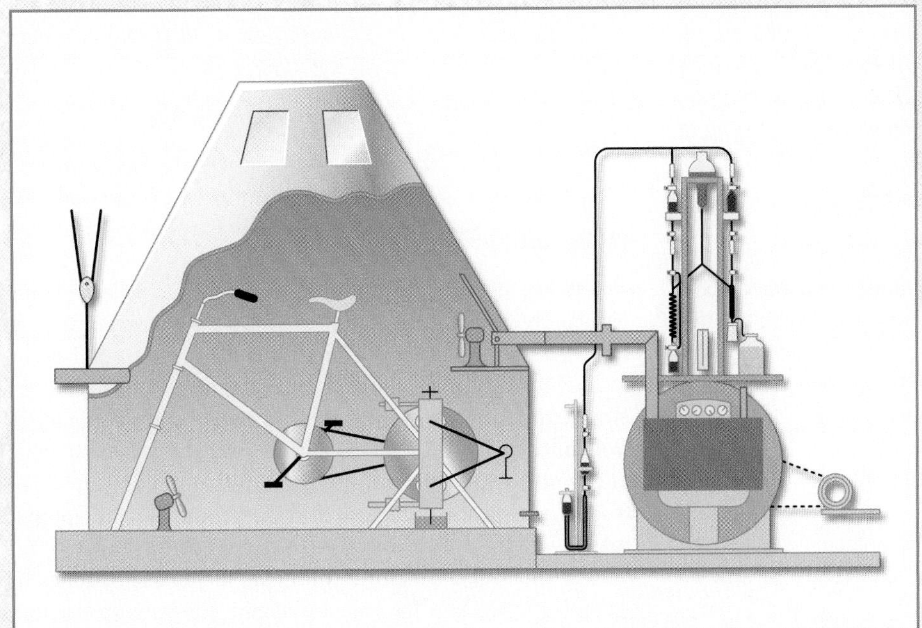

Unique enclosed chamber containing a cycle ergometer and two fans. The gas collection apparatus, situated outside the chamber, is connected to the chamber via small-bore tubing. The chamber sat in water to ensure an airtight seal.

period. Oxygen consumption is easily estimated on the basis of CO_2 production and an assumed (or measured) RQ value of 0.85 (see next section).

Under normal circumstances, analysis of the subject's urine or saliva before ingestion of the doubly labeled water provides the control baseline values for ^{18}O and ^{2}H. Ingested isotopes require about 5 hours to distribute throughout the body water. The researchers then measure the enriched urine or saliva sample initially and then every day (or week) thereafter for the study's duration, which is usually up to 2 or 3 weeks. The progressive decrease in the sample concentrations of the two isotopes permits computation of the CO_2 production rate.[25] Accuracy of the doubly labeled water technique versus directly measured energy expenditure in controlled settings averages between 3 and 5%. This magnitude of error probably increases in field studies, particularly among physically active individuals.[29]

The doubly labeled water technique provides an ideal way to assess total energy expenditure of individuals over prolonged periods including bed rest and extreme activities like climbing Mt. Everest, cycling the Tour de France, trekking across Antarctica, military activities, extravehicular activities in space, and endurance running and swimming.[16,27] Drawbacks to the method include the cost of enriched ^{18}O and expense incurred in spectrometric analysis of both isotopes.

THE RESPIRATORY QUOTIENT

Research in the early part of the 20th century uncovered a way to evaluate the metabolic mixture metabolized during rest and exercise from measures of pulmonary gas exchange (see Focus on Research).[13] Because of inherent chemical differences in carbohydrate, fat, and protein composition, they require different amounts of oxygen to effect complete oxidation of each molecule's carbon and hydrogen atoms to the carbon dioxide and water end products. Thus, carbon dioxide produced per unit of oxygen consumed varies with the type of substrate (carbohydrate, fat, protein) metabolized. The **respiratory quotient (RQ)** describes this ratio of metabolic gas exchange as follows:

$$RQ = CO_2 \text{ produced} \div O_2 \text{ consumed}$$

The RQ provides a convenient guide for approximating the nutrient mixture catabolized for energy during rest and aerobic exercise.[8,14] Also, because the caloric equivalents for oxygen differ somewhat depending on the nutrient oxidized, precise determination of the body's heat production by indirect calorimetry requires measuring both RQ and oxygen consumption.

RQ for Carbohydrate

The complete oxidation of one glucose molecule requires six oxygen molecules and produces six molecules of carbon dioxide and water as follows:

$$C_6H_{12}O_6 + 6\ O_2 \div \rightarrow 6\ CO_2 + 6\ H_2O$$

$$RQ = 6\ CO_2 \div 6\ O_2 = 1.00$$

Gas exchange during glucose oxidation produces a number of CO_2 molecules equal to the number of O_2 molecules consumed; therefore, the RQ for carbohydrate equals 1.00.

RQ for Fat

The chemical composition of fats differ from that of carbohydrates because fats contain considerably more hydrogen and carbon atoms compared with the number of oxygen atoms. Consequently, fat catabolism requires more oxygen in relation to carbon dioxide production. For example, palmitic acid, a typical fatty acid, oxidizes to carbon dioxide and water, producing 16 carbon dioxide molecules for every 23 oxygen molecules consumed. The following equation summarizes this exchange to compute the RQ:

$$C_{16}H_{32}O_2 + 23\ O_2 \rightarrow 16\ CO_2 + 16\ H_2O$$

$$RQ = 16\ CO_2 \div 23\ O_2 = 0.696$$

Generally, a value of 0.70 represents the RQ for fat, with values ranging between 0.69 and 0.73, depending on the oxidized fatty acid's carbon-chain length.

RQ for Protein

Proteins do not simply oxidize to carbon dioxide and water during energy metabolism in the body. Rather, the liver first deaminates the amino acid molecule. The body then excretes the nitrogen and sulfur fragments in the urine, sweat, and feces. The remaining keto acid fragment then oxidizes to carbon dioxide and water to provide energy for biologic work. To achieve complete combustion, these short-chain keto acids, as in fat catabolism, require more oxygen in relation to carbon dioxide produced. The protein albumin oxidizes as follows:

$$C_{72}H_{112}N_2O_{22}S + 77\ O_2 \rightarrow 63\ CO_2 + 38\ H_2O + SO_3 + 9\ CO(NH_2)_2$$

$$RQ = 63\ CO_2 \div 77\ O_2 = 0.818$$

The general value 0.82 characterizes the RQ for protein.

Nonprotein RQ

The RQ computed from the compositional analysis of expired air usually reflects the catabolism of a blend of carbohydrates, fats, and proteins. One can determine the precise contribution of each of these nutrients to the metabolic mixture. For example, the kidneys excrete approximately 1 g of urinary nitrogen for every 5.57 (modern value) to 6.25 g (classic value) of protein metabolized for energy.[10] Each gram of excreted nitrogen represents a carbon dioxide production of approximately 4.8 L and an oxygen consumption of about 6.0 L. Within this framework, the following example illustrates the stepwise procedure for calculating the elements in the **nonprotein RQ**; that is, that portion of the respiratory exchange attributed not to the combustion of protein, but *only* to carbohydrate and fat.

This example considers data from a subject who consumes 4.0 L of oxygen and produces 3.4 L of carbon dioxide during a 15-minute rest period. During this time, the kidneys excrete 0.13 g of nitrogen in the urine.

Step 1. 4.8 L CO_2 per g protein metabolized × 0.13 g = 0.62 L CO_2 produced in protein catabolism

Step 2. 6.0 L O_2 per g protein metabolized × 0.13 g = 0.78 L O_2 consumed in protein catabolism

Step 3. Nonprotein CO_2 produced = 3.4 L CO_2 – 0.62 L CO_2 = 2.78 L CO_2

Step 4. Nonprotein O_2 consumed = 4.0 L O_2 – 0.78 L O_2 = 3.22 L O_2

Step 5. Nonprotein RQ = 2.78 ÷ 3.22 = 0.86

Table 8.1 presents the thermal (energy) equivalents for oxygen consumption for different nonprotein RQ values and the actual percentage of fat and carbohydrate used for energy. For the nonprotein RQ of 0.86 computed in the previous example, each liter of oxygen consumed liberates 4.875 kcal. Also, for this RQ, 54.1% of the nonprotein calories derive from carbohydrate, and 45.9% derive from fat. The total 15-minute heat production at rest attributable to fat and carbohydrate catabolism equals 15.70 kcal (4.875 kcal · L^{-1} × 3.22 L O_2); the energy from the breakdown of protein equals 3.51 kcal (4.5 kcal · L^{-1} × 0.78 L O_2). Consequently, the total energy from both the protein and nonprotein macronutrients during the 15-minute period equals 19.21 kcal (15.70 kcal nonprotein + 3.51 kcal protein).

Interestingly, if the thermal equivalent for a mixed diet (RQ = 0.82) had been used in the caloric transformation, or if RQ had been computed from total respiratory gas exchange and applied to Table 8.1 without considering the protein component, the estimated energy expenditure would be 19.3 kcal (4.825 kcal · L^{-1} × 4.0 L O_2; assuming a mixed diet). This cor-

TABLE 8.1 ➤ THERMAL EQUIVALENTS OF OXYGEN FOR THE NONPROTEIN RQ, INCLUDING PERCENTAGE KILOCALORIES AND GRAMS DERIVED FROM CARBOHYDRATES AND FAT

		Percentage kcal Derived from		Grams per LO_2	
Nonprotein RQ	kcal per LO_2	Carbohydrate	Fat	Carbohydrate	Fat
0.707	4.686	0.0	100.0	0.000	0.496
0.71	4.690	1.1	98.9	0.012	0.491
0.72	4.702	4.8	95.2	0.051	0.476
0.73	4.714	8.4	91.6	0.090	0.460
0.74	4.727	12.0	88.0	0.130	0.444
0.75	4.739	15.6	84.4	0.170	0.428
0.76	4.750	19.2	80.8	0.211	0.412
0.77	4.764	22.8	77.2	0.250	0.396
0.78	4.776	26.3	73.7	0.290	0.380
0.79	4.788	29.9	70.1	0.330	0.363
0.80	4.801	33.4	66.6	0.371	0.347
0.81	4.813	36.9	63.1	0.413	0.330
0.82	4.825	40.3	59.7	0.454	0.313
0.83	4.838	43.8	56.2	0.496	0.297
0.84	4.850	47.2	52.8	0.537	0.280
0.85	4.862	50.7	49.3	0.579	0.263
0.86	4.875	54.1	45.9	0.621	0.247
0.87	4.887	57.5	42.5	0.663	0.230
0.88	4.899	60.8	39.2	0.705	0.213
0.89	4.911	64.2	35.8	0.749	0.195
0.90	4.924	67.5	32.5	0.791	0.178
0.91	4.936	70.8	29.2	0.834	0.160
0.92	4.948	74.1	25.9	0.877	0.143
0.93	4.961	77.4	22.6	0.921	0.125
0.94	4.973	80.7	19.3	0.964	0.108
0.95	4.985	84.0	16.0	1.008	0.090
0.96	4.998	87.2	12.8	1.052	0.072
0.97	5.010	90.4	9.6	1.097	0.054
0.98	5.022	93.6	6.4	1.142	0.036
0.99	5.035	96.8	3.2	1.186	0.018
1.00	5.047	100.0	0	1.231	0.000

From Zuntz N. Ueber die Bedeutung der verschiedenen Nährstoffe als Erzeuger der Muskelkraft. Arch Gesamte Physiol, Bonn, Germany: 1901;LXXXIII: 557–571; Pflügers Arch Physiol,1901;83:557.

In a Practical Sense

➤➤ The Weir Method to Calculate Energy Expenditure

In 1949, J.B. Weir, a Scottish physician and physiologist from Glasgow University, presented a simple method to estimate caloric expenditure ($kcal \cdot min^{-1}$) from measures of pulmonary ventilation and expired oxygen percentage, accurate to within ±1% of the traditional respiratory quotient (RQ) method.

Basic Equation

Weir showed that the following formula calculated energy expenditure if total energy production from protein breakdown equaled 12.5% (a reasonable percentage for most people):

$$kcal \cdot min^{-1} = \dot{V}_{E(STPD)} \times (1.044 - 0.0499 \times \%\ O_{2E})$$

where $\dot{V}_{E(STPD)}$ represents expired minute ventilation corrected to STPD conditions, and $\%O_{2E}$ represents expired oxygen percentage. The value in parenthesis ($1.044 - 0.0499 \times \%O_{2E}$) represents the "Weir factor." The table displays Weir factors for different $\%O_{2E}$ values.

To use the table, locate the $\%O_{2E}$ and corresponding Weir factor. Compute energy expenditure in $kcal \cdot min^{-1}$ by multiplying the Weir factor by $\dot{V}_{E(STPD)}$.

Example

A person runs on a treadmill and $\dot{V}_{E(STPD)} = 50\ L \cdot min^{-1}$ and $\%O_{2E} = 16.0\%$. One computes energy expenditure by the Weir method as follows:

$$kcal \cdot min^{-1} = \dot{V}_{E(STPD)} \times (1.044 - [0.0499 \times \%O_{2E}])$$
$$kcal \cdot min^{-1} = 50 \times (1.044 - [0.0499 \times 16.0])$$
$$kcal \cdot min^{-1} = 50 \times 0.2456$$
$$kcal \cdot min^{-1} = 12.3$$

Weir also derived the following equation to calculate $kcal \cdot min^{-1}$ from RQ and $\dot{V}O_2$ in $L \cdot min^{-1}$:

$$kcal \cdot min^{-1} = [(1.1 \times RQ) + 3.9] \times \dot{V}O_2.$$

Weir Factors

$\%O_{2E}$	Weir Factor	$\%O_{2E}$	Weir Factor
14.50	0.3205	17.00	0.1957
14.60	0.3155	17.10	0.1907
14.70	0.3105	17.20	0.1857
14.80	0.3055	17.30	0.1807
14.90	0.3005	17.40	0.1757
15.00	0.2955	17.50	0.1707
15.10	0.2905	17.60	0.1658
15.20	0.2855	17.70	0.1608
15.30	0.2805	17.80	0.1558
15.40	0.2755	17.90	0.1508
15.50	0.2705	18.00	0.1468
15.60	0.2656	18.10	0.1408
15.70	0.2606	18.20	0.1368
15.80	0.2556	18.30	0.1308
15.90	0.2506	18.40	0.1268
16.00	0.2456	18.50	0.1208
16.10	0.2406	18.60	0.1168
16.20	0.2366	18.70	0.1109
16.30	0.2306	18.80	0.1068
16.40	0.2256	18.90	0.1009
16.50	0.2206	19.00	0.0969
16.60	0.2157	19.10	0.0909
16.70	0.2107	19.20	0.0868
16.80	0.2057	19.30	0.0809
16.90	0.2007	19.40	0.0769

If $\%O_{2E}$ does not appear in the table, compute individual Weir factors as $1.044 - 0.0499 \times \%O_{2E}$. From Weir JB. New methods for calculating metabolic rates with special reference to protein metabolism. J Physiol 1949;109:1.

responds to a difference of only 0.5% from the value obtained with the more-elaborate and time-consuming method requiring urinary nitrogen analysis. *In most cases, use of the gross metabolic RQ calculated from pulmonary gas exchange and applied to Table 8.1 without measures of urinary and other nitrogen sources introduces only minimal error, because the contribution of protein to energy metabolism is usually small.*

How Much Food Is Metabolized for Energy?

The last two columns of Table 8.1 present conversions for the nonprotein RQ to grams of carbohydrate and fat metabolized per liter of oxygen consumed. For the subject with an RQ of 0.86, this represents approximately 0.62 g of carbohydrate and 0.25 g of fat. For the 3.22 L of oxygen consumed during the 15-minute rest period, this represents 2.0 g of carbohydrate (3.22 L O_2 × 0.62) and 0.80 g of fat (3.22 L O_2 × 0.25) metabolized for energy.

RQ for a Mixed Diet

The RQ seldom reflects the oxidation of pure carbohydrate or pure fat during activities ranging from complete bed rest to mild aerobic exercise (walking or slow jogging). Instead, catabolism of a mixture of these nutrients occurs, with an RQ intermediate between 0.70 and 1.00. *For most purposes, we assume an RQ of 0.82 (metabolism of a mixture of 40% carbohydrate and 60% fat) and apply the caloric equivalent of 4.825 kcal per liter of oxygen for energy transformations.* In using 4.825, the maximum error possible in estimating energy expenditure from steady-rate oxygen consumption averages about 4%. Of course, when requiring greater precision, one must compute the actual RQ and consult Table 8.1 to obtain the exact caloric transformation and percentage contribution of carbohydrate and fat to the metabolic mixture.

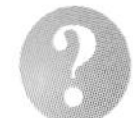

INTEGRATIVE QUESTION

How have exercise physiologists been able to determine that between 70% and 80% of the energy is derived from the combustion of fat during the last phases of a marathon run?

RESPIRATORY EXCHANGE RATIO

Use of the RQ assumes that the exchange of O_2 and CO_2 measured at the lungs reflects the actual gas exchange from macronutrient catabolism in the cell. This assumption remains reasonably valid during rest and steady-rate exercise conditions with little reliance on anaerobic metabolism. However, factors spuriously alter the exchange of oxygen and carbon dioxide in the lungs, so that the ratio of gas exchange no longer reflects only the substrate mixture in energy metabolism. Respiratory physiologists refer to the ratio of carbon dioxide produced to oxygen consumed under such conditions as the **respiratory exchange ratio** (**R**, or **RER**). In this case, the pulmonary exchange of oxygen and carbon dioxide no longer reflects cellular oxidation of specific foods. One computes this exchange ratio in exactly the same manner as the RQ.

For example, carbon dioxide elimination increases during hyperventilation, because breathing increases to disproportionately high levels compared with actual metabolic demands (see Chapter 14). Overbreathing decreases the blood's normal level of carbon dioxide because this gas "blows off" from the lungs in the expired air without a corresponding increase in oxygen consumption. This creates a rise in the respiratory exchange ratio (usually above 1.00) that does not reflect macronutrient oxidation.

Exhaustive exercise presents another situation in which R rises significantly above 1.00. Sodium bicarbonate in the blood buffers, or neutralizes, the lactate generated during anaerobic metabolism, to maintain proper acid–base balance. Lactate buffering produces carbonic acid, a weaker acid. In the pulmonary capillaries, carbonic acid degrades to its component carbon dioxide and water molecules, and carbon dioxide readily exits the lungs in the reaction:

$$\text{HLa} + \text{NaHCO}_3 \rightarrow \text{NaLa} + \text{H}_2\text{CO}_3 \rightarrow \text{H}_2\text{O} + \text{CO}_2 \rightarrow \text{Lungs}$$

The R increases above 1.00 because buffering adds "extra" carbon dioxide to the expired air, above the quantity normally released during energy metabolism. In rare instances, the exchange ratio exceeds 1.00 when a person gains body fat through excessive dietary carbohydrate intake. In this lipogenic situation, the conversion of carbohydrate to fat liberates oxygen as the excess calories accumulate in adipose tissue. The released oxygen then supplies energy metabolism; this reduces the lungs' uptake of atmospheric oxygen despite the normal carbon dioxide production.

Relatively low R values can also occur. For example, the cells and bodily fluids retain carbon dioxide following exhaustive exercise to replenish the sodium bicarbonate that buffered the accumulating lactate. This action to replenish alkaline reserve decreases the expired carbon dioxide level without affecting oxygen consumption and may cause the respiratory exchange ratio to dip below 0.70.

METABOLIC CALCULATIONS

Much of the study of exercise physiology involves assessment of energy metabolism. Measurement of the oxygen and carbon dioxide content of expired air, together with either the inspired or expired breathing volume, provides the basic data for determining respiratory gas exchange and oxygen consumption for inferring energy expenditure. Appendix D presents the step-by-step method and rationale for metabolic calculations based on experimental data obtained from open-circuit spirometry.

Summary

1. Direct and indirect calorimetry represent two methods for determining human energy expenditure. Direct calorimetry measures heat production in an appropriately insulated calorimeter. Indirect calorimetry infers energy expenditure from measurements of oxygen consumption and carbon dioxide production, using either closed-circuit spirometry or open-circuit spirometry.
2. The doubly labeled water technique estimates energy expenditure of children and adults in free-living conditions without the normal constraints imposed by laboratory procedures. It serves as a "gold standard" to validate other long-term energy expenditure estimates. Drawbacks include the cost of enriched ^{18}O and the expense of spectrometric analysis of both isotopes.
3. The complete oxidation of each nutrient requires a different quantity of oxygen consumption for comparable carbon dioxide production. The ratio of carbon dioxide produced to oxygen consumed, the respiratory quotient (RQ), provides quantitative information about the macronutrient mixture catabolized for energy. The RQ equals 1.00 for carbohydrate, 0.70 for fat, and 0.82 for protein.
4. For each RQ, a corresponding caloric value exists per liter of oxygen consumed. The RQ–kcal relationship provides an accurate way to determine energy expenditure during exercise.
5. The respiratory exchange ratio (R) reflects the pulmonary exchange of carbon dioxide and oxygen under differing physiologic and metabolic conditions; R does not fully mirror the gas exchange of the macronutrient mixture catabolized.

References

1. Atwater WO, Rosa EB. Description of a new respiration calorimeter and experiments on the conservation of energy in the human body. US Department of Agriculture, Office of Experiment Stations, Bulletin no. 63. Washington, DC: Government Printing Office, 1899.
2. Brooks GA, et al. Estimation of anaerobic energy production and efficiency in rats during exercise. J Appl Physiol 1984;56:520.
3. Crandall CG, et al. Evaluation of the Cosmed K2 portable telemetric oxygen uptake analyzer. Med Sci Sports Exerc 1994;26:108.
4. Dulloo AG, et al. A low-budget and easy-to-operate room respirometer for measuring daily energy expenditure in man. Am J Clin Nutr 1988;48:1367.
5. Ferraro R, et al. Energy cost of physical activity on a metabolic ward in relationship to obesity. Am J Clin Nutr 1991;53:1368.
6. Fogelholm M, et al. Assessment of energy expenditure in overweight women. Med Sci Sports Exerc 1998;30:1191.
7. Haldane JS, Priestley JG. Respiration. New York: Oxford University Press, 1935.
8. Jansson E. On the significance of the respiratory exchange ratio after different diets during exercise in man. Acta Physiol Scand 1982;114:103.
9. Jéquier E, Schutz Y. Long-term measurements of energy expenditure in humans using a respiration chamber. Am J Clin Nutr 1983;38:989.
10. Jungas RL, et al. Quantitative analysis of amino acid oxidation and related gluconeogenesis in humans. Physiol Rev 1992;72:419.
11. Kannagi T, et al. An evaluation of the Beckman Metabolic Cart for measuring ventilation and aerobic requirements during exercise. J Cardiac Rehab 1983;3:38.
12. Koffranyi E, Michaelis HF. Ein tragbarer Apparat zur Bestimmung des Gasstoffwechsels. Arbeitsphysiologie 1940;11:148.
13. Krogh A, Lindhard J. The relative value of fat and carbohydrate as sources of muscular energy. Biochem J 1920;14:290.
14. Livesey G, Elia M. Estimation of energy expenditure, net carbohydrate utilization and net fat oxidization and synthesis by indirect calorimetry: evaluation of errors with special reference to detailed composition of fuels. Am J Clin Nutr 1988;47:608.
15. Montoye HJ, et al. Measuring physical activity and energy expenditure. Boca Raton, FL: Human Kinetics, 1996.
16. Mudambo KS, et al. Adequacy of food rations in soldiers during exercise in hot, day-time conditions assessed by double labeled water and energy balance methods. Eur J Appl Physiol 1997;76:346.
17. Murgatroyd RR, James WPT. Energy measurement in man by direct calorimetry. In: Björntorp P, et al., eds. Recent advances in obesity research. London: John-Libby, 1982.
18. Ravussin E, et al. Determinants of 24-hour energy expenditure in man: methods and results using a respiratory chamber. J Clin Invest 1986;78:1568.
19. Rumpler W, et al. Repeatability of 24-hour energy expenditure measurements in humans by indirect calorimetry. Am J Clin Nutr 1990;51:147.
20. Scholander PF. Analyzer for accurate estimation of respiratory gases in one-half cubic centimeter samples. J Biol Chem 1947;167:235.
21. Schutz Y, Deurenberg P. Energy metabolism: overview of recent methods used in human studies. Ann Nutr Metab 1996;40:183.
22. Snellen JW. Studies in human calorimetry. In: Assessment of energy in health and disease. Columbus, OH: Ross Laboratories, 1980.
23. Snellen JW, et al. Technical description and performance characteristics of a human whole-body calorimeter. Med Biol Eng Comput 1983;21:9.
24. Speakman JR. The history and theory of the doubly labeled water technique. Am J Clin Nutr 1998;68(suppl):932S.
25. Speakman JR, et al. Revised equations for calculating CO_2 production from doubly labeled water in humans. Am J Physiol 1993;61:1200.
26. Starling RD, et al. Energy requirements and physical activity in free-living older women and men: a doubly labeled water study. J Appl Physiol 1998;85:1063.
27. Stroud MA, et al. Energy expenditure using isotope-labeled water ($^2H^{18}O$), exercise performance, skeletal muscle enzyme activities and plasma biochemical parameters in humans during 95 days of endurance exercise with inadequate energy intake. Eur J Appl Physiol 1997;76:243.
28. Webb P. Human calorimeters. Endocrinology and Metabolism Series, vol 7. New York: Praeger Scientific, 1985.
29. Westerterp KR, et al. Comparison of doubly labeled water with respirometry at low-and high-activity levels. J Appl Physiol 1988;65:53.
30. Wideman L, et al. Assessment of the Aerosport TEEM 100 portable metabolic measurement system. Med Sci Sports Exerc 1996;28:509.
31. Wilmore JH, et al. An automated system for assessing metabolic and respiratory function during exercise. J Appl Physiol 1976;40:619.
32. Withers RT, et al. Energy metabolism in sedentary and active 49- to 70-yr-old women. J Appl Physiol 1998;84:1333.

CHAPTER 9

Human Energy Expenditure During Rest and Physical Activity

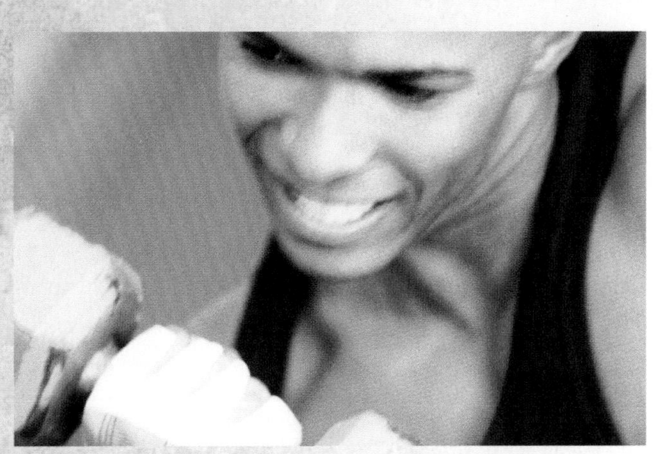

Chapter Objectives

- Define basal metabolic rate and list the factors that affect it
- Discuss important factors that affect the total daily energy expenditure
- Outline different classification systems for rating the strenuousness of physical activity
- Explain the role of body weight in the energy cost of different physical activities
- Present advantages and limitations of using heart rate to estimate exercise energy expenditure

Metabolism involves all of the chemical reactions of biomolecules within the body encompassing both synthesis (anabolism) and breakdown (catabolism). Figure 9.1 illustrates the three general factors that determine **total daily energy expenditure (TDEE)**:

1. Resting metabolic rate, consisting of basal and sleeping conditions plus the added metabolic cost of arousal.
2. Thermogenic effect of the food consumed.
3. Energy expended during physical activity and recovery.

➤ PART 1 • Energy Expenditure at Rest

BASAL METABOLIC RATE

Each person requires a minimum level of energy to sustain vital functions in the waking state. This energy requirement, called the **basal metabolic rate**, or simply **BMR** (sometimes referred to as **basal energy expenditure** [BEE]), reflects the body's heat production. Measuring oxygen consumption under stringent conditions indirectly determines the BMR. For example, measurement takes place while the subject rests in the postabsorptive state—having eaten no food for at least the 12 previous hours, to avoid increases in metabolism from digestion, absorption, and assimilation of ingested nutrients. To reduce other calorigenic influences, the subject cannot perform any physical activity for several hours prior to the test. The subject rests supine for about 30 minutes in a comfortable, thermoneutral environment; then oxygen consumption is measured for 10 minutes. Oxygen consumption values for

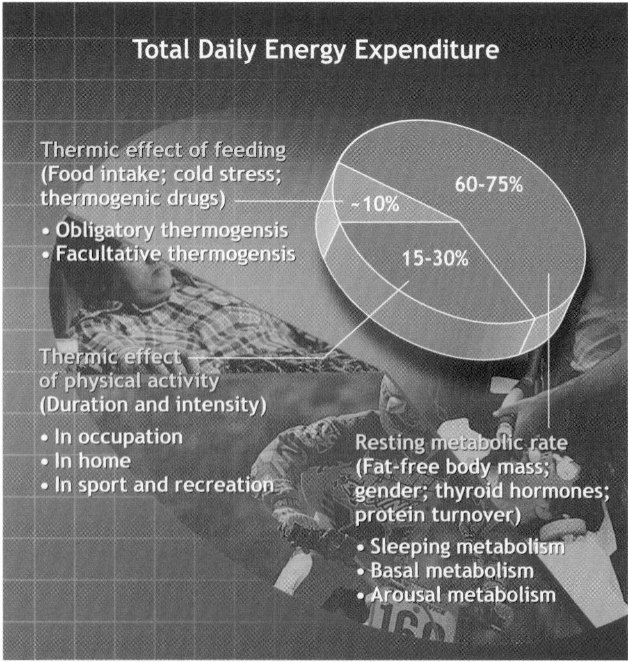

FIGURE 9.1 • Components of total daily energy expenditure (TDEE).

BMR usually range between 160 and 290 mL · min^{-1} (0.8 to 1.43 kcal · min^{-1}), depending on such factors as gender, age, overall body size, and fat-free body mass (FFM).

Knowledge of BMR establishes the important energy baseline for constructing a sound program of weight control through food restriction, exercise, or a combination of both. In most instances, so-called basal values measured under controlled laboratory conditions fall only slightly below values for **resting metabolic rate (RMR)** measured 3 to 4 hours after a light meal without prior physical activity. For this reason the term RMR sometimes substitutes for BMR in many situations. Essentially, RMR refers to the sum of the metabolic processes of the active cell mass required to maintain normal regulatory balance and body functions at rest. For the typical person, RMR accounts for about 60 to 75% of TDEE, while thermic effects from eating account for approximately 10%, and physical activity accounts for the remaining 15 to 30%.

An equation to predict TDEE in elderly women (67 ± 6 y) and men (70 ± 7 y) uses estimated resting daily energy expenditure (RDEE; see p 191) and $\dot{V}O_{2peak}$ as follows:

$$\text{TDEE (kcal} \cdot \text{d}^{-1}) = [1.95 \times \text{RDEE (kcal} \cdot \text{d}^{-1})] + [217.3 \times \dot{V}O_{2peak}\ (\text{L} \cdot \text{min}^{-1})] - 825.5$$

The equation, formulated from doubly labeled water determinations of daily energy expenditure of 51 women and 48 men, explained 62% of the total variance in TDEE with a standard error of estimate of ±348 kcal · d^{-1}.[32]

METABOLISM AT REST

Experiments in the late 1800s indicated that resting energy metabolism varied in proportion to the body's surface area. This led to a "surface area law" to account for individual differences in energy metabolism. A series of careful experiments determined energy metabolism of a dog and a man over a 24-hour period. The total heat generated by the larger man exceeded the energy metabolism of the dog by about 200%. However, expressing heat production in relation to surface area reduced the metabolic difference between man and dog to only about 10%. This result provided the basis for the common practice of expressing basal metabolic rate (energy expenditure) by body surface per hour (kcal · m^{-2} · h^{-1}).

Later research in the 1920s provided evidence that the surface-area formulation did not apply universally to different species of temperature-regulating animals (homeotherms). One classic monograph proposed the concept of *metabolic size* that related basal metabolism to body mass raised to the 0.75 power (body $\text{mass}^{0.75}$).[12] The value of body mass raised to the 0.75 power holds true for humans and a wide variety of mammals and birds that differ considerably in size and shape. Figure 9.2 illustrates the logarithmic plot of body mass (range, 0.01 kg to 10,000 kg) and metabolic rate (range, 0.1 to 1000 W). The best-fitting straight line describing this relationship truly represents one of the more striking biologic observations related to animal size and metabolic and physiologic functions. Chapter 22 discusses the use of allometric scaling as a mathematical procedure to establish a proper re-

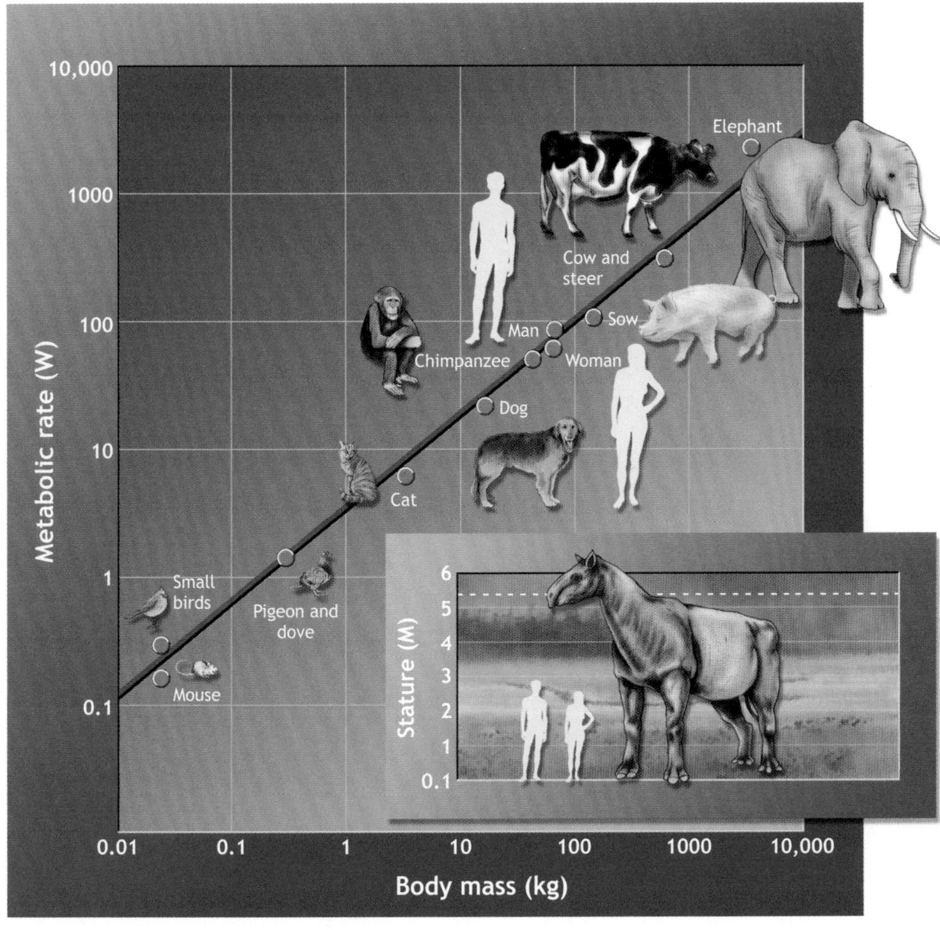

FIGURE 9.2 • Metabolic rate from mouse to elephant. Logarithmic plot of body mass and metabolic rate for a variety of birds and mammals differing considerably in body size and shape. Numerous experiments have confirmed the "mouse-to-elephant curve" for metabolism using body mass to the 0.75 power, whereas metabolic rate relates to body surface area to the 0.67 power. The schematic inset figure compares the body size of the world's tallest male (2.89 m [9 ft 5 3/4 in]) and female (2.48 m [8 ft 1 3/4 in]) with the world's largest land mammal (*Baluchitherium,* predecessor of the rhinoceros), whose body mass approximated 30 tons at a stature of 5.26 m (17 ft 3 in) Comparisons between a microorganism (amoeba; mass, 0.1 mg) and a 100-ton blue whale (or the smallest shrew at one-tenth the size of a mouse or one-millionth the size of an elephant) illustrate the importance of appropriate scaling procedures when relating physiologic variables such as oxygen consumption, heart size, and blood volume to body mass.

lationship between a body size variable (e.g., stature, body mass, FFM) and some other variable of interest, such as muscular strength or aerobic capacity. This permits comparisons among individuals or groups that exhibit large individual differences in body size.

Many subsequent studies have shown that indexing RMR to lean body mass (representing the nonadipose tissue component of the body) and FFM (representing nonlipid mass) provides the overall best method to account for intergender differences in energy expenditure (see inset Fig. 9.3). However, for an individual or group of individuals of the same gender, body surface area provides as good an index of RMR as lean body mass. This results because of the strong within-gender association between body surface area and lean body mass. A pitfall in comparing males and females with regard to RMR per unit body surface area arises because females have a smaller lean body mass, which reflects a smaller muscle mass component, not necessarily an implied lower proportion of active protoplasmic tissues. Having less protoplasmic tissues implies clinical ramifications, including the promulgation of what has been termed the "myth of feminine metabolism."[6]

Numerous experiments have provided data on average BMR values for men and women over a wide range of age and body weight. Figure 9.3 presents BMR data expressed as hourly values of heat production per square meter of body surface ($kcal \cdot m^{-2} \cdot h^{-1}$). Whereas the values represent averages from measurements of large numbers of men and women, an individual's BMR (RMR) estimated from the curves generally falls within $\pm 10\%$ of the actual value obtained from laboratory measurements. The inset figure illustrates the relatively strong association between FFM and daily resting metabolic rate for men and women.

Figure 9.3 also reveals that BMR averages 5 to 10% lower in women than in men. This does not necessarily reflect a true "sex difference" in the metabolic rate of specific tissues. Rather, it results largely because women generally possess more body fat (and less fat-free tissue) than men of similar size, and fat tissue has lower metabolic activity than muscle. Changes in body composition, either a decrease in FFM and/or increase in body fat during adulthood,[10] usually explain the 2 to 3% per decade BMR reduction observed for adult men and women.[3,11,27] Some depression of the metabolic activity of the lean tissue components also may progress as one ages,[24] which could contribute to an age-related increase in body fat.

Effects of Regular Exercise

Remarkably similar BMR measures emerged in comparisons of young and middle-aged endurance-trained men who showed no group difference for FFM.[20] Moreover, resting me-

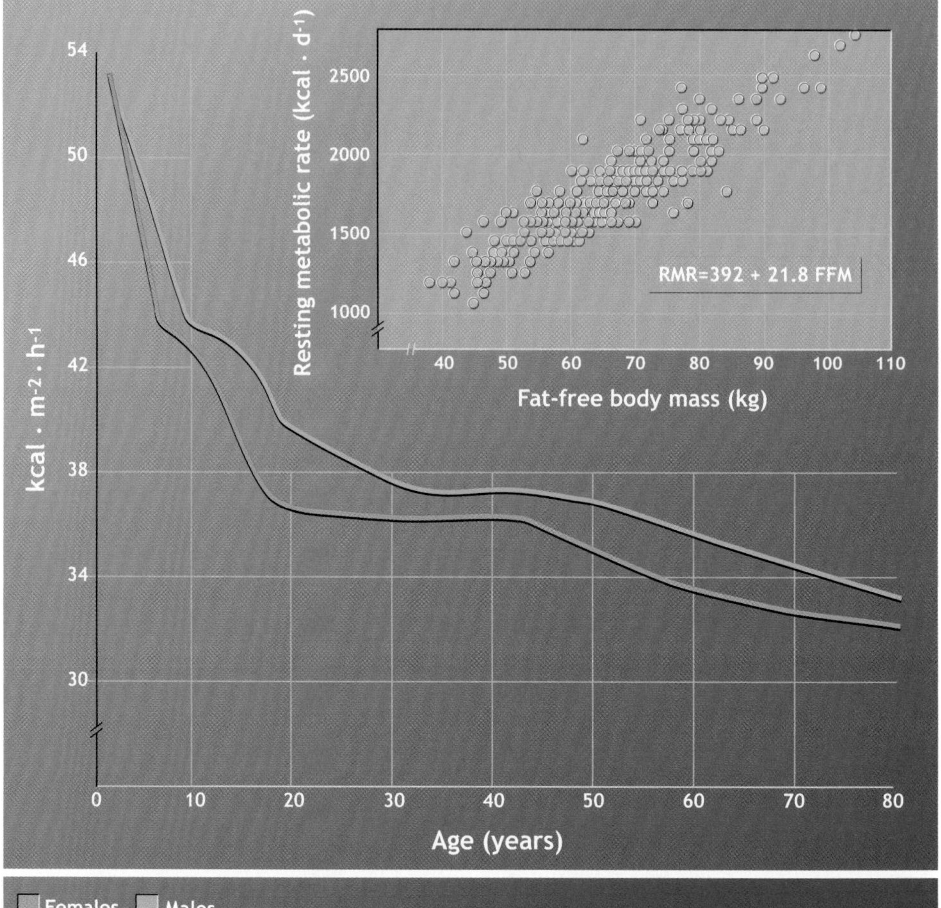

FIGURE 9.3 • Basal metabolic rate (BMR) as a function of age and gender. (Data from Altman PL, Dittmer D. Metabolism. Bethesda, MD: Federation of American Societies for Experimental Biology, 1968.) Inset graph shows the relatively strong relationship between fat-free body mass (FFM) and resting metabolic rate (RMR) for men and women. (From Ravussin E, et al. Determination of 24-hour energy expenditure in man. Methods and results using a respiratory chamber. J Clin Invest 1986; 78:1568.)

tabolism increased by 8% when 50- to 65-year-old men increased their FFM with heavy resistance training.[28] In addition, an 8-week aerobic training program for older individuals caused a 10% increase in resting metabolism despite *no change* in FFM.[25] This suggests that regular exercise also affects factors other than body composition to stimulate resting metabolism. *Research indicates that regular endurance and resistance exercise offsets the decrease in resting metabolism that usually accompanies aging.*

The curves in Figure 9.3 adequately estimate a person's resting metabolic rate. For example, between the ages of 20 and 40 years, the BMR of men averages about 38 kcal per m^2 per hour, whereas for women the corresponding value equals 35 kcal. For greater precision, read the specific age-related value directly from the appropriate curve. To estimate total metabolic rate per hour, multiply the BMR value by the person's surface area. This hourly total provides important information for estimating the daily energy baseline requirement for caloric intake.

Figure 9.4 illustrates a simple method to determine body surface area from body stature and mass. To determine surface area from the nomogram, locate stature on scale I and mass on scale II. Connect these two points with a straightedge; the intersection on scale III gives the surface area in square meters (m^2). For example, if stature equals 185 cm and mass equals 75 kg, surface area from scale III on the nomogram equals 1.98 m^2.

Accurate measurement of the body surface area poses a considerable challenge. Experiments in the early 1900s provided the data used to formulate Figure 9.4. The studies clothed 8 men and 2 women in very tight whole-body underwear and applied melted paraffin and paper strips to prevent modification of the surface. The treated cloth was then removed and cut into flat pieces to allow precise measurements of body surface area (length × width). The close relationship between height (stature) and body weight (mass) and body surface area enabled derivation of the following empirical formula to predict body surface area (BSA):

$$\text{BSA} = H^{0.725} \times W^{0.425} \times 71.84$$

where H = stature in cm and W = mass in kg. This formula yields results similar to the nomogram values in Figure 9.4.

"Normalcy" of BMR Values

BMR and RMR are typically expressed as kcal or kJ per squared meter of body surface area or per kilogram body mass or FFM, per min, per hour, or per day. Classical clini-

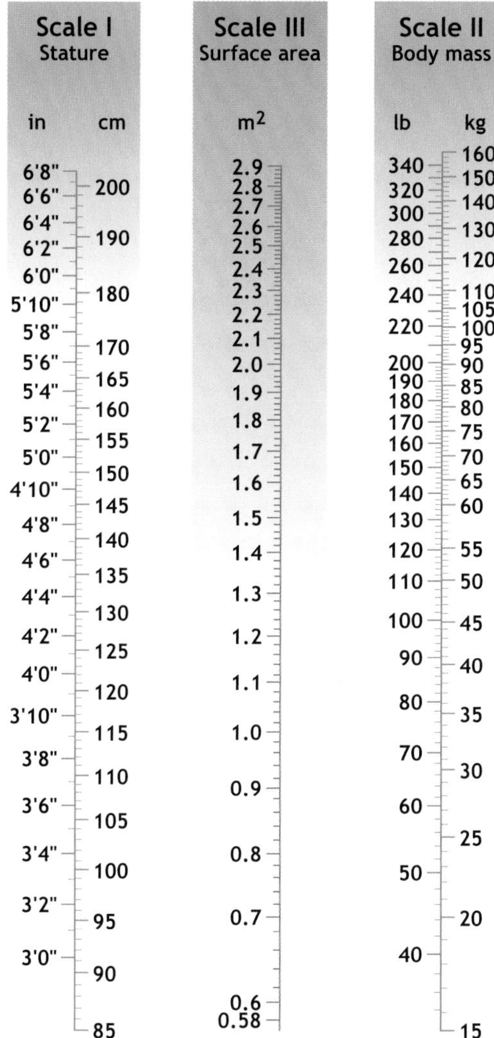

FIGURE 9.4 • Nomogram to estimate body surface area from stature and mass. (Reproduced from "Clinical spirometry," prepared by Boothby and Sandiford of the Mayo Clinic, through the courtesy of Warren E. Collins, Inc., Braintree, MA.); based on work of Dubois, EF. Basal metabolism in health and disease. Philadelphia: Lea & Febiger, 1936.

cal assessment of the normalcy of thyroid function compares a person's measured BMR with "standard metabolic rates" based on age and gender (Table 9.1 and Fig. 9.3). Any value within ±10% of the standard represents a normal BMR. The following formula computes the deviation expressed as a percentage:

$$\Delta \text{ BMR} = (\text{measured BMR} - \text{standard BMR}) \times 100 \div \text{standard BMR}$$

For example, a BMR of 35 kcal · m^{-2} · h^{-1} for a 19-year-old male, determined by indirect calorimetry falls 10.7% below the standard BMR.

$$\Delta \text{ BMR} = (35 - 39.2) \times 100 \div 39.2$$
$$\Delta \text{ BMR} = -10.7\%$$

Estimating Resting Daily Energy Expenditure

To estimate a person's resting daily energy expenditure, multiply the appropriate BMR value in Table 9.1 by the surface area computed from stature and mass. For a 50-year-old woman, for example, the estimated BMR equals 34 kcal per m^2 per hour. For a surface area of 1.40 m^2, the hourly energy expenditure would equal 47.6 kcal per hour (34 kcal × 1.40 m^2). On a daily basis, this amounts to an energy expenditure of 1142 kcal (47.6 kcal × 24).

Table 9.2 provides an estimate of RDEE from FFM estimated from several indirect procedures described in Chapter 28. The data in the table were computed from the following generalized equation, applicable to males and females over a wide range of body weights:

$$\text{RDEE (kcal)} = 370 + 21.6 \text{ (FFM, kg)}$$

For example, a male who weighs 90.9 kg at 21% body fat has an estimated FFM of 71.7 kg. Rounding to 72 kg translates to an RDEE of 1,925 kcal, or 8047 kJ (8.08 MJ).

TABLE 9.1 ➤ STANDARD BASAL METABOLIC RATES

AGE	KCAL · M^{-2} · H^{-1}		KJ · M^{-2} · H^{-1}	
(YEARS)	MEN	WOMEN	MEN	WOMEN
1	53.0	53.0	222	222
2	52.4	52.4	219	219
3	51.3	51.2	215	214
4	50.3	49.8	211	208
5	49.3	48.4	206	203
6	48.3	47.0	202	197
7	47.3	45.4	198	190
8	46.3	43.8	194	183
9	45.2	42.8	189	179
10	44.0	42.5	184	178
11	43.0	42.0	180	176
12	42.5	41.3	178	173
13	42.3	40.3	177	169
14	42.1	39.2	176	164
15	41.8	37.9	175	159
16	41.4	36.9	173	154
17	40.8	36.3	171	152
18	40.0	35.9	167	150
19	39.2	35.5	164	149
20	38.6	35.3	162	148
25	37.5	35.2	157	147
30	36.8	35.1	154	147
35	36.5	35.0	153	146
40	36.3	34.9	152	146
45	36.2	34.5	152	144
50	35.8	33.9	150	142
55	35.4	33.3	148	139
60	34.9	32.7	146	137
65	34.4	32.2	144	135
70	33.8	31.7	141	133
75+	33.2	31.3	139	131

From Fleish A. Le Metabolisme basal standard et sa determination au moyen du "Metabocalculator." Helv Med Acta 1951;18:23.

TABLE 9.2 ➤ ESTIMATION OF RESTING DAILY ENERGY EXPENDITURE (RDEE) BASED ON FAT-FREE BODY MASS

FFM (KG)	RDEE[a] (KCAL)[b]	FFM (KG)	RDEE (KCAL)[b]	FFM (KG)	RDEE (KCAL)[b]
30	1018	58	1623	86	2228
31	1040	59	1644	87	2249
32	1061	60	1666	88	2271
33	1083	61	1688	89	2292
34	1104	62	1709	90	2314
35	1126	63	1731	91	2336
36	1148	64	1752	92	2357
37	1169	65	1774	93	2379
38	1191	66	1796	94	2400
39	1212	67	1817	95	2422
40	1234	68	1839	96	2444
41	1256	69	1860	97	2465
42	1277	70	1882	98	2487
43	1299	71	1904	99	2508
44	1320	72	1925	100	2530
45	1342	73	1947	101	2552
46	1364	74	1968	102	2573
47	1385	75	1990	103	2595
48	1407	76	2012	104	2616
49	1428	77	2033	105	2638
50	1450	78	2055	106	2660
51	1472	79	2076	107	2681
52	1493	80	2098	108	2703
53	1515	81	2120	109	2724
54	1536	82	2141	110	2746
55	1558	83	2163	111	2768
56	1580	84	2184	112	2789
57	1601	85	2206	113	2811

[a]Prediction equation for RDEE derived as the weighted mean of regression constants from studies of large samples of males and females.[6]
[b]To convert kcal to kJ, multiply by 4.18; to convert kcal to MJ, multiply by 0.0042.

TABLE 9.3 ➤ OXYGEN CONSUMPTION OF VARIOUS BODY TISSUES AT REST FOR A 65-KG MAN

ORGAN	OXYGEN CONSUMPTION (ML · MIN^{-1})	PERCENTAGE OF RESTING METABOLISM
Liver	67	27
Brain	47	19
Heart	17	7
Kidneys	26	10
Skeletal muscle	45	18
Remainder	48	19
	250	100

Contribution of Diverse Tissues

Table 9.3 shows estimates of the absolute and relative energy needs, expressed in terms of oxygen consumption, of various organs and tissues of adults at rest. Note that the brain and skeletal muscles consume about the same total quantity of oxygen, even though the brain weighs only 1.6 kg (2.3% of body mass), while muscle constitutes almost 50% of the body mass. For children, brain metabolism represents nearly 50% of total resting energy expenditure. This similarity in metabolism, however, does not transfer to maximal exercise because the energy generated by active muscle increases nearly 100 times, whereas the total energy expended by the brain increases only slightly.

INTEGRATIVE QUESTION

Discuss the weight control advantage for middle-aged men and women of maintaining or even increasing muscle mass.

FACTORS THAT AFFECT ENERGY EXPENDITURE

Important factors that affect TDEE include physical activity, diet-induced thermogenesis, climate, and pregnancy and lactation.

Physical Activity

As we discuss and illustrate throughout this text, *physical activity has by far the most profound effect on human energy expenditure.* World-class athletes, for example, nearly double their TDEE with 3 or 4 hours of hard training. Most people can sustain metabolic rates 10 times the resting value during continuous "big muscle" exercise such as fast walking, running, bicycling, and swimming. Under normal circumstances, physical activity accounts for between 15 and 30% of a person's TDEE.

Diet-Induced Thermogenesis

Food consumption generally increases energy metabolism. **Diet-induced thermogenesis (DIT)** consists of two components. One component called **obligatory thermogenesis** (formerly called specific dynamic action, or SDA), results from the energy required digesting, absorbing, and assimilating food nutrients. The second component, called **facultative thermogenesis**, relates to the activation of the sympathetic nervous system and its stimulating effect on metabolic rate.

The first experiment on DIT (indirect calorimetry), purportedly performed by Max Rubner in 1891,[17] established the 24-hour energy expenditure of a fasting dog at 742 kcal. Rubner then fed the dog 2 kg of meat containing 1926 kcal. Food consumption increased the dog's daily energy expenditure to 1046 kcal. The 41% increase of 304 kcal was attributed to the "chemical work of glands in metabolizing absorbed nutrients," or the "work of digestion." The increased metabolism represented 16% of the total energy ingested. Numerous subsequent experiments indicate that factors such as the size and macronutrient composition of the meal, time elapsed since the previous meal, nutritional status, and health status affect the magnitude of DIT.

The thermic effect of food generally reaches maximum within 1 hour after a meal. While considerable variability exists among individuals, the magnitude of DIT usually varies between 10 and 30% of the ingested food energy, depending on the quantity and type of food eaten.[2,12] A meal of pure protein, for example, elicits a thermic effect nearly 25% of the meal's total caloric value.[9] This large thermic effect results largely from activation of digestive processes. It also includes extra energy required by the liver to assimilate and synthesize protein and/or to deaminate amino acids and convert them to glucose or triglycerides.

The relatively large calorigenic effect of ingested protein has been used by some to advocate a high-protein diet for weight reduction. It is maintained that because of protein's relatively high thermic effect, fewer calories ultimately become available to the body compared with a meal of similar caloric value consisting mainly of lipid or carbohydrate. Although this point has some merit, one must consider other factors in formulating a prudent and effective program for weight loss—not to mention the potentially harmful strain on kidney and liver function from inordinate protein intake. Well-balanced nutrition requires a blend of carbohydrate, lipid, and protein combined with appropriate quantities of vitamins and minerals. In addition, when physical activity combines with dietary modification for weight loss, adequate carbohydrate intake maintains glycogen reserves to power diverse forms of exercise.

Research indicates that overweight individuals often have a blunted thermic response to eating that contributes to accumulation of excess body fat.[29–31] Interestingly, the magnitude of DIT may also be lower in endurance-trained individuals than in their untrained counterparts.[15,26,34] Any "training effect" probably reflects a calorie-sparing adaptation to conserve energy and glycogen during periods of increased physical activity. Energy conservation in any form seems counterproductive to the potential of increased physical activity for weight control. However, for a physically active person, DIT represents only a small portion of TDEE, compared with the energy expended through regular physical activities.

Calorigenic Effect of Food on Exercise Metabolism

Researchers have compared DIT in resting and exercising subjects after consuming meals of identical macronutrient composition and caloric content. In one study, six men performed moderate exercise on a bicycle ergometer before breakfast on 1 day; then on separate days, they performed exercise for 30 minutes after a breakfast containing either 350, 1000, or 3000 kcal.[4] The results indicated that (1) breakfast increased resting metabolism by 10%, (2) variations in the caloric value of the meal exerted no influence on the thermic effect, and (3) performing exercise following a meal of 1000 or 3000 kcal produced a larger energy expenditure than exercise without prior food. The calorigenic effect of food on exercise metabolism nearly doubled the food's thermic effect at rest. Apparently, exercise augments DIT. This agrees with previous findings in which the thermic response to a 1000-kcal meal averaged 28% of the basal requirement at rest, yet increased to 56% of the basal requirement when subjects exercised after eating.[21] Like their response during rest, some obese men and women exhibit a blunted DIT when they exercise after eating (see Chapter 4, "Focus on Research").[30,35] For most individuals, however, it seems reasonable to encourage moderate exercise after eating to possibly augment a diet-induced increase in caloric expenditure for weight control.

Climate

Environmental factors influence resting metabolic rate. For example, the resting metabolism of people in a tropical climate is generally 5 to 20% higher than values for counterparts living in more-temperate areas. Exercise performed in hot weather also imposes a small additional metabolic load, causing about 5% higher oxygen consumption than a thermoneutral environment. This probably results from the thermogenic effect of an elevated core temperature per se, including additional energy required for sweat gland activity and altered circulatory dynamics during work in the heat.

Cold environments significantly increase energy metabolism during rest and exercise. The magnitude of the effect depends largely on a person's body fat content and effectiveness of the clothing ensemble. Metabolic rate can increase up to fivefold at rest during extreme cold stress, because shivering generates body heat to maintain a stable core temperature. The effects of cold stress during exercise become most evident in cold water because of the great difficulty maintaining a stable core temperature in such a stressful environment.[33]

Pregnancy

One area of interest concerns the degree that pregnancy affects the metabolic cost and physiologic strain imposed by exercise.[5] One investigation studied 13 women from the sixth month of pregnancy to 6 weeks after gestation.[13] Physiologic measures taken every 4 weeks included heart rate and oxygen consumption during bicycle and treadmill exercise. Heart rate and oxygen consumption during walking (weight-bearing exercise) increased progressively during the measurement period, whereas exercise heart rate and oxygen consumption remained unchanged during weight-supported bicycle exercise at a constant intensity. These findings indicate that the added energy cost to weight-bearing locomotion like walking, jogging, and stair climbing during pregnancy results *primarily* from the additional weight transported (and reduced economy of effort from encumbrance of fetal tissue) with a relatively small effect from the developing fetus per se.

IN A PRACTICAL SENSE

PREDICTING $\dot{V}O_{2MAX}$ During Pregnancy From Submaximum Exercise Heart Rate and Oxygen Consumption

Authorities recommend that a woman participate in regular physical activity during an uncomplicated pregnancy. Most agree that an individualized exercise prescription should guide exercise because of concern for fetal well-being. The exercise prescription typically specifies intensity, duration, and frequency of activity. Exercise intensity usually represents some percentage of the maximal oxygen consumption (%$\dot{V}O_{2max}$) obtained from equations relating heart rate (HR) to % $\dot{V}O_{2max}$. The direct determination of $\dot{V}O_{2max}$ necessitates that subjects perform near-exhaustive exercise, an unacceptable requirement for most pregnant women.

Predicting $\dot{V}O_{2max}$ from Submaximal Exercise

Predicting $\dot{V}O_{2max}$ during pregnancy involves a three-stage, submaximum cycle-ergometer exercise test. Oxygen consumption ($\dot{V}O_2$) and HR, measured toward the end of the final exercise stage, predict $\dot{V}O_{2max}$ via regression analyses.

SUBMAXIMUM CYCLE ERGOMETER TEST

Subject rests for 10 minutes and then performs a continuous three-stage, 6-minute per stage, cycle ergometer test as follows:

Stage 1: 0 watts (W) (unloaded cycling)
Stage 2: 30 W (184 kg-m · min^{-1})
Stage 3: 60 W (367 kg-m · min^{-1})

Prediction Equations

Measure $\dot{V}O_2$ (L · min^{-1}) and HR (b · min^{-1}) for each of the last 3 minutes of the final exercise stage. Average the three HR values to predict % $\dot{V}O_{2max}$ in the following equation:

$$\text{Predicted } \% \dot{V}O_{2max} = (0.634 \times HR\ [b \cdot min^{-1}]) - 30.79$$

Use the predicted $\dot{V}O_{2max}$ and the measured $\dot{V}O_2$ (L · min^{-1}) during the last exercise stage to predict $\dot{V}O_{2max}$ (L · min^{-1}) in the following equation:

$$\text{Predicted } \dot{V}O_{2max} = \dot{V}O_2 \div \text{predicted } \% \dot{V}O_{2max} \times 100$$

EXAMPLE

A woman 20 weeks pregnant, weighing 70.4 kg, performs the three-stage cycle-ergometer test. The average value for final-stage exercise HR equals 155 b · min^{-1}; the average value for $\dot{V}O_2$ equals 1.80 L · min^{-1}.

$$\begin{aligned}
\text{Predicted } \% \dot{V}O_{2max} &= (0.634 \times HR\ [b \cdot min^{-1}]) - 30.79 \\
&= (0.634 \times 155) - 30.79 \\
&= 67.5\% \\
\text{Predicted } \dot{V}O_{2max} &= \dot{V}O_2 \div \text{predicted } \% \dot{V}O_2 \times 100 \\
&= 1.80 \div 67.5 \times 100 \\
&= 2.67\ L \cdot min^{-1}\ (2670\ mL \cdot min^{-1}) \\
&= 2670\ mL \cdot min^{-1} \div 70.4\ kg \\
&= 37.9\ mL \cdot kg^{-1} \cdot min^{-1}
\end{aligned}$$

Sady SP, et al. Prediction of $\dot{V}O_{2max}$ during cycle exercise in pregnant women. J Appl Physiol 1988;65:657.

Chapter 21 discusses more fully the physiologic and metabolic impact of exercise on both mother and fetus during pregnancy.

Summary

1. Total daily energy expenditure equals the sum of resting metabolism, thermogenic influences (e.g., thermic effect of food), and the energy generated in physical activity.
2. The BMR represents the minimum energy required to maintain vital functions in the waking state, measured under controlled laboratory conditions. The BMR averages only slightly lower than the resting metabolic rate (RMR) and closely relates to body surface area.
3. RMR (like BMR) decreases with age. Owing to variations in FFM, the RMR for men generally exceeds values for women of similar body size. One can accurately predict RMR from FFM in men and women who vary considerably in body size.
4. Different organs expend different amounts of energy during rest and exercise. At rest, muscles generate about 20% of the body's total energy expenditure. In contrast, the energy expended by skeletal muscles during all-out exercise can increase more than 100 times above its resting value.
5. In addition to body size, four major factors affect a person's metabolic rate: physical activity, DIT, climate, and pregnancy. The greatest influence comes from physical activity.

PART 2 • Energy Expenditure in Physical Activity

CLASSIFICATION OF PHYSICAL ACTIVITIES BY ENERGY EXPENDITURE

Most individuals have performed some type of physical work they would classify as "exceedingly difficult." This might include walking up a long flight of stairs, shoveling snow for 60

TABLE 9.4 ➤ **FIVE-LEVEL CLASSIFICATION OF PHYSICAL ACTIVITY BASED ON EXERCISE INTENSITY**

LEVEL	ENERGY EXPENDITURE[a]			
	Men			
	kcal · min^{-1}	L · min^{-1}	mL · kg^{-1} · min^{-1}	METs
Light	2.0–4.9	0.40–0.99	6.1–15.2	1.6–3.9
Moderate	5.0–7.4	1.00–1.49	15.3–22.9	4.0–5.9
Heavy	7.5–9.9	1.50–1.99	23.0–30.6	6.0–7.9
Very heavy	10.0–12.4	2.00–2.49	30.7–38.3	8.9–9.9
Unduly heavy	≥12.5	≥ 2.50	≥38.4	≥10.0
	Women			
Light	1.5–3.4	0.30–0.69	5.4–12.5	1.2–2.7
Moderate	3.5–5.4	0.70–1.09	12.6–19.8	2.8–4.3
Heavy	5.5–7.4	1.10–1.49	19.9–27.1	4.4–5.9
Very heavy	7.5–9.4	1.50–1.89	27.2–34.4	6.0–7.5
Unduly heavy	≥ 9.5	≥1.90	≥34.5	≥7.6

[a]L · min^{-1} based on 5 kcal per liter of oxygen; mL · kg^{-1} · min^{-1} based on 65-kg man and 55-kg woman; one MET equals the average resting oxygen consumption.

minutes, running to catch a bus, digging a deep trench, skiing through a blizzard, or hiking up a steep mountain. *Intensity and duration represent two important factors affecting the strenuousness of a particular physical task.* For example, it requires about the same number of calories to complete a 26.2-mile marathon at various running speeds. One person, however, might expend a considerable rate of energy expenditure running at maximum steady-rate pace (e.g., 80% $\dot{V}O_{2max}$) and complete the race in a little more than 2 hours. Another runner of equal fitness might select a slower, more comfortable pace (e.g., 55% $\dot{V}O_{2max}$) and complete the run in 3 hours. In this example, the *intensity* of effort distinguishes the physical demands of the task. In another example, two people of equal fitness may run at the same speed, but one person runs for twice as long as the other. In this situation, exercise *duration* becomes the important consideration in classifying the strenuousness of physical effort.

Several classification systems rate sustained physical activity for its strenuousness. One system recommends classification of work by the ratio of energy required for the task to the resting energy requirement.[1] This system uses the **physical activity ratio (PAR)**. **Light work** for men elicits an oxygen consumption (or energy expenditure) up to 3 times the resting requirement. **Heavy work** encompasses physical activity requiring 6 to 8 times resting metabolism, whereas **maximal work** includes any task requiring metabolism to increase 9 times or more above rest. As a frame of reference, most industrial jobs and household tasks require less than 3 times resting energy expenditure. These work classifications (in multiples of resting metabolism) average slightly lower for women because of their generally lower aerobic capacity. Work classification based on the PAR model rates the strenuousness of occupational tasks at a somewhat lower level than typical classifications for general exercise. Occupational and industrial work usually extends for much longer periods than exercise training, often requiring the use of a small muscle mass and performed under varying and often stressful environmental conditions and physical constraints.

The MET

Table 9.4 presents a five-level classification system based on the energy (kcal) required by untrained men and women performing different physical activities including a broad range of occupational tasks.[8] Because 5 kcal equals approximately 1 L of oxygen consumed, one can transpose these values into liters of oxygen consumed per minute (L · min^{-1}) or milliliters of oxygen per kilogram of body mass per minute (mL · kg^{-1} · min^{-1}), or **METs**, *defined as multiples of the resting metabolic rate.* Thus, 1 MET equals resting oxygen consumption, or about 250 mL · min^{-1} for an average man and 200 mL · min^{-1} for an average woman. Exercise performed at 2 METs requires twice the resting metabolism (about 500 mL · min^{-1} for a man), 3 METs equals three times rest, and so on. For a different but usually more accurate classification that considers variations in body size, one should express the MET in terms of oxygen consumption per unit body mass: *1 MET equals 3.5 mL · kg^{-1} · min^{-1}.*

Table 9.5 presents a classification system for characterizing the intensity of leisure-time physical activity in absolute (METs) and relative (%$\dot{V}O_{2max}$) intensity for various age categories. Categorization for exercise intensity in METs adjusts lower with age to account for the general aging effect on aerobic capacity.

TABLE 9.5 ➤ CHARACTERIZATION OF THE INTENSITY OF LEISURE-TIME PHYSICAL ACTIVITY IN RELATION TO AGE

		ABSOLUTE INTENSITY (METs)			
CATEGORIZATION	RELATIVE INTENSITY (% $\dot{V}O_{2MAX}$)	YOUNG	MIDDLE-AGED	OLD	VERY OLD
Rest	<10	1.0	1.0	1.0	1.0
Light	<35	<4.5	<3.5	<2.5	<1.5
Fairly light	<50	<6.5	<5.0	<3.5	<2.0
Moderate	<70	<9.0	<7.0	<5.0	<2.8
Heavy	>70	>9.0	>7.0	>5.0	>2.8
Maximal	100	13.0	10.0	7.0	4.0

From Bouchard C, et al. Exercise, fitness, and health: a consensus of current knowledge. Champaign, IL: Human Kinetics, 1990.

DAILY RATES OF AVERAGE ENERGY EXPENDITURE

Table 9.6 shows averages for stature and body mass and daily energy expenditure for males and females living in the United States. The average man aged 19 to 50 years expends 2900 kcal per day, whereas his female counterpart expends 2200 kcal. As shown at the bottom of the table, these men and women spend nearly 75% of the day in activities requiring only light energy expenditure. Energy expenditure for most individuals rarely rises substantially above the resting level, with walking the most prevalent physical activity. Indeed, the term *homo sedentarius* all too appropriately describes our citizens.

ENERGY COST OF HOUSEHOLD, INDUSTRIAL, AND RECREATIONAL ACTIVITIES

Appendix C lists examples of energy expenditures, expressed by body mass, for common household activities, selected industrial tasks, and popular recreational and sports activities. These data illustrate the large variation in energy expenditure with participation in diverse physical activities. The caloric values also represent averages, with values for an individual varying considerably, depending on skill, pace, and fitness level.

The values listed in the column for body mass represent the activity's caloric cost for 1 minute. This equals the gross energy value (see Chapter 10) because it includes the cost of rest for the 1-minute period. Estimate the total cost of performing an activity by multiplying the caloric value in the table by the number of minutes of participation. For example, if a 70-kg man spends 30 minutes vacuuming (carpet sweeping), his total energy expenditure for this household task equals 102 kcal (3.4 kcal × 30 min). The same individual expends approximately 690 kcal during a 50-minute judo workout, but only 90 kcal while sitting quietly watching television for 2 hours. Golf requires about 6.0 kcal each minute, or 360 kcal · h^{-1}, for a person weighing 70 kg. The same person expends almost twice this energy, or 708 kcal · h^{-1}, while swimming backstroke. Viewed somewhat differently, 25 minutes of swimming backstroke requires about the same number of calories as playing golf for 1 hour. Increasing the pace of either the swim or the golf game proportionally increases energy expenditure.

Effect of Body Mass

Body mass significantly increases the energy expended in many physical activities (see Appendix C), particularly in **weight-bearing exercise** like walking and running, in which persons must transport their body mass during the activity. Figure 9.5 clearly illustrates that the energy cost of walking increases directly with body mass. For persons with the same body mass, such a small variation in oxygen consumption exists that body mass will accurately predict the energy expended walking.

The influence of body mass on energy metabolism in weight-bearing exercise occurs whether a person gains weight naturally as body fat or as an acute added load such as sports equipment or a weighted vest on the torso.[7,22] With **weight-supported** exercise (e.g., stationary cycling), the influence of body mass on energy cost decreases considerably. It averages only about 5% higher in cycling among heavy people, because of extra energy required to lift heavier lower limbs.[14,16] This weight effect in stationary cycling exercise slightly lowers energy cost values for women compared to men. For overweight people desiring to use exercise for weight loss, weight-bearing exercise generates a considerable caloric expenditure.

Appendix C also shows that the energy cost for cross-country running ranges between 8.2 kcal per minute for a 50-kg person and almost twice as much (16.0 kcal) for a person weighing 98 kg. However, expressing the energy requirement by body mass as kcal · kg^{-1} · min^{-1} essentially eliminates this variation. In this case, energy cost averages about 0.164 kcal · kg^{-1} · min^{-1}. Expressing energy cost per unit body mass reduces differences between individuals, regardless of age, race, gender, and body mass. The heavier person still expends more *total* calories than a lighter person for an equivalent exercise period, mainly because the activity requires transport of body mass—and this requires proportionately more energy.

TABLE 9.6 ➤ **REFERENCE HEIGHTS, WEIGHTS, AND ENERGY EXPENDITURES OF CHILDREN AND ADULTS LIVING IN THE UNITED STATES**

HEIGHT, WEIGHT, AND BODY MASS INDEX

GENDER	AGE	MEDIAN BODY MASS INDEX[a]	REFERENCE HEIGHT (CM [IN])	REFERENCE WEIGHT,[b] (KG [LB])
Male, female	2–6 mo	—	64 (25)	7 (16)
	7–11 mo	—	72 (28)	9 (20)
	1–3 y	—	91 (36)	13 (29)
	4–8 y	15.8	118 (46)	22 (48)
Male	9–13 y	18.5	147 (58)	40 (88)
	14–18 y	21.3	174 (68)	64 (142)
	19–30 y	24.4	176 (69)	76 (166)
Female	9–13 y	18.3	148 (58)	40 (88)
	14–18 y	21.3	163 (64)	57 (125)
	19–30 y	22.8	163 (64)	61 (133)

[a]In kg/m^2.
[b]Calculated from median body mass index and median heights for ages 4–8 years and older.
Adapted from Dietary reference intakes: a risk assessment model for establishing upper intake levels for nutrients. Food and Nutrition Board. Institute of Medicine. Washington, DC: National Academy Press, 1998.

GENDER, AGE, AND ENERGY EXPENDITURE

	AGE (Y)	ENERGY EXPENDITURE (KCAL)
Males	15–18	3000
	19–24	2900
	25–50	2900
	51+	2300
Females	15–18	2200
	19–24	2200
	25–50	2200
	50+	1900

AVERAGE TIME SPENT DURING THE DAY

ACTIVITY	TIME (H)
Sleeping and lying down	8
Sitting	6
Standing	6
Walking	2
Recreational activity	2

Data from Food and Nutrition Board, National Research Council. Recommended dietary allowances, revised. Washington, DC: National Academy of Sciences, 1989.

HEART RATE TO ESTIMATE ENERGY EXPENDITURE

For each person, heart rate and oxygen consumption relate linearly throughout a large range of aerobic exercise intensities. By knowing this relationship, the exercise heart rate provides an estimate of oxygen consumption (and thus energy expenditure) during aerobic exercise. This approach has proved useful when the oxygen consumption could not be measured during the actual activity.

Figure 9.6 presents data for two members of a women's basketball team during a laboratory treadmill running test. For each woman, heart rate increased linearly with oxygen consumption—a proportionate increase in exercise heart rate (HR) accompanied each increase in oxygen consumption ($\dot{V}O_2$). Even though both HR–$\dot{V}O_2$ lines displayed linearity, the same heart rate does not correspond to the same oxygen consumption for both women because the slope (rate of change) of the line differs. Heart rate of subject B increases less than that of subject A for a given increase in oxygen consumption. Chapters 11, 17, and 21 discuss the significance of the difference in heart rate increase with exercise and its relation to cardiovascular fitness. For the current discussion, exercise heart rate can estimate exercise oxygen consumption with reasonable accuracy. For player A, an exercise heart rate of 140 b · min^{-1} corresponds to an

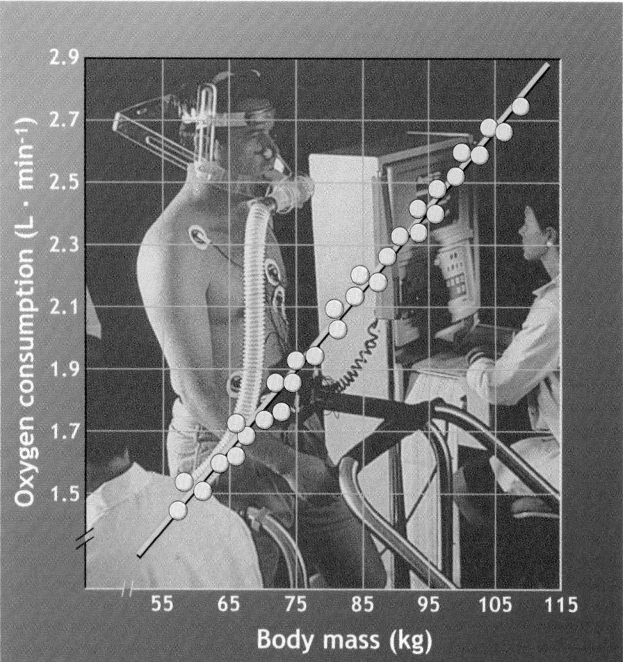

FIGURE 9.5 • Relationship between body mass and oxygen consumption measured during submaximal, brisk treadmill walking. (From Laboratory of Applied Physiology Queens College, NY.)

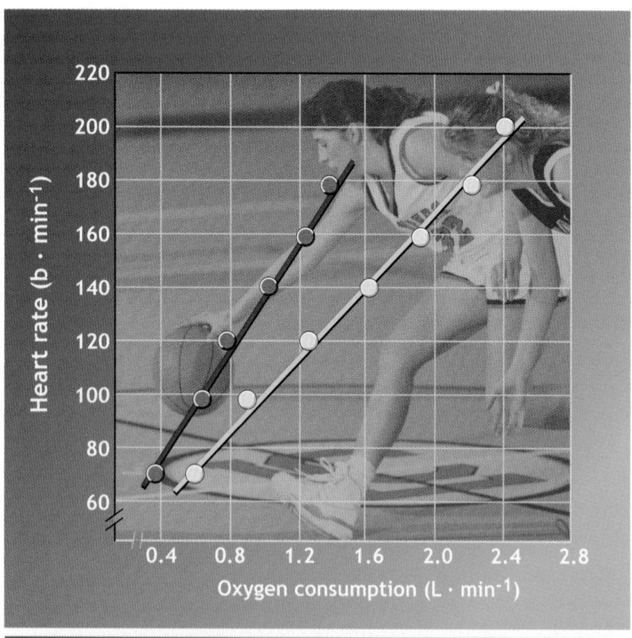

FIGURE 9.6 • Linear relationship between heart rate and oxygen consumption for two women collegiate basketball players of different aerobic fitness levels. Measurements made during a graded exercise test on a motor-driven treadmill. (From Laboratory of Applied Physiology, Queens College, NY.)

oxygen consumption of 1.08 L · min^{-1}, whereas the same heart rate for player B corresponds to a 1.60 L · min^{-1} oxygen consumption. Heart rates obtained by radiotelemetry during actual basketball competition were then applied to each player's HR–$\dot{V}O_2$ line to estimate energy expenditure under game conditions.[19]

Although the use of heart rate to estimate energy expenditure appears practical, it offers limited use for research purposes because it has been validated for only a few general activities. One major problem concerns the degree of similarity between the laboratory exercise test to establish the HR–$\dot{V}O_2$ line and the specific activities to which it applies. For example, factors other than oxygen consumption influence the exercise heart rate response. These include environmental temperature, emotions, previous food intake, body position, muscle groups exercised, continuous or discontinuous (stop-and-go) exercise, or whether the muscles act statically or more dynamically. In aerobic dance, for example, heart rates while dancing at a specific oxygen consumption significantly exceed heart rates at the same oxygen consumption during treadmill exercise.[23] Consistently higher heart rates occur in upper-body exercise or when muscles act statically in straining-type exercise than in dynamic leg exercise at any submaximal oxygen consumption. Consequently, applying heart rate during upper-body or static exercise to an HR–$\dot{V}O_2$ line developed during running or cycling *overpredicts* the actual oxygen consumption.[18]

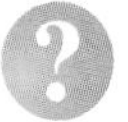

INTEGRATIVE QUESTION

A high-tech computer company asks you to validate a wrist-mounted device to measure exercise energy expenditure. The person exhales one breath onto the top of the instrument while exercising. The device's electronic components and microprocessor analyze expired air to compute oxygen consumption and energy expenditure. Outline the steps necessary to establish the instrument's validity.

Summary

1. Different classification systems exist to rate the strenuousness of physical activities. These include ratings based on (1) the ratio of the energy cost of the task to the resting energy requirement, (2) the oxygen requirement in mL · kg^{-1} · min^{-1}, or (3) multiples of resting metabolism as METs.
2. Average total daily energy expenditure averages 2900 kcal for men and 2200 for women ages 19 to 50 years. Considerable variability among people exists for daily energy expenditure, with the largest variation determined by one's physical activity level.
3. Daily energy expenditure provides a framework for classifying different occupations. Within any classification, energy expended during leisure time recre-

Focus on Research

Factors That Affect Recovery Oxygen Consumption

Margaria R, et al. The possible mechanisms of contracting and paying the oxygen debt and the role of lactic acid in muscular contraction. Am J Physiol 1933;106:689.

➤ A. V. Hill and colleagues had theorized that the increased oxygen consumption in recovery from exhaustive exercise ("oxygen debt") resulted largely from the delayed oxidation of a portion of the lactic acid (LA) that accumulated during exercise. These researchers, however, did not provide direct evidence to quantify the relationship between the oxygen debt and LA accumulation to confirm their hypothesis.

Margaria and his group at the prestigious Harvard Fatigue Laboratory provided the first quantitative assessment of Hill's theory. The researchers determined the time-course characteristics of LA removal, described as an exponential function of time. They also related LA removal rate to recovery oxygen consumption ($\dot{V}O_2$). The $\dot{V}O_2$ recovery curve subdivided into two parts that the researchers attributed to distinctly different metabolic events during exercise. The terms *alactacid* and *lactacid* described these components of recovery $\dot{V}O_2$.

One subject, observed during 10-minute runs on different occasions at varied exercise intensities, provided the experimental data. LA, measured from the femoral vein and brachial artery at different times throughout exercise, indicated rapid and uniform diffusion of LA throughout the body. Blood LA concentration varied directly with the body's total LA content. The figure illustrates the relationship between exercise blood LA concentrations and the magnitude of recovery $\dot{V}O_2$. Note that the curve does not deviate from baseline LA until the oxygen debt reaches 3 to 4 L. This coincided with the subject's exercise $\dot{V}O_2$ of about 3.0 L · min^{-1}. Blood LA concentration (and corresponding oxygen debt) then increased linearly with exercise intensity ($\dot{V}O_2$). The researchers reasoned that when the total oxygen debt remained below 3.0 L, the LA mechanism in exercise remained inactive. They termed this level of exercise *alactic* to signify work production without significant LA accumulation. Under these conditions, recovery $\dot{V}O_2$ proceeds rapidly to the resting level. LA began to accumulate with exercise at about 65% of the maximum aerobic metabolism ($\dot{V}O_{2max}$), accumulating rapidly thereafter. LA removal, a slow process, progressed at a velocity constant of 0.02—one-half removed each 15 minutes.

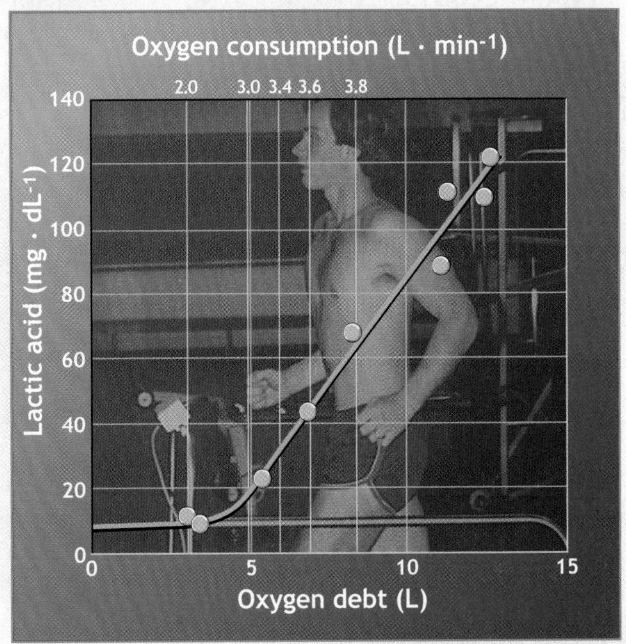

Relation between blood lactic acid concentration and oxygen debt (calculated after A. V. Hill) and oxygen consumption at various levels of exercise. Exercise duration equaled 10 minutes in each case.

Margaria and colleagues concluded that LA production became important only during strenuous exercise. They postulated that the total recovery $\dot{V}O_2$ consisted of the combined effects of two distinct components: (1) lactacid oxygen debt attributable to oxidation of LA produced in exercise and (2) alactacid oxygen debt, unrelated to LA accumulation and repaid early and rapidly in recovery. This important experiment in the early history of exercise physiology provided insight into why different $\dot{V}O_2$ recovery patterns emerged for different exercise intensities. Subsequent research in the 1970s further clarified factors contributing to the excess postexercise oxygen consumption.

ational pursuits often contributes considerable additional variability.

4. Heavier individuals generally expend more total energy in physical activity than their lighter counterparts, particularly in weight-bearing walking and running activities.
5. Heart rate serves as a valid indicator of the relative strenuousness of physical activity. However, it has only limited use in predicting oxygen consumption and caloric expenditure in diverse forms of physical activities.

References

1. Ainsworth BE, et al. Compendium of physical activities: classification of energy costs of human physical activities. Med Sci Sports Exerc 1993;25:71.
2. Belko, A, et al. Effect of energy and protein intake and exercise intensity on the thermic effect of food. Am J Clin Nutr 1986;43:863.
3. Bemben MG, et al. Age-related patterns in body composition for men aged 20–79 yr. Med Sci Sports Exerc 1995;27:264.
4. Bray G. The acute effects of food intake on energy expenditure during cycle ergometry. Am J Clin Nutr 1974;27:254.
5. Brenner IK, et al. Physical conditioning effects on fetal heart rate responses to graded maternal exercise. J Appl Physiol 1999;32:792.
6. Cunningham JJ. Body composition and resting metabolic rate: the myth of feminine metabolism Am J Clin Nutr 1982;36:721.

7. Cureton KJ, Sparling PB. Distance running performance and metabolic responses to running in men and women with excess weight experimentally equated. Med Sci Sports 1908;12:288.
8. Durnin JVGA, Passmore R. Energy, work and leisure. London: Heinmann, 1967.
9. Flatt JB. Energetics of intermediary metabolism. In: Assessment of energy metabolism in health and disease. Columbus, OH: Ross Laboratories, 1980.
10. Going S, et al. Aging and body composition: biological changes and methodological issues. Exerc Sport Sci Rev 1995;23:459.
11. Keys A, et al. Basal metabolism and age of adult men. Metabolism 1973;22:579.
12. Kleiber M. The fire of life: an introduction to animal energetics. Huntington, NY: Krieger, 1975.
13. Knuttgen HG, Emerson K Jr. Physiological response to pregnancy at rest and during exercise. J Appl Physiol 1974;36:549.
14. Latin RW, Berg KE. The accuracy of the ACSM and a new cycle ergometry equation for young women. Med Sci Sports Exerc 1994;26:642.
15. LeBlanc J, et al. Hormonal factors in reduced post prandial heat production of exercise trained subjects. J Appl Physiol 1984;56:772.
16. Londeree BR, et al. Oxygen consumption of cycle ergometry is nonlinearly related to work rate and pedal rate. Med Sci Sports Exerc 1997;29:775.
17. Lusk G. The elements of the science of nutrition. 4th ed. Philadelphia: WB Saunders, 1928.
18. Maas S, et al. The validity of the use of heart rate in estimating oxygen consumption in static and in combined static/dynamic exercise. Ergonomics 1989;32:141.
19. McArdle WD, et al. Aerobic capacity, heart rate, and estimated energy cost during women's competitive basketball. Res Q 1971;42:178.
20. Meredith CN, et al. Body composition and aerobic capacity in young and middle-aged endurance-trained men. Med Sci Sports Exerc 1987;19:557.
21. Miller DS, et al. Gluttony 2: thermogenesis in overeating man. Am J Clin Nutr 1967;20:1223.
22. Montgomery DL, et al. The effect of added weight on ice hockey performance. Phys Sportsmed 1982;10:91.
23. Parker SB, et al. Failure of target heart rate to accurately monitor intensity during aerobic dance. Med Sci Sports Exerc 1989;21:230.
24. Piers LS, et al. Is there evidence for an age-related reduction in BMR related to quantitative or qualitative change in components of lean tissue. J Appl Physiol 1998;85:2196.
25. Poehlman ET, Danforth E Jr. Endurance training increases metabolic rate and norepinephrine appearance rate in older individuals. Am J Physiol 1991;261:E233.
26. Poehlman ET, et al. Resting metabolic rate and post prandial thermogenesis in highly trained and untrained males. Am J Clin Nutr 1988;47:793.
27. Poehlman ET, et al. Endurance exercise in aging humans: effects on energy metabolism. Exerc Sport Sci Rev 1994;22:751.
28. Pratley R, et al. Strength training increases resting metabolic rate and norepinephrine levels in healthy 50- to 65-yr-old men. J Appl Physiol 1994;73:133.
29. Schutz Y, et al. Diet-induced thermogenesis measured over a whole day in obese and non-obese women. Am J Clin Nutr 1984;40:542.
30. Segal KR, et al. Thermic effects of food and exercise on lean and obese men of similar lean body mass. Am J Physiol 1987;252:E110.
31. Shetty PS, et al. Post prandial thermogenesis in obesity. Clin Sci 1981;60:519.
32. Starling RD, et al. Energy requirements and physical activity in free-living older women and men: a doubly labeled water study. J Appl Physiol 1998;85:1063.
33. Toner MM, McArdle WD. Human thermoregulatory responses to acute cold stress with special reference to water immersion. In: Fregly MJ, Blatteis CM, eds. Handbook of physiology, environmental physiology, section 4, vol. 1. New York: Oxford University Press, 1996.
34. Trembly A, et al. Diminished dietary thermogenesis in exercise-trained human subjects. Eur J Appl Physiol 1983;52:1.
35. Zahorska-Markiewicz B. Thermic effect of food and exercise in obesity. Eur J Appl Physiol 1980;44:231.

CHAPTER 10

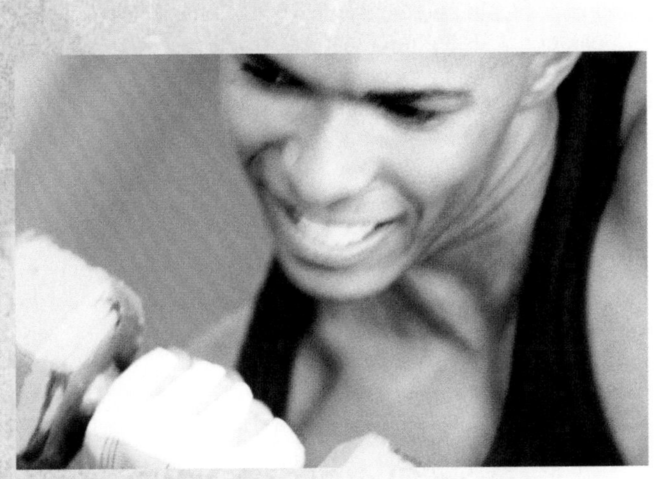

Energy Expenditure During Walking, Jogging, Running, and Swimming

Chapter Objectives

- Differentiate between gross energy expenditure and net energy expenditure of physical activity
- Explain the concepts of exercise economy and mechanical efficiency, including the differences in running economy between trained and untrained children and adults
- Graph the relationship between walking velocity and energy expenditure up to velocities achieved during competitive racewalking
- Discuss the influence of body mass, exercise surface, and footwear on energy expenditure during walking and running
- Describe the advantages and disadvantages of ankle weights and handheld weights for increasing energy expenditure during walking and running
- Graph the relationship between running velocity and energy expenditure
- Explain the association between running velocity and energy cost per unit distance traveled
- Outline the interactions between stride length and stride frequency, and linear velocity during running and competitive racewalking
- Quantify the influence of drafting on energy expenditure during running, swimming, and bicycling
- Identify factors that contribute to the significantly lower exercise economy of swimming compared with running

Total energy expended each day depends largely on the type and duration of one's physical activity. The following sections detail energy expenditure for walking, running, and swimming. Aside from being competitive sports, these activities take on special significance to the general population for their roles in weight control, physical conditioning, and health maintenance and rehabilitation.

GROSS VERSUS NET ENERGY EXPENDITURE

The following example illustrates the use of oxygen consumption to estimate the energy expenditure in swimming. A 25-year-old man swimming for 40 minutes at a moderate, steady pace requiring 2.0 L per minute oxygen consumption consumes a total of 80 L of oxygen. One can transpose this oxygen consumption to an energy value by using the approximate calorific transformation of 5.0 kcal per liter of oxygen consumed (assumes carbohydrate is sole energy fuel). Thus, the swimmer expends about 400 kcal (80 L $O_2 \times$ 5 kcal) during the swim. This, however, does not assess the energy cost of the swim per se, because the measured total or **gross energy expenditure** also includes energy that would have been expended if the person only rested and did not swim for the period. To obtain the true requirement of just exercise—the **net energy expenditure**—one must subtract resting metabolism from the gross energy expenditure of the exercise as follows:

Net energy expenditure = Gross energy expenditure − Resting energy expenditure (for equivalent time)

Knowing the swimmer's size (mass, 65 kg; stature, 174 cm) permits computation of the surface area of 1.78 m^2 from the nomogram in Figure 9.4. Multiplying this value by the average basal metabolic rate (BMR) for young men, 38 kcal $\cdot$ $m^{-2} \cdot h^{-1}$ (Fig. 9.3), gives an estimated resting energy expenditure of 67.6 kcal per hour (1.78 $m^2 \times$ 38 kcal) or about 45 kcal for the 40-minute swim. The energy expended solely for the swim then computes as gross energy expenditure (400 kcal) minus the 40-minute resting value (45 kcal), or a net energy expenditure of 355 kcal just for swimming.

In Figure 7.3 of Chapter 7, we showed that oxygen consumption during constant-load light-to-moderate exercise rises rapidly during the first several minutes, then levels off and remains stable thereafter. Thus, one can estimate total energy expenditure from only one or two oxygen consumption measures during steady-rate exercise. Activities with considerable variation in pace such as tennis, soccer, lacrosse, field hockey, or basketball, require more frequent measures for accurate estimates of total energy expenditure. Strenuous exercise, when energy requirements considerably exceed aerobic energy transfer, derives considerable energy anaerobically with accompanying blood lactate accumulation. Energy expenditure estimates in this situation become virtually impossible.

MECHANICAL EFFICIENCY AND ECONOMY OF HUMAN MOVEMENT

The concept of **mechanical efficiency** considers the relationship between energy input and output. In a figurative comparison to economics, efficiency of operation parallels the cost required to produce goods relative to the money generated from the sale of such goods. We might also liken human efficiency of operation to the auto industry, which always strives to optimize vehicle aerodynamic design to improve efficiency of operation and the important miles-per-gallon rating. Efficiency of human movement relates the amount of energy required performing a particular task to the actual work accomplished. **Movement economy**, in contrast to mechanical efficiency, refers to the energy required (usually measured as oxygen consumption) to maintain a constant velocity of movement.

In a sense, an evaluation of efficiency and economy of movement occurs when assessing the ease of movement of elite athletes. One does not need a trained eye to qualitatively discriminate the ease, efficiency, or economy of physical effort when comparing elite swimmers, skiers, tennis players, gymnasts, basketball players, cyclists, and dancers with less-skilled counterparts who seemingly expend considerable "wasted energy" performing the same task.

Economy of Movement

Assessing economy of movement requires evaluating the oxygen consumed while a subject performs an exercise at a set power output or velocity.[94] This approach only applies to steady-rate exercise in which oxygen consumption closely mirrors energy expenditure. For example, at an established submaximal speed of running, cycling, or swimming, an individual with greater movement economy consumes *less* oxygen (lower steady-rate $\dot{V}O_2$). African women who balance heavy loads on their heads have mastered a subtle adjustment in walking technique that enables them to carry up to 20% of their body weight with no increase in energy expenditure. A group of Europeans, on the other hand, exerted proportionately more effort (increased oxygen consumption) as the added weight on their head increased. Economy takes on considerable importance during longer-duration exercise, in which success largely depends on the individual's aerobic capacity and ability to maintain as low a $\dot{V}O_2$ as possible relative to the work rate. For children and adults, any training adjustment that improves the economy of effort usually improves performance.[26,44] Figure 10.1 shows the strong association between running economy and endurance performance in elite athletes of comparable aerobic fitness. Clearly, athletes with greater running economies achieve better race times. In a statistical sense, variation in running economy among this homogeneous group explains approximately 64% of the total variation in 10-km running performance.[64]

No single biomechanical factor accounts for individual differences in running economy.[17,53] Even among trained runners,

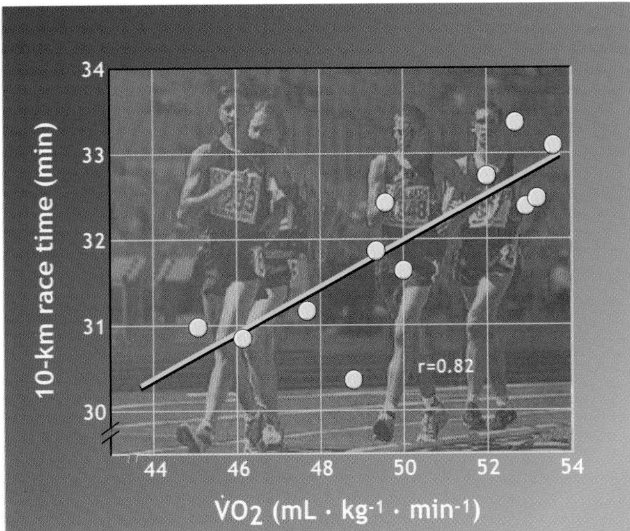

FIGURE 10.1 • Relationship between submaximal oxygen consumption at 268 m · min^{-1} and 10-km race time in elite male runners of comparable aerobic capacity. (From Morgan DW, Craib M. Physiological aspects of running economy. Med Sci Sports Exerc 1992;24:456.)

significant variation in economy emerges at a submaximal running speed.[21,65,69] In general, long-term programs of run training improve running economy,[22,86] which relates partly to training-induced reductions in pulmonary ventilation during submaximal exercise.[14,35] It remains unclear whether the early stages of run training (first 6 weeks) affect running mechanics or economy despite significant improvements in performance and physiologic function.[35,48] Short-term training that emphasizes "proper" running techniques (i.e., arm movements and body alignment) probably does not improve running economy.[45] On the other hand, distance runners lacking an economical stride-length pattern benefit from a short-term audiovisual feedback program that focuses on optimizing stride length,[68] and biofeedback and relaxation psychophysiologic interventions.[14]

Indirect evidence from studies of cycling indicates that muscle fiber-type distribution affects the economy of effort. During submaximal cycling, exercise economies of well-trained cyclists vary by as much as 15%.[23] Differences in muscle fiber type in the active muscles represented an important component of variation in economy. Cyclists exhibiting greater economy possessed a larger percentage of slow-twitch (type I) muscle fibers in their vastus lateralis muscle. These observations suggests that aerobic, type I muscle fibers act with greater mechanical efficiency than faster-contracting, highly anaerobic type II fibers.[24]

Mechanical Efficiency

Mechanical efficiency represents another strategy for evaluating the relationship between energy input and exercise power output. *Mechanical efficiency reflects the percentage of total chemical energy expended that contributes to external work, with the remainder lost as heat.* Within this context:

$$\text{Mechanical efficiency (\%)} = \text{External work accomplished (energy output)} \div \text{Energy input} \times 100$$

The external work accomplished (energy output) equals force acting through a vertical distance (F × D), usually recorded as foot-pounds (ft-lb) or kilogram-meters (kg-m), and then expressed in kcal units (1 kcal = 3087 ft-lb, or 426.4 kg-m in a perfect machine without loss in efficiency). External work is easily determined during cycle ergometry or an exercise such as stair climbing or bench stepping, which requires lifting the body mass (see "In A Practical Sense," Chapter 5). One cannot compute mechanical efficiency during horizontal walking or running because technically no external work is accomplished; reciprocal arm and leg movements negate each other, and the body achieves no net gain in vertical distance. If a person walks or runs up a grade, the work component can be estimated from body mass and the vertical distance (lift) achieved during the exercise. Total oxygen consumed provides the means to infer the denominator (energy input) of the efficiency equation. Oxygen consumption converts to energy units—roughly 1.0 L O_2 = 5.0 kcal (see Table 8.1 for precise calorific transformations based on RQ).

For example, suppose a 15-minute ride on a stationary bicycle generates 13,300 kg-m of work, and the net oxygen consumed to produce the work totals 25 L (RQ = 0.88). To create common units of measurement, convert the oxygen consumed to a corresponding kcal value. At an RQ of 0.88, each liter of oxygen consumption generates an energy equivalent of 4.9 kcal (Table 8.1). Therefore, 25 L of oxygen consumption during the 15-minute ride generates 122.5 kcal of energy (25 × 4.9 kcal). The energy equivalent of 13,300 kg-m of external work equals 31.19 kcal (13,300 kg-m ÷ 426.4 kg-m per kcal). Mechanical efficiency computes as follows:

$$\begin{aligned}\text{Mechanical efficiency} &= 31.19 \text{ kcal} \div 122.5 \text{ kcal} \times 100\\ &= 25.5\%\end{aligned}$$

As with all machines, the efficiency of the human body for mechanical work falls considerably below 100%. The energy required to overcome internal and external friction is the largest factor affecting efficiency. This constitutes wasted energy because it does not accomplish work; consequently, work input *always* exceeds work output.

Delta Efficiency

Extensive research permits estimates of mechanical efficiencies for different large-muscle physical activities. On average, efficiency ranges between 20 and 25% for walking, running, and stationary cycling. Of course factors such as body size, gender, fitness level and skill affect individual differences in efficiency. For activities with substantial drag force that resists movement (e.g., road cycling, cross-country skiing, ice skating, rowing, and swimming), mechanical efficiency falls considerably below 20%. Competitors in these sports focus attention on reducing drag by improving aerodynamics and/or hydrodynamics through alterations in equipment and technique. For an elite athlete, a small improvement in efficiency significantly influences the likelihood of success.

An alternative approach to determining mechanical efficiency (not affected by body mass or changes in body weight)[6,74] involves calculating **delta efficiency** as follows:

$$\text{Delta efficiency} = \frac{\Delta \text{ Work production}}{\Delta \text{ Energy expenditure}} \times 100$$

where Δ work production equals the calculated difference in work output at two different exercise levels, and Δ energy expenditure equals the difference in the energy expenditure between the two exercise levels. Like traditional calculations for mechanical efficiency, the delta efficiency equation expresses both terms in the same measurement unit.

For example, suppose an individual cycles at 100 W at a $\dot{V}O_2$ of 1.50 L · min^{-1} and RQ of 0.89. Work intensity then increases to 200 W, with a corresponding $\dot{V}O_2$ of 2.88 L · min^{-1} and RQ of 0.95. Delta efficiency computes as follows, where 1 W = 0.014 kcal · min^{-1}; RQ of 0.89 = 4.911 kcal · LO_2^{-1}; RQ of 0.95 = 4.985 kcal · LO_2^{-1}:

$$\begin{aligned}
\text{Delta efficiency} &= 200\text{ W} - 100\text{ W} \div 2.88\text{ L} \cdot \text{min}^{-1} - 1.50\text{ L} \cdot \text{min}^{-1} \times 100 \\
&= (200 \times 0.014) - (100 \times 0.014) \div (2.88 \times 4.985) - (1.50 \times 4.911) \times 100 \\
&= 1.4\text{ kcal} \cdot \text{min}^{-1} \div 6.99\text{ kcal} \cdot \text{min}^{-1} \times 100 \\
&= 0.2003 \times 100 = 20.0\% \\
&= 20.0\%
\end{aligned}$$

ENERGY EXPENDITURE DURING WALKING

For most people, walking represents their major daily physical activity. Figure 10.2 displays research from five countries on the energy expenditure of men who walked at speeds ranging from 1.5 to 9.5 km · h^{-1} (0.9 to 5.9 mph). The relationship between walking speed and oxygen consumption remains approximately linear between speeds of 3.0 and 5.0 km · h^{-1} (1.9 and 3.1 mph); at faster speeds, walking economy decreases, and the relationship curves upward, indicating a disproportionate increase in energy expenditure with increasing speed. This explains why, per unit distance traveled, faster, less-efficient walking speeds expend greater total calories.[9,33]

Influence of Body Mass

One can accurately predict energy expenditure of horizontal walking at speeds between 3.2 and 6.4 km · h^{-1} (2.0 and 4.0 mph) for men and women who differ in body mass, using an equation based on the combined data in Figure 10.2 and other studies.[1,32] These values, listed in Table 10.1, generally achieve an accuracy to within 15% of the actual energy expenditure. On a daily basis, therefore, error estimates of energy expended in walking would generally range from 50 to 100 kcal, assuming the person walks 2 hours daily. The data in the table provide reasonable accuracy for assessing the caloric cost of walking at the speeds indicated and for body masses up to 91 kg. One can extrapolate for heavier individuals, but accuracy is lost.

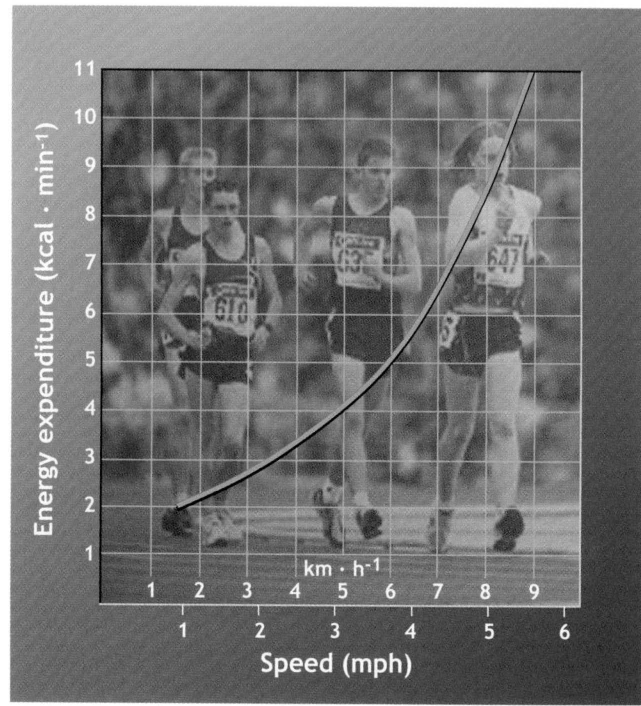

FIGURE 10.2 • Energy expenditure while walking on a level surface at different speeds. The *yellow line* represents a compilation of average values from various studies reported in the literature.

Terrain and Walking Surface

Table 10.2 summarizes the influence of terrain and surface on the energy cost of walking. Similar economies exist for level walking on a grass track or paved surface. Walking in the sand, however, requires almost twice as much energy as walking on a hard surface, in large part due to sand's hindering effects on the forward movement of the foot and the added force required by the calf muscle to compensate for foot slippage. Walking in soft snow triples metabolic cost compared with similar walking on a treadmill.[85] A brisk walk (or run) along a beach or in freshly fallen snow provides excellent exercise stress to "burn" additional calories or improve physiologic fitness.[83]

Another series of experiments showed no differences between energy cost of treadmill walking at 2.93 km · h^{-1} and 5.86 km · h^{-1} and normal walking on a hard surface at the same speeds.[78] These and other data indicate that people generate essentially the same physiologic stress by walking on a level surface or walking on a treadmill at an equivalent speed and distance. Such results also lend support to the use of laboratory data to quantify human energy expenditure in real-life situations. From a mechanical perspective, however, small but significant differences exist in force patterns between treadmill and overground walking.[48]

TABLE 10.1 ➤ PREDICTION OF ENERGY EXPENDITURE (KCAL · MIN^{-1}) FROM SPEED OF LEVEL WALKING AND BODY MASS[a]

WALKING SPEED		BODY MASS						
	KG	36	45	54	64	73	82	91
MPH	KM · H^{-1} / LB	80	100	120	140	160	180	200
2.0	3.22	1.9	2.2	2.6	2.9	3.2	3.5	3.8
2.5	4.02	2.3	2.7	3.1	3.5	3.8	4.2	4.5
3.0	4.83	2.7	3.1	3.6	4.0	4.4	4.8	5.3
3.5	5.63	3.1	3.6	4.2	4.6	5.0	5.4	6.1
4.0	6.44	3.5	4.1	4.7	5.2	5.8	6.4	7.0

[a]How to use the table: A 120-lb (54-kg) person who walks at 3.0 mph (4.83 km · h^{-1}) expends 3.6 kcal · min^{-1}. This person expends 216 kcal in a 60-minute walk (3.6 × 60).
Data from Passmore R, Durnin JVGA. Human energy expenditure. Physiol Rev 1955;35:801.

Downhill Walking

For most individuals, walking the downhill portion of a mountain hike or golf course provides a welcome relief, compared with the uphill portion of the exercise. Downhill walking (or running) represents a form of **negative work**, in which the body's center of mass moves in a downward vertical direction with each step cycle. This decreases the total potential energy of the system. Consequently, at the same speed and elevation, it requires less energy to perform eccentric muscle actions (negative work) than the concentric actions of positive work.

Figure 10.3 illustrates the net oxygen requirement of both level and negative grade walking at constant speeds of either 6.3 or 5.4 km · h^{-1}.[93] Compared with walking on level ground, progressive negative grade walking decreases oxygen cost down to a −9% grade for speeds of 5.4 km · h^{-1} and −12% for speeds of 6.3 km · h^{-1}. Energy cost, however, begins to increase at the more-severe negative grades. The increase in oxygen cost for walking down the steeper grades probably results from additional energy to resist, or "brake," the body from the pull of gravity while attempting to maintain a proper and safe walking rhythm.

Footwear

It requires considerably more energy to carry weight on the feet or ankles than to carry similar weight on the torso. For example, a weight equal to 1.4% of body mass, placed on the ankles, increases the energy cost of walking an average of 8%, or nearly 6 times more than with the same weight on the torso.[43] In a practical sense, wearing boots increases the energy cost of walking and running disproportionately compared with the cost when wearing lighter running shoes. Simply adding an additional 100 g to each shoe increases oxygen consumption during moderate running by 1%. Clear implications exists for these findings in the design of running shoes, hiking and climbing boots, and work boots traditionally required in professions such as mining, forestry, fire fighting, and the military—small changes in shoe weight produce meaningful changes in movement economy. The cushioning properties of shoes also affect exercise economy.[72] A softer-soled running shoe reduces the oxygen cost of running at a moderate speed by 2.4% compared with that for a similar shoe with a firmer cushioning system, even though the pair of softer-soled shoes weigh an additional 31 g.[36]

Handheld and Ankle Weights

The impact force on the legs while running averages about three times body mass, whereas the level of leg shock walking equals only 30% of this value. Thus, individuals desiring to increase energy expenditure using only walking as the exercise mode often add extra weight to the body. This modification has also been applied to running activities.

Walking

Ankle weights increase the energy expenditure of walking to values usually observed for running.[61] The effect benefits individuals who desire to use only walking as a low-impact training modality, yet require greater energy expenditures than occur during normal walking. Also, use of handheld weights, walking poles (simulate arm action in cross-

TABLE 10.2 ➤ EFFECT OF DIFFERENT TERRAIN ON THE ENERGY EXPENDITURE OF WALKING BETWEEN 5.2 AND 5.6 KM · H^{-1}

TERRAIN	CORRECTION FACTOR[a]
Paved road (similar to grass track)	0.0
Plowed field	1.5
Hard snow	1.6
Sand dune	1.8

[a]The correction factor is a multiple of the energy expenditure for walking on a paved road or grass track. For example, the energy cost of walking in a plowed field equals 1.5 times that of walking on a paved road.
First entry from Passmore R, Durnin JVGA. Human energy expenditure. Physiol Rev 1955; 35:801. Last three entries from Givoni B, Goldman RF. Predicting metabolic energy cost. J Appl Physiol 1971; 30:429.

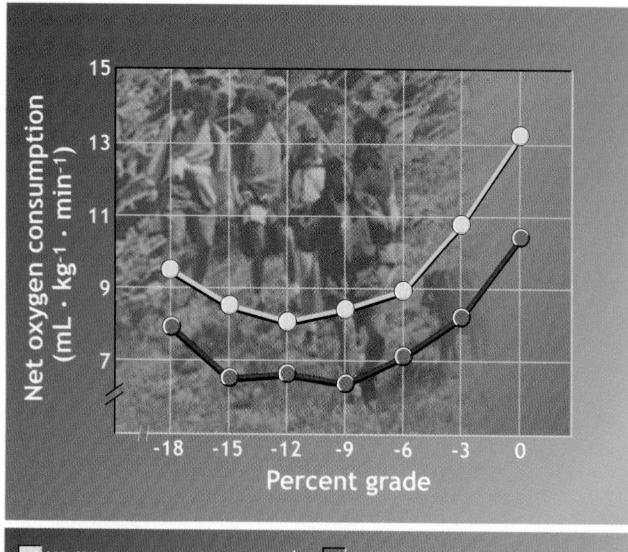

FIGURE 10.3 • Net oxygen costs of level (0%) and downhill walking at grades between −3 and −18% and speeds between 5.4 and 6.3 km · h^{-1}. *Percent grade* reflects the vertical distance moved downward per unit horizontal distance traversed. (From Wanta DM, et al. Metabolic response to graded downhill walking. Med Sci Sports Exerc 1993;25:159.)

country skiing), power belts (worn around waist with resistance cords with handles for arm action), and upper-body exercise such as swinging the arms significantly increase the energy expenditure of walking.[13,31,75,80,95] However, use of handheld weights and walking poles may disproportionately increase exercise systolic blood pressure, perhaps from the blood pressure–elevating effects of (1) upper-body exercise (see Chapter 15, p. 319) and (2) increased intramuscular tension from gripping the object. An augmented blood pressure response contraindicates use of handheld weights for individuals with existing hypertension or coronary heart disease.

INTEGRATIVE QUESTION

What recommendations would you make for exercise mode–specific physical activities for aerobic training of individuals with osteoarthritis of the knees.

Running

Considering the relatively small increase in energy expenditure with hand or ankle weights in running, it seems more practical to simply increase the unweighted running speed or distance. This reduces the injury potential from the added impact force caused by weights and eliminates discomfort from carrying the weights.[20] For individuals with orthopedic limitations that could worsen with leg impact shock from running, in-line skating offers a less-stressful alternative for an equivalent aerobic demand.[49,59]

Competition Walking

Researchers studied the energy expenditures of five Olympic-caliber walkers at various walking and running speeds on a treadmill.[60] Walking speed during competition averaged 13.0 km · h^{-1} (11.5 to 14.8 km · h^{-1} [7.1 to 9.2 mph]) over distances ranging from 1.6 to 50 km. This represents a relatively fast speed, because the world-record walk, set in 1994 by Bernardo Segura of Mexico, averaged 15.1 km · h^{-1} (9.38 mph, or 6 min:24 s per mile)! Figure 10.4 illustrates that the break point in the economy of locomotion between walking and running for these race-walkers ranged between 8.0 and 9.0 km · h^{-1}. These data, plus biomechanical evidence, indicate about the same crossover speed—when running becomes more economical than walking—for conventional and competitive styles of walking (Fig. 10.5).[16] In addition, treadmill walking at competition speeds produced only a slightly lower oxygen consumption for race-walkers than their highest oxygen consumptions during treadmill running. A linear relationship existed between oxygen consumption and walking at speeds greater than 8 km per hour (5.0 mph), but the slope of the line was *twice* as steep than that for running at the same speeds. The athletes could walk at velocities of nearly 16 km · h^{-1} (9.9 mph). *However, the economy of walking faster than 8 km · h^{-1} equaled only one-half the economy for running at the same speeds.* The attainment of similar values for $\dot{V}O_{2max}$ during race-walking and running by elite competitors further supports the model for aerobic training specificity because $\dot{V}O_{2max}$ in untrained subjects during walking generally falls from 5 to 15% below values for running.[37,56]

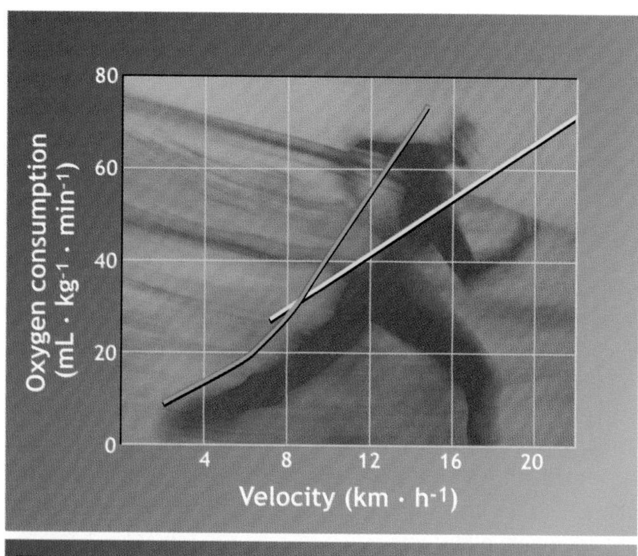

FIGURE 10.4 • Relationship between oxygen consumption and horizontal velocity for walking and running in competition walkers. (Adapted from Menier DR, Pugh LGCE. The relation of oxygen intake and velocity of walking and running in competition walkers. J Physiol 1968;197:717.)

IN A PRACTICAL SENSE

PREDICTING ENERGY EXPENDITURE DURING TREADMILL WALKING AND RUNNING

A linear relationship exists between oxygen consumption (energy expenditure) and walking speeds between 3.0 and 5.0 km · h^{-1} (1.9 and 3.1 mph), and running at speeds faster than 8.0 km · h^{-1} (5 to 10 mph). Adding the resting oxygen consumption to the oxygen requirements of the horizontal and vertical components of the walk or run makes it possible to estimate total (gross) exercise oxygen consumption ($\dot{V}O_2$) and energy expenditure.

Basic Equation

$\dot{V}O_2$ (mL · kg^{-1} · min^{-1}) = Resting component (1 MET [3.5 mL O_2 · kg^{-1} · min^{-1}]) + Horizontal component (speed, [m · min^{-1}] × oxygen cost of horizontal movement) + Vertical component (percent grade × speed [m · min^{-1}] × oxygen cost of vertical movement).

[To convert mph to m · min^{-1}, multiply by 26.82; to convert m · min^{-1} to mph, multiply by 0.03728.]

Walking: Oxygen cost of the horizontal component of movement equals 0.1 mL · kg^{-1} · min^{-1}, and 1.8 mL · kg^{-1} · min^{-1} for the vertical component.

Running: Oxygen cost of the horizontal component of movement equals 0.2 mL · kg^{-1} · min^{-1}, and 0.9 mL · kg^{-1} · min^{-1} for the vertical component.

Predicting Energy Cost of Treadmill Walking

PROBLEM

A 55-kg person walks on a treadmill at 2.8 mph (2.8 × 26.82 = 75 m · min^{-1}) up a 4% grade. Calculate (1) $\dot{V}O_2$ (mL · kg^{-1} · min^{-1}), (2) METs, and (3) energy expenditure (kcal · min^{-1}). ***[Note: express % grade as a decimal value; i.e., 4% grade = 0.04]***

SOLUTION

1. $\dot{V}O_2$ (mL · kg^{-1} · min^{-1}) = Resting component + Horizontal component + Vertical component
   $\dot{V}O_2$ = Resting $\dot{V}O_2$ (mL · kg^{-1} · min^{-1}) + [speed (m · min^{-1}) × 0.1 mL · kg^{-1} · min^{-1}] + [% grade × speed (m · min^{-1}) × 1.8 mL · kg^{-1} · min^{-1}]
   = 3.5 + (75 × 0.1) + (0.04 × 75 × 1.8)
   = 3.5 + 7.5 + 5.4
   = 16.4 mL · kg^{-1} · min^{-1}
2. METs = $\dot{V}O_2$ (mL · kg^{-1} · min^{-1}) ÷ 3.5 mL · kg^{-1} · min^{-1}
   = 16.4 ÷ 3.5
   = 4.7
3. Kcal · min^{-1} = $\dot{V}O_2$ (mL · kg^{-1} · min^{-1}) × Body mass (kg) × 5.05 kcal · LO_2^{-1}
   = 16.4 mL · kg^{-1} · min^{-1} × 55 kg × 5.05 kcal · L^{-1}
   = 0.902 L · min^{-1} × 5.05 kcal · L^{-1}
   = 4.6

Predicting Energy Cost of Treadmill Running

PROBLEM

A 55-kg person runs on a treadmill at 5.4 mph (5.4 × 26.82 = 145 m · min^{-1}) up a 6% grade. Calculate (1) $\dot{V}O_2$ in mL · kg^{-1} · min^{-1}, (2) METs, and (3) energy expenditure (kcal · min^{-1}).

SOLUTION

1. $\dot{V}O_2$ (mL · kg^{-1} · min^{-1}) = Resting component + Horizontal component + Vertical component
   $\dot{V}O_2$ = Resting $\dot{V}O_2$ (mL · kg^{-1} · min^{-1}) + [speed (m · min^{-1}) × 0.2 mL · kg^{-1} · min^{-1}] + [% grade × speed (m · min^{-1}) × 0.9 mL · kg^{-1} · min^{-1}]
   = 3.5 + (145 × 0.2) + (0.06 × 145 × 0.9)
   = 3.5 + 29.0 + 7.83
   = 40.33 mL · kg^{-1} · min^{-1}
2. METs = $\dot{V}O_2$ (mL · kg^{-1} · min^{-1}) ÷ 3.5 mL · kg^{-1} · min^{-1}
   = 40.33 ÷ 3.5
   = 11.5
3. Kcal · min^{-1} = $\dot{V}O_2$ (mL · kg^{-1} · min^{-1}) × Body mass (kg) × 5.05 kcal · LO_2^{-1}
   = 40.33 mL · kg^{-1} · min^{-1} × 55 kg × 5.05 kcal · L^{-1}
   = 2.22 L · min^{-1} × 5.05 kcal · L^{-1}
   = 11.2

Competition walkers achieve high yet uneconomical rates of movement, unattainable with conventional walking, with a distinctive modified walking technique that constrains the athlete to certain movement patterns regardless of walking speed. The athlete must maintain this gait despite progressive decreases in walking economy as exercise duration progresses and fatigue increases.[11,12] Among elite race-walkers, variations in walking economy contribute more to successful performance than in competitive running.[37]

ENERGY EXPENDITURE DURING RUNNING

Primary biomechanical factors that determine the energy cost of running in relation to velocity in mammals include the magnitude and rate of muscular force generation to counteract the effect of gravity and to operate the spring-like properties of the muscle-tendon system.[46] Energy expenditure for running has been quantified in two ways: (1) during performance of the actual activity and (2) on a treadmill with precise control of speed

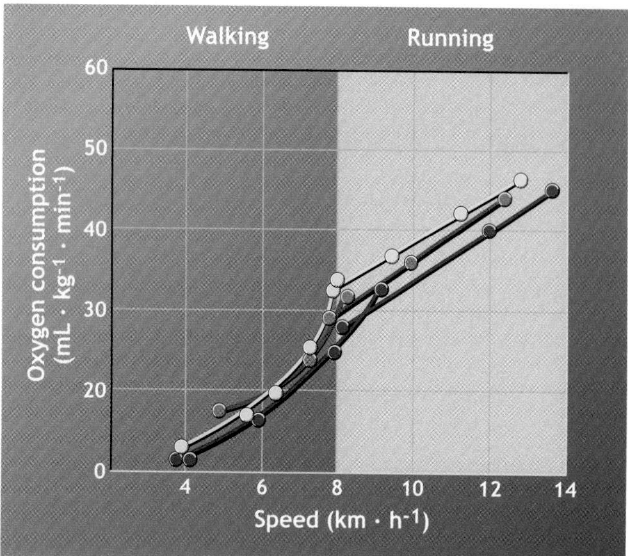

FIGURE 10.5 • Relationship between oxygen consumption and speed of horizontal walking and running in men and women. Different symbols represent values from various research studies. (From Falls HB, Humphrey LD. Energy cost of running and walking in young women. Med Sci Sports 1976;8:9.)

and grade. The terms *jogging* and *running* reflect qualitative assessments related to speed and relative strenuousness. At identical submaximal speeds, an endurance athlete runs at a lower percentage of his or her $\dot{V}O_{2max}$ than an untrained person, even though both maintain similar oxygen consumptions while running. Thus, the demarcation between a jog and a run relates more to the participant's fitness level; a jog for one person would represent a run for another.

Independent of fitness, however, it becomes more economical from an energy standpoint to discontinue walking and begin running at speeds above about 8 km · h^{-1}. Figure 10.5 illustrates the relationship between oxygen consumption and horizontal walking and running for men and women at speeds between 4 and 14 km · h^{-1}. For the data depicted in purple and yellow,[51] the lines relating oxygen consumption and speed intersect at a running speed of 8.0 km · h^{-1}; the breakpoint in locomotion economy for competition walkers (shown in red) occurs at about 8.7 km · h^{-1}.[60]

Economy of Running Fast or Slowly

The data for running in Figure 10.5 illustrate an important principle about running speed and energy expenditure. *Because of the linear relationship between oxygen consumption and running speed, the total energy requirement for running a given distance (in steady rate) is about the same regardless of speed.* Simply stated, running a mile at 10 mph requires about twice the energy per minute as running a mile at 5 mph; however, at the faster speed completing the mile requires 6 minutes, while running at the slower speed takes twice as long or 12 minutes. Consequently, the net energy cost to traverse the mile remains about the same. Equivalent energy costs per mile (regardless of running speed) occur not only for horizontal running but also for running at a specific grade that ranges from −45 to +15%.[28,51] *During horizontal running, the net energy cost (i.e., excluding the resting requirement) per kilogram of body mass per kilometer traveled averages 1 kcal or 1 kcal · kg^{-1} · km^{-1}.* Thus, the net energy cost of running 1 km for individuals weighing 78 kg averages 78 kcal, regardless of running speed. Expressed in terms of oxygen consumption (5 kcal = 1 L O_2), this amounts to 15.6 L of oxygen consumed per kilometer. Comparisons of net energy cost of locomotion per unit distance traveled for walking and running indicate greater energy expenditure when running a given distance.[7]

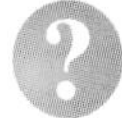

INTEGRATIVE QUESTION

An elite 140-lb runner claims that she consistently consumes 12,000 kcal daily simply to maintain body weight owing to the strenuousness of her training. Using examples of exercise energy expenditures, discuss whether this level of intake could reflect a plausible energy intake requirement.

Net Energy Cost Values

Table 10.3 presents values for net energy expenditure during running for 1 hour at various speeds—expressed in kilometers per hour, miles per hour, and the number of minutes required to complete 1 mile at a specific speed. Bolded values indicate net calories expended running 1 mile for a given body mass. As mentioned above, the energy requirement per mile remains fairly constant regardless of running speed. *Thus, a person who weighs 62 kg requires approximately 2600 kcal (net) to run a 26.2-mile marathon regardless of whether the run takes just over 2 hours, 3 hours, or 4 hours!*

Table 10.3 also indicates that the energy cost per mile increases proportionately with body mass. A lower energy cost (less heat production) in lighter runners at any given speed partly explains why small stature (and relatively larger surface area for heat dissipation) provides an advantage in distance running, particularly in warm, humid environments.[30] The influence of body mass on exercise energy expenditure certainly supports the role of weight-bearing exercise as additional caloric stress for the overly fat person who wishes to increase daily energy expenditure for weight control (see Focus on Research). For example, a 102-kg person who runs 5 miles each day at a comfortable pace expends 163 kcal for each mile completed, or a total of 815 kcal for the 5-mile run. Increasing or decreasing the speed (within the broad range of steady-rate paces) simply alters the duration of the 5-mile run; it has little effect on the total energy (calories) expended.

Table 10.4 summarizes data from various studies of energy expenditure for horizontal and grade walking and running on a firm surface. The energy requirement represents multiples of the resting metabolic rate or METs (3.5 mL O_2 kg^{-1} · min^{-1}).

TABLE 10.3 ➤ **NET ENERGY EXPENDITURE PER HOUR OF HORIZONTAL RUNNING RELATED TO VELOCITY AND BODY MASS**[a]

Body Mass		KM · H⁻¹[b]	8	9	10	11	12	13	14	15	16
		MPH	**4.97**	**5.60**	**6.20**	**6.84**	**7.46**	**8.08**	**8.70**	**9.32**	**9.94**
		MIN PER MILE	**12:00**	**10:43**	**9:41**	**8:46**	**8:02**	**7:26**	**6:54**	**6:26**	**6:02**
(KG)	(LB)	KCAL PER MILE									
50	110	**80**	400	450	500	550	600	650	700	750	800
54	119	**86**	432	486	540	594	648	702	756	810	864
58	128	**93**	464	522	580	638	696	754	812	870	928
62	137	**99**	496	558	620	682	744	806	868	930	992
66	146	**106**	528	594	660	726	792	858	924	990	1056
70	154	**112**	560	630	700	770	840	910	980	1050	1120
74	163	**118**	592	666	740	814	888	962	1036	1110	1184
78	172	**125**	624	702	780	858	936	1014	1092	1170	1248
82	181	**131**	656	738	820	902	984	1066	1148	1230	1312
86	190	**138**	688	774	860	946	1032	1118	1204	1290	1376
90	199	**144**	720	810	900	990	1080	1170	1260	1350	1440
94	207	**150**	752	846	940	1034	1128	1222	1316	1410	1504
98	216	**157**	784	882	980	1078	1176	1274	1372	1470	1568
102	225	**163**	816	918	1020	1122	1224	1326	1428	1530	1632
106	234	**170**	848	954	1060	1166	1272	1378	1484	1590	1696

[a]Interpret the table as follows: For a 50-kg person, the *net* energy expenditure for running for 1 hour at 8 km · h⁻¹ or 4.97 mph equals 400 kcal; this speed represents a 12-minute per mile pace. Thus, 5 miles would be run in 1 hour and 400 kcal would be expended. Increasing the pace to 12 km · h⁻¹, expends 600 kcal during the hour of running.

[b]Running speeds are expressed as kilometers per hour (km · h⁻¹), miles per hour (mph), and minutes required to complete each mile (min per mile). The values in **boldface type** are the *net* calories expended to run 1 mile for a given body mass, independent of running speed.

TABLE 10.4 ➤ **ENERGY REQUIREMENTS (METs) FOR HORIZONTAL AND GRADE WALKING AND RUNNING ON A SOLID SURFACE**

HORIZONTAL AND GRADE WALKING

% GRADE	MPH	1.7	2.0	2.5	3.0	3.4	3.75
	M · MIN⁻¹	**45.6**	**53.7**	**67.0**	**80.5**	**91.2**	**100.5**
0		2.3	2.5	2.9	3.3	3.6	3.9
2.5		2.9	3.2	3.8	4.3	4.8	5.2
5.0		3.5	3.9	4.6	5.4	5.9	6.5
7.5		4.1	4.6	5.5	6.4	7.1	7.8
10.0		4.6	5.3	6.3	7.4	8.3	9.1
12.5		5.2	6.0	7.2	8.5	9.5	10.4
15.0		5.8	6.6	8.1	9.5	10.6	11.7
17.5		6.4	7.3	8.9	10.5	11.8	12.9
20.0		7.0	8.0	9.8	11.6	13.0	14.2
22.5		7.6	8.7	10.6	12.6	14.2	15.5
25.0		8.2	9.4	11.5	13.6	15.3	16.8

HORIZONTAL AND GRADE JOGGING/RUNNING

% GRADE	MPH	5	6	7	7.5	8	9	10
	M · MIN⁻¹	**134**	**161**	**188**	**201**	**215**	**241**	**268**
0		8.6	10.2	11.7	12.5	13.3	14.8	16.3
2.5		10.3	12.3	14.1	15.1	16.1	17.9	19.7
5.0		12.0	14.3	16.5	17.7	18.8		
7.5		13.9	16.4	18.9				
10.0		15.5	18.5					

Modified from ACSM guidelines for exercise testing and prescription, 6th ed. Baltimore: Williams & Wilkins, 2000.

Stride Length, Stride Frequency, and Speed

Running

One can increase running speed in three ways: (1) increase the number of steps each minute (*stride frequency*), (2) increase the distance between steps (*stride length*), or (3) increase *both* the length and frequency of strides. Although the third option may seem obvious for increasing running speed, several experiments have provided objective data concerning this alternative.

Research in 1944 evaluated the stride pattern for the Danish champion in the 5- and 10-km running events.[9] At a running speed of 9.3 km · h^{-1}, this athlete's stride frequency equaled 160 per minute, with a corresponding stride length of 97 cm. When running speed increased 91% to 17.8 km · h^{-1}, stride frequency increased only 10%, to 176 per minute, whereas stride length increased 83%, to 168 cm. Figure 10.6A displays the interaction between stride frequency and stride length as running speed increases. Doubling the speed from 10 to 20 km · h^{-1} increases stride length by 85%, whereas stride frequency increases only about 9%. Running at speeds above 23 km · h^{-1}, however, occurs mainly by increasing stride frequency. *As a general rule, running speed increases mainly by lengthening the stride. Only at faster speeds does stride frequency become important.* Relying on increasing the length of the "stroke" cycle, not the frequency, to achieve more rapid speeds in endurance performance also occurs among top-flight kayakers, rowers, cross-country skiers, and speed skaters.

Competition Walking

The competitive walker does not increase speed the same way a runner does. Figure 10.6B illustrates the stride length–stride frequency relationship for an Olympic 10-km medal winner walking at speeds from 10 to 14.4 km · h^{-1}. When walking speed increased within this range, stride frequency increased by 27%, and stride length increased by 13%. Faster speeds produced an even greater increase in stride frequency. Unlike running, in which the body glides through the air, competitive racewalking requires that the back foot remain on the ground until the front foot makes contact. Thus, lengthening the stride becomes a difficult and ineffective way to increase speed. Consequently, involvement of the trunk and arm musculature to move the leg forward rapidly requires additional energy expenditure; this explains the poorer economy for walking than for running at speeds above 8 or 9 km · h^{-1} (see Fig. 10.4).

Optimum Stride Length

Each person runs at a constant speed with an optimum combination of stride length and stride frequency. This optimum depends largely on the person's mechanics, or "style" of running, and cannot be determined from body measurements.[18] Nevertheless, energy expenditure increases more for overstriding than for understriding. Figure 10.7 relates oxygen consumption to different stride lengths, altered by a subject running at the relatively fast speed of 14 km · h^{-1}.

For this runner, a stride length of 135 cm produced the lowest oxygen consumption (3.35 L · min^{-1}). When stride length decreased to 118 cm, oxygen consumption increased 8%; lengthening the distance between steps to 153 cm increased oxygen consumption by 12%. The inset graph shows a similar pattern for oxygen consumption when running speed increased to 16 km · h^{-1} and stride lengths varied between 135 and 169 cm. Decreasing this runner's stride length from the optimum of 149 cm to 135 cm increased oxygen consumption by 4.1%; lengthening the stride to 169 cm increased the aero-

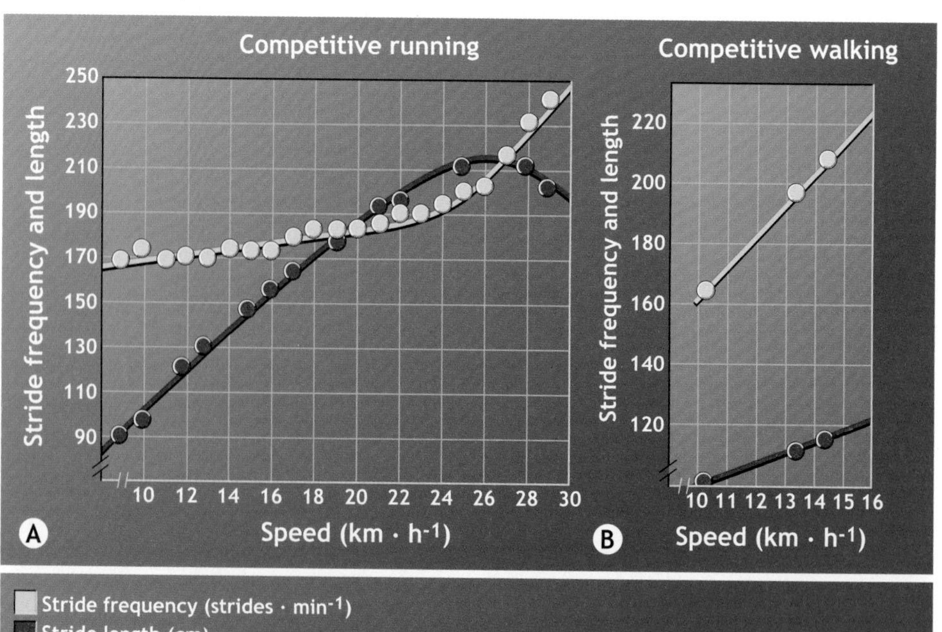

FIGURE 10.6 • **A**. Stride frequency and stride length plotted as a function of running speed. **B**. Data for an Olympic walker during race-walking. (From Hogberg P. Length of stride, stride frequency, flight period and maximum distance between the feet during running with different speeds. Int Z Angew Physiol 1952;14:431.)

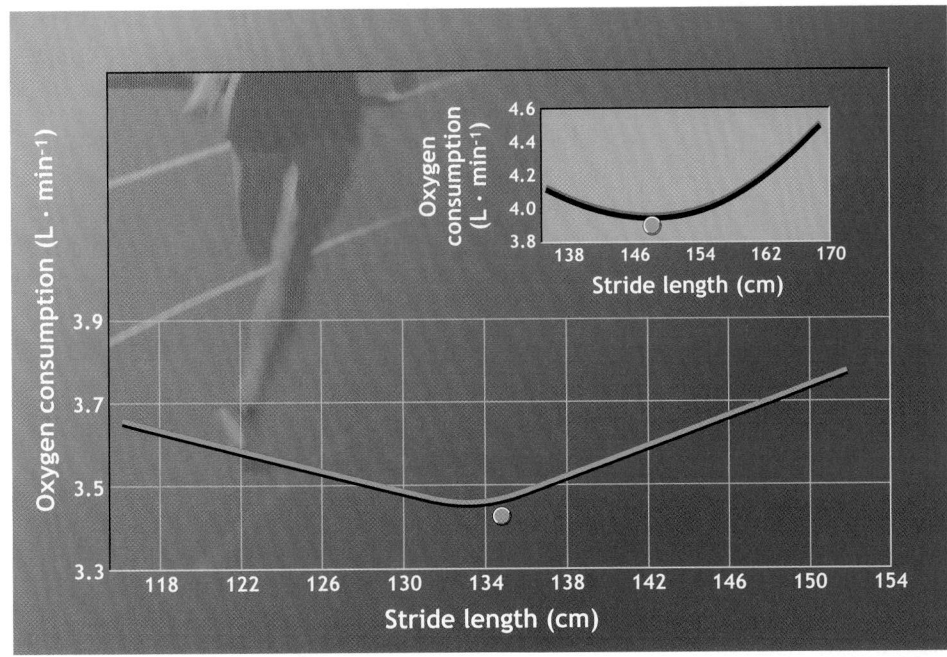

FIGURE 10.7 • Oxygen consumption while running at 14 km · h^{-1} as affected by different stride lengths. The inset graph plots oxygen consumption at a faster speed of 16 km · h^{-1}. (From Hogberg P. Length of stride, stride frequency, flight period and maximum distance between the feet during running with different speeds. Int Z Angew Physiol 1952;14:431.)

bic energy expenditure nearly 13%. As one might expect, the stride length selected by the subject (marked in the figure by the solid orange circle) produced the most economical stride length (lowest $\dot{V}O_2$). Lengthening the stride above the optimum caused a larger increase in oxygen consumption than a shorter-than-optimum length. Thus, urging a runner who shows signs of fatigue to "lengthen your stride!" to maintain speed actually proves counterproductive in terms of economy of effort.

Well-trained runners should run at the stride length they have selected through years of running.[40] In keeping with the concept that the body attempts to achieve a **level of minimum effort**, the self-selected length and frequency generally produce the most economical running performance. This reflects an individual's unique body size, inertia of limb segments, and anatomic development.[17,62,63] *No "best" style characterizes elite runners.* Biomechanical analysis may help the athlete correct minor irregularities in movement patterns while running.[71] For the competitive runner, any minor improvement in movement economy generally translates into improved performance.

Running Economy: Children and Adults, Trained and Untrained

Boys and girls are less economical runners than adults because they require 20 to 30% more oxygen per unit body mass to run at a particular speed.[2,27,45] Consequently, use of adult models to predict energy cost in weight-bearing locomotion fails to account for the increased (and changing) energy costs in children and adolescents. Figure 10.8 illustrates the relationship between walking and running speeds (speeds between 2 and 8 mph) and (A) oxygen consumption and (B) energy expenditure in 47 male and 35 female adolescent volunteers.[92] Despite the higher oxygen consumption and energy expenditure values during walking and running for adolescents compared to the data for the adults depicted in Figure 10.5, the shape of the curves for both groups remains remarkably similar.

Increased energy expenditure (reduced economy) among children and adolescents in weight-bearing exercise has been attributed to a larger ratio of surface area to mass, greater stride frequencies, and shorter stride lengths and to differences in anthropometric variables and body mechanics that could reduce movement economy.[34,81] Figure 10.9B shows that running economy improves steadily during years 10 through 18. Poor running economy among young children partly explains their inferior performance in distance running, compared with adults, and their progressive performance improvement through adolescence, even though aerobic capacity (mL O_2 · kg^{-1} · min^{-1}; Fig. 10.9A) remains relatively constant throughout this period.[25,27] Consequently, improvements during the growth years in scores in weight-bearing exercise tests such as the 1-mile walk-run do not necessarily infer concomitant improvement in $\dot{V}O_{2max}$.[26]

INTEGRATIVE QUESTION

Discuss the practical implications for knowing that children demonstrate significantly lower economy for walking and running than adults.

When running at a particular speed, elite adolescent and adult endurance runners generally have lower oxygen consumptions than less-trained or less-successful age-matched counterparts.[44,54,69] Distance athletes as a group run 5 to 10% more economically than well-trained middle-distance runners.[21] For trained runners, economy values and biomechanical characteristics during running remain fairly stable from day to day, even during high-intensity exercise,[66,67] with probably no difference between genders.[29]

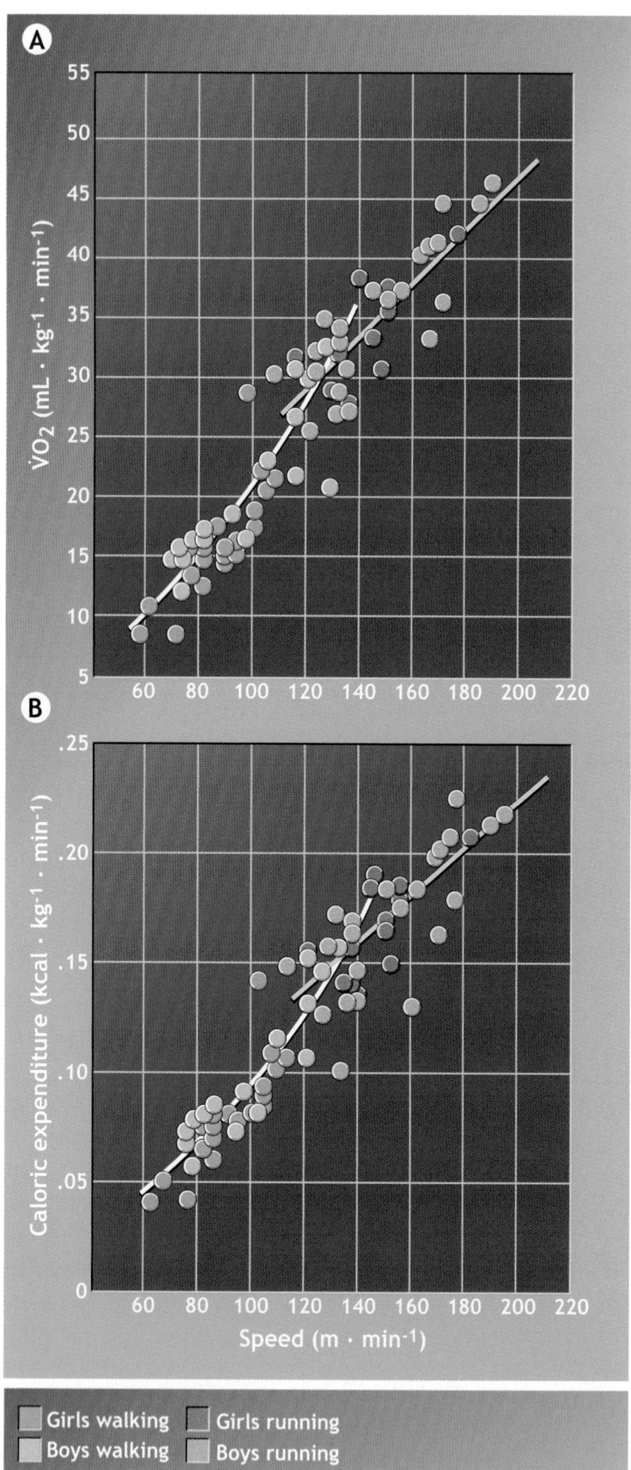

FIGURE 10.8 • Relationship between speed of walking and running and (**A**) oxygen consumption, and (**B**) energy expenditure in adolescent boys and girls. The *white line* represents the curve-of-best-fit for walking; the *yellow line* represents the line for running. (From Walker JL, et al. The energy cost of horizontal walking and running in adolescents. Med Sci Sports Exerc 1999;31:311.)

Air Resistance

Anyone who has run into a headwind knows that it requires greater energy to maintain a given pace than running in calm air or with the wind at one's back. The effect of air resistance on the energy cost of running varies with three factors: (1) air density, (2) the runner's projected surface area, and (3) the square of the runner's velocity. Depending on speed, overcoming air resistance can require 3 to 9% of the total energy cost of running in calm air.[41,76] Running into a headwind creates an additional energy expense. Figure 10.10 shows that the oxygen consumption while running at 15.9 km · h^{-1} in calm conditions averaged 2.92 L · min^{-1}. This increased 5.5% to 3.09 L · min^{-1} against a 16-km · h^{-1} headwind, and further to 4.1 L · min^{-1} when running against the strongest wind (66 km · h^{-1}; 41 mph)—an additional 41% expenditure of energy to maintain running velocity!

Some may argue that the negative effects of running into a headwind become counterbalanced during one's return with the tailwind. This does not occur, however, because the energy cost of cutting through a headwind significantly exceeds the reduced oxygen consumption with an equivalent wind velocity at one's back. Wind tunnel tests have shown that clothing modification or even trimming one's hair improves aerodynamics and reduces the effects of air resistance up to 6%. A reduction of this magnitude could translate into improved running performance.[4] This fact has not escaped the elite athlete, as witnessed in the Sydney 2000 Olympics where many athletes wore modern running suits to take advantage of any reduction in air resistance. At higher altitudes, wind velocity has less effect on energy expenditure than at sea level because of the reduced air density at higher

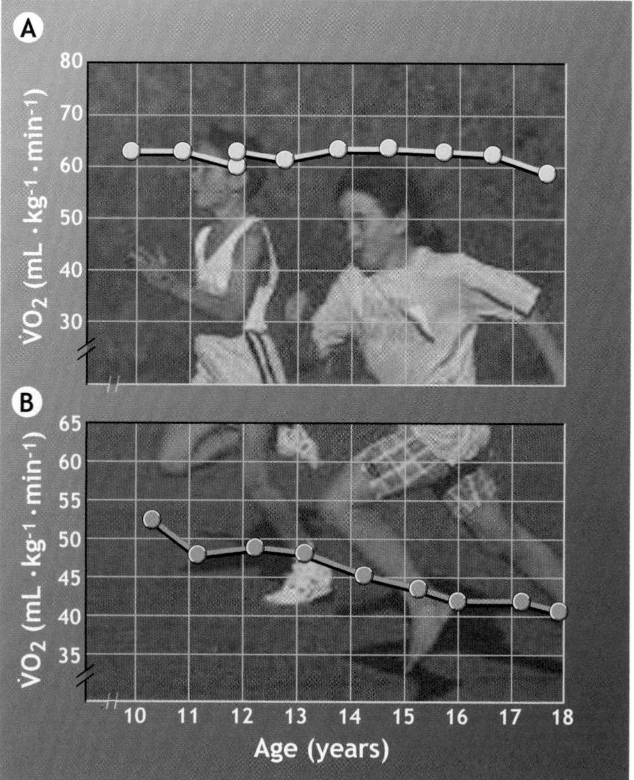

FIGURE 10.9 • Effects of growth on (**A**) aerobic capacity and (**B**) submaximal oxygen consumption during running at 202 m · min^{-1}. (Adapted from Daniels J, et al. Differences and changes in $\dot{V}O_2$ among runners 10 to 18 years of age. Med Sci Sports 1978;10:200.)

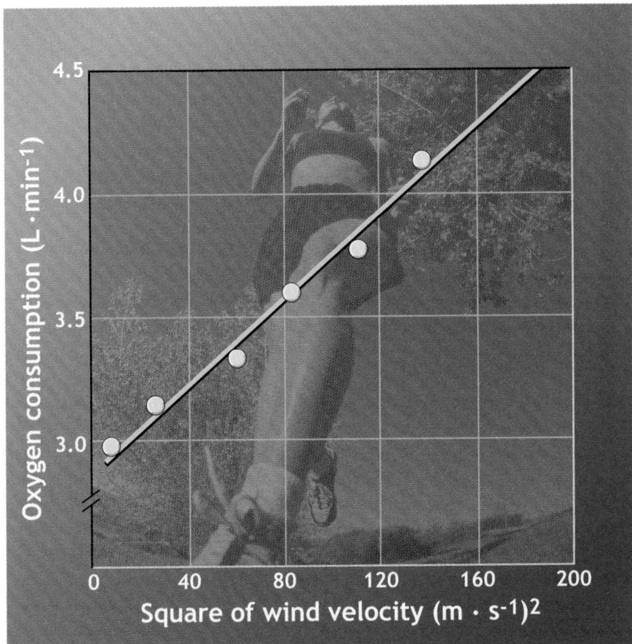

FIGURE 10.10 • Oxygen consumption as a function of the square of the wind velocity while running at 15.9 km · h^{-1} against various headwinds. (From Pugh LGCE. Oxygen intake and treadmill running with observations on the effect of air resistance. J Physiol 1970;207:823.)

elevations. For example, moderate altitude always lowers the oxygen cost of competitive skating at a given speed compared with sea level.[3] In all likelihood, an altitude effect also applies to the energy cost of running, cross-country skiing, and cycling.

Drafting: Often a Wise Position

The negative effect of air resistance and headwind on the energy cost of running confirms the wisdom of athletes who choose to run in a more aerodynamically desirable position directly behind a competitor, a technique called **drafting**, or maintaining a sheltered position. For example, running 1 m behind another runner at a speed of 21.6 km · h^{-1} decreases total energy expenditure by about 7%.[76] The beneficial effect of drafting on economy of effort also occurs for cross-country skiing, short-track speed skating, and bicycling.[8,57,82] Bicycling at 40 km · h^{-1} on a calm day requires application of about 90% of the total power generated simply to overcome air resistance. At this speed, energy expenditure decreases 26 to 38% when a competitor closely follows another cyclist.[47] For elite speed skaters, drafting (within 1 m of the leader) during controlled-pace 4-minute skating trials significantly lowered exercise heart rate and blood lactate concentration.[82] A reduced level of exercise stress with drafting should theoretically give the competitor an additional energy reserve for the sprint to the finish. Furthermore, when triathletes maintained the drafting position during the cycling leg of a sprint-distance triathlon (0.75-km swim, 20-km bike, 5-km run), oxygen consumptions, heart rates, and blood lactate concentrations remained significantly lower than when the athletes cycled at the same speed without drafting.[39] These physiologic benefits translated into improved subsequent performance as maximal running speed after biking in the drafting situation was faster than performance in no-draft trials.

Treadmill Versus Track Running

The treadmill has provided the primary exercise mode for evaluating the physiology of running, yet one might question the validity of this procedure for determining energy metabolism during running and relating it to competitive track performance. For example, does the energy required to run at a given treadmill speed equal that required to run on a track in calm weather? To answer this question, eight distance runners ran on a treadmill and track under calm air conditions at three submaximal speeds of 180 m · min^{-1}, 210 m · min^{-1}, and 260 m · min^{-1}.[58] Graded exercise tests determined possible differences between treadmill and track running on maximal oxygen consumption. Table 10.5 summarizes the results for one running speed and maximal exercise.

From a practical standpoint, no measurable differences emerged in the aerobic requirements of submaximal running (up to 286 m · min^{-1}) on the treadmill and track, either on level or up a grade, or between the $\dot{V}O_{2max}$ measured in both forms of exercise.[4,58] The possibility exists that at the faster speeds achieved by elite endurance runners, the impact of air resistance on a calm day increases the oxygen cost of track running, compared with "stationary" treadmill running at the same fast speed. This certainly occurs in activities requiring the athlete to move at high velocities such as cycling and speed skating, in which the retarding effects of air resistance become considerable. This causes these athletes to focus on factors that improve aerodynamics—clothing, equipment, and body position.

Marathon Running

In 1988, the Ethiopian Belayneh Densimo set the world record in the marathon with a time of 2 h:06 min:50 s. His average speed of just under 4 min:53 s per mile over the

TABLE 10.5 ➤ COMPARISON OF AVERAGE METABOLIC RESPONSES DURING TREADMILL AND TRACK RUNNING

MEASUREMENT	TREADMILL	TRACK	DIFFERENCE
Submaximal Exercise			
Oxygen consumption, mL · kg^{-1} · min^{-1}	42.2	42.7	0.5
Respiratory exchange ratio	0.89	0.87	−0.02
Running speed, m · min^{-1}	213.7	216.8	3.1
Maximal Exercise			
Oxygen consumption, L · min^{-1}	4.40	4.44	0.04
mL · kg^{-1} · min^{-1}	66.9	66.3	−0.6
Ventilation, L · min^{-1}, BTPS	142.5	146.5	4.0
Respiratory exchange ratio	1.15	1.11	−0.04

Adapted from McMiken DF, Daniels JT. Aerobic requirements and maximum aerobic power in treadmill and track running. *Med Sci Sports* 1976;8:14.

Focus on Research — It Costs More to Move More

Mahadeva K, et al. Individual variations in the metabolic cost of standardized exercises: the effects of food, age, sex and race. J Physiol 1953;121:225.

➤ Few early experiments in human energy metabolism dealt with energy requirements during exercise, particularly the influence of body size, age, gender, and skill. We now know that such contributing factors serve an important purpose for exercise prescription and estimating energy expenditure to adjust energy balance for weight loss and weight maintenance.

Mahadeva and colleagues conducted one of the first large-scale energy cost studies that focused attention on energy expenditure in two common exercise forms: (1) stepping that produces measurable external work in raising body mass and (2) walking on the level at a constant speed. The researchers made multiple observations on 50 men and women aged 13 to 79 years, of diverse ethnic backgrounds, whose body mass ranged from 48 to 110 kg. Measurements included basal and resting metabolism with the Douglas bag method of open-circuit spirometry. Exercise studies used the portable Kofranyi-Michaelis spirometer (see Fig 8.3). Subjects stepped to a metronome cadence of 15 up-and-down cycles per minute for 10 minutes on a 25.4-cm stool and walked on an indoor track for 10 minutes at 4.8 km · h^{-1}.

The two graphs show the relationship and corresponding prediction (regression) line between energy expenditure and body mass for each activity (*C*, energy expenditure in kcal per 10 min; *W*, body mass in kg). Energy expenditure in walking and stepping varied directly with body mass. Separate analyses showed that age, gender, ethnicity, and previous diet contributed little to predicting energy cost of the activities. This pioneering work showed that body mass primarily determines the energy expended in nonskilled physical activities that require transporting one's body mass (i.e., weight-bearing exercise). Consequently, we now accurately predict energy cost during steady-rate walking, running, and stepping exercise simply from knowledge of exercise intensity and body mass.

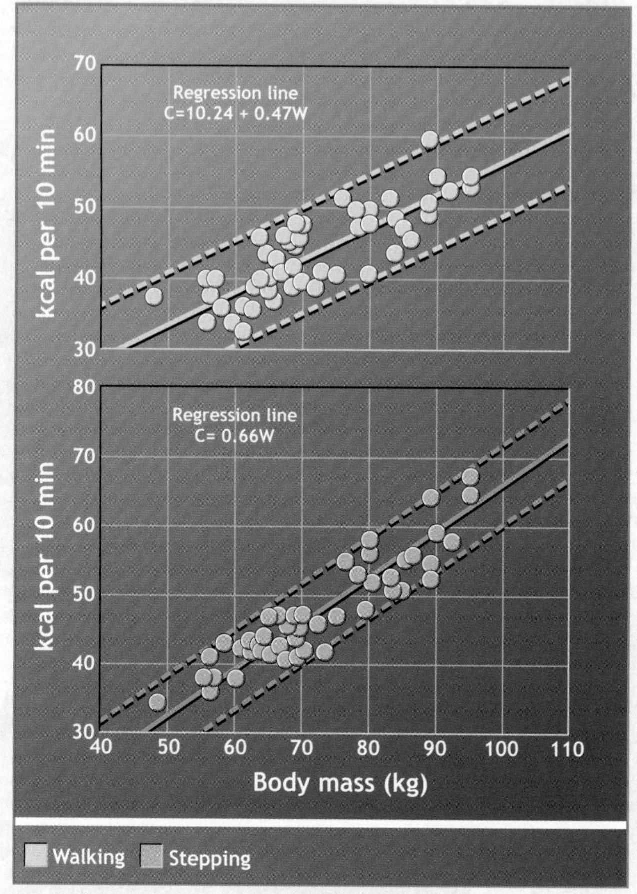

Top. Energy expenditure in kilocalories per 10 minutes as a function of body mass during walking at 3 mph. *Bottom.* Energy expenditure in kilocalories per 10 minutes as a function of body mass during stepping. The *dashed lines* show twice the standard error of estimate.

26.2-mile course represents a truly outstanding achievement in human exercise capacity. Not only does this blistering pace require a steady-rate oxygen consumption that exceeds the aerobic capacity of most male college students, it also demands that the marathoner sustain 80 to 90% of $\dot{V}O_{2max}$ for just over 2 hours!

Researchers measured two distance runners during a marathon to assess energy expenditure each minute and the total caloric cost of the run.[52] They determined oxygen consumption every 3 miles using open-circuit spirometry (see Fig. 8.4). Marathon times were 2 h:36 min:34 s ($\dot{V}O_{2max}$ = 70.5 mL · kg^{-1} · min^{-1}) and 2 h:39 min:28 s ($\dot{V}O_{2max}$ = 73.9 mL · kg^{-1} · min^{-1}). The first runner maintained an average speed of 16.2 km · h^{-1}, requiring an oxygen consumption equal to 80% of his $\dot{V}O_{2max}$. For the second runner, who averaged a slower speed of 16.0 km · h^{-1}, the aerobic component averaged 78.3% of maximum. For both men, the total energy required to run the marathon ranged between 2300 and 2400 kcal.

SWIMMING

Swimming differs in several important aspects from walking or running. One obvious difference entails the expenditure of energy to maintain buoyancy while simultaneously generating horizontal movement by using arms and legs, either in combination or separately. Other differences include the requirements for overcoming the **drag forces** that impede a swimmer's forward movement. The amount of drag depends on the fluid medium and the swimmer's size, shape, and velocity. These factors contribute to a mechanical efficiency in front-crawl swimming that ranges between only 5 and 9.5%.[90]

A significantly lower mechanical efficiency makes the energy cost of swimming a given distance average about four times more than the energy cost of running the same distance.

Methods of Measurement

For short swims of 25 yards at different velocities, subjects need not breathe, and estimates of energy expenditure can derive from oxygen consumption during a 20- to 40-minute recovery. For longer swims, including 12- to 14-hour endurance events, one can compute energy expenditure from oxygen consumption measured with open-circuit spirometry during portions of the swim. In studies conducted in the pool, the researcher walks alongside the swimmer and carries portable gas-collection equipment (Fig. 10.11E).[55] For another form of swimming exercise, illustrated in Figure 10.11A, the subject remains stationary, attached or tethered to a cable and pulley system by a belt worn around the waist.[50] Periodic increases in the weight stack attached to the cable force the swimmer to exert greater effort to maintain a

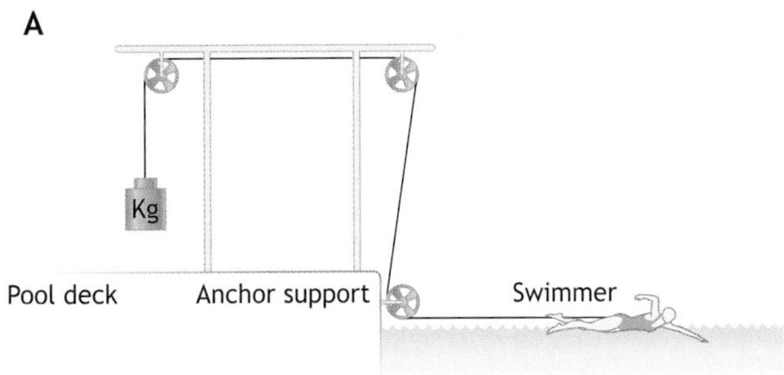

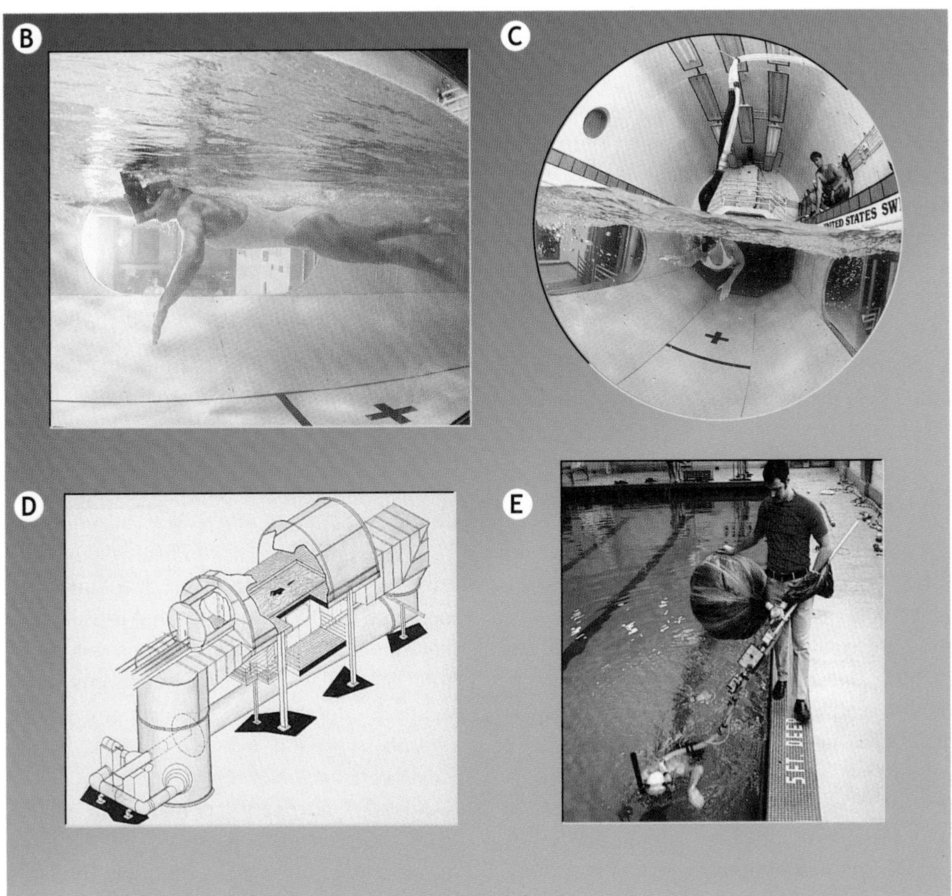

Figure 10.11 • **A**. Tethered swimming apparatus. **B–D**. Swimming treadmill. An environmental chamber surrounding the swimming treadmill controls atmospheric pressure (and other environmental conditions) during swimming. Using the swimming treadmill, researchers conduct physiologic and biomechanical experiments during swimming that simulate actual performance conditions. The underwater viewing area provides a convenient means for directly observing swimming performance related to stroke mechanics. **E**. Open-circuit spirometry (bag technique) to measure oxygen consumption during front-crawl swimming. (Schematic and photos of swimming treadmill courtesy of the United States Swimming International Center for Aquatic Research, Colorado Springs, CO.)

constant body position. Figure 10.11, B–D shows a swimmer in a flume, or "swimming treadmill." Water circulates at velocities varying from a slow swimming speed to near-record pace for a freestyle sprint. Aerobic capacity measurements using tethered, free, or flume swimming techniques produce essentially identical values.[10] Any of these modes of measurement can objectively evaluate metabolic and physiologic dynamics during swimming.

Energy Cost and Drag

The total drag force encountered by the swimmer consists of three components:

- **Wave drag**—caused by waves that build up in front of, and form hollows behind, the swimmer moving through the water. This component of drag does not significantly affect swimming at slow velocities, but its influence increases at faster swimming speeds.
- **Skin friction drag**—produced as the water slides over the skin surface. Even at relatively fast swimming velocities, the quantitative contribution of skin friction drag to the total drag remains small. However, research supports the common practice of swimmers "shaving down" to reduce skin friction drag, thereby decreasing energy cost.[84]
- **Viscous pressure drag**—caused by the pressure differential created in front of, and behind, the swimmer, which substantially counters propulsive efforts at slow velocities. Viscous pressure drag, caused by the separation of the thin sheet of water or boundary layer, forms adjacent to the swimmer. Its effect is reduced for highly skilled swimmers who learn to streamline stroke mechanics, reducing the separation region by moving it closer to the trailing edge of the water. This effect resembles an oar slicing through water with the blade parallel rather than perpendicular to the water flow.

Ways to Reduce Effects of Drag Force

Figure 10.12 depicts a curvilinear relationship between body drag and swimming velocity when towing a swimmer through the water. As velocity increases above 0.8 $m \cdot s^{-1}$, drag decreases by supporting the legs with a flotation device that places the body in a more hydrodynamically desirable horizontal position. Generally, the drag force increases about 2 to 2.5 times more during swimming than in passive towing.[88]

Wet suits worn by triathletes during swimming reduce body drag by about 14%,[89] thus lowering oxygen consumption at a given speed.[91] Improved swimming economy largely explains the faster swim times of athletes using wet suits. As in running, cross-country skiing, and cycling, drafting in swimming (following closely behind the wake of a lead swimmer) reduces physiologic demands.[5] This enables an endurance swimmer (e.g., triathlete or ocean racer) to conserve energy and possibly improve performance toward the end of the competition. Triathletes swimming 400 m swam the total distance 3% faster in a drafting position with lower blood lactate levels and stroke rates than in the lead position.[19] Performance changes related to large reductions in passive drag force in the drafting position; faster and leaner swimmers showed the greatest drag force reduction and performance improvement.

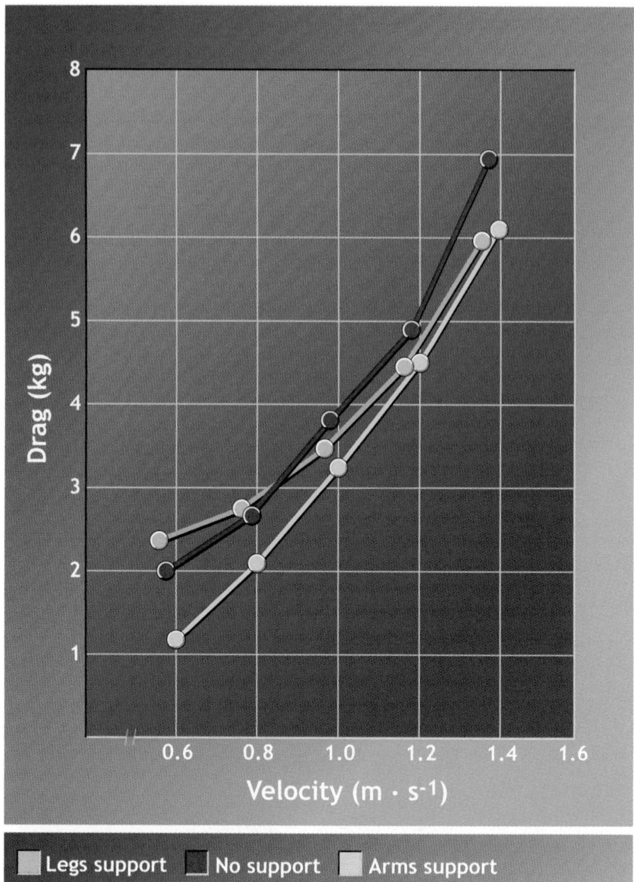

FIGURE 10.12 • Drag force in three different prone positions related to towing velocity. (From Holmér I. Energy cost of arm stroke, leg kick, and the whole stroke in competitive swimming styles. Eur J Appl Physiol 1974;33:105.)

The influence of swimsuit design on swimming economy has led to the use of neck-to-ankle body suits by swimmers in the 2000 Olympics in Australia. Proponents maintain that the technology-driven approach to competitive swimming maximizes swimming economy to a degree that allows swimmers to achieve 3% faster times compared to standard swimsuits.

KAYAKING. The energy demands of kayaking largely result from the resistance provided by the water to the forward movement of the craft. Consequently, drafting (wash riding) behind the leader reduces the energy requirements of paddling between 18 and 32%.[73] Improved kayaking economy results from the assist to forward movement provided by the wash generated by the boat in front. This effect decreases resistance and pressure of the water through which the boat moves.

Energy Cost, Swimming Velocity, and Skill

Elite swimmers swim a particular stroke at a given velocity with a lower oxygen consumption (greater economy) than relatively untrained or recreational swimmers. Highly skilled swimmers use more of the energy they generate per stroke to overcome drag forces. Consequently, they cover a greater distance per stroke than less-skilled swimmers, who waste considerable energy ineffectively moving water.[87] Figure 10.13A compares the oxygen consumptions and velocities for the breaststroke, back crawl, and front crawl at three levels of swimming ability. One subject, a recreational swimmer, did not participate in swim training; the trained subject, a top Swedish swimmer, swam on a daily basis; the elite swimmer was a European champion. Except during the breaststroke, the elite swimmer had a lower oxygen consumption at a given speed than his trained and untrained counterparts. Figure 10.13B shows that the breaststroke required a greater oxygen consumption for the trained swimmers at any speed, followed by the backstroke, with the front crawl being the least "expensive" of the three strokes. Because of marked accelerations and decelerations within the stroke cycle, energy ex-

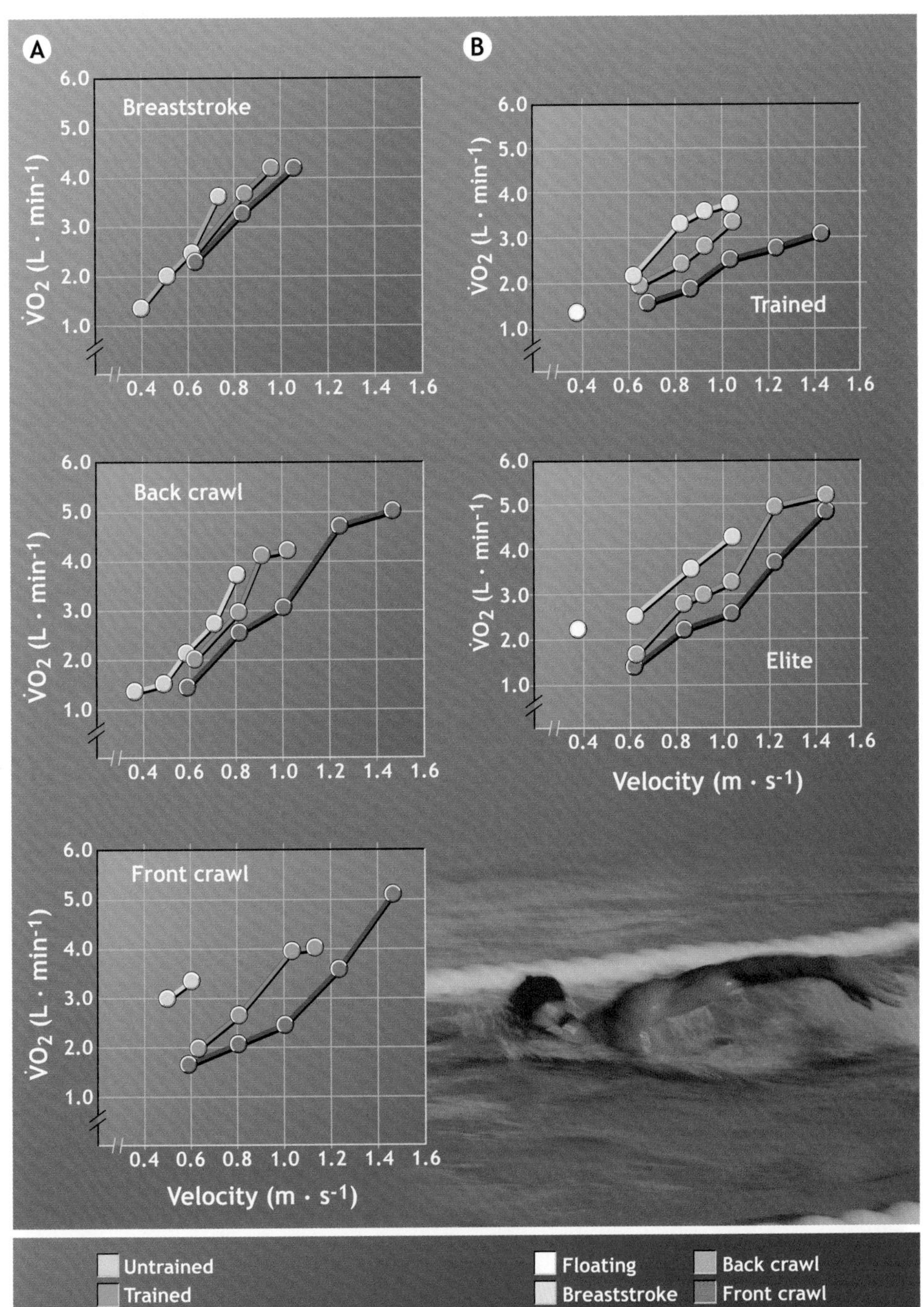

FIGURE 10.13 • **A**. Oxygen consumption related to speed for the breaststroke, front crawl, and back crawl in subjects at three levels of skill ability. **B**. Oxygen consumption for two trained swimmers during three competitive strokes. (From Holmér I. Oxygen uptake during swimming in man. J Appl Physiol 1972;33:502.)

pended for the butterfly and breaststroke is nearly double that for the front and back crawl at the same speeds.[87]

Effects of Water Temperature

Relatively cold water places the swimmer under thermal stress, initiating metabolic and cardiovascular adjustments different from swimming in warmer water.[42] These adaptive responses primarily serve to maintain a stable core temperature by compensating for a considerable heat loss from the body, particularly at water temperatures below 25°C (77°F). Body heat loss occurs most readily in lean swimmers, who benefit less from the insulatory effects of greater subcutaneous fat accumulation.[70]

Figure 10.14 illustrates oxygen consumption during breaststroke swimming at water temperatures of 18°, 26°, and 33°C. Regardless of swimming speed, the highest oxygen consumption occurred in cold water. The extra oxygen cost of swimming in cold water results primarily from energy expended in shivering as the body attempts to regulate core temperature. For individuals of average body composition, optimal water temperature for competitive swimming ranges between 28° and 30°C (82° to 86°F). Within this temperature range, the metabolic heat generated during exercise transfers readily to the water, yet the heat flow gradient from the body does not stimulate increased energy metabolism (shivering) or reduce core temperature from cold stress.

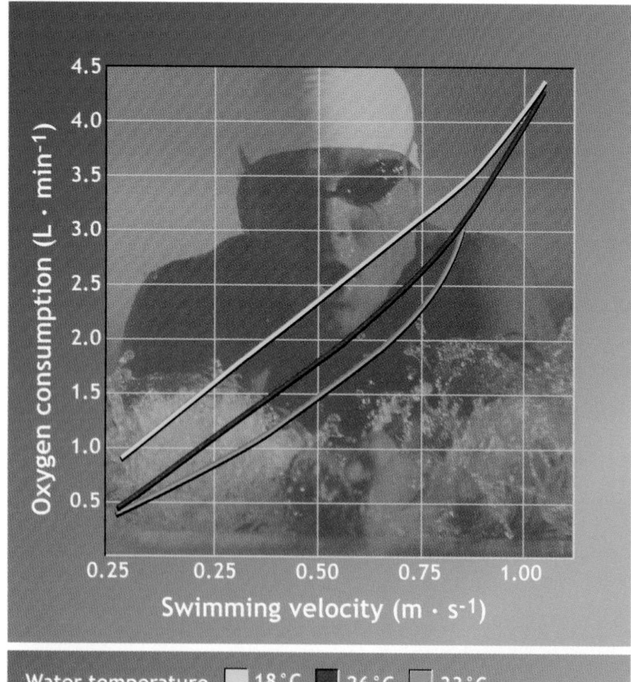

FIGURE 10.14 • Energy expenditure for the breaststroke at three water temperatures related to swimming velocity. (From Nadel ER, et al. Energy exchanges of swimming man. J Appl Physiol 1974;36:465.)

Effects of Buoyancy: Men Versus Women

Women of all ages possess, on average, a significantly higher body fat percentage than men. Because fat floats and muscle and bone sink in water, the average woman gains a hydrodynamic lift and expends less energy to stay afloat than her male counterpart. More than likely, gender differences in percentage body fat and thus body buoyancy partially explain the greater swimming economy for women.[79] For example, women swim a given distance at about a 30% lower total energy cost than men. Expressed another way, women achieve higher swimming velocities than men for the same energy expenditure.

Greater peripheral body fat distribution in women than in men causes their legs and arms to float relatively high in water, making them more horizontal (streamlined), whereas the leaner legs of men tend to swing down and float lower in the water.[15] Lowering the legs to a deeper position increases body drag and reduces swimming economy (see Fig. 10.12). Enhanced flotation and the females' smaller body size, which also reduces drag, contribute to the gender difference in swimming economy.[87,88] The potential hydrodynamic benefits that women possess become noteworthy at longer-distance ocean swims because swimming economy and body insulation contribute significantly to success. The world record for swimming the English Channel by female champion Penny Dean (1978; 7 h:40 min) remained intact until 1994, when it was lowered 23 minutes by male swimmer Chad Hundeby.

Endurance Swimmers

Distance swimming in ocean water poses a severe metabolic and physiologic challenge. A study of nine English Channel swimmers included measurements taken under race conditions in a salt-water pool at swimming speeds ranging from 2.6 to 4.9 km · h^{-1}.[77] During the race, competitors maintained a constant stroke rate and pace until the last few hours when fatigue set in. From detailed observations of one male subject, the average speed of 2.85 km · h^{-1} during a 12-hour swim required an average oxygen consumption of 1.7 L O_2 · min^{-1}, or an equivalent energy expenditure of 8.5 kcal · min^{-1}. Consequently, the gross caloric requirement for the 12-hour swim was about 6120 kcal (8.5 kcal × 60 min × 12 h). The net energy cost of swimming the English Channel, assuming a resting energy expenditure of 1.2 kcal · min^{-1} (0.260 L O_2 · min^{-1}), exceeded 5200 kcal, or approximately twice the number of calories expended running a marathon.

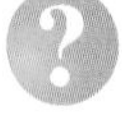

INTEGRATIVE QUESTION

Discuss whether swimming economy should improve to a greater extent with swim training than running economy with a comparable run-training program.

Summary

1. One can express energy expenditure in gross and net terms. Total or gross values include the resting

energy requirement, whereas net energy expenditure represents the energy cost of the activity per se, excluding the resting value.

2. Economy of movement refers to the submaximum oxygen consumption during steady-rate exercise; mechanical efficiency evaluates the relationship between work accomplished and energy expended doing the work.
3. Typical walking, running, and cycling produce mechanical efficiencies between 20 and 25%. For activities with considerable resistance to movement (drag), efficiencies decrease below 20%.
4. A linear relationship exists between walking speed and oxygen consumption at normal walking speeds. Walking surface also affects energy cost, because walking on sand requires about twice the energy as walking on firm surfaces. A proportionately larger energy cost exists for heavier people during such weight-bearing exercises.
5. At speeds exceeding 8 $km \cdot h^{-1}$, running becomes more economical than walking from an energy standpoint.
6. Handheld and ankle weights can increase the energy cost of walking to values usually observed for running. This factor benefits those wanting to use walking alone as a low-impact form of exercise training.
7. The total caloric cost of running a given distance at a steady-rate oxygen consumption remains essentially the same regardless of running speed. Net energy expenditure during horizontal running approximates 1 $kcal \cdot kg^{-1} \cdot km^{-1}$.
8. It generally requires less energy to shorten running stride and increase stride frequency to maintain a constant running speed than to lengthen stride and reduce its frequency. An individual subconsciously "selects" the combination of stride length and frequency that favors optimal economy of movement.
9. Energy expended to overcome air resistance accounts for 3 to 9% of the energy cost of running in calm air. This percentage increases considerably if a runner attempts to maintain pace while running into a brisk headwind.
10. Children generally require significantly more oxygen while running to transport their body mass than adults. A relatively lower running economy accounts for the poor endurance performance of children, compared with that of adults of similar aerobic capacity.
11. Running a given distance or speed on a treadmill requires about the same energy as running on a track under identical environmental conditions.
12. A person expends about four times more energy to swim a given distance than to run the same distance, because the swimmer expends considerable energy maintaining buoyancy and overcoming drag forces that impede forward movement.
13. Elite swimmers expend fewer calories to swim a given stroke at any velocity than less skilled counterparts. The optimal water temperature for most competitive swimming ranges from 28° to 30°C.
14. Significant gender differences exist in body drag, mechanical efficiency, and net oxygen consumption during swimming. Women swim a given distance at about a 30% lower energy cost than men.

References

1. ACSM's guidelines for exercise testing and prescription. 6th ed. Baltimore: Williams & Wilkins, 2000.
2. Ariëns GA, et al. The longitudinal development of running economy in males and females aged between 13 and 27 years: The Amsterdam Growth and Health Study. Eur J Appl Physiol 1998;4.
3. Åstrand PO, Rodahl K. Textbook of work physiology. 3rd ed. New York: McGraw-Hill, 1986.
4. Bassett DR, et al. Aerobic requirements of overground versus treadmill running. Med Sci Sports Exerc 1985;17:477.
5. Bassett DR Jr, et al. Metabolic responses to drafting during front crawl swimming. Med Sci Sports Exerc 1991;23:744.
6. Berry M, et al. Effects of body mass on exercise efficiency and $\dot{V}O_2$ during steady-state cycling. Med Sci Sports Exerc 1993;25:1031.
7. Bhambhani Y, Singh M. Metabolic and cinematographic analysis of walking and running in men and women. Med Sci Sports Exerc 1985;17:131.
8. Bilodeau B, et al. Effect of drafting on heart rate in cross-country skiing. Med Sci Sports Exerc 1994;26:637.
9. Bøje O. Energy production, pulmonary ventilation, and length of steps in well-trained runners working on a treadmill. Acta Physiol Scand 1944;7:362.
10. Bonen A, et al. Maximal oxygen uptake during free, tethered, and flume swimming. J Appl Physiol 1980;48:232.
11. Brisswalter J, et al. Effect of three hours race walk on energy cost, cardiorespiratory parameters and stride duration in elite race walkers. Int J Sports Med 1996;17:182.
12. Brisswalter J, et al. Variability in energy cost and walking gait during race walking in competitive race walkers. Med Sci Sports Exerc 1998;30:1451.
13. Butts NK, et al. Energy costs of walking on a dual-action treadmill in men and women. Med Sci Sports Exerc 1995;27:121.
14. Caird SJ, et al. Biofeedback and relaxation techniques improve running economy in sub-elite long distance runners. Med Sci Sports Exerc 1999;31:717.
15. Campaigne BN. Body fat distribution in females: metabolic consequences and implications for weight loss. Med Sci Sports Exerc 1990;22:291.
16. Cavagna GA, Franzetti P. Mechanics of competition walking. J Physiol (London) 1981;315:243.
17. Cavanagh PR, Kram R. Mechanical and muscular factors affecting the efficiency of human movement. Med Sci Sports Exerc 1985;17:326.
18. Cavanagh PR, Kram R. Stride length in distance running: velocity, body dimensions, and added mass effects. Med Sci Sports Exerc 1989;21:467.
19. Chatard J-C, et al. Performance and drag during drafting swimming in highly trained triathletes. Med Sci Sports Exerc 1998;30:1276.
20. Claremont AP, Hall SJ. Effects of extremity loading on energy expenditure and running mechanics. Med Sci Sports Exerc 1988;20:161.
21. Conley DL, Krahenbuhl GS. Running economy and distance running performance of highly trained athletes. Med Sci Sports Exerc 1980;12:357.
22. Conley DL, et al. Training for aerobic capacity and running economy. Phys Sportsmed 1981;9:107.
23. Coyle EF, et al. Physiological and biomechanical factors associated with elite endurance cycling performance. Med Sci Sports Exerc 1991;23:93.
24. Coyle EF, et al. Cycling efficiency is related to the percentage of type I muscle fibers. Med Sci Sports Exerc 1992;24:782.

25. Cunningham DA. Development of cardiorespiratory function in circumpubertal boys: a longitudinal study. J Appl Physiol 1984;56:302.
26. Cureton KJ, et al. Metabolic determinants of the age-related improvement in one-mile run/walk performance in youth. Med Sci Sports Exerc 1997;29:259.
27. Daniels J, et al. Differences and changes in $\dot{V}O_2$ among runners 10 to 18 years of age. Med Sci Sports 1978;10:200.
28. Davies CTM, et al. The physiological responses to running downhill. Eur J Appl Physiol 1974;32:187.
29. Davies MJ, et al. Running economy: comparison of body mass adjustment methods. Res Q Exerc Sport 1997;68:177.
30. Dennis SC, Noakes TD. Advantages of a smaller body mass in humans when distance-running in warm, humid conditions. Eur J Appl Physiol 1999;79:280.
31. Evans BW, et al. Metabolic and hemodynamic responses to walking with hand weights in older individuals. Med Sci Sports Exerc 1994;26:1047.
32. Falls HB, Humphrey LD. Energy cost of running and walking in young women. Med Sci Sports 1976;8:9.
33. Fellingham GW, et al. Calorie cost of walking and running. Med Sci Sports 1978;10:132.
34. Fortney VL. The kinematics of the running pattern of two, four, and six year old children. Res Q Exerc Sport 1983;54:126.
35. Franch J, et al. Improved running economy following intensified training correlates with reduced ventilatory demands. Med Sci Sports Exerc 1998;30:1250.
36. Frederick EC, et al. Lower oxygen demands of running in soft-soled shoes. Res Q Exerc Sport 1986;57:174.
37. Hagberg JM, Coyle EF. Physiological determinants of endurance performance as studied in competitive race walkers. Med Sci Sports Exerc 1983;15:287.
38. Hamill J, et al. Effects of shoe type on cardiorespiratory responses and rear foot motion during treadmill running. Med Sci Sports Exerc 1988;20:515.
39. Hausswirth C, et al. Effects of cycling alone or in a sheltered position on subsequent running performance during a triathlon. Med Sci Sports Exerc 1999;31:599.
40. Heinert LD, et al. Effect of stride length variation on oxygen uptake during level and positive grade treadmill running. Res Q Exerc Sport 1988;59:127.
41. Hill AV. The air resistance to a runner. Proc R Soc Lond (Biol) 1927;102:380.
42. Holmér I. Physiology of swimming man. In Exercise and sport sciences reviews, vol 7, Hutton RS, Miller DI, eds. Philadelphia: Franklin Institute Press, 1980.
43. Jones BH, et al. Energy cost of walking and running in boots and shoes. Ergonomics 1984;27:895.
44. Joyner MJ. Physiological limiting factors and distance running: influence of gender and age on record performance. Exerc Sport Sci Rev 1993;21:103.
45. Krahenbuhl GS, Pangrasi R. Characteristics associated with running performance in young boys. Med Sci Sports Exerc 1983;5:488.
46. Kram, R. Muscular force or work: what determines the metabolic energy cost of running? Exer Sport Sci Rev 2000;28:138.
47. Kyle CR. Ergogenics of bicycling. In: Lamb DR, Williams MH, eds. Perspectives in exercise science and sports medicine, vol 4: ergogenics: enhancement of performance in exercise and sport. Madison, WI: Brown and Benchmark, 1991:.
48. Lake MJ, Cavanagh PR. Six weeks of training does not change running mechanics or improve running economy. Med Sci Sports Exerc 1996;28:860.
49. Mahar AT, et al. Impact shock and attenuation during in-line skating. Med Sci Sports Exerc 1997;29:1069.
50. Magel JR, et al. The specificity of swim training on maximum oxygen uptake. J Appl Physiol 1974;36:753.
51. Margaria R, et al. Energy cost of running. J Appl Physiol 1963;18:367.
52. Maron M, et al. Oxygen uptake measurements during competitive marathon running. J Appl Physiol 1976;40:836.
53. Martin PE, Morgan DW. Biomechanical considerations for economical walking and running. Med Sci Sports Exerc 1992;24:467.
54. Mayers N, Gutin B. Physiological characteristics of elite prepubertal cross-country runners. Med Sci Sports 1979;11:172.
55. McArdle WD, et al. Metabolic and cardiorespiratory response during free swimming and treadmill walking. J Appl Physiol 1971;30:733.
56. McArdle WD, et al. Comparison of continuous and discontinuous treadmill and bicycle tests for $\dot{V}O_{2max}$. Med Sci Sports 1973;5:156.
57. McCole SD, et al. Energy expenditure during bicycling. J Appl Physiol 1990;68:748.
58. McMiken DF, Daniels JT. Aerobic requirements and maximum aerobic power in treadmill and track running. Med Sci Sports 1976;8:14.
59. Melanson EL, et al. Changes in $\dot{V}O_{2max}$ and maximal treadmill time after nine weeks of running or in-line skate training. Med Sci Sports Exerc 1996;28:1422.
60. Menier DR, Pugh LGCE. The relation of oxygen intake and velocity of walking and running in competition walkers. J Physiol (London) 1968;197:717.
61. Miller JE, Stamford BA. Intensity and energy cost of weighted walking vs. running for men and women. J Appl Physiol 1987;62:1947.
62. Minetti AE, et al. Mechanical determinants of the minimum energy cost of gradient running in humans. J Exp Biol 1994;195:211.
63. Minetti AE, et al. Effects of stride frequency on mechanical power and energy expenditure of walking. Med Sci Sports Exerc 1995;27:1195.
64. Morgan DW, Craib M. Physiological aspects of running economy. Med Sci Sports Exerc 1992;24:456.
65. Morgan DW, et al. Ten kilometer performance and predicted velocity at $\dot{V}O_{2max}$ among well-trained male runners. Med Sci Sports Exerc 1989;21:78.
66. Morgan DW, et al. Variability in running economy and mechanics among trained runners. Med Sci Sports Exerc 1991;23:378.
67. Morgan DW, et al. Daily variability in running economy among well-trained male and female distance runners. Res Q Exerc Sport 1994;65:72.
68. Morgan DW, et al. Effect of step length optimization on the aerobic demand of running. J Appl Physiol 1994;77:245.
69. Morgan DW, et al. Variation in the aerobic demand of running among trained and untrained subjects. Med Sci Sports Exerc 1995;27:404.
70. Nadel E, et al. Energy exchanges of swimming man. J Appl Physiol 1974;36:465.
71. Nelson RC, Gregor RJ. Biomechanics of distance running: a longitudinal study. Res Q 1976;47:471.
72. Nigg BM, Anton A. Energy aspects for elastic and viscous shoe soles and playing surfaces. Med Sci Sports Exerc 1995;27:92.
73. Pérez-Landaluce J, et al. Importance of wash riding in kayaking training and competition. Med Sci Sports Exerc 1998;30:1721.
74. Poole DC, et al. Pulmonary and leg $\dot{V}O_2$ during submaximal exercise: applications for muscular efficiency. J Appl Physiol 1992;72:805.
75. Porcari J. Pump up your walk. ACSM Health Fitness J 1999;3(1):25.
76. Pugh LGCE. Oxygen uptake in track and treadmill running with observations on the effect of air resistance. J Physiol (London) 1970;207:823.
77. Pugh LGCE, Edholm OG. The physiology of channel swimmers. Lancet 1955;2:761.
78. Ralston HJ. Comparison of energy expenditure during treadmill walking and floor walking. J Appl Physiol 1960;15:1156.
79. Rennie DW, et al. Energetics of swimming in man. In: Lewille L, Clarys J, eds. Swimming II. Baltimore: University Park Press, 1975.
80. Rogers C, et al. Energy expenditure during submaximal walking with Exerstriders. Med Sci Sports Exerc 1995;28:607.
81. Rowland TW, et al. Physiologic responses to treadmill running in adult and prepubertal males. Int J Sports Med 1987;8:292.
82. Rundell KW. Effects of drafting during short-track speed skating. Med Sci Sports Exerc 1996;29:765.
83. Semih SY, Feluni T. A comparison of the endurance training responses to road and sand running in high school and college students. J Strength Cond Res 1998;12:79.
84. Sharp RL, Costill DL. Influence of body hair removal on physiological responses during breaststroke swimming. Med Sci Sports Exerc 1989;21:576.
85. Smolander J, et al. Cardiorespiratory strain during walking in snow with boots of differing weights. Ergonomics 1989;32:319.
86. Svedenhag J, Sjodin B. Physiological characteristics of elite male runners in and off season. Can J Appl Sport Sci 1985;10:127.
87. Toussaint HM, Hollander AP. Energetics of competitive swimming: implications for training programs. Sports Med 1994;18:384.
88. Toussaint HM, et al. Active drag related to velocity in male and female swimmers. J Biomechanics 1988;21:435.
89. Toussaint HM, et al. Effect of triathlon wet suit on drag during swimming. Med Sci Sports Exerc 1989;21:325.

90. Toussaint HM, et al. The mechanical efficiency of front crawl swimming. Med Sci Sports Exerc 1990;22:402.
91. Trappe TA, et al. Thermal responses to swimming in three water temperatures: influence of a wet suit. Med Sci Sports Exerc 1995;27:1014.
92. Walker JL, et al. The energy cost of horizontal walking and running in adolescents. Med Sci Sports Exerc 1999;31:311.
93. Wanta DM, et al. Metabolic response to graded downhill walking. Med Sci Sports Exerc 1993;25:159.
94. Williams KR, Cavanagh PR. Relationship between distance running mechanics, running economy, and performance. J Appl Physiol 1987;63:1236.
95. Zedaker JM, et al. Physiological responses to walking and running with a Powerbelt. Med Sci Sports Exerc 1998;30(suppl):S168.

CHAPTER 11

Individual Differences and Measurement of Energy Capacities

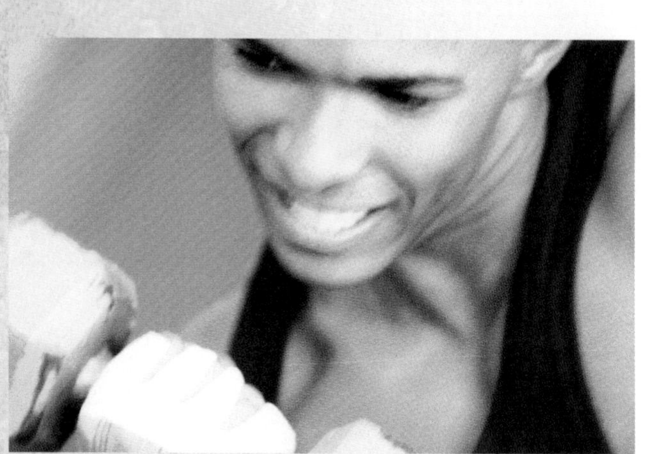

Chapter Objectives

- Explain specificity and generality as applied to exercise performance and physiologic function
- Outline the anaerobic-to-aerobic exercise energy transfer continuum related to exercise intensity and duration
- Review procedures for administering two practical "field tests" to evaluate power output capacity of the high-energy intramuscular phosphates (immediate energy system)
- Describe a commonly used test procedure to evaluate power output capacity of the glycolytic energy pathway (short-term energy system)
- Explain the influence of motivation, buffering, and exercise training on capacity to generate energy via the glycolytic pathway
- Define maximal oxygen consumption ($\dot{V}O_{2max}$); discuss the physiologic significance of this measure of aerobic fitness
- Differentiate between maximal oxygen consumption and peak oxygen consumption
- Define the term graded exercise test, and list criteria that indicate attainment of a "true" $\dot{V}O_{2max}$ during graded exercise testing
- Outline three common treadmill protocols for assessing $\dot{V}O_{2max}$
- Indicate the influence of each of the following on $\dot{V}O_{2max}$: (1) mode of exercise, (2) heredity, (3) state of training, (4) gender, (5) body composition, and (6) age
- Describe procedures for administering a submaximal walking field test to predict $\dot{V}O_{2max}$
- List three assumptions when using submaximal exercise heart rate to predict $\dot{V}O_{2max}$
- Outline procedures for administering a step test for college-age men and women

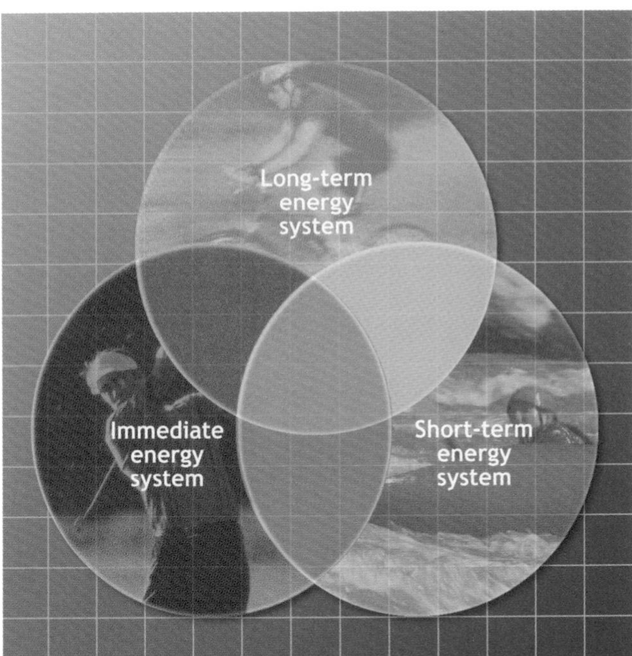

FIGURE 11.1 • Specificity–generality of the three systems for energy transfer. When considering only two systems, their overlap represents generality and the remainder specificity.

We derive useful energy from anaerobic and aerobic energy metabolic pathways. However, the capacity for each form of energy transfer varies considerably among individuals. This between-person variability underlies the concept of **individual differences** in metabolic capacity for exercise. Highly specific physiologic and energy transfer capacities do not simply represent general fitness components; rather, they depend on the specific mode of exercise for training and evaluation.[62,63,70,82] **Specificity** of metabolic capacity dictates that a high $\dot{V}O_{2max}$ in running does not necessarily ensure a similar metabolic power level using different muscle groups as in swimming and rowing. However, some individuals with high aerobic power in one activity also possess above average aerobic power in other activities. This illustrates the **generality** principle of metabolic function. Often, considerable specificity emerges when comparing the body's distinct energy transfer systems. The nonoverlapped areas in Figure 11.1 represent specificity of metabolic function, while the three overlapped portions represent generality. For each energy system, specificity exceeds generality. For example, most people do not possess high energy-generating capacity for activities as different as running (lower-body exercise) or swimming (upper-body exercise) or a particular sport's sprint, middle-distance, and long-distance competitions. Hence, it is unusual to identify an athlete who excels in sporting events like high jumping, 200-m swimming, and the 3000-m steeplechase.

Because of exercise specificity, training to achieve a high $\dot{V}O_{2max}$ contributes little to one's capacity to generate energy anaerobically, and vice versa. A high degree of specificity also exists for the effects of exercise training on neuromuscular patterning and demands. *Terms such as "speed," "power," and "endurance" must be applied precisely within the context of the specific movement patterns and specific metabolic and physiologic requirements of the activity.*

This chapter evaluates the capacity of the three energy-transfer systems discussed in Chapters 6 and 7, with emphasis on individual differences, specificity, and measurement.

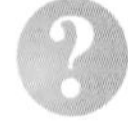

INTEGRATIVE QUESTION

Respond to a potential triathlete who asks: "Why is it important to train in each of the sport's three events? Since they all require a high level of aerobic fitness, why can't I train aerobically for just one of the events?"

OVERVIEW OF ENERGY-TRANSFER CAPACITY DURING EXERCISE

The immediate and short-term energy systems largely power all-out exercise for up to 2 minutes. Both systems operate anaerobically because their transfer of chemical energy does not require molecular oxygen. Generally, a greater reliance on anaerobic energy exists for fast, short-duration movements, or during increasing resistance to movement at a given speed.[56] Figure 11.2 illustrates the relative activation of the anaerobic and aerobic energy-transfer systems for different durations of all-out exercise. When movement begins at either fast or slow speed, the intramuscular high-energy phosphates adenosine triphosphate (ATP) and phosphocreatine (PCr) provide immediate, nonaerobic energy to power muscle actions. Following the first few seconds of movement, glycolytic pathways

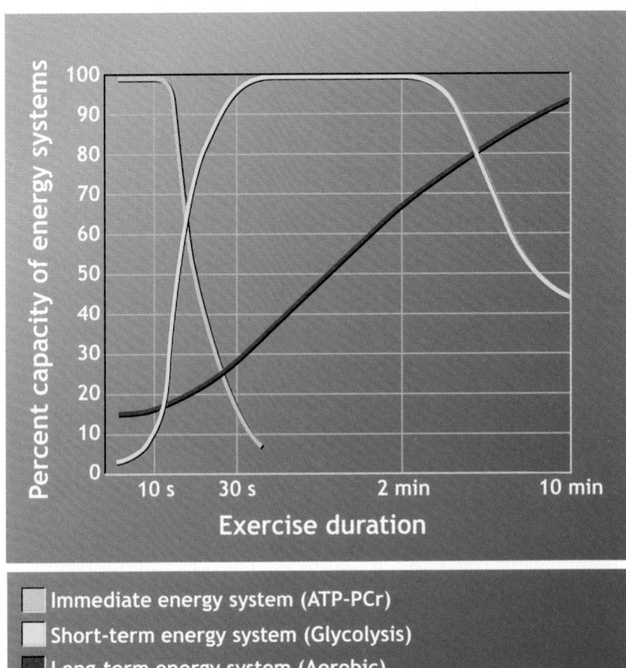

FIGURE 11.2 • The three systems of energy transfer and their percentage contributions to total energy output during all-out exercise of different durations.

generate an increasingly greater percentage of energy for ATP resynthesis. Continued exercise places progressively greater demands on the long-term system of aerobic metabolism. All physical activities and sports lend themselves to classification on an anaerobic-to-aerobic continuum. Some activities rely predominantly on a single system of energy transfer, whereas most require activation of more than one energy system, depending on exercise intensity and duration. When performing at a higher intensity but shorter duration of effort, the demand placed on anaerobic energy transfer increases markedly.

ANAEROBIC ENERGY TRANSFER: THE IMMEDIATE AND SHORT-TERM ENERGY SYSTEMS

Evaluation of the Immediate Energy System: Performance Tests

Football, weight lifting, and other brief, maximal-effort physical activities that require an almost instantaneous energy release rely almost exclusively on energy derived from the intramuscular high-energy phosphates.[45,93] Performance tests that maximally activate the ATP–PCr energy system serve as practical field tests to evaluate the capacity for "immediate" energy transfer. Two assumptions underlie the use of performance test scores to infer the power-generating capacity of the high-energy phosphates: (1) all ATP at maximal power output regenerates via ATP–PCr hydrolysis and (2) enough ATP and PCr exist to support maximal performance for about 6 seconds. The term *power test* generally describes these measures of brief, maximal exercise capacity. Power in this context refers to the time-rate of accomplishing work, computed as follows:

$$P = (FD) \div T$$

where F equals force generated, D equals distance the force moves, and T represents exercise duration. Power is expressed in watts—1 watt equals 0.73756 ft-lb $\cdot$ s^{-1}, 0.01433 kcal $\cdot$ min^{-1}, 1.341×10^{-3} hp (or 0.0013 hp), or 6.12 kg-m $\cdot$ min^{-1}.

Stair-Sprinting Power Tests

Researchers have evaluated high-energy phosphate power output by the time required to run up a staircase as fast as possible, taking three steps at a time (Fig. 11.3). External work accomplished consists of the total vertical distance traversed up the stairs; this distance for six stairs usually equals 1.05 m. For example, the power output of a 65-kg woman who traverses six steps in 0.52 second computes as follows:

$$\begin{aligned} F &= 65 \text{ kg} \\ D &= 1.05 \text{ m} \\ T &= 0.52 \text{ s} \\ \text{Power} &= (65 \text{ kg} \times 1.05 \text{ m}) \div 0.52 \text{ s} \\ &= 131.3 \text{ kg-m} \cdot \text{s}^{-1} \text{ (1287 watts)} \end{aligned}$$

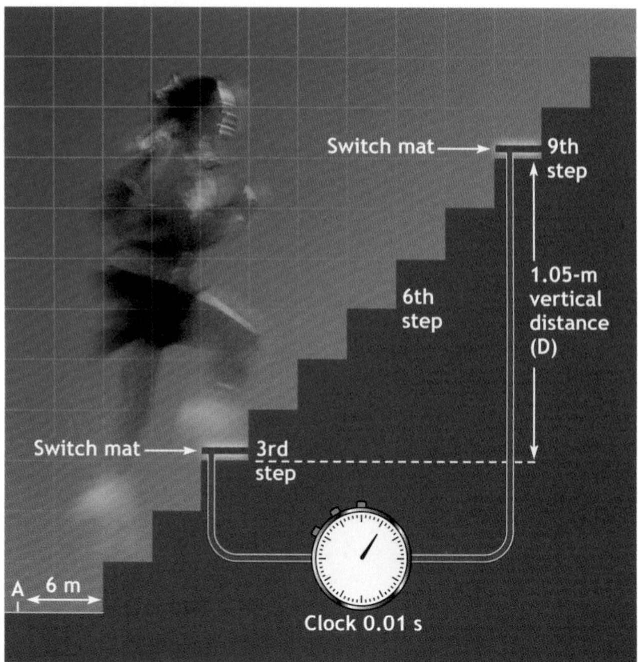

FIGURE 11.3 • Stair-sprinting power test. The subject begins at point *A* and runs as fast as possible up a flight of stairs, taking three steps at a time. Electric switch mats placed on the steps record the time needed to cover the distance between stairs 3 and 9 to the nearest 0.01 second. Power output equals the product of the subject's mass (*F*) and vertical distance covered (*D*), divided by the time (*T*).

Because the person's body mass significantly influences the power score in the stair-sprinting test, a heavier person who achieves the same speed as a lighter counterpart necessarily achieves a higher power score. This implies that the heavier person possesses a more highly developed immediate energy system. Because no direct evidence justifies this conclusion, one must use care interpreting differences in stair-sprinting power scores and inferring individual differences in ATP–PCr energy-transfer capacity. *The test should be used with individuals of similar body mass or the same individuals before and after specific training designed to develop leg power output from the immediate energy system (assuming no change in body mass).*

INTEGRATIVE QUESTION

Within the framework of training specificity, describe how you would test the power output capacity of the immediate energy system of (1) volleyball players, (2) swimmers, and (3) soccer players.

Jumping-Power Tests

Jump tests such as the popular Sargent jump-and-reach test or a standing broad jump often appear in physical fitness test batteries. The Sargent jump score reflects the difference between a person's standing reach and the maximum vertical jump-and-touch height.[94,103] The broad jump score consists of the horizontal distance covered in a leap from a semicrouched

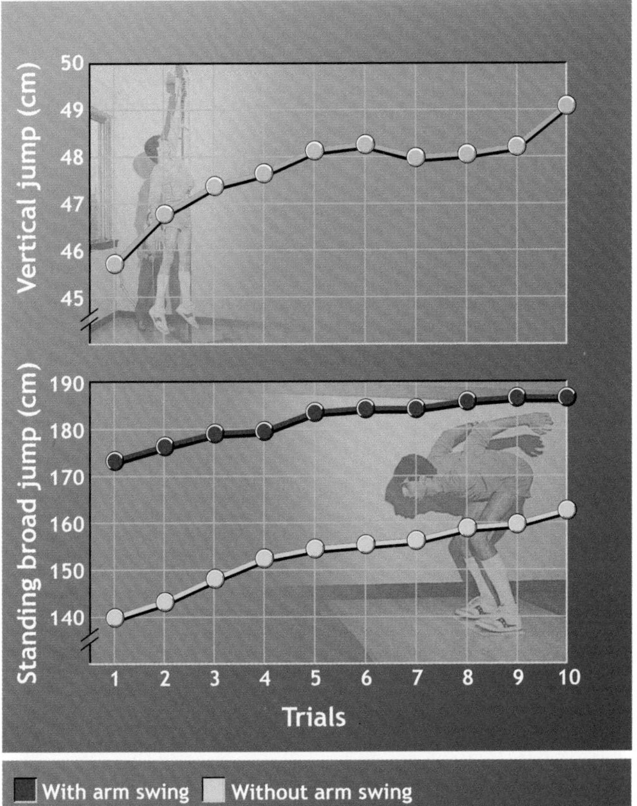

FIGURE 11.4 • *Top.* Ten consecutive vertical jump trials (no arm swing) of male collegiate baseball players and (*bottom*) long-jump performances (with and without arm swing) of female collegiate soccer players. Prior to testing, subjects stretched for 3 minutes and performed light calisthenics. Subjects were exhorted to make a maximal effort in all jumps. A 7.5% improvement in vertical jump occurred between trials 1 and 10; improvement for the standing broad jump averaged 7.0% from trial 1 to trial 10 with arm swing and 15.5% without arm swing. (Vertical jump data courtesy of Jeff Smith; standing long-jump data courtesy of Jesse Sutella, Human Performance Laboratory, Exercise Science Department, University of Massachusetts, Amherst, 1996.)

position. Although both tests purport to measure leg power, they probably fail to achieve this goal. For example, jump tests generate power to propel the body from the crouched position *only* while the feet maintain contact with the surface. *This extremely brief period of muscle activation probably does not adequately evaluate a person's ATP and PCr energy transfer capacity.* Also, no data exist to show a relationship (correlation) between jump-test scores and actual ATP–PCr levels or depletion patterns in the primary muscles activated during the jump.

When using jump tests to assess the immediate generation of anaerobic power, attention should focus on the methodology to obtain such information. Figure 11.4 displays data for subjects who performed both consecutive multiple vertical jumps and standing broad jumps. Vertical jump trials consisted of 10 jumps with a 1-minute rest between jumps. Subjects stood with their hands on hips during the crouch before the jump to eliminate arm swing that augments vertical displacement. A significant underestimation of peak power occurs using the scores from only the first 2 or 3 jumps. Whether the progressive increase in power with repeated jumps results from a warming-up effect or improved neuromuscular activation has not been established. From a testing perspective, however, the important consideration requires administering sufficient trials to establish a person's true power score. This is best achieved by using an average of 2 or 3 jumps after the performance curve plateaus. However, a plateau achieved after 6 or 7 jumps does not guarantee continued stabilization in performance. Additional subject motivation and arousal can boost performance to a higher level.

Other Power Performance Tests

Figure 11.2 suggests that any all-out exercise of 6 to 8 seconds probably reflects a person's capacity for immediate power from the high-energy phosphates in the specific muscles activated. In addition to stair-sprinting and jump tests, other tests include sprint running or cycling, brief shuttle runs, and localized movements produced by arm cranking.

Interrelationships Among Power Performance Tests

If the various power tests measure the same "general" metabolic capacity, then individuals who perform best on one test should rank correspondingly high on a second or third different test. Unfortunately, this does not usually occur to any great extent. While some individuals who score well on one power performance test tend to score well on another test, a poor relationship generally exists.[103] Table 11.1 shows the interrelationship (expressed statistically as a correlation coefficient) between several tests intended to measure immediate power output. The relationship ranges from poor to good, depending on the nature of the test, indicating some commonality among tests for measuring metabolic capacity. The fairly strong relationship between stair-sprinting power test scores and 40-yard dash scores ($r = -0.88$) indicates that one can obtain almost the same information on short-term power performance through sprint running on a track as in the more elaborate procedures required in the stair sprint.

Several factors explain the relatively low relationships among the other test scores. *First, human exercise perfor-*

TABLE 11.1 ➤ **CORRELATIONS AMONG TESTS PURPORTED TO MEASURE IMMEDIATE ANAEROBIC POWER OUTPUT FROM THE INTRAMUSCULAR HIGH-ENERGY PHOSPHATES ATP AND PCr**

VARIABLE	JUMP & REACH	STAIR-SPRINTING
40-yard dash	−0.48[a]	−0.88[a]
Jump and reach	—	−0.31[a]

[a]Negative correlations mean faster times (lower scores) associate with higher jumps or greater power outputs.
From the Applied Physiology Laboratory, University of Michigan (n = 31 males).

mance remains highly task specific. From a metabolic and performance perspective, this means that the best sprint runner does not necessarily rank as the best sprint swimmer, sprint cyclist, "stair sprinter," or "arm cranker." While identical metabolic reactions generate energy to power each performance, these reactions occur within the specific muscles activated by the exercise. Each specific test also requires different neuromuscular and skill components that introduce variability and specificity into test scores.

Besides evaluating changes in an athlete's performance from specific training, power tests offer an excellent means for self-testing and motivation. The tests can serve as exercise for training the immediate energy system. For example, football coaches often use the 40-yard dash both for power training and as a criterion to evaluate horizontal movement speed. Forty-yard dash test scores *may* provide relevant information concerning "speed" in football, even though no data exist to quantify how a 40-yard sprint in a straight line relates to all of the complex skills involved in game performance, let alone some general factor of overall football ability. A run test of shorter distance (up to 20 yd) and/or with multiple changes in direction and pacing may provide a more reasonable, task-specific performance criterion to evaluate football personnel.

Evaluation of the Immediate Energy System: Physiologic Tests

In addition to exercise performance, several physiologic and biochemical measures can evaluate the energy-generating capacity of the immediate energy system. These include estimating the (1) size of the intramuscular ATP–PCr pool, (2) depletion rates of ATP and PCr in all-out, short-duration exercise, (3) oxygen deficit calculated from the initial phase of the exercise oxygen consumption curve, and (4) alactic portion (fast component) of recovery oxygen consumption.[50,122] Of these measures, ATP and PCr depletion rate provides the most direct estimate and correlates highly with physical performance assessments of the immediate energy system. For example, one experiment determined muscle PCr depletion at different intervals of a 100-m sprint using the muscle biopsy technique.[40] Compared with resting values (22 mmol · kg wet weight^{-1}), PCr decreased by 60% during the first 40 m (<6 s) and only another 20% for the remainder of the sprint. Because of time delays and other technical difficulties, it remains nearly impossible with current technology to readily obtain precise biochemical data during all-out exercise of brief duration. Consequently, we still rely on the "face validity" of the various specific performance measures as satisfactory markers of one's capacity for ATP–PCr energy transfer.

Evaluation of the Short-Term Energy System

Figure 11.2 showed that when all-out exercise continues for longer than a few seconds, the short-term energy system (anaerobic glycolysis) generates increasingly more of the energy for ATP resynthesis. This does not mean that aerobic metabolism is unimportant at this stage of exercises or that oxygen-consuming reactions have not "switched on." To the contrary, the contribution of aerobic energy transfer increases early in the exercise (Fig. 11.2).[98] During short duration, maximal exercise, however, the energy requirement significantly exceeds the energy generated by hydrogen oxidation in the respiratory chain. Consequently, anaerobic glycolysis predominates, and large quantities of lactate accumulate in active muscle, and ultimately in blood. *The level of blood lactate provides the most common indicator of activation of the short-term energy system.*

Unlike tests for maximal oxygen consumption, no specific criteria exist to indicate that a person has attained maximal anaerobic effort. More than likely, self-motivation and the testing environment greatly influence performance on such tests.[118] Despite difficulty in validly assessing a person's true anaerobic power capacity, performance test scores show good reproducibility from day to day, particularly under standardized conditions.[5]

Anaerobic Power Performance and Capacity Tests

Performances that substantially activate the short-term energy system require maximal exercise for up to 3 minutes.[5,45] All-out runs and stationary cycling have usually assessed anaerobic capacity, as have shuttle runs and repetitive weight lifting of a certain percentage of maximum capacity. The influence of age, gender, skill, motivation, and body size creates difficulty selecting a suitable criterion test or developing appropriate norms to evaluate anaerobic power capacity. Above-normal intramuscular glycogen levels do not affect exercise test performance or the final level of blood lactate accumulation.[106] Also, because of exercise specificity, one cannot use a test requiring maximum activation of the leg musculature to assess short-term anaerobic capacity for an upper-body activity like rowing or swimming. *The performance test must closely resemble the activity that requires energy capacity assessment.* In most cases, the activity itself best serves as the performance test.

In 1973, the **Katch test** of all-out stationary cycling of short duration estimated the power and capacity of the anaerobic energy systems.[50] Subsequent extension of this work resulted in a stationary bicycle test with frictional resistance against the flywheel preset at a high load (6 kg for men; 5 kg for women).[52] Subjects turned as many revolutions as possible in 40 seconds with pedal rate continuously recorded with a microswitch assembly. Peak cycling power represented the subject's anaerobic power, while total work accomplished indicated anaerobic capacity. A later modification, the **Wingate test**, involves 30 seconds of supermaximal exercise on either an arm-crank or leg-cycle ergometer.[5,123] Body mass determines resistance to pedaling (originally set to 0.075 kg per kg body mass, but now can exceed 0.12 kg in athletes), applied within 3 seconds after overcoming the initial inertia and unloaded frictional resistance of the ergometer. **Peak power** represents the highest mechanical power generated during any 3- to 5-second period of the test; **relative power** represents peak power di-

TABLE 11.2 ➤ **PERCENTILE NORMS FOR AVERAGE POWER AND PEAK POWER FOR PHYSICALLY ACTIVE YOUNG ADULT MEN AND WOMEN**

	Average Power Watts (W)		Peak Power Watts (W)	
% Rank	Male	Female	Male	Female
90	662	470	822	560
80	618	419	777	527
70	600	410	757	505
60	577	391	721	480
50	565	381	689	449
40	548	367	671	432
30	530	353	656	399
20	496	336	618	376
10	471	306	570	353
	W · kg BM^{-1a}		W · kg BM^{-1}	
	Male	Female	Male	Female
90	8.24	7.31	10.89	9.02
80	8.01	6.95	10.39	8.83
70	7.91	6.77	10.20	8.53
60	7.59	6.59	9.80	8.14
50	7.44	6.39	9.22	7.65
40	7.14	6.15	8.92	6.96
30	7.00	6.03	8.53	6.86
20	6.59	5.71	8.24	6.57
10	5.98	5.25	7.06	5.98

From Maud PJ, Schultz BB. Norms for the Wingate anaerobic test with comparisons in another similar test. Res Q Exerc Sport 1989;60:144.
[a]W · kg BM^{-1}, watts per kilogram of body mass.

vided by body mass. **Anaerobic fatigue** is the percentage decline in power output during the test, and **anaerobic capacity** is the total work accomplished over the 30 seconds. **Rate of fatigue** represents the decline in power in relation to the peak value. The Katch and Wingate tests assume that peak power output represents the energy-generating capacity of the high-energy phosphates, while average power reflects glycolytic capacity.[43] "In a Practical Sense" provides the step-by-step procedure for determining anaerobic power and capacity on the Wingate cycle ergometer test. Table 11.2 presents normative standards for average and peak power outputs in young, physically active men and women during the Wingate cycling test. Performance scores, blood lactate concentrations, and peak heart rates show high test-retest reproducibility and moderate validity compared with other anaerobic capacity criteria.[80,114] Elite volleyball and ice hockey players have achieved some of the highest Wingate power scores.

Figure 11.5A and B present the relative contributions of each energy system during three cycle ergometer anaerobic power tests of different durations. The lower figure (B) gives estimated kilojoules of total energy; the upper figure presents the percentage contribution of each system to total work accomplished. Note the progressive change in the percentage contribution of each energy system as a function of increasing duration of effort.

LOWER IN CHILDREN. The reason for the relatively poor performance of children on the Wingate test compared with that of adolescents and young adults, remains unclear. Possible explanations include children's relatively lower intramuscular glycogen concentrations and their slower rate of glycogen use during exercise.[24,43]

GENDER DIFFERENCES. As with most measures of physiologic capacity and exercise performance, large gender differences exist in anaerobic power capacity when comparing test scores on an absolute basis.[25,91] These observations seem readily explained by the clear gender differences in factors that affect absolute anaerobic power-output capacity—body

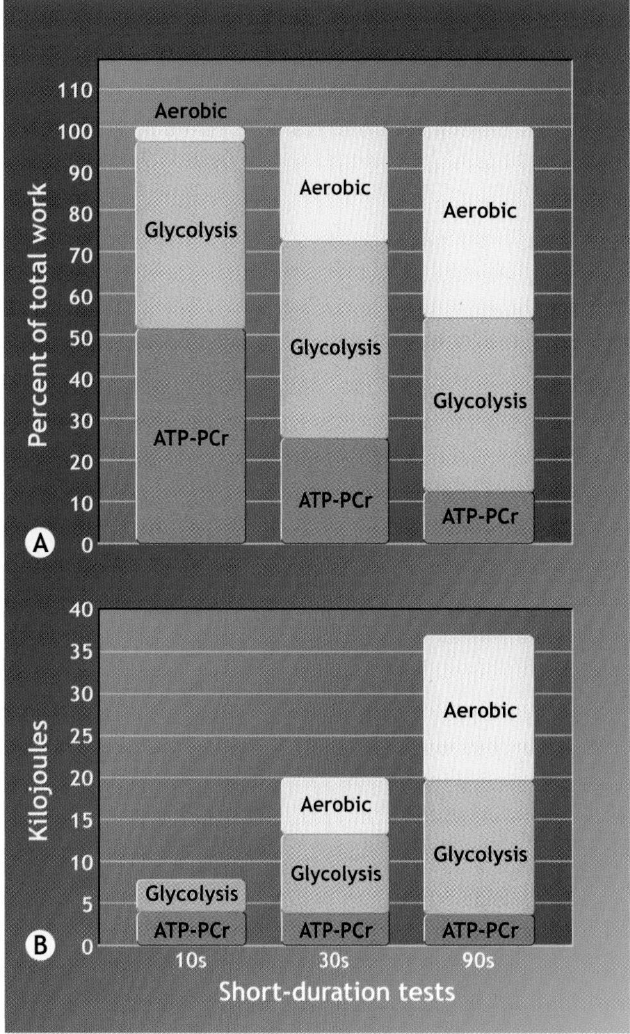

FIGURE 11.5 • Relative contribution of each of the energy systems to total work accomplished in three short-duration exercise tests. **A**. Percentage of total work output. **B**. Total kilojoules of energy. Test results based on Katch test protocol (see page 226). (Data from Applied Physiology Laboratory, University of Michigan, Ann Arbor).

IN A PRACTICAL SENSE

➤➤ DETERMINING ANAEROBIC POWER AND CAPACITY: THE WINGATE CYCLE ERGOMETER TEST

Many sport and daily activities occur with rapid rest-to-exercise transitions or at high intensities using anaerobic metabolic processes. The Wingate cycle ergometer test represents the most popular test to assess anaerobic capacity. Developed at the Wingate Institute in Israel in the 1970s, test scores can reliably determine peak anaerobic power, anaerobic fatigue, and total anaerobic capacity.

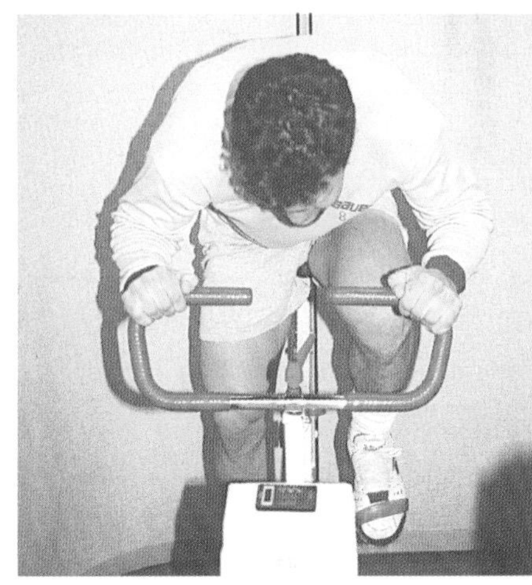

The Test

A mechanically braked bicycle ergometer serves as the testing device. After warmup (3 to 5 min), the subject begins pedaling as fast as possible without resistance. Within 3 s, a fixed resistance is applied to the flywheel; the subject continues to pedal "all out" for 30 s. An electrical or mechanical counter continuously records flywheel revolutions in 5-s intervals.

Resistance

Flywheel resistance equals 0.075 kg per kg body mass. For a 70-kg person, the flywheel resistance would equal 5.25 kg (70 kg × 0.075). Resistance often increases to 0.10 kg per kg body mass or higher (up to 0.12 kg) when testing power- and sprint-type athletes.

Test Scores

1. **Peak power output (PP)**—The highest power output, observed during the first 5-s exercise interval, indicates the energy-generating capacity of the immediate energy system (intramuscular high-energy phosphates ATP and PCr). PP, expressed in watts (1 W = 6.12 kg-m · min^{-1}), computes as Force × Distance (number of revolutions × distance per revolution) ÷ Time in minutes (5 s = 0.0833 min).
2. **Relative peak power output (RPP)**—Peak power output relative to body mass: PP ÷ Body mass (kg).
3. **Anaerobic fatigue (AF)**—Percentage decline in power output during the test; AF represents the total capacity to produce ATP via the immediate and short-term energy systems. AF computes as (Highest 5-s PP − Lowest 5-s PP) ÷ Highest 5-s PP × 100.
4. **Anaerobic capacity (AC)**—Total work accomplished over 30 s; AC computes as the sum of each 5-s PP, or Force × Total distance in 30 s.

Example

A male weighing 73.3 kg performs the Wingate test on a Monark cycle ergometer (6.0 m traveled per pedal revolution) with an applied resistance of 5.5 kg (73.3-kg body mass × 0.075 = 5.497, rounded to 5.5 kg); pedal revolutions for each 5-s interval equal 12, 10, 8, 7, 6, and 5 (48 total revolutions in 30 s).

Calculations

1. Peak power output
   PP = Force × Distance ÷ Time
   = 5.5 kg × (12 rev × 6 m) ÷ 0.0833 min
   = 396 kg-m ÷ 0.0833 min
   = 4753.9 kg-m · min^{-1} or 776.8 W
2. Relative peak power output
   RPP = PP ÷ Body mass, kg
   = 776.8 W ÷ 73.3 kg
   = 10.6 W · kg^{-1}
3. Anaerobic fatigue
   AF = (Highest PP − Lowest PP) ÷ Highest PP × 100
   [Highest PP = Force × Distance ÷ Time: 5.5 kg × (12 rev × 6 m) ÷ 0.0833 min = 4753.9 kg-m · min^{-1} or 776.8 W]
   [Lowest PP = Force × Distance ÷ Time: 5.5 kg × (5 rev × 6 m) ÷ 0.0833 min = 1980.8 kg-m · min^{-1} or 323.7 W]
   AF = 776.8 W − 323.7 W ÷ 776.8 W × 100 = 58.3%
4. Anaerobic capacity
   AC = Force × Total Distance (in 30 s)
   = 5.5 × [(12 rev + 10 rev + 8 rev + 7 rev + 6 rev + 5 rev) × 6 m]
   = 1584 kg-m · min^{-1} (258.8 W)

mass, active muscle mass, and fat-free body mass (FFM). Consequently, expressing power output capacity in relation to a component of body mass or composition should minimize or even eliminate the gender difference in anaerobic capacity. This adjustment should offer insight into whether true gender effects exist in a muscle's capacity to generate energy anaerobically.

Available data indicate that gender differences in body composition, physique, muscular strength, or neuromuscular factors do not fully explain the significantly lower anaerobic performance of women.[67,81] For example, for a given fat-free leg volume, the peak oxygen deficit (a measure of anaerobic capacity)[4,72] during supermaximal cycling remained significantly higher in men than in women.[115] These differences averaged about 20%, even after adjusting for the estimated difference in active muscle mass between the genders. Similar gender differences in anaerobic exercise capacity exist for children and adolescents.[78,91] The gender effect among adolescents remains apparent for the lower body musculature, even after correction for differences in body composition.[81] Possible inequities in the relative areas and metabolic capacities of the two fiber types and the catecholamine response to exercise may contribute to males' generally superior anaerobic capacity.

Available evidence suggests a biologic difference in anaerobic exercise capacity between the genders. If correct, physical testing that focuses on this fitness component would inflate the typically observed performance differences between men and women. Even adjusting the performance score to body size or body composition would not eliminate this difference. In the occupational setting, the justifiable concern when using all-out anaerobic exercise relates to the potential to exacerbate gender differences in performance scores and magnify adverse impact on females. It does not appear that variations in menstrual cycle phase affect maximal anaerobic performance.[33]

Maximally Accumulated Oxygen Deficit

Determination of the **maximally accumulated oxygen deficit (MAOD)** provides another indirect measure of anaerobic metabolic capacity.[72,73,96] MAOD determination relies on an extrapolation procedure using the linear exercise intensity–oxygen consumption relationship established from several levels of submaximal treadmill exercise. From these data, a regression line predicts the individual's supramaximal oxygen consumption, usually set at 125% of the subject's directly measured $\dot{V}O_{2max}$. MAOD calculates as the difference between the predicted supramaximal oxygen consumption from the exercise intensity–oxygen consumption relationship and the actual oxygen consumption during a 2- to 3-minute all-out treadmill run to fatigue. The measure correlates positively with other anaerobic performance tests (e.g., Wingate test, sprint running, stair climbing); it demonstrates independence from aerobic energy estimates, differentiates between aerobically and anaerobically trained individuals, and remains unchanged with high-intensity exercise of varying durations.

Biologic Indicators for Anaerobic Power

Blood Lactate Levels

Traditionally, physiologists have interpreted the appearance of "excess" lactate in muscle and blood following exercise to indicate the contribution of anaerobic metabolism to the exercise energy requirement. Thus, measurements of muscle or venous blood lactate routinely served to verify steady-rate exercise or the magnitude of glycolytic activity consequent to non–steady-rate exercise. This view now appears overly simplified in light of recent research showing lactate's role as a metabolic intermediate rather than a "dead end," whose only fate involves reconversion to pyruvate. As much as 50% of glucose catabolized for energy converts to lactate, which then serves as an important substrate in energy-storing *and* energy-generating pathways in different tissues. As such, lactate measures during or following exercise do not necessarily reflect absolute levels of anaerobic energy transfer via glycolysis.[14,21,34,35] Nevertheless, with increasing exercise intensity, including near-maximal and supramaximal levels, greater lactate production reflects increasing ATP resynthesis from anaerobic pathways.[99] About 70% of the total energy yield for 30 seconds of all-out exercise derives from anaerobic glycolysis and PCr degradation, with the remaining energy generated from aerobic pathways (Fig. 11.5).

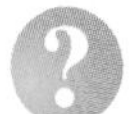

INTEGRATIVE QUESTION

Discuss why females generally score poorly when graded on an absolute score basis for "average power" and "peak power" on the Wingate leg-cycle ergometer test.

Glycogen Depletion

The pattern of glycogen depletion indicates the glycolytic contribution to exercise, because glycogen stored in the specific muscles activated by exercise chiefly powers the short-term energy system. Figure 11.6 illustrates the close connection between glycogen depletion rate in the quadriceps femoris muscle during bicycle exercise and exercise intensity. During prolonged but relatively light exercise (30% $\dot{V}O_{2max}$), a considerable muscle glycogen reserve remains even after 180 minutes. This occurs because relatively large quantities of fatty acids provide fuel for exercise with only minimal reliance on stored glycogen. The two heaviest supermaximal workloads produced the most rapid and pronounced glycogen depletion. This outcome makes sense from a metabolic standpoint because glycogen (1) provides the most rapid phosphorylation of ATP of the three macronutrients and (2) is the only stored macronutrient that anaerobically resynthesizes ATP. Clearly, this important substrate receives high priority as energy substrate in the "metabolic mill" during strenuous exercise.

Changes in *total* muscle glycogen, like those illustrated in Figure 11.6, do not necessarily indicate the precise degree of glycogen catabolism in specific fibers within an active muscle. Depending on exercise intensity, glycogen depletion progresses selectively in either fast- or slow-twitch muscle fibers.[85] All-out exercise (e.g., repeated 1-min sprints on a bicycle ergometer at a heavy load) activates fast-twitch fibers to provide most of the power requirement. Because of the exercise's anaerobic nature, the glycogen content of these fibers becomes almost totally depleted. In contrast, during moderately heavy, but more prolonged aerobic exercise, the slow-twitch fibers become glycogen depleted first.[37] Specificity in

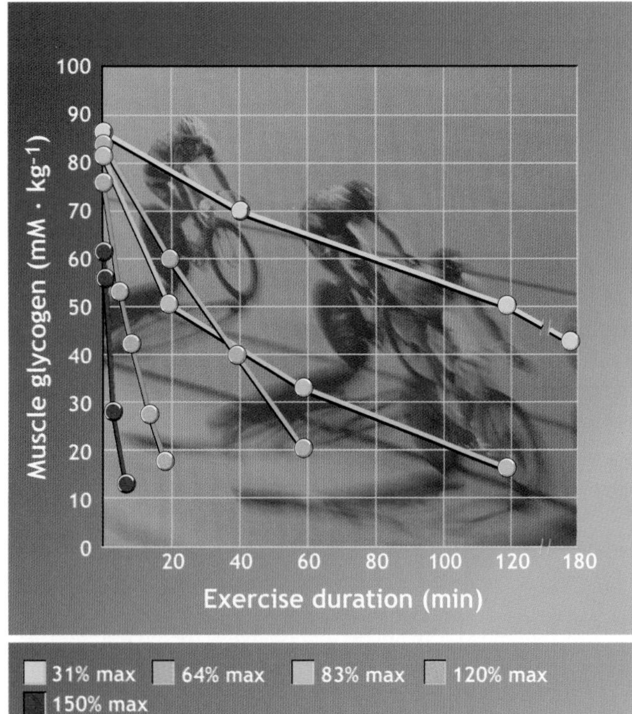

FIGURE 11.6 • Glycogen depletion from the vastus lateralis of the quadriceps femoris muscles during bicycle exercise of different intensities and durations. Exercise at 31% of $\dot{V}O_{2max}$ (the lightest workload) caused some depletion of muscle glycogen, but the most rapid and largest depletion occurred during exercise between 83 and 150% of $\dot{V}O_{2max}$. (Adapted from Gollnick PD. Selective glycogen depletion pattern in human muscle fibers after exercise of varying intensity and at varying pedaling rates. J Physiol 1974;241:45.)

glycogen use (and depletion) makes it difficult to evaluate the anaerobic involvement of specific fibers from changes in a muscle's total glycogen content before and after exercise.

Individual Differences in Anaerobic Energy-Transfer Capacity

Several factors contribute to differences among individuals in their capacity to generate short-term anaerobic energy. These include the effects of previous training, the capacity to buffer acid metabolites, and motivation.

Effects of Training

Figure 11.7 compares biochemical factors of anaerobic metabolism for trained and untrained subjects. After short-term maximal bicycle ergometer exercise, trained subjects always exhibited higher levels of muscle and blood lactate and greater depletion of muscle glycogen. These cross-sectional comparisons suggest that training for short-term, all-out exercise enhances the capacity to generate energy from anaerobic sources.[29] In sprint- and middle-distance activities, individual differences in anaerobic capacity can help to explain the considerable variations in exercise performance.

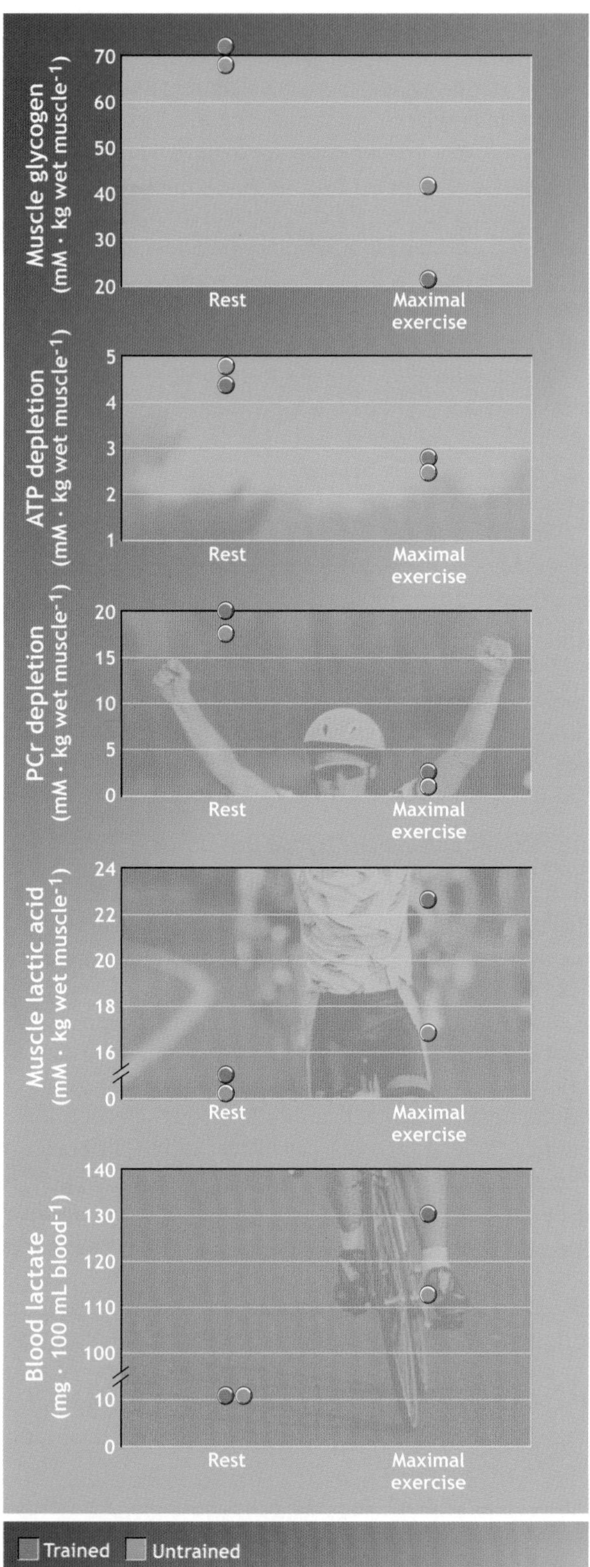

FIGURE 11.7 • Depletion of anaerobic substrates (ATP, PCr, and glycogen) and increases in muscle and blood lactate during short-term maximal exercise by trained and untrained subjects. Trained subjects exhibited a greater increase in anaerobic metabolism (higher lactate levels) and more-pronounced muscle glycogen depletion, while reductions in the intramuscular high-energy phosphates remained essentially the same as for the nontrained subjects. (From Karlsson J, et al. Muscle metabolites during submaximal and maximal exercise in man. Scand J Clin Invest 1971;26:382.)

Buffering of Acid Metabolites

Buffering capacity refers to how well different substances resist increases in free hydrogen ion concentration by binding free protons to blunt a decrease in pH. When anaerobic energy transfer predominates, lactate accumulates and muscle and blood acidity increase and negatively affect the intracellular environment and the contractile capacity of active muscles.[36] Such alterations with maximal exercise led to speculation that anaerobic training might enhance short-term energy capacity by improving the body's alkaline reserve for buffering. This training adaptation would theoretically enable greater lactate production through more-effective buffering. Although such reasoning seems appealing, athletes have only a slightly larger alkaline reserve than sedentary counterparts. Furthermore, no appreciable change in alkaline reserve occurs following hard physical training. *Training most likely confers a buffering capability within the range expected for healthy untrained individuals.*

Altering acid-base balance in the direction of alkalosis temporarily enhances high-intensity anaerobic exercise performance. For example, ingesting a buffering solution of sodium bicarbonate prior to an 800-m race significantly improved running performance.[117] Higher blood lactate levels and extracellular H^+ concentrations suggested an increased anaerobic energy transfer that contributed to the faster run times. Chapter 23 discusses the potential ergogenic effects of preexercise-induced alkalosis.

Motivation

Individuals with a higher "pain tolerance," "toughness," or ability to "push" beyond the discomforts of fatiguing exercise can accomplish more work anaerobically. They usually exhibit higher blood lactate concentrations and greater glycogen depletion. They also score higher on tests of short-term energy capacity.[118] Motivational factors that are sometimes difficult to categorize or quantify undoubtedly play an integral role in achieving superior performance at most levels of competition.

AEROBIC ENERGY: THE LONG-TERM ENERGY SYSTEM

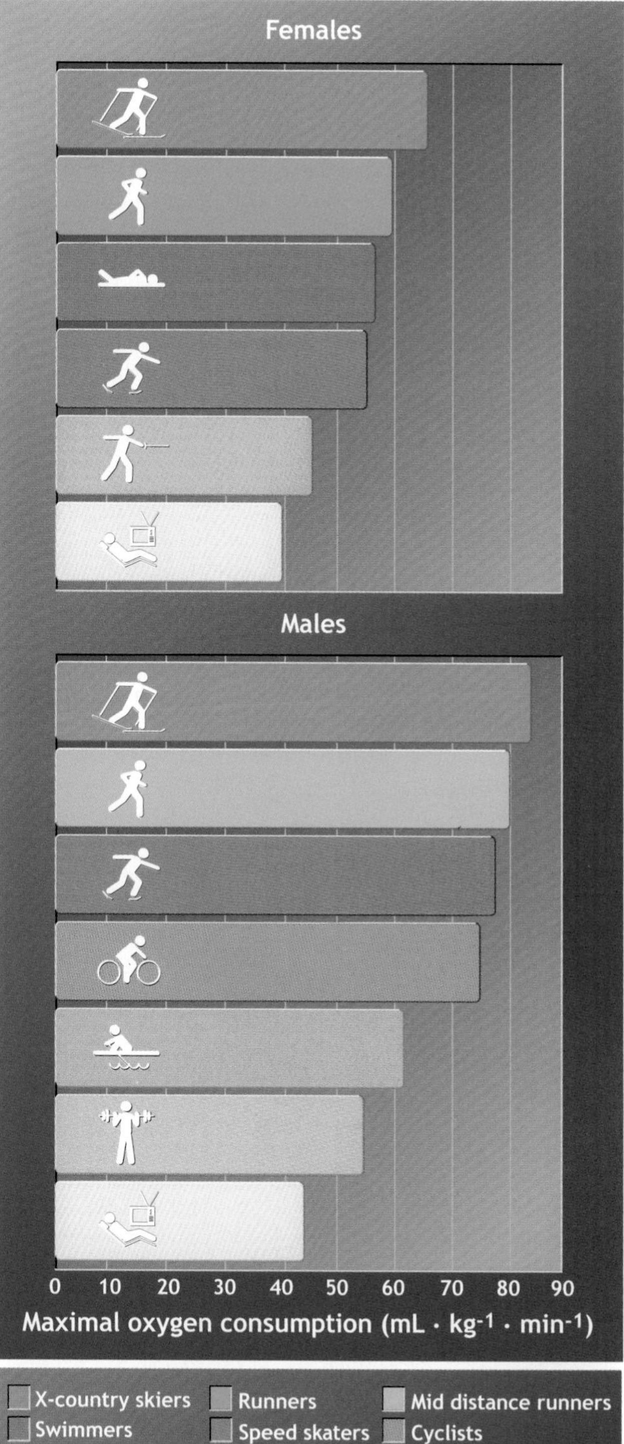

FIGURE 11.8 • Maximal oxygen consumption of male and female Olympic-caliber athletes in different sports categories compared with those of healthy sedentary subjects. (Adapted from Saltin B, Åstrand PO. Maximal oxygen consumption in athletes. J Appl Physiol 1967;23:353.)

Figure 11.8 illustrates that athletes who excel in endurance sports generally have a large capacity for aerobic energy transfer. The maximal oxygen consumption recorded for competitors in distance running, swimming, bicycling, and cross-country skiing exceeds that of sedentary men and women by almost twofold.[2,44] This does not mean that $\dot{V}O_{2max}$ makes up the sole determinant of endurance performance. Other factors, principally those at the local tissue level, such as capillary density, enzymes, mitochondrial size and number, and muscle fiber type, strongly influence a muscle's capacity to sustain a high level of aerobic exercise.[41] However, $\dot{V}O_{2max}$ does provide important information about the capacity of the long-term energy system. This measure also conveys important physiologic meaning, because attaining a high $\dot{V}O_{2max}$ requires integration of high levels of pulmonary, cardiovascular, and neuromuscular function (see Fig. 7.6). *This makes $\dot{V}O_{2max}$ a fundamental measure of physiologic functional capacity for exercise.*

Focus on Research

An Important Measure of Cardiorespiratory Functional Capacity

Mitchell JH, et al. The physiological meaning of the maximal oxygen intake test. J Clin Invest 1958;37:538.

➤ In the 1920s, A. V. Hill and colleagues—and in latter years other scientists—considered maximal oxygen consumption ($\dot{V}O_{2max}$) the single best measure of cardiorespiratory capacity. Hill asserted that $\dot{V}O_{2max}$ "was physiologically restricted owing to the limitation of the circulatory and respiratory systems." This assertion, however, had not been tested experimentally because the interplay among physiologic parameters had not yet been established. Mitchell and coworkers directly examined the relationships among $\dot{V}O_{2max}$ and various cardiovascular–pulmonary measures to objectify the physiologic significance of $\dot{V}O_{2max}$.

Sixty-five men performed graded, discontinuous treadmill exercise to $\dot{V}O_{2max}$. Subgroups ran in several different protocols to volitional exhaustion. Measurements included cardiac output and a-$\bar{v}$ O_2 difference by the dye dilution technique, blood gas pressures, and central blood volume. Two significant findings emerged that related to test methodology: First, $\dot{V}O_{2max}$ provides a highly reproducible measure of aerobic capacity "if rigid criteria for determining the point at which the maximal value has been attained are applied." The reproducibility of test scores (i.e., test–retest reliability coefficient) for 15 subjects was $r = 0.92$, with a standard error of measurement of $\pm 7\%$ for determining an individual's maximal value. Second, a "peaking over" or "plateauing" criterion (when relating oxygen consumption to exercise intensity) provided an important conceptual standard to establish attainment of $\dot{V}O_{2max}$ in diverse forms of exercise as follows:

> Plots of oxygen intake against workload for the entire material showed that, until a maximal value was attained, oxygen intake rose 142 ±44 mL with each increase in workload. If the rise was less than 142 minus 88 (twice the standard deviation), or 54 mL, the final value was accepted as the maximal intake, the assumption being that the subject had attained his true maximal value or had reached the beginning of a plateau and could not increase his intake very much more.

The physiologic findings from this study endorsed the view that the $\dot{V}O_{2max}$ depended almost exclusively on the functional capacity of the cardiovascular system (cardiac output and a-$\bar{v}$ O_2 difference) and not accommodation of left ventricular output by the peripheral vascular bed. No significant change occurred in arterial oxygen pressure from rest to heavy work; the slight arterial desaturation often observed in heavy exercise resulted from a blood pH decrease and the resulting Bohr effect on hemoglobin saturation. Maintenance of high arterial oxygen pressures during heavy exercise argued against the possibility that pulmonary factors provided a "weak link" in limiting $\dot{V}O_{2max}$. In essence, the researchers maintained that in healthy individuals an adequate arterial oxygen diffusion gradient always exits from the alveoli to the blood and from the blood to active tissues.

This study confirmed the importance of $\dot{V}O_{2max}$ to indicate central circulatory function (cardiac capacity) and, to a lesser degree, the capacity of peripheral or local factors as reflected by the a-$\bar{v}$ O_2 difference. This and subsequent research by other laboratories firmly established $\dot{V}O_{2max}$ as a "benchmark" to quantify cardiovascular functional capacity and aerobic fitness.

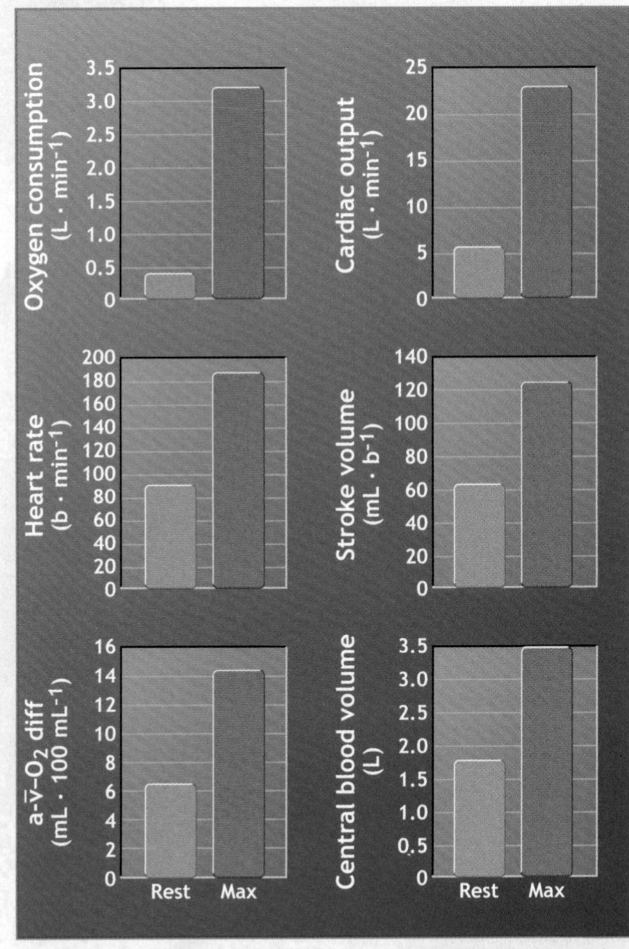

Magnitude of changes in cardiovascular dynamics (arteriovenous oxygen difference, heart rate, oxygen consumption, stroke volume, and blood volume) in 15 normal subjects, between rest and exercise at the maximal oxygen consumption.

Assessment of Maximal Oxygen Consumption

Considerable research effort has developed and standardized tests to assess maximal aerobic power and provided normative standards related to age, gender, state of training, and body size.

Criteria for Maximal Oxygen Consumption

The plot in Figure 11.9 relates oxygen consumption and exercise intensity during progressive increases in treadmill effort. The test terminated when the subject would not complete the full duration of a particular exercise interval. The highest oxygen consumption (average of 18 subjects) occurred before subjects attained their maximum exercise level. *Demonstration of a leveling off or peaking over in oxygen consumption with increasing exercise intensity generally provides assurance that a person has reached maximum capacity for aerobic metabolism (i.e., achieved "true" $\dot{V}O_{2max}$; see Focus on Research).* However, agreement on a precise standard for the criterion remains controversial.[23,42] Less stringent criteria, besides an absolute failure for oxygen consumption to increase in graded exercise, also establish attainment of $\dot{V}O_{2max}$. For example, oxygen consumption that fails to increase by the value expected on the basis of previous observations with the specific test protocol often serves as an appropriate criterion.[1,42,76,102]

Oxygen consumption at the higher exercise levels does not readily plateau, particularly among children,[89] except in treadmill running. The term **peak oxygen consumption**, or $\dot{V}O_{2peak}$, applies when leveling off does not occur or test performance appears to be limited by local muscular factors rather than central circulatory dynamics. *$\dot{V}O_{2peak}$ refers to the highest value of oxygen consumption measured during a graded exercise test.* Often, the highest oxygen consumption occurs in the last minute of exercise. Secondary criteria that objectify $\dot{V}O_{2peak}$ include attainment of the age-predicted maximum heart rate (see Fig. 21.19) or a respiratory exchange ratio (R) above 1.15. Some also argue that to accept an oxygen consumption value as near maximum, blood lactate levels should attain 70 or 80 mg per dL of blood (8 to 10 mmol) or higher.[23]

Maximal Oxygen Consumption Tests

One can determine $\dot{V}O_{2max}$ using a variety of exercises that activate the body's large muscle groups, provided the intensity and duration of effort are sufficient to maximize aerobic energy transfer. The usual exercise modes include treadmill running or walking, bench stepping, and stationary cycling. Other forms of testing use free, tethered, and flume swimming[9,61]; swim-bench ergometry[32]; in-line skating[110]; roller skiing[90]; simulated arm-leg climbing[13]; rowing[17]; ice skating[27]; and arm-crank and wheelchair exercise.[95,105,107] Such performance tests generally remain unaffected by a subject's strength, speed, body size, and skill, with the exception of specialized tests that measure aerobic capacity in sport-specific activities.

The $\dot{V}O_{2max}$ test may require a single, continuous 3- to 5-minute supermaximal effort but usually consists of progressive increments in effort (**graded exercise**) to a point at which the subject simply refuses to continue exercising. Some researchers have termed this end point "exhaustion." However, the person exercising terminates the test—a decision often influenced by psychologic or motivational factors that do not necessarily reflecting true physiologic strain. Bringing the subject to the point of acceptable criteria for either $\dot{V}O_{2max}$ or $\dot{V}O_{2peak}$ often requires considerable urging and prodding.[109] Practical experience indicates that attaining a plateau in oxygen consumption during a graded exercise test requires a high level

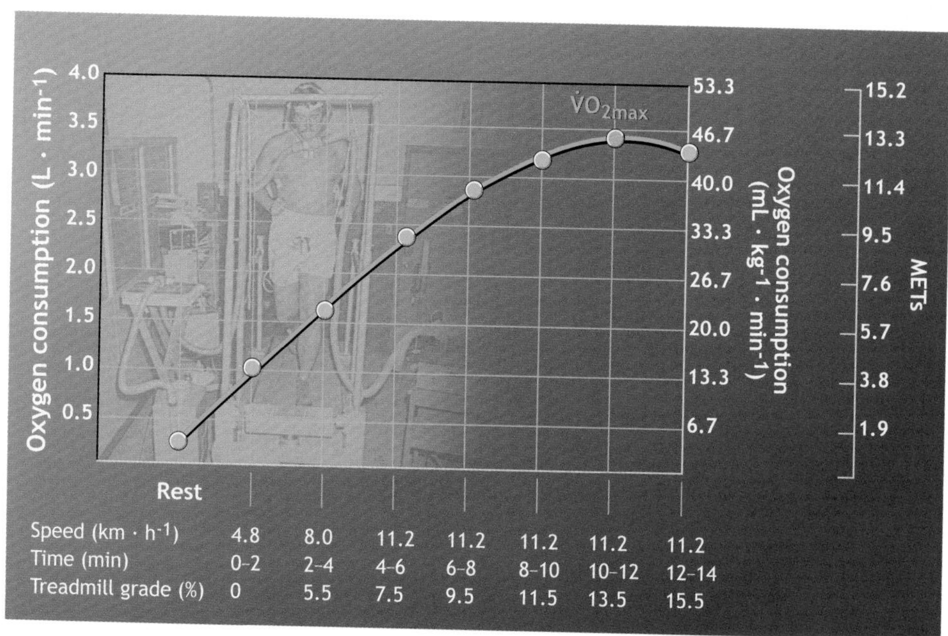

FIGURE 11.9 • Peaking over in oxygen consumption with increasing treadmill exercise intensity. Each point represents the average oxygen consumption of 18 sedentary males. The region where oxygen consumption fails to increase the expected amount or even decreases slightly with increasing exercise intensity represents the $\dot{V}O_{2max}$. (Data from the Applied Physiology Laboratory, University of Michigan, Ann Arbor.)

TABLE 11.3 ➤ AVERAGE $\dot{V}O_{2max}$ FOR 15 MALE COLLEGE STUDENTS DURING CONTINUOUS AND DISCONTINUOUS TESTS ON THE TREADMILL AND BICYCLE ERGOMETER[a]

VARIABLE	BIKE, DISCONTINUOUS	BIKE, CONTINUOUS	TREADMILL, DISCONTINUOUS RUN-WALK	TREADMILL, CONTINUOUS WALK	TREADMILL, DISCONTINUOUS RUN	TREADMILL, CONTINUOUS RUN
$\dot{V}O_{2max}$, mL · min^{-1}	3691 ± 453	3683 ± 448	4145 ± 401	3944 ± 395	4157 ± 445	4109 ± 424
$\dot{V}O_{2max}$, mL · kg^{-1} · min^{-1}	50.0 ± 6.9	49.9 ± 7.0	56.6 ± 7.3	53.7 ± 7.6	56.6 ± 7.6	55.5 ± 6.8

Adapted from McArdle WD, et al. Comparison of continuous and discontinuous treadmill and bicycle tests for max $\dot{V}O_2$. Med Sci Sports 1973;5:156.
[a]Values are means ± standard deviations.

of anaerobic energy output. This poses some difficulty, particularly for untrained and elderly people who normally do not perform strenuous exercise with its associated discomforts.

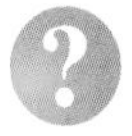

INTEGRATIVE QUESTION

In what specific ways does $\dot{V}O_{2max}$ provide important insights about the functional capacities of diverse physiologic systems?

Test Comparisons

Maximal oxygen consumption tests are usually:

- Continuous—no rest between exercise increments
- Discontinuous—several minutes of recovery between exercise increments

Both test protocols give similar $\dot{V}O_{2max}$ values.[23,70] The data in Table 11.3 show a systematic comparison of $\dot{V}O_{2max}$ scores

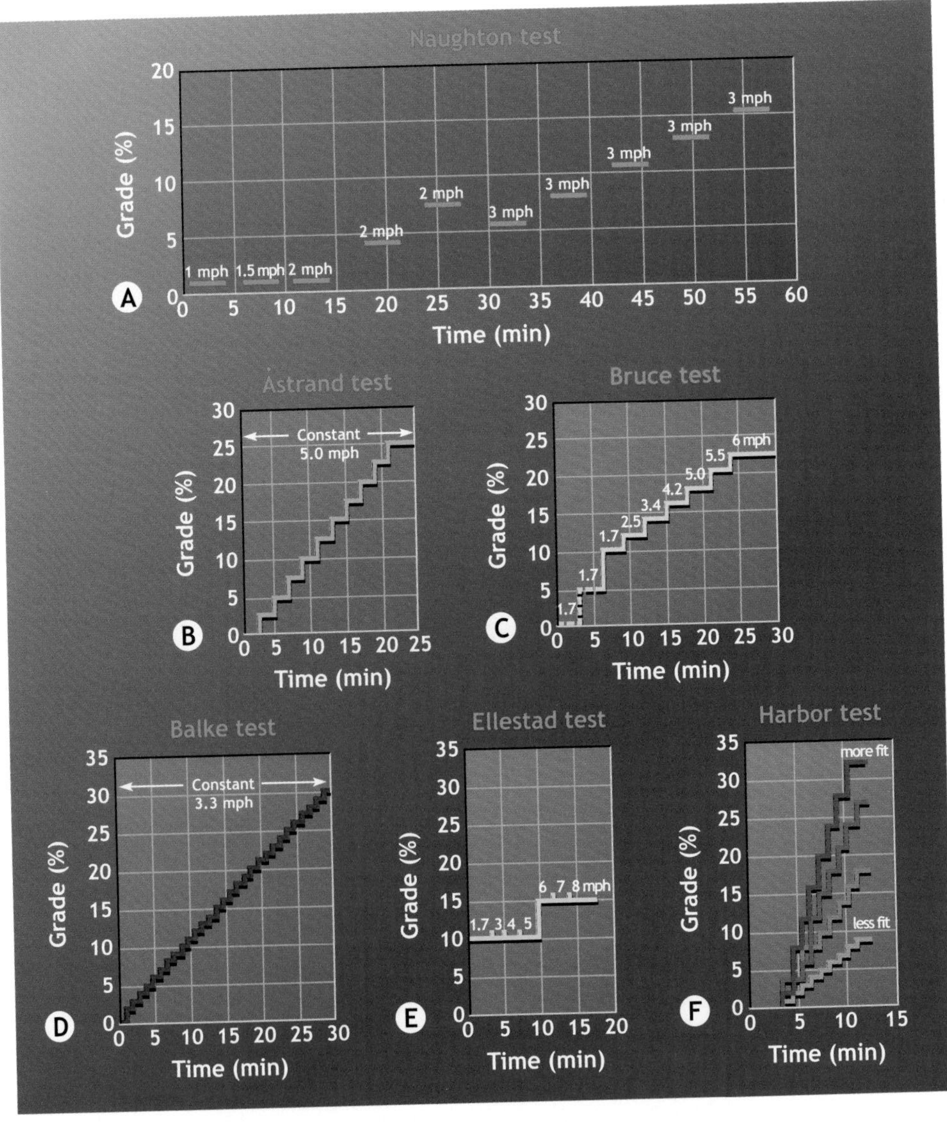

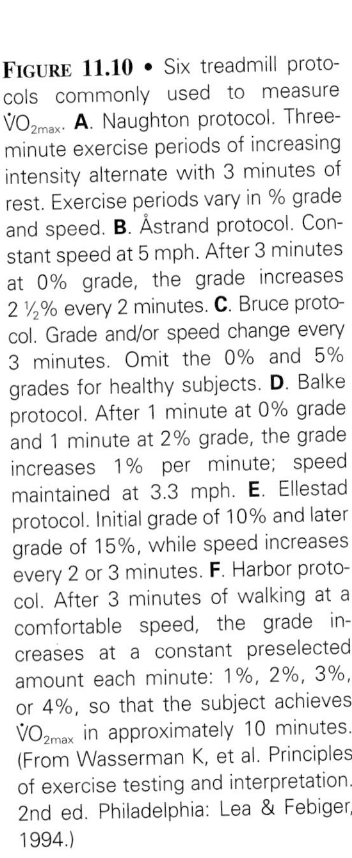

FIGURE 11.10 • Six treadmill protocols commonly used to measure $\dot{V}O_{2max}$. **A**. Naughton protocol. Three-minute exercise periods of increasing intensity alternate with 3 minutes of rest. Exercise periods vary in % grade and speed. **B**. Åstrand protocol. Constant speed at 5 mph. After 3 minutes at 0% grade, the grade increases 2 ½% every 2 minutes. **C**. Bruce protocol. Grade and/or speed change every 3 minutes. Omit the 0% and 5% grades for healthy subjects. **D**. Balke protocol. After 1 minute at 0% grade and 1 minute at 2% grade, the grade increases 1% per minute; speed maintained at 3.3 mph. **E**. Ellestad protocol. Initial grade of 10% and later grade of 15%, while speed increases every 2 or 3 minutes. **F**. Harbor protocol. After 3 minutes of walking at a comfortable speed, the grade increases at a constant preselected amount each minute: 1%, 2%, 3%, or 4%, so that the subject achieves $\dot{V}O_{2max}$ in approximately 10 minutes. (From Wasserman K, et al. Principles of exercise testing and interpretation. 2nd ed. Philadelphia: Lea & Febiger, 1994.)

measured using six common continuous and discontinuous treadmill and bicycle protocols. Although only an 8-mL difference in $\dot{V}O_{2max}$ emerged between the continuous and discontinuous bicycle tests, $\dot{V}O_{2max}$ during cycling averaged 6.4 to 11.2% below treadmill values. The largest difference among the three treadmill running tests equaled only 1.2%. The walking test, on the other hand, elicited $\dot{V}O_{2max}$ scores nearly 7% higher than values on the bicycle, but 5% lower than the three running tests.

Subjects commonly complained of intense local discomfort in the thigh muscles during heavy exercise (which limited their ability to continue) in both continuous and discontinuous bicycle tests. Subjects experienced local discomfort in the lower back and calf muscles during treadmill walking, notably at the higher treadmill elevations. Running tests rarely produced local discomfort; subjects complained more of general fatigue, usually categorized as feeling "winded." For ease of administration, the continuous treadmill run provides a practical test of aerobic capacity for most healthy subjects. The total time to administer the test averaged about 12 minutes, compared with 65 minutes for the discontinuous running test. Subjects tolerated the continuous test well and preferred the shorter time. Research also indicates achievement of $\dot{V}O_{2max}$ with a continuous protocol that increases exercise intensity progressively in 15-second intervals.[26] With this approach, the total test time for either bicycle or treadmill exercise averages only about 5 minutes.

COMMON TREADMILL PROTOCOLS. Figure 11.10 summarizes six common treadmill protocols for assessing aerobic capacity in normal individuals and cardiac patients.[79] Manipulation of exercise duration and treadmill speed and grade share common features. The Harbor treadmill test (example *F*), referred to as a ramp test, depicts a unique application. With this protocol, treadmill grade increases by a constant amount (between 1 and 4%) each minute for up to 10 minutes, depending on the person's fitness. This relatively quick procedure—well tolerated by both healthy subjects and cardiac patients—elicits a linear increase in oxygen consumption up to maximum.[15,20,112]

Can Manipulation of Test Protocol Increase $\dot{V}O_{2max}$?

When a person completes a maximal oxygen consumption test, we assume that the tester has made every attempt to "push" the subject to the near-limits of performance. This can involve verbal encouragement and/or monetary incentive. If proper criteria are met, one assumes that the test score represents "true" $\dot{V}O_{2max}$. Figure 11.11 shows data for 44 either sedentary or trained men and women who performed a continuous treadmill $\dot{V}O_{2max}$ test *(Peak 1)* to volitional "exhaustion." After the test, the subjects recovered actively for 2 minutes and then performed a second $\dot{V}O_{2max}$ test *(Peak 2)*.

Treadmill speed increased to the *Peak 1* test speed for 30 seconds, and percentage grade then increased to the final grade of *Peak 1*. Treadmill grade increased every 2 minutes thereafter until the subject once again terminated the test,

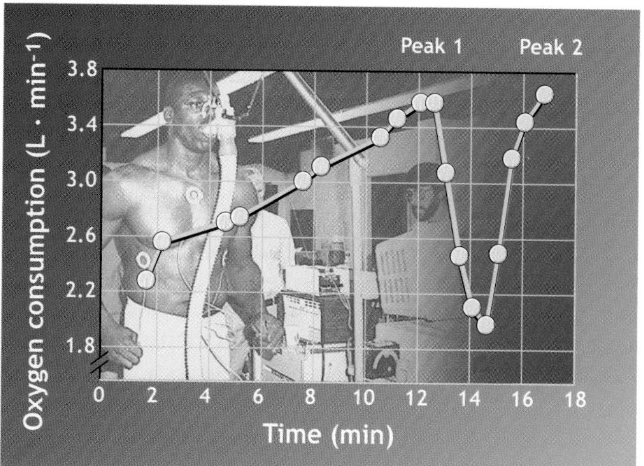

FIGURE 11.11 • Oxygen consumption plotted in relation to time during repeat treadmill $\dot{V}O_{2max}$ tests in 44 men and women. *Peak 1* refers to the highest oxygen consumption during the first test and *Peak 2* equals the highest oxygen consumption during the repeat test. (From Keller B, Katch FI. It is not valid to adjust gender differences in aerobic capacity and strength for body mass or lean body mass. Med Sci Sports Exerc 1991;23:S167.)

believing that he or she had exercised maximally. The researchers provided strong verbal encouragement during both tests, particularly in the last minutes, when the endpoint appeared near. The $\dot{V}O_{2max}$ score averaged 1.4% higher (statistically significant) on the second test (Peak 2). This difference of 48 mL (0.7 mL · kg^{-1} · min^{-1} for a typical subject), while small, nearly doubled the difference normally obtained between the two final oxygen consumption values of single, continuous or discontinuous tests. Thus, a "booster" test following a typically administered test of aerobic capacity can slightly increase the final oxygen consumption. This observation points out the need to pay considerable attention to test standardization and administration.

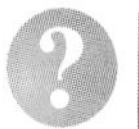

INTEGRATIVE QUESTION

Discuss the importance for training studies to demonstrate objectively attainment of true $\dot{V}O_{2max}$ in both pre- and posttest measures. How can this goal be verified?

Factors That Affect Maximal Oxygen Consumption

The most important factors that influence the maximal oxygen consumption score include mode of exercise, heredity, state of training, gender, body size and composition, and age.

Mode of Exercise

Variations in $\dot{V}O_{2max}$ with different forms of exercise generally reflect the quantity of muscle mass activated.[8,58] Studies that determined $\dot{V}O_{2max}$ for the same subjects during different exercise modes indicate that treadmill exercise usually produces the highest values. Bench-stepping has produced $\dot{V}O_{2max}$ scores identical to treadmill values and significantly higher than values on a cycle ergometer.[46] During arm-crank exercise, aerobic capacity averages only about 70% of one's treadmill score.[105] For skilled but untrained swimmers, the $\dot{V}O_{2max}$ during swimming usually equals about 80% of treadmill values.[61,71] A definite test specificity emerges for this form of exercise because trained collegiate swimmers achieve $\dot{V}O_{2max}$ values swimming only 11% below treadmill values,[68] and some elite swimmers equal or even exceed their treadmill scores during swimming tests.[61] Similarly, a distinct exercise specificity exists for competitive racewalkers who achieve a similar $\dot{V}O_{2max}$ during treadmill walking and running.[74] When competitive cyclists pedal at the rapid frequencies of competition, they too achieve $\dot{V}O_{2max}$ values equivalent to their treadmill $\dot{V}O_{2max}$ scores.[38,101]

Treadmill exercise proves highly desirable for determining $\dot{V}O_{2max}$ in healthy subjects in the laboratory. One can easily quantify and regulate exercise intensity. Compared with other forms of exercise, the treadmill allows subjects to more easily meet one or more of the criteria for attaining $\dot{V}O_{2max}$ or $\dot{V}O_{2peak}$. Outside the laboratory setting, in field experiments, bench-stepping and cycle ergometry become suitable alternatives.

Heredity

The interaction between inherited factors (DNA sequence variation; see Section 8, "A Look to the Future") and exercise enhances our understanding of individual variations in training responsiveness, including anticipated health-related benefits derived from regular physical activity.[10,39,77,88] Frequent questions concern the relative contribution of natural endowment (**genotype**) to physiologic function and exercise performance (**phenotype**).[30,60] For example, to what extent does heredity determine the extremely high aerobic capacities of the endurance athletes in Figure 11.8? Do these exceptionally high levels of functional capacity simply result from intensive training? Although the answer remains incomplete, researchers have focused on the genetic contribution to individual differences in physiologic and metabolic capacity.

In general, most physical fitness characteristics demonstrate high heritability. Earlier research studied 15 pairs of identical twins (monozygous; same heredity from a single fertilized ovum) and 15 pairs of fraternal twins (dizygous; like ordinary siblings, derived from two separate fertilized ovum) raised in the same city and with parents of similar socioeconomic backgrounds. The results indicated that heredity alone accounted for up to 93% of observed differences in $\dot{V}O_{2max}$. In addition, the capacity of the short-term glycolytic energy system indicated a genetic determination of approximately 81%, and maximum heart rate showed an approximate 86% genetic determination.[55] Subsequent studies of larger groups of brothers, fraternal twins, and identical twins showed a significant but smaller effect of inherited factors on aerobic capacity and endurance performance.[11,12] Figure 11.12 presents data for $\dot{V}O_{2max}$ for identical twin and fraternal twin brothers. The least variation in aerobic capacity between brother pairs emerged for identical twins with identical genetic constitutions. Chapters 21 and Section 8, "A Look to the Future" discuss the potential contribution of genetic makeup to one's responsiveness to aerobic exercise training.

Researchers currently estimate the genetic effect at about 25 to 40% for $\dot{V}O_{2max}$, 50% for maximum heart rate, and 70% for physical working capacity.[10,11,84] Combining the estimated effects of genetics and familial environment raises the upper limit of genetic determination to about 50% for $\dot{V}O_{2max}$, when adjusted for age, gender, and body mass and/or body composition.[12] Identical twins have similar muscle fiber type composition, whereas fiber type varies widely between fraternal twins and brothers.[59] About 40% of the variation in muscular strength among individuals probably results from genetic factors.[83] Table 11.4 summarizes current estimations of the genetic contribution to some important health-related physical fitness components. Future research may determine a precise upper limit of genetic determination; at this time, we can assume that inherited factors contribute significantly to physiologic function, exercise performance, training responsiveness, and specific components of health-related physical fitness.[30,60,87,88]

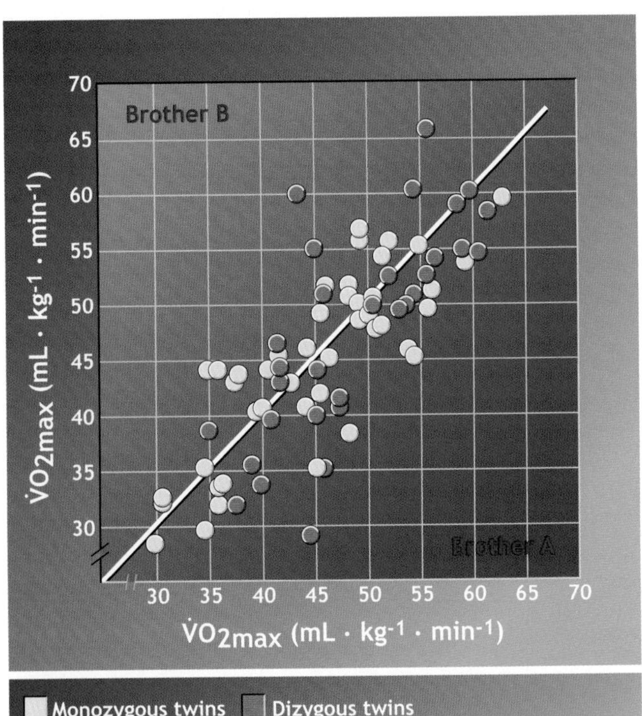

FIGURE 11.12 • Maximal oxygen consumptions ($\dot{V}O_{2max}$) for pairs of monozygotic and dizygotic twin brothers. (From Bouchard C, et al. Aerobic performance in brothers, dizygotic and monozygotic twins. Med Sci Sports Exerc 1986;18:639.)

TABLE 11.4 ➤ **ESTIMATED GENETIC CONTRIBUTION TO INDIVIDUAL DIFFERENCES IN IMPORTANT COMPONENTS OF HEALTH-RELATED PHYSICAL FITNESS**

FITNESS COMPONENT	GENETIC CONTRIBUTION
• $\dot{V}O_{2max}$	20–30%
• Submaximal exercise response	20–30%
• Muscular fitness	20–30%
• Blood lipid profile	30–50%
• Resting blood pressure	30%
• Total body fat	25%
• Regional fat distribution	30%
• Habitual activity level	30%

Modified from Bouchard C, Perusse L. Heredity, activity level, fitness, and health. in Physical activity, fitness, and health. Champaign, IL: Human Kinetics, 1994.

State of Training

A person's state of aerobic training contributes significantly to the $\dot{V}O_{2max}$; it normally varies between 5 and 20% depending on a person's fitness at the time of testing. Chapter 21 further discusses the influence of training on aerobic capacity.

Gender

Women typically achieve $\dot{V}O_{2max}$ scores 15 to 30% below values of male counterparts.[107] Even among trained endurance athletes, gender differences range between 15 and 20%.[6] These differences are considerably larger for $\dot{V}O_{2max}$ expressed in absolute units ($L \cdot min^{-1}$) rather than in relation to body mass ($mL \cdot kg^{-1} \cdot min^{-1}$).[112] Among world-class cross-country skiers, for example, a 43% lower $\dot{V}O_{2max}$ absolute value for women (6.54 versus 3.75 $L \cdot min^{-1}$) becomes 15% lower when expressed relative to body mass (83.8 versus 71.2 $mL \cdot kg^{-1} \cdot min^{-1}$).

The gender difference in $\dot{V}O_{2max}$ has generally been ascribed to differences in body composition (discussed in the next section) and hemoglobin concentration. Untrained young adult women generally average about 25% body fat, whereas men average 15%.[48] Thus, the average male generates more total aerobic energy simply because he possesses more muscle mass and has less fat than the average female. Trained athletes have lower percentages of fat than average individuals, although trained women still possess significantly more body fat than their male counterparts. Also, perhaps because of higher testosterone levels, men also have a 10 to 14% greater hemoglobin concentration than women. This difference in the blood's oxygen-carrying capacity enables men to circulate more oxygen during exercise, thus increasing their aerobic capacities above that of women.[120]

Factors other than lower body fat and higher hemoglobin concentrations may also explain male-female aerobic capacity differences. For example, normal physical activity levels differ between the average male and average female. One could argue that social constraints reduce opportunities for females of all ages to participate in extracurricular athletic activities and recreational pursuits. Among prepubertal children, boys show significantly more daily physical activity than girls of the same age. Despite these fitness-inhibiting factors, the aerobic capacities of physically active females generally exceed those of sedentary males. The $\dot{V}O_{2max}$ of female cross-country skiers, for example, exceeds scores of untrained males by 40%.[6] Even among the so-called normal population, considerable variability exists within each gender, and the $\dot{V}O_{2max}$ scores for many women exceed average values for men.

ARE GENDER DIFFERENCES SHRINKING FOR ENDURANCE PERFORMANCE? Figure 11.13A illustrates the decline in running speed over increasing race distances for men and women in events that place a predominant demand on aerobic energy transfer.[97] The average of the top 50 race times for the 1996 world rankings for the 1500-m, 10-km, and marathon events provided the data points to construct the curves. Despite the decline in running speed with increasing race distance, a nearly identical gender difference emerged for each race. Men ran on average 14.5% faster than women, with no narrowing of the gender difference as race distance increased, despite a 37-fold greater duration for the marathon than for the 1500-m run. Clearly, this analysis does not support the contention that gender differences in endurance diminish as distance increases. In addition, analysis of annual world rankings (world best and 100th best times) from 1980 to 1996 indicates that the gender difference in competitive distance running plateaued and remained stable for both the 1500-m and marathon for more than a decade (Fig. 11.13, B and C). These findings run counter to current speculation that women's endurance should improve at a faster rate than men's to a point at which gender differences in performance vanish or reverse.[116]

Body Size and Composition

Variations in body mass may explain nearly 70% of the differences in $\dot{V}O_{2max}$ scores among individuals.[121] This limits interpretations of exercise performance or absolute values for oxygen consumption when comparing individuals who differ in body size or composition. The effect of body size on aerobic capacity has led to the common practice of expressing oxygen consumption in relation to body-size variables such as surface area, body mass, FFM, or limb volume. Table 11.5 shows a 43% difference in $\dot{V}O_{2max}$ ($L \cdot min^{-1}$) for an untrained man and woman differing considerably in body mass. When expressed per unit of body mass ($mL \cdot kg^{-1} \cdot min^{-1}$), the $\dot{V}O_{2max}$ of the woman still remains about 20% lower than that of the man. Expressing aerobic capacity in terms of FFM reduces the between-subject difference even more. In addition to total FFM, adjusting for variation in muscle mass activated in exercise provides additional information to

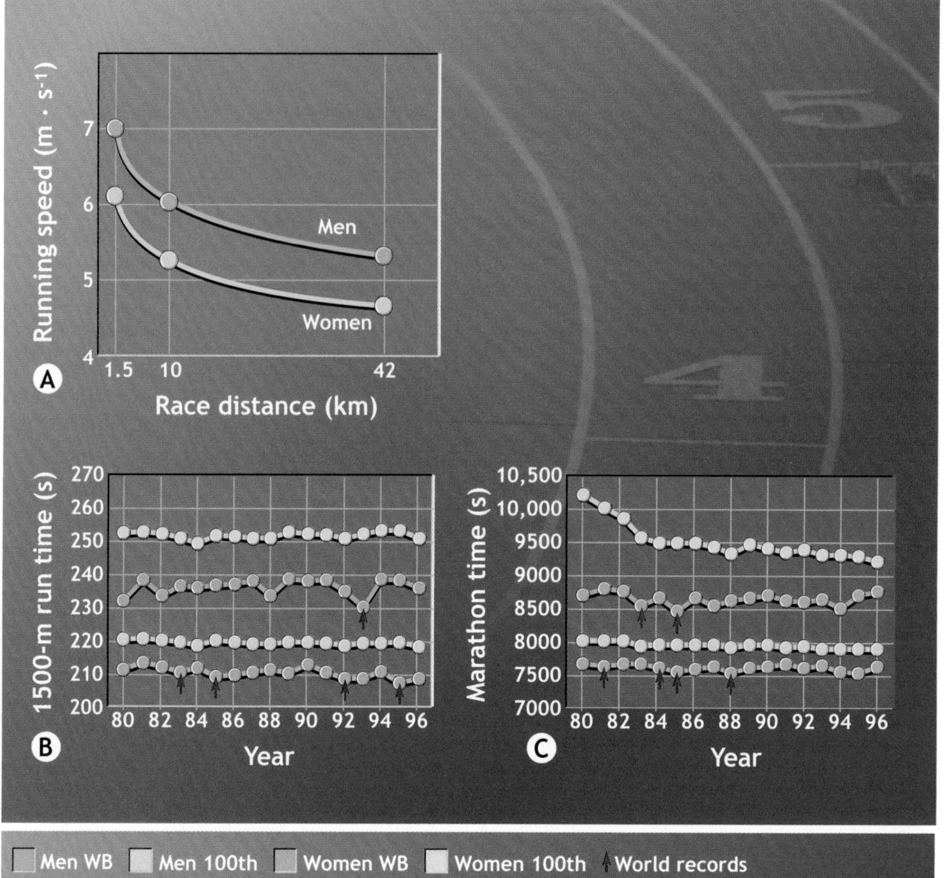

FIGURE 11.13 • A. Decline in running pace over increasing race distance for men and women. Performance represents the average of the top 50 times for the 1996 world rankings for the 1500-m (1.5-km), 10-km, and marathon (42-km) events. Annual world best *(WB)* and 100th ranked 1500-m times (**B**) and marathon times (**C**) for men and women from 1980 to 1996. *Red arrows* indicate world records. (From Sparling PB, et al. The gender difference in distance running performance has plateaued: an analysis of world rankings from 1980 to 1996. Med Sci Sports Exerc 1998; 30:1725.)

TABLE 11.5 ➤ DIFFERENT WAYS TO EXPRESS OXYGEN CONSUMPTION

VARIABLE	FEMALE	MALE	FEMALE VS. MALE % DIFFERENCE
$\dot{V}O_{2max}$, L · min⁻¹	2.00	3.50	−43
$\dot{V}O_{2max}$, mL · kg⁻¹ · min⁻¹	40.0	50.0	−20
$\dot{V}O_{2max}$, mL · kgFFM⁻¹ · min⁻¹	53.3	58.8	−9
Body mass, kg	50	70	−29
Percent body fat	25	15	+67
Fat-free body mass, kg	37.5	59.5	−37

explain interindividual variation in $\dot{V}O_{2max}$. For example, adjusting oxygen consumption values obtained during maximal arm-cranking exercise for variations in estimated arm and shoulder size *eliminates* the gender difference in $\dot{V}O_{2peak}$.[111] Similarly, expressing oxygen consumption per unit of appendicular skeletal muscle mass often negates the difference in $\dot{V}O_{2max}$ between men and women of similar training status.[16,86] *These findings suggest that the size of the contracting muscle mass largely accounts for the gender difference in aerobic capacity.* On the other hand, one should not believe that simply expressing aerobic or endurance performance capacity by some body composition measure automatically adjusts these measures to a gender-neutral state.

AN ARGUMENT FOR BIOLOGIC DIFFERENCES BETWEEN GENDERS. The traditional ways to express oxygen consumption, presented in Table 11.5, do not necessarily answer whether gender differences in $\dot{V}O_{2max}$ remain biologically inherent or merely reflect differences in muscle mass and body composition.[119] Uncertainty exists because ratio adjustments may not truly "eliminate," "equate," or "normalize" gender differences: they simply express the criterion trait (e.g., aerobic capacity or muscular strength) relative to a specific divisor (e.g., body mass, FFM, or muscle cross-sectional area). Justification of which divisor best expresses an individual's $\dot{V}O_{2max}$ for comparison purposes makes certain assumptions that are not always met. For example, creating a ratio score such as $\dot{V}O_2$ divided by FFM implies a direct and proportional relationship between the two variables, a condition not achieved for any of the variables mentioned above.[51] Any deviation in linearity in the relationship between numerator and denominator in the ratio expression either underestimates or overestimates an individual's "true" $\dot{V}O_2$.

An experimental approach to this important topic would compare physiologic responses and capacities of men and women of near-similar body size, body composition, and training history. The comparison eliminates the need to express oxygen consumption as a ratio score relative to body size or body composition. If gender exerts no effect on aerobic capacity, then men and women should achieve similar $\dot{V}O_{2max}$ scores. One study tested this hypothesis in 10 pairs of sedentary and endurance-trained men and women matched for age, stature, body mass, FFM, and prior training history. The researchers also adjusted aerobic capacity for the gender difference in hemoglobin concentration. Figure 11.14 illustrates the effect of gender matching for body mass and FFM on the percentage difference in aerobic capacity during incremental treadmill running. The $\dot{V}O_{2max}$ differences between men and women matched for body mass equaled 25.3% (sedentary) and 22.1% (trained). Gender differences persisted after adjustment for hemoglobin concentration *(adjusted $\dot{V}O_{2max}$)*; they decreased only slightly to 18.4% for the sedentary group and 12.8% for the trained group. Matching the groups for FFM did not minimize substantial gender differences that averaged 18.4% for the sedentary group and 20.5% for the trained group. Adjusting these differences in aerobic capacity further for hemoglobin concentration reduced the gender differences somewhat, but they still averaged about 11% for each group.[53]

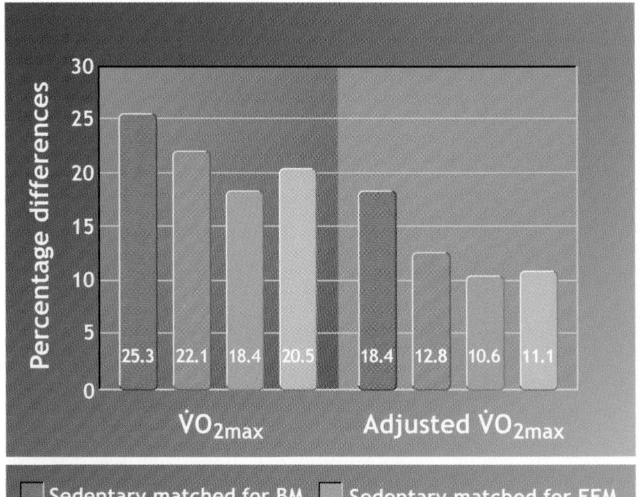

FIGURE 11.14 • Percentage differences in $\dot{V}O_{2max}$, including the adjustment for hemoglobin (*adjusted $\dot{V}O_{2max}$*), in sedentary and trained men and women matched for body mass (BM) and fat-free body mass (FFM). (From Keller BA, Katch FI. It is not valid to adjust gender differences in aerobic capacity and strength for body mass or lean body mass. Med Sci Sports Exerc 1991;23:S167.)

These findings suggest a biologically inherent and unalterable component to the gender difference in aerobic capacity. This does not mean that aerobic capacity cannot be significantly and equally affected for men and women by training or body composition alterations. Rather, the results suggest that a person should not necessarily expect gender-free differences in aerobic capacity. Chapter 22 presents data on gender differences in muscular strength from experiments with equally trained men and women with the same body size and composition.

Age

Age does not spare its effect on maximal oxygen consumption.[47,86,100] Although one can draw only limited inferences from cross-sectional studies of people of different ages, available data provide insight into the possible effects of aging on physiologic function. Figure 11.15 summarizes data from various studies on age trends in aerobic capacity of children and adults.

CHILDREN. Figure 11.15A and B illustrates age trends in the absolute and relative aerobic capacities of boys and girls aged 6 to 16 years.

- **Absolute values**—$\dot{V}O_{2max}$ values in $L \cdot min^{-1}$ (Fig. 11.15A) for boys and girls remain the same until about age 12; at age 14, $\dot{V}O_{2max}$ for boys averages 25% higher than that for girls, and by age 16 the difference exceeds 50%. The difference generally relates to the combined effect of the development of a greater muscle mass in boys and their greater daily physical activity levels.
- **Relative values**—For boys, average aerobic capacity in $mL \cdot kg^{-1} \cdot min^{-1}$ (Fig. 11.15B) remains level at about 52 $mL \cdot kg^{-1} \cdot min^{-1}$ from ages 6 to 16; for girls, the line slopes downward with age, reaching about 40 $mL \cdot kg^{-1} \cdot min^{-1}$ at age 16, a value 32% below that of their male counterparts. These lower values probably result from the greater accumulation of body fat in adolescent females; they must transport this extra fat that does not enhance the capacity for aerobic metabolism.[7,57]

ADULTS. $\dot{V}O_{2max}$ declines steadily after age 25 at a rate of about 1% per year, so at age 55 it averages about 27% below values reported for 20-year-olds (Fig. 11.15C). The data in the inset graph indicate that while active adults retain a relatively high $\dot{V}O_{2max}$ at all ages, it still progressively declines with advancing years. For eight women nearly 80 years of age, $\dot{V}O_{2max}$ averaged 13.4 $mL \cdot kg^{-1} \cdot min^{-1}$, or about 3.7 METs.[28] Despite this apparent significant aging effect, strong evidence indicates that a person's habitual level of physical activity exerts far greater influence on aerobic capacity than chronological age per se.[75] Chapter 31 more fully discusses age-related influences on physiologic function.

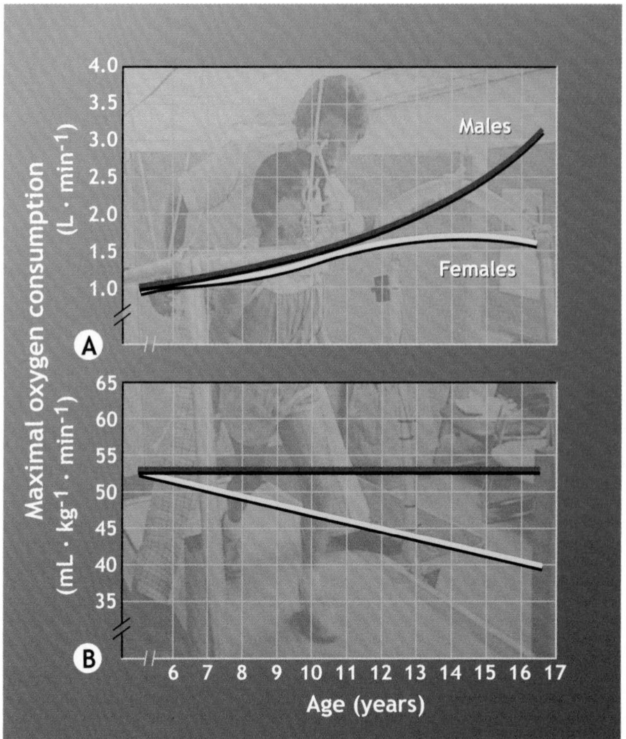

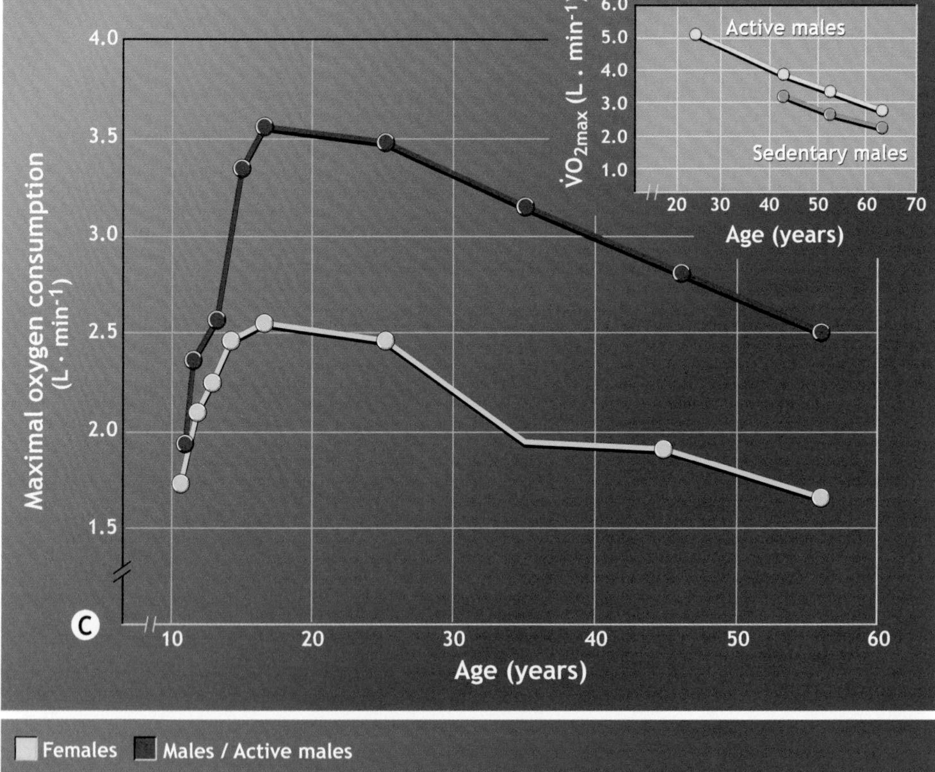

FIGURE 11.15 • Maximal oxygen consumption in relation to age in boys and girls (**A** and **B**) and men and women (**C**). (**A** and **B** from Krahenbuhl GS, et al. Developmental aspects of maximal aerobic power in children. Exerc Sport Sci Rev. Terjung RL, ed. vol 13, New York: Macmillan, 1985, **C** modified from Hermansen L. Individual differences. In: Larson LA, ed. Fitness, health, and work capacity. International standards for assessment. New York: Macmillan, 1974. Inset graph in **C** redrawn from tabled data of Åstrand PO, Rodahl KR. Textbook of work physiology. New York: McGraw-Hill, 1970.)

Aerobic Capacity Prediction Tests

The direct measurement of $\dot{V}O_{2max}$ requires an extensive laboratory, specialized equipment, and considerable subject motivation. Consequently, laboratory tests are impractical for measuring large groups of untrained subjects. In addition, strenuous exercise could prove risky to adults who do not receive proper medical clearance and appropriate safeguards or supervision. These considerations increase the importance of submaximal exercise testing to *predict* $\dot{V}O_{2max}$ from performance during walking and running or from heart rate measured during or immediately after exercise.

A Word of Caution About Predictions

All predictions contain error, referred to as the **standard error of estimate** (**SEE**), derived from the original equation for the prediction. Errors of estimate are expressed in measurement units of the predicted variable (e.g., kg, mL, s) or as a percentage. For example, suppose the $\dot{V}O_{2max}$ ($mL \cdot kg^{-1} \cdot min^{-1}$) predicted from time on a walking test equals 55 $mL \cdot kg^{-1} \cdot min^{-1}$, and the SEE is ± 10 $mL \cdot kg^{-1} \cdot min^{-1}$. This means that the actual $\dot{V}O_{2max}$ probably (68% confident) lies within ± 10 $mL \cdot kg^{-1} \cdot min^{-1}$ (between 45 and 65 $mL \cdot kg^{-1} \cdot min^{-1}$) of the predicted value. This represents a very large error.

Some predictions are associated with small errors (SEE $\leq 5\%$) and others with larger errors. Obviously, the larger the error, the less useful the predicted score, since the likely true score encompasses such a large range of possible values. Without knowing the magnitude of the SEE, one cannot judge the usefulness of a predicted score. Moreover, using some prediction methods on repeated occasions for the same individual (e.g., pre-, mid-, and posttraining) can introduce large and sometimes unknown errors. Whenever predictions are made, one must interpret the predicted score in light of the magnitude of the prediction error. With a relatively small prediction error, prediction of $\dot{V}O_{2max}$ can be useful in appropriate situations in which direct measurement is not possible.

Walking Tests

Walking tests can be used to predict $\dot{V}O_{2max}$. The following equation predicts $\dot{V}O_{2max}$ in $L \cdot min^{-1}$ from walking speed and other variables in men and women:[54]

$$\dot{V}O_{2max} = 6.9652 + (0.0091 \times Wt) - (0.0257 \times Age) + (0.5955 \times Gender) - (0.224 \times T1) - (0.0115 \times HR1\text{-}4)$$

where Wt is body weight in pounds; Age is in years; Gender is 0 for females, 1 for males; T1 is time for the 1-mile track walk, expressed as minutes and hundredths of a minute; and HR1-4 is heart rate in beats per minute measured immediately at the end of the last quarter-mile.

The following equation predicts $\dot{V}O_{2max}$ in $mL \cdot kg^{-1} \cdot min^{-1}$:

$$\dot{V}O_{2max} = 132.853 - (0.0769 \times Wt) - (0.3877 \times Age) + (6.315 \times Gender) - (3.2649 \times T1) - (0.1565 \times HR1\text{-}4)$$

The multiple correlation for predicting $\dot{V}O_{2max}$ from 1-mile walking performance for both equations is R = 0.92, with a standard error of prediction of 0.335 $L \cdot min^{-1}$, or 4.4 $mL \cdot kg^{-1} \cdot min^{-1}$. This means that about 68% of the people tested have an actual $\dot{V}O_{2max}$ within 0.335 $L \cdot min^{-1}$ (4.4 $mL \cdot kg^{-1} \cdot min^{-1}$) of the predicted value. Because the group studied ranged in age from 30 to 69 years, this prediction method applies to a large segment of the adult population.

The following data for a 30-year-old female illustrate the test's use:

Body weight = 155.5 lb
T1 = 13.56 min
HR1-4 = 145 $b \cdot min^{-1}$

Substituting in the equation to predict $\dot{V}O_{2max}$ in $mL \cdot kg^{-1} \cdot min^{-1}$:

$$\dot{V}O_{2max} = 132.853 - (0.0769 \times 155.5) - (0.3877 \times 30.0) + (6.315 \times 0) - (3.2649 \times 13.56) - (0.1565 \times 145)$$

$$\dot{V}O_{2max} = 132.853 - (11.96) - (11.63) + (0) - (44.27) - (22.69)$$

$$\dot{V}O_{2max} = 42.3\ mL \cdot kg^{-1} \cdot min^{-1}$$

Endurance Runs

Like walking tests, runs of various durations or distances can evaluate aerobic fitness.[3,18,49] Test use reasonably assumes that a person's ability to maintain a high, steady-rate oxygen consumption largely determines the distance run over at least 5 minutes' duration. This ability, in turn, depends on the maximum capacity to generate energy aerobically, that is, the $\dot{V}O_{2max}$. This rationale provided the framework for a field performance test devised in 1959 to evaluate aerobic fitness of military personnel.[3] The test required subjects to run as far as possible in 15 minutes. A 1968 study by Cooper shortened run time to 12 minutes.[18]

In his original validation of the 12-minute test, Cooper observed a strong association between $\dot{V}O_{2max}$ of Air Force personnel and the distances they could run-walk in 12 minutes. The correlation coefficient was $r = 0.90$ between 12-minute run-walk distance and $\dot{V}O_{2max}$ ($mL \cdot kg^{-1} \cdot min^{-1}$) in 47 men who varied considerably in age (17 to 54 y), body mass (52 to 123 kg), and $\dot{V}O_{2max}$ (31 to 59 $mL \cdot kg^{-1} \cdot min^{-1}$). Other researchers reported the same correlation for 9 ninth-grade boys.[22] However, subsequent studies have been unable to demonstrate as strong a connection between "Cooper test" scores and aerobic capacity. For example, one study measured 11- to 14-year-old boys and reported a correlation of $r = 0.65$.[64] For a group of 26 female athletes, the correlation between the run-walk scores and $\dot{V}O_{2max}$ was $r = 0.70$,[65] and for 36 untrained college women, a similar correlation of $r = 0.67$ emerged.[49]

Importantly, a simple correlation between run-walk scores and $\dot{V}O_{2max}$ does not consider the interacting effects of such factors as age and body mass. These variables themselves relate to both run-walk times and $\dot{V}O_{2max}$ scores. When restricting the original data of Cooper to the same age range as subjects in the preceding study of 36 untrained women, the computed correlation coefficient decreased dramatically from $r = 0.90$ to $r = 0.59$.

One must view with caution $\dot{V}O_{2max}$ predictions based on running performance. The need to establish a consistent level of motivation and effective pacing while running becomes critical with inexperienced subjects. Some individuals achieve an optimal pace throughout the run. Others may run too fast early in the run and be forced to slow down or even stop before completing the test. Other individuals may begin too slowly and continue this way, so that their final performance scores reflect inappropriate pacing or lack of motivation rather than poor physiologic capacity. In addition, $\dot{V}O_{2max}$ does not singularly determine endurance running performance. Body mass and fatness, running economy, and the percentage of aerobic capacity that one sustains without blood lactate buildup contribute significantly to successful running. *Generally, the SEE of predicting $\dot{V}O_{2max}$ from field tests such as walk-run performance averages about 8 to 10% of the predicted value.*

LIMITATIONS FOR USE WITH CHILDREN. Maximum 1-mile run or walk times serve only limited use for $\dot{V}O_{2max}$ prediction in growing children because the documented age-related exercise performance improvements in youth relate poorly to changes in aerobic capacity.[19] Rather, the largest contributions to test score improvement in children as they grow older result from (1) increased percentage of $\dot{V}O_{2peak}$ sustained during the exercise (i.e., increased blood lactate threshold) and (2) improved running economy. Both factors contribute significantly to faster times independent of any improvement in $\dot{V}O_{2max}$.

Predictions Based on Heart Rate

Tests to predict $\dot{V}O_{2max}$ use exercise or postexercise heart rate during a standardized regimen of submaximal exercise performed either on a bicycle ergometer or treadmill or in a step test. These tests apply the essentially linear relationship between heart rate (HR) and oxygen consumption ($\dot{V}O_2$) during increasing intensities of light to relatively heavy aerobic exercise. The slope of the line describing the HR–$\dot{V}O_2$ relationship (i.e., rate of heart rate increase) reflects the adequacy of the cardiovascular response and aerobic fitness capacity. The test administrator estimates $\dot{V}O_{2max}$ by drawing a best-fit straight line through several submaximal points that relate heart rate and oxygen consumption (or exercise intensity) and extends this **HR–$\dot{V}O_2$ line** to an assumed maximum heart rate for the subject's age.

Figure 11.16 illustrates the **extrapolation procedure** for an untrained and an endurance-trained college student. Four submaximal measures during graded exercise provided the data points to construct the HR–$\dot{V}O_2$ line. Although each person's HR–$\dot{V}O_2$ line tends toward linearity, the slope of the line often differs considerably. A person of relatively high aerobic fitness performs more-intense exercise (achieves higher $\dot{V}O_2$) before reaching a heart rate of 140 or 160 b · min^{-1} than does a less-fit person. Also, because heart rate increases linearly with exercise intensity ($\dot{V}O_2$), the person with the smallest heart rate increase tends to achieve the highest exercise capacity and, hence, the highest $\dot{V}O_{2max}$. Extrapolation of the HR–$\dot{V}O_2$ line to a heart rate of 195 b · min^{-1}—the assumed maximum heart rate for subjects of college age— predicted the $\dot{V}O_{2max}$ of the two subjects depicted in Figure 11.16.

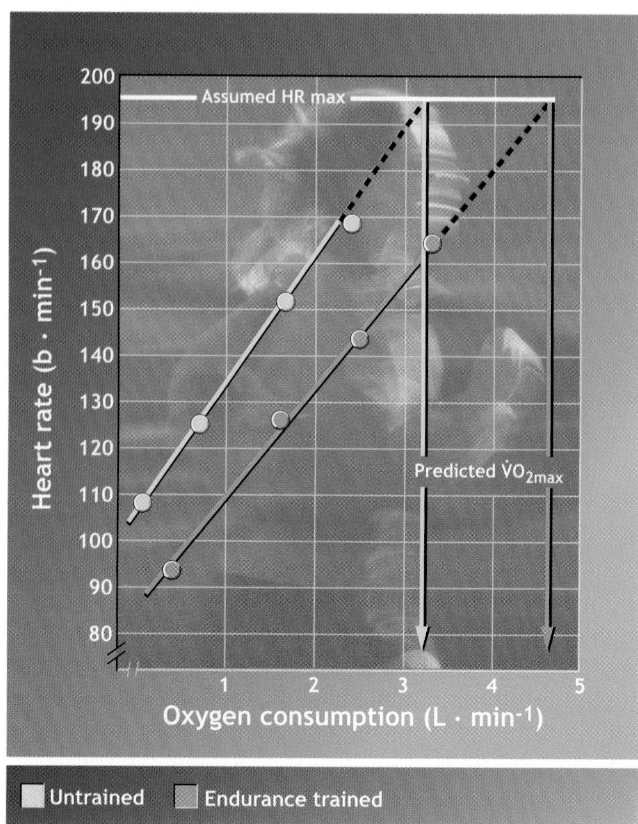

FIGURE 11.16 • Extrapolating the linear relationship between submaximal heart rate and oxygen consumption up to $\dot{V}O_{2max}$ during graded exercise by an untrained and an endurance-trained subject.

The following assumptions limit the accuracy of the $\dot{V}O_{2max}$ prediction from submaximal exercise heart rate:

- *Linearity of heart rate–oxygen consumption (exercise intensity) relationship.* This assumption generally holds, particularly during light-to-moderate exercise. In some subjects, however, the HR–$\dot{V}O_2$ line curves (asymptotes) at more-intense workloads in a direction that indicates a larger-than-expected increase in oxygen consumption per unit increase in heart rate. Oxygen consumption actually increases more than predicted by linear extrapolation of the HR–$\dot{V}O_2$ line. This underestimates the $\dot{V}O_{2max}$ of these subjects.
- *Similar maximum heart rates for all subjects.* One standard deviation from the average maximum heart rate for individuals of the same age equals ±10 b · min^{-1}. Therefore, extrapolating the HR–$\dot{V}O_2$ line of a young adult to 195 b · min^{-1} overestimates the $\dot{V}O_{2max}$ of a person whose actual maximum heart rate is 185 b · min^{-1}. The opposite occurs for a subject with an actual maximum heart rate of 210 b · min^{-1}. Maximum heart rate also decreases with age. Failure to consider this age effect (i.e., extrapolating to a heart rate of 195 b · min^{-1}, the average heart rate for 25-year-olds) consistently overestimates $\dot{V}O_{2max}$ in

older subjects. Chapter 31 discusses the effect of age on maximum heart rate.

- *Assumed constant economy and mechanical efficiency during exercise.* Variations in exercise economy contribute to $\dot{V}O_{2max}$ prediction errors with tests that estimate submaximal oxygen consumption from the external workload (rather than measuring $\dot{V}O_2$ directly). More specifically, an underestimation of $\dot{V}O_{2max}$ results for a subject with poor exercise economy whose submaximal oxygen consumption increases more than assumed on the basis of estimates from exercise intensity. This occurs because of an elevated heart rate from the added oxygen cost of uneconomical exercise. Variation in walking or cycling economy among individuals usually does not exceed 6%; for bench-stepping, the variation can equal about 10%, a value unrelated to age, leg length, aerobic fitness, or body fat.[104] Seemingly small modifications in test procedures also profoundly affect the economy of exercise. Simply allowing individuals to support themselves with the treadmill handrails reduces the oxygen cost of exercise by as much as 30%.[124]
- *Day-to-day heart rate variation.* Even under highly standardized conditions, the day-to-day variation in heart rate averages about 5 b · min^{-1} during submaximal exercise.

Within the framework of these limitations, $\dot{V}O_{2max}$ predicted from submaximal heart rate generally falls within 10 to 20% of the person's actual value. While this accuracy level remains unacceptable for research purposes, the prediction tests can effectively screen and classify individuals for aerobic fitness. The technique also has proved useful for estimating aerobic capacity during pregnancy (see "In a Practical Sense," Chapter 9).[92]

The Step Test

A practical way to classify people for aerobic fitness uses heart rate during recovery from a standardized stepping exercise. "Prediction equations," applied to step-test results, have estimated $\dot{V}O_{2max}$ with reasonable accuracy.

We used a simple 3-minute step test to evaluate exercise heart rate responses of thousands of college men and women.[69] The test used gymnasium bleachers (16¼ in high) to test large numbers of students at the same time. Subjects performed each stepping cycle to a four-step cadence, "up-up-down-down." The women performed 22 complete step-ups per minute, regulated by a metronome set at 88 beats per minute. Because males tended to be "fitter" for step-up exercise than females, their cadence was 24 step-ups per minute or 96 beats per minute on the metronome. The step test began after a brief demonstration and practice period. At the completion of stepping, students remained standing while pulse rate was measured for 15 seconds, 5 to 20 seconds into recovery. Recovery heart rate was converted to beats per minute (15-s HR × 4) and compared with the established percentile rankings presented in Table 11.6.

INTEGRATIVE QUESTION

Respond to a student who asks: "I've had my $\dot{V}O_{2max}$ measured directly in the laboratory and predicted with a 12-minute run. Why don't both values agree?"

TABLE 11.6 ➤ **PERCENTILE RANKINGS FOR STEP TEST RECOVERY HEART RATE (HR) AND PREDICTED $\dot{V}O_{2max}$ FOR UNTRAINED MALE AND FEMALE COLLEGE STUDENTS**

Percentile Ranking	Recovery HR, Female	Predicted $\dot{V}O_{2max}$ (mL · kg^{-1} · min^{-1})	Recovery HR, Male	Predicted $\dot{V}O_{2max}$ (mL · kg^{-1} · min^{-1})
100	128	42.2	120	60.9
95	140	40.0	124	59.3
90	148	38.5	128	57.6
85	152	37.7	136	54.2
80	156	37.0	140	52.5
75	158	36.6	144	50.9
70	160	36.3	148	49.2
65	162	35.9	149	48.8
60	163	35.7	152	47.5
55	164	35.5	154	46.7
50	166	35.1	156	45.8
45	168	34.8	160	44.1
40	170	34.4	162	43.3
35	171	34.2	164	42.5
30	172	34.0	166	41.6
25	176	33.3	168	40.8
20	180	32.6	172	39.1
15	182	32.2	176	37.4
10	184	31.8	178	36.6
5	196	29.6	184	34.1

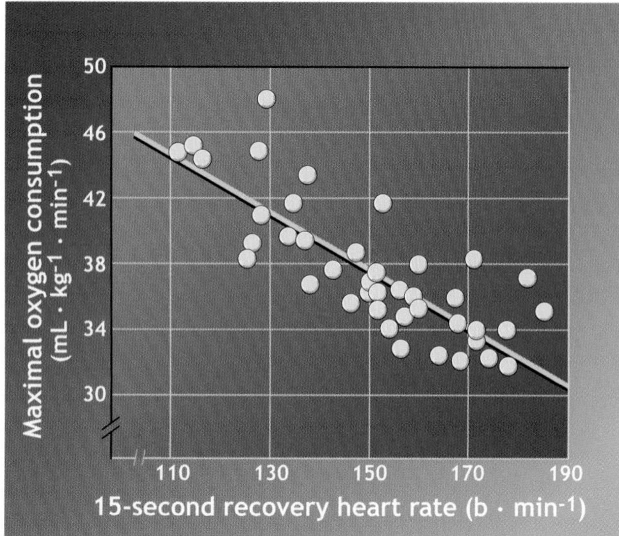

FIGURE 11.17 • Scattergram and line of "best fit" relating step-test heart rate score and maximal oxygen consumption in untrained college women.

Based on the essentially linear relationship between heart rate and oxygen consumption during submaximal exercise, one would expect a person with a low step-test heart rate (i.e., farther from maximum) to experience less exercise stress than someone performing the identical exercise with a relatively high heart rate. In other words, a lower heart rate during a standard exercise corresponds to a higher $\dot{V}O_{2max}$. To determine the validity of the step test for estimating aerobic capacity, we measured the $\dot{V}O_{2max}$ for a group of untrained, young adult men and women who also performed the step test.[69] Figure 11.17 illustrates the relationship between $\dot{V}O_{2max}$ and the women's step-test scores. The results clearly indicated that step-test heart rate provided significant information about $\dot{V}O_{2max}$. Subjects with a high recovery heart rate tended to have a lower $\dot{V}O_{2max}$, whereas a faster recovery (lower heart rate) related to a relatively high $\dot{V}O_{2max}$. The following equations predict $\dot{V}O_{2max}$ (mL · kg^{-1} · min^{-1}) from step-test results for similar groups of young adult men and women:

Men:
$\dot{V}O_{2max}$ = 111.33 – (0.42 × step-test pulse rate [b · min^{-1}])

Women:
$\dot{V}O_{2max}$ = 65.81 – (0.1847 × step-test pulse rate [b · min^{-1}])

To simplify these conversions, the "Predicted $\dot{V}O_{2max}$" columns of Table 11.6 present the maximal oxygen consumption values for men and women, based on recovery heart rate scores. For predictive accuracy, one can be 95% confidant that the predicted $\dot{V}O_{2max}$ falls within 16% of the person's true $\dot{V}O_{2max}$. For a high degree of accuracy, one must measure $\dot{V}O_{2max}$ directly in the laboratory using an appropriate, graded exercise test. If this proves impractical or if accuracy can be compromised somewhat, prediction tests provide reasonable alternatives but *not* precise benchmarks.

Predictions From Nonexercise Data

A unique approach to $\dot{V}O_{2max}$ prediction for quick screening of large groups of individuals involves collecting specific nonexercise data from a questionnaire.[31] The SEE for a predicted score equals ±3.44 mL O_2 · kg^{-1} · min^{-1}.

Data input to predict $\dot{V}O_{2max}$:

1. **Sex** (female = 0; male = 1)
2. **Body mass index (BMI; kg · m^{-2})**. Self-reported body mass (kg) and body stature (m) used to compute BMI as follows:

   BMI = Body mass (kg) ÷ Stature (m^2)

3. **Physical activity rating (PA-R)**. A point value between 0 and 10 representing overall physical activity level for the previous 6 months (Table 11.7A)
4. **Perceived functional ability (PFA)**. Sum of the point values between 0 and 13 for questions about current level of perceived functional ability to maintain a continuous pace on an indoor track for 1 mile and perceived pace to cover a distance of 3 miles without becoming breathless or overly fatigued (Table 11.7B).

Equation

$\dot{V}O_{2max}$ (mL · kg^{-1} · min^{-1}) = 44.895 + (7.042 × Sex) – (0.823 × BMI) + (0.738 × PFA) + (0.688 × PA-R)

Example

1. Sex, female
2. BMI = 22.66 (self-reported body mass = 136 lb [61.7 kg]; self-reported height = 5 feet 5 inches [1.65 m]);
   BMI = 61.7 ÷ (1.65 × 1.65) = 22.66
3. PA-R score = 5 (see Table 11.7A)
4. PFA score = 15 (sum of 7 scored on first set of questions and 8 on second set; see Table 11.7B.)

Computation

$\dot{V}O_{2max}$ = 44.895 + (7.042 × Sex) – (0.823 × BMI) + (0.738 × PFA) + (0.688 × PA-R)
= 44.895 + (7.042 × 0) – (0.823 × 22.66) + (0.73 × 15 + (0.688 × 5)
= 44.895 + 0 – 18.65 + 11.07 + 3.77
= 41.1 mL · kg^{-1} · min^{-1}

TABLE 11.7 ➤ **INPUT INFORMATION ON LEVEL OF PHYSICAL ACTIVITY AND PERCEIVED FUNCTIONAL CAPACITY FOR PREDICTING $\dot{V}O_{2MAX}$ FROM NON-EXERCISE DATA.**

A. PHYSICAL ACTIVITY RATING (PA-R)

SELECT THE NUMBER THAT BEST DESCRIBES YOUR OVERALL LEVEL OF PHYSICAL ACTIVITY FOR THE PREVIOUS 6 MONTHS:

Points	Description
0	**inactive:** avoid walking or exertion; e.g., always use elevator, drive when possible instead of walking
1	**light activity:** walk for pleasure, routinely use stairs, occasionally exercise sufficiently to cause heavy breathing or perspiration
2	**moderate activity:** 10 to 60 minutes per week of moderate activity such as golf, horseback riding, calisthenics, table tennis, bowling, weight lifting, yard work, cleaning house, walking for exercise
3	**moderate activity:** over 1 hour per week of moderate activity described above
4	**vigorous activity:** run less than 1 mile per week or spend less than 30 min per week in comparable activity such as running or jogging, lap swimming, cycling, rowing, aerobics, skipping rope, running in place, or engaging in vigorous aerobic-type activity such as soccer, basketball, tennis, racquetball, or handball
5	**vigorous activity:** run 1 mile to less than 5 miles per week or spend 30 min to less than 60 min per week in comparable physical activity as described above
6	**vigorous activity:** run 5 miles to less than 10 miles per week or spend 1 hour to less than 3 hours per week in comparable physical activity as described above
7	**vigorous activity:** run 10 miles to less than 15 miles per week or spend 3 hours to less than 6 hours per week in comparable physical activity as described above
8	**vigorous activity:** run 15 miles to less than 20 miles per week or spend 6 hours to less than 7 hours per week in comparable physical activity as described above
9	**vigorous activity:** run 20 to 25 miles per week or spend 7 to 8 hours per week in comparable physical activity as described above
10	**vigorous activity:** run over 25 miles per week or spend over 8 hours per week in comparable physical activity as described above

B. PERCEIVED FUNCTIONAL ABILITY (PFA) QUESTIONS

SUPPOSE YOU EXERCISE CONTINUOUSLY ON AN INDOOR TRACK FOR 1 MILE. WHICH EXERCISE PACE IS RIGHT FOR YOU—NOT TOO EASY OR NOT TOO HARD? CIRCLE THE APPROPRIATE NUMBER FROM 1 TO 13.

Points	Description
1	Walking at a slow pace (18-min mile or more)
2	
3	Walking at a medium pace (16-min mile)
4	
5	Walking at a fast pace (14-min mile)
6	
7	Jogging at a slow pace (12-min mile)
8	
9	Jogging at a medium pace (10-min mile)
10	
11	Jogging at a fast pace (8-min mile)
12	
13	Running at a fast pace (7-min mile or less)

HOW FAST COULD YOU COVER A DISTANCE OF 3 MILES AND NOT BECOME BREATHLESS OR OVERLY FATIGUED? BE REALISTIC. CIRCLE THE APPROPRIATE NUMBER FROM 1 TO 13.

Points	Description
1	I could walk the entire distance at a slow pace (18-min per mile or more)
2	
3	I could walk the entire distance at a medium pace (16-min per mile)
4	
5	I could walk the entire distance at a fast pace (14-min per mile)
6	
7	I could jog the entire distance at a slow pace (12-min per mile)
8	
9	I could jog the entire distance at a medium pace (10-min per mile)
10	
11	I could jog the entire distance at a fast pace (8-min per mile)
12	
13	I could run the entire distance at a fast pace (7-min per mile or less)

From George JD, et al. Non-exercise $\dot{V}O_{2max}$ estimation for physically active college students. Med Sci Sports Exerc 1997;29:415.

Summary

1. The concepts of individual differences and exercise specificity provide an important framework for understanding anaerobic and aerobic power capacities. The term individual differences refers to real differences among individuals in contrast to the instability of a measure for any one person. Specificity refers to metabolic and physiologic functions that do not apply generally to all forms of exercise but rather depend on multiple factors.
2. Precise contributions of anaerobic and aerobic energy transfer depend largely on exercise intensity and duration. During strength and power–sprint activities, energy transfer primarily involves the immediate and short-term (anaerobic) energy systems. The long-term (aerobic) energy system becomes progressively more active during exercise lasting longer than 2 minutes.
3. Appropriate physiologic measurements and performance tests evaluate the capacity of each energy-transfer system. These tests can (1) evaluate energy-transfer capacity at a particular point in time or (2) show changes consequent to a specific exercise training program.
4. The stair-sprinting test commonly measures the power capacity of the intramuscular high-energy phosphates ATP and PCr. The 30-second, all-out Wingate test evaluates peak power and average power output capacity from the glycolytic pathway. Interpretations of test results must consider body size and the exercise specificity principle.
5. The maximal accumulated oxygen deficit (MAOD) positively correlates with other anaerobic performance tests, demonstrates independence from aerobic energy sources, and differentiates between aerobically and anaerobically trained individuals.
6. Training status, acid-base regulation, and motivation contribute to individual differences in the capacities of the immediate and short-term energy systems.
7. Maximal oxygen consumption ($\dot{V}O_{2max}$) provides important, reproducible information on the power capacity of the long-term energy system, including the functional capacity of the physiologic support systems. Consideration of the dynamics of metabolic and physiologic functions during the test helps determine whether the result represents true $\dot{V}O_{2max}$.
8. Heredity, state and type of training, age, gender, and body composition contribute uniquely to an individual's $\dot{V}O_{2max}$
9. Expressing aerobic capacity by some ratio of body size or composition (e.g., $mL \cdot kg^{-1} \cdot min^{-1}$ or $mL \cdot kgFFM^{-1} \cdot min^{-1}$) reduces the gender difference in $\dot{V}O_{2max}$. However, such ratio manipulation does not answer the question whether true gender differences exist in $\dot{V}O_{2max}$.
10. Tests to predict $\dot{V}O_{2max}$ from submaximal physiologic and performance data often prove useful for classification purposes. However, the quality of the inferences relies on the validity of the test's assumptions. These assumptions include (1) linearity of the HR–$\dot{V}O_2$ relationship, (2) constancy in maximum heart rates, (3) relatively constant exercise economy, and (4) minimal day-to-day variation in exercise heart rate.
11. When used and interpreted properly, field methods provide useful information about cardiovascular-aerobic function in the absence of more-valid laboratory methods.
12. $\dot{V}O_{2max}$ can be predicted from nonexercise data with accuracy acceptable for screening and classification purposes.

References

1. Armstrong N, Welsman JR. Assessment and interpretation of aerobic fitness in children and adolescents. Exerc Sport Sci Rev 1994;22:435.
2. Åstrand PO, Saltin B. Maximal oxygen uptake and heart rate in various types of muscular activity. J Appl Physiol 1961;16:977.
3. Balke B, Ware RW. An experimental study of fitness of Air Force personnel. US Armed Forces Med J 1959;10:675.
4. Bangsbo J, et al. Anaerobic energy production and O_2 deficit-debt relationship during exhaustive exercise in humans. J Physiol (Lond) 1990;422:539.
5. Bar-Or O. The Wingate anaerobic test: an update on methodology, reliability, and validity. Sports Med 1987;4:381.
6. Bergh V. The influence of body mass in cross-country skiing. Med Sci Sports Exerc 1987;19:324.
7. Beunen G, Malina R. Growth and physical performance relative to timing of the adolescent spurt. Exercise and Sport Sciences Reviews. Pandolf KB, ed. vol 16. New York: Macmillan, 1988.
8. Blomquist CG, et al. Similarity of the hemodynamic responses to static, and dynamic exercise of small muscle groups. Circ Res 1982;48(suppl I):87.
9. Bonen A, et al. Maximal oxygen uptake during free, tethered, and flume swimming. J Appl Physiol 1980;48:232.
10. Bouchard C, Pérusse L. Heredity, activity level, fitness, and health. In: Bouchard C, et al., eds. Physical activity, fitness, and health. Champaign, IL: Human Kinetics, 1994.
11. Bouchard C, et al. Genetics of aerobic and anaerobic performance. Exerc Sport Sci Rev 1992;20:27.
12. Bouchard C, et al. Familial resemblance for $\dot{V}O_{2max}$ in the sedentary state: the HERITAGE family study. Med Sci Sports Exerc 1998;30:252.
13. Brahler CJ, Blank SE. VersaClimbing elicits higher $\dot{V}O_{2max}$ than does treadmill running or rowing ergometry. Med Sci Sports Exerc 1995;27:249.
14. Brooks GA. Intra- and extra-cellular lactate shuttles. Med Sci Sports Exerc 2000;32:790.
15. Buchfuhrer MJ, et al. Optimizing the exercise protocol for cardiopulmonary assessment. J Appl Physiol 1983;55:1558.
16. Buskirk ER, Hodgson JL. Age and aerobic power: the rate of change in men and women. Fed Proc 1997;46:1824.
17. Carey P, et al. Comparison of oxygen uptake during maximal work on the rowing ergometer. Med Sci Sport 1974;6:101.
18. Cooper K. Correlation between field and treadmill testing as a means for assessing maximal oxygen intake. JAMA 1968;203:201.
19. Cureton KJ, et al. Metabolic determinants of the age-related improvement in one-mile run/walk performance in youth. Med Sci Sports Exerc 1997;29:259.
20. Davis JA, et al. Effect of ramp slope on measurement of aerobic parameters from the ramp exercise test. Med Sci Sports Exerc 1982;14:339.
21. Donovan CM, Pagliassotti MJ. Quantitative assessment of pathways for lactate disposal in skeletal muscle fiber types. Med Sci Sports Exerc 2000;32:772.
22. Doolittle TL, Bigbee R. The twelve-minute run-walk: a test of cardiorespiratory fitness of adolescent boys. Res Q 1968;39:41.

23. Duncan GE, et al. Applicability of $\dot{V}O_{2max}$ criteria: discontinuous versus continuous protocols. Med Sci Sports Exerc 1997;29:273.
24. Eriksson BO. Muscle metabolism in children: a review. Acta Paediatr Scand 1980;283 (suppl):20.
25. Esbjornsson B, et al. Fast-twitch fibers may predict anaerobic performance in both females and males. Int J Sports Med 1993;14:257.
26. Fairshter RD, et al. A comparison of incremental exercise tests during cycle and treadmill ergometry. Med Sci Sports Exerc 1983;15:549.
27. Ferguson RJ, et al. A maximal oxygen uptake test during ice skating. Med Sci Sport 1969;1:207.
28. Foster VL, et al. The reproducibility of $\dot{V}O_{2max}$, ventilatory, and lactate threshold in elderly women. Med Sci Sports Exerc 1986;18:425.
29. Fournier M. Skeletal muscle adaptation in adolescent boys: endurance training and detraining. Med Sci Sports Exerc 1982;14:453.
30. Gayagay G, et al. Elite endurance athletes and the ACE I allele—the rose of genes in athletic performance. Hum Genet 1998;103:48.
31. George JD, et al. Non-exercise $\dot{V}O_{2max}$ estimation for physically active college students. Med Sci Sports Exerc 1997;29:415.
32. Gergley T, et al. Specificity of arm training on aerobic power during swimming and running. Med Sci Sports Exerc 1984;16:349.
33. Giacomoni M, et al. Influence of the menstrual cycle phase and menstrual symptoms on maximal anaerobic performance. Med Sci Sports Exerc 2000;32:486.
34. Gladden LB. The role of skeletal muscle in lactate exchange during exercise: introduction. Med Sci Sports Exerc 2000;32:753.
35. Gladden LB. Muscle as a consumer of lactate. Med Sci Sports Exerc 2000;32:764.
36. Gollnick PD, Saltin B. Significance of skeletal muscle oxidative enzyme enhancement with endurance training. Clin Physiol 1982;2:1.
37. Gollnick PD, et al. Glycogen depletion pattern in human skeletal muscle fiber after heavy exercise. J Appl Physiol 1973;34:615.
38. Hagberg JM, et al. Comparison of three procedures for measuring $\dot{V}O_{2max}$ in competitive cyclists. Eur J Appl Physiol 1978;39:47.
39. Hagberg JM, et al. Specific genetic markers of endurance performance and $\dot{V}O_{2max}$. Exerc Sport Sci Rev 2001;29:15.
40. Hirvonen J, et al. Breakdown of high-energy phosphate compounds and lactate accumulation during short supramaximal exercise. Eur J Appl Physiol 1987;56:253.
41. Holloszy JO, Coyle EF. Adaptations of skeletal muscle to endurance exercise and their metabolic consequences. J Appl Physiol 1984;56:831.
42. Howley ET, et al. Criteria for maximal oxygen uptake: review and commentary. Med Sci Sports Exerc 1995;27:1292.
43. Inbar O, Bar-Or O. Anaerobic characteristics in male children and adolescents. Med Sci Sports Exerc 1986;18:264.
44. Joyner MJ. Physiological limiting factors and distance running: influence of gender and age on record performances. Exerc Sport Sci Rev 1993;21:103.
45. Karlsson J, et al. Muscle metabolites during submaximal and maximal exercise in man. Scand J Clin Lab Invest 1971;26:385.
46. Kasch FW, et al. A comparison of maximal oxygen uptake by treadmill and step test procedures. J Appl Physiol 1966;21:1387.
47. Kasch FW, et al. A longitudinal study of cardiovascular stability in active men aged 45 to 65 years. Phys Sportsmed 1988;16:117.
48. Katch FI, McArdle WD. Introduction to nutrition, exercise, and health. 4th ed. Philadelphia: Lea & Febiger, 1993.
49. Katch FI, et al. Maximal oxygen intake, endurance running performance, and body composition in college women. Res Q 1973;44:301.
50. Katch VL. Kinetics of oxygen uptake and recovery for supramaximal work of short duration. Int Z Angew Physiol 1973;31:197.
51. Katch VL. Use of the oxygen/body weight ratio in correlational analyses: spurious correlations and statistical considerations. Med Sci Sports 1973;5:253.
52. Katch VL, et al. Optimal test characteristics for maximal anaerobic work on the bicycle ergometer. Res Q 1977;48:319.
53. Keller B, Katch FI. It is not valid to adjust gender differences in aerobic capacity and strength for body mass or lean body mass. Med Sci Sports Exerc 1991;23:S167.
54. Kline G, et al. Estimation of $\dot{V}O_{2max}$ from a one-mile track walk, gender, age, and body weight. Med Sci Sports Exerc 1987;19:253.
55. Klissouras V, et al. Adaptation to maximal effort: genetics and age. J Appl Physiol 1973;35:288.
56. Koziris LB, et al. Relationship of aerobic power to anaerobic performance indices. J Strength Cond Res 1996;10:35.
57. Krahenbuhl GS, et al. Developmental aspects of maximal aerobic power in children. Exercise and Sport Sciences Reviews. RL Terjung, ed. vol. 13. New York: Macmillan, 1985.
58. Lewis SF, et al. Cardiovascular responses to exercise as functions of absolute and relative work load. J Appl Physiol 1983;54:1314.
59. Lortie G, et al. Muscle fiber type composition and enzyme activities in brothers and monozygotic twins. In: Malina RM, Bouchard C, eds. Proceedings of the 1984 Olympic Scientific Congress, vol. 4: Sport and human genetics. Champaign, IL: Human Kinetics, 1986.
60. Maes HH, et al. Inheritance of physical fitness in 10-yr-old twins and their parents. Med Sci Sports Exerc 1996;28:1479.
61. Magel JR, Faulkner JA. Maximum oxygen uptake of college swimmers. J Appl Physiol 1967;22:929.
62. Magel JR, et al. Specificity of swim training on maximum oxygen uptake. J Appl Physiol 1975;38:151.
63. Magel JR, et al. Metabolic and cardiovascular adjustment to arm training. J Appl Physiol 1978;45:75.
64. Maksud MG, Coutts KD. Application of the Cooper twelve-minute run-walk to young males. Res Q 1971;42:54.
65. Maksud MG, et al. Energy expenditure and $\dot{V}O_{2max}$ of female athletes during treadmill exercise. Res Q 1976;47:692.
66. Margaria R, et al. Measurement of muscular power (anaerobic) in man. J Appl Physiol 1966;21:1662.
67. Mayhew JL, Salm PC. Gender differences in anaerobic power tests. Eur J Appl Physiol 1990;60:133.
68. McArdle WD, et al. Metabolic and cardiorespiratory response during free swimming and treadmill walking. J Appl Physiol 1971;30:733.
69. McArdle WD, et al. Reliability and inter-relationships between maximal oxygen intake, physical work capacity, and step-test scores in college women. Med Sci Sport 1972;4:182.
70. McArdle WD, et al. Comparison of continuous and discontinuous treadmill and bicycle tests for max $\dot{V}O_2$. Med Sci Sport 1973;5:156.
71. McArdle WD, et al. Specificity of run training on $\dot{V}O_{2max}$ and heart rate changes during running and swimming. Med Sci Sport 1978;10:16.
72. Medbo JL, et al. Anaerobic capacity determined by maximal accumulated oxygen deficit. J Appl Physiol 1988;64:50.
73. Medbo JL, et al. Relative importance of aerobic and anaerobic energy release during short-lasting exhausting exercise. J Appl Physiol 1989;67:1881.
74. Menier DR, Pugh LGCE. The relation of oxygen intake and velocity of walking in competition walkers. J Physiol (Lond) 1968;197:717.
75. Meredith CN, et al. Body composition and aerobic capacity in young and middle-aged endurance-trained men. Med Sci Sports Exerc 1987;19:557.
76. Mitchell J, et al. The physiological meaning of the maximal oxygen intake test. J Clin Invest 1958;37:538.
77. Montgomery HE, et al. Human gene for physical performance. Nature 1998;393:221.
78. Naughton GA, et al. Accumulated oxygen deficit measurements during and after high-intensity exercise in trained male and female adolescents. Eur J Appl Physiol 1997;76:525.
79. Naughton J, et al. Treadmill exercise in assessment of patients with cardiac disease. Am J Cardiol 1972;30:757.
80. Nebelsick-Gullett LJ, et al. A comparison between methods of measuring anaerobic work capacity. Ergonomics 1988;31:1413.
81. Nindl BC, et al. Lower and upper body anaerobic performance in male and female adolescent athletes. Med Sci Sports Exerc 1995; 27:235.
82. Pechar GS, et al. Specificity of cardiorespiratory adaptation to bicycle and treadmill training. J Appl Physiol 1974;36:753.
83. Pérusse L, et al. Inter-generation transmission of physical fitness in the Canadian population. Can J Sport Sci 1988;13:8.
84. Pérusse L, et al. Genetic and environmental influences on level of habitual physical activity and exercise participation. Am J Epidemiol 1989;129:1012.
85. Piehl K. Glycogen storage and depletion in human skeletal muscle fibers. Acta Physiol Scand 1974:402(suppl):1.
86. Proctor DN, Joyner MJ. Skeletal muscle mass and the reduction of $\dot{V}O_{2max}$ in trained older subjects. J Appl Physiol 1997;82:1411.
87. Prud'homme D, et al. Sensitivity of maximal aerobic power to training is genotype-dependent. Med Sci Sports Exerc 1994;16:489.
88. Rivera MA, et al. Linkage between a muscle-specific CK gene marker and $\dot{V}O_{2max}$ in the HERITAGE Family Study. Med Sci Sports Exerc 1999;31:698.

89. Rowland TW. Does peak $\dot{V}O_2$ reflect $\dot{V}O_{2max}$ in children? Med Sci Sports Exerc 1993;25:689.
90. Rundell KW. Treadmill roller ski test predicts biathlon roller ski race results of elite U.S. biathlon women. Med Sci Sports Exerc 1995;27:1677.
91. Saavedra C, et al. Maximal anaerobic performance of the knee extensor muscles during growth. Med Sci Sports Exerc 1991;23:1083.
92. Sady SP, et al. Prediction of $\dot{V}O_{2max}$ during cycle exercise in pregnant women. J Appl Physiol 1988;65:657.
93. Saltin B. Metabolic fundamentals in exercise. Med Sci Sport 1973;5:137.
94. Sargent DA. Physical test of man. Am Phys Ed Rev 1921;26:188.
95. Sawka MN. Physiology of upper body exercise. Exerc Sport Sci Rev 1986;14:175.
96. Scott B, et al. The maximally accumulated oxygen deficit as an indicator of anaerobic capacity. Med Sci Sports Exerc 1991;23:618.
97. Sparling PB, et al. The gender difference in distance running performance has plateaued: an analysis of world rankings from 1980 to 1996. Med Sci Sports Exerc 1998;30:1725.
98. Spencer MR, Gastin PB. Energy system contribution during 200-m to 1500-m running in highly trained athletes. Med Sci Sports Exerc 2001;33:157.
99. Spriet LL, et al. An enzymatic approach to lactate production in human skeletal muscle during exercise. Med Sci Sports Exerc 2000;32:756.
100. Stamford BA. Exercise in the elderly. Exercise and Sport Sciences Reviews. Pandolf KB, ed. vol. 16. New York: Macmillan, 1988.
101. Strømme SB, et al. Assessment of maximal aerobic power in specially trained athletes. J Appl Physiol 1977;42:833.
102. Taylor HL, et al. Maximal oxygen intake as an objective measure of cardiorespiratory performance. J Appl Physiol 1955;8:73.
103. Thomas M, et al. Leg power in young women: relationship to body composition, strength, and function. Med Sci Sports Exerc 1996;28:1321.
104. Thomas SG, et al. Sources of variation in oxygen consumption during a stepping task. Med Sci Sports Exerc 1993;25:139.
105. Toner MN, et al. Cardiorespiratory responses to exercise distributed between the upper and lower body. J Appl Physiol 1983;54:1403.
106. Vandenberghe K, et al. No effect of glycogen level on glycogen metabolism during high intensity exercise. Med Sci Sports Exerc 1995;27:1278.
107. Veeger HEJ, et al. Peak oxygen uptake and maximal power output of Olympic wheelchair-dependent athletes. Med Sci Sports Exerc 1991;23:1201.
108. Vogel JA, et al. An analysis of aerobic capacity in a large United States population. J Appl Physiol 1986;60:494.
109. Wagner PD. New ideas on limitations to $\dot{V}O_{2max}$. Exer Sport Sci Rev 2000;1:10.
110. Wallick ME, et al. Physiological responses to in-line skating compared to treadmill running. Med Sci Sports Exerc 1995;27:242.
111. Washburn RA, Seals DR. Peak oxygen uptake during arm cranking in men and women. J Appl Physiol 1984;56:954.
112. Wasserman K, et al. Principles of exercise testing and interpretation. 3rd ed, Baltimore: Lipincott Williams & Wilkins, 1999.
113. Wells CL, Plowman SA. Sexual differences in athletic performance: biological or behavioral? Phys Sportsmed 1983;11:52.
114. Weinstein Y, et al. Reliability of peak-lactate, heart rate, and plasma volume following the Wingate test. Med Sci Sports Exerc 1998;30:1456.
115. Weyand PG, et al. Peak oxygen deficit during one- and two-legged cycling in men and women. Med Sci Sports Exerc 1993;25:584.
116. Whipp BJ, Ward SA. Will women soon outrun men? Nature 1992;355:25.
117. Wilkes D, et al. Effect of acute induced metabolic alkalosis on 800-m racing time. Med Sci Sports Exerc 1983;4:277.
118. Wilmore JH. Influence of motivation on physical work capacity and performance. J Appl Physiol 1968;24:459.
119. Winter EM, et al. Maximal exercise performance and lean leg volume in men and women. J Sports Sci 1991;9:3.
120. Woodson RD. Hemoglobin concentration and exercise capacity. Am Rev Respir Dis 1984;129(suppl):72.
121. Wyndham CH, Hegns AJA. Determinants of oxygen consumption and maximum oxygen intake of Caucasians and Bantu males. Int Z Angew Physiol 1969;27:51.
122. Yamamoto SH, et al. Quantitative estimation of anaerobic and oxidative energy metabolism and contraction characteristics in intact human skeletal muscle in response to electrical stimulation. Clin Physiol 1983;3:227.
123. Zajac A, et al. The diagnostic value of the 10- and 30-second Wingate test for competitive athletes. J Strength Cond Res 1999;13:16.
124. Zeimetz GA, et al. Quantifiable changes in oxygen uptake, heart rate, and time to target heart rate when hand support is allowed during treadmill exercise. J Cardiac Rehabil 1985;11:525.

SECTION

3

Systems of Energy Delivery and Utilization

Many sports, recreational, and occupational activities require a moderately intense and sustained energy release. The aerobic breakdown of carbohydrates, fats, and proteins provides energy for exercise by phosphorylating adenosine diphosphate (ADP) to adenosine triphosphate (ATP). Without a steady rate between oxidative phosphorylation of ADP to ATP and the energy requirements of exercise, an anaerobic–aerobic energy imbalance develops, tissue acidity increases, and fatigue eventually ensues. Sustaining a high level of physical activity with minimal fatigue depends on two factors:

- Capacity and integration of the physiologic systems for oxygen delivery
- Capacity of the specific muscle fibers to generate ATP aerobically

Individual differences in aerobic exercise capacity depend on the functions of the ventilatory, circulatory, muscular, and endocrine systems during exercise described in this section. Knowledge about the energy requirements and corresponding physiologic adjustments to exercise also provides a sound basis to formulate a proper training program and evaluate its effectiveness.

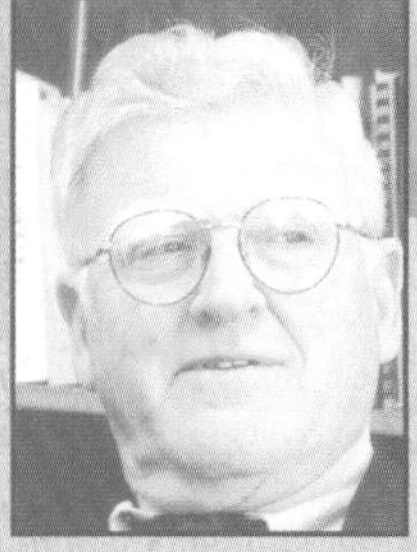

Interview with Dr. Loring B. Rowell

Education: BS (Springfield College, Springfield, MA); PhD (Physiology, University of Minnesota, MN); Postgraduate Training (Senior Fellow, Department of Physiology and Biophysics, and of Medicine in Cardiology, University of Washington School of Medicine, St. Louis, MO)

Current Affiliation: Professor Emeritus, University of Washington

Honors and Awards: See Appendix E.

Research Focus: Human cardiovascular system control and adjustments to exercise.

Memorable Publication: Rowell LB. Neural control of muscle blood flow. Importance during dynamic exercise. Clin & Exper Pharm & Physiol 1997; 24:117–125.

Statement of Contributions: ACSM Honor Award

In recognition of his having achieved excellence in his contributions to cardiovascular physiology, as a scientist, as a teacher and mentor and as an author and editor.

Dr. Rowell's contributions have focused on the regulation of the human cardiovascular system in response to the stresses imposed by exercise, heat, gravity and hypoxia. Included among a long list of landmark findings:

Demonstration that decrements in visceral organ blood flow were proportionate to relative exercise intensity. Evidence that the sympathetically mediated redistribution of blood flow, blood volume and filling pressures was a critical regulatory response to exercise in the heat. Proof of teh dominant reflex role of systemic baroreceptors in the regulation of blood pressure under stress. Evidence that muscle chemoreflexes and baroreceptors were reset during exercise and that this was crucial in the matching of cardiovascular responses to metabolic requirements.

Tracing Dr. Rowell's scientific achievements over the past three decades reveals a fascinating progression of discovery, with one study springing from the questions raised by its predecessor. The questions become more and more difficult and the methods and experimental designs more complex and ingenious. Thus, as the years progressed the risk of failure was often high, but this was overridden by the excitement of producing truly novel and significant advances. He demonstrated how important basic physiologic understandings could be uncovered in healthy human subjects, but did not hesitate to use animal or disease models when necessary to further knowledge. The same thoroughness in scientific inquiry has been perpetuated by the many leading scientists he has mentored.

Larry Rowell's writing has had a major impact on the field. He wrote the first Physiological Reviews on the topic of exercise physiology over twenty years ago. More recently he has provided two landmark reference texts concerned with human cardiovascular regulation and was editor in chief of the first APS sponsored Handbook of Exercise Physiology. As an author he was never merely an information broker; rather his writings constantly challenged the reader to criticize accepted dogma, to tackle the toughest questions and to advance the field.

Larry Rowell has been especially valuable to his students, his colleague, his professional societies and his science, because he never trivialized any task or problem. His approach to life's challenges has always been intense and thorough, whether the problem was of a scientific or humanistic nature. Thus, he tackled the mysteries of baroreceptor resetting with the same zeal and dedication and work ethic that he applied to the editing of a handbook, or to traversing the steep terrain of a snow covered mountain, or in the preparation of a single lecture, or debating a controversial point of science, or in solving the predicaments of friends or colleagues whom he felt were dealt with unfairly. In short, Larry Rowell is indeed "good value"! He is well deserving of the College's highest distinction.

➤ What first inspired you to enter the exercise science field? What made you decide to pursue your advanced degree and/or line of research?

Dr. Peter V. Karpovich at Springfield College (MA) provided my first exposure to the science of physiology. His precise and demanding teaching provided the motivation to seek an advanced degree in physiology and to do research in that field.

➤ What influence did your undergraduate education have on your final career choice?

Again, the undergraduate teaching of Dr. Karpovich, my experience working in his laboratory, and his urging and support paved the way. His influence led me to the Department of Physiology at the University of Minnesota Medical School and the laboratories of Ancel Keys, Henry L. Taylor, and Francisco Grande and colleagues.

➤ Who were the most influential people in your career, and why?

First, Drs. Henry L. Taylor and Francisco Grande guided my graduate education and taught me how to do research. They became lifelong models for an approach to research and scholarship that I admire greatly. Second, my scientific colleagues, students, and fellows have all provided me with constant stimulation and education, and have enriched my career.

➤ What has been the most interesting/enjoyable aspect of your involvement in science? What was the least interesting/enjoyable aspect?

Regarding the most interesting and enjoyable aspects: First, are the wonderful colleagues from all over the world who became lifelong friends and enormous positive influences on my life. Second was the research, the excitement of developing methods to answer a scientific question, getting an answer, having it accepted by peers, and seeing it published. The least enjoyable aspects were not having our answers accepted by our peers and any breakdown or failure of our developed methods.

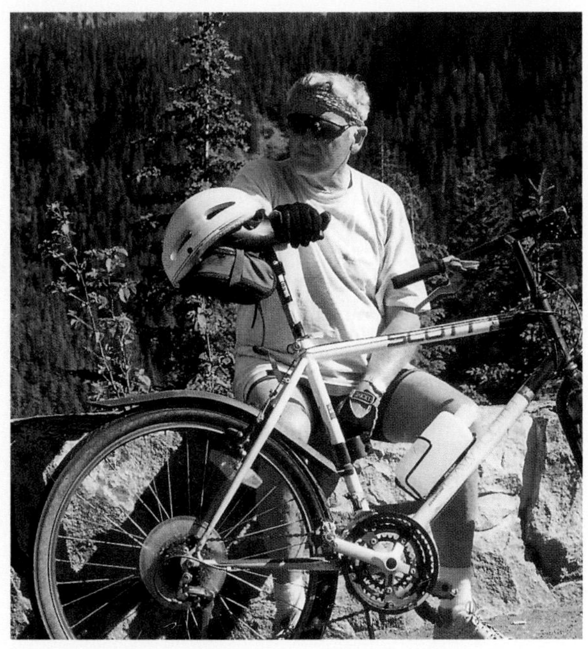

➤ **What is your most meaningful contribution to the field of exercise science, and why is it so important?**

Time and history must judge. I think it is the collection of experiments (1964-1974) in which we quantified the reductions in regional organ blood flow, which were closely related to exercise intensity expressed as percent of $\dot{V}O_{2max}$ *and heart rate. They revealed the quantitative significance of this regional vasoconstriction to blood pressure regulation and to the redistribution of oxygen from resting organs to active muscle. And they showed how this regional vasoconstriction determines the volume of blood available to fill the heart (and thus stroke volume) in exercising humans and how this crucial adjustment is upset by skin vasodilation during heat stress.*

➤ **What advice would you give to students who express an interest in pursuing a career in exercise science research?**

My advice is based on physiology, because that is what I do. I am a cardiovascular physiologist who has used exercise as a powerful precision tool to understand how the cardiovascular system works. Acquisition of a strong background in general physics, mathematics, and chemistry (inorganic, analytical, organic, and especially basic physical chemistry) is essential. In as much as the physiology of exercise is actually the total physiology of a nonresting, nonsupine individual, all areas of physiology are essential because there is no physiological function, regulation, or control that is not vital (i.e., exercise physiology = physiology in toto). Thus, the broader and deeper the training in physiology, the more likely the research will yield basic new information. To quote Sir Joseph Barcroft (1934), "The condition of exercise is not a mere variant of the condition of rest, it is the essence of the machine."

➤ **What interests have you pursued outside your professional career?**

Competitive and recreational Alpine skiing, plus coaching and instruction; Alpinism (glacier and rock climbing); road and mountain bicycling; tennis; landscape painting (oil); and historical literature.

➤ **Where do you see the exercise science field (particularly your area of greatest interest) heading in the next 20 years?**

This field may play a more vital role in the biological sciences than we had once imagined. If the basic life scientist's rush to apply their expertise to provide functional meaning to the genetic code, as is expected, who will be left to teach basic human biology and physiology? Who will explore the functional consequences of aging, for example? Who will discover what controls breathing and the circulation during exercise? Who will do the systematic, integrative science that reveals how whole organ systems and organisms actually work? These questions are not likely to be answered by reductionists (e.g., molecular biologists) working upward from molecules to cells to systems – this is in the wrong direction!

➤ **You have the opportunity to give a "last lecture." Describe its primary focus.**

Its primary focus would be on the question, "What reflexes govern cardiovascular function in exercise?" This century-old, unanswered question concerns what is being controlled (and how), and what signals or errors are being sensed (and how) and corrected (and how) by the autonomic nervous system. The lecture would present the currently dominant ideas and would argue which ones do not seem feasible (and why), and which ones seem feasible based on current knowledge. It would ask where we turn next. And, finally, it would warn us of the great danger of ignoring history – a danger now encouraged by exclusion of all literature published before 1970 from the computer indexing services.

CHAPTER 12

Pulmonary Structure and Function

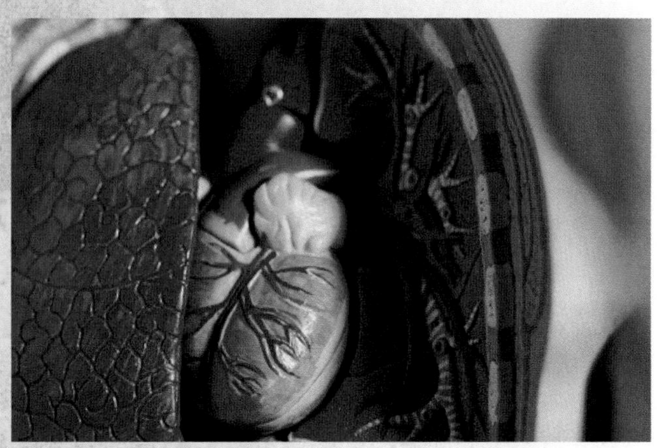

Chapter Objectives

- Diagram the ventilatory system showing the glottis, trachea, bronchi, bronchioles, and alveoli
- Discuss the mechanical and muscular aspects of inspiration and expiration during rest and exercise
- Define and quantify static and dynamic lung function measures and their relation to exercise performance
- Define minute ventilation, alveolar ventilation, ventilation-perfusion ratio, and anatomic and physiologic dead space
- Explain the four phases of the Valsalva and discuss the physiologic consequences of this maneuver
- Describe the effects of cold-weather exercise on the respiratory tract

SURFACE AREA AND GAS EXCHANGE

If oxygen supply to humans depended only on diffusion through the skin, one could not sustain the basal energy requirement, let alone the 4- to 5-L per minute oxygen consumption and carbon dioxide elimination necessary to run a world-class, 5 minute per mile marathon pace. The relatively compact and remarkably effective **ventilatory system** meets the requirements for gas exchange. This system, depicted in Figure 12.1, regulates the gaseous state of the body's "external" environment to effectively aerate body fluids.

ANATOMY OF VENTILATION

Pulmonary ventilation describes the process in which ambient air moves into and exchanges with the air in the lungs. Air entering the nose and mouth flows into the conductive portions of the ventilatory system, where it becomes adjusted to body temperature, filtered, and almost completely humidified as it passes through the **trachea**. Air conditioning continues as inspired air passes into two **bronchi**, the large first-generation of airways that serve as primary conduits into each of the lungs. The bronchi further subdivide into numerous **bronchioles** that conduct inspired air through a tortuous and narrow route

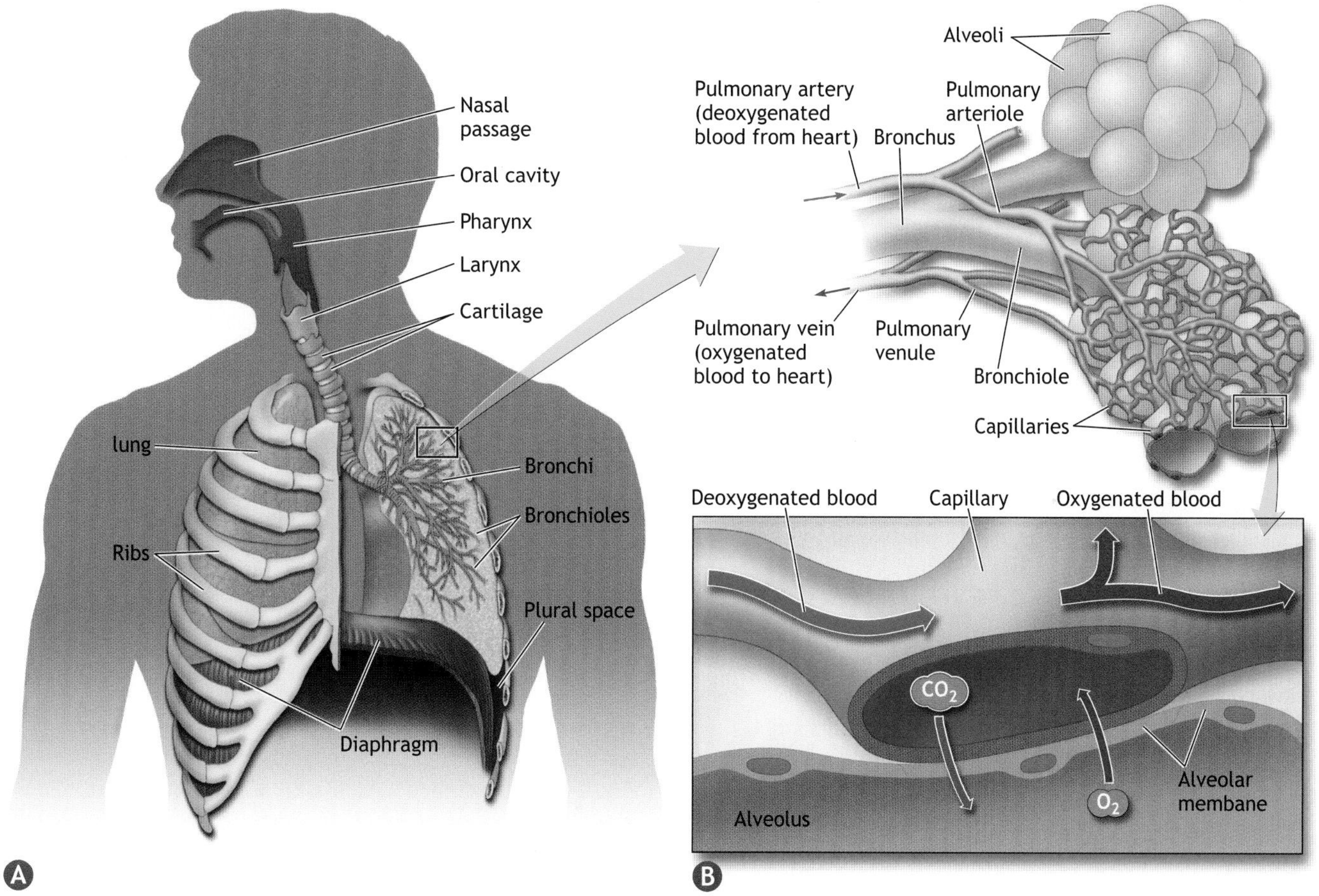

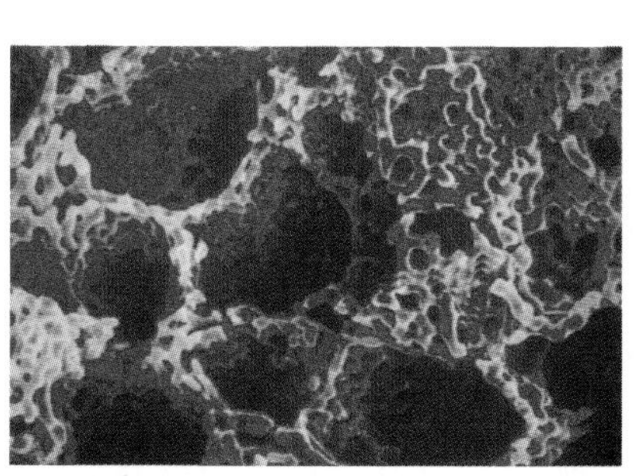

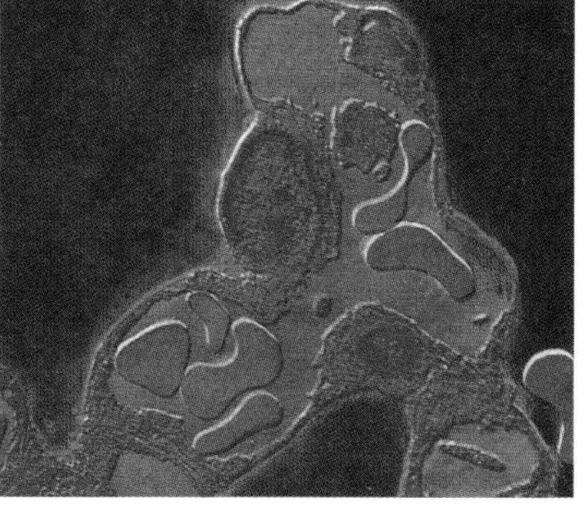

Figure 12.1 • **A**. Major pulmonary structures within the thoracic cavity. **B**. General view of the ventilatory system showing the respiratory passages, alveoli, and gas exchange function in an alveolus. **C**. A section of lung tissue showing individual alveoli; the holes in the alveolar wall are the pores of Kohn. **D**. The pulmonary capillaries run within the walls of the alveoli. (Bottom images from West JB. Respiratory physiology—the essentials. 5th ed. Baltimore: Williams & Wilkins, 1995.)

until it eventually mixes with the existing air in the alveolar ducts. Microscopic **alveoli**, the terminal branches of the respiratory tract, completely envelop these ducts.

The Lungs

The lungs provide the **gas exchange** surface separating blood from the surrounding alveolar gaseous environment. Oxygen transfers from alveolar air into alveolar capillary blood; simultaneously, the blood's carbon dioxide moves into the alveolar chambers where it subsequently flows into ambient air. An average-sized adult's lungs weigh approximately 1 kg, and the volume varies between 4 and 6 L (the amount of air in a basketball), yet the lungs provide a considerable surface area. If spread out, lung tissue would cover an area of 50 to 100 m^2, an area 20 to 50 times larger than the body's external surface, or about one-half of a tennis court or an entire badminton court (Fig. 12.2).

The highly vascularized, moist surface of the lungs fits within the confines of the chest cavity with numerous infoldings—the lung membranes actually fold over onto themselves to provide a considerable interface to aerate blood. At rest, a single red blood cell remains in a pulmonary capillary for only about 0.5 to 1.0 second as it traverses past two to three individual alveoli. During any 1 second of maximal exercise, no more than 1 pint of blood flows within the fine network of lung tissue blood vessels.

The Alveoli

The lungs contain more than 300 million **alveoli**. These elastic, thin-walled, membranous sacs (approximately 0.3 mm in diameter) provide the vital surface for gas exchange between lung tissue and blood. Alveolar tissue receives the largest blood supply of any of the body's organs. Millions of short, thin-walled capillaries and alveoli lie side by side; air moves along one side and blood along the other. Gases diffuse across the extremely thin barrier of alveolar and capillary cells (~ 0.3 μm); the diffusion distance remains relatively constant throughout varying levels of exercise. For most individuals, the integrity of the extremely thin pulmonary blood–gas barrier does not change during sustained exercise. The surface remains as thin as possible (without compromising structural integrity) to facilitate rapid exchange of respiratory gases. In elite athletes, however, alveolar mechanical stress in near-maximal exercise (large ventilation and accompanying pulmonary blood flow) may impair the barrier's permeability. Increased concentrations of red blood cells, total protein, and leukotriene B_4 in bronchoalveolar lavage fluid reflect the increased permeability.[27]

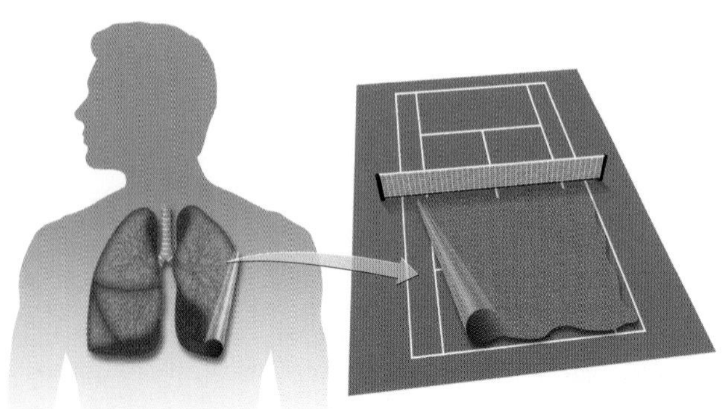

FIGURE 12.2 • The lungs provide an exceptionally large surface for gas exchange.

Also, small **pores of Kohn** within each alveolus allow for even dispersion of surfactant (see page 257) over the respiratory membranes to reduce surface tension for easier alveolar inflation. The pores also provide for gas interchange between adjacent alveoli. Mixing in this manner sustains the indirect ventilation of alveoli damaged or blocked from chronic obstructive lung diseases such as emphysema (see Chapter 32).

Each minute at rest, approximately 250 mL of oxygen leaves the alveoli and enters the blood, and 200 mL of carbon dioxide diffuses in the opposite direction. When endurance athletes exercise intensely, nearly 25 times this quantity of oxygen readily transfers across the alveolar–capillary membrane. *Pulmonary ventilation primarily functions to maintain a fairly constant and favorable concentration of oxygen and carbon dioxide in the alveolar chambers during rest and exercise.* Adequate ventilation ensures complete gaseous exchange before the blood leaves the lungs for transport throughout the body.

MECHANICS OF VENTILATION

Figure 12.3 illustrates the physical principle that underlies breathing dynamics. Note the two lung-shaped balloons suspended in a jar with its glass bottom replaced by a thin rubber membrane. Pulling the membrane down increases jar volume. This reduces air pressure within the jar compared with that of ambient air outside the jar. This imbalance causes air to rush in and inflate the balloons. Conversely, as the elastic membrane recoils, pressure within the jar temporarily increases, and air rushes out. Increasing the depth and rate of descent and ascent of the rubber membrane exchanges a considerable air volume within the balloons in a given time. This depicts essentially how ambient air and alveolar air exchange within the lungs.

Figure 12.4 illustrates the ventilatory system subdivided into two parts: (1) **conducting zone** that includes the trachea and terminal bronchioles and (2) transitional and **respiratory zones** comprising respiratory bronchioles, alveolar ducts, and alveoli. Because the structures of the conducting zone contain no alveoli, the term anatomic dead space describes this area (see page 262). The respiratory zone, representing the location of gas exchange, occupies about 2.5 to 3.0 L and constitutes the largest portion of the total lung volume. Air moving into the lungs literally flows down the trachea to the terminal bronchi, much like water flowing through a hose. As air reaches the smaller air passages in the transitional zone, the tremendous increase in surface area significantly slows airflow into the alveoli.

The two ventilatory zones serve functions more diverse than the simple conduction and exchange of gases between

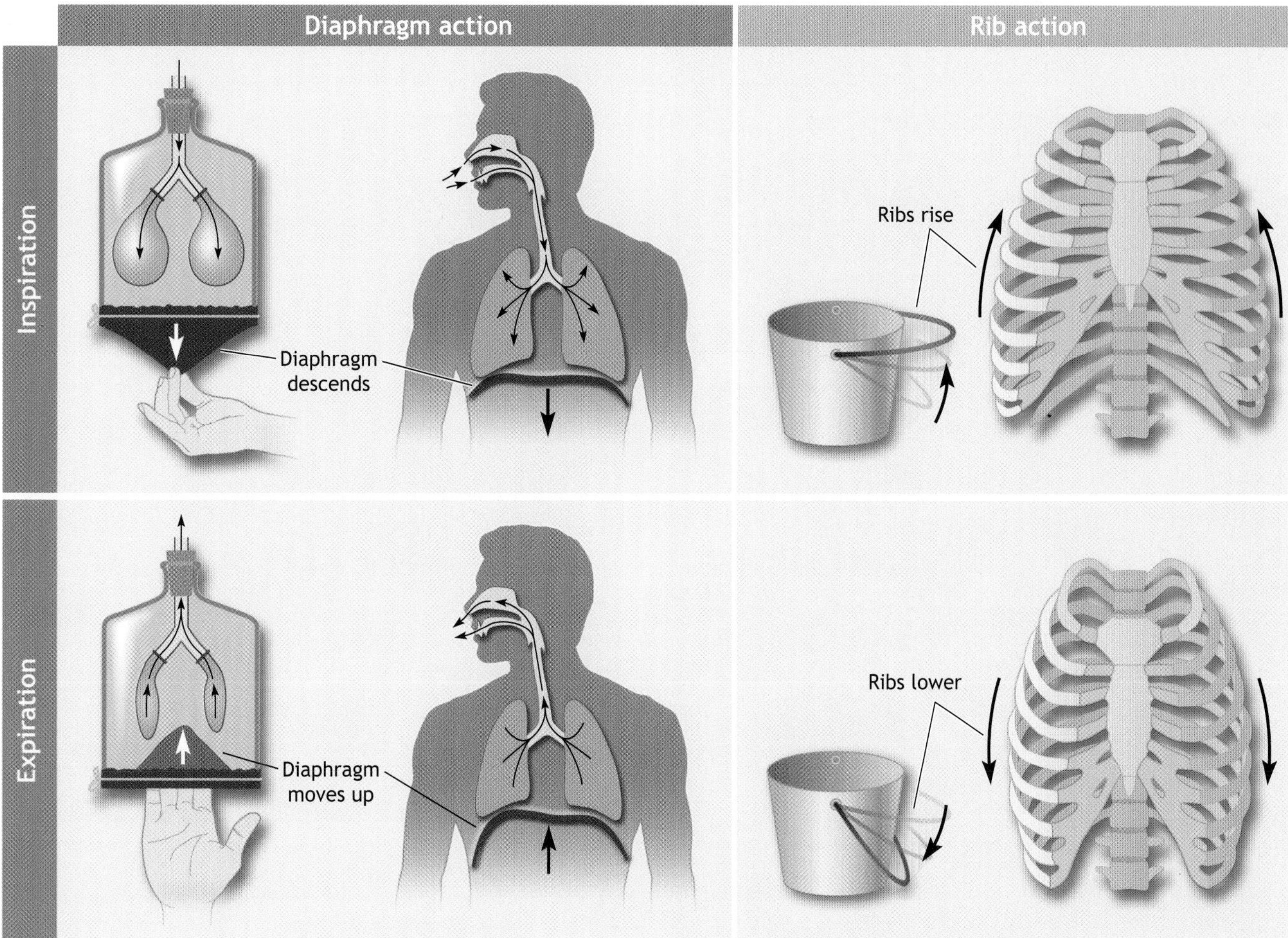

FIGURE 12.3 • Mechanics of breathing. During *inspiration*, the chest cavity increases in size because the ribs raise and the diaphragm descends, causing air to move into the lungs. Inhalation increases in the anterior-posterior (A-P) and vertical diameters of the rib cage. Approximately 70% of lung expansion results from A-P enlargement and 30% from diaphragmatic descent. In addition to diaphragmatic action, the external intercostal muscles become active, and the internal intercostal muscles relax during inhalation. During *exhalation,* the ribs swing down, and the diaphragm returns to a relaxed position. This reduces thoracic cavity volume, and air rushes out. The movement of the jar's rubber bottom causes air to enter and exit the two balloons, simulating the action of the diaphragm. The movement of the bucket handle simulates rib action. The diaphragm, external intercostals, sternocleidomastoids, scapular elevators, anterior serrati scleni, and spinal erector muscles compose the inspiratory muscles that elevate and enlarge the thorax; muscles of expiration depress the thorax and reduce its size (rectus abdominis, internal intercostals, posterior inferior serrati muscles).

blood and alveoli. Conducting-zone functions include air transport, humidification, warming, particle filtration, vocalization, and immunoglobulin secretion. In addition to providing the surface for gaseous exchange, respiratory zone functions encompass surfactant production (in the alveolar endothelium), molecule activation and inactivation (in the capillary endothelium), blood clotting regulation, and endocrine function.

Figure 12.5 depicts the relationship between airway generation (forward velocity) and total cross-sectional area of the conducting passages of various lung segments. Airway cross-section increases considerably (and velocity slows) as air moves through the conducting zone to the terminal bronchioles. At this stage, diffusion provides the primary means for gas movement and distribution. In the alveoli, gas pressures rapidly equilibrate on each side of the alveolar–capillary membrane. **Fick's law** governs gas diffusion through the alveolar membrane. This law states that a gas diffuses through a sheet of tissue at a rate (1) directly proportional to the tissue area, a diffusion constant, and the pressure differential of the gas on each side of the membrane and (2) inversely proportional to the tissue's thickness. The diffusion constant (D) relates directly to gas solubility (S) and inversely to the square root of the molecular weight (MW) of the gas ($D \propto S \div \sqrt{MW}$). On a per-molecule basis, carbon dioxide (MW = 44) diffuses about 20 times faster through thin membranous tissues than oxygen (MW = 32), because of carbon dioxide's higher solubility, despite the relatively similar MWs of the two gases.

The lungs do not merely suspend in the chest cavity like the balloons in Figure 12.3. Instead, the pressure differential between the air in the lungs and the lung–chest wall interface causes the lungs to adhere to the chest wall and literally follow its every movement. Therefore, any change in thoracic cavity volume correspondingly alters lung volume. The lungs

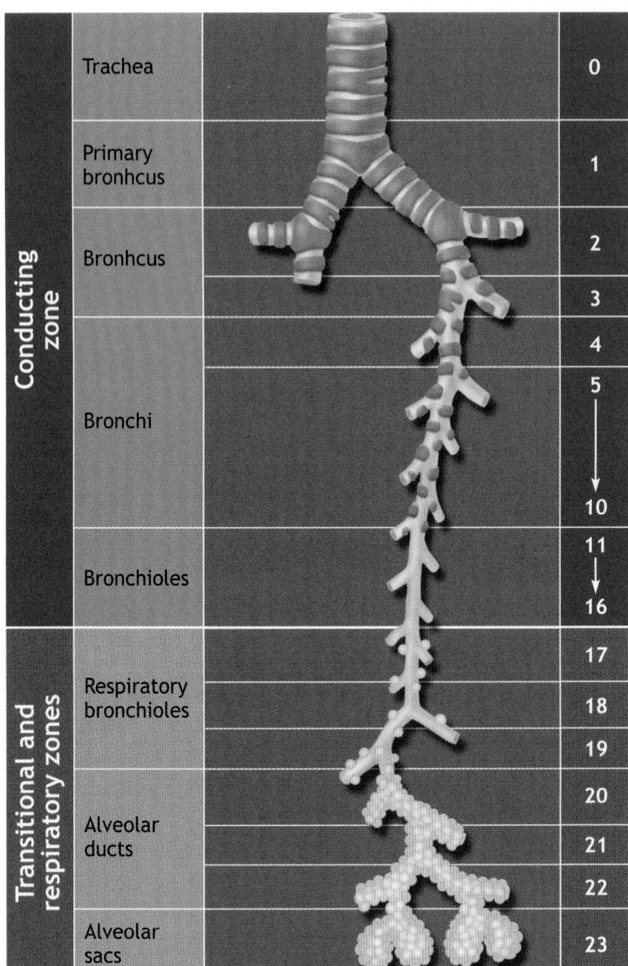

FIGURE 12.4 • Separation of human lung tissue into a series of discrete zones designated as conduction zones (zones 1 through 16) and transitional and respiratory zones (zones 17 through 23).

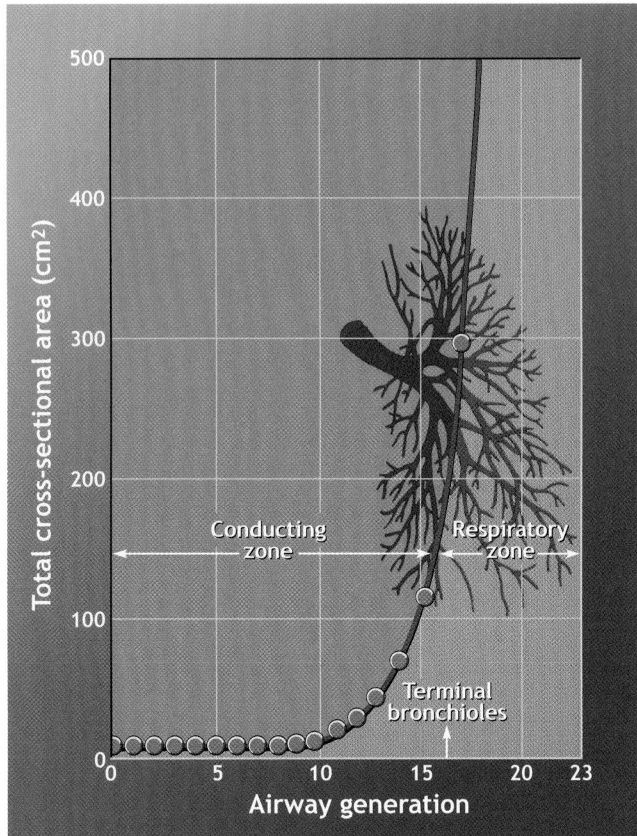

FIGURE 12.5 • Airflow in the lungs in relation to the total cross-sectional tissue area. Forward airflow velocity during inspiration decreases significantly because of the large increase in tissue cross-sectional area beginning in the region of the terminal bronchioles. (Modified from West JB. Respiratory physiology—the essentials. 5th ed. Baltimore: Williams & Wilkins, 1995.)

depend on accessory means for altering their volume because they contain no skeletal muscles. The action of a highly versatile, **multimuscle respiratory pump system** alters the volume of the lungs during inspiration and expiration.

Inspiration

The **diaphragm**, a large, dome-shaped sheet of striated, musculofibrous tissue, serves the same purpose as the jar's rubber membrane in Figure 12.3. This primary ventilatory muscle creates an airtight separation between the abdominal and thoracic cavities but provides a series of openings through which the esophagus, blood vessels, and nerves pass. The diaphragm possesses high oxidative potential and the greatest capacity of all the respiratory muscles for shortening and volume displacement.[16,43] During **inspiration**, the diaphragm muscle contracts, flattens, and moves downward toward the abdominal cavity by as much as 10 cm. Elongation and enlargement of the chest cavity expands the air in the lungs, causing its pressure, referred to as **intrapulmonic pressure**, to decrease to slightly below atmospheric pressure. The lungs inflate as air literally becomes sucked in through the nose and mouth. The degree of filling depends on the magnitude of inspiratory movements. Maximal activation of the inspiratory muscles of healthy individuals produces maximal pressures that range between 80 and 140 mm Hg.[32] Inspiration ends when thoracic cavity expansion ceases, causing intrapulmonic pressure to increase to equal ambient atmospheric pressure.

During exercise, the highly efficient movements of the diaphragm, rib cage (ribs and sternum), and abdominal muscles synchronize to contribute to inspiration and expiration.[2,29] During inspiration, contraction of the **scaleni** and **external intercostal** muscles between the ribs causes the ribs to rotate and lift up and away from the body. This action corresponds somewhat to the movement of the handle lifted up and away from the side of a bucket (see Fig. 12.3, *right*). Inspiration increases during exercise when the diaphragm descends, the ribs swing upward, and the sternum thrusts outward to increase the lateral and anterior-posterior diameter of the thorax. Athletes often bend forward from the waist to facilitate breathing following exhausting exercise. This probably serves two purposes: (1) it promotes blood flow back to the heart and (2) it minimizes any antagonistic effects of gravity on the usual upward direction of inspiratory movements.

Expiration

Expiration during rest and light exercise represents a predominantly passive process of air movement out of the lungs. It results from two factors: (1) natural recoil of the stretched lung tissue and (2) relaxation of the inspiratory muscles. This causes the sternum and ribs to swing down and the diaphragm to rise toward the thoracic cavity. These movements decrease chest cavity volume and compress alveolar gas so that air moves out of the respiratory tract into the atmosphere. Expiration ends when the compressive force of the expiratory musculature ceases and intrapulmonic pressure decreases to atmospheric pressure. During strenuous exercise, **internal intercostal** and **abdominal muscles** act powerfully on the ribs and abdominal cavity to reduce thoracic dimensions.[18] Thus, exhalation is rapid and more extensive.

No major differences exist in ventilatory mechanics between men and women of different ages. At rest in the supine position, most people breathe diaphragmatically ("abdominal breathers"), whereas in the upright position rib and sternum actions become more apparent.[50] Rib cage movement largely accounts for the rapid alterations in thoracic volume required during heavy exercise. Evidence that the rib musculature acts more rapidly than the diaphragm and abdominal muscles derives from distinct biochemical differences among muscles that compose the respiratory pump.[44] The position of the head and back naturally adopted by distance runners—forward lean from the waist, neck flexed, and head extended forward with mandible parallel to the ground—favors pulmonary ventilation during heavy exercise.[25]

Surfactant

Pressures vary continually within the alveolar and pleural spaces throughout the ventilatory cycle. Resistance to normal expansion of lung cavity and alveoli progressively increases during inspiration, owing to the effect of **surface tension**, primarily in the alveoli. Surface tension relates to a resisting force created at the surface of a liquid in contact with a gas, structure, or another liquid. The tension or force created causes the liquid to assume a shape that presents the smallest surface area to the surrounding medium. The greater the surface tension surrounding a spherical object such as an alveolus, the greater the force required to overcome the pressure within the sphere and cause it to enlarge (inflate). **Surfactant**, a lipoprotein mixture of phospholipids, proteins, and calcium ions produced by alveolar epithelial cells, mixes with the fluid that encircles the alveolar chambers. Its action interrupts the surrounding water layer to reduce the alveolar membrane's surface tension. This effect greatly reduces the energy required for alveolar inflation and deflation.

LUNG VOLUMES AND CAPACITIES

Figure 12.6 illustrates various lung volume measurements that affect the ability to increase breathing depth, including average values for men and women. To obtain these measurements, the subject rebreathes through a water-sealed, volume-displacement recording spirometer similar to the one described in Chapter 8 (Fig. 8.2) for measuring oxygen consumption by the closed-circuit method. As with many anatomic and physiologic measures, lung volumes vary with age, gender, and body size and composition, but particularly with stature. *Therefore, common practice evaluates lung volumes in relation to established standards that consider these factors.*[3]

Static Lung Volumes

The spirometer bell falls and subsequently rises during inhalation and exhalation, to provide a record of ventilatory volume and breathing rate. **Tidal volume (TV)** describes air volume moved during either inspiratory or expiratory phase of each breathing cycle (first portion of the record). Under resting conditions, TV usually ranges between 0.4 and 1.0 L of air per breath.

After recording several representative tracings for TV, the subject inspires as deeply as possible following a normal inspiration. The additional 2.5- to 3.5-L volume above inspired tidal air represents the reserve ability for inhalation, referred to as the **inspiratory reserve volume (IRV)**. Following IRV measurement, the subject reestablishes the normal breathing pattern. After a normal exhalation, the subject continues to exhale and forces as much air as possible from the lungs. This additional volume represents **expiratory reserve volume (ERV)**, which ranges between 1.0 and 1.5 L for an average-sized man. *During exercise, encroachment on both IRV and ERV, particularly IRV, produces a considerable increase in TV.*

The total volume of air voluntarily moved in one breath, from full inspiration to maximum expiration, represents the vital capacity (VC), or, more precisely, **forced vital capacity (FVC)**. FVC includes TV plus IRV and ERV. This value varies considerably with body size and composition (negatively associated with % body fat[31]) and with body position during measurement. FVC usually ranges between 4 and 5 L in healthy young men and between 3 and 4 L in young women. Values of 6 to 7 L are not uncommon for tall individuals, and unusually large FVC values have been reported for a professional football player (7.6 L) and an Olympic gold medalist in cross-country skiing (8.1 L).[5,57] These athletes' large lung volumes generally reflect genetic influences and body size characteristics, because exercise training does *not* appreciably change static lung volumes.

Residual Lung Volume

An air volume remains in the lungs even after exhaling as deeply as possible. This volume, termed the **residual lung volume (RLV)**, averages between 0.8 and 1.2 L for college-aged, healthy women and between 0.9 and 1.4 L for men. RLV for apparently healthy professional football players ranges between 0.96 and 2.46 L.[57] RLV increases with age, whereas IRV and ERV decrease proportionally. A decline in the elasticity of lung tissue components probably induces a decrease in breathing reserve and concomitant increase in

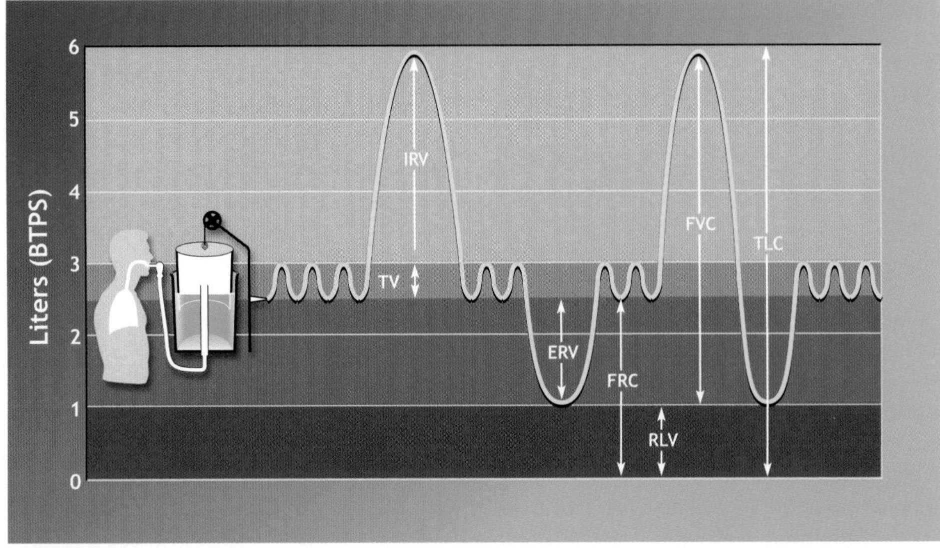

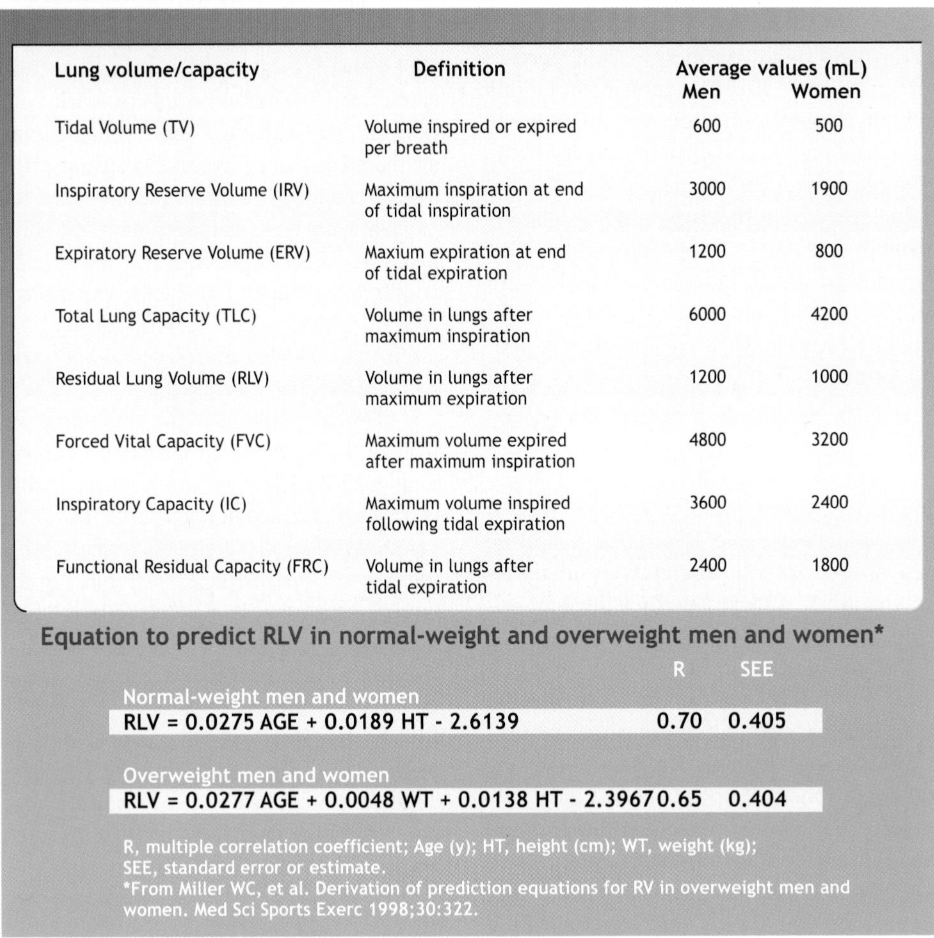

Lung volume/capacity	Definition	Average values (mL) Men	Women
Tidal Volume (TV)	Volume inspired or expired per breath	600	500
Inspiratory Reserve Volume (IRV)	Maximum inspiration at end of tidal inspiration	3000	1900
Expiratory Reserve Volume (ERV)	Maxium expiration at end of tidal expiration	1200	800
Total Lung Capacity (TLC)	Volume in lungs after maximum inspiration	6000	4200
Residual Lung Volume (RLV)	Volume in lungs after maximum expiration	1200	1000
Forced Vital Capacity (FVC)	Maximum volume expired after maximum inspiration	4800	3200
Inspiratory Capacity (IC)	Maximum volume inspired following tidal expiration	3600	2400
Functional Residual Capacity (FRC)	Volume in lungs after tidal expiration	2400	1800

Equation to predict RLV in normal-weight and overweight men and women*

	R	SEE
Normal-weight men and women: RLV = 0.0275 AGE + 0.0189 HT - 2.6139	0.70	0.405
Overweight men and women: RLV = 0.0277 AGE + 0.0048 WT + 0.0138 HT - 2.3967	0.65	0.404

R, multiple correlation coefficient; Age (y); HT, height (cm); WT, weight (kg); SEE, standard error or estimate.

*From Miller WC, et al. Derivation of prediction equations for RV in overweight men and women. Med Sci Sports Exerc 1998;30:322.

FIGURE 12.6 • Static measurements of lung volumes.

residual lung volume with aging. Importantly, alterations in pulmonary function may not entirely reflect an aging phenomenon, because regular aerobic training blunts the typical age-related decline in static and dynamic lung functions.[21] The RLV allows an uninterrupted exchange of gas between the blood and alveoli, thus preventing fluctuations in blood gases during phases of the breathing cycle, including deep breathing. RLV plus FVC constitutes **total lung capacity** (**TLC**).

HELIUM DILUTION AND OXYGEN DILUTION METHODS. RLV cannot be measured directly from spirographic tracings. Instead, indirect determinations involve rebreathing a known gas volume containing either helium or pure oxygen. With the **helium dilution method**, the subject expires normally. Air remaining in the lungs at this end-normal expiration position, termed the **functional residual capacity** (**FRC**), includes the known ERV and unknown RLV. The subject then rebreathes a known helium mixture for approximately 5 minutes. Absorbents remove expired carbon dioxide, while an external oxygen supply continually replaces consumed oxygen to maintain a constant rebreathing volume within the spirometer. FRC computes easily from the dilution of the original helium rebreathing mixture. FRC minus ERV equals RLV. The **oxygen dilution method** provides a more rapid RLV assessment than the helium dilution method.[56] Oxygen dilution determines RLV from dilution of the lung's original nitrogen concentration, achieved by rapidly rebreathing a volume of approximately 5 L of 100% oxygen. Figure 12.7 illustrates the dilution principle used to measure RLV via the rebreathing of a helium-containing gas mixture.

EFFECTS OF PREVIOUS EXERCISE. The RLV temporarily increases from an acute bout of either short-term or prolonged exercise.[17,38] In one study, RLV increased during recovery from a maximal treadmill test by 21% after 5 minutes, 17% after 15 minutes, and 12% after 30 minutes.[8] RLV generally reverts to its original value within 24 hours. Possible factors that increase RLV with exercise include (1) closure of the small peripheral airways and (2) increase in thoracic blood volume. The added blood volume does not alter the lungs' mechanical properties, but it does displace air, thus preventing complete exhalation (reduced FVC).[11] Any temporary increase in RLV would significantly impact subsequent computations of body volume by hydrostatic weighing for body composition studies (see Chapter 28). When measurement of RLV becomes impractical, prediction equations based on the relation between RLV and age, stature, gender, and body mass provide reasonably accurate estimates (see inset table, Fig. 12.6).[41]

Dynamic Lung Volumes

Adequacy of pulmonary ventilation depends on ability to sustain high airflow levels rather than air movement in a single breath. Dynamic ventilation depends on two factors: (1) maximum "stroke volume" of the lungs (FVC) and (2) speed of

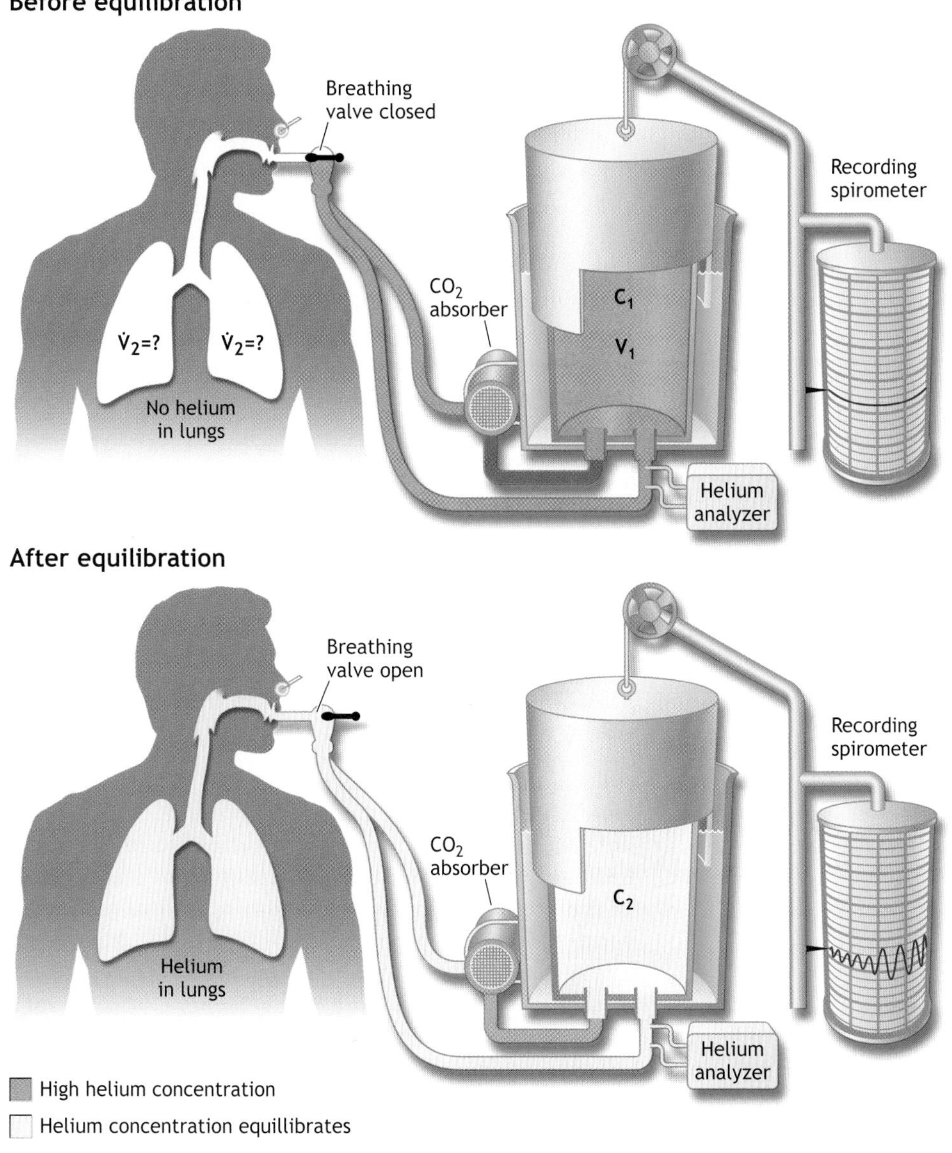

FIGURE 12.7 • Application of the dilution principle to assess residual lung volume. The subject exhales to the unknown functional residual capacity or residual lung volume and then breathes from a known volume and concentration of a gas such as oxygen or helium. In this example, a small concentration of helium represents the dilution gas. After a short period of deep, rapid breathing, the unknown, initially helium-free volume in the subject's lungs mixes with the known concentration of helium in the known volume that the subject rebreathes. Equilibrium occurs between the gases in the spirometer and the gases in the subject's lung volume. During rebreathing, oxygen is continually added to the spirometer to replace that consumed by the subject. An absorbent continually removes carbon dioxide from the system. Residual lung volume computes from the concentration–volume relationship, in which initial helium volume (V_1) × initial helium concentration (C_1) = final gas volume (V_2) × final helium concentration (C_2). The residual lung volume (V_2) is determined from the relationship $V_1 (C_1 - C_2) \div C_2$. The final gas volume is corrected to body temperature and pressure saturated (BTPS), using the constants from Appendix D.

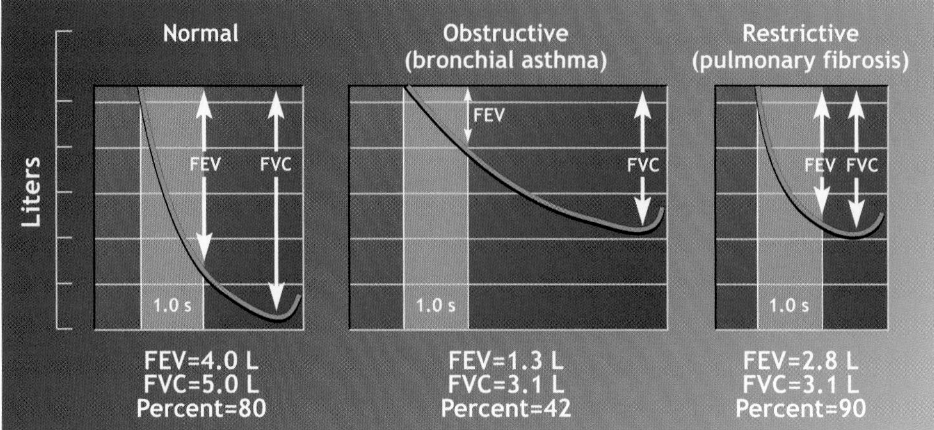

FIGURE 12.8 • Examples of spirometric tracings during standard pulmonary function tests for $FEV_{1.0}$ and FVC in individuals with normal dynamic lung function and in patients with either obstructive or restrictive lung disease.

moving a volume of air (breathing rate). Airflow velocity, in turn, depends on the resistance of the respiratory passages to the smooth flow of air, and the "stiffness" imposed by the mechanical properties of the chest and lung tissue to a change in shape during breathing, termed **lung compliance**. Owing to a normally large pulmonary reserve, patients with lung disease rarely experience symptoms of distress until a large part of their ventilatory capacity decreases. Individuals with mild airway obstruction regularly and successfully engage in competitive distance running.[35]

FEV-to-FVC Ratio

Some individuals with severe lung disease achieve near-normal FVC values if measured with no time limit for this maneuver. For this reason, clinicians prefer a "dynamic" measurement of lung function such as the **forced expiratory volume** (**FEV**), usually measured over 1 second (**$FEV_{1.0}$**). $FEV_{1.0}$ divided by the FVC (**$FEV_{1.0} \div FVC$**) indicates pulmonary airflow capacity. It reflects pulmonary expiratory power, or driving pressure, and overall resistance to air movement upstream in the lungs. Healthy individuals normally expel about 85% of the vital capacity in 1 second. Severe obstructive lung disease such as emphysema or bronchial asthma—with accompanying reduced airway caliber and loss of elastic recoil of lung tissue—considerably reduces $FEV_{1.0}$/FVC, often to values less than 40% of the vital capacity.[37,52] *Usually, the demarcation point for airway obstruction during dynamic spirometry represents an $FEV_{1.0}$/FVC of 70% or less.*[47] Figure 12.8 presents pulmonary function test results for $FEV_{1.0}$ and FVC in individuals with normal lung function and with obstructive and restrictive lung diseases. Clinicians also compute other values from portions of the curve generated in the forced spirometry maneuver (e.g., mid-50% of the expiratory curve or instantaneous flows at 25, 50, or 75% FVC) to assess airflow dynamics in the small airways of the pulmonary tract.[54]

Maximum Voluntary Ventilation

The **maximum voluntary ventilation** (**MVV**) evaluates ventilatory capacity with rapid and deep breathing for 15 seconds. The 15-second volume, extrapolated to the volume if the subject continued for 1 minute, represents MVV and typically ranges between 35 and 40 times the $FEV_{1.0}$.[55] MVV also averages 25% higher than ventilation during maximal exercise, because exercise does not maximally stress a healthy person's ability to breathe. For healthy, college-aged men, MVV ranges between 140 and 180 $L \cdot min^{-1}$, with values for women ranging between 80 and 120 $L \cdot min^{-1}$. MVV in male members of the United States Nordic Ski Team averaged 192 $L \cdot min^{-1}$; the individual high was 239 $L \cdot min^{-1}$.[22] Conversely, patients with obstructive lung disease achieve only about 40% of MVV considered normal for their age and size.[33]

Specific exercise training of the ventilatory muscles improves their strength and endurance and increases MVV.[1,52] Ventilatory training in patients with chronic pulmonary disease can enhance exercise capacity and reduce physiologic strain.[12,42,48] Progressive desensitization to the feeling of breathlessness, and greater self-control of respiratory symptoms, represent important benefits of ventilatory muscle training and regular exercise to patients with chronic obstructive lung disease.

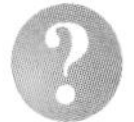

INTEGRATIVE QUESTION

How might regular resistance and aerobic exercise training blunt the typical decline in measures of lung function with advancing age?

Exercise Implications of Gender Differences in Static and Dynamic Lung Function Measures

Adult women consistently show smaller static and dynamic lung function measures than men, even with correction for difference in stature.[3] This disparity produces expiratory flow limitations and greater use of ventilatory reserve during maximal exercise, particularly for highly trained women, compared with trained men and less-fit women.[39] A relatively smaller lung volume plus a high expiratory flow rate requirement in trained women during heavy exercise places considerable demand on the maximum flow–volume envelope of the airways (i.e., mechanical constraint of TV and pulmonary minute ventilation). The gender difference in lung volumes and maximal flow rates adversely affects how highly fit women maintain adequate alveolar-to-arterial oxygen exchange, which could compromise arterial oxygen saturation.[24]

LUNG FUNCTION, AEROBIC FITNESS, AND EXERCISE PERFORMANCE

Different dynamic lung function tests can indicate the severity of obstructive and restrictive lung diseases. However, such tests generally provide little information about aerobic fitness or exercise performance if the values fall within the normal range. For example, no difference emerges when comparing the average FVC of prepubescent and Olympic wrestlers, middle-distance athletes, and untrained, healthy subjects.[45,46] Professional football players averaged only 94% of their predicted FVC; the defensive backs achieved only 83% of predicted "normal" values for their body size (see "In a Practical Sense").[61] Somewhat surprisingly, comparable values emerged for static and dynamic lung function of accomplished marathon runners and other endurance-trained athletes compared with untrained controls of similar body size.[21,36]

Swimming and diving stimulate development of larger-than-normal static lung volumes. These sports strengthen the inspiratory muscles that work against additional resistance of the mass of water compressing the thorax. Enhanced ventilatory muscle strength and power explain the relatively large FVC reported for skin divers and competitive swimmers.[7,9,13,14]

Little relationship exists among diverse lung volumes and capacities and various track performances, including distance running, for a large group of teenage boys and girls, even after adjusting for body size.[15] Similarly, for marathon runners versus sedentary subjects of similar body size, no difference existed for lung function values (Table 12.1).[30] For healthy, untrained individuals, no relationship exists between maximal oxygen consumption and either FVC or MVV (adjusted for body size).[20] *Whereas fatigue from strenuous exercise frequently relates to feeling "out of breath," or "winded," the normal capacity for pulmonary ventilation does not limit maximal aerobic exercise performance for most individuals.* The larger-than-normal lung volumes and breathing capacities of certain athletes probably reflect genetic endowment. Some increase in pulmonary function may reflect strengthened respiratory muscles from specific exercise training.

TABLE 12.1 ➤ ANTHROPOMETRIC DATA, PULMONARY FUNCTION, AND RESTING MINUTE VENTILATION IN 20 MARATHON RUNNERS AND HEALTHY CONTROLS

MEASURE	RUNNERS	CONTROLS	DIFFERENCE[a]
ANTHROPOMETRIC			
Age, y	27.8	27.4	0.4
Stature, cm	175.8	176.7	0.9
Surface area, m^2	1.82	1.89	0.07
PULMONARY FUNCTION			
FVC, L	5.13	5.34	0.21
TLC, L	6.91	7.13	0.22
$FEV_{1.0}$, L	4.32	4.47	0.15
$FEV_{1.0}$ / FVC, %	84.3	83.8	0.5
MVV, $L \cdot min^{-1}$	179.8	176.0	3.8
RESTING VENTILATION			
$\dot{V}_E$, $L \cdot min^{-1}$	11.9	11.9	0.9
Breathing rate, breaths $\cdot min^{-1}$	10.9	11.1	0.2
Tidal volume, L	1.16	1.06	0.10

From Mahler DA, et al. Ventilatory responses at rest and during exercise in marathon runners. J Appl Physiol 1982;52:388.
[a]All differences not statistically significant.

PULMONARY VENTILATION

One can view pulmonary ventilation from two perspectives: (1) the volume of air moved into or out of the total respiratory tract each minute and (2) the air volume that ventilates only the alveolar chambers each minute.

Minute Ventilation

The normal breathing rate during quiet breathing at rest in a thermoneutral environment averages 12 breaths per minute, and TV averages 0.5 L of air per breath. Consequently, the volume of air breathed each minute, referred to as **minute ventilation**, equals 6 L.

$$\text{Minute ventilation } (\dot{V}_E) = \text{Breathing rate} \times \text{Tidal Volume}$$
$$= 12 \times 0.5 \text{ L}$$
$$= 6 \text{ L} \cdot \text{min}^{-1}$$

An increase in either the rate or depth of breathing or both significantly increases minute ventilation. During strenuous exercise, healthy young adults readily increase their breathing rate to 35 to 45 breaths per minute, although elite endurance athletes breathe as rapidly as 60 to 70 times each minute during maximal exercise. TVs of 2.0 L and above commonly occur during exercise. Such increases in breathing rate and TV readily increase exercise minute ventilation to 100 L or more (about 17 to 20 times the resting value). In male endurance athletes, ventilation may increase to 160 L · min^{-1} during maximal exercise. Several research studies have reported minute ventilation volumes of 200 L, with a high

TYPICAL VALUES FOR PULMONARY VENTILATION DURING REST AND MODERATE AND VIGOROUS EXERCISE

Condition	Breathing Rate (breaths $\cdot min^{-1}$)	Tidal Volume (L $\cdot breath^{-1}$)	Pulmonary Ventilation (L $\cdot min^{-1}$)
Rest	12	0.5	6
Moderate exercise	30	2.5	75
Vigorous exercise	50	3.0	150

IN A PRACTICAL SENSE

PREDICTING PULMONARY FUNCTION VARIABLES IN MALES AND FEMALES

Although pulmonary function variables do not directly relate to measures of physical fitness in healthy individuals, their measurement often forms part of a standard medical/health/fitness examination, particularly for individuals at risk for limited pulmonary function (e.g., chronic cigarette smokers, asthmatics). Measurement of diverse components of pulmonary dimension and lung function with a water-filled spirometer (see figure) or electronic spirometer also provides the framework for discussions of pulmonary dynamics during rest and exercise. Proper evaluation of measured values for pulmonary function requires comparison to "expected" values (norms) from the clinical literature.

Equations

Because pulmonary function scores associate closely with stature and age, these two variables can predict the expected average lung function value (normal) for an individual.

DATA

Man: Age (A), 22 y; stature (ST), 182.9 cm (72 in)

Woman: A, 22 y; ST, 165.1 cm (65 in)

Examples

WOMAN

1. *Forced vital capacity (FVC)*

$$\text{FVC (L)} = (0.0414 \times \text{ST [cm]}) - (0.0232 \times \text{A [y]}) - 2.20$$
$$= 6.835 - 0.5104 - 2.20$$
$$= 4.12 \text{ L}$$

2. *Forced expiratory volume in 1 s ($FEV_{1.0}$)*

$$FEV_{1.0} \text{ (L)} = (0.0268 \times \text{ST [cm]}) - 0.0251 \times \text{A [y]}) - 0.38$$
$$= 4.425 - 0.5522 - 0.38$$
$$= 3.49 \text{ L}$$

3. *Percentage forced vital capacity in 1 s ($FEV_{1.0}/FVC$):*

$$FEV_{1.0}/FVC \text{ (\%)} = (-0.2145 \times \text{ST [cm]}) - 0.1523 \times \text{A [y]}) + 124.5$$
$$= -35.41 - 3.35 + 124.5$$
$$= 85.7\%$$

4. *Maximum voluntary ventilation (MVV)*

$$\text{MVV (L} \cdot \text{min}^{-1}) = 40 \times FEV_{1.0}$$
$$= 40 \times 3.49 \text{ (from \#2)}$$
$$= 139.6 \text{ L} \cdot \text{min}^{-1}$$

volume of 208 L observed in a professional football player during maximal bicycle exercise.[57] *Despite such large minute ventilations, TVs for trained and untrained individuals rarely exceed 60% of vital capacity.*

Alveolar Ventilation

A portion of the air in each breath does not enter the alveoli and, therefore, does not take part in gaseous exchange with the blood. The term **anatomic dead space** describes this air that fills the nose, mouth, trachea, and other nondiffusable conducting portions of the respiratory tract. In healthy individuals, the anatomic dead space generally ranges between 150 and 200 mL (about 30% of the resting TV). The composition of dead-space air remains almost identical to that of ambient air, except for its full saturation with water vapor.

The dead-space volume permits about 350 mL of the 500 mL inspired TV at rest to enter into and mix with existing alveolar air. This does not mean that only 350 mL of air enters and leaves the alveoli with each breath. Instead, if TV equals 500 mL, then 500 mL of air enters the alveoli but only 350 mL of this is fresh air. This represents about one-seventh of total alveolar air. Such relatively small and seemingly inefficient **alveolar ventilation**—that portion of inspired air reaching the alveoli and participating in gas exchange—prevents drastic changes in alveolar air composition; this ensures consistency in arterial blood gases throughout the breathing cycle.

Table 12.2 indicates that minute ventilation does not always reflect alveolar ventilation. The first example of shallow breathing shows that one can reduce TV to 150 mL, yet still maintain a 6-L minute ventilation by increasing breathing rate to 40 breaths per minute. The same 6-L minute volume results

IN A PRACTICAL SENSE

PREDICTING PULMONARY FUNCTION VARIABLES IN MALES AND FEMALES—CONT'D

MAN

1. *Forced vital capacity (FVC)*

$$FVC\ (L) = (0.0774 \times ST\ [cm] - (0.0212 \times A\ [y] - 7.75$$
$$= 14.156 - 0.4664 - 7.75$$
$$= 5.49\ L$$

2. *Forced expiratory volume in 1 s ($FEV_{1.0}$)*

$$FEV_{1.0}\ (L) = (0.0566 \times ST\ [cm]) - 0.0233 \times A\ [y]) - 0.491$$
$$= 10.35 - 0.5126 - 4.91$$
$$= 4.93\ L$$

3. *Percentage forced vital capacity in 1 s ($FEV_{1.0}/FVC$)*

$$FEV_{1.0}/FVC\ (\%) = (-0.1314 \times ST\ [cm]) - 0.1490 \times A\ [y)] + 110.2$$
$$= -24.03 - 3.35 + 110.2$$
$$= 82.8\%$$

4. *Maximum voluntary ventilation (MVV)*

$$MVV\ (L \cdot min^{-1}) = 40 \times FEV_{1.0}$$
$$= 40 \times 4.93\ L\ (\text{from \#2})$$
$$= 197.2\ L \cdot min^{-1}$$

EQUATIONS TO PREDICT PULMONARY FUNCTION VARIABLES

VARIABLE	MEN <25 y	Men >25 y	Female <25 y	Female >25 y
Forced vital capacity (FVC): Maximum volume expired following a maximum inspiration	FVC (L) = (0.0774 × ST) − (0.0212 × A) − 7.75	FVC (L) = (0.065 × ST) + (0.029 × A) − 5.459	FVC, (L) = (0.0414 ST) − (0.0232 A) − 2.20	FVC (L) = (0.037 × ST) + (0.092 × A) − 3.469
Forced expiratory volume in 1 s ($FEV_{1.0}$): Volume forcibly expired in 1 s following a maximum inspiration	$FEV_{1.0}$ (L) = (0.0566 × ST) − 0.0233 × A) − 0.491	$FEV_{1.0}$ (L) = (0.052 × ST) + (0.027 × A) − 4.203	$FEV_{1.0}$, (L) = (0.0268 × ST) − 0.0251 × A) − 0.38	$FEV_{1.0}$ (L) = (0.027 × ST) − (0.021 × A) − 0.794
$FEV_{1.0}/FVC$: Percentage of forced vital capacity expired in 1 s	$FEV_{1.0}/FVC$, (%) = (−0.1314 × ST) − 0.1490 × A) + 110.2	$FEV_{1.0}/FVC$, (%) = 103.64 0 (0.087 × ST) − (0.14 × A)	$FEV_{1.0}/FVC$, (%) = (−0.2145 × ST) − (0.1523 × A) + 124.5	$FEV_{1.0}/FVC$, (%) = 107.38 − (0.111 × ST) − (0.109 × A)
Maximum voluntary ventilation (MVV): Maximum amount of air forcibly breathed in 1 min	MMV ($L \cdot min^{-1}$) = 40 × $FEV_{1.0}$	MMV ($L \cdot min^{-1}$) = (1.15 × H) − (1.27 × A) + 14	MMV ($L \cdot min^{-1}$) = 40 × FEV	MMV ($L \cdot min^{-1}$) = (0.55 × ST) − (0.72 × A) + 50

ST, stature (height) in centimeters; A, age in years

Comroe JH, et al. The lung. Chicago: Year Book Medical Publishers, 1962.
Miller A. Pulmonary function tests in clinical and occupational disease. Philadelphia: Grune & Stratton, 1986.
Taylor AE, et al. Clinical respiratory physiology. Philadelphia: WB Saunders, 1989.
Wasserman K, et al. Principles of exercise testing. Baltimore: Lippincott Williams & Wilkins, 1999.

from decreasing breathing rate to 12 breaths per minute and increasing TV to 500 mL. In contrast, doubling TV and halving the breathing rate, as in the example of deep breathing, also produces a 6-L minute ventilation. Each of these ventilatory adjustments drastically affects alveolar ventilation. In the example of shallow breathing, dead-space air represents the only air volume moved without any alveolar ventilation. In the other examples, deeper breathing causes a larger portion of each breath to enter into and mix with alveolar air. Alveolar ventilation determines the gaseous concentrations at the alveolar–capillary membrane.

TABLE 12.2 ➤ RELATIONSHIPS AMONG TIDAL VOLUME, BREATHING RATE, AND BOTH TOTAL AND ALVEOLAR MINUTE VENTILATION

CONDITION	TIDAL VOLUME (mL)	×	BREATHING RATE (BREATHS · MIN^{-1})	=	TOTAL MINUTE VENTILATION (mL · MIN^{-1})	−	DEAD SPACE MINUTE VENTILATION (mL · MIN^{-1})	=	ALVEOLAR MINUTE VENTILATION (mL · MIN^{-1})
Shallow breathing	150		40		6000		(150 mL × 40)		0
Normal breathing	500		12		6000		(150 mL × 12)		4200
Deep breathing	1000		6		6000		(150 mL × 6)		5100

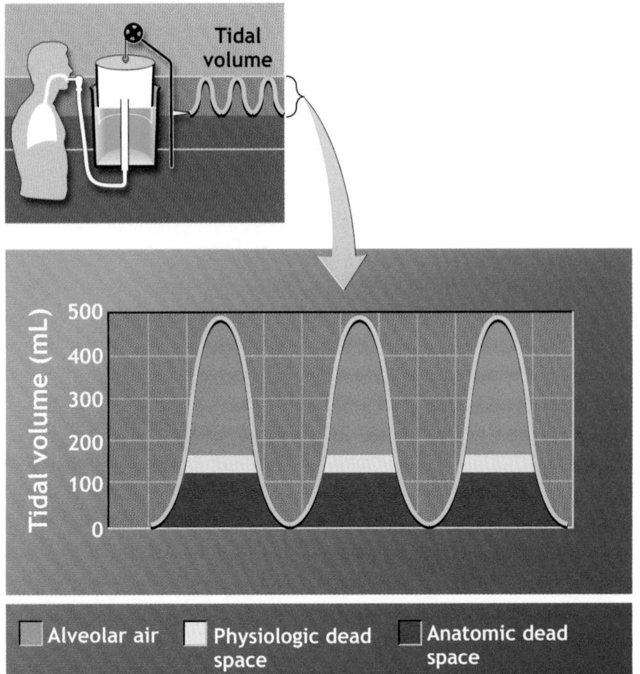

FIGURE 12.9 • Distribution of tidal volume (TV) in a healthy subject at rest. TV includes about 350 mL of ambient air that mixes with alveolar air, 150 mL of ambient air that remains in the larger air passages (anatomic dead space), and a small portion of air distributed to either poorly ventilated or poorly perfused alveoli (physiologic dead space).

Dead Space Versus Tidal Volume

The preceding examples of alveolar ventilation represent oversimplifications because they assumed a constant dead space despite changes in TV. Actually, anatomic dead space increases as TV becomes larger; it often doubles during deep breathing from some stretching of the respiratory passages with a fuller inspiration.[4] Importantly, any increase in dead space still represents proportionately less volume than the accompanying increase in TV. *Consequently, deeper breathing provides more effective alveolar ventilation than a similar minute ventilation achieved through an increased breathing rate.*

Ventilation–Perfusion Ratio

Adequate gas exchange between alveoli and blood requires effective matching of alveolar ventilation to the blood perfusing the pulmonary capillaries. Approximately 4.2 L of air normally ventilates the alveoli each minute at rest, whereas an average of 5.0 L of blood flows through the pulmonary capillaries. In this instance, the ratio of alveolar ventilation to pulmonary blood flow, termed the **ventilation–perfusion ratio**, equals 0.84 (4.2 ÷ 5.0). This ratio means that alveolar ventilation of 0.84 L matches each liter of pulmonary blood flow. In light exercise, the ventilation–perfusion ratio remains approximately 0.8, whereas heavy exercise produces a disproportionate increase in alveolar ventilation. In healthy individuals, the ventilation–perfusion ratio may increase to more than 5.0; this still provides a fairly uniform pulmonary blood flow distribution to ensure adequate aeration of venous blood.

Physiologic Dead Space

Sometimes, the alveoli may not function adequately in gas exchange because of either (1) underperfusion of blood or (2) inadequate ventilation relative to the alveolar surface. The term **physiologic dead space** describes the portion of the alveolar volume with a ventilation–perfusion ratio that approaches zero. Figure 12.9 shows the negligible physiologic dead space in the healthy lung. In certain situations, physiologic dead space can increase to 50% of the TV. This occurs with either *inadequate perfusion* from hemorrhage or blockage of the pulmonary circulation by an embolism or with *inadequate ventilation* in emphysema, asthma, and pulmonary fibrosis. An increased physiologic dead space from decreased functional alveolar surface in emphysema, for example, produces excessive ventilation even at low exercise intensities. Many of these patients cannot achieve maximal circulatory capacity because of ventilatory muscle fatigue from excessive breathing. When the dead space of the lung exceeds 60% of total lung volume, adequate gas exchange becomes impossible.

Rate Versus Depth

Increasing both rate and depth of breathing increases alveolar ventilation in exercise. In moderate exercise, well-trained athletes maintain alveolar ventilation by increasing TV (with only a small increase in breathing rate).[20] As breathing becomes deeper during exercise, alveolar ventilation increases from 70% of the total minute ventilation at rest to more than 85% of the exercise ventilation. Figure 12.10 shows that the increased exercise TV results largely from encroachment on the IRV, with a smaller decrease in the end-expiratory level. With more-intense exercise, the increase in TV begins to plateau at approximately 60% of

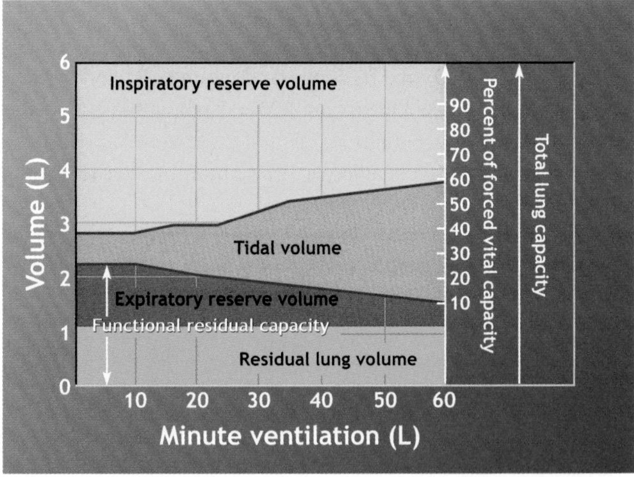

FIGURE 12.10 • Tidal volume and subdivisions of pulmonary air during rest and exercise.

the vital capacity; minute ventilation increases further through increases in breathing rate. These adjustments occur unconsciously. Each person develops a "style" of breathing in which breathing rate and TV blend to provide effective alveolar ventilation. Conscious manipulation of breathing usually disturbs the exquisitely regulated physiologic adjustments to exercise. Attempts to modify breathing during general physical activities such as running offer no benefit to exercise performance. *At rest and during all levels of exercise, a healthy person should breathe in the manner that seems most natural.*

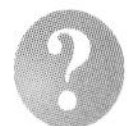

INTEGRATIVE QUESTION

One technique during "natural" childbirth requires the woman to breathe rapidly to effectively "work with" the normal ebb and flow of uterine contractions. How can a person accelerate breathing rate at rest without disrupting the normal alveolar ventilation?

VARIATIONS FROM NORMAL BREATHING PATTERNS

Breathing patterns during exercise generally progress in an effective and highly economical manner, yet some pulmonary responses potentially adversely affect exercise performance and/or physiologic balance.

Hyperventilation

Hyperventilation refers to an increase in pulmonary ventilation that exceeds the oxygen needs of metabolism. This "overbreathing" quickly lowers normal alveolar carbon dioxide concentration, causing excess carbon dioxide to leave bodily fluids via the expired air. An accompanying decrease in hydrogen ion (H^+) concentration increases plasma pH. Several seconds of hyperventilation generally produce lightheadedness; prolonged hyperventilation can sometimes lead to unconsciousness from excessive carbon dioxide unloading.

Dyspnea

Dyspnea refers to an inordinate shortness of breath or subjective distress in breathing. The sense of breathing incapacity during exercise, particularly in novice exercisers, usually accompanies significantly elevated arterial carbon dioxide and H^+ concentrations. Both chemicals excite the inspiratory center to increase breathing rate and depth. Failure to regulate arterial carbon dioxide and H^+ concentrations adequately most likely relates to low aerobic fitness levels and a poorly conditioned ventilatory musculature. The normal strong neural drive to breathe during exercise causes poorly conditioned respiratory muscles to fatigue, unable to maintain normal plasma carbon dioxide and H^+ levels. This produces an accelerated pattern of shallow, ineffective breathing, and the individual senses an inability to breathe sufficient air.

Valsalva Maneuver

The expiratory muscles, besides their normal role in pulmonary ventilation, provide for the ventilatory maneuvers of coughing and sneezing. They also contribute to stabilizing the abdominal and chest cavities during heavy lifting. In quiet breathing, intrapulmonic pressure decreases only about 3 mm Hg during inspiration and rises a similar amount above atmospheric pressure in exhalation. However, closing the **glottis** (narrowest part of the larynx through which air passes into the trachea) following a full inspiration while maximally activating the expiratory muscles causes compressive forces to increase **intrathoracic pressure** more than 150 mm Hg above atmospheric pressure. Pressures increase to somewhat higher levels within the abdominal cavity during a maximal exhalation against a closed glottis.[23] Forced exhalation against a closed glottis, termed the **Valsalva maneuver**, occurs commonly in weight lifting and other similar activities that require a rapid, maximum application of force of short duration. The Valsalva stabilizes the abdominal and thoracic cavities, enhancing the action of the chest muscles.

Physiologic Consequences of the Valsalva Maneuver

An acute drop in blood pressure represents the primary hemodynamic consequence of a prolonged Valsalva maneuver. Increased intrathoracic pressure during a Valsalva maneuver becomes transmitted through the thin walls of the veins that pass through the thoracic region. Because venous blood remains under relatively low pressure, thoracic veins collapse, considerably reducing blood flow to the heart. Reduced venous return sharply reduces the heart's stroke volume, triggering a significant fall in blood pressure below the resting level.[10,30] Performing a prolonged Valsalva maneuver during static, straining-type exercise, dramatically reduces venous return and arterial blood pressure. These effects diminish blood supply to the brain, often producing dizziness, "spots before the eyes," or fainting. Once the glottis reopens and intrathoracic pressure normalizes, blood flow reestablishes with an "overshoot" in arterial blood pressure.[51,53]

Figure 12.11 illustrates four phases of the typical blood pressure response (heart beat by heart beat) during the Valsalva maneuver in a healthy subject.[26] Aortic pulse pressure presented on the vertical axis represents the difference between systolic and diastolic pressures. Aortic pulse pressure increases slightly as the Valsalva begins (Phase I), probably from the mechanical effect of elevated intrathoracic pressure that expels blood from the left ventricle into the aorta. A biphasic response occurs within six heartbeats of the Valsalva onset, consisting of a large reduction in aortic pulse pressure (Phase IIa) followed by a relatively small gradual rise (Phase IIb) and secondary decrease (Phase III) during the continued Valsalva strain. When the maneuver ceases (release of strain), blood pressure rises rapidly and overshoots the resting value (Phase IV).

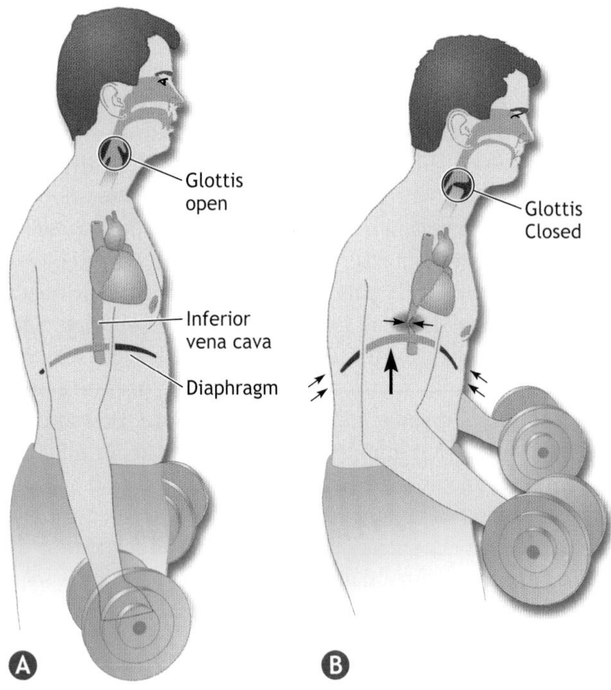

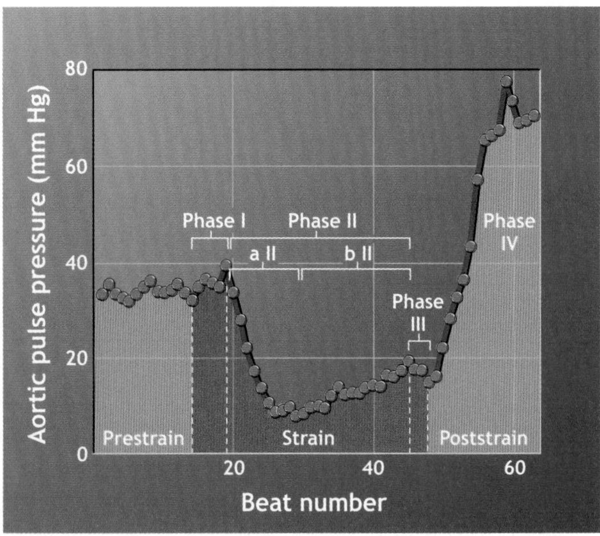

Figure 12.11 • The Valsalva maneuver significantly reduces the return of blood to the heart because increased intrathoracic pressure collapses the inferior vena cava that passes through the chest cavity. **A**. Normal breathing. **B**. Straining exercise with accompanying Valsalva maneuver. **C**. Typical normal response of aortic pulse pressure with a Valsalva maneuver during calibrated muscle strain. The figure illustrates 63 consecutive heartbeats (●). High-fidelity aortic pressure recordings were obtained at the aortic root level. Pulse pressure represents systolic pressure minus diastolic pressure. (Data from Hébert J-L, et al. Pulse pressure response to the strain of the Valsalva maneuver in humans with preserved systolic function. J Appl Physiol 1998;85:817.)

A Common Misconception. Many individuals believe incorrectly that the Valsalva maneuver *causes* the relatively large increases in blood pressure consistently observed with heavy resistance training exercises. Recall from the preceding figure that a prolonged Valsalva dramatically *reduces* blood pressure. Confusion arises because a Valsalva maneuver of insufficient duration to cause a prolonged lowering of blood pressure usually accompanies straining muscular efforts common during isometric and dynamic resistance exercise. These exercises (with or without Valsalva) greatly increase resistance to blood flow in active muscle.[19] For example, intramuscular fluid pressure increases linearly with all levels of isometric force up to maximum.[49] Increased peripheral vascular resistance significantly increases the arterial blood pressure *and* workload of the heart throughout exercise.[34] These responses (not the Valsalva, which, if prolonged, produces the opposite effect) pose potential danger to individuals with cardiovascular disease; they form the basis for advising cardiac patients to refrain from heavy resistance training. On the other hand, performing rhythmic muscular activity, including moderate weight lifting, promotes a steadier blood flow with only a modest increase in blood pressure and work of the heart. Chapter 15 more fully discusses the blood pressure response to different exercise modes.

INTEGRATIVE QUESTION

After completing a maximum-lift standing press, a person exclaims: "I feel slightly dizzy and see spots before my eyes." Provide a plausible physiologic explanation.

THE RESPIRATORY TRACT DURING COLD-WEATHER EXERCISE

Cold ambient air normally does not pose a danger for damaging the respiratory passages. Even in extreme cold weather, the incoming air generally warms to 26.5 to 32.2°C by the time it reaches the bronchi, and values as low as 20°C can occur during breathing large volumes of cold, dry air.[40] Airway warming of inspired air greatly increases its capacity to hold moisture, which produces considerable water loss from the respiratory passages. Thus, in cold weather, the respiratory tract loses a significant amount of water and heat, most notably during strenuous exercise and its accompanying large ventilatory volumes. Fluid loss from the airways often contributes to overall dehydration, dry mouth, burning sensation in the throat, and generalized irritation of the respiratory passages. Wearing a scarf or cellulose mask-type "balaclava" that covers the nose and mouth traps the water in exhaled air and subsequently warms and moistens the next incoming breath of air. This effect greatly reduces the symptoms of respiratory discomfort.

Postexercise Coughing

Exercise, particularly in cold weather, frequently dries the throat and triggers coughing during the recovery period. The response becomes prevalent following exercise in cold weather, when the respiratory tract loses considerable water. Postexercise coughing relates directly to the overall respiratory water loss (rather than respiratory heat loss)

Focus on Research

Physiologic Control of Pulmonary Ventilation

Dejours P. The regulation of breathing during muscular exercise in man. A neuro-humoral theory. In: Cunningham DJC, Lloyd BB, eds. The regulation of human respiration. Oxford, England: Blackwell, 1963.

➤ Early theories about pulmonary ventilation regulation during exercise centered singularly on arterial P_{CO_2}, arterial blood pH, or reflex stimulation originating from muscle receptors. Dejours believed that no factor by itself, but rather a multiplicity of interacting factors, regulated breathing during exercise. He hypothesized that exercise hyperpnea depended on humoral (chemical) and neurogenic stimuli that varied their contributions depending on the phase of exercise and recovery.

The figure presents Dejours' observations that the time course of pulmonary minute ventilation ($\dot{V}_E$) during the transitions from rest to exercise to recovery followed a consistent pattern. $\dot{V}_E$ increases within the same ventilatory cycle coinciding with the start of exercise. Some 10 to 20 seconds later, ventilation volumes slowly increase to an eventual steady state. Minute ventilation declines abruptly when exercise stops, remains fairly constant for 20 to 30 seconds, and then decreases progressively to the resting value.

Dejours concluded that ventilatory dynamics in exercise consist of a combination of rapid (fast component) and slow (slow component) responses that progress in defined stages during exercise and recovery. He proposed that different physiologic factors control the fast and slow components. Two factors contribute to the fast component: (1) cerebral input from afferent impulses from the brain's psychomotor area to the respiratory center in the medulla and (2) extrathoracic mechanoreceptor stimulation from "proprioceptors" in active body segments. Two mechanisms also modulate the slower component of the ventilatory response. The first, a reflex, originates from muscle chemoreceptors sensitive to progressive physiochemical changes within active muscle as exercise progresses. The second factor is a humoral mechanism. Dejours' belief in humoral control developed from experiments that occluded leg blood flow. Restricting venous return during leg exercise caused $\dot{V}_E$ to decline below resting levels, thus demonstrating ventilatory dependence on blood-borne (humoral) chemicals produced in active tissues.

Dejours stressed the interrelationship between the fast and slow components in exercise ventilation. Reflex and cortical factors initiated the rapid rise in ventilation at the start of exercise. Subsequently, humoral factors, and possibly progressive neurogenic output, modulated the slower rise in ventilation during the first minutes of exercise. The latter steady-state response during exercise probably related to (1) increases in reflex drive through local physical and chemical changes at the peripheral mechanoreceptors and (2) positive interactions between neurogenic and humoral drives. When exercise stops and neurogenic input ceases, ventilation decreases precipitously. Ventilation then becomes regulated exclusively by humoral factors from the recovering musculature.

The studies of Dejours formed the basis for explaining pulmonary ventilation during exercise and recovery. Subsequent research (see Fig. 14.4) provides additional factors to explain exercise hyperpnea and offers a more comprehensive model for ventilatory control.

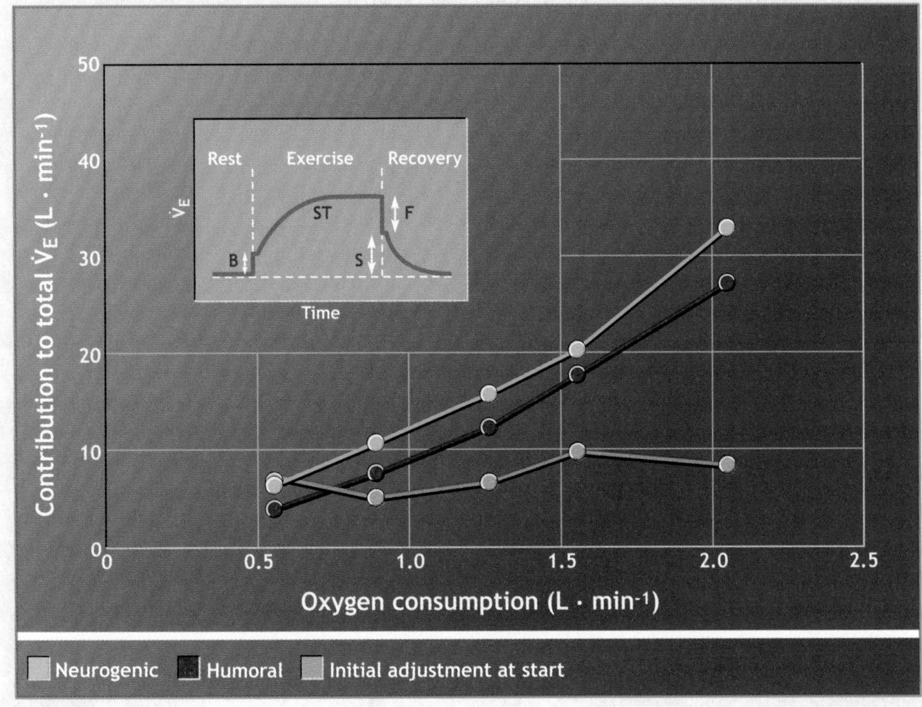

Pulmonary minute ventilation ($\dot{V}_E$) during mild exercise and recovery (inset graph). Portion *B* represents the immediate, rapid increase at the onset of exercise; *ST* reflects the more gradual rise to a steady state; *F* is the quick fall when exercise stops; and *S* represents the slower return of ventilation to the preexercise level. The main graph shows the magnitude of the contribution of each of these ventilatory response components related to oxygen consumption. Both neurogenic and humoral components increase with the intensity of the preceding exercise; the fast component at the start of exercise increases with exercise intensity much less than the progressive increase in neurogenic and humoral controls relative to exercise intensity.

associated with the large ventilatory volumes breathed during exercise.[6]

Summary

1. The lungs provide a large surface between the body's internal fluid environment and the gaseous external environment. During any 1 second of exercise, no more than 1 pint of blood flows in the pulmonary capillaries.
2. Normal regulation of pulmonary ventilation maintains a favorable concentration of alveolar oxygen and carbon dioxide, to ensure adequate aeration of blood flowing through the lungs.
3. Pulmonary airflow depends on small pressure differentials between ambient air and air within the lungs. Muscle actions that alter thoracic cavity dimensions produce these pressure differences.
4. Lung volumes vary with age, gender, and body size (particularly stature) and should only be evaluated with established norms based on these factors.
5. The residual lung volume represents air remaining in the lungs following maximal exhalation. This air volume allows uninterrupted exchange of gas during all phases of the breathing cycle.
6. Forced expiratory volume and maximum voluntary ventilation dynamically measure the ability to sustain a high level of airflow. These lung function measures serve as excellent screening tests to detect lung disease.
7. Measures of static and dynamic lung function within the normal range poorly predict aerobic fitness and exercise performance.
8. Breathing rate and tidal volume (TV) determine pulmonary minute ventilation. Minute ventilation averages 6 $L \cdot min^{-1}$ at rest and can increase to 200 $L \cdot min^{-1}$ during maximal exercise.
9. Alveolar ventilation reflects the portion of minute ventilation that enters the alveoli for gaseous exchange with the blood.
10. The ventilation–perfusion ratio describes the association between alveolar minute ventilation and pulmonary blood flow. At rest, alveolar ventilation of 0.8 L matches each liter of pulmonary blood flow. During heavy exercise, alveolar ventilation in healthy individuals increases disproportionately to increase the ventilation–perfusion ratio, often to 5.0.
11. TV increases during exercise by encroachment into inspiratory and expiratory reserve volumes. As exercise becomes more intense, TV begins to plateau at approximately 60% of the vital capacity; minute ventilation increases further through increases in breathing rate.
12. A healthy person should breathe in a manner that seems most natural during rest, exercise, and recovery.
13. Hyperventilation refers to an increase in pulmonary ventilation that exceeds the oxygen needs of metabolism. This "overbreathing" quickly lowers normal alveolar carbon dioxide concentration, causing excess carbon dioxide to leave body fluids via the expired air.
14. A Valsalva maneuver describes a forced exhalation against a closed glottis. This action causes large pressure increases within the chest and abdominal cavities that compress the thoracic veins, thereby reducing venous return to the heart.
15. The straining muscular effort that usually accompanies the Valsalva temporarily elevates blood pressure and adds to the heart's workload. Individuals with heart and vascular disease should refrain from exercises such as heavy weight lifting and isometric muscle actions.
16. Cold ambient air normally does not pose a risk for damaging the respiratory passages.

References

1. Akabas SR, et al. Metabolic and functional adaptation of the diaphragm to training with resistive loads. J Appl Physiol 1989;66:529.
2. Aliverti A, et al. Human respiratory muscle actions and control during exercise. J Appl Physiol 1997;83:1256.
3. American Thoracic Society. Lung function testing: selection of reference values and interpretative strategies. Am Rev Respir Dis 1991;144:1202.
4. Asmussen E, Nielsen M. Physiological dead-space and alveolar gas pressures at rest and during muscular exercise. Acta Physiol Scand 1956;38:1.
5. Åstrand P-O, Rodahl K. Textbook of work physiology. New York: McGraw-Hill, 1986.
6. Banner AS, et al. Relation of respiratory water loss to coughing after exercise. N Engl J Med 1984;311:883.
7. Bjurström RL, Schoene RB. Control of ventilation in elite synchronized swimmers. J Appl Physiol 1987;63:1019.
8. Buno MJ, et al. The effect of an acute bout of exercise on selected pulmonary function measurements. Med Sci Sports Exerc 1981;13:290.
9. Carey CR, et al. Effects of skin diving on lung volumes. J Appl Physiol 1955;8:19.
10. Clifford PS, et al. Arterial blood pressure response to rowing. Med Sci Sports Exerc 1994;26:715.
11. Coast JR, et al. Effects of lower body pressure changes on pulmonary function. Med Sci Sports Exerc 1998;30:1035.
12. Cooper CB. Determining the role of exercise in patients with chronic pulmonary disease. Med Sci Sports Exerc 1995;27:147.
13. Cordain L, et al. Lung volumes and maximal respiratory pressures in collegiate swimmers and runners. Res Q Exerc Sport 1990;61:70.
14. Courteix D, et al. Effects of intensive swimming training on lung volumes, airway resistances and the maximal expiratory flow-volume relationship in prepubertal girls. Eur J Appl Physiol 264, 1997.
15. Cummings GR. Correlation of athletic performance with pulmonary function in 13 to 17 year old boys and girls. Med Sci Sports Exerc 1969;1:140.
16. Farkas GA, et al. Contractility of the ventilatory pump muscles. Med Sci Sports Exerc 1996;28:1106.
17. Farrell PA, et al. The course of lung volume changes during prolonged treadmill exercise. Med Sci Sports Exerc 1983;15:319.
18. Fuller D, et al. Expiratory muscle endurance performance after exhaustive submaximal exercise. J Appl Physiol 1996;80:1495.
19. Gaffney FA, et al. Cardiovascular and metabolic responses to static contraction in man. Acta Physiol Scand 1990;138:249.
20. Grimby G. Respiration in exercise. Med Sci Sports Exerc 1969;1:9.
21. Hagberg JM, et al. Pulmonary function in young and older athletes and untrained men. J Appl Physiol 1988;65:101.
22. Hanson JS. Maximal exercise performance in members of the U.S. Nordic Ski Team. J Appl Physiol 1973;33:592.

23. Harman EA, et al. Intra-abdominal and intra-thoracic pressures during lifting and jumping. Med Sci Sports Exerc 1988;20:195.
24. Harms CA, et al. Exercise induced arterial hypoxemia in healthy young women. J Physiol (Lond) 1998;507:619.
25. Hass F, et al. Effect of upper body posture on forced inspiration and expiration. J Appl Physiol 1982;52:879.
26. Hébert J-L, et al. Pulse pressure response to the strain of the Valsalva maneuver in humans with preserved systolic function. J Appl Physiol 1998;85:817.
27. Hopkins SR, et al. Sustained submaximal exercise does not alter the integrity of the lung blood-gas barrier in elite athletes. J Appl Physiol 1998;84:1185.
28. Kaufmann DA, et al. Pulmonary function of marathon runners. Med Sci Sports Exerc 1974;6:114.
29. Kenyon CM, et al. Rib cage mechanics during quiet breathing and exercise in humans. J Appl Physiol 1997;83:1242.
30. Lassen A, et al. Cardiovascular responses to static contractions in man with topical nerve blockade. J Physiol (Lond) 1989;409:333.
31. Lazarus R, et al. Effects of body composition and fat distribution on ventilatory function in adults. Am J Clin Nutr 1998;68:35.
32. Leech JA, et al. Respiratory pressures and function in young adults. Am Rev Respir Dis 1983;128:17.
33. Levison H, Cherniack R. Ventilatory cost of exercise in chronic obstructive pulmonary disease. J Appl Physiol 1968;25:21.
34. MacDougall JD, et al. Arterial blood pressure response to resistance exercise. J Appl Physiol 1985;58:785.
35. Mahler DA, et al. Exercise performance in marathon runners with airway obstruction. Med Sci Sports Exerc 1981;13:284.
36. Mahler DA, et al. Ventilatory responses at rest and during exercise in marathon runners. J Appl Physiol 1982;52:388.
37. Mahler DA, Harper A. Prediction of peak oxygen consumption in obstructive airway disease. Med Sci Sports Exerc 1988;20:574.
38. Maron MB, et al. Alterations in pulmonary function consequent to competitive marathon running. Med Sci Sports Exerc 1979;11:244.
39. McClaran SR, et al. Smaller lungs in women affect exercise hyperpnea. J Appl Physiol 1998;84:1872.
40. McFadden ER Jr. Respiratory heat and water exchange: physiological and clinical implications. J Appl Physiol 1984;54:331.
41. Miller WC, et al. Derivation of prediction equations for RV in overweight men and women. Med Sci Sports Exerc 1998;30:322.
42. Pardy RL, et al. Respiratory muscle training compared with physiotherapy in chronic airflow limitation. Am Rev Respir Dis 1981;123:421.
43. Poole DC, et al. Diaphragm structure and function in health and disease. Med Sci Sports Exerc 1997;29:738.
44. Powers S, et al. Diaphragmatic fiber type specific adaptation to endurance exercise. Respir Physiol 1992;89:195.
45. Rasch PJ, Brandt JWA. Measurement of pulmonary function in United States Olympic free style wrestlers. Res Q 1957;28:279.
46. Sady S, et al. Physiological characteristics of high-ability prepubescent wrestlers. Med Sci Sports Exerc 1984;6:72.
47. Schapira RM, et al. The value of expiratory time in the physical diagnosis of obstructive airway disease. JAMA 1993;270:731.
48. Scherer TA, et al. Respiratory muscle endurance training in chronic obstructive pulmonary disease. Impact on exercise capacity, dyspnea, and quality of life. Am J Respir Crit Care Med 2000;162:1709.
49. Sejersted ON, et al. Intramuscular fluid pressure during isometric contraction of human skeletal muscle. J Appl Physiol 1984;56:287.
50. Sharp JT, et al. Relative contributions of rib cage and abdomen to breathing in normal subjects. J Appl Physiol 1975;39:609.
51. Smith MA, et al. Assessment of beat to beat changes in cardiac output during the Valsalva maneuver using bioimpedence cardiology. Clin Sci 1987;72:423.
52. Sonne LJ, Davis JA. Increased exercise performance in patients with severe COPD following inspiratory resistive training. Chest 1982;81:436.
53. Ten Harkel ADJ, et al. Assessment of cardiovascular reflexes: influence of posture and period of preceding rest. J Appl Physiol 1990;68:147.
54. Wagner J. Pulmonary function testing: a practical approach. 2nd ed, Baltimore: Williams & Wilkins, 1996.
55. Weisman IM, Zevallos RJ. An integrated approach to the interpretation of cardiopulmonary exercise testing. Clin Chest Med 1994;15:421.
56. Wilmore JH. A simplified method for the determination of residual lung volume. J Appl Physiol 1969;27:96.
57. Wilmore JH, Haskell WL. Body composition and endurance capacity of professional football players. J Appl Physiol 1972;33:564.

CHAPTER 13

Gas Exchange and Transport

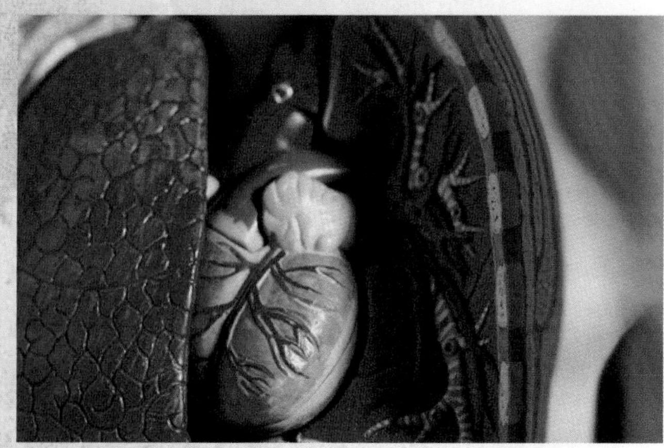

Chapter Objectives

- List the partial pressures of the respired gases during rest and maximal exercise in the alveoli, arterial blood, active muscles, and mixed-venous blood
- Explain the impact of Henry's law on pulmonary gas exchange
- Quantify oxygen transport (1) in arterial plasma and (2) combined with hemoglobin under sea-level, ambient conditions
- Discuss the physiologic advantages of oxyhemoglobin's S-shaped dissociation curve
- Describe factors that produce the "Bohr effect," and outline the benefit of this effect in physical activity
- Explain the role of myoglobin during high-intensity, physical activity
- List and quantify three ways for carbon dioxide transport in blood

The body's supply of oxygen depends on its *concentration* and *pressure* in ambient air. Ambient air remains relatively constant in composition, containing 20.93% oxygen, 79.04% nitrogen (including small quantities of other inert gases that behave physiologically like nitrogen), 0.03% carbon dioxide, and usually small quantities of water vapor. The gas molecules move at relatively high speeds and exert a pressure against any surface they contact. At sea level, the pressure of air molecules raises a column of mercury in a barometer to a height of 760 mm (29.9 in) or 1 torr. The **torr**—named for the Italian physicist and mathematician Evangelista Torricelli (1608–1647), who invented the barometer—is not an SI unit but expresses gas pressure. One torr equals the pressure sufficient to raise a 1-mm column of mercury 1 mm high at 0°C against the standard acceleration of gravity at 45° north latitude ($980.6 \text{ cm} \cdot \text{s}^{-2}$). One standard atmosphere equals 760 torr. The barometric reading varies with changing weather conditions and becomes considerably lower at higher altitudes (see Chapter 24).

➤ PART 1 • Gaseous Exchange in the Lungs and Tissues

CONCENTRATIONS AND PARTIAL PRESSURES OF RESPIRED GASES

The molecules of each specific gas in a mixture of gases exert their own **partial pressure**. The mixture's total pressure then equals the sum of the partial pressures of the individual gases in the mixture (**Dalton's law**). Partial pressure computes as follows:

$$\text{Partial pressure} = \text{Percentage concentration} \times \text{Total pressure of gas mixture}$$

COMMON SYMBOLS FOR GAS PRESSURE IN RESPIRATORY PHYSIOLOGY

- **P_AO_2**: Partial pressure of oxygen in alveolar chambers
- **PaO_2**: Partial pressure of oxygen in arterial blood
- **SaO_2%**: Percent saturation of arterial blood with oxygen
- **$P\bar{v}O_2$**: Partial pressure of oxygen in venous blood
- **P_ACO_2**: Partial pressure of carbon dioxide in alveolar chambers
- **$PaCO_2$**: Partial pressure of carbon dioxide in arterial blood
- **$P\bar{v}CO_2$**: Partial pressure of carbon dioxide in venous blood
- **$S\bar{v}O_2$%**: Percent saturation of venous blood with oxygen
- **a-v O_2 diff**: Arteriovenous oxygen difference; difference between oxygen carried in arterial blood and carried in venous blood
- **a-$\bar{v}$ O_2 diff**: Arterial–mixed-venous oxygen difference; difference between oxygen carried in arterial blood and carried in mixed-venous blood
- **$\bar{v}$**: mixed-venous blood

TABLE 13.1 ➤ **PARTIAL PRESSURE AND VOLUME OF GASES IN DRY AMBIENT AIR AT SEA LEVEL**

Gas	Percentage	Partial Pressure[a] (mm Hg)	Volume of Gas ($\text{mL} \cdot \text{L}^{-1}$)
Oxygen	20.93	159	209.3
Carbon dioxide	0.03	0.2	0.4
Nitrogen	79.04[b]	600	790.3

[a]At 760 mm Hg ambient air pressure.
[b]Includes 0.93% argon and other trace rare gases.

Ambient Air

Table 13.1 lists the volumes, percentages, and partial pressures of the gases in dry ambient air at sea level. The partial pressure of oxygen equals 20.93% of the total 760 mm Hg pressure exerted by air, or 159 mm Hg (20.93 ÷ 100 × 760 mm Hg). Carbon dioxide exerts a small pressure of only 0.23 mm Hg (0.03 ÷ 100 × 760 mm Hg), whereas the molecules of nitrogen exert a pressure that raises the mercury in a manometer about 600 mm (79.04 ÷ 100 × 760 mm Hg). A *P* in front of the gas symbol usually denotes partial pressure. The partial pressures at sea level for the principal components of ambient air average: oxygen (PO_2) = 159 mm Hg, carbon dioxide (PCO_2) = 0.2 mm Hg, and nitrogen (PN_2) = 600 mm Hg.

Tracheal Air

Air completely saturates with water vapor as it enters the nasal cavities and mouth and passes down the respiratory tract. The vapor dilutes the inspired air mixture somewhat. At a body temperature of 37°C, for example, the pressure of water molecules in humidified air equals 47 mm Hg; this leaves 713 mm Hg (760 – 47 mm Hg) as the total pressure exerted by the inspired dry air molecules. Consequently, the effective PO_2 in **tracheal air** decreases by about 10 mm Hg from its ambient value of 159 mm Hg to 149 mm Hg [0.2093 × (760 – 47 mm Hg)]. Humidification exerts little effect on the inspired PCO_2 because of carbon dioxide's negligible contribution to inspired air.

Alveolar Air

Alveolar air composition differs considerably from the incoming breath of moist ambient air because carbon dioxide continually enters the alveoli from the blood, whereas oxygen flows from the lungs into the blood for transport throughout the body. Table 13.2 shows that alveolar air contains on average 14.5% oxygen, 5.5% carbon dioxide, and 80.0% nitrogen. After subtracting the vapor pressure from moist alveolar gas, the average alveolar PO_2 becomes 103 mm Hg [0.145 × (760 – 47 mm Hg)] and 39 mm Hg [0.055 × (760 – 47 mm Hg)] for PCO_2. *These values represent average pressures exerted by oxygen and carbon dioxide molecules against the alveolar*

TABLE 13.2 ➤ PARTIAL PRESSURE AND VOLUME OF DRY ALVEOLAR GASES AT SEA LEVEL (37° C)

GAS	PERCENTAGE	PARTIAL PRESSURE[a] (MM HG)	VOLUME OF GAS (ML · L^{-1})
Oxygen	14.5	103	145
Carbon dioxide	5.5	39	55
Nitrogen[b]	80.0	571	800
Water vapor		47	

[a]At 760–47 mm Hg alveolar gas pressure.
[b]Nitrogen occupies a slightly greater percentage of alveolar air than ambient air because energy metabolism generally produces less carbon dioxide than oxygen consumed (i.e., the respiratory quotient [RQ = $\dot{V}CO_2 \div \dot{V}O_2$] equals less than 1.00). Because of this exchange imbalance, the nitrogen percentage increases.

side of the alveolar–capillary membrane. They do not remain physiologic constants; rather, they vary somewhat with the ventilatory cycle phase and the adequacy of ventilation in various lung regions. Recall that after each normal exhalation a relatively large volume of air remains in the lungs. This functional residual capacity serves as a damper, so each incoming breath exerts only a small effect on the composition of alveolar air. This explains why the partial pressures of alveolar gases remain relatively stable.

MOVEMENT OF GAS IN AIR AND FLUIDS

In accordance with **Henry's law** (named for English chemist William Henry [1775–1836]), gases diffuse from high-pressure areas to low-pressure areas. The rate of gas diffusion into a fluid depends on two factors:

1. The **pressure differential** between the gas above the fluid and the gas dissolved in the fluid.
2. The **solubility** of the gas in the fluid.

Pressure Differential

Oxygen molecules continually strike the surface of the water in the three chambers illustrated in Figure 13.1. The pure water in chamber *A* contains no oxygen (P = 0 mm Hg), and a large number of oxygen molecules enter the water and become dissolved in it. Because dissolved gas molecules also move randomly, some oxygen molecules leave the water. In chamber *B*, oxygen still shows a net movement into the fluid from the gaseous state. Eventually, the number of molecules entering and leaving the fluid equalizes, as occurs in chamber *C*. When this happens, the gas pressures equilibrate, with no net oxygen diffusion into or out of the water. Conversely, if the pressure of dissolved oxygen molecules exceeds the pressure of the free gas in air, oxygen leaves the fluid until it attains a new pressure equilibrium. In humans, the pressure *difference* between alveolar and pulmonary blood gases creates the driving force for gas diffusion across the pulmonary membrane.

Solubility

For two different gases at identical pressure differentials, the solubility (dissolving power) of each gas determines the number of molecules moving into or out of a fluid. One expresses gas solubility as mL of a gas per 100 mL (dL) of a fluid. Oxygen, carbon dioxide, and nitrogen have different solubility coefficients in whole blood. Carbon dioxide dissolves most readily, with a solubility coefficient of 57.03 mL of carbon dioxide per dL of fluid at 760 mm Hg and 37°C. Oxygen, with a solubility coefficient of 2.26 mL, remains relatively insoluble, and nitrogen is least soluble, with a coefficient of 1.30 mL.

The amount of gas dissolved in a fluid calculates as:

$$\text{Quantity of gas} = \text{Solubility coefficient} \times (\text{Gas partial pressure} \div \text{Total barometric pressure})$$

For example, the amount of oxygen dissolved in 1 dL of arterial whole blood (Po_2 = 100 mm Hg) at sea level (760 mm Hg) computes as:

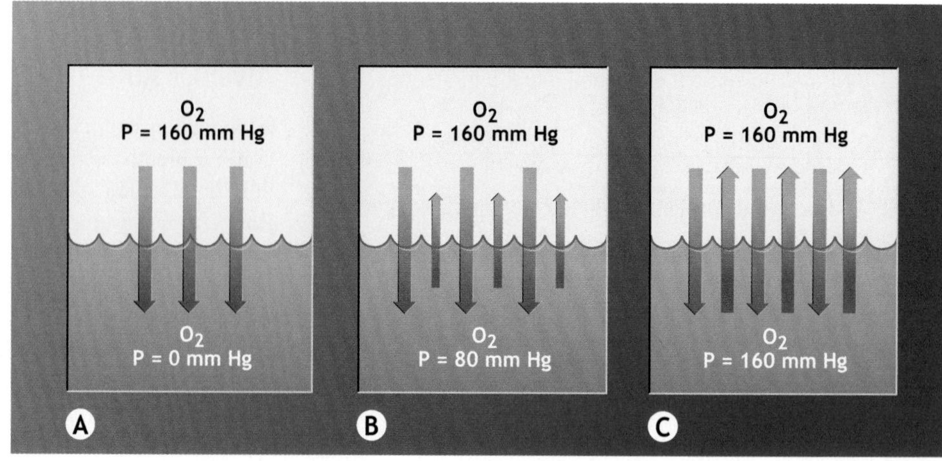

FIGURE 13.1 • Solution containing oxygen in water. **A**. When oxygen first comes in contact with pure water. **B**. Dissolved oxygen halfway to equilibrium with gaseous oxygen. **C**. Equilibrium between oxygen in air and in water.

$$\text{Quantity of gas} = 2.26 \times (100 \div 760) = 0.3 \text{ mL} \cdot \text{dL}^{-1}$$

For each unit of pressure favoring diffusion, approximately 25 times more carbon dioxide than oxygen moves into (or from) a fluid. Viewed another way, equal quantities of oxygen and carbon dioxide enter or leave a fluid under significantly different pressure gradients for each gas. This represents the precise situation in the body.

APPROXIMATE SOLUBILITY COEFFICIENT OF GASES IN PHYSIOLOGIC FLUIDS

Gas	Water	Plasma	Blood (quantity dissolved per dL)
Oxygen	2.39	2.14	2.26 (0.3 mL)
Carbon dioxide	56.7	51.5	57.03 (3.0 mL)
Nitrogen	1.23	1.18	1.30 (0.8 mL)

Dissolved oxygen contributes about 4% of the total oxygen consumed by the body each minute during rest; in maximal exercise, it provides less than 2% of the total requirement. Even increasing arterial Po_2 by breathing 100% oxygen (ambient Po_2 = 760 mm Hg), dissolved oxygen (1.5 to 2.0 mL · dL of blood) still supplies only 40% of the total oxygen for rest and about 10% during maximal exercise. However, the physiologic significance of dissolved oxygen and carbon dioxide comes not from its role as a vehicle for transport, but rather in determining the partial pressures of these gases. Partial pressure plays a central role in loading and unloading oxygen and carbon dioxide in the lungs and tissues.

GAS EXCHANGE IN THE LUNGS AND TISSUES

Exchange of gases between the lungs and blood, and gas movement at the tissue level, progresses passively by diffusion, depending on the pressure gradients established. Figure 13.2 illustrates the pressure gradients favoring gas transfer in different areas of the body at rest.

Gas Exchange in the Lungs

At rest, the 100-mm Hg pressure of oxygen molecules in the alveoli exceeds by about 60 mm Hg the 40-mm Hg oxygen pressure in blood entering the pulmonary capillaries. Consequently, oxygen dissolves and diffuses through the alveolar membranes into the blood. In contrast, carbon dioxide exists under a slightly greater pressure in returning venous blood than it does in the alveoli; this causes a net diffusion of carbon dioxide from the blood into the lungs. Despite the relatively small pressure gradient of 6 mm Hg for carbon dioxide diffusion (compared with a 60-mm Hg gradient for oxygen), carbon dioxide transfer occurs rapidly owing to its high solubility in plasma. Nitrogen, neither used nor produced in metabolic reactions, remains essentially unchanged in alveolar–capillary gas.

Gas exchange occurs so rapidly in the healthy lung that alveolar gas–blood gas equilibrium takes place in about 0.25 second, or within one-third of the blood's transit time through the lungs. Even in high-intensity exercise, a red blood cell's velocity through a pulmonary capillary generally does not exceed its velocity at rest by 50%. With increasing exercise intensity, the pulmonary capillaries increase the blood volume within them by about 3 times the resting value.[2] The larger pulmonary blood volume helps to maintain a relatively slow pulmonary blood flow velocity during physical activity. With complete aeration, the blood leaving the lungs contains oxygen at an average pressure of 100 mm Hg and carbon dioxide at 40 mm Hg. These values vary little during vigorous exercise for most healthy people.

The Po_2 of arterial blood usually remains slightly lower than the alveolar Po_2 because some blood in the alveolar capillaries passes through poorly ventilated alveoli; also, the blood leaving the lungs joins venous blood from the bronchial and cardiac circulations. The term **venous admixture** defines this small amount of poorly oxygenated blood. Although venous admixture exerts a small effect in healthy individuals, it does reduce the arterial Po_2 slightly below the value in pulmonary end-capillary blood.

Pulmonary Disease

Two factors can impair gas transfer capacity at the alveolar–capillary membrane in pulmonary disease: (1) buildup of a pollutant layer that "thickens" the alveolar membrane and/or (2) reduction in alveolar surface area. Each factor extends the time before alveolar–capillary gas attains equilibration. For individuals with impaired lung function, the added demand for rapid gas exchange in exercise compromises aeration, ultimately affecting exercise performance adversely.

INTEGRATIVE QUESTION

Why is it that just minute amounts of impurities like CO_2 and CO in a breathing mixture exert such profound physiologic effects?

Gas Transfer in the Tissues

In the tissues, where energy metabolism consumes oxygen and produces an almost equal amount of carbon dioxide, gas pressures differ considerably from those in arterial blood. At rest, the Po_2 in the fluid immediately outside a muscle cell averages 40 mm Hg, and the intracellular Pco_2 averages 46 mm Hg. In vigorous exercise, oxygen pressure within muscle tissue falls toward 0 mm Hg,[17] while the pressure of carbon dioxide approaches 90 mm Hg. *Pressure differences between gases in plasma and tissues establish diffusion gradients.* Oxygen leaves the blood and diffuses toward the cell, while carbon dioxide flows from the cell into the blood. Blood then passes into the venous circuit (venules and veins) for return to the heart and delivery to the lungs. Diffusion occurs rapidly as blood enters the dense pulmonary capillary network. The

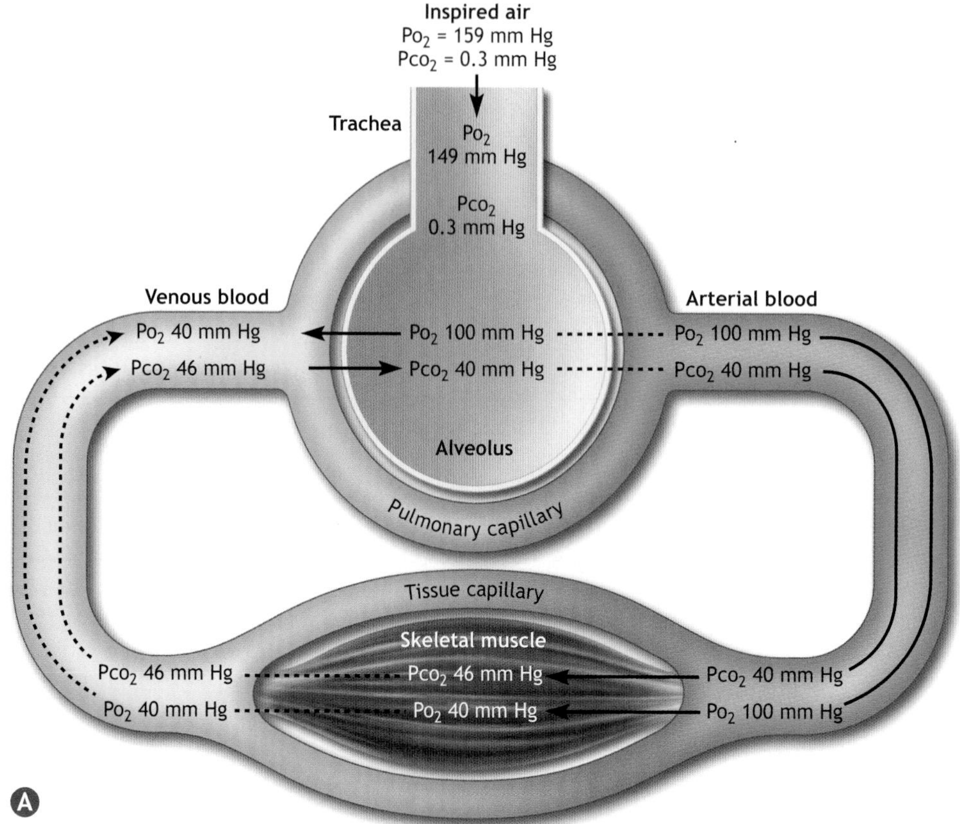

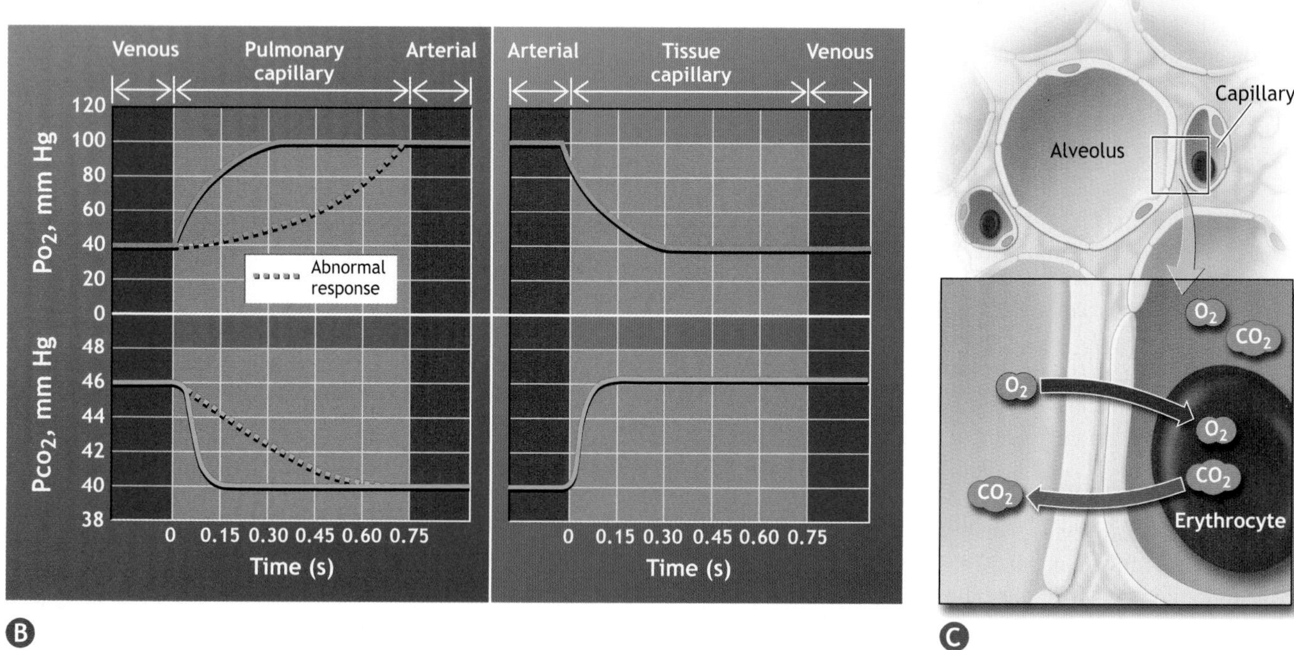

FIGURE 13.2 • Pressure gradients for gas transfer within the body at rest. **A**. The Po_2 and Pco_2 of ambient, tracheal, and alveolar air and these gas pressures in venous and arterial blood and muscle tissue. Gas movement at the alveolar–capillary and tissue–capillary membranes always progresses from an area of higher partial pressure to lower partial pressure. **B**. The time required for gas exchange. At rest, blood remains in the pulmonary and tissue capillaries for about 0.75 s. Pulmonary disease (*dashed line*) impairs the rate of gas transfer across the alveolar–capillary membrane, thus prolonging the time for equilibration of gases. Blood's transit time through the pulmonary capillaries during maximal exercise decreases to about 0.4 s, but this still remains adequate for complete aeration in the healthy lung. **C**. Gas exchange (diffusion) between a capillary and its adjacent alveolus.

body does not attempt to rid itself completely of carbon dioxide. To the contrary, each liter of blood leaving the lungs with a PCO_2 of 40 mm Hg contains about 50 mL of carbon dioxide. As discussed in Chapter 14, this small "background level" of carbon dioxide provides the chemical basis for ventilatory control through its stimulating effect on the neurons of the pons and medullary centers of the brainstem. The term **respiratory center** describes this collection of neural tissue.

If we could not breathe, diffusion would cease as alveolar and blood gases reached some average pressure. Inhaling another breath of air increases alveolar oxygen content and dilutes carbon dioxide concentration. *Alveolar ventilation couples tightly to metabolic demands, keeping alveolar gas composition remarkably constant. Stability in alveolar gas concentrations persists even during strenuous exercise that increases oxygen consumption and carbon dioxide output 25 times the values at rest.*

Summary

1. Gas molecules diffuse in the lungs and tissues down their concentration gradients from an area of higher concentration (higher pressure) to lower concentration (lower pressure).
2. The partial pressure of a specific gas in a mixture of gases varies directly with the concentration of the gas and the mixture's total pressure.
3. Henry's law states that pressure gradient and solubility determine how much gas dissolves in a fluid. Oxygen, carbon dioxide, and nitrogen exhibit different solubilities in whole blood. Carbon dioxide dissolves most readily, while oxygen and nitrogen show relatively low solubility.
4. Because carbon dioxide solubility in plasma exceeds oxygen solubility in plasma by 25 times, carbon dioxide moves into and from body fluids down a relatively small diffusion (pressure) gradient.
5. Pulmonary ventilation adjusts during rest and exercise to maintain a remarkably constant alveolar gas composition. Alveolar ventilation maintains PO_2 at about 100 mm Hg and PCO_2 at 40 mm Hg. Oxygen diffuses into the blood and carbon dioxide diffuses into the lungs because venous blood contains oxygen at lower pressure and carbon dioxide at higher pressure than alveolar gas.
6. Alveolar–blood gas exchange reaches equilibrium in the healthy lung at about the midpoint of the blood's transit through the pulmonary capillaries. Even in high-intensity exercise, blood flow velocity through the lungs generally does not compromise full loading of oxygen and unloading of carbon dioxide.
7. Diffusion gradients favor oxygen movement from the capillaries to the tissues and carbon dioxide from the cells to the blood. Oxygen and carbon dioxide diffuse rapidly as their pressure gradients expand during exercise.

➤ PART 2 • Oxygen Transport

TRANSPORT OF OXYGEN IN THE BLOOD

The blood carries oxygen in two ways:

1. In physical solution dissolved in the fluid portion of blood.
2. In loose combination with hemoglobin, the iron-protein molecule within the red blood cell.

Oxygen in Solution

As pointed out previously, oxygen's relative insolubility in water keeps its concentration low in bodily fluids. At an alveolar PO_2 of 100 mm Hg, only about 0.3 mL of gaseous oxygen dissolves in each dL of blood (0.003 mL for each additional 1-mm Hg increase). This equals 3 mL of oxygen per liter of blood. The blood volume of a 70-kg person averages about 5 L; thus, 15 mL of oxygen dissolves in the fluid portion of the blood (3 mL per L $\times$ 5). This small amount of oxygen would sustain life for about 4 seconds. Viewed from a different perspective, if oxygen in physical solution provided the sole oxygen source to the body, about 80 L of blood would need to circulate each minute to supply the resting oxygen requirements—a blood flow about twice the maximum ever recorded for an exercising human!

As with carbon dioxide, the small quantity of oxygen transported in physical solution serves important functions. The random movement of dissolved oxygen molecules establishes the PO_2 of the plasma and tissue fluids. The pressure of oxygen in solution helps to regulate breathing, particularly at an altitude when ambient PO_2 decreases considerably; it also determines the oxygen loading of hemoglobin in the lungs and subsequent release in tissues.

Oxygen Combined with Hemoglobin

Metallic compounds exist in the blood of many animal species and serve to augment the blood's oxygen-carrying capacity. Figure 13.3 illustrates the iron-containing globular protein pigment **hemoglobin** carried within the red blood cells of humans. About 280 million hemoglobin molecules pack into each of the body's more than 25 trillion red blood cells. This concentration carries 65 to 70 times more oxygen than normally dissolves in plasma. Thus, hemoglobin temporarily "captures" and transports about 197 mL of oxygen in each liter of blood. Each of the four iron atoms in the hemoglobin molecule can loosely bind one oxygen molecule in the reversible reaction:

$$Hb_4 + 4\ O_2 \leftrightarrows Hb_4O_8$$

The reaction requires no enzymes; it proceeds without a change in the valence of Fe^{2+}, as occurs in the more permanent process of oxidation. *The partial pressure of oxygen dissolved in physical solution dictates the oxygenation of hemoglobin to oxyhemoglobin.*

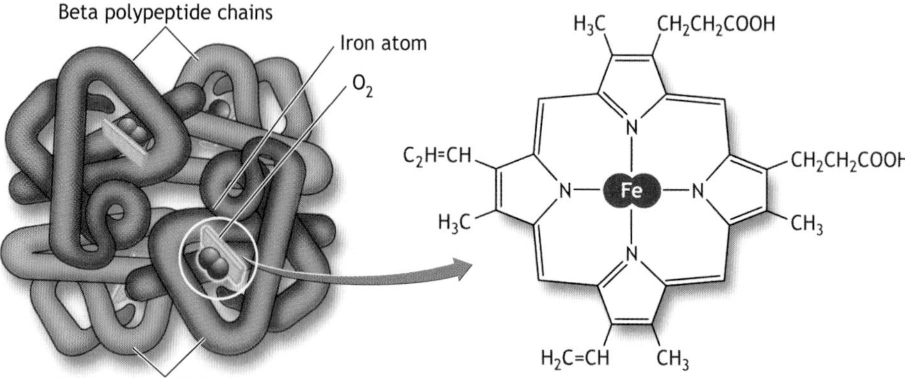

FIGURE 13.3 • The hemoglobin molecule consists of the protein globin, which is composed of four subunit polypeptide chains. Each of these polypeptides contains a single heme group with its single iron atom that acts as a "magnet" for oxygen.

Oxygen-Carrying Capacity of Hemoglobin

In men, each dL of blood contains about 15 g of hemoglobin. The value decreases 5 to 10% for women and averages about 14 g per dL of blood. This gender difference helps to explain the lower aerobic capacity of women relative to men, even when considering differences in body mass and body fat. The reason for higher hemoglobin concentrations in men relates to the stimulating effects on red blood cell production of the "male" hormone testosterone.

Each gram of hemoglobin combines loosely with 1.34 mL of oxygen. Thus, if one knows the hemoglobin content of the blood, its oxygen-carrying capacity readily computes as follows:

$$\text{Blood's oxygen capacity } (\text{mL} \cdot \text{dL blood})^{-1} = \text{Hemoglobin } (\text{g} \cdot \text{dL blood})^{-1} \times \text{Oxygen capacity of hemoglobin}$$

$$20 \text{ mLO}_2 = 15 \times 1.34 \text{ mL} \cdot \text{g}^{-1}$$

With full saturation with oxygen (i.e., when all hemoglobin converts to HbO_2) and with normal hemoglobin levels, hemoglobin carries nearly 20 mL of oxygen in each dL of whole blood.

ALTITUDE EFFECTS. Physiologists often use the term **volume percent (vol%)** to describe blood's oxygen content. In this regard, volume percent refers to the milliliters of oxygen extracted (in a vacuum) from a 100-mL sample of either whole blood (with plasma) or packed red blood cells (without plasma). The oxygen capacity of a 100-mL sample of packed human red blood cells averages 45.7 vol%, but it averages significantly higher for species of mammals (including humans) that reside at high altitudes. For example, packed red blood cells contain 58 vol% oxygen for the llama and vicuña, two members of the camel family that work regularly at altitudes between 15,000 and 17,000 feet. Increased oxygen-carrying capacity of blood confers a particular advantage at high altitudes where arterial Po_2 may equal only 40 mm Hg. In this environment, human whole blood carries oxygen at 14 vol%, while the capacity of the vicuña's blood averages 29% higher at 18 vol%.

ANEMIA AFFECTS OXYGEN TRANSPORT. The blood's oxygen transport capacity changes only slightly with normal variations in hemoglobin content. On the other hand, a significant decrease in the iron content of red blood cells reduces the blood's oxygen-carrying capacity. **Iron-deficiency anemia** diminishes a person's capacity to sustain even mild-intensity aerobic exercise.[1,6,7]

Table 13.3 presents data from 29 iron-deficient anemic men and women with low hemoglobin levels. They formed two groups; one received intramuscular iron injections over an 80-day period, while the placebo group received similar intramuscular injections of a colored saline solution. A third group with normal hemoglobin levels served as controls. The researchers tested all groups during exercise prior to the experiment and after 80 days of either iron therapy or placebo treatment. The results clearly show that the anemic group given iron supplements improved significantly in exercise response compared with their nonsupplemented counterparts. Peak heart rate during 5 minutes of stepping exercise decreased from 155 to 113 $b \cdot min^{-1}$ for men and from 152 to 123 $b \cdot min^{-1}$ for women. This translates into an average of 15% more oxygen delivered per heartbeat.

Po_2 and Hemoglobin Saturation

The term **cooperative binding** describes the union of oxygen with hemoglobin. The binding of an oxygen molecule to the iron atom in one of the four globin chains shown in Figure 13.3 progressively facilitates the binding of subsequent molecules. The cooperative binding phenomenon explains hemoglobin's sigmoid or S-shaped oxygen saturation curve.

The **oxyhemoglobin dissociation curve** (Fig. 13.4) illustrates the saturation of hemoglobin with oxygen at various

TABLE 13.3 ➤ HEMOGLOBIN (HB) LEVELS AND EXERCISE HEART RATE RESPONSES OF NORMAL SUBJECTS AND ANEMIC SUBJECTS PRIOR TO AND FOLLOWING SUPPLEMENTAL IRON TREATMENT

SUBJECTS	HB (G PER dL BLOOD)	PEAK EXERCISE HEART RATE
Normal		
Men	14.3	119
Women	13.9	142
Iron-deficient men		
Pretreatment	7.1	155
Posttreatment	14.0	113
Iron-deficient women		
Pretreatment	7.7	152
Posttreatment	12.4	123
Iron-deficient men		
Preplacebo	7.7	146
Postplacebo	7.4	137
Iron-deficient women		
Preplacebo	8.1	154
Postplacebo	8.4	144

Values represent averages
From Gardner GW, et al. Cardiorespiratory, hematological, and physical performance responses of anemic subjects to iron treatment. Am J Clin Nutr 1975; 28:982.

Po_2 values, including alveolar–capillary gas at sea level (Po_2, 100 mm Hg). The right ordinate gives the quantity of oxygen carried in each dL of normal blood at a particular plasma Po_2 value. Physical chemists establish dissociation curves (oxygen content and percentage saturation) by exposing about 200 mL of blood in a sealed glass vessel (tonometer) to various pressures of oxygen at a given pH in a water bath of known temperature. Percentage saturation computes as follows:

$$\text{Percent saturation} = \frac{O_2 \text{ combined with hemoglobin}}{O_2 \text{ capacity of hemoglobin}} \times 100$$

For example, if an individual's hemoglobin oxygen-carrying capacity in whole blood equals 20 vol% and only 12 vol% oxygen actually combines with hemoglobin, then

$$\begin{aligned}\text{Percent saturation} &= 12 \text{ vol\%} \div 20 \text{ vol\%} \times 100 \\ &= 60\%\end{aligned}$$

One hundred percent saturation indicates that the oxygen actually combined with hemoglobin equals the oxygen carrying capacity of hemoglobin.

Figure 13.4B depicts the **oxygen transport cascade** for Po_2 as oxygen moves from ambient air at sea level to the mitochondria of maximally active muscle tissue.

Po_2 in the Lungs

So far, we have assumed that hemoglobin fully saturates with oxygen when exposed to alveolar gas. *This does not occur, however, because at the sea-level alveolar Po_2 of 100 mm Hg, hemoglobin achieves 98% oxygen saturation.* The right ordinate of Figure 13.4 shows that at a Po_2 of 100 mm Hg the hemoglobin in each dL of blood leaving the lungs carries about 19.7 mL of oxygen. Clearly, any additional increase in alveolar Po_2 contributes little to how much more oxygen can combine with hemoglobin. In addition to the oxygen bound to hemoglobin, the plasma of each dL of arterial blood contains 0.3 mL of oxygen in solution. Thus, in healthy individuals who breathe ambient air at sea level, each dL of blood leaving the lungs carries approximately 20.0 mL of oxygen—19.7 mL bound to hemoglobin and 0.3 mL dissolved in plasma. Figure 13.5 shows the percentage composition of centrifuged whole blood for red blood cells (termed **hematocrit**) and plasma, including representative values for the quantity of oxygen carried in each component.

On television one frequently sees competitive athletes breathing a gas mixture of concentrated oxygen following strenuous exercise. This makes no sense from an oxygen-transport perspective. The oxyhemoglobin dissociation curve shows little or no potential for increased hemoglobin loading from additional pressure of supplemental oxygen inhaled at sea level or low altitude. We discuss the topic of breathing hyperoxic gas mixtures and exercise performance in more detail in Chapter 23.

Figure 13.4 also shows that hemoglobin saturation with oxygen changes little until the pressure of oxygen declines to about 60 mm Hg. This flat upper portion of the oxyhemoglobin dissociation curve provides a margin of safety to ensure adequate saturation of arterial blood with oxygen despite significant fluctuations in ambient Po_2. Even if alveolar Po_2 decreases to 75 mm Hg, as occurs in lung disease or traveling to higher altitudes, the saturation of hemoglobin lowers by only about 6%. At an alveolar Po_2 of 60 mm Hg, hemoglobin still remains 90% saturated with oxygen! Below this pressure, however, the quantity of oxygen combined with hemoglobin declines precipitously.

INTEGRATIVE QUESTION

How would you respond to a high-school football coach who asks about the advisability of having players breathe from a tank of oxygen on the sidelines during time-outs or rest breaks to improve game performance?

Po_2 in the Tissues

At rest, the Po_2 in the cell fluids averages 40 mm Hg. Dissolved oxygen from the plasma diffuses across the capillary membrane through the tissue fluids into the cells. This reduces plasma Po_2 below the Po_2 in the red blood cell, de-

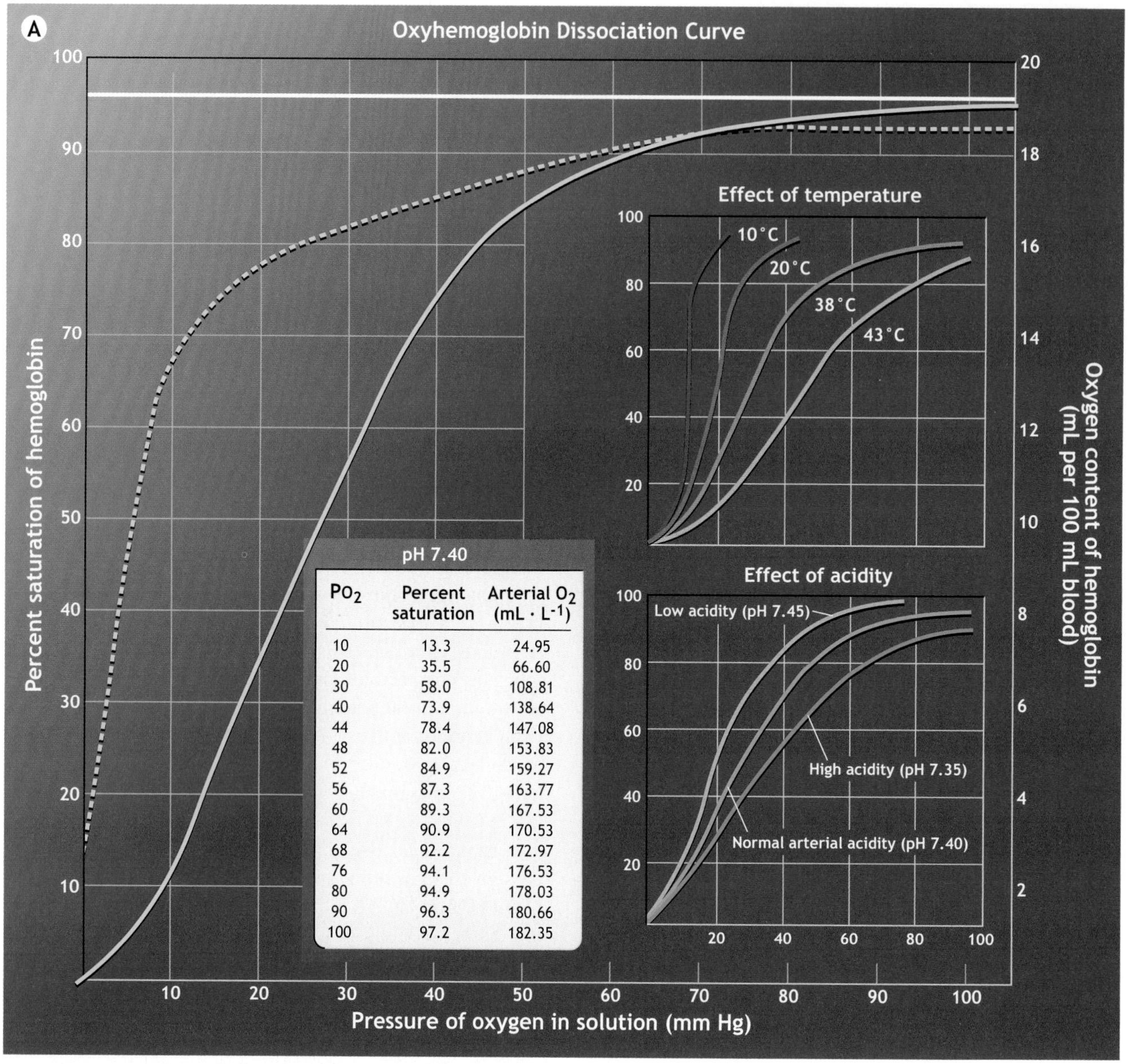

A

Oxyhemoglobin Dissociation Curve

Percent saturation of hemoglobin

Oxygen content of hemoglobin (mL per 100 mL blood)

Effect of temperature

10°C 20°C 38°C 43°C

Effect of acidity

Low acidity (pH 7.45)

High acidity (pH 7.35)

Normal arterial acidity (pH 7.40)

pH 7.40

Po_2	Percent saturation	Arterial O_2 ($mL \cdot L^{-1}$)
10	13.3	24.95
20	35.5	66.60
30	58.0	108.81
40	73.9	138.64
44	78.4	147.08
48	82.0	153.83
52	84.9	159.27
56	87.3	163.77
60	89.3	167.53
64	90.9	170.53
68	92.2	172.97
76	94.1	176.53
80	94.9	178.03
90	96.3	180.66
100	97.2	182.35

Pressure of oxygen in solution (mm Hg)

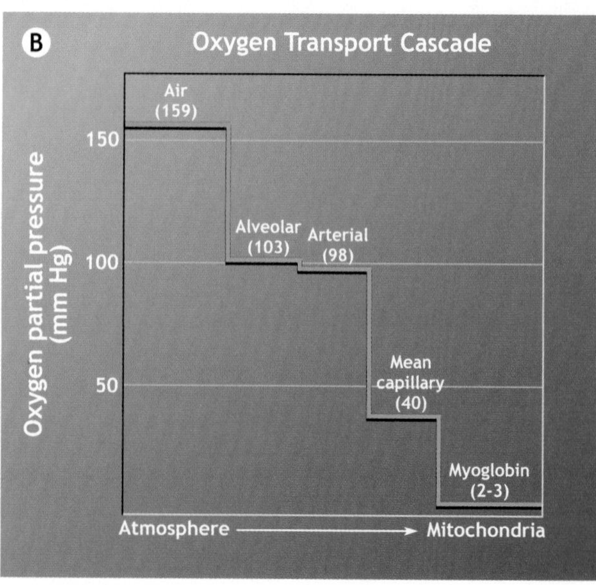

FIGURE 13.4 • A. The oxyhemoglobin dissociation curve. The lines indicate the percent saturation of hemoglobin (*solid line*) and myoglobin (*dashed line*) in relation to oxygen pressure. The *right ordinate* shows the quantity of oxygen carried in each dL of blood under normal conditions. The *inset curves within the figure* illustrate the effects of temperature and acidity in altering hemoglobin's affinity for oxygen (Bohr effect). *Inset box* presents oxyhemoglobin saturation and arterial blood's oxygen-carrying capacity for different Po_2 values with hemoglobin concentration of 14 $g \cdot dL\ blood^{-1}$. The *white horizontal line at the top of the graph* indicates percentage saturation of hemoglobin at the average sea-level alveolar Po_2 of 100 mm Hg. **B**. Partial pressures as oxygen moves from ambient air at sea level to the mitochondria of maximally active muscle tissue (oxygen transport cascade).

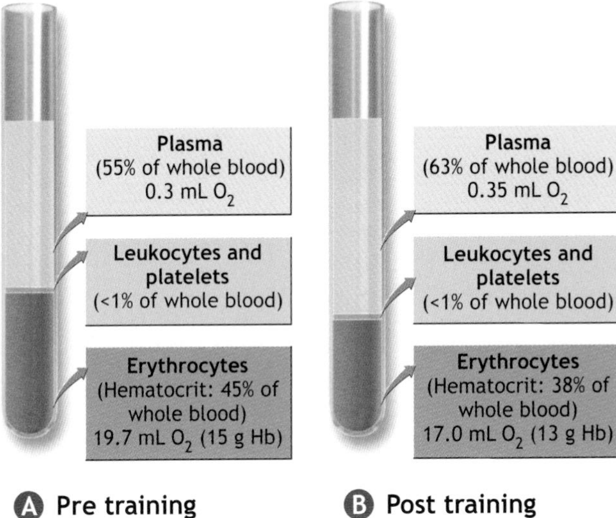

FIGURE 13.5 • **A**. Major components of centrifuged whole blood, including the quantity of oxygen carried in each dL of blood (Hb = hemoglobin). **B**. Changes in constituents of whole blood following 4 days of aerobic exercise training. Note that the significant increase in plasma volume (hemodilution) early in training decreases red blood cell concentration toward borderline anemia (see Chapter 2 and Chapter 21). Oxygen transport capacity does not decrease with training because total erythrocyte mass remains constant or increases slightly.

creasing hemoglobin's high oxygen saturation level. The released oxygen ($HbO_2 \rightarrow Hb + O_2$) moves out of the blood cells through the capillary membrane into the tissues.

At the tissue–capillary Po_2 at rest (Po_2 = 40 mm Hg), hemoglobin holds about 70% of its original oxygen (Fig. 13.4). Thus, when blood leaves the tissues and returns to the heart, it carries about 15 mL of oxygen in each dL of blood, giving up 5 mL of oxygen to the tissues.

Arteriovenous Oxygen Difference

The **arteriovenous oxygen difference (a-$\bar{v}$ O_2 difference)** describes the difference in the oxygen content of arterial and mixed-venous blood. The a-$\bar{v}$ O_2 difference at rest normally averages 4 to 5 mL of oxygen per dL of blood. The large quantity of oxygen still remaining with hemoglobin provides an "automatic" reserve so the cells can immediately obtain oxygen should metabolic demands suddenly increase. As the cell's use of oxygen increases in exercise, tissue Po_2 becomes reduced causing hemoglobin to rapidly release a larger quantity of oxygen. During high-intensity exercise, when extracellular Po_2 decreases to nearly 15 mm Hg, only about 5 mL of oxygen remains bound to hemoglobin. The a-$\bar{v}$ O_2 difference increases to 15 mL of oxygen per 100 mL of blood. When active muscle Po_2 falls to 2 or 3 mm Hg during exhaustive exercise, the blood perfusing these tissues releases virtually all its oxygen.[15] Oxygen release from hemoglobin can occur without any increase in local tissue blood flow. The amount of oxygen released to the muscles increases almost three times above that normally supplied at rest—just by a more complete unloading of hemoglobin, particularly as it flows through endurance-trained muscles (see Focus on Research). *Many researchers would argue that active muscles' uncompromising capacity to use available oxygen in their large blood supply supports the position that oxygen supply (blood flow), not muscle oxygen use, limits aerobic exercise capacity.*[14]

The Bohr Effect

The sigmoid-shaped yellow line in Figure 13.4 represents the oxyhemoglobin dissociation curve under resting physiologic conditions at an arterial pH of 7.4 and tissue temperature of 37°C. The **inset curves** depict other important characteristics of hemoglobin's affinity for oxygen. For example, any increase in plasma acidity (including carbon dioxide concentration) and temperature causes the dissociation curve to shift significantly downward and to the right. This phenomenon, called the **Bohr effect** after its discoverer, Danish physiologist Christian Bohr (1855–1911; father of Nobel physicist Niels Bohr), indicates an altered hemoglobin molecular structure.[4] It describes the reduced effectiveness of hemoglobin to hold oxygen, particularly in the Po_2 range between 20 and 50 mm Hg. The Bohr effect is particularly evident during high-intensity exercise as even more oxygen releases to the tissues because of associated increases in metabolic heat, carbon dioxide, and increased acidity owing to blood lactate accumulation.[13] At normal alveolar Po_2, however, the Bohr effect exerts almost no effect on pulmonary capillary blood, even during maximal exercise, so that hemoglobin can load (bind) fully with oxygen as blood flows through the lungs.

Red Blood Cell 2,3-DPG

Because the red blood cell contains no mitochondria, it derives its energy solely from the anaerobic reactions of glycolysis; this establishes the normal plasma lactate levels at rest. Red blood cells produce the compound **2,3-diphosphoglycerate (2,3-DPG**; also referred to as 2,3-biphosphoglycerate [2,3 BPG]) during glycolysis. 2,3-DPG binds loosely with subunits of the hemoglobin molecule, reducing its affinity for oxygen. This causes greater oxygen release to the tissues for a given decrease in Po_2.[3,4]

Individuals with cardiopulmonary disorders and those who live at high altitudes have an increased level of red blood cell 2,3-DPG.[9] This provides compensatory adjustments to facilitate oxygen release to the cells. During strenuous exercise, 2,3-DPG also aids in oxygen transfer to the muscles.[8] Conflicting results emerge in comparison of 2,3-DPG levels of trained and untrained subjects.[5,10,13] One study reported significantly higher resting levels of 2,3-DPG in two groups of athletes than in untrained subjects.[18] The level of this metabolic intermediate increased by 15% for the middle-distance runners following maximal exercise of short duration. Prolonged steady-rate exercise, on the other hand, produced a small decrease in 2,3-DPG in endurance athletes. These data support the proposition that increases in 2,3-DPG concentration with intense exercise (and perhaps training) reflect an adaptive response to augment oxygen delivery to more metabolically active tissues. More than likely, the effect of different types of exercise on erythrocyte 2,3-DPG level reflects the specific metabolic demands of exercise. Furthermore, females have significantly higher levels of red blood cell 2,3-DPG than males of similar fitness status and activity level. This possible gender difference might compensate for the lower hemoglobin levels in females.[12]

Focus on Research — A Remarkably Adaptable Tissue

Holloszy JO. Biochemical adaptations in muscle: effects of exercise on mitochondrial oxygen uptake and respiratory enzyme activity in skeletal muscle. J Biol Chem 1967;242:2278.

➤ For years prior to the mid-1960s, conventional wisdom maintained that increases in endurance performance with aerobic training *exclusively* resulted from central cardiovascular adaptations that increased capacity to deliver oxygen to active muscle. Proponents of this view argued that training-induced improvements in $\dot{V}O_{2max}$ resulted from an increase in maximal cardiac output because of an increase in the heart's maximal stroke volume. Central to this concept was the belief that working muscle becomes hypoxic during high-intensity exercise, and improved oxygen delivery results in less hypoxia after training. Virtually no data were available demonstrating adaptive changes in a muscle's metabolic machinery with regular exercise, although thyroxine feeding in rats had been shown to induce changes in mitochondrial composition and number.

The study by Holloszy was the first to show that endurance exercise training increased skeletal muscle mitochondrial content in rats. The author hypothesized that local (peripheral) changes in muscle (primarily in mitochondria) contribute significantly to the improved endurance performance with training. This work and subsequent research by Holloszy and colleagues ushered in a burgeoning in exercise biochemistry research.

In the exercise training program rats ran on a treadmill 5 days per week for 12 weeks. Running speed and duration gradually increased so that after 12 weeks, the animals ran for 120 minutes daily on an 8% incline at 31 m · min^{-1}, including 12, 30-second intervals at 42 m · min^{-1} interspersed at 10-min intervals. The protocol was the most strenuous reported in the exercise literature of that time. The animals were placed into one of four groups of 12: (1) exercise trained; (2) exercise control–pair weighted, who performed only mild daily exercise (10 min, 5 d per wk) with food intake adjusted to maintain the same body weight as group 1; (3) sedentary control–pair weighted, with food intake adjusted to maintain the same body weight as group 1; and (4) sedentary, freely eating.

The dependent variables were measured from the gastrocnemius and soleus muscles to show evidence for exercise training adaptations in muscle mitochondria and mitochondrial enzymes. These measures included succinate dehydrogenase, NADH dehydrogenase, NADH-cytochrome c reductase, level of respiratory control, mitochondrial protein, and succinate and cytochrome oxidase activity per gram of muscle.

The table shows that the capacity of the mitochondrial fraction from gastrocnemius muscle to oxidize pyruvate doubled in the trained rats. Succinate dehydrogenase, NADH dehydrogenase, NADH-cytochrome c reductase, and cytochrome oxidase activities per gram of muscle also increased approximately twofold. The near doubling of cytochrome c activity provided evidence that increases in respiratory chain enzyme activities resulted from increased mitochondrial enzyme activity. The total protein content of the mitochondrial fraction of trained muscle increased about 60%. The high level of mitochondrial respiratory control and tightly-coupled oxidative phosphorylation provided evidence that the increase in electron transport capacity with training accompanied a concomitant rise in the capacity to generate ATP via oxidative phosphorylation.

Subsequent investigations with animals and humans soon confirmed the findings of an increase in respiratory capacity and mitochondrial enzyme levels in trained muscle. This pioneering work by Holloszy served as a catalyst for ensuing research demonstrating the profound effect of exercise training on muscle biochemistry. The research also helped to explain why regular aerobic overload increases an individual's ability to exercise at a higher percentage of $\dot{V}O_{2max}$ (i.e., increased blood actate threshold) and provided an important component to verify the specificity of training principle for aerobic exercise.

EFFECTS OF ENDURANCE EXERCISE ON RAT MUSCLE MITOCHONDRIA

Variable	Trained	Sedentary Control
Body mass, g	353 ± 17	491 ± 21.9
Gastrocnemius muscle weight, g	2.1 ± 0.06	2.62 ± 0.12
Treadmill run to exhaustion (min) at 31 m · min^{-1}	186 ± 18	29.0 ± 3
$\dot{V}O_2$, mL · h^{-1} · g^{-1}	1022 ± 118	506 ± 53
Respiratory control index	16.1 ± 2.2	14.7 ± 2.6
Cytochrome oxidase, mL O_2 · min^{-1} · g muscle^{-1}		
Gastrocnemius	551 ± 31	305 ± 15
Soleus	691 ± 52	427 ± 16
Succinate oxidase, mL O_2 · min^{-1} · g muscle^{-1}		
Gastrocnemius	117 ± 8	73 ± 5
Soleus	160 ± 8	95 ± 10
Succinate dehydrogenase activity, mmol · g muscle^{-1}	15.1 ± 1.4	8.3 ± 0.7
Cytochrome c concentration, mmol · g muscle^{-1}	6.46 ± 0.58	3.47 ± 0.18
DPNH dehydrogenase, mmol · g muscle^{-1}	11.8 ± 1.5	5.6 ± 0.6
Mitochondrial protein, mmol · min^{-1} · mg protein^{-1}	4.67 ± 0.30	2.97 ± 0.20
DPNH cytochrome c reductase, mmol · g muscle^{-1}	0.60 ± 0.09	0.25 ± 0.05

Myoglobin, the Muscle's Oxygen Store

Myoglobin, an iron-containing globular protein in skeletal and cardiac muscle fibers, provides for intramuscular oxygen storage. X-ray crystallography first described myoglobin's structural details. The molecule contains a peptide backbone embedded with the heme group and its metallic Fe^{2+}. Reddish muscle fibers have a high concentration of this respiratory pigment, whereas myoglobin-deficient fibers appear pale or white.[11] Myoglobin resembles hemoglobin because it also combines reversibly with oxygen; however, each myoglobin molecule contains only one iron atom while hemoglobin, in contrast, contains four. Myoglobin adds additional oxygen to the muscle in the following chemical reaction:

$$Mb + O_2 \longrightarrow MbO_2$$

Oxygen Released at Low Pressures

Aside from its function as an "extra" source of oxygen in muscle, myoglobin facilitates the transfer of oxygen to the mitochondria, particularly when exercise begins and during intense exercise when cellular Po_2 rapidly declines.[19] The dissociation curve for myoglobin (Fig. 13.4; *dashed yellow line*) does not form an S-shaped line as does hemoglobin, but instead plots as a rectangular hyperbola. At the low end of Po_2 values, the curve form shows an abrupt, significant increase in percentage myoglobin saturation, with a relatively small increase in Po_2 until the asymptote. Little further change in saturation occurs over a broad Po_2 range. Compared with the oxygen saturation curve for hemoglobin, the curve for myoglobin shows that it binds and retains oxygen at low oxygen pressures much more readily. During rest and moderate exercise, myoglobin maintains high oxygen saturation. For example, at a Po_2 of 40 mm Hg, myoglobin holds 95% of its oxygen. The greatest quantity of oxygen releases from MbO_2 when tissue Po_2 drops below 5 mm Hg. Unlike hemoglobin, acidity, carbon dioxide, and temperature do not affect the oxygen-binding affinity of myoglobin, so it does not exhibit a Bohr effect. Chapter 21 presents the effects of aerobic exercise training on the muscles' myoglobin content.

Summary

1. Hemoglobin, the iron-protein pigment in the red blood cell, increases the amount of oxygen carried in whole blood to about 65 times that carried in physical solution in plasma.
2. The small amount of oxygen dissolved in plasma exerts molecular movement and establishes the partial pressure of oxygen (Po_2) in the blood. Plasma Po_2 determines the loading of hemoglobin at the lungs (oxygenation) and its unloading at the tissues (deoxygenation).
3. The blood's oxygen-transport capacity varies only slightly with normal variations in hemoglobin content. Iron-deficiency anemia significantly lowers hemoglobin concentration, thus decreasing the blood's oxygen-carrying capacity. Lowered hemoglobin concentration impairs aerobic exercise performance.
4. The shape of the oxyhemoglobin dissociation curve indicates that hemoglobin saturation changes little until Po_2 falls below 60 mm Hg. Consequently, the quantity of oxygen bound to hemoglobin falls sharply as oxygen moves from capillary blood to the tissues when metabolic demands increase.
5. Arterial blood releases only about 25% of its total oxygen to the tissues at rest; the remaining 75% returns "unused" to the heart in venous blood. The difference in oxygen content of arterial and venous blood—the arteriovenous oxygen difference—under resting conditions indicates that an automatic reserve of oxygen exists for rapid use should metabolism suddenly increase.
6. The Bohr effect reflects alterations in the molecular structure of hemoglobin from increased acidity, temperature, carbon dioxide concentration, and red blood cell 2,3-DPG that reduce its effectiveness to hold oxygen. Exercise accentuates these factors, further facilitating oxygen's release to the tissues.
7. The iron-protein pigment myoglobin in skeletal and cardiac muscle acts as an "extra" oxygen store to release oxygen at low Po_2. During strenuous exercise, myoglobin facilitates oxygen transfer to the mitochondria when the intracellular Po_2 in active muscle decreases dramatically.

➤ PART 3 • Transport of Carbon Dioxide

TRANSPORT OF CARBON DIOXIDE IN THE BLOOD

Once carbon dioxide forms in the cell, diffusion and subsequent transport in the venous blood provides the only means for its "escape" through the lungs. The blood carries carbon dioxide in three ways:

1. In physical solution in plasma (small amount).
2. Combined with hemoglobin within the red blood cell
3. As plasma bicarbonate.

Figure 13.6 illustrates the three ways for transporting carbon dioxide from the tissues to the lungs.

Carbon Dioxide in Solution

Approximately 5% of the carbon dioxide formed during energy metabolism moves into solution in the plasma as free carbon dioxide. *The random movement of this small quantity of dissolved carbon dioxide molecules establishes the* Pco_2 *of the blood.*

Carbon Dioxide Transport As Bicarbonate

Carbon dioxide in solution combines with water to form carbonic acid in the following reversible reaction:

$$CO_2 + H_2O \rightleftarrows H_2CO_3$$

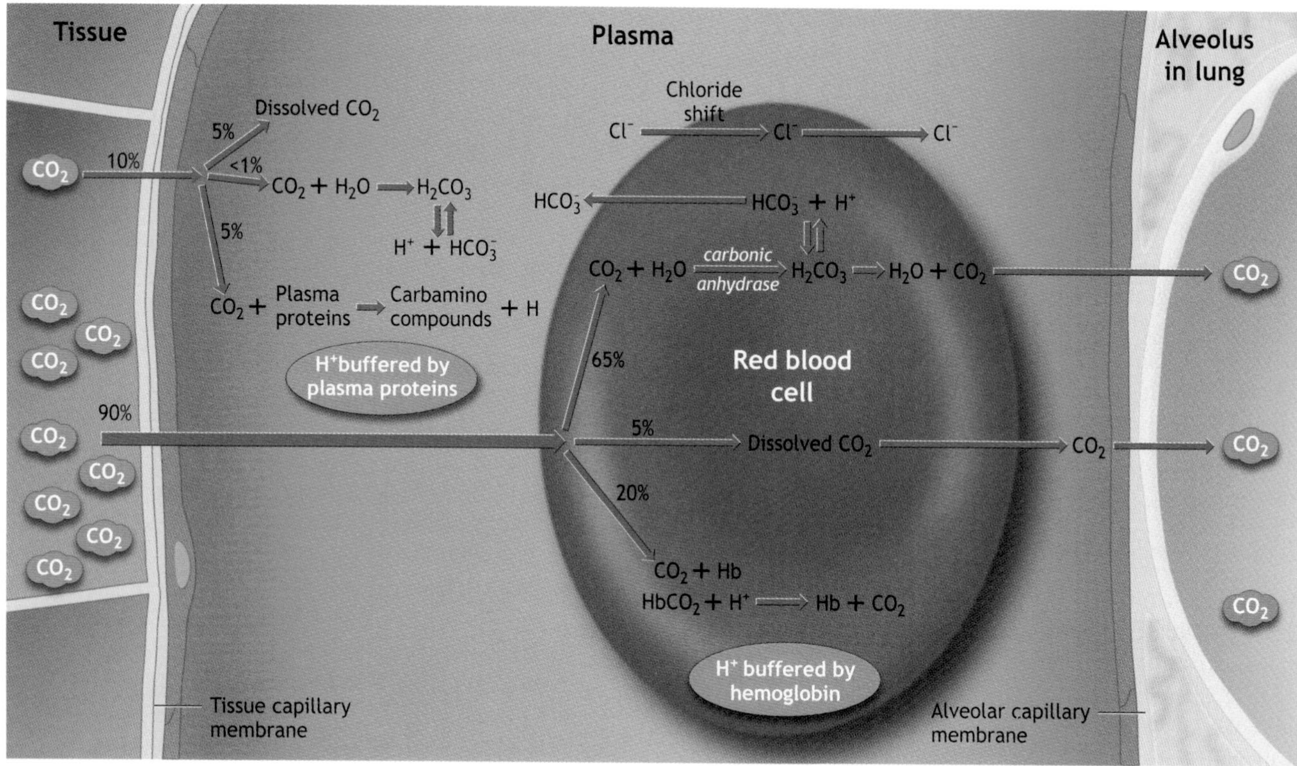

FIGURE 13.6 • Transport of carbon dioxide in the plasma and red blood cells as dissolved CO_2, bicarbonate, and carbamino compounds. By far, the greatest amount of carbon dioxide combines with water to form carbonic acid.

This reaction proceeds slowly, and little carbon dioxide transport as carbonic acid would take place without **carbonic anhydrase**, a zinc-containing enzyme within the red blood cell. One mole of this catalyst accelerates the union of a mole of carbon dioxide and water to a rate of about 800,000 times a second, or 5,000 times faster than occurs without enzymatic action. The reaction reaches equilibrium while the blood cell moves through the tissue's capillary.

Once carbonic acid forms in the tissues, most of it ionizes into hydrogen ions (H^+) and bicarbonate ions (HCO_3^-) as follows:

In tissues

$$CO_2 + H_2O \xrightarrow{\text{carbonic anhydrase}} H_2CO_3 \rightarrow H^+ + HCO_3^-$$

Buffering of the H^+ by the protein portion of hemoglobin maintains blood pH within relatively narrow limits (see "Acid-Base Regulation," Chapter 14). Because HCO_3^- remains soluble, it diffuses from the red blood cell into the plasma. There it exchanges for a chloride ion (Cl^-) that moves into the blood cell to maintain ionic equilibrium. This phenomenon, termed the **chloride shift**, causes the Cl^- content of erythrocytes in venous blood to exceed that in arterial red blood cells, particularly during exercise.

Sixty to 80% of the total carbon dioxide exists as ***plasma bicarbonate***. Bicarbonate forms in accordance with the law of mass action; carbonic acid formation accelerates as tissue P_{CO_2} increases. Carbon dioxide leaves the blood via the lungs, thus lowering the plasma P_{CO_2}. This disturbs the equilibrium between carbonic acid and bicarbonate ion formation. As a result, H^+ and HCO_3^- recombine to form carbonic acid. In turn, carbon dioxide and water re-form and carbon dioxide exits through the lungs as follows:

In lungs

$$H^+ + HCO_3^- \rightarrow H_2CO_3 \xrightarrow{\text{carbonic anhydrase}} CO_2 + H_2O$$

Because plasma HCO_3^- decreases in the pulmonary capillaries, the Cl^- moves from the red blood cell back into the plasma.

Carbon Dioxide Transport As Carbamino Compounds

At the tissue level, carbon dioxide reacts directly with the amino acid molecules of blood proteins to form **carbamino compounds**. The globin portion of hemoglobin, which carries about 20% of the body's carbon dioxide, forms a carbamino compound as follows:

$$CO_2 + \underset{\text{(Hemoglobin)}}{HbNH} \longrightarrow \underset{\text{(Carbaminohemoglobin)}}{HbNHCOOH}$$

Carbamino formation reverses as the plasma P_{CO_2} decreases in the lungs. This causes carbon dioxide to move into solution and enter the alveoli. Concurrently, oxygenation of hemoglobin reduces its ability to bind carbon dioxide. The interaction between oxygen loading and carbon dioxide release, termed the **Haldane effect**, facilitates carbon dioxide removal in the lung.

IN A PRACTICAL SENSE

➤➤ FACTORS THAT CONTRIBUTE TO THE SMOKING HABIT

Cigarette smoking represents the single greatest cause of death worldwide. Each year, more than 450,000 people in the United States die from smoking-related diseases—heart disease, cancer, stroke, aortic aneurysm, chronic bronchitis, emphysema, and peptic ulcers. Chronic cigarette smokers live an average of 18 years less than nonsmokers, and each cigarette smoked shortens life by 7 minutes! In addition to its significant effects on health, cigarette smoking (both acute and chronic) has the potential to negatively impact exercise performance (see Chapter 14).

Why People Start Smoking

People usually start smoking without realizing its detrimental effects. Cigarette smoking usually begins during the teen years or earlier. Health problems resulting from smoking begin to accrue quickly in young smokers. Three reasons generally explain why youths begin smoking: (1) peer pressure, (2) desire to appear "grown up," and (3) rebellion against authority.

Cigarettes Cause Addiction

Tobacco smoke contains more than 1200 toxic chemicals; tar alone contains nearly 30 known carcinogens. Within seconds of inhalation, nicotine affects the central nervous system to act simultaneously as a tranquilizer *and* stimulant. Nicotine's stimulating effect produces a strong physiologic and psychologic dependency. Estimates place the physiologic addiction to nicotine at about 6 to 8 times the addictive power of alcohol. Psychologic dependency develops over a longer time and associates with calming and pleasurable activities such as drinking coffee or alcohol, participating in social gatherings, relaxing after a meal, talking on the telephone, driving, reading, and watching television.

The "Why-Do-You-Smoke Test"

The Why-Do-You-Smoke Test identifies reasons for smoking, which provides the important first step in behavioral approaches to smoking cessation.

The Why-Do-You-Smoke Test lists 18 statements about why people smoke. A score between 1 and 5 indicates the strength of agreement with the statement, with 5 representing the strongest agreement. The responses to each of the statements provide input about one of six factors most frequently related to a person's smoking behavior. The information obtained provides (1) insight as to why a person smokes and (2) possible behavioral substitutes to aid in cessation.

WHY-DO-YOU-SMOKE TEST

Question	*Always*	*Frequently*	*Occasionally*	*Seldom*	*Never*
A. I smoke in order to keep myself from slowing down.	5	4	3	2	1
B. Handling a cigarette is part of the enjoyment of smoking it.	5	4	3	2	1
C. Smoking is pleasant and relaxing.	5	4	3	2	1
D. I light up when I feel angry about something.	5	4	3	2	1
E. When I have run out of cigarettes, I find it almost unbearable until I can get them.	5	4	3	2	1
F. I smoke automatically without even being aware of it.	5	4	3	2	1
G. I smoke to stimulate myself, to perk myself up.	5	4	3	2	1
H. Part of the enjoyment of cigarettes comes from the steps I take to light up.	5	4	3	2	1
I. I find cigarettes pleasurable.	5	4	3	2	1
J. When I feel uncomfortable or upset about something, I light up.	5	4	3	2	1
K. I am very much aware of the act when I am not smoking.	5	4	3	2	1
L. I light up without realizing I still have one burning in the ashtray.	5	4	3	2	1
M. I smoke to give myself a "lift."	5	4	3	2	1
N. When I smoke, part of the enjoyment is watching the smoke as I exhale it.	5	4	3	2	1
O. I want a cigarette most when I am comfortable and relaxed.	5	4	3	2	1
P. When I feel "blue" or want to take my mind off cares and worries, I smoke.	5	4	3	2	1
Q. I get a real gnawing hunger for a cigarette when I haven't smoked for a while.	5	4	3	2	1
R. I've found a cigarette in my mouth and didn't remember putting it there.	5	4	3	2	1

SCORING

Enter the number you circled on the test questions in the spaces provided below, putting the number you circled to question A on line A, to question B on line B, etc. Add the three scores on each line to get a total for each factor. For example, the sum of your scores over lines A, G, and M gives the score on "Stimulation"; lines B, H, and N give the score on "Handling," etc. Scores can vary between 3 and 15. Any score above 11 is high; any score 7 and below is low and indicates greater likelihood for successful smoking cessation.

A_____ + G_____ + M_____ = _____ Stimulation
B_____ + H_____ + N_____ = _____ Handling
C_____ + I_____ + O_____ = _____ Pleasure Relaxation
D_____ + J_____ + P_____ = _____ Crutch: tension reduction
E_____ + K_____ + Q_____ = _____ Craving: psychological addiction
F_____ + L_____ + R_____ = _____ Habit

From A self-test for smokers. *U.S. Department of Health and Human Services,* 1983.

IN A PRACTICAL SENSE

➤➤ FACTORS THAT CONTRIBUTE TO THE SMOKING HABIT, CONT'D

- Stimulation ("cigarettes are stimulating"): you feel that they help wake you up, organize your energies, and keep you going. Choose a safe substitute—a brisk walk or moderate exercise.
- Handling ("keep my hands busy"): toy with a pen or pencil or doodle, play with a coin, piece of jewelry, or some other harmless object while quitting.
- Accentuation of pleasure/pleasurable relaxation ("makes me feel good"): substitute social and physical activities or other relaxing activities to accentuate pleasure.
- Reduction of negative feelings/crutch ("gets me through the tough times"): learning to handle stress helps with quitting.
- Craving or dependence ("can't get through the day without them"): "cold turkey" is the most effective way to quit; biofeedback has shown some success.
- Habit ("don't even know when I'm smoking"): need to break the habitual smoking pattern; being more aware of conditions and situations when smoking occurs aids in quitting.

Scores for each factor can vary between 3 and 15. A score of 11 or higher indicates that for this factor smoking represents an important source of satisfaction. Scoring low (< 7) on a factor indicates a greater likelihood of successful smoking cessation.

Summary

1. A small amount (5%) of carbon dioxide travels in the plasma as free carbon dioxide in physical solution. Dissolved carbon dioxide establishes the P_{CO_2} of the blood, which modulates important physiologic functions.
2. The major quantity of carbon dioxide (80%) transports in chemical combination with water to form bicarbonate as follows:

$$CO_2 + H_2O \rightarrow H_2CO_3 \rightarrow H^+ + HCO_3^-$$

   In the lungs, the reaction reverses and carbon dioxide exits the blood into the alveoli.
3. About 20% of the body's carbon dioxide combines with blood proteins, including hemoglobin, to form carbamino compounds.

References

1. Beard J, Tobin B. Iron status and exercise. Am J Clin Nutr 2000;72:594S.
2. Dempsey JA. Is the lung built for exercise? Med Sci Sports Exerc 1986;18:143.
3. Dempsey JA, et al. Muscular exercise, 2,3-DPG and oxy-hemoglobin affinity. Int J Physiol 1971;30:34.
4. Fang TY, et al. Assessment of roles of surface histidyl residues in the molecular basis of the Bohr effect and of beta 143 histidine in the binding of 2,3-biphosphoglycerate in human normal adult hemoglobin. Biochemistry 1999;38:13423.
5. Fornaini G, et al. Glucose utilization in human erythrocytes during physical exercise. Med Sci Sports Exerc 1981;13:323.
6. Gardner GW, et al. Cardiorespiratory, hematological and physical performance responses of anemic subjects to iron treatment. Am J Clin Nutr 1975;28:982.
7. Hinton PS, et al. Iron supplementation improves endurance after training in iron-depleted women. J Appl Physiol 2000;88:1103.
8. Klein JP, et al. Hemoglobin affinity for oxygen during short-term exhaustive exercise. J Appl Physiol 1980;48:236.
9. Lenfant C, et al. Effect of altitude on oxygen binding by hemoglobin and on organic phosphate levels. J Clin Invest 1968;47:2652.
10. Lijnen P, et al. Erythrocyte 2,3-diphosphoglycerate and serum enzyme concentrations in trained and sedentary men. Med Sci Sports Exerc 1986;18:174.
11. Nemeth PM, Lowry OH. Myoglobin in individual human skeletal muscle fibers of different types. J Histochem Cytochem 1984;32:1211.
12. Pate RR, et al. A physiological comparison of performance-matched female and male distance runners. Res Q Exerc Sport 1985;56:245.
13. Rand PW, et al. Influence of athletic training on hemoglobin-oxygen affinity. Am J Physiol 1973;224:1334.
14. Richardson RS. Oxygen transport: air to muscle cell. Med Sci Sports Exerc 1998;30:53.
15. Richardson RS, et al. Myoglobin O_2 desaturation during exercise: evidence of a limited oxygen transport. J Clin Invest 1995;96:1916.
16. Severinghaus JW. Exercise O_2 transport model assuming zero cytochrome P_{O_2} at $\dot{V}O_{2max}$. J Appl Physiol 1994;77:671.
17. Stainsby WN, Otis AB. Blood flow, blood oxygen tension, oxygen uptake and oxygen transport in skeletal muscle. Am J Physiol 1964;206:858.
18. Taunton JE, et al. Alterations in 2,3-DPG and P_{50} with maximal and submaximal exercise. Med Sci Sports 1974;6:238.
19. Wittenberg BA, et al. Role of myoglobin in the oxygen supply to red skeletal muscle. J Biol Chem 1975;250:9038.

CHAPTER 14

Dynamics of Pulmonary Ventilation

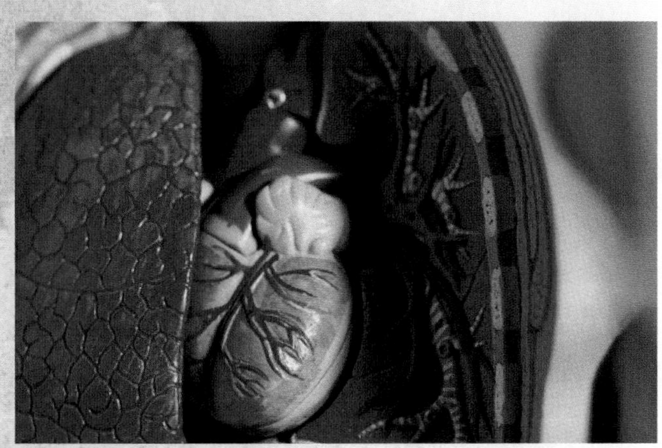

Chapter Objectives

- Describe the role of the hypothalamic neural command center in the control of pulmonary ventilation
- Identify the major chemical and nonchemical factors that regulate pulmonary ventilation during rest and exercise
- Describe how hyperventilation extends breath-holding time but also poses a danger in sport diving
- Outline the dynamic phases of minute ventilation at the onset, early phase, and late stage of moderate exercise and recovery
- Graph the relationships among pulmonary ventilation, blood lactate, and oxygen consumption during incremental exercise, indicating the point of onset of blood lactate accumulation (OBLA)
- Explain the increase in the ventilatory equivalent during the transition from steady-rate to non–steady-rate exercise
- Give the rationale for the blood lactate threshold or OBLA rather than $\dot{V}O_{2max}$ to predict performance in endurance activities
- Quantify the energy cost of breathing at rest and during strenuous exercise in health and pulmonary disease
- Describe the acute effects of cigarette smoking on heart rate and the energy cost of breathing during exercise
- Outline the endurance training adaptations in pulmonary ventilation during submaximal and maximal exercise
- Discuss the pros and cons to the argument that pulmonary ventilation represents the "weak link" in oxygen supply during maximal exercise
- Summarize the actions of the chemical and physiologic buffer systems that regulate the acid–base quality of body fluids at rest and during exercise

PART 1 • Regulation of Pulmonary Ventilation

VENTILATORY CONTROL

Complex mechanisms exquisitely adjust breathing rate and depth in response to metabolic needs. Intricate neural circuits relay information from higher centers in the brain, from the lungs, and from other sensors throughout the body to contribute to ventilatory control.[6,74] In addition, the gaseous and chemical states of the blood that bathes the medulla and aortic and carotid artery chemoreceptors mediate alveolar ventilation. In healthy individuals, these control mechanisms maintain relatively constant alveolar (and arterial) gas pressures throughout a broad range of exercise intensities. Figure 14.1 presents a schematic view of the input for ventilatory control.

Neural Factors

The inherent activity of inspiratory neurons with cell bodies located in the medial portion of the **medulla** governs the normal respiratory cycle. These neurons activate the diaphragm and intercostal muscles, causing the lungs to inflate. The inspiratory neurons cease firing because of their self-limitations and because of the inhibitory influence of expiratory neurons also located in the medulla. Inhibitory and excitatory signals from throughout the body influence the normal rhythm of medullary neurons. For example, inflation of the lungs stimulates stretch receptors, particularly in the bronchioles. These receptors act through afferent fibers to inhibit inspiration and stimulate expiration. As the inspiratory muscles relax, exhalation occurs by passive recoil of the stretched lung tissue and raised ribs. Activation of expiratory neurons and associated muscles that facilitate expiration synchronize with this passive phase. As expiration proceeds, the inspiratory center becomes progressively less inhibited and once again becomes active.

The inherent activity of the respiratory center alone cannot account for the smooth pattern of ventilatory adjustment to metabolic demands. A neural center in the hypothalamus integrates input from descending neurons in the higher locomotor areas of the cerebral hemispheres, the pons, and other brain regions to affect the duration and intensity of the inspiratory cycle. At the same time, ascending neural signals initiated by mechanical and/or chemical changes within active

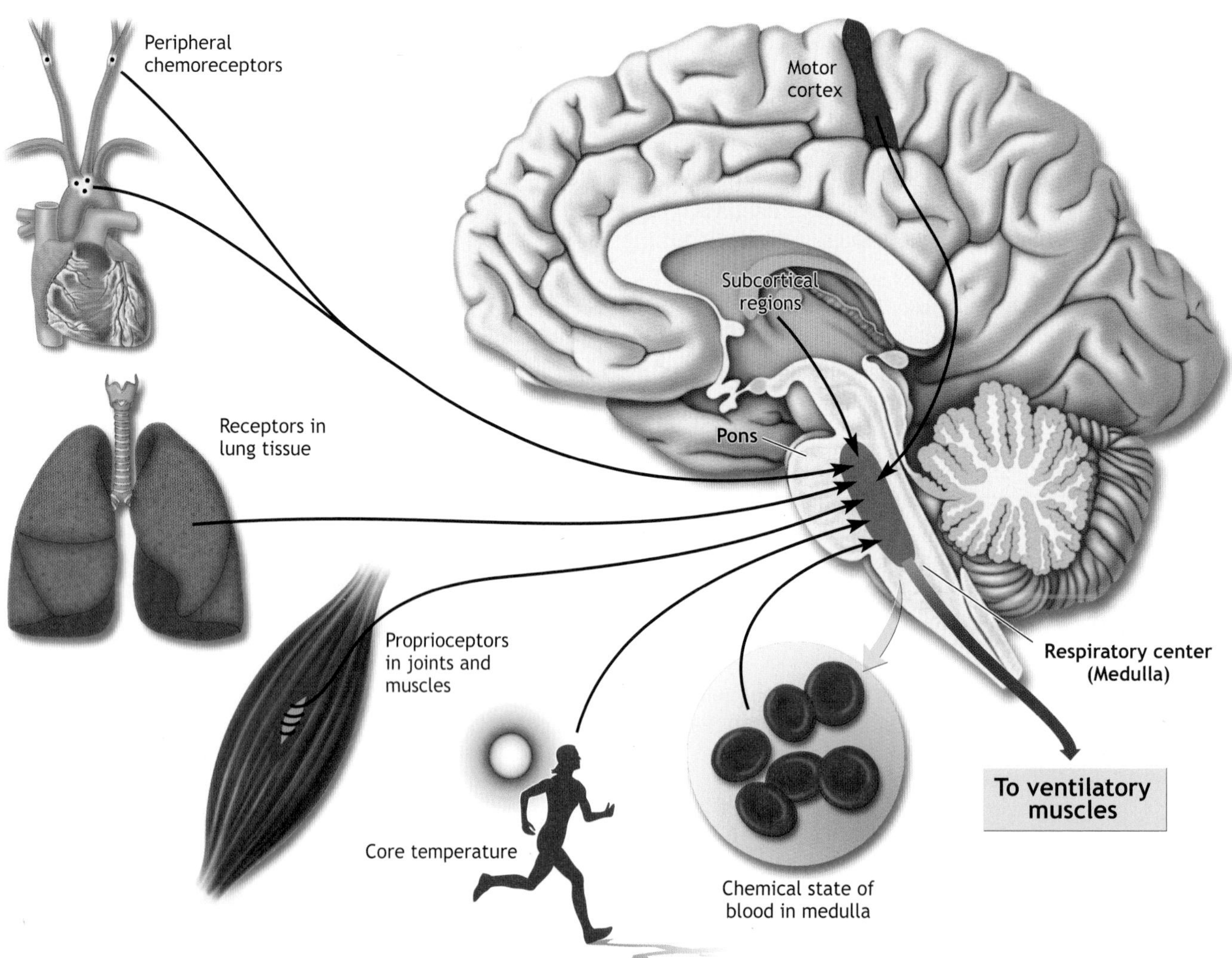

FIGURE 14.1 • Schematic representation of factors that affect medullary control of pulmonary ventilation.

muscles provide peripheral feedback control via the cerebellum to the respiratory center to modulate ventilatory adjustments to exercise.

The lungs contain sensory receptors that communicate with the respiratory center via vagal nerve afferents. Activation of these receptors by diverse irritants initiates a cough reflex. Irritation of the tracheal or bronchial mucosa by dust, air pollutants, cigarette smoke, noxious fumes, inhaled debris, or accumulated mucus promotes coughing, while the same irritants in the nasal cavity cause sneezing. Both reflexes help keep the airways clear, because bronchial irritation often leads to constriction of these conduits.

Humoral Factors

At rest, the chemical state of the blood exerts the greatest control of pulmonary ventilation. Variations in arterial Po_2, Pco_2, acidity, and temperature activate sensitive neural units in the medulla and arterial system to adjust ventilation and maintain arterial blood chemistry within narrow limits.

Plasma Po_2 and Peripheral Chemoreceptors

Inhalation of a gas mixture containing 80% oxygen greatly increases alveolar Po_2 and causes a 20% reduction in minute ventilation. Conversely, ventilation increases if the inspired oxygen concentration decreases below ambient levels, particularly if the alveolar Po_2 falls below 60 mm Hg. Hemoglobin saturation at this Po_2 begins to decrease considerably (see Fig. 13.4).

Sensitivity to reduced oxygen pressure does not reside in the respiratory center. Instead, peripheral **chemoreceptors** provide the primary site for detecting arterial hypoxia and initiating a ventilatory response.[74] Figure 14.2 shows these specialized neurons, weighing only a few milligrams, located in the arch of the aorta and branching of the carotid arteries in the neck. The strategic positioning of the **carotid bodies** enables them to monitor the state of arterial blood just before it perfuses the brain. A decrease in arterial Po_2, as occurs in pulmonary disease or when one ascends to high altitude, activates the aortic and carotid chemoreceptors to increase alveolar ventilation. These receptors *alone* protect the organism against reduced oxygen pressure in inspired air.

In addition to providing an early warning system against reduced arterial Po_2, peripheral chemoreceptor afferents also stimulate ventilation in exercise, even though reductions in arterial Po_2 do not normally occur.[58] The stimulating effects of exercise on carotid afferent chemoreceptor discharge most likely results from increases in temperature, acidity, and carbon dioxide and potassium concentrations.[24,81]

Plasma Pco_2 and H^+ Concentration

Carbon dioxide pressure in arterial plasma provides the most important respiratory stimulus at rest. Small increases in Pco_2 in inspired air trigger large increases in minute ventilation. For example, the resting ventilation nearly doubles by increasing inspired Pco_2 to just 1.7 mm Hg (0.22% CO_2 in inspired air).

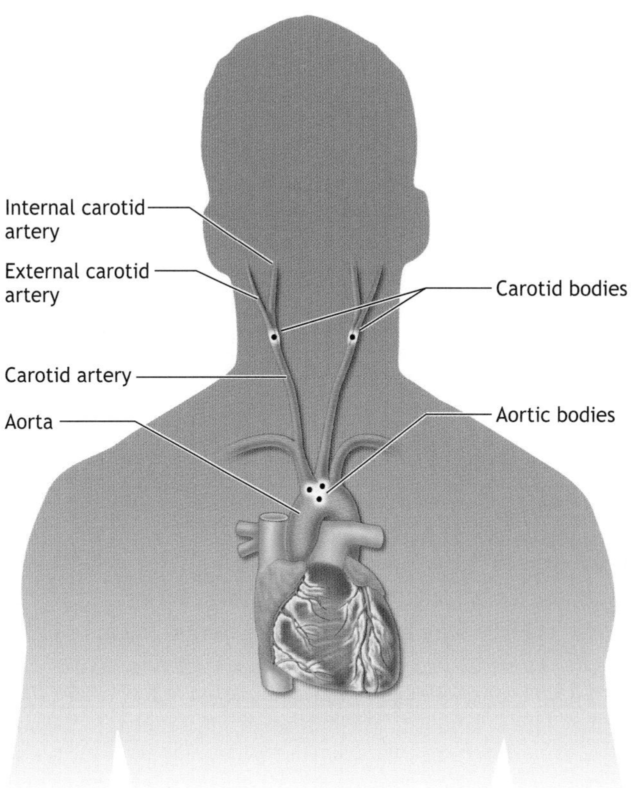

FIGURE 14.2 • The aortic arch and bifurcation of the carotid arteries contain cell bodies sensitive to reduced Po_2 and increased Pco_2 and H^+ and potassium concentrations in arterial blood. These peripheral chemoreceptors provide the body's first line of defense against arterial hypoxia that occurs in pulmonary disease and ascent to high altitude. The chemoreceptors also help regulate exercise hyperpnea through the stimulating effects of increased arterial carbon dioxide and H^+ concentrations.

The action of molecular carbon dioxide per se does not mediate the ventilatory response to arterial Pco_2. Instead, plasma acidity, which varies directly with the blood's carbon dioxide content, exerts a significant command over minute ventilation. A fall in blood pH (signaling acidosis) usually reflects carbon dioxide retention and subsequent carbonic acid formation. It may also result from metabolic causes such as lactate accumulation in strenuous exercise or fatty acid (ketone) accumulation in diabetes. Regardless of cause, as the arterial pH declines and hydrogen ions accumulate, inspiratory activity increases to eliminate carbon dioxide and thus reduce arterial levels of carbonic acid (see Chapter 13).

Hyperventilation and Breath-Holding

If a person breath-holds after a normal exhalation, it takes approximately 40 seconds before the urge to breathe becomes strong enough to initiate inspiration. The stimulus to breathe mainly results from the effects of increased arterial Pco_2 and H^+ concentration and *not* to decreased Po_2 in the breath-holding condition.[20] The break point for a breath-hold corresponds to an increase in arterial Pco_2 to approximately 50 mm Hg.

If one consciously increases ventilation above the normal level (**hyperventilation**) before breath-holding, alveolar air composition becomes more like ambient air. This decreases alveolar PCO_2 from its normal value of 40 mm Hg to as low as 15 mm Hg. This creates a considerable diffusion gradient for carbon dioxide runoff into the alveoli from venous blood entering the pulmonary capillaries. Consequently, a larger-than-normal quantity of carbon dioxide leaves the blood, and arterial PCO_2 decreases. Hyperventilation extends breath-hold duration until arterial PCO_2 and/or H^+ concentration rise to levels that again stimulate the urge to breathe.

Swimmers and divers use hyperventilation and subsequent breath-holding to improve performance. In sprint swimming, for example, it is mechanically undesirable to roll the body and turn the head during the stroke's breathing phase. Consequently, many sprinters hyperventilate on the starting blocks to prolong the breath-hold during the swim. In sport diving, hyperventilation offers an effect similar to that in competitive swimming—to extend breath-holding time. In diving, however, extended breath-holding from hyperventilation can be tragic.[19] As the length and depth of the dive increase, the blood's oxygen content decreases to critically low values before arterial PCO_2 rises sufficiently to stimulate breathing and signal ascent to the surface. This can cause the diver to lose consciousness before reaching the surface. Chapter 26 discusses hyperventilation and other important factors related to sport diving.

REGULATION OF VENTILATION DURING EXERCISE

Chemical Control

Neither chemical stimuli nor any other single mechanism entirely explains the increase in ventilation (**hyperpnea**) in physical activity. For example, the classic feedback control of resting ventilation via oxygen– and carbon dioxide–mediated mechanisms does not adequately explain exercise hyperpnea.[24] Inducing maximum changes in plasma acidity and inspired PO_2 and PCO_2 does not increase minute ventilation to values observed during vigorous exercise.

Figure 14.3 illustrates the relationship between oxygen consumption during graded exercise and venous and alveolar PCO_2 and alveolar PO_2. As exercise intensity increases, alveolar (arterial) PO_2 does not decrease to an extent that increases ventilation through chemoreceptor stimulation. The large ventilatory volumes during intense exercise cause alveolar PO_2 to rise *above* the average resting value of 100 mm Hg. Any increase in alveolar PO_2 in exercise hastens oxygenation of blood in the alveolar capillaries. Pulmonary ventilation during light and moderate exercise closely couples with metabolism in a manner proportional to oxygen consumption and carbon dioxide production.[76] Under these conditions, alveolar (and arterial) PCO_2 generally averages 40 mm Hg. During strenuous exercise with its relatively large anaerobic component, carbon dioxide and subsequent H^+ concentrations increase to provide an additional ventilatory stimulus. The resulting hyperventilation *reduces* alveolar and arterial PCO_2, sometimes to as low as 25 mm Hg.[39] Any reduction in arterial PCO_2 would decrease the ventilatory drive from carbon dioxide during exercise.

On the basis of alterations in alveolar and arterial gas pressures during exercise, one might question how peripheral chemoreceptors exert their influence on exercise ventilation. A possible explanation considers the pattern of ventilation that causes alveolar–capillary PCO_2 to reach slightly lower values at the end of inhalation and higher values at the end of exhalation. Even though *average* levels of arterial oxygen, carbon dioxide, and pH remain well regulated during moderate exercise, the chemoreceptors may detect cyclic plasma oscillations in these variables during breathing to influence exercise ventilation. Any increase in chemoreceptor sensitivity would also facilitate chemoreceptor control of exercise ventilation.

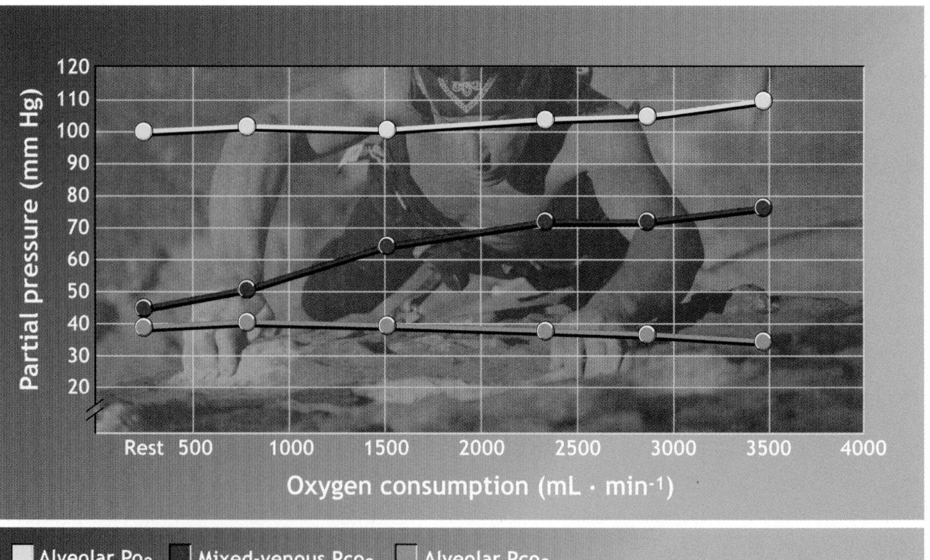

FIGURE 14.3 • Relationship between oxygen consumption during graded exercise and values for PCO_2 in mixed-venous blood entering the lungs, and alveolar PO_2 and PCO_2. Alveolar PO_2 and PCO_2 remain near resting levels throughout a broad range of exercise intensities, despite relatively large increases in mixed-venous PCO_2. (Data from the Laboratory of Applied Physiology, Queens College, Flushing, NY.)

Nonchemical Control

The rapidity of the ventilatory response at the onset and cessation of exercise strongly suggests that input other than changes in arterial PCO_2 and H^+ concentration mediate these phases of exercise hyperpnea.

Neurogenic Factors

Neurogenic factors for ventilatory control include cortical and peripheral influences.

- *Cortical influence:* Neural outflow from regions of the motor cortex and cortical activation in anticipation of exercise stimulate respiratory neurons in the medulla to initiate the abrupt increase in exercise ventilation.
- *Peripheral influence:* Sensory input from joints, tendons, and muscles influence the ventilatory adjustments throughout exercise. Experiments involving passive limb movements, electrical muscle stimulation, and voluntary exercise with the muscle's blood flow occluded support the contribution of local mechanoreceptors and chemoreceptors to reflex exercise hyperpnea.

Influence of Temperature

Except perhaps for extreme hyperthermia, an increase in body temperature exerts little effect on the regulation of ventilation during exercise. In most exercise conditions, the rise in ventilation at exercise onset and its decline upon cessation occurs too quickly to reflect control from changes in core temperature.

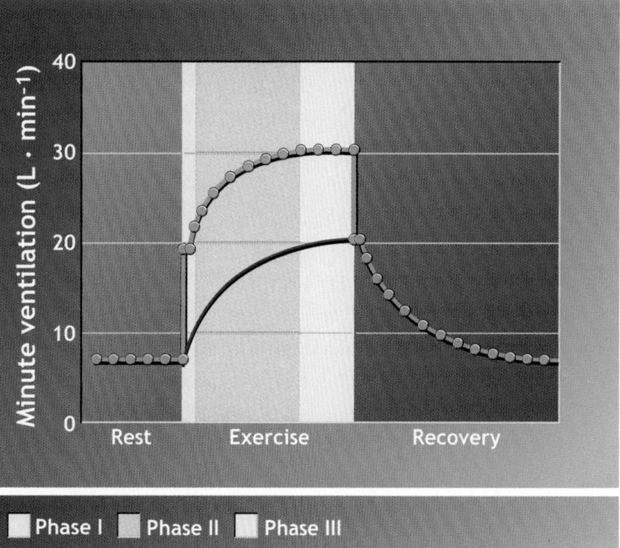

FIGURE 14.4 • The three phases of exercise hyperpnea. *Phase I:* rapid increase from rest and brief plateau from central command drive and input from active muscles. *Phase II:* slower exponential rise begins approximately 20 seconds after onset of exercise. Central command continues, along with feedback from active muscles plus the added effect of short-term potentiation of respiratory neurons. *Phase III:* major regulatory mechanisms reach stable values; added input from peripheral chemoreceptors provide the fine tuning of the ventilatory response. The *lower graph* (red line) depicts the contribution of central neuronal short-term potentiation and rising arterial H^+ concentration to the respiratory response. (Modified from Eldridge FL. Central integration of mechanisms in exercise hyperpnea. Med Sci Sports Exerc 1994;26:319.)

Integrated Regulation

During Exercise

No single factor controls ventilation during exercise. Rather the combined and perhaps simultaneous effects of several chemical and neural stimuli initiate and modulate exercise alveolar ventilation.[74] Figure 14.4 shows the dynamic phases of minute ventilation during moderate exercise and recovery. In **phase I** at the start of exercise, neurogenic stimuli from the cerebral cortex (**central command**), combined with feedback from the active limbs, stimulate the medulla to increase ventilation abruptly. Cortical and locomotor peripheral input continues throughout the exercise period. After a short plateau (approximately 20 s), minute ventilation then rises exponentially (in **phase II**) to reach a steady level related to the demands for metabolic gas exchange. Central command input, including factors intrinsic to neurons of the respiratory control system, regulates this phase of exercise ventilation. Continued activity of the respiratory neurons in the medulla causes short-term potentiation that augments their responsiveness to the same continuing stimulation. This brings minute ventilation to a new, higher level. In all likelihood, input from the peripheral chemoreceptors in the carotid bodies also contributes to regulation during phase II.[81] The final phase of control (**phase III**) involves a fine tuning of the steady-state ventilation through peripheral sensory feedback mechanisms. Modulation of alveolar gas pressures in this phase results from central and reflex stimuli from the main by-products of increased muscle metabolism—carbon dioxide and H^+ concentration. These factors stimulate chemoreceptor group IV unmyelinated neurons that communicate with regions of the central nervous system to regulate cardiorespiratory function.[56] The lactate anion itself, apart from lactic acidosis, contributes an additional stimulus to increase ventilation in strenuous exercise.[28] Reflexes related to pulmonary blood flow and the mechanical movement of the lung and respiratory muscles also provide regulatory input.

In Recovery

The abrupt decline in ventilation when exercise stops reflects the removal of both the central command drive and the sensory input from previously active muscles. More than likely, the slower recovery phase results from (1) gradual diminution of the short-term potentiation of the respiratory center and (2) reestablishment of the body's normal metabolic, thermal, and chemical milieu.

Summary

1. The normal respiratory cycle results from the inherent activity of medullary neurons in the medulla. Input from higher brain centers, from the lungs, and from other sensors throughout the body interacts with medullary neural output to regulate ventilation.
2. Chemical factors that act directly on the respiratory center or modify its activity through chemoreceptors control alveolar ventilation at rest. Arterial P_{CO_2} and H^+ concentration are the most important regulatory factors. A drop in arterial oxygen pressure, as occurs during ascent to high altitude or in severe pulmonary disease, also stimulates breathing.
3. Hyperventilation significantly lowers arterial P_{CO_2} and H^+ concentration. This prolongs breath-holding time until levels of carbon dioxide and acidity increase to stimulate breathing. One should not attempt to extend breath-holding by hyperventilating before underwater swimming because of potentially deadly consequences.
4. Nonchemical regulatory factors augment the ventilatory adjustments to exercise. These factors include (1) cortical activation in anticipation of exercise and outflow from the motor cortex when exercise begins, (2) peripheral sensory input from chemoreceptors and mechanoreceptors in joints and muscles, and (3) increased body temperature.
5. The ventilatory response to exercise occurs in three phases. Cortical stimulus plus feedback for active limbs cause the abrupt increase in ventilation as exercise begins (phase I); ventilation then rises exponentially in phase II to reach a steady level in relation to exercise demands; phase III involves fine tuning the steady-state ventilation through peripheral sensory feedback mechanisms.

PART 2 • Pulmonary Ventilation During Exercise

VENTILATION AND ENERGY DEMANDS

Physical activity affects oxygen consumption and carbon dioxide production more than any other physiologic stress. With exercise, oxygen diffuses from the alveoli into the venous blood returning to the lungs while about the same quantity of carbon dioxide moves from the blood into the alveoli. Concurrently, alveolar ventilation increases to maintain the proper gas concentrations for rapid gas exchange.

Ventilation in Steady-Rate Exercise

Figure 14.5 shows the relationship between oxygen consumption and minute ventilation during increasing levels of exercise up to maximal oxygen consumption ($\dot{V}O_{2max}$). During light-to-moderate exercise, ventilation increases *linearly* with oxygen consumption and carbon dioxide production, averaging between 20 and 25 L of air for each liter of oxygen consumed. In this case, ventilation increases mainly through an

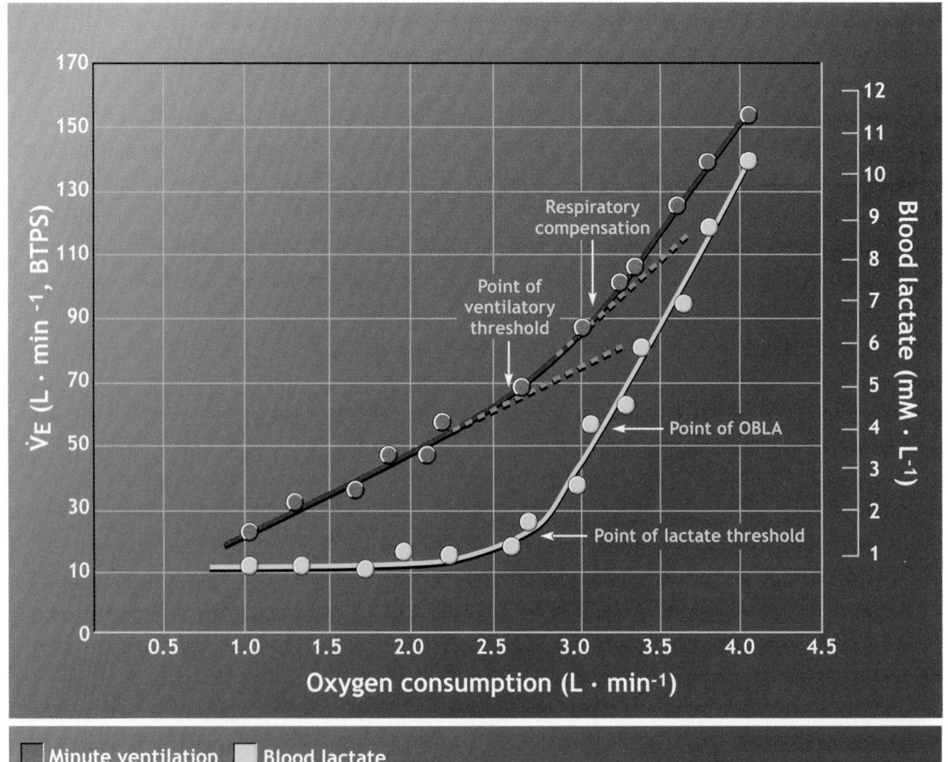

FIGURE 14.5 • Pulmonary ventilation, blood lactate concentration, and oxygen consumption during graded exercise to maximum. The *dashed line* represents the extrapolation of the linear relationship between $\dot{V}_E$ and $\dot{V}O_2$ during submaximal exercise. The lactate threshold (not necessarily the threshold for anaerobic metabolism) represents the highest exercise intensity (oxygen consumption) not associated with an elevated blood lactate concentration. It occurs at the point at which the relationship between $\dot{V}_E$ and $\dot{V}O_2$ deviates from linearity, indicated as the point of ventilatory threshold. OBLA represents the point of lactate increase just above a 4.0 mM baseline. Respiratory compensation represents a further increase in ventilation to counter the decrease in plasma pH in heavy exercise.

increase in tidal volume; at higher exercise intensities, breathing frequency takes on a more important role. Such ventilatory adjustments provide for complete aeration of blood because alveolar Po_2 and Pco_2 remain near resting values. Transit time for blood in the pulmonary capillaries remains long enough for complete equilibration of the lung–blood gases (see Fig. 13.2).

The term **ventilatory equivalent** (symbolized $\dot{V}_E/\dot{V}O_2$) describes the ratio of minute ventilation to oxygen consumption. Healthy young adults usually maintain this ratio at 25 (i.e., 25 L of air breathed per liter of O_2 consumed) during submaximal exercise up to approximately 55% of the $\dot{V}O_{2max}$.[75] Higher ventilatory equivalents occur in children, with values averaging 32.[64] Exercise mode also affects the ventilatory equivalent. For example, prone swimming generates significantly lower $\dot{V}_E/\dot{V}O_2$ ratios than running, at all levels of energy expenditure.[49] The lower ventilatory equivalent results from the restrictive nature of swimming on breathing; this could constrain adequate gas exchange at maximal swimming velocities. This may partly explain the lower $\dot{V}O_{2max}$ achieved during swimming compared with $\dot{V}O_{2max}$ during running.[46]

Ventilation in Non–Steady-Rate Exercise

At higher levels of progressively more intense submaximal exercise, minute ventilation moves sharply upward and increases disproportionately in relation to oxygen consumption. The ventilatory equivalent can attain values as high as 35 or 40 L of air per liter of oxygen consumed.

Ventilatory Threshold

The term **ventilatory threshold** ($\mathbf{V_T}$) describes the point at which pulmonary ventilation increases disproportionately with oxygen consumption during graded exercise (see Fig. 14.5 and "In a Practical Sense"). At this exercise intensity, pulmonary ventilation no longer links tightly to oxygen demand at the cellular level. In fact, the "excess" ventilation (in relation to the oxygen consumed) results directly from carbon dioxide's increased output from buffering of the lactate that begins to accumulate partly from increased anaerobic glycolysis. Sodium bicarbonate in the blood buffers almost all of the lactate generated in anaerobic metabolism to sodium lactate in the following reaction:

$$\text{Lactic acid} + NaHCO_3 \longrightarrow \text{Na Lactate} + H_2CO_3$$
$$H_2CO_3 \rightleftharpoons H_2O + CO_2$$

The excess, nonmetabolic carbon dioxide released in the buffering reaction stimulates pulmonary ventilation that disproportionately increases $\dot{V}_E/\dot{V}O_2$. Additional carbon dioxide exhaled because of acid buffering causes the respiratory exchange ratio (R;$\dot{V}CO_2/\dot{V}O_2$) to exceed 1.00. Traditionally, researchers incorrectly believed that the disproportionate increase in $\dot{V}_E$ and increase in R above 1.00 indicated that the oxygen demands of the active muscles exceeded mitochondrial oxygen supply with a resulting increase in anaerobic energy transfer. They maintained that the $\dot{V}_T$ thus indicated the threshold for anaerobiosis and was termed the anaerobic threshold, or simply A_T, to indicate reliance on anaerobic glycolysis (see "Focus on Research"). Figure 14.6 outlines the underlying factors related to A_T detected from pulmonary gas exchange dynamics during graded exercise.

Attempts to validate linkage between ventilatory changes and glycolytic events at the cellular level have proved elusive. Nevertheless, use of an anaerobic threshold concept to indicate endurance exercise performance and physiologic response to exercise persists.

Onset of Blood Lactate Accumulation

In lieu of using ventilatory markers to indicate anaerobic metabolic events, researchers directly measure lactate's appearance in muscle and blood. During steady-rate exercise, aerobic metabolism matches the energy requirements of the active muscles. Under these conditions, little or no blood lactate accumulates because lactate production equals lactate disappearance. *The term* ***lactate threshold*** *describes the highest oxygen consumption or exercise intensity with less than a 1.0 mM per liter increase in blood lactate concentration above the preexercise level.*[78] Lactate is expressed in millimoles (mM) per liter of whole blood ($mM \cdot L^{-1}$), or as $mg \cdot dL^{-1}$ of whole blood, also termed volume percent (vol%); 1.0 $mM \cdot L^{-1}$ equals 9.0 vol%. By convention, blood lactate concentration is usually expressed in millimoles.

Onset of blood lactate accumulation (OBLA) signifies when blood lactate concentration shows a systematic increase equal to 4.0 mM.[66,83] Researchers often use the terms lactate threshold and *OBLA* interchangeably (as we do below), although each represents an operationally different precise point in terms of exercise intensity and blood lactate level. To some, the 4.0-mM value for OBLA implies the maximum exercise intensity that a person can sustain for a prolonged duration. In reality, however, the maximum stable lactate level shows considerable variability among individuals.[15]

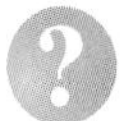

INTEGRATIVE QUESTION

In what ways are the terms lactate threshold and onset of blood lactate accumulation biochemically more precise than the term anaerobic threshold?

The exact cause of OBLA remains controversial. Some assume that it represents a distinct point for the onset of muscle anaerobiosis. However, blood lactate values do not always reflect the lactate concentration in specific muscles.[34] Lactate may accumulate not only from muscle anaerobiosis, but also from a decreased total lactate clearance or increased lactate production in specific muscle fibers.

Focus on Research

Detecting the Onset of Anaerobic Metabolism

Wasserman K, McIlroy MB. Detecting the threshold of anaerobic metabolism in cardiac patients during exercise. Am J Cardiol 1964;14:844.

➤ The onset of anaerobiosis during exercise powerfully predicts a person's capability for sustained aerobic exercise. The pioneering work of Wasserman and colleagues presented their rationale and methodology using simple respiratory gas exchange data in an attempt to detect the threshold of anaerobic metablolism; they named this point the "anaerobic threshold." These researchers argued that one could detect the threshold of anaerobic metabolism during exercise in one of three ways: (1) increased blood lactate concentration, (2) decreased arterial blood bicarbonate and pH, and (3) increased respiratory gas exchange ratio (R). A method that assesses R has the advantage of avoiding blood-sampling procedures while at the same time using equipment common to exercise physiology laboratories.

Subjects performed a graded exercise test by either pedaling a cycle ergometer or walking on a treadmill for 4-minute exercise intervals. Measurements included heart rate, minute ventilation, oxygen consumption, and end-tidal CO_2 and N_2 concentrations. End-tidal oxygen and carbon dioxide concentrations provided data for computing R. The *upper figure* shows a sigmoid curve results from plotting R from the last 30 seconds of each exercise level against $\dot{V}O_2$. The inflection point at the onset of the steepest part of this curve, called by these researchers the *threshold* of anaerobic metabolism, was believed to indicate the $\dot{V}O_2$ level at which anaerobic metabolism became significant. The anaerobic threshold also corresponded to the exercise intensity at which arterial blood bicarbonate concentration decreased and blood lactate increased.

The *lower figure* displays the anaerobic threshold data for 37 patients with heart disease. Subjects with the poorest fitness attained anaerobic threshold at a lower $\dot{V}O_2$ (i.e., lower exercise intensity). From a clinical perspective, the researchers postulated that the respiratory exchange ratio during exercise provides a useful measure of cardiovascular function, to indicate how much exercise a patient could perform before cardiovascular dynamics failed to meet the tissues' oxygen requirements. Although current research indicates factors other than the onset of exercise anaerobiosis affect pulmonary and gas exchange dynamics, the initial research of Wasserman and coworkers provided an important impetus to study interactions among pulmonary, cardiovascular, and metabolic dynamics during graded exercise.

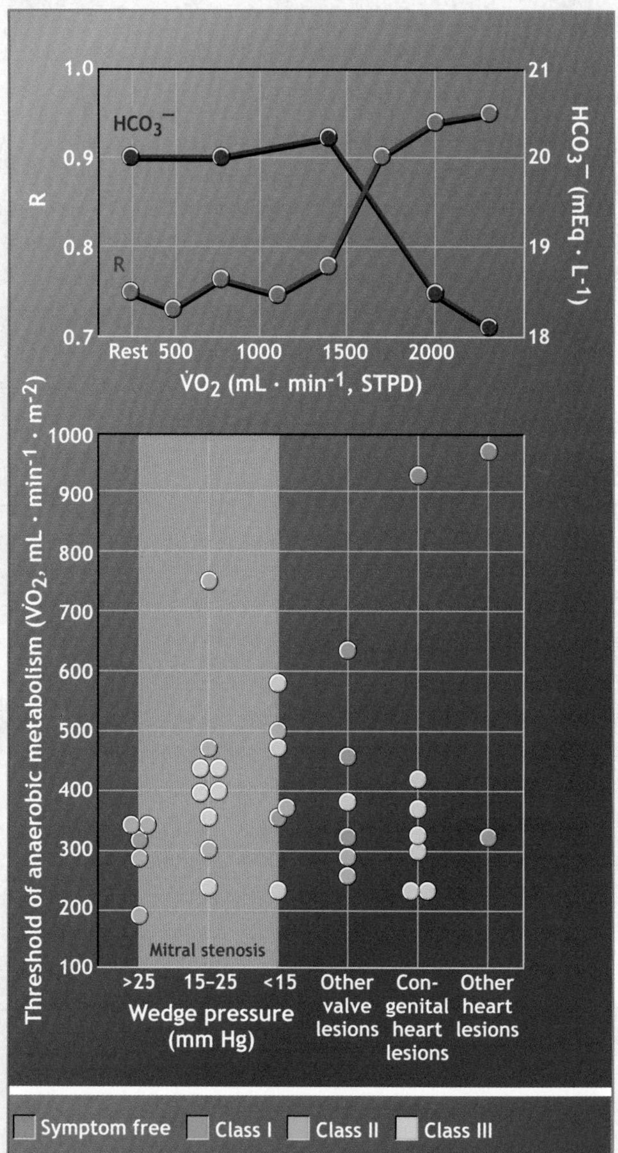

Top. Respiratory exchange ratio (R) and plasma bicarbonate (HCO_3^-) during rest and continuous graded exercise in one subject. *Bottom.* Threshold for anaerobic metabolism in 37 heart disease patients.

Moreover, a threshold of lactate appearance could result from (1) imbalance between the rate of glycolysis and mitochondrial respiration, (2) decreased redox potential (increased NADH relative to NAD^+), (3) lowered blood oxygen content, or (4) lowered blood flow to skeletal muscle. Because of possible different causes, caution should temper interpretations of the specific metabolic significance (and cause) of OBLA. However, it probably does signify initiation of an exponential accumulation of lactate in active muscle.[37]

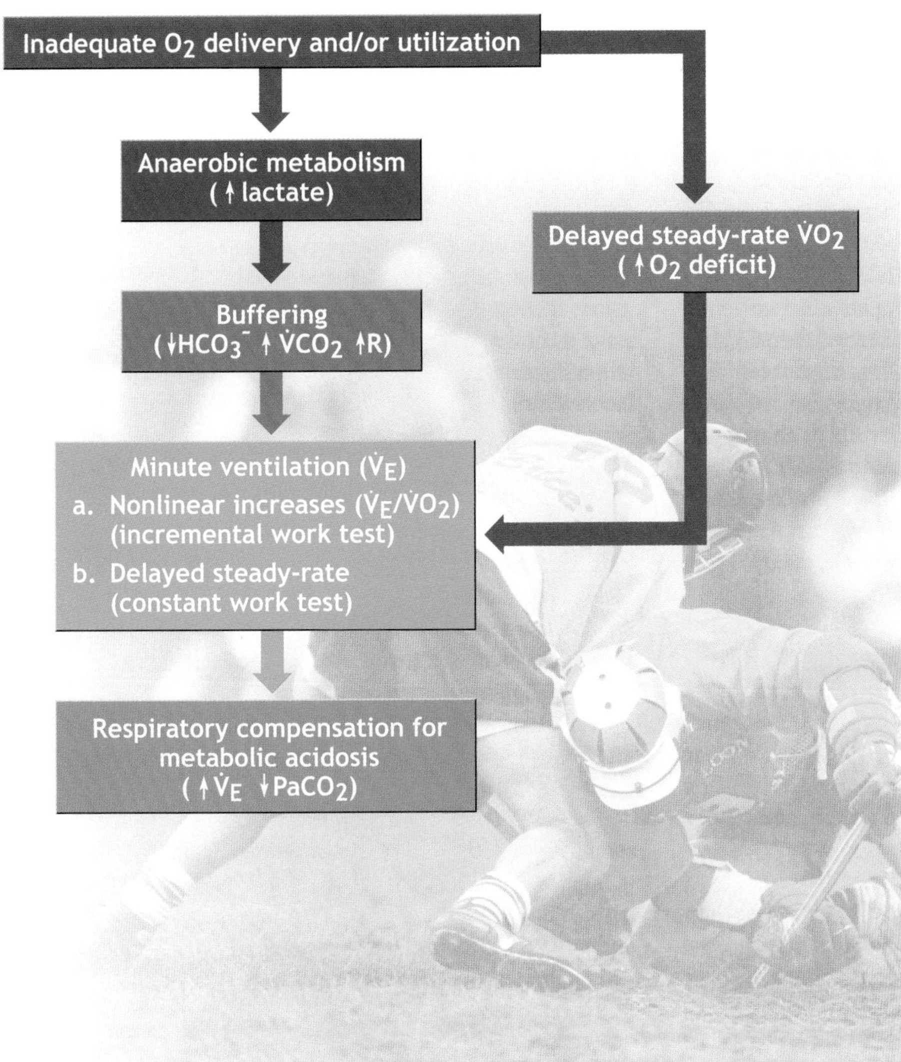

FIGURE 14.6 • Factors that relate to pulmonary gas exchange dynamics for detecting the lactate threshold.

Because blood lactate accumulation reflects plasma changes in pH, bicarbonate and H^+ concentrations, and carbon dioxide production via buffering, these variables provide an indirect assessment of OBLA.[39,75] Changes in these measures do indeed relate to OBLA, but they probably cannot serve independently to denote precisely the onset of anaerobic metabolism in muscle. Even if metabolic events and ventilatory dynamics in exercise do not relate causally, practical information about exercise performance results from these indirect evaluation procedures. "In a Practical Sense" illustrates several methods commonly used to indicate tissue hypoxia and an imbalance between lactate formation and its clearance during exercise.

SPECIFICITY OF OBLA. As with many measures of physiologic function and exercise performance, OBLA demonstrates exercise task specificity. Differences in OBLA relative to oxygen consumption occur in comparing bicycle, treadmill, and arm-crank exercise.[82] These differences likely result from variations in the muscle mass activated in each form of exercise. At a particular exercise intensity or submaximal oxygen consumption, a higher metabolic rate per unit of active muscle mass exists in arm-crank and bicycle exercise than in treadmill walking or running. Therefore, OBLA occurs at a lower exercise level (oxygen consumption) during bicycling and arm-crank exercise.[43] *Diverse exercise modes cannot interchangeably define the point of OBLA during graded exercise testing.*

SOME INDEPENDENCE BETWEEN OBLA AND $\dot{V}O_{2MAX}$. Chapter 7 indicated that blood lactate in a trained individual accumulates not only at a higher submaximal oxygen consumption than in an untrained person, but also at a higher percentage of $\dot{V}O_{2max}$.[82] For children and adults, endurance training often improves the exercise intensity for OBLA *without* a concomitant increase in $\dot{V}O_{2max}$.[5,21,42,48] This indicates that different factors influence OBLA and $\dot{V}O_{2max}$. Muscle fiber type, capillary density, mitochondrial size and number, and enzyme concentrations play major roles in establishing the percentage of aerobic capacity sustainable without lactate accumulation.[13,36,77]

IN A PRACTICAL SENSE

➤➤ MEASURING LACTATE THRESHOLD

Conceptually, the lactate threshold (LT) represents an exercise level (power output, $\dot{V}O_2$, or energy expenditure) in which tissue hypoxia triggers an imbalance between lactate formation and its clearance, with a resulting increase in blood lactate concentration. All of the following terms refer essentially to the same LT phenomenon: expiratory compensation threshold, anaerobic threshold, onset of blood lactate accumulation, optimal ventilatory efficiency, aerobic–anaerobic threshold, onset of plasma lactate accumulation, individual anaerobic threshold, and point of metabolic acidosis.

The measurement of LT serves several important functions:

- Provides a sensitive indicator of aerobic training status
- Predicts endurance performance, often with greater accuracy than $\dot{V}O_{2max}$
- Establishes an effective training intensity geared to the active muscles' aerobic metabolic dynamics

Different Indicators of LT

1. Fixed blood lactate concentration
2. Ventilatory threshold
3. Blood lactate–exercise $\dot{V}O_2$ response

Fixed Blood Lactate Concentration

During low-intensity, steady-rate exercise, blood lactate concentration does not increase beyond the normal biologic variation observed at rest. As exercise intensity increases, blood lactate levels exceed normal variation. The exercise intensity (or $\dot{V}O_2$) associated with a fixed blood lactate concentration that exceeds normal resting variation denotes the LT. This often coincides with a 2.5 millimole (mM) value. A 4.0 mM lactate value indicates the onset of blood lactate accumulation (OBLA). The top figure illustrates LT and OBLA computations from fixed blood lactate concentrations during incremental, 4-minute exercise stages on a bicycle ergometer. Interpolation from a visual plot of power output ($\dot{V}O_2$) versus blood lactate determines the exercise level associated with the fixed blood lactate concentrations. The decision regarding stage duration, number of stages, and interval between stages becomes important. Stages 4 minutes or longer provide better predictability than shorter ones. For the data illustrated, LT occurred at an exercise power output of 205 W, while 225 W predicted the fixed blood lactate concentration for OBLA.

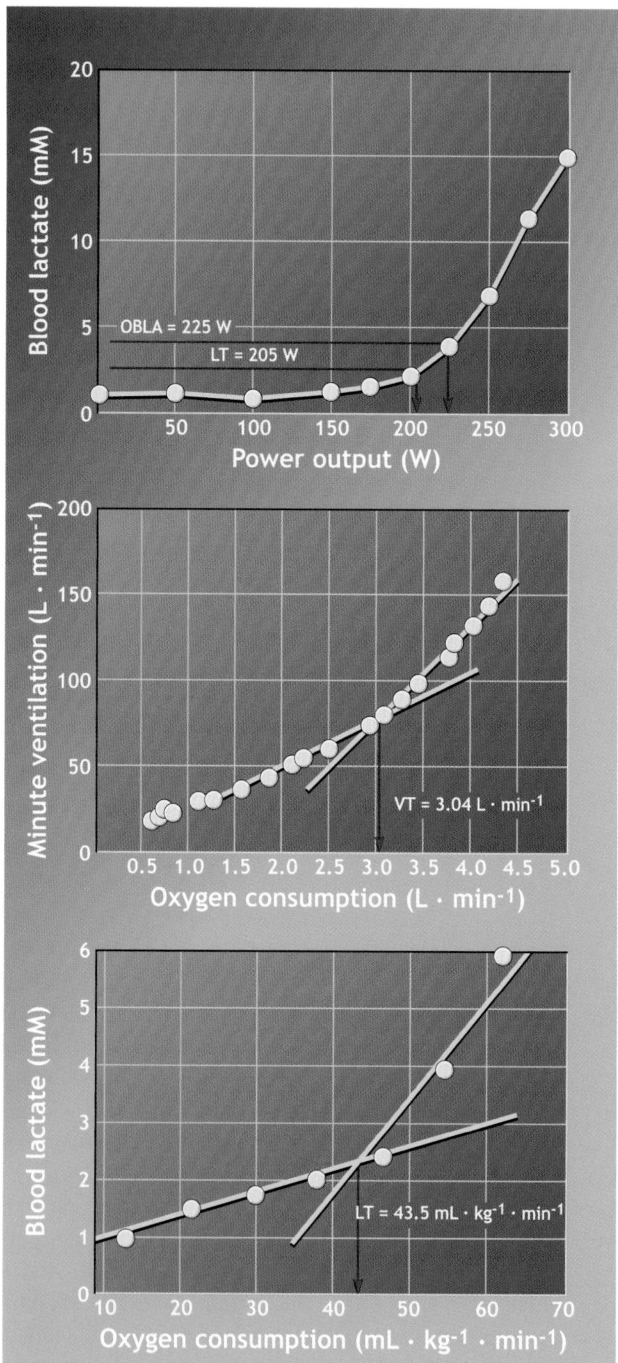

Top. Fixed blood lactate concentration method for determining lactate threshold (LT) and onset of blood lactate accumulation (OBLA). This example shows LT at a fixed blood lactate of 2.5 mM and OBLA at a fixed blood lactate of 4.0 mM. *Middle.* Determination of LT from the relationship between pulmonary minute ventilation and oxygen consumption during incremental exercise. *Bottom.* Determination of LT from relationship between blood lactate concentration and oxygen consumption during incremental exercise.

Ventilatory Threshold

Pulmonary minute ventilation ($\dot{V}_E$) during exercise increases disproportionately in its relationship to oxygen consumption at about the same time blood lactate begins to accumulate. This ventilatory threshold (VT) permits prediction of LT from the $\dot{V}_E$ response during graded exercise. The mechanistic link of lactate buffering by plasma bicarbonate to produce

IN A PRACTICAL SENSE

MEASURING LACTATE THRESHOLD—CONT'D

additional CO_2 (and respiratory stimulus unrelated to $\dot{V}O_2$) justifies the use of VT on a physiologic basis.

The test involves exercise with increments of short duration (a ramp test of 1- or 2-min increments) with continuous measurement of $\dot{V}_E$ (breath-by-breath or every 10, 20, or 30 s) to the point of fatigue (usually within 8 to 12 min). The point of nonlinear increase in $\dot{V}_E$ versus $\dot{V}O_2$ represents VT, expressed as a specific $\dot{V}O_2$ value rather than as running speed or power output common with the fixed blood lactate concentration method. The middle figure shows the relationship between $\dot{V}_E$ and $\dot{V}O_2$ during incremental exercise; VT occurs at an exercise $\dot{V}O_2$ of 3.04 L · min^{-1}. It is common to express the $\dot{V}O_2$ at LT as a percentage of $\dot{V}O_{2max}$. This represents 71% in this example.

Blood Lactate–Exercise $\dot{V}O_2$ Response

This protocol plots blood lactate concentration versus either $\dot{V}O_2$ or exercise intensity in a manner similar to that described for determination of fixed blood lactate concentration. The person exercises for 3- or 4-minute increments on a bicycle ergometer or treadmill. With treadmill exercise, blood is sampled for lactate determination during a brief pause at the end of each stage, or without pause when using stationary cycling exercise. The bottom figure plots blood lactate versus oxygen consumption throughout the test. A best-fitting straight line depicts the linear portion of the curve; a second line describes the upward-trending curve after it "breaks" from linearity. The intersection of the two lines represents LT.

On the other hand, two important factors help to achieve a high $\dot{V}O_{2max}$:

1. Functional capacity of the cardiovascular system for oxygen transport.
2. Absolute quantity of muscle mass activated in exercise.

A unique comparison among trained and untrained cardiac patients and trained healthy counterparts demonstrated the lack of close association between aerobic capacity and OBLA.[16] The patients showed impaired cardiac function (i.e., a blunted capacity for maximal blood flow) that significantly lowered $\dot{V}O_{2max}$ below the levels attained by healthy individuals. However, the trained patients could run at the same speed (and achieve essentially the same endurance performance) as the healthy individuals, without accumulating blood lactate. Figure 14.7 shows that these patients maintained nearly a metabolic steady rate while running at a speed that elicited $\dot{V}O_{2max}$. In fact, the point of OBLA represented 100% of $\dot{V}O_{2max}$!

OBLA AND ENDURANCE PERFORMANCE. Figure 14.8 illustrates the major variables that contribute to oxygen transport and use. They ultimately determine the maximum velocity a person can maintain in prolonged exercise. Two important factors influence endurance performance in a specific exercise mode:

1. Maximum capacity to consume oxygen ($\dot{V}O_{2max}$).
2. Maximum level for steady-rate exercise (OBLA).

Traditionally, exercise physiologists have used $\dot{V}O_{2max}$ as the yardstick to gauge capacity for endurance exercise. Although this measure generally relates to exercise performance, it does not fully explain success, because one does not perform endurance exercise at $\dot{V}O_{2max}$. *The exercise intensity at the point of OBLA consistently and powerfully predicts endurance exercise performance of men and women.*[7,17,54,69,71] A study of competitive racewalkers clearly illustrates this point.[27] Racewalking velocity at the point of lactate accumulation correlated highly to 20-km run times. Racewalking velocity at OBLA predicted race performance to within ± 0.6% of the actual time. Similar results occurred in elite cyclists. Cycling power output at the lactate threshold showed a strong relationship ($r = 0.93$) to the average absolute power output maintained during a 1-hour ride in the laboratory.[18] The laboratory measurement, in turn, predicted performance in a 40-km road race. Improved endurance performance with training more closely relates to training-induced improvement in the exercise level for OBLA than to changes in $\dot{V}O_{2max}$.[2,72,83]

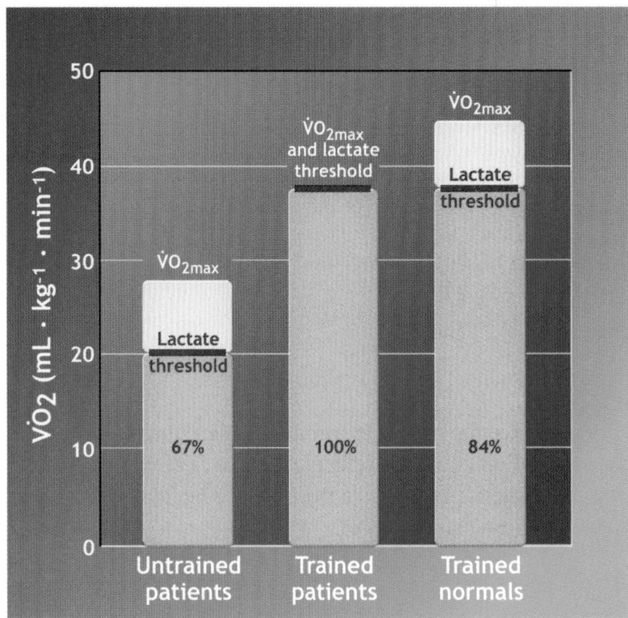

FIGURE 14.7 • Lactate threshold in relation to the $\dot{V}O_{2max}$ in trained and untrained patients with coronary artery disease and in healthy, trained subjects. (Modified from Coyle EF, et al. Blood lactate threshold in some well-trained ischemic heart disease patients. J Appl Physiol 1983;54:18.)

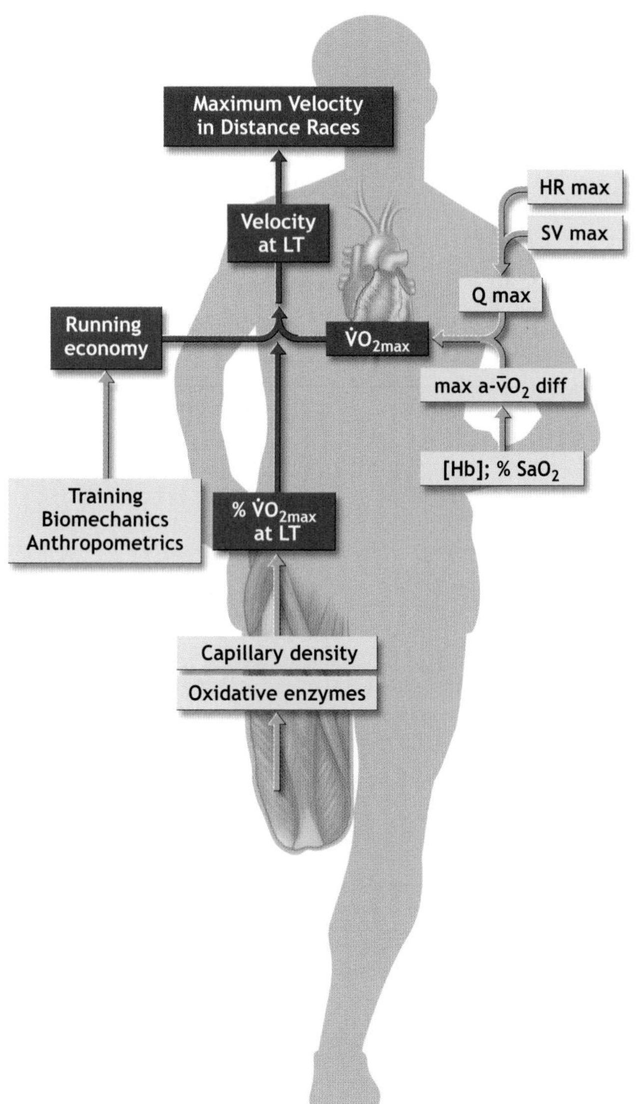

FIGURE 14.8 • Major variables related to maximal oxygen consumption, OBLA, and maximal running velocity during sustained exercise. Q, cardiac output; [Hb], hemoglobin concentration; max a-$\bar{v}O_2$ diff, maximum arteriovenous oxygen difference; OBLA, onset of blood lactate accumulation. (Modified from Bassett DR Jr, Howley ET. Maximal oxygen uptake: "classical" versus "contemporary" viewpoints. Med Sci Sports Exerc 1997;29:591.)

INTEGRATIVE QUESTION

Give the rationale for measuring pulmonary ventilation and gas exchange dynamics during graded exercise to indicate the onset of lactic acid buildup at the cellular level.

Racial Differences. The overwhelming dominance of East African athletes in competitive, high-intensity endurance running events between 3,000 and 10,000 m has stimulated research into the possibility of racial differences in resistance to fatigue, blood lactate accumulation, and intramuscular oxidative enzyme capacity. Research in this area consistently shows that African and South African endurance runners show greater resistance to fatigue at the same percentage of peak treadmill running velocity than their Caucasian counterparts, despite similar values for $\dot{V}O_{2max}$ and peak treadmill velocity.[12,65,79] The African athletes can sustain a relatively higher percentage of maximal exercise capacity (i.e., superior fatigue resistance) because of significantly higher oxidative enzyme profiles (citrate synthase and 3-hydroxyacyl-CoA dehydrogenase) and lower plasma lactate concentrations during sustained submaximal exercise. In addition to a higher fractional utilization of $\dot{V}O_{2max}$, greater running economy may also contribute to superior endurance performance of African runners at the elite level.[80]

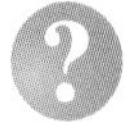

INTEGRATIVE QUESTION

What biochemical rationale exists for measuring oxygen consumption and carbon dioxide production to infer the onset of metabolic anaerobiosis (lactate accumulation) during exercise?

ENERGY COST OF BREATHING

Figure 14.9 shows the generalized relationship between pulmonary ventilation and oxygen consumption during rest and submaximal exercise and its division into ventilatory and

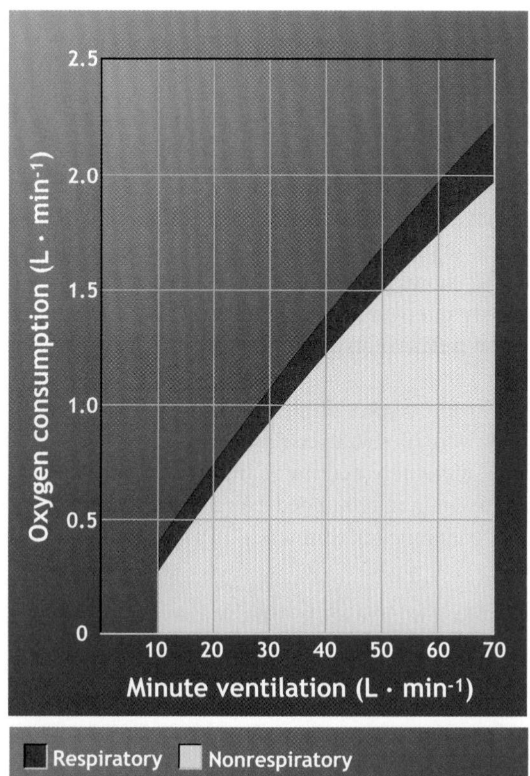

FIGURE 14.9 • Relationship between minute ventilation and total oxygen consumption (partitioned into respiratory and nonrespiratory components) during submaximal exercise in healthy subjects. (From Levison H, Cherniak R. Ventilatory cost of exercise in chronic obstructive pulmonary disease. J Appl Physiol 1968;25:21.)

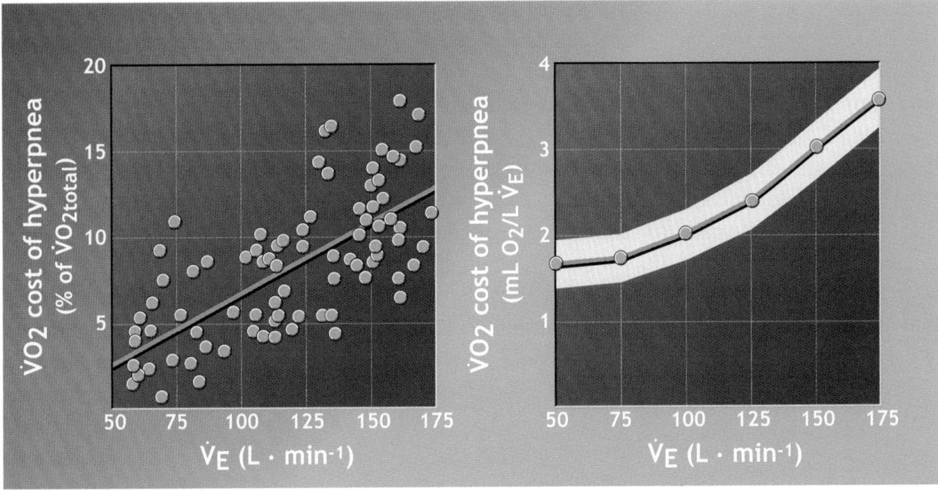

FIGURE 14.10 • Oxygen cost of breathing during whole-body graded exercise up to maximum. *Left panel,* Effects of increasing minute ventilation ($\dot{V}_E$) on the total oxygen cost of breathing expressed as a percentage of total exercise oxygen consumption. *Right panel,* Effects of increasing minute ventilation on the oxygen cost per liter air breathed per minute. (From Dempsey JA, et al. Respiratory muscle perfusion and energetics during exercise. Med Sci Sports Exerc 1996;28:1123.)

nonventilatory components.[45] At rest and during light-to-moderate exercise, the oxygen requirement of breathing remains relatively small.[11] Figure 14.10 specifies the oxygen cost of breathing during whole-body, graded exercise up to maximum.[23] The left panel indicates the effects of increasing minute ventilation on the oxygen cost of breathing expressed as a percentage of the total exercise oxygen consumption. The right panel illustrates the influence of increasing minute ventilation on the oxygen cost per liter of air breathed per minute. During exercise ventilations up to about 100 L · min^{-1}, oxygen cost averaged between 1.5 and 2.0 mL per liter of air breathed each minute (right panel). This represented from 3 to 5% of the total oxygen consumption in moderate exercise and 8 to 11% for minute ventilations at $\dot{V}O_{2max}$ values typical for most individuals (left panel). Among highly trained endurance athletes in whom maximum exercise minute ventilations reach 150 L · min^{-1} and higher, the cost of exercise hyperpnea may exceed 15% of the total oxygen consumption. At this exercise level, the inspiratory muscles operate at 40 to 60% of their maximum capacity to generate pressure (force).[1] The rate of blood flow to these muscles may equal flow to the limb locomotor muscles.[23]

The metabolic demands of respiratory muscles during maximal exercise require a significant portion of the total blood flow. Recent evidence from healthy, fit individuals indicates a "competition" for blood flow and oxygen between the respiratory muscles and locomotor muscles during heavy exercise. The respiratory muscles receive as much as 15% of the exercise cardiac output.[29–31] Altering respiratory muscle work during maximal exercise to increase the energy cost of breathing caused vasoconstriction in the locomotor muscles. Redirection of cardiac output to the respiratory musculature compromised perfusion of the active, nonrespiratory muscles. This reduced the total percentage of $\dot{V}O_{2max}$ used by the active locomotor muscles. Conversely, easing the work of breathing during maximal exercise with an assist ventilator elicited a corresponding increase in oxygen consumption (greater $\%\dot{V}O_{2max}$) of the active leg muscles.

Respiratory Disease

The healthy person rarely senses the effort to breathe, even during moderate exercise. In respiratory disease, however, the work of breathing often becomes an exhaustive exercise in itself. In chronic obstructive pulmonary disease (COPD), the added expiratory resistance can triple the normal cost of breathing at rest; during light exercise, ventilatory cost may reach 10 mL of oxygen for each liter of air breathed.[45] In severe pulmonary disease, the cost of breathing easily attains 40% of the total exercise oxygen consumption. Competition between the oxygen–blood flow needs of the locomotor muscles and the respiratory muscles encroaches on the oxygen available to the active, nonrespiratory muscle mass.[29] The increased cost of breathing severely limits the exercise capacity of individuals with COPD. Unfortunately, only small improvements in measures of pulmonary function or disease status generally accrue from exercise training. Other important positive results of regular exercise include improved exercise capacity, reduced dyspnea, decreased ventilatory equivalents for oxygen, improved respiratory and peripheral muscle function, and enhanced psychologic state.[10,52,67] Chapter 32 more fully discusses the role of regular physical activity in the rehabilitation of COPD patients.

Cigarette Smoking

The research relating smoking habits to exercise performance remains meager, yet most endurance athletes avoid cigarettes for fear of hindering performance because of a "loss of wind." Chronic cigarette smokers tend toward more-sedentary lifestyles and have lower fitness levels than their nonsmoking counterparts.[68] For some unknown reason, cigarette smoking increases one's dependence on carbohydrate for energy during rest and sustained exercise.[14] Smokers also have decreased dynamic lung function, which in severe instances manifests itself in COPD. For adolescent smokers, relatively little chronic cigarette smoking obstructs the airways and slow normal lung function development, with greater deficits in girls than boys.[25] Children who smoked had higher rates of asthma and wheezing and reduced dynamic lung function capacity in a dose-response relationship to their smoking habits. Female smokers who trained vigorously for 12 weeks significantly improved measures of aerobic capacity and endurance performance compared to smokers who remained sedentary.[3] In addition, females who exercised and quit smoking made greater fitness improvements than counterparts who trained similarly but continued to smoke. "In a Practical Sense," Chapter 13, provides an objective means to uncover factors that contribute to a person's smoking behavior.

Acute Effects

Airway resistance at rest increases as much as threefold in chronic smokers and nonsmokers following 15 puffs on a cigarette during a 5-minute period.[53] Added resistance to breathing lasts an average of 35 minutes; it probably exerts only a minor effect during light exercise, when breathing cost remains small. However, the residual effect of smoking could prove detrimental during vigorous exercise because of the significant additional oxygen cost for moving large air volumes. Increased peripheral airway resistance with smoking results mainly from the vagal reflex—possibly triggered from sensory stimulation by minute particles in cigarette smoke—and partially from stimulation of parasympathetic ganglia by nicotine.

Researchers determined the oxygen cost of breathing in six habitual smokers immediately after they smoked two cigarettes and 1 day after abstinence from tobacco.[63] The subjects ran on a treadmill at a speed and grade requiring 80% of $\dot{V}O_{2max}$. Two methods increased ventilation during the "smoking" and "nonsmoking" runs: (1) subjects voluntarily hyperventilated during the run (voluntary HV) and (2) researchers induced hyperventilation by increasing alveolar P_{CO_2} by having subjects breathe through a large-diameter tube that increased anatomic dead space by 1400 mL (dead space HV). The oxygen cost of the "extra" breathing equaled the difference between the normal oxygen consumption and the oxygen consumption in the hyperventilation experiments.

Table 14.1 shows that the oxygen cost of breathing decreased between 13 and 79% with smoking abstinence. During exercise, the energy requirement of breathing averaged 14% of the total exercise oxygen consumption after smoking, but only 9% in the nonsmoking trials for the heaviest smokers. Also, heart rates averaged 5 to 7% lower during exercise following 1 day of cigarette abstinence, and all subjects reported feeling better exercising in the nonsmoking condition. These findings indicate a substantial reversibility of the increased cost of breathing with smoking in chronic smokers with only 1 day of abstinence. *From a practical standpoint, an athlete who cannot eliminate smoking completely should at least abstain the day before a competition.* Recent research complements these findings and indicates that a 7-day smoking abstinence period in young men produced significant reductions in submaximal exercise heart rate and enhanced exercise performance as measured by time to exhaustion during graded exercise testing on a treadmill.[33]

Blunted Heart Rate Response

A paradox exists between the maximal exercise capacity of cigarette smokers and their submaximal heart rate response to exercise. Chronic smokers exhibit significantly less endurance during graded exercise to maximum than nonsmokers.[68] Despite their poorer performance in maximal testing (i.e., shorter time to fatigue), the smokers showed a significantly longer submaximal graded exercise test duration to reach a heart rate of 130 b · min^{-1}. A longer time to reach a predetermined submaximal heart rate during graded exercise testing indicates a *relatively higher* fitness level (i.e., more exercise accomplished before reaching the submaximal heart rate value). An altered sensitivity in autonomic neural control from cigarette smoking may blunt the heart rate response of smokers to submaximal exercise.[44] These findings emphasize the need to consider smoking status when evaluating fitness

TABLE 14.1 ➤ OXYGEN COST OF HYPERVENTILATION (HV) IN "SMOKING" AND "NONSMOKING" EXERCISE AT APPROXIMATELY 80% OF EACH SUBJECT'S $\dot{V}O_{2MAX}$

	Smoking				Nonsmoking			
	Voluntary HV		Dead Space HV		Voluntary HV		Dead Space HV	
Subject	$\dot{V}_E$ (L · min^{-1})	Cost (mL · L^{-1})	$\dot{V}_E$ (L · min^{-1})	Cost (mL · L^{-1})	$\dot{V}_E$ (L · min^{-1})	Cost (mL · L^{-1})	$\dot{V}_E$ (L · min^{-1})	Cost (mL · L^{-1})
1	26.4	15.1	18.9	12.7	22.7	11.4	23.0	6.5
2	39.0	10.3	28.1	5.9	42.6	11.3	41.3	4.8
3	22.8	7.9	27.2	7.0	23.8	7.2	22.8	5.7
4	36.3	5.0	28.7	5.6	44.7	3.8	18.6	−1.6[a]
5	52.7	13.5	26.7	12.4	75.2	6.1	22.8	5.7
6	22.4	8.5	27.3	1.1	23.2	3.4	30.1	3.0
Average	32.6	10.1	26.2	7.4	38.7	7.2	26.5	4.0

Note: The implication of the "negative" cost of $\dot{V}_E$ in this subject is that the added dead space reduced the cost of the normal exercise ventilation.
From Rode A, Shephard RJ. The influence of cigarette smoking upon the oxygen cost of breathing in near-maximal exercise. Med Sci Sports Exerc 1971;3:51.

data from submaximal heart rate response to standard exercise such as a step test or heart rate prediction test. Failure to consider cigarette smoking would inflate fitness estimates, because the lower heart rate (blunted response) of the smokers would erroneously predict higher aerobic fitness.

DOES VENTILATION LIMIT AEROBIC POWER AND ENDURANCE?

Aerobic training produces considerably less adaptation in pulmonary structure and function than in the cardiovascular and neuromuscular systems. Current interest concerns how the lack of pulmonary system "plasticity" affects aerobic exercise performance, particularly at the extreme exercise levels routinely performed by elite endurance athletes.

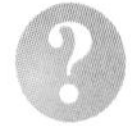

INTEGRATIVE QUESTION

Advise a person who performs specific breathing exercises rather than an endurance training program to increase "wind" and eliminate the feelings of breathlessness when running continuously for 20 to 30 minutes.

If ability to breathe during graded exercise becomes inadequate, the relationship between pulmonary ventilation and oxygen consumption would curve in a direction opposite to that indicated in Figure 14.5. In this case, the ventilatory equivalent would decrease. Such a response, common in COPD patients, indicates a *failure* of ventilation to keep pace with oxygen consumption;[4] in this situation, one truly would "run out of breath." During strenuous exercise, healthy individuals actually overbreathe at higher levels of oxygen consumption. The hyperventilation response generally produces a *decrease* in alveolar PCO_2 (see Fig. 14.3) and a concomitant but small *increase* in alveolar PO_2. Even during maximal exercise, a considerable **breathing reserve** exists because minute ventilation at $\dot{V}O_{2max}$ equals only 60 to 85% of a healthy person's maximum voluntary ventilation (MVV).[8,47] Most individuals demonstrate a reserve of 20 to 40% of the MVV during high-intensity exercise. *Such findings indicate that pulmonary function does not form a "weak link" in the oxygen transport system of healthy individuals with average to moderately high aerobic capacities.*

An Important Exception

For endurance athletes, the pulmonary system may lag behind their exceptional cardiovascular and aerobic muscular adaptations to training. The potential for inequality in alveolar ventilation relative to pulmonary capillary blood flow (i.e., impaired ventilation perfusion ratio) during high-intensity exercise may actually compromise arterial saturation and oxygen transport capacity—a condition termed **exercise-induced arterial hypoxemia (EIH)**.[32,51,59–61] EIH among trained individuals remains variable. It sometimes occurs at exercise levels as low as 40% $\dot{V}O_{2max}$ at sea level and mild and moderate altitudes.[9,26,65] When some highly trained endurance athletes exercise at near $\dot{V}O_{2max}$ (>65 mL · kg^{-1} · min^{-1}; Fig. 14.11), pressure differentials between alveolar and arterial oxygen widen to more than 30 mm Hg.[38] This causes arterial oxygen saturation to fall below 90%, with a corresponding arterial PO_2 below 75 mm Hg. These findings indicate that some elite aerobic athletes cannot achieve complete aeration of the blood in the pulmonary capillaries in high-intensity exercise; arterial desaturation becomes more apparent as exercise duration progresses.

It does not appear that alterations in pulmonary structure at the alveolar–capillary interface produce EIH.[70] Possible functionally based causes for arterial desaturation include:

1. Inequality in ventilation-perfusion ratio within the lungs or specific portions of the lungs.
2. Shunting of blood between venous and arterial circulations, thus bypassing areas for diffusion.
3. Failure to achieve end-capillary equilibrium between alveolar oxygen pressure and pressure of oxygen in blood perfusing the pulmonary capillaries; interstitial pulmonary edema or rapid blood flow in endurance athletes through a relatively normal-sized pulmonary capillary volume could produce this diffusion limitation.

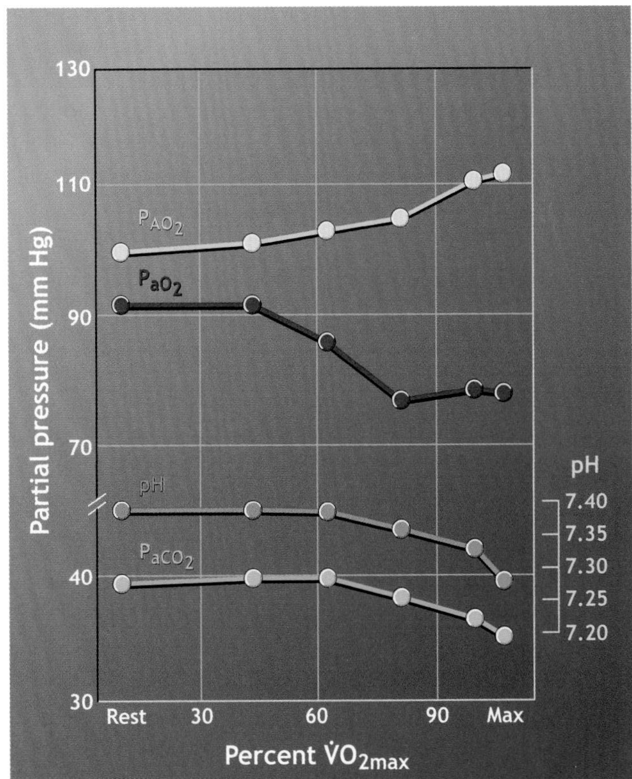

FIGURE 14.11 • Average values for blood gas pressures (PaO_2 and $PaCO_2$), acid–base status (pH), and difference between alveolar (PAO_2) and arterial (PaO_2) oxygen pressure in eight male athletes during graded exercise up to $\dot{V}O_{2max}$. Note the widening of the (A-a)O_2 gradient and the fall in PaO_2 during maximal exercise. (From Johnson BD, et al. Mechanical constraints on exercise hyperpnea in endurance athletes. J Appl Physiol 1992;73:874.)

To some extent, mechanical constraints on expiratory flow volumes of highly trained individuals during heavy exercise contribute to their relative lack of hyperventilation.[50] This can cause inadequate compensation for an excessively widened alveolar–arterial Po_2 difference, which contributes to arterial hypoxemia and a limitation in systemic oxygen transport and aerobic capacity. The reason for the potentiation of the desaturation effect during intense exercise among older endurance athletes remains unknown,[60] although venous–arterial shunting remains an unlikely explanation.[22]

INTEGRATIVE QUESTION

Present arguments to justify that pulmonary ventilation does not limit aerobic exercise performance for most healthy people.

Summary

1. In light-to-moderate exercise, pulmonary ventilation increases linearly with oxygen consumption. During this period, the ventilatory equivalent ($\dot{V}_E/\dot{V}O_2$) generally averages 20 to 25 L of air breathed per liter of oxygen consumed.
2. In non–steady-rate exercise, ventilation increases disproportionately with increases in oxygen consumption, and the ventilatory equivalent may exceed 35 L.
3. A sharp rise in minute ventilation during incremental exercise provides a "bloodless" means to estimate the onset of blood lactate accumulation (OBLA). This submaximal exercise measure of aerobic fitness relates to the beginning of anaerobiosis in the active muscles. OBLA occurs without significant metabolic acidosis or severe cardiovascular strain.
4. The oxygen cost of breathing for healthy individuals remains relatively small throughout a broad range of submaximal exercise. The work of breathing becomes excessive for individuals with respiratory disease, often producing inadequate alveolar ventilation.
5. Cigarette smoking causes airway resistance to rise significantly. This increases the cost of breathing, and can adversely affect prolonged exercise performance. Substantial reversibility occurs with just 1 day of smoking abstinence.
6. Exercise training generally reduces the ventilatory equivalent in submaximal exercise. This "conserves" oxygen because the cost of breathing decreases during a particular exercise task.
7. For individuals of average aerobic fitness, maximal exercise does not tax pulmonary ventilation to a point that limits optimal alveolar gas exchange and arterial saturation. In contrast, pulmonary function improvements for the endurance athlete may lag behind their exceptional adaptations in cardiovascular and muscle function, thereby compromising aeration of blood during maximal effort.

➤ PART 3 • Acid–Base Regulation

BUFFERING

Acids are substances that dissociate in solution and release H^+, whereas **bases** pick up or accept H^+ to form hydroxide ions (OH^-). The term **buffering** designates reactions that minimize changes in H^+ concentration; **buffers** refer to the chemical and physiologic mechanisms that prevent this change.

The symbol **pH** designates a quantitative measure of acidity or alkalinity (basicity) of a liquid solution. Specifically, pH refers to the concentration of protons or H^+. Acid solutions have more H^+ than OH^- at a pH below 7.0, and vice versa for basic solutions, whose pH exceeds 7.0. Chemically pure (distilled) water, considered neutral, has equal amounts of H^+ and OH^- and thus has a pH of 7.0. The pH scale shown in Figure 14.12, devised in 1909 by Danish chemist Sören Sörensen, ranges from 1.0 to 14.0. An inverse relation exists between pH and H^+ concentration. Because of the logarithmic nature of the pH scale, a 1-unit change in pH produces a 10-fold change in H^+ concentration. For example, lemon juice and gastric juice (pH = 2.0) have 1000 times the H^+ concentration of black coffee (pH = 5.0), whereas hydrochloric acid (pH = 1.0) has approximately 1 million times the H^+ concentration of blood at a pH of 7.4.

The pH of bodily fluids ranges from a low of 1.0 for the digestive acid hydrochloric acid to a slightly basic pH between 7.35 and 7.45 for arterial and venous blood and most other bodily fluids. An increase in pH above the normal average of 7.4 results directly from a decrease in H^+ concentration (increased pH, or **alkalosis**). Conversely, **acidosis** refers to increased H^+ concentration (decreased pH). The acid–base characteristics of bodily fluids fluctuate within narrow limits, because metabolism is highly sensitive to H^+ concentrations in the reacting medium. Three mechanisms regulate the pH of the internal environment:

1. Chemical buffers
2. Pulmonary ventilation
3. Renal function

Chemical Buffers

The chemical buffering system consists of a weak acid and the salt of that acid. Bicarbonate buffer, for example, consists of the weak acid, **carbonic acid**, and the salt of that acid, **sodium bicarbonate**. Carbonic acid forms when bicarbonate binds H^+. As long as the H^+ concentration remains elevated, the reaction produces the weak acid because the excess H^+ ions bind in accord with the general reaction:

$$H^+ + \text{Buffer} \rightarrow \text{H-Buffer}$$

In contrast, if the concentration of H^+ decreases—as occurs during hyperventilation, when plasma carbonic acid decreases because carbon dioxide leaves the blood and exits

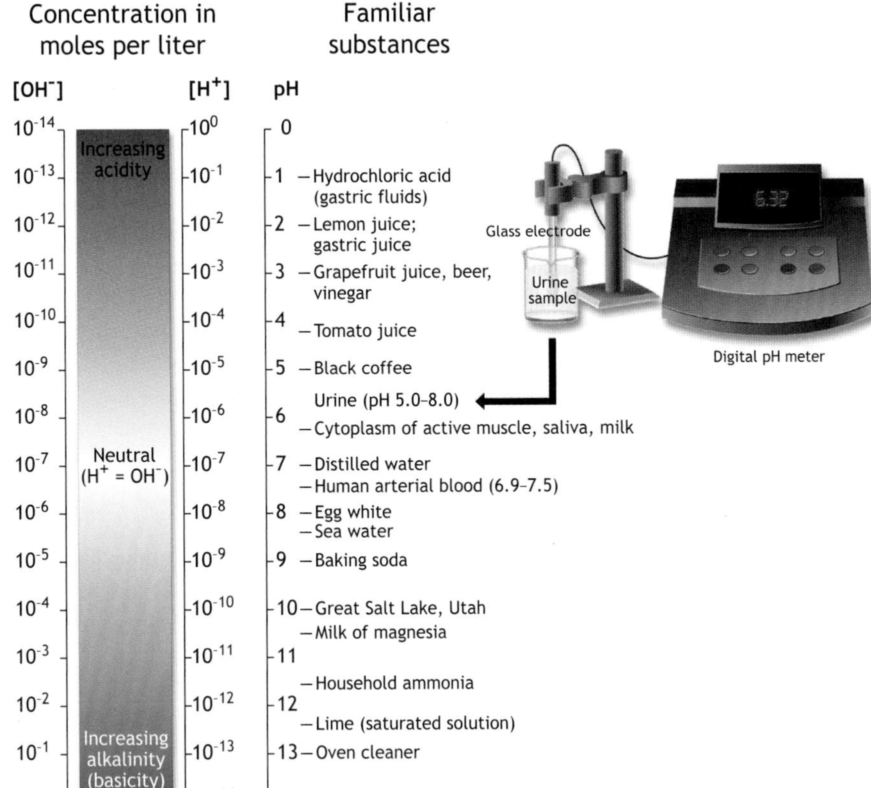

FIGURE 14.12 • The pH scale represents a quantitative measure of the acidity or alkalinity (basicity) of a liquid solution. Blood pH normally stabilizes at the slightly alkaline pH of 7.4. Values for blood pH rarely fall below a pH of 6.9, even during the most strenuous exercise. The digital pH meter accurately determines the pH of any substance. The example shows a pH of 6.32 for the urine sample.

through the lungs—the buffering reaction moves in the opposite direction and releases H^+:

$$H^+ + \text{Buffer} \leftarrow \text{H-Buffer}$$

Much of the carbon dioxide generated in energy metabolism reacts with water to form the relatively weak carbonic acid. The latter dissociates into H^+ and HCO_3^-. Likewise, the stronger lactic acid reacts with sodium bicarbonate to form sodium lactate and carbonic acid; in turn, carbonic acid dissociates and increases the H^+ concentration of the extracellular fluids. Other organic acids such as fatty acids dissociate and liberate H^+, as do sulfuric and phosphoric acids produced during protein catabolism.

Bicarbonate, phosphate, and protein chemical buffers provide the rapid first line of defense to maintain consistency in the acid–base character of the internal environment.

Bicarbonate Buffer

The bicarbonate buffer system consists of carbonic acid and sodium bicarbonate in solution. During buffering, hydrochloric acid (a strong acid) converts to the much weaker carbonic acid by combining with sodium bicarbonate in the following reaction:

$$HCl + NaHCO_3 \rightarrow NaCl + H_2CO_3 \leftrightarrows H^+ + HCO_3^-$$

The buffering of hydrochloric acid results in only a slight reduction in pH. As mentioned previously, sodium bicarbonate in plasma exerts a strong buffering action on lactic acid to form sodium lactate and carbonic acid. Any additional increase in H^+ concentration from carbonic acid dissociation causes the dissociation reaction to move in the opposite direction. This releases carbon dioxide into solution as follows:

Result of acidosis

$$H_2O + CO_2 \leftarrow H_2CO_3 \leftarrow H^+ + HCO_3^-$$

An increase in plasma carbon dioxide or H^+ concentration immediately stimulates ventilation to eliminate "excess" carbon dioxide.

Conversely, a decrease in plasma H^+ concentration (bodily fluids become more alkaline) inhibits the ventilatory drive. This causes retention of carbon dioxide. Carbon dioxide retained in this manner combines with water to increase acidity and normalize pH.

Result of alkalosis

$$H_2O + CO_2 \rightarrow H_2CO_3 \rightarrow H^+ + HCO_3^-$$

Phosphate Buffer

The phosphate buffering system consists of phosphoric acid and sodium phosphate. These chemicals act similarly to those in the bicarbonate system. Phosphate buffer exerts an important effect on acid–base balance in the kidney tubules and intracellular fluids where phosphate concentration remains high.

TABLE 14.2 ➤ RELATIVE BUFFERING POWER OF THE CHEMICAL BUFFERS

CHEMICAL BUFFER	BLOOD	BLOOD PLUS INTERSTITIAL FLUIDS
Bicarbonate	1.0	1.0
Phosphate	0.3	0.3
Proteins (excluding Hb)	1.4	0.8
Hemoglobin	5.3	1.5

Protein Buffer

Venous blood buffers the H^+ released from the dissociation of relatively weak carbonic acid (produced from $H_2O + CO_2$). *By far, hemoglobin provides the most important H^+ acceptor for this buffering function.* Hemoglobin is almost six times more potent in regulating acidity than the other plasma proteins. In addition, hemoglobin's release of oxygen to the cells makes hemoglobin a weaker acid, increasing its affinity to bind H^+. The H^+ generated from the formation of carbonic acid in the erythrocyte combines readily with deoxygenated hemoglobin (Hb^-) in the reaction

$$H^+ + Hb^- \text{ (Protein)} \longrightarrow HHb$$

Intracellular tissue proteins also regulate plasma pH. Some amino acids possess free acidic radicals that, when dissociated, form OH^-, which readily reacts with H^+ to form water.

Relative Power of Chemical Buffers

Table 14.2 lists the relative power of the blood's chemical buffers and those in blood and interstitial fluids combined. As a frame of reference, the buffering power of the bicarbonate system receives the value 1.00.

PHYSIOLOGIC BUFFERS

The pulmonary and renal systems present the second line of defense in acid–base regulation. Their buffering function comes into play only when a change in pH has already occurred.

Ventilatory Buffer

Any increase in the quantity of free H^+ in extracellular fluid and plasma directly stimulates the respiratory center, immediately increasing alveolar ventilation. This rapid adjustment reduces alveolar P_{CO_2} causing carbon dioxide to be "blown off" from the blood. Reduced plasma carbon dioxide levels accelerate recombination of H^+ and HCO_3^-, thus lowering free H^+ concentration in plasma. For example, doubling alveolar ventilation by hyperventilation at rest increases blood alkalinity and pH by 0.23 units, from 7.40 to 7.63. Conversely, reducing normal alveolar ventilation (hypoventilation) by one-half increases blood acidity by approximately 0.23 pH units. The potential magnitude of ventilatory buffering equals twice the combined effect of all the body's chemical buffers.

Renal Buffer

Chemical buffers only temporarily affect excess acid buildup. Excretion of H^+ by the kidneys, although time consuming, provides an important longer-term defense to maintain the body's buffer reserve (**alkaline reserve**). To this end, the kidneys stand as the final sentinel. The renal tubules regulate acidity through complex chemical reactions that secrete ammonia and H^+ into the urine and then reabsorb alkali, chloride, and bicarbonate.

EFFECTS OF SHORT- AND LONG-TERM EXERCISE

During strenuous exercise, pH regulation becomes progressively more difficult because of increased H^+ concentration from carbon dioxide production and lactate formation. Acid–base regulation becomes exceedingly more difficult during repeated, brief bouts of all-out exercise that elevate blood lactate values to 30 mM (270 mg of lactate per dL of blood) or higher.[35] Figure 14.13 illustrates the inverse linear relationship between blood lactate concentration and blood pH.[57] In these experiments, blood lactate concentration varied between 0.8 mM at rest (pH 7.43) and 32.1 mM during exhaustive exercise (pH 6.80). In active muscle, pH reaches even lower values, falling to 6.4 or lower at exhaustion.[73]

These data indicate that humans *temporarily* tolerate pronounced disturbances in acid–base balance during maximal exercise, at least to a blood pH as low as 6.80—one of the lowest values ever reported. A plasma pH below 7.00 does not occur without consequences; this level of acidosis often produces nausea, headache, and dizziness, in addition to discomfort and pain within active muscles.

Summary

1. The chemical and physiologic buffer systems normally regulate the acid–base character of the bodily fluids within narrow limits.
2. The bicarbonate, phosphate, and protein chemical buffers provide the rapid first line of defense in acid–base regulation. These buffers consist of a weak acid and the salt of that acid. Their action during acidosis converts a strong acid to a weaker acid and a neutral salt.
3. When the chemical buffer system becomes stressed, the lungs and kidneys contribute to pH regulation. Changes in alveolar ventilation rapidly alter the free H^+ concentration in extracellular fluids. In response to increased acidity, the renal tubules act as the body's final defense by secreting H^+ into the urine and reabsorbing bicarbonate.

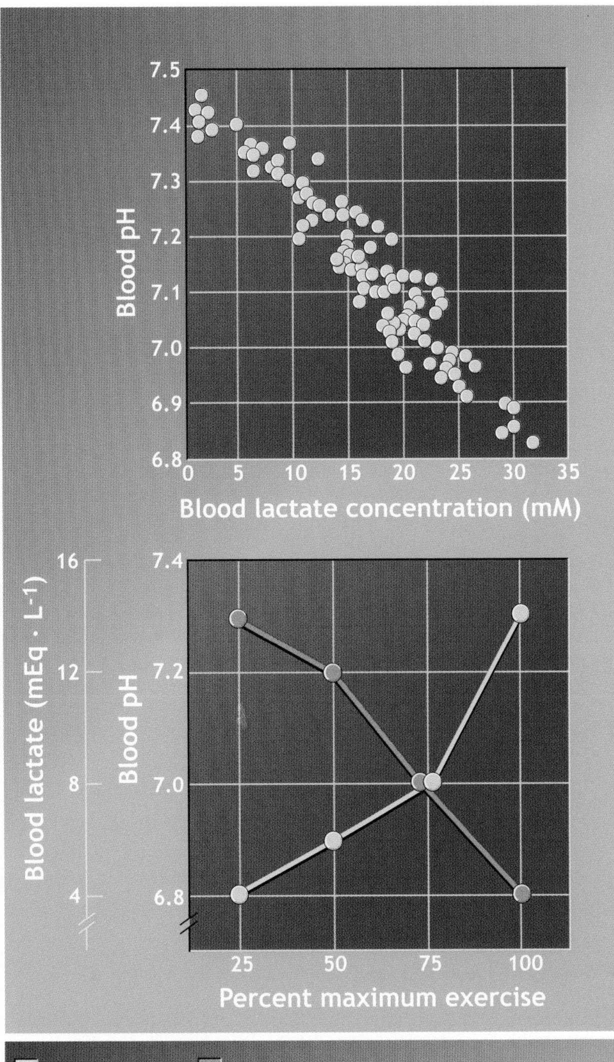

FIGURE 14.13 • *Top.* Relationship between blood pH and blood lactate concentration at rest and during increasing intensities of short-duration exercise up to maximum. (From Osnes JB, Hermansen L. Acid–base balance after maximal exercise of short duration. J Appl Physiol 1972;32:59.) *Bottom.* Blood pH and blood lactate concentration in relation to exercise intensity expressed as a percentage of maximum. A decrease in blood pH accompanies an increase in blood lactate concentration.

4. Anaerobic exercise increases the demand for buffering, and pH regulation becomes progressively more difficult.

References

1. Aaron EA, et al. Oxygen cost of exercise hyperpnea: implications for performance. J Appl Physiol 1992;75:1818.
2. Acevedo EO, Goldfarb AH. Increased training intensity effects on plasma lactate, ventilatory threshold, and endurance. Med Sci Sports Exerc 1989;21:563.
3. Albrecht AE, et al. Effect of smoking cessation on exercise performance in female smokers participating in exercise training. Am J Cardiol 1998;82:950.
4. Babb TG. Mechanical ventilatory constraints in aging, lung disease and obesity: perspectives and brief review. Med Sci Sports Exerc 1999;31(suppl 1):S12.
5. Bassett DR Jr, Howley ET. Limiting factors for maximum oxygen uptake and determinants of endurance performance. Med Sci Sports Exerc 2000;32:270.
6. Bianchi AL, et al. Central control of breathing in mammals: neuronal circuitry, membrane properties, and neurotransmitters. Physiol Rev 1995;75:1.
7. Bishop D, et al. The relationship between plasma lactate parameters, Wpeak and 1-h cycling performance in women. Med Sci Sports Exerc 1998;30:1270.
8. Bye PTP, et al. Ventilatory muscles during exercise in air and oxygen in normal men. J Appl Physiol 1984;56:464.
9. Chapman RF, et al. Degree of arterial desaturation in normoxia influences $\dot{V}O_{2max}$ decline in mild hypoxia. Med Sci Sports Exerc 1999;31:658.
10. Clark CJ, et al. Low intensity peripheral muscle conditioning improves exercise tolerance and breathlessness in COPD. Eur Respir J 1996;9:2590.
11. Coast JR, et al. Ventilatory work and oxygen consumption during exercise and hyperventilation. J Appl Physiol 1993;74:793.
12. Coetzer P, et al. Superior fatigue resistance of elite black South African distance runners. J Appl Physiol 1993;75:1822.
13. Coggan AR, et al. Plasma glucose kinetics during exercise in subjects with high and low lactate thresholds. J Appl Physiol 1992;73:1873.
14. Colberg SR, et al. Increased dependence on blood glucose in smokers during rest and sustained exercise. J Appl Physiol 1994;76:26.
15. Coyle EF. Integration of the physiological factors determining endurance performance in athletes. Exerc Sport Sci Rev 1995;23:25.
16. Coyle EF, et al. Blood lactate threshold in some well-trained ischemic heart disease patients. J Appl Physiol 1983;54:18.
17. Coyle EF, et al. Determinants of endurance in well trained cyclists. J Appl Physiol 1988;64:2622.
18. Coyle EF, et al. Physiological and biomechanical factors associated with elite endurance cycling performance. Med Sci Sports Exerc 1991;23:93.
19. Craig AB Jr. Principles and problems of underwater swimming and diving. Med Sci Sports Exerc 1976;8:171.
20. Craig AB Jr. Principles and problems of underwater diving. Phys Sportsmed 1980;8(3):72.
21. Davis C, et al. Effect of 40 weeks of endurance training on anaerobic threshold. Int J Sports Med 1982;3:208.
22. Dempsey, JA, et al. Exercise-induced arterial hypoxemia in healthy persons at sea level. J Physiol 1984;355:161.
23. Dempsey JA, et al. Respiratory muscle perfusion and energetics during exercise. Med Sci Sports Exerc 1996;28:1123.
24. Eldridge FL. Central integration of mechanisms in exercise hyperpnea. Med Sci Sports Exerc 1994;26:319.
25. Gold DR, et al. Effects of cigarette smoking on lung function in adolescent boys and girls. N Engl J Med 1996;331:335.
26. Gore TP, et al. Increased arterial desaturation in trained cyclists during maximal exercise at 580m altitude. J Appl Physiol 1996;80:2204.
27. Hagberg JM, Coyle EF. Physiological determinants of endurance performance as studied in competitive racewalkers. Med Sci Sports Exerc 1983;15:287.
28. Hardarson T, et al. Importance of the lactate anion in control of breathing. J Appl Physiol 1998;84:411.
29. Harms CA, et al. Respiratory muscle work compromises leg blood flow during maximal exercise. J Appl Physiol 1997;82:1573.
30. Harms CA. Effect of skeletal muscle demand on cardiovascular function. Med Sci Sports Exerc 2000;32:94.
31. Harms CA, et al. Effect of respiratory muscle work on cardiac output and its distribution during maximal exercise. J Appl Physiol 1998;85:609.
32. Harms CA, et al. Exercise induced arterial hypoxemia in healthy young women. J Physiol (Lond) 1998;507:619.
33. Hashizume K, et al. Effects of abstinence from cigarette smoking on the cardiorespiratory capacity. Med Sci Sports Exerc 2000;32:386.
34. Hermansen L. Lactate production during exercise. In: Pernow B, Saltin B, eds. Muscle metabolism during exercise. New York: Plenum, 1971.
35. Hermansen L. Effect of metabolic changes on force generation in skeletal muscle during maximal exercise. In: Human muscle fatigue: physiological mechanisms. London: Pitman Medical, 1981.

36. Holloszy JO, Coyle EF. Adaptations of skeletal muscle to endurance exercise and their metabolic consequences. J Appl Physiol 1984;56:834.
37. Ivy JL, et al. Progressive metabolite changes in individual muscle fibers with increasing work rates. Am J Physiol 1987;252:C630.
38. Johnson BD, et al. Mechanical constraints on exercise hyperpnea in endurance athletes. J Appl Physiol 1992;73:874.
39. Jones NL. Dyspnea in exercise. Med Sci Sports Exerc 1984;16:14.
40. Jones NL, Ehrsam RE. The anaerobic threshold. Exercise and Sport Sciences Reviews. Terjung RL, ed. vol 10. Philadelphia: Franklin Institute, 1982.
41. Katch FI, et al. The influence of the estimated oxygen cost of ventilation on oxygen deficit and recovery oxygen intake for moderately heavy bicycle ergometer exercise. Med Sci Sports Exerc 1972;4:71.
42. Kohrt WM, et al. Longitudinal assessment of responses by triathletes to swimming, cycling, and running. Med Sci Sports Exerc 1989;21:569.
43. Koyal SN, et al. Ventilatory responses to the metabolic acidosis of treadmill and cycle ergometry. J Appl Physiol 1976;40:864.
44. Laustiola KE, et al. Cigarette smoking alters sympathoadrenal regulation by decreasing the density of beta 2-adrenoceptors. A study of monitored smoking cessation. J Cardiovasc Pharmacol 1991;17:923.
45. Levison H, Cherniack R. Ventilatory cost of exercise in chronic obstructive pulmonary disease. J Appl Physiol 1968;25:21.
46. Magel JR, et al. Specificity of swim training on maximum oxygen uptake. J Appl Physiol 1975;38:151.
47. Mahler DA, et al. Ventilatory responses at rest and during exercise in marathon runners. J Appl Physiol 1982;52:388.
48. Mahon AD, Vaccaro P. Ventilatory threshold and $\dot{V}O_{2max}$ changes in children following endurance training. Med Sci Sports Exerc 1989;21:425.
49. McArdle WD, et al. Metabolic and cardiorespiratory response during free swimming and treadmill walking. J Appl Physiol 1971;30:733.
50. McClaran S, et al. Role of expiratory flow limitation in determining lung volumes and ventilation during exercise. J Appl Physiol 1999;86:1357.
51. McKenzie DC, et al. The effect of repeat exercise on pulmonary diffusing capacity and EIH in trained athletes. Med Sci Sports Exerc 1999;31:99.
52. Mink BD. Exercise and chronic obstructive pulmonary disease: modest fitness gains pay big dividends. Phys Sportsmed 1997;25(11):43.
53. Nadel JA, Comroe JH. Acute effects of inhalation of cigarette smoke on airway resistance. J Appl Physiol 1961;16:713.
54. Nicholson RM, Sleivert GG. Indices of lactate threshold and their relationship with 10-km running velocity. Med Sci Sports Exerc 2001;33:339.
55. Nye PCG. Identification of peripheral chemoreceptor stimuli. Med Sci Sports Exerc 1994;26:311.
56. Oleberg DA, et al. Skeletal muscle chemoreflex and pH in exercise ventilatory control. J Appl Physiol 1998;84:676.
57. Osnes JB, Hermansen L. Acid–base balance after maximal exercise of short duration. J Appl Physiol 1972;32:59.
58. Pan LG, et al. Important role of carotid afferents in control of breathing. J Appl Physiol 1998;85:1299.
59. Powers SK, et al. Effects of incomplete pulmonary gas exchange on $\dot{V}O_{2max}$. J Appl Physiol 1989;66:2491.
60. Préfaut C, et al. Exercise-induced hypoxemia in older athletes. J Appl Physiol 199476:120.
61. Rasmussen J, et al. Muscle mass effect on arterial desaturation after maximal exercise. Med Sci Sports Exerc 1991;23:1349.
62. Rice AJ, et al. Exercise-induced hypoxaemia in highly trained cyclists at 40% peak oxygen uptake. Eur J Appl Physiol 1999;79:353.
63. Rode A, Shephard RJ. The influence of cigarette smoking upon the oxygen cost of breathing in near-maximal exercise. Med Sci Sports Exerc 1971;3:51.
64. Rowland TW, Green GM. Physiological responses to treadmill exercise in females: adult-child differences. Med Sci Sports Exerc 1988;20:474.
65. Saltin B, et al. Morphology, enzyme activities and buffer capacity in leg muscles of Kenyan and Scandinavian runners. Scand J Med Sci Sports 1995;5:222.
66. Seip RL, et al. Perceptual responses and blood lactate concentration: effect of training state. Med Sci Sports Exerc 1991;23:80.
67. Serres I, et al. Skeletal muscle abnormalities in patients with COPD: contribution to exercise intolerance. Med Sci Sports Exerc 1998;30:1019.
68. Sidney S, et al. Cigarette smoking and submaximal exercise test duration in a biracial population of young adults: the CARDIA study. Med Sci Sports Exerc 1993;25:911.
69. Speechly DP, et al. Difference in ultra-endurance exercise in performance-matched male and female runners. Med Sci Sports Exerc 1996;28:359.
70. St. Croix CM, et al. Effects of prior exercise on exercise-induced hypoxemia in young women. J Appl Physiol 1998;85:1556.
71. Tanaka K, et al. Relationship of anaerobic threshold and onset of blood lactate accumulation with endurance performance. Eur J Appl Physiol 1983;52:51.
72. Tanaka K, et al. A longitudinal assessment of anaerobic threshold and distance-running performance. Med Sci Sports Exerc 1984;16:278.
73. Taylor DJ, et al. Energetics of human muscle: exercise-induced ATP depletion. Magn Reson Med 1986;3:44.
74. Ward SA. Control of exercise hyperpnea in humans: a modeling perspective. Respir Physiol 2000;122(2–3):149.
75. Wasserman K, et al. Respiratory physiology of exercise: metabolism, gas exchange and ventilatory control. In: Widdicombe JG, ed. Respiratory physiology III, vol 23. International Review of Physiology. Baltimore: University Park Press, 1981.
76. Wasserman K, et al. Principles of exercise testing and interpretation. 2nd ed. Philadelphia: Lea & Febiger, 1994.
77. Weltman A. The blood lactate response to exercise. Champaign, IL: Human Kinetics, 1995.
78. Weltman A, et al. Reliability and validity of a continuous incremental treadmill protocol for the determination of lactate threshold, fixed blood lactate concentrations and $\dot{V}O_{2max}$. Int J Sports Med 1990;11:26.
79. Weston A, et al. African runners exhibit greater fatigue resistance, lower lactate accumulation, and higher oxidative enzyme activity. J Appl Physiol 1999;86:915.
80. Weston AR, et al. Running economy of African and Caucasian distance runners. Med Sci Sports Exerc 2000;32:1110.
81. Whipp BJ. Peripheral chemoreceptor control of exercise hyperpnea in humans. Med Sci Sports Exerc 1994;26:337.
82. Wyatt FB. Comparison of lactate and ventilatory threshold to maximal oxygen consumption: a meta-analysis. J Strength Cond Res 1999;13:67.
83. Yoshida T, et al. Blood lactate parameters related to aerobic capacity and endurance performance. Eur J Appl Physiol 1987;56:7.

CHAPTER 15

The Cardiovascular System

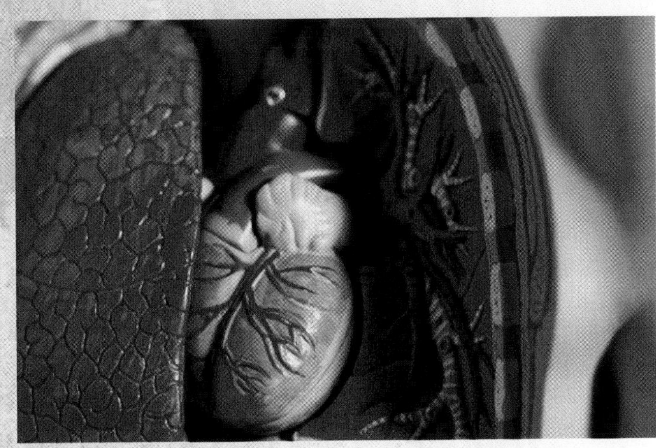

Chapter Objectives

- List important functions of the cardiovascular system
- Describe the interactions among cardiac output, total peripheral resistance, and arterial blood pressure
- Discuss the role of the venous system as an active blood reservoir
- Describe the auscultatory method to measure blood pressure, and quantify the typical response for systolic and diastolic blood pressures during rest and moderate-intensity aerobic exercise
- Discuss the blood pressure response during (1) resistance exercise, (2) upper-body exercise, and (3) exercise in the inverted position
- Define the "hypotensive response" in recovery from exercise, and give possible explanations for its occurrence
- Diagram the major vessels of the coronary circulation
- Describe the pattern of myocardial blood flow, oxygen consumption, and substrate use during rest and various levels of physical activity
- Explain the rate-pressure product and the rationale for its use in clinical exercise physiology.

The **cardiovascular system** integrates the body as a unit. It provides the active muscles with a continuous stream of nutrients and oxygen to sustain a high level of energy transfer. The circulation also removes byproducts of metabolism from the site of energy release.

Chapters 15, 16, and 17 explore the dynamics of circulation, particularly its role in oxygen delivery during exercise. Oxygen transport and delivery during exercise, coupled with the active muscles' capacity to generate adenosine triphosphate (ATP) aerobically, sets the maximum level for aerobic energy transfer.

CARDIOVASCULAR SYSTEM COMPONENTS

The cardiovascular system consists of a continuous linkage of a pump, a high-pressure distribution circuit, exchange vessels, and a low-pressure collection and return circuit. If stretched out in a line, the 100,000 miles of blood vessels of an average-sized adult would encircle the earth four times. Figure 15.1 presents a schematic view of the cardiovascular system, including the major arteries. The tabular inset shows the distribution of blood in absolute and percentage terms. Note that small arteries, veins, and capillaries of the systemic circulation contain approximately 75% of the total blood volume, whereas heart muscle contains only 7%.

The Heart

The heart provides the impetus for blood flow. Situated in the midcenter of the chest cavity, about two thirds of its mass lies to the left of the body's midline. Although this four-chambered muscular organ weighs less than 0.5 kg, it beats so steadily and powerfully that the force generated during its approximately 40 million beats per year could lift its owner 100 miles above the earth. At rest, the heart's output of blood averages 1400 gallons daily, or 38.3 million gallons over a 75-year lifetime. Even for a person of average physical fitness, the maximum output of blood from this remarkable organ in 1 minute exceeds the fluid output from a household faucet turned wide open.

Figure 15.2 summarizes general functional and structural characteristics and mode of activation of the body's three types of muscle—skeletal, cardiac, and smooth. The heart muscle, or **myocardium**, represents a form of striated muscle similar to skeletal muscle. However, the multinucleated, individual cells (fibers) interconnect in latticework fashion. Consequently, the stimulation or depolarization of one cell spreads the action potential through the myocardium to all cells to make the heart function as a unit.

Figure 15.3 shows the structural details of the heart as a pump. Functionally, one can view the heart as two separate pumps. The hollow chambers on the right side of the heart (right heart) perform two crucial functions:

1. Receive blood returning from throughout the body.
2. Pump blood to the lungs for aeration through the **pulmonary circulation**.

The left side of the heart (left heart) also performs two crucial functions:

1. Receive oxygenated blood from the lungs.
2. Pump blood into the thick-walled, muscular aorta for distribution throughout the body in the **systemic circulation**.

A thick, solid muscular wall, or interventricular septum, separates the heart's left and right sides. The **atrioventricular valves** situated within the heart provide a one-way flow of blood from the right atrium to the right ventricle via the **tricuspid valve** and from the left atrium to the left ventricle through the **mitral** or **bicuspid valve**. The **semilunar valves**, located in the arterial wall just outside the heart, prevent blood from flowing back into the heart between contractions. The relatively thin-walled, saclike atrial chambers serve as primer or "booster" pumps to receive and store blood during ventricular contraction. Approximately 70% of the blood returning to the atria flows directly into the ventricles before the atria contract. The simultaneous contraction of both atria then forces the remaining blood into their respective ventricles directly below. Almost immediately after atrial contraction, the ventricles contract and propel blood into the arterial system.

As ventricular pressure builds, the atrioventricular valves snap closed. All heart valves remain closed for 0.02 to 0.06 seconds. This brief interval of rising ventricular tension, during which heart volume and muscle fiber length remain unchanged, represents the heart's **isovolumetric contraction period**. When ventricular pressure exceeds arterial pressure, blood ejects from the heart. The spiral and circular arrangement of bands of cardiac muscle literally "wrings out" blood from the ventricles with each contraction.

The Arterial System

The arteries compose the high-pressure tubing that propels oxygen-rich blood to the tissues. Figure 15.4 illustrates that arteries consist of layers of connective tissue and smooth muscle. No gaseous exchange takes place between arterial blood and the surrounding tissues because of the thickness of these vessels. Blood pumped from the left ventricle into the highly muscular yet elastic **aorta** distributes throughout the body via a network of arteries and smaller arterial branches called **arterioles**. The walls of arterioles contain circular layers of smooth muscle that either constrict or relax to regulate blood flow to the periphery. These "resistance vessels" dramatically alter their internal diameter to rapidly regulate blood flow through the vascular circuit. This redistribution function takes on added importance during exercise, because blood diverts to active muscles from areas that temporarily compromise their blood supply. The inset table of Figure 15.4 lists average values for the diameter of the various blood vessels and corresponding velocities of blood flowing through them.

INTEGRATIVE QUESTION

What advantage does a "closed" circulatory system provide to the physically active individual?

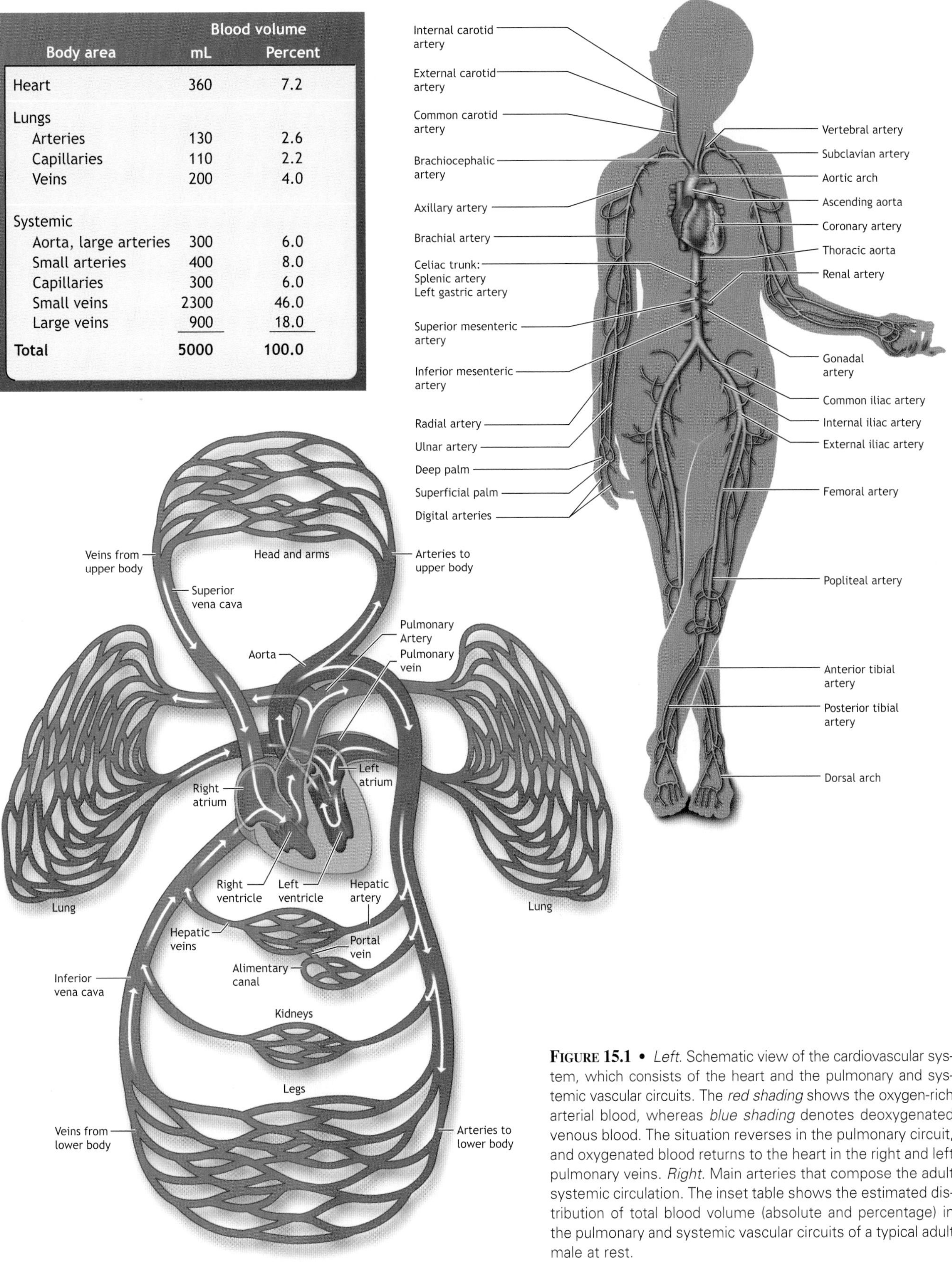

Body area	Blood volume mL	Blood volume Percent
Heart	360	7.2
Lungs		
Arteries	130	2.6
Capillaries	110	2.2
Veins	200	4.0
Systemic		
Aorta, large arteries	300	6.0
Small arteries	400	8.0
Capillaries	300	6.0
Small veins	2300	46.0
Large veins	900	18.0
Total	**5000**	**100.0**

FIGURE 15.1 • *Left.* Schematic view of the cardiovascular system, which consists of the heart and the pulmonary and systemic vascular circuits. The *red shading* shows the oxygen-rich arterial blood, whereas *blue shading* denotes deoxygenated venous blood. The situation reverses in the pulmonary circuit, and oxygenated blood returns to the heart in the right and left pulmonary veins. *Right.* Main arteries that compose the adult systemic circulation. The inset table shows the estimated distribution of total blood volume (absolute and percentage) in the pulmonary and systemic vascular circuits of a typical adult male at rest.

Muscle type	Location	Appearance	Type of activity	Stimulation
Skeletal ("striated" or "voluntary") muscle 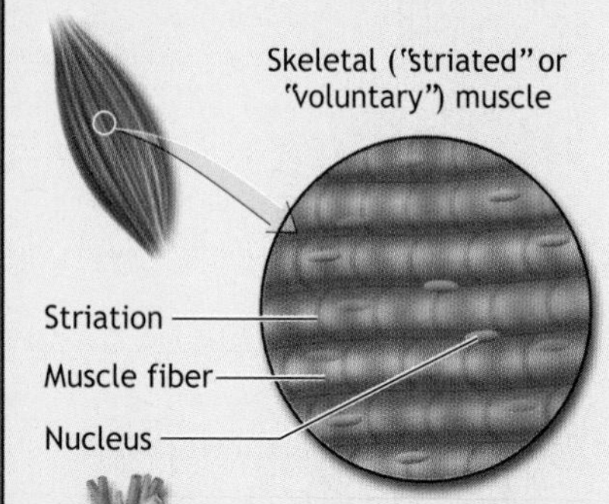 Striation Muscle fiber Nucleus	Named muscle (e.g., the biceps of the arm) attached to the skeleton and fascia of limbs, body wall, and head/neck	Large, long, unbranched, cylindrical fibers with transverse striations (stripes) arranged in parallel bundles; multiple, peripherally located nuclei	Strong, quick intermittent (phasic) contraction above a baseline tonus; acts primarily to produce movement or resist gravity	Voluntary (or reflexive) by the somatic nervous system
Cardiac muscle 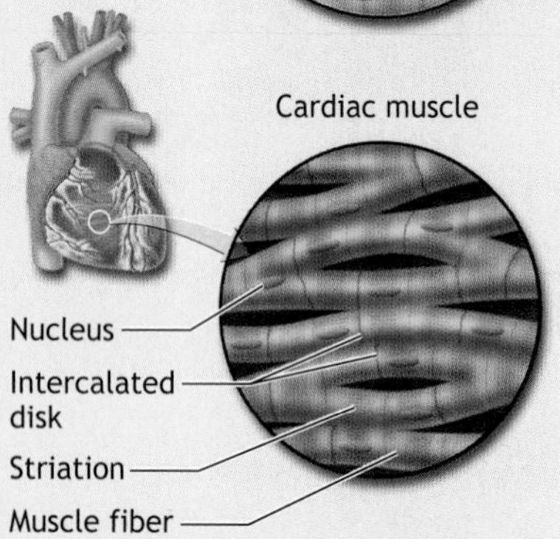 Nucleus Intercalated disk Striation Muscle fiber	Muscle of heart (myocardium) and adjacent portions of the great vessels (aorta, vena cava)	Branching and anastomosing shorter fibers with transverse striations (stripes) running parallel and connected end-to-end by complex junctions (intercalated disks); single, central nucleus	Strong, quick continuous rhythmic contraction; pumps blood from the heart	Involuntary; intrinsically (myogenically) stimulated and propagated; rate and strength of contraction modified by the autonomic nervous system
Smooth ("unstriated" or "involuntary") muscle 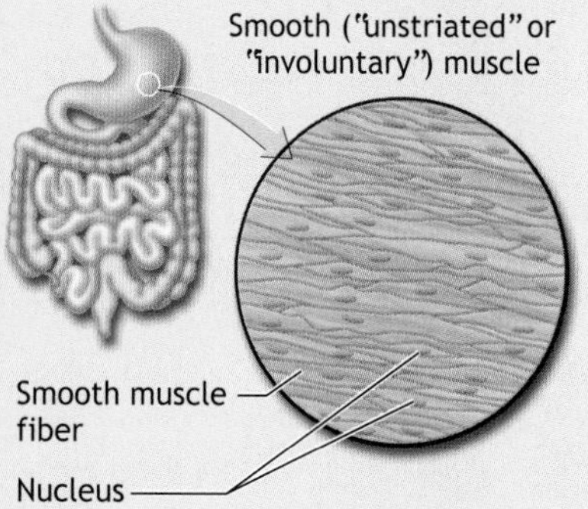 Smooth muscle fiber Nucleus	Walls of hollow viscera and blood vessels, iris, and ciliary body of eye; attached to hair follicles of skin (arrector muscle of hair)	Single or agglomerated small, spindle-shaped fibers without striations; single, central nucleus	Weak, slow, rhythmic, or sustained tonic contraction; acts mainly to propel substances (peristalsis) and to restrict flow (vasoconstriction and sphincteric activity)	Involuntary by autonomic nervous system

FIGURE 15.2 • Functional and structural characteristics and mode of activation of skeletal, cardiac, and smooth muscle. (From Moore KL, Dalley AF. Clinically oriented anatomy. 4th ed. Baltimore: Lippincott Williams & Wilkins, 1999.)

Blood Pressure

Each contraction of the left ventricle forces a surge of blood through the aorta. Peripheral vessels do not permit blood to "run off" into the arterial system as rapidly as it ejects from the heart, allowing the distensible aorta to "store" a portion of the blood. This creates pressure within the entire arterial system, causing a pressure wave to travel down the aorta to the remote branches of the arterial tree. The characteristic "pulse" in superficial arteries occurs from the stretch and subsequent recoil of the arterial wall during a cardiac cycle. Identical values exist for pulse rate and heart rate in healthy individuals. *In essence, arterial blood pressure reflects the combined effects of arterial blood flow per minute (i.e., cardiac output) and the resistance to that flow offered by the peripheral vasculature.* The following equation expresses this relationship:

$$\text{Blood pressure} = \text{Cardiac output} \times \text{Total peripheral resistance}$$

SYSTOLIC BLOOD PRESSURE. At rest in normotensive individuals, the highest pressure generated by the heart averages 120 mm Hg during left ventricular contraction (**systole**). The brachial artery at the level of the right atrium usually provides the point of reference for this measurement. **Systolic blood pressure** provides an estimate of the work of the heart and the force that blood exerts against the arterial walls during ventricular systole. During the heart's relaxation phase when the aortic valves close, the natural elastic recoil of the arterial system provides a continuous head of pressure. This maintains a steady flow of blood into the periphery until the next surge of blood.

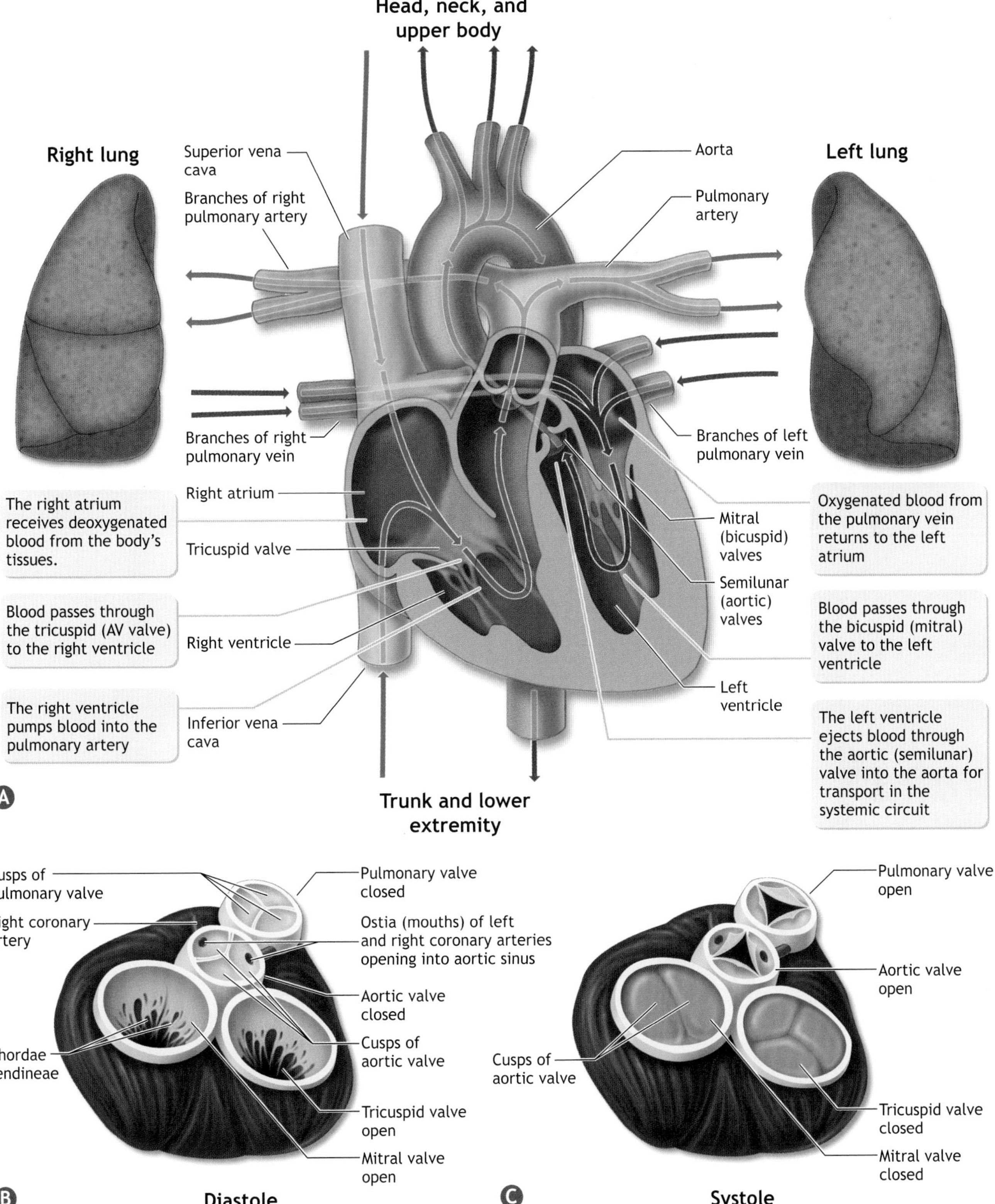

FIGURE 15.3 • **A**. The heart, its great vessels, and the action of its valves. The valves provide for the one-way flow of blood as indicated by the *arrows*. **B**. In diastole, the aortic and pulmonary valves snap close; shortly thereafter, the mitral and tricuspid valves open and blood flows into the ventricular cavities. **C**. With the initiation of systole and ventricular emptying, the tricuspid and mitral valves close and the aortic and pulmonary valves open.

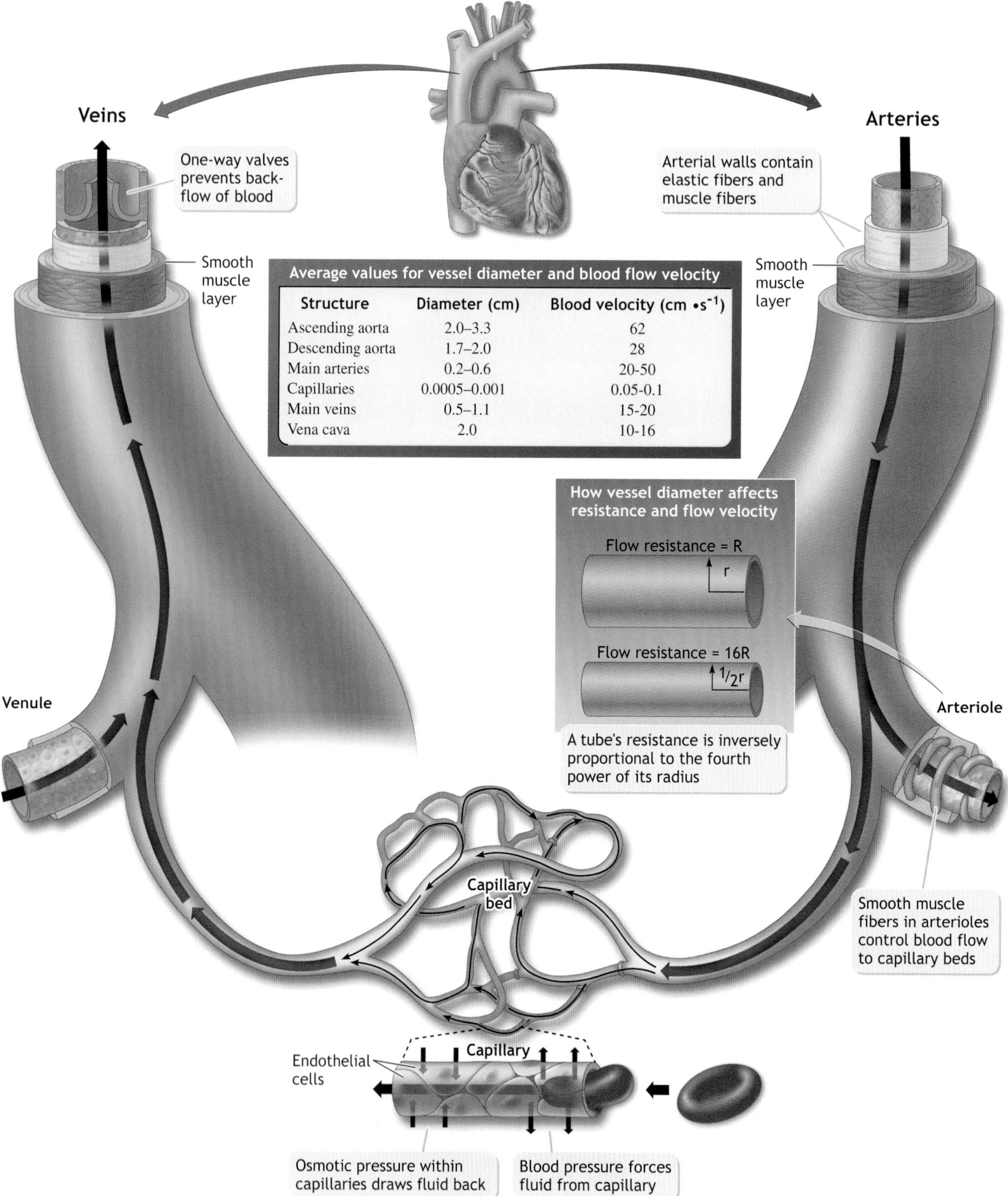

Average values for vessel diameter and blood flow velocity

Structure	Diameter (cm)	Blood velocity (cm $\cdot s^{-1}$)
Ascending aorta	2.0–3.3	62
Descending aorta	1.7–2.0	28
Main arteries	0.2–0.6	20-50
Capillaries	0.0005–0.001	0.05-0.1
Main veins	0.5–1.1	15-20
Vena cava	2.0	10-16

FIGURE 15.4 • The structure of the walls of the various blood vessels. A single layer of endothelial cells lines each vessel. Fibrous tissue, wrapped in several layers of smooth muscle surrounds the arterial walls. A single layer of muscle cells sheathes the arterioles; capillaries consist of only one layer of endothelial cells. In the venule, fibrous tissue encases the endothelial cells; veins also possess a layer of smooth muscle. The *inset table* displays the average values for vessel diameter and corresponding values for blood flow velocity. A vessel's resistance to flow depends on its diameter. Decreasing vessel diameter by one-half increases resistance 16-fold.

DIASTOLIC BLOOD PRESSURE. During the relaxation phase of the cardiac cycle (**diastole**), arterial blood pressure typically decreases to 70 or 80 mm Hg. **Diastolic blood pressure** indicates **peripheral resistance**, or the ease that blood flows from the arterioles into the capillaries. With high peripheral resistance, the pressure within the arteries after systole does not rapidly dissipate. Instead, it remains elevated for a larger portion of the cardiac cycle. "In a Practical Sense" illustrates the measurement of systolic and diastolic blood pressure by the **auscultation method**.

IN A PRACTICAL SENSE

Blood Pressure Measurement, Classifications, and Recommended Follow-Up

Blood pressure represents the force (pressure) exerted by blood against the arterial walls during a cardiac cycle. Systolic blood pressure, the higher of the two pressure measurements, occurs during ventricular contraction (systole) as the heart propels 70 to 100 mL of blood into the aorta. After systole, the ventricles relax (diastole), the arteries recoil, and arterial pressure continually declines as blood flows into the periphery and the heart refills with blood. The lowest pressure reached during ventricular relaxation represents diastolic blood pressure. Normal systolic blood pressure in an adult varies between 110 and 140 mm Hg, and diastolic pressure varies between 60 and 90 mm Hg. Elevated systolic or diastolic blood pressure (termed hypertension) is defined as a resting systolic blood pressure greater than 140 mm Hg and diastolic pressure exceeding 90 mm Hg. Pulse pressure refers to the difference between systolic and diastolic pressures.

CLASSIFICATION AND RECOMMENDED FOLLOW-UP OF INITIAL SCREENING BLOOD PRESSURE IN ADULTS[a]

SYSTOLIC (MM HG)	DIASTOLIC (MM HG)	CATEGORY	FOLLOW-UP
<120	<80	Optimal	—
<130	<85	Normal	Recheck in 2 y
130–139	85–89	High-normal	Recheck in 1 y
140–159	90–99	Stage 1 hypertension	Confirm within 2 months
160–179	100–109	Moderate (Stage 2) hypertension	Begin treatment within 1month if blood pressure is consistently high
180–209	110–119	Severe (Stage 3) hypertension	Begin treatment within 1 week
>210	120	Very severe (Stage 4) hypertension	Treat immediately

[a] Not taking antihypertensive drugs and not acutely ill. When systolic and diastolic blood pressure categories vary, the higher reading determines the blood pressure classification. For example, a reading of 152/82 mm Hg is classified as Stage 1 hypertension.
From National Institutes of Health. The sixth report of the Joint National Committee on Detection, Evaluation, and Treatment of High Blood Pressure. NIH Pub. no. 98-4080, 1997.

Measurement Procedures

Blood pressure, measured indirectly by auscultation (listening to sounds; described in 1902 by Russian physician N.S. Korotkoff; 1874–1920), uses a stethoscope and sphygmomanometer, consisting of a blood pressure cuff and an aneroid or mercury column pressure gauge.

1. Subject, seated in a quiet room, exposes upper arm.
2. Locate the brachial artery at the inner side of the upper arm, approximately 1 inch above the bend in the elbow.

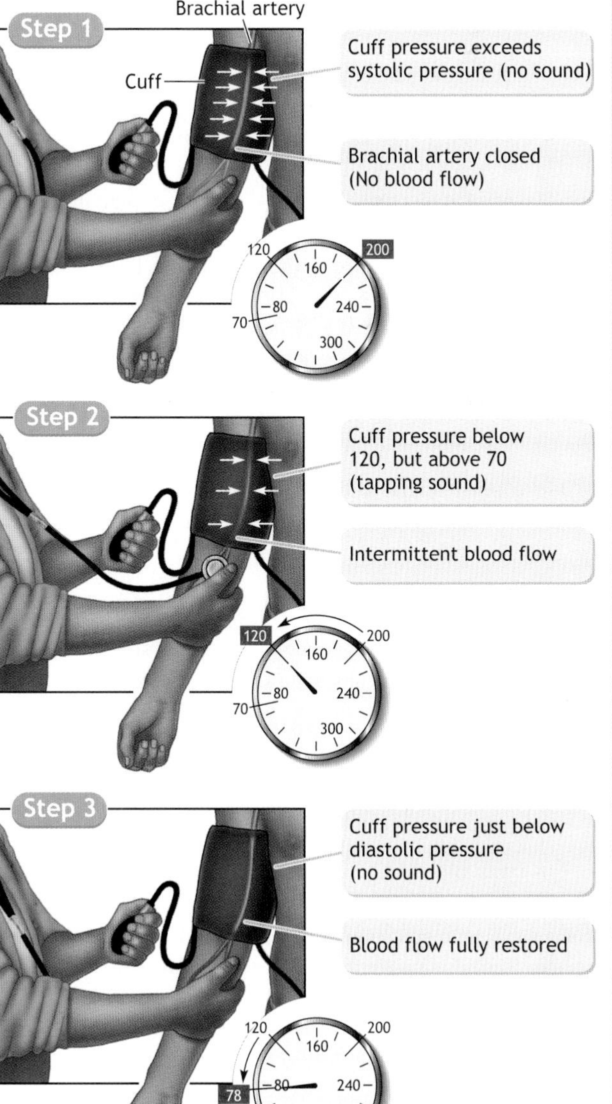

IN A PRACTICAL SENSE

➤➤ BLOOD PRESSURE MEASUREMENT, CLASSIFICATIONS, AND RECOMMENDED FOLLOW-UP, CONT'D

3. Take the free end of the cuff and gently slide it through the metal loop (or wrap over exposed Velcro), and flap it back over so the cuff wraps around the upper arm at heart level. Align the arrows on the cuff with the brachial artery. Secure the Velcro parts of the cuff. The sphygmomanometer cuff should fit snugly (but not tightly) to obtain accurate readings. Use appropriate-sized cuffs for children and the obese.
4. Place the stethoscope bell below the antecubital space over the brachial artery.
5. The cuff should now have the connecting tube (from the sphygmomanometer bulb and gauge) exiting the cuff toward the arm.
6. Before inflating the cuff, make sure the air-release switch remains closed (turn the knob clockwise).
7. Inflate the cuff with quick, even pumps to 180 to 200 mm Hg.
8. Gradually release cuff pressure (about 3–5 mm per s) by slowly opening the air-release knob (counterclockwise turn), noting the first sound. This sound results from turbulence from the rush of blood as the formerly closed artery briefly opens during the highest pressure in the cardiac cycle. This represents systolic blood pressure.
9. Continue to reduce pressure, noting when the sound becomes muffled *(4th phase diastolic pressure)* and when the sound disappears *(5th phase diastolic pressure).* Clinicians usually record the 5th phase as diastolic blood pressure.
10. If the measured pressure exceeds 140/90 mm Hg, allow a 10-minute rest and repeat the procedure.

MEAN ARTERIAL PRESSURE. Systolic blood pressure typically averages 120 mm Hg, and the diastolic pressure equals 80 mm Hg in young, healthy adults at rest. The average or **mean arterial pressure (MAP)** is slightly lower than simply the arithmetic average of the systolic and diastolic pressures, because the heart remains in diastole longer than in systole. MAP averages 93 mm Hg at rest; this represents the average force exerted by the blood against the arterial walls during the entire cardiac cycle. The following formula estimates MAP:

$$\text{MAP} = \text{Diastolic BP} + [0.333\ (\text{Systolic} - \text{Diastolic BP})]$$

For a person with a diastolic blood pressure of 89 mm Hg and a systolic pressure of 127 mm Hg, MAP equals 89 + [0.333 (127 − 89)] or 102 mm Hg.

CARDIAC OUTPUT AND TOTAL PERIPHERAL RESISTANCE. The hemodynamic equation that relates blood pressure to cardiac output and total peripheral resistance rearranges as follows to illustrate factors that determine either cardiac output or total peripheral resistance:

$$\text{Cardiac output} = \text{MAP} \div \text{Total peripheral resistance}$$
$$\text{Total peripheral resistance} = \text{MAP} \div \text{Cardiac output}$$

For example, MAP (computed from systolic and diastolic blood pressures) and cardiac output estimate the change in total resistance to blood flow in the transition from rest to exercise. Suppose systolic blood pressure at rest equals 120 mm Hg, diastolic pressure equals 80 mm Hg (MAP = 93.3 mm Hg), and cardiac output averages 5.0 $L \cdot min^{-1}$. Substituting these values in the formula for total peripheral resistance yields 18.7 mm Hg per liter of blood flow (93.3 mm Hg ÷ 5.0 $L \cdot min^{-1}$). During strenuous exercise, when systolic pressure increases considerably more than diastolic pressure, and cardiac output increases six or seven times the resting value in an elite endurance athlete, resistance to peripheral blood flow *decreases* dramatically. For example, if exercise cardiac output equals 35.0 $L \cdot min^{-1}$ and MAP equals 130 mm Hg (systolic = 210 mm Hg; diastolic = 90 mm Hg), then resistance to blood flow in the systemic circulation would average 3.71 mm Hg per liter per minute, or five times *less* than the resting value.

Capillaries

The arterioles continue to branch and form smaller and less muscular vessels called **metarterioles**. These vessels end in a network of microscopic blood vessels approximately 0.01 mm in diameter called **capillaries**, which generally contain 6% of the total blood volume. The average capillary diameter is 7 to 10 μm (approximately $^1/_{100}$th of a millimeter). Figure 15.4 shows that the capillary wall usually consists of a single layer of endothelial cells. Some capillaries are so narrow that only one blood cell at a time can squeeze through. In many instances, the extensive proliferation of capillaries actually causes their walls to abut the membranes of the surrounding cells. Capillary density of human skeletal muscle averages between 2000 and 3000 capillaries per square millimeter of tissue. Greater capillary density exists in heart muscle, where no cell lies farther than 0.008 mm from its nearest capillary.

Blood Flow in Capillaries

The **precapillary sphincter**, a ring of smooth muscle that encircles the vessel at its origin, controls capillary diameter. Constriction and relaxation of this sphincter provides an extremely important local means for blood flow regulation

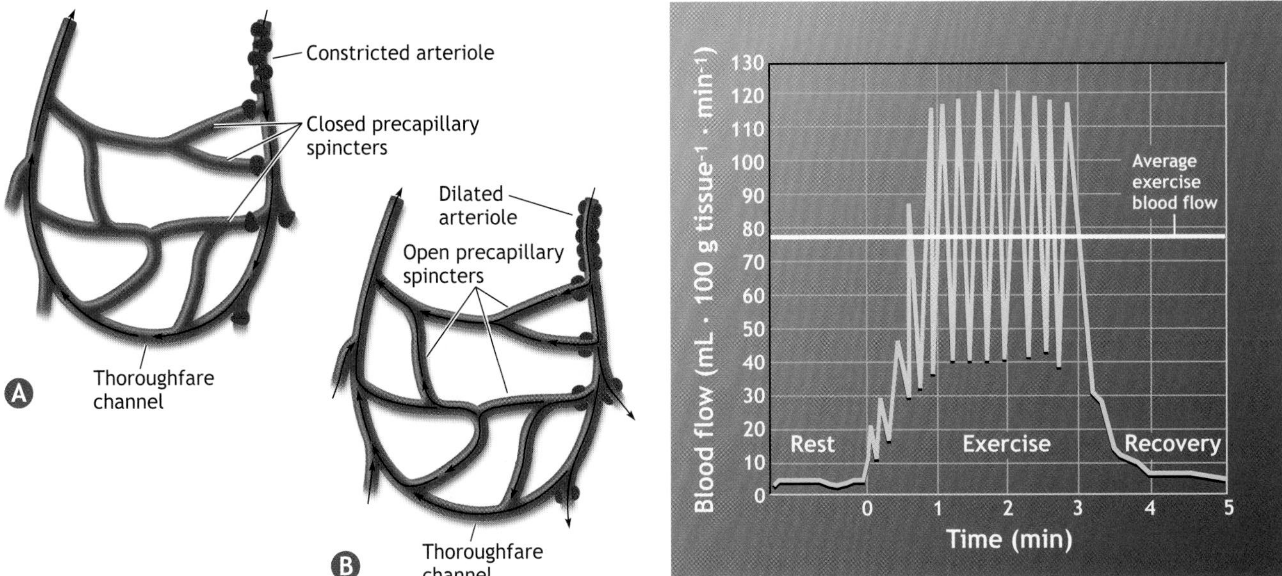

FIGURE 15.5 • Capillary blood flow during rest (**A**) and exercise (**B**). Capillary diameter, red blood cell size, and blood viscosity all affect capillary blood flow. The *right figure* shows the pulsatile pattern of blood flow at rest, during exercise, and when exercise stops. Dilation of the active muscle's arterioles provides the major mechanism for augmenting local blood flow.

within a specific tissue to meet metabolic requirements. Chapter 16 discusses specific factors for autoregulation of local blood supply.

Figure 15.5 depicts a generalized view of the dynamics of capillary blood flow within muscle during rest and exercise. Fewer capillaries function at rest than are actually available. In this example for the gastrocnemius muscle, blood flow each minute at rest averages 5 mL for every 100 g of muscle tissue. Thus, if the muscle weighs 600 g, then approximately 30 mL of blood flows through it each minute. During exercise, blood flow increases rapidly as previously "unused" capillaries open. Two factors trigger the relaxation of precapillary sphincters: (1) the driving force of increased local blood pressure plus intrinsic neural control and (2) local metabolites produced in exercise. During strenuous exercise, a sustained local blood flow increases 15 to 20 times the resting value. For the gastrocnemius muscle, it averages about 80 mL per 100 g of tissue each minute.

Branching of the capillary microcirculation increases its cross-sectional area to about 800 times the 1-inch-diameter aorta. Because blood flow velocity relates inversely to the vasculature's cross section (Velocity [$cm \cdot s^{-1}$] = Volume of flow [$cm^3 \cdot s^{-1}$] ÷ Cross-sectional area [cm^2]), velocity progressively decreases as blood moves toward and enters the capillaries. As a result, it takes approximately 1.5 seconds for a blood cell to pass through an average-sized capillary. The total surface area of the capillary walls exceeds the external body surface of the average adult by 100 times. An extremely effective means for exchange between the blood and the tissues derives from a huge surface area combined with a slow rate of blood flow (approximately 0.5 to 1.0 $mm \cdot sec^{-1}$ at rest).

The Venous System

The continuity of the vascular system progresses as the capillaries feed deoxygenated blood at almost a trickle into the small veins (**venules**) with which they merge. Blood flow velocity then increases somewhat because the cross-sectional area of the venous system is smaller than that of the capillaries. The smaller veins in the lower portion of the body eventually empty into the body's largest vein, the **inferior vena cava** (Fig. 15.6). This large vessel returns blood to the right atrium from the abdomen, pelvis, and lower extremities. Venous blood from tributary vessels in the head, neck, shoulder regions, thorax, and part of the abdominal wall flows into the 7-cm–long **superior vena cava** and joins the inferior vena cava at heart level. This mixture of blood draining the upper and lower body, called **mixed-venous blood**, then enters the right atrium. From there it descends into the right ventricle for pumping through the pulmonary artery to the lungs. Gas exchange takes place in the alveolar–capillary network of the lungs; oxygenated blood then returns in the pulmonary veins to the left side of the heart to begin again its passage throughout the body.

Figure 15.7 illustrates that blood pressure and blood flow vary considerably in the systemic circulation. In the aorta and large arteries, blood pressure fluctuates between 120 and 80 mm Hg during the cardiac cycle. The pressure then falls in direct proportion to the resistance encountered in the vascular circuit. For example, blood at the arteriole end of the capillaries exerts an average pressure of only 30 mm Hg. As blood enters the venules, it loses nearly all its impetus for forward movement. The pressure falls to approximately 0 mm Hg by the time blood reaches the right atrium. Because the venous

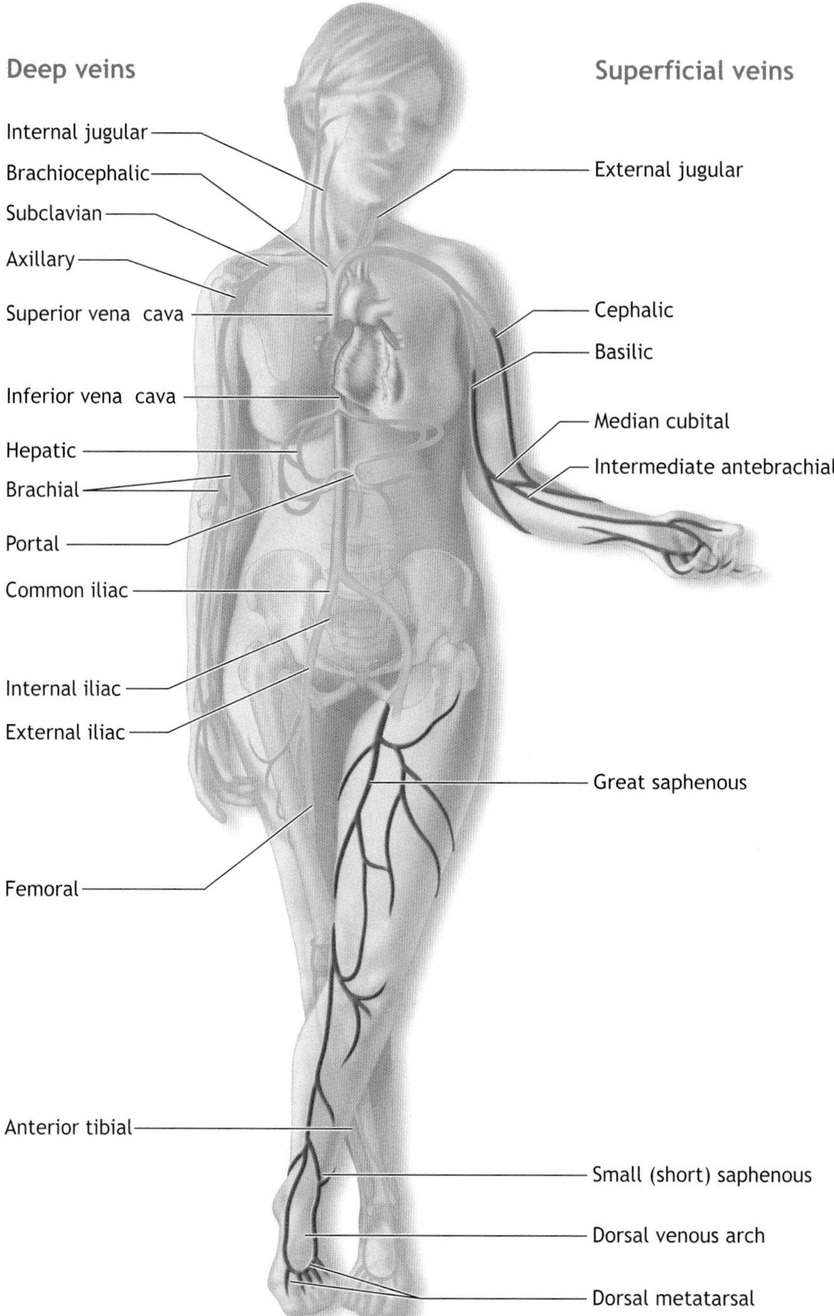

FIGURE 15.6 • Distribution of the superficial (dark blue) and deep (light blue) veins.

system operates under relatively low pressure, the veins possess much thinner and less muscular walls than the thicker-walled and less distensible arteries (see Fig. 15.4).

Venous Return

The low pressure of blood in the venous system poses a special problem that a unique characteristic of veins partly solves. Figure 15.8 shows that thin, membranous, flaplike **valves** spaced at short intervals within the vein permit blood to flow one way toward the heart. Owing to the low pressure in the venous circuit, the smallest muscular contractions or even minor pressure changes within the thoracic cavity with breathing readily compress the veins.[19] The alternate compression and relaxation of the veins and the one-way action of their valves provide a "milking" action similar to heart action. Compressing the veins imparts considerable energy for blood flow, whereas "diastole" of these vessels lets them refill as blood flows to the heart. Without valves, blood would pool as it sometimes does in veins of the extremities. People would faint every time they stood up because of reduced venous return and cerebral blood flow.

An Active Vasculature?

Physiologists have debated the role of the venous system as an active vasculature for mobilizing blood volume. For example, the systemic venous vessels normally contain 65% of the total

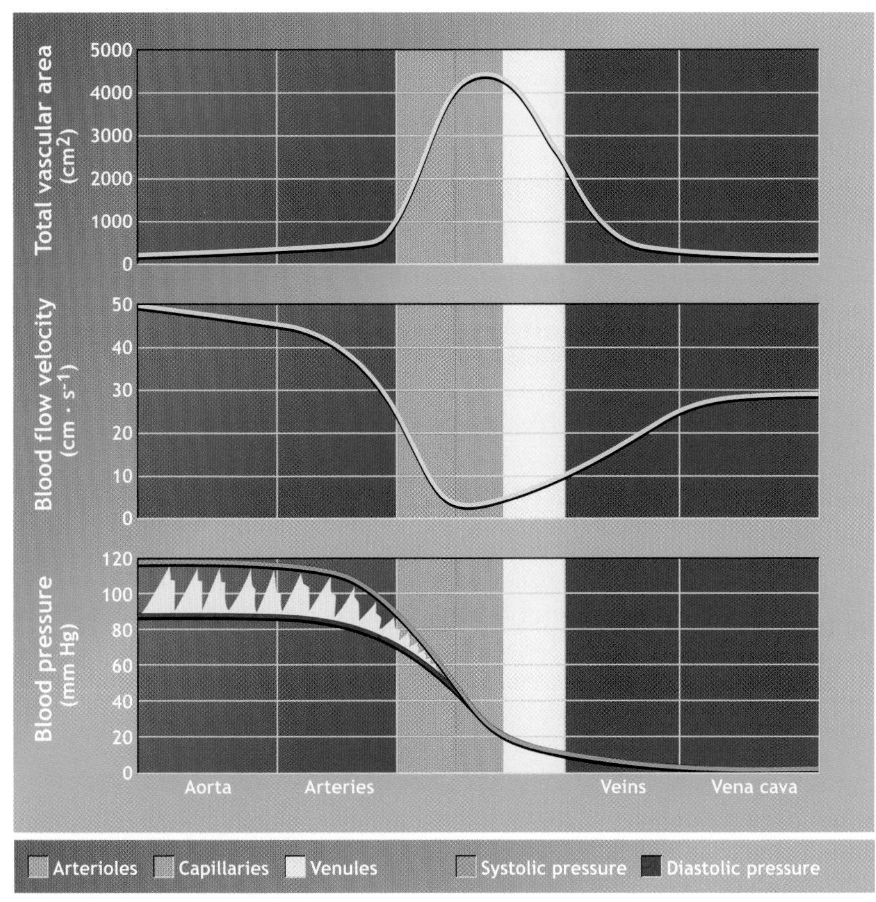

FIGURE 15.7 • Blood flow and blood pressure in the systemic circulation. Note that blood pressure within each portion of the arterial system inversely relates to the total area (resistance) in that section of the vascular tree.

blood volume at rest; therefore, the veins represent **capacitance vessels** that serve as blood reservoirs. This has caused some physiologists to speculate on the role of the veins as an active blood reservoir to either retard or facilitate delivery of blood to the systemic circulation. They maintain that any increase in tension or tone of the vessels' smooth muscle layer alters the diameter of the venous tree. This initiates rapid redistribution of blood from peripheral veins toward the central blood volume returning to the heart. Physiologists who have the opposing position point out that only the veins in the splanchnic and cutaneous regions are innervated richly enough to contribute to blood mobilization. In fact, skeletal muscle veins do not receive neural input, and whatever brief venoconstriction occurs in other regions does little to contribute to blood redistribution. Current opinion maintains that the major contribution to blood mobilization in exercise occurs by the action of active muscle pump and the passive effect of arterial vasoconstriction (not visceral venoconstriction), which reduces downstream venous pressure. As much as 80% of the blood volume mobilized from all veins results from the passive effect of vasoconstriction and not active venoconstriction.[44]

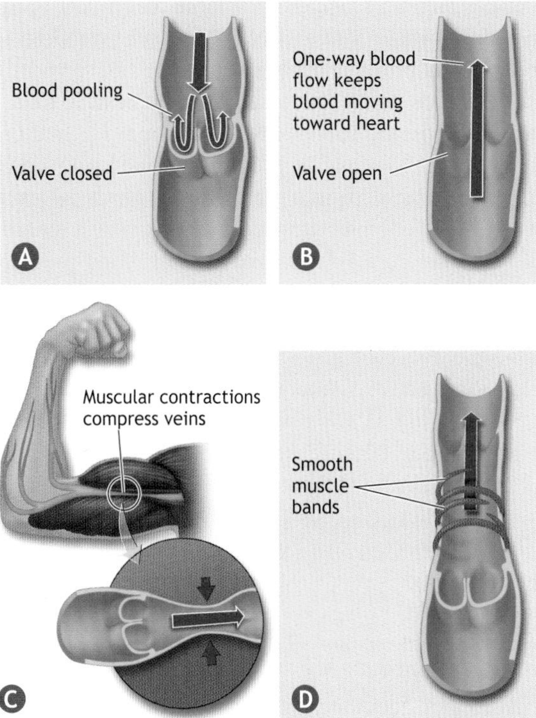

FIGURE 15.8 • The valves in veins (**A**) prevent the back flow of blood but (**B**) do not hinder the normal one-way flow of blood. Blood moves through veins by the action of nearby active muscle (**C**) or by the contraction of smooth muscle bands within the veins themselves (**D**).

Varicose Veins

Sometimes the valves within a vein become defective and fail to maintain their one-way blood flow, a condition termed **varicose veins**. This valvular deformity usually occurs in the surface veins of the lower extremities, owing to the force of gravity that retards blood flow in the upright posture.[8] The surface veins have little external support from surrounding tissues. Consequently, blood gathers in them and they become excessively distended and painful, impairing circulation from the affected area. In severe cases, the venous wall becomes inflamed and progressively deteriorates—a condition called **phlebitis**. This necessitates vessel removal either surgically or nonsurgically by use of injected solutions that irritate the vessel's surface membranes, causing a portion of the vein to collapse, fuse, and eventually shrivel up. Blood then reroutes to the deeper veins.

Individuals with varicose veins should avoid straining-type exercises that often accompany resistance training. During sustained, nonrhythmic muscle actions, the muscle and ventilatory "pumps" contribute little to venous return. Increased intrathoracic and abdominal pressures with straining (Valsalva maneuver) also impede venous return. These factors act to pool blood in the veins of the lower body, which can aggravate an existing varicose-vein condition. Exercise training does not prevent varicose veins, but regular and rhythmic physical activity may minimize complications because repeated muscle actions continually propel blood toward the heart.[45]

Venous Pooling

The rhythmic action of muscular activity and consequent compression of the vascular tree (i.e., the **muscle pump**) contribute so much to venous return that many people faint when forced to maintain an upright posture without movement. The classic "tilt table" experiment demonstrates this point. A subject lies supine, strapped on a table that pivots to different positions. Heart rate and blood pressure stabilize if the person remains horizontal. When the table tilts vertically, an uninterrupted column of blood exists from heart to toes. This creates a hydrostatic force of 80 to 100 mm Hg that causes blood to pool in the lower extremities. Fluid backs up in the capillary bed and seeps into the surrounding tissues, causing them to swell (**edema**). Reduced venous return simultaneously reduces cardiac output and arterial blood pressure; at the same time, heart rate accelerates and blood is mobilized from the splanchnic region by upstream vasoconstriction (causing passive mobilization from downstream veins) and perhaps some active venoconstriction to counter the effects of venous pooling. Forcing the person to maintain the upright position induces fainting because of insufficient cerebral blood supply. Tilting the person either horizontally or head down immediately restores circulation and consciousness.

The pressurized suits worn by test pilots and special support stockings for individuals with varicose veins reduce hydrostatic shifts of blood to the veins of the lower extremities in the upright position. A swimming pool provides a similar supportive effect in upright exercise because the water's external support facilitates venous return.

THE ACTIVE "COOL DOWN." The preceding discussion of venous pooling provides a sound rationale for continuing to walk or jog at a slow pace after strenuous exercise. Moderate exercise in recovery, popularly known as "**cooling down**," facilitates blood flow through the vascular circuit, including myocardial vessels. In Chapter 7, we discussed how active recovery removes lactate from the blood. Continuation of mild exercise in recovery also may blunt potential deleterious effects on cardiac function from elevated levels of catecholamines (epinephrine and norepinephrine) released during exercise.[7,9]

INTEGRATIVE QUESTION

The Romans executed criminals by tying their arms and legs to a cross mounted in the vertical position. Discuss the physiologic responses that would cause death under these circumstances.

HYPERTENSION

Systolic pressure at rest can exceed 300 mm Hg in individuals whose arteries (1) have become "hardened" with fatty materials deposited within their walls or because the vessel's connective tissue layer has thickened or (2) offer excessive resistance to peripheral blood flow because of neural hyperactivity

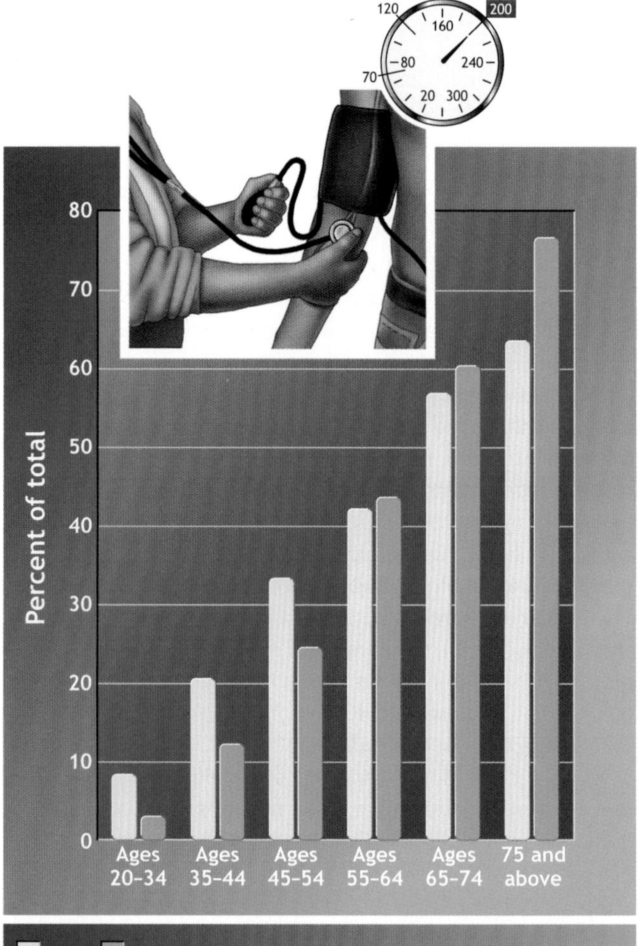

FIGURE 15.9 • Prevalence of hypertension in the United States. Figures based on studies from 1988 to 1994. (Data from National Center for Health Statistics and the American Heart Association.)

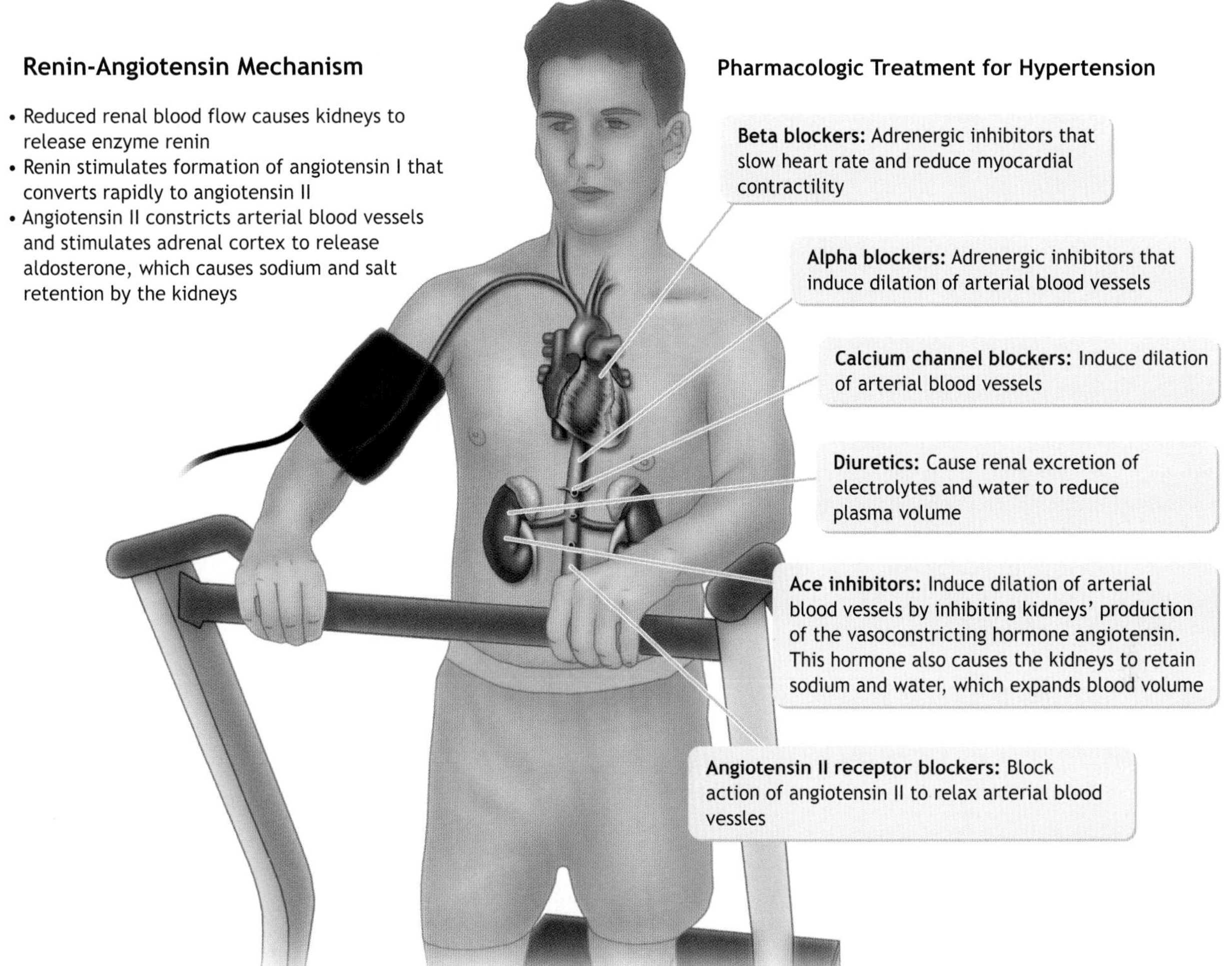

FIGURE 15.10 • Recommended pharmacologic therapies for the treatment of hypertension following an initial 6 to 12 months of treatment with diet, weight loss, reduced alcohol intake, and regular exercise. Also illustrated is the renin–angiotensin mechanism that when chronically overactive causes certain forms of high blood pressure.

or kidney malfunction. Diastolic pressure can also exceed 100 mm Hg under these conditions. Abnormally high blood pressure, termed **hypertension**, imposes chronic strain on the cardiovascular system. The cause of 95% of reported hypertension remains unknown. Untreated, chronic hypertension damages arterial vessels and leads to arteriosclerosis, heart disease, stroke, and kidney failure. Figure 15.9 shows the percentages of the United States population with hypertension (systolic pressure >140 mm Hg; diastolic pressure >90 mm Hg) and its increased prevalence with age. Recent evidence indicates that an elevated systolic blood pressure is a more reliable and accurate predictor of the risk associated with hypertension (and need for treatment) than diastolic blood pressure, particularly in middle age.[30]

A Prevalent Disorder

One out of every three to four persons experiences chronic, high blood pressure some time during his or her life. A high prevalence of hypertension exists among African Americans, who as a group exhibit a two- to threefold higher risk of hypertension and ischemic stroke than Caucasians. Their predisposition for hypertension reflects reduced sensitivity to the vasodilating action of nitric oxide (see Chapter 16, p. 335).[6,47] Presently, about 50 million Americans have systolic pressures that exceed 140 mm Hg or diastolic pressures above 90 mm Hg—values generally considered **borderline for hypertension**. Only two-thirds of hypertensives have knowledge of their disease, only one-half are being treated, and only one-quarter have their blood pressure under control. Each year, an additional 2 million people become hypertensive.[46] An individual on medication for hypertension still classifies as hypertensive, even if blood pressure remains within the normal range. Uncorrected hypertension often leads to congestive heart failure, kidney disease, myocardial infarction, or stroke. Just a 2–mm Hg lowering of systolic blood pressure reduces deaths from stroke by 6% and heart disease by 4%. Figure 15.10 shows recommended pharmacologic therapies for treating hypertension after initial nonpharmacologic approaches. Also illustrated is the renin-angiotensin mechanism. Chapter 20 discusses that prolonged overresponse of this mechanism with a resulting excess aldosterone output causes hypertension.

Effectively Treated

Preventing a chronic rise in blood pressure serves a crucial function because even when elevated blood pressure normalizes (through lifestyle changes or medication), the disease risk remains higher than if the person had never become hypertensive in the first place. Blood pressure should be checked periodically because hypertension progresses unnoticed for years. Effective prevention strategies apply lifestyle changes—regular physical activity, modest weight loss, stress management, smoking cessation, reduced sodium and alcohol consumption, and adequate potassium, calcium, and magnesium intake.[41,50,51] Hypertension treatment also uses lifestyle changes in addition to medications that reduce either extracellular fluid volume or peripheral resistance to blood flow. Prudent diet, weight control, and regular, moderate exercise should precede pharmacologic treatment for **mild hypertension** (140 to 159 mm Hg systolic; 90 to 99 mm Hg diastolic) and **moderate hypertension** (160 to 179 mm Hg systolic; 100 to 109 mm Hg diastolic) because of possible harmful side effects of drug therapy on other coronary artery disease risk factors.[24]

The inset table for "In a Practical Sense" gives classifications and recommended follow-up in initial blood pressure screening for adults. Chapter 32 discusses the role of regular aerobic exercise and resistance exercise to treat moderate hypertension.

BLOOD PRESSURE RESPONSE TO EXERCISE

The blood pressure response to exercise varies with the exercise mode.

Resistance Exercise

Straining exercise, particularly during the concentric (shortening) or static phase of muscle action, mechanically compresses the peripheral arterial vessels that supply active muscles. Vascular compression dramatically increases total peripheral resistance and reduces muscle perfusion. In fact, muscle blood flow decreases in direct proportion to the percentage of the maximum force capacity exerted. Consequently, in an attempt to restore muscle blood flow, sympathetic nervous system activity, cardiac output, and MAP increase substantially.[16,20] The magnitude of the hypertensive response relates directly to the intensity of effort and amount of muscle mass activated.[15,22,36] The acute hemodynamic responses to resistance exercise appear to be similar in healthy young and older adults.[33,34]

Research has focused on comparing blood pressure responses during static and dynamic resistance exercise.[12,32] A study from one of our laboratories measured blood pressure of normotensive subjects directly with a pressure transducer connected to a catheter inserted into the femoral artery.[14] Measurements were made during three forms of exercise: (1) isometric bench press performed at 25, 50, 75, and 100% of the maximal voluntary contraction (MVC); (2) free-weight bench press performed at 25 and 50% of the isometric MVC; and (3) hydraulic resistance bench press exercise performed "all out" for 20 seconds at slow and fast speeds. The results, displayed in Table 15.1, show clearly that the three exercise modes substantially increased blood pressure and the heart's corresponding workload (see "Rate-Pressure Product," page 321). Other studies also show that exercise that activates a large muscle mass and requires relatively great muscle strain elicits rather dramatic blood pressure increases.[12,28,37] As we point out in Chapter 16, this exacerbated pressure response results from the combined effect of (1) greater stimulation of the cardiovascular center by the active areas of the motor cortex and (2) large peripheral feedback to this center from the contracting muscle mass.

The acute cardiovascular strain with heavy resistance exercise could prove harmful to individuals with heart and vascular disease, particularly individuals untrained in this form of exercise. For them, more-rhythmic moderate exercise provides less strain and greater health-related benefits. Figure 15.11 presents generalized responses for blood pressure during rhythmic aerobic exercise and heavy resistance exercises that activate either a relatively small or relatively large muscle mass.

TABLE 15.1 ➤ COMPARISON OF PEAK SYSTOLIC AND DIASTOLIC BLOOD PRESSURE AT VARIOUS PERCENTAGES OF A MAXIMUM VOLUNTARY CONTRACTION (MVC) DURING ISOMETRIC EXERCISE AND FREE-WEIGHT AND HYDRAULIC BENCH PRESS EXERCISE

	Isometric[a] (% MVC)				Free-Weight Bench Press[b] (% MVC)		Hydraulic Bench Press[c]	
Condition	25	50	75	100	25	50	Slow	Fast
Peak systolic, mm Hg	172	179	200	225	169	232	237	245
Peak diastolic, mm Hg	106	116	135	156	104	154	101	160

[a]Open glottis (no Valsalva maneuver); average of two trials; contraction time 2 to 3 seconds; arm position that of bench-press exercise with hands slightly above chest.
[b]The weight lifted was either 25 or 50% of previously determined isometric maximum action.
[c]Performed on Hydra-Fitness chest-press apparatus at dial setting 3 (slow) and 5 (fast) for 20 seconds of repeated maximal actions.
Values are averages for seven subjects. Data from reference 14 and unpublished data, Human Performance Laboratory, Department of Exercise Science, University of Massachusetts, Amherst, MA.

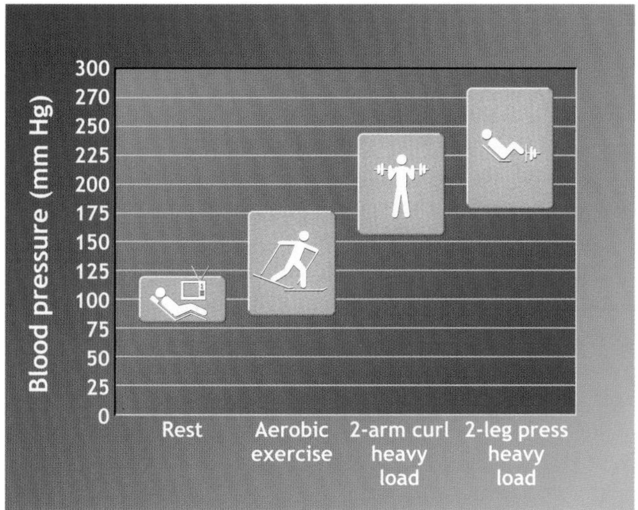

FIGURE 15.11 • Heavy resistance exercise magnifies the exercise blood pressure response (higher with legs than arms) compared with rhythmic, continuous aerobic exercise. Height of bar indicates pulse pressure.

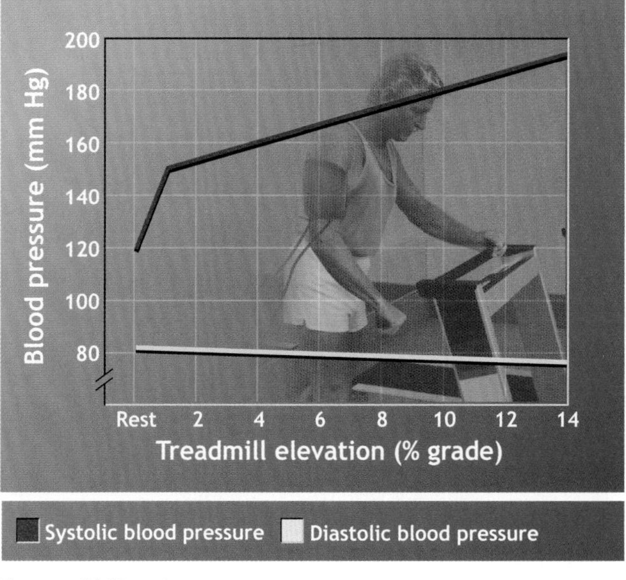

FIGURE 15.12 • Generalized response for systolic and diastolic blood pressures during continuous, graded treadmill exercise testing.

Steady-Rate Exercise

During rhythmic muscular activity (e.g., jogging, swimming, bicycling), vasodilation in the active muscles reduces total peripheral resistance, thus enhancing blood flow through large portions of the peripheral vasculature. Alternate muscle contraction and relaxation also provide an effective force to propel blood through the vascular circuit and return it to the heart. Increased blood flow during rhythmic, steady-rate exercise rapidly increases systolic pressure during the first few minutes of exercise. Blood pressure then generally levels off at 140 to 160 mm Hg for healthy men and women.[11] As exercise continues, systolic pressure may gradually decline as the arterioles in the active muscles continue to dilate, further reducing peripheral resistance to blood flow. Diastolic blood pressure remains relatively unchanged throughout exercise.

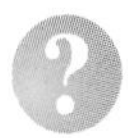

INTEGRATIVE QUESTION

How can regular resistance exercise training that disproportionately elevates blood pressure during resistance exercise ultimately blunt the blood pressure response to a standard lift (e.g., 80-lb, 2-arm curl)?

Graded Exercise

Figure 15.12 reveals the general pattern for systolic and diastolic blood pressures during continuous, graded treadmill exercise. After the initial rapid rise from the resting level, systolic blood pressure increases linearly with exercise intensity, while diastolic pressure remains stable or decreases slightly at the higher exercise levels. Both sedentary and endurance-trained subjects demonstrate similar blood pressure responses. During maximum exercise by healthy, fit men and women, systolic blood pressure may increase to 200 mm Hg or higher, despite significantly reduced total peripheral resistance.[36] This level of blood pressure most likely reflects the heart's large output of blood during maximal exercise by individuals with high aerobic capacity.

Blood Pressure in Upper-Body Exercise

Exercise with the arms produces considerably higher systolic and diastolic blood pressures than leg exercise at a given percentage of $\dot{V}O_{2max}$ (Table 15.2).[40,48] This occurs because the smaller arm muscle mass and vasculature offer greater resistance to blood flow than the larger leg mass and blood supply.[4] Upper-body exercise (and the accompanying elevated blood pressure responses) clearly produces a greater cardiovascular strain because the work requirement of the myocardium

TABLE 15.2 ➤ **COMPARISON OF SYSTOLIC AND DIASTOLIC BLOOD PRESSURE DURING ARM AND LEG EXERCISE AT SIMILAR PERCENTAGES OF MAXIMAL OXYGEN CONSUMPTION**

Percentage of $\dot{V}O_{2max}$	Systolic Pressure (mm Hg) Arms	Systolic Pressure (mm Hg) Legs	Diastolic Pressure (mm Hg) Arms	Diastolic Pressure (mm Hg) Legs
25	150	132	90	70
40	165	138	93	71
50	175	144	96	73
75	205	160	103	75

From Åstrand, P.-O, et al. Intra-arterial blood pressure during exercise with different muscle groups. J Appl Physiol 1965;20:253.

increases considerably. For individuals with cardiovascular dysfunction, these observations support the use of exercise requiring relatively large muscle groups, as in walking, bicycling, and running, in contrast to exercise that engages a limited muscle mass, such as shoveling, overhead hammering, or arm-crank exercise.[13,35] Upper-body exercise to train coronary heart disease patients requires that the proper exercise levels emanate from the person's response to upper-body exercise and not from an exercise stress test prescription based on bicycling or running. Chapter 17 further discusses the cardiovascular adjustments to upper-body exercise.

In Recovery

Upon completion of submaximal exercise, systolic blood pressure temporarily falls below preexercise levels for both normotensive and hypertensive individuals.[21,25,41] This **hypotensive response to previous exercise** can last up to 12 hours. It occurs in response to either low- and moderate-intensity aerobic exercise or resistance exercise.[31,40] One explanation for postexercise hypotension proposes that a significant quantity of blood remains pooled in the visceral organs and/or lower limbs during recovery.[5] Venous pooling reduces central blood volume, which in turn decreases atrial filling pressure and lowers systemic arterial blood pressure. A prolonged increase in cutaneous blood flow in recovery may also contribute to the hypotensive response. Release of atrial natriuretic peptide hormone, a potent vasodilator, does not account for postexercise hypotension.[31] Observations of significant postexercise reductions in blood pressure provide further support for moderate exercise as nonpharmacologic treatment for hypertension. Relatively prolonged reductions in postexercise blood pressure justify recommending multiple periods of physical activity interspersed throughout the day.

BODY INVERSION. Individuals use gravity-inversion devices to hang in the upside-down position, believing that this maneuver offers relaxation, facilitates a strength-training response, or relieves lower back pain. While objective evidence for either practical or physiologic benefits of inverting the body remains elusive, body inversion significantly elevates systolic and diastolic blood pressures. In one study of 50 normotensive men and women, body inversion elevated systolic blood pressure from an average of 114 mm Hg to nearly 140 mm Hg, while diastolic pressure increased from 76 to 91 mm Hg.[27] The elevated blood pressure continued throughout the 3-minute inversion maneuver. The hypertensive response raises concern about possible negative consequences of inversion for individuals with hypertension.

THE HEART'S BLOOD SUPPLY

Each day, more than 2000 gallons of blood flow through the heart's chambers. However, none of the blood's nourishment passes directly into the myocardium because no direct circulatory channels lead from the chambers into the tissues. Instead, the heart muscle maintains an elaborate circulatory network of its own. Figure 15.13 shows that these vessels form a visible, crownlike network (**coronary circulation**) that arises from the top portion of the heart.

The right and left coronary arteries emerge from the upper part of the ascending aorta. Their openings form just above the semilunar valves at a point where oxygenated blood leaves the left ventricle. These arteries then curl around the heart's surface. The right coronary artery supplies predominantly the right atrium and ventricle. *The greatest volume of blood flows in the left coronary artery to the left atrium and ventricle and a small portion of the right ventricle.* These vessels divide and eventually form a dense capillary network within the myocardium. Blood leaves the tissues of the left ventricle through the **coronary sinus**; blood from the right ventricle exits via the **anterior cardiac veins**, which empty directly into the right atrium.

The driving force of each ventricular systole pushes some blood into the coronary arteries. Normal blood flow to the myocardium at rest equals 200 to 250 mL per minute; this represents approximately 5% of the heart's total output.

Myocardial Oxygen Use

At rest, the myocardium uses considerable oxygen in relation to its blood flow; it extracts about 70 to 80% of the oxygen from the blood in the coronary vessels. The magnitude of myocardial oxygen extraction contrasts significantly to that of most other tissues, which use only about one-fourth of their available oxygen at rest. Consequently, a proportionate increase in coronary blood flow in exercise provides essentially the *sole mechanism* for increasing myocardial oxygen supply. During vigorous exercise, coronary blood flow may increase four to six times above the resting level. Blood flow increases because elevated myocardial metabolism stimulates the coronary vessels to dilate. For example, tissue hypoxia provides a potent stimulus to myocardial blood flow. Adenosine, a byproduct of ATP breakdown, also mediates autoregulation of myocardial blood flow.[3] In addition to local regulatory factors, sympathetic nervous system hormones released during exercise cause coronary dilation. Arterial blood pressure further facilitates coronary blood flow. Increased aortic pressure during exercise forces a proportionately greater volume of blood into the coronary circulation. The ebb and flow of blood in the coronary vessels fluctuates with each phase of the cardiac cycle. On average, about 2.5 times more blood flows during diastole than systole.

Effects of Impaired Blood Supply

The myocardium depends on an adequate oxygen supply because, unlike skeletal muscle, this tissue has limited anaerobic energy-generating capacity. Extensive vascular perfusion supplies at least one capillary to each of the heart's muscle fibers. Impaired coronary blood flow usually produces chest pains termed **angina pectoris**. More-pronounced pain occurs

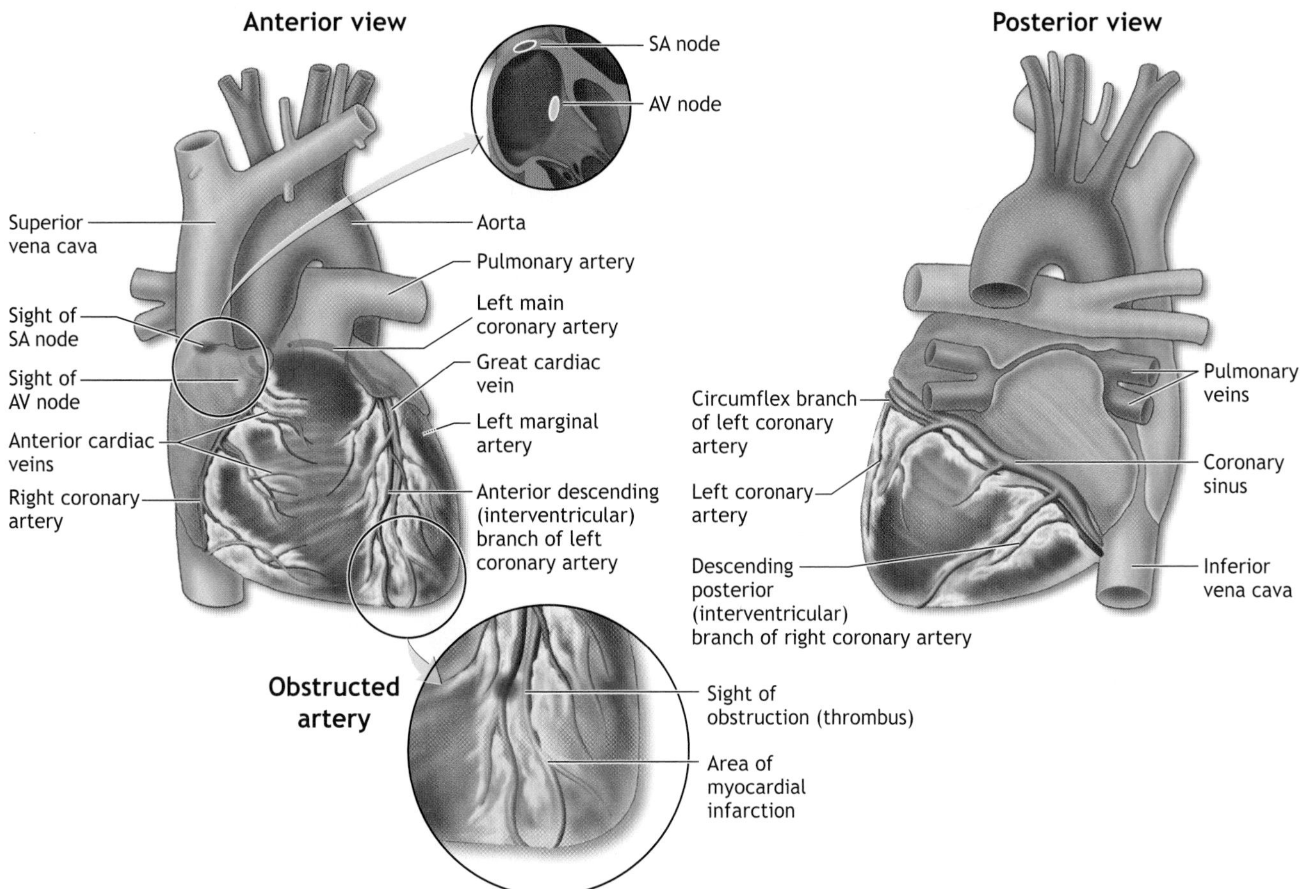

FIGURE 15.13 • Anterior and posterior views of the coronary circulation including site of SA and AV nodes (upper inset). Arteries are *shaded red* and veins *blue*, with the exception of the pulmonary circulation where colors reverse. The *lower inset* illustrates a myocardial infarction from the blockage of a coronary vessel.

during exercise because the heart's energy requirements increase significantly. In fact, the stress of exercise provides a unique way to evaluate adequacy of myocardial blood flow. A blood clot (**thrombus**) lodged in a coronary vessel usually impairs normal heart function. This form of "heart attack," or more specifically **myocardial infarction**, may be mild; a more complete blockage causes severe damage to the myocardium and death. Chapters 31 and 32 provide the details about coronary heart disease, stress testing, and the possible role of regular exercise as preventive medicine.

Rate-Pressure Product: An Estimate of Myocardial Work

Interactions between several mechanical factors—most importantly, the development of tension within the myocardium and its contractility, and heart rate—determine myocardial oxygen consumption. With increases in each of these factors during exercise, myocardial blood flow adjusts to balance oxygen supply with demand. One common estimate of myocardial workload (and resulting oxygen consumption) uses the product of peak systolic blood pressure (SBP), measured at the brachial artery, and heart rate (HR). *This index of relative cardiac work, termed the* ***double product****, or* ***rate-pressure product (RPP)****, relates closely to directly measured myocardial oxygen consumption and coronary blood flow in healthy subjects over a wide range of exercise intensities.*[26,39] RPP computes as follows:

$$\text{RPP} = \text{SBP} \times \text{HR}$$

Changes in heart rate and blood pressure contribute equally to changes in RPP. Typical values for RPP range from 6,000 at rest (HR = 50 b · min^{-1}; SBP = 120 mm Hg) to 40,000 (HR = 200 b · min^{-1}; SBP = 200 mm Hg) or higher, depending on intensity and mode of exercise. Resistance training and upper-body exercise produce substantially higher heart rate and blood pressure responses (hence higher RPPs) than more rhythmic exercise with the lower body. This added myocardial work poses an unnecessary risk for coronary heart disease patients with compromised myocardial oxygen supply.

Research with heart disease patients has shown a physiologic correlation between the RPP and the onset of angina pectoris and electrocardiographic abnormalities during exercise. In this regard, the RPP provides an objective yardstick to evaluate the effects on cardiac performance of various clinical, surgical, or exercise interventions. The well-documented

Focus on Research

Required Exercise Intensity to Improve Fitness

Karnoven MJ, et al. The effects of training on heart rate: a longitudinal study. Ann Med Exp Biol Fenn 1957; 35:307

➤ For many years, research focused on the best ways to develop and maintain cardiorespiratory fitness. Exercise frequency, intensity, type, and time (FITT) all influence the exercise prescription, but the most important variable remains exercise intensity. Experts cannot agree about which method best determines optimal exercise intensity for inducing a training response. The study by Karvonen and colleagues provided a simple method using heart rate to gauge the minimum training threshold.

The researchers used different exercise intensities to determine the influence of resting, exercise, and maximal heart rate on the training response of six young adult (20- to 23-y-old) male medical students. The study's unique aspect included constancy of exercise mode (treadmill running), duration (30 min), frequency (4 or 5 d per week), and length of training (4 wk). Three different heart rates served as criterion measures: (1) training heart rate (THR), heart rate measured during each exercise session; (2) resting heart rate (RHR), measured every morning in bed before rising; and (3) maximal heart rate (MHR), determined before and after the 4-week training period.

Because the study aimed to keep relative training intensity constant, running speed increased periodically, so THR did not decrease as cardiovascular fitness improved. The researchers' method for calculating THR, now known as the "**Karvonen method**," or "**HR reserve method**," applies the subject's exercise HR increase above RHR in relation to the range between the MHR and RHR. The following formula applies these data to establish THR at a given percentage training intensity ($\%T_{INT}$):

$$THR = [(MHR - RHR) \times \%T_{INT}] + RHR$$

The following formula computes $\%T_{INT}$ at a known THR as follows:

$$\%T_{INT} = (THR - RHR) \div (MHR - RHR) \times 100$$

For example, if a woman wished to know her THR at $\%T_{INT} = 70\%$ and knows that her MHR equals 170 $b \cdot min^{-1}$ and RHR equals 52 $b \cdot min^{-1}$, then THR equals 135 $b \cdot min^{-1}$: $[(170 - 52) \times 0.70] + 52 = 135$. Conversely, knowing THR enables one to calculate the $\%T_{INT}$: $(135 - 52) \div (170 - 52) \times 100 = 70\%$.

The researchers showed that when heart rate was used for training intensity, the "borderline" between effective and ineffective training slightly exceeded the 60% of the percentage training intensity. They therefore recommended that THR must reach *at least* $60\%T_{INT}$ and preferably $70\%T_{INT}$. The inset figure for a representative subject graphically shows that THR averaged 136 $b \cdot min^{-1}$, or 71% of the available heart rate range. The *top panel* displays the change in running speed required to maintain a constant THR throughout the 4-week training period.

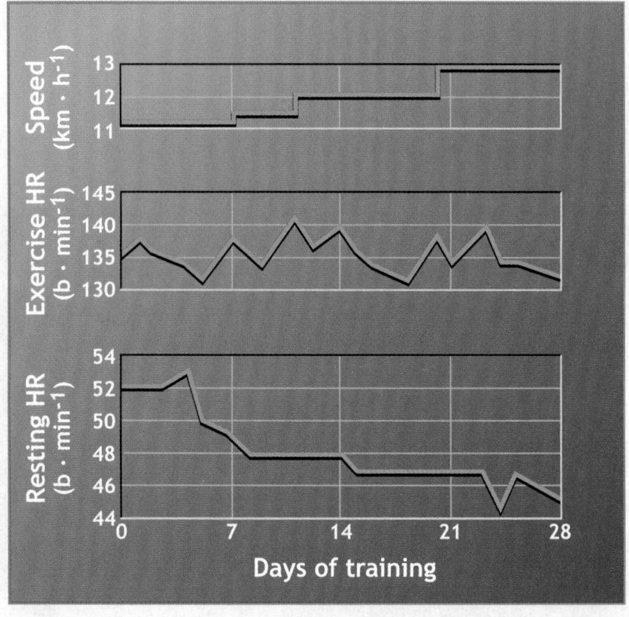

The concept and computations developed by Karvonen for establishing effective training intensity threshold using HR significantly impacted the study of exercise training.

lowering of exercise heart rate and systolic blood pressure (hence lower RPP and myocardial oxygen requirement) with training helps to explain the improved exercise capacity of cardiac patients following exercise training. Several research studies show that prolonged, high-intensity aerobic training enables cardiac patients to achieve a higher exercise RPP.[10,18] In nine patients followed over a 7-year training period, RPP increased by 11.5% before ischemic symptoms appeared during graded exercise testing.[43] These important findings provide *indirect* evidence for improved myocardial oxygenation, perhaps owing to greater coronary vascularization or reduced obstruction from the training adaptation.

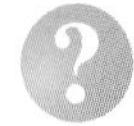

INTEGRATIVE QUESTION

Why would a training-induced increase in the rate-pressure product before a person experiences angina during exercise imply enhanced myocardial oxygenation?

MYOCARDIAL METABOLISM

As with all tissue, the myocardium uses the chemical energy stored in food to generate ATP to power its work. The myocardium, however, relies almost totally on energy released

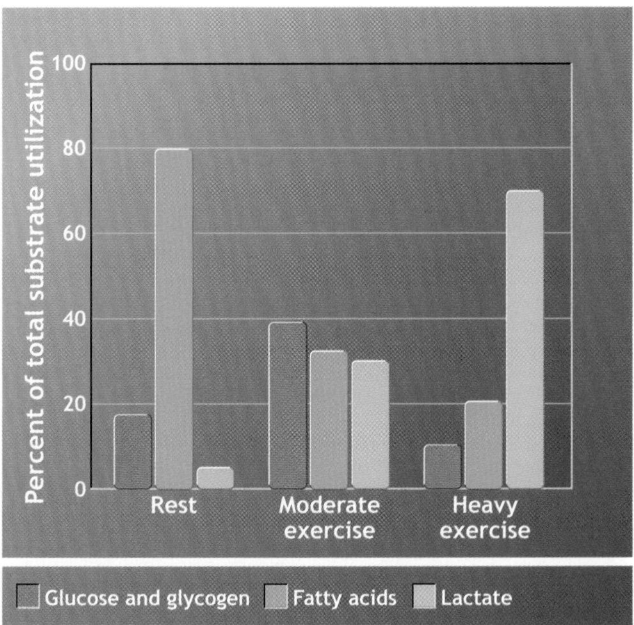

FIGURE 15.14 • Generalized pattern of substrate use by the myocardium at rest and in relation to exercise intensity.

in aerobic reactions; it has a threefold higher oxidative capacity than skeletal muscle.[23] Myocardial fibers contain the greatest mitochondrial concentration of all tissues, with exceptional capacity for fat catabolism as a primary means for ATP resynthesis.[49]

Figure 15.14 shows the specific substrate use (on a percentage basis) by the myocardium during rest and moderate and heavy exercise. Glucose, fatty acids, and lactate formed from glycolysis in skeletal muscle provide the energy for proper myocardial functioning.[2] At rest, these three substrates contribute to ATP resynthesis, with the greatest energy derived from free fatty acid breakdown.[17] In essence, the heart uses for energy whatever substrate it "sees" on a physiologic level—so during heavy exercise, when lactate efflux from active skeletal muscle into the blood increases significantly, the heart derives its major energy from oxidizing circulating lactate. In more-moderate exercise, equal amounts of fat and carbohydrate provide the energy fuel. During prolonged submaximal exercise (not illustrated), myocardial metabolism of free fatty acids rises to almost 70% of the total energy requirement. Similar patterns of myocardial metabolism exist for trained and untrained individuals. However, an endurance-trained person demonstrates considerably greater myocardial reliance on fat catabolism in submaximal exercise. This difference, similar to the effect for skeletal muscle, again illustrates the "carbohydrate-sparing effect" of aerobic training.

Summary

1. The striated fibers of the myocardium interconnect so that portions of the heart contract in a unified manner. The heart functions as two separate pumps: one pump receives blood from the body and pumps it to the lungs for aeration (pulmonary circulation) while the other receives oxygenated blood from the lungs and pumps it throughout the body (systemic circulation).
2. Pressure changes created during the cardiac cycle act on the heart's valves to provide a one-way flow of blood in the vascular circuit.
3. The surge of blood with ventricular contraction (and subsequent run-off of blood in relaxation) creates pressure changes within the arterial vessels. Ventricular contraction generates systolic blood pressure, the highest pressure during the cardiac cycle. Diastolic pressure represents the lowest pressure before the next ventricular contraction.
4. The dense capillary network provides a large and effective surface for exchange between the blood and tissues. These minute-diameter blood vessels possess autoregulatory capacity to adjust blood flow in response to the tissue's metabolic activity.
5. Although the venous tree contains the largest portion of central blood volume at rest, an increase in venous tone (venoconstriction) probably contributes little to the redistribution of blood during exercise.
6. Compression and relaxation of the veins by skeletal muscle action impart considerable energy to facilitate venous return. The "muscle pump" provides additional justification for active recovery immediately following vigorous exercise.
7. One of every three to four persons experiences chronic, abnormally high blood pressure sometime during his or her life. Hypertension imposes a chronic stress on the cardiovascular system that eventually damages arterial vessels and leads to arteriosclerosis, heart disease, stroke, and kidney failure.
8. Systolic blood pressure increases in proportion to oxygen consumption and blood flow during graded exercise, whereas diastolic pressure remains relatively unchanged or decreases slightly. At the same relative and absolute exercise levels, upper-body exercise produces a greater rise in systolic pressure than leg exercise.
9. After exercising, blood pressure decreases below the preexercise level and may remain lower for up to 12 hours.
10. During isometric, free-weight, and hydraulic resistance exercises, peak systolic and diastolic blood pressures mirror a hypertensive state. Performing high-intensity resistance exercises pose a risk to individuals with hypertension or heart disease.
11. The myocardium extracts approximately 80% of the oxygen flowing through the coronary arteries at rest. The high level of oxygen extraction means that an increase in coronary blood flow provides the primary means to meet myocardial oxygen demands in exercise.

12. The myocardium relies on a continual supply of oxygen. Impairment of coronary blood flow initiates chest (angina) pains; blockage of a coronary artery (myocardial infarction) causes irreversible damage to the heart muscle.
13. The product of heart rate and systolic blood pressure, termed rate-pressure product (RPP), estimates myocardial workload. RPP proves useful in studying the effects of exercise training on cardiac performance.
14. The myocardium metabolizes glucose, fatty acids, and circulating lactate for energy. Their percentage use varies with the severity and duration of exercise and the individual's training status.

References

1. Baglivo HP, et al. Effect of moderate physical training on left ventricular mass in mild hypertensive persons. Hypertension 1990;15(suppl I):1.
2. Baher SK, et al. Training-intensity dependent and tissue-specific increases in lactate uptake and MCT-1 in heart muscle. J Appl Physiol 1998;84:987.
3. Berne RM. The role of adenosine in the regulation of coronary blood flow. Circ Res 1980;47:807.
4. Blomqvist CG, et al. Similarity of the hemodynamic responses to static and dynamic exercise of small muscle groups. Circ Res 1982;1:87.
5. Brown SP, et al. Blood pressure, hemodynamic, and thermal responses after cycling exercise. J Appl Physiol 1993;75:240.
6. Cardillo C, et al. Racial differences in nitric oxide-mediated vasodilator response to mental stress in the forearm circulation. Hypertension 1998;31:1235.
7. Dimsdale JE, et al. Postexercise peril: plasma catecholamines and exercise. JAMA 1987;251:630.
8. Donaldson MC. Varicose veins in active people. Phys Sportsmed 1990;18:46.
9. Duncan JJ, et al. The effects of aerobic exercise on plasma catecholamines and blood pressure in patients with mild hypertension. JAMA 1985;254:2609.
10. Ehsani AA, et al. Improvement of left ventricular contractile function by exercise training in patients with coronary artery disease. Circulation 1986;74:350.
11. Fagard RH, et al. The effect of gender on aerobic power and exercise hemodynamics in hypertensive adults. Med Sci Sports Exerc 1995;27:29.
12. Fleck SJ. Cardiovascular adaptations to resistance training. Med Sci Sports Exerc 1988;20:S146.
13. Franklin BS, et al. Cardiac demands of heavy snow shoveling. JAMA 1995;273:880.
14. Freedson PF, et al. Intra-arterial blood pressure during free weight and hydraulic resistive exercise. Med Sci Sports Exerc 1984;16:131.
15. Friedman DB, et al. Cardiovascular response to voluntary and nonvoluntary static exercise in humans. J Appl Physiol 1992;73:1982.
16. Gaffney FA, et al. Cardiovascular and metabolic responses to static contraction in man. Acta Physiol Scand 1990;138:249.
17. Gertz EW, et al. Myocardial substrate utilization during exercise in humans: dual carbon-labeled carbohydrate isotope experiments. J Clin Invest 1988;82:2017.
18. Hagberg JM, et al. Effect of 12 months of intense exercise training on stroke volume in patients with coronary artery disease. Circulation 1983;67:1194.
19. Harms CA, Dempsey JA. Cardiovascular consequences of exercise hyperpnea. Exerc Sport Sci Rev 1999;27:37.
20. Hill DW, Butler SD. Haemodynamic responses to weight lifting exercise. Sports Med 1991;12:1.
21. Holtzhausen L-M, Noakes TD. The prevalence and significance of post-exercise (postural) hypotension in ultramarathon runners. Med Sci Sports Exerc 1995;27:1595.
22. Iellamo F, et al. Role of muscular factors in cardiorespiratory responses to static exercise: contribution of reflex mechanisms. J Appl Physiol 1999;86:174.
23. Jansson E, Sylven E. Myoglobin in human heart and skeletal muscle in relation to oxidative potential as estimated by citrate synthase. Clin Physiol 1981;1:596.
24. Kaplan MN. Clinical hypertension. 5th ed. Baltimore: Williams & Wilkins, 1990.
25. Kaufman FL, et al. Effect of exercise on recovery blood pressure in normotensive and hypertensive subjects. Med Sci Sports Exerc 1987;19:17.
26. Kitamura K, et al. Hemodynamic correlates of myocardial oxygen consumption during upright exercise. J Appl Physiol 1972;32:516.
27. Le Marr JD, et al. Cardiorespiratory responses to inversion. Phys Sportsmed 1983;11:51.
28. Lentini AC, et al. Left ventricular response in healthy young men during heavy-intensity, weight-lifting exercise. J Appl Physiol 1993;75:2703.
29. Lightfoot JT, et al. Ambient noise interferes with auscultatory blood pressure measurement during exercise. Med Sci Sports Exerc 1996;28:502.
30. Lloyd-Jones DM, et al. Differential impact of systolic and diastolic blood pressure on JNC-VI staging. Hypertension 1999;34:381.
31. MacDonald JR, et al. Hypotension following mild bouts of resistance exercise and submaximal dynamic exercise. Eur J Appl Physiol 1999;79:148.
32. MacDougall JD, et al. Arterial blood pressure response to heavy resistance exercise. J Appl Physiol 1985;58:785.
33. Mayo JJ, Kravitz L. A review of the acute cardiovascular responses to resistance exercise of healthy young and older adults. J Strength Cond Res 1999;13:90.
34. McCartney N. Acute responses to resistance training and safety. Med Sci Sports Exerc 1999;31:31.
35. Miles DS. Cardiovascular responses to upper body exercise in normals and cardiac patients. Med Sci Sports Exerc 1989;21:S126.
36. Mitchell JH, Raven PB. Cardiovascular adaptation to physical activity. In: Bouchard C, et al., eds. Physical activity, fitness, and health. Champaign, IL: Human Kinetics, 1994.
37. Narloch JA, Brandstater ME. Influence of breathing technique on arterial blood pressure during heavy weight lifting. Arch Phys Med Rehabil 1995;76:457.
38. Nelson L, et al. Effect of changing levels of physical activity on blood pressure and haemodynamics in essential hypertension. Lancet 1986;2:473.
39. Nelson RR, et al. hemodynamic predictors of myocardial oxygen consumption during static and dynamic exercise. Circulation 1974;50:1179.
40. Pescatello LS, et al. Short-term effect of dynamic exercise on arterial blood pressure. Circulation 1991;83:1557.
41. Raglin JS, Morgan WP. Influence of exercise and quiet rest on state anxiety and blood pressure. Med Sci Sports Exerc 1987;19:456.
42. Report on Secretary's Task Force on Black and Minority Health. U.S. Dept. of Health and Human Services publication 0-174-719. Washington, DC: Government Printing Office, August 1985.
43. Rogers MA, et al. The effects of 7 years of intense exercise training on patients with coronary artery disease. J Am Coll Cardiol 1987;10:321.
44. Rowell LB. Human cardiovascular control. Cary, NC: Oxford University Press, 1994.
45. Smith ML, et al. Effect of muscle tension on the cardiovascular responses to lower body negative pressure in man. Med Sci Sports Exerc 1987;19:436.
46. The fifth report of the Joint National Committee on Detection, Evaluation, and Treatment of High Blood Pressure (JNCV). Arch Intern Med 1993;153:154.
47. The sixth report of the Joint National Committee on Prevention, Detection, Evaluation, and Treatment of High Blood Pressure. Arch Intern Med 1997;157:2413.
48. Toner MM, et al. Cardiovascular adjustment to exercise distributed between the upper and lower body. Med Sci Sports Exerc 1990;22:773.
49. Vary TC, et al. Control of energy metabolism of heart muscle. Annu Rev Physiol 1981;43:419.
50. Whelton PK, et al. Effects of oral potassium on blood pressure: meta-analysis of randomized controlled clinical trials. JAMA 1997;277:1624.
51. Whelton PK, et al. Sodium reduction and weight loss in the treatment of hypertension in older persons: a randomized controlled trial of nonpharmacologic interventions in the elderly (TONE). JAMA 1998;279:839.

CHAPTER 16

Cardiovascular Regulation and Integration

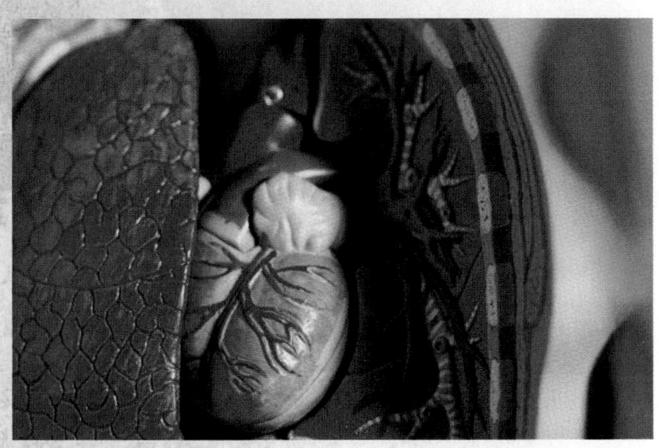

Chapter Objectives

- Discuss the influence of intrinsic and extrinsic factors that regulate heart rate during rest and exercise
- Draw a normal electrocardiogram (ECG) tracing, and identify and describe its major components
- Describe local metabolic factors that regulate blood flow during rest and exercise
- Explain the role of "central command" in cardiovascular regulation during exercise
- Describe the effects of aerobic exercise training on neural regulation of heart rate
- Outline the contributions of chemoreceptors, mechanoreceptors, and the metaboreflex in exercise cardiovascular regulation
- Indicate how each component of Poiseuille's law affects blood flow
- Summarize the dynamics of blood flow to diverse tissues at the onset of exercise and as exercise progresses in duration and intensity
- Describe the proposed mechanisms for nitric oxide's regulation of local blood flow
- Outline the dynamics of the cardiovascular response to exercise in the heart transplant patient

The vascular system demonstrates exceptional capacity for expansion. For example, the vessels of the skin, viscera, and skeletal muscles have the potential to conduct blood that is three to four times the pumping capacity of the normal heart.[52] Consequently, complex mechanisms continually interact to maintain a dynamic balance between systemic blood pressure and blood flow to various tissues under different conditions. Neurochemical factors regulate heart rate and the internal opening of the blood vessels. An exquisite level of cardiovascular regulation provides rapid control of heart function and effective distribution of blood flow throughout the body. When a person rests, for example, approximately 5% of the 5 L of blood pumped by the heart each minute goes to the skin. This contrasts to exercise in a hot, humid environment when as much as 20% of the total blood flow diverts to the body's surface to dissipate heat. "Shunting" of blood and maintenance of blood pressure occur only within a closed vascular system. Such a system demonstrates the capability for immediate redistribution of blood to meet changing metabolic and physiologic needs.

INTRINSIC REGULATION OF HEART RATE

Cardiac muscle, unlike other tissues, maintains its own rhythm. If left to this inherent rhythmicity, the heart would beat steadily at about 100 times each minute. Situated within the posterior wall of the right atrium lies a small (3-mm wide and 1-cm long) mass of specialized muscle tissue called the **sinoatrial node** or (**SA node**). This node spontaneously depolarizes and repolarizes to provide the innate stimulus for heart action. For this reason, the term **pacemaker** describes the SA node. Figure 16.1 *(left)* shows the normal route for impulse transmission within the myocardium.

Heart's Electrical Activity

Electrochemical rhythms originating at the SA node spread across the atria to another small knot of tissue called the **atrioventricular node** or **AV node**. Figure 16.1 *(right)* illustrates the time sequence of the propagation of the electrical impulse from the SA node throughout the myocardium.

A 0.10-second delay occurs after the electrical impulse spreads through the atria to allow them to contract and propel blood into the ventricles. The AV node gives rise to the 1-cm long **AV bundle**, also called the **bundle of His**, named for the German physician Wilhelm His, Jr. (1863–1934), who first described this tissue in 1893. The AV bundle transmits the impulse rapidly through the ventricles over specialized conducting fibers referred to as the **Purkinje system** (named for German anatomist–physiologist Johannes Von Purkinje [1787–1869]). These fibers form distinct bundle branches that penetrate the right and left ventricles. Purkinje system fibers transmit the impulse about 6 times faster than normal ventricular muscle fibers. Each ventricular cell becomes stimulated within 0.06 second from the passage of the impulse into the ventricles; this per-

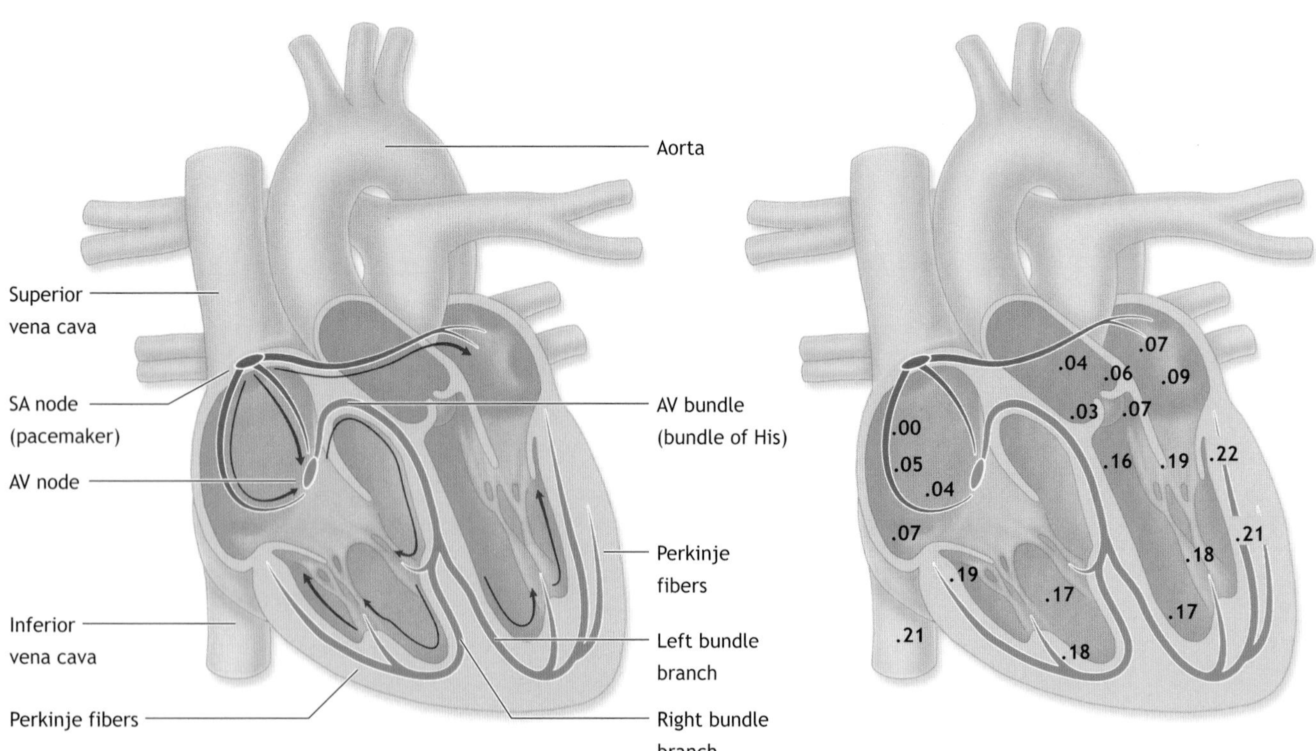

FIGURE 16.1 • *Left.* Normal route for excitation and conduction of the cardiac impulse denoted by the red arrows. The impulse originates at the SA node, travels to the AV node, and then spreads throughout the ventricular mass. *Right.* Time sequence in seconds for electrical impulse transmission from the SA node throughout the myocardium.

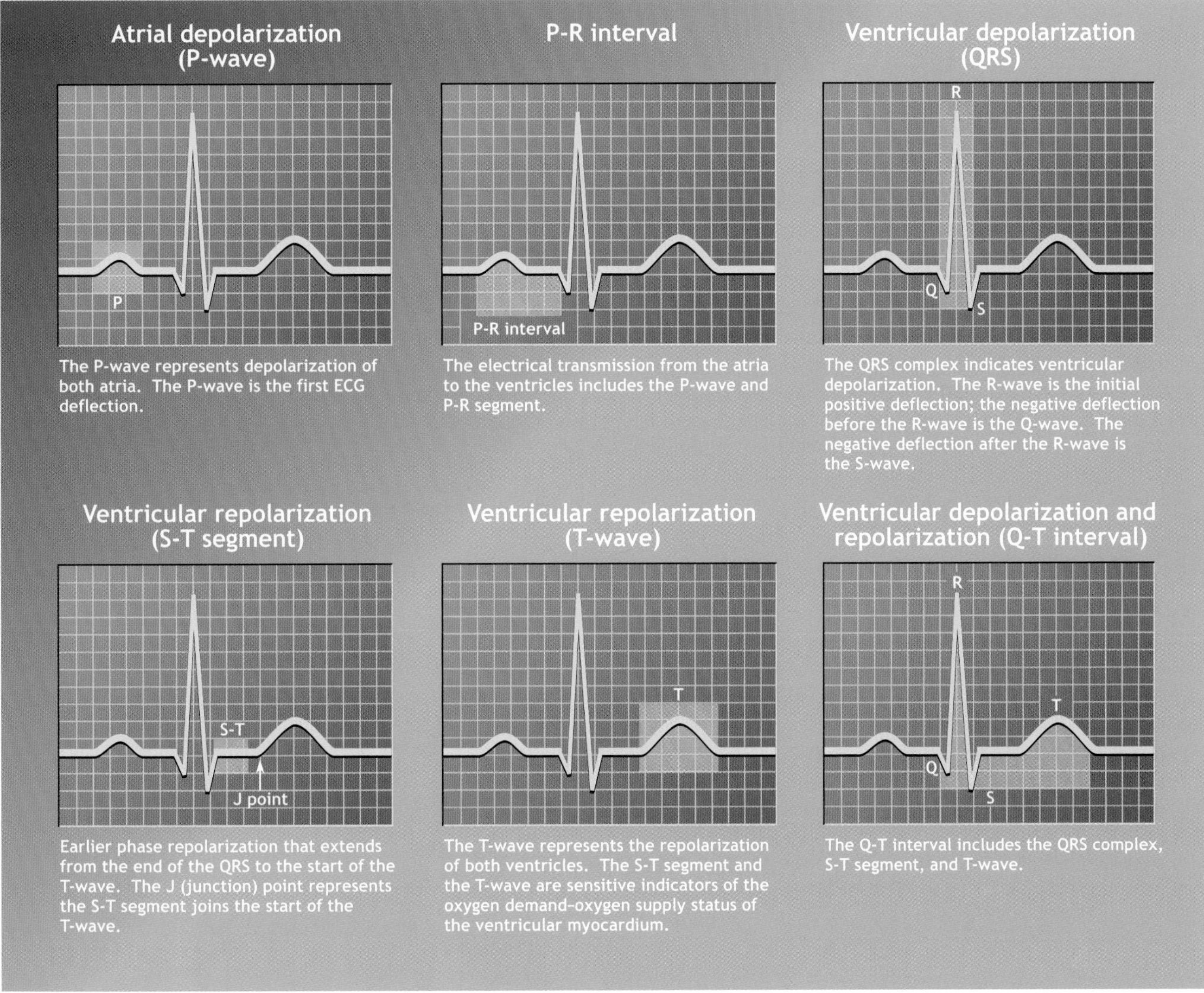

FIGURE 16.2 • The different phases of the normal ECG from atrial depolarization (*upper left*) to ventricular repolarization (*lower middle*).

mits a unified and simultaneous subsequent contraction of both ventricles. The transmission of the cardiac impulse flows as follows:

SA node → Atria → AV node → AV bundle
(Purkinje fibers) → Ventricles

Electrocardiogram

Like all nerve and muscle tissue, the outer surface of myocardial cells (fibers) maintains a more positive electrical charge than the inside. Upon stimulation prior to contraction, polarity reverses and the myocardial cells' inside becomes more positive than outside. During the diastolic phase of the cardiac cycle, the membranes repolarize to reestablish the normal resting membrane potential.

The myocardium's electrical activity creates an electrical field throughout the body. The sequence of electrical events before and during each cardiac cycle is readily detected as voltage changes by electrodes on the skin's surface, because the salty bodily fluids provide an excellent conducting medium. Figure 16.2 graphically displays the normal cycle of the heart's electrical activity by the **electrocardiogram**, or simply **ECG** (see also "In a Practical Sense").

Recording the heart's electrical activity began in 1842 when Italian physicist Carlo Matteuci (1811–1868) showed that an electric current accompanied each heart beat in dogs. One year later, German physiologist Emil Dubois-Reymond (1818–1868) confirmed Matteucci's findings doing experiments with fish. In 1887, British physiologist Augustus D. Waller (1816–1870), of St Mary's Hospital Medical School, London, published the first human electrocardiodiagram (J Physiol [London] 1887;8:229–223), and demonstrated his unique technique at the First International Congress of Physiologists in 1889. Several years later, British physiologists Sir William Maddock Bayliss (1860–1924) and Edward Starling (1866–1927), of University College London, connected the terminals from a capillary electrometer (invented by French physicist Gabriel

In a Practical Sense

➤➤ Placing Electrodes for Bipolar and 12-Lead ECG Recordings

The electrocardiogram (ECG) represents a composite record of the heart's electrical events during a cardiac cycle. These events provide a means of monitoring heart rate during different physical activities and exercise stress testing. The ECG can detect contraindications to exercise, including previous myocardial infarction, ischemic S-T segment changes, conduction defects, and left ventricular enlargement (hypertrophy). A valid ECG tracing requires proper electrode placement. The term **ECG lead** indicates the specific placement of a *pair* of electrodes on the body that transmits the electrical signal to a recorder. The record of electrical differences across diverse ECG leads creates the composite electrical "picture" of myocardial activity.

Skin Preparation

Proper skin preparation reduces extraneous electrical "noise" (interference and skeletal muscle artifact). Abrade the skin with fine sandpaper or commercially available pads and alcohol to remove surface epidermis and oil; the skin should appear red, slightly irritated, dry, and clean.

Bipolar (3-electrode) Configuration

The *top figure* shows the typical electrode placement for a 3-lead bipolar configuration. This positioning provides less sensitivity for diagnostic testing but proves useful for routine ECG monitoring in functional exercise testing and radiotelemetry of the ECG during physical activity. The ground (green or black) electrode attaches over the sternum, the positive (red) electrode attaches on the left side of the chest in the V_5 position (level of the 5th intercostal space adajcent to the midaxillary line), and the positive (white) electrode attaches on the right side of the chest, just below the nipple at the level of the 5th intercostal space. Placement of the positive electrode can be altered to optimize the recording (e.g., 3rd and 4th intercostal spaces, anterior portion of the right shoulder, or near the clavicle). Correct electrode placement can be remembered as follows: *white to right, green to ground, red to left.*

Modified 12-Lead (10-electrode torso-mounted) Configuration for Exercise Stress Testing

The standard 12-lead ECG consists of three limb leads, three augmented unipolar leads, and six chest leads. For improved exercise ECG recordings, electrodes mounted on the torso (abdominal level) replace the conventional ankle (leg) and wrist electrodes. This "torso-mounted limb lead system" *(bottom figure)* reduces electrical artifact introduced by limb movement during exercise.

Electrode Positioning in the Modified 10-Electrode, Torso-Mounted System

1. RL (right leg): just above right iliac crest on midaxillary line
2. LL (left leg): just above left iliac crest on midaxillary line
3. RA (right arm): just below right clavicle medial to deltoid muscle
4. LA (left arm): just below left clavicle medial to deltoid muscle
5. V_1: on right sternal border in 4th intercostal space
6. V_2: on left sternal border in 4th intercostal space
7. V_3: at midpoint of a straight line between V_2 and V_4
8. V_4: on midclavicular line in 5th intercostal space
9. V_5: on anterior axillary line and horizontal to V_4
10. V_6: on midaxillary line and horizontal to V_4 and V_5

Reference

Phibbs B, Buckels L. Comparative yields of ECG leads in multistage stress testing. Am Heart J 1985;90:275.

Bipolar configuration

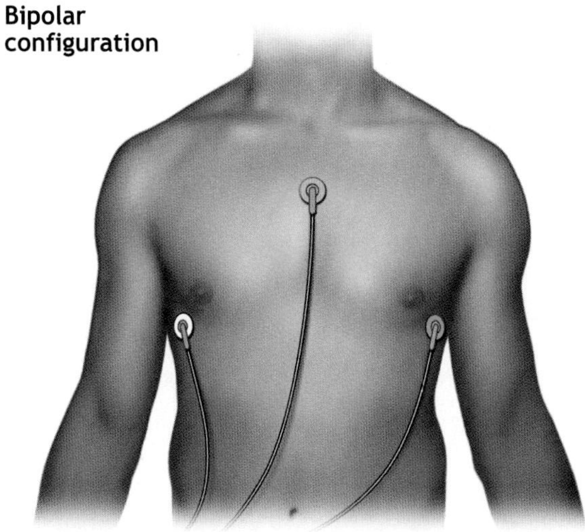

Modified 12-Lead configuration

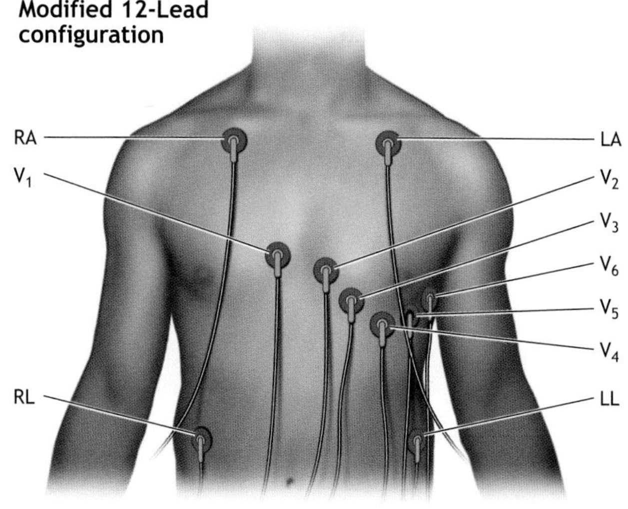

Lippmann [1845–1921] in 1872, later 1908 Physics Nobel Prize for producing colors photographically based on the phenomenon of interference) to the right hand and to the skin over the apex beat. The pattern showed a "triphasic variation accompanying (or rather preceding) each beat of the heart." These patterns of electrical deflections are now referred to as the P, QRS, and T.

The **P wave** represents depolarization of the atria. It lasts approximately 0.15 second and heralds atrial contraction. The relatively large **QRS complex** follows the P wave; it signals electrical changes from ventricular depolarization. At this point, the ventricles contract. Atrial repolarization follows the P wave; it produces a wave so small that the large QRS complex usually obscures it. The **T wave** represents ventricular repolarization and occurs during ventricular diastole. The heart's relatively long depolarization period prevents initiation of the next myocardial impulse (and subsequent contraction) for 0.20 to 0.30 second. This rest, or brief time-out **refractory period**, allows sufficient time for ventricular filling between beats.

The ECG objectively monitors heart rate during exercise. Radiotelemetry (using wireless telephony) transmits the ECG while a person freely performs such physical activities as football, weight lifting, basketball, ice hockey, dancing, swimming and diving, and space exploration. As discussed in Chapter 31, electrocardiography furnishes a vital diagnostic tool to uncover abnormalities in heart function, particularly abnormalities related to cardiac rhythm, electrical conduction, myocardial oxygenation, and tissue damage.

EXTRINSIC REGULATION OF HEART RATE AND CIRCULATION

Changes in heart rate occur rapidly through nerves that directly supply the myocardium and chemical "messengers" that circulate in blood. These **extrinsic controls** of cardiac function accelerate the heart in anticipation, before exercise begins, and then rapidly adjust to the intensity of physical effort. To a large extent, extrinsic regulation can decrease heart rate to 25 to 30 b · min^{-1} under normal ambulatory conditions in highly trained endurance athletes[8] and exceed 200 b · min^{-1} in maximum exercise.

Figure 16.3 illustrates neural mechanisms for cardiovascular regulation before and during exercise. Continual input from the brain and peripheral nervous system impinges upon the cardiovascular control center in the **ventrolateral medulla**. This center regulates the heart's output of blood and its preferential distribution to tissues throughout the body.

Sympathetic and Parasympathetic Neural Input

Neural influences superimpose on the inherent rhythm of the myocardium. These influences originate in the cardiovascular center and flow through the **sympathetic** and **parasympathetic** components of the autonomic nervous system (see Chapter 19). These divisions operate in parallel but act by distinctly different structural pathways and transmitter systems. Figure 16.4 illustrates the distribution of sympathetic and parasympathetic nerve fibers within the myocardium. Large numbers of sympathetic and parasympathetic neurons innervate the atria, whereas the ventricles receive sympathetic fibers almost exclusively.

Sympathetic Influence

Stimulation of the sympathetic cardioaccelerator nerves releases the **catecholamines** epinephrine and norepinephrine. These neural hormones accelerate SA node depolarization, causing the heart to beat faster (**chronotropic effect**). The term **tachycardia** describes heart rate acceleration, usually to rates greater than 100 b · min^{-1}. Catecholamines also increase myocardial contractility (**inotropic effect**) to augment the amount of blood the heart pumps with each beat. Maximum sympathetic stimulation nearly doubles the force of ventricular contraction. Epinephrine, released from the medullary portion of the adrenal glands during general sympathetic activation, also produces a similar but slower-acting tachycardia effect on cardiac function.

In addition to its potent effect on the myocardium, sympathetic stimulation profoundly affects blood flow throughout the body. Sympathetic stimulation produces vasoconstriction, except in the coronary vasculature. Figure 16.5 presents a schematic view of the distribution of sympathetic and parasympathetic outflow. Preganglionic axons of the sympathetic system emerge *only* from the thoracic and lumbar segments of the spinal cord. The preganglionic neurons of the sympathetic nervous system lie within the cord's gray matter. Their axons emerge through the ventral roots to synapse in the ganglia of the sympathetic chain adjacent to the spinal column. Postganglionic sympathetic nerve fibers end in the smooth muscle layers of small arteries, arterioles, and precapillary sphincters. Norepinephrine acts as a general vasoconstrictor released by specific sympathetic neurons termed **adrenergic fibers**. No consistent evidence supports the existence of **cholinergic sympathetic fibers** in humans that release acetylcholine to cause vasodilation—as contrasted to the spillover of acetylcholine from the myoneural junction that probably causes a small vasodilation effect. Some adrenergic constrictor nerves remain continually active. Consequently, some blood vessels always exhibit a state of constriction referred to as **vasomotor tone**, even within active muscle during intense exercise.[10] Dilation of blood vessels under adrenergic influence results more from reduced vasomotor tone (decreased adrenergic activity) than from increased activity of either cholinergic sympathetic or parasympathetic dilator fibers (see next section). In addition, powerful vasodilation induced by byproducts of local metabolism (see "Factors Within Active Muscle," p. 335) rapidly overrides any sympathetically activated vasoconstriction in active tissue. Humoral feedback from blood-borne factors (e.g., metabolites) released to the circulation from active muscles accelerates heart rate during exercise.[29]

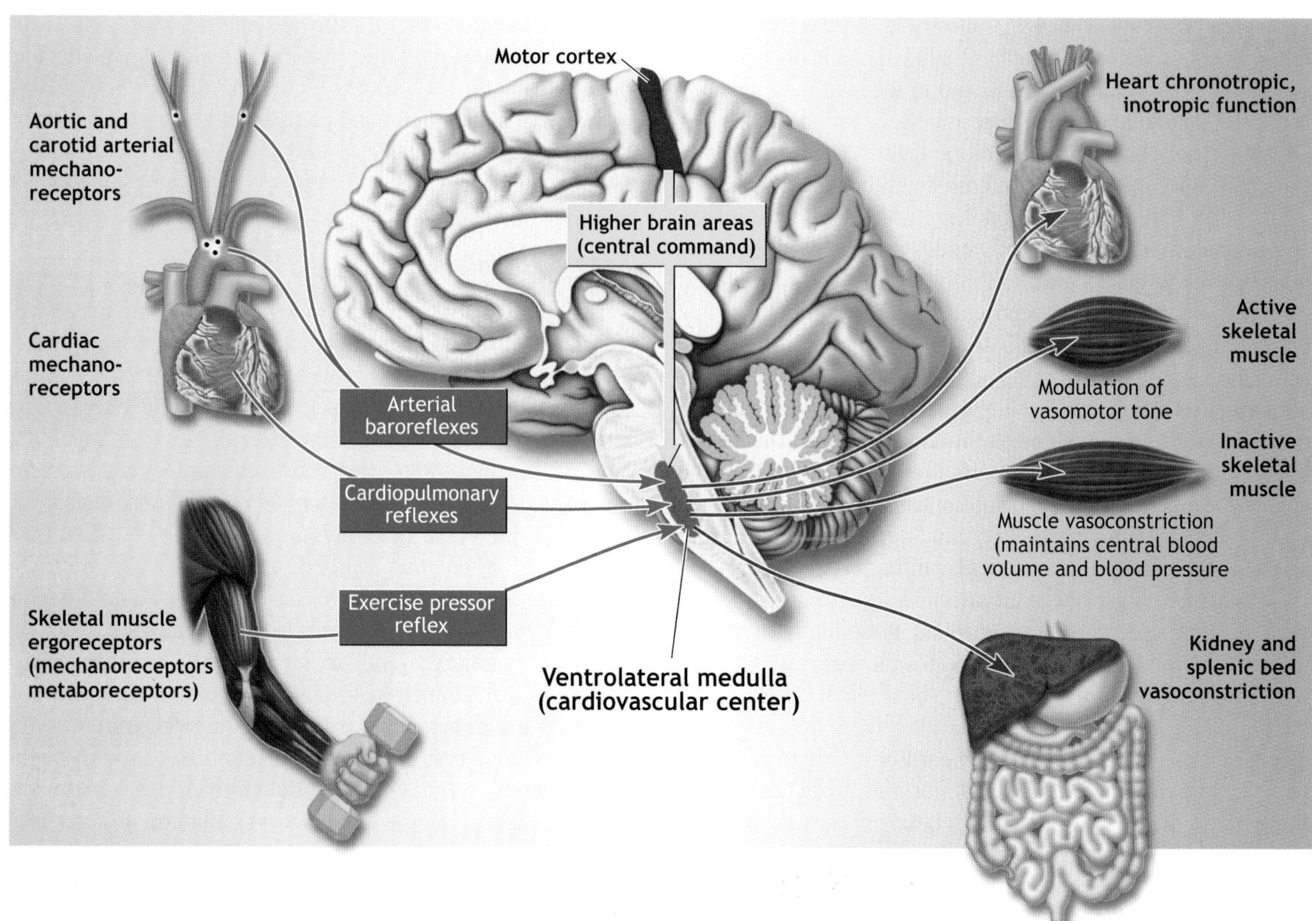

Condition	Activator	Response
Preexercise "anticipatory" response	Activation of central command from motor cortex and higher area of the brain increase in sympathetic outflow and reciprocal inhibitions of parasympathetic activity.	Acceleration of heart rate; increased myocardial contractility; vasodilation in skeletal and heart muscle (cholinergic fibers); vasoconstriction in other areas, especially skin, gut, spleen, liver, and kidneys (adrenergic fibers); increase in arterial blood pressure.
Exercise	Parasympathetic withdrawal at onset and during low-intensity exercise; progressive sympathetic stimulation in more-intense exercise; reflex feed-back from peripheral mechanical and chemical receptors that monitor muscle action; alterations in local metabolic conditions due to hypoxia, ↓pH, ↑Pco_2, ↑ADP, ↑Mg^{2+}, ↑Ca^{2+}, and ↑temperature cause autoregulatory vasodilation in active muscle.	Further dilation of muscle vasculature.
	Continued sympathetic adrenergic outflow in con-junction with epinephrine and norepinephrine from the adrenal medullae.	Concomitant constriction of vasculature in inactive tissues to maintain adequate perfusion pressure throughout arterial system. Action of the muscle pump and visceral vasoconstiction combine to facilitate venous return and maintain central blood volume.

FIGURE 16.3 • Neural regulation of the cardiovascular system during exercise. (Modified from Mitchell JH, Raven PB. Cardiovascular adaptation to physical activity. (In: Bouchard C, et al., eds. Physical activity, fitness, and health. Champaign, IL: Human Kinetics, 1994.)

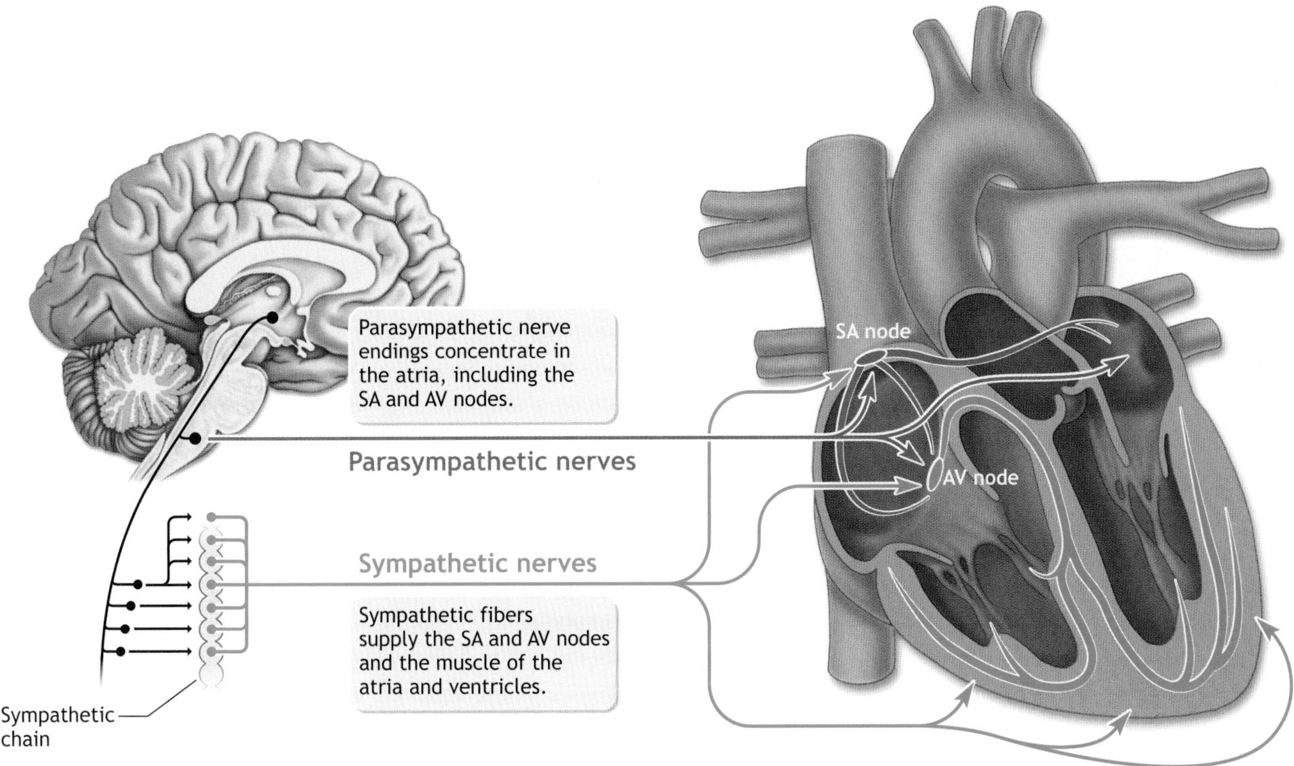

FIGURE 16.4 • Distribution of sympathetic and parasympathetic nerve fibers to the myocardium. Sympathetic nerve fiber endings secrete the neurohormone epinephrine. Sympathetic fibers supply the SA and AV nodes and the muscle of the atria and ventricles. Parasympathetic nerve endings secrete acetylcholine. These fibers concentrate in the atria, including the SA and AV nodes.

Parasympathetic Influence

Whereas preganglionic sympathetic axons emerge *only* from the thoracic and lumbar segments of the spinal cord (and distribute to all vascularized portions of the body), preganglionic axons of the parasympathetic division emerge *only* from the brainstem and the cord's sacral segments. Consequently, the parasympathetic and sympathetic systems complement each other anatomically. The preganglionic parasympathetic neurons lie within brainstem tissue and lower spinal cord. Their axons travel farther than sympathetic axons because their ganglia typically locate adjacent to or within target organs. Parasympathetic fibers distribute to the head, neck, and body cavities (except for erectile tissues of genitalia) and never emerge in the body wall and limbs. When stimulated, parasympathetic neurons release the neurohormone acetylcholine, which retards the rate of sinus discharge and slows heart rate. Reduced heart rate (**bradycardia**) results largely from stimulation of the pair of **vagus nerves**, whose cell bodies originate in the medulla's cardioinhibitory center. The vagus nerves are the only cranial nerves that exit the head and neck region and descend to the thorax and abdominal regions. These nerves carry approximately 80% of all parasympathetic fibers. Vagal stimulation exerts no effect on myocardial contractility. Aside from slowing heart rate, parasympathetic nerve fibers leave the brainstem and spinal cord to affect diverse body areas. Like sympathetic function, parasympathetic stimulation excites some tissues (e.g., muscles of the iris, gallbladder and bile ducts, bronchi, coronary arteries) and inhibits others (muscles of gut sphincters, intestines, skin vasculature). Except for sweat glands, parasympathetic stimulation induces glandular secretion.

At the start of and during low- to moderate-intensity exercise, heart rate increases by inhibition of parasympathetic stimulation, largely through central command activation (see next section). During strenuous exercise, heart rate increases by additional parasympathetic inhibition and direct activation of sympathetic cardioaccelerator nerves. The magnitude of heart rate acceleration relates directly to physical activity intensity and duration.[41,54]

Central Command: Input From Higher Centers

Impulses originating in the brain's higher somatomotor **central command** center continually modulate medullary activity. The motor center recruits muscles required for physical activity. Impulses from the "feed-forward" central command descend via small afferent nerves through the cardiovascular center in the medulla. This neural input coordinates the rapid adjustment of the heart and blood vessels to optimize tissue perfusion and maintain central blood pressure in relation to motor cortex involvement. This type of neural control oper-

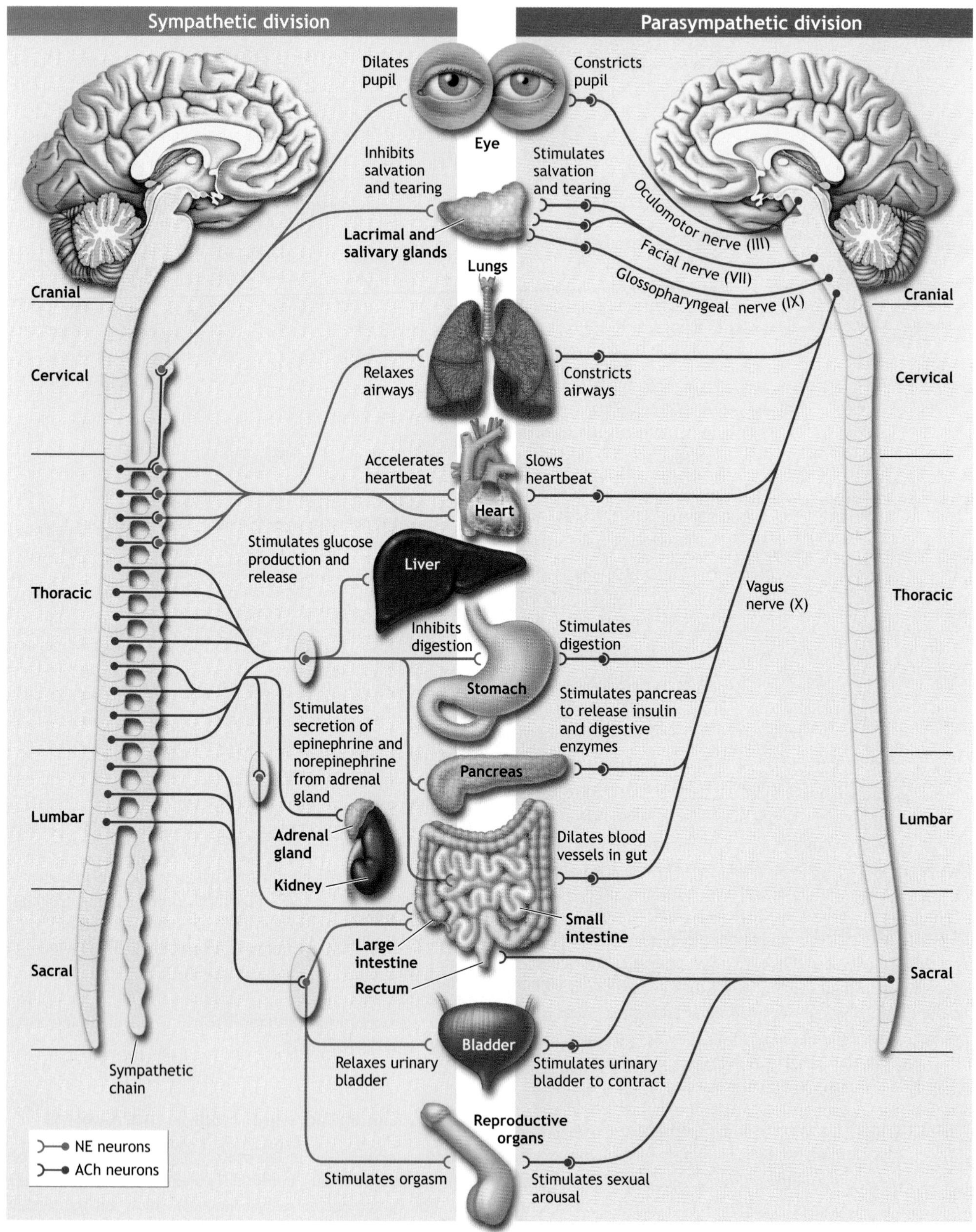

FIGURE 16.5 • Schematic view of the chemical, anatomic, and functional organization of the sympathetic and parasympathetic divisions of the autonomic nervous system. The preganglionic inputs of both divisions use acetylcholine (ACh; colored red) as neurotransmitter. The postganglionic parasympathetic innervation to the visceral organs also uses ACh, but postganglionic sympathetic innervation uses norepinephrine (NE; colored blue), with the exception of innervation of the sweat glands, which use ACh. The adrenal medulla receives preganglionic sympathetic innervation and secretes epinephrine into the bloodstream when activated. In general, sympathetic stimulation produces catabolic effects that prepare the body to "fight" or "flee," while parasympathetic stimulation produces anabolic responses that promote normal function and conserve energy. (Modified from Bear MF, et al. Neuroscience: exploring the brain. Baltimore: Williams & Wilkins, 1996.)

ates during exercise as well as in the preexercise anticipatory period. Motor cortex stimulation of the medulla increases with the size of the muscle mass activated in exercise. *Central command provides the greatest control over heart rate during exercise.*[21,42,69]

Figure 16.6 shows the influence of the central command on heart rate at the beginning of exercise.[35] Radiotelemetry continuously monitored the heart rate of trained sprint runners at rest, at the starting commands, and during 60-, 220-, and 440-yard races. Heart rate averaged 148 b · min^{-1} at the starting commands in anticipation of the 60-yard sprint; this represented 74% of the total heart rate adjustment to the run before exercise even began. The longer sprint events elicited successively lower anticipatory heart rates. This pattern of anticipatory heart rate also occurred for longer duration events. For example, anticipatory heart rates of four athletes trained for the 880-yard run averaged 122 b · min^{-1}, whereas heart rates averaged 118 b · min^{-1} during the starting commands of the 1-mile run and 108 b · min^{-1} immediately before the 2-mile run. A high level of neural outflow from central command in anticipation of exercise and immediately at the start seems desirable for intense sprint activity to mobilize physiologic reserves rapidly. On the other hand, "revving the body's engine" might prove wasteful before distance events. Interestingly, muscle blood flow also increases in anticipation of exercise. The response demonstrates training specificity, because the magnitude of the preexercise increases in mean arterial pressure and decreases in skeletal muscle vascular resistance varies with exercise intensity, duration, *and* specific mode of prior training.[3,16]

The heart rapidly "turns on" in exercise by decreased parasympathetic and increased stimulating input from the brain's central command. Accelerator input as exercise begins also comes from activation of receptors in active joints and muscles (see following section). The much slower contribution to heart rate increase from the sympathetic nervous system—triggered by reflex activity and *not* central command—does not occur until a moderate intensity of exercise is acheived. Even in so-called nonsprint events, heart rate reaches 180 b · min^{-1} within 30 seconds of 1- and 2-mile runs. Further heart rate increases progress gradually, with several plateaus during the run. Almost identical results occur for heart rate measured by telemetry during competitive swimming events, except for lower maximum heart rates during swimming.[33,35]

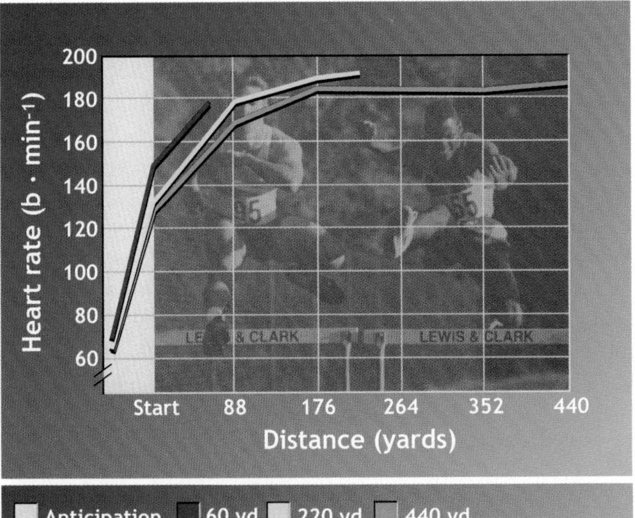

Figure 16.6 • Heart rate response of sprint-trained runners. The largest increase in anticipatory heart rate (HR immediately before exercising) increased most in the short-sprint events and was successively smaller before the longer sprints. (From McArdle WD, et al. Telemetered cardiac response to selected running events. J Appl Physiol 1967;23:566.)

Central command involvement in cardiovascular regulation also explains how variations in emotional state significantly affect cardiovascular response. Such neural input creates difficulty obtaining "true" resting values for heart rate and blood pressure.[6]

INTEGRATIVE QUESTION

Give a physiologic rationale for biofeedback and relaxation techniques to treat hypertension and stress-related disorders.

Peripheral Input

The cardiovascular center receives reflex sensory input (feedback) from peripheral receptors in blood vessels, joints, and muscles. **Chemoreceptors** and **mechanoreceptors** within muscle monitor its chemical and physical state. Afferent impulses from these receptors—slow-conducting, thin-fiber group III and IV afferents from pacinian corpuscles and unencapsulated nerve-ending receptors—provide rapid feedback. This input modifies either vagal (parasympathetic) or sympathetic outflow to bring about appropriate cardiovascular responses to various intensities of physical activity.[1,18,41,52,60,62] Activation of chemically sensitive afferents within the interstitium of muscle plays an important role in regulating sympathetic neural activation of muscle during typical submaximal exercise. This **metaboreflex** arises from stimulation by metabolites produced primarily during the concentric phase of muscular activity.[13] Three mechanisms continually assess the nature and intensity of exercise and the mass of muscle activated:

1. Reflex neural input from mechanical deformation of type III afferents.
2. Chemical stimulation of type IV afferents within active muscles (**exercise pressor reflex**).
3. Feed-forward outflow from the motor areas of the central command.

Input from specific mechanoreceptors provides feedback for the central nervous system's regulation of blood flow and blood pressure during dynamic exercise.[45,64] The aortic arch and carotid sinus contain pressure-sensitive **baroreceptors**, while cardiopulmonary mechanoreceptors assess mechanical activity in the left ventricle, right atrium, and large veins. These receptors function as a negative feedback controller to

(1) inhibit sympathetic outflow from the cardiovascular center and (2) blunt an inordinate rise in arterial blood pressure.[50,53] As blood pressure increases, the stretch of the arterial vessels activates the baroreceptors to slow the heart reflexly and dilate the peripheral vasculature. This *decreases* blood pressure toward more normal levels. During exercise, blood pressure becomes effectively regulated but at higher levels. This probably results from overriding of the arterial baroreflex feedback mechanism or an upward resetting of its threshold and/or sensitivity (i.e., reduced baroreflex gain).[37a,45] More than likely, the baroreceptors brake abnormally high blood pressure levels during exercise.

Carotid Artery Palpation

External pressure against the carotid artery sometimes slows the heart rate from direct baroreceptor stimulation at the bifurcation of the carotid artery. The potential for bradycardia from **carotid artery palpation** is important to exercise specialists because palpation is commonly used to determine exercise heart rate. Consistently low heart rate estimation with carotid artery palpation in susceptible individuals would push the person to a higher exercise level—certainly an undesirable effect in exercise prescription for cardiac patients.

Research in the late 1970s showed that carotid artery palpation significantly slowed postexercise heart rate and occasionally produced electrocardiographic abnormalities.[68] Several later reports indicated, rather convincingly for healthy adults and cardiac patients, that carotid artery palpation caused little or no heart rate alteration at rest or during exercise and recovery.[14,44,55] However, vascular disease can affect carotid sinus sensitivity to give a falsely low heart rate reading. If this occurs, an excellent substitute method uses pulse rate at the radial artery (thumb side of wrist) or temporal artery (side of head at temple) because even firm palpation of these vessels does not affect heart rate. In addition, commercially available, wrist-worn monitors and watches readily provide valid heart rate measurements under many exercise conditions, including space shuttle missions and the earliest manned suborbital flights.[17a,38]

Local Factors

The byproducts of energy metabolism provide an autoregulatory mechanism within the muscle to augment perfusion during physical activity. We discuss the local control of circulation in the following sections.

DISTRIBUTION OF BLOOD

If fully dilated, the body's blood vessels could hold approximately 20 L of blood, four times more than the total blood volume of 5 L. Thus, maintenance of blood flow and blood pressure, particularly during exercise, requires a finely regulated balance between vascular dilation and vascular constriction. *The capacity of large portions of the vasculature to either constrict or dilate provides rapid blood redistribution to meet the tissue's metabolic requirements. At the same time, it optimizes blood pressure throughout the vascular circuit.*

Physical Factors Affecting Blood Flow

Blood flows through the vascular circuit generally following physical laws of hydrodynamics applied to rigid, cylindrical vessels. However, blood is not a homogeneous fluid, and blood vessels are not rigid tubes; thus, such mathematical relationships exist mainly in a qualitative sense. The volume of flow in any vessel relates:

- Directly to the pressure gradient between the two ends of the vessels, *not* to the absolute pressure within the vessel
- Inversely to the resistance encountered to fluid flow

Friction between the blood and internal vascular wall creates resistance or force that impedes blood flow. Three factors determine resistance: (1) blood thickness or viscosity, (2) length of the conducting tube, and, most importantly, (3) blood vessel radius. The equation, referred to as **Poiseuille's law**, expresses the general relationship among pressure differential, resistance, and flow as follows:

$$\text{Flow} = \text{Pressure gradient} \times \text{Vessel radius}^4 \div \text{Vessel length} \times \text{Viscosity}$$

In the body, the transport vessel length remains constant, while blood viscosity varies only slightly under most circumstances. The radius of the conducting tube affects blood flow the most, because resistance to flow changes with the vessel's radius raised to the fourth power. For example, halving a vessel's radius decreases flow by 16 times. Conversely, doubling the radius increases volume 16-fold. Without changing the pressure differential within the vascular circuit, only a small change in vessel radius dramatically alters blood flow. *On a physiologic basis, constriction and dilation of the smaller arterial blood vessels provide the crucial mechanism for regulating regional blood flow.*

Effect of Exercise

Any increase in energy expenditure requires rapid adjustments in blood flow that affect the entire cardiovascular system. For example, nerves and local metabolites act on the smooth muscle bands of arteriole walls, altering their internal diameter almost instantaneously to meet blood flow demands. In addition, visceral vasoconstriction and the action of the muscle pump divert a large flow of blood into the central circulation.

At the onset of exercise, the vascular component of active muscles increases by dilation of local arterioles.[11] These small, feed arteries to skeletal muscle normally possess well-developed flow-mediated and myogenic regulatory mechanisms. Thus, they need little modification through exercise training to adequately supply the blood flow requirements of vigorous physical activity.[22] Concurrently, other vessels that can temporarily compromise their blood supply constrict, or "shut down." Two examples include splanchnic and renal areas.

Here, blood flow decreases in proportion to relative exercise intensity (i.e., $\%\dot{V}O_{2max}$). Blood flow shifts significantly from the abdominal viscera to active muscles even during relatively light exercise (HR $\leq$90 b · min^{-1}).[48] Two factors contribute to reduced blood flow to nonactive tissues: (1) increased sympathetic nervous system outflow (central and peripheral mechanisms) and (2) local chemicals that directly stimulate vasoconstriction or enhance the effects of other vasoconstrictors.[32,34,40]

The kidneys vividly illustrate an ability to adjust regional blood flow and conserve bodily fluid via sympathetic vasoconstriction of the renal vasculature.[70] Renal blood flow at rest normally averages 1100 mL per minute (20% of the total cardiac output), among the highest blood flows to any organ as either a percentage of cardiac output or relative to organ weight. During maximal exercise, renal blood flow decreases to 250 mL per minute or only 1% of the total exercise cardiac output. A large, temporary reduction in blood flow during strenuous exercise also occurs in tissues of the liver, pancreas, and gastrointestinal tract.[52]

Factors Within Active Muscle

At rest, only 1 of every 30 to 40 capillaries in muscle tissue remains open.[71] Keeping the remaining dormant capillaries open in exercise serves three important functions:

1. Increases total muscle blood flow.
2. Delivers a large blood volume with only a minimal increase in blood flow velocity.
3. Increases the effective surface for gas and nutrient exchange between the blood and muscle fibers.

Vasodilation occurs from local factors related to tissue metabolism that act directly on the smooth muscle bands of small arterioles and precapillary sphincters. This rapid response adjusts precisely to the muscle's force output and metabolic needs.[7] Decreased tissue oxygen supply serves as a potent local stimulus for vasodilation in skeletal and cardiac muscle. Additionally, local increases in blood flow, temperature, carbon dioxide, acidity, adenosine, magnesium and potassium ions, and nitric oxide production (see next section) by the endothelial cells lining the blood vessels trigger the discharge of relaxing factors that enhance regional blood flow.[17,31,37,59] These **autoregulatory mechanisms** for blood flow make sense physiologically because they reflect elevated tissue metabolism and increased oxygen need. Local regulation provides such strong control that it maintains adequate regional blood flow even for patients whose nerves to the blood vessels have been surgically removed. Local metabolite stimulation of chemoreceptors also provides the peripheral neural reflex input for medullary control of the heart and vasculature.

NITRIC OXIDE: AN IMPORTANT FACTOR IN AUTOREGULATION OF TISSUE BLOOD FLOW. **Nitric oxide (NO)** serves as an important signal molecule to facilitate dilation of blood vessels and decrease vascular resistance.[24] This gas, a common, unstable industrial and automotive air pollutant, forms when nitrogen burns or is produced naturally by most living organisms from its precursor L-arginine. Stimuli from diverse signal chemicals (including neurotransmitters) and sheering stress and vessel stretch from increased blood flow through the vessel lumen provoke NO synthesis and release by the vascular endothelium to serve its role as a vascular gatekeeper. Formerly termed *endothelium-derived relaxing factor* by 1998 Physiology or Medicine Nobel Prize recipient Robert F. Furchgott, NO rapidly spreads through underlying cell membranes to muscle cells within the arterial wall. Here it binds with and activates the enzyme guanylyl cyclase. This initiates a cascade of reactions that induce arterial smooth muscle relaxation to increase blood flow in neighboring blood vessels. NO exerts its potent vasodilation effect in skeletal muscle (including the diaphragm), skin, and myocardial tissue (Fig. 16.7).[5,25,28,49,56,58,65,66]

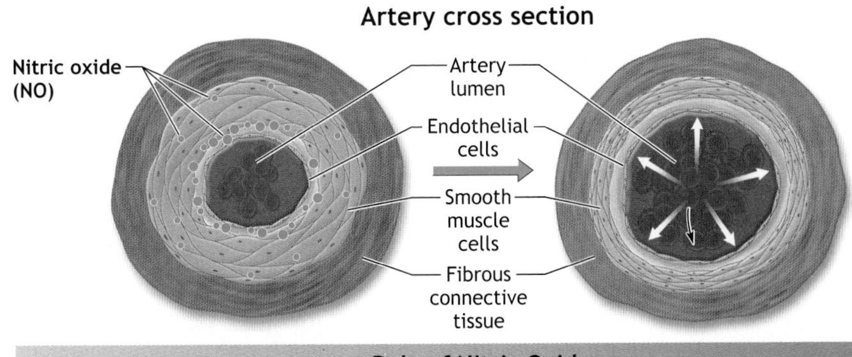

FIGURE 16.7 • Mechanism for the role of nitric oxide in regulating local blood flow.

NO mediates bodily functions as diverse as olfaction, inhibition of blood clot formation, and enhanced immune response regulation and acts as an interneuron or signaling messenger. It contributes to cutaneous active vasodilation during heat stress[26] and facilitates rapid dilation of the coronary vasculature as an early coronary circulation adaptation to moderate exercise training.[57,63] Vascular wall receptors for NO contribute to blood pressure regulation in response to central cardiovascular stimulation during emotionally stressful situations and exercise. Racial differences in resting blood pressure relate to decreased sensitivity to NO's dilating action in blacks compared with whites.[12] In coronary artery disease, the endothelium produces less NO. This explains the potent beneficial effect of exogenous nitroglycerin treatment (which releases NO gas) in blunting the effects of angina pectoris.

Research must determine how NO affects cardiovascular dynamics in exercise. Figure 16.8 illustrates a proposed mechanism for how hemoglobin molecules provide vascular control of blood flow to individual tissues via NO transport and release.[17b,23] The model proposes that hemoglobin oxygenation in the lungs changes the hemoglobin molecule's shape, enabling it to accept a different form of NO (*S*-nitrosohemoglobin, or SNO) that does not affix to hemoglobin's iron. Oxygen release in the local tissues again alters hemoglobin's shape, liberating NO and causing vasodilation. Greater oxygen release from hemoglobin (greater tissue oxygen need) should induce greater NO release and a more-pronounced vasodilation and oxygen delivery. Thus, hemoglobin plays an active role in the autoregulation and homeostatic control of tissue blood flow in relation to oxygen needs. If the model proves correct, exogenous enriched SNO-hemoglobin could serve as a potent blood substitute to treat oxygen-deficiency diseases such as atherosclerosis, stroke, septic shock, and sickle cell disease.

Hormonal Factors

Sympathetic nerves terminate in the medullary portion of the adrenal glands. With sympathetic activation, this glandular tissue secretes large quantities of epinephrine and a smaller amount of norepinephrine into the blood. These hormones act as chemical messengers to bring about a generalized constrictor response, except in blood vessels of the heart and skeletal muscles. Hormonal control of regional blood flow plays a relatively minor role during exercise compared with the more local, rapid, and potent sympathetic neural drive.

INTEGRATED EXERCISE RESPONSE

The neural command center above the medullary region initiates cardiovascular changes immediately before and at the onset of exercise. Heart rate and myocardial contractility increase owing to feed-forward input from this center, which suppresses parasympathetic activation. Concurrently, predictable alterations in regional blood flow occur in proportion to exercise severity. Modulation of dilation and constriction optimizes blood flow to areas in need while maintaining blood pressure throughout the arterial system. As exercise continues, reflex feedback to the medulla from peripheral mechanical and chemical receptors in active tissue appraises tissue metabolism and circulatory needs. Local metabolic factors also act directly to dilate resistance vessels in active muscles. Vasodilation reduces peripheral resistance, permitting greater blood flow in these areas. Arterial blood flow through active muscles progresses in pulsatile oscillations that favor enhanced flow during eccentric muscle actions and/or the recovery phases of a concentric action.[51] Centrally mediated constrictor adjustments also occur in the vasculature of nonexercising tissues (skin, kidneys, splanchnic region, and inactive muscle). Constrictor action maintains adequate perfusion pressure within exercising muscle, while simultaneously increasing blood supply to meet metabolic demands.

Factors that affect venous return are as important as those that regulate arterial blood flow. Muscle and ventilatory pump actions and visceral vasoconstriction (mediated by sympathetic activity) immediately return blood to the right ventricle when exercise begins, and continue to facilitate venous return as cardiac output increases. These adjustments balance venous return with cardiac output. In upright exercise, regulation of venous blood flow becomes particularly important because gravity tends to impede the return of blood from the extremities.

INTEGRATIVE QUESTION

Discuss the following statement: "Task-specific, regular aerobic exercise not only trains the cardiovascular system, but also 'trains' the neuromuscular system to facilitate physiologic adjustments to the specific exercise mode."

EXERCISING AFTER CARDIAC TRANSPLANTATION

Patients with left ventricular dysfunction—ejection fraction less than 20%, referred to as end-stage heart disease—show poor long-term prognosis. Even though some asymptomatic and minimally symptomatic patients show near-normal function and survive for several years, most symptomatic patients die within 1 year of diagnosis. For these patients, cardiac transplantation becomes their only hope of survival. Figure 16.9A shows the number of transplants per calendar year reported to the registry of heart transplantations of the International Society for Heart and Lung Transplantation, beginning with the first human transplant nearly 35 years ago.[19] The plateau at between 3,500 to 4,000 annual transplants after 1990 (2,500 yearly in United States) results largely from limitations in donor availability. Prior to 1985, 1-year survival rate averaged 70% (Fig. 16.9B). With the introduction of the immunosuppressive drug cyclosporine in the early 1980s, overall 1-year survival rates increased to approximately 80%, with

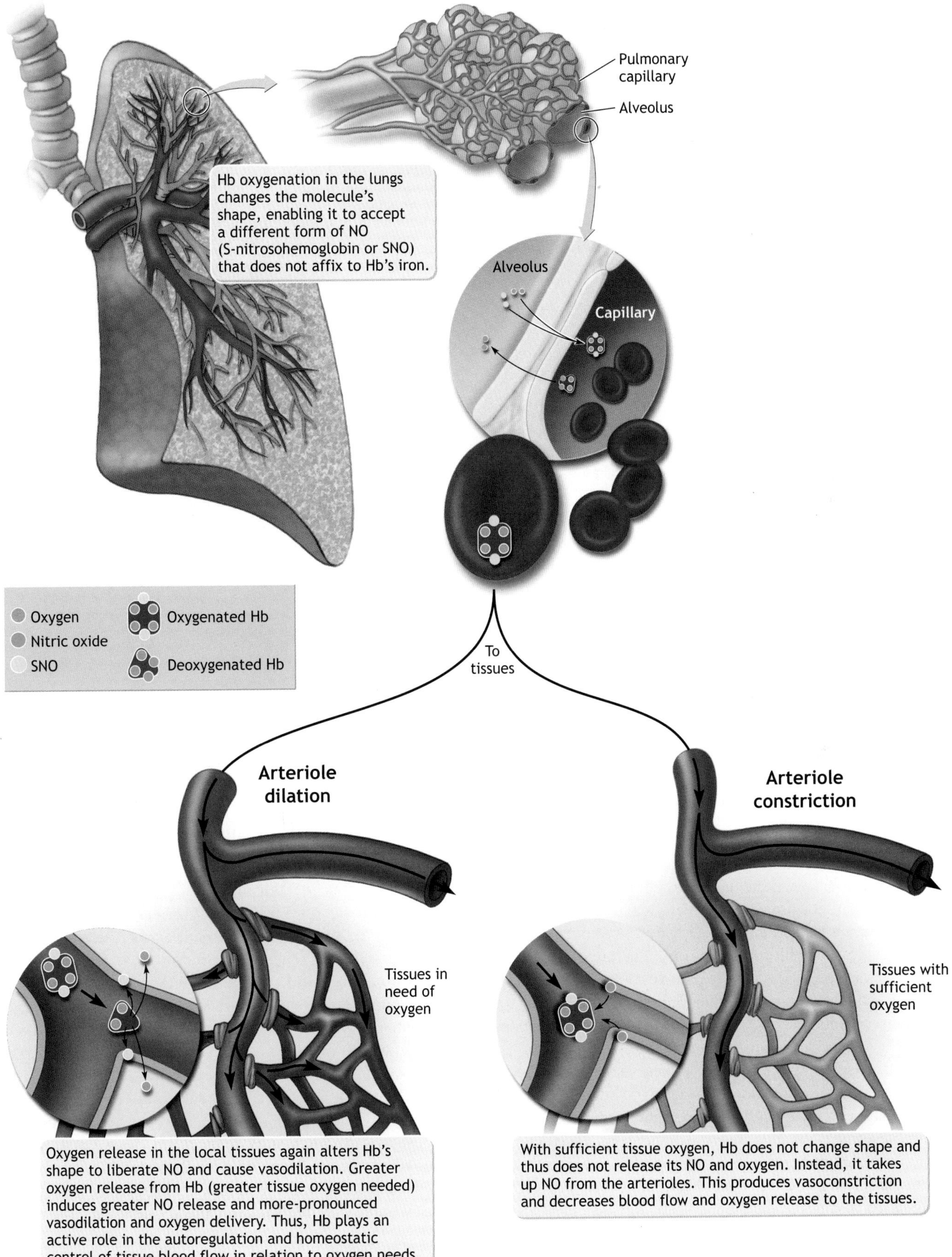

FIGURE 16.8 • Proposed mechanism for hemoglobin (Hb)–nitrous oxide (NO) interaction for vascular control of blood flow to individual tissues.

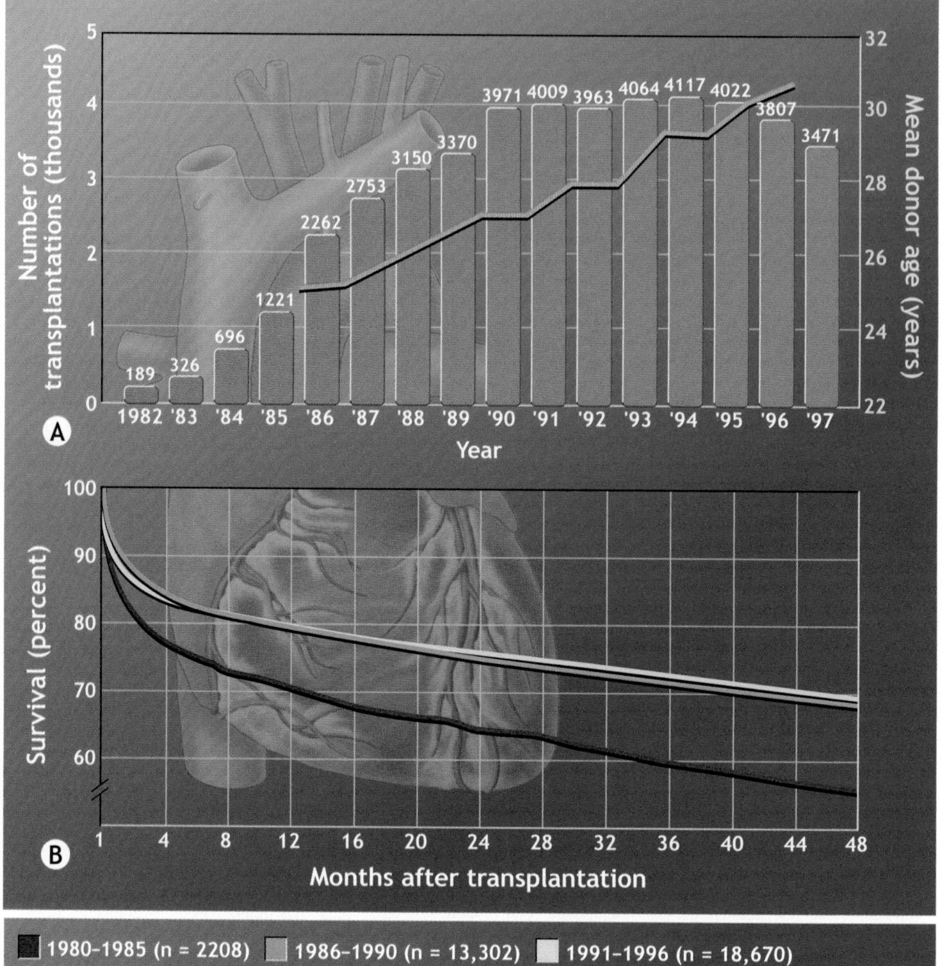

FIGURE 16.9 • A. Number of cardiac transplantations *(purple bars)* and mean donor age *(green line)* per calendar year worldwide. **B**. Actuarial survival of adult heart transplantation patients by era. Survival improved significantly after 1986. The half-life survival (time when one-half of those who underwent transplantation had died) was 8.0 years for 1991 through 1996, compared with 5.4 years for 1980 through 1985. (From Hosenpud JD, et al. The registry of the International Society for Heart and Lung Transplantation: 15th official report—1998. J Heart Lung Transplant 1998;17:656.)

4-year survival approaching 70%. In 1990, the 5-year survival rate for the 12,000 reported transplant patients averaged 72%.[30] Current postoperative therapy uses improved immunosuppressive drug combinations and applies the transvenous endomyocardial biopsy technique for early detection of tissue rejection.

Cardiac transplantation, also called **orthotopic transplantation**, clearly illustrates extrinsic neural control of exercise heart rate. The procedure removes donor and recipient hearts by transection at the midatrial level—preserving the pulmonary venous connections of the posterior wall of the left atrium of the recipient—and transection of the aortas just above their respective semilunar valves.[20,47] Transplantation eliminates neural innervation of the myocardium, although hormonal feedback from circulating catecholamines, largely from the adrenal medulla, remains intact (Fig. 16.10A). Selected patients may receive a "piggyback" or **heterotropic transplant** that places the donor heart in the recipient's chest without removing the recipient's heart. Regardless of transplantation form, significant complications occur in recovery (e.g., donor heart rejection and infection), often requiring recurrent hospitalization and prolonged, costly medical care.

Improved Function but Altered Circulatory Dynamics

Following successful transplantation, patients generally report a favorable quality of life, and approximately 50% of individuals return to work. Successful pregnancy and vaginal delivery have also occurred, as well as completion of a full marathon in less than 6 hours. In general, a transplant patient demonstrates impaired exercise capacity and diminished physiologic and hemodynamic function, which rarely exceeds 45 to 70% of normal.[2,9,15,39,43] For younger patients, this does not necessarily represent the rule; the 1998 United States' top-ranked junior golfer (18 years old) received a heart transplant at age 12 years, when dilated congestive cardiomyopathy reduced his heart function below 30% of normal. Depressed levels of aerobic fitness and exercise tolerance become magnified in heart transplant patients who also suffer from impaired pulmonary diffusion capacity.[65]

Figure 16.11(A–C) illustrates the peak oxygen consumption ($\dot{V}O_{2peak}$) for an initial pool of 140 patients evalu-

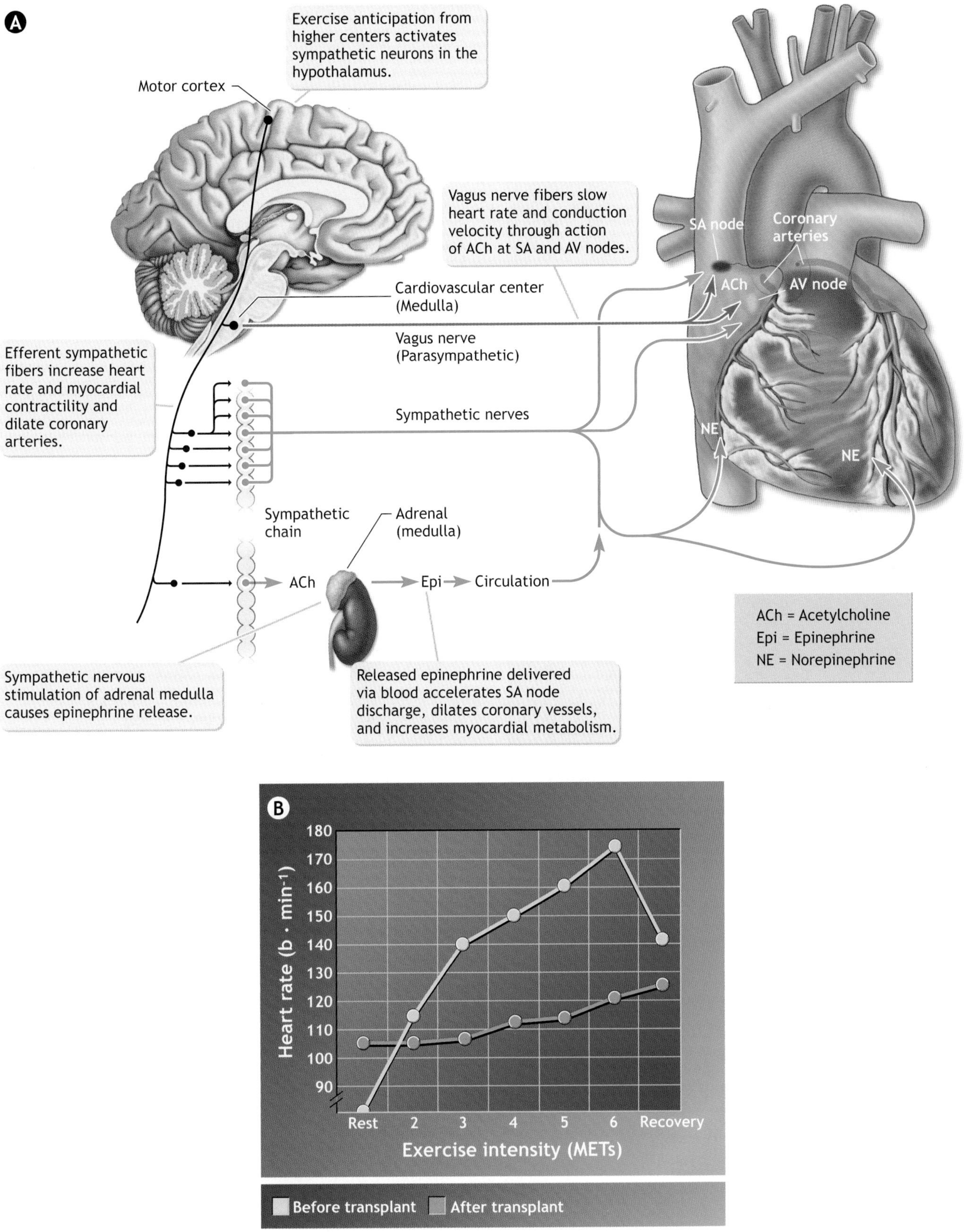

A

Exercise anticipation from higher centers activates sympathetic neurons in the hypothalamus.

Motor cortex

Vagus nerve fibers slow heart rate and conduction velocity through action of ACh at SA and AV nodes.

SA node

Coronary arteries

ACh

AV node

Cardiovascular center (Medulla)

Vagus nerve (Parasympathetic)

Efferent sympathetic fibers increase heart rate and myocardial contractility and dilate coronary arteries.

Sympathetic nerves

NE

NE

Sympathetic chain

Adrenal (medulla)

ACh

Epi

Circulation

ACh = Acetylcholine
Epi = Epinephrine
NE = Norepinephrine

Sympathetic nervous stimulation of adrenal medulla causes epinephrine release.

Released epinephrine delivered via blood accelerates SA node discharge, dilates coronary vessels, and increases myocardial metabolism.

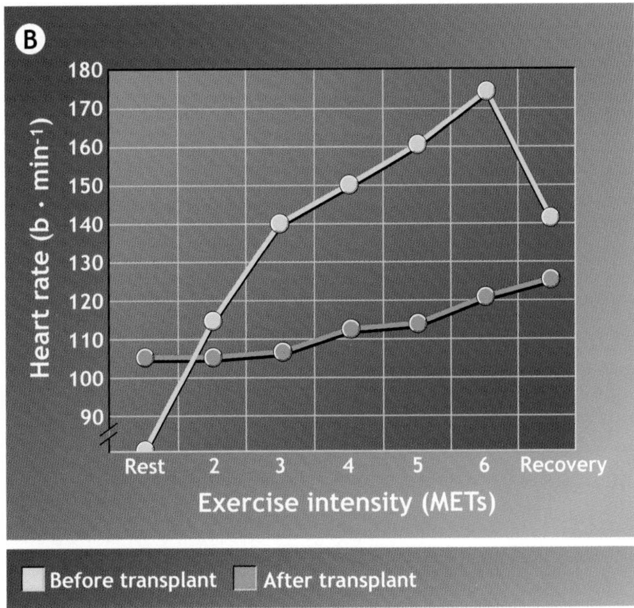

FIGURE 16.10 • **A**. Regulation of heart rate under normal conditions. Heart transplantation results in cardiac denervation. This removes vagal and sympathetic efferent stimulation to the myocardium. Consequently, circulating epinephrine from the adrenal medulla provides the primary mechanism to regulate exercise heart rate. **B**. Heart rate response of a patient during graded exercise before and after orthotopic cardiac transplantation. Note the elevated resting heart rate and the delayed and blunted heart rate after transplantation. (Figure B from Squirers RW. Exercise training after cardiac transplantation. Med Sci Sports Exerc 1991;23:686.)

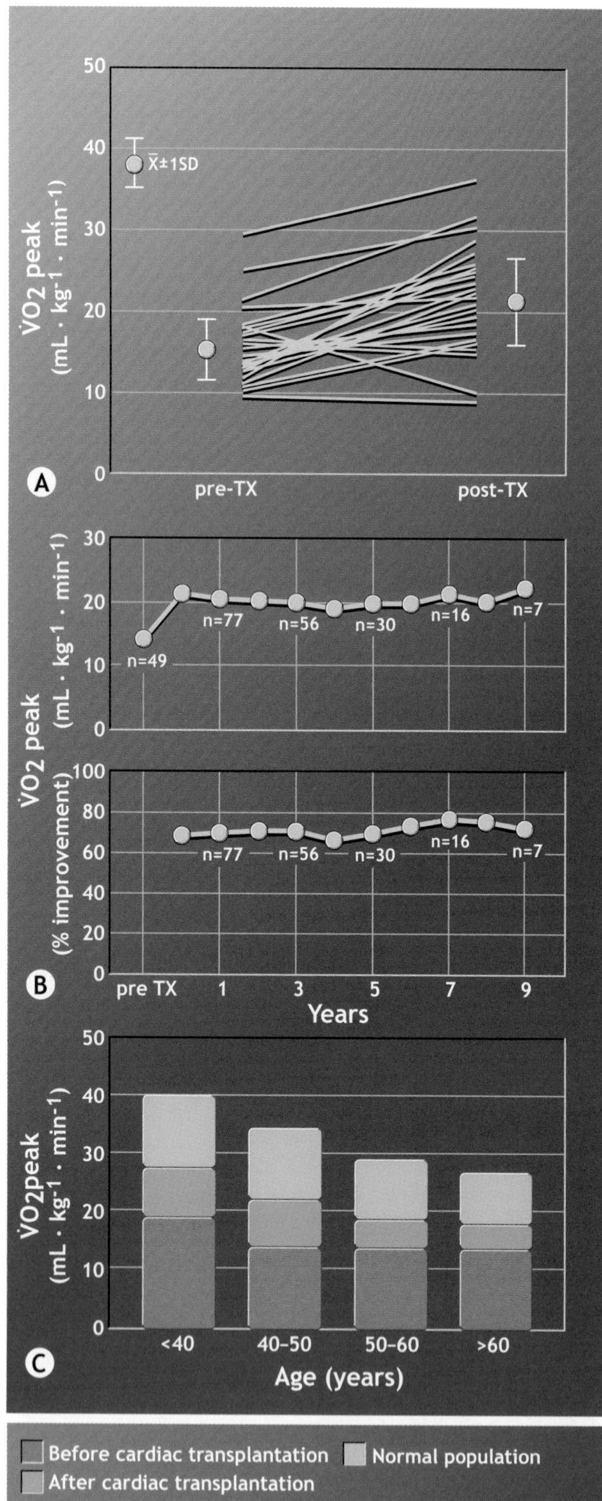

Figure 16.11 • Long-term effects of heart transplantation (TX) on aerobic functional capacity. **A**. $\dot{V}O_{2peak}$ before and 11.2 months after cardiac transplantation in 43 patients who underwent testing at both intervals. Post-TX average significantly higher than pre-TX. **B**. Significant improvements in peak oxygen consumption ($\dot{V}O_{2peak}$) and percentage improvement occurred as early as 6 months after transplantation and remained improved up to 9 years after the transplant procedure. **C**. Impact of age on improvement in $\dot{V}O_{2peak}$ in 43 patients who underwent exercise testing before and 1 year after cardiac transplantation. (From Osada N, et al. Long-term cardiopulmonary exercise performance after heart transplantation. Am J Cardiol 1997;79:451.)

ated prior to transplantation and up to 9 years after the procedure.[46] Cardiac transplantation produced an average 50% improvement in $\dot{V}O_{2peak}$ (Fig. 16.11A) from 14.2 mL · kg^{-1} · min^{-1} before to 21.4 · kg^{-1} · min^{-1} an average of 11.2 months after surgery. In comparing $\dot{V}O_{2peak}$ with that of the typical healthy population, 44% of the patients achieved 50 to 70% of the predicted value, 31% reached 70 to 90%, and several patients achieved more than 90%. The patients maintained improved aerobic capacity up to 9 years postsurgery (Fig. 16.11B). Figure 16.11C shows that the younger patients exhibited the greatest improvement following transplantation.

Sluggish Circulatory Response

An elevated resting heart rate characterizes the denervated heart because the intrinsic activity of the donor SA node governs heart rate. Without extrinsic neural control, the SA node generally depolarizes about 100 times each minute. The short-term exercise response for transplant patients classifies as abnormal. These patients demonstrate limited cardiac output and oxygen consumption during exercise, with accompanying reduced left ventricular ejection capacity. Figure 16.10B reveals that circulatory sluggishness results from the denervated heart's inability to accelerate significantly with increasing exercise demands (often by only 20 to 40 b · min^{-1}).[4,36,61] The exercise response of the denervated transplanted heart does improve over the 12-month postsurgery period. However, the adaptations exert no meaningful effect on submaximal or peak exercise oxygen consumption. In healthy individuals, stroke volume increases up to approximately 50% of $\dot{V}O_{2max}$ and then plateaus; further increases in cardiac output result mainly from heart rate increases. Transplant patients, on the other hand, show an absence of a stroke volume plateau during graded exercise; stroke volume progressively increases by the Frank-Starling mechanism throughout the exercise range. Stroke volume increases represent the primary mechanism for these patients to increase cardiac output during more-intense exercise.[27]

Recent evidence indicates possible reinnervation of the donor heart with parasympathetic cardiac fibers.[67] Thirty-two months after transplantation, two P waves at somewhat different rates were recorded from the hearts of two young, fit transplant patients. These waves appeared to arise from donor *and* recipient SA nodes. They accompanied rapid heart rate acceleration at the start of exercise for both patients. Chapter 32 discusses the effects of exercise training for the heart transplant patient.

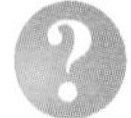

INTEGRATIVE QUESTION

If heart transplantation surgically removes all nerves to the myocardium, explain why heart rate increases for these patients during physical activity.

Focus on Research

Age-Related Changes in Exercise Physiology

Robinson S. Experimental studies of physical fitness in relation to age. Arbeitsphysiologie 1938;10:18.

➤ Robinson's classic research, a comprehensive cross-sectional study, documents the relationship of aging to physiologic responses during rest and exercise in 93 healthy, nonathletic males aged 6 to 91 years. Measurement variables included resting and exercise oxygen consumption ($\dot{V}O_2$), lung volumes, heart rate (HR), arterial blood pressure, submaximal treadmill walking performance at 5.6 km · h^{-1} at an 8.6% incline for 15 minutes, and a 2- to 5-minute treadmill run to exhaustion.

The *top figure* shows that HR_{max} in older men is nearly 20% lower than in young boys. The younger individuals also showed greater variability in HR response to exercise and more-rapid HR acceleration at the start of exercise; their HRs returned to baseline more rapidly in recovery than older subjects. In the *middle figure,* $\dot{V}O_{2peak}$ increased from age 8 to 10 years, declined significantly for the next few years, then increased further until about age 17, and decreased steadily thereafter. Interestingly, Robinson suggested that the $\dot{V}O_{2peak}$ decrease with age probably related to a reduced level of general physical activity and was not necessarily true "aging." Thus, recognition of the deleterious effects of a sedentary lifestyle on cardiovascular function occurred as early as 1938. The *bottom figure* shows pulmonary ventilation relative to body mass (BM; $\dot{V}_E$ · $kgBM^{-1}$ · min^{-1}), breathing rate (breaths · min^{-1}), and tidal air volume (TV) expressed as a percentage of forced vital capacity (TV × 100 ÷ FVC) during maximal exercise. Measures of ventilatory function declined with age, and older men used a greater fraction of FVC as TV than younger men. Boys increased ventilation over resting values principally by increasing breathing frequency; adults increased ventilation by increasing breathing rate and tidal volume.

This pioneering cross-sectional study demonstrated an age–and sedentary lifestyle–related decline in cardiovascular and pulmonary function variables during rest and the full range of exercise intensity. Subsequent research verified Robinson's assertion that a significant component of the functional capacity decline with aging coincides more with lifestyle characteristics than with chronologic age per se.

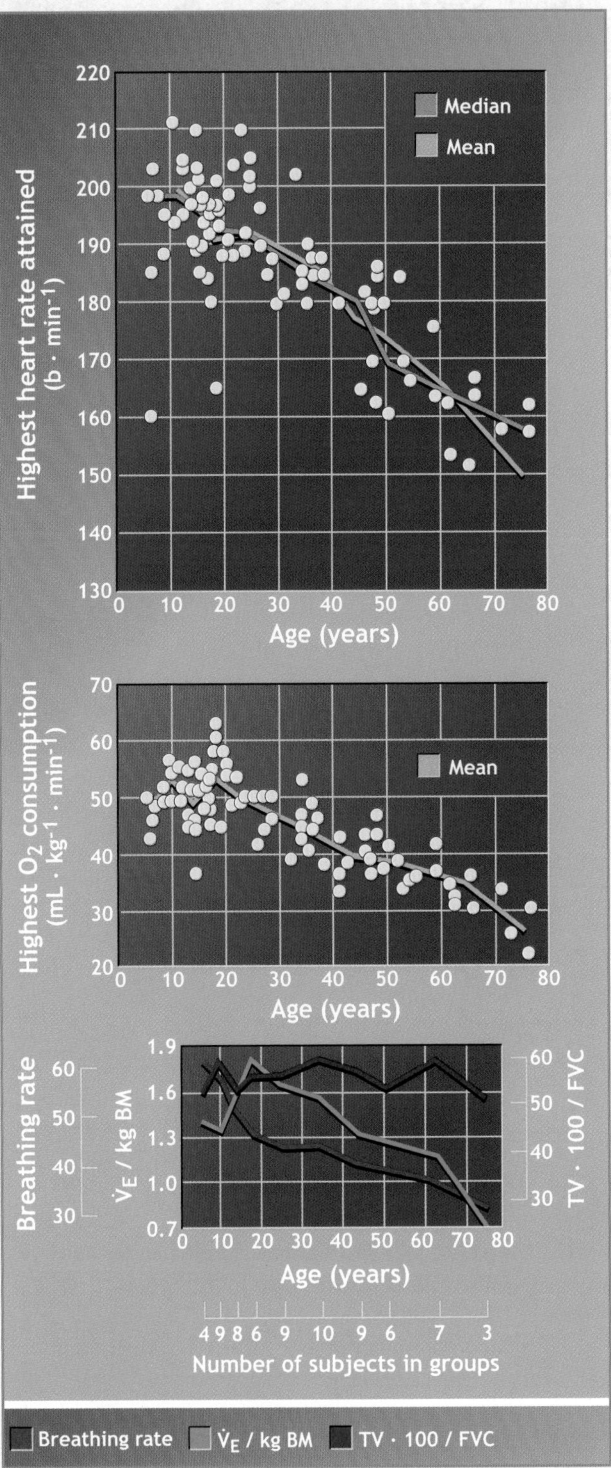

Top. HR_{max} (b · min^{-1}) versus age. *Middle.* $\dot{V}O_{2peak}$ versus age. *Bottom.* Pulmonary minute ventilation ($\dot{V}_E$), breathing rate, and tidal volume (TV) versus age.

Summary

1. The cardiovascular system provides rapid heart rate regulation and effective distribution of blood through the vascular circuit (while maintaining blood pressure) in response to overall metabolic and physiologic needs.
2. The cardiac rhythm originates at the SA node. The impulse then travels across the atria to the AV node. After a brief delay, it spreads across the large ventricular mass. This normal conduction pattern initiates atrial and ventricular contractions to provide impetus for blood flow.
3. The electrocardiogram (ECG) records the sequence of the heart's electrical events during the cardiac cycle. The ECG detects various heart function abnormalities during rest and exercise of increasing intensity.
4. The sympathetic catecholamines epinephrine and norepinephrine accelerate heart rate and increase myocardial contractility. The parasympathetic neurotransmitter hormone acetylcholine acts through the vagus nerve to slow heart rate.
5. The heart "turns on" in the transition from rest to exercise from increased sympathetic and decreased parasympathetic activity integrated with central command input.
6. Cortical influence in anticipation before and during the initial stage of physical activity governs a substantial part of the heart rate adjustment to exercise.
7. Reflex sensory input from peripheral receptors in blood vessels, joints, and muscles provides the cardiovascular center with continual feedback about the physical and chemical state of active muscles.
8. Neural and hormonal extrinsic factors modify the heart's inherent rhythm. The heart rate accelerates in anticipation of exercise and reaches about 200 $b \cdot min^{-1}$ in maximum exercise.
9. Carotid artery palpation usually accesses heart rate accurately during and immediately after exercise.
10. Nerves, hormones, and local metabolic factors act on the smooth muscle bands in blood vessels to alter their internal diameter and regulate blood flow in response to metabolic demands.
11. Blood flow in the vascular circuit changes with the vessels' radius raised to the fourth power in accord with Poiseuille's law. Adrenergic sympathetic fibers release norepinephrine (causes vasoconstriction); no consistent evidence supports the existence of cholinergic sympathetic dilator neurons.
12. Nitric oxide, an extraordinarily important and potent endothelium-derived relaxing factor, facilitates blood vessel dilation and decreases vascular resistance.
13. The kidneys and splanchnic regions can dramatically compromise their blood flow in exercise to augment delivery of blood to the muscles and maintain systemic blood pressure.
14. Patients who successfully undergo orthotopic transplantation have a depressed cardiovascular response to exercise, owing to the denervated heart's inability to accelerate rapidly to meet the demands of physical activity.

References

1. Adreani CM, Kaufman MC. Effect of arterial occlusion on responses of group III and IV afferents to dynamic exercise. J Appl Physiol 1998;84:1827.
2. Aravot D, et al. Functional status and quality of life of heart transplant recipients surviving beyond 5 years. Transplant Proc. 2000;32:731.
3. Armstrong RB, et al. Blood flow distribution in rat muscles during preexercise anticipatory response. J Appl Physiol 1989;67:1855.
4. Badenhop DT. The therapeutic role of exercise in patients with orthotopic heart transplant. Med Sci Sports Exerc 1995;27:975.
5. Balon TW. Integrative biology of nitric oxide and exercise. Exerc Sport Sci Rev 1999;27:219.
6. Bellomo G, et al. Prognostic value of 24-hour blood pressure in pregnancy. JAMA 1999;282:1447.
7. Bevegård BS, Shepherd JT. Regulation of the circulation during exercise in man. Physiol Rev 1967;47:178.
8. Bjornstad H, et al. Ambulatory electrocardiographic findings in top athletes, athletic students and control subjects. Cardiology 1994;84:42.
9. Brubaker PH, et al. Relationship of lactate and ventilatory thresholds in cardiac transplant patients. Med Sci Sports Exerc 1993;25:191.
10. Buckwalter JB, et al. Sympathetic vasoconstriction in active skeletal muscle during dynamic exercise. J Appl Physiol 1997;83:1575.
11. Buckwalter JB, et al. Skeletal muscle vasodilation at the onset of exercise. J Appl Physiol 1998;85:1649.
12. Cardillo C, et al. Racial differences in nitric-oxide mediated vasodilator response to mental stress in forearm circulation. Hypertension 1998;31:1235.
13. Carrasco DI, et al. Effect of concentric and eccentric muscle actions on muscle sympathetic nerve activity. J Appl Physiol 1999;86:558.
14. Couldry WC, et al. Carotid vs. radial pulse counts. Phys Sportsmed 1982;10:67.
15. Daida H, et al. Sequential assessment of exercise tolerance in heart transplantation compared with coronary artery bypass surgery after phase II cardiac rehabilitation. Am J Cardiol 1996;77:696.
16. Delp MD. Differential effects of training on the control of skeletal muscle perfusion. Med Sci Sports Exerc 1998;30:361.
17. Delp MD. Control of skeletal muscle perfusion at the onset of dynamic exercise. Med Sci Sports Exerc 1999;31:1011.

17a. Gandsas A, et al. In-flight continuous vital signs telemetry via the internet. Aviat Space Environ Med 2000;71:68.

17b. Gladwin MT, et al. Role of circulating nitrite and S-nitrosohemoglobin in the regulation of regional blood flow in humans. Proc Natl Acad Sci USA. 2000; 97:11482.

18. Herr MD, et al. Characteristics of the muscle mechanoreflex during quadriceps contractions in humans. J Appl Physiol 1999;86:767.
19. Hosenpud JD, et al. The registry of the International Society for Heart and Lung Transplantation: 15th official report—1998. J Heart Lung Transplant 1998;17:656.
20. Hunt SA. Current status of cardiac transplantation. JAMA 1998;280:1692.
21. Innes JA, et al. Central command influences cardiorespiratory response to dynamic exercise in humans with unilateral weakness. J Physiol (Lond) 1992;448:551.
22. Jasperse JL, Laughlin MH. Vasomotor response of soleus feed arteries from sedentary and exercise-trained rats. J Appl Physiol 1999;86:41.
23. Jia L, et al. *S*-Nitrosohaemoglobin: a dynamic activity of blood involved in vascular control. Nature 1996;380:221.
24. Joannides R, et al. Nitric oxide is responsible for flow-mediated vasodilation is largely responsible for flow-dependent dilatation of human peripheral conduit arteries in vivo. Circulation 1995;91:1314.
25. Joyner MJ, Dietz NM. Nitric oxide and vasodilation in human limbs. J Appl Physiol 1997;83:1785.
26. Kellog DL Jr, et al. Nitric oxide and cutaneous active vasodilation during heat stress in humans. J Appl Physiol 1998;85:824.
27. Keteyain SJ, et al. Cardiovascular responses to submaximal arm and leg exercise in cardiac transplant patients. Med Sci Sports Exerc 1994;26:420.

28. King-Van Vlack CE, et al. Endothelial modulation of neural sympathetic vascular tone in canine skeletal muscle. J Appl Physiol 1998;85:1362.
29. Kjaer M, et al. Heart rate during exercise with leg vascular occlusion in spinal cord-injured patients. J Appl Physiol 1999;86:806.
30. Kriett JM, Kaye MP. The registry of the International Society for Heart Transplantation: seventh official report—1990. J Heart Transplant 1990;9:323.
31. Laughlin MH, et al. Control of blood flow to cardiac and skeletal muscle during exercise, In: Rowell LB, Sheperd JT, eds. Handbook of physiology, exercise: regulation and integration of multiple systems. Bethesda, MD: American Physiological Society, 1996.
32. Maeda S, et al. Exercise causes tissue-specific enhancement of endothelin-1 mRNA expression in internal organs. J Appl Physiol 1998;85:425.
33. Magel JR, et al. Telemetered heart rate response to selected competitive swimming events. J Appl Physiol 1969;26:764.
34. McAllister RM. Adaptations in control of blood flow with training: splanchnic and renal blood flows. Med Sci Sports Exerc 1998;30:375.
35. McArdle WD, et al. Telemetered cardiac response to selected running events. J Appl Physiol 1967;23:566.
36. Mettauer B. $\dot{V}O_2$ kinetics reveal a central limitation at the onset of subthreshold exercise in heart transplant patients. J Appl Physiol 2000;88:1228.
37. Miller VM, Burnett JCJ. Modulation of NO and endothelin by chronic increases in blood flow in canine femoral arteries. Am J Physiol 1992;263:H103.
37a. Monahon KD, et al. Regular aerobic exercise modulates age-associated lines in cardiovagal baroreflex sensitivity in healthy men. J Physiol 2000;529 (Pt1):263
38. Moore AD, et al. Validity of a heart rate monitor during work in the laboratory and on the space shuttle. AIHA J 1997;58:299.
39. Mottaver B, et al. Persistent exercise intolerance following cardiac transplantation despite normal oxygen transport. J Sports Med 1996;17:277.
40. Mueller P, et al. Renal hemodynamic responses to dynamic exercise in rabbits. J Appl Physiol 1998;85:1605.
41. Nóbrega ACL, Araújo CGS. Heart rate transient at the onset of active and passive dynamic exercise. Med Sci Sports Exerc 1993;25:37.
42. Nóbrega ACL, et al. Cardiovascular responses to active and passive cycling movements. Med Sci Sports Exerc 1994;26:709.
43. Notaricus CF, et al. Cardiac versus noncardiac limits to exercise after heart transplantation. Am Heart J 1998;135(2 Pt 1):339.
44. Oldridge NB, et al. Carotid palpation, coronary heart disease, and exercise rehabilitation. Med Sci Sports Exerc 1981;13:6.
45. O'Leary DS. Heart rate control during exercise by baroreceptors and skeletal muscle afferents. Med Sci Sports Exerc 1996;28:210.
46. Osada N, et al. Long-term cardiopulmonary exercise performance after heart transplantation. Am J Cardiol 1997;79:451.
47. Osada N, et al. Cardiopulmonary exercise testing identifies low risk patients with heart failure and severely impaired exercise capacity considered for heart transplantation. J Am Coll Cardiol 1998;31:577.
48. Osada T, et al. Reduced blood flow in abdominal viscera measured by Doppler ultrasound during one-legged knee extension. J Appl Physiol 1999;86:709.
49. Poole DC, et al. Diaphragm structure and function in health and disease. Med Sci Sports Exerc 1997;29:738.
50. Raven PB, et al. Baroreflex regulation of blood pressure during dynamic exercise. Exerc Sport Sci Rev 1997;25:365.
51. Robergs RA, et al. Temporal inhomogeneity in brachial artery blood flow during forearm exercise. Med Sci Sports Exerc 1997;29:1021.
52. Rowell LB. Human cardiovascular control. Cary, NC: Oxford University Press, 1994.
53. Seals DR, Victor RG. Regulation of muscle sympathetic nerve activity during exercise in humans. Exerc Sport Sci Rev 1991;19:313.
54. Seals DR, et al. Exercise and aging: autonomic control of the circulation. Med Sci Sports Exerc 1994;26:568.
55. Sedlock DA, et al. Accuracy of subject-palpated carotid pulse after exercise. Phys Sportsmed 1983;11:106.
56. Segal SS. Communication among endothelial and smooth muscle cells coordinates blood flow control during exercise. News Physiol Sci 1992;7:152.
57. Sessa WC, et al. Chronic exercise in dogs increases coronary vascular nitric oxide production and endothelial cell nitric oxide synthase gene expression. Circ Res 1994;74:349.
58. Shastry S, et al. Effects of nitric oxide synthase inhibition on cutaneous vasodilation during body heating in humans. J Appl Physiol 1998;85:830.
59. Shen W, et al. Nitric oxide production and NO synthase gene expression contribute to vascular regulation during exercise. Med Sci Sports Exerc 1995;27:1125.
60. Shepherd JT, et al. Static (isometric) exercise. Retrospection and introspection. Circ Res 1981;48(suppl I):179.
61. Squirers RW. Exercise training after cardiac transplantation. Med Sci Sports Exerc 1991;23:686.
62. Stebbins CL, et al. Reflex effect of skeletal muscle mechanoreceptor stimulation on the cardiovascular system. J Appl Physiol 1988;65:1539.
63. Stewart JM, et al. Exercise reduces epicardial coronary artery wall stiffness: roles of cGMP and CAMP. Med Sci Sports Exerc 1998;30:220.
64. Strange S, et al. Neural control of cardiovascular responses and of ventilation during dynamic exercise in man. J Physiol (Lond) 1993;70:693.
65. Ville N, et al. Exercise tolerance in heart transplant patients with altered pulmonary diffusion capacity. Med Sci Sports Exerc 1998;30:339.
66. Wang J, et al. Chronic exercise enhances endothelium-mediated dilation of epicardial coronary artery in conscious dogs. Circ Res 1993;73:829.
67. Wesche J, et al. Electrophysiological evidence of reinnervation of the transplanted human heart. Cardiology 1998;89:73.
68. White JR. EKG changes using carotid artery for heart rate monitoring. Med Sci Sports Exerc 1977;9:88.
69. Williamson JW, et al. Instantaneous heart rate increase with dynamic exercise: central command and muscle-heart reflex contributions. J Appl Physiol 1995;78:1273.
70. Zambraski EJ. Body fluid balance. Boca Raton, FL: CRC Press, 1996.
71. Zweifach BJ. The microcirculation of the blood. Sci Am Jan 1959.

CHAPTER 17

Functional Capacity of the Cardiovascular System

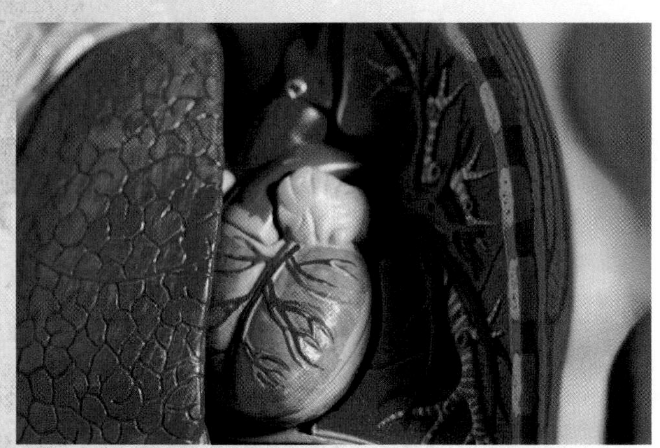

Chapter Objectives

- Describe the direct Fick, indicator dilution, and CO_2 rebreathing techniques to measure cardiac output, and list advantages and disadvantages of each method
- Compare average values for cardiac output during rest and maximal exercise for an endurance-trained and sedentary person
- Explain the influence of each of the components of the Fick equation on $\dot{V}O_{2max}$
- Discuss two physiologic mechanisms that influence stroke volume during exercise
- Contrast the components of cardiac output during rest and maximal exercise for sedentary and endurance-trained individuals
- Discuss the contribution of the Frank-Starling mechanism to augment cardiac output during different exercise modes
- Outline the dynamics of cardiovascular drift and proposed mechanisms for this phenomenon
- Outline the distribution of cardiac output to body tissues during rest and intense aerobic exercise
- Describe the relationship between maximal cardiac output and maximal oxygen consumption among individuals with varied aerobic fitness
- Indicate the factors that contribute to the expansion of the a-$\bar{v}$ O_2 difference during graded exercise
- Contrast cardiovascular and metabolic dynamics during upper-body versus lower-body graded exercise

CARDIAC OUTPUT

Cardiac output ($\dot{Q}$) refers to the amount of blood pumped by the heart during a 1-minute period. The maximal value for cardiac output reflects the functional capacity of the cardiovascular system to meet physical activity demands. Output from the heart, as with any pump, depends on its rate of pumping (**heart rate**; **HR**) and the quantity of blood ejected with each stroke (**stroke volume**; **SV**). Cardiac output computes as follows:

$$\text{Cardiac output} = \text{Heart rate} \times \text{Stroke volume}$$

Measuring Cardiac Output

One can easily determine output from a hose, pump, or faucet by simply opening the valve and collecting and measuring the volume of fluid ejected over a given time. For obvious reasons, this technique does not apply in animals or humans. In addition, any invasive "opening" of the main output vessel in a closed circulatory system dramatically alters normal flow. Three common methods assess cardiac output in humans: (1) direct Fick, (2) indicator dilution, and (3) CO_2 rebreathing.

Direct Fick Method

Knowledge of two factors can determine the output of fluid from a pump in a closed circuit: (1) change in concentration of a substance between the outflow and inflow ports of the pump and (2) total quantity of that substance taken up (or given off) by the fluid in a given time. For cardiovascular dynamics, calculating cardiac output requires knowledge of two factors: (1) average difference between the oxygen content of arterial and mixed-venous blood (**a-$\bar{v}$ O_2 difference**) and (2) oxygen consumption during 1 minute ($\dot{V}O_2$). The question then becomes how much blood circulates during the minute to account for the observed oxygen consumption, given the observed a-$\bar{v}$ O_2 difference. The **Fick equation**, derived by influential German physiologist Adolph Fick in 1870, expresses the relationships among cardiac output, oxygen consumption, and a-$\bar{v}$ O_2 difference.

$$\underset{(\text{mL} \cdot \text{min}^{-1})}{\text{Cardiac output}} = \frac{\dot{V}O_2, \text{ mL} \cdot \text{min}^{-1}}{\underset{(\text{mL per 100 mL blood})}{\text{a-}\bar{v}\ O_2 \text{ difference}}} \times 100$$

Figure 17.1 illustrates the Fick principle for determining cardiac output. In this example, the person consumes 250 mL

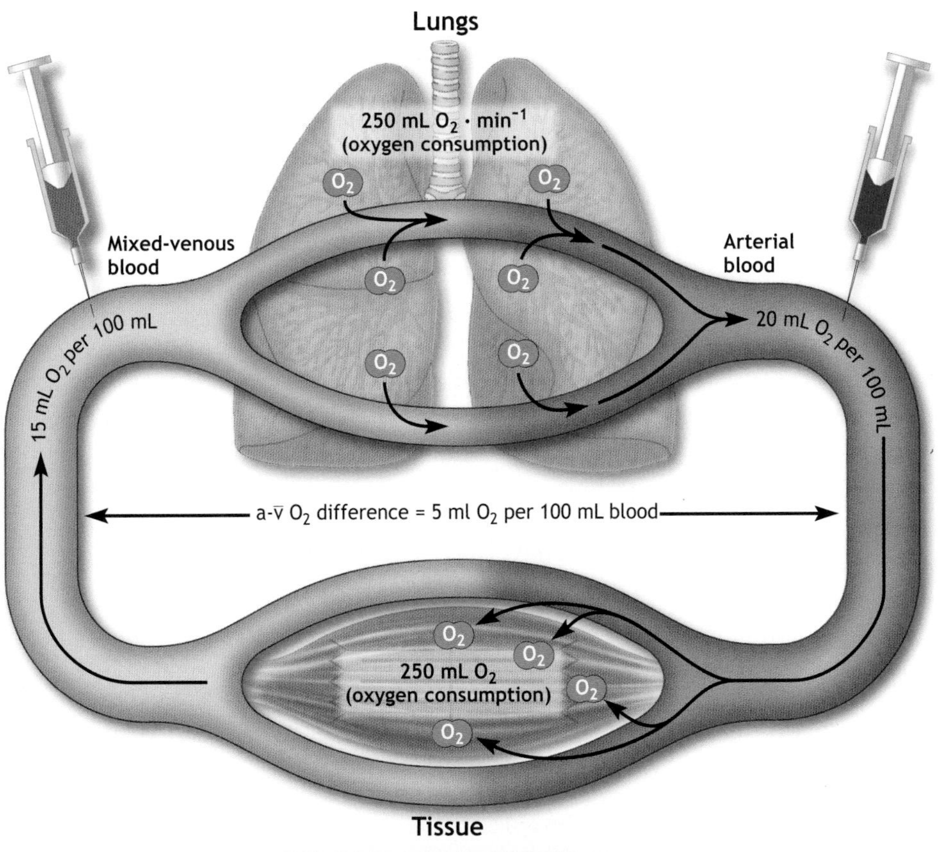

FIGURE 17.1 • The Fick principle for measuring cardiac output per minute ($\dot{Q}$).

of oxygen during 1 minute at rest, and the a-$\bar{v}$ O_2 difference during this time averages 5 mL of oxygen per 100 mL (deciliter, or dL) of blood. Substituting these values in the Fick equation computes cardiac output as follows:

$$\text{Cardiac output } (\text{mL} \cdot \text{min}^{-1}) = \frac{250 \text{ mL } O_2}{5 \text{ mL } O_2} \times 100 = 5000 \text{ mL blood}$$

Although straightforward in principle, the actual Fick method for determining cardiac output requires complex methodology usually limited to a clinical setting where the benefits of measurement exceed any potential risk. Measuring oxygen consumption involves open-circuit spirometry methods summarized in Chapter 8. The more difficult task is determining a-$\bar{v}$ O_2 difference. One can obtain a representative sample of arterial blood from any convenient systemic artery (e.g., femoral, radial, brachial). These arteries are easily located, but the arterial puncture has some risk. Sampling mixed-venous blood presents additional difficulties because the blood in each vein only reflects the metabolic activity of the specific area it drains. An accurate estimate of the average oxygen content of all venous blood requires sampling from an anatomic "mixing chamber" such as the right atrium, right ventricle, or most accurately, the pulmonary artery. Such sampling requires threading a small flexible tube (catheter) through the antecubital vein in the arm into the superior vena cava that leads into the right heart. Arterial and mixed-venous blood are then sampled simultaneously with measurement of oxygen consumption.

Numerous studies of cardiovascular dynamics under various experimental conditions have applied the direct Fick method. The method generally serves as the criterion standard to validate other techniques for cardiac output measurement. The main criticism of the Fick method concerns its *invasiveness*. This most likely alters normal cardiovascular dynamics during the measurement period so that they may not reflect the person's usual cardiovascular response.

Indicator Dilution Method

The **indicator dilution method** involves venous and arterial punctures but does not require cardiac catheterization. A large vein is injected with a known quantity of an inert dye (e.g., indocyanine green) or radioactive substance. The indicator material remains in the vascular stream, usually bound to plasma proteins or red blood cells. It then mixes in the blood as the blood travels to the lungs and back to the heart before ejection throughout the systemic circuit. A radioactive counter or photosensitive device continually assesses arterial blood samples. The area under the dilution-concentration curve (obtained by repetitive sampling) shows the average concentration of indicator material in blood leaving the heart. From the dilution of a known quantity of dye in an unknown quantity of blood, cardiac output computes as follows:

$$\text{Cardiac output} = \frac{\text{Quantity of dye injected}}{\text{Average dye concentration blood for duration of curve} \times \text{Duration of curve}}$$

CO_2 Rebreathing Method

One can determine cardiac output by substituting CO_2 values for O_2 values in the Fick equation.[58] The same open-circuit spirometry method for determining oxygen consumption in the typical Fick technique determines CO_2 production in the rebreathing method. Using a rapid CO_2 gas analyzer and making certain reasonable assumptions concerning gas exchange, one can obtain valid estimates of mixed-venous and arterial CO_2 levels. This noninvasive or "bloodless" technique requires breath-by-breath CO_2 analysis.[2] Values for CO_2 production and mixed-venous and arterial CO_2 concentrations (derived from expired CO_2 obtained during different times) provide the data to compute cardiac output in accordance with the Fick principle as follows:

$$\text{Cardiac output} = \frac{\dot{V}CO_2}{\bar{v}\text{-a } CO_2 \text{ difference}} \times 100$$

The **CO_2 rebreathing method** offers obvious advantages over the direct Fick and indicator dilution methods. It does not require blood sampling or close medical supervision and only minimally interferes with the subject during bicycle ergometer or treadmill exercise. Because the method is noninvasive, it may provide more-accurate estimates of the "real" cardiovascular dynamics during exercise than those obtained with invasive strategies. One limitation of the CO_2 rebreathing method is the requirement that subjects exercise under conditions of steady-rate aerobic metabolism. This restricts the method's use during maximal and "supermaximal" exercise and in the transition from rest to exercise.

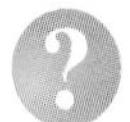

INTEGRATIVE QUESTION

In what ways does the Fick equation fully explain the physiologic components that determine VO_{2max}?

CARDIAC OUTPUT AT REST

Cardiac output varies considerably at rest. Influencing factors include emotional conditions that alter cortical outflow (central command) to the cardioaccelerator nerves and to nerves that modulate the arterial resistance vessels. Each minute, the left ventricle pumps the entire 5-L blood volume of a representative adult male weighing 70 kg. A 5-L cardiac output at rest represents an average value for both trained and untrained males. Resting cardiac output for a representative 56-kg woman averages nearly 4.0 L · min^{-1} (see next section).

Untrained

For the average sedentary person at rest, an average heart rate of 70 b · min^{-1} usually sustains the 5-L cardiac output. Substituting this heart rate value in the cardiac output equation, the heart's calculated stroke volume equals 0.714 L, or 71.4 mL (SV = $\dot{Q} \div$ HR). Stroke volume and cardiac output for women average about 25% below values for men; in women, the stroke volume at rest averages 50 to 60 mL. This "gender difference" generally relates to the average woman's smaller body size.

Endurance Athletes

Endurance training brings the heart's sinus node under greater influence of acetylcholine, the parasympathetic hormone that slows heart rate.[54] At the same time, resting sympathetic activity decreases. This training adaptation partially explains the low resting heart rates of many endurance athletes. However, relatively brief training periods exert little lowering effect on resting heart rate.[65] Heart rates in healthy endurance athletes generally average 50 b · min^{-1} at rest, although heart rates below 30 b · min^{-1} have been reported. Consequently, in athletes, a resting cardiac output of 5 L · min^{-1} circulates with the proportionately larger stroke volume of 100 mL. The following summarizes average values for cardiac output, heart rate, and stroke volume for endurance-trained and untrained men at rest:

Rest

	Cardiac output	=	Heart rate	×	Stroke volume
Untrained:	5000 mL · min^{-1}	=	70 b · min^{-1}	=	71 mL
Trained:	5000 mL · min^{-1}	=	50 b · min^{-1}	=	100 mL

Although straightforward, these computations do not clarify the underlying physiologic mechanisms for the different response patterns of trained and untrained persons. For example, does bradycardia with endurance training "cause" a larger stroke volume or vice versa, because the myocardium itself may respond more forcefully in response to regular aerobic exercise? Two factors probably operate with endurance-trained athletes:

1. Increased vagal tone and decreased sympathetic drive, both of which slow the heart
2. Increased blood volume, myocardial contractility, and compliance of the left ventricle, which augment the heart's stroke volume

CARDIAC OUTPUT DURING EXERCISE

Systemic blood flow increases directly with exercise intensity. Cardiac output increases rapidly during the transition from rest to steady-rate exercise. Thereafter, cardiac output rises gradually until it reaches a plateau when blood flow meets the exercise metabolic requirements.

In sedentary, college-aged males, cardiac output during maximal exercise increases four times above the resting level to an average maximum of 20 to 22 L · min^{-1}. Maximum heart rate for these young adults averages 195 b · min^{-1}. Consequently, the stroke volume generally ranges between 103 and 113 mL (20,000 mL · min^{-1} ÷ 195 b · min^{-1} = 103 mL · b^{-1}; 22,000 mL · min^{-1} ÷ 195 b · min^{-1} = 113 mL). In contrast, world-class endurance athletes achieve maximum cardiac outputs of 35 to 40 L · min^{-1}. This high value assumes greater significance when one considers that the trained person generally achieves a slightly *lower* maximum heart rate than the sedentary person of similar age.[32,37] *Thus, the endurance athlete achieves a large maximal cardiac output solely through a large stroke volume.* For example, the cardiac output of an Olympic medal winner in cross-country skiing increased to 40 L · min^{-1} in maximum exercise (almost 8 times above rest); the stroke volume was 210 mL. This is nearly double the maximum volume of blood pumped per beat by a sedentary counterpart. As a point of comparison among species, cardiac outputs of 600 L · min^{-1} (accompanying 120 to 150 mL · kg^{-1} · min^{-1} $\dot{V}O_{2max}$) have been reported in thoroughbred racehorses.[13,39]

The following summarizes average values for cardiac output, heart rate, and stroke volume of endurance-trained and untrained men during maximal exercise.

Maximum Exercise

	Cardiac output	=	Heart rate	×	Stroke volume
Untrained:	22,000 mL	=	195 b · min^{-1}	=	113 mL
Trained:	35,000 mL	=	195 b · min^{-1}	=	179 mL

Stroke Volume: Diastolic Filling Versus Systolic Emptying

Three physiologic mechanisms increase the heart's stroke volume during exercise. The first, intrinsic to the myocardium, involves enhanced cardiac filling in diastole, followed by a more forceful systolic contraction. Neurohormonal influence governs the second mechanism, which involves normal ventricular filling with a subsequent forceful ejection and emptying during systole. The third mechanism for increased stroke volume results from training adaptations that expand blood volume and reduce resistance to blood flow in peripheral tissues.[14,15,23,57,59]

Enhanced Diastolic Filling

Any factor that increases venous return or slows the heart produces greater ventricular filling (**preload**) during the cardiac cycle's diastolic phase. An increase in **end-diastolic volume** stretches myocardial fibers and initiates a powerful ejection stroke during contraction. This ejects the normal stroke volume plus any additional blood that entered the ventricles and stretched the myocardium.

Two researchers, German physiologist Otto Frank (1865–1944) and British physiologist Ernest Starling (1866–1927), described the relationship between contractile force and the resting length of the heart's muscle fibers. This phenomenon, **Starling's law of the heart**, always operates during the cardiac cycle and applies to all of the heart's chambers. For years, physiologists taught that the Frank-Starling mechanism

TABLE 17.1 ➤ MAXIMAL VALUES FOR OXYGEN CONSUMPTION, HEART RATE, STROKE VOLUME, AND CARDIAC OUTPUT IN THREE GROUPS WITH VERY LOW, NORMAL, AND HIGH AEROBIC CAPACITIES

GROUP	$\dot{V}O_{2MAX}$ (L · MIN^{-1})	MAX HEART RATE (B · MIN^{-1})	MAX STROKE VOLUME (ML)	MAX CARDIAC OUTPUT (L · MIN^{-1})
Mitral stenosis	1.6	190	50	9.5
Sedentary	3.2	200	100	20.0
Athlete	5.2	190	160	30.4

Modified from Rowell LB: Circulation. Med Sci Sports 1969;1:15.

provided the modus operandi for *all* stroke volume increases during exercise. They believed that venous return in exercise facilitated greater cardiac filling. This preload stretched the ventricles in diastole, producing a more forceful ejection. More than likely, this response pattern for stroke volume operates during the transition from rest to exercise or as a person moves from an upright to a recumbent position. Enhanced diastolic filling also occurs in swimming because the body's horizontal position optimizes venous return. A more optimal arrangement of the sarcomere's myofilaments as the muscle fiber stretches probably enhances contractility.

The data in Table 17.1 show the clear effect of body position on circulatory dynamics.[3] The horizontal position produces the largest and most stable cardiac output and stroke volume. Stroke volume remains near maximum in this position at rest and increases only slightly during exercise. In contrast, in the upright position, gravity counters the return flow of blood to the heart (decreased preload), diminishing stroke volume and cardiac output. During upright exercise of increasing intensity, stroke volume increases and approaches the maximum stroke volume in the supine position.

Greater Systolic Emptying

In most forms of upright exercise, the heart does not fill to increase cardiac volume significantly, as it does in the recumbent position. Despite research inconsistencies on this topic, the progressive increase in stroke volume during graded upright exercise results from the *combined effect* of enhanced diastolic filling and more-complete emptying during systole.[8,15,34,52] Greater systolic ejection occurs despite increased resistance to blood flow in the arterial circuit from exercise-induced elevation of systolic blood pressure (**afterload**), which acts to reduce ventricular contraction velocity.[38]

Enhanced systolic ejection, with or without increased end-diastolic volume, occurs because the ventricles always contain a **functional residual volume of blood**. At rest in the upright position, approximately 40% of the total end-diastolic blood volume (50 to 70 mL) remains in the left ventricle after systole. Catecholamine release in exercise enhances myocardial contractile force, which augments stroke power to facilitate systolic emptying.

More than likely, endurance training increases compliance of the left ventricle (reduced cardiac stiffness) to facilitate its ability to accept blood in the diastolic phase of the cardiac cycle.[27,28,35,67] Whether endurance training enhances the myocardium's innate contractile state remains unclear.[39] If this adaptation does occur, it too would contribute to a larger stroke volume.

Cardiovascular Drift: Reduced Stroke Volume and Increased Heart Rate During Prolonged Exercise

Submaximal exercise for more than 15 minutes, particularly in the heat, produces progressive water loss through sweating and a fluid shift from plasma to tissues. A rise in core temperature also causes redistribution of blood to the periphery for body cooling. At the same time, the progressive fall in plasma volume decreases central venous cardiac filling pressure (preload), which reduces stroke volume. A reduced stroke volume initiates a compensatory heart rate increase to maintain a nearly constant cardiac output as exercise progresses. The term **cardiovascular drift** describes the gradual time-dependent downward "drift" in several cardiovascular responses, most notably stroke volume (with concomitant heart rate increase), during prolonged steady-rate exercise. Under these circumstances, a person must exercise at a lower intensity than if cardiovascular drift did not occur.[4,9,20,44]

One explanation for cardiovascular drift suggests the effects of a progressive increase in cutaneous blood flow with a core temperature rise in prolonged exercise. Increased redistribution of blood to the periphery for heat dissipation increases the skin's venous volume, ultimately reducing ventricular filling pressure and stroke volume. Recent evidence provides an alternative explanation for the stroke volume decline during cardiovascular drift in prolonged exercise.[12] Figure 17.2 shows responses for heart rate, stroke volume, and cutaneous blood flow for seven active men during 60 minutes of cycling at 57% of $\dot{V}O_{2peak}$ in a thermoneutral environment. In one exercise trial the men received a placebo; in the other trial they received, at the onset of exercise, a small dose of the β_1-adrenoceptor blocker atenolol to prevent the increase in heart rate that occurs after 15 minutes of exercise to the end. Fifteen minutes into exercise, heart rate and stroke volume remained similar during control and β_1-adrenoceptor blockade conditions. From 15 to 55 minutes during the control trial, a 13% decrease in stroke volume accompanied an 11% heart rate increase, while cutaneous blood flow did not increase from 20 to 60 minutes of exercise. However, from 15 to 55 minutes of exercise under blockade conditions (when atenolol prevented a heart rate increase), stroke volume failed to decline compared with control conditions, despite similar levels of cutaneous blood flow in both trials. Cardiac output remained stable at about 16 L · min^{-1} under both conditions. These observations confirm that a stroke volume decline during prolonged exercise in a thermoneutral environment relates to increased exercise heart rate and *not* increased cutaneous blood flow. More than likely, the progressive increase in heart rate with cardiovascular drift during exercise decreases end-diastolic volume, subsequently reducing the heart's stroke volume.

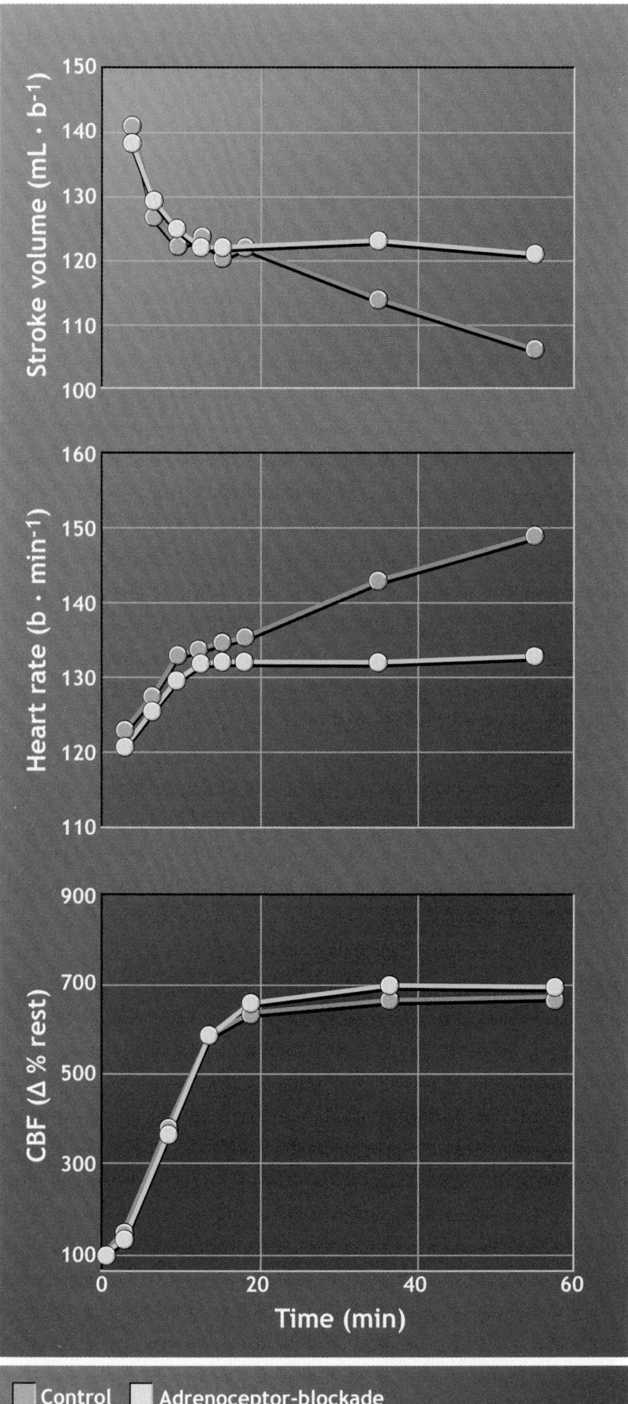

FIGURE 17.2 • Stroke volume, heart rate, and laser Doppler cutaneous blood flow (CBF) during 60 minutes of exercise under β_1-adrenoceptor blockade and control treatments. (From Fritzsche RG, et al. Stroke volume decline during prolonged exercise is influenced by the increase in heart rate. J Appl Physiol 1999;86:799.)

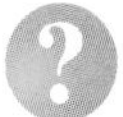

INTEGRATIVE QUESTION

Moderate increases in hemoglobin concentration increase $\dot{V}O_{2max}$ during maximal exercise at sea level. This effect supports the contention that what component of the Fick equation limits maximal oxygen consumption? Discuss.

CARDIAC OUTPUT DISTRIBUTION

Blood generally flows to tissues in proportion to their metabolic activity. Blood flow to the kidneys, skin, and splanchnic areas, however, also varies with the metabolic demands of skeletal muscle during physical activity.

Blood Flow at Rest

At rest in a comfortable environment, the typical 5-L cardiac output generally distributes in the proportions shown in Figure 17.3A. Approximately one-fifth of the cardiac output flows to muscle tissue, while the digestive tract, liver, spleen, brain, and kidneys receive major portions of the remaining blood.

Blood Flow During Exercise

Figure 17.3B illustrates the percentage distribution of cardiac output during light, moderate, and strenuous exercise. *Environmental stress, level of fatigue, and exercise mode and intensity affect regional blood flow, but the major portion of the exercise cardiac output diverts to the active muscles.* Approximately 4 to 7 mL of blood flows each minute to each 100 g of muscle at rest. This flow increases steadily in graded exercise, with active muscle receiving up to 50 to 75 mL per 100 g of tissue during each minute of maximum exertion.[46] Blood flow within active muscle is highly regulated. The greatest quantity of blood diverts to the oxidative portions of the muscle at the expense of those areas with high glycolytic capacity.[7,25] Thus, peak blood flow values in a small portion of active quadriceps muscle achieves a perfusion as high as 300 to 400 mL · 100 g^{-1} · min^{-1}.[41–43] During "big muscle" activities such as running and cycling at maximum intensity, muscle blood flow accounts for 80 to 85% of the total cardiac output.[47]

Redistribution of Blood

Increases in cardiac output contribute greatly to increased muscle blood flow during exercise. In addition, blood flow to muscle increases disproportionately relative to flow to other tissues. For trained individuals, blood redistribution—from one organ

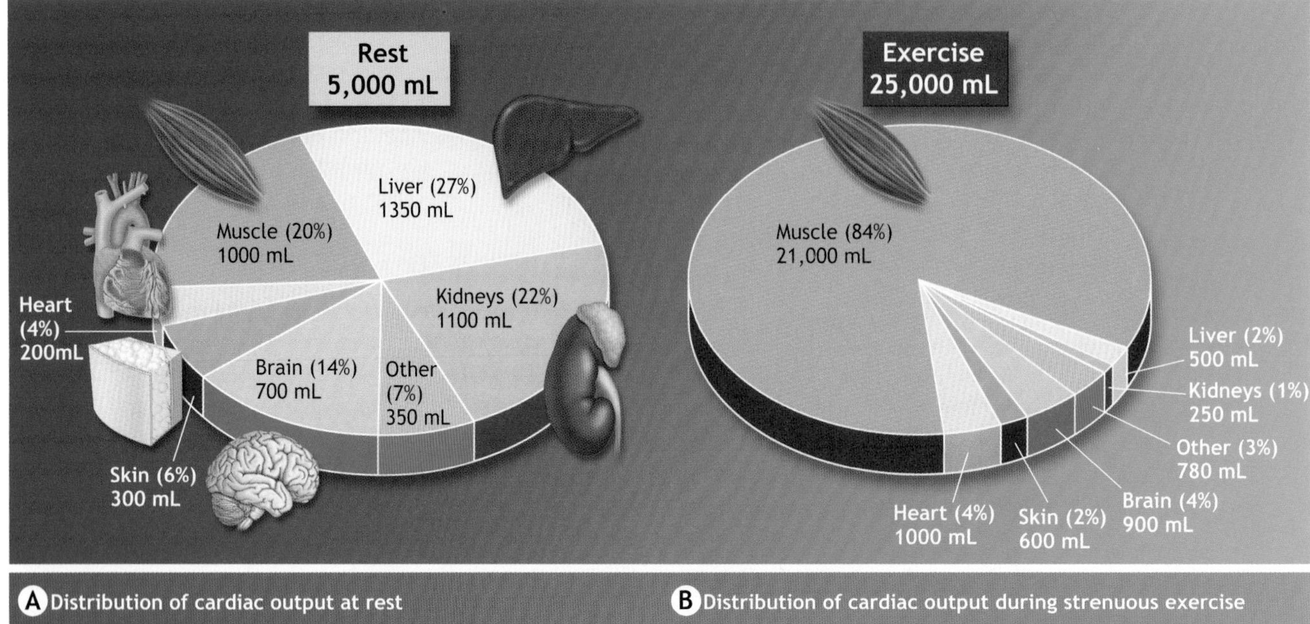

FIGURE 17.3 • Relative distribution of cardiac output during rest (**A**) and strenuous endurance exercise (**B**). The number in parentheses indicates percentage of the total cardiac output. Note that despite its large absolute mass, muscle tissue at rest receives about the same quantity of blood as the much smaller kidneys. In strenuous exercise, however, approximately 84% of the cardiac output diverts to the active muscles.

to another by vasoconstriction in one and vasodilation in the other—actually begins in the anticipatory period just prior to exercise.[7] Two factors, hormonal vascular regulation and local metabolic conditions, cause blood to route through active muscles from areas that temporarily tolerate compromised blood flow.[31] Blood redistribution among specific tissues occurs primarily during high-intensity exercise. For example, blood flow to the skin, the primary heat-exchange organ, increases during light and moderate exercise in relation to the rise in core temperature.[19,68] During near-maximal effort, however, the skin restricts its blood flow, redirecting it to active muscle, even in a hot environment.[43] The kidneys and splanchnic tissues consume only 10 to 25% of the oxygen in their normal blood supply. Consequently, these tissues tolerate a considerably reduced blood flow before oxygen demand exceeds supply and compromises function.[36] Renal blood flow can decrease up to four-fifths of the blood supply at rest. Increased oxygen extraction from the available blood supply generally maintains the oxygen needs of tissues with reduced blood flow. The visceral organs sustain a substantially reduced blood supply for more than 1 hour during heavy exercise. Redistribution of 2 to 3 L of blood away from these tissues "frees" up to 600 mL of oxygen each minute for use by active muscles.[43] Sustained blood flow reduction to the liver and kidneys, however, may contribute to fatigue often experienced during prolonged submaximal exercise. Regular aerobic training blunts the typical vasoconstrictor response to splanchnic and renal tissues.[31] Capacity to maintain blood flow to the liver and kidneys during sustained exercise probably contributes to improved endurance.

Blood Flow to the Heart and Brain

Some tissues cannot compromise their blood supply (Fig. 17.3). At rest, the myocardium normally uses approximately 75% of the oxygen in the blood flowing through the coronary circulation. With such a limited margin of reserve, increased coronary blood flow during exercise primarily supplies the increased myocardial oxygen needs. Thus, a four- to fivefold increase in coronary circulation accompanies a similar increase in myocardial work during exercise; this amounts to a blood flow of about 1 L · min^{-1} during maximum exercise. Cerebral blood flow also increases during exercise by approximately 25 to 30%, compared with the resting flow.[16,60]

CARDIAC OUTPUT AND OXYGEN TRANSPORT

Rest

Arterial blood carries approximately 200 mL of oxygen per liter in a person with a normal hemoglobin level (see Chapter 13). If resting cardiac output each minute equals 5 L, potentially 1000 mL of oxygen becomes available to the body (5 L blood × 200 mL O_2). Because the resting oxygen consumption typically averages 250 to 300 mL · min^{-1}, 750 mL of oxygen returns unused to the heart. This does not reflect an unnecessary waste of cardiac output. Instead, the extra oxygen circulating above the resting requirement represents oxygen in reserve—a margin of safety should a tissue's metabolism suddenly increase dramatically.

Exercise

A healthy, young adult with a maximum heart rate of 200 b · min^{-1} and stroke volume of 80 mL (0.08 L) generates a maximum cardiac output of 16 L · min^{-1} (200 × 0.08 L). Even during maximum exercise, hemoglobin saturation with oxygen remains nearly complete, so each liter of arterial blood carries about 200 mL of oxygen. Consequently, 3200 mL of oxygen circulates each minute via a 16-L cardiac output (16 L × 200 mL O_2 · L^{-1}). Even if the tissues could extract all of the oxygen from all of the blood as it traveled throughout the body, the $\dot{V}O_{2max}$ could not exceed 3200 mL. This represents a purely theoretical value because the oxygen needs of some tissues such as the brain and skin do not increase markedly with exercise, even though they still require a substantial blood supply.

Based on the preceding example, increasing the heart's stroke volume from 80 to 200 mL while maintaining the maximum heart rate at 200 b · min^{-1} dramatically increases maximum cardiac output to 40 L · min^{-1}. This represents a 2.5-fold increase in oxygen circulated during each minute of exercise (from 3200 to 8000 mL). *An increase in maximum cardiac output clearly produces a proportionate increase in capacity to circulate oxygen and profoundly affects an individual's maximal oxygen consumption.*

Close Association Between Maximum Cardiac Output and $\dot{V}O_{2max}$

Figure 17.4 shows the close relationship between maximum cardiac output and the capacity to achieve a high level of aerobic exercise metabolism. $\dot{V}O_{2max}$ values represent averages for the sedentary person to the elite endurance athlete. An unmistakable association exists—a low maximal oxygen consumption corresponds closely with a low maximum cardiac output, whereas ability to generate a 5- or 6-L $\dot{V}O_{2max}$ invariably accompanies a 30- to 40-L cardiac output.

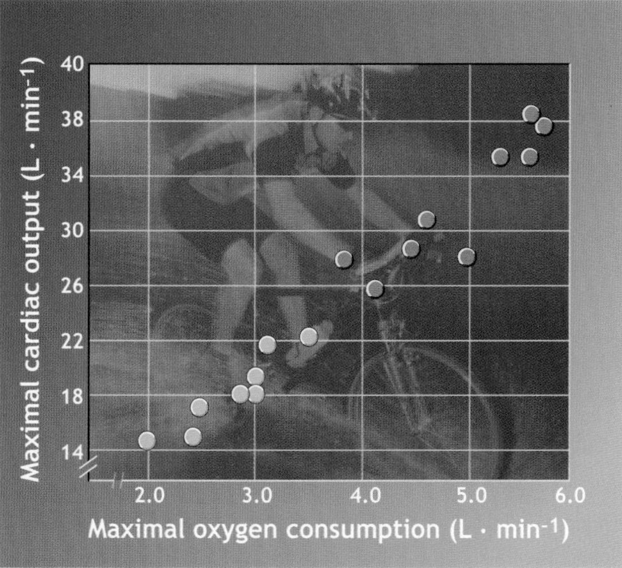

FIGURE 17.4 • Relationship between maximal cardiac output and maximal oxygen consumption ($\dot{V}O_{2max}$) in trained and untrained individuals. Maximal cardiac output relates to $\dot{V}O_{2max}$ in the ratio of about 6:1.

A 5- to 6-L increase in blood flow accompanies each 1-L increase in oxygen consumption above the resting value; this relationship remains essentially unchanged regardless of exercise mode over a broad range of dynamic exercises.[29] *High levels of maximal oxygen consumption and cardiac output provide distinguishing characteristics for preadolescent and adult endurance athletes.*[50,56] An almost proportionate increase in maximum cardiac output accompanies increases in $\dot{V}O_{2max}$ with endurance training (see Chapter 21).

Cardiac Output Differences Among Men and Women and Children

Cardiac output and oxygen consumption remain linearly related during graded exercise for boys and girls and men and women. However, teenage and adult females exercise at any level of *submaximal* oxygen consumption with a 5 to 10% *larger* cardiac output than males,[1,54] although this difference does not emerge consistently.[40] Any apparent gender difference in submaximal cardiac output most likely results from the 10% lower hemoglobin concentration in women than in men. A proportionate increase in submaximal cardiac output compensates for this small decrease in the blood's oxygen-carrying capacity.

Higher heart rates in children than in adults during submaximal treadmill and cycle ergometer exercise do not fully compensate for their smaller stroke volume. This produces a smaller cardiac output for children at a given submaximal exercise oxygen consumption.[22,49,63] Consequently, the a-$\bar{v}$ O_2 difference expands to satisfy the oxygen requirements. The biologic significance remains unclear of this difference in central circulatory function between children and adults. Comparisons of cardiac responses (stroke volume, aortic peak blood flow velocity, systolic ejection time) between prepubertal children and adults fail to demonstrate any age-related exercise impairment.[48]

Oxygen Extraction: The a-$\bar{v}$ O_2 Difference

If only blood flow increased a tissue's oxygen supply, then increasing cardiac output from 5 L · min^{-1} at rest to 100 L · min^{-1} during maximum exercise would achieve the 20-fold oxygen consumption increase common among endurance athletes. Fortunately, strenuous exercise does not require this large cardiac output. Instead, hemoglobin releases a considerable quantity of its "reserve" oxygen from blood perfusing active tissues. Exercise oxygen consumption increases by two mechanisms:

1. Increase in the total quantity of blood pumped by the heart (i.e., increased cardiac output).
2. Greater use of the relatively large quantity of oxygen already carried by the blood (i.e., expanding the a-$\bar{v}$ O_2 difference).

Rearranging the Fick equation summarizes the important relationship among cardiac output, a-$\bar{v}$ O_2 difference, and $\dot{V}O_2$ as follows:

$$\dot{V}O_2 = \dot{Q} \times \text{a-}\bar{v}\ O_2 \text{ difference}$$

a-$\bar{v}$ O_2 Difference During Rest

Resting metabolism uses an average of 5 mL of oxygen from the 20 mL of oxygen in each deciliter of arterial blood (50 mL per liter) that passes through the tissue capillaries. This represents an a-$\bar{v}$ O_2 difference of 5 mL of oxygen per every deciliter of blood perfusing the tissue-capillary bed. Thus, 15 mL of oxygen, or 75% of the blood's original oxygen load, still remains bound to hemoglobin.

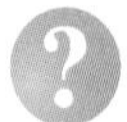

INTEGRATIVE QUESTION

How would factors that influence the a-$\bar{v}$ O_2 difference in maximal exercise explain the specificity of $\dot{V}O_{2max}$ improvement with different modes of aerobic training?

a-$\bar{v}$ O_2 Difference During Exercise

Figure 17.5 shows a progressive expansion of the a-$\bar{v}$ O_2 difference from rest to maximum exercise for physically active men. A similar pattern emerges for women, except that the arterial oxygen content averages 5 to 10% lower because of their lower hemoglobin concentrations. The figure includes values for the oxygen content of arterial and mixed-venous blood during different exercise oxygen consumptions. Arterial blood oxygen content varies little from its value of 20 mL · dL^{-1} at rest throughout the full exercise intensity range. In contrast, mixed-venous oxygen content varies between 12 and 15 mL · dL^{-1} during rest to a low of 2 to 4 mL · dL^{-1} during maximum exercise. The difference between arterial and mixed-venous blood oxygen content at any time (i.e., the a-$\bar{v}$ O_2 difference) represents oxygen extraction from arterial blood as it circulates throughout the body.

The progressive expansion of the a-$\bar{v}$ O_2 difference to at least three times resting value occurs from a reduced venous oxygen content, which in maximal exercise approaches 20 mL · 100 mL^{-1} in active muscle (all oxygen extracted). The oxygen content of a true mixed-venous sample from the pulmonary artery rarely falls below 2 to 4 mL · dL^{-1} because blood returning from active tissues mixes with oxygen-rich venous blood from metabolically less active regions.

As shown in Figure 17.5, the capacity of each 100 mL of arterial blood to carry oxygen actually increases during exercise. This results from an increased concentration of red blood cells (hemoconcentration) owing to the progressive movement of fluid from the plasma to the interstitial space with (1) increases in capillary hydrostatic pressure as blood pressure rises and (2) metabolic byproducts of exercise metabolism that create an osmotic pressure that draws fluid from the plasma into tissue spaces.

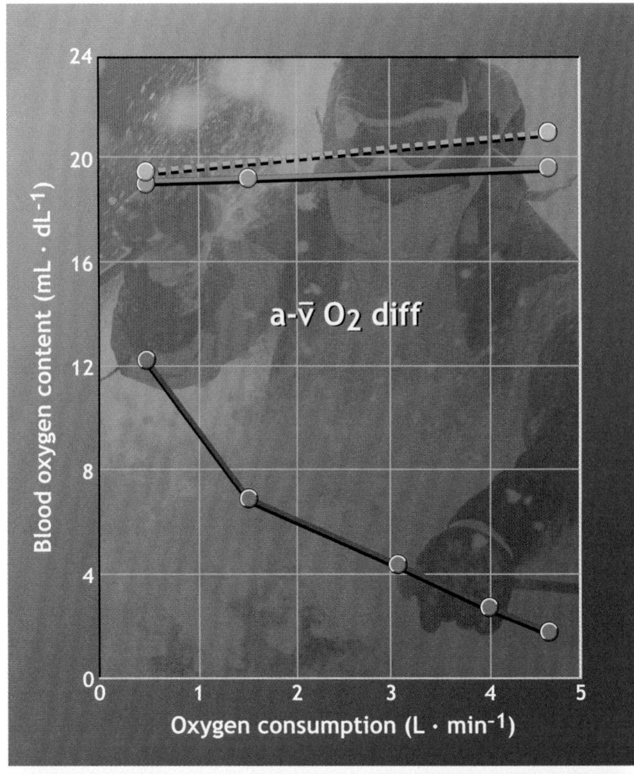

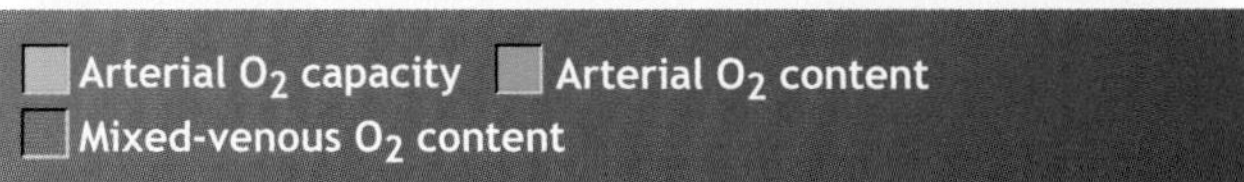

FIGURE 17.5 • Changes in a-$\bar{v}$ O_2 difference from rest to maximal exercise in physically active men.

Severe Heart Disease

The myocardium of patients with advanced coronary artery disease shows impaired capacity to perform work or to improve its function with regular exercise. These individuals exhibit negligible training adaptations in maximal stroke volume and cardiac output. Nevertheless, they can improve exercise tolerance and $\dot{V}O_{2max}$ because regular aerobic exercise increases skeletal muscles' ability to receive, extract, and metabolize oxygen. These adaptations expand the a-$\bar{v}$ O_2 difference, enabling patients to exercise at higher intensities or at submaximal levels with a lower cardiac output. A reduced submaximal exercise cardiac output also decreases myocardial workload, which greatly benefits patients with exertional angina.

Factors Affecting the Exercise a-$\bar{v}$ O_2 Difference

Central and peripheral factors interact to increase oxygen extraction in active tissue during exercise. Diverting a large portion of the cardiac output to active muscles influences the magnitude of the a-$\bar{v}$ O_2 difference in maximal exercise. As mentioned previously, some tissues temporarily compromise their blood supply during exercise by redistributing blood to make more oxygen available for muscle metabolism. Exercise training facilitates redirection of the central circulation to active muscle.

Focus on Research

Consequences of Stopping Regular Exercise

Coyle EF, et al. Time course of loss of adaptations after stopping prolonged intense endurance training. J Appl Physiol 1984;57:1857.

➤ Considerable research frames our understanding about physiologic and metabolic adaptations to diverse types of exercise training. Much less attention has focused on what happens when training stops. A clearer picture of the dynamics of "detraining" would clarify the importance of regular physical activity and the consequences of adapting a sedentary lifestyle.

Coyle and colleagues studied cessation of exercise training in seven highly trained runners or cyclists. Subjects had trained for 10 to 12 months at least 5 days per week for 60 minutes daily at 70 to 80% of $\dot{V}O_{2max}$. Fifty-seven sedentary subjects served as controls. Testing included muscle biopsies on the last day of training and on days 12, 21, 56, and 84 of detraining. Physiologic variables included oxygen consumption ($\dot{V}O_2$), cardiac output ($\dot{Q}$), heart rate (HR), stroke volume (SV), and arteriovenous oxygen difference (a-$\bar{v}$ O_2 diff) during 15 minutes of exercise at 75% of $\dot{V}O_{2max}$ and at $\dot{V}O_{2max}$. The muscle biopsy included the left gastrocnemius for runners and vastus lateralis for cyclists.

Except for exercise during testing, the subjects limited their physical activity to the minimal level required in their sedentary jobs and walked less than 500 m a day at a slow pace. The inset figure shows average changes in physiologic variables at each testing session. $\dot{V}O_{2max}$ decreased in all subjects, declining 7% below training levels after 12 days, 14% after 56 days, and 16% by day 84. ($\dot{Q}$), SV, and a-$\bar{v}$ O_2 $diff_{max}$ each declined significantly while HR_{max} increased during detraining. Stroke volume decreased by 11% during the first 12 days and stabilized at 86% of the trained value by day 56. No further decreases occurred in the final 4 weeks. The increase in HR_{max} partially compensated for the decrease in SV_{max}. Thus, $\dot{Q}_{max}$ declined by only 8% during the initial 3 weeks of detraining, with an average total decrease of 10% over 84 days.

The muscle biopsy data also indicated impressive detraining changes. Citrate synthase and succinate dehydrogenase, major enzymes of aerobic respiration, declined in parallel to reach their lowest levels at day 56. However, detraining did not affect myoglobin levels or muscle capillarization. Because capillary density did not change with detraining, the researchers attributed the decreased oxygen extraction (a-$\bar{v}$ O_2 $diff_{max}$) to reduced mitrochondrial capacity reflected in depressed respiratory enzyme levels.

This study confirmed that decreases in maximum SV (central factor) and a-$\bar{v}$ O_2 diff (peripheral factor) contributed to reductions in $\dot{V}O_{2max}$ with detraining. The results thus support the age-old dictum, "use it or lose it."

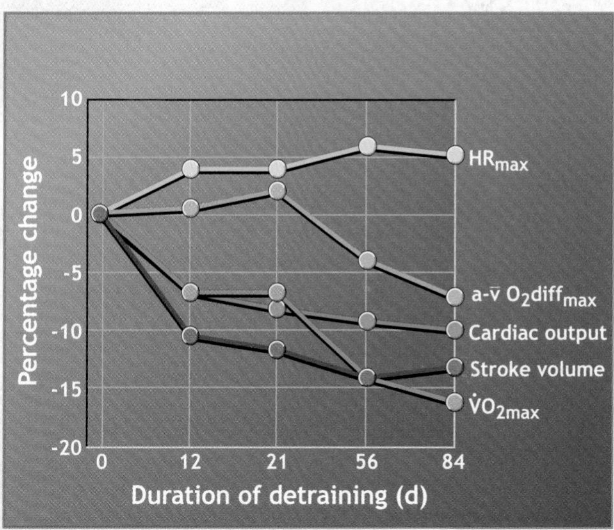

Average changes in maximum heart rate (HR_{max}), stroke volume, arteriovenous oxygen differences (a-$\bar{v}$ O_2 $diff_{max}$), cardiac output, and $\dot{V}O_{2max}$ over 84 days of detraining.

Increases in skeletal muscle microcirculation also increase tissue oxygen extraction.[5,24] Muscle biopsy specimens from the quadriceps femoris show a relatively large ratio of capillaries to muscle fibers in individuals who exhibit large a-$\bar{v}$ O_2 differences in intense exercise. An increase in the capillary to fiber ratio reflects a positive adaptation that enlarges the interface for nutrient and metabolic gas exchange during exercise. Individual muscle cells' ability to generate energy aerobically represents another important factor governing oxygen extraction capacity.

Other factors such as increasing the size and number of mitochondria as well as increasing aerobic enzyme activity also improve a muscle's metabolic capacity in exercise.[17,18] Finally, local vascular and metabolic improvements within muscle ultimately enhance its capacity to produce ATP aerobically,[66] which translates to an increased oxygen extraction capacity.

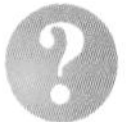

INTEGRATIVE QUESTION

Present a physiologic rationale to support or refute the contention that either (1) central circulatory factors or (2) peripheral factors residing within the active muscle mass limit $\dot{V}O_{2max}$.

CARDIOVASCULAR ADJUSTMENTS TO UPPER-BODY EXERCISE

Exercise with the upper body produces significantly different metabolic and cardiovascular responses than exercise requiring predominantly activation of the leg musculature.

Maximal Oxygen Consumption

The highest oxygen consumption achieved during arm exercise generally averages 20 to 30% lower than that with leg exercise.[34,51] Similarly, arm exercise produces significantly lower maximal values for heart rate and pulmonary ventilation.[30,64] The relatively smaller muscle mass activated in arm exercise compared with that activated in leg exercise accounts for such differences in maximal physiologic variables.

In a Practical Sense

Predicting $\dot{V}O_{2max}$ Using Running and Swimming Tests

The 1.5-mile run and the 12-minute swim provide two reliable and valid tests to predict $\dot{V}O_{2max}$. The tests have proved effective for mass testing in schools and for use with recreational runners and swimmers. These tests are not recommended for unconditioned beginners, men over age 40, and women over age 50 without proper medical clearance, symptomatic individuals, and those with known disease or coronary heart disease risk factors. The swim test assumes at least relatively high-level swimming skill to minimize the effects of variations in exercise economy in swimming.

The Tests

1.5-Mile Run Test

1. Testing site: a school track (each lap usually measures 1/4 mile) or premeasured 1.5-mile course.
2. Warm-up with easy stretching, mild calisthenics, and jogging in place.
3. Cover the 1.5-mile distance as fast as possible by walking, jogging, and/or running.
4. Record run time with a stop watch (min:s).
5. Five-minute cool-down upon test completion.
6. Refer to Table 1 for predicted $\dot{V}O_{2max}$ from run time.

Cooper KH. A means of assessing maximal oxygen uptake. JAMA 1968;203:201.

Pollock ML, et. al. Health and fitness through physical activity. New York: John Wiley & Sons, 1978.

Table 1

Predicted $\dot{V}O_{2max}$ (mL · kg^{-1} · min^{-1}) for the 1.5-Mile Walk/Run Test (min:s).

Time	$\dot{V}O_{2max}$	Time	$\dot{V}O_{2max}$	Time	$\dot{V}O_{2max}$
6:10	80.0	10:30	48.6	14:50	34.0
6:20	79.0	10:40	48.0	15:00	33.6
6:30	77.9	10:50	47.4	15:10	33.1
6:40	76.7	11:00	46.6	15:20	32.7
6:50	75.5	11:10	45.8	15:30	32.2
7:00	74.0	11:20	45.1	15:40	31.8
7:10	72.6	11:30	44.4	15:50	31.4
7:20	71.3	11:40	43.7	16:00	30.9
7:30	69.9	11:50	43.2	16:10	30.5
7:40	68.3	12:00	42.3	16:20	30.2
7:50	66.8	12:10	41.7	16:30	29.8
8:00	65.2	12:20	41.0	16:40	29.5
8:10	63.9	12:30	40.4	16:50	29.1
8:20	62.5	12:40	39.8	17:00	28.9
8:30	61.2	12:50	39.2	17:10	28.5
8:40	60.2	13:00	38.6	17:20	28.3
8:50	59.1	13:10	38.1	17:30	28.0
9:00	58.1	13:20	37.8	17:40	27.7
9:10	56.9	13:30	37.2	17:50	27.4
9:20	55.9	13:40	36.8	18:00	27.1
9:30	54.7	13:50	36.3	18:10	26.8
9:40	53.5	14:00	35.9	18:20	26.6
9:50	52.3	14:10	35.5	18:30	26.3
10:00	51.1	14:20	35.1	18:40	26.0
10:10	50.4	14:30	34.7	18:50	25.7
10:20	49.5	14:40	34.3	19:00	25.4

12-Minute Swim Test

Individuals swim as far as possible in 12 minutes, with distance measured in yards. Differences in skill level, swimming conditioning, and body composition greatly affect oxygen consumption (exercise economy), thus making $\dot{V}O_{2max}$ predictions less valid than those based on walking and running tests (with smaller variation in economy).

1. Warm up with easy stretching, mild calisthenics, and several laps of easy swimming.
2. Swim as many laps as possible in 12 minutes; paced swimming is preferred to intervals of fast and slow effort.
3. Determine total distance swam in yards during the 12 minutes; if the test ends in the middle of the pool, estimate distance; find the corresponding swim fitness category in Table 2.

Cooper KH. The aerobics program for total well-being. New York: Bantam Books, 1982.

Table 2

12-Minute Swim Test Fitness Categories (Age 18–29 y)

		Estimated $\dot{V}O_{2max}$ (mL · kg^{-1} · min^{-1})	
Distance (yd)	Fitness Category	Males	Females
≥ 700	Excellent	>52.5	>41.0
500–700	Good	46.5–52.4	37.0–40.0
400–500	Average	42.5–46.4	33.0–36.9
200–400	Fair	36.5–42.4	29.0–32.9
≤ 200	Poor	33.0–36.4	23.6–28.9

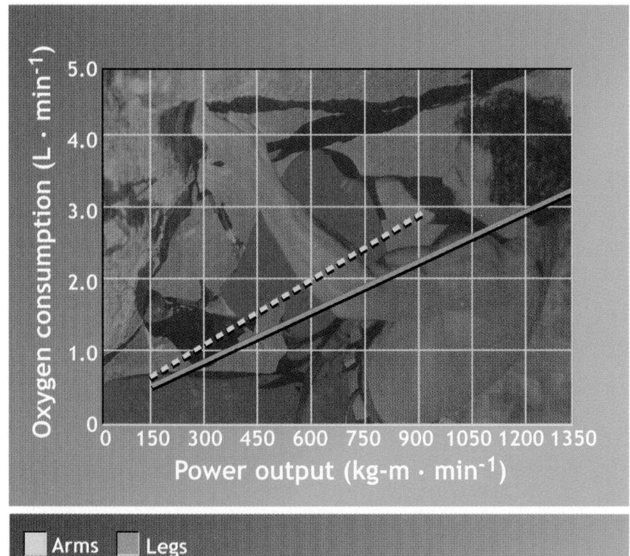

FIGURE 17.6 • Arm exercise requires greater oxygen consumption than leg exercise at any submaximal power output throughout the comparison range. The largest differences occur during heavy exercise. Data represent averages for men and women. (From Laboratory of Applied Physiology, Queens College, Flushing, NY.)

Submaximal Oxygen Consumption

Submaximal exercise reverses the pattern for oxygen consumption between upper- and lower-body exercise observed in maximal effort.[11,21,60] Figure 17.6 shows higher oxygen consumption at all submaximal power outputs during arm exercise. The small differences during light exercise become progressively larger as intensity increases. This results from (1) lower mechanical efficiency in upper-body exercise from the additional cost of static muscle actions that do not contribute to external work and (2) recruitment of additional musculature to stabilize the torso during arm exercise.[53]

Physiologic Response

Any level of submaximal oxygen consumption (or percentage $\dot{V}O_{2max}$) with upper-body exercise provides greater physiologic strain than the same power output in lower-body exercise.[50,62] More specifically, submaximal arm exercise produces higher heart rates, pulmonary ventilations, and perceptions of effort than comparable intensities of leg exercise. This also applies to blood pressure during arm and leg exercise (see Chapter 15). Even varying arm position either at, above, or below heart level does not reduce the differences in physiologic strain between arm and leg work.[6]

The elevated heart rate response in submaximal arm exercise probably results from two factors: (1) greater feedforward stimulation from the brain's central command to the medullary control center and (2) increased feedback stimulation to the medulla from peripheral receptors in active tissue. Upper-body exercise places a greater strain (i.e., greater force per unit muscle, greater percentage of maximum capacity, and more metabolic byproducts) on the relatively smaller upper-body musculature for any submaximum exercise level. Added strain augments peripheral feedback to the medulla, which increases heart rate and blood pressure. More than likely, activating a significantly smaller muscle mass than leg exercise accounts for the lower maximum heart rate in upper-body exercise. This reduces input to the medullary cardiovascular control center from the motor cortex, with less peripheral feedback from the smaller upper-body muscle mass.

IMPLICATIONS. *A standard submaximal exercise load (power output or oxygen consumption) with the upper body produces greater metabolic and physiologic strain than leg exercise.* For this reason, exercise prescriptions based on running and bicycling do *not* apply to arm exercise. Because low correlations often emerge between $\dot{V}O_{2max}$ in arm versus leg exercise, one should not expect to accurately predict aerobic capacity for arm exercise from a test using the legs and vice versa.[10,26] This lack of strong association between the two forms of exercise further amplifies the specificity concept applied to aerobic fitness.

Summary

1. Cardiac output reflects the functional capacity of the cardiovascular system. Heart rate and stroke volume determine the heart's output capacity expressed as follows: Cardiac output = Heart rate × Stroke volume.
2. Several invasive and noninvasive methods measure cardiac output in humans. Each has specific advantages and disadvantages during exercise.
3. Cardiac output increases proportionally with exercise intensity, starting from approximately 5 L · min^{-1} at rest to a maximum of 20 to 25 L · min^{-1} in untrained, college-aged men and 35 to 40 L · min^{-1} in elite male endurance athletes. The large stroke volumes of athletes explain the difference in maximum cardiac outputs compared with untrained persons.
4. Stroke volume increases during upright exercise from the interaction between greater ventricular filling during diastole and more-complete systolic emptying.
5. Sympathetic hormones augment systolic ejection by increasing stroke power during systole.
6. Blood flows to specific tissues in proportion to their metabolic activity. Most cardiac output diverts to active muscles during exercise. The kidneys and splanchnic regions temporarily compromise their blood supply to redistribute blood to exercising muscles.
7. Maximum cardiac output and a-$\bar{v}$ O_2 difference determine maximal oxygen consumption. A large cardiac output clearly differentiates endurance athletes from their untrained counterparts.

8. Arm exercise generates a 25% lower $\dot{V}O_{2max}$ than leg exercise.
9. Any level of submaximal oxygen consumption (or % $\dot{V}O_{2max}$) with upper-body exercise provides greater physiologic strain than the same power output in lower-body exercise.

References

1. Bar-Or O, et al. Cardiac output of 10- to 13-year old boys and girls during submaximal exercise. J Appl Physiol 1971;30:219.
2. Beekman RH, et al. Validity of CO_2-rebreathing cardiac output during rest and exercise in young adults. Med Sci Sports Exerc 1984;16:306.
3. Bevegård S, et al. Circulatory studies in well-trained athletes at rest and during heavy exercise, with special reference to stroke volume and the influence of body position. Acta Physiol Scand 1963;57:26.
4. Coyle EF. Cardiovascular drift during prolonged exercise and the effects of dehydration. Int J Sports Med 1998;19(suppl 2):S121.
5. Coyle EF, et al. Time course of loss of adaptations after stopping prolonged intense endurance training. J Appl Physiol 1984;57:1857.
6. Cummins TD, Gladden LB. Responses to submaximal and maximal arm cycling above, at, and below heart level. Med Sci Sports Exerc 1983;15:295.
7. Delp MD. Differential effects of training on control of skeletal muscle perfusion. Med Sci Sports Exerc 1998;30:361.
8. DiBello V, et al. Left ventricular function during exercise in athletes and in sedentary men. Med Sci Sports Exerc 1996;28:190.
9. Ekelund L-G. Circulatory and respiratory adaptation during prolonged exercise of moderate intensity in the sitting position. Acta Physiol Scand 1967;69:327.
10. Franklin BA, et al. Aerobic requirements of arm ergometry: implications for exercise testing and training. Phys Sportsmed 1983;11:81.
11. Franklin BA, et al. Trainability of arms versus legs in men with previous myocardial infarction. Chest 1994;105:262.
12. Fritzsche RG, et al. Stroke volume decline during prolonged exercise is influenced by the increase in heart rate. J Appl Physiol 1999;86:799.
13. Gauvreau GM, et al. Comparison of aerobic capacity between racing standardbred horses. J Appl Physiol 1995;78:1447.
14. Gledhill N, et al. Endurance athletes' stroke volume does not plateau: major advantage is diastolic function. Med Sci Sports Exerc 1994;26:1116.
15. Hagberg JM, et al. Expanded blood volumes contribute to increased cardiovascular performance of endurance-trained older men. J Appl Physiol 1998;85:484.
16. Herlhoz K, et al. Regional cerebral blood flow in man at rest and during exercise. J Neurol 1987;234:9.
17. Hickson RC. Skeletal muscle cytochrome c and myoglobin, endurance, and frequency of training. J Appl Physiol 1981;51:746.
18. Holloszy JO, Coyle EF. Adaptations of skeletal muscle to endurance training and their metabolic consequences. J Appl Physiol 1984;56:831.
19. Johnson JM. Physical training and the control of skin blood flow. Med Sci Sports Exerc 1998;30:382.
20. Johnson JM, Rowell LB. Forearm and skin vascular responses to prolonged exercise in man. J Appl Physiol 1975;39:920.
21. Kang J, et al. Metabolic efficiency during arm and leg exercise at the same relative intensities. Med Sci Sports Exerc 1997;29:277.
22. Katsura T. Influences of age and sex on cardiac output during submaximal exercise. Ann Physiol Anthropol 1986;5:39.
23. Krip B, et al. Effect of alterations in blood volume on cardiac function during maximal exercise. Med Sci Sports Exerc 1997;29:1469.
24. Lash JM, et al. Exercise training effects on collateral and microvascular resistance in rat model of arterial insufficiency. Am J Physiol 1995;28:H125.
25. Laughlin MH, et al. Physical activity and the microcirculation in cardiac and skeletal muscle. In: Bouchard C, et al., eds. Physical activity, fitness, and health. Champaign, IL: Human Kinetics, 1994.
26. Lazarus B, et al. Comparison of the reproducibility of arm and leg exercise tests in men with angina pectoris. Am J Cardiol 1981;47:1074.
27. Levine BD, et al. Left ventricular pressure–volume and Frank–Starling relations in endurance athletes: implications for orthostatic tolerance and exercise performance. Circulation 1991;84:1016.
28. Levy WC, et al. Endurance exercise training augments diastolic filling at rest and during exercise in healthy young and older men. Circulation 1993;88:116.
29. Lewis SF, et al. Cardiovascular responses to exercise as a function of absolute and relative work load. J Appl Physiol 1983;54:1314.
30. Magel JR, et al. Metabolic and cardiovascular adjustment to arm training. J Appl Physiol 1978;45:75.
31. McAllister RM. Adaptations in control of blood flow with training: splanchnic and renal blood flows. Med Sci Sports Exerc 1998;30:375.
32. McArdle WD, et al. Specificity of run training on $\dot{V}O_{2max}$ and heart rate changes during running and swimming. Med Sci Sports Exerc 1978;10:16.
33. Mier CM, et al. Cardiovascular adaptations to 10 days of cycle exercise. J Appl Physiol 1997;83:1900.
34. Miles DS, et al. Cardiovascular responses to upper body exercise in normals and cardiac patients. Med Sci Sports Exerc 1989;21:S126.
35. Mitchell JH, Raven PB. Cardiovascular adaptation to physical activity. In: Bouchard C, et al., eds. Physical activity, fitness, and health. Champaign, IL: Human Kinetics, 1994.
36. Mueller P et al. Renal hemodynamic responses to dynamic exercise in rabbits. J Appl Physiol 1998;85:1605.
37. Pechar GS, et al. Specificity of cardio-respiratory adaptation to bicycle and treadmill training. J Appl Physiol 1974;36:753.
38. Poliner LR, et al. Left ventricular performance in normal subjects: a comparison of the responses to exercise in upright and supine positions. Circulation 1980;62:528.
39. Potard US, et al. Force, speed, and oxygen consumption in thoroughbred and draft horses. J Appl Physiol 1998;84:2052.
40. Proctor DN, et al. Influence of age and gender on cardiac output-$\dot{V}O_2$ relationship during submaximal cycle ergometry. J Appl Physiol 1998;84:599.
41. Richardson RS, et al. High muscle blood flow in man: is maximal O_2 extraction compromised? J Appl Physiol 1993;75:1911.
42. Richardson RS, et al. Determinants of maximal exercise $\dot{V}O_2$ during single leg knee extensor exercise in man. Am J Physiol 1995;268:1453.
43. Robergs RA, et al. Temporal inhomogeneity in brachial artery blood flow during forearm exercise. Med Sci Sports Exerc 1997;29:1021.
44. Rowell LB. Human circulation, regulation during physical stress. New York: Oxford University Press, 1986.
45. Rowell LB. Human cardiovascular control. Cary, NC: Oxford University Press, 1994.
46. Rowell LB, et al. Is peak quadriceps blood flow in humans even higher during exercise with hypoxemia? Am J Physiol 1986:251:H1038.
47. Rowell LB, et al. Integration of cardiovascular control systems in dynamic exercises. In: Rowell LB, Shepard J, eds. Handbook of physiology. New York: Oxford University Press, 1996.
48. Rowland T, et al. Cardiac responses to maximal upright cycle exercise in healthy boys and men. Med Sci Sports Exerc 1997;29:1146.
49. Rowland T, et al. Cardiac responses to exercise in normal children: a synthesis. Med Sci Sports Exercise 2000;32:253.
50. Saltin B. Physiological effects of physical conditioning. Med Sci Sports Exerc 1969;1:50.
51. Sawka MN. Physiology of upper body exercise. Exerc Sport Sci Rev 1986;14:175.
52. Schulman SP, et al. Continuum of cardiovascular performance across a broad range of fitness levels in healthy older men. Circulation 1996;94:359.
53. Schwade J, et al. A comparison of the response to arm and leg work in patients with ischemic heart disease. Am Heart J 1977;94:203.
54. Seely JE, et al. Heart and lung function at rest and during exercise in adolescence. J Appl Physiol 1974;36:34.
55. Shin K, et al. Autonomic differences between athletes and nonathletes: spectral analysis approach. Med Sci Sports Exerc 1997;29:1482.
56. Soto KI, et al. Cardiac output in preadolescent competitive swimmers and in untrained normal children. J Sports Med Phys Fitness 1983;23:291.
57. Stevenson ET, et al. Maximal aerobic capacity and total blood volume in highly trained middle-aged and older female endurance athletes. J Appl Physiol 1994;77:1691.
58. Sun XG et al. Comparison of exercise cardiac output by the Fick prinicple using oxygen and carbon dioxide. Chest 2000;118:631.
59. Tate CA, et al. Mechanism for the responses of cardiac muscle to physical activity in old age. Med Sci Sports Exerc 1994;26:561.
60. Thomas SN, et al. Cerebral blood flow during submaximal and maximal dynamic exercise in humans. J Appl Physiol 1989:67:744.

61. Toner MM, et al. Cardiorespiratory responses to exercise distributed between the upper and lower body. J Appl Physiol 1983;54:1403.
62. Toner MM, et al. Cardiovascular adjustment to exercise distributed between the upper and lower body. Med Sci Sports Exerc 1990;22:773.
63. Turley KR, Wilmore JH. Cardiovascular responses to treadmill and cycle ergometer exercise in children and adults. J Appl Physiol 1997;83:948.
64. Vokac Z, et al. Oxygen uptake/heart rate relationship in leg and arm exercise, sitting and standing. J Appl Physiol 1975;39:54.
65. Wilmore JH, et al. Endurance exercise training has a minimal effect on resting heart rate: the HERITAGE Study. Med Sci Sports Exerc 1996;28:829.
66. Wilson DF. Energy metabolism in muscle approaching maximal rates of oxygen utilization. Med Sci Sports Exerc 1995;27:54.
67. Woodiwiss AJ, et al. Reduced cardiac stiffness following exercise is associated with preserved myocardial collagen characteristics in the rat. Eur J Appl Physiol 1998;78:148.
68. Yoshida E, et al. Relationship between aerobic power, blood volume, and thermoregulatory responses to exercise-heat stress. Med Sci Sports Exerc 1997;29:867.

CHAPTER 18

Skeletal Muscle: Structure and Function

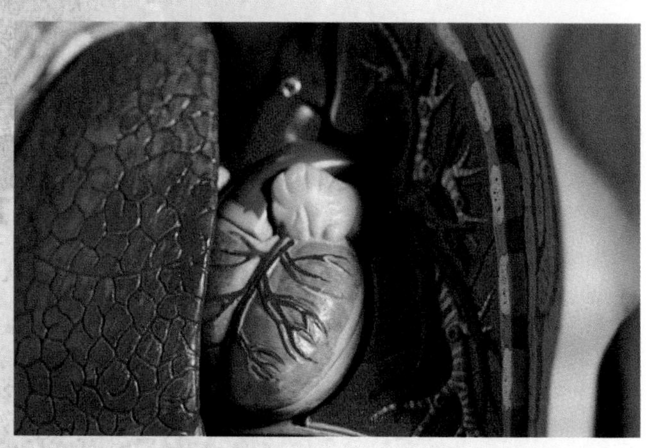

Chapter Objectives

- Outline the levels of organization in the gross structure of skeletal muscle
- List four major protein constituents of skeletal muscle and their functions
- Draw and label the structures that characterize a skeletal muscle fiber's striated appearance under the light microscope at low magnification
- Describe different arrangements of individual muscle fibers along the long axis of skeletal muscle and explain the biomechanical advantage of each
- Draw and label a skeletal muscle fiber's ultrastructural components
- Summarize the major aspects of the sliding filament model of muscle contraction
- Outline the sequence of chemical and mechanical events during skeletal muscle excitation–contraction coupling and relaxation
- Discuss the function of the triad and T-tubule system
- Contrast slow-twitch and fast-twitch (including subdivisions) muscle fiber characteristics
- Outline muscle fiber type distribution patterns among diverse groups of elite athletes
- Discuss modifications in muscle fibers and fiber types with specific exercise training

Human movement requires conversion of the chemical energy in adenosine triphosphate (ATP) to mechanical energy through the action of skeletal muscles, the body's most abundant tissue. Muscle forces act on the body's bony lever system and cause one or more bones to move about their joint axis to propel an object, move the body itself, or do both simultaneously. The following sections present the architectural organization of skeletal muscle, with focus on its gross and microscopic structures. Discussion centers on the sequence of chemical and mechanical events in muscle action and relaxation, including differences in muscle fiber characteristics among sedentary and elite athletes in different sports.

GROSS STRUCTURE OF SKELETAL MUSCLE

Each of the more than 660 skeletal muscles in the body contains various wrappings of fibrous connective tissue. Figure 18.1 illustrates the gross structural details of a skeletal muscle and its thousands of cylindrical cells called **fibers**. These long, slender, multinucleated fibers (whose number probably remains fixed by the second trimester of fetal development) lie parallel to each other, with the force of action directed along the fiber's long axis. Individual fiber length varies from a few mm in the eye muscles to nearly 30 cm in the large antigravity muscles of the leg, with width reaching 0.15 mm.

Levels of Organization

A fine layer of connective tissue, the **endomysium**, wraps each muscle fiber and separates it from neighboring fibers. Another layer of connective tissue, the **perimysium**, surrounds a bundle of up to 150 fibers called a **fasciculus**. A fascia of fibrous connective tissue, the **epimysium**, surrounds the entire muscle. This protective sheath tapers at its distal and proximal ends as it blends into and joins the intramuscular tissue sheaths to form the dense, strong connective tissue of the **tendons**. The tendons connect both ends of the muscle to the **periosteum**, the outermost covering of the bone.

The tissues of the tendon intermesh with the collagenous fibers within the bone. This forms a powerful link between muscle and bone, which remains inseparable except during severe stress, when it can sever or literally pull away from the bone. When the tendon attaches to the end of a long bone, the bone adapts by enlarging at that end to create a more stable union. Depending on bone size, the terms *tubercle, tuberosity,* or *trochanter* describe this overgrowth.

The force of muscle action transmits directly from the connective tissue harness to the tendons, which then pull on the bones at their points of attachment. The force exerted on the tendinous attachments under various conditions of muscular exertion ranges from 20 to 50 newtons (197 to 492 kg) per cm^2 of cross-sectional area—forces often much larger than can be tolerated by the muscle fibers themselves. The muscle's **origin** refers to the location at which the tendon joins a relatively stable skeletal part, generally the proximal or fixed end of the lever system or that nearest the body's midline; the point of distal attachment to the moving bone represents the **insertion**. Figure 18.1B illustrates the tendon's ultrastructural details. The protein collagen comprises about 70% of the tendon's dry mass.

Beneath the endomysium and surrounding each muscle fiber lies the **sarcolemma**, a thin, elastic membrane enclosing the fiber's cellular contents. It contains a plasma membrane (plasmalemma) and a basement membrane. The plasma membrane, a bilayer lipid structure, conducts the electrochemical wave of depolarization over the surface of the muscle fiber. The membrane also insulates one fiber from another during depolarization. The basement membrane contains proteins and strands of collagen fibrils that fuse with the collagenous fibers in the outer covering of the tendon. Between the basement and plasma membranes lie myogenic stem cells known as **satellite cells**, the normally quiescent myoblasts that function in regenerative cellular growth, possible adaptations to exercise training, and recovery from injury.[51,72] In fact, incorporation of satellite cell nuclei into existing muscle fibers seems a likely explanation for exercise-induced muscle fiber hypertrophy. The fiber's aqueous protoplasm (**sarcoplasm**) contains enzymes, fat and glycogen particles, nuclei (approximately 250 per mm of fiber length) that contain the genes, mitochondria, and other specialized organelles. Figure 18.1C details the **sarcoplasmic reticulum**, an extensive longitudinal lattice-like network of tubular channels and vesicles. This highly specialized system provides structural integrity to the cell. This allows the wave of depolarization to spread rapidly from the fiber's outer surface to its inner environment through the T-tubule system to initiate muscle action. The sarcoplasmic reticulum that surrounds each myofibril contains calcium pumps that take up Ca^{2+} from the fiber's sarcoplasm. This produces a calcium concentration gradient between the sarcoplasmic reticulum (higher Ca^{2+}) and the sarcoplasm surrounding the filaments (lower Ca^{2+}).

Chemical Composition

Water makes up approximately 75% of skeletal muscle, and protein comprises 20%. The remaining 5% contains salts and other substances, including high-energy phosphates; urea; lactate; the minerals calcium, magnesium, and phosphorus; various enzymes; sodium, potassium, and chloride ions; amino acids, fats, and carbohydrates. **Myosin** (approximately 60% of muscle protein), **actin**, and **tropomyosin** are the most abundant muscle proteins. Also, each 100-g of muscle tissue contains about 700 mg of the oxygen-binding, conjugated protein **myoglobin**, the molecular relative of hemoglobin, shown for comparison in the unnumbered figure inset, as revealed by x-ray diffraction, a technique commonly used to study muscle structures. Chapter 13 discusses the specific functions of myoglobin.

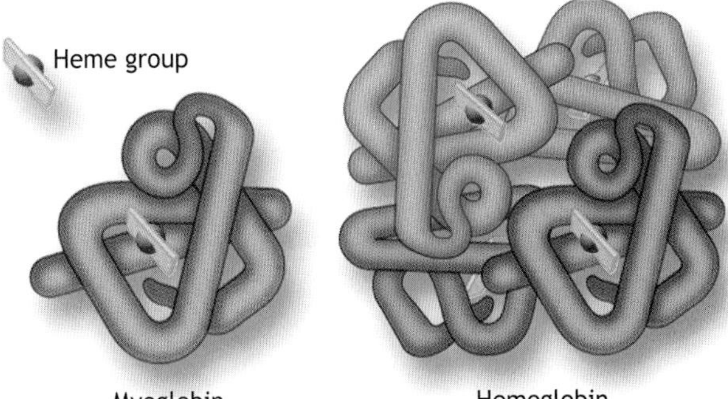

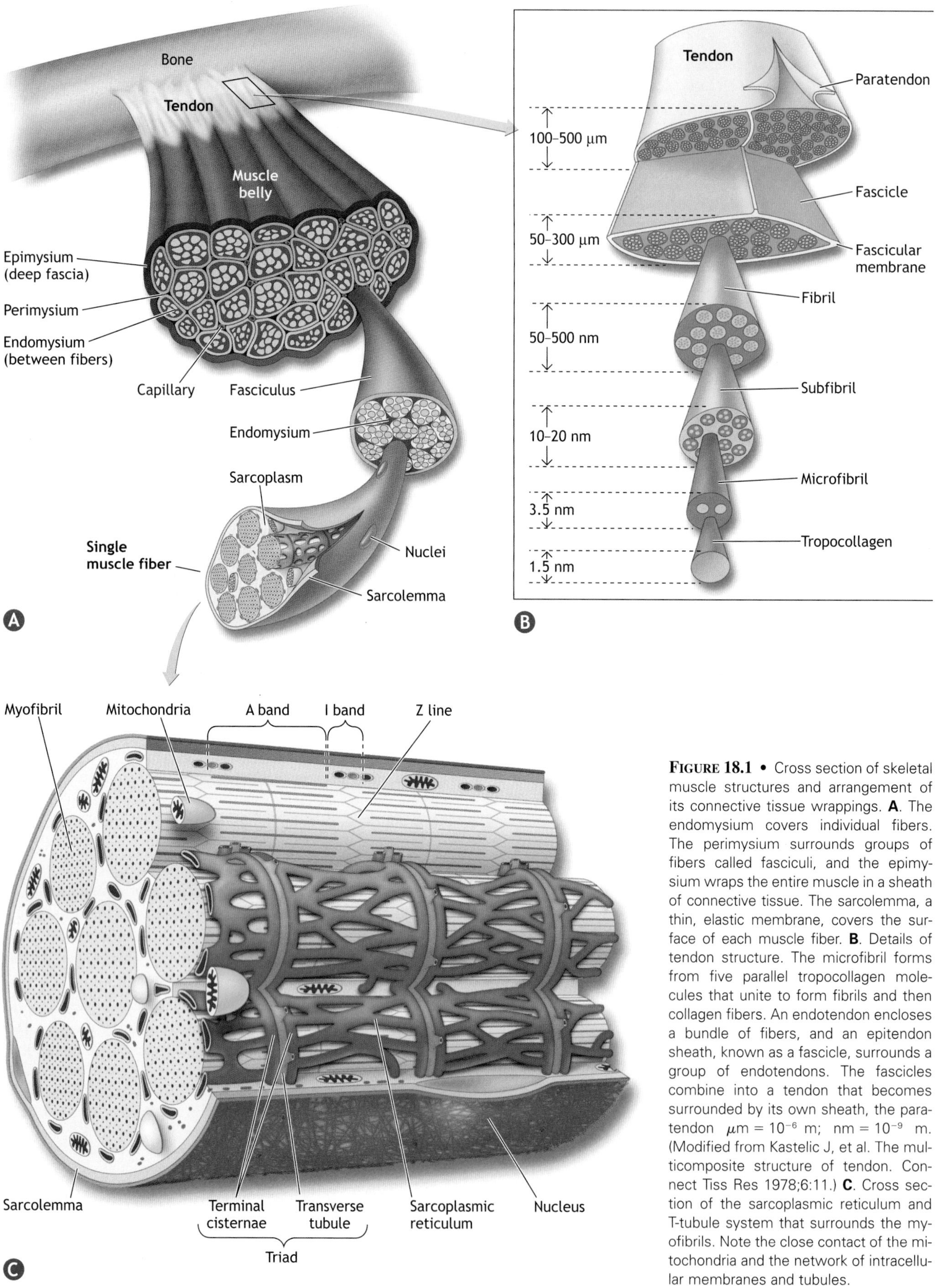

Bone
Tendon
Muscle belly
Epimysium (deep fascia)
Perimysium
Endomysium (between fibers)
Capillary
Fasciculus
Endomysium
Sarcoplasm
Single muscle fiber
Nuclei
Sarcolemma
A

Tendon
Paratendon
100–500 μm
Fascicle
50–300 μm
Fascicular membrane
Fibril
50–500 nm
Subfibril
10–20 nm
Microfibril
3.5 nm
Tropocollagen
1.5 nm
B

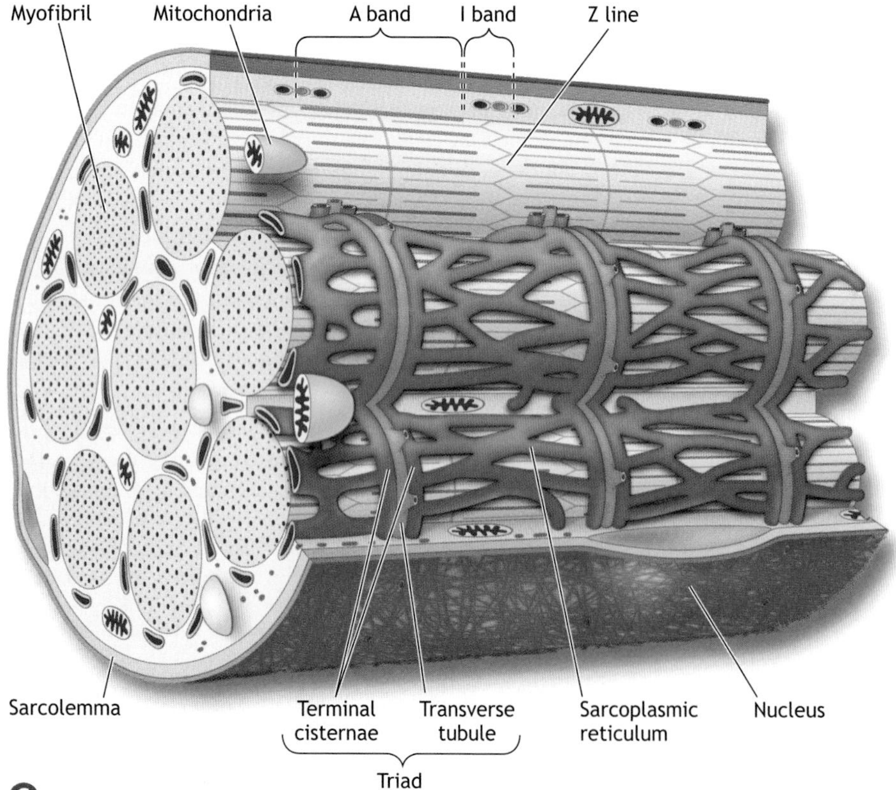

Figure 18.1 • Cross section of skeletal muscle structures and arrangement of its connective tissue wrappings. **A**. The endomysium covers individual fibers. The perimysium surrounds groups of fibers called fasciculi, and the epimysium wraps the entire muscle in a sheath of connective tissue. The sarcolemma, a thin, elastic membrane, covers the surface of each muscle fiber. **B**. Details of tendon structure. The microfibril forms from five parallel tropocollagen molecules that unite to form fibrils and then collagen fibers. An endotendon encloses a bundle of fibers, and an epitendon sheath, known as a fascicle, surrounds a group of endotendons. The fascicles combine into a tendon that becomes surrounded by its own sheath, the paratendon $\mu m = 10^{-6}$ m; $nm = 10^{-9}$ m. (Modified from Kastelic J, et al. The multicomposite structure of tendon. Connect Tiss Res 1978;6:11.) **C**. Cross section of the sarcoplasmic reticulum and T-tubule system that surrounds the myofibrils. Note the close contact of the mitochondria and the network of intracellular membranes and tubules.

Focus on Research: A Tissue Responsive to Regular Exercise

Tipton CM, et al. Influence of exercise on strength of medial collateral knee ligaments of dogs. Am J Physiol 1970;218:894.

➤ Exercise has been considered important for rehabilitating injured ligaments, despite the lack of understanding of precise mechanism(s) for the beneficial effects of exercise on connective tissues. This has not always been the case, however. Prior to 1970, evidence showing that exercise improved connective tissue strength came from studies using laboratory animals (e.g., mice, rats). The pioneering study by Tipton and colleagues provided direct experimental evidence of exercise training benefits on the strength of either intact or surgically repaired medial collateral ligaments of dogs. These data provided an important framework to justify the current commonly accepted use of exercise, not immobilization, to rehabilitate soft tissue injury and surgical repair.

Tipton studied more than 100 male mongrel dogs (age >1 y) to answer several questions, including the effects of 6 weeks (w) of increased or decreased physical activity (exercise training, immobilization, normal cage activity, and sham surgical procedures) on intact knee ligament strength. A second goal was describing the effects of variations in exercise training, immobilization, and normal cage activity on the strength of surgically repaired ligaments, a question of primary interest in sports medicine.

In all evaluations of ligament strength, the plantaris, gastrocnemius, and extensor digitorum longus muscles were removed (along with the joint's surrounding soft tissue), leaving the capsule and ligaments intact. A testing apparatus held the bone-capsule-bone preparation as the tibia was pulled from the femur at a constant speed of 0.25 mm · s^{-1}. The force (kg) necessary to separate the ligament from the bone—stress-strain measurement—represented the separation force (SF). The SF ÷ body mass ratio (SFR) adjusted for the animals' differences in body mass. Exercise training included treadmill running at different speeds, grades, and durations for a maximum of 6 d weekly for 6 w; 3 d endurance and 3 d of "wind sprint" training. By week 3, the animals were exercising 1 h daily.

Immobilization involved fixing one of the hind legs with the knee flexed at 60 to 80° using pins placed through the femur and one through the tibia. A fast-drying plaster cast then secured the leg. Surgical repair of the left medial collateral ligament involved exposing the ligament by making an incision through its superficial and deep portions along the joint line while preserving the blood supply. Two steel-wire sutures were used to reattach the ligament at its original location. Sham operations (no ligament cut) included pin insertion, skin incision, ligament exposure, and wound closure.

Figure 1 shows that strength of the intact knee ligament relates to the animal's level of physical activity, with immobilization (Group 2) producing the least strength (lowest SF) and 6 weeks of treadmill running (Group 4) yielding the greatest strength. Strength of the surgically repaired ligaments (Fig. 2) depended on the time interval before sacrifice and the amount of activity performed by the experimental leg. Location of separation also varied between intact and repaired ligaments; intact ligaments separated from their tibial attachment, while surgically repaired ligaments invariably separated at the repair site.

The data indicate that physical activity markedly affects ligament strength. These important findings showed that connective tissue responds to the mechanical stress of exercise.

Tipton's innovative work provided the first experimental verification that ligaments from immobilized legs were weaker and weighed less than ligaments from normal control and exercised legs. The study also provided evidence that cast doubt on the efficacy of immobilization following ligament surgery. Instead, they support exercise training as a first line of rehabilitation following soft tissue surgery.

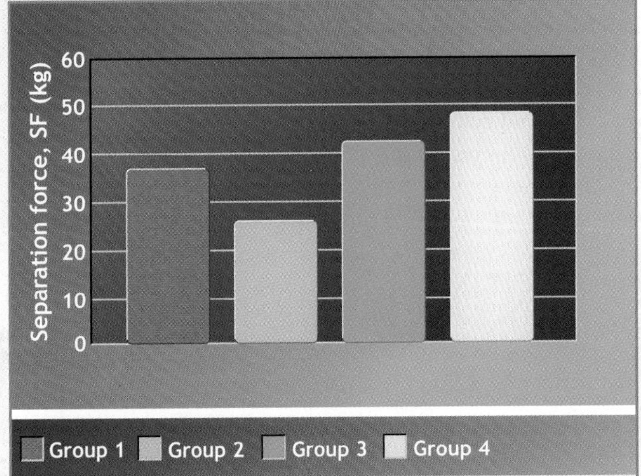

Figure 1. Physical activity levels and strength (separation force) of intact knee ligaments. Group 1, sham procedure on left leg: Group 2, decreased physical activity by leg immobilization; Group 3, normal cage activity; Group 4, increased physical activity with exercise training. Group 2 data are significantly lower than other group means.

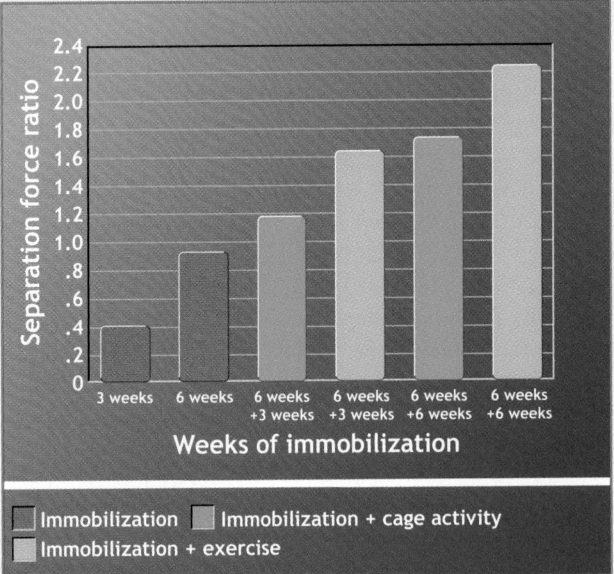

Figure 2. Strength of surgically repaired ligaments in relation to duration of immobilization and level of physical activity.

Blood Supply

Arteries and veins, oriented parallel to individual muscle fibers, provide muscles with a rich vascular supply. These vessels divide into numerous arterioles, capillaries, and venules to form a vast network in and around the endomysium. Extensive branching of blood vessels assures each muscle fiber of an adequate supply of oxygenated blood from the arterial system and rapid removal of carbon dioxide in the venous circulation. During exercise at an oxygen consumption of 4.0 $L \cdot min^{-1}$, the muscle's oxygen uptake increases nearly 70 times to approximately 11 mL per 100 g per minute (total of 3400 $mL \cdot min^{-1}$ for an elite encurance athlete). To accommodate this oxygen requirement, the local vascular bed channels large quantities of blood through the active tissues. Blood flow distribution fluctuates in rhythmic activities such as running, swimming, or cycling. It decreases during the muscle's contraction phase and increases during relaxation to provide a "milking action" that moves blood through the muscles and propels it back to the heart. The rapid dilation of previously dormant capillaries complements the pulsatile blood flow. Consequently, between 200 and 500 capillaries deliver blood to each square millimeter of active muscle cross-section, with up to four capillaries directly contacting each fiber. In endurance athletes, five to seven capillaries surround each fiber, ensuring greater local blood flow when needed (see next section).

Muscular activities that require straining present a somewhat different picture for muscle blood flow.[21] When a muscle generates about 60% of its force-generating capacity for several seconds, elevated intramuscular pressure occludes local blood flow during the contraction. With a sustained contraction, the intramuscular high-energy phosphates and glycolytic anaerobic reactions provide the main energy for muscular effort.

Capillarization

Improved exercise capacity with endurance training may partly result from trained muscles' increased capillary-to-muscle fiber ratio.[1,8] An enhanced capillary microcirculation expedites the removal of heat and metabolic byproducts from active tissues in addition to facilitating delivery of oxygen, nutrients, and hormones. In one study, electron microscopy revealed that the total number of capillaries per muscle (and capillaries per mm^2 of muscle tissue) averaged about 40% higher in endurance-trained athletes than in untrained counterparts. This almost equaled the 41% difference in $\dot{V}O_{2max}$ between the two groups. A positive association also exists between $\dot{V}O_{2max}$ and one's average number of muscle capillaries.[56] Enhanced vascularization on the capillary level proves particularly beneficial during exercise requiring a high level of steady-rate aerobic metabolism. Vascular stretch and shear stress on the vessel walls caused by the increased blood flow during aerobic exercise may stimulate capillary development with intense aerobic training.[41]

SKELETAL MUSCLE ULTRASTRUCTURE

Electron microscopy, x-ray diffraction, histochemical staining, helium–neon laser diffraction, and in vitro motility assays[60] and optical tweezers technologies[68] (see Chapter 33) have revealed the microscopic anatomy (ultrastructure) of skeletal muscle. Figure 18.2 shows the different levels of gross and subcellular organization within a skeletal muscle fiber. A single multinucleated muscle fiber contains smaller functional units that lie parallel to the fiber's long axis. These **fibrils** or **myofibrils**, approximately 1 μm (1 μm = 1/1000 mm) in diameter, contain even smaller subunits (**filaments** or **myofilaments**) that lie parallel to the long axis of the myofibril. The myofilaments chiefly consist of ordered assemblages of two proteins, **actin** and **myosin**, which account for about 85% of the myofibrilar complex. Twelve to 15 other proteins either have a structural function or significantly affect protein filament interaction during muscle action. Examples include (1) **tropomyosin**, located along the actin filaments (5%); (2) **troponin** (which consists of troponin-1, T, C), located in the actin filaments (3%); (3) **α-actinin**, distributed in the Z band region (7%); (4) **β-actinin**, found in the actin filaments (1%); (5) **M protein**, identified in the region of the M lines within the sarcomere (less than 1%); and (5) **C protein** (less than 1%), which probably contributes to the sarcomere's structural integrity.

The Sarcomere

At low magnification, the alternating light and dark bands along the length of the muscle fiber give it a characteristic **striated** appearance. Figure 18.3 *(top)* illustrates the structural details of this cross-striation pattern within a myofibril. The lighter area is the *I band,* and the darker zone, the *A band.* The *Z line* bisects the I band and adheres to the sarcolemma to give stability to the entire structure. Optical properties denote the specific bands. When polarized light passes through the I band, it moves at the same velocity in all directions (isotropic). Light passing through the A band does not scatter equally (anisotropic). The letter *Z* indicates between (from German, *zwischenscheibe*); the letter *M (mittelscheibe),* middle; and the letter *H (hellerscheibe),* clear disk or zone.

*The **sarcomere** consists of the basic repeating unit between two Z lines. This structural entity makes up the functional unit of a muscle fiber.* The actin and bipolar myosin filaments within the sarcomere contribute primarily to the mechanical process of muscle contraction. Sarcomeres lie in series, and their filaments have a parallel configuration within a given fiber. In the resting state, the length of each sarcomere averages 2.5 μm. Thus, a myofibril 15-mm long contains about 6000 sarcomeres joined end to end. The size (length) of the sarcomere largely determines a muscle's functional properties.

The position of thin actin and thicker myosin proteins in the sarcomere results in an interdigitating overlap of the two filaments. The center of the A band contains the *H zone,* a region of lower optical density because of the absence of actin filaments in this area. The *M band* bisects the central portion of the H zone, which delineates the sarcomere's center. The

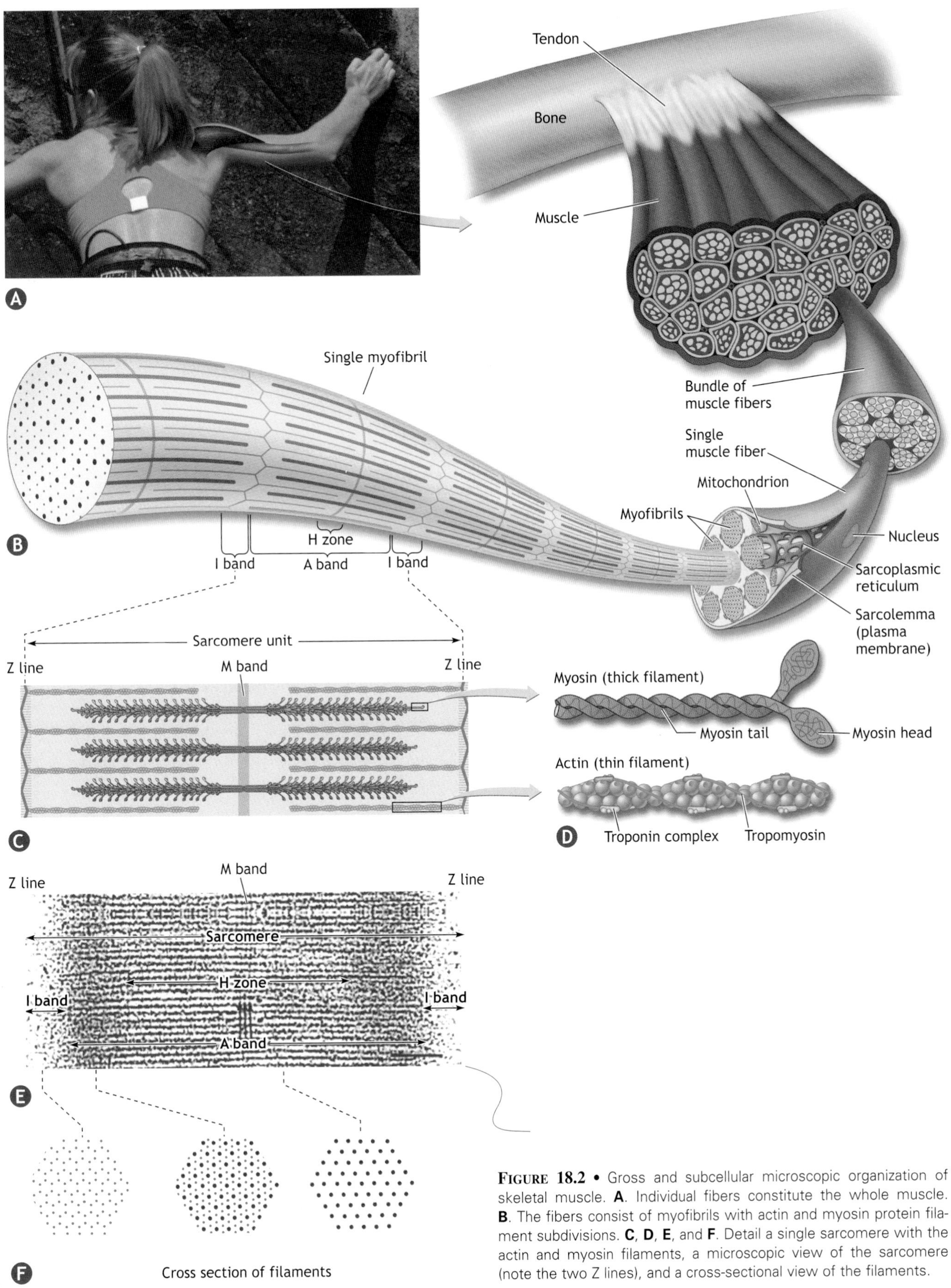

FIGURE 18.2 • Gross and subcellular microscopic organization of skeletal muscle. **A**. Individual fibers constitute the whole muscle. **B**. The fibers consist of myofibrils with actin and myosin protein filament subdivisions. **C**, **D**, **E**, and **F**. Detail a single sarcomere with the actin and myosin filaments, a microscopic view of the sarcomere (note the two Z lines), and a cross-sectional view of the filaments.

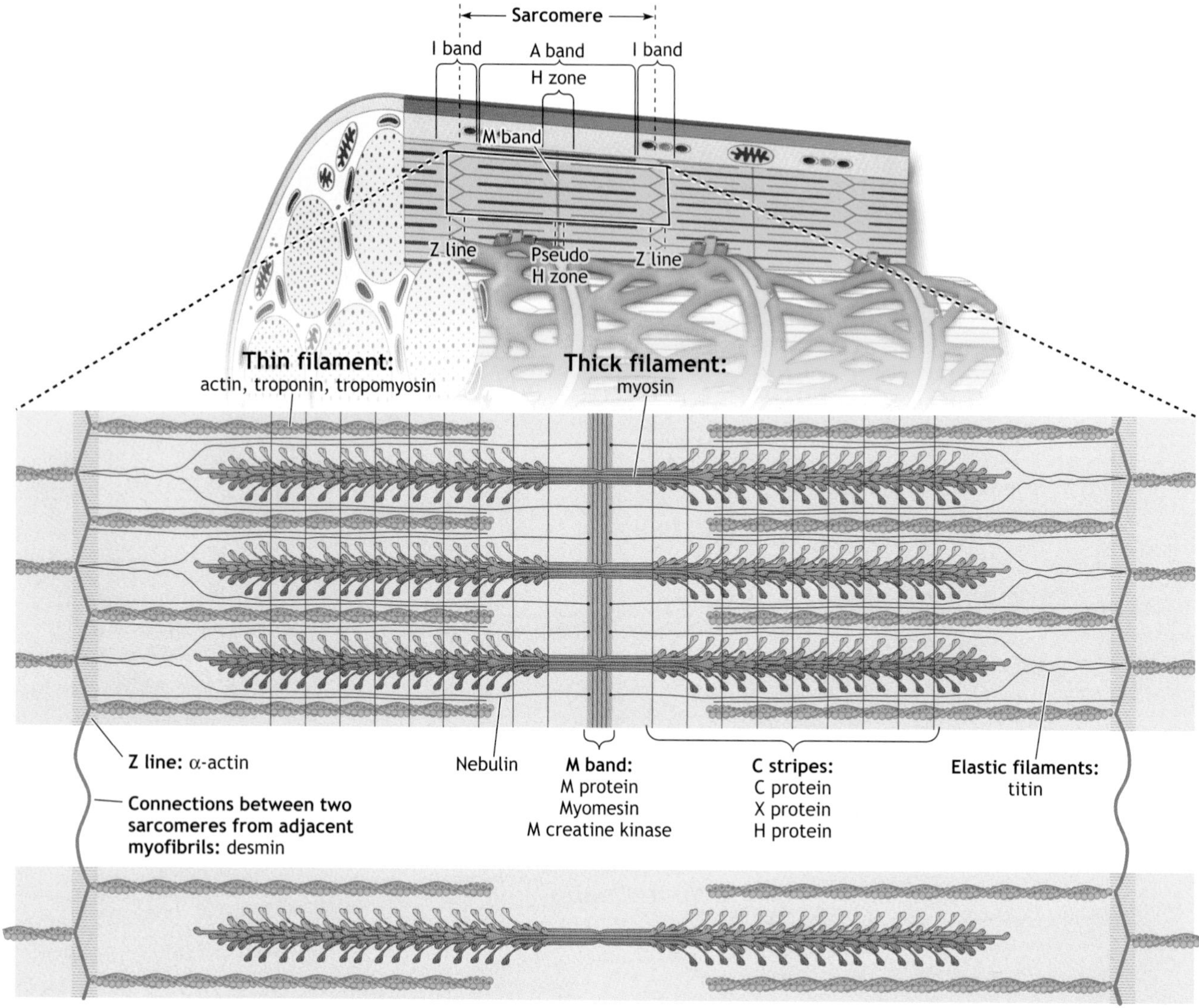

FIGURE 18.3 • *Top.* Structural position of the filaments in a sarcomere. The Z line bounds a sarcomere at both ends. *Bottom.* Detailed view of a sarcomere, including the proteins listed in Table 18.1.

M band consists of the protein structures that support the arrangement of the myosin filaments. Figure 18.3 *(bottom)* shows a detailed view of a sarcomere and Table 18.1 lists proteins and their proposed functions identified within a sarcomere.

MUSCLE FIBER ALIGNMENT

The long axis of the muscle determines the arrangement of individual fibers; it is determined from an imaginary line drawn through the origin and insertion, or the fiber angle relative to the force-generating axis. Differences in sarcomere alignment and length strongly affect a muscle's force- and power-generating capacity (Fig. 18.4). **Fusiform**, or spindle-shaped, fibers run parallel to the muscle's long axis (e.g., biceps brachii) and taper at the tendinous attachment. In contrast, **pennate**, or fan-shaped fibers' fasciculi (bundles of fibers) lie at an oblique pennation angle that varies up to 30°. In the soleus muscle, for example, the pennation angle averages 25°, whereas the pennation angle for the vastus medialis equals 5°, and no angle of pennation exists for the sartorius muscle. Of functional significance, the degree of pennation directly affects the number of sarcomeres per cross-sectional muscle area (no fibers run full length). In essence, pennation allows individual muscle fibers to remain short while the overall muscle may reach considerable length. In a fusiform fiber (no pennation), the cross-sectional area of the fiber represents the true anatomic cross section. In pennate muscle, on the other hand, the complex arrangement of connective tissue, tendons, and relatively short fibers creates a larger cross-sectional area because more sarcomeres "pack" into a given volume of muscle. The term **physiologic cross-sectional area (PCSA)** refers to the sum of the cross-sectional areas of all of the fibers within a particular muscle. (PCSA, cm^2 = Muscle mass (g) × cos θ/muscle density [g × cm^{-3}] × fiber length [cm], where muscle density = 1.056 g · cm^{-3}, and θ is the surface pennation angle.) An unusually large pennation angle of 30° results in a loss of only 13% in an individual fiber's force capacity, for a huge increase in total fiber packing ability.[42] Thus, pennation per se allows packing of a large number of fibers into a smaller cross-sectional area. Pennate muscles tend to generate considerable

TABLE 18.1 ➤ TWELVE PROTEINS ASSOCIATED WITH A MUSCLE FIBER'S SARCOMERE AND THEIR PROPOSED FUNCTIONS

STRUCTURE	PROTEIN	FUNCTION
Thin filament	Actin	The main protein of actin that interacts with myosin during excitation–contraction coupling
	Tropomyosin	Transduces the conformational change of the troponin complex to actin
	Troponin	Binds Ca^{2+} and affects tropomyosin. Represents the "switch" that transforms the Ca^{2+} signal into a molecular signal that induces crossbridge cycling
	Nebulin	Present next to actin and believed to control the number of actin monomers joined to each other in a thin filament
Thick filament	Myosin	Splits ATP and is responsible for the "power stroke" of the myosin head
C stripes	C protein	Holds the myosin thick filaments in a regular array; may hold the H protein of adjacent thick filaments at an even distance during force generation; may also control the number of myosin molecules in a thick filament
M line	M protein	Helps hold thick filaments in a regular array
	Myomesin	Provides a strong anchoring point for the protein titin
	M-CK	Provides ATP from phosphocreatine; located proximal to the myosin heads
Z line	α-actinin	Holds the thin filaments in place spatially
	Desmin	Forms the connection between adjacent Z lines from different myofibrils; helps to keep the sarcomeres in register so they maintain their striated appearance
Elastic filament	Titin	Helps keep the thick filament centered between two Z lines during contraction; believed to control the number of myosin molecules contained in the thick filament

power. Figure 18.4 (*bottom*) illustrates the effect of pennation on fiber packing and force-generating capacity.

The fibers in a fusiform muscle run parallel to the muscle's long axis. In this situation, fiber length equals muscle length, and a fiber's force generation transmits directly to the tendon. *This arrangement facilitates rapid muscle shortening.* A unipennate fiber arrangement, in which muscle fibers lie at an oblique angle to the tendon, produces a larger effective cross-sectional area than that in the fusiform muscle. *Muscles with greater pennation, although slower in contractile velocity, generate greater force and power than fusiform muscles (other factors being equal), because a greater number of sarcomeres contribute to the muscle action.*[54] A bipennate muscle has two sets of fibers that lie obliquely on both sides of a common tendon (e.g., gastrocnemius and rectus femoris muscles), whereas a multipennate muscle (e.g., human deltoid) contains

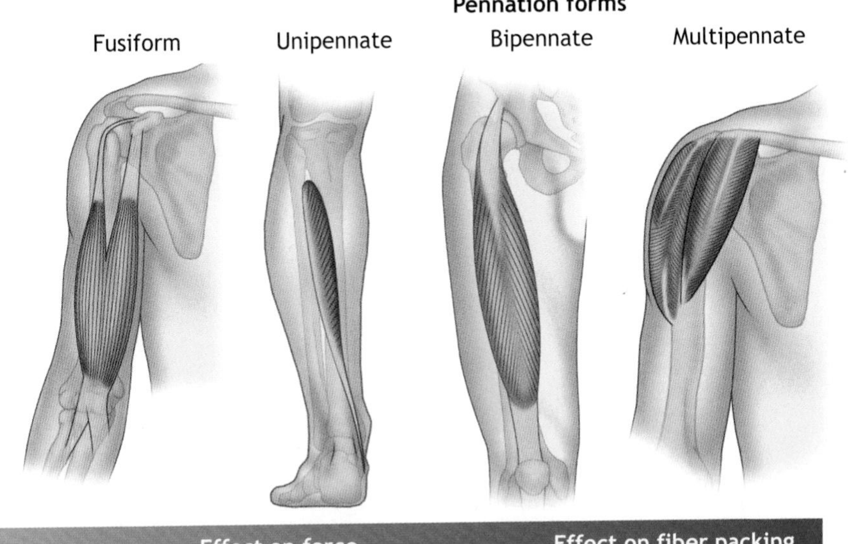

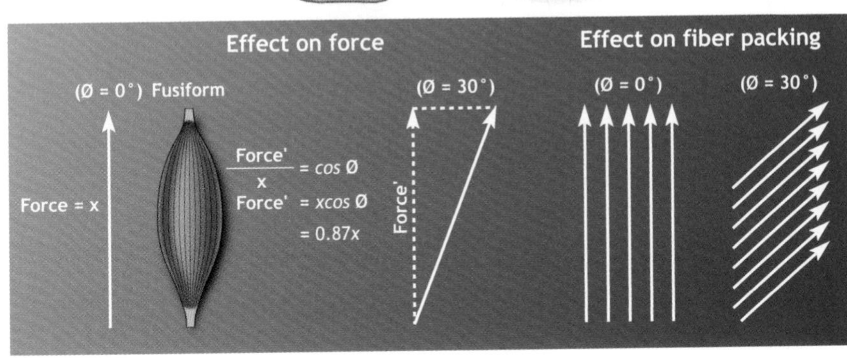

FIGURE 18.4 • *Top.* Various forms of fiber arrangement in human skeletal muscle. *Bottom.* Force development in a fusiform muscle with no angle of pennation ($\theta = 0°$) and when $\theta = 30°$. A 30° angle of pennation results in a 13% loss of each fiber's maximum force on the tendon, solely a result of muscle mechanics. However, pennation angle increases the number of fibers that pack into a given volume of muscle (bottom right). Muscle mass and the contractile capacity relate proportionately for a given muscle in comparisons among individuals. Because of the effect of pennation angle, however, it does not necessarily follow that muscle mass per se relates to an equivalent tension output in comparisons among different muscle groups. (Modified from Lieber RL. Skeletal muscle structure and function. Baltimore: Williams & Wilkins, 1992.)

more than two sets of fibers that converge at different angles and insert directly into tendons at both their ends. Pennate muscles contain generally shorter fibers than fusiform muscles, possess a greater number of individual fibers, and do not produce as great a range of motion as fusiform fibers.

Complex Fusiform Arrangement

The **complex parallel** or **series-fibered muscle** features individual fibers that run parallel to the muscle's line of pull. Unlike the simple fusiform arrangement in which a fiber runs the entire muscle length, the complex parallel arrangement features muscle fibers that terminate midbelly and taper to interact with the connective tissue matrix and/or adjacent muscle fibers. This arrangement enables parallel packing of relatively short fibers within in a long muscle (e.g., the 50-cm long human sartorius). However, this structural specialization with diverse intrafascicular terminations also creates lateral tension—either through connective tissue into tendon or through adjacent and series fibers into connective tissue—at various points along the fiber's surface. Future research must determine (1) how length and activation level of specific fibers in the series-fibered arrangement affects the velocity and magnitude of tension development and (2) how motor unit recruitment modulates force output.[61]

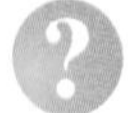

INTEGRATIVE QUESTION

List the advantages of a skeletal muscle organ system composed of muscles whose fibers vary in architectural design.

Fiber Length:Muscle Length Ratio

The ratio of individual fiber length to a muscle's total length usually varies between 0.2 and 0.6. This means that individual fibers in the longest muscles (e.g., muscles of the upper and lower limbs) are still significantly shorter than the muscle's overall length.[42] Figure 18.5 (*left*) illustrates the architectural properties of four lower limb muscles. On average,

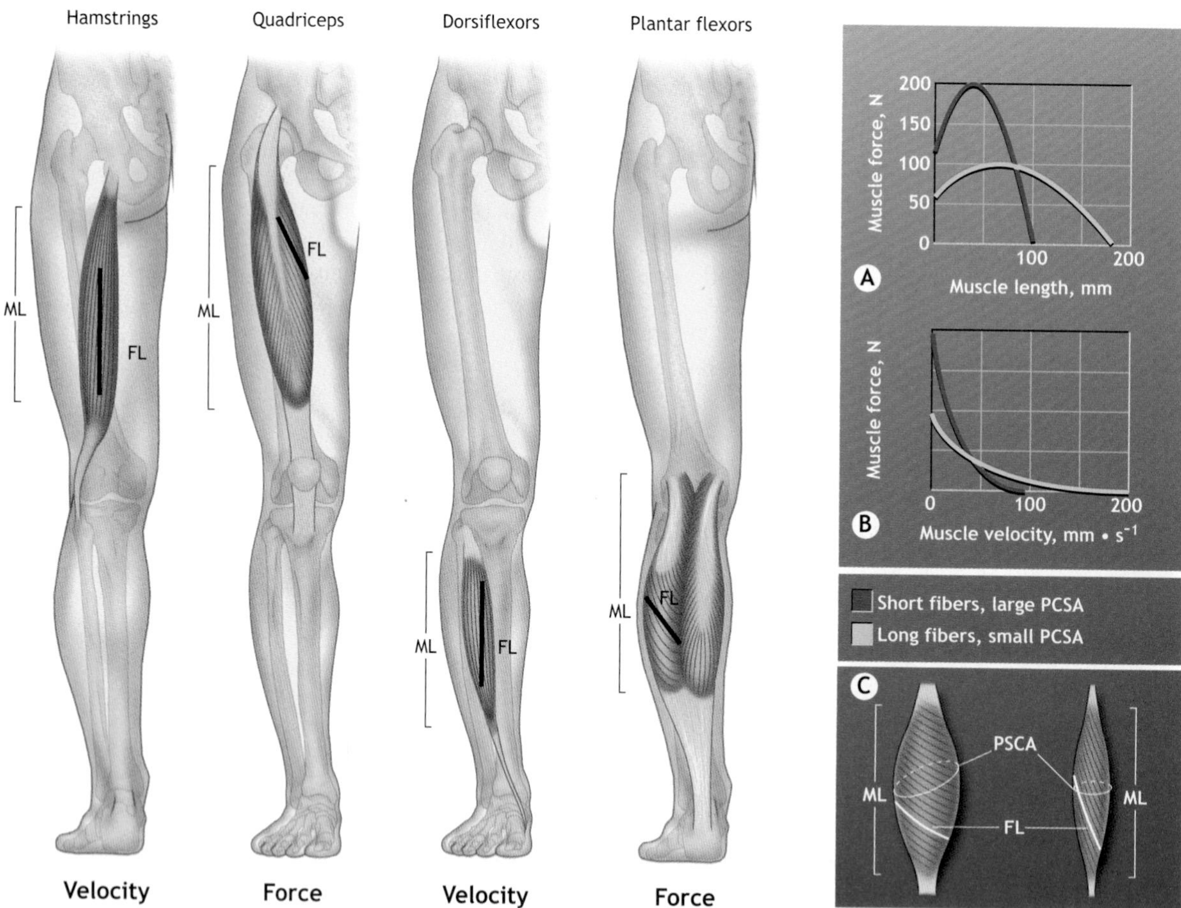

FIGURE 18.5 • *Left.* Muscle architectural properties in the lower limb. The quadriceps and plantar flexors show design for high force production because of their low fiber length-to-muscle length (FL:ML) ratios and relatively large physiologic cross-sectional areas (PCSA). The hamstrings and dorsiflexor muscles, on the other hand, show architecture designed for high contractile velocity because of their relatively high FL:ML and long FL. *Right.* Hypothetical pennate (short fibers) and fusiform (long fibers) muscles of the same length and with the same amount of contractile machinery. The muscle force–muscle length curve (**A**) shows the fusiform muscle with a longer working range and lower maximum force output than the pennate muscle. Lower force capacity (dorsiflexors and hamstrings) results because for a given change in muscle length, the individual sarcomeres lengthen less, with the change in muscle length distributed over more sarcomeres. A greater force output (quadriceps and plantar flexors) results from a greater PCSA (**C**). The muscle force–muscle velocity curve (**B**) shows that the fusiform muscle with longer fibers exhibits higher contractile velocity but a lower maximum force output. (Modified from Lieber RL. Skeletal muscle structure and function. Baltimore: Williams & Wilkins, 1992.)

quadriceps muscle fibers maintain pennation angles that average 4.6°, a PCSA of approximately 21.7 cm^2, and a fiber length that averages 68 mm. This contrasts with the biceps femoris (hamstring) muscle with relatively long fibers (111 mm) and an intermediate PCSA (11.7 cm^2). Quadriceps muscles exhibit approximately 50% greater force capacity than the hamstrings, whose design provides for rapid shortening. These design differences suggest susceptibility of the hamstrings to tearing should a rapid force output imbalance occur between the quadriceps and hamstrings, as often occurs in sprint running.

Figure 18.5 (*right inset, A and B*) shows the generalized muscle force–muscle length and muscle force–muscle velocity relationships for fusiform and pennate muscles with the same quantity of contractile protein and identical muscle fiber type. In this hypothetical example, the muscle force–muscle length curve for fusiform muscle shows a longer working range and lower maximum force output because of longer individual fibers and a smaller PCSA (Fig. 18.5C). The opposite occurs for pennate muscle with its shorter fibers and larger PCSA—these fibers generate force about double that of fusiform muscles. For the muscle force–muscle velocity curve, the fusiform muscle with longer fibers exhibits a higher contractile velocity but lower force-output capacity.

ACTIN–MYOSIN ORIENTATION

Thousands of myosin filaments lie along the actin filaments in a muscle fiber. Figure 18.6A illustrates the actin–myosin orientation within a sarcomere at resting length; Figure 18.6B

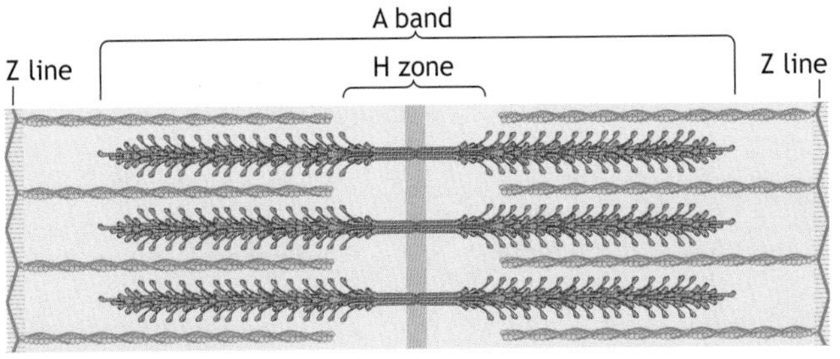

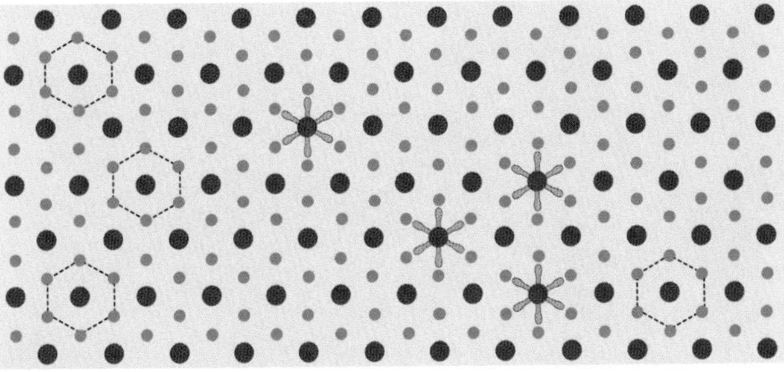

FIGURE 18.6 • **A**. Ultrastructure of actin–myosin orientation within a resting sarcomere. **B**. Representation of electron micrograph through a cross-section of myofibrils in a single muscle fiber. Note the hexagonal orientation of the smaller actin and larger myosin filaments, including crossbridges that extend from a thick to thin filament.

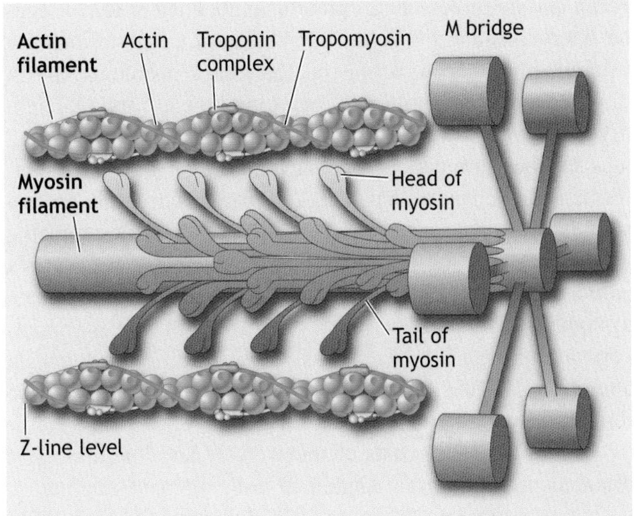

FIGURE 18.7 • Details of the thick and thin protein filaments including tropomyosin, troponin complex, and the M bridge. The globular heads of the myosin contain myosin ATPase; this "active" head frees the energy from ATP for use in muscle action.

shows the hexagonal arrangement of myosin and actin filaments. Myosin filaments consist of bundles of molecules with polypeptide tails and globular heads. Actin filaments, in contrast, have two twisted chains of monomers bound by tropomyosin polypeptide chains. Six relatively thin actin filaments, each about 50 Å in diameter and 1 μm long, encircle the thicker myosin filament (150 Å in diameter and 1.5 μm long). This represents an extremely impressive substructural configuration. For example, a myofibril 1 μm in diameter contains approximately 450 thick filaments in the sarcomere's center and 900 thin filaments at each end. A muscle fiber 100 μm in diameter and 1-cm long contains approximately 8000 myofibrils; each myofibril consists of 4500 sarcomeres on average. In a single fiber, this arrangement consists of 16 billion thick filaments and 64 billion thin filaments.[67]

Figure 18.7 illustrates the spatial orientation of various components of contractile filaments. Projections, or "crossbridges," spiral around the myosin filament in the region where actin and myosin filaments overlap. The crossbridges repeat at intervals of approximately 450 Å along the filament. Globular "lollipop-like" myosin heads extend perpendicularly to latch onto the thinner double-twisted actin strands to create structural and functional links between myofilaments. The unique feature of myosin's two heads concerns their opposite orientation at the ends of the thick filament. ATP hydrolysis activates the two heads, placing them in an orientation to bind actin's active sites, thus pulling the thin filaments and Z lines of the sarcomere toward the middle.

Tropomyosin and troponin are two other important constituents of the actin helical structure. These proteins regulate the make-and-break contacts between the myofilaments during muscle action. Tropomyosin distributes along the length of the actin filament in a groove formed by the double helix. Tropomyosin probably inhibits actin and myosin interaction (coupling) and thus prevents their permanent bonding. Troponin and its three-subunit proteins embedded at fairly regular intervals along the actin strands exhibit a high affinity for calcium ions (Ca^{2+}), a mineral that plays a crucial role in muscle action and fatigue.[38] For example, Ca^{2+} and troponin trigger myofibrils to interact and slide past each other. During muscle fiber stimulation, troponin molecules undergo a conformational change that "tugs" on tropomyosin protein strands. This causes tropomyosin to move deeper into the groove between the two actin strands, "uncovering" actin's active sites so muscle action proceeds. Muscle fatigue relates to significant reductions in Ca^{2+} concentration in the transverse tubules during heavy exercise, in addition to intrinsic alterations in the contractile apparatus and sarcoplasmic reticulum function.[10,71]

The M band consists of transversely and longitudinally oriented proteins that maintain myosin filament orientation within a sarcomere. As Figure 18.7 illustrates, the perpendicularly oriented M bridges connect with six adjacent thick (myosin) filaments in a hexagonal pattern.

An exciting area of muscle biochemistry, physiology, and mechanics involves the study of cytoskeletal proteins and structures that serve as an intermediate intracellular filament system.[48] The intracellular cytoskeleton provides for (1) structural integrity in the inactive muscle cell, (2) lateral force transmission to adjacent sarcomeres through interaction with actomyosin during muscle action, and (3) connections to the cell's surface membrane. A better understanding of the role of the cytoskeleton, its diverse proteins, and the myofibrilar lattice structure should enhance current understanding of muscle action, including processes in muscle injury, repair, and overload.

Intracellular Tubule Systems

Figure 18.8 illustrates the complex tubule system within a muscle fiber. The lateral end of each tubule channel terminates in a saclike vesicle that stores Ca^{2+}. Another network of tubules, the transverse tubule system, or (**T-tubule system**), runs perpendicular to the myofibril. T tubules lie between the most lateral portion of two sarcoplasmic channels; vesicles of these structures abut the T tubule. The term **triad** describes this repeating pattern of two vesicles and a T tubule in each Z line region**.** Each sarcomere contains two triads, with the pattern repeated regularly along the myofibril's length.

The T tubules pass through the fiber and open externally from the inside of the muscle cell. *The triad and T-tubule system function as a microtransportation network to spread the action potential (wave of depolarization) from the fiber's outer membrane inward to deeper regions of the cell.* This releases Ca^{2+} from the triad sacs, which diffuses a short distance to "activate" the actin filaments. Muscle action begins when myosin filament crossbridges momentarily attach to active sites on the actin filaments. When electrical excitation ceases, Ca^{2+} concentration in cytoplasm decreases; this relates to muscle relaxation. To some extent, the ability to propagate an action potential (and counter fatigue in exercise) depends on maintenance of continued steep gradients of Na^+ and K^+ across the sarcolemma. A decrease in the chemical gradients of these electrolytes (from a reduction in Na^+/K^+ pump activity) can severely impact muscle fiber excitability and consequent contractile performance of active muscles.[47]

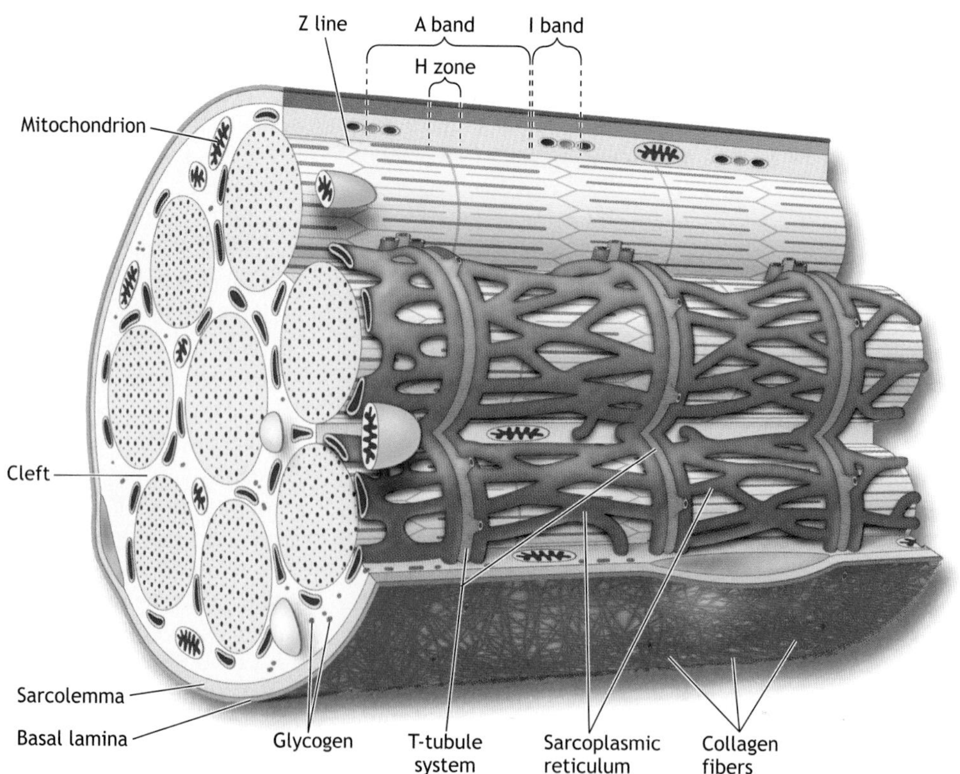

FIGURE 18.8 • The complex T-tubule system within a muscle fiber.

CHEMICAL AND MECHANICAL EVENTS DURING MUSCLE ACTION AND RELAXATION

Electron microscopy, x-ray diffraction, and biochemical methods have unraveled many secrets of cellular structure and kinetics, providing testable hypotheses about chemical and mechanical events during muscle activation and relaxation. Many pieces of the puzzle remain unanswered, but considerable evidence supports the **sliding-filament model** to explain muscle contraction. Proposed nearly 50 years ago to explain the molecular movements that underlie muscle action, the model still fits nicely with the ever-expanding details about muscle ultrastructure and function.[27]

Mechanism of Muscle Action: The Sliding-Filament Model

In the early 1950s, two British biologists, Hugh and Andrew Huxley (unrelated and working independently), proposed a sliding-filament model of muscle contraction. In 1957, A. Huxley extended the theory to include specifics of crossbridge behavior.[28,29] *The theory proposes that a muscle shortens or lengthens because the thick and thin filaments slide past each other, without actually changing length. The myosin crossbridges, which cyclically attach, rotate, and detach from the actin filaments with energy from ATP hydrolysis, provide the* ***molecular motor*** *to drive fiber shortening.*[52] This causes a major conformational change in relative size within the sarcomere's zones and bands and produces a force at the Z bands.[3] Figure 18.9 shows that the thin actin filaments move past the myosin myofilaments (translate over them by a preset amount)[7] and into the A band region

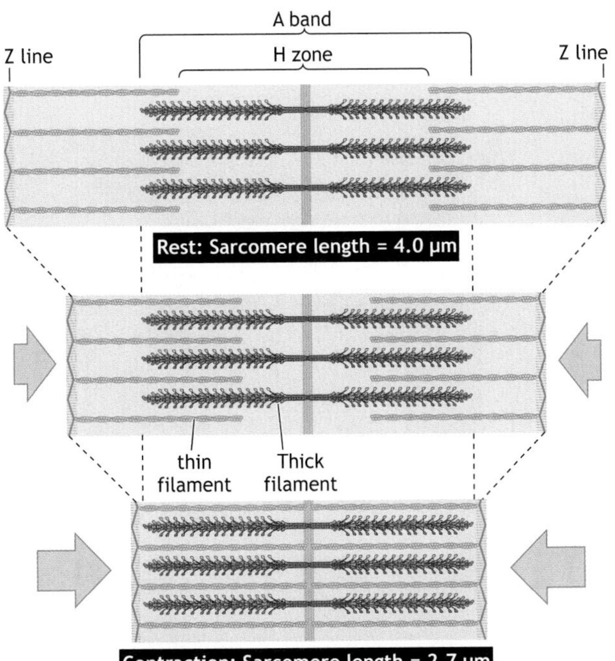

FIGURE 18.9 • Structural rearrangement of actin and myosin filaments at rest (sarcomere length, 4.0 μm) and during muscle shortening (contracted sarcomere length, 2.7 μm).

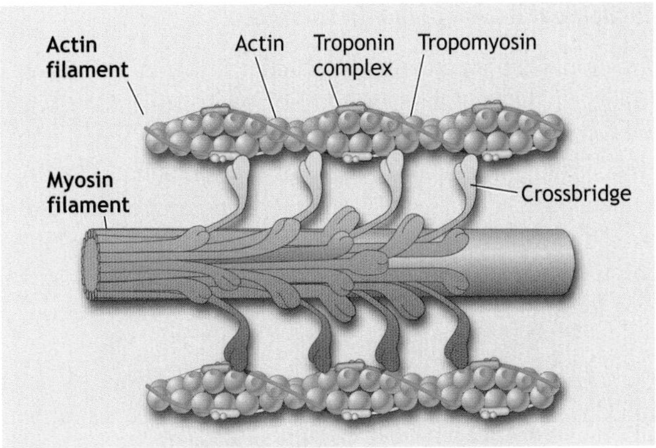

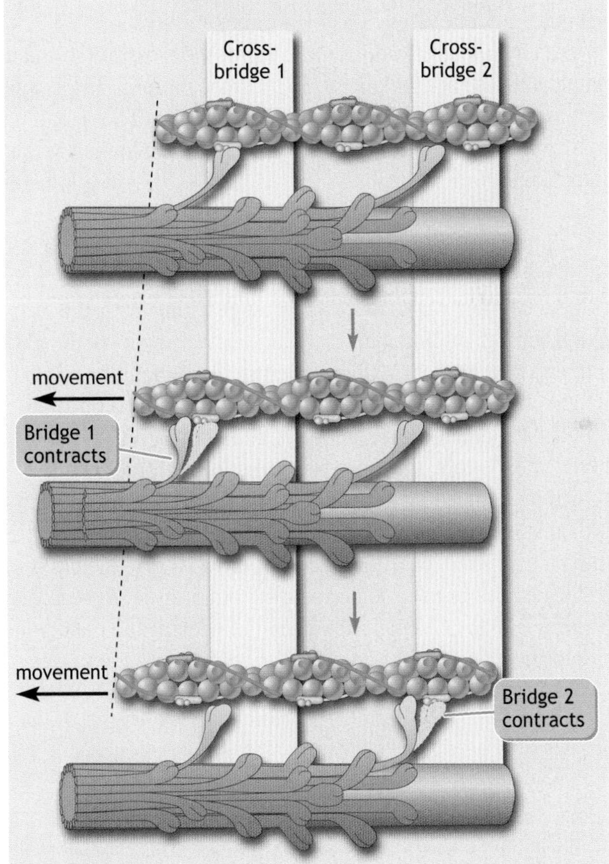

FIGURE 18.10 • Relative positioning of actin and myosin filaments during crossbridge oscillation. The action of each crossbridge contributes a small displacement of movement. For clarity, we show only one actin strand.

during shortening (and move out during relaxation). Thus, the major structural rearrangement during shortening occurs in the region of the I band, which decreases significantly as the Z bands are pulled toward the center of each sarcomere. No change occurs in the width of the A band, although the H zone can disappear when the actin filaments make contact at the sarcomere center. A static muscle action (isometric) generates force, but the fiber's length remains unchanged, and the relative spacing of I and A bands stays constant. In this case, the same molecular groups interact repeatedly. The A band widens in an eccentric action as the fiber lengthens during force generation.

Mechanical Action of the Crossbridges

Myosin plays both an enzymatic and a structural role in muscle action. The globular head of the myosin crossbridge, which contains an actin-activated ATPase in its actin binding site, provides the mechanical power stroke for the actin and myosin filaments to slide past each other.[26,44] The cyclic, oscillating, to-and-fro motion of the crossbridges (powered by ATP hydrolysis) moves in a manner similar to that of oars slicing through water (Fig. 18.10). Unlike oars, however, crossbridges do not all move synchronously. If they did, the muscle action would produce a series of uneven actions instead of finely graded, smoothly modulated movements and force outputs. During shortening, each crossbridge undergoes many repeated but independent cycles of asynchronous movement.

At any one time, only about 50% of the crossbridges make contact with the actin filaments to form the protein complex **actomyosin**, which exhibits contractile properties. The remaining crossbridges move through some other position in their vibrating cycle. Figure 18.10 shows that each crossbridge action contributes only a small longitudinal displacement to the filament's total sliding action. The process resembles the action of a person climbing a rope. The arms and legs represent the crossbridges. Climbing progresses by first reaching with the arms; then grabbing, pulling, and breaking contact while the legs extend; and then repeating this procedure throughout the climb as the person traverses from point A to point B and so on.

The biochemical technique of *in vitro* motility assays has played a key role in quantifying the behavior of actin and myosin molecules.[38] Careful experiments have determined that myosin elicits a 1 to 10 piconewton (pN; 10^{-2} N) force, in which myosin movement ranges from 1 to 20 nanometers (nm; 10^{-9} m) over a brief time period of about 5 msec. Researchers have devised four elegant approaches to determine the chemical and mechanical properties of the actomyosin complex.

1. *Microneedles*. A glass needle placed in contact with myosin molecules and an actin filament records the mechanical movements of the molecules. Researchers then deduce the forces produced by the myosin heads as they slide along the actin strand.[30]
2. *Optical tweezers*. This technique interfaces powerful laser technology with a microscope to isolate individual molecules and measure molecular movement one at a time.[17]
3. *Atomic force microscope*. The displacement and forces from a probe (with actin and myosin molecules attached) interfaced with a microscope yields quantitative data about actin–myosin interaction.[35]
4. *Fluorescent probes*. Light-emitting probes quantify the kinetics of molecular binding and release between myosin and actin and how ATP releases energy when degraded to ADP and inorganic phosphate.[20] The technique also has revealed how actin rotates slightly as it moves along myosin[58] and the behavior of the myosin heads during their power stroke.[69]

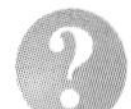

INTEGRATIVE QUESTION

Discuss the meaning of *molecular motor* to describe how the myofilament crossbridges contribute to muscle fiber action.

Sarcomere Length–Isometric Tension Curve in an Isolated Fiber

Figure 18.11 displays the interactions between actin and myosin during isometric tension development in an isolated skeletal muscle preparation. British and Swedish researchers obtained this length–tension curve approximately 35 years ago by electrically stimulating a single frog muscle fiber (8 mm long and 75 μm in diameter) and plotting maximum

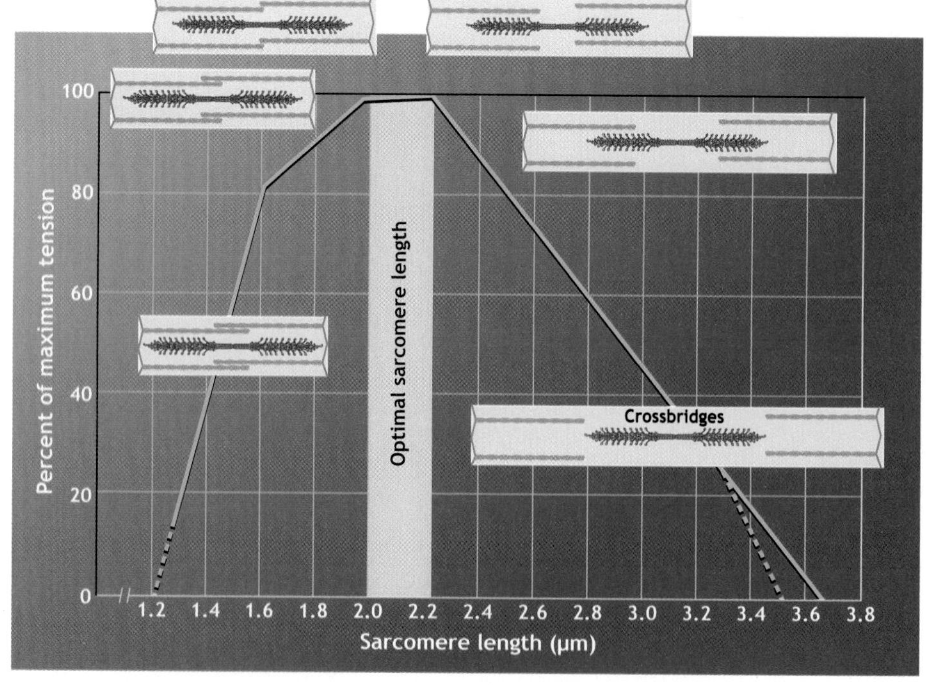

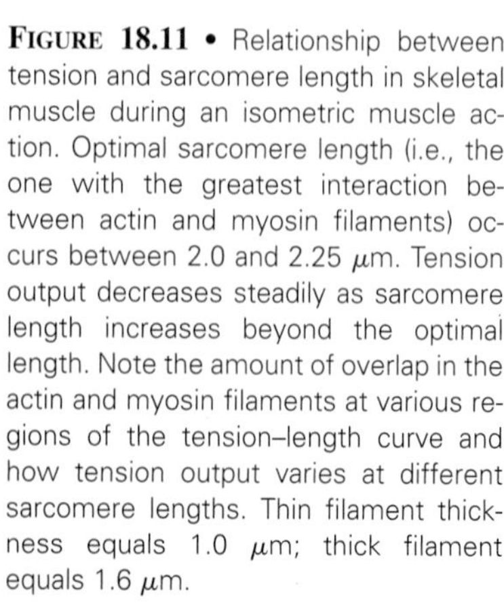

FIGURE 18.11 • Relationship between tension and sarcomere length in skeletal muscle during an isometric muscle action. Optimal sarcomere length (i.e., the one with the greatest interaction between actin and myosin filaments) occurs between 2.0 and 2.25 μm. Tension output decreases steadily as sarcomere length increases beyond the optimal length. Note the amount of overlap in the actin and myosin filaments at various regions of the tension–length curve and how tension output varies at different sarcomere lengths. Thin filament thickness equals 1.0 μm; thick filament equals 1.6 μm.

tension output at selected muscle sarcomere lengths.[14,24] The length of the sarcomere (horizontal axis) ranged from 1.6 μm at maximum overlap of the actin filaments (approximately 70% of maximum tension) to 3.6 μm when fully relaxed. Note that the crest of the upward curve for tension occurred at a sarcomere length between 2.0 and 2.25 μm; this length for maximal tension represents the region of maximum actin and myosin filament interaction. Interestingly, the difference of 0.2 μm at this part of the curve equals precisely the width of the region in which no change takes place in actin–myosin interaction. As the sarcomere stretches beyond 2.2 μm, the curve shifts downward, showing a decline in peak tension. This occurs because of reduced overlap between actin and myosin filaments; less overlap produces less crossbridge interaction and, therefore, diminished active tension development. The fiber fails to develop tension at the maximum point of stretch of 3.65 μm (maximum actin filament length, 2.0 μm; maximum myosin filament length, 1.65 μm). Crossbridge interaction cannot take place at a sarcomere length of 3.65 μm and greater.

Sarcomere Length–Isometric Tension Curve in Human Muscle Fibers in Vivo

An elegant procedure has determined the range over which sarcomeres in intact human muscle operate on their length–tension curve. Figure 18.12 illustrates sarcomere action during different wrist position angles in patients undergoing surgery to correct chronic lateral epicondylitis ("tennis elbow").[43] Observations during surgery provided for a comparison of the length–tension characteristics of an animal preparation (Fig. 18.11) with those of human muscle *in vivo*. Figure 18.12 *(top right)* depicts the use of an intraoperative helium–neon laser to quantify sarcomere length. The laser, positioned beneath the lateral end of the extensor carpi radialis brevis muscle (ECRB), quantified sarcomere lengths at three different wrist positions: full flexion to increase sarcomere length, neutral, and full extension to decrease sarcomere length. Figure 18.12 *(top left)* shows an example of the laser diffraction pattern for computing sarcomere length. Biopsy specimens from

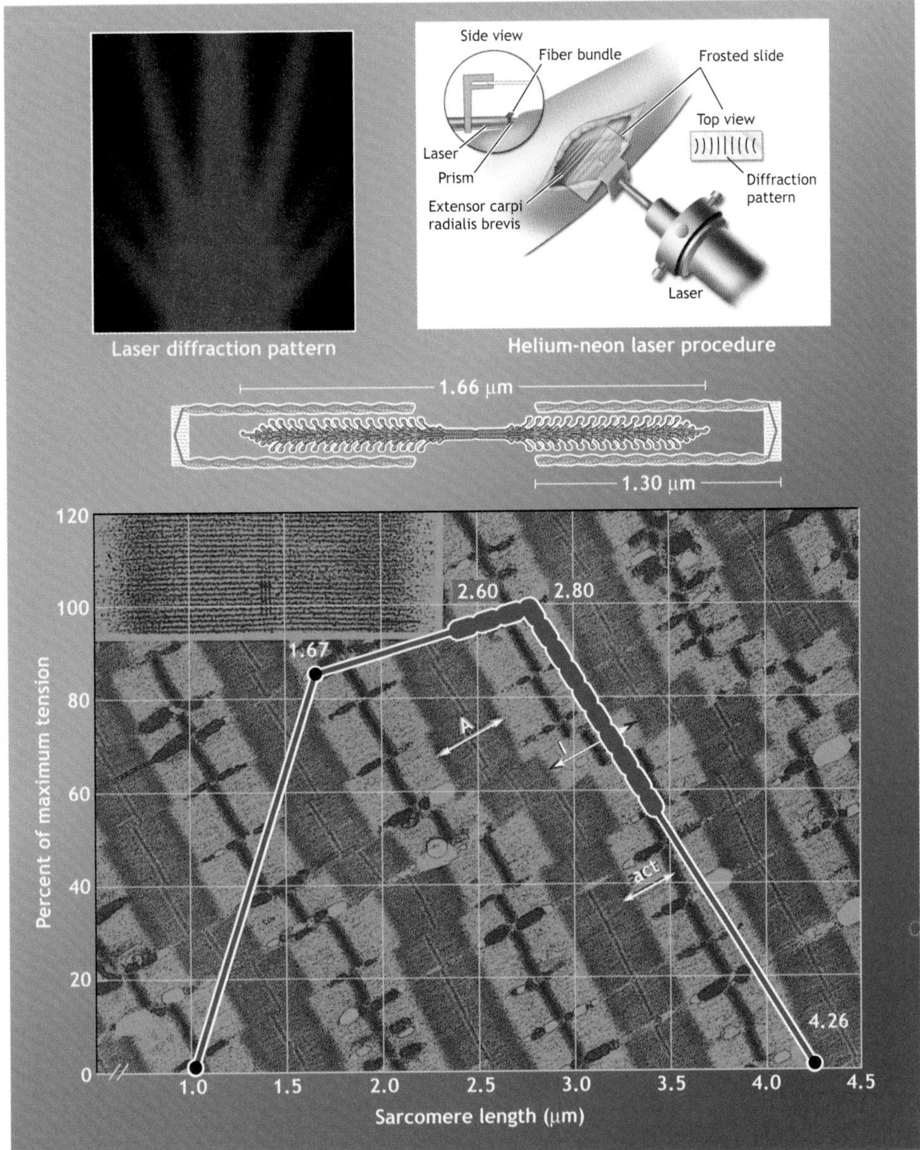

FIGURE 18.12 • Changes in the length–tension curve for sarcomeres *in vivo* during human wrist flexion and extension. The *top insets* illustrate the helium-neon laser procedure (and view of the illumination prism) used during the surgery. The electron micrograph depicted behind the length–tension curve shows the actin and myosin filaments and the A and I bands from biopsy samples of the extensor carpi radialis brevis muscle, used to verify the sarcomere lengths. The *thickened blue portion* of a hypothetical length–tension curve represents sarcomere length change during wrist flexion (causing a sarcomere length increase) and wrist extension (causing a sarcomere length decrease). The numbers over the curve represent the inflection points based on the measured filament lengths. (Modified from Lieber RL, et al. In vivo measurement of human wrist extensor muscle sarcomere length changes. J Neurophysiol 1994;71:874. Illustration of the experimental procedure, including the example of the laser diffraction pattern and electron micrograph courtesy of Dr. R. L. Lieber, Professor of Orthopaedics and Bioengineering, Muscle Physiology Laboratory, University of California and Veterans Administration Medical Centers, San Diego, CA.)

the same muscle verified the laser determinations. An electron micrograph displayed behind the length–tension curve shows the actin and myosin filaments and A and I bands from a muscle biopsy sample. In this experiment, actin filament length equaled 1.30 μm while the myosin filaments were 1.66 μm long. The thicker blue portion for the plateau and downward parts of the curve show the operating range of the ECRB sarcomeres during both passive (2.6 to 3.4 μm) and active (2.44 to 3.33 μm) muscle actions. These data objectify the intrinsic relation between sarcomere length and muscle fiber force capacity (length–tension curve) measured *in vivo* in human muscle.

Link Between Actin, Myosin, and ATP

The interaction and movement of the protein filaments during muscle action necessitate that myosin crossbridges continually undergo oscillatory movements by combining, detaching, and recombining with new sites along the actin strands (or the same sites in a static action). The myosin crossbridges detach from the actin filament when ATP molecules join the actomyosin complex. In this chemical reaction, the myosin crossbridge returns to its original state ready to bind to a new active actin site. The dissociation of actomyosin occurs as follows:

Actomyosin + ATP ⟶ Actin + Myosin-ATP

Energy from ATP hydrolysis transduces into mechanical force during formation of ADP and inorganic phosphate end products. One of the reacting sites on the globular head of the myosin crossbridge binds to an actin reactive site. The other myosin active site serves as the actin-activated enzyme **myofibrilar adenosinetriphosphatase (myosin ATPase)**. This enzyme splits ATP to yield energy for muscle action. The rate of ATP splitting is relatively slow if myosin and actin remain apart; when they join, however, myosin ATPase reaction rates increase substantially. Energy released from ATP splitting activates the crossbridges, causing them to oscillate. This course of energy transfer produces a conformational change in the shape of myosin's globular head so that it interacts with the appropriate actin molecule. Conformational change at multiple points of contact between myosin and actin slides the actin filament forward.

Prior to muscle action, the elongated, pear-shaped, flexible myosin head literally bends around the energy-carrying ATP molecule and becomes cocked, almost like a spring. The myosin then interacts with the adjacent actin filament, splits a phosphate from ATP, and releases its stored mechanical energy as it straightens. This forces the sliding motion that generates muscle tension.[53,54] The actin and myosin filaments slide past each other at speeds up to 15 $\mu m \cdot s^{-1}$.[5]

Excitation–Contraction Coupling

Excitation—contraction coupling *provides the physiologic mechanism whereby an electrical discharge at the muscle initiates chemical events at the cell surface, releasing intracellular Ca^{2+} and ultimately causing muscle action.* Intracellular Ca^{2+} plays an intimate role in regulating a muscle fiber's contractile and metabolic activity.[37] Ca^{2+} concentration within a nonactive muscle fiber remains relatively low compared with that of the extracellular fluid bathing the cell. Muscle fiber stimulation causes an immediate, small increase in intracellular Ca^{2+}, which precedes contractile activity. Cellular Ca^{2+} increases when the action potential at the transverse tubules causes Ca^{2+} release from the lateral sacs of the sarcoplasmic reticulum. The inhibitory action of troponin (which prevents actin–myosin interaction) rapidly dissipates when Ca^{2+} binds with this and other proteins in the actin filaments. In a sense, the muscle "turns on" for action.

Actin + Myosin ATPase ⟶ Actomyosin + ATPase

Joining the active sites on actin and myosin activates myosin ATPase to split ATP. The energy generated causes myosin crossbridge movement to produce muscle tension.

Actomyosin ATP ⟶ Actomyosin + ADP + P + Energy

The crossbridge uncouples from actin when ATP binds to the myosin crossbridge. Coupling and uncoupling continue as long as Ca^{2+} concentration remains high enough to inhibit the troponin–tropomyosin system. When neural stimulation ceases, Ca^{2+} moves back into the lateral sacs of the sarcoplasmic reticulum. This restores the inhibitory action of troponin–tropomyosin, and actin and myosin stay apart as long as ATP concentration remains adequate. In rigor mortis, the muscles stiffen and become rigid soon after death because the cell no longer contains ATP. Without ATP, the myosin crossbridges and actin remain attached and do not separate. Figure 18.13 illustrates the interaction between actin and myosin filaments, Ca^{2+}, and ATP in both a relaxed and a shortened muscle fiber.

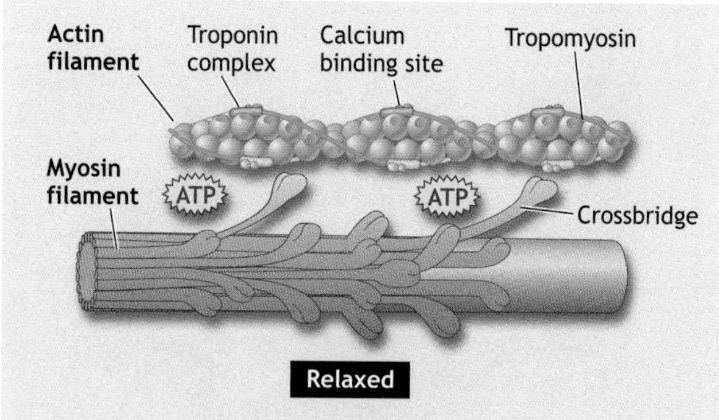

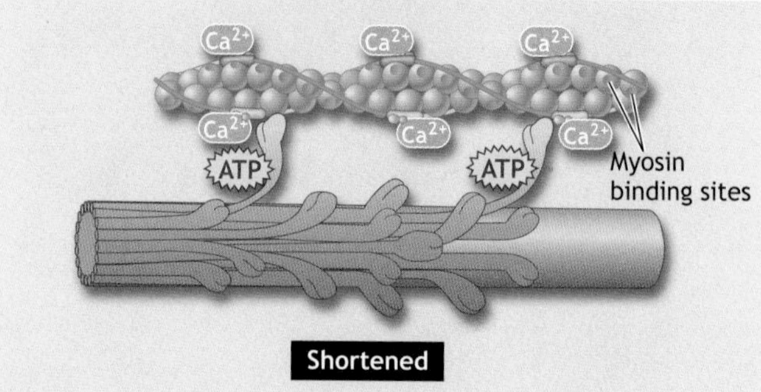

FIGURE 18.13 • Interaction between the actin–myosin filaments, Ca^{2+}, and ATP in relaxed and shortened muscle. In the relaxed state, troponin and tropomyosin interact with actin, preventing the myosin crossbridge from coupling to actin. During muscle action, the crossbridge couples with actin because of Ca^{2+} binding with troponin–tropomyosin.

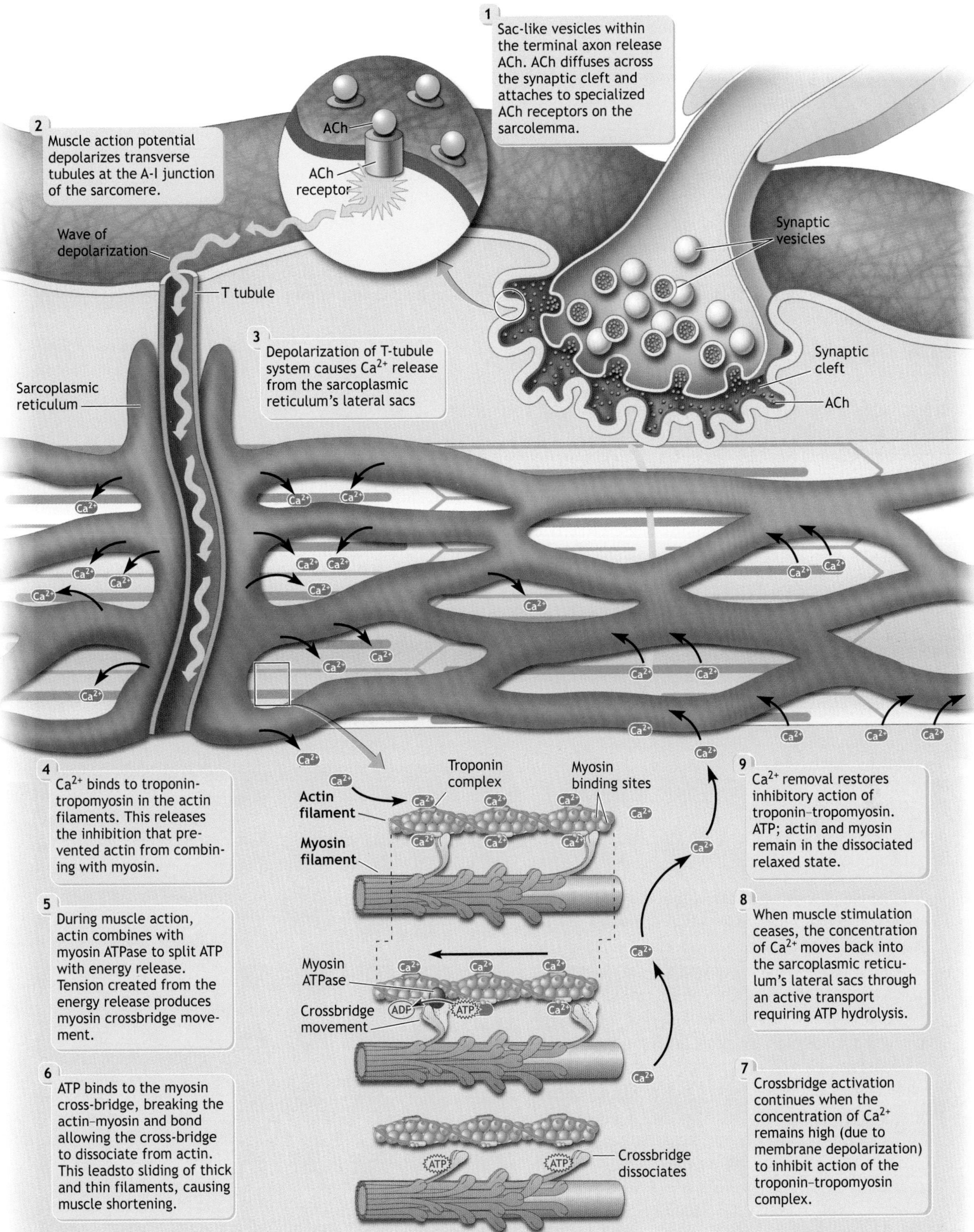

FIGURE 18.14 • Schematic view of the main events in muscle contraction and relaxation. The *numbers* correspond to the sequence of nine steps outlined in the text. The neurotransmitter acetylcholine (ACh), released from saclike vesicles within the terminal axon, facilitates nerve transmission at the myoneural junction. Here, the electrochemical signal "jumps" across the 0.05-μm cleft between neuron and muscle fiber. The electrical impulse, traveling at a velocity of 1 $m \cdot s^{-1}$ or more, spreads through the fiber's tubule system to the inner contractile "machinery" of the myofibrils.

Stimulation produces a threefold rise in Ca^{2+} concentration and an accompanying increase in the magnitude of the action potential in type II (fast-twitch) muscle fibers, compared with type I (slow-twitch) muscle fibers in isolated muscle preparations.[55] Such differences may reflect faster Ca^{2+} transport through the sarcoplasmic reticulum and ultimately to the contractile proteins in type II fibers. During excitation–contraction coupling, electrochemical events occur within the cell membrane at the site of excitation. The common pathway for precisely targeting the chemical signal to the contractile proteins depends mostly on ion channel regulators. These structures serve as selective "gates," or "sensors," to modulate ion passage between the intracellular and extracellular fluids before myofilament activation.

Relaxation

When muscle stimulation ceases, Ca^{2+} flow stops and troponin frees up to inhibit actin–myosin interaction. Recovery involves active pumping of Ca^{2+} into the sarcoplasmic reticulum, where it concentrates in the lateral vesicles. Retrieval of Ca^{2+} from the troponin–tropomyosin protein complex "turns off" the active sites on the actin filament. Deactivation serves two purposes: (1) it prevents any mechanical link between the myosin crossbridges and actin filaments and (2) it inhibits the activity of myosin ATPase, which curtails ATP splitting. Muscle relaxation takes place when the actin and myosin filaments return to their original states.

Sequence of Events in Muscle Action

Figure 18.14 summarizes the main events in muscle activation, contraction, and relaxation. The sequence begins with the initiation of an action potential by the motor nerve. The impulse then propagates over the entire fiber surface (sarcolemma) as it depolarizes. The following nine steps correspond to the numbered sequence in Figure 18.14:

Step 1: Small, saclike vesicles within the terminal axon release acetylcholine (ACh). ACh diffuses across the synaptic cleft and attaches to specialized ACh receptors on the sarcolemma. Almost perfect symmetry exists between the "imprint" of the presynaptic vesicles that contain ACh and the "imprint" of the postsynaptic receptors that capture ACh.

Step 2: The muscle action potential depolarizes the transverse tubules at the A-I junction of the sarcomere.

Step 3: Depolarization of the T-tubule system causes Ca^{2+} release from the lateral sacs (terminal cisternae) of the sarcoplasmic reticulum.

Step 4: Ca^{2+} binds to troponin–tropomyosin in the actin filaments. This releases the inhibition that prevented actin from combining with myosin.

Step 5: During muscle action, actin combines with myosin–ATP. Actin also activates the enzyme myosin ATPase, which then splits ATP. The energy from this reaction produces myosin crossbridge movement and creates tension.

Step 6: ATP binds to the myosin crossbridge, which breaks the actin–myosin bond and allows the crossbridge to dissociate from actin. This enables the thick and thin filaments to slide past each other, and the muscle shortens.

Step 7: Crossbridge activation continues as long as Ca^{2+} concentration remains high enough (on account of membrane depolarization) to inhibit the troponin–tropomyosin system.

Step 8: When muscle stimulation ceases, intracellular Ca^{2+} concentration rapidly decreases because Ca^{2+} moves back into the lateral sacs of the sarcoplasmic reticulum through active transport requiring ATP hydrolysis.

Step 9: Ca^{2+} removal restores the inhibitory action of troponin–tropomyosin. In the presence of ATP, actin and myosin remain in the dissociated, relaxed state.

MUSCLE FIBER TYPE

Skeletal muscle does not simply contain a homogeneous group of fibers with similar metabolic and contractile properties. Despite continuing discussion concerning the method, terminology, and criteria for classifying human skeletal muscle, researchers have identified and classified *two* distinct fiber types by their *contractile* and *metabolic* characteristics.[2] A common technique for establishing the specific muscle fiber type assesses the myosin molecule's heavy chain, which exists in three different forms (isoforms). Assessment evaluates a fiber's differential sensitivity to an altered pH of the enzyme myosin ATPase (a measure of myosin phenotype).[37,40,49] The different characteristics of this enzyme determine the rapidity of ATP hydrolysis in the myosin heavy chain region and thus the velocity of sarcomere shortening. More specifically, an acid pH inactivates the activity of the specific myosin ATPase in fast-twitch fibers, but this enzyme remains fairly stable with pH in the alkaline range; these fibers stain *dark* for this enzyme. In contrast, specific myosin ATPase activity for slow-twitch fibers remains high at an acid pH but becomes inactive in an alkaline medium; these fibers stain *light* for myosin ATPase. Figure 18.15 illustrates serial cross sections of the human vastus lateralis muscle with identification of type I and type II muscle fibers and subdivisions. Table 18.2 lists different classification schemes for skeletal muscle fiber types on the basis of morphology, histochemistry and biochemistry, function, and contractility.

Fast-Twitch Fibers

Fast-twitch muscle fibers exhibit the following characteristics:

- High capability for electrochemical transmission of action potentials.
- High myosin ATPase activity.
- Rapid Ca^{2+} release and uptake by an efficient sarcoplasmic reticulum.
- High rate of crossbridge turnover.

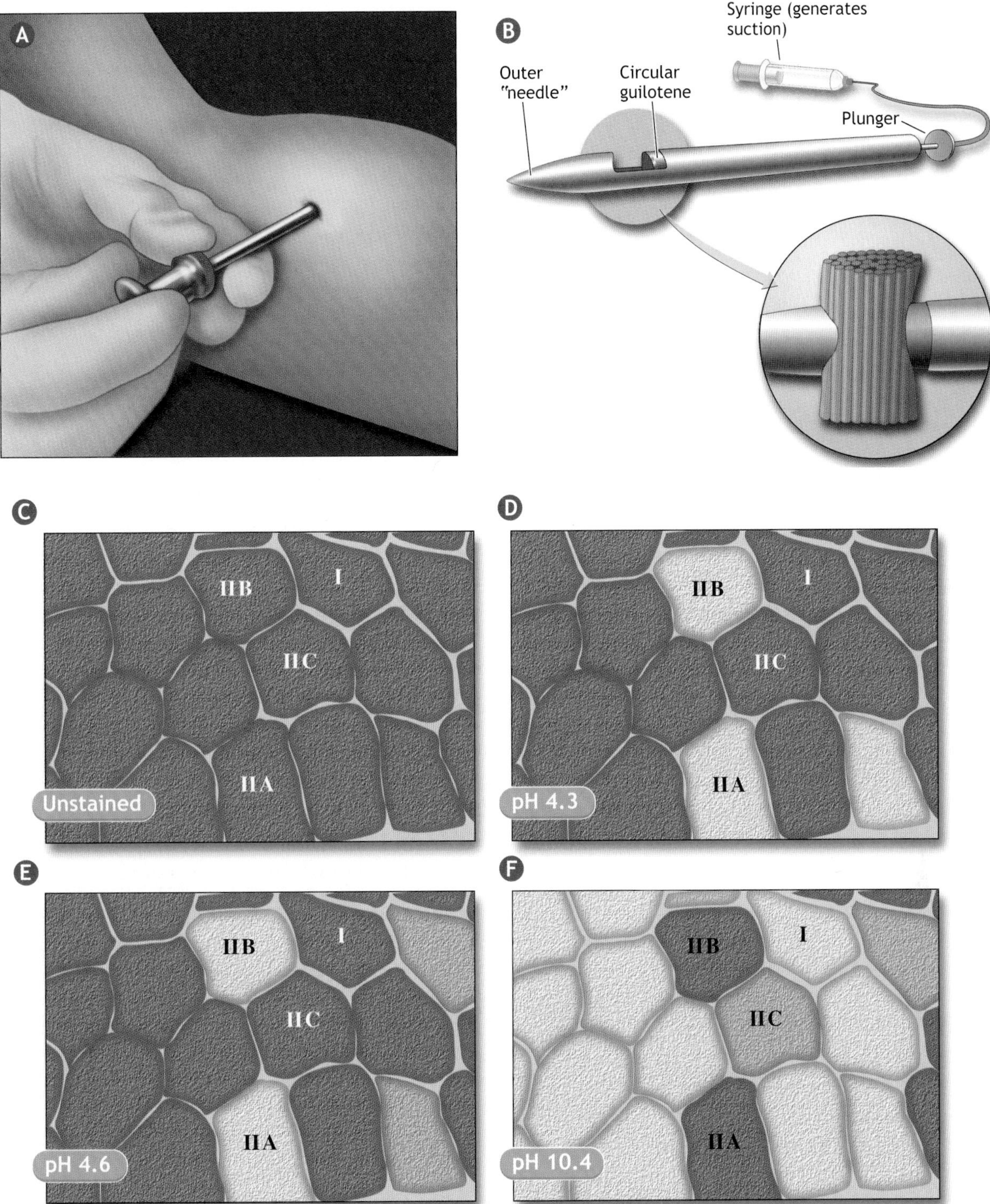

FIGURE 18.15 • Serial cross sections of human vastus lateralis muscle obtained by muscle biopsy (**A** and **B**) with identification of type I and type IIA, B, and C fiber subdivisions. **C**. Thick unstained section (40–50 μm) where all fibers appear similar. Three other panels indicate same fibers stained for myosin–ATPase activity at a preincubation pH of (**D**) 4.3 (highly acidic), (**E**) 4.6 (intermediate acidity), and (**F**) 10.6 (alkaline). *Bar in bottom right of panel C* indicates distance of 100 μm.

All of these factors contribute to this fiber's rapid energy generation for quick, powerful actions. The fast-twitch fiber's intrinsic speed of shortening and tension development ranges three to five times faster than fibers classified as slow twitch (see following section).[18] Fast-twitch fibers often rely on a well-developed, short-term glycolytic system for energy transfer. *This explains why activation of these fibers predominates in anaerobic-type sprint activities and other forceful muscle actions that depend almost entirely on anaerobic energy metabolism.*[23,34] Activation of fast-twitch fibers plays an important role in the stop-and-go or change-of-pace sports such as basketball, soccer, lacrosse, or field hockey. These ac-

TABLE 18.2 ➤ CLASSIFICATION SCHEMES OF SKELETAL MUSCLE FIBER TYPES

	Fiber Types		
	Fast-Twitch		Slow-Twitch
Characteristic	**Type IIB**	**Type IIA**	**Type I**
Electrical activity patterns	Phasic; high frequency		Tonic; low frequency
Morphology	**FTb**	**FTa**	**ST**
Color	White	White/red	Red
Fiber diameter	Large	Intermediate	Small
Capillaries/mm²	Low	Intermediate	High
Mitochondrial volume	Low	Intermediate	High
Histochemistry and biochemistry	**Type IIb** **FG**	**Type IIa** **FOG**	**Type I** **SO**
Myosin ATPase	High	High	Low
Calcium capacity	High	Medium/high	Low
Glycolytic capacity	High	High	Low
Oxidative capacity	Low	Medium/high	High
Function and contractility	**FF** **FT**	**FR** **FT**	**S** **ST**
Speed of action	Fast	Fast	Slow
Speed of relaxation	Fast	Fast	Slow
Fatigue resistance	Low	Moderate/high	High
Force capacity	High	Intermediate	Low

FT, fast twitch; FG, fast, glycolytic; FOG, fast, oxidative, glycolytic; SO, slow, oxidative; FF, fast contracting, fast fatigue; FR, fast contracting, fatigue resistant; S, slow contracting.

From Kraus W. Skeletal muscle adaptation to chronic low-frequency motor nerve stimulation. Exerc Sport Sci Rev, 1994;22:313.

tivities often demand rapid energy that only anaerobic pathways generate. "In a Practical Sense" describes a popular jumping test for inferring the immediate power output from the intramuscular high-energy phosphates ATP and phosphocreatine (PCr). Theoretically, individuals with a predominance of fast-twitch muscle fibers should achieve relatively high scores on such a test.

Slow-Twitch Fibers

Slow-twitch fibers generate energy for ATP resynthesis predominantly through the aerobic system of energy transfer. Their distinguishing characteristics include:

- Relatively low myosin ATPase activity
- Slower calcium handling ability and shortening speed
- Glycolytic capacity less well developed than that of fast-twitch fibers
- Relatively large and numerous mitochondria

Large, numerous mitochondria (and accompanying iron-containing cytochromes) combined with high myoglobin levels give slow-twitch fibers their characteristic red pigmentation. A high concentration of mitochondrial enzymes (needed to sustain aerobic metabolism) links closely to a slow-twitch fiber's enhanced metabolic machinery.[16,22,31] *These characteristics make slow-twitch fibers highly fatigue resistant and ideally suited for prolonged aerobic exercise.* The fibers have been labeled **SO (slow-oxidative) fibers** to describe their slow shortening speed and reliance on oxidative metabolism. Unlike fast-twitch fibers that fatigue readily, SO fibers (more precisely, motor units) become selectively recruited in aerobic activities.[33] Muscle glycogen depletion patterns indicate that prolonged, high-intensity exercise demands almost exclusive reliance on slow-twitch muscle fibers. Even after exercising for 12 hours, the limited glycogen remaining in active muscle exists mostly in the relatively "unused" fast-twitch fibers.[57] Differences in oxidative capacity of the two fiber types also determine the magnitude of blood flow through muscle, with slow-twitch fibers receiving the largest quantity.[41,63]

Most researchers classify slow-twitch fibers as **type I**, and fast-twitch fibers (and proposed subdivisions) as **type II.** *Both fiber types contribute during near-maximum aerobic and anaerobic exercise as in middle-distance running or swimming or basketball, field hockey, or soccer, which combine high levels of aerobic and anaerobic energy transfer.*

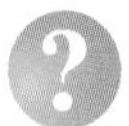

INTEGRATIVE QUESTION

Present the pros and cons for muscle fiber typing of children to "guide" them into sports to increase their likelihood of future success.

Fast-Twitch Subdivisions

Several subdivisions characterize fast-twitch muscle fibers. The intermediate **type IIa fiber** exhibits a fast shortening speed and a moderately well-developed capacity for energy transfer from both aerobic (high level of aerobic enzyme succinic dehydrogenase, or SDH) and anaerobic (high level of anaerobic enzyme phosphofructokinase, or PFK) sources. These fibers represent the **fast–oxidative–glycolytic (FOG)**

IN A PRACTICAL SENSE

PREDICTING PEAK ANAEROBIC POWER OUTPUT USING A VERTICAL JUMP TEST

Peak anaerobic power output underlies success in many sports activities. The vertical jump test is often used to infer "explosive" peak anaerobic power output from the intramuscular high-energy phosphates.

Vertical Jump Test

The vertical jump test measures the highest distance jumped from a semicrouched position by use of the following protocol:

1. Establish standing reach height. The subject, standing with preferred shoulder adjacent to a wall and feet flat on the floor, reaches as high as possible to touch the wall. Starting point (standing reach height) represents the distance from the wall mark (middle finger) to the floor, recorded in centimeters (cm) (Fig. *A*).
2. Bend knees to about a 90° angle while moving arms back in a winged position (Fig. *B*).
3. Thrust forward and upward, touching as high as possible on the wall (Fig. *C*).
4. Perform three trials of the jump test; use the highest score as the vertical height.
5. Compute vertical jump height (cm) as the difference between standing reach height and vertical height achieved in the jump.

Predicting Immediate Anaerobic Power Output

The following equation predicts peak anaerobic power output in watts (PAP_w) from vertical jump height in cm (VJ_{cm}) and body mass in kilograms (BM_{kg}). This equation applies to males and females:

$$PAP_w = 60.7\ (VJ_{cm}) + 45.3\ (BM_{kg}) - 2055$$

EXAMPLE

A 21-year-old male weighing 78 kg records a vertical jump of 43 cm (standing reach height, 185 cm; vertical height, 228 cm); predict peak anaerobic power output in watts.

COMPUTATIONS

$$\begin{aligned} PAP_w &= 60.7\ (VJ_{cm}) + 45.3\ (BM_{kg}) - 2055 \\ &= 60.7\ (43\ \text{cm}) + 45.3\ (78\ \text{kg}) - 2055 \\ &= 4088.5\ \text{W} \end{aligned}$$

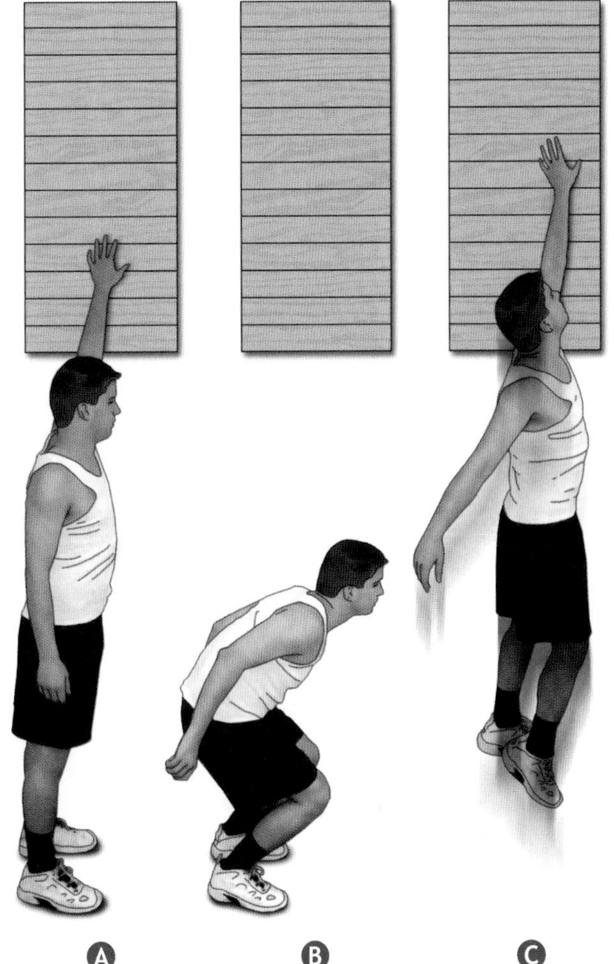

Figure. *(A)* Starting point (standing reach height), *(B)* just prior to jumping, and *(C)* final point in determining vertical jump height.

COMPARISONS

As a frame of reference, average peak power output measured with this vertical jump protocol averages 4620.2 (SD ± 822.5) W for males, and 2993.7 (SD ± 542.9) W for females.

Sayers S, et al. Cross-validation of three jump power equations. Med Sci Sports Exerc 1999;31:572.

fibers. Another subdivision, the **type IIb fiber** (also termed type IIx), possesses the greatest anaerobic potential and most rapid shortening velocity, and represents the "true" **fast–glycolytic (FG) fiber**. The **type IIc fiber**, normally rare and undifferentiated, may contribute to reinnervation and motor unit transformation.[39]

SPECIES DIFFERENCES: A COMPARATIVE LOOK AT MUSCLE METABOLISM AND DYNAMICS

The study of comparative physiology provides an appreciation for the diversity of function and adaptation among species and insight into a better understanding of human physiology and muscle metabolism. Throughout the animal kingdom—from the elephant who weighs 100,000 times more than a mouse to the smallest shrew, about one-millionth the elephant's size—extraordinary examples of muscular strength, power, and endurance make the athletic feats of humans pale by comparison. For example, the world's fastest humans run 200 m at an average velocity of 10.4 $m \cdot s^{-1}$ (23.3 mph; 1994 World Record pace), yet the greyhound dog covers the same distance at 60% greater velocity (16.6 $m \cdot s^{-1}$). For elite human endurance athletes, aerobic metabolism during sustained exercise exceeds the resting requirement by 25 times. However, the muscle machines of other animal species have adapted over millions of years to perform extraordinary metabolic and performance feats. Figure 18.16 shows the maximal rates of oxygen consumption during treadmill running for 22 species of African mammals, both wild and domestic. On average, a 10-fold difference occurs in the ratio of resting to maximal oxygen consumption. The ratio, termed the **factorial aerobic scope** or **metabolic scope**[59] displays considerable intraspecies variation. For example, in four species of canids with different body masses (gray fox, 4.7 kg; coyote, 12.4 kg; timber wolf, 23.3 kg; dog, 25.3 kg) the metabolic scope ranged from 24 for the gray fox to 32 for the dog,[62] a value about the same as that for a champion human endurance athlete.

Contractile Dynamics

From the perspective of muscle fiber dynamics, consider the hummingbird, a super avian athlete that sustains a wing beat frequency of 80 Hz, with an ATP turnover rate of 500 mmol per gram of muscle per minute (500 times the value at rest). This represents the highest metabolic rate in the vertebrate world, accomplished from the resting state to full wing activity in less than 15 ms! Intuitively, one might expect the hummingbird to have an advanced chemical system to fuel a multifaceted network of different muscle fiber types. Some might argue that unique metabolic pathways would sustain high-intensity fiber activity without the negative, fatiguing consequences of anaerobic metabolism characteristic of the human response to all-out effort. In actuality, the hummingbird's flight muscles show a simple architecture consisting of only FOG fibers. The homogeneity of the internal metabolic machinery of these fast-acting fibers shows tremendous upregulation of aerobic functions. For example, fibers have five to seven times the mitochondrial density of human muscle fibers. Capillaries literally wrap around each fiber. Fibers also contain a large sarcoplasmic reticulum volume, a larger-than-normal mitochondrial cristae surface area, reduced diameter of individual fibers (to facilitate diffusion), and high concentrations of key aerobic enzymes. Even fat droplets lie against

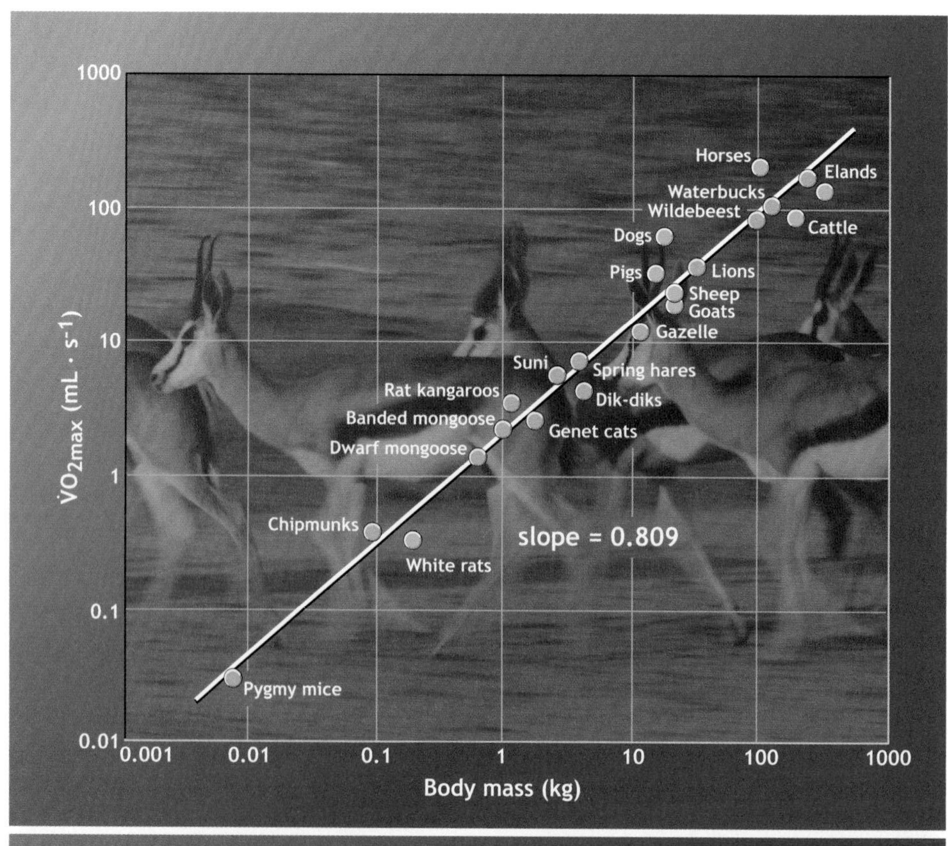

FIGURE 18.16 • Maximal oxygen consumption ($\dot{V}O_{2max}$) during running for 22 species of African mammals, ranging in body mass from 0.007 kg (pygmy mouse) to 263 kg (horse). (From Taylor CR, et al. Design of the mammalian respiratory system. III. Scaling maximum aerobic capacity to body mass: wild and domestic mammals. Resp Physiol 1981;44:25.)

the mitochondria for immediate uptake as aerobic fuel along with glucose. To accentuate these remarkable aerobic adaptations, the fibers possess essentially no capacity for anaerobic metabolism. For most mammals, total muscle mass represents about 40 to 45% of body mass, regardless of body size. In flying birds, pectoral muscles average 15% of body mass, except in the hummingbird, where the value increases to nearly 30%. This makes sense from a standpoint of muscle because the power output requirement for hovering flight exceeds that for forward flight.[70]

Other species in the animal and insect world also show remarkable adaptation in muscle functions to support tasks required for survival.[11] The fast-twitch muscle fibers of "sprint-type" fish (e.g., pike and white tuna) demonstrate homogeneity in cellular architecture and function. Such tremendous upregulation emphasizes glycolytic and high-energy phosphate–driven power performance with a corresponding blunting of aerobic function. At a different extreme, the muscle machinery of the electric eel creates a 2000-fold increase in ATP production to generate a paralyzing electric charge within 300 ms.[6]

Force and Power

For generating muscle power, the limiting factor in humans and animals depends on the energy-producing capacity of the muscle's protein filaments. Maximal force of any muscle (roughly 3 to 4 kg · cm^{-2} cross section of muscle [300 to 400 kN · m^{-2}]) relates to its cross-sectional area, independent of total body size, and thus is about the same for a mouse and an elephant (and human). The reason for the narrow intraspecies range relates to the similarity in dimensions of the actin and myosin filaments and quantitative similarity in crossbridge number. A microscopist would have difficulty distinguishing between the muscular ultrastructure of an elephant and mouse, except for the larger number of mitochondria in the muscles of smaller animals and the relative length of individual fibers.[59] This gives smaller animals a tremendous advantage in endurance activities, whether moving horizontally or vertically.

Compared with a human, the small animal would win by large margin any speed and power contest. Anyone who has run on a treadmill at 20% grade knows the difficulty in sustaining power output for a minute or two, even at a relatively slow speed of 6 mph. If it were possible to triple the treadmill elevation to 60%, how long could a human maintain the 6 mph velocity? Although the answer remains unknown, the task would clearly tax the cardiovascular, metabolic, and muscular systems beyond their limits. The small mammal, however, performs this task with relative ease. Mice trained to run on a treadmill up a 15° incline exhibited no difference in oxygen consumption between uphill and level running.[62] For chimpanzees and horses, the energy expenditure more than doubles as it does for humans when running up the same incline. Thus, the smaller animal "athlete" such as a squirrel runs up and down tall trees rapidly with relative ease for extended durations. The best-conditioned human endurance or strength athletes would offer no match in uphill climbing competition against a small, furry mammal.

The same would hold true for jumping events. The world's high-jump champion (Javier Sotomayor; 2.45 m) exceeded his own length (stature) in jumping height by a relatively small amount. In contrast, the galago—a 1.3-m bush baby prosimian primate found in many regions south of the Sahara desert and characterized by a hopping gait similar to that of a kangaroo—can leap vertically (2.25 m) more than 70% of its stature![25] The galago's jumping ability relates to its large muscles for jumping (10% of body mass), nearly double that of humans. On a relative basis, the maximal vertical jumping ability of a human, properly scaled to body size (see Chapter 22, Allometric Scaling), falls far short of that of a flea (*Pulex;* body mass of 50 mg). The 2 mm-long flea leaps more than 100 times its body length or twice as far as its human "competition," when appropriately adjusted for the large body size differences. The flea, a remarkable "athlete" in its own right, has a muscular system perfectly adapted to its needs, as do most locomotor and flying members of the animal kingdom.

FIBER TYPE DIFFERENCES AMONG ATHLETIC GROUPS

Several observations concern muscle fiber type and the possible influence of specific training on fiber composition and metabolic capacity.[31,32] Men, women, and children possess 45 to 55% slow-twitch fibers in their arm and leg muscles.[13] The fast-twitch fibers probably distribute equally between type IIa and type IIb subdivisions. While no gender differences exist in fiber distribution, large interindividual variation occurs. Generally, the trend in one's muscle fiber type distribution remains consistent among the body's major muscle groups.

Certain patterns of muscle fiber distribution appear readily in comparisons among highly proficient athletes.[64] For example, successful endurance athletes have predominantly slow-twitch fibers in the major muscles activated in their specific sport. In contrast, fast-twitch fibers predominate for elite sprint athletes.[4] Figure 18.17 illustrates fiber-type distribution for top Scandinavian competitors in different sports. Athletic groups with the highest aerobic and endurance capacities (e.g., distance runners and cross-country skiers) possess the highest percentage of slow-twitch fibers, often as high as 90 to 95% in the leg's gastrocnemius muscle. Weight lifters, ice hockey players, and sprinters tend to have more fast-twitch fibers and relatively lower aerobic capacities. As might be expected, men and women who perform in middle-distance events display approximately equal percentages of the two fiber types. The same distribution also occurs in power athletes—throwers, jumpers, and high jumpers.[12]

The relatively clear-cut distinctions between exercise performance and muscle fiber composition pertain mainly to elite athletes with prominence in a sport category. Even among this group, muscle fiber composition does not solely determine performance success.[9,39] This seems reasonable because successful performance reflects blending of many physiologic, biochemical, neurologic, and biomechanical "support systems," not simply a single factor such as muscle fiber type.[36]

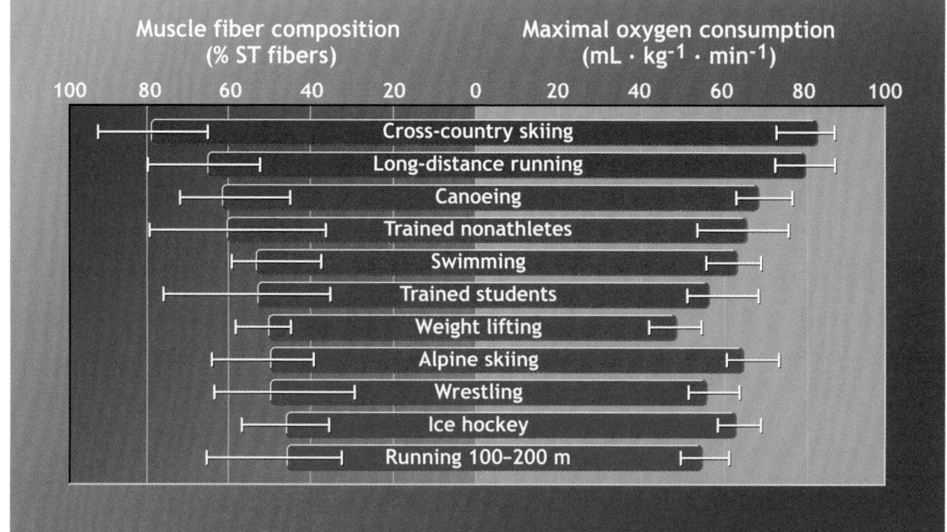

FIGURE 18.17 • Muscle fiber composition (% slow-twitch fibers, *left side*) and maximal oxygen consumption *(right side)* in athletes representing different sports. The *outer, white bars* denote the range. (From Bergh U, et al. Maximal oxygen uptake and muscle fiber types in trained and untrained humans. Med Sci Sports 1978;10:151.)

Endurance athletes have relatively normal-sized muscle fibers, with a tendency toward enlargement of the slow twitch fibers.[15] Conversely, weight lifters and other power athletes show definite enlargement in both fiber types, particularly fast-twitch fibers,[65,66] that may exceed by 45% those of endurance athletes or sedentary people of the same age.[15] Strength and power training induce a definite enlargement of the fiber's contractile apparatus—specifically the actin and myosin filaments—and total glycogen content.[45,46] *Larger muscle fibers in male athletes and a larger total muscle mass are the principal gender differences in muscle morphology.* Chapter 22 discusses the potential for exercise training to alter the metabolic and fiber-type characteristics and size of skeletal muscle.

Summary

1. Various connective tissue wrappings that encase skeletal muscle blend into and join the tendinous attachment to bone. This harness enables muscles to act on the bony levers to transform the chemical energy of ATP into the mechanical energy of motion.
2. A skeletal muscle fiber consists of 75% water, 20% protein, and the remainder as inorganic salts, enzymes, pigments, fats, and carbohydrates.
3. The muscle's oxygen consumption during vigorous exercise increases up to 70 times the resting level. Immediate adjustments and longer-term training adaptations that increase the size or the local vascular bed support this elevated metabolic requirement.
4. The sarcomere provides the functional unit of the muscle fiber. It contains the contractile proteins actin and myosin. An average muscle fiber contains 4500 sarcomeres and 16 billion thick (myosin) and 64 billion thin (actin) filaments.
5. Myosin projections, or crossbridges, serve as structural links between the thick and thin contractile filaments. During a muscle action, the myofibrilar proteins tropomyosin and troponin regulate the make-and-break contacts between the filaments. Tropomyosin inhibits actin and myosin interaction; troponin plus Ca^{2+} triggers the myofibrils to interact and slide past each other.
6. The triad and T-tubule system function as a microtransportation network to spread the action potential from the fiber's outer membrane inward to deeper cell regions. Muscle action takes place when Ca^{2+} activates actin, causing the myosin crossbridges to attach to active sites on the actin filaments. Relaxation occurs when Ca^{2+} concentration decreases.
7. The sliding filament model proposes that a muscle shortens or lengthens because the protein filaments slide past each other without changing their length. The mechanism of excitation–contraction coupling links electrochemical and mechanical events to achieve muscle action.
8. Contractile and metabolic characteristics classify the two types of muscle fibers: (1) fast-twitch, which generate energy predominantly anaerobically for quick, powerful actions (FG fibers, to signify their fast shortening speed and high glycolytic capacity) and (2) slow-twitch, which shorten relatively slowly and generate energy predominantly by aerobic metabolism (SO fibers, to signify their slow shortening speed and reliance on oxidative metabolism). An intermediate, fast–oxidative–glycolytic (FOG) fiber also exists.
9. Significant interindividual differences exist in the percentage of fiber type distribution. Most likely, the variation results from genetic factors, although some modification may result from specific training.

References

1. Andersen P, Henrickson J. Capillary supply of the quadriceps femoris muscle of man: adaptive response to exercise. J Physiol (Lond) 1977;270:677.
2. Armstrong RB. Muscle fiber recruitment patterns and their metabolic correlates. In: Horton ES, Terjung RL, eds. Exercise, nutrition, and energy metabolism. New York: Macmillan, 1988.
3. Borovikov YS. Conformational changes of contractile proteins and their role in muscle contraction. (Review.) Int Rev Cytol 1999;189:267.
4. Bergh U, et al. Maximal oxygen uptake and muscle fiber types in trained and untrained humans. Med Sci Sports 1978;10:151.
5. Billeter R, Hoppeler H. Muscular basis of strength. In: Komi P, ed. Strength and power in sport. London: Blackwell Scientific, 1992.
6. Blum H, et al. Coupled in vivo activity of the membrane band Na^+K^+ ATPase in resting and stimulated electric organ of the electric fish *Narcine brasiliensis.* J Biol Chem 1991;266:1054.
7. Blyakhamn FA, et al. Quantal length changes in single contraction sarcomeres. J Muscle Res Cell Motil 1999;20:529.
8. Brodal P, et al. Capillary supply of skeletal muscle fibers in untrained and endurance trained men. Acta Physiol Scand 1976;440(suppl):1.
9. Campbell CJ, et al. Muscle fiber composition and performance capacities of women. Med Sci Sports 1979;11:260.
10. Carins SP, et al. Role of extracellular $[Ca^{2+}]$ in fatigue of isolated mammalian skeletal muscle. J Appl Physiol 1998;84:1395.
11. Casey TM, et al. Allometric scaling of muscle performance and metabolism: insects. Adv Biosci 1992;84:152.
12. Costill DL, et al. Skeletal muscle enzyme and fiber composition in male and female track athletes. J Appl Physiol 1976;40:149.
13. Dudley GA, et al. Muscle fiber composition and blood ammonia levels after intense exercise in humans. J Appl Physiol 1983;54:582.
14. Edman KAP. The relation between sarcomere length and active tension in isolated semitendinosus fibers of the dog. J Physiol (Lond) 1966;183:407.
15. Edström L, Ekblom B. Differences in sizes of red and white muscle fibers in vastus lateralis of musculus quadriceps of normal individuals and athletes: relation to physical performance. Scand J Clin Lab Invest 1972;30:175.
16. Faulkner JA, et al. Contractile properties of isolated human muscle preparation. Clin Sci 1979;57:20.
17. Finer JT, et al. Single myosin molecule mechanics: piconewton forces and nanometre steps. Nature 1994;368:113.
18. Fitts RH, et al. Effect of swim exercise training on human muscle fiber function. J Appl Physiol 1989;66:465.
19. Foster DN, et al. Effect of training frequency on lumbar extension strength. Med Sci Sports Exerc 1989;21:S88.
20. Funatsu T, et al. Imaging of single fluorescent molecules and individual ATP turnovers by single myosin molecules in aqueous solution. Nature 1995;374:555.
21. Gaffney FA. Cardiovascular and metabolic responses to static contraction in man. Acta Physiol Scand 1990;138:249.
22. Gollnick PD. Effects of training on enzyme activity and fiber composition of human skeletal muscle. J Appl Physiol 1973;34:107.
23. Gollnick PD, et al. Fiber number and size in overloaded chicken anterior latissimus dorsi muscle. J Appl Physiol 1983;54:1292.
24. Gordon AM, et al. The variation in isometric tension with sarcomere length in vertebrate muscle fibers. J Physiol (Lond) 1966;184:170.
25. Hall-Craggs ECB. An analysis of the jump of the lesser galago (Galago senegalensis). J Zool 1965;147:20.
26. Hochachka PW. Muscles as molecular and metabolic machines. Boca Raton, FL: CRC Press, 1994.
27. Holmes KC, Geeves MA. The structural basis of musce contraction (Review.) Philos Trans R Soc Lond B Biol Sci 2000 Apr 29;355(1396):419.
28. Huxley HE. The mechanism of muscular contraction. Science 1969;164:1356.
29. Huxley HE, Hanson J. Changes in the cross-striations of muscle during contraction and stretch, and their structural interpretation. Nature 1954;173:973.
30. Ishijima A, et al. Sub-piconewton force fluctuations of actomyosin in vitro. Nature 1991;352:113.
31. Jansson E, Kaijser L. Muscle adaptation to extreme endurance training in man. Acta Physiol Scand 1977;100:315.
32. Jansson E, et al. Changes in muscle fiber type distribution in man after physical training. Acta Physiol Scand 1978;104:235.
33. Karlsson J, Jacobs I. Onset of blood lactate accumulation during muscular exercise as a threshold concept. I. Theoretical considerations. Int J Sports Med 1982;3:190.
34. Karlsson JB, et al. LDH isozymes in skeletal muscles of endurance and strength trained athletes. Acta Physiol Scand 1975;93:150.
35. Kitmura K, et al. A single myosin head moves along an actin filaments with regular steps of 5.3 nanometers. Nature 1999;397:129.
36. Klausen K, et al. Adaptative changes in work capacity, skeletal muscle capillarization and enzyme levels during training and detraining. Acta Physiol Scand 1981;113:9.
37. Klug GA, Tibbits GF. The effects of activity on calcium-mediated events in striated muscle. Exerc Sport Sci Rev 1988;16:1.
38. Knight AE, Molloy JE. Muscle, myosin, and single molecules. In: Higgins SJ, Banting G, eds. Essays in biochemistry, vol 35. Molecular motors. London: Portland Press, 2000.
39. Komi PV, Karlsson J. Skeletal muscle fiber types, enzyme activities and physical performance in young males and females. Acta Physiol Scand 1978;103:210.
40. Kraus WE, et al. Skeletal muscle adaptation to chronic low-frequency motor nerve stimulation. Exerc Sport Sci Rev 1994;22:313.
41. Laughlin MH, et al. Physical activity and the microcirculation in cardiac and skeletal muscle. In: Bouchard C, et al, eds. Physical activity, fitness, and health. Champaign, IL: Human Kinetics, 1994.
42. Lieber RL. Skeletal muscle structure and function. Baltimore: Williams & Wilkins, 1992.
43. Lieber RL, et al. In vivo measurement of human wrist extensor muscle sarcomere length changes. J Neurophysiol 1994;71:874.
44. Lutz GJ, Lieber RL. Skeletal muscle myosin II structure and function. Exerc Sport Sci Rev 1999;27:63.
45. MacDougall JD, et al. Biochemical adaptation of human skeletal muscle to heavy resistance training and immobilization. J Appl Physiol 1977;43:700.
46. MacDougall JD, et al. Mitrochondrial volume density in human skeletal muscle following heavy resistance training. Med Sci Sports 1979;11:164.
47. Nielsen OB, Clausen T. The Na^+/K^+-pump protects muscle excitability and contractility during exercise. Exerc Sport Sci Rev 2000;28:159.
48. Patel TJ, Lieber RL. Force transmission in skeletal muscle: from actomyosin to external tendons. Exerc Sport Sci Rev 1997;25:321.
49. Pette D, Staron RS. Cellular and molecular diversities of mammalian skeletal muscle fibers. Rev Physiol Biochem Pharmacol 1990;116:1.
50. Pette Q, Vrbova G. Invited review: neural control of phenotypic expression in mammalian muscle fiber. Muscle Nerve 1985;8:676.
51. Putman CT, et al. Satellite cell content and myosin isoforms in low-frequency-stimulated fast muscle of hypothyroid rat. J Appl Physiol 1999;86:40.
52. Rayment I, et al. Three-dimensional structure of myosin subfragment-1: a molecular motor. Science 1993;261:50.
53. Rayment I, et al. Structure of the actin-myosin complex and its implications for muscle contraction. Science 1993;261:58.
54. Roy RR, Edgerton VR. Skeletal muscle architecture and performance. Komi PV, ed. Strength and power in sport. Boston: Blackwell Scientific, 1992.
55. Rugg JC. Calcium in muscle activation. A comparative approach. Berlin: Springer-Verlag, 1986.
56. Saltin B, Gollnick PD. Skeletal muscle adaptability: significance for metabolism. In: Handbook of physiology. Skeletal muscle. Bethesda, MD: American Physiological Society, 1983.
57. Saltin B, et al. Fiber types and metabolic potentials of skeletal muscles in sedentary man and endurance runners. Ann NY Acad Sci 1977;301:3.
58. Sase I, et al. Axial rotation of sliding actin filaments revealed by single-fluorophore imaging. Proc Natl Acad Sci USA 1997;94:5646.
59. Schmidt-Nielsen K. Scaling. Why is animal size so important? Cambridge: Cambridge University Press, 1991.
60. Scholey JM. Motility assays for motor proteins. Wilson L, Matsudaria P, eds. Methods in cell biology, vol 39. San Diego: Academic Press, 1993.
61. Sheard PW. Tension delivery from short fibers in long muscles. Exerc Sport Sci Rev 2000;28:51.
62. Taylor CR, Weibel ER. Design of the mammalian respiratory system. 1. Problem and strategy. Respir Physiol 1981;44:1.
63. Terjung RL, Engbretson BM. Blood flow to different rat skeletal muscle fiber type sections during isometric contractions in situ. Med Sci Sports Exerc 1988;20:S124.

64. Tesch PA, Karlsson J. Muscle fiber type and size in trained and untrained muscles of elite athletes. J Appl Physiol 1985;59:1716.
65. Tesch PA, Larsson L. Muscle hypertrophy in body builders. Eur J Appl Physiol 1982;49:301.
66. Thorstensson A. Muscle strength, fiber types and enzyme activities in man. Acta Physiol Scand 1976;443(suppl):1.
67. Vander AJ, et al. Human physiology: the mechanisms of body function. 7th ed. New York: William C Brown, 1997.
68. Veigel C, et al. The stiffness of rabbit skeletal actomyosin crossbridges determined with an optical tweezers transducer. Biophysical J 1998;75:1424.
69. Warshaw DM, et al. Myosin conformational states determined by single fluorophore polarization. Proc Natl Acad Sci USA 1998;95:8034.
70. Weis-Fogh T. Energetics of hovering flight in hummingbirds and in Drosophila. J Exp Biol 1972;56:79.
71. Williams JH. Contractile apparatus and sarcoplasmic reticulum function: effects of fatigue, recovery, and elevated Ca^{2+}. J Appl Physiol 1997;83:444.
72. Yan Z. Skeletal muscle adaptation and cell cycle regulation. Exerc Sport Sci Rev 2000;1:24.

CHAPTER 19

Neural Control of Human Movement

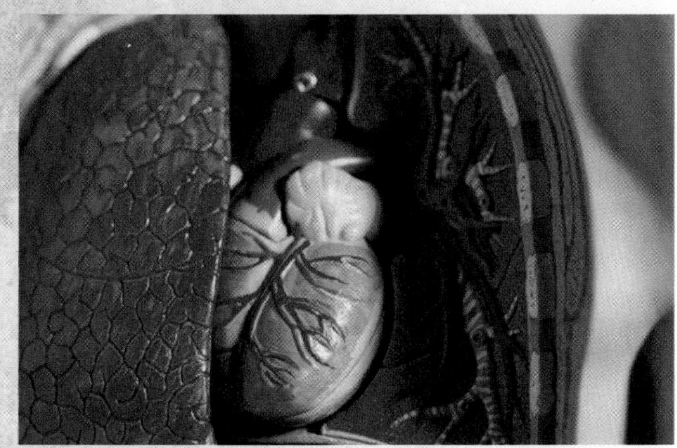

Chapter Objectives

- Draw the major structural components of the brain including the four lobes of the cerebral cortex
- Discuss specific functions of the pyramidal and extrapyramidal tract
- Diagram the anterior motoneuron and discuss its role in human movement
- Draw and label the basic components of a reflex arc
- Define the terms (1) motor unit, (2) neuromuscular junction, and (3) autonomic nervous system
- Summarize the events in motor unit excitation prior to muscle action
- Outline motor unit facilitation and inhibition and the contribution of each to exercise performance and responsiveness to resistance training
- Discuss variations in twitch characteristics, resistance to fatigue, and tension development in the diverse motor units
- Describe mechanisms that adjust force of muscle action from slight to maximum
- Define fatigue and discuss factors that act and interact to bring about neuromuscular fatigue
- List and describe functions of the specific proprioceptors within joints, muscles, and tendons

The effective application of force during relatively complex, learned movements (e.g., tennis serve, shot put, golf swing) depends on a series of coordinated neuromuscular patterns, not just on the strength of muscle groups recruited for the activity. Neural control mechanisms linked together by diverse pathways regulate such movements. The neural circuitry in the brain, spinal cord, and the periphery functions like a modern computer network, although the integrative and organizational structure of the nervous system far exceeds a computer's complexity. In response to changing internal and external stimuli, millions of bits of sensory input automatically synchronize for rapid processing by central neural control mechanisms. The input becomes properly organized, routed, and transmitted at high speed to the effector organs, the skeletal muscles.

The following sections present a general outline of the neural control of human movement, including:

- Structural organization for motor control
- Neuromuscular transmission
- Motor unit function and activation
- Sensory input from muscle activity

NEUROMOTOR SYSTEM ORGANIZATION

The human nervous system consists of two major parts: (1) the **central nervous system (CNS)** consisting of the brain and spinal cord and (2) the **peripheral nervous system (PNS)** containing nerves that transmit information to and from the CNS. Figure 19.1 presents an overview of these two subdivisions of the human nervous system.

Central Nervous System—The Brain

The human brain exhibits great complexity, with selective growth of different anatomic areas. From a comparative perspective, mammalian brains share similarities in structure and function but differ in size and intricacy (Fig. 19.2). Notably, the size of the human brain exceeds that of most (but not all) mammals. A larger brain (A and B of Fig. 19.2) permits more complexity, but factors other than size also explain variations in functional differentiation. Figure 19.2C shows the lateral view of the cerebral cortex in three mammalian species (human, cat, and rat), with primary sensory and motor areas identified. Note expansion of the human cortex that serves neither strict primary sensory nor motor functions. Evolution of the cortex, particularly the frontal and temporal lobes coincides with such unique human functions as use of spoken and written language, reasoning, and abstract thinking. Such differentiation in structure and function has framed the hypothesis that larger, more-complex brains allow greater neural circuitry within the cortex and, hence, increased intellectual function.

For decades, conventional wisdom maintained that the number of brain cells was fixed at birth, unlike the cells of other organ systems that continually renew themselves throughout life. Neurobiologists now believe that brain cells (and perhaps spinal neurons) and neural circuits are created throughout life with elimination of unneeded or redundant synapses in developing neural tissues. From birth through late adolescence, the brain probably adds billions of new cells, literally constructing new circuits from the newly formed cells.[8,9,21] After adolescence, the plasticity of neuronal addition and formation of new circuits slows but does not stop, even into old age. Regular physical activity appears to play a contributory role in the development and maintenance of optimal neural circuitry in middle and old age.

Figure 19.3 categorizes the brain into six main areas: **medulla oblongata**, **pons**, **midbrain**, **cerebellum**, **diencephalon**, and **telencephalon**. Figure 19.3C depicts four lobes of the cerebral cortex and associated sensory areas. As a frame of reference, roughly 10 million sensory (afferent) neurons, 50 billion central neurons, and 500,000 motor (efferent) neurons exist within the body. This represents a ratio of about 20 to 1 between the sensory and motor circuits.

Brainstem

The medulla, pons, and midbrain compose the **brainstem**. The medulla, located immediately above the spinal cord, extends into the pons and serves as a bridge between the two hemispheres of the cerebellum. The midbrain, only 1.5 cm long, attaches to the cerebellum and forms a connection between the pons and the cerebral hemispheres. The midbrain contains parts of the extrapyramidal motor system, specifically the red nucleus and substantia. The **reticular formation** integrates various incoming and outgoing signals that flow through it. These signals originate from the stretching of sensors in joints and muscles, from pain receptors in the skin, and as visual signals from the eye and auditory impulses from the ear. Once activated, the reticular system produces either inhibitory or facilitory effects on other neurons. Twelve pairs of cranial nerves innervate predominantly the head region. Each cranial nerve has a name and associated number, originally derived by Galen some 1800 years ago.

Cerebellum

The cerebellum, made up of two lateral hemispheres and a central vermis, functions by means of intricate feedback circuits to monitor and coordinate other areas of the brain and spinal cord involved in motor control. The cerebellum receives motor output signals from the central command in the cortex. This specialized brain tissue also obtains sensory information from peripheral receptors in muscles, tendons, joints, and skin and from visual, auditory, and vestibular end organs. *The cerebellum serves as the major comparing, evaluating, and integrating center for postural adjustments, locomotion, maintenance of equilibrium, perceptions of speed of body movement, and other diverse reflex functions related to movement.*[36] In essence, the cerebellum serves as the motor control center providing "fine tuning" for all forms of muscular activity.

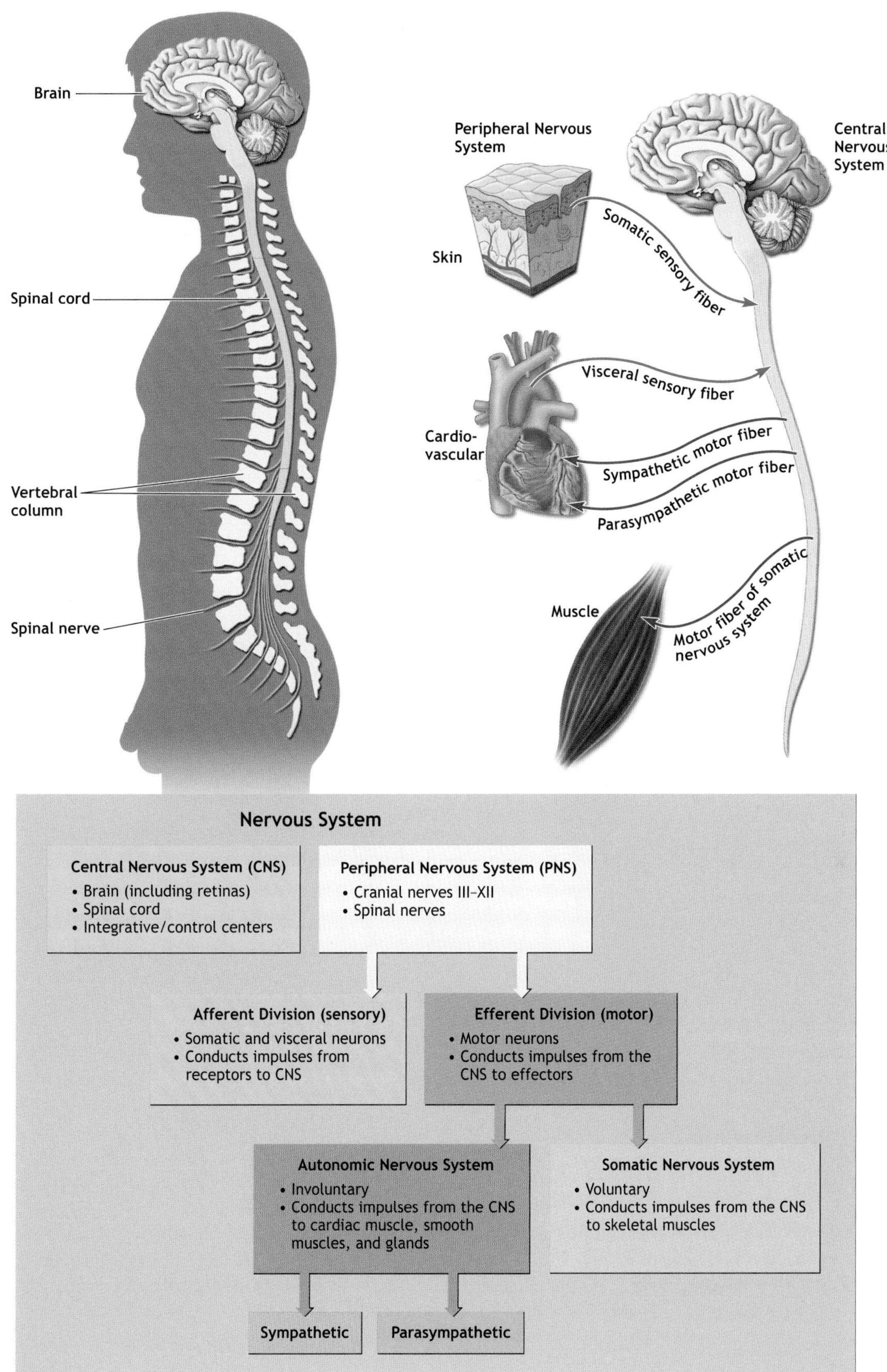

FIGURE 19.1 • The human nervous system has two divisions. The central nervous system (CNS) contains the brain (including retinas), spinal cord, and integrating and control centers; the cranial nerves and spinal nerves compose the peripheral nervous system (PNS). The PNS further subdivides into the afferent (sensory) and efferent (motor) divisions. The somatic nervous system and autonomic nervous system (sympathetic and parasympathetic divisions) make up the efferent division.

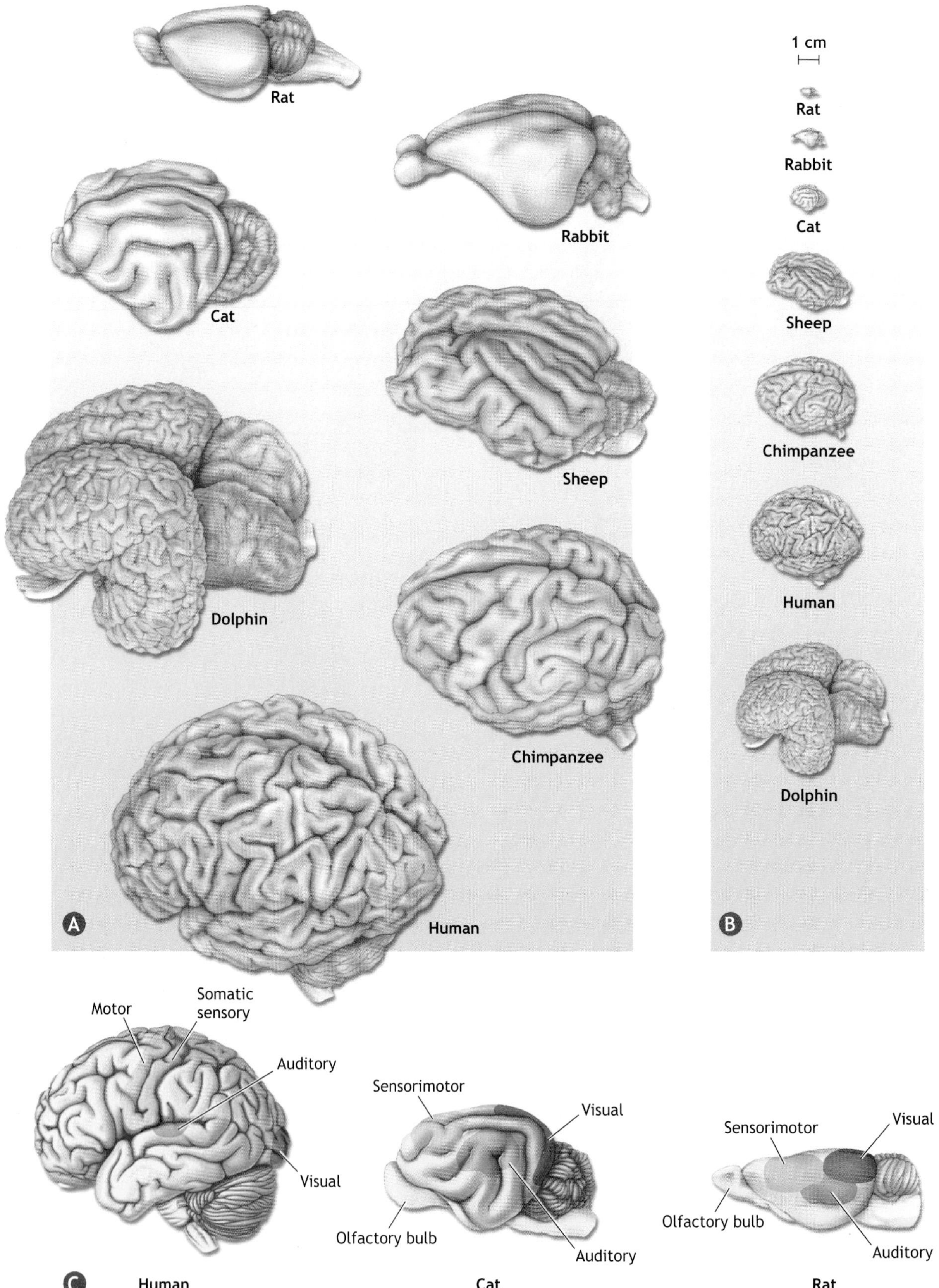

FIGURE 19.2 • **A**. Brains of different mammals drawn to the same size. **B**. Relative brain sizes. **C**. Lateral view of the cerebral cortex in three species, showing expansion of the human cortex that is neither strictly primarily sensory nor motor. (From Bear MF, et al. Neuroscience: exploring the brain. Baltimore: Williams & Wilkins, 1996.)

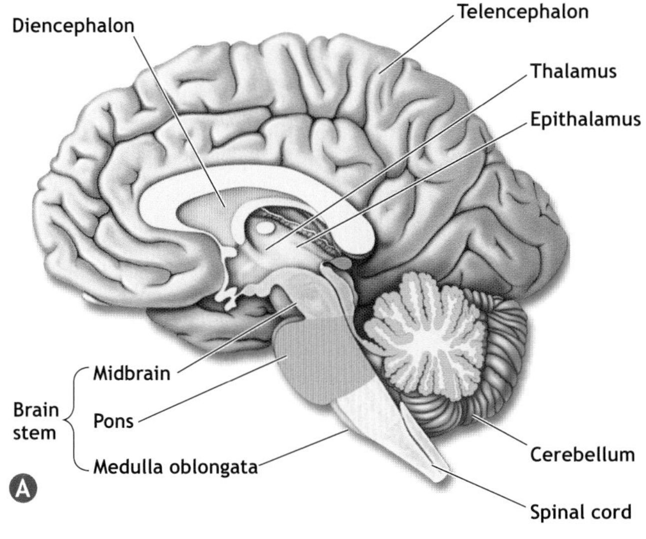

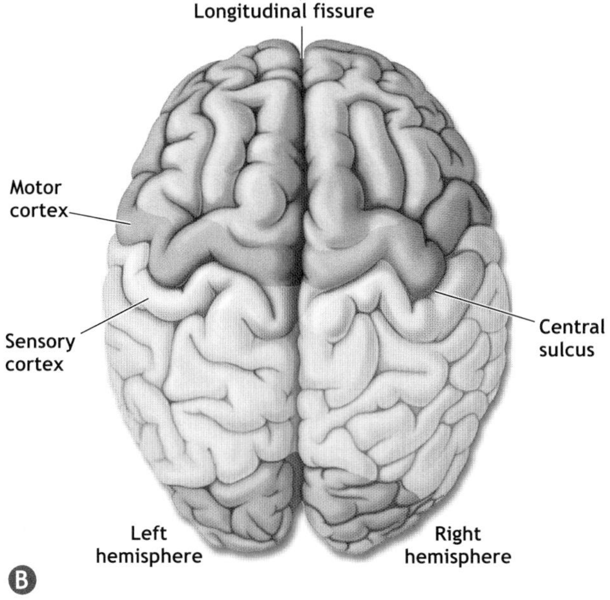

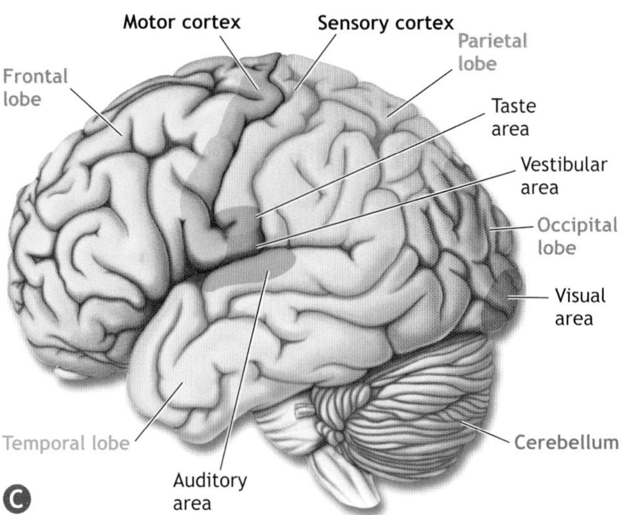

FIGURE 19.3 • **A**. Side (medial) view of the brain and brainstem. **B**. Superior view of the brain. **C**. Four lobes of the cerebral cortex.

Diencephalon

The diencephalon, located immediately above the midbrain, forms part of the cerebral hemispheres. The thalamus, hypothalamus, epithalamus, and subthalamus are the major structures of the diencephalon. The **hypothalamus**, situated below the thalamus, regulates functions ranging from metabolic rate to body temperature. The hypothalamus also influences activity of the autonomic nervous system (see page 392); it receives regulatory input from the thalamus and limbic brain system and responds to the effects of diverse hormones (see Chapter 20). Changes in arterial blood pressure and blood gas tensions influence hypothalamic activity via peripheral receptors located in the aortic arch and carotid arteries.

Telencephalon

The telencephalon contains the two hemispheres of the **cerebral cortex**, in addition to the corpus striatum and medulla. The cerebral cortex makes up approximately 40% of the total brain weight and is divided into four lobes: frontal, temporal, parietal, and occipital. Neurons in the cortex provide specialized sensory and motor functions. Beneath each cerebral hemisphere and in close association with the thalamus lie the basal ganglia, which play an important role in the control of motor movements.

Limbic System

In 1878, French surgeon and neurologist Pierre Broca (1824–1880) described a group of areas on the medial surface of the cerebrum that were distinctly different from the surrounding cortex. Using the Latin word for "border" *(limbus)*, Broca named the area the **limbic lobe** because its structures formed a ring or border around the brainstem and corpus callosum on the medial surface of the temporal lobe.[4]

Work in the 1930s suggested that a number of limbic structures (or parts of structures) linked by a major nerve tract were responsible for sensations and expressions of emotion. These limbic structures were thought to include the anterior nuclei of the thalamus, hypothalamus, hippocampus, cingulate cortex, and neocortex. Damage to portions of these cortical areas produced profound deficits in emotional behavior, with little change in perception or intelligence, which suggested a structure–function relationship. Also, tumors located near the cingulate cortex were associated with emotional disturbance including fear and irritability. More-recent evidence however, points to no one "system" responsible for specific human emotions. Although the term limbic system retains common usage in describing this configuration of neurons around the brainstem, neuroscience continues to reveal the intricacies of how the brain contributes to emotions, "feelings," and learning.

Central Nervous System—The Spinal Cord

Figure 19.4 illustrates the spinal cord, about 45 cm in length and 1 cm in diameter, encased by 33 vertebrae (7 cervical, 12 thoracic, 5 lumbar, 5 sacral, and 4 coccygeal). The bony vertebral

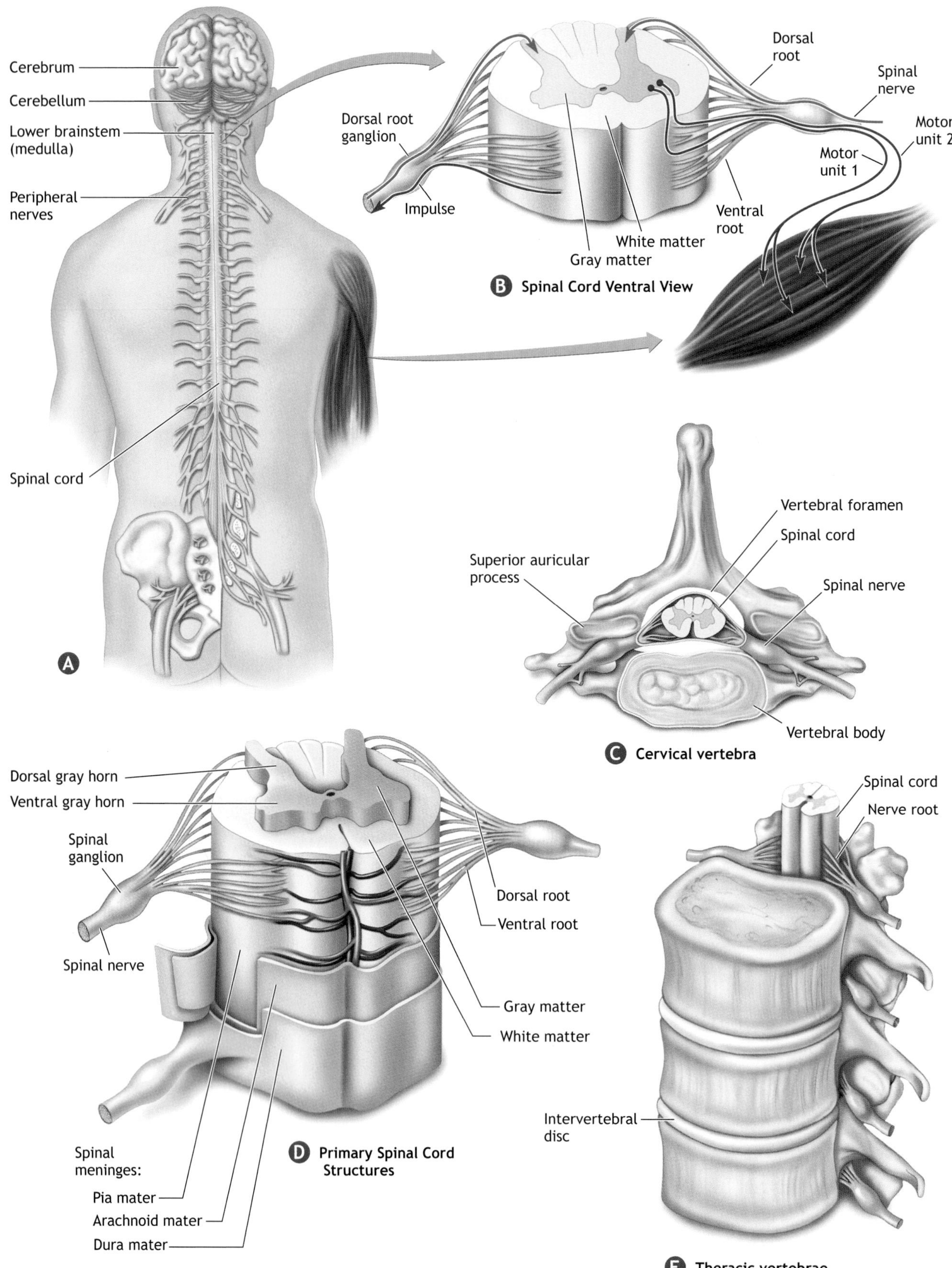

FIGURE 19.4 • Human central nervous system anatomy. **A**. Spinal cord showing the peripheral nerves. **B**. Ventral view of spinal cord section illustrates dorsal and ventral root neural pathways and nerve impulse direction. **C**. Cross-section through one cervical vertebra. **D.** Primary spinal cord structures. **E**. Enlarged view of the junction of three thoracic vertebral bodies.

TABLE 19.1 ➤ COMMON NAMES DESCRIBING NEURONS AND AXONS OF THE SPINAL CORD

NAME	DESCRIPTION/EXAMPLE
Neurons	
Gray matter	Generic term for a collection of neuronal cell bodies in the CNS (neurons appear gray in a freshly dissected brain)
Cortex	Collection of neurons forming a thin sheet, usually at the brain's surface; example: *cerebral cortex,* the sheet of neurons found just under the surface of the cerebrum
Nucleus	Distinguishable mass of neurons, usually deep in the brain (not to be confused with the nucleus of a cell); example: *lateral geniculate nucleus,* a cell group in the brainstem relaying information from the eye to the cerebral cortex
Substantia	Related neurons deep within the brain, but with less distinct borders than those of nuclei; example: *substantia nigra,* a brainstem cell group involved in voluntary movement control
Locus (plural—loci)	Small, well-defined group of cells; example: *locus coeruleus,* a brainstem group of cells involved in control of wakefulness and behavioral arousal
Ganglion (plural—ganglia)	From the Greek term for knot; collection of neurons in the peripheral nervous system; example: *dorsal root ganglia* that contain the cell bodies of sensory axons entering the spinal cord in the dorsal roots; only one cell grouping, the *basal ganglia,* in the CNS goes by this name; the basal ganglia that lie deep within the cerebrum control movement
Axons	
Nerve	A bundle of axons in the peripheral nervous system; the optic nerve is the only collection of CNS axons termed *nerve*
White matter	Generic term for a collection of CNS axons (neurons appear white in a freshly dissected brain)
Tract	Collection of CNS axons having a common site of origin and a common destination; example: *corticospinal tract* that originates in the cerebral cortex and ends in the spinal cord
Bundle	Collection of axons running together but not necessarily having the same origin and destination; example: *medial forebrain bundle* that connects the brainstem with the cerebral cortex
Capsule	Collection of axons that connect the cerebrum with the brainstem; example: *internal capsule* that connects the brainstem with the cerebral cortex
Commissure	Any collection of axons that connect one side of the brain to the other side
Lemniscus	A tract that meanders through the brain in ribbonlike fashion; example: *medial lemniscus* that brings tactile information from the spinal cord through the brainstem

From Bear MF, et al. Neuroscience: exploring the brain. Baltimore: Williams & Wilkins, 1996.

column encases and protects the spinal cord, which attaches to the brainstem. The spinal cord provides the major conduit for the two-way flow of information from the skin, joints, and muscles to the brain. It provides for communication throughout the body via spinal nerves of the PNS (see page 390). These nerves exit the cord through small openings or notches between the vertebrae. Each spinal nerve connects to the spinal cord by means of two branches, the dorsal root and ventral root. Table 19.1 lists common names that describe the collections of spinal cord neurons and axons.

When viewed in cross section, the spinal cord shows an H-shaped core of gray matter (see Fig. 19.5). The **ventral** (anterior) and **dorsal** (posterior) **horns** describe the limbs of this core. The spinal cord core contains principally three types of neurons: **motor neurons**, **sensory neurons**, and **interneurons**. The motoneurons **(efferent)** run through the ventral horn to supply the extrafusal and intrafusal skeletal muscle fibers (see pages 401-402). Sensory **(afferent)** nerve fibers enter the spinal cord from the periphery by way of the dorsal horn. The white matter, containing the ascending and descending nerve tracts, surrounds the gray matter within the cord.

Ascending Nerve Tracts

Ascending nerve tracts in the spinal cord forward sensory information from peripheral receptors to the brain for processing. Three neurons typically make up the sensory pathway. The dorsal root ganglion contains the cell body of the first neuron whose axon relays information into the spinal cord. The cell body of the second neuron lies within the spinal cord itself; its axon passes up the cord to the thalamus, which contains the third neuron's cell body. The axon of this third neuron passes up to the central command center in the cerebral cortex.

SENSORY RECEPTORS. *Peripheral sensory nerve endings serve as specialized receptors that detect both conscious and subconscious sensory information.* The "conscious" receptors show sensitivity to such input as body position (kinesthesia and proprioception), temperature, and the sensations of light, sound, smell, taste, touch, and pain. Receptors also monitor subconscious changes in the body's internal environment; these include **chemoreceptors** that respond to changes in blood gas tension (PO_2, PCO_2) and pH, and **baroreceptors** that react rapidly to changes in arterial blood pressure.

Descending Nerve Tracts

Axons from the brain move downward through the spinal cord along two major pathways displayed in Figure 19.5. One pathway, the lateral or **pyramidal tract**, activates the skeletal musculature in voluntary movement under direct cortical control. The other pathway, the ventromedial or **extrapyramidal tract**, involves control of posture and muscle tone via the brainstem.

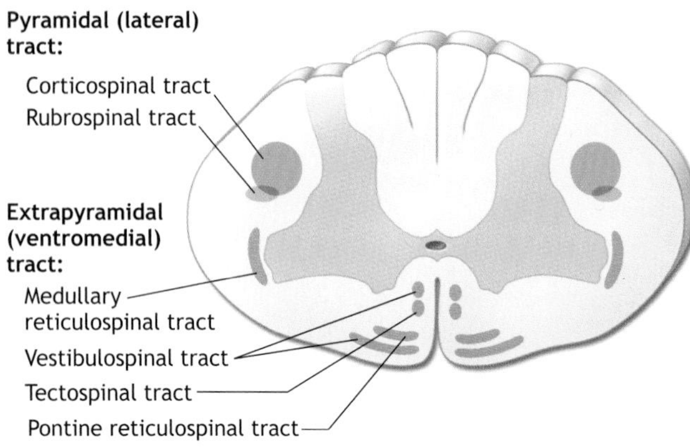

FIGURE 19.5 • Descending spinal cord tracts from the brain. (From Bear MF, et al. Neuroscience: exploring the brain. Baltimore: Williams & Wilkins, 1996.)

PYRAMIDAL (LATERAL) TRACT. Neurons in the pyramidal tract (which includes corticospinal and rubrospinal tracts) transmit impulses downward through the spinal cord. By means of direct routes and interconnecting neurons in the cord, these nerves eventually excite the **alpha** (α) **motor neurons** that control skeletal muscle activity. The corticospinal tract, the longest and one of the largest CNS tracts in the body, has two-thirds of its axons originating from the frontal lobe, collectively called the **motor cortex**.

EXTRAPYRAMIDAL (VENTROMEDIAL) TRACT. The extrapyramidal neurons (which include the reticulospinal, vestibulospinal, and tectospinal tracts) originate in the brainstem and connect at all levels of the spinal cord. These neurons control posture and provide a continual background level of neuromuscular tone.

Reticular Formation

The reticular formation provides an extensive and intricate neural network running through the core of the brainstem that integrates the spinal cord, cerebral cortex, basal ganglia, and cerebellum. It receives a continuous flow of sensory data. Once activated, the reticular system produces either an inhibitory or a facilitory effect on other neurons. For example, the reticular formation contributes to postural control by regulating the sensitivity of neurons to the antigravity muscles. Excitation of peripheral sensory neurons arouses the reticular nerve cells, which excite the cerebral cortex. This initiates transmission of signals back to the reticular system to maintain appropriate cortical arousal and wakefulness. The reticular formation also exerts a powerful influence on vital functions such as cardiovascular and pulmonary regulation.

The modulating influences of other feedback networks superimpose on reticular formation activity. For example, increased neural outflow to the postural muscles augments the tension of these muscles. An increase in neuromuscular tone also stimulates the muscle's own set of internal sensors, the spindles (see page 402), to redirect impulses back to the CNS to maintain the proper activation level of the reticular formation. This level of integrated response provides an example of **multiple feedback control**, one of the most complex aspects of nervous system function.

Peripheral Nervous System

The peripheral nervous system consists of 31 pairs of spinal nerves and 12 pairs of cranial nerves. Figure 19.6 shows the distribution of the 12 pairs of cranial nerves numbered I through XII. Cranial nerves I and II serve visual and olfactory functions and are part of the CNS. Cranial nerves emerge through foramina or fissures in the skull (cranium). Like their spinal counterparts, cranial nerves contain fibers that transmit either sensory and/or motor information. Their neurons innervate muscles or glands or transmit impulses from sensory areas into the brain. The spinal nerves consist of 8 pairs of cervical nerves, 12 pairs of thoracic nerves, 5 pairs of lumbar nerves, 5 pairs of sacral nerves, and 1 pair of coccygeal nerves. A specific letter and number identifies these nerves (e.g., C-1, first nerve from the cervical region; T-4, fourth nerve in thoracic region). Careful research has traced the exact location of the spinal nerves by mapping the tissues they innervate. Therefore, an injury to a specific area of the spinal cord produces predictable neurologic damage. For example, severe damage to the upper thoracic vertebra and the corresponding descending nerve tract usually results in quadriplegia. Figure 19.7 maps the distribution of the different spinal nerves in relation to the sensory innervation of the skin. The term **dermatome** defines the skin area (delineated by a set of stripes on the body surface) innervated by the dorsal roots of a single spinal segment; one-to-one correspondence exists between dermatomes and spinal segments.

The peripheral nervous system includes the afferent neurons that relay sensory information from receptors in the periphery *toward* the CNS, and efferent neurons that transmit information *away from* the brain to peripheral tissues. **Somatic** and **autonomic** nerves are the two types of efferent neurons. Somatic nerve fibers (also called *motor neurons* or *motoneurons*) innervate skeletal muscle. Their firing always produces an excitatory response to activate muscle. The autonomic nerves (also called *visceral, involuntary,* or *vegetative* nerves) activate cardiac muscle, sweat and salivary glands, some endocrine glands, and smooth muscle cells (also called *involuntary muscle*) in the intestines and walls of blood vessels. Autonomic activity produces either an excitatory or inhibitory effect, depending on the specific neurons activated.

Whereas tissues of the heart and viscera display significant autonomic excitability, conscious control also affects these tissues. For example, individuals who practice yoga or meditation control their heart rate and blood flow "on command." Such conscious control of the autonomic system has some application as an alternative treatment in medicine (e.g., GI disturbances, hypertension) and for enhancing sports performance. Competitors in archery and biathlon control cardiovascular activity and respiratory movements to temporarily halt normal breathing cycle and pulse rate during the

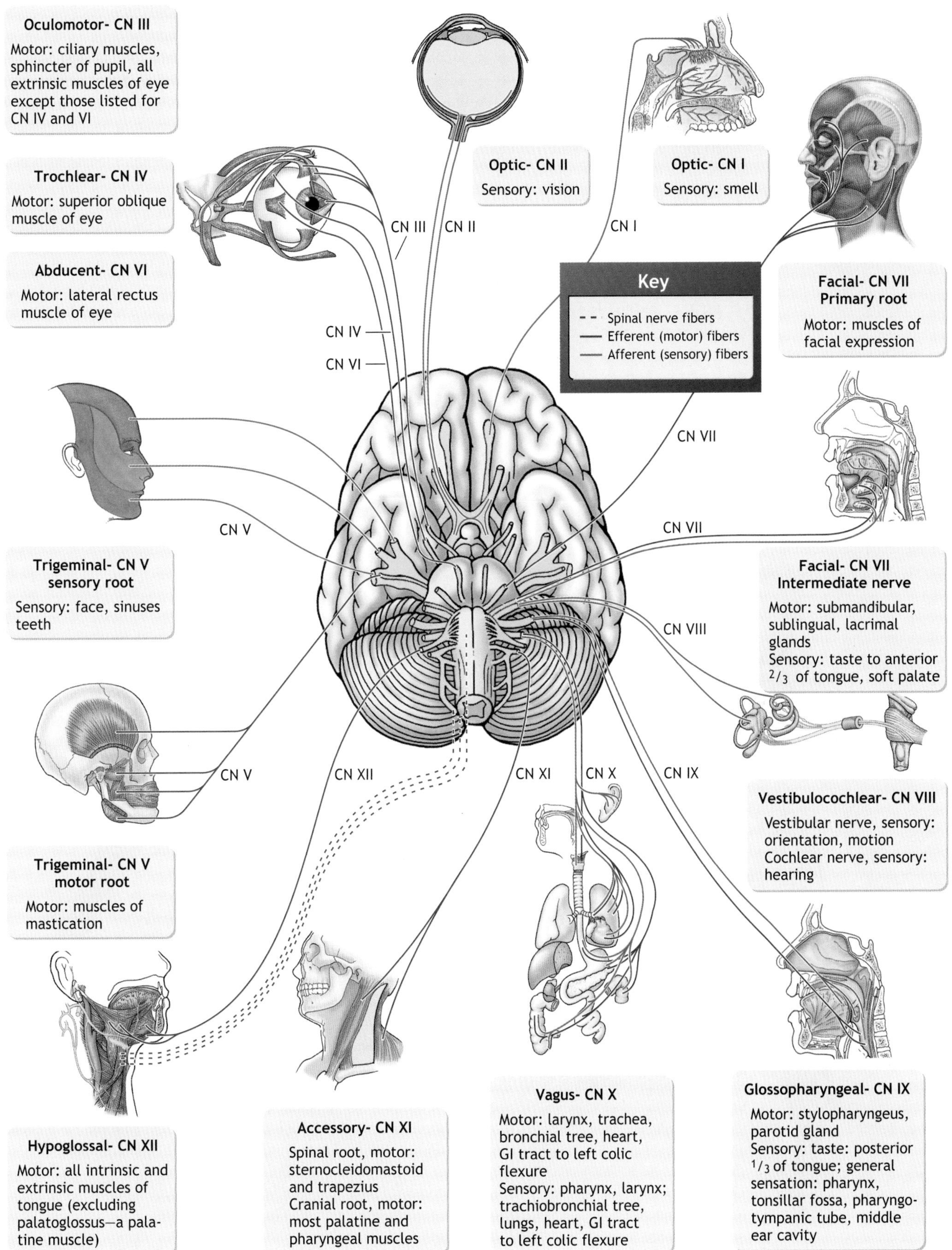

FIGURE 19.6 • Distribution of the 12 cranial nerves (CN) (From Moore KL, Dalley AF, eds. Clinically oriented anatomy. 4th ed. Baltimore: Lippincott Williams & Wilkins, 1999.)

crucial phase of the performance (i.e., immediately prior to releasing the bowstring or firing the rifle).

Sympathetic and Parasympathetic Nervous Systems

Based on anatomic and physiologic differences, the **autonomic nervous system** subdivides into **sympathetic** and **parasympathetic** components. These neurons operate in parallel but use structurally distinct pathways and differ in their transmitter systems. Recall from Figure 16.5 that axons of the sympathetic division emerge only from the middle third of the spinal cord (thoracic and lumbar segments); in contrast, preganglionic axons of the parasympathetic division emerge only from the brainstem and the lowest (sacral) spinal cord segments. Thus, the two systems complement each other anatomically.

Sympathetic fiber distribution, while displaying some overlap with parasympathetic fibers, supply the heart, smooth muscle, sweat glands, and viscera. Fibers of the parasympathetic nervous system leave the brainstem and sacral segments of the spinal cord to supply the thorax, abdomen, and pelvic regions.

Regions of the medulla, pons, and diencephalon control the autonomic nervous system. For example, fibers that originate in the medullary region of the lower brainstem control blood pressure, heart rate, and pulmonary ventilation, whereas nerve fibers of upper hypothalamic origin regulate body temperature.

The Reflex Arc

Figure 19.8 diagrams the neural arrangement for a typical **reflex arc** in one of the 31 spinal cord segments. Afferent neurons that enter the spinal cord through the dorsal (sensory) root transmit sensory input from peripheral receptors. These neurons interconnect (**synapse**) in the cord through **interneurons** that relay information to various levels of the cord. The impulse then passes over the **motor root pathway** via anterior motor neurons to the effector organ, the muscles.

Operation of the reflex arc becomes evident when one unknowingly touches a hot object. Stimulation of pain receptors in the fingers sends sensory information rapidly over afferent fibers to the spinal cord. This activates efferent motor fibers to elicit an appropriate muscular response (rapidly re-

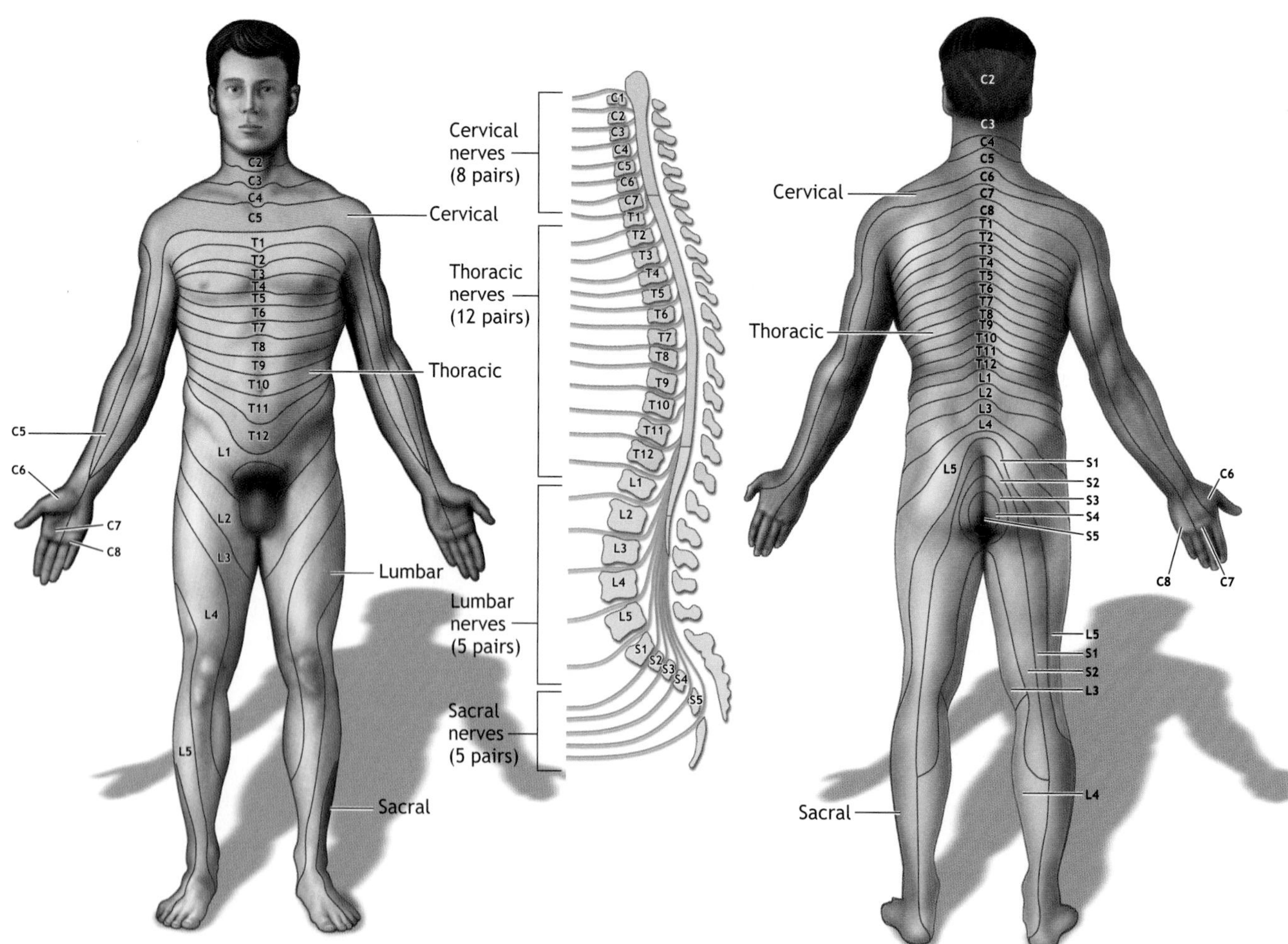

FIGURE 19.7 • Distribution of the spinal nerves in relation to the sensory innervation of the skin. The term *dermatome* defines the skin area (delineated by a set of *stripes on the body surface*) innervated by the dorsal roots of a single spinal segment. *Center inset,* lateral view of vertebral column, spinal cord, spinal ganglia, and outflow of spinal nerves in the adult.

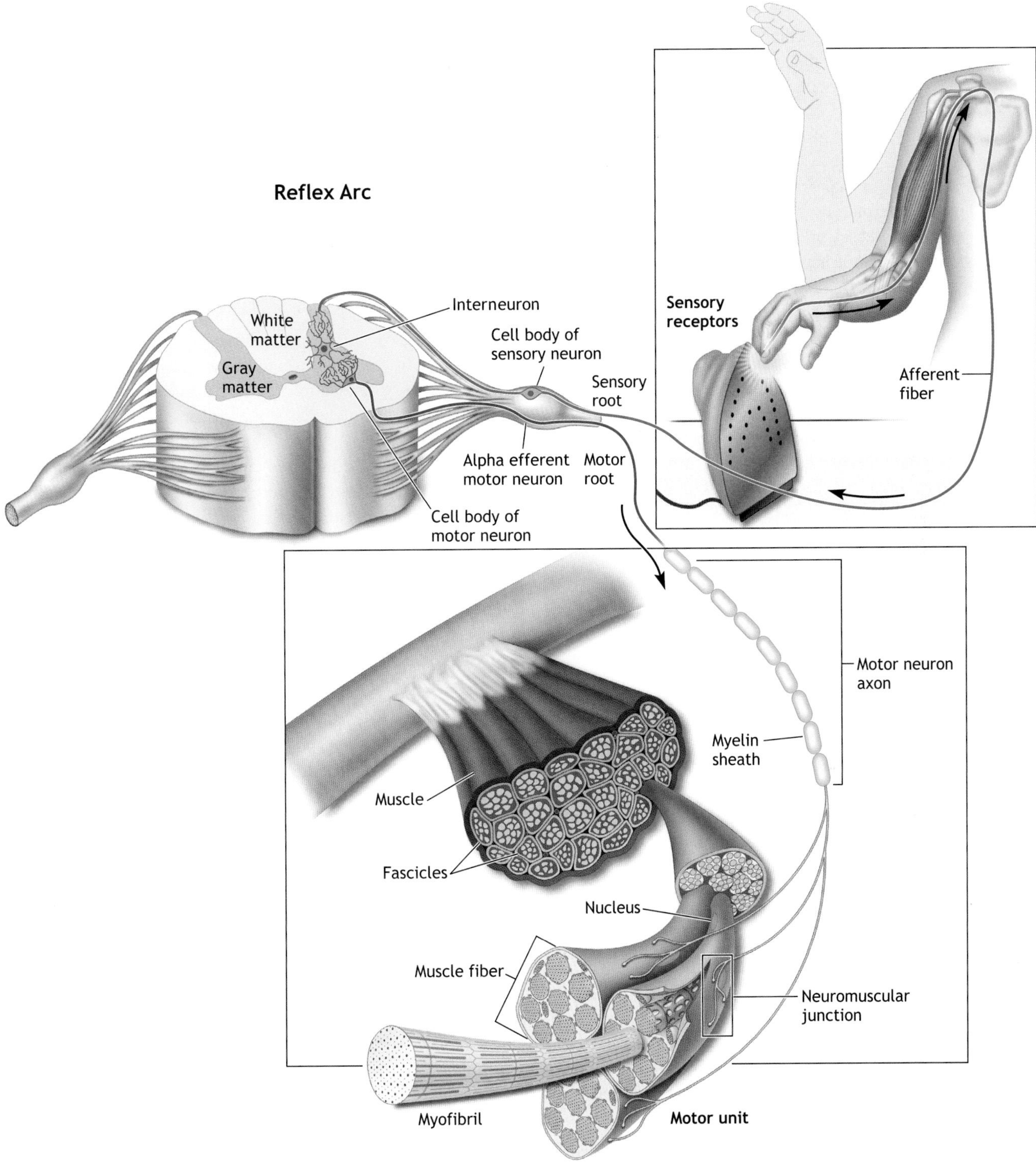

FIGURE 19.8 • Reflex arc showing the afferent and efferent neurons plus an interneuron in a spinal cord segment. The darker shaded or gray matter contains the neuron cell bodies; longitudinal columns of nerve fibers make up the white matter. Stimulation of a single α-motor neuron activates as many as 3000 muscle fibers. The motor neuron and the fibers it innervates collectively make up the motor unit. The figure shows only one side of the spinal nerve complex.

moving the hand). Concurrently, the signal transmits through interneuron activity up the cord to sensory areas in the brain, the area that actually "feels" the pain. These various levels of operation for sensory input, processing, and motor output, including the reflex action just described, cause removal of the hand from the hot object before the actual perception of pain. Reflex actions in the spinal cord and other subconscious areas of the CNS control many muscle functions. Hundreds of hours of practicing a particular skill "grooves" the neuromuscular movements to become automatic, requiring little or no conscious control. Of course, improper practice also can automate a task to produce less than optimal neuromuscular actions. The adage "practice makes perfect" should be amended to "perfect practice makes perfect."

NERVE SUPPLY TO MUSCLE

One nerve or its terminal branches innervate at least one of the body's approximately 250 million muscle fibers. Because a person possesses only about 420,000 motor neurons, this means that a single nerve usually supplies many individual muscle fibers. *The number of muscle fibers per motor neuron generally relates to a muscle's particular movement function.* Delicate and precise work of the eye muscles, for example, requires that a neuron control fewer than 10 muscle fibers. For less-complex movements of the large muscle groups, a motor neuron may innervate as many as 2,000 or 3,000 fibers. For muscular activity, the spinal cord is the major processing and distribution center for motor control. The next sections take a closer look at how information processed in the CNS activates the muscles to bring about an appropriate motor response.

Motor Unit Anatomy

The ***motor unit*** *makes up the functional unit of movement; this anatomic unit consists of the anterior motor neuron and the specific muscle fibers it innervates.* Muscle action results from the individual and combined actions of motor units. Although each muscle fiber generally receives input from only one neuron, a motor neuron may innervate many muscle fibers because the terminal end of an axon forms numerous branches. **Motor neuron pool** describes the collection of α motor neurons that innervates a single muscle (e.g., triceps or biceps) (Fig.19.9). Diverse motor points exist within the muscle to allow neural stimulation throughout the muscle's length.[32] Some motor units contain up to 1000 or more muscle fibers, whereas motor units of the larynx, fingers, or eyeball contain relatively few. For example, the first dorsal interosseous muscle of the finger contains 120 motor units that control 41,000 fibers; the medial gastrocnemius (calf) muscle has 580 motor units and 1,030,000 muscle fibers. The average ratio of muscle fibers to motor unit is 340 for the finger muscle and about 1,800 for the gastrocnemius muscle.[13]

The Anterior Motoneuron

The anterior motor neuron, illustrated in Figure 19.10, consists of a **cell body**, **axon**, and **dendrites**. Its unique design enables it to transmit an electrochemical impulse from the spinal cord to the muscle. The cell body houses the control center—the structures involved in replication and transmission of the genetic code. The spinal cord's gray matter contains this part of the motor neuron. The axon extends from the cord to deliver the impulse to the muscle; the dendrites consist of the short neural branches that receive impulses through numerous connections and conduct them toward the cell body. Nerve cells conduct impulses in one direction only—down the axon, away from the point of stimulation.

The **myelin sheath**, a lipoprotein membrane that wraps around the axon over most of its length, encases the larger nerve fibers. A specialized cell known as a **Schwann cell** covers the bare axon and then spirals around it, sometimes up to 100 times in the biggest fibers. Myelin forms a large part of this sheath and insulates the axon. A thinner membrane, the **neurilemma**, covers the myelin sheath. The **nodes of Ranvier** interrupt the Schwann cells and myelin every 1 or 2 mm along the axon's length. Whereas the myelin sheath insulates the axon to the flow of ions, the nodes of Ranvier permit depolarization of the axon. This alternating sequence of myelin sheath and node of Ranvier allows impulses to "jump" from node to node (saltatory conduction) as the electrical current travels toward the terminal branches at the **motor endplate**. This means of conduction causes faster transmission velocities in myelinated than in unmyelinated fibers. Conduction speed in a nerve fiber increases in direct proportion to a fiber's diameter and the thickness of its myelin sheath. Large, myelinated neurons conduct impulses at speeds exceeding 100 $m \cdot s^{-1}$ (224 mph).

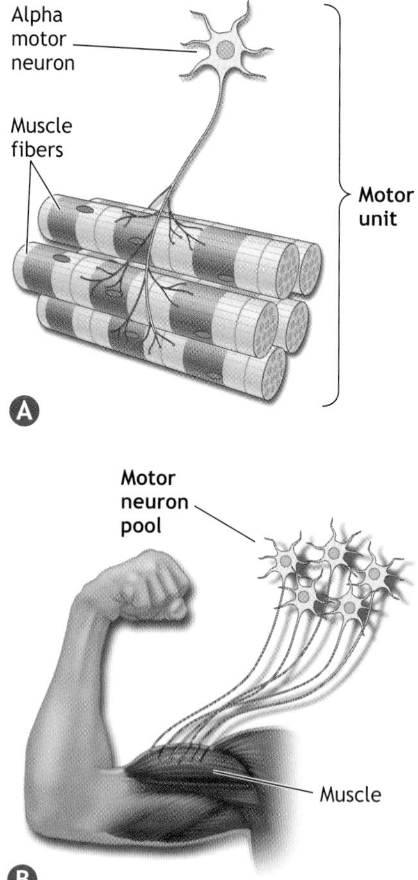

FIGURE 19.9 • Motor unit and motor neuron pool. **A.** Motor unit represents an α-motoneuron and the fibers it innervates. **B.** Motor neuron pool represents all the α motor neurons that innervate one muscle.

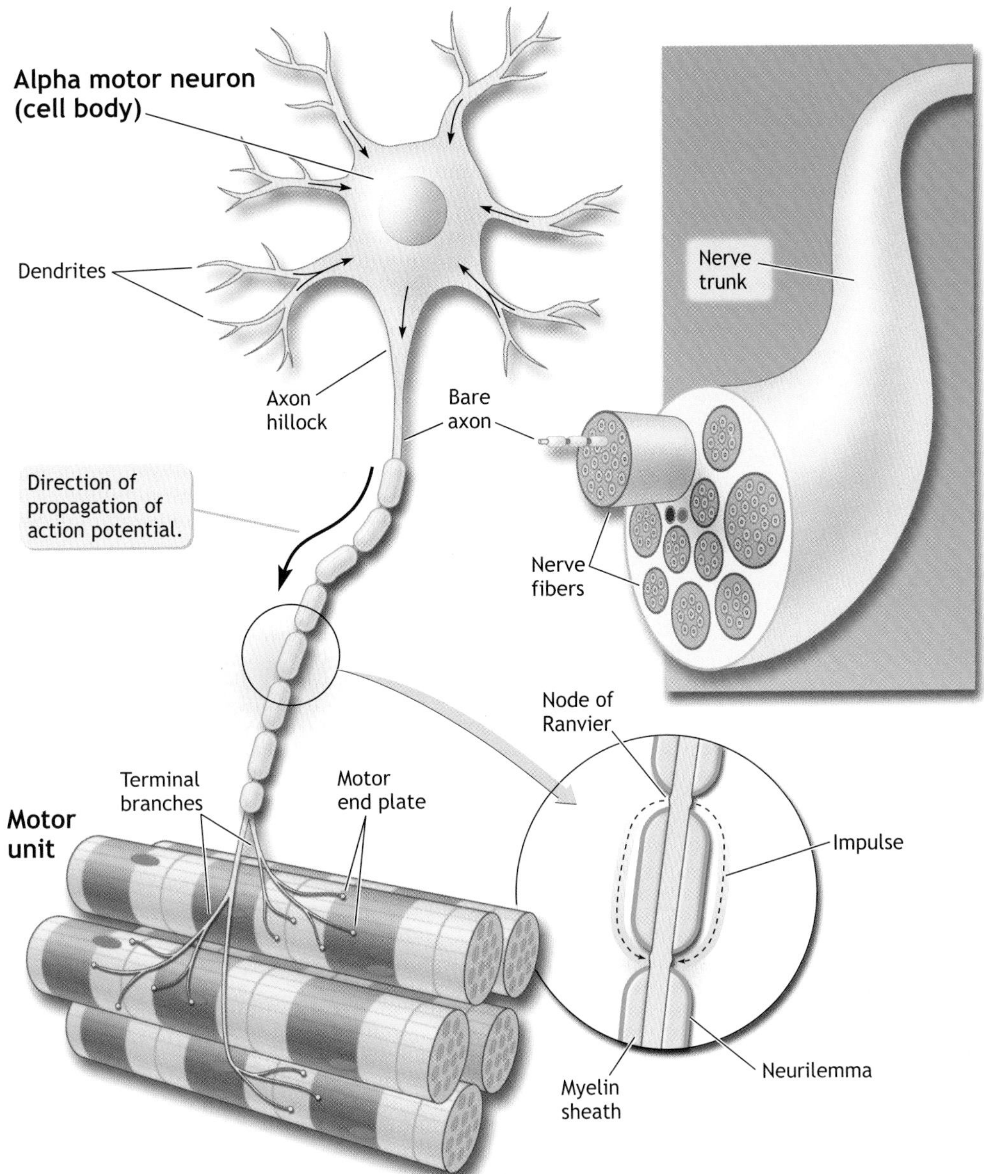

FIGURE 19.10 • The anterior (α) motor neuron consists of a cell body, axon, and dendrites. *Top inset* shows a nerve trunk containing numerous individual nerve fibers, including a bare axon. *Bottom inset* shows a node of Ranvier on the bare axon, which permits impulses to jump from one node to another as the electrical current travels toward the terminal branches at the motor endplate.

The anterior motor neurons, also known as **type A** (α) **nerve fibers** (α motor neurons) possess large diameters, ranging from about 8 to 20 μm. Other smaller type A fibers (**gamma** [γ] **efferent motor neurons**) have diameters no larger than about 10 μm and a conduction velocity about one-half that of the larger α fibers. As discussed in the section on proprioception, the γ efferent fibers connect with special stretch sensors in skeletal muscle that detect minute changes in muscle fiber length.

All muscle action ultimately depends on three primary sources of input to α motor neurons (motor units): (1) dorsal root ganglion cells with axons that innervate specialized muscle spindle sensory units embedded within the muscle, (2) motor neurons in the brain, primarily in the cerebral cortex's precentral gyrus, and (3) the largest input from excitatory and inhibitory spinal cord interneurons.

NEUROMUSCULAR JUNCTION (MOTOR ENDPLATE). The **neuromuscular junction** (**NMJ**) or **motor endplate** represents the interface between the end of a myelinated motor neuron and a muscle fiber (Fig. 19.11). It functions to transmit the nerve impulse to initiate a muscle action. Each skeletal muscle fiber usually contains just one NMJ.

Five common features describe the NMJ:[7]

1. Presence of Schwann cells.
2. The terminal section of the neuron contains the neurotransmitter substance acetylcholine (ACh).
3. A basement membrane that lines the synaptic space.

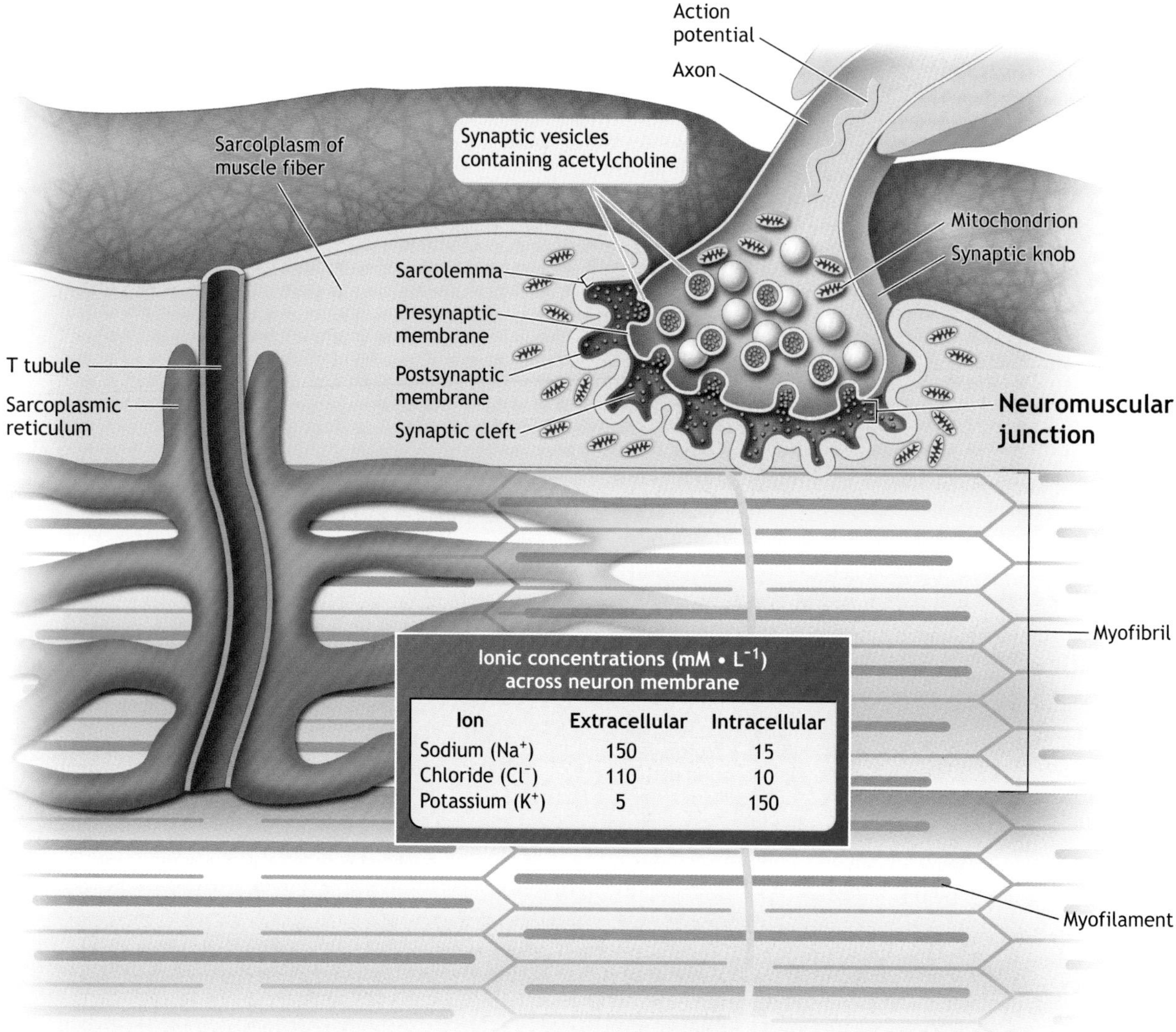

Ionic concentrations (mM • L^{-1}) across neuron membrane		
Ion	Extracellular	Intracellular
Sodium (Na^+)	150	15
Chloride (Cl^-)	110	10
Potassium (K^+)	5	150

FIGURE 19.11 • Microanatomy of the neuromuscular junction, including details of the presynaptic and postsynaptic contact area between the motor neuron and the muscle fiber it innervates. *Inset table* shows representative values for ionic concentrations across the motor neuron membrane.

4. A membrane across from the synaptic space (the postsynaptic membrane) that contains ACh receptors
5. Connector microtubules at the postsynaptic membrane that transmit the electrical signal deep within the muscle fiber

The terminal portion of the axon below the myelin sheath forms several smaller axon branches whose endings become the **presynaptic terminals**. This region possesses approximately 50 to 70 ACh-containing vesicles per square micrometer.[6,15] They lie close to, but not in contact with, the muscle fiber's sarcolemma. The invaginated region of the **postsynaptic membrane** (also called the *synaptic gutter*) provides many infoldings that increase the membrane's surface area. The **synaptic cleft**, between the synaptic gutter and the presynaptic terminal of the axon, provides the region for transmission of the neural impulse between nerve and muscle fiber.

EXCITATION. *Excitation normally occurs only at the NMJ.* Arrival of an impulse at the NMJ releases ACh from saclike vesicles in the terminal axons into the synaptic cleft. ACh, which changes a basically electrical neural impulse into a chemical stimulus, then combines with a transmitter–receptor complex in the postsynaptic membrane. The resulting change in the electrical properties of the postsynaptic membrane elicits an **endplate potential** that spreads from the motor endplate to the extrajunctional sarcolemma. This causes an **action potential** (wave of depolarization) to travel the length of the fiber, enter the T-tubule system, and spread to the inner structures of the muscle fiber to prime the contractile machinery.

The enzyme **cholinesterase** (concentrated at the borders of the junctional folds at the synaptic cleft) degrades ACh within 5 ms of its release from the synaptic vesicles. ACh hydrolysis by cholinesterase allows the postsynaptic membrane to repolarize rapidly. The axon resynthesizes the end products of cholinesterase action (acetic acid and choline) to ACh so the entire process can begin again with the arrival of another neural impulse.

Facilitation. Release of ACh from the synaptic vesicles excites the postsynaptic membrane of its connecting neuron. This changes the membrane permeability and permits sodium ions to diffuse rapidly into the stimulated neuron. An action potential generates if the change in transmembrane microvoltage (influx of extracellular sodium and/or efflux of intracellular potassium) reaches the **threshold for excitation**. The term **excitatory postsynaptic potential** (**EPSP**) describes this change in membrane potential at the junction between two neurons (Fig. 19.12A). The arrival of a subthreshold EPSP does not cause the neuron to discharge. Instead, the flow of positive charges into

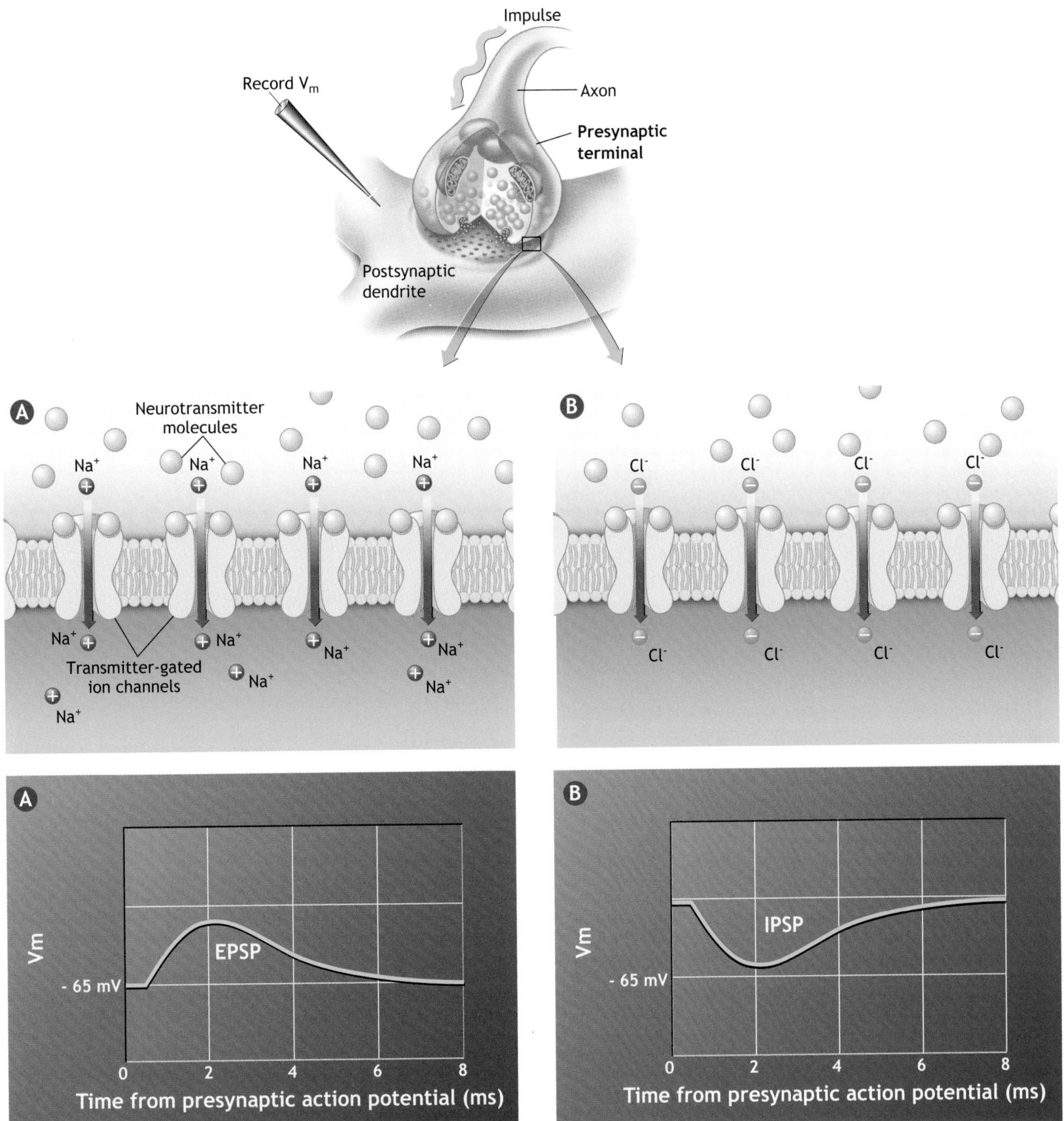

FIGURE 19.12 • **A**. Generation of an excitatory postsynaptic potential (EPSP). An impulse arriving in the presynaptic terminal (top inset) causes neurotransmitter release. The molecules bind to transmitter-gated ion channels in the postsynaptic membrane. If Na^+ enters the postsynaptic cell through the open channels, the membrane becomes hypopolarized. The EPSP represents the resulting change in membrane potential (V_m) as recorded by a microelectrode in the cell. **B**. Generation of an inhibitory postsynaptic potential (IPSP). An impulse arriving in the presynaptic terminal (top inset) causes neurotransmitter release. The molecules bind to transmitter-gated ion channels in the postsynaptic membrane. If Cl^- enters the postsynaptic cell through the open channels, the membrane becomes hyperpolarized. The IPSP represents the resulting change in V_m as recorded by a microelectrode in the cell. (From Bear MF, et al. Neuroscience: exploring the brain. Baltimore: Williams & Wilkins, 1996.)

the cell increases, lowering its **resting membrane potential** (usually an electrical potential of 65 mV between outside and inside the cell) and temporarily increasing its tendency to "fire." The neuron fires when many subthreshold excitatory impulses arrive in rapid succession and the resting membrane potential lowers to about 50 mV. **Temporal summation** describes this condition of repeated subthreshold stimulation. Simultaneous stimulation of different presynaptic terminals of the same neuron produces **spatial summation**. This can induce an action potential from the "summing" of each individual effect.

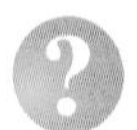

INTEGRATIVE QUESTION

Describe neuromuscular factors accounting for performance differences among individuals who spend the same time practicing a specific sports skill?

The phenomenon of neural facilitation (disinhibition) affects neurons within the CNS rather than electrochemical events at the NMJ because the NMJ does not release inhibitory neurotransmitters.[11] Neuronal facilitation can result from (1) decreased sensitivity of the motor neuron to inhibitory neurotransmitters, (2) reduced quantity of inhibitory neurotransmitter substance transported to the motor neuron, or (3) the combined effect of both mechanisms.

Neural facilitation exerts an important influence under certain exercise conditions. In all-out strength and power activities, for example, ability to disinhibit and maximally activate all motor neurons required for a movement becomes crucial to topflight performance.[22,30] *Enhanced facilitation (disinhibition) leads to full activation of muscle groups during all-out effort and largely accounts for the rapid and highly specific strength increases during the early stages of resistance training.*[17,18,31,34] Chapter 22 discusses the potential for augmenting maximal strength performance through CNS facilitation with intense concentration, or "psyching."

Inhibition. Some presynaptic terminals produce inhibitory impulses. The inhibitory transmitter substance increases the postsynaptic membrane's permeability to the efflux of potassium and chloride ions. This increases the cell's resting membrane potential, creating an **inhibitory postsynaptic potential (IPSP**; Fig. 19.12B). The IPSP hyperpolarizes the neuron, making it more difficult to fire. A large IPSP prevents initiation of an action potential when a motor neuron receives both excitatory and inhibitory stimulation. For example, one usually can override (inhibit) the reflex to pull the hand away when removing a splinter and so steady the hand to expedite this usually painful task.

The precise neurochemical that provokes an IPSP remains unknown, although γ-aminobutyric acid (GABA) and the amino acid glycine exert inhibitory effects. Neural inhibition serves protective functions and reduces the input of unwanted stimuli to produce a smooth, purposeful response.

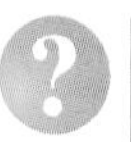

INTEGRATIVE QUESTION

How can drugs that mimic neurotransmitters affect physiologic response and performance in exercise?

MOTOR UNIT FUNCTIONAL CHARACTERISTICS

A motor unit contains only one specific muscle fiber type (type 1 or type 2) or a subdivision of the type 2 fiber with the same metabolic profile.[25] In addition to anatomic distinctions, Table 19.2 indicates classification of motor units on the basis of the physiologic and mechanical properties of the muscle fibers they innervate:

- Twitch characteristics
- Tension characteristics
- Fatigability

Twitch Characteristics

Early experiments in motor unit physiology revealed that motor units developed high, low, or intermediate tension in response to a single electrical stimulus. Additionally, motor units with low force capacity exhibited a slow shortening time (and time to peak force) but remained fatigue resistant, whereas units with higher force capacity shortened rapidly but fatigued earlier. Figure 19.13 illustrates the major characteristics for the three categories of motor units:

1. Fast twitch, high force, and fast fatigue (type IIb).
2. Fast twitch, moderate force, and fatigue resistant (type IIa).
3. Slow twitch, low tension, and fatigue resistant (type I).

TABLE 19.2 ➤ CHARACTERISTICS AND CORRESPONDENCE BETWEEN MOTOR UNITS AND MUSCLE FIBER TYPES

Motor Unit Designation	Force Production	Contraction Speed	Fatigue Resistance	Sag[a]	Muscle Fiber Type in the Motor Unit
Fast fatigable (FF)	High	Fast	Low	Yes	Fast glycolytic (FG)
Fast fatigue-resistant (FR)	Moderate	Fast	High	Yes	Fast oxidative–glycolytic (FOG)
Slow (S)	Low	Slow	High	No	Slow oxidative (SO)

[a]Under repetitive stimuli, some motor units respond smoothly with a systematic increase in tension, while others first increase tension and then decrease, or "sag" slightly in response to the same tetanic stimulus. These sag characteristics can be used to classify the different motor units. Only the slow motor units do not exhibit sag, which is probably related more to their diminished force-generating capabilities than to their fatigue characteristic.

Modified from Lieber RL. Skeletal muscle structure and function: implications for rehabilitation and sports medicine. Baltimore: Williams & Wilkins, 1992.

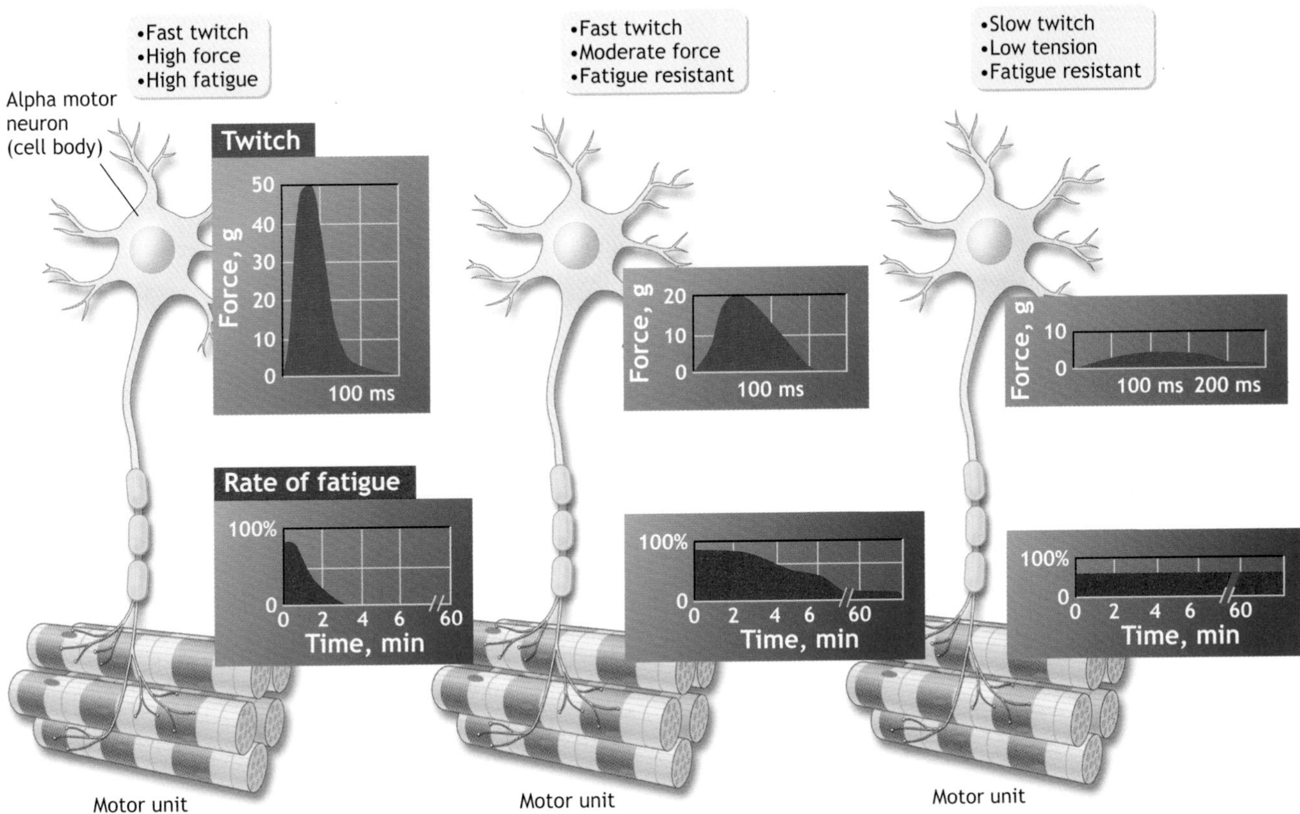

FIGURE 19.13 • Speed, force, and fatigue characteristics of motor units. "Phasic" motor neurons fire rapidly with short bursts; "tonic" motor neurons fire slowly but continuously.

Relatively large motor neurons with fast conduction velocities innervate the two major subdivisions of fast-twitch muscle fibers. These motor units generally contain between 300 and 500 muscle fibers. The fast-fatigable (FF) and fast–fatigue-resistant (FR) units reach greater peak tension and develop it faster than slow-twitch (S) motor units that receive innervation from smaller motor neurons with slow conduction velocities. The slower-contracting units, however, exhibit more fatigue resistance than fast-twitch motor units. As discussed in Chapter 22, specific exercise training can modify the particular metabolic characteristics of each specific muscle fiber type. *With prolonged aerobic training, fast-twitch muscle fibers become almost as fatigue resistant as their slow-twitch counterparts.*

Evidence indicates that motor neurons themselves have a trophic or stimulating effect on the muscle fibers they innervate in a way that modulates the fibers' properties and adaptive response to stimuli.[16] Surgically innervating fast-twitch muscle fibers with the neuron from a slow-twitch motor unit eventually alters the twitch characteristics of the fast-contracting fibers. Furthermore, application of long-term, low-frequency stimulation to intact fast-twitch motor units induces conversion of the muscle fibers to the slow-twitch type.[22,28] This neurotrophic effect suggests that the myoneural junction has much greater significance than just being the site of muscle fiber depolarization. It suggests a remarkable plasticity of skeletal muscle that may indeed be altered through long-term use.

Tension Characteristics

A stimulus strong enough to trigger an action potential in the motor neuron activates all of the accompanying muscle fibers in the motor unit to contract synchronously. A motor unit does not exert a force gradation—either the impulse elicits an action or it does not. After the neuron fires and the impulse reaches the NMJ, all fibers of the motor unit act simultaneously. This embodies the principle of **"all-or-none"** as related to the normal action of skeletal muscle.

Gradation of Force

The force of muscle action varies from slight to maximal via two mechanisms:

1. Increased *number* of motor units recruited.
2. Increased *frequency* of their discharge.

A muscle generates considerable force upon activation of all of its motor units. Also, repetitive stimuli that reach a muscle before it relaxes further increase the total tension. By blending these two factors, recruitment of motor units and modification of their firing rate, optimal patterns of neural discharge permit a wide variety of graded muscle actions—from the delicate touch required in eye surgery to the maximal effort in throwing a baseball from deep center field to home plate.

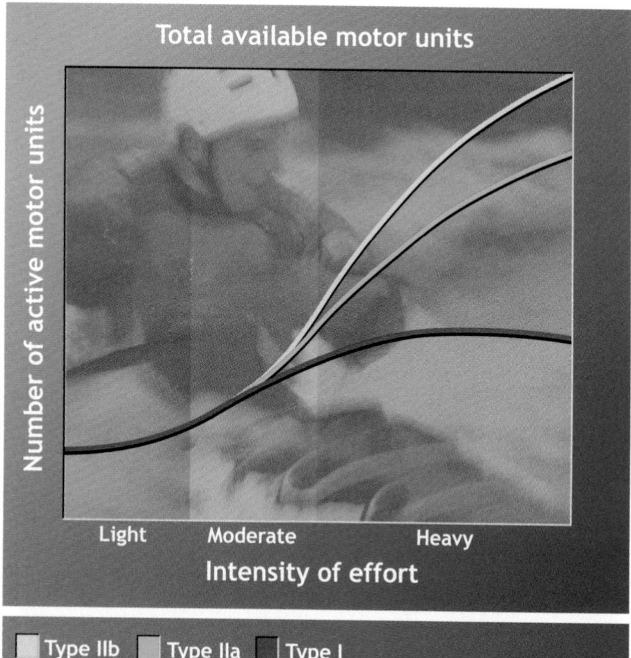

FIGURE 19.14 • Recruitment of slow-twitch (type I) and fast-twitch (type IIa and b) muscle fibers (motor units) in relation to exercise intensity. More-intense exercise progressively recruits more fast-twitch fibers.

MOTOR UNIT ACTIVITY. Low-force muscle actions activate only a few motor units; a higher force requirement progressively enlists more motor units. **Motor unit recruitment** describes adding motor units to increase muscle force. As muscle force increases, motor neurons with progressively larger axons are recruited. This exemplifies the **size principle**, which provides an anatomic basis for the orderly recruitment of specific motor units to produce a smooth muscle action.

All of the motor units in a muscle do not fire at the same time (Fig. 19.14). If they did, it would be virtually impossible to control muscle force output. Consider the tremendous gradation of forces and speeds that muscles generate. For example, when lifting a barbell, specific muscles act to move the limb at a particular speed under a particular rate of tension development. One can lift a relatively light weight at a number of speeds. As weight increases, however, the speed options decrease accordingly. With a light object such as a pencil, one generates the proper force to lift the pencil regardless of how fast or slowly the arm moves. *From the standpoint of neural control, the selective recruitment and firing pattern of the fast-twitch and slow-twitch motor units provide the mechanism to produce the desired response.*

In accordance with the size principle, slow-twitch motor units, with the lowest threshold for activation, become selectively recruited during light-to-moderate effort. Activation of slow-twitch units occurs during sustained activities like jogging or cycling on a level grade or during slow swimming or slowly lifting a light weight. More-rapid, powerful movements progressively activate fast-twitch fatigue-resistant (type IIa) units up through the fast-twitch fatigable (type IIb) units at peak force.[14,33] As a runner or cyclist reaches a hill during a distance race, some fast-twitch units become activated to maintain a fairly constant pace over varying terrain. Large single muscles such as the deltoid, with broad origins and/or insertions, may actually contain smaller, independently controlled "muscles within muscles" that become activated depending on the segment's line of action and the direction of intended motion. Such an arrangement allows for CNS flexibility to fine tune skeletal muscle activity to fit the demands of the imposed motor task.[37]

The differential control of motor unit firing patterns represents a major factor distinguishing not only skilled from unskilled performances, but also specific athletic groups.[10] For example, weight lifters generally demonstrate a synchronous pattern of motor unit firing (i.e., many motor units recruited simultaneously during lifting), whereas the firing pattern of endurance athletes becomes more asynchronous (i.e., some units fire while others recover). As discussed previously, a muscle's composition of specific motor units (muscle fibers) also contributes to an athlete's performance.[2,35] Furthermore, the synchronous firing of fast-twitch motor units certainly aids the weight lifter in generating force quickly for the desired lift. For the endurance athlete, on the other hand, the asynchronous firing of predominantly slow-twitch, fatigue-resistant units provides a built-in recuperative period so performance can continue with minimal fatigue as motor units share the burden of multiple movements and intensities during exercise.

INTEGRATIVE QUESTION

How can knowledge of neuromuscular exercise physiology help to enhance an athlete's (1) strength and power and (2) sports skill performance?

Neuromuscular Fatigue

Fatigue represents the decline in muscle tension (force) capacity with repeated stimulation. This definition also includes perceptual alterations of increased difficulty for achieving a desired submaximal or maximal exercise outcome. Motor unit fatigue results from many complex factors, each of which relates to the specific demands of the exercise that produces it.[1,23,24] These factors interact to ultimately affect either excitation, contraction, or both.

Voluntary muscle actions exhibit four main components listed in the following order of nervous system hierarchy:

1. Central nervous system
2. Peripheral nervous system
3. Neuromuscular junction
4. Muscle fiber

Fatigue results from an interruption in the chain of events between the CNS and the muscle fiber, regardless of the reason. Example include:

- Exercise-induced alterations in levels of CNS neurotransmitters such as serotonin, 5-hydroxytryptamine (5-HT), dopamine, and ACh in various brain regions,

Focus on Research — Muscular Fatigue: A Complex Phenomenon

Merton PA. Voluntary strength and fatigue. J Physiol (Lond) 1954;123:553.

➤ Since the turn of the century, scientists have tried to explain why repeated maximal muscular activity produced decreased tension output in muscle (fatigue). The debate over the site of fatigue focuses on the existence of either a central or a peripheral mechanism. *Central mechanism* refers to a location proximal to the motor neuron (i.e., mainly the brain); a *peripheral mechanism* involves the motor units (i.e., anterior motor neurons, motor endplates, and muscle fibers). Merton reasoned that he could distinguish central and peripheral mechanisms by inducing fatigue in a muscle group by use of maximal voluntary contractions (MVCs) and then stimulating the motor unit electrically. "Extra" localized electrical stimulation's failure to increase force production (i.e., no change in fatigue pattern) would indicate a purely peripheral fatigue site. In contrast, an increase in muscle tension (i.e., pattern of fatigue decreased) with electrical stimulation would support a central site for muscular fatigue hypothesis.

Merton experimented mainly on himself, using an apparatus (modified from one used to measure force recordings of excized muscle from animals [left inset figure]) that measured muscle tension output of the isolated adductor pollicis, a muscle that produces thumb adduction. The upper arm remained fixed in a flexed position with the hand rotated outward and stabilized in a grasping position. The arm and hand rested in a splint-type device that allowed only thumb abduction/adduction movement. This hand and arm position enabled isolation and recording of muscle tension by either voluntary muscle action or by electrical stimulation via the ulnar nerve.

Subjects performed maximal isometric actions to fatigue. Merton then delivered a series of single twitches (evoked by stimulation of the ulnar nerve) at approximately 12-second intervals preceding and following fatigue. The *top tracing* in the right figure below shows the fatigue curve for the muscles during the sustained isometric MVC. Tension declined linearly over time, reaching one-half its initial value in 1 minute. The *lower tracing* shows the corresponding action potentials in response to repeated nerve stimulation. Stimulating the motor nerve electrically did not alter the pattern of fatigue. Merton reasoned that some part of the peripheral apparatus directly affected fatigue during MVC. Because nerve stimulation did not diminish the amplitude of the action potential during fatigue *(lower tracing)*, the site of fatigue must have been within the muscle fiber itself, rather than at the neuromuscular junction. Merton's classic experiments provided the first strong support for the role of peripheral factors in muscular fatigue.

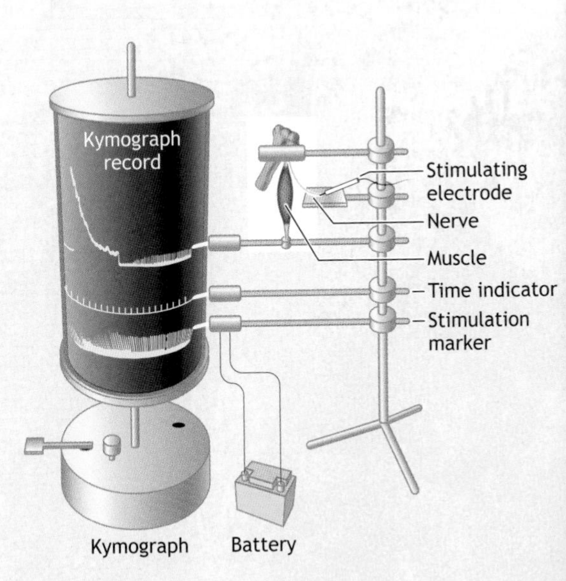

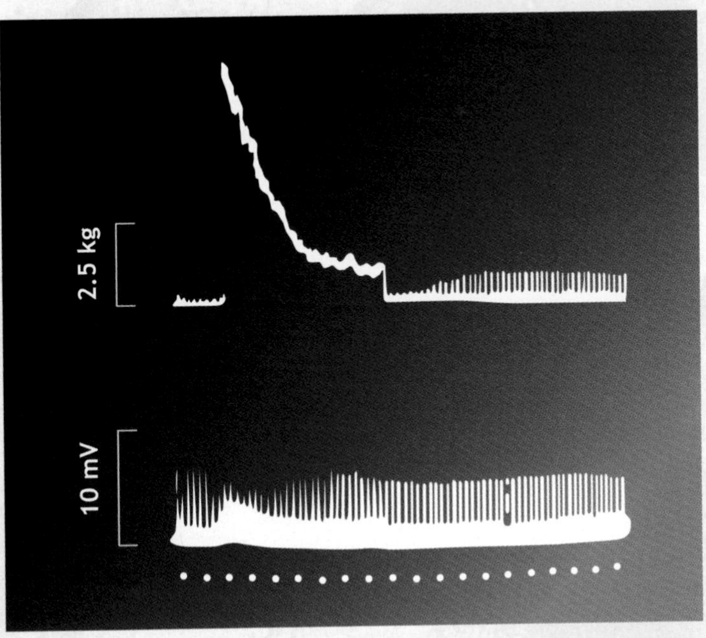

Left. Laboratory apparatus for use with excised muscle preparation from small animals to record magnitude of muscle action in response to repeated electrical nerve stimulation. *Right.* Results from modification by Merton of technique on left for use on intact muscle of humans to show fatigue curve during sustained isometric maximal voluntary muscle action (*top*) and the corresponding action potentials in response to repeated electrical stimulation of the motor nerve (*bottom*).

along with the neuromodulators ammonia and cytokines secreted by immune cells probably alter one's psychic or perceptual state to cause deterioration in ability to exercise.[5,26]

- Significant reduction in the glycogen content of the active muscle fibers relates to fatigue in both endurance-trained and untrained individuals during prolonged high-intensity exercise.[3,12] This "nutrient fatigue" occurs even with sufficient oxygen available to generate energy through aerobic pathways. Depletion of phosphocreatine (PCr) and decline in the total adenine nucleotide pool (ATP + ADP + AMP) that reflects a mismatch between ATP supply and demand (decreased ATP synthesis and/or increased ATP degradation) also accompanies the fatigue state in prolonged submaximal exercise in untrained individuals.[3]

- Oxygen lack and an increased level of blood and muscle lactate relate to muscle fatigue in short-term, maximal exercise. The dramatic increase in H^+ concentration in the active muscle, which accompanies lactate accumulation, dramatically disrupts the intracellular environment.[20,29] Alterations in contractile function in anaerobic exercise also relate to PCr depletion, changes in myosin ATPase, an impaired glycolytic energy transfer capacity from reduced activity of the key enzymes phosphorylase and phosphofructokinase, a disturbance in the T-tubule system for transmitting the impulse throughout the cell, and ionic imbalances.[19] Certainly a change in intracellular Ca^{2+} release, distribution, and uptake would alter the activity of the myofilaments and impair muscular performance. This local disturbance produces fatigue even though nerve impulses continue to bombard the muscle fiber.
- Fatigue also occurs at the NMJ when an action potential fails to cross from the motor neuron to the muscle fiber. The precise mechanism for this aspect of "neural fatigue" remains unknown.

As muscle function deteriorates during prolonged submaximal exercise, additional motor-unit recruitment maintains the force output required for the activity. In all-out exercise, which presumably activates all motor units, a decrease in neural activity (as measured by the electromyogram, or EMG) accompanies fatigue. Reduced neural activity supports the contention that fatigue in maximal effort results from failure in neural or myoneural transmission.

INTEGRATIVE QUESTION

In terms of neuromuscular physiology, discuss the validity of the adage "Perfect practice makes perfect."

RECEPTORS IN MUSCLES, JOINTS, AND TENDONS: THE PROPRIOCEPTORS

Muscles and tendons contain specialized sensory receptors sensitive to stretch, tension, and pressure. These end organs, known as **proprioceptors**, rapidly relay information about muscular dynamics and limb movement to conscious and subconscious portions of the CNS. Proprioception allows continual monitoring of the progress of any sequence of movements and serves as a basis for modifying subsequent motor behavior.[27]

Muscle Spindles

The **muscle spindles** provide sensory information about changes in muscle fiber length and tension of muscle fibers. They primarily respond to any stretch of a muscle and, through reflex response, initiate a stronger muscle action to reduce this stretch.

Structural Organization

Figure 19.15 shows a fusiform muscle spindle aligned in parallel to the regular muscle fibers, or **extrafusal fibers**. Consequently, when the muscle stretches, the spindle stretches as well. The number of spindles within a quantity of muscle

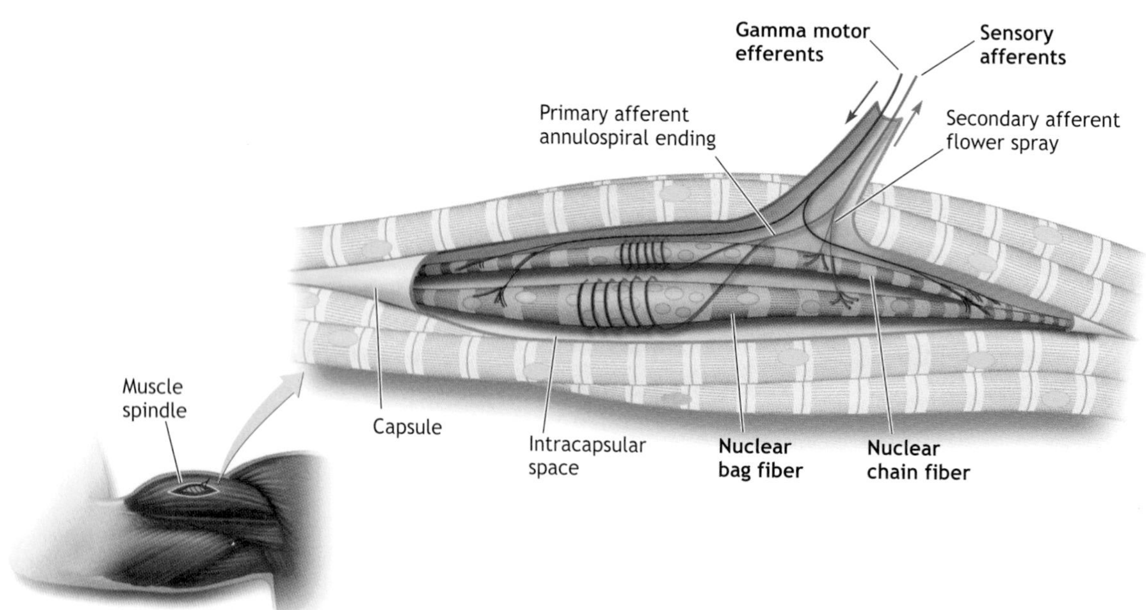

FIGURE 19.15 • Structural organization of the muscle spindle, with an enlarged view of the equatorial region of the spindle.

IN A PRACTICAL SENSE

➤➤ DETERMINATION OF UPPER-ARM MUSCLE AND FAT AREAS

Girth measurements include bone surrounded by a mass of muscle tissue ringed by a layer of subcutaneous fat (Fig. A). Because muscle represents the largest component of the girth (except in the obese and elderly), girth indicates one's relative muscularity. The procedure for estimating limb muscle area assumes similarity between a limb and a cylinder, with subcutaneous fat evenly distributed around the cylinder (Fig. A).

Measurements

Determine the following:

1. Upper-arm girth (relaxed triceps; G_{arm}): Measure with arm extended relaxed at the side (or parallel to the ground in an abducted position). Measure girth (cm) midway between the acromial and olecranon process (Fig. B).
2. Triceps skinfold (Sf_{tri}): Measure in decimeters (dm; mm ÷ 10) on the back of the arm, over the triceps muscle, as a vertical fold at the same level as the relaxed arm girth (Fig. C).

EXAMPLE

Data

Upper-arm girth (G_{arm}) in cm = 30.0; Sf_{tri} = 2.5 dm (25 mm).

COMPUTATIONS

1. Arm muscle girth, cm $= G_{arm} - (\pi Sf_{tri})$
   $= 30.0\text{ cm} - (\pi 2.5\text{ dm})$
   $= 30.0 - 7.854$
   $= 22.1\text{ cm}$
2. Arm muscle area, cm² $= [G_{arm} - (\pi Sf_{tri})] \div 4\pi$
   $= (30.0\text{ cm}) - (\pi 2.5\text{ dm})^2 \div 4\pi$
   $= 488.4 \div 12.566$
   $= 38.9\text{ cm}^2$
3. Arm area (A), cm² $= (G_{arm})^2 \div 4\pi$
   $= (30.0\text{ cm})^2 \div 4\pi$
   $= 900 \div 12.566$
   $= 71.6\text{ cm}^2$
4. Arm fat area, cm² = arm area − arm muscle area
   $= 71.6\text{ cm}^2 - 38.9\text{ cm}^2$
   $= 32.7\text{ cm}^2$
5. Arm fat index, % fat area = (arm fat area ÷ arm area) × 100
   $= (32.7\text{ cm}^2 \div 71.6\text{ cm}_2) \times 100$
   $= 45.7\%$

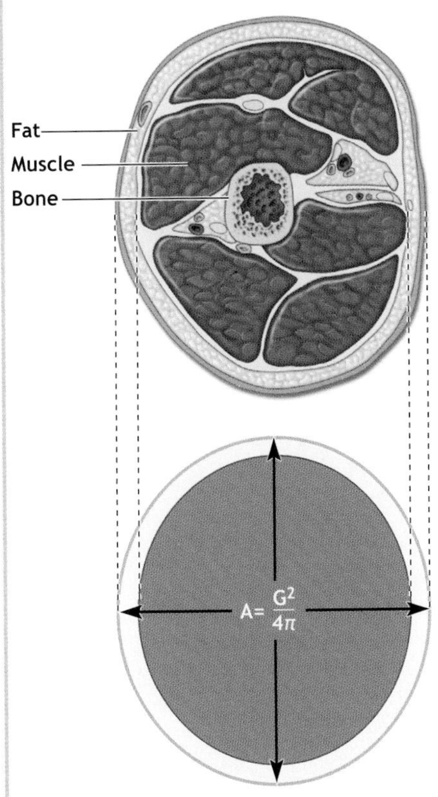

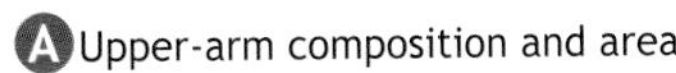
Ⓐ Upper-arm composition and area

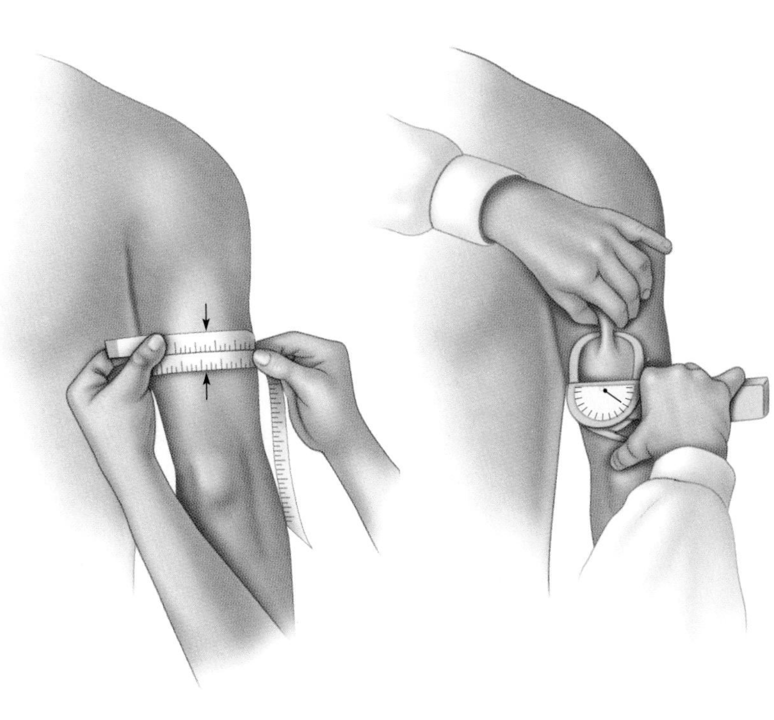

Ⓑ Relaxed triceps arm girth, cm

Ⓒ Triceps skinfold, mm

varies depending on the muscle group. On a relative basis, muscles involved in complex movements contain more spindles per gram than muscles that perform gross movement patterns. The spindle, covered by a sheath of connective tissue, contains two specialized types of muscle fiber called **intrafusal fibers**. One type of intrafusal fiber, the fairly large **nuclear bag fiber**, contains numerous nuclei packed centrally through its diameter. Each spindle usually contains two nuclear bag fibers. The other type of intrafusal fiber, the **nuclear chain fiber**, contains many nuclei along its length. These fibers attach to the surface of the longer nuclear bag fibers. Each spindle usually contains four to five chain fibers. The ends of the intrafusal fibers contain actin and myosin filaments and exhibit shortening capability.

Two sensory afferent fibers and one motor efferent fiber service the spindles. A primary afferent nerve fiber, the **annulospiral nerve fiber**, entwines about the midregion of the bag fiber. This fiber responds directly to the stretch of the spindle; its firing frequency increases in proportion to the stretch. A second group of smaller sensory nerve fibers, the **flower-spray endings**, makes connections mainly on the chain fibers but also attaches to the bag fibers. These endings show less sensitivity to stretch than the annulospiral fibers. Activation of the annulospiral and flower-spray sensors relays impulses through the dorsal root into the cord to cause reflex activation of the motor neurons to the stretched muscle. This causes the muscle to act more forcefully and shorten, which reduces the stretch stimulus from the spindles.

The third type of spindle nerve fiber, the thin **γ efferent fiber** that innervates the contractile, striated ends of the intrafusal fibers, serves a motor function. These fibers, activated by higher centers in the brain, provide the mechanism to maintain optimal sensitivity of the spindle at all muscle lengths. Gamma-efferent stimulation activates the intrafusal fibers, thereby regulating their length and sensitivity regardless of the overall length of the muscle itself. This mechanism prepares the spindle for other lengthening actions, even though the muscle itself may remain shortened. Adjustments in γ-efferent activation enable the spindle to continuously monitor the length of the muscles that contain them.

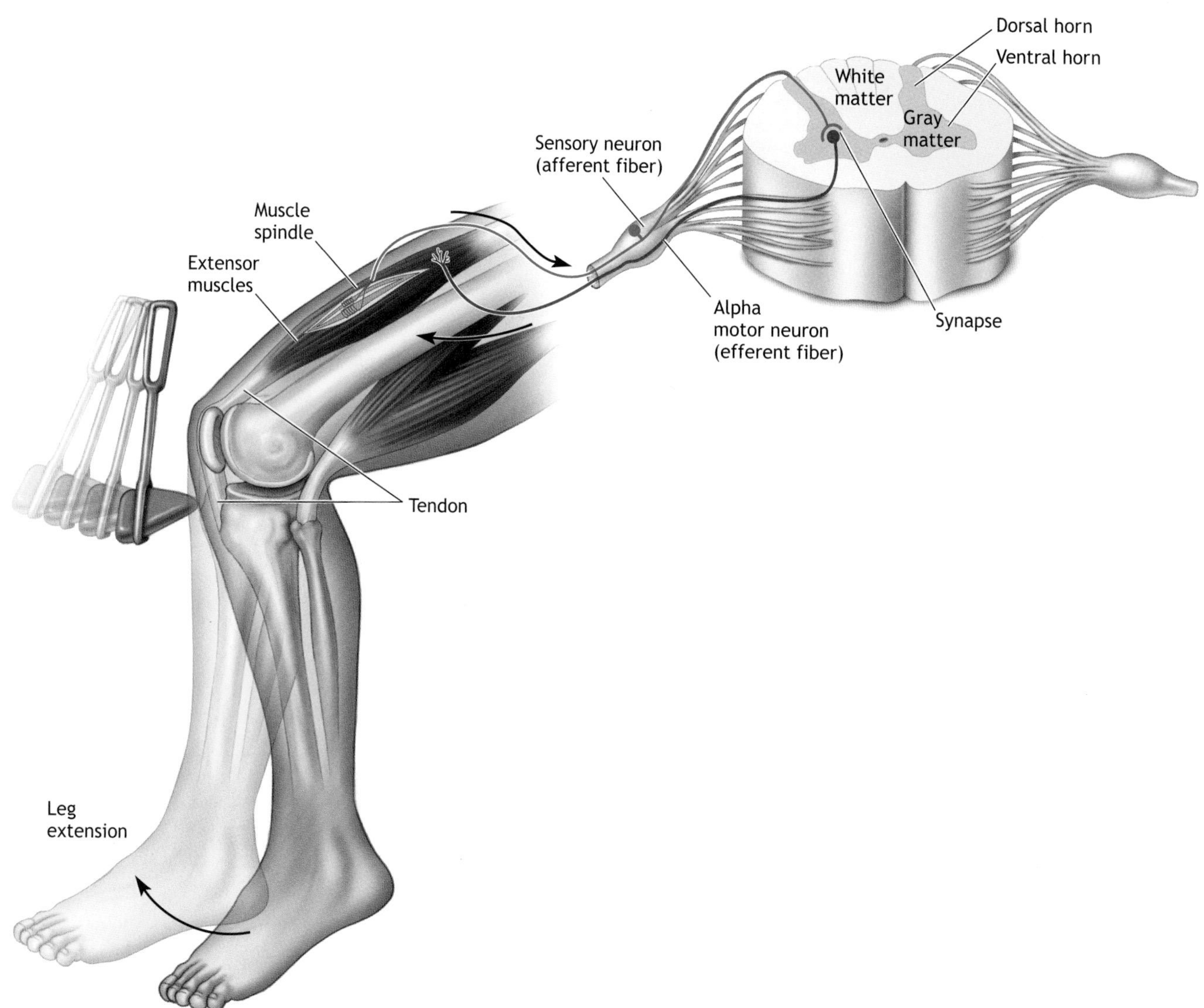

FIGURE 19.16 • The patella tendon stretch reflex. The diagram shows only one side of the spinal nerve complex.

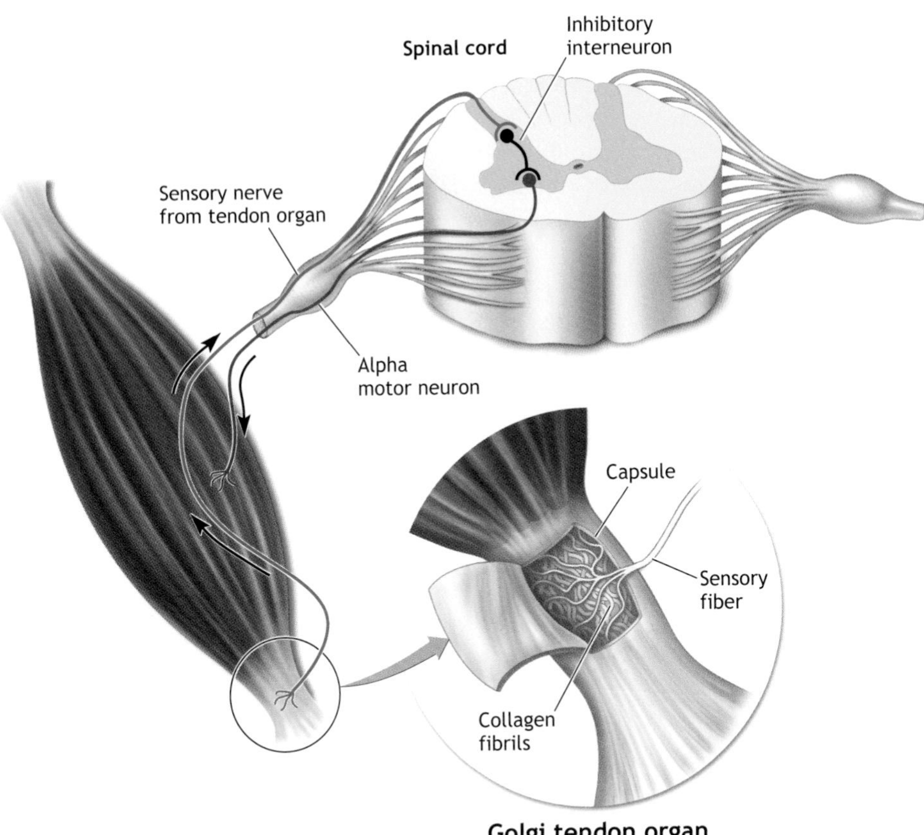

FIGURE 19.17 • The Golgi tendon organ, named for the Italian anatomist and Nobel laureate Camillo Golgi (1843-1926), who first described them in the late 1800s. Excessive tension or stretch on a muscle activates the tendon's Golgi receptors, which brings about a reflex inhibition of the muscles they supply. In this way, the Golgi tendon organ functions as a protective sensory mechanism to detect and subsequently inhibit undue strain within the muscle–tendon structure.

The Stretch Reflex

The functional significance of the muscle spindle lies in its ability to detect, respond to, and modulate changes in the length of the extrafusal muscle fibers. This provides important regulatory function for movement and maintenance of posture. Postural muscles continuously receive neural input to maintain their readiness to respond to conscious (voluntary) movements. These muscles also require a continual degree of subconscious activity to adjust to the pull of gravity in upright posture. To this end, the stretch reflex provides a fundamental controlling mechanism.

Three main components make up the stretch reflex: (1) the muscle spindle that responds to stretch, (2) an afferent nerve fiber that carries the sensory impulse from the spindle to the spinal cord, and (3) an efferent spinal cord motor neuron that activates the stretched muscle fibers.

Figure 19.16 illustrates the patella tendon stretch reflex (knee-jerk reflex), the simplest autonomic reflex arc involving only one synapse (monosynaptic). Because the spindles lie parallel to the extrafusal fibers, they become stretched when these fibers elongate as the hammer strikes the patella tendon. The spindle's sensory receptors fire when its intrafusal fibers stretch. This directs impulses through the dorsal root into the spinal cord to directly activate the anterior motor neurons. The gray matter contains neuron cell bodies; the white matter carries longitudinal columns of nerve fibers. Stimulation of a single α motor neuron can affect up to 3000 muscle fibers. The reflex also activates interneurons within the cord to facilitate the appropriate motor response. For example, excitatory impulses activate synergistic muscles that support the desired movement, while inhibitory impulses flow to motor units that normally act counter to the movement. In this way, the stretch reflex acts as a self-regulating, compensating mechanism; it enables the muscle to adjust automatically to differences in load (and length) without requiring immediate information processing through higher centers of the CNS.

Golgi Tendon Organs

In contrast to the muscle spindles that lie parallel to the extrafusal muscle fibers, the **Golgi tendon organs** connect to up to 25 extrafusal fibers near the tendon's junction to the muscle. These sensory receptors detect differences in the tension generated by active muscle rather than muscle length. Figure 19.17 shows that the Golgi tendon organs respond as a feedback monitor to discharge impulses under either of two conditions: (1) in response to tension created in the muscle when it shortens and (2) in response to tension when the muscle stretches passively.

When stimulated by excessive tension, the Golgi receptors conduct their signals rapidly into the spinal cord to elicit reflex inhibition of the muscles they supply. This occurs because of the overriding influence of the inhibitory spinal interneuron on the motor neurons supplying the muscle. Therefore, the Golgi tendon organ functions as a *protective* sensory mechanism much like a "governor" mechanism that prevents motorized go-carts from moving too fast. Excessive change in muscle tension increases the Golgi sensor's discharge; this depresses motor neuron activity and reduces force output. If muscle action produces little tension, Golgi receptors remain relatively inactive and exert little influence. *Ultimately, the Golgi tendon organs protect the muscle and its connective tissue harness from injury from excessive load.*

Pacinian Corpuscles

The **Pacinian corpuscles** are small, ellipsoidal bodies located close to the Golgi tendon organs and embedded in a single, unmyelinated nerve fiber. These sensory receptors are sensitive to quick movement and deep pressure. Deformation or compression of the onionlike capsule by a mechanical stimulus transmits pressure to the sensory nerve ending within its core. This produces a change in the electric potential of the sensory nerve ending. If this **generator potential** reaches sufficient magnitude, a sensory signal propagates down the myelinated axon that leaves the corpuscle.

Pacinian corpuscles classify as fast-adapting mechanical sensors because they discharge a few impulses at the onset of a steady stimulus and then remain electrically silent or may discharge a second volley of impulses when the stimulus ceases. Consequently, they detect *changes* in movement or pressure, rather than the magnitude of movement or the quantity of pressure applied.

Summary

1. Neural control mechanisms located in the central nervous system (CNS) finely regulate human movement. In response to internal and external stimuli, bits of sensory input automatically become coded, routed, organized, and transmitted to the effector organ, the skeletal muscles.
2. Tracts of neural tissue descend from the brain to influence spinal cord neurons. Neurons in the extrapyramidal tract control posture and provide a continual background level of neuromuscular tone; the pyramidal tract neurons stimulate discrete muscular movements.
3. The cerebellum provides the fine-tuning for muscle activity through its function as the major comparing, evaluating, and integrating center.
4. The spinal cord and other subconscious areas of the CNS control diverse muscle functions. The reflex arc provides the basic mechanism for processing these automatic muscle actions.
5. The motor unit makes up the functional unit of movement. The number of muscle fibers in a motor unit depends on a muscle's movement function. Intricate movement patterns require a small fiber-to-neuron ratio, whereas a single neuron may innervate a thousand muscle fibers for gross movements.
6. The anterior motor neuron (cell body, axon, and dendrites) transmits electrochemical nerve impulses from the spinal cord to the muscle. The dendrites receive impulses and conduct them toward the cell body, whereas the axon transmits the impulse in one direction only—down the axon to the muscle.
7. The neuromuscular junction (NMJ) establishes the interface between the motor neuron and the muscle fiber. Acetylcholine (ACh) release at the NMJ provides the chemical stimulus that activates the muscle fiber.
8. Stimulation of a muscle fiber progresses in the following sequence: (1) the action potential propagates down the motor neuron's axon; (2) calcium channels open at the end of the nerve terminal; (3) calcium moves into the nerve terminal; (4) ACh becomes primed for release; (5) ACh traverses the synapse and binds to ACh receptors on the postsynaptic membrane at the sarcolemma; and (6) an endplate potential generates and a depolarization wave spreads throughout the T-tubular network.
9. Both excitatory and inhibitory impulses continually bombard the synaptic junctions between neurons. These impulses alter a neuron's threshold for excitation by either increasing or decreasing its tendency to fire. During all-out power exercise, a high degree of neural facilitation (disinhibition) proves beneficial because it enables maximal activation of a muscle's motor units.
10. Motor units classify into three types depending upon the speed of muscle action, the force generated, and fatigability: (1) fast twitch, high force, high fatigue; (2) fast twitch, moderate force, fatigue resistant; and (3) slow twitch, low tension, fatigue resistant.
11. Muscle force gradation progresses through the interaction of factors that regulate the number and type of motor units recruited and their frequency of discharge. Low-intensity exercise recruits predominantly slow-twitch motor units, followed by activation of fast-twitch units when more powerful forces are required.
12. Alterations in motor unit recruitment and firing pattern probably explain much of the rapid strength improvement during the early stages of resistance training.
13. Special sensory receptors in muscles, tendons, and joints relay information about muscular dynamics and limb movement to specific portions of the CNS. This provides important sensory feedback during physical activity.

References

1. Asmussen E. Muscle fatigue. Med Sci Sports Exerc 1993;25:412.
2. Bergh U, et al. Maximal oxygen uptake and muscle fiber types in trained and untrained humans. Med Sci Sports 1978;10:151.
3. Baldwin J, et al. Muscle IMP accumulation during fatiguing submaximal exercise in endurance trained men. Am J Physiol 1999;277:R295.
4. Broca P. Anatomie compare de circonvolutions cerebrales. Le grand lobe limbique et la scissure limbique dans le serie des mammiferes. Rev Anthropol 1878;1:385.

5. Davis JM, Bailey SP. Possible mechanisms of central nervous system fatigue during exercise. Med Sci Sports Exerc 1997;29:45.
6. DeCamilli P, et al. Synapsin I (protein I), a nerve-terminal-specific phosphoprotein. II. Its specific association with synaptic vesicles demonstrated by immunocytochemistry in agarose-embedded synaptosomes. J Cell Biol 1983;96:1355.
7. Deschenes MR, et al. The neuromuscular junction: structure, function, and its role in the excitation of muscle. J Strength Cond Res 1994;8:103.
8. Diamond M. Enriching heredity: the impact of the environment on the anatomy of the brain. New York: Macmillan, 1988.
9. Diamond M, et al. Increases in cortical depth and glial numbers in rats subjected to enriched environment. J Comp Neurol 1966;128:117.
10. Edgerton VR, et al. The matching of neuronal and muscular physiology. In: Borer KT, et al., eds. Frontiers of exercise biology. Champaign, IL: Human Kinetics, 1991.
11. Engle AG. The neuromuscular junction. In: Engle G, Banker B, eds. Myology, basic and clinical. New York: McGraw-Hill, 1986.
12. Febbraio MA, Dancey J. Skeletal muscle energy metabolism during prolonged, fatiguing exercise. J Appl Physiol 1999;87:2341.
13. Feinstein B, et al. Morphologic studies of motor units in normal human muscle. Acta Anat (Basel) 1955;23:127.
14. Freund HJ. Motor unit and muscle activity in voluntary motor control. Physiol Rev 1983;63:387.
15. Gershon MD, et al. Morphology of chemical synapses and patterns of interconnection. In: Kandel ER, Schwartz JH, eds. Principles of neural science. New York: Elsevier North Holland, 1985.
16. Gordon T, Pattullo MC. Plasticity of muscle fiber and motor unit types. Exerc Sport Sci Rev 1993;21:331.
17. Häkkinen K, Komi PV. Electromyographic changes during strength training and detraining. Med Sci Sports Exerc 1983;15:455.
18. Häkkinen K, et al. Effect of combined concentric and eccentric strength training and detraining on force-time, muscle fiber, and metabolic characteristics of leg extensor muscles. Scand J Sports Sci 1981;3:50.
19. Hermansen L. Effect of metabolic changes on force generation in skeletal muscle during maximal exercise. In: Human muscle fatigue: physiological mechanisms. London: Pitman Medical, 1981.
20. Hogan MC, et al. Increased [lactate] in working dog muscle reduces tension development independent of pH. Med Sci Sports Exerc 1995;27:371.
21. Kakizawa S, et al. Critical period for activity-dependent synapse elimination in developing cerebellum. J Neurosci 2000;20:4954.
22. Kraus WE, et al. Skeletal muscle adaptation to chronic low-frequency motor nerve stimulation. Exerc Sport Sci Rev 1994;22:313.
23. Lewis SF, Fulco CS. A new approach to studying muscle fatigue and factors affecting performance during dynamic exercise in humans. Exerc Sport Sci Rev 1998;26:91.
24. MacLaren CP, et al. A review of metabolic and physiologic factors in fatigue. Exerc Sport Sci Rev 1989;17:29.
25. Nemete P, et al. Comparison of enzyme activities among single muscle fibers within defined motor units. J Physiol 1985;311:489.
26. Newsholme EA, et al. Physical and mental fatigue: metabolic mechanisms and importance of plasma amino acids. Br Med Bull 1992;48:477.
27. Nichols TR, et al. Rapid spinal mechanisms of motor coordination. Exerc Sport Sci Rev 1999;27:255.
28. Pette D, Vrbova G. Invited review: neural control of phenotypic expression in mammalian muscle fibers. Muscle Nerve 1985;8:676.
29. Sahlin K. Intracellular pH and energy metabolism in skeletal muscle of man. Acta Physiol Scand 1978;455(suppl):1.
30. Sale DG. Influence of exercise and training on motor unit activation. Exerc Sport Sci Rev 1987;15:95.
31. Sale DG, et al. Neural adaptation to resistance training. Med Sci Sports Exerc 1988;20:S135.
32. Sheard PW. Tension delivery from short fibers in long muscles. Exerc Sport Sci Rev 2000;28:51.
33. Spectar SA, et al. Muscle architecture and force-velocity characteristics of cat soleus and medial gastrocnemius: implications for motor control. J Neurobiol 1980;44:951.
34. Tesch PA, et al. Effects of strength training on G tolerance. Aviat Space Environ Med 1984;54:691.
35. Tesch PA, Karlsson J. Muscle fiber type and size in trained and untrained muscles of elite athletes. J Appl Physiol 1985;59:1716.
36. The cerebellum: the brain's engine of agility. Science 1998;281:1588.
37. Wickham JB, Brown JM. Muscles within muscles: the neuromotor control of intra-muscular segments. Eur J Appl Physiol 1998;78:219.

CHAPTER 20

The Endocrine System: Organization and Acute and Chronic Responses to Exercise

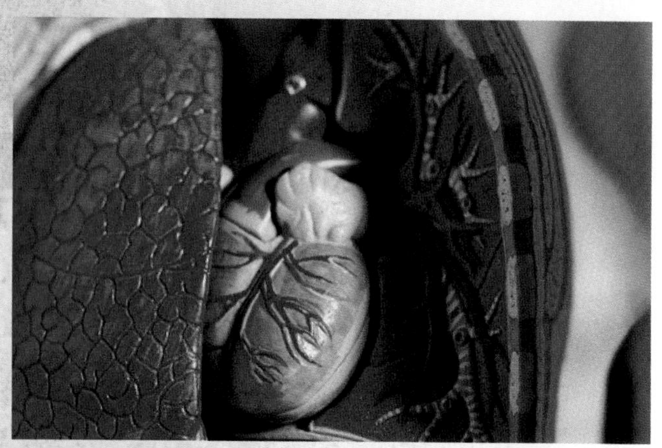

Chapter Objectives

- Draw the locations of the body's major endocrine glands
- List the sequence of events by which hormones affect specific "target cell" functions
- Outline the specific role of the intracellular messenger cyclic 3'5'-adenosine monophosphate (cyclic AMP)
- Discuss the role of hormones on enzyme activity and enzyme-mediated membrane transport
- Describe the influence of hormonal, humoral, and neural stimulation on endocrine gland activity
- List the hormones secreted by the anterior and posterior pituitary glands, their functions, and how short- and long-term physical activity affect their release
- List the thyroid gland hormones, their functions, and how short- and long-term physical activity affect their release
- List hormones of the adrenal medulla and adrenal cortex, their functions, and how short- and long-term physical activity affect their release
- List hormones of the α- and β-cells of the pancreas, their functions, and how short- and long-term physical activity affect their release
- Define the terms type 1 and type 2 diabetes and outline symptoms and effects of each disorder
- Describe three test options for diagnosing diabetes mellitus
- List the fasting blood glucose classification categories for diabetes
- Give the risk factors for type 2 diabetes and the benefits of regular exercise for the prevention and treatment of this disease
- Outline the overall effects of exercise training on endocrine function
- Describe the proposed effect of resistance training on testosterone and growth hormone release
- Characterize the functions of opioid peptides, their response to short- and long-term exercise, and their possible role in the phenomenon of the "exercise high"
- Outline the interactions among acute moderate and exhaustive exercise, exercise training, susceptibility to illness, and overall immune function

The endocrine system helps to integrate and regulate bodily functions and thus provides stability to the internal environment. Hormones produced by endocrine glands affect almost all aspects of human function; they activate enzyme systems, alter cell membrane permeability, cause muscular contraction and relaxation, stimulate protein and fat synthesis, initiate cellular secretion, and augment the body's ability to respond to physical and psychologic stress. The following sections provide a general overview of the endocrine system, its functions during rest and physical activity, and responses to acute exercise and chronic training.

ENDOCRINE SYSTEM OVERVIEW

Relatively small compared with other organs, the combined weight of the endocrine organs averages 0.5 kg. Figure 20.1 shows the location of the major endocrine organs—the pituitary, thyroid, parathyroid, adrenal, pineal, and thymus

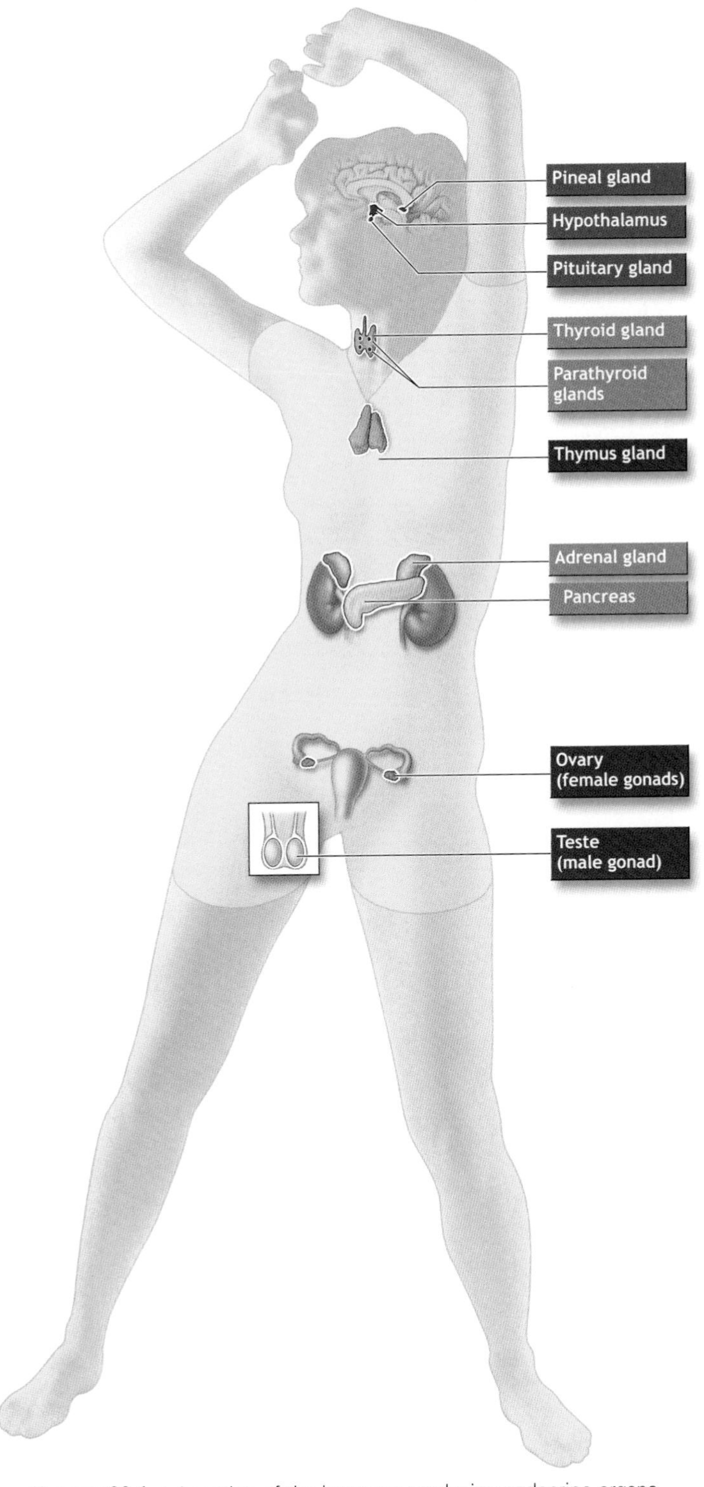

FIGURE 20.1 • Location of the hormone-producing endocrine organs.

glands. Several other organs contain discrete areas of endocrine tissue that also produce hormones. These include the pancreas, gonads (ovaries and testes), and hypothalamus. The hypothalamus also serves as a major organ of the nervous system; thus it functions as a **neuroendocrine organ**. Pockets of hormone-producing cells also form in the walls of the small intestine, stomach, kidneys, and heart, although these organs exert little influence on hormone production per se.

ENDOCRINE SYSTEM ORGANIZATION

The endocrine system consists of a host organ (gland), minute quantities of chemical messengers (hormones), and a target or receptor organ. Glands classify as either **endocrine** or **exocrine**. Some glands serve both functions.

Because endocrine glands possess no ducts (referred to as *ductless glands*), they secrete substances directly into the extracellular spaces around the gland. Figure 20.2 shows that these hormones then diffuse into the blood for transport throughout the body to fulfill their intercellular communication functions. The term *endocrine* means the same as *hormone secreting*. Exocrine glands, on the other hand, contain secretory ducts that carry substances directly to a specific compartment or surface. The nervous system controls almost all exocrine glands. Examples of exocrine glands include sweat glands and glands of the upper digestive tract.

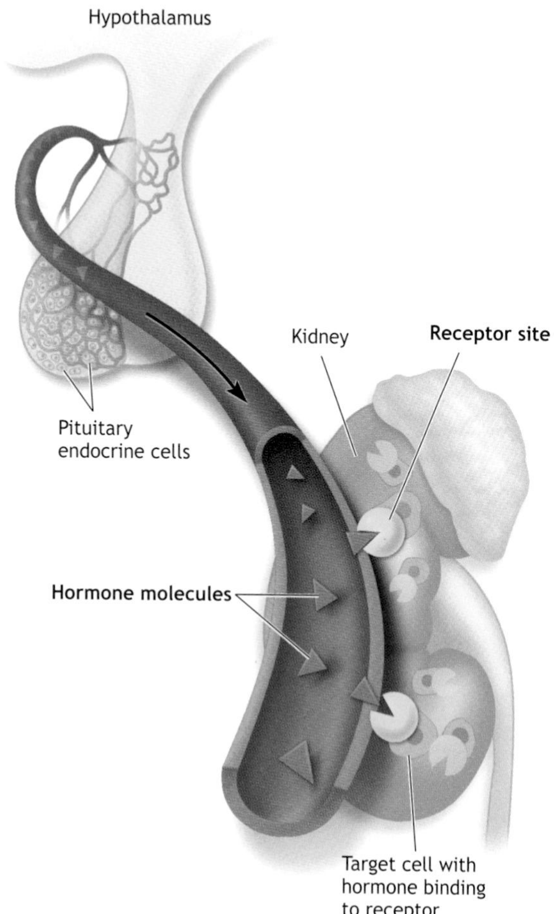

FIGURE 20.2 • Hormones secreted from endocrine glands travel in the bloodstream to exert their influence on various tissues throughout the body.

Types of Hormones

***Hormones** are the chemical substances synthesized by specific host glands, secreted into the blood, and carried throughout the body.* Hormones generally fit into one of two categories: (1) **steroid-derived hormones** and (2) hormones synthesized from amino acids, **amine** and **polypeptide hormones**. In contrast to steroid hormones, amine and peptide hormones are soluble in blood plasma. This allows easy uptake at target sites. The term **half-life** describes the time required to reduce a hormone's blood concentration by one-half. For example, the half-life of epinephrine is slightly less than 3 minutes. A hormone's half-life gives a good indication of how long its effect persists.

Table 20.1 lists eight different hormones produced by organs other than the major endocrine glands. Of these, **prostaglandins** constitute a third chemical class of hormones; they represent biologically active lipids found in the plasma membrane of nearly all cells. **Erythropoietin**, a glycoprotein, stimulates production of red blood cells by the bone marrow.

Although most hormones circulate in the blood as messengers that affect tissues a distance from the specific gland, other hormones (e.g., prostaglandins and the gastrointestinal hormone **gastrin**) exert local effects in their region of synthesis.

Hormone–Target Cell Specificity

Hormones alter cellular reactions of specific "target cells" by:

- Modifying the rate of intracellular protein synthesis by stimulating DNA in the nucleus.
- Changing the rate of enzyme activity.
- Altering plasma membrane transport via a second messenger system.
- Inducing secretory activity.

A target cell's ability to respond to a hormone depends largely on the presence of specific protein receptors that bind the hormone in a complementary way. These target cell receptors occur either (1) on the plasma membrane (up to 10,000 receptors per cell) or (2) in the cell's interior (usually for fat-soluble steroid hormones that pass through the plasma membrane). Hormone receptors exist in specific local areas or more diffusely throughout the body. For example, certain adrenal cortex cells normally contain receptors for **adrenocorticotropic hormone (ACTH)**. In contrast, all cells contain receptors for **thyroxine**, the principal hormone that stimulates cellular metabolism.

Hormone–Receptor Binding

***Hormone–receptor binding** is the first step in initiating hormone action.* The extent of a target cell's activation by a hormone depends on three factors: (1) hormone concentration in

TABLE 20.1 ➤ **HORMONES PRODUCED BY ORGANS OTHER THAN THE MAJOR ENDOCRINE ORGANS**

Hormone	Composition	Source and Stimulus for Secretion	Target and Outcome
Prostaglandins	20-carbon fatty acid synthesized from arachidonic acid	*Source:* plasma membrane of different body cells *Stimulus:* local irritation, different hormones	*Target:* multiple sites *Outcome:* controls local hormone response; stimulates arterioles to increase blood pressure; increases uterine contractions, HCl and pepsin secretion in stomach, platelet aggregation, blood clotting, constriction of bronchioles, inflammation, pain, and fever
Gastrin	Peptide	*Source:* stomach *Stimulus:* food	*Target:* stomach *Outcome:* release of HCl
Enterogastrin	Peptide	*Source:* duodenum *Stimulus:* food (especially lipids)	*Target:* stomach *Outcome:* inhibits HCl secretion and gastrointestinal motility
Secretin	Peptide	*Source:* duodenum *Stimulus:* food	*Target:* pancreas *Outcome:* release of bicarbonate-rich juice *Target:* liver *Outcome:* release of bile *Target:* stomach *Outcome:* inhibits secretion
Cholecystokinin	Peptide	*Source:* duodenum *Stimulus:* food	*Target:* pancreas *Outcome:* release of bicarbonate-rich juice *Target:* gallbladder *Outcome:* expulsion of bile *Target:* sphincter of Oddi *Outcome:* relaxes sphincter and allows bile to enter duodenum
Erythropoietin	Glycoprotein	*Source:* kidneys[a] *Stimulus:* hypoxia	*Target:* bone marrow *Outcome:* production of red blood cells
Active vitamin D_3	Steroid	*Source:* kidneys activate vitamin D made by epidermal skin cells *Stimulus:* parathyroid hormone	*Target:* intestine *Outcome:* active transport of dietary Ca^{2+} across intestinal membranes
Atrial natriuretic hormone	Peptide	*Source:* atrium of heart *Stimulus:* atrial stretching	*Target:* kidneys *Outcome:* inhibits Na^+ reabsorption and renin release *Target:* adrenal cortex *Outcome:* inhibits secretion of aldosterone

[a]The kidneys release an enzyme that modifies a circulating blood protein to produce erythropoietin.

the blood, (2) number of target cell receptors for the hormone, and (3) sensitivity (strength) of the union between hormone and receptor. Consider cell hormone receptors as dynamic structures that continually adjust to physiologic demands. **Upregulation** describes the state in which target cells form more receptors in response to increasing hormone levels. In contrast, prolonged exposure to high hormone concentrations desensitizes target cells in a manner that blunts their response to hormonal stimulation. This **downregulation** also involves a loss of receptors, which prevents target cells from overresponding to persistently high hormone levels.

CYCLIC AMP: THE INTRACELLULAR MESSENGER. The binding of a hormone with its specific receptor in the plasma membrane alters the target cell's permeability to a particular chemical (e.g., insulin's effect on cellular glucose uptake) or modifies the target cell's manufacture of intracellular substances, primarily proteins. Such actions ultimately affect cellular function. Figure 20.3 shows that for nonsteroid hormones (e.g., epinephrine and glucagon), the binding hormone acts as **first messenger** to react with the enzyme **adenylate cyclase** found in the plasma membrane. This forms the compound **cyclic 3′5′-adenosine monophosphate (cyclic AMP)** from an original ATP molecule. Cyclic AMP then acts as a ubiquitous **second messenger** to activate a specific protein kinase, which then activates a target enzyme to alter cellular function.

The sequence of reactions set into motion by cyclic AMP depends on three factors: (1) type of target cell, (2) specific enzymes contained in the target cell, and (3) specific hormone that acts as first messenger. In thyroid cells, for example, the cyclic AMP generated in response to the binding of thyroid-stimulating hormone promotes thyroxine synthesis. In bone and muscle cells, on the other hand, the cyclic AMP produced via growth-hormone binding activates anabolic reactions to synthesize amino acids into tissue proteins.

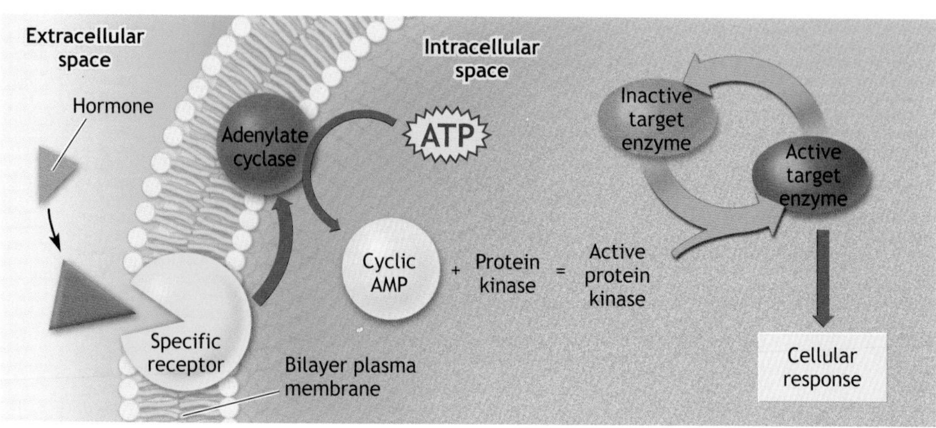

Figure 20.3 • Action of non-steroid hormones. Circulating hormone (first messenger) binds to a specific receptor in the cell's plasma membrane to trigger production of cyclic AMP from ATP. The enzyme adenylate cyclase catalyzes this reaction. Cyclic AMP then acts as second messenger to activate a protein kinase within the cell. This in turn activates a target enzyme to elicit the cellular response.

Effects on Enzymes

Altering enzyme activity and enzyme-mediated membrane transport are major hormone actions. A hormone increases enzyme activity in one of three ways:

1. Stimulating enzyme production
2. Combining with the enzyme to alter its shape and ability to act, a process known as **allosteric modulation**, which either increases or decreases the enzyme's catalytic effectiveness
3. Activating inactive forms of the enzyme, thus increasing the total amount of active enzyme

In addition to altering enzyme activity, hormones either facilitate or inhibit the uptake of substances by cells. Insulin, for example, facilitates glucose transport into the cell by combining with extracellular glucose and a glucose carrier within the plasma membrane. In contrast, epinephrine inhibits insulin release, thus slowing cellular glucose uptake.

Hormone action can exert potent, although often indirect, secondary effects. For instance, insulin release increases glucose uptake by muscle fibers (primary effect), which increases synthesis of muscle glycogen (secondary effect). This effect of insulin on glucose uptake (and glycogen synthesis) maintains fuel homeostasis during exercise. In insulin-deficient individuals, depressed glucose metabolism impairs exercise performance. Inadequate cellular glucose uptake caused by chronic insulin deficiency abnormally increases blood glucose concentrations. In the extreme, glucose eventually spills into the urine. We discuss the conditions of insulin insufficiency and/or insulin resistance in more detail on page 431.

Factors That Determine Hormone Levels

Hormone secretion rarely occurs at a constant rate. As with nervous system activity, hormone secretion usually adjusts rapidly to meet the demands of changing bodily conditions. For this reason, all protein hormones secrete in a pulsatile manner (see next section). Four factors determine plasma concentration of a particular hormone: (1) quantity synthesized in the host gland, (2) rate of either catabolism or secretion into the blood, (3) quantity of transport proteins present (for some hormones), and (4) plasma volume changes.

The rate at which endocrine glands secrete hormones depends on the magnitude of chemical stimulatory or inhibitory input from more than one source. For example, insulin secretion from the pancreas responds directly to plasma changes in glucose and amino acids, norepinephrine (from sympathetic neurons) and circulating epinephrine, and acetylcholine released from parasympathetic neurons. Each of these chemical messengers supplies inhibitory or excitatory input that determines whether insulin secretion increases or decreases. Over an extended time, hormone synthesis tends to equal hormone release. For a short period, however, hormone release can exceed its synthesis. The term **secreted amount** describes the plasma concentration of a hormone. In reality, this represents the sum of both hormone synthesis and release by the host gland, in addition to its uptake by receptor tissues and its removal by the liver and kidneys.

Hormone concentration depends on its rate of secretion into the blood and/or the rate of its metabolism (i.e., it becomes inactive). Hormone inactivation takes place at or near receptors or in the liver or kidneys. Since blood flow to splanchnic and renal areas decreases during exercise (blood distributes to active muscle), hormone inactivation rate decreases and plasma hormone concentration rises.

Steroid hormones must dissociate from their plasma protein carriers before exerting their influence. The quantity and affinity of the transport protein affects the amount of free hormone and its potential effect on tissue. Changes in plasma volume also alter hormone concentrations, independent of the host organ's secretion rate. For example, decreased plasma volume during prolonged exercise concurrently increases plasma hormone concentration, even without any absolute change in the amount of hormone.

Figure 20.4 shows three factors—hormonal, humoral, and neural—that stimulate endocrine gland activity.

- *Hormonal stimulation:* Hormones influence secretion of other hormones. For example, release-inhibiting hormones produced by the hypothalamus regulate the secretion of most anterior pituitary hormones. Anterior pituitary hormones, in turn, stimulate other endocrine organs to release their hormones into the blood. The increased blood levels of a hormone produced by the final target gland provide feedback to *inhibit* the release of anterior pituitary hormones and ultimately their own release.

- *Humoral stimulation:* Changing levels of certain ions and nutrients in blood, bile, and other body fluids stimulate hormone release. The term **humoral stimuli** describes these chemicals to distinguish them from hormonal stimuli, which also are fluid-borne chemicals. For example, an increase in blood sugar concentration (the humoral agent) prompts insulin release from the pancreas. Because insulin promotes glucose entry into cells, blood sugar levels soon decline, thus ending the stimulus for insulin release.
- *Neural stimulation:* Neural activity affects hormone release. For example, activation of the adrenal medulla by sympathetic neurons during stress releases catecholamines (epinephrine and norepinephrine). In certain cases, the nervous system overrides normal endocrine control to maintain homeostasis. Insulin action normally maintains blood sugar levels between 80 to 120 mg per 100 mL (dL) of blood. During exercise, however, activation of the hypothalamus and sympathetic nervous system blunts insulin release. This attenuates a further decline in blood sugar and ensures sufficient carbohydrate to fuel neural tissue and active muscle.

Patterns of Hormone Release

Most hormones respond to peripheral stimuli on an as-needed basis, but others are released at regular intervals during a 24-hour cycle, referred to as **diurnal variation**. Some secretory cycles span several weeks, while others follow daily cycles. Cycling patterns are not confined to one category of hormones. Figure 20.5 shows the pulsatile release profiles during a normal day for the peptide luteinizing hormone (LH) and cortisol, a steroid hormone. Graph A illustrates two different LH pulsatile patterns: (1) during acute anorexia nervosa and (2) following clinical remission with return of body weight to normal. The data points during anorexia resemble a prepubertal or early puberty pattern, while the remission data show a

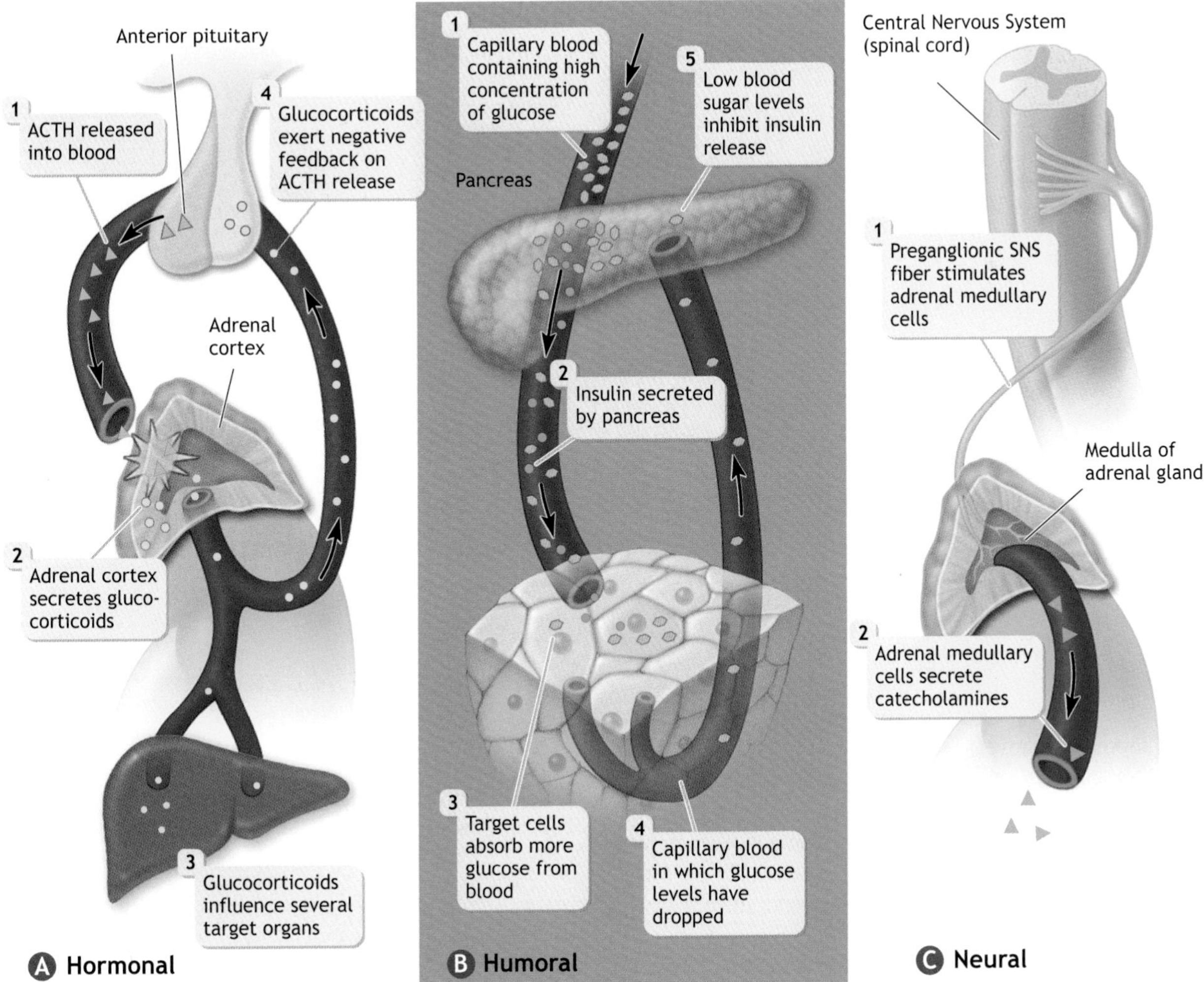

FIGURE 20.4 • Endocrine gland stimulation. **A**. Hormonal. Adrenocorticotropic hormone (ACTH) stimulates release of glucocorticoid hormones by the adrenal cortex. **B**. Humoral. High blood glucose concentrations trigger insulin release, causing rapid cellular glucose uptake. The subsequent decrease in blood glucose removes the stimulus for insulin release. C. Neural. Sympathetic nervous system (SNS) fibers trigger catecholamine release to blood. (From Marieb E. Anatomy and physiology. Redwood City, CA: The Benjamin/Cummings Company, 1989.)

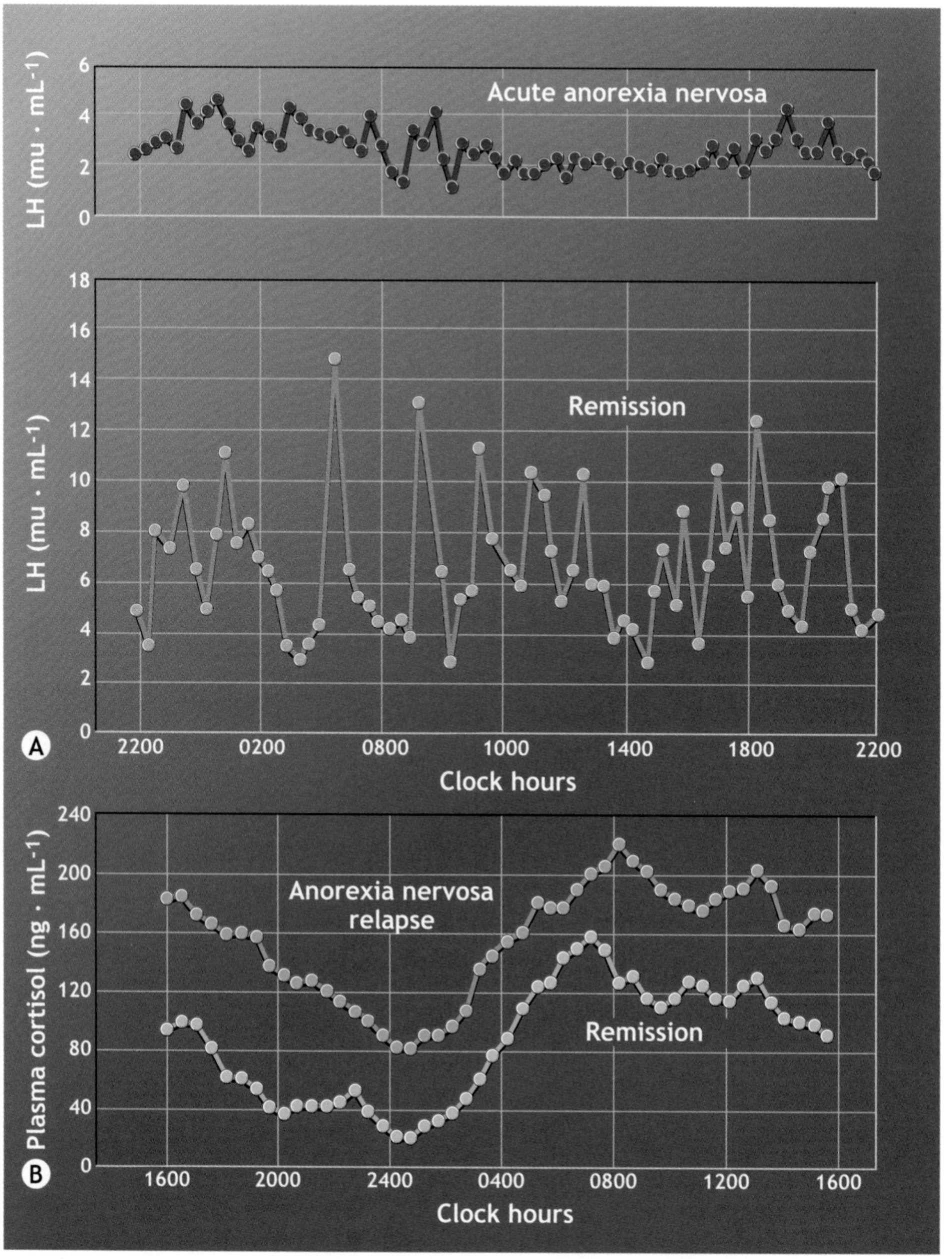

FIGURE 20.5 • **A**. Cycling pattern of LH release during acute episode of anorexia nervosa *(upper graphic)* and after clinical remission, with body weight return to normal *(lower graphic)*. **B**. Pattern of cortisol release during relapse *(upper data points)* and after subsequent recovery *(lower data points)* in patients with anorexia nervosa. (From Boyar R, et al. Anorexia nervosa: immaturity of the 24-hour luteinizing hormone secretory pattern. N Engl J Med 1974; 291:861; Doerr P, et al. Relationship between weight gain and hypothalamic pituitary adrenal function in patients with anorexia nervosa. J Steroid Biochem 1980;13:529.)

near-normal pulsatile pattern. The two sets of data points in part B of the figure show pulsatile patterns for plasma cortisol, an adrenocortical hormone, during relapse and after recovery in anorectic patients. Similar pulsatile patterns emerge under both conditions, but absolute hormone concentrations differ significantly between conditions.

Pulsatile hormone release patterns reveal information not available from a single blood sample that fails to show potentially significant variation in hormone levels during a daily cycle. Patterns of release and/or amplitude and frequency of discharge provide more-meaningful information about hormone dynamics than simply examining mean concentration at any single time.

INTEGRATIVE QUESTION

Discuss the meaning of the following statement: "Hormones act as silent messengers to integrate the body as a unit."

RESTING AND EXERCISE-INDUCED ENDOCRINE SECRETIONS

Table 20.2 lists the different endocrine host organs, specific hormones secreted, control factors, hormone functions, effects of hyposecretion and hypersecretion, and the influence of exercise on hormone output. The following sections review

TABLE 20.2 ➤ ENDOCRINE GLANDS AND THEIR SECRETIONS, FUNCTIONS, CONTROL FACTORS, EFFECTS OF HYPOSECRETION AND HYPERSECRETION, AND THE ACUTE EFFECTS OF EXERCISE ON HORMONE OUTPUT

Host Gland	Hormone	Hormone Effects	Control of Hormone Secretion	Effects of Hyposecretion and Hypersecretion	Exercise Effects on Hormone Secretion
Anterior pituitary	Growth hormone (GH; somatotropin)	Stimulates tissue growth; mobilizes fatty acids for energy; inhibits CHO metabolism	Hypothalamic releasing factor (GHRF)	*Hypo-*: dwarfism in children; *Hyper-*: gigantism in children, acromegly in adults	↑ with increasing exercise
	Thyrotropin (TSH)	Stimulates production and release of thyroxine from thyroid gland	Hypothalamic TSH-releasing factor; thyroxine	*Hypo-*: cretinism in children (stunted growth, mental retardation); myxedema in adults (low BMR, constipation, dry skin, puffy eyes, edema, lethargy) *Hyper-*: Graves' disease (autoimmune disease—elevated BMR, weight loss, irregular heartbeat); heart disease	↑ with increasing exercise
	Corticotropin (ACTH)	Stimulates production and release of cortisol, aldosterone, and adrenal hormones	Hypothalamic ACTH-releasing factor; cortisol	*Hypo-*: rarely seen *Hyper-*: Cushing's disease (persistant hyperglycemia, dramatic losses in muscle and bone protein, and water and salt retention leading to hypertension)	Unknown
	Gonadotropic (FSH and LH)	FSH works with LH to stimulate production of estrogen by ovaries; LH works with FSH to stimulate production of estrogen and progesterone by ovaries and testosterone by testes	Hypothalamic FSH and LH releasing factor; female—estrogen and progesterone; male—testosterone	*Hypo-*: Failure of sexual maturation *Hyper-*: none	No change
	Prolactin (PRL)	Inhibits testosterone; mobilizes fatty acids	Hypothalamic PRL-inhibiting factor	*Hypo-*: poor milk production in nursing women *Hyper-*: galactorrhea, cessation of menses in females; impotence in males	↑ with increasing exercise
	Endorphins	Blocks pain; promotes euphoria; affects feeding and female menstrual cycle	Stress—emotional/physical (may be intensity related)	Unknown	↑ with long-duration exercise
Posterior pituitary	Vasopressin (ADH)	Controls water excretion by kidneys	Hypothalamic secretory neurons	*Hypo-*: diabetes *Hyper-*: unknown	↑ with increasing exercise
	Oxytocin	Stimulates muscles in uterus and breast; important in birthing and lactation	Hypothalamic secretory neurons	Unknown	Unknown
Adrenal cortex	Cortisol Corticosterone	Promotes fatty acid and protein catabolism; conserves blood sugar/insulin antagonist; has anti-inflammatory effects with epinephrine	ACTH; stress	*Hypo-*: Addison's disease (weight loss; glucose and sodium levels decline and potassium levels rise, resulting in hypotension and dehydration) *Hyper-*: Cushing's disease	↑ in heavy exercise only

Continued

TABLE 20.2—*continued*

HOST GLAND	HORMONE	HORMONE EFFECTS	CONTROL OF HORMONE SECRETION	EFFECTS OF HYPOSECRETION AND HYPERSECRETION	EXERCISE EFFECTS ON HORMONE SECRETION
	Aldosterone	Promotes kidney's retention of sodium, potassium, and water	Angiotensin and plasma potassium concentration; renin	*Hypo-:* Addison's disease *Hyper-:* aldosteronism (excessive sodium and water retention and accelerated excretion of potassium)	↑ with increasing exercise
Adrenal medulla	Epinephrine Norepinephrine	Facilitates sympathetic activity, increases cardiac output, regulates blood vessels, increases glycogen catabolism and fatty acid release	Stress stimulated hypothalamic sympathetic nerves	*Hypo-:* unimportant *Hyper-:* hypertension, increased metabolism	Epinephrine, ↑ in heavy exercise Norepinephrine, ↑ with increasing exercise
Thyroid	Thyroxine (T_4) Triiodothyronine (T_3)	Stimulates metabolic rate; regulates cell growth and activity	TSH; whole body metabolism	*Hypo-:* decreased BMR and body temperature, cold intolerance, decreased appetite, weight gain, decreased glucose metabolism, elevated cholesterol, decreased protein synthesis, hypotension, muscle cramps, growth retardation, depressed ovarian function *Hyper-:* increased BMR, temperature, heat intolerance, increased appetite, weight loss, hypertension, enhanced glucose, lipid, and protein catabolism, loss of muscle, muscle atrophy, depressed ovarian function	↑ with increasing exercise
Pancreas	Insulin	Promotes CHO transport into cells; increases CHO catabolism and decreases blood glucose; promotes fatty acid and amino acid transport into cells	Plasma glucose levels	*Hypo-:* diabetes *Hyper-:* hypoglycemia, anxiety, nervousness, weakness	↓ with increasing exercise
	Glucagon	Promotes liver's release of glucose to blood; increases lipid metabolism, reduces amino acid levels	Plasma glucose levels	*Hypo-:* chronic hypoglycemia, low circulating amino acids *Hyper-:* hyperglycemia	↑ with increasing exercise
Parathyroid	Parathormone (PTH)	Raises blood calcium; lowers blood phosphate	Plasma calcium concentration	*Hypo-:* hypocalcemia, respiratory paralysis, uncontrolled spasms and convulsions *Hyper-:* hypercalcemia, extreme leaching of calcium from bones, depression of nervous system activity, muscle weakness, formation of kidney stones	↑ with long-term exercise

TABLE 20.2—*continued*

Host Gland	Hormone	Hormone Effects	Control of Hormone Secretion	Effects of Hyposecretion and Hypersecretion	Exercise Effects on Hormone Secretion
Ovaries	Estrogen Progesterone	Controls menstrual cycle; increased fat deposition; promotes female sex characteristics	FSH, LH	*Hypo-:* (estrogen) *Hyper-:* (progesterone) masculinization or virilization	↑ with exercise; depends on menstrual phase
Testes	Testosterone	Controls muscle size; increases RBC; decreases body fat; promotes male sex characteristics		*Hypo-:* feminization; *Hyper-:* masculinization or virilization	↑ with exercise
Kidneys	Renin	Simulates aldosterone secretion	Plasma sodium	*Hypo-:* hypertension *Hyper-:* hypotension	↑ with increasing exercise

these hormones, with special emphasis on their immediate response to exercise and adaptations to physical training.

Anterior Pituitary Hormones

Figure 20.6 illustrates the pituitary gland (also called the **hypophysis**), its secretions, and various target glands and their hormone secretions. Located beneath the base of the brain, the pituitary secretes at least six different polypeptide hormones. Because of its widespread influence, the anterior pituitary gland was often called the *master gland;* we now know, however, that the hypothalamus actually controls anterior pituitary activity; therefore, the hypothalamus should truly claim that title. Each of the primary pituitary hormones has its own hypothalamic releasing hormone, called a **releasing factor**. Neural input to the hypothalamus from stimuli such as anxiety, stress, and physical activity controls output of these releasing factors. In addition to the hormones displayed in Figure 20.6, the pituitary secretes **proopiomelanocortin (POMC)**, a large precursor molecule of other active molecules by enzymatic cleavage. POMC is the source of a number of neurotransmitters and hormones including ACTH, melanocortin peptides, and some of the naturally produced opiates such as β-endorphin (see page 444). These hormones exert a remarkable range of influence, including effects on pigmentation, adrenocortical function, food intake and fat storage, and nervous and immune system functions.

Growth Hormone

Growth hormone–releasing factor from the hypothalamus influences resting **growth hormone (GH)** secretion by directly stimulating the anterior pituitary gland. GH (also called **somatotropin**) exerts widespread physiologic activity because

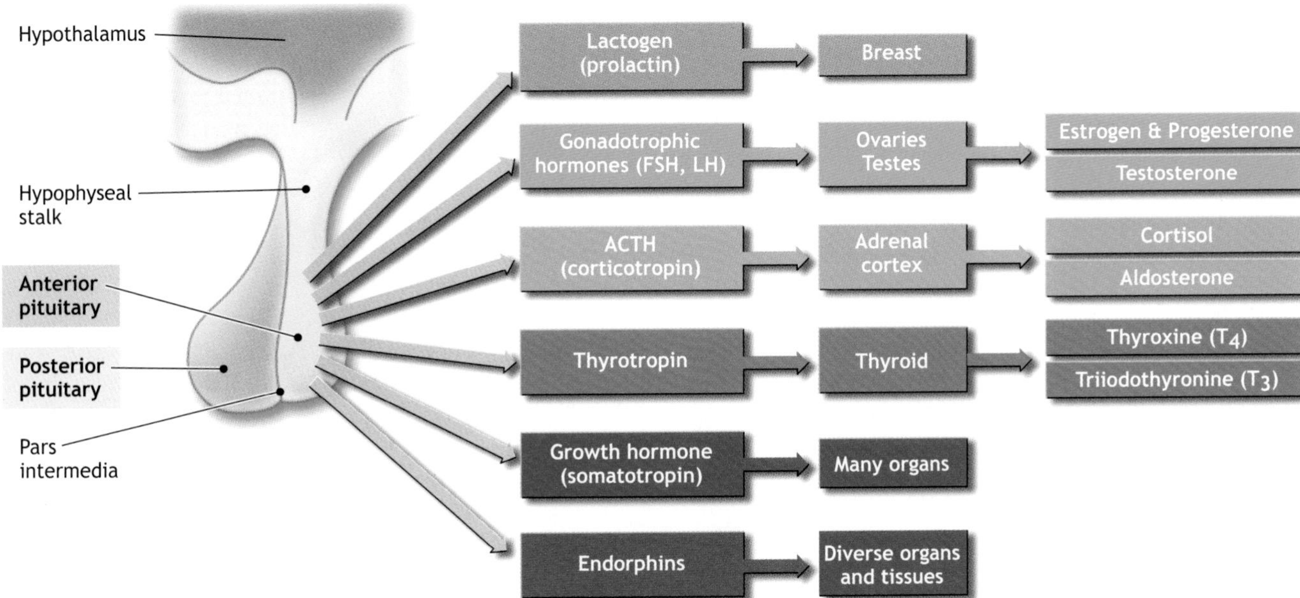

FIGURE 20.6 • The pituitary gland, its secretions, and target organs.

it promotes cell division and cellular proliferation throughout the body. In adults, GH facilitates protein synthesis by (1) increasing amino acid transport through the plasma membrane, (2) stimulating RNA formation, or (3) activating cellular ribosomes that increase protein synthesis.[64] GH also slows carbohydrate breakdown and initiates subsequent mobilization and use of fat as an energy source.

GROWTH HORMONE, EXERCISE, AND TISSUE SYNTHESIS. Short-term physical activity stimulates a sharp rise in GH pulse amplitude and the amount of hormone secreted per pulse.[16,117] Augmented GH release represents a beneficial response for muscle, bone, and connective tissue growth and also optimizes the fuel mixture during exercise, principally decreasing tissue glucose uptake, increasing free fatty acid mobilization, and enhancing liver gluconeogenesis. The net metabolic effect of increased exercise-induced GH production preserves plasma glucose concentration for central nervous system and muscle functions. GH also stimulates the liver's production of **insulin-like growth factors** (IGF-1 and IGF-II; see next section) that exert potent peripheral effects on motor units and other tissues.[130]

How exercise stimulates GH release to augment protein synthesis (and subsequent muscle hypertrophy), cartilage formation, skeletal growth, and cell proliferation remains unclear.[144,153] Concurrent measurements of circulating lactate, alanine, and pyruvate; blood glucose; and body temperature reveal no association with GH secretory patterns during exercise.[121] One hypothesis suggests that exercise directly stimulates GH release (or release of somatomedins from the liver or kidneys), which in turn stimulates anabolic processes.[15] Exercise may also indirectly affect GH by stimulating cholinergic pathways to trigger GH release. Furthermore, exercise stimulates endogenous opiate production that facilitates GH release by inhibiting the liver's production of somatostatin, a hormone that blunts GH release.[22,230]

Figure 20.7 outlines the overall metabolic actions of GH. GH modulates the metabolic mixture during exercise by stimulating fatty acid release from adipose tissue while simultaneously inhibiting cellular glucose uptake. This glucose-sparing action maintains blood glucose at relatively high levels, thus augmenting performance in prolonged exercise.

Both fit and sedentary individuals show similar increases in GH concentration when exercising to exhaustion, although the sedentary person maintains higher GH levels for several hours into recovery. During a standard bout of submaximal exercise, however, sedentary individuals show a greater GH response. Because this absolute submaximal exercise level represents greater stress for the less fit person, GH release generally relates more to the relative strenuousness of physical effort.

Insulin-like Growth Factors

IGFs (or somatomedins) mediate many of GH's effects.[39] In response to GH stimulation, liver cells synthesize **IGF-I** (a 70–amino acid polypeptide) and **IGF-II** (a 67–amino acid polypeptide), a process requiring between 8 and 30 hours. IGFs travel in the blood attached to one of five types of binding proteins and are then released as free hormones to interact with specific receptors. The diverse factors that influence IGF transport include binding proteins within muscle, nutritional status, and plasma insulin levels.

Because of the time required for IGF synthesis in response to GH stimulation, any IGF appearance during or immediately following exercise suggests that its release resulted from disruption of cells already containing IGF. Also, GH-mediated release of IGF with exercise may reflect a different time course than that typically observed in nonexercise conditions.[106]

Thyrotropin

Thyrotropin, also known as **thyroid-stimulating hormone (TSH)**, controls hormone secretion by the thyroid gland. TSH also acts to maintain growth and development of the thyroid gland and to increase thyroid cell metabolism. Considering the important role of thyroid hormones in regulating overall body metabolism, one would expect TSH output from the pituitary to increase during exercise, but this response does not occur consistently.

Adrenocorticotropic Hormone

ACTH, also known as **corticotropin**, functions as part of the **hypothalamic-pituitary-adrenal axis** to regulate output of hormones secreted by the adrenal cortex in a manner similar to TSH control of thyroid gland secretion. ACTH acts directly to (1) enhance fatty acid mobilization from adipose tissue, (2) increase gluconeogenesis, and (3) stimulate protein catabolism. Owing to difficulty in assay methods and the rapid disappearance of this hormone from the blood, data remain scarce concerning ACTH response during exercise. Available data suggest that ACTH concentrations increase proportionately with exercise intensity and duration if intensity exceeds 25% of aerobic capacity.[55,64,101] Corticotropin-releasing hormone (CRH) and arginine vasopressin (AVP) mediate ACTH release. CRH exhibits a definite diurnal rhythm, with highest levels in early morning just after rising. As the day progresses, CRH levels decline, essentially blocking ACTH release. Factors that alter the normal ACTH rhythm by triggering CRH release include fever, hypoglycemia, and other forms of stress. Because CRH represents both an ACTH regulator and a central nervous system neurotransmitter, it is often termed the *stress response integrator*. Speculation suggests that high-intensity exercise favors AVP release while prolonged exercise favors release of CRH, both resulting in ACTH inhibition.[103]

Prolactin

Prolactin (PRL) initiates and supports milk secretion from the mammary glands. PRL levels increase at high exercise intensities and return toward baseline within 45 minutes during recovery.[23] Owing to its important role in female sexual function, re-

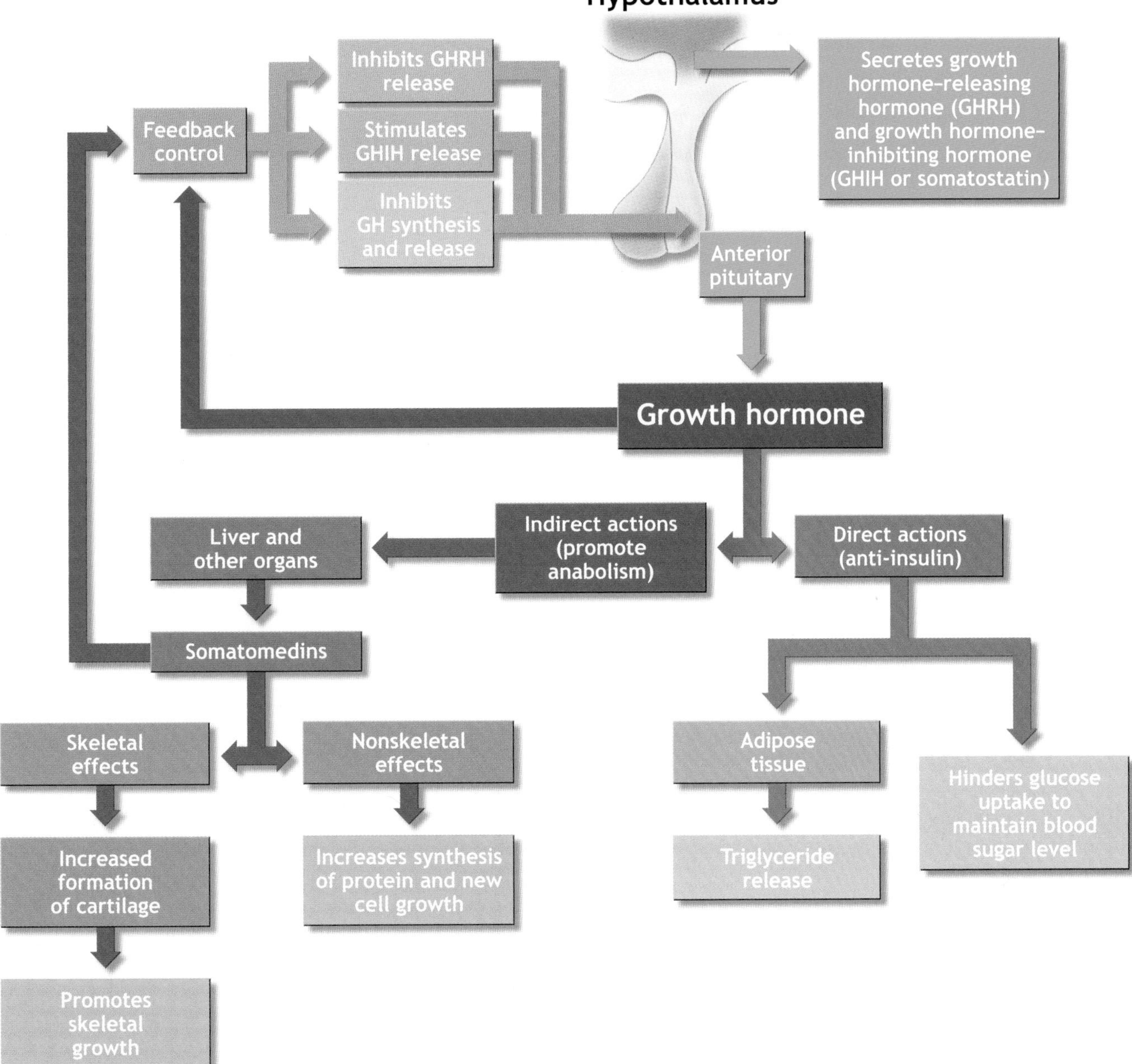

FIGURE 20.7 • Overview of growth hormone (GH) actions. GH stimulates the breakdown and release of triglycerides from adipose tissue and hinders glucose uptake by the cells (anti-insulin effect) to maintain a relatively high blood glucose level. Somatomedins mediate the indirect anabolic effects of GH. Elevated GH levels and somatomedins provide feedback to promote GH-inhibiting hormone (GHIH) release and depress the release of GH-releasing hormone (GHRH) by the hypothalamus; this further inhibits GH release by the anterior pituitary gland.

peated exercise-induced PRL release may possibly inhibit ovarian function and contribute to menstrual cycle alterations in athletic women.[18,152] Greater increases in PRL occur in women who run without wearing a bra; either fasting or consuming a high-fat diet also enhances release of this hormone.[110,180] PRL concentration increases in men following maximal exercise.[38]

Gonadotropic Hormones

Gonadotropic hormones stimulate the male and female sex organs to grow and secrete their hormones at a faster rate. **Follicle-stimulating hormone (FSH)** and **luteinizing hormone (LH)** are the two gonadotropic hormones. FSH initiates follicle growth in the ovaries and stimulates these organs to secrete estrogen, one type of female sex hormone. LH complements FSH action in causing estrogen secretion and rupture of the follicle, which allows the ovum to pass through the fallopian tube for fertilization. In the male, FSH stimulates germinal epithelium growth in the testes to promote sperm development. LH also stimulates the testes to secrete the male sex hormone testosterone.

Inconsistent reports describe short-term exercise–associated alterations in FSH and LH.[220] Because LH release is normally pulsatile, it becomes difficult to separate any specific exercise-related change from the normal pulsatile pattern (see Fig. 20.5). Generally, LH concentration rises even before exercise begins and reaches its peak during recovery.

Posterior Pituitary Hormones

The posterior pituitary gland forms as an outgrowth of the hypothalamus and actually resembles true neural tissue (Fig. 20.6). This tissue, often called the **neurohypophysis**, stores two hormones, **antidiuretic hormone (ADH** or **vasopressin)** and **oxytocin.** The posterior pituitary does not synthesize its hormones. Instead, the hypothalamus produces these hormones and secretes them to the neurohypophysis for release as needed via neural stimulation. Because of this important hypothalamic function, damage or surgical removal of the posterior pituitary does not dramatically affect ADH or oxytocin production.

ADH influences water excretion by the kidneys. Its action limits the production of large volumes of urine by stimulating reabsorption of water in the kidney tubules. Oxytocin initiates muscle contraction in the uterus and stimulates ejection of milk from the breasts during lactation. These functions make oxytocin important during birthing and nursing.

Exercise provides a potent stimulus for ADH secretion.[214,222] Increased ADH release, probably stimulated by sweating, helps the body conserve fluids, particularly during hot-weather exercise when dehydration becomes a real risk.[47] This water-conserving effect of ADH also contributes to the efficient modulation of the cardiovascular response to exercise.[156] ADH release decreases in response to a fluid overload, thus increasing urine volume and resulting in more dilute urine (i.e., lighter color urine). Little information exists about the effects of short-term exercise on oxytocin release.

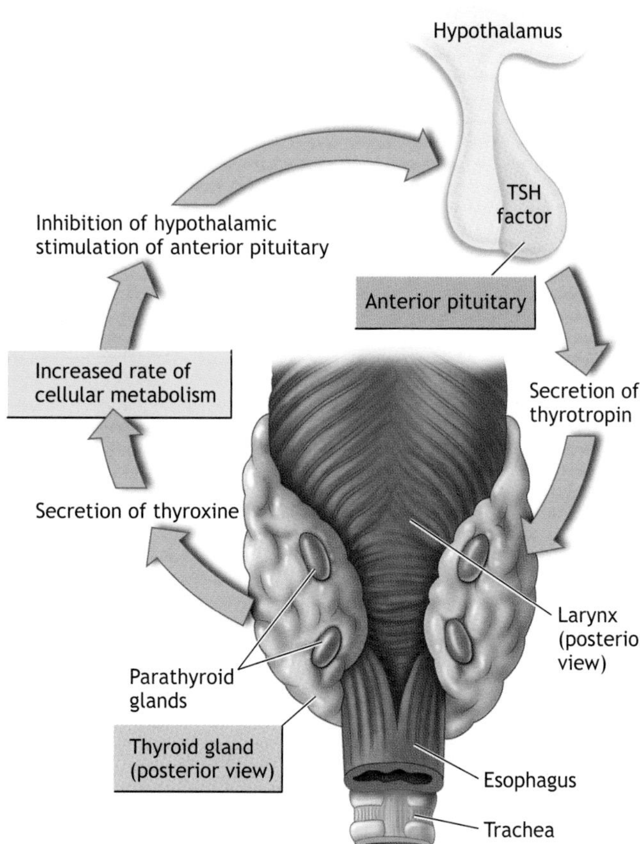

FIGURE 20.8 • Feedback system that controls the release of thyroid hormone.

Thyroid Hormones

The thyroid gland, located in the neck, just below the larynx, comes under the influence of TSH produced by the anterior pituitary gland. The thyroid gland secretes two protein-iodine–bound hormones, **thyroxine (T_4)**, and **triiodothyronine (T_3**, the active form of thyroid hormone), often referred to as the *major metabolic hormones.* T_4 is secreted in greater quantities than T_3; although less abundant, T_3 acts several times faster than T_4. Most receptor cells for T_4 metabolize it to T_3.

T_4 secretion raises the metabolism of all cells except the brain, spleen, testes, uterus, and thyroid itself through its stimulating effect on enzyme activity. For example, abnormal T_4 secretion raises the basal metabolic rate (BMR) up to four times. Because of this potent thermogenic effect, significant BMR deviations often indicate thyroid gland abnormality (see Chapter 9). A person may lose weight rapidly with abnormally high thyroid activity. In contrast, depressed thyroid production blunts BMR, which usually leads to gains in body weight and body fat. *Because fewer than 3% of obese people show abnormal thyroid function, depressed thyroid activity cannot explain excessive body fat gain in most individuals.*[21] In terms of nervous system function, T_3 release facilitates neural reflex activity, whereas decreased T_4 levels cause sluggishness, often inducing people to sleep for as long as 15 hours a day. Thyroid hormones also provide important regulation for tissue growth and development, skeletal and nervous system formation, and maturation and reproductive capabilities. They also play an important role in maintaining blood pressure by provoking an increase in adrenergic receptors in blood vessels.

Whole-body metabolism influences the synthesis of thyroid hormones. Depressing the metabolic rate to some critical value directly stimulates hypothalamic release of TSH. This increases thyroid output and increases resting metabolism. Conversely, a chronic increase in metabolism reduces TSH production, causing metabolism to slow. Figure 20.8 illustrates this exquisite feedback system.

During exercise, blood levels of *free T_4* (thyroxine not bound to plasma proteins) increase by approximately 35%.[68] This increase could result from an exercise-induced elevation in core temperature, which alters the protein binding of several hormones, including T_4. Whereas liver concentrations of T_4 increase during exercise, muscle concentrations remain unchanged.[237] The importance of these transient exercise-induced alterations in thyroid hormone dynamics requires further study.[191]

Parathyroid Hormones

Normally, four parathyroid glands, measuring 6-mm long, 4-mm wide, and 2-mm deep embed in the posterior aspect of the thyroid gland (Fig. 20.8). However, as many as eight glands have been reported, and some have been found in other regions of the neck or in the thorax. **Parathyroid hormone (PTH**, or parathormone) controls blood calcium balance. PTH release is triggered by a decrease in blood calcium levels and inhibited by increasing calcium concentrations. PTH's major effect increases ionic calcium levels by stimulating three target organs—bone, kidneys, and small intestine (Fig 20.9).

PTH release results in the following:

- Activation of osteoclasts (bone-reabsorbing cells) to digest some of the bone matrix to release ionic calcium and phosphate to the blood
- Enhancement of calcium ion reabsorption and decreased retention of phosphate by the kidneys
- Increased calcium absorption by intestinal mucosa

Plasma calcium ion homeostasis provides important modulation for numerous bodily functions such as nerve impulse conduction, muscle contraction, and blood clotting. Limited evidence suggests that physical activity increases PTH release in young, middle-aged, and older individuals, an effect that may contribute to the positive effects of exercise on bone mass.[8,78,126,140,218] For example, one study exercised six subjects on bicycle ergometers at different intensities for 10 minutes.[20] Blood samples were analyzed for ionized calcium, total calcium, calcitonin, pH, and plasma PTH. Moderate exercise (50% $\dot{V}O_{2max}$) initially depressed PTH levels, whereas near-maximal effort elevated hormone concentration during and in recovery from exercise. PTH release and subsequent calcium mobilization may provide the osteogenic raw material that allows the mechanical forces from exercise to produce positive effects on skeletal mass and density.

Adrenal Hormones

The adrenal glands appear as flattened, caplike tissues situated just above each kidney (Fig. 20.10). They have two distinct parts: (1) the **medulla** (inner portion) and (2) the **cortex** (outer portion). Each part secretes different types of hormones; consequently, the cortex and medulla are generally considered two distinct glands.

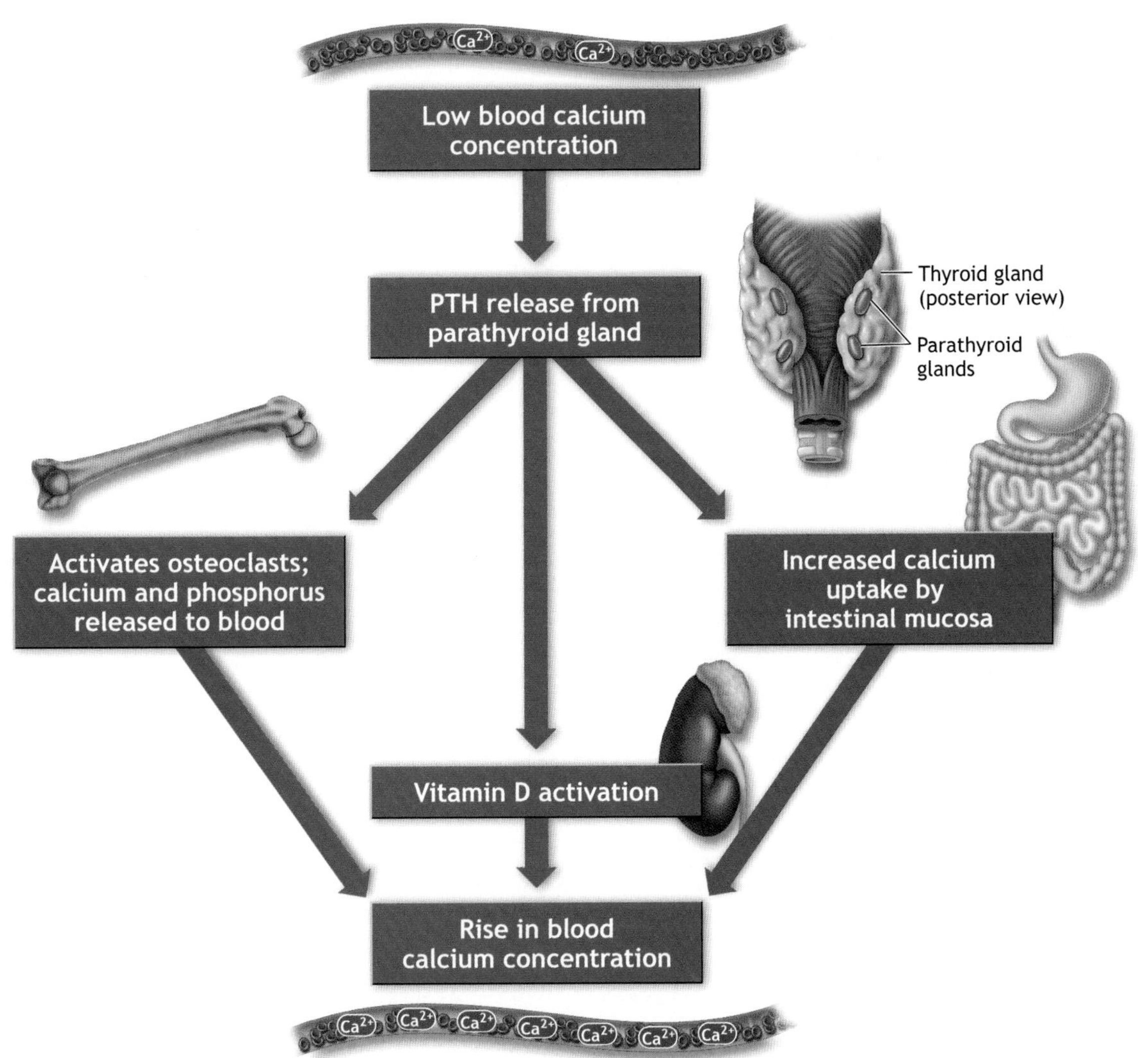

FIGURE 20.9 • Dynamics of parathyroid hormone (PTH) release and its actions.

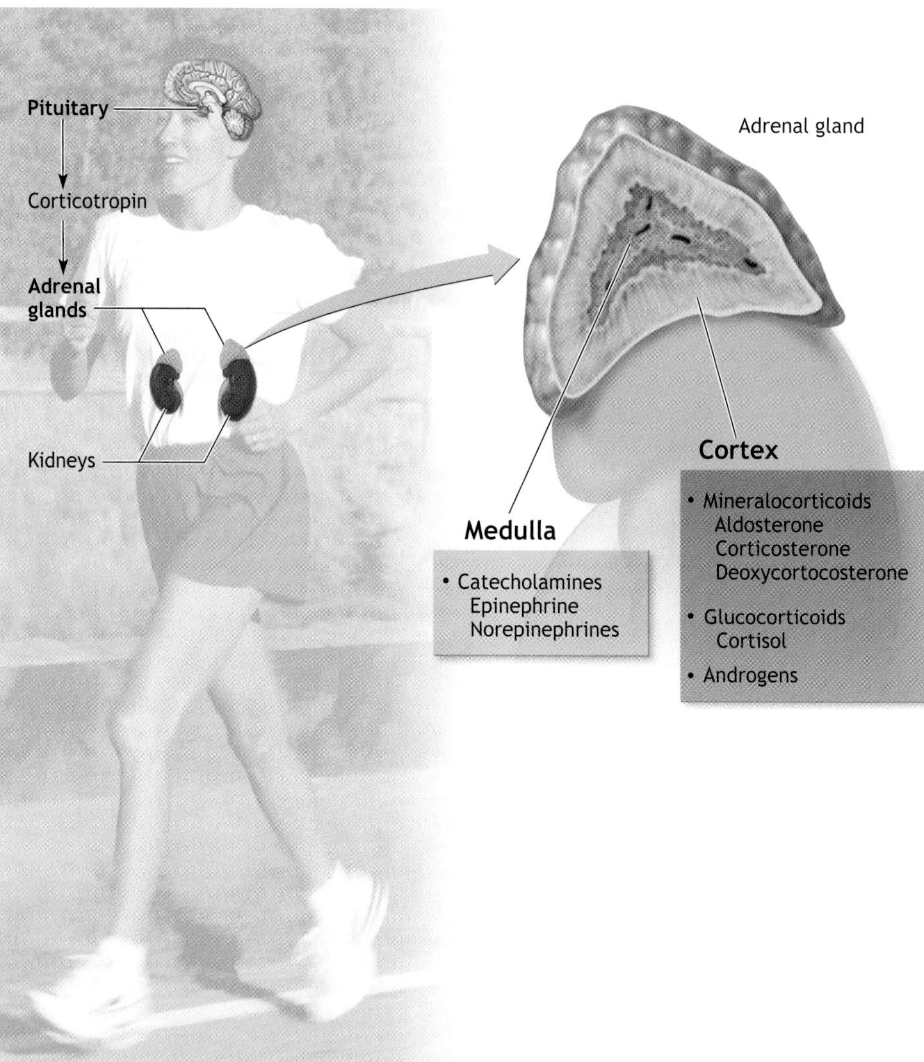

FIGURE 20.10 • Adrenal gland secretions.

Adrenal Medulla Hormones

The adrenal medulla makes up part of the sympathetic nervous system. It acts to prolong and augment sympathetic effects by secreting two hormones, **epinephrine** and **norepinephrine**, collectively called **catecholamines**. Figure 20.11 shows the chemical structure of epinephrine and norepinephrine and the role of each in substrate mobilization. Norepinephrine, a hormone in its own right, serves as a precursor of epinephrine. It also acts as a neurotransmitter when released by sympathetic nerve endings. *Epinephrine represents 80% of adrenal medulla secretions, whereas norepinephrine provides the principal neurotransmitter released from the sympathetic nervous system.* An outflow of neural impulses from the hypothalamus stimulates the adrenal medulla to increase catecholamine release. These hormones then affect the heart, blood vessels, and glands in the same, albeit slower-acting, way as direct sympathetic nervous system stimulation. Epinephrine's primary function in energy metabolism is to stimulate glycogenolysis (in the liver and active muscles) and lipolysis (in adipose tissue and active muscles); norepinephrine provides powerful lipolytic stimulation in adipose tissue.[57,211] Because sympathetic nerve endings (including those to the adrenal gland) secrete both epinephrine and norepinephrine, it is more appropriate to discuss the "sympathoadrenal" response to exercise and training rather than simply the adrenal gland response. *The sympathoadrenal response to exercise most closely relates to relative rather than absolute exercise intensity.*[238]

Figure 20.12 illustrates the catecholamine response at various exercise intensities (expressed as $\%\dot{V}O_{2max}$) in 10 male subjects. Norepinephrine increases markedly at intensities exceeding 50% $\dot{V}O_{2max}$, whereas epinephrine levels remain unchanged until exercise intensity exceeds about 60% $\dot{V}O_{2max}$. At maximum effort, an approximate two- to sixfold increase in norepinephrine release takes place. More than likely, increased secretion occurs from sympathetic postganglionic nerve endings and relates to cardiovascular and metabolic adjustments in active tissues. Epinephrine output from the adrenal medulla also increases with exercise, with the magnitude of increase directly related to intensity and duration of effort.[32,135–137,158] Athletes involved in sprint–power training show greater sympathoadrenergic activation during maximal exercise than counterparts trained in aerobic exercise.[212] This difference relates to the higher anaerobic contribution to maximal exercise energy supply by the sprint–power athletes. Age does not affect the catecholamine response to exercise among individuals equated for aerobic fitness.[122,150] The effects of increased adrenal medulla activity on blood flow distribution, cardiac contractility, and substrate mobilization all benefit the exercise response.[125]

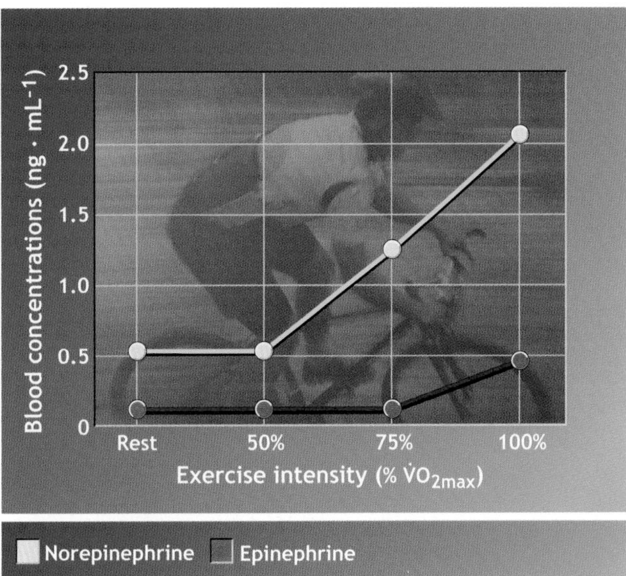

FIGURE 20.12 • Catecholamine response to exercise of increasing intensity in 10 male subjects. (From Applied Physiology Laboratory, University of Michigan, Ann Arbor.)

Adrenocortical Hormones

The adrenal cortex, stimulated by corticotropin from the anterior pituitary, secretes **adrenocortical hormones**. These corticosteroid hormones fit functionally into one of three groups: (1) **mineralocorticoids**, (2) **glucocorticoids**, and (3) **androgens**—each produced in a different zone (layer) of the adrenal cortex.

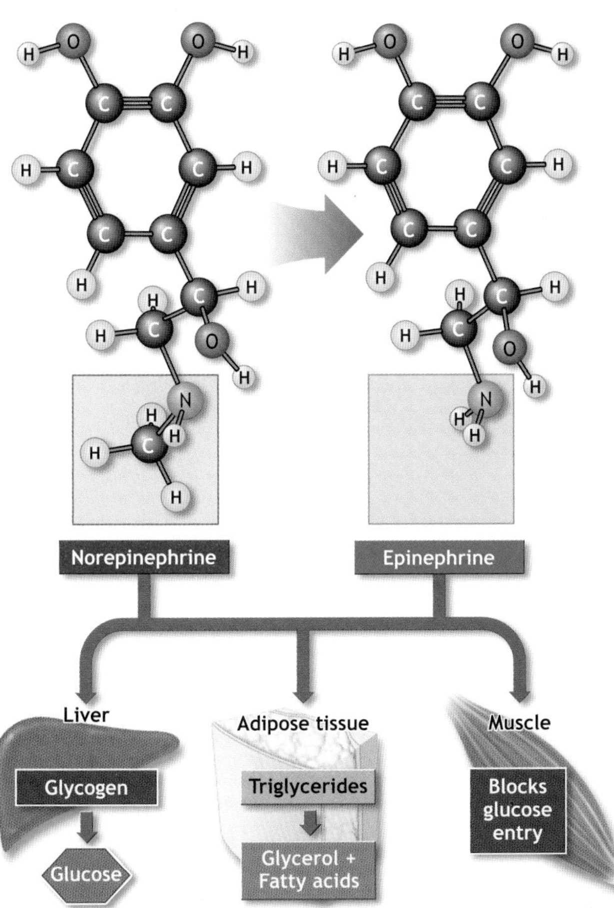

FIGURE 20.11 • Chemical structure of the catecholamines epinephrine and norepinephrine and their role in substrate use (e.g., mobilizing glucose from the liver and free fatty acids from adipose tissue and blunting glucose uptake by skeletal muscle). Norepinephrine serves both as a hormone and as a precursor of epinephrine. It also functions as a neurotransmitter when released by sympathetic nerve endings.

MINERALOCORTICOIDS. As the name suggests, mineralocorticoids regulate the mineral salts sodium and potassium in the extracellular fluid. **Aldosterone** is the most physiologically important of the three mineralocorticoids, representing almost 95% of all mineralocorticoids produced.

Figure 20.13 shows four major controlling factors for aldosterone release from the adrenal cortex. *Aldosterone secretion provides control of total sodium concentration and extracellular fluid volume. It stimulates sodium ion reabsorption (along with fluid) in the distal tubules of the kidneys by increasing the synthesis of sodium transporter proteins by the epithelial cells of the tubules and collecting duct.*[36,48] Consequently, little sodium (and fluid) voids in the urine. An increase in cardiac output and arterial blood pressure also accompanies an increase in plasma volume with aldosterone secretion. In contrast, sodium and water literally flow into the urine when aldosterone secretion ceases. Aldosterone also contributes to maintenance of serum potassium and pH because the kidneys exchange either a K^+ or H^+ for each Na^+ reabsorbed. Proper mineral balance maintains nerve transmission and muscle function. Neuromuscular activity would cease without effective regulation of sodium and potassium exchange. As with all steroid hormones, cellular response to increased aldosterone production is slow. It would require relatively prolonged exercise (<45 min) for aldosterone's effect to emerge; hence, its major effects occur during recovery.

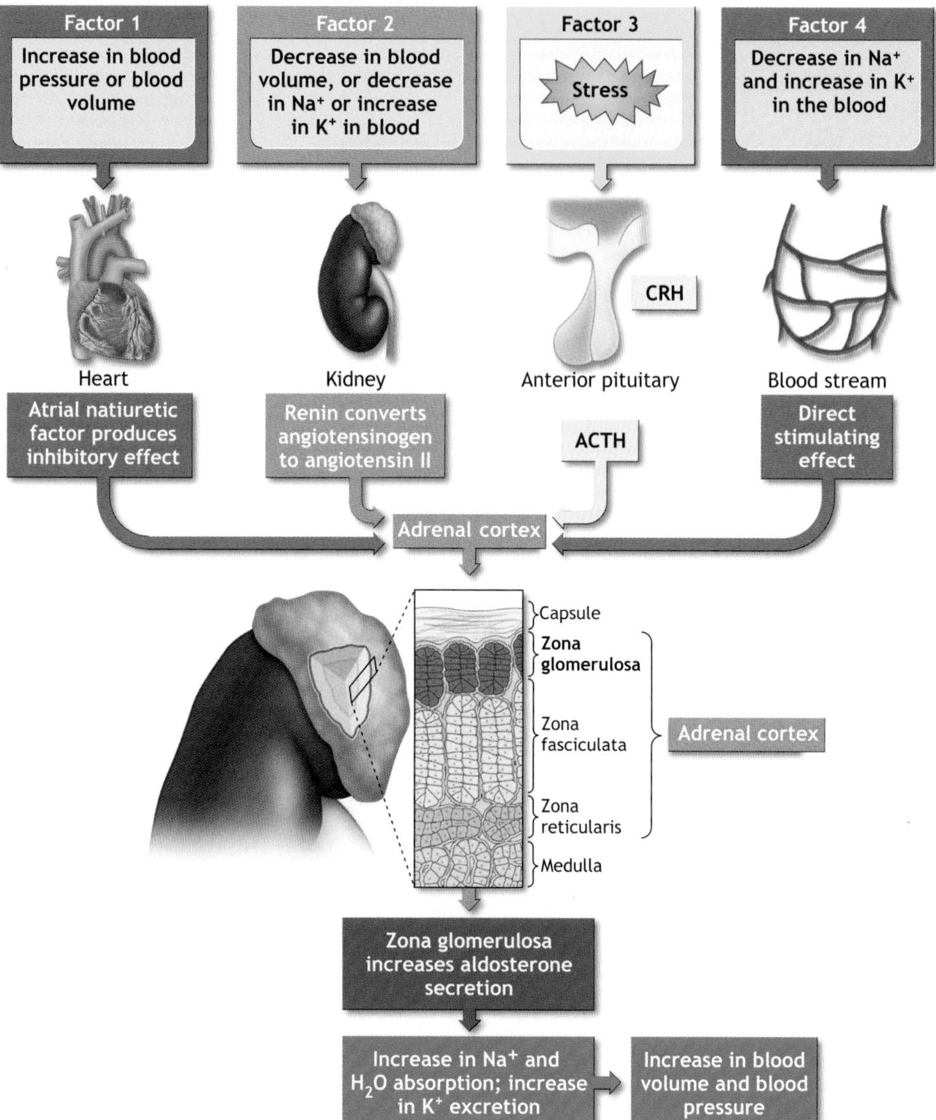

FIGURE 20.13 • Four major factors that control aldosterone release from the adrenal cortex. *CRH,* corticotropin-releasing hormone; *ACTH,* adrenocorticotropic hormone.

Renin–Angiotensin Mechanism. Increased sympathetic nervous system activity during exercise constricts blood vessels to the kidneys. Reduced renal blood flow stimulates the kidneys to release the enzyme **renin** into the blood. Increased renin concentration activates production of two kidney hormones, **angiotensin II** and **angiotensin III**. These hormones stimulate both arterial constriction and adrenocortical secretion of aldosterone, which causes the kidneys to retain sodium and excrete potassium.[47] Renal absorption of sodium also conserves water, causing plasma volume to expand and blood pressure to increase. Aldosterone secretion rises progressively during exercise, with peak plasma levels reaching as high as six times resting values.

A chronic reduction in renal blood flow at rest, perhaps from abnormal sympathetic stimulation, activates the **renin–angiotensin system**. Prolonged over-response of this mechanism with a resulting excess aldosterone output can trigger hypertension. High blood pressure associated with increased aldosterone production is prevalent in teenage obesity.[187] Teenage hypertension relates to (1) decreased salt sensitivity (hence increased water retention), (2) increased sodium intake, and (3) decreased sensitivity to the effects of insulin (hyperinsulinemia). These interrelationships suggest a direct link between obesity as a disease and development of hypertension. Similar relationships have been reported for adults.[45,46,84]

GLUCOCORTICOIDS. Emotionally charged situations or the stressful demands of physical activity stimulate the hypothalamus to secrete **corticotropin-releasing factor** that causes the anterior pituitary to release ACTH. In turn, ACTH promotes glucocorticoid release by the adrenal cortex. **Cortisol** (hydrocortisone), the major glucocorticoid of the adrenal cortex, significantly affects glucose, protein, and free fatty acid metabolism as follows (Fig. 20.14):

- Promotes the breakdown of protein to amino acids in all cells of the body except the liver; the circulation delivers these "liberated" amino acids to the liver for synthesis to glucose via gluconeogenesis

- Supports the action of other hormones, primarily glucagon and GH, in the gluconeogenic process
- Serves as an insulin antagonist by inhibiting cellular glucose uptake and oxidation
- Promotes triglyceride breakdown in adipose tissue to glycerol and fatty acids

Long-standing, high serum concentrations of cortisol initiate excessive protein breakdown, tissue wasting, and negative nitrogen balance. Cortisol secretion also accelerates fat mobilization for energy during starvation and intense, prolonged exercise. With rapid and large increases in cortisol output, the liver splits mobilized fat into its simple ketoacid components. Excess ketoacid concentrations in the extracellular fluid can lead to the potentially dangerous condition of **ketosis** (a form of acidosis). Individuals who subsist on very low carbohydrate, low-calorie weight-loss diets (termed *ketogenic diets*; see Chapter 30) often experience ketosis, augmented by elevated cortisol secretion.

Cortisol turnover, the difference between its production and removal, provides a convenient means to study cortisol response to exercise. Considerable variability exists in cortisol turnover with exercise, depending on such factors as exercise intensity and duration, fitness level, nutritional status, and even circadian rhythm.[41,213] Most research indicates that cortisol output increases with exercise intensity; this accelerates lipolysis, ketogenesis, and proteolysis. In addition, extremely high cortisol levels occur following long-duration exercise such as marathon running.[34,179] Even during more-moderate exercise, plasma cortisol concentration rises with prolonged exercise. Data for cortisol turnover indicate that highly trained runners maintain a state of hypercortisolism that heightens before competition or heavy training.[86,143] Cortisol levels also remain elevated for as long as 2 hours following exercise, suggesting that cortisol plays a role in tissue recovery and repair. Unlike the direct, active metabolic effect of epinephrine and glucagon on fuel homeostasis during exercise, cortisol exerts a more facilitating effect on substrate use.

GONADOCORTICOIDS. The reproductive organs (gonads) provide the major source of the so-called sex steroids, but the adrenal cortex produces androgen hormones (gonadocorticoids) with similar actions. For example, the adrenal cortex produces **dehydroepiandrosterone**, which exerts effects similar to those of the dominant male hormone testosterone. Also, the adrenal cortex produces small amounts of the "female" hormones estrogen and progesterone.

GONADAL HORMONES

The testes in the male and the ovaries in the female are the reproductive glands. These endocrine glands produce the hormones that promote sex-specific physical characteristics and initiate and maintain reproductive function. No distinctly "male" or "female" hormones exist, but rather, general differences in hormone concentrations between the sexes. **Testosterone** is the most important androgen secretion from the interstitial cells of the testes. Figure 20.15 shows that testosterone is important in initiating sperm production and stimulating the development of male secondary sex characteristics. In addition, testosterone's anabolic, tissue-building role contributes to the male–female differences in muscle mass and strength that emerge at the onset of puberty. As

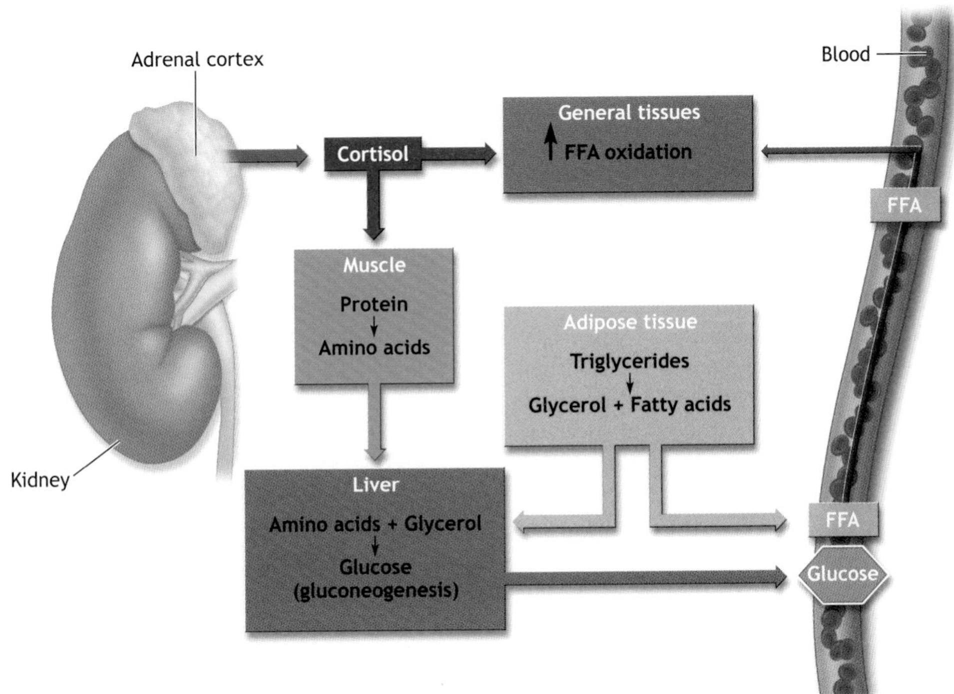

FIGURE 20.14 • Cortisol's role in energy metabolism.

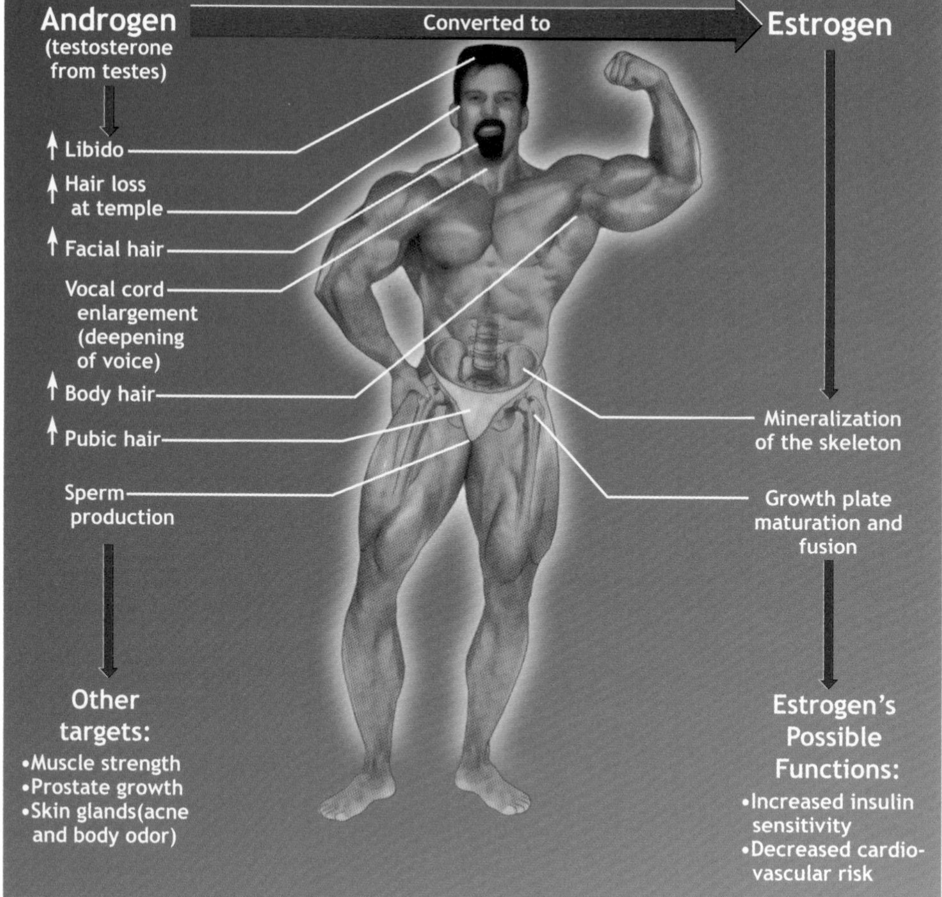

Figure 20.15 • Androgen's effects in men. Binding with special receptor sites in muscle and various other tissues, androgen (testosterone) contributes greatly to the male secondary sex characteristics and to the sex differences in muscle mass and strength that begin to develop at the onset of puberty. Some androgen converts to estrogen in peripheral tissues and gives males a significant edge over females in maintaining bone mass throughout life.

noted in Chapter 2, testosterone conversion to estrogen in peripheral tissues, under control of the enzyme aromatase, provides the male with significant protection in maintaining bone structure throughout life.

The ovaries provide the primary source of estrogens, particularly **estradiol** and **progesterone**. Estrogens regulate ovulation, menstruation, and the physiologic adjustments during pregnancy. Estrogen, both circulating in the bloodstream and generated locally in peripheral tissues, also exerts effects on blood vessels, bone, lungs, liver, intestine, prostate, and testes through action on α- and β-receptor proteins. Progesterone contributes specific regulatory input to the female reproductive cycle, uterine smooth muscle action, and lactation. Controversy exists concerning the role of estrogen and progesterone in substrate metabolism, particularly during exercise.[5,160] Estradiol-17β (biologically active estrogen synthesized from cholesterol) increases free fatty acid mobilization from adipose tissue and inhibits glucose uptake by peripheral tissues. In this way, the increases in estradiol-17β and GH during exercise exert similar metabolic effects.[193]

Testosterone

Plasma testosterone concentration commonly serves as a physiologic marker of anabolic status. In addition to its direct effects on muscle tissue synthesis, testosterone may indirectly affect a muscle fiber's protein content by promoting GH release, which leads to IGF synthesis and release from the liver.[77] Testosterone also interacts with neural receptors to increase neurotransmitter release and initiate structural protein changes that alter the size of the neuromuscular junction. These neural effects enhance the force-production capabilities of skeletal muscle.

Testosterone's effect on the cell nucleus remains controversial. More than likely, a transport protein (sex-hormone–binding globulin) delivers testosterone to target tissues, after which testosterone associates with a membrane-bound or cytosolic receptor. It subsequently migrates to the cell nucleus where it interacts with nuclear receptors that initiate protein synthesis.[60,61]

Plasma testosterone concentration in females, although only one-tenth that of males, increases with exercise. Exercise also elevates estradiol and progesterone levels.[114] In untrained males, both resistance exercise and moderate aerobic exercise significantly increase serum and free testosterone levels after approximately 15 to 20 minutes. The mechanism for this increase remains unclear.[38] Findings remain equivocal concerning the effect of strenuous endurance exercise on testosterone levels.[179,220]

Figure 20.16 shows the pattern of plasma cortisol and testosterone 48 hours before swimming, immediately following 15 × 200-m freestyle at the swimmer's competitive velocity with a 20-second rest between swims, and 1 hour into

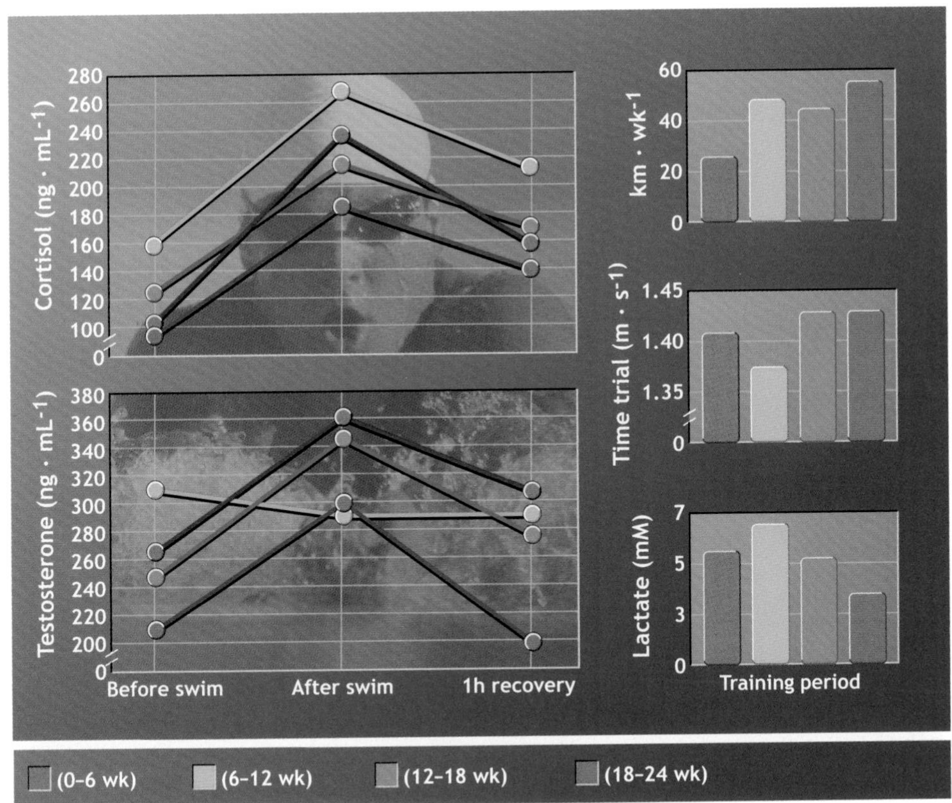

FIGURE 20.16 • Pattern of plasma cortisol and testosterone concentrations measured at three time intervals (4 h before swimming, immediately after multiple sprint swims, and after 1-h recovery) over a 24-week swim-training season. *Bar graphs on right show* values for swim volume, time-trial performance, and blood lactate during the four 6-week training periods. (Modified from Bonifazi M, et al. Blood levels of exercise during the training season. In: Miyashita M. et al, eds. Medicine and science in aquatic sports. Basel: Karger, 1994.)

recovery. Four 6-week periods formed the training program, with careful monitoring of training volume. The bar graphs (right) show values for swim volume during the four training periods, along with average performance during time trials. The results show clearly that cortisol and testosterone are significantly higher after exercise. Values remained elevated 1 hour after exercise except for testosterone levels in training weeks 6–12 and 18–24. The generalized decrease in cortisol and testosterone concentrations when the swimmers "peaked" for the championships (weeks 18–24) indicates a long-term adaptation for these hormones, not the immediate result of excess stress induced by overtraining and subsequent poor performance. The depressed performance during weeks 18–24 might indicate overtraining; this period corresponded to a large increase in training volume. Chapter 21 provides an in-depth discussion of overtraining and its related syndrome.

INTEGRATIVE QUESTION

Hormones play crucial roles in normal growth and development and the regulation of physiologic function. Give specific examples why "more is not necessarily better" for these chemicals.

Pancreatic Hormones

The pancreas gland, approximately 14-cm long and weighing about 60 g, lies just below the stomach. Two different types of tissues, **acini** and **islets of Langerhans** (Fig. 20.17) compose the pancreas. The islets contain **α-cells** that secrete glucagon and **β-cells** that secrete insulin. The acini serve an exocrine function and secrete digestive enzymes.

Insulin

Insulin regulates glucose entry into all tissues (primarily muscle and adipose cells) except the brain. Insulin's action mediates **facilitated diffusion**, in which glucose combines with a carrier protein on the cell's plasma membrane for transport into cells. In this way, insulin actually regulates glucose metabolism. Any glucose not immediately catabolized for energy becomes stored as glycogen for later use. Without insulin, only trace amounts of glucose enter the cells. Figure 20.18 outlines insulin's role in overall metabolism.

Insulin-mediated glucose uptake by the cells (and correspondingly reduced hepatic glucose output) following a meal decreases blood glucose levels. In essence, insulin exerts a hypoglycemic effect by reducing blood glucose concentration. Conversely, with insufficient insulin secretion, blood glucose concentration increases, sometimes from a normal level of about 90 mg · dL^{-1} to a high of 350 mg · dL^{-1}. When blood glucose levels remain high, glucose ultimately spills into the urine. In the absence of insulin, fatty acids mobilize for use as the primary energy substrate.

Insulin also exerts a pronounced effect on fat synthesis. A rise in blood glucose levels (as normally occurs after a meal) stimulates insulin release, which causes some glucose uptake by fat cells for synthesis to triglyceride. Insulin's ac-

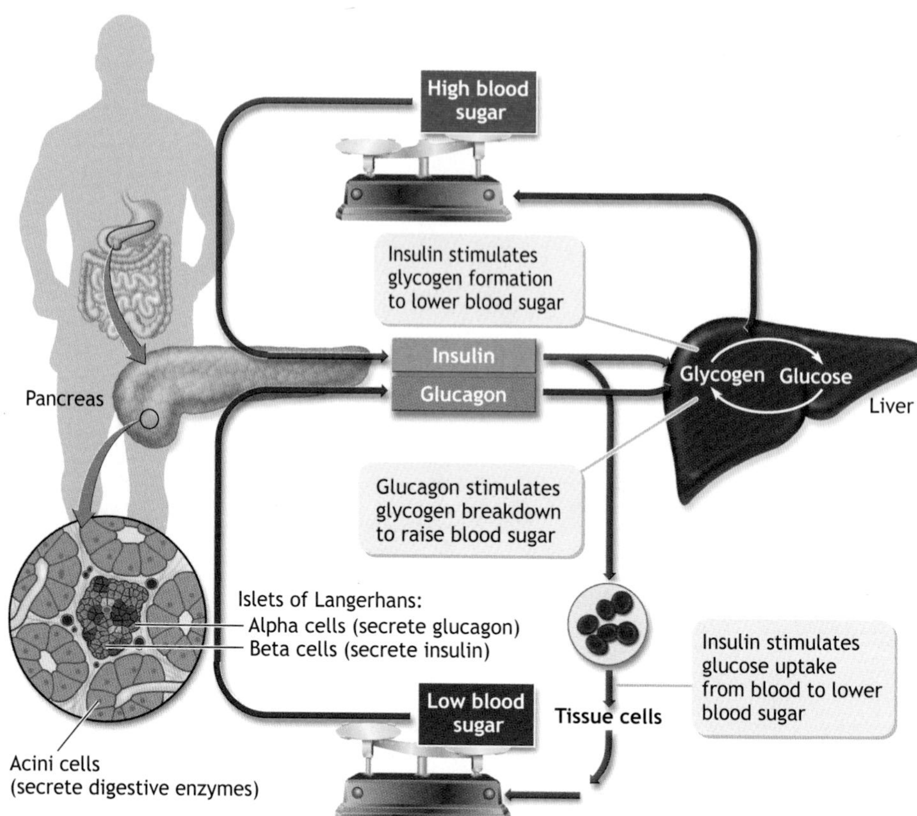

FIGURE 20.17 • The pancreas, its secretions, and their actions.

tion also triggers intracellular enzyme activity that facilitates protein synthesis. This occurs by one or all of the following actions: (1) increasing amino acid transport through the plasma membrane, (2) increasing cellular levels of RNA, and (3) increasing protein formation by ribosomes.

INSULIN TRANSPORT INTO CELLS: GLUCOSE TRANSPORTERS. Cells possess different glucose transport proteins (termed **glucose transporters**, or **GLUTs**), which vary in response to insulin and glucose concentrations (non–insulin transporter, GLUT-1 transporter, and insulin-mediated GLUT-4 transporter, that largely depends upon intracellular calcium concentrations).[148] Muscle fibers contain GLUT-1 and GLUT-4, with most glucose entering by the GLUT-1 carrier during rest. With high blood glucose or insulin concentrations, as occur after eating or during exercise, muscle cells receive glucose via the insulin-dependent GLUT-4 transporter. GLUT-4 action is mediated through a second messenger, perhaps stimulated by muscle action, which permits migration of the intracellular GLUT-4 protein to the surface to promote glucose uptake. The fact that GLUT-4 moves to the cell surface through a separate, *insulin-independent* mechanism is consistent with observations that active muscles can take up glucose without insulin.[186]

GLUCOSE–INSULIN INTERACTION. *Blood glucose levels within the pancreas directly control insulin secretion.* Elevated blood glucose levels cause insulin release. This, in turn, induces glucose entry into the cells, lowers blood glucose, and removes the stimulus for insulin release. A decrease in blood glucose concentration, on the other hand, dramatically lowers blood insulin levels, thus providing a favorable milieu for increasing blood glucose. The interaction between glucose and insulin provides a feedback mechanism that normally maintains blood glucose concentration within narrow limits. Insulin secretion also increases in response to rising levels of plasma amino acids.

Figure 20.19 relates plasma insulin concentration to exercise duration for cycling exercise at 70% $\dot{V}O_{2max}$. The inset graph shows insulin response as a function of exercise intensity (%$\dot{V}O_{2max}$). The decreased insulin concentration (below rest values) as exercise duration extends or intensity increases results from inhibitory effects on the pancreatic β-cell activity from an exercise-induced catecholamine release.[67] *Catecholamine suppression of insulin relates directly to exercise intensity. Exercise blunting of insulin output helps explain why no excessive insulin release (and possible rebound hypoglycemia) occurs with a concentrated glucose feeding during exercise.* Prolonged exercise derives progressively more energy from free fatty acids mobilized from the adipocytes because of reduced insulin output and decreased carbohydrate reserves. Blood glucose lowering with prolonged exercise directly enhances hepatic glucose output and sensitizes the liver to the glucose-releasing effects of glucagon and epinephrine, whose actions contribute to maintaining blood glucose levels.

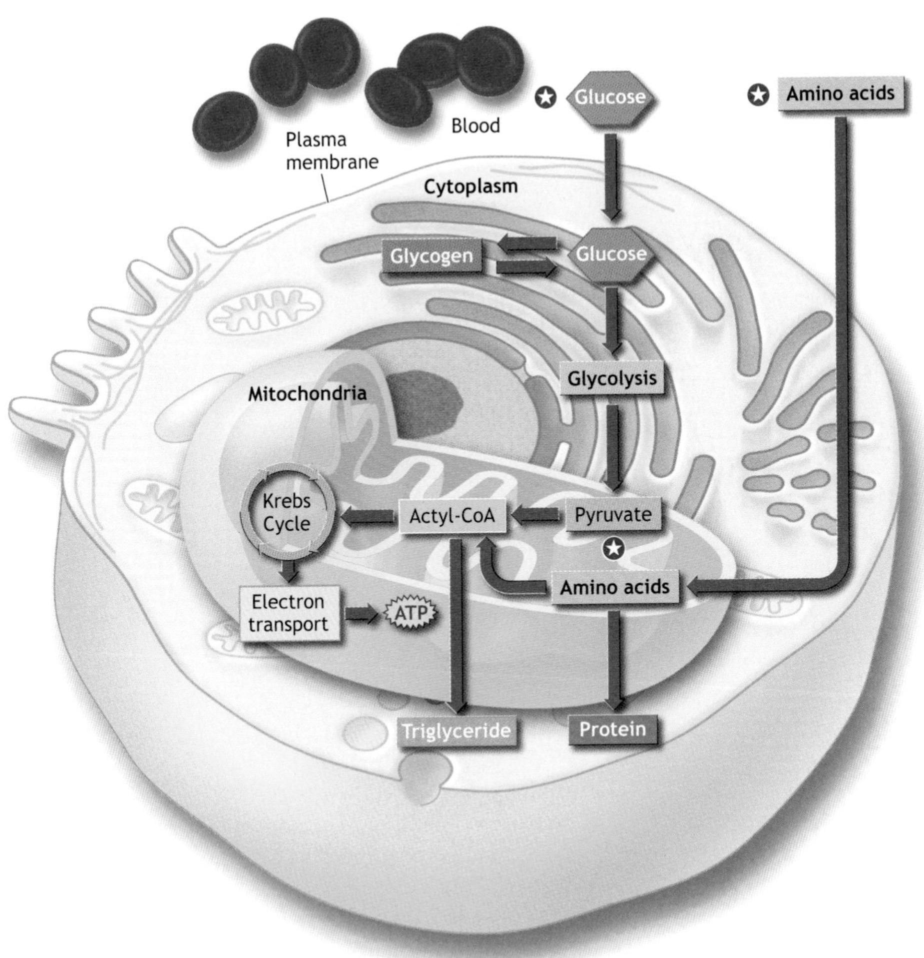

FIGURE 20.18 • Primary functions of insulin in the body. The ✪ show where insulin exerts its influence in metabolism.

DIABETES MELLITUS. Diabetes mellitus consists of subgroups of disorders (with different pathophysiologies) that currently afflict 16 million Americans, with the number expected to rise to 23 million Americans by 2025 (Fig. 20.20). Diabetes is the sixth leading cause of death by disease in the United States (195,000 diabetes-related deaths annually) and the leading cause of blindness, kidney failure, and limb amputations. Researchers believe that diabetes represents an inde-

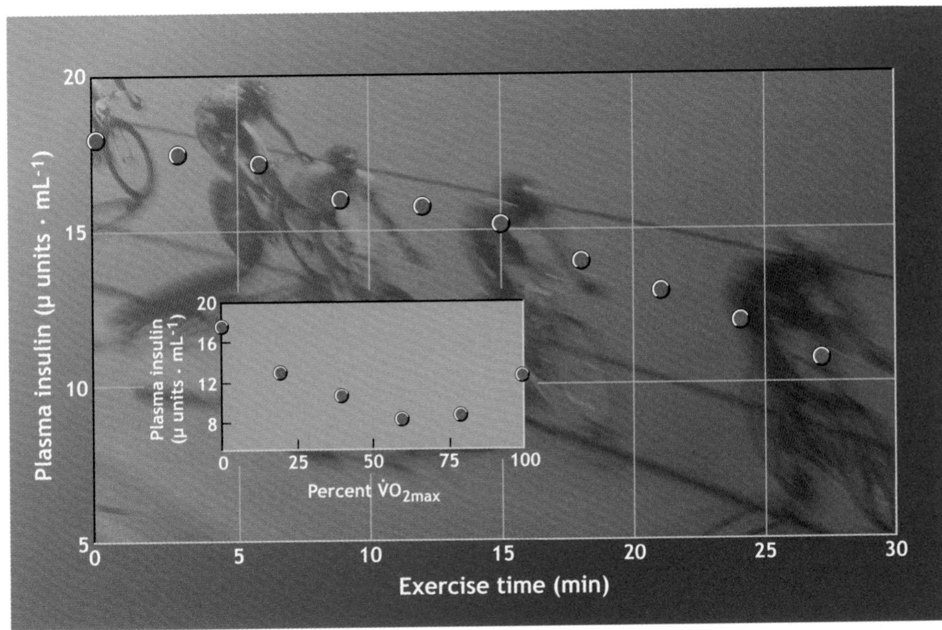

FIGURE 20.19 • Plasma insulin levels during cycle ergometer exercise at 70% $\dot{V}O_{2max}$. *Inset,* data show insulin concentrations related to exercise intensity (%$\dot{V}O_{2max}$). (From Applied Physiology Laboratory, University of Michigan, Ann Arbor.)

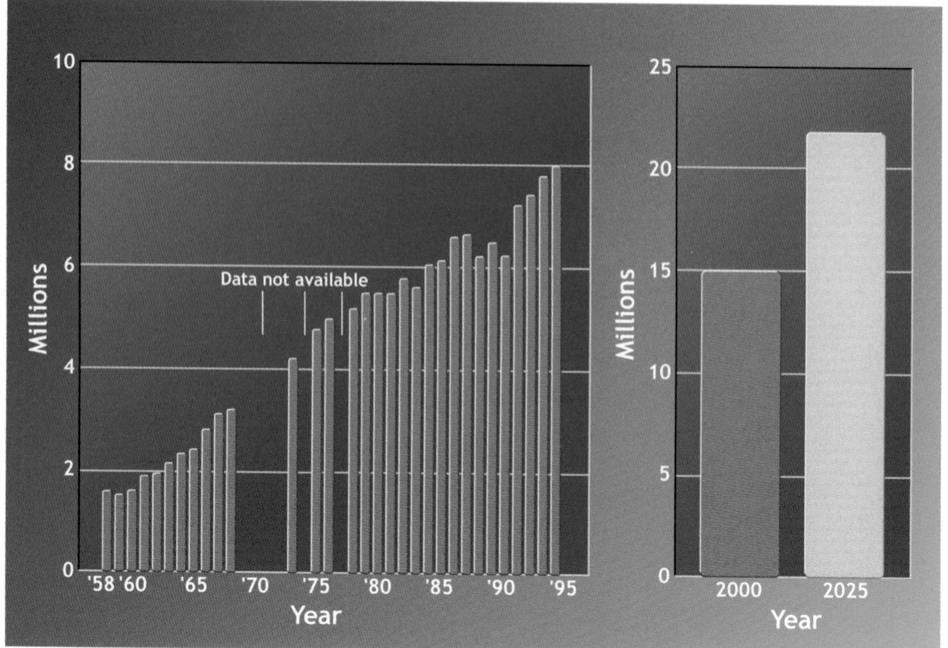

FIGURE 20.20 • Rates of diagnosed cases of type 1 and type 2 diabetes between 1958 and 1995, and projected increases in new cases to the year 2025. Type 2 diabetes represents nearly 95% of all cases. (Source: National Institutes of Health)

pendent risk factor for cardiovascular disease.[80] The terms **type 1** and **type 2** identify the two largest diabetes subgroups. Use of the terms *insulin-dependent diabetes mellitus* (type 1) and *non–insulin-dependent diabetes mellitus* (type 2), in addition to Roman numerals I and II for subgroup identification, respectively, has been discontinued because they indicate treatments that overlap and vary, rather than reflecting an underlying etiology. For example, many people with type 2 diabetes require exogenous insulin.

Tests for Diabetes Mellitus. Different tests diagnose diabetes, including the laboratory-based glucose and insulin clamp methodology, an oral glucose-tolerance test, and a simple 8-hour fasting plasma glucose test.

- The clamp procedure involves maintaining insulin at a constantly above-normal blood concentration using infusion technology (termed **hyperinsulinemic clamp**). Once insulin stabilizes at the higher level, the body's use of glucose can be measured by infusing a known amount of glucose into the patient's blood. A **euglycemic clamp** maintains blood glucose at near-normal concentration with insulin production measured. A **euglycemic-hyperinsulinemic clamp** combines both clamp procedures.[42] A large glucose uptake for a given insulin concentration reflects increased **insulin sensitivity**, while increased insulin release to a constant glucose condition relates to augmented **insulin responsiveness**. Decreased insulin sensitivity indicates inability of cells to respond adequately to insulin to increase glucose uptake. Type 2 diabetes commonly reflects inadequacies in either insulin receptors or cellular response to insulin binding. Decreased insulin responsiveness indicates impaired β-cell function evident in some type 2 diabetics and is the primary cause of type 1 diabetes.
- The **oral glucose-tolerance test** evaluates blood sugar levels 2 hours after drinking a concentrated glucose-containing solution. Delayed removal of ingested glucose indicates diabetes.
- The **fasting plasma glucose (FPG) test** simply measures plasma glucose following an 8-hour fast. The American Diabetes Association currently recommends the FPG test.

CLASSIFICATION CATEGORIES FOR FASTING BLOOD GLUCOSE

Category	*Fasting Plasma Glucose*
Normal	<110 mg · dL^{-1}
Impaired range	110–125 mg · dL^{-1}
Suspected diabetes	>125 mg · dL^{-1}

Significant risks exist for impaired glucose homeostasis—probably a genetic trait that can manifest itself in adolescence—in which blood glucose remains elevated but not high enough for diabetic classification. Nondiabetic middle-aged men whose FPG falls in the upper range of normal show a higher risk of death from heart disease than those in the low-normal range.[10] Men with fasting blood glucose levels above 85 mg · dL^{-1} have a 40% higher risk of cardiovascular death than men with lower values, even after adjusting for age, smoking habits, blood pressure, and fitness status. The current plasma glucose cutoff for suspected diabetes—FPG of 126 mg · dL^{-1}, down from the previous standard of 140 mg · dL^{-1}

set in 1979—acknowledges that patients can remain asymptomatic despite microvascular complications (damaged small blood vessels) with FPG values in the low- to mid-120 mg · dL^{-1} range. The *impaired range* represents a transition between normal and overt diabetes. In this situation, the body no longer responds properly to insulin and/or secretes inadequate amounts of insulin.

Metabolic Syndrome X

Metabolic syndrome X (or simply metabolic syndrome), first mentioned in the late 1980s,[62,120,181–183] represents a multifaceted grouping of coronary artery disease risks.[11] This "disease of modern civilization" afflicts a large number of adults (more common in men than women) in western industrialized countries. Disease occurrence relates to genetic, hormonal, and lifestyle factors such as obesity, physical inactivity, and nutrient excesses, including high intakes of saturated and *trans* fatty acids. The syndrome is characterized by the clustering of insulin resistance and hyperinsulinemia; it also coincides with dyslipidemia (atherogenic plasma lipid profile), essential hypertension, abdominal (visceral) obesity, and glucose intolerance. Abnormalities of blood coagulation (higher plasminogen activator inhibitor type 1 and fibrinogen levels), hyperuricemia, and microalbuminuria also emerge in the metabolic syndrome. Because these individuals are at higher risk for coronary artery disease, they should receive special attention in terms of diagnosis and treatment.

Psychosocial stress, socioeconomic disadvantage, and abnormal psychiatric traits have also been linked to the syndrome's pathogenesis.[11,12] Such factors, in all likelihood, relate to a central neuroendocrine origin in the form of enhanced activation of the hypothalamic–pituitary–adrenal axis, with endpoints of hyperinsulinemia, obesity, coronary artery disease, type 2 diabetes, stroke, and increased colorectal cancer risk.[196]

METABOLIC SYNDROME X

- Insulin resistance
- Glucose intolerance
- Dyslipidemia (high triglycerides, low HDL, high LDL)
- Stroke
- Upper-body obesity
- Type 2 diabetes mellitus
- Hypertension
- Coronary artery disease
- Reduced ability to dissolve blood clots

Insulin Actions and Impaired Glucose Homeostasis

Figure 20.21 summarizes insulin's normal response and the response under insulin-resistant and type 2 diabetes conditions. The increase in blood glucose concentration following a meal induces insulin release from the β-cells in the islets of Langerhans. Insulin then migrates in the blood to target cells throughout the body, where it binds to receptor molecules on the cell surface. Insulin–receptor interaction triggers a series of events within the cell that enhance glucose uptake and its subsequent catabolism or storage as glycogen and/or fat. A defect anywhere along the pathway for glucose uptake signals diabetes. Possible causes include (1) destruction of β-cells, (2) abnormal synthesis of insulin, (3) depressed insulin release, (4) inactivation of insulin in the blood by antibodies or other blocking agents, (5) altered insulin receptors or a decreased number of receptors on peripheral cells, (6) defective processing of the insulin message within the target cells, and (7) abnormal glucose metabolism.

Type 1 Diabetes. Type 1 diabetes, formerly called juvenile-onset diabetes, typically occurs in younger individuals and represents between 5 and 10% of all diabetes cases. This diabetes form results from an autoimmune response, possibly the result of a single protein that stimulates the body's immune system to render the β-cells incapable of producing insulin and often other pancreatic hormones.[244] Type 1 diabetic patients present a more severe abnormality for glucose homeostasis than those in the type 2 subgroup. Exercise exerts more-pronounced effects on the metabolic state in these individuals, and the management of exercise-related problems requires greater attention (see In a Practical Sense, p. 442).

Type 2 Diabetes. Type 2 diabetes tends to occur after age 40 except in overweight children. A sharp increase has occurred in the number of children with type 2 diabetes, some younger than age 10. This alarming new health trend signals that type 2 diabetes probably represents a "pediatric disease."[75] So ingrained is the belief that type 2 diabetes occurs primarily in overweight, middle-aged men and women that it is frequently called adult-onset diabetes. Recent estimates indicate that the disease has more than tripled in children over the last 3 to 5 years. Many physicians consider the spiraling rate of childhood obesity—particularly among African American, Native American, and Hispanics (most notably children of Mexican descent)—to be the predominant factor in the rising number of children with type 2 diabetes. Type 2 diabetes accounts for nearly 95% of all diabetes cases in the United States, and represents the leading cause of death because of the disease.[138] Treatment costs exceed $1 billion yearly.

Type 2 diabetes relates to three factors: (1) the body's inability to respond properly to insulin, and links closely with a significant resistance to insulin's actions (particularly in skeletal muscle), (2) an abnormal but relatively well-maintained insulin secretion, and (3) normal-to-high plasma insulin levels.[105] A dysregulation in glycolytic and oxidative capacities of skeletal muscle also relates to insulin resistance in type 2 diabetes.[205] The disease probably results from the interaction of genes and lifestyle factors—physical inactivity, weight gain, and possibly a high-fat diet heighten the risk, which increases with age. This most likely accounts for the 70% increase in the disorder among people in their 30s during the last decade of the 20th century and a 33% overall increase nationally, to 6.5% of the population. Also, the form of insulin

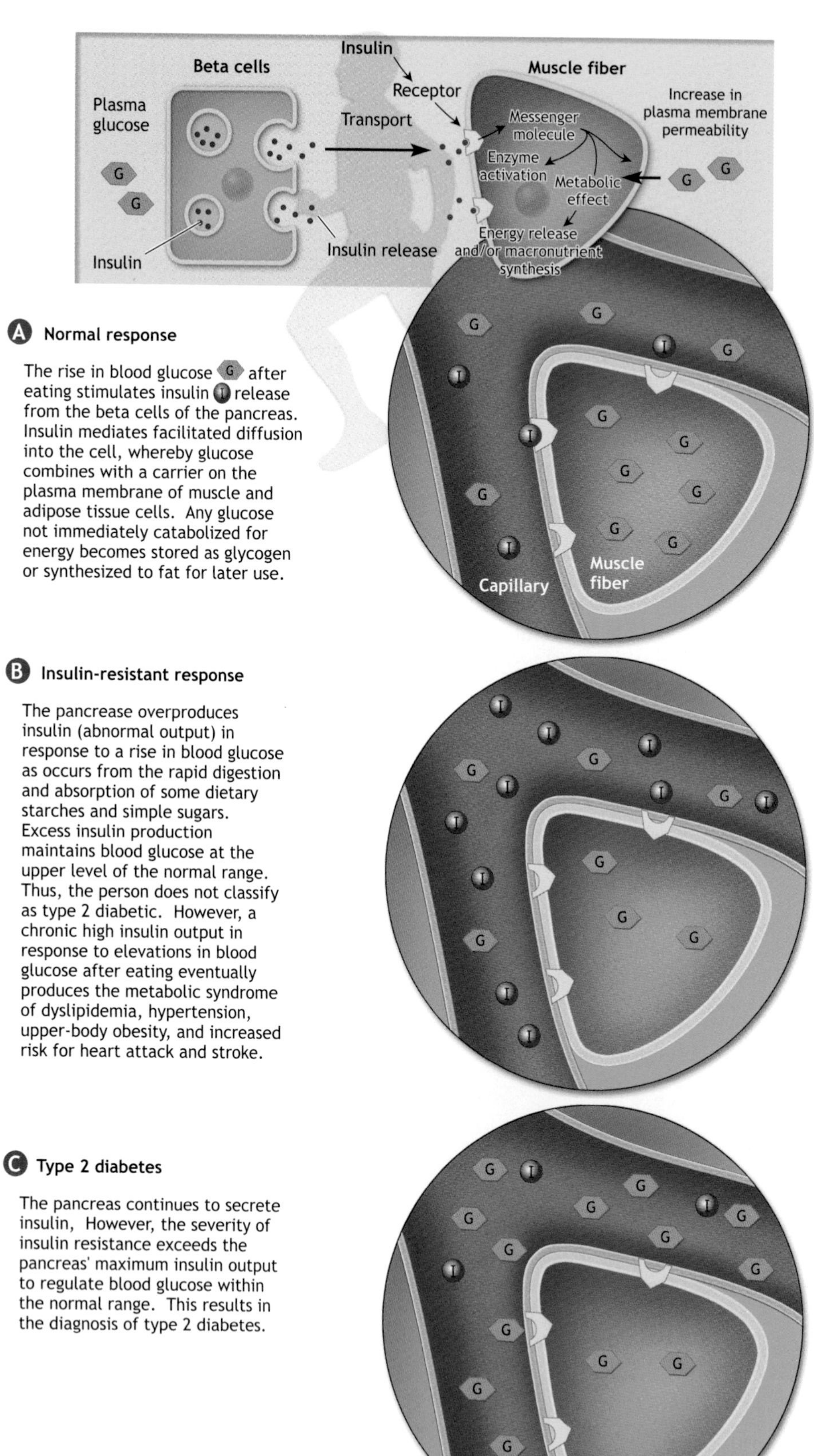

FIGURE 20.21 • Normal insulin–glucose interaction (**A**) and with insulin resistance (**B**) and in type 2 diabetes (**C**).

resistance in type 2 diabetes has a strong genetic component. The gene directs synthesis of a protein that inhibits insulin's action in cellular glucose transport.

Obesity, particularly upper-body fat distribution, and lack of regular physical activity are major risks for type 2 diabetes in adults and children. An estimated 60 to 80 million Americans show insulin resistance but have not developed overt symptoms of type 2 diabetes. One-third of these individuals will eventually become full-blown diabetics, and many of the others are at increased risk of cardiovascular disease. The term **insulin-resistant** means that the pancreas overproduces insulin (abnormal output) when blood glucose rises, as occurs from the rapid digestion and absorption of dietary high-glycemic carbohydrates (Fig. 20.21). Increased blood glucose levels in many of these individuals are not high enough for a type-2 diabetes classification. Failure of insulin to exert its normal effect increases glucose conversion to and storage as body fat. For the insulin-resistant individual, a diet high in simple sugars and refined carbohydrates (with a relatively high glycemic index) facilitates body fat accumulation. Fat cell enlargement further exacerbates the situation, since these cells exhibit insulin resistance because of their reduced insulin receptor density.

AT RISK FOR TYPE 2 DIABETES

- Body mass exceeds 20% of ideal
- First-degree relative with diabetes (genetic influence)
- Member of a high-risk ethnic group (black, Hispanic American, Pacific Islander, American Indian, Asian)
- Delivered a baby weighing more than 9 pounds or developed gestational diabetes
- Blood pressure at or above 140/90 mm Hg
- HDL-cholesterol level of 35 mg · dL^{-1} or below and/or a triglyceride level of 250 mg · dL^{-1} or above
- Impaired fasting plasma glucose or impaired glucose tolerance on previous testing

As with type 1 diabetes, adequate glucose fails to enter the cells of a person with type 2 diabetes. This causes abnormally high levels of blood glucose that ultimately are filtered by the kidney tubules and voided in the urine (**glycosuria**). Excessive glucose particles in renal filtrate create an osmotic effect that diminishes water reabsorption so the diabetic person loses large amounts of fluid (**polyuria**). With decreased cellular glucose uptake, a diabetic person relies largely on fat catabolism for energy. This produces an excess of ketoacids and a tendency toward acidosis. In extreme situations, plasma pH falls as low as 7.0, eventually resulting in diabetic coma. Medical conditions such as arteriosclerosis, small blood vessel and nerve disease, and susceptibility to infection occur at increased rates in type 2 diabetes.[119] Obese diabetic women also face an almost three times greater risk of endometrial cancer than diabetic women of normal weight, perhaps from their persistently high insulin levels (insulin insensitivity).[197]

CHARACTERISTICS OF TYPE 1 AND TYPE 2 DIABETES

Characteristics	Type 1 Diabetes	Type 2 Diabetes
Age at onset	Usually <20 y	Usually >40 y (but increasing in children)
Proportion of all diabetics	<10%	>90%
Appearance of symptoms	Acute or subacute	Slow
Metabolic ketoacidosis	Frequent	Rare
Obesity at onset	Uncommon	Common
β-cells	Decreased	Variable
Insulin	Decreased	Variable
Inflammatory cells in islets	Present initially	Absent
Family history	Uncommon	Common

Whereas heart disease mortality has fallen by 36% in nondiabetic males and 27% in nondiabetic females since 1970, it has decreased only 13% in diabetic males and has increased by 23% in women with diabetes.[81] The discrepancy in heart disease reduction between diabetic and nondiabetic persons may result from more-limited reductions in risk factors over time among those with diabetes or a blunted response to risk factor reduction.

DIABETES AND EXERCISE. Hypoglycemia represents the most common disturbance in glucose homeostasis during exercise in diabetics who take exogenous insulin. Hypoglycemia is particularly severe in patients who undergo intensive insulin therapy to normalize plasma glucose levels throughout the day. Under normal conditions, hypoglycemia can occur during prolonged, intense exercise when hepatic glucose release does not match increased glucose use by active muscle. Persons with type 2 diabetes often demonstrate reduced exercise tolerance independent of glycemic control. Contributing factors include genetics, undesirable lifestyle characteristics, excessive body fat, and poor physical fitness.

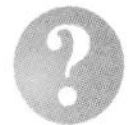

INTEGRATIVE QUESTION

What would account for the sweet-smelling breath of individuals suffering from (1) poorly regulated diabetes mellitus and (2) malnutrition due to starvation?

Glucagon

The α-cells of the islets of Langerhans secrete **glucagon**, the "insulin antagonist" hormone. In contrast to insulin's effect in lowering blood sugar levels, glucagon's primarily stimulates both glycogenolysis and gluconeogenesis by the liver.

The glucose generated in this process then moves into the blood. Glucagon exerts its effect by activating the enzyme adenylate cyclase. This stimulates cyclic AMP in the liver cells and causes hepatic glycogen breakdown to glucose (glycogenolysis). Glucagon also exerts a stimulating effect on gluconeogenesis by promoting amino acid uptake by the liver.

As with insulin, plasma glucose concentration controls glucagon output by the pancreas. A decrease in blood glucose concentration, as occurs in prolonged high-intensity exercise or food (or carbohydrate) restriction, stimulates the α-cells of the pancreas to release glucagon. However, glucagon release in exercise does not always link to decreased plasma glucose.[215] Glucagon elicits an almost instantaneous release of glucose from the liver.[58]

Unlike its effects on insulin secretion, autonomic nervous stimulation does not mediate glucagon release because neither α- nor β-autonomic receptor blockade affects glucagon secretion in prolonged exercise.[66] Also, no gender differences exist in the glucagon response to exercise when individuals exercise at the same percentage of aerobic capacity.[41,216] Because glucagon release occurs later in exercise, this hormone probably exerts little influence in the early regulation of hepatic glycogenolysis.[9] More than likely, it primarily contributes to blood glucose regulation as exercise progresses and glycogen reserves deplete.

TABLE 20.3 ➤ HORMONES AND THEIR RESPONSES TO ENDURANCE TRAINING

HORMONE	TRAINING RESPONSE
Hypothalamus-pituitary hormones	
Growth hormone	No effect on resting values; less dramatic rise during exercise
Thyrotropin	No known training effect
ACTH	Increased exercise values
Prolactin	Some evidence that training lowers resting values
FSH, LH, and Testosterone	Trained females have depressed values; reduced testosterone in males (testosterone levels may increase in males with long-term resistance training)
Posterior pituitary hormones	
Vasopressin (ADH)	Slightly reduced ADH at a given workload
Oxytocin	No research results available
Thyroid hormones	
Thyroxine (T_4)	Reduced concentration of total T_3 and increased free thyroxine at rest
Triiodothyronine (T_3)	Increased turnover of T_3 and T_4 during exercise
Adrenal hormones	
Aldosterone	No significant training adaptation
Cortisol	Slight elevations during exercise
Epinephrine and Norepinephrine	Decreased secretion at rest and at same absolute exercise intensity after training
Pancreatic hormones	
Insulin	Increased sensitivity to insulin; normal decrease in insulin during exercise greatly reduced with training
Glucagon	Smaller increase in glucose levels during exercise at absolute and relative workloads
Kidney enzyme and hormone	
Renin and Angiotensin	No apparent training effect

Other Glands and Hormones

Other hormones also influence bodily functions. The liver, for example, secretes somatomedins, which affect the growth of muscle, cartilage, and other tissues. The mucosal lining of the small intestine secretes **secretin**, **gastrin**, and **cholecystokinin**, which promote and coordinate digestive processes. As discussed previously, the hypothalamus itself constitutes an important endocrine gland that secretes several stimulating or releasing hormones that activate or release diverse anterior pituitary hormones. The hypothalamus also releases **somatoliberin**, which stimulates somatotropin secretion from the anterior pituitary gland.

EXERCISE TRAINING AND ENDOCRINE FUNCTION

Table 20.3 lists the different hormones and their general response to exercise training. Because of the complex interactions between endocrine secretions and the nervous system, only limited research has evaluated multiple hormone secretions and changes consequent to exercise training. *The magnitude of hormonal response to a standard exercise load generally declines with endurance training.* For example, when highly trained athletes perform at the same absolute exercise level as sedentary subjects, hormonal responses remain lower in the athletes. Much of this "efficiency" in response probably results from improved target tissue sensitivity and/or responsiveness to a given amount of hormone.[35,99,188] A similar level of hormonal response results regardless of state of training when subjects exercise at the same relative exercise intensity (i.e., the same percentage of maximum [lower absolute load for the untrained]).[185] With maximal exercise, trained subjects show an identical or somewhat greater hormonal response than untrained subjects.

Anterior Pituitary Hormones

Growth Hormone

Because GH stimulates lipolysis and inhibits carbohydrate breakdown, one could hypothesize that training enhances GH secretion and conserves glycogen reserves. However, this does not occur. Compared with untrained counterparts, endurance-trained individuals show *less* rise in blood GH levels at a given exercise intensity—a response attributed to a reduction in the stress of exercise as training progresses and fitness improves.[14,15] Regardless of training status, women typically maintain higher GH levels at rest than men; this difference disappears during prolonged exercise.[25] Figure 20.22A illustrates the significant training-induced blunting of the GH response of a representative subject from a group of six men during 20 minutes of constant-load, high-intensity exercise before and after 3 and 6 weeks of endurance training.[231] Integrated GH concentrations (exercise plus recovery) for the group averaged 45% lower than pretraining values at both training measures. Responses for the plasma catecholamines (Fig. 20.22B and C) and blood lactate (Fig. 20.22D) paralleled the decrease in GH. Because the constant-load exercise test represented significantly less physiologic demand after training (reflected by lower catecholamine and lactate levels), a similar release of GH after training probably requires higher absolute exercise intensity. Also, the effect of exercise training on GH release may also become apparent under nonexercise conditions. For example, aerobic training above the lactate threshold level amplified the 24-hour pulsatile GH release during rest (see Focus on Research).[230]

ACTH

ACTH provides potent stimulation to the adrenal cortex and thus increases free fatty acid mobilization for energy. Training increases release of ACTH during exercise—a response that stimulates adrenal gland activity to promote fat catabolism and spare glycogen. This would certainly benefit prolonged, high-intensity exercise performance.[17,94]

PRL

Little information exists concerning exercise training changes in PRL. It does appear that resting PRL levels of male runners averaged below values for sedentary nonrunners.[83,233]

FSH, LH, and Testosterone

Regular exercise depresses reproductive hormone responses in women and men.[37,49,234] Male endurance athletes generally maintain resting testosterone levels between 60 and 85% of values for sedentary men. The implications of these findings remain unclear.

WOMEN. Women with a long history of exercise participation have altered FSH and LH levels at different times in their menstrual cycles, which may contribute to menstrual dysfunction.[18] For example, FSH levels are depressed in trained females throughout an abbreviated anovulatory menstrual cycle, whereas LH and progesterone concentrations rise in the follicular phase of the cycle. Several concomitant factors other than exercise per se may alter reproductive function. These include energy drain, weight loss, dietary changes, alterations in the lean-to-fat ratio, the physical and emotional

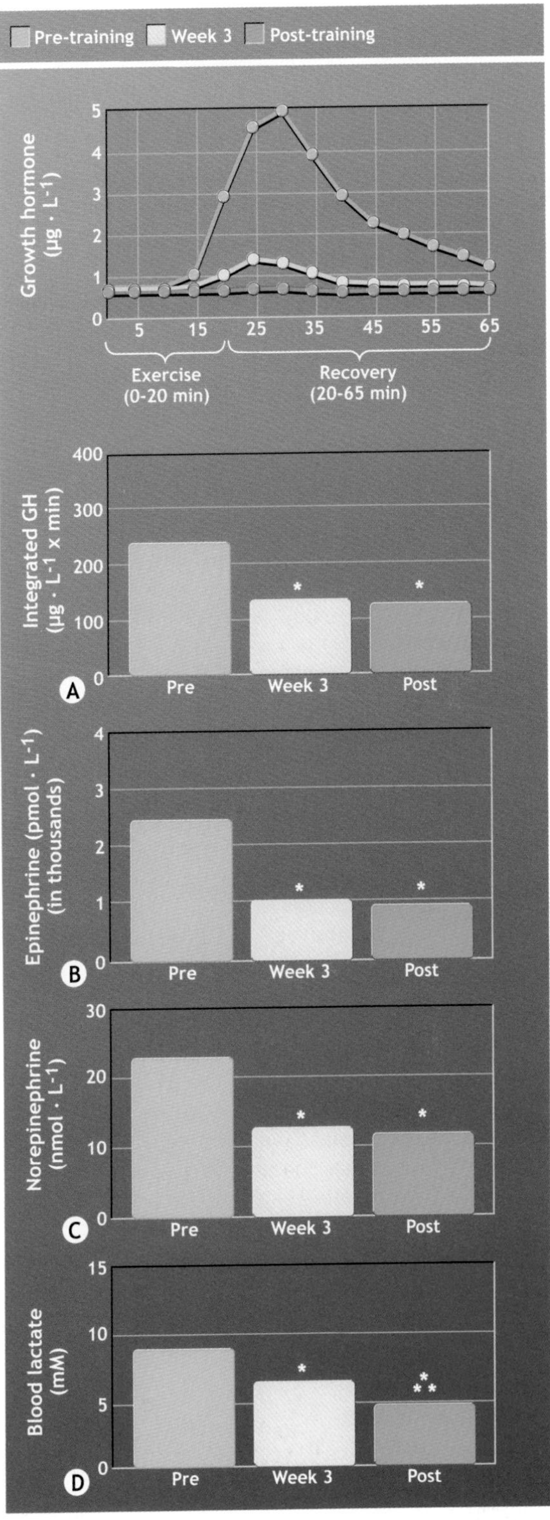

FIGURE 20.22 • *Top.* Serum growth hormone (GH) concentrations during 20 minutes of constant-load exercise and 45 minutes of recovery pretraining, after 3 weeks of training and after 6 weeks of training in a representative subject. *Bottom.* The effects of 6 weeks of training on integrated GH concentration (**A**), and end exercise concentrations of epinephrine (**B**), norepinephrine (**C**), and blood lactate (**D**) in response to constant-load cycle ergometry exercise ($n = 6$, mean). Pretraining; week 3, after 3 weeks of training; Post, after 6 weeks of training. * $P < 0.05$ versus pretraining; ** < 0.05 versus week 3. (From Weltman A, et al. Exercise training decreases the growth hormone (GH) response to acute constant-load exercise. Med Sci Sports Exerc 1997;29:669.)

Focus on Research

Training Intensity Affects Growth Hormone Release

Weltman A, et al. Endurance training amplifies the pulsatile release of growth hormone: effects of training intensity. J Appl Physiol 1992;72:2188.

➤ Research has focused on growth hormone (GH) responses to a single session of exercise and long-term training. While most investigators report that an intense exercise bout increases plasma GH concentration, less information exists about GH levels with prolonged training. The dynamics of GH secretions during exercise training takes on clinical importance because of the causal relationship between GH availability and maintenance of lean body tissue during aging and weight loss.

Weltman and colleagues studied GH dynamics with 52 weeks of aerobic run training in two groups of 21 healthy, eumenorrheic women. One group ran at a speed corresponding to lactate threshold (@LT) and the other at a faster speed, above the lactate threshold level (>LT). Nontraining women served as controls (C). Both training groups completed similar weekly mileage. The distance covered during the first week was 5 miles. Weekly mileage then gradually increased to 24 miles by week 20 and continued at 24 miles per week until week 40. Thereafter, weekly mileage increased by 1.25 miles for three of the weeks. Subjects ran between 35 and 40 miles per week by the end of the study.

Yearlong training increased $\dot{V}O_{2max}$ by 9.9% for the @LT group and 11.8% for the >LT group. In addition, the @LT group increased the exercise $\dot{V}O_2$ at LT ($\dot{V}O_{2\text{-}LT}$) by 21.5%, while the >LT group's $\dot{V}O_{2\text{-}LT}$ increased by 28%. The C group remained unchanged on all measures. No differences in body mass, fat mass, or percentage body fat emerged within or among groups, although the >LT group showed a trend toward body fat reduction. Both exercise groups increased fat-free body mass with training.

The figure illustrates the effects of the run training program on 24-hour integrated serum GH concentrations. Training induced a 50% increase in resting GH concentration for the >LT group. GH concentrations remained unchanged for the C and @LT groups. The investigators speculated that the release of endogenous opiates and catecholamines and inhibition of somatostatin release in more intense exercise performed by the >LT group facilitated GH release.

This research showed that exercise training augments resting pulsatile GH release by amplitude enhancement, but only with training intensity above LT. Training at intensities above the LT may provide a natural and healthful means to increase pulsatile GH secretion under conditions that depress GH release, as in aging. Increased GH release through regular physical activity may also conserve the lean tissue mass during weight loss.

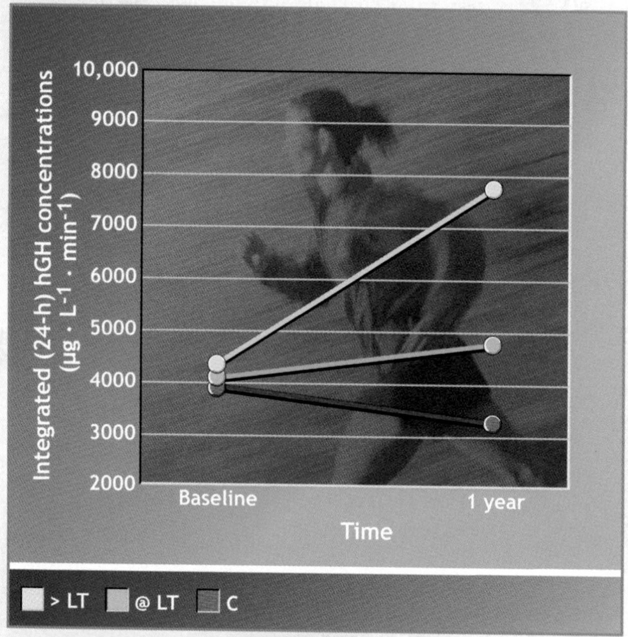

Integrated 24-hour GH concentrations for the control groups (C) and groups that exercised either at an intensity equivalent to the lactate threshold (@LT) or greater than the lactate threshold (>LT). Note the large (50%) increase in GH concentration for the >LT group compared with the @LT and C groups.

stress of strenuous training and competition, and alterations in clearance rates of gonadal steroid hormones. However, variations in the menstrual cycle do not significantly affect metabolic and hormonal responses to acute bouts of physical activity.[70,116]

MEN. Endurance training affects a man's pituitary-gonadal function, including levels of testosterone and PRL.[98] Figure 20.23 shows comparisons among 46 male runners (average weekly running distance, 64 km) and 18 nonrunners matched for age, stature, and body mass. The runners showed lower testosterone than the nonrunners, with no significant differences in the levels of LH and FSH. The reduced testosterone concentration (both increased clearance and lower production) in endurance-trained men parallels the sex-steroid reductions observed in women who undergo endurance training and associated reductions in body fat.[18,210] Because no difference exists in LH and FSH levels between trained and untrained men, impaired gonadotropin release from the anterior pituitary does not cause the lower testosterone levels during standard exercise in the trained state.

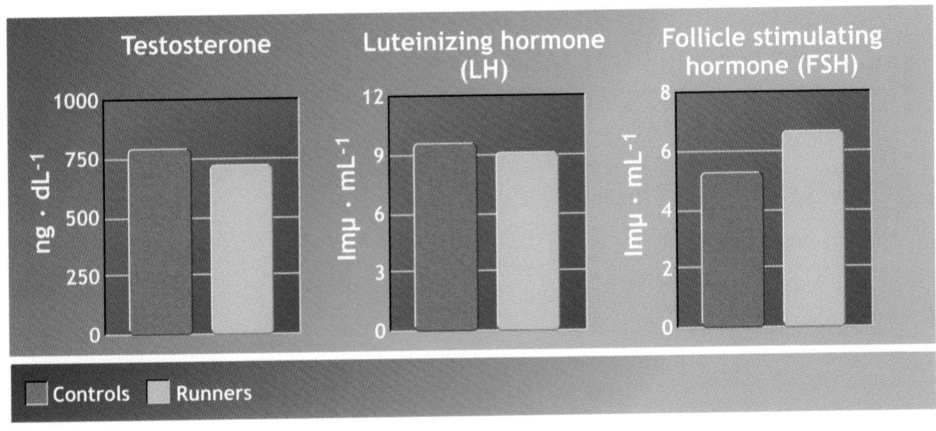

FIGURE 20.23 • Comparison of testosterone, LH, and FSH levels in trained runners and untrained controls. Runners show significantly lower testosterone levels and no significant difference in LH and FSH compared with controls. (From Wheeler GD, et al. Reduced serum testosterone and prolactin levels in male distance runners. JAMA 1984;252:514.)

Posterior Pituitary Hormones

ADH

High-intensity exercise to exhaustion or prolonged submaximal exercise at the same relative intensity produces no difference in ADH levels between trained and untrained individuals.[33] Some evidence suggests that ADH concentration decreases with training in response to pre- and posttraining exercise at the same absolute submaximal intensity.[222]

Oxytocin

We are unaware of research on training-induced changes in oxytocin.

Parathyroid Hormone

Endurance training enhances the exercise-related increase in PTH in young and elderly adults.[194,245] The significance of an augmented rise in PTH with exercise following training for preserving bone mass with aging awaits further study.

Thyroid Hormones

Exercise training produces a coordinated pituitary–thyroid response that reflects increased turnover of thyroid hormones. Increased thyroid turnover often reflects excessive hormonal action that ultimately leads to hyperthyroidism. However, no evidence indicates a higher incidence of hyperthyroidism in highly trained individuals.[65] For example, inordinately high BMR levels and basal body temperatures rarely occur in the trained state. Consequently, the greater T_4 turnover accompanying physical training occurs through a mechanism that differs from "normal" thyroid hormone dynamics.

Research on women who endurance train reveals interesting results regarding thyroid turnover. Changing from a baseline of relatively sedentary living to running 48 km per week produced a mild thyroid impairment reflected by a decrease in T_3 and T_4 levels.[19] On the other hand, nearly doubling the weekly distance significantly increased plasma hormone levels. To explain these apparent conflicting effects of regular exercise, the researchers suggested that greater body fat loss with heavier training in females produced an exercise-induced increase in thyroid output. Six months of resistance training in men slightly reduced the concentrations of T_4 and plasma-free T_4, with no change in TSH. However, the magnitude of the change was of no clinical or physiologic significance.[172] The importance of any changes in thyroxine levels in adapting to training remains unclear.

Adrenal Hormones

Aldosterone

The renin–angiotensin–aldosterone system contributes significantly to homeostatic control of body fluid volumes, electrolytes, and blood pressure,[223] but exercise training does not affect resting levels of these compounds or their normal response to exercise.[71]

Cortisol

Plasma cortisol levels tend to increase less in trained subjects than in sedentary subjects who perform the same absolute level of submaximal exercise.[202] Adrenal gland enlargement can result from both cellular hypertrophy and hyperplasia with repeated bouts of high-intensity exercise training and correspondingly high cortisol output.[208]

Epinephrine and Norepinephrine

Sympathoadrenal activity (principally norepinephrine) in response to an *absolute* submaximum workload remains lower in trained than in untrained individuals.[54,85] Output of epinephrine and norepinephrine in a standard exercise bout falls dramatically during the first several weeks of training. *The appearance of bradycardia and a smaller rise in blood pressure during submaximal exercise represent the most familiar consequences of the sympathoadrenal training adaptation.* Reductions in exercise heart rate and blood pressure reflect favorable training adaptations because they lower myocardial oxygen demands during exercise and possibly during other forms of stress.[142] For equivalent *relative* exercise intensities,

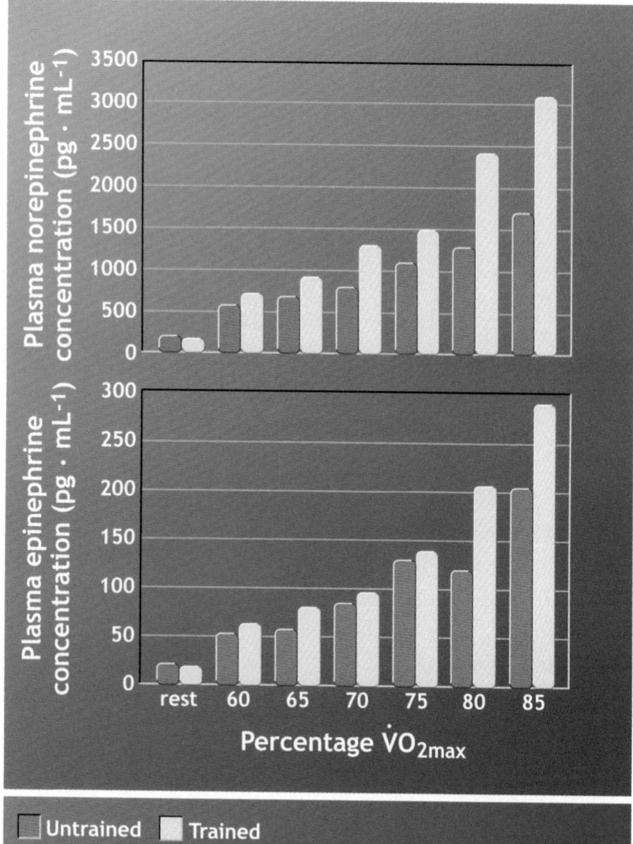

FIGURE 20.24 • Plasma norepinephrine *(top)* and epinephrine concentrations *(bottom)* at rest and after 15 minutes of exercise at the same relative exercise intensity (%$\dot{V}O_{2max}$) before and after 10 weeks of endurance exercise training. (From Greiwe JS, et al. Norepinephrine response to exercise at the same relative intensity before and after endurance training. J Appl Physiol 1999;86:531.)

on the other hand, a *higher* sympathoadrenal response occurs following aerobic training.[76] Figure 20.24 illustrates norepinephrine and epinephrine responses during exercise performed at 60 to 85% of aerobic capacity by three adult men and six women prior to and following 10 weeks of aerobic cycle ergometry and run training that increased $\dot{V}O_{2max}$ by an average of 20%. Plasma norepinephrine levels (Fig. 20.24, *top*) increased progressively with exercise intensity before and after training. However, training produced significantly higher plasma norepinephrine during exercise intensities continually adjusted to range between 65 and 85% of aerobic capacity. Consistently higher epinephrine values also emerged following training (Fig. 20.24, *bottom*), although the differences did not reach statistical significance. More than likely, the greater catecholamine output at the same relative exercise intensity following training reflects three factors requiring greater sympathetic nervous system activation: (1) greater absolute demand for substrate use via glycogenolysis and lipolysis, (2) increased overall cardiovascular response (e.g., cardiac output), and (3) larger muscle mass activation. Whether exercise training alters resting catecholamine levels remains unclear.[176]

Pancreatic Hormones

Studies of training-induced changes in the response patterns for insulin and glucagon reveal several interesting findings. Endurance training maintains the blood levels of insulin and glucagon during exercise closer to resting values. *In essence, the trained state requires less insulin at any stage from rest through light-to-moderately intense exercise.* Figure 20.25 shows insulin and glucagon responses in 10 young males before and after 20 weeks of training at 60 to 80% $\dot{V}O_{2max}$, 4 days per week. Aerobic training blunted the response to exercise of both hormones, with glucagon showing the most pronounced effect. These findings agree with previous reports for adults who trained for 10 weeks by running and cycling.[82]

Regular Physical Activity and Type 2 Diabetes Risk

Data from cross-sectional, retrospective, prospective, and interventional epidemiologic research including studies of enforced inactivity provide strong evidence that regular exercise reduces type 2 diabetes risk with or without concomitant changes in body composition[2,221,227,235] (see LWW's connection website @ http://connection/lww.com/go/mcardle for ACSM position stand on exercise and type 2 diabetes). More than

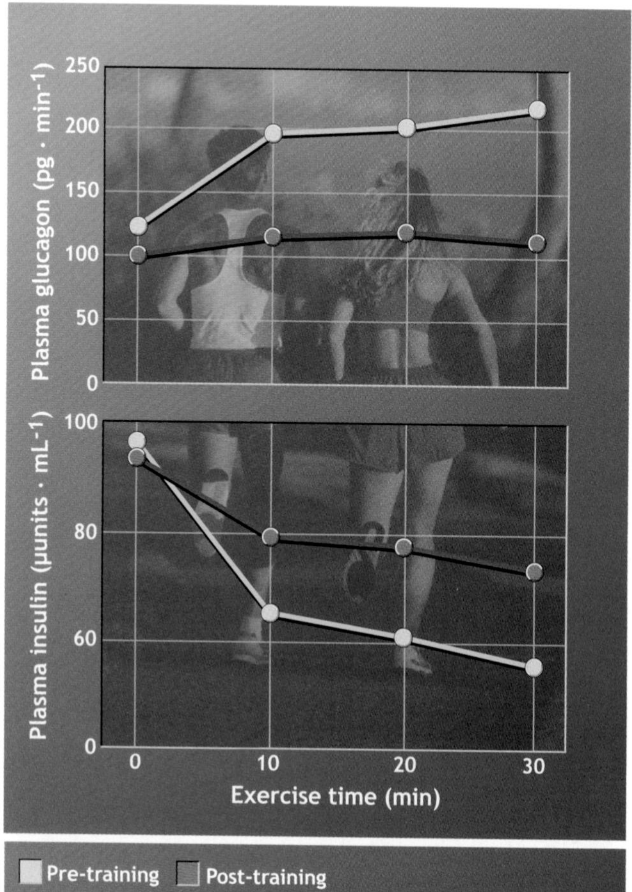

FIGURE 20.25 • Pre–post differences in plasma glucagon and insulin responses to exercise before and after a 20-week exercise training program. (From Applied Physiology Laboratory, University of Michigan.)

likely, those individuals at greatest risk for type 2 diabetes (obese, hypertensive, family history, sedentary lifestyle) reap the greatest benefit from regular exercise.[1,75,139,151,173] For adult men and women, low fitness levels coincide with increased clustering of the metabolic abnormalities associated with the **insulin-resistant syndrome** (see "Metabolic Syndrome X," page 431), the "deadly quartet" of insulin resistance, glucose intolerance, upper-body obesity, and dyslipidemia.[50,232] For sedentary, middle-aged men, aerobic exercise plus weight loss lowers blood pressure and improves glucose and fat metabolism.[44] A 6-year clinical trial evaluated the effects of dietary and exercise lifestyle interventions on the occurrence of type 2 diabetes in individuals with impaired glucose tolerance.[242] Some 577 men and women were randomly assigned to either control, diet-only, exercise-only, or diet plus exercise groups. Diet modification consisted of 25 to 30 kcal per kg of body mass (55–60% carbohydrate, 25–30% lipid, and 10–15% protein) for individuals with a BMI below 25; individuals with a BMI above 25 maintained the same macronutrient mixture as the leaner group while gradually losing weight at a rate of 0.5 to 1.0 kg per month until they reached a BMI of 23. Exercise intervention required a progressive increase in the quantity of mild-to-moderate, regular physical activity. The diet–exercise intervention combined the major components of both diet and exercise treatments. Figure 20.26 shows that diet, exercise, and combined diet–exercise interventions significantly decreased the incidence of diabetes after the 6-year intervention.

A large prospective study evaluated diabetes risk of a cohort of 70,102 female nurses aged 40 to 65 years who did not have diabetes, cardiovascular disease, or cancer at baseline measurements in 1986. In agreement with previous prospective research on men, an 8-year follow-up found increased physical activity associated with a substantially reduced relative risk for type 2 diabetes.[102] Figure 20.27 indicates that after adjustment for smoking, alcohol use, history of hypertension, and elevated cholesterol levels, relative risk across physical activity quintiles (20-%ile units) related inversely to diabetes risk in both lean and overweight women. The dose–response relationship remained consistent in those at low or high risk for diabetes and stayed significant after adjustment for BMI. Women who walked regularly showed greater benefits with a brisker walking pace; the most vigorous exercise lowered diabetes risk by 46%. Equivalent energy

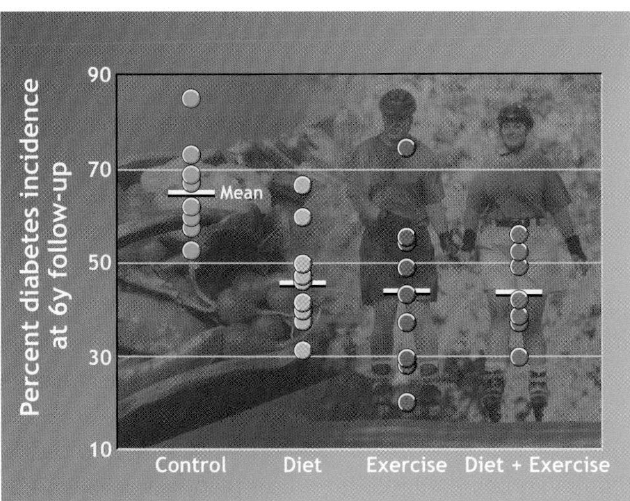

FIGURE 20.26 • Effects of dietary and exercise lifestyle interventions on the occurrence of type 2 diabetes in individuals with impaired glucose tolerance. (From Xiao-ren P, et al. Effects of diet and exercise in preventing NIDDM in people with impaired glucose tolerance. Diabetes Care 1997;20:537.)

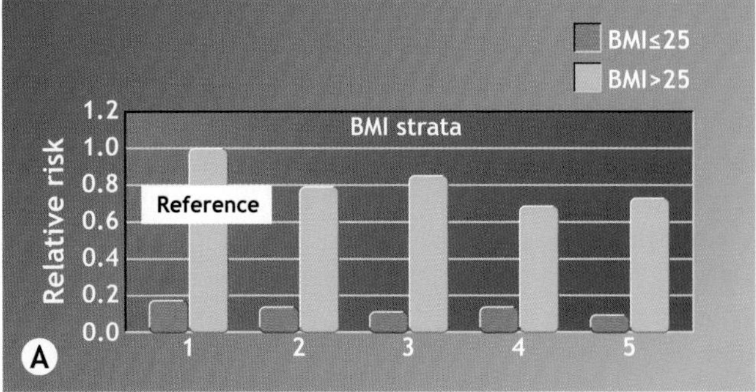

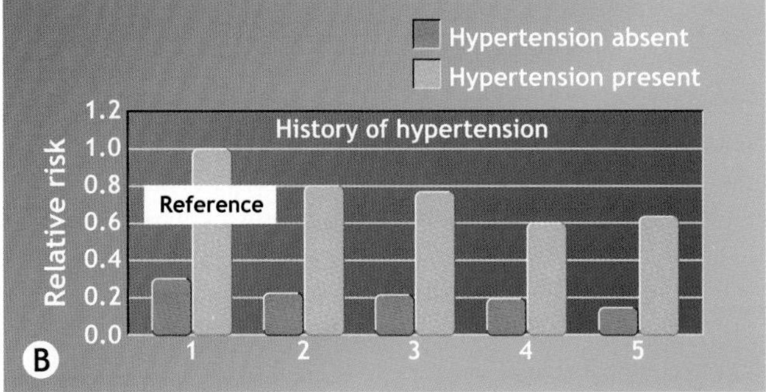

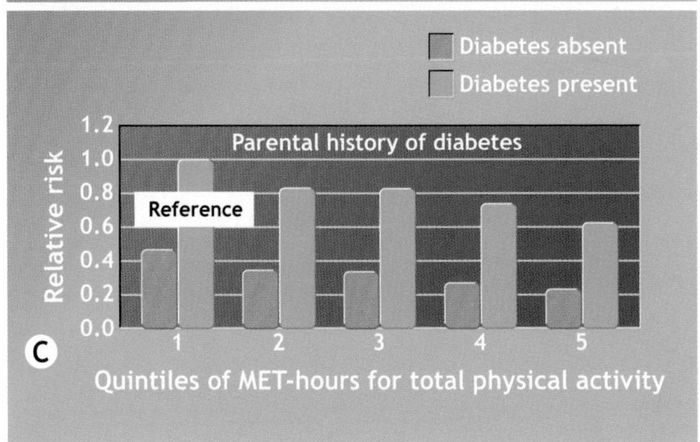

FIGURE 20.27 • Multivariate relative risks of type 2 diabetes according to MET-hours for total physical activity quintile (ascending 20-percentile units) within strata of (**A**) body mass index (BMI), (**B**) history of hypertension, and (**C**) parental history of diabetes. *MET-hours for total physical activity* represents average time per week spent in each of eight physical activities multiplied by the MET value of each activity. The MET value equals energy need per kilogram of body mass per hour of activity divided by the energy need per kilogram of body mass per hour at rest. (From Hu GB, et al. Walking compared with vigorous physical activity and the risk of type 2 diabetes in women: a prospective study. JAMA 1999;282:1433.)

expenditures from waking or other forms of physical activity resulted in comparable risk reduction.

Adult Native Americans of the Pima tribe in Arizona, a group with 10 to 15 times more type 2 diabetes than the typical U.S. population, retrospectively rated their participation in various sports and leisure activities at various stages of their lives.[138] Regardless of gender, individuals with diabetes consistently reported less physical activity over their lifetime than disease-free individuals. This relationship existed even after accounting for age, body mass, body fat distribution, family history, and current physical activity level. These retrospective data agree with prospective data obtained over a 5-year follow-up of more than 21,000 healthy U.S. male physicians aged 40 to 85 years (Fig. 20.28).[149] Clearly, physicians reporting more physical activity, regardless of body mass, experienced a lower incidence of type 2 diabetes. Figure 20.29 outlines the possible mechanisms by which exercise training—via its effects on skeletal muscle, adipose tissue, liver, and pancreatic output—improves insulin action and blood glucose control in type 2 diabetes.

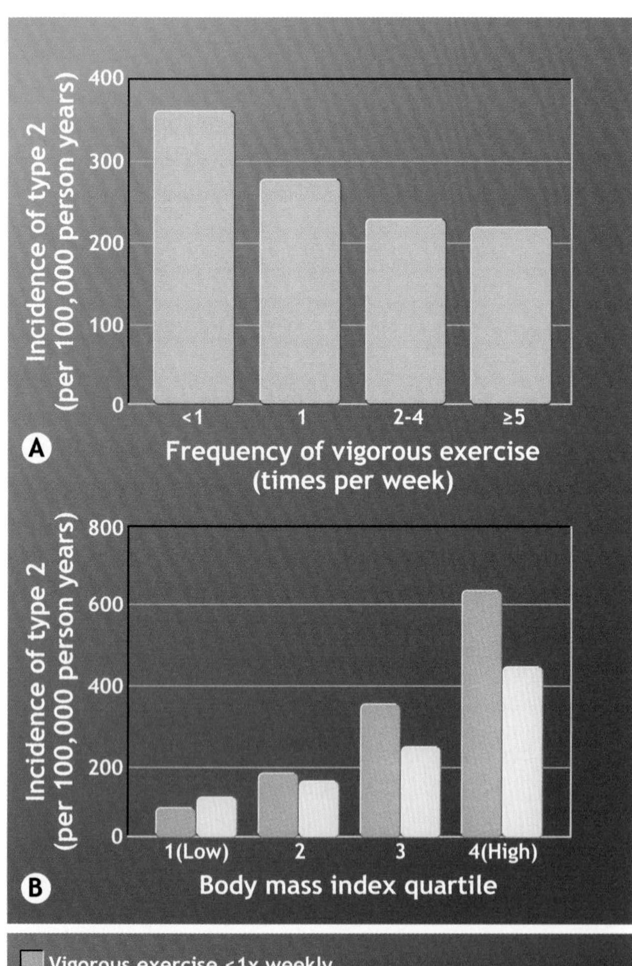

FIGURE 20.28 • **A**. Age-adjusted incidence rates of type 2 diabetes in relation to frequency of vigorous exercise, and (**B**) for individuals with similar values for body size as measured by the body mass index. (From Manson JE, et al. A prospective study of exercise and incidence of diabetes among US male physicians. JAMA 1993;268:63.)

EXERCISE BENEFITS FOR TYPE 2 DIABETES. Exercise training provides the following benefits for persons with type 2 diabetes:

Glycemic Control. Skeletal muscle consumes a significant amount of glucose transported in the blood. For example, muscle generally clears between 70 and 90% of the glucose in an oral or intravenous glucose challenge. A single bout of moderate- or high-intensity exercise abruptly decreases plasma glucose levels, an effect that persists for up to several days.[118,124] Most likely, the immediate effects of each exercise session on the active muscles' **insulin sensitivity** (decrease in insulin concentration required to cause 50% of the maximal response) causes the long-term improvement in glycemic control with regular exercise, rather than any exercise-induced long-term adaptations in tissue function. On resumption of a sedentary lifestyle, the muscle's sensitivity to insulin decreases, thus requiring more insulin to clear a given quantity of blood glucose.[157] *Improved insulin sensitivity with exercise training gives type 2 diabetics important "therapy" that ultimately lowers their insulin requirement.* Improved insulin sensitivity for glucose transport in skeletal muscle and adipose tissue after a short exercise bout results from (1) translocation of the glucose transporter protein GLUT-4 from the endoplasmic reticulum to the cell surface and (2) an increase in the total quantity of GLUT-4.[59,90,96] For example, 4 days of vigorous training increased skeletal muscle GLUT-4 content and insulin-stimulated glucose transport by up to 100%.[184] The hyperinsulinemic patient who requires the largest insulin release for glucose regulation derives the greatest benefits from regular exercise.[52,124,225] This observation remains consistent with the theory that exercise acts by reversing insulin resistance (i.e., exercise increases insulin sensitivity). *Improved insulin sensitivity is one of the most important health benefits that regular physical activity provides to the diabetic.*[151] Combining resistance exercise *and* endurance training improves markers of insulin resistance and body composition for insulin-resistant individuals more than endurance training alone.[224] Benefits of resistance plus endurance training for hyperinsulinemia most likely derive from the specific effects of activating a relatively larger muscle mass (than that with endurance training alone) and the additional caloric expenditure. Improvements in blood glucose homeostasis with regular exercise rapidly dissipate once training ceases and are completely lost within several weeks of inactivity.[3] Exercise training also increases the liver's insulin sensitivity.[51]

Cardiovascular Disease. Excess morbidity and mortality in type 2 diabetes results from coronary heart disease, stroke, and peripheral vascular disease from accelerated atherosclerosis.[207] Disease risk factors that improve with regular exercise include hyperinsulinemia, hyperglycemia, abnormal

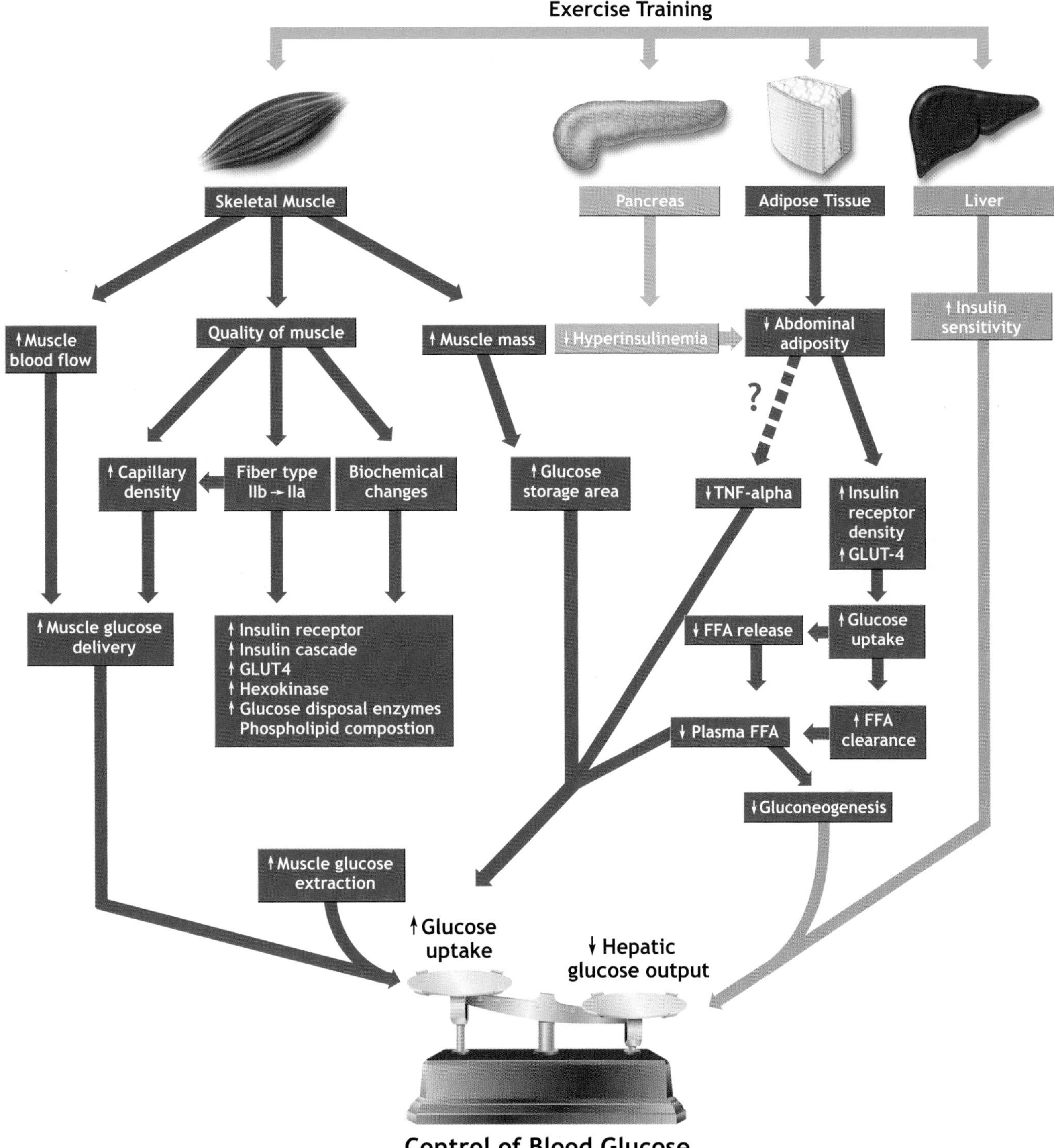

FIGURE 20.29 • Possible mechanisms by which regular physical activity improves insulin action and blood glucose homeostasis in type 2 diabetes. TNF-alpha, tumor necrosis factor-alpha, a hormonelike substance released from active adipocytes in the abdominal region, which may depress insulin-regulated glucose transport. (From Ivy JL, et al. Prevention and treatment of non-insulin-dependent diabetes mellitus. Exerc Sport Sci Rev 1999;27:1.)

plasma lipoproteins, some blood coagulation parameters, and hypertension.

Weight Loss. Weight loss and the accompanying reduction in body fat and its distribution enhance glucose tolerance and insulin sensitivity.[138,139] The beneficial effects of exercise on fat loss often are underestimated because body weight changes with exercise do not always reflect even more favorable, exercise-induced body composition changes (fat loss and muscle gain). As with nondiabetic persons, combining

IN A PRACTICAL SENSE

➤➤ DIABETES, HYPOGLYCEMIA, AND EXERCISE

Persons with type 1 or type 2 diabetes can and should exercise regularly as part of a comprehensive treatment regimen. Hypoglycemia represents the major risk of exercise for individuals who take insulin or oral hypoglycemic agents. A physically active diabetic person needs to pay particular attention to the following:

- Warning signs of hypoglycemia
- Immediate response to a hypoglycemia attack
- Treatment of late-onset hypoglycemia

Hypoglycemia Warning Signs

Symptoms of moderate and severe hypoglycemia (see Table) result from an inadequate glucose supply to the brain. In general, hypoglycemic symptoms appear only after blood glucose concentration drops below 60 mg · dL^{-1}.

Symptoms of low blood glucose vary considerably. Some diabetic persons with autonomic neuropathy who lose the ability to secrete adrenaline-like hormones in response to hypoglycemia experience *hypoglycemic unawareness.* These individuals require regular blood glucose monitoring during and after exercise. Individuals who take β-blocker medication also have increased risk for developing hypoglycemic unawareness.

WARNING SIGNS OF HYPOGLYCEMIA

Mild hypoglycemic reaction
- Trembling or shakiness
- Nervousness
- Rapid heart rate
- Palpitations
- Increased sweating
- Excessive hunger

Moderate hypoglycemic reactions
- Headache
- Irritability and abrupt mood changes
- Impaired concentration and attentiveness
- Mental confusion
- Drowsiness

Severe hypoglycemic reactions
- Unresponsiveness
- Unconsciousness and coma
- Convulsions

Hypoglycemia Attack: What to Do

1. *Respond quickly:* Hypoglycemic reactions appear suddenly and progress rapidly.
2. *Stop exercising:* Test blood glucose to confirm hypoglycemia.
3. *Eat or drink carbohydrate:* Immediately consume 10 to 15 g of simple sugar. A diabetic person should always carry high-glycemic carbohydrate while exercising (e.g., hard candy, sugar cubes, raisins, juice). Consuming ice cream or chocolates is a poor choice; their high fat content depresses the glycemic index and impedes glucose absorption.
4. *Rest 10 to 15 minutes:* This allows for intestinal absorption of glucose. Test blood glucose levels before resuming exercise. If blood glucose registers below 100 mg · dL^{-1}, do not exercise but eat more sugar.
5. *Remonitor during exercise:* After resuming exercise, pay close attention to further signs of hypoglycemia. If possible, measure blood glucose within 30 to 45 minutes.
6. *Replenish carbohydrate immediately after exercise:* Consume complex carbohydrates. If carbohydrate intake does not increase blood glucose concentration, be prepared to administer glucagon subcutaneously to boost glucose levels.

Late-Onset Hypoglycemia

Late-onset hypoglycemia describes the condition of excessively low blood glucose occurring more than 4 hours (and up to 48 h) after exercise. It occurs more frequently in new exercisers or after a strenuous workout. Since insulin sensitivity remains high for 24 to 48 hours after exercise, late-onset hypoglycemia poses a particular problem for many medicated diabetics. The following precautions can guard against late-onset hypoglycemia:

- Adjust insulin dosage or other medication before exercising. If needed, increase food intake before and during exercise.
- If exercise lasts beyond 45 minutes, monitor blood glucose at 2-hour intervals for 12 hours into recovery or until sleep. Consider reducing insulin or oral hypoglycemic agents until bedtime. Before retiring, eat some low-glycemic food to increase blood glucose levels.
- Use caution when initiating an exercise program. Start slowly and gradually increase exercise intensity and duration over a 3- to 6-week period.
- If planning to exercise longer than 45 to 60 minutes, exercise with a friend who can assist in an emergency. Always carry snacks and important phone numbers (doctor, hospital, home) and wear a medical ID bracelet.

Adjusting Insulin Levels

For intense exercise, consider the following:

- Intermediate-acting insulin: Decrease dose by 30 to 35% on the day of exercise.
- Intermediate- and short-acting insulin: Omit dose if it normally precedes exercise.
- Multiple doses of short-acting insulin: Reduce dose before exercise by 30% and supplement with carbohydrate-rich food.
- Continuous subcutaneous insulin infusion: Eliminate mealtime bolus or insulin increment that precedes or follows exercise.
- For 1 hour, avoid exercising muscles that receive the short-acting insulin injection.
- Avoid exercising in late evening.

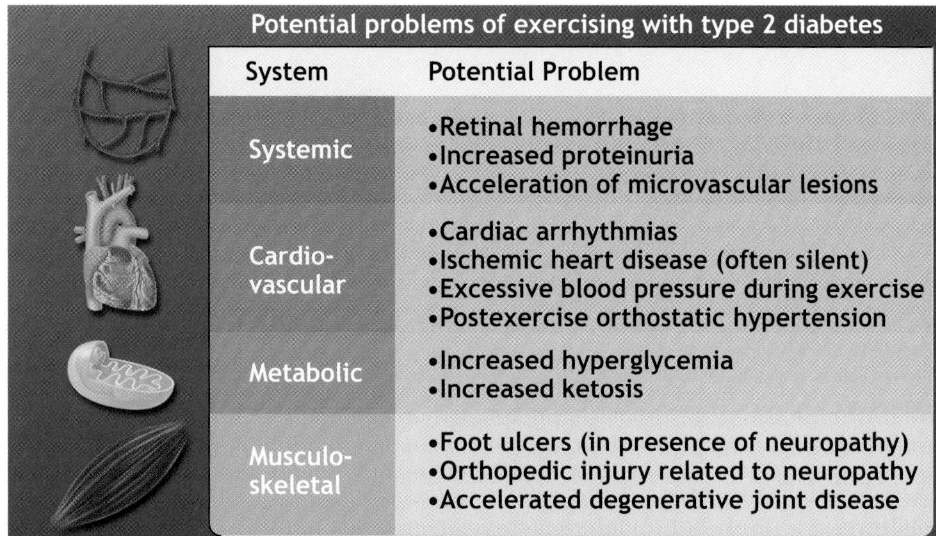

FIGURE 20.30 • Potential physical and physiologic problems faced by type 2 diabetics who begin an exercise program.

diet and regular exercise reduces body fat in diabetic persons more effectively than either treatment alone.[239]

Psychologic Profile. Improved exercise capacity in diabetic persons relates to decreased anxiety, improved mood and self-esteem, increased sense of well-being and psychologic control, enhanced socialization, and improved quality of life.[159]

Occurrence of Type 2 Diabetes. Regular exercise contributes to delaying and even preventing the onset of insulin resistance and type 2 diabetes in persons at high risk for developing this disease. Exercise benefits are particularly pronounced for obese individuals and perhaps all persons with increased abdominal fat deposition.[139,149]

EXERCISE RISKS FOR TYPE 2 DIABETES. One must consider the possible complications from exercise for patients with diabetes Figure 20.30 lists potential adverse effects of exercise in type 2 diabetics. One can minimize these risks by properly screening patients before they start an exercise program and carefully monitoring them during exercise when the program begins.

EXERCISE GUIDELINES FOR TYPE 1 DIABETES. The clinical utility of regular exercise for improving glucose control in type 1 diabetes remains uncertain.[97] To complicate matters for type 1 diabetics, exercise can trigger a potentially dangerous dual response: (1) enhanced glucose uptake by active muscles and (2) greater-than-anticipated exogenous insulin distributed by the rapid circulation that accompanies exercise. These two factors could *worsen* the imbalance between glucose supply and use, possibly increasing the risk of serious complications from hypoglycemia. "In a Practical Sense" offers exercise guidelines for the diabetic patient engaging in exercise. The guidelines also apply to patients with well-controlled type 1 diabetes who wish to perform prolonged and strenuous exercise while minimizing the principal risk of hypoglycemia.[75,219]

RESISTANCE TRAINING AND ENDOCRINE FUNCTION

Muscle remodeling in resistance training reflects a complex process of cell receptor interaction with different hormones and the DNA-mediated production of new contractile proteins. The specific exercise response to muscular overload initially links to configuration of the exercise stimulus—intensity, frequency, volume, sequence, mode, and recovery interval. Figure 20.31 proposes how resistance exercise training improves overall muscular size, strength, and power. Factors responsible for exercise-induced changes in muscle size and function include changes in hepatic and extrahepatic hormone clearance rates, differential rates of hormone secretion (and accompanying fluid shifts around the receptor sites), and altered receptor-site activation via neurohumoral control.[129] Further research must piece together the myriad factors that interact to induce cellular and performance adaptations with resistance training. In general, however, early-phase adaptations to resistance training in men and women reflect a response that mediates neuromuscular system adaptations that improve muscle strength.[87,133]

Testosterone and GH are two primary hormones that affect resistance training adaptations.[77,132] Testosterone augments GH release and interacts with nervous system function to increase muscle force production. These roles may be more important than any direct anabolic effect of testosterone per se. A single session of resistance training generally elicits a short-term rise in serum testosterone and a decrease in cortisol, with a greater response in men than women.[41,134,198,209] Concurrently, catecholamine release from the adrenal medulla increases in response to the acute stress of both high-force and high-power exercise protocols.[26] Whether these hormone response patterns exceed those observed with short-term aerobic exercise remains unclear.[109]

Researchers believe that resistance training in men increases frequency and amplitude of testosterone and GH se-

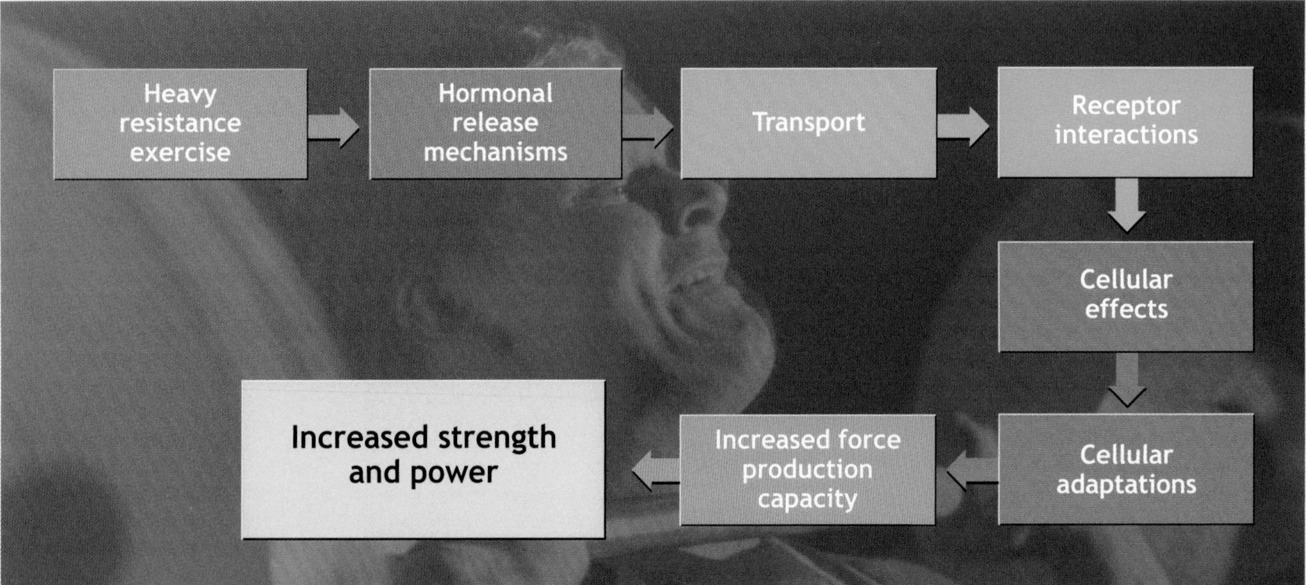

FIGURE 20.31 • Schematic model of how heavy resistance training produces favorable adaptations in muscle structure and maximal strength performance. (Modified from Kraemer WJ. Endocrine responses and adaptations to strength training. In: Komi PV, ed. Strength and power in sport. London: Blackwell Scientific, 1992.)

cretion, thereby creating a favorable hormonal environment for muscular growth (hypertrophy). On the other hand, most studies fail to demonstrate changes in testosterone and GH concentrations with training in females. Thus, gender differences in hormone output with chronic resistance training may ultimately explain any variation in responsiveness of muscle strength and muscle size to long-term muscular overload in men and women.

Testosterone response to resistance exercise reveals several factors that increase its release. These include activation of large-muscle groups with such activities as dead lifts, power cleans and squats, and other forms of heavy resistance exercise (i.e., 85 to 95% 1-RM) or moderate- to high-volume (total quantity) training with multiple sets and/or exercises with less than 1-minute rest intervals.[135] Long-term resistance training in men increases resting testosterone levels, which correlates with the pattern of strength improvement over time.[86]

OPIOID PEPTIDES AND EXERCISE

Scientists studying the pain-relieving effects of opioid peptides (e.g., morphine) on brain function in the 1970s reported that these substances exhibited neurotransmitter effects that reflected activation of specific opioid receptor sites in the brain. With this finding came the realization that perhaps the brain itself produced endogenous opioid, mood-altering substances.[159] Evidence for the existence of endogenous substances with opiate-like behavior first emerged with the isolation and purification of two opioid pentapeptides, methionine and leucine enkephalin (Greek, meaning *in the brain*). These opioids form part of a larger propiocortin precursor molecule produced in the anterior part of the pituitary gland. Other opioid substances include **β-lipotropin**, **β-endorphin**, and **dynorphin**, the most potent of the opioid peptides.

The various endogenous opioids exert widespread effects and range in function from neurohormones to neurotransmitters. Endogenous opiates strongly inhibit hormonal release from the anterior pituitary, principally the release of LH and FSH.[79,128] This inhibition may play a key role in menstrual cycle disturbances—delay in menarche, dysfunctional uterine bleeding, secondary amenorrhea, and inadequacy of the luteal phase—observed among many physically active women.[6] On the other hand, the opioid peptides stimulate release of GH and PRL.

Endorphins also appear to regulate other hormones, including ACTH, the catecholamines, and cortisol.[152] Serum concentrations of endogenous opioids, primarily β-endorphin and/or β-lipotropin, generally increase in response to exercise to a similar degree in men and women, although the response varies among individuals and varies inversely with exercise intensity.[53,73,131] Exercise increases β-endorphin by as much as five times the resting level and probably even more in the brain itself.[72,91,112] With resistance exercise, β-endorphin release varies with the exercise protocol; longer duration (lighter resistance) and longer interset rest intervals elicit the greatest response.[132]

The precise physiologic significance of the various endogenous opioid peptides' response to exercise remains unclear, but several noteworthy effects emerge. These include the postulated opioid effect in triggering the so-called **exercise high**, a state described by some as euphoria and exhilaration as the duration of moderate-to-intense aerobic exercise increases. Endorphin secretion also may relate to increased pain tolerance, improved appetite control, and reduced anxiety, tension, anger, and confusion. Interestingly, these effects generally reflect the proposed psychologic benefits of regular exercise.[159,243]

The effect of exercise training on endorphin response remains controversial, partly because of limited data and partly from variations in training and testing protocols.[91,100] One study reported no significant change in β-endorphin response to prolonged exercise following 8 weeks of endurance training. In contrast, other research showed that general physical conditioning augmented β-endorphin and β-lipotropin release in exercise.[28] Augmented endorphin release also occurs with heavy sprint-type training, suggesting that anaerobic factors affect endorphin dynamics.[131]

Exercise training may also increase an individual's sensitivity to opioid effects, thus reducing the amount of hormone required to induce a specific effect. Furthermore, regular exercise causes the opioids produced during exercise to degrade more slowly than in the pretraining condition.[107] Certainly, a slower rate of hormone disposal would facilitate and prolong an opioid response and possibly augment one's tolerance for extended exercise. Taken in total, one could view the endogenous opioid response to regular exercise as a type of "positive addiction."

INTEGRATIVE QUESTION

List supplements at your local health food store that claim to enhance exercise performance. Which supplements purport to simulate hormonal release? Based on hormonal regulation and function, can any of these products deliver on their claims?

EXERCISE, INFECTIOUS ILLNESS, CANCER, AND IMMUNE RESPONSE

"Don't exercise when fatigued or you'll get sick" reflects the common perception of many parents, athletes, and coaches that excessive high-intensity exercise increases susceptibility to certain illnesses. In contrast, some also believe that regular, more-moderate exercise improves health and reduces susceptibility to such infectious illnesses as the common cold.

Studies as early as 1918 reported that most cases of pneumonia in boys in boarding school occurred among athletes, and respiratory infections seemed to progress toward pneumonia after intense sports training. Anecdotal reports also related the severity of poliomyelitis to participation in heavy physical activity at the critical time of infection. Current epidemiologic and clinical findings from the now flourishing field of **exercise immunology**—the study of the interactions of physical, environmental, and psychologic factors on immune function—support the contention that short-term, unusually strenuous physical activity affects immune function to increase susceptibility to illness, particularly upper respiratory tract infection (URTI). Repeated URTI may signal a state of overtraining (see Chapter 21).[175]

The immune system comprises a highly complex and well-regulated grouping of cells, hormones, and interactive modulators that defend the body from invasion from outside microbes (bacterial, viral, and fungal), foreign macromolecules, and abnormal cancerous cell growth. If infection does occur, an optimal immune system aids greatly in blunting the severity of illness and speeding recovery.

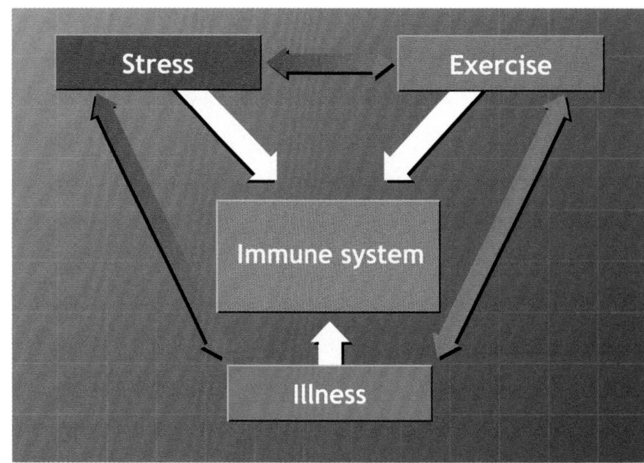

FIGURE 20.32 • Theoretical model of the interrelationships between stress, exercise, illness, and the immune system. (From MacKinnon LT. Current challenges and future expectations in exercise immunology: back to the future. Med Sci Sports Exerc 1994;26:191.)

Figure 20.32 shows a proposed model for the interactions of exercise, stress, illness, and the immune system. Within this framework, exercise, stress, and illness interact, each with its own effect on immunity. For example, exercise affects susceptibility to illness, while certain illnesses clearly affect exercise capacity. Likewise, psychologic factors (via links between the hypothalamus and immune function) and other forms of stress, including nutritional deficiencies and acute alterations in normal sleep schedule, influence resistance to illness. Concurrently, exercise can either positively or negatively modulate the response to stress. Each factor—stress, illness, and short- and long-term exercise—exerts an independent effect on immune status, immune function, and resistance to disease.

Upper Respiratory Tract Infections

Figure 20.33 shows the general J-shaped curve that describes the relationship between acute short-term exercise (or unusually heavy training) and susceptibility to URTI. Diverse markers of immune function also generally follow an inverted J-shaped curve.[241] While implications drawn from this relationship may be simplistic, light-to-moderate physical activity does appear to offer more protection against URTI and possibly diverse cancers than a sedentary lifestyle.[113,145,146,201] In addition, moderate exercise does not exacerbate the severity and duration of illness if infection does occur.[228] In contrast, a bout of intense physical activity (e.g., a marathon run or heavy training session) provides an "open window" (3 to 72 h) that decreases antiviral and antibacterial resistance and increases risk of URTI that manifests itself within 1 to 2 weeks.[40,177] For example, approximately 13% of the participants in a Los Angeles

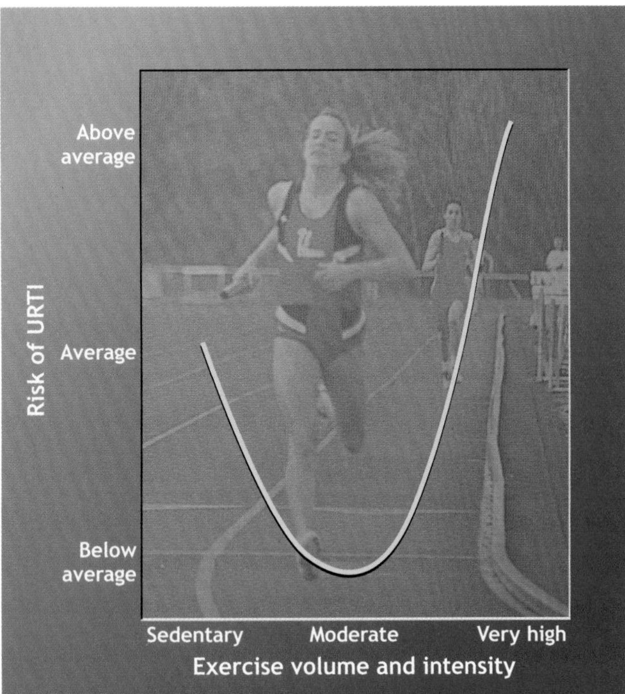

FIGURE 20.33 • General model for the relationship between intensity of physical activity and susceptibility to upper respiratory tract infection (URTI). Moderate exercise reduces risk of URTI, whereas exhaustive competition or training places the participant at increased risk. (From Nieman DC. Exercise, upper respiratory tract infection, and the immune system. Med Sci Sports Exerc 1994;26:128.)

marathon reported an episode of infectious URTI during the week following the race. For runners of comparable ability who did not compete for reasons other than illness, the infection rate approximated just 2%.[165] Future research must establish a precise causal link between the magnitude of immunosuppression following a bout of heavy exertion and subsequent occurrence of infection.

Acute Exercise Effects

- Moderate exercise: *A bout of moderate exercise boosts natural immune functions and host defenses for up to several hours.* [123] Noteworthy effects include the increase in **natural killer (NK) cell** activity. These phagocytic lymphocyte subpopulations enhance the cytotoxic capacity of the blood and provide the body's first line of defense against diverse pathogens. The NK cell does not require prior or specific sensitization to foreign bodies or neoplastic cells. Rather, these cells demonstrate spontaneous cytolytic activity that ultimately ruptures and/or inactivates viruses and the metastatic potential of tumor cells.[175,236]
- Exhaustive exercise: *Whereas moderate exercise heightens immune functions, a period of exhaustive exercise (and other forms of extreme stress or increased training) produces the opposite effect and severely blunts the body's first line of defense against infection.*[24,115,127,147,203,229] Elevated temperature, cytokines, and various stress-related hormones (epinephrine, GH, cortisol, β-endorphins) in exhaustive exercise may mediate the transient depression of the body's innate (NK cell and neutrophil activity) and adaptive immune defenses (T- and B-cell function).[7,166] Diminished immunity after strenuous exercise becomes particularly apparent in the mucosal immune system of the upper respiratory tract.[162] This negative effect on immune response clearly supports the wisdom of advising individuals with URTI symptoms to refrain from physical activity (or at least "go easy") to optimize normal immune mechanisms that combat infection. Table 20.4 summarizes components of the immune system that exhibit transient changes after prolonged, heavy exertion.

Long-Term Exercise Effects

Limited data indicate that aerobic exercise training affects natural immune functions positively in young and old individuals and in obese persons during weight loss.[56,195,200] Areas of improvement include (1) enhanced functional capacity of natural cytotoxic immune mechanisms (e.g., antitumor actions of NK cell activity) and (2) blunted age-related decrease in T-cell function and associated cytokine production.[111,167] The cytotoxic T cells defend directly against viral

TABLE 20.4 ➤ IMMUNE SYSTEM COMPONENTS THAT EXHIBIT CHANGE AFTER PROLONGED, HEAVY EXERTION

- High neutrophil and low lymphocyte blood counts, induced by high concentrations of plasma cortisol
- Increase in blood granulocyte and monocyte phagocytosis (engulfing of infectious agents and of breakdown products of muscle fiber); decrease in nasal neutrophil phagocytosis
- Decrease in granulocyte oxidative-burst activity (killing activity)
- Decrease in nasal mucociliary clearance (sweeping movement of cilia)
- Decrease in NK-cell cytotoxic activity (the ability to kill infected cells or cancer cells)
- Decrease in mitogen-induced lymphocyte proliferation (a measure of T-cell function)
- Decrease in the delayed-type hypersensitivity skin response (the ability of the immune system to produce hard red lumps after the skin is pricked with antigens)
- Increase in plasma concentrations of pro- and anti-inflammatory cytokines (e.g., interleukin-6 and interleukin-1 receptor antagonist)
- Decrease in *ex vivo* production of cytokines (interferon-8, interleukin-1, and interleukin-6) to mitogens and endotoxin
- Decrease in nasal and salivary IgA concentration (an important antibody)
- Blunted expression of major histocompatibility complex (MHC) II in macrophages (an important step in recognition of foreign agents by the immune system)

From Nieman DC. Immunity in athletes: current issues. Sports Sci Exchange, Gatorade Sports Science Institute 1998; 11(2).

and fungal infections and contribute to regulating other immune mechanisms.

If exercise training enhances immune function, one might ask why trained individuals show increased susceptibility to URTI after intense competition. The **open window hypothesis** maintains that an inordinate increase in training or actual competition exposes the highly conditioned athlete to non-normal stress that transiently but severely depresses NK cell function. This period of immunodepression (open window) decreases natural resistance to infection. Speculation is that the inhibitory effect of strenuous exercise on ACTH and cortisol's maintenance of optimal blood glucose concentrations negatively affects the immune process. For individuals who exercise regularly but only at moderate levels, the window of opportunity for infection remains "closed," thus maintaining the protective benefits of regular exercise on immune function.[175]

RESISTANCE TRAINING. In contrast to the beneficial effect of regular aerobic exercise on immune function, 9 years of prior resistance exercise training exerted no effect on resting NK cell activity or number in comparisons between experienced weight trainers and sedentary controls.[168] The comparison also indicated that resistance training activated monocytes more than typically observed for aerobic training. Monocyte activation releases prostaglandins that downregulate NK cells following exercise, thus blunting the long-term positive effect of exercise on NK cells.[174] Earlier these same investigators had shown a substantial 225% increase in NK cells following an acute bout of resistance exercise,[169] a response similar to the short-term effect of moderate aerobic exercise.[63,89]

PERHAPS A ROLE FOR NUTRITIONAL SUPPLEMENTS. Nutrition may optimize immune system function in response to strenuous exercise.[31,93] Supplementing with a 6% carbohydrate beverage (0.71 L before; 0.25 L every 15 min during; 500 mL every h throughout a 4.5-h recovery) blunted cytokine levels in the inflammatory cascade after 2.5 hours of running at 77% $\dot{V}O_{2max}$.[164] Subsequent research by the same laboratory showed that ingesting carbohydrates (4 mL per kg of body mass) every 15 minutes during 2.5 hours of high-intensity running or cycling maintained higher plasma glucose levels in 10 triathletes during exercise than a placebo.[171] A blunted cortisol response and diminished pro- and anti-inflammatory cytokine responses accompanied the higher plasma glucose levels with supplementation in both forms of exercise. This suggests a carbohydrate-induced reduction in overall physiologic stress in prolonged high-intensity exercise.

Combined supplementation with the antioxidant vitamins C and E produces more-prominent immunopotentiating effects (enhanced cytokine production) in young, healthy adults than supplementation with either vitamin alone.[108] In other research, a 200-mg daily vitamin E supplement enhanced several clinically relevant indices of T-cell–mediated function in healthy elderly subjects.[154] Additional research must determine whether intake of vitamins C and E (and other antioxidants such as β-carotene) above recommended levels upgrades immune function to protect the general population against URTI. However, daily supplementation with vitamin C appears to benefit individuals engaged in heavy exercise, particularly those predisposed to frequent viral URTI.[92,178] Runners who received a 600-mg daily vitamin C supplement before and for 3 weeks after a 90-km ultramarathon competition experienced significantly fewer symptoms of URTI—running nose, sneezing, sore throat, coughing, fever—than runners receiving a placebo.[177] Interestingly, infection risk inversely related to race performance; those with the fastest times suffered more symptoms. URTI also appeared most frequently in runners with strenuous training regimens. For these individuals, additional vitamin C and E and perhaps carbohydrate ingestion before, during, and after a prolonged stressful exercise bout may boost normal immune mechanisms for combating this type of infection.[166,170] More than likely, other stressors such as sleep deficit, mental stress, poor nutrition, or weight loss magnify the stress on the immune system from a single bout (or repeated bouts) of exhaustive exercise.[31,166]

Glutamine and the Immune Response. The nonessential amino acid glutamine plays an important role in normal immune function. One protective aspect concerns glutamine's role as an energy fuel for nucleotide synthesis by disease-fighting cells, particularly the lymphocytes and macrophages that defend against infection.[4,204] In humans, sepsis, injury, burns, surgery and endurance exercise lowers plasma and skeletal muscle glutamine levels. Lowered plasma glutamine levels most likely occur because glutamine demand by the liver, kidneys, gut, and immune system exceeds its supply from the diet and skeletal muscle. The lowered plasma glutamine concentration contributes, at least in part, to the immunosuppression that accompanies situations of extreme physical stress.[13,95,192,206] Thus, speculation is that glutamine supplementation might reduce susceptibility to URTI following prolonged competition or a bout of exhaustive training.[199]

Marathoners who ingested a glutamine drink (5 g L-glutamine in 330 mL mineral water) at the end of a race and then 2 hours later reported fewer URTI symptoms than unsupplemented athletes.[29] More specifically, 65% more athletes reported no symptoms of infection. In subsequent studies by the same researchers to determine a possible protective mechanism, glutamine's effect on postexercise infection risk did not relate to any change in blood lymphocyte distribution.[30] Also, appearance of URTI in athletes during intense training does not fluctuate with changes in plasma glutamine concentration. Furthermore, preexercise glutamine supplementation does not affect the immune response following repeated bouts of intense exercise.[190,226] Glutamine supplements taken 0, 30, 60, and 90 minutes after a marathon race prevented the drop in glutamine concentrations following the race but had *no influence* on the lymphokine-activated killer cell activity, the proliferative responses, or the exercise-induced changes in leukocyte subpopulations.[189] At this time, insufficient data exist to recommend use of glutamine supplements to reliably blunt immunosuppression from exhaustive exercise.

The Exercise–Cancer Connection

Epidemiologic studies generally demonstrate a protective association between regular physical activity and risk of cancers of the breast, colon, lung, and prostate (see Chapter 31).[141,155] In addition to exercise's beneficial effect on NK cell activity, long-term enhancement of other natural immune functions may contribute to the cancer-protective effect of regular exercise. Upgraded defenses include augmented phagocytic capacity of the monocyte–macrophage lineage combined with more robust cytotoxic and intracellular killing capacities (T-cell activity) that inhibit tumor growth and destroy cancer cells.[236,240] Other potential effects of regular exercise on aspects of cancer development include beneficial changes in the body's antioxidant functions, endocrine profiles, prostaglandin metabolism, body composition, and, in the case of colon cancer, a beneficial increase in intestinal transit time with physical activity. In Chapter 31, we review the role of exercise in the prevention and treatment of different cancers.

Summary

1. The endocrine system consists of a host organ, a transmitted substance (hormone), and a target or receptor organ. Steroids or amino acid (polypeptide) derivatives make up the hormones.
2. Hormones primarily alter the rate of cellular reactions by acting at specific receptor sites to either enhance or inhibit enzyme function.
3. The amount of hormone synthesized, the amount released, the amount taken up by the target organ, and the removal rate from the blood all influence blood hormone concentration.
4. Most hormones respond to peripheral stimulus on an as-needed basis; others are released at regular intervals. Some secretory cycles span several weeks; others pattern on a 24-hour cycle.
5. The anterior pituitary secretes at least six hormones: PRL, the gonadotropic hormones FSH and LH, corticotropin, TSH, and GH.
6. GH promotes cell division and cellular proliferation. IGFs (or somatomedins) mediate many of GH's effects.
7. TSH controls the amount of hormone secreted by the thyroid gland; ACTH regulates output of hormones from the adrenal cortex; PRL affects reproduction and the development of secondary sex characteristics of females; FSH and LH stimulate the ovaries to secrete estrogen in females and testosterone in males.
8. The posterior pituitary secretes ADH, which controls water excretion by the kidneys. It also secretes oxytocin, an important hormone in birthing and lactation.
9. PTH controls blood calcium balance; a decrease in blood calcium concentration triggers its release. Its major effect increases ionic (free) calcium levels by stimulating three target organs: bone, kidneys, and the small intestine.
10. TSH stimulates metabolism of all cells and increases carbohydrate and fat breakdown in energy metabolism.
11. The inner (medulla) and outer (cortex) regions of the adrenal gland secrete two different types of hormones. The medulla secretes the catecholamines epinephrine and norepinephrine. The adrenal cortex secretes mineralocorticoids that regulate extracellular sodium and potassium levels, glucocorticoids (that stimulate gluconeogenesis and serve as insulin antagonists), and androgens that control male secondary sex characteristics.
12. The testes in the male and the ovaries in the female (the gonads) produce testosterone (testes) and the estrogens estradiol and progesterone (ovaries).
13. Moderate aerobic exercise and resistance training increase testosterone in untrained males. For females, plasma testosterone and estrogens levels increase during exercise.
14. Secreted by the β-cells of the pancreas' islets of Langerhans, insulin increases glucose transport into cells. Thus, insulin controls blood glucose levels and carbohydrate metabolism. Total lack of insulin or decreased sensitivity or increased resistance to this hormone produces diabetes mellitus.
15. The α-cells of the pancreas secrete glucagon, an insulin antagonist that raises blood sugar levels.
16. Exercise training exerts differential effects on resting and exercise-induced hormone production and release. Trained persons generally show elevated hormone response during exercise for ACTH and cortisol; depressed values for GH, PRL, FSH, LH, testosterone, ADH, thyroxine, catecholamines, and insulin; and no training response for aldosterone, renin, and angiotensin.
17. Exercise-induced elevation of β-endorphins and associated opioid-like hormones may contribute to the euphoria, increased pain tolerance, the "exercise high," and altered menstrual function associated with exercise and training.
18. Unusually heavy physical activity affects immune function in a manner that increases susceptibility to URTI. In contrast, moderate exercise upgrades immune responses to protect against URTI.
19. Regular exercise training exerts a desirable effect on natural immune functions. An enhanced immune profile can protect against not only URTI but various cancers.

References

1. ADA/ACSM. Diabetes mellitus and exercise joint position paper. Med Sci Sports Exerc 1997;29:I.
2. American College of Sports Medicine. Position Stand. Exercise and type 2 diabetes. Med Sci Sports Exerc 32:1345;2000.

3. Arciero PJ, et al. Effects of short-term inactivity on glucose tolerance, energy expenditure, and blood flow in trained subjects. J Appl Physiol 1998;84:1365.
4. Ardawi MSN, Newsholme EA. Metabolism in lymphocytes and its importance in the immune response. Essays Biochem 1985;21:1.
5. Ashley CD, et al. Estrogen and substrate metabolism: a review of contradictory research. Sports Med 2000;29(4):221.
6. Baker ER. Menstrual dysfunction and hormonal status in athletic women: a review. Fertil Steril 1981;36:391.
7. Baum M, et al. Moderate and exhaustive endurance exercise influences the interferon-γ levels in whole-blood culture supernatants. Eur J Appl Physiol 1997;76:165.
8. Bischoff HA, et al. Relationship between muscle strength and vitamin D metabolites: are there therapeutic possibilities in the elderly? Z Rheumatol 2000;59:Suppl 1.
9. Bjorkman O, et al. Influence of hypoglucagonemia on splanchnic glucose output during leg exercise in man. Clin Physiol 1981;1:43.
10. Bjørnholt JV, et al. Fasting blood glucose: an underestimated risk factor for cardiovascular death. Diabetes Care 1999;22:45.
11. Björntorp P, et al. Hypertension and the metabolic syndrome: closely related central origin? Blood Press 2000;9:71.
12. Björntorp P, Rosmond R. Hypothalamic origin of the metabolic syndrome X. Ann NY Acad Sci 1999;892:297.
13. Blanchard MA, et al. The influence of diet and exercise on muscle and plasma glutamine concentrations. Med Sci Sports Exerc 2001;33:69.
14. Bloom SR, et al. Differences in the metabolic and hormonal responses to exercise between racing cyclists and untrained individuals. J Physiol (Lond) 1976;258:1.
15. Borer KT. Exercise-induced facilitation of pulsatile growth hormone (GH) secretion and somatic growth. In: Laron Z, Rogol AD, eds. Hormones and sport, vol 55. New York: Raven Press, 1989.
16. Bonifazi M, et al. Influence of training on the response to exercise of adrenocorticotropin and growth hormone plasma concentrations in human swimmers. Eur J Appl Physiol 1998;78:394.
17. Bosco C, et. al. Monitoring strength training: neuromuscular and hormonal profile. Med Sci Sports Exerc 2000;32:202.
18. Boyden TW, et al. Prolactin responses, menstrual cycles and body composition of women runners. J Clin Endocrinol Metab 1982;58:711.
19. Boyden TW, et al. Thyroidal changes associated with endurance training in women. Med Sci Sports Exerc 1984;16:234.
20. Brahm H, et al. Bone metabolism during exercise and recovery: the influence of plasma volume and physical fitness. Calcif Tissue Int 1997;61:192.
21. Bray, G. The obese patient. Major problems in internal medicine, vol. 9. Philadelphia: WB Saunders, 1976.
22. Brillon D, et al. Cholinergic but not serotonergic mediation of exercise-induced growth hormone secretion. Endocr Res 1986;12:137.
23. Brisson D, et al. Exercise-induced dissociation of the blood prolactin response in young women according to their sports habits. Horm Metab Res 1980;12:201.
24. Bruunsgaard H, et al. In vivo cell-mediated immunity and vaccination response following prolonged, intense exercise. Med Sci Sports Exerc 1997;29:1176.
25. Bunt JC, et al. Sex and training differences in human growth hormone levels during prolonged exercise. J Appl Physiol 1986;61:1796.
26. Bush JA, et al. Exercise and recovery responses of adrenal medullary neurohormones to heavy resistance exercise. Med Sci Sports Exerc 1999;31:554.
27. Calder PC, Yaqoob P. Glutamine and the immune system. Amino Acids 1999;17:227.
28. Carr CB, et al. Physical conditioning facilitates exercise induced secretion of beta-endorphins and beta-lipotrophin in women. N Engl J Med 1981;305:560.
29. Castell LM, et al. Does glutamine have a role in reducing infections in athletes? Eur J Appl Physiol 1996;73:488.
30. Castell LM, et al. Some aspects of the acute phase response after a marathon race, and the effects of glutamine supplementation. Eur J Appl Physiol 1997;75:47.
31. Chandra RK. Nutrition and the immune system: an introduction. Am J Clin Nutr 1997;60(suppl):460S.
32. Coggan AR, et al. Fat metabolism during high-intensity exercise in endurance-trained and untrained men. Metabolism 2000;49:122.
33. Convertino VA, et al. Exercise induced hypervolemia: role of plasma albumin, renin and vasopressin. J Appl Physiol 1980;48:665.
34. Cook NJ, et al. Changes in adrenal and testicular activity monitored by salivary sampling in males throughout marathon runs. J Appl Physiol 1986;55:634.
35. Crampes F, et al. Effect of physical training in humans on the response of isolated fat cells to epinephrine. J Appl Physiol 1991;61:25.
36. Criswell D, et al. Fluid replacement beverages and maintenance of plasma volume during exercise: role of aldosterone and vasopressin. Eur J Appl Physiol 1992;65:445.
37. Cumming DC, et al. Defects in pulsatile LH release in normally menstruating runners. J Clin Endocrinol Metab 1985;60:810.
38. Cumming DC, et al. Reproductive hormone increases in response to acute exercise in men. Med Sci Sports Exerc 1986;18:369.
39. Czech MP. Signal transmission by the insulin-like growth factors. Cell 1989;59:235.
40. Davis JM, et al. Exercise, alveolar macrophage function, and susceptibility to respiratory infection. J Appl Physiol 1997;83:1461.
41. Davis SN, et al. Effects of gender on neuroendocrine and metabolic counterregulatory responses to exercise in normal man. J Clin Endocrinol Metab 2000;85:224.
42. DeFronzo RA, et al. Glucose clamp technique: a method for quantifying insulin secretion and resistance. Am J Physiol 1979;237:E214.
43. Del Corral P, et al. Metabolic effects of low cortisol during exercise in humans. J Appl Physiol 1998;84:939.
44. Dengel DR, et al. Improvements in blood pressure, glucose metabolism, and lipoprotein lipids after aerobic exercise plus weight loss in obese, hypertensive middle-aged men. Metabolism 1998;47:1075.
45. Dengel DR, et al. Effect of dietary sodium on insulin sensitivity in older, obese, sedentary hypertensives. Am J Hypertens 1997;10(9 Pt 1):964.
46. Dengel DR, et al. Insulin sensitivity is associated with blood pressure response to sodium in older hypertensives. Am J Physiol 1998;274:E403.
47. De Sousa MJ, et al. Menstrual status and plasma vasopressin, renin activity, aldosterone and exercise responses. J Appl Physiol 1989;67:736.
48. DeSousa MJ, et al. Menstrual status and plasma vasopressin, renin activity, aldosterone, and exercise response. J Appl Physiol 1990;68:520.
49. DeSousa MJ, et al. Gonadal hormones and semen quality in male runners. Int J Sports Med 1994;15:383.
50. Després J-P. Visceral obesity, insulin resistance, and dyslipidemia: contribution of endurance exercise training to the treatment of the plurimetabolic syndrome. Exerc Sport Sci Rev 1997;25:271.
51. Devlin JT, et al. Enhanced peripheral and splanchnic insulin sensitivity in NIDDM men after a single bout of exercise. Diabetes 1987;36:434.
52. Dolkas CB, et al. Effect of body weight gain on insulin sensitivity after retirement from exercise training. J Appl Physiol 1990;68:520.
53. Dorion BA, et al. Beta-endorphin response to high intensity exercise and music in college-age women. J Strength Cond Res 1999;13:24.
54. Duncan JJ, et al. The effects of aerobic exercise on plasma catecholamines and blood pressure in patients with mild hypertension. JAMA 1985;254:2609.
55. Fabbri A, et al. Body-fat distribution and responsiveness of the pituitary-adrenal axis to corticotropin-releasing-hormone stimulation in sedentary and exercising women. J Endocrinol Invest 1999;22:377.
56. Fahlman M, et al. Effects of endurance training on selected parameters of immune function in elderly women. Gerontology 2000;46:97.
57. Febbario MA, et al. Effect of epinephrine on muscle glycogenolysis during exercise in trained men. J Appl Physiol 1998;84:465.
58. Felig P, et al. Plasma glucagon levels in exercising man. N Engl J Med 1972;287:184.
59. Ferrara CM, et al. Short-term exercise enhances insulin-stimulated GLUT-4 translocation and glucose transport into adipose cells. J Appl Physiol 1998;85:2106.
60. Florini JR. Hormonal control of muscle cell growth. J Anim Sci 1985:61:21.
61. Florini JR. Hormonal control of muscle growth. Muscle Nerve 1987;10:577.
62. Foster DW. Insulin resistance—a secret killer? N Engl J Med 1989;320:733.
63. Gabriel HA, et al. Circulating leukocyte and lymphocyte subpopulations before and after intensive endurance exercise to exhaustion. J Appl Physiol 1991;63:449.
64. Galbo H. Hormonal and metabolic adaptation to exercise. New York: GT Verlag, 1983.
65. Galbo H. Exercise physiology: humoral function. Sport Sci Rev 1992;1:65.

66. Galbo H, et al. Glucagon and plasma catecholamine responses to graded and prolonged exercise in man. J Appl Physiol 1975;38:70.
67. Galbo H, et al. Catecholamines and pancreatic hormones during autonomic blockade in exercising man. Acta Physiol Scand 1977;101:428.
68. Galbo H, et al. Thyroid and testicular hormone response to graded and prolonged exercise in man. Eur J Appl Physiol 1977;36:101.
69. Galbo H, et al. The effect of fasting on the hormonal response to graded exercise. J Clin Endocrinol Metab 1981;52:1106.
70. Galliven EA, et al. Hormonal and metabolic responses to exercise across time of day and menstrual cycle phase. J Appl Physiol 1997;83:1822.
71. Geyssant A, et al. Plasma vasopressin, renin activity, and aldosterone: effects of exercise and training. Eur J Appl Physiol 1980;46:21.
72. Goldfarb AH, Jamurtas AZ. Beta-endorphins response to exercise: an update. Sports Med 1997;24:8.
73. Goldfarb AH, et al. Gender effect on beta-endorphin response to exercise. Med Sci Sports Exerc 1998;30:1672.
74. Gotshalk LA, et al. Hormonal response of multiset versus single-set heavy-resistance exercise protocol. Can J Appl Physiol 1997;22:244.
75. Gower BA, et al. Fat distribution and insulin response in prepubertal African American and white children, Am J Clin Nutr 1998;67:821.
76. Greiwe JS, et al. Norepinephrine response to exercise at the same relative intensity before and after endurance training. J Appl Physiol 1999;86:531.
77. Griggs RC, et al. Effect of testosterone on muscle mass and muscle protein synthesis. J Appl Physiol 1989;66:498.
78. Grimston SK, et al. The calciotropic hormone response to changes in serum calcium during exercise in female long distance runners. J Clin Endocrinol Metab 1993;76:867.
79. Grossman A, Sutton JR. Endorphins: what are they? How are they measured? What is their role in exercise? Med Sci Sports Exerc 1985;17:74.
80. Grundy SM, et al. Diabetes and cardiovascular disease: a statement for health professionals from the American Heart Association. Circulation 1999;100:1134.
81. Gu K, et al. Diabetes and decline in heart disease mortality in US adults. JAMA 1999;281:1291.
82. Gyntelberg FM, et al. Effect of training on the response of plasma glucagon to exercise. J Appl Physiol: Respir Environ Exerc Physiol 1977;43:302.
83. Hackney AC, et al. Basal reproductive hormonal profiles are altered in endurance trained men. J Sports Med Phys Fitness 1998;38:138.
84. Hagberg JM, et al. Exercise training-induced blood pressure and plasma lipid improvements in hypertensives may be genotype dependent. Hypertension 1999;34:18.
85. Haggendal L, et al. Arterial noradrenaline concentration during exercise in relation to the relative work levels. Scand J Clin Lab Invest 1970;26:337.
86. Hakkinen KA, et al. Basal concentrations and acute responses of serum hormones and strength development during heavy resistance training in middle-aged and elderly men and women. J Gerontol A Biol Sci Med Sci 2000;55:B95.
87. Hakkinen KA, et al. Neuromuscular and hormonal adaptations in athletes to strength training in two years. J Appl Physiol 1988;65:2406.
88. Hallmark MA, et al. Effects of chromium and resistive training on muscle strength and body composition. Med Sci Sports Exerc 1996;28:139.
89. Hansen JB, et al. Biphasic changes in leukocytes induced by strenuous exercise. Eur J Appl Physiol 1991;62:157.
90. Hansen PA, et al. Increased GLUT-4 translocation mediates enhanced insulin sensitivity of muscle glucose transport after exercise. J Appl Physiol 1998;85:1218.
91. Heitkamp HC, et al. Endurance training in females: changes in beta-endorphin and ACTH. Int J Sports Med 1998;19:260.
92. Hemilä H. Vitamin C and common cold incidence: a review of studies with subjects under heavy physical stress. Int J Sports Med 1996;17:379.
93. Henson DA, et al. Carbohydrate supplementation and lymphocyte proliferative response to long endurance running. Int J Sports Med 1998;19:574.
94. Heitkamp HC, et al. Endurance training in females: changes in beta-endorphin and ACTH. Int J Sports Med 1998;19:260.
95. Hickson RC, et al. Glutamine prevents down-regulation of myosin heavy-chain synthesis and muscle atrophy from glucocorticoids. Am J Physiol 1995;31:E730.
96. Hirshman MF, et al. Exercise training increases GLUT-4 protein in rat adipose cells. Am J Physiol 1993;264:E882.
97. Holm G, Stromblad G. Type I diabetes and physical exercise. Acta Med Scand 1983;671(suppl):95.
98. Houmard JA, et al. Testosterone, cortisol, and creatine kinase levels in male distance runners during reduced training. Int J Sports Med 1990;11:41.
99. Houmard JA, et al. Elevated skeletal muscle glucose transporter levels in exercise-trained middle-aged men. Am J Physiol 1991;261:E437.
100. Howlett TA, et al. Release of beta-endorphin and met-enkephalin during exercise in normal women: response to training. Br Med J 1984;288:1950.
101. Howlett TA. Hormonal responses to exercise and training: a short review. Clin Endocrinol 1987;26:723.
102. Hu GB, et al. Walking compared with vigorous physical activity and the risk of type 2 diabetes in women: a prospective study. JAMA 1999;282:1433.
103. Inder WJ, et al. Prolonged exercise increases peripheral plasma ACTH, CRH, and AVP in male athletes. J Appl Physiol 1998;85:835.
104. Ivy JL. Muscle glycogen synthesis before and after exercise. Sports Med 1991;11:6.
105. Ivy JL, et al. Prevention and treatment of non-insulin-dependent diabetes mellitus. Exerc Sport Sci Rev 1999;27:1.
106. Jahreis G, et al. Effect of endurance exercise on somatomedin-C/insulin-like growth factor I concentration in male and female runners. Exp Clin Endocrinol 1989;94:89.
107. Jaskowski MA, et al. Enkephalin metabolism: effect of acute exercise stress and cardiovascular fitness. Med Sci Sports Exerc 1989;21:154.
108. Jeng K-CG, et al. Supplementation with vitamins C and E enhances cytokine production by peripheral blood mononuclear cells in healthy adults. Am J Clin Nutr 1996;64:960.
109. Jensen J, et al. Comparison of changes in testosterone after strength and endurance exercise in well trained men. Eur J Appl Physiol 1991;63:467.
110. Johannessen A, et al. Prolactin, growth hormone, thyrotropin, 3,5,3-triiodothyronine, and thyroxine response to exercise after fat and carbohydrate enriched diet. J Clin Endocrinol Metab 1981;52:56.
111. Jonsdottir IH, et al. Voluntary chronic exercise augments in vivo natural immunity in rats. J Appl Physiol 1997;80:1799.
112. Jonsdottir IH, et al. Physical exercise, endogenous opioids and immune function. Acta Physiol Scand Suppl 1997;640:47.
113. Jonsdottir IH, et al. Enhancement of natural immunity seen after voluntary exercise in rats. Role of central opioid receptors. Life Sci 2000;66:1231.
114. Jurkowski J, et al. Ovarian hormone response to exercise. J Appl Physiol 1978;44:109.
115. Kajuura JS, et al. Immune responses to changes in training intensity and volume in runners. Med Sci Sports Exerc 1995;27:1111.
116. Kanaley JA, et al. Substrate oxidation and GH responses to exercise are independent of menstrual phase and status. Med Sci Sports Exerc 1992;24:873.
117. Kanaley JA, et al. Human growth hormone response to repeated bouts of aerobic exercise. J Appl Physiol 1997;83:1756.
118. Kang J, et al. Substrate utilization and glucose turnover during exercise of varying intensities in individuals with NIDDM. Med Sci Sports Exerc 1999;31:82.
119. Kannel WB, McGee DL. Diabetes and cardiovascular risk factors: the Framingham Study. Circulation 1979;59:8.
120. Kaplan NM. The deadly quartet: upper body obesity, glucose intolerance, hypertriglyceridemia, and hypertension. Arch Intern Med 1989;149:1514.
121. Karagiorgos A, et al. Growth hormone response to continuous and intermittent exercise. Med Sci Sports 1979;11:302.
122. Kastello GM, et al. Young and old subjects matched for aerobic capacity have similar noradrenergic responses to exercise. J Appl Physiol 1993;74:49.
123. Keast D, et al. Exercise and the immune response. Sports Med 1988;5:248.
124. King DS, et al. Time course for exercise-induced alterations in insulin action and glucose tolerance in middle aged people. J Appl Physiol 1995;78:17.
125. Kjaer M. Regulation of hormonal and metabolic responses during exercise in humans. Exerc Sport Sci Rev 1992;20:161.
126. Klausen T, et al. Plasma levels of parathyroid hormone, vitamin D, calcitonin, and calcium in association with endurance exercise. Calcif Tissue Int 1993;52:205.

127. Koppel M, et al. Effects of elevated plasma noradrenaline concentration on the immune system in humans. Eur J Appl Physiol 1998;79:93.
128. Kraemer WJ. Endocrine responses and adaptations to strength training. In: Komi PV, ed. Encyclopedia of sports medicine: strength and power. London: Blackwell Scientific, 1992.
129. Kraemer WJ. Endocrine responses and adaptations to strength training. In: Komi PV, ed. Encyclopedia of sports medicine: strength and power. London: Blackwell Scientific, 1993.
130. Kraemer WJ. Hormonal mechanisms related to the expression of muscular strength and power. Kraemer WJ. Endocrine responses and adaptations to strength training. In: Komi PV, ed. Encyclopedia of sports medicine: strength and power. London: Blackwell Scientific, 1993.
131. Kraemer WJ, et al. Training responses of plasma beta-endorphin, adrenocorticotropin, and cortisol. Med Sci Sports Exerc 1989;21:146.
132. Kraemer WJ, et al. Effects of different heavy-resistance exercise protocols on plasma β-endorphin concentrations. J Appl Physiol 1993;74:450.
133. Kraemer WJ, et al. The effects of short-term resistance training on endocrine function in men and women. Eur J Appl Physiol 1998;78:69.
134. Kraemer WJ, et al. Acute hormonal responses to a single bout of heavy resistance exercise in trained power lifters and untrained men. Can J Appl Physiol 1999;24:524.
135. Kramer WJ. Endocrine responses to resistance exercise. Med Sci Sports Exerc 1988;29:S152.
136. Kreisman SH, et al. Epinephrine infusion during moderate intensity exercise increases glucose production and uptake. Am J Physiol 2000;278:E949.
137. Kreisman SH, et al. Glucoregulatory responses to intense exercise performed in the postprandial state. Am J Physiol 2000;278:E786.
138. Kriska AM, et al. The association of physical activity with obesity, fat distribution and glucose intolerance in Pima Indians. Diabetologia 1993;36:863.
139. Kriska AM, et al. The potential role of physical activity in the prevention of non-insulin-dependent diabetes mellitus: the epidemiological evidence. Exerc Sport Sci Rev 1994;22:21.
140. Kroll MH. Parathyroid hormone temporal effects on bone formation and resorption. Bull Math Biol 2000;62:163.
141. Lee I-M. Physical activity, fitness and cancer. In: Bouchard C, et al, eds. Physical activity, fitness, and health. Champaign, IL: Human Kinetics, 1994:.
142. Lockette W, et al. Endurance training and human α_2-adrenergic receptors on platelets. Med Sci Sports Exerc 1987;19:7.
143. Luger A, et al. Acute hypothalamic-pituitary-adrenal responses to the stress of treadmill exercise: physiologic adaptations to physical training. N Engl J Med 1987;316:1309.
144. MacIntyre JG. Growth hormone and athletes. Sports Med 1987;4:129.
145. Mackinnon LT. Future directions in exercise and immunology: regulation and integration. Int J Sports Med 1998;19:S205.
146. Mackinnon LT, Hooper Sl. Plasma glutamine and upper respiratory tract infection during intensified training in swimmers. Med Sci Sports Exerc 1996;28:285.
147. Mackinnon LT, Jenkins DG. Decreased salivary immunoglobins after intense interval exercise before and after training. Med Sci Sports Exerc 1993;25:678.
148. Maclean PS, et al. Muscle glucose transporter (GLUT 4) gene expression during exercise. Exer Sport Sci Rev 2000;28:148.
149. Manson JD, et al. A prospective study of exercise and incidence of diabetes among US male physicians. JAMA 1992;268:63.
150. Marliss EB, et al. Gender differences in glucoregulatory responses to intense exercise. J Appl Physiol 2000;88:457.
151. Mayer-Davis EJ, et al. Intensity and amount of physical activity in relation to insulin sensitivity. JAMA 1998;279:669.
152. McArthur JW. Endorphins and exercise in females: possible connection with reproductive dysfunction. Med Sci Sports Exerc 1985;17:82.
153. McCall GE, et al. Maintenance of mononuclear domain size in rat soleus after overload and growth hormone/IGF-I treatment. J Appl Physiol 1998;84:1407.
154. Meydani SN, et al. Vitamin E supplementation and in vivo immune response in healthy elderly subjects. JAMA 1997;277:1380.
155. Mezzetti M, et al. Population attributable risk for breast cancer: diet, nutrition, and physical exercise. J Natl Cancer Inst 1998;90:389.
156. Michelini LC, Morris M. Endogenous vasopressin modulates the cardiovascular responses to exercise. Ann NY Acad Sci 1999; 897:198.
157. Mikines KJ, et al. Seven days of bed rest decreases insulin action on glucose uptake in leg and whole body. J Appl Physiol 1991;70:1245.
158. Mora-Rodriguez R, Coyle EF. Effects of plasma epinephrine on fat metabolism during exercise: interactions with exercise intensity. Am J Physiol 2000;278:E669.
159. Morgan WP. Affective beneficence of vigorous physical activity. Med Sci Sports Exerc 1985;17:94.
160. Morris FL, et al. Prospective decrease in progesterone concentrations in female lightweight rowers during the competition season compared with the off season: a controlled study examining weight loss and intensive exercise. Br J Sports Med 1999;33:417.
161. Mujika I, et al. Physiological responses to a 6-d taper in middle-distance runners: influence of training intensity and volume. Med Sci Sports Exerc 2000;32:511.
162. Müns G, et al. Impaired nasal mucociliary clearance in long-distance runners. Int J Sports Med 1995;16:209.
163. Naveri H, et al. Metabolic and hormonal changes in moderate and intense long-term running exercises. Int J Sports Med 1985;6:276.
164. Nehlsen-Cannarella SL, et al. Carbohydrate and cytokine response to 2.5 hr of running. J Appl Physiol 1997;82:1662.
165. Nieman DC. Physical activity, fitness, and infection. In: Bouchard C, et al, eds. Physical activity, fitness, and health. Champaign, IL: Human Kinetics, 1994: .
166. Nieman DC. Immune response to heavy exertion. J Appl Physiol 1997;82:1385.
167. Nieman DC, et al. Physical activity and immune function in elderly women. Med Sci Sports Exerc 1993;25:823.
168. Nieman DC, et al. Natural killer cell cytotoxic activity in weight trainers and sedentary controls. J Strength Cond Res 1994;8:251.
169. Nieman DC, et al. The acute immune response to exhaustive resistance exercise. Int J Sports Med 1995;16:322.
170. Nieman DC, et al. Carbohydrate supplementation affects blood granulocyte and monocyte trafficking but not function following 2.5 h of running. Am J Clin Nutr 1997;66:153.
171. Nieman DC, et al. Influence of mode and carbohydrate on the cytokine response to heavy exertion. Med Sci Sports Exerc 1998;30:671.
172. Pakarinen A, et al. Serum thyroid hormones, thyrotropin and thyroxine binding globulin during prolonged strength training. Eur J Appl Physiol 1988;57:394.
173. Pan X, et al. Effects of diet and exercise in preventing NIDDM in people with impaired glucose tolerance: the DaQuing and Diabetes Study. Diabetes Care 1997;20:537.
174. Pedersen BK. Influence of physical activity on the cellular immune system: mechanism of action. Int J Sports Med 1991;12:S23.
175. Pedersen BK, et al. Exercise and the immune system—influence of nutrition and aging. J Sci Med Sport 1999;2:234.
176. Peronnet F, et al. Plasma norepinephrine response to exercise before and after training in humans. J Appl Physiol 1992;51:812.
177. Peters EM, et al. Vitamin C supplementation reduces the incidence of postrace symptoms of upper-respiratory-tract infection in ultramarathon runners. Am J Clin Nutr 1993;57:170.
178. Peters-Futre EM. Vitamin C, neutrophil function, and URTI risk in distance runners: the missing link. Exerc Immunol Rev 1997;3:32.
179. Ponjee GAE, et al. Androgen turnover during marathon running. Med Sci Sports Exerc 1994;26:1274.
180. Prior JC, et al. Prolactin changes with exercise vary with breast motion: analysis of running versus cycling. Fertil Steril 1981;36:268.
181. Reaven GM. Syndrome X: 6 years later. J Intern Med 1994;736 (suppl):13.
182. Reaven GM. The kidney: an unwilling accomplice in syndrome X. Am J Kidney Dis 1997;30:928.
183. Reaven GM. Insulin resistance and human disease: a short history. J Basic Clin Physiol Pharmacol 1998;9:387.
184. Reynolds TH, et al. Effects of exercise training on insulin- and hypoxia-stimulated glucose transport in isolated rat epitrochlearis muscle: assessment of cell-surface GLUT-4 using ATB-BMPA photolabeling. Am J Physiol 1997;264:E320.
185. Richter EA, Sutton JR. Hormonal adaptation to physical activity. In: Bouchard C, et al, eds. Physical activity, fitness, and health. Champaign, IL: Human Kinetics, 1994: .
186. Richter EA, et al. Muscle glycogenolysis during exercise: dual control by epinephrine and contractions. Am J Physiol 1982;242:E25.
187. Rocchini AP, et al. The effects of weight loss on the sensitivity of blood pressure to sodium in obese adolescents. N Engl J Med 1989;321:580.

188. Rodnick K, et al. Improved insulin action in muscle, liver and adipose tissue in physically trained human subjects. Am J Physiol 1987;253: E489.
189. Rohde T, et al. Competitive sustained exercise in humans, lymphokine activated killer cell activity, and glutamine—an intervention study. Eur J Appl Physiol 1998;78:448.
190. Rohde T, et al. Effect of glutamine supplementation on changes in the immune system induced by repeated exercise. Med Sci Sports Exerc 1998;30:856.
191. Rosolowska-Huszcz D. The effect of exercise training intensity on thyroid activity at rest. J Physiol Pharmacol 1998;49:457.
192. Rowbottom DG, et al. The emerging role of glutamine as an indicator of exercise stress and overtraining. Sports Med 1996;21:80.
193. Ruby BC, et al: Effects of estradiol on substrate turnover during exercise in amenorrheic females. Med Sci Sports Exerc 1977;29:1160.
194. Salvesen H, et al. Intact serum parathyroid hormone levels increase during running exercise in well-training men. Calcif Tissue Int 1994;54:256.
195. Scanga CB, et al. Effects of weight loss and exercise training on natural killer cell activity in obese women. Med Sci Sports Exerc 1998;30:1668.
196. Schoen RE, et al. Increased blood glucose and insulin, body size, and incidence of colorectal cancer. J Natl Cancer Inst 1999;91:1147.
197. Schoff SM, Newcomb PA. Diabetes, body size, and risk of endometrial cancer. Am J Epidemiol 1998;148:234.
198. Schwab R, et al. Acute effects of different intensities of weight lifting on serum testosterone. Med Sci Sports Exerc 1993;25:1381.
199. Sharp NCC, Koutedakis Y. Sport and the overtraining syndrome: Immunological aspects. Br Med Bull 1992;48:518.
200. Shephard RJ, Shek PN. Exercise, aging and immune function. Int J Sports Med 1995;16:1.
201. Shephard RJ, Shek PN. Exercise, immunity, and susceptibility to infection. Phys Sportsmed 1999;27(6):47.
202. Shephard RJ, Sidney KH. Effects of physical exercise on plasma growth hormone and cortisol levels in human subjects. In: Wilmore JH, ed. Exercise and sport sciences reviews, vol 3. New York: Academic Press, 1975.
203. Shephard RJ, et al. The impact of exercise on the immune system: NK cells, interleukins 1 and 2, and related responses. Exerc Sport Sci Rev 1995;23:215.
204. Shewchuk LD, et al. Dietary L-glutamine does not improve lymphocyte metabolism or function in exercise-trained rats. Med Sci Sports Exerc 1997;29:474.
205. Simoneau J-A, et al. Altered glycolytic and oxidative capacities of skeletal muscle contribute to insulin resistance in NIDDM. J Appl Physiol 1997;83:166.
206. Smith DJ, Norris SR. Changes in glutamine and glutamate concentrations for tracking training tolerance. Med Sci Sports Exerc 2000;32:684.
207. Solomon C. Diabetes mellitus and risk of cardiovascular disease in women. Med Sci Sports Exerc 1996;28:15.
208. Song MK, et al. The mode of adrenal gland enlargement in the rat in response to exercise training. Pflügers Arch 1973;339:59.
209. Staron RS, et al. Skeletal muscle adaptations during the early phase of heavy-resistance training in men and women. J Appl Physiol 1994;76:1247.
210. Strauss RH, et al. Weight loss in amateur wrestlers and its effects on serum testosterone levels. JAMA 1985;254:3337.
211. Stich V, et al. Adipose tissue lipolysis is increased during a repeated bout of aerobic exercise. J Appl Physiol 2000;88:1277.
212. Strobel G, et al. Effect of severe exercise on plasma catecholamines in differently trained athletes. Med Sci Sports Exerc 1999;31:560.
213. Suay F, et al. Effects of competition and its outcome on serum testosterone, cortisol and prolactin. Psychoneuroendocrinology 1999;24:551.
214. Sutton JR, et al. Plasma vasopressin, catecholamines and lactate during exhaustive exercise at extreme simulated altitude: "Operation Everest II." Can J Appl Sports Sci 1986;11:43P.
215. Tadjoré M, et al. Effects of dietary manipulations and glucose infusion on glucagon response during exercise in rats. J Appl Physiol 1997;83:148.
216. Tarnopolsky L, et al. Gender differences in hormonal and metabolic responses to prolonged exercise in males and females. J Appl Physiol 1990;68:650.
217. Taylor-Tolbert NS, et al. Ambulatory blood pressure after acute exercise in older men with essential hypertension. Am J Hypertens 2000;13:44.
218. Tsai KS, et al. Effect of exercise and exogenous glucocorticoid on serum level of intact parathyroid hormone. Int J Sports Med 1997;18:583.
219. Vitug A, et al. Exercise and type I diabetes mellitus. In: Pandolf KB, ed. Exercise and sport sciences reviews, vol. 16. New York: Macmillan, 1988.
220. Vogel RB, et al. Increase of free and total testosterone during submaximal exercise in normal males. Med Sci Sports Exerc 1985;17:119.
221. Vukovich MD, et al. Changes in insulin action and GLUT-4 with 6 days of inactivity in endurance runners. J Appl Physiol 1996;80:240.
222. Wade CE. Response, regulation, and actions of vasopressin during exercise: a review. Med Sci Sports Exerc 1984;16:506.
223. Wade CE, et al. Plasma aldosterone and renal function in runners during a 20-day road race. Eur J Appl Physiol 1985;54:456.
224. Wallace MB, et al. Effects of cross-training on markers of insulin resistance/hyperinsulinemia. Med Sci Sports Exerc 1997;29:1170.
225. Wallberg-Henriksson H. Exercise and diabetes mellitus. Exerc Sport Sci Rev 1992;20:339.
226. Walsh NP, Blannin AK. Effect of oral glutamine supplementation on human neutrophil lipopolysaccharide-stimulated degranulation following prolonged exercise. Int J Sport Nutr Exerc Metab 2000;1:39.
227. Wannamethee, S.G., et al.: Physical activity, metabolic factors, and the incidence of coronary heart disease and type 2 diabetes. Arch Intern Med 160:2108, 2000.
228. Weidner TG, et al. The effect of exercise training on the severity and duration of a viral upper respiratory illness. Med Sci Sports Exerc 1998;30:1578.
229. Weinstock C, et al. Effect of exhaustive exercise stress on the cytokine response. Med Sci Sports Exerc 1997;29:345.
230. Weltman A, et al. Endurance training amplifies the pulsatile release of growth hormone: effects of training intensity. J Appl Physiol 1992;72:2188.
231. Weltman A, et al. Exercise training decreases the growth hormone (GH) response to acute constant-load exercise. Med Sci Sports Exerc 1997;29:669.
232. Whaley MH, et al. Physical fitness and clustering of risk factors associated with the metabolic syndrome. Med Sci Sports Exerc 1999;31:287.
233. Wheeler GD. Reduced serum testosterone and prolactin levels in male distance runners. JAMA 1984;252:514.
234. Wheeler GD. Endurance training decreases serum testosterone levels in men without change in luteinizing hormone pulsatile release. J Clin Endocrinol Metab 1991;72:422.
235. White RD, Sherman C. Exercise in diabetes management: maximizing benefits, controlling risks. Phys Sportsmed 1999;27(4):63.
236. Whiteside TL, Herberman RB. Short analytical review: the role of natural killer cells in human diseases. Clin Immunol Immunopathol 1989;53:1.
237. Winder WW, Heninger V. Effect of exercise on tissue levels of thyroid hormones in the rat. Am J Physiol 1971;221:1139.
238. Winder WE, et al. Time course of sympatho-adrenal adaptation to endurance exercise training in man. J Appl Physiol 1978;45:370.
239. Wing RR, et al. Exercise in a behavioral weight control programme for obese patients with type II (non-insulin-dependent) diabetes. Diabetologia 1988;31:902.
240. Woods JA, Davis JM. Exercise, monocyte/macrophage function, and cancer. Med Sci Sports Exerc 1994;26:147.
241. Woods JA, et al. Exercise and cellular innate immune function. Med Sci Sports Exerc 1999;31:57.
242. Xiao-ren P, et al. Effects of diet and exercise in preventing NIDDM in people with impaired glucose tolerance. Diabetes Care 1997;20:537.
243. Yates A, et al. Running—an analogue of anorexia. N Engl J Med 1983;308:251.
244. Yoon J-W, et al. Control of autoimmune diabetes in NOD mice by GAD expression or suppression in cells. Science 1999;284:1183.
245. Zerath E, et al. Effect of endurance training on postexercise parathyroid hormone levels in elderly men. Med Sci Sports Exerc 1997;29:1139.

PART *Two*

APPLIED EXERCISE PHYSIOLOGY

SECTION

4

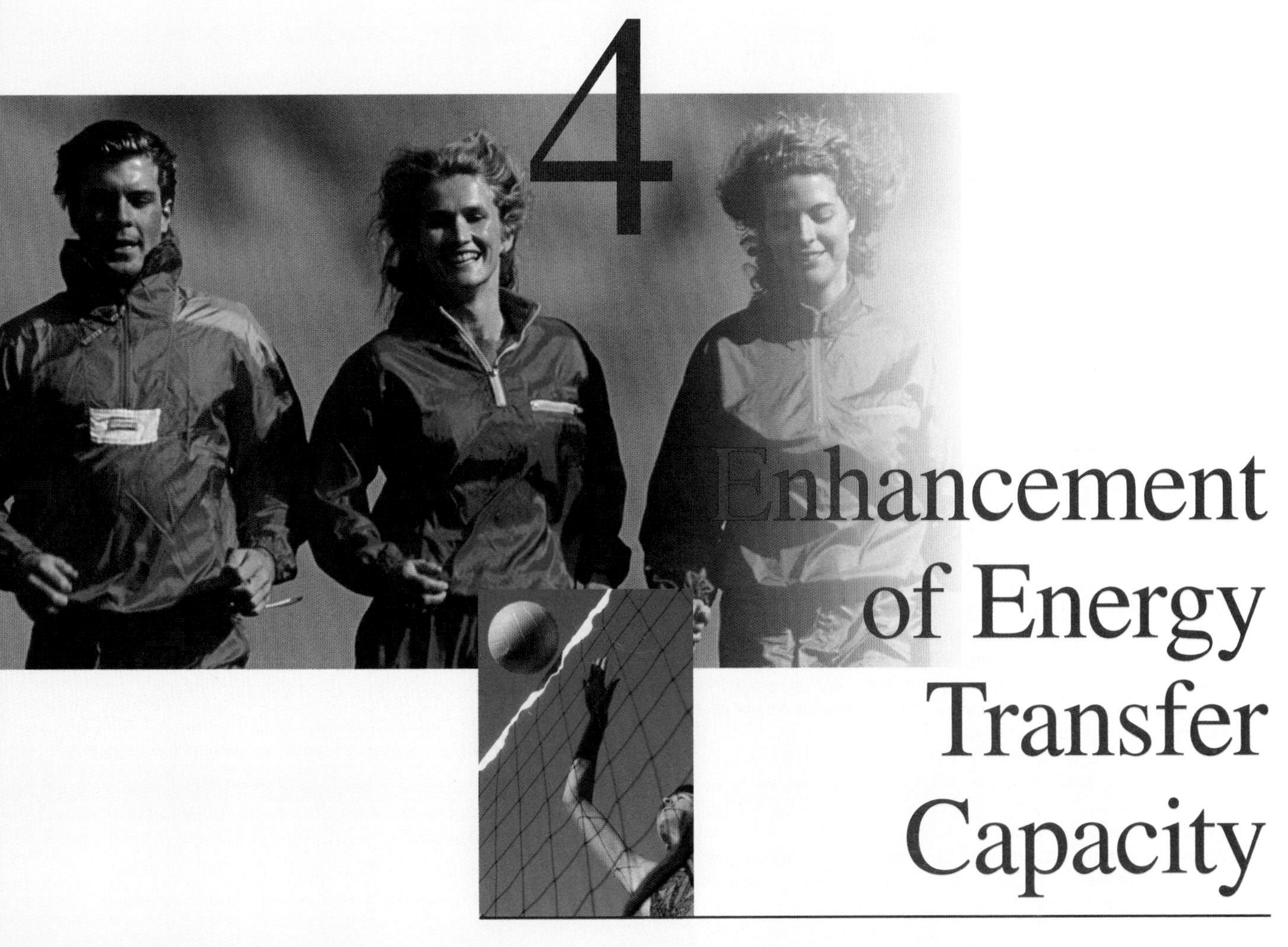

Enhancement of Energy Transfer Capacity

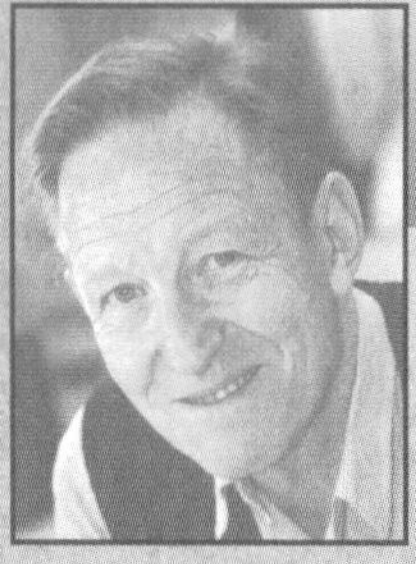

Interview with Bengt Saltin

Name: Bengt Saltin

Education: Södertälje Gymnasium (1955); Medical School, Karolinska Institute, Stockholm (1956–62); Thesis in physiology, Karolinksa Institute, Stockholm (1964).

Current Affiliation: Director, Copenhagen Muscle Research Centre at Rigshospitalet and the University of Copenhagen; Adjunct professor, August Krogh Institute, University of Copenhagen

Honors and Awards: See Appendix E.

Research Focus: Exploration of integrative cardiovascular and metabolic response to physical exercise, including studies on skeletal muscle in humans by direct needle biopsy.

Memorable Publication: Saltin B, et al. Response to exercise after bed rest and after training: A longitudinal study of adaptive changes in oxygen transport and body composition. Circulation. 1968;38:VIII-79.

Statement of Contributions: ACSM Honor Award
In recognition of his studies which provide a better understanding of maximal oxygen uptake in human subjects under different physiological and patho-physiological conditions, particularly thermal stress and dehydration.

His classic study on exercise after bed rest and after training was the scientific foundation for the current early ambulation and exercise treatment of patients with coronary heart disease and the understanding of deconditioning that occurs in space travel.

In the late 1960s, he began his seminal studies on skeletal muscle in humans obtained by direct needle biopsy. This pioneering work has had a profound influence on our understanding of the anatomical, physiological, and biochemical behavior of skeletal muscle and its interactions with the cardiovascular system. His recent work has determined the maximal flow capacity in active skeletal muscle, and shows that the limiting factor in maximal oxygen uptake is the pumping capacity of the heart.

Dr. Saltin has provided training for many of the current leaders in exercise and sports science and they have greatly benefited from his unique ability to acquire new knowledge by studying at all levels of integration.

➤ What first inspired you to enter the exercise science field? What made you decide to pursue your advanced degree and/or line of research?

In January of 1958, I had my oral examination in physiology as part of my medical studies. The examiner was Professor Ulf von Euler (later the 1970 Nobel Prize winner in Physiology and Medicine for discoveries concerning humoral transmitters in the nerve terminal and the mechanisms for their storage, release, and inactivation). At the end of the examination I was asked whether I would be interested in staying on as a student instructor. My answer was yes. As I had an interest in orienteering (a common sport in Scandinavia), I wanted to be associated with exercise-related research. Professor Euler called Erik Hohwü-Christensen, who was the professor of physiology at the Royal School of Gymnastics. The week after I met with Professor Hohwü-Christensen in the summer of 1958, I started to work with him on a project that evaluated energy demands in intermittent exercise. During the semesters, I helped with teaching while at the same time continuing my medical studies. In the fall of 1961, I decided to go for a doctoral thesis in physiology, which I defended in May 1964.

➤ Who were the most influential people in your career, and why?

Two people played a very important role in my scientific career. I would like to acknowledge Professor Erik Hohwü-Christensen and Professor Per-Olof Åstrand. Professor Hohwü-Christensen had been a student of Johannes Lindhard, the first Docent of the equivalent of an endowed Chair in Anatomy, Physiology, and Theory of Gymnastics at the University of Copenhagen, and had also done cooperative research with 1920 Nobel Prize winner August Krogh. Professor Per-Olof Åstrand at the Karolinska Institute was the equivalent of my PhD dissertation research advisor. My projects were concerned with trying to better understand maximal oxygen uptake in human subjects and its determinants under different physiological and pathophysiological conditions, particularly thermal stress and dehydration. The knowledge and passion of these two pioneer scientists encouraged a younger generation of researchers-to-be to focus on human integrative physiology.

➤ What has been the most interesting/enjoyable aspect of your involvement in science? What was the least interesting/enjoyable aspect?

This is a difficult question to answer. I have been very fortunate to work with many scientists from all over the world. For example, in 1965, I spent 1 year in the Department of Medicine at the University of Texas in Dallas. Later, I worked for 5 months at the John B. Pierce Institute and Department of Physiology at Yale University in New Haven, Connecticut. In 1972, I spent 2 months in the Department of Medicine at the University of California, San Francisco, and then in 1976, I spent 3 months working with David Costill in The Human Performance Laboratory at Ball State University in Muncie, Indiana. I also spent 4 months at Cumberland College and the Department of Physiology at New South Wales University in Sydney, Australia. For my interest in high-altitude physiology and temperature regulation, I was fortunate to spend from 1 to 5 months between the years

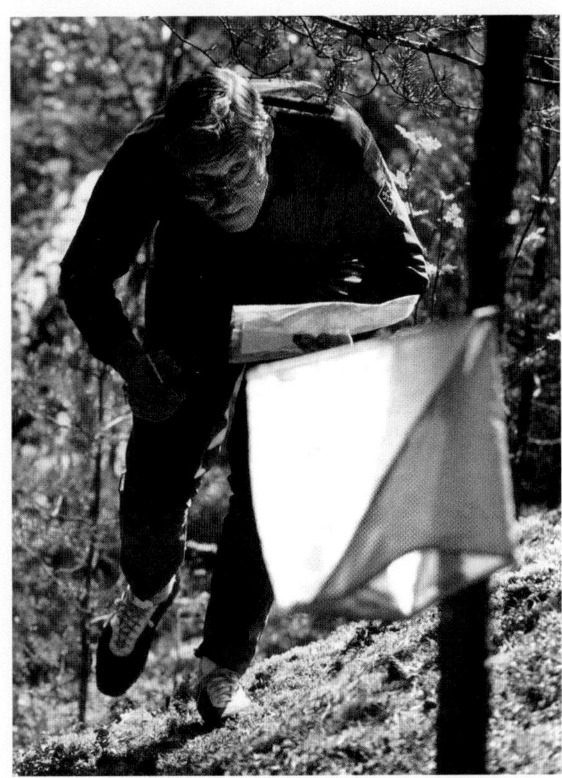

of 1960 and 1989 in laboratories in Northern Norway studying the physical profile and health of Nomadic Lapps, and at the following locations studying high-altitude physiology: Mt. Evans (Colorado), Mexico City, the Andes and Himalayan mountains, and Kenya. I also had a wonderful experience studying the physiological responses to exercise in racing camels in the Arabian desert.

➤ What is your most meaningful contribution to the field of exercise science, and why is it so important?

To try to better understand, not only to describe, basic phenomena concerned with physiological responses to exercise under various environmental conditions. Exercise science was a key area in science in the latter part of the 19th century and in the first three decades of the 20th century. There are many reasons for the lack of major contributions since then. One reason could be that the majority of exercise scientists describe a phenomenon, but they do not try hard enough to penetrate the mechanisms and thereby contribute to the fundamental understanding of the phenomenon.

➤ What advice would you give to students who express an interest in pursuing a career in exercise science research?

Become very focused and learn basic techniques. Today, exercise science is to a large extent the study of acute and chronic adaptations. Thus, one route I would highlight is to identify the exercise stimulus and the intracellular signalling of genes of importance for muscle adaptation. In a recent article in Scientific American *(September 2000), we pointed out that Olympic athletes depend on how well their muscles adapt to the stress of high-intensity aerobic, anaerobic, and resistance training. However, recent research suggests that the ratio of fast-to-slow-twitch muscle fibers depends on inherited characteristics. Unfortunately, future genetic technologies could change even that as athletes experiment with methods to enhance muscle performance.*

➤ What interests have you pursued outside your professional career?

I have been heavily involved in the sport of orienteering, both as a runner and administrator. From 1982 to 1988, I served as a Board Member and President of the International Orienteering Federation. I am a theater freak and have an interest in literature. Ibsen and Strindberg are my favorites, but most classical plays from antique Greece onwards will bring me to the theater. Throughout life my "reading companions" have been Katherine Mansfield, Albert Camus, Joseph Brodsky, and to name a Dane, J.P. Jacobsen.

➤ You have the opportunity to give a last lecture. Describe its primary focus.

I have given my "last" lecture. It focused on how young exercise physiologists could best serve an area in research and also make a major contribution to science. A major point was to identify an important phenomenon. If there are ample methods to study it, then stay with it until it has been solved. In other words, be mechanistic, carefully explain the phenomena, and then do whatever you can to understand it.

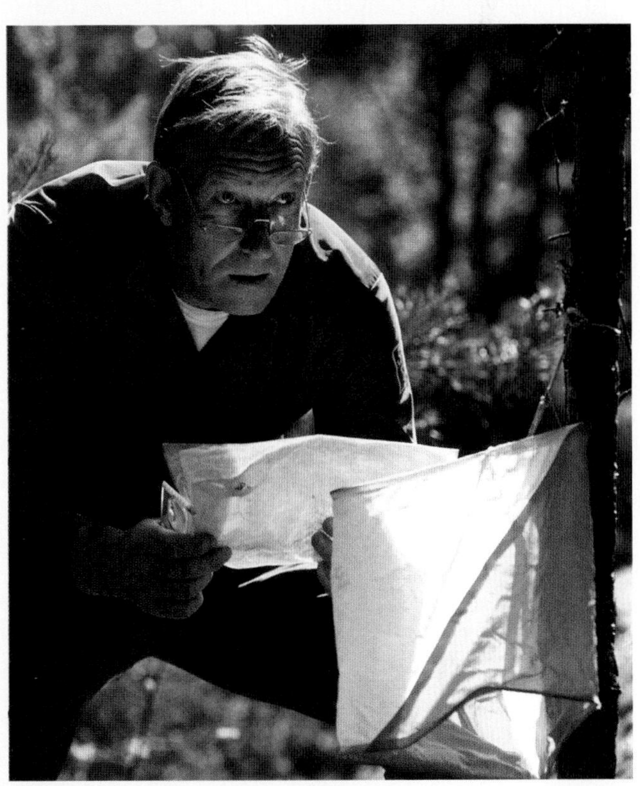

CHAPTER 21

Training for Anaerobic and Aerobic Power

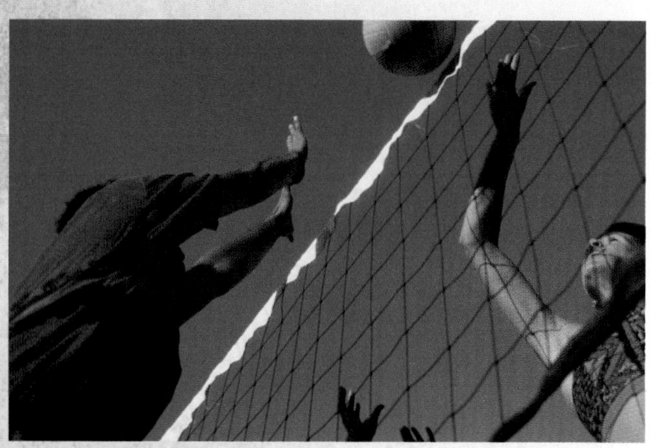

Chapter Objectives

- Discuss and provide examples of the exercise training principles of (1) overload, (2) specificity, (3) individual differences, and (4) reversibility
- Outline the metabolic adaptations from anaerobic exercise training
- Outline the metabolic, cardiovascular, and pulmonary adaptations from aerobic exercise training
- Discuss factors that contribute to expansion of the a-$\bar{v}$ O_2 difference during graded exercise, and how endurance training affects each component
- Explain the effects of endurance training on regional blood flow
- Explain the term athlete's heart; contrast structural and functional characteristics of an endurance athlete's heart and a resistance-trained athlete's heart
- Describe the influence of (1) initial fitness level, (2) genetics, (3) training frequency, (4) training duration, and (5) training intensity on the response to aerobic training
- Discuss the rationale for using heart rate to establish exercise intensity for aerobic training
- Discuss the term *training-sensitive zone,* including its rationale, advantages, limitations, and use for men and women of different ages
- Give the reason for adjusting the "training-sensitive zone" for swimming and other forms of upper-body exercise
- Justify the use of "rating of perceived exertion" to establish exercise intensity for aerobic training
- Outline advantages of training at the lactate threshold
- Contrast continuous and intermittent aerobic exercise training and give the advantages and disadvantages of each
- Summarize the latest recommendations by the American College of Sports Medicine concerning the recommended quantity and quality of exercise for developing and maintaining cardiorespiratory and muscular fitness and flexibility in healthy adults
- Outline the application of the overload principle to train the (1) intramuscular high-energy phosphates and (2) glycolytic energy system
- Summarize important factors that compose the exercise prescription for interval training
- Describe the most common form of overtraining syndrome and summarize the interacting factors that initiate overtraining in endurance athletes
- Summarize current opinion concerning recommendations for regular physical activity during pregnancy

Throughout this book we emphasize that different physical activities, depending on duration and intensity, activate specific energy transfer systems. Figure 21.1 illustrates exercise broadly classified for duration and predominant energy pathways. We realize the difficulty in placing certain activities into one category. For example, as a person increases aerobic fitness, an activity previously classified as anaerobic may become aerobic. In many cases, all three energy-transfer systems—the adenosine triphosphate–phosphocreatine (ATP-PCr) system, the lactic acid system, and the aerobic system—operate predominantly at different times during exercise. Their relative contributions to the energy continuum directly relate to the duration and intensity (power output) of the specific activity.

Brief power activities lasting up to 6 seconds rely almost exclusively on "immediate" energy generated from breakdown of the stored intramuscular high-energy phosphates, ATP and PCr. Consequently, power athletes (e.g., sprinters, football players, shot-putters, pole vaulters) must gear training toward improving this energy-transfer capacity. As all-out exercise progresses to 60-second duration and power output decreases somewhat, most energy still arises through anaerobic pathways. These metabolic reactions, however, also involve the short-term energy system of glycolysis, with subsequent lactate accumulation. As exercise intensity diminishes and duration extends to 2 to 4 minutes, reliance on energy from the intramuscular phosphagens and anaerobic glycolysis decreases, and aerobic ATP production becomes increasingly more important. Prolonged exercise progresses on a "pay-as-you-go" basis, with aerobic metabolism generating more than 99% of the energy requirement. Clearly, an efficient training program allocates a proportionate commitment to proper training of the specific energy and physiologic systems activated in the activity. In the sections that follow, we discuss anaerobic and aerobic conditioning, with emphasis on principles, methods, and acute responses and longer-term training adaptations. *The basic approach to physiologic conditioning applies similarly to men and women within a broad age range: both respond and adapt to training in essentially the same manner.*

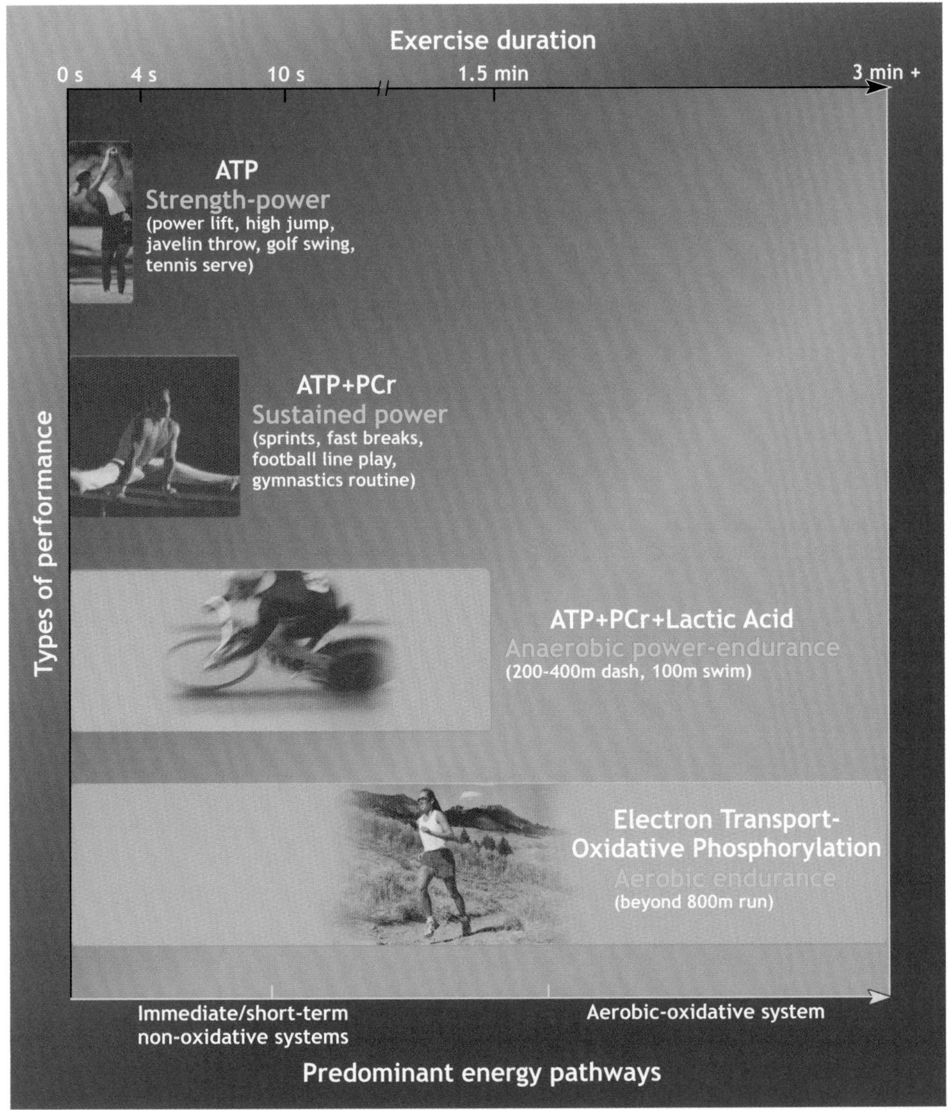

FIGURE 21.1 • Classification of physical activity on the basis of duration of all-out exercise and the corresponding predominant intracellular energy pathways.

TRAINING PRINCIPLES

Stimulating structural and functional adaptations that improve performance in specific tasks is the major objective of exercise training. These adaptations require adherence to carefully planned programs, with attention focused on frequency and length of workouts, type of training, speed, intensity, duration, and repetition of the activity, rest intervals, and appropriate competition. Application of these factors varies, depending on the performance and fitness goals. However, several principles of physiologic conditioning are common to improving performance in the diverse physical activity classifications illustrated in Figure 21.1.

Overload Principle

The regular application of a specific exercise ***overload*** *enhances physiologic function to bring about a training response.* Exercising at intensities greater than normal induces a variety of highly specific adaptations that enable the body to function more efficiently. Achieving the appropriate overload requires manipulating combinations of training *frequency, intensity,* and *duration,* with focus on exercise *mode.*

The concept of individualized and progressive overload applies to athletes, sedentary persons, disabled persons, and even cardiac patients. An increasing number in this latter group have applied appropriate exercise rehabilitation to walk, jog, and eventually run marathons. As we discuss in Chapter 31, achieving significant health-related benefits of regular exercise (e.g., metabolic parameters, lipid profile, blood pressure) requires lower exercise intensity (but greater volume) than required to improve cardiovascular fitness.[6,16,50,51]

Specificity Principle

Exercise training specificity refers to adaptations in metabolic and physiologic functions that depend upon the type of overload imposed. A specific anaerobic exercise stress (e.g., strength–power training) induces specific strength–power adaptations, while specific endurance exercise stress elicits specific aerobic system adaptations—with only a limited interchange of benefits derived between strength–power and aerobic training.[92,219] However, the specificity principle extends beyond this broad demarcation. For example, aerobic training does not represent a singular entity requiring *only* cardiovascular overload. Aerobic training using the specific muscles in the desired performance most effectively improves aerobic fitness for such activities as swimming,[135] bicycling,[160] running,[138] or upper-body exercise.[121] Some evidence even suggests a temporal specificity in training response such that indicators of training improvement peak when measured at the time of day when training regularly occurred.[86] Furthermore, the most effective evaluation of sport-specific performance results when the laboratory measurement most closely simulates the actual sport activity and/or uses the muscle mass required by the sport.[14,66,188] *Simply stated, specific exercise elicits specific adaptations creating specific training effects.*

Specificity of $\dot{V}O_{2max}$

Table 21.1 presents results from research in one of our laboratories, concerning the specificity of endurance swim training on aerobic capacity improvements. Fifteen men trained 1 hour daily, 3 days per week, for 10 weeks. For all subjects, treadmill running and tethered swimming tests measured $\dot{V}O_{2max}$ before and after training. Because vigorous swimming elicits a general circulatory overload, we had expected at least some improvement (or "transfer") in aerobic power from swimming to running. This did not occur, however, as almost total specificity accompanied the $\dot{V}O_{2max}$ improvement with swim training. If treadmill running alone had evaluated swim-training effects, we would have mistakenly concluded no swim training effect!

When training for specific aerobic activities such as cycling, swimming, rowing, or running, the overload must (1) en-

TABLE 21.1 ➤ EFFECTS OF 10 WEEKS OF INTERVAL SWIM TRAINING ON CHANGES IN $\dot{V}O_{2MAX}$ AND ENDURANCE PERFORMANCE DURING RUNNING AND SWIMMING

		Running Test			Swimming Test		
Subjects	Measure	Pretraining	Posttraining	% Change	Pretraining	Posttraining	% Change
Swim Training							
	$\dot{V}O_{2max}$						
	$L \cdot min^{-1}$	4.05	4.11	+1.5	3.44	3.82	+11.0
	$mL \cdot kg^{-1} \cdot min^{-1}$	54.9	55.7	+1.5	46.6	51.8	+11.0
	Max work time						
	min	19.6	20.5	+4.6	11.9	15.9	+34.0
Nontraining Controls							
	$\dot{V}O_{2max}$						
	$L \cdot min^{-1}$	4.12	4.18	+1.5	3.51	3.40	+3.1
	$mL \cdot kg^{-1} \cdot min^{-1}$	55.1	55.5	+0.7	46.8	45.0	−3.8
	Max work time						
	min	20.7	19.7	−4.8	11.5	11.5	0

From Magel JR, et al. Specificity of swim training on maximum oxygen uptake. J Appl Physiol 1975;38:151.

gage the appropriate muscles required by the activity and (2) provide exercise stress for the cardiovascular system.[60,160] Little improvement occurs when measuring aerobic capacity with dissimilar exercise, yet the greatest improvement results when the test exercise duplicates the training exercise.[66,138] These results also emerge in exercise rehabilitation of patients with coronary artery disease.[154] The data in Table 21.1 also indicate that while swimming $\dot{V}O_{2max}$ improved 11% with swim training, maximum exercise time increased 34% during the swim test. Improvements in $\dot{V}O_{2max}$ probably reach a peak in training; thereafter, other mechanisms (only partly related to the capacity of the oxygen transport system) support performance improvements. These adaptations most likely take place within the active musculature rather than in relation to central circulatory factors (see "Focus on Research").

Whereas aerobic exercise training induces a highly specific $\dot{V}O_{2max}$ improvement, general improvements take place in cardiac function. For example, ventricular contractility that improves with one mode of exercise training also shows improvement when exercising the untrained limbs.[223] This finding indicates that one can condition the myocardium per se with diverse "big-muscle" exercise modes.

Specificity of Local Changes

Overloading specific muscle groups with endurance training enhances exercise performance and aerobic power by facilitating oxygen transport *and* use at the local level of the trained muscles.[88,129,184] For example, the vastus lateralis muscle of well-trained cyclists has greater oxidative capacity than that of endurance runners; oxidative capacity in these muscles improves significantly following training on a bicycle ergometer.[70] Such local adaptations would certainly increase the capacity of the trained muscles to generate ATP aerobically before the onset of lactate accumulation. The specificity of aerobic improvement may also result from greater regional blood flow in active tissues because of either (1) increased microcirculation, (2) more-effective distribution of cardiac output, or (3) the combined effect of both factors. Regardless of the mechanism, such adaptations would take place *only* in the specifically trained muscles and *only* manifest in exercise that activates this musculature.

Individual Differences Principle

Many factors contribute to individual variation in the training response. For example, a person's relative fitness level at the start of training exerts an influence. Even when a relatively homogenous group starts exercise training at the same time, one cannot expect each person to reach the same state of fitness (or exercise performance) after 10 or 12 weeks. Consequently, a coach should not insist that all athletes on the same team (or even in the same event) train the same way or at the same relative or absolute exercise intensity. It is unrealistic to expect all individuals to respond to a given training stimulus in the same manner.

Figure 21.2 shows the heart rate curves of two college varsity forwards during warm-up and four consecutive 15-minute quarters of a basketball game. The heart rate for player A *(yellow line)* averaged 174 b · min^{-1} during each of the four quarters. Player B *(red line)* showed a similar heart rate response pattern, except heart rate averaged 163 b · min^{-1} during the game, with relatively small heart rate variation for both players. This difference in the magnitude of heart rate response during the hour-long game illustrates that two individuals can perform at approximately equivalent intensity but at a 6.3% different level of cardiovascular strain as reflected by average exercise heart rate. *Optimal training benefits result with exercise programs geared to the individual needs and capacities of the participants.* As discussed in Chapter 11 and page 484 of this chapter, genetic factors clearly interact to influence the training response.

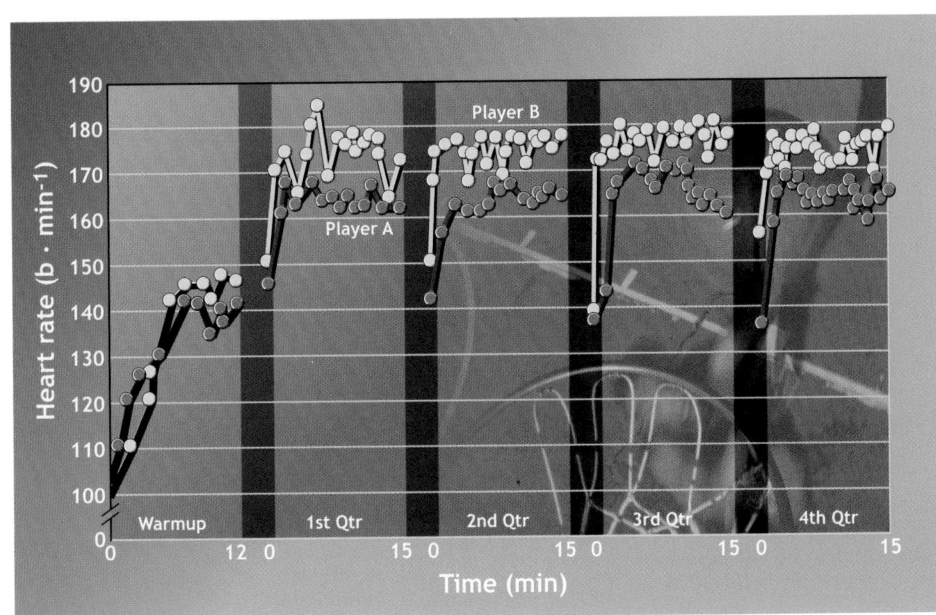

FIGURE 21.2 • Individual differences in heart rate response in two forwards during a 60-minute basketball game. For player A *(yellow line)*, the heart rate averaged 174 b · min^{-1}, and for player B *(red line)*, 163 b · min^{-1}. A miniature telemetry transmitter taped to each player's lower back monitored heart rate continuously throughout the game. (Data from F. Katch, Department of Exercise Science, University of Massachusetts, Amherst.)

Focus on Research

Highly Specific Nature of the Training Response

Saltin B, et al. The nature of the training response: peripheral and central adaptations to one-legged exercise. Acta Physiol Scand 1976;96:289.

➤ Research has focused on the specific versus general nature of exercise training adaptations. In 1976, Saltin and colleagues performed one of the first studies to show that regular exercise induces marked local adaptations in the trained muscles. Importantly, these adjustments not only enhance local blood flow and metabolism in response to physical activity, but also contribute significantly to general cardiovascular function during exercise.

In an elegant series of experiments the investigators separated local and general training effects. They applied different combinations of one-legged bicycle exercise to study simultaneously the adaptations of skeletal muscles and adaptations of central circulatory functions with training. Healthy but otherwise sedentary males with pretraining $\dot{V}O_{2max}$ of 46 $mL \cdot kg^{-1} \cdot min^{-1}$ (range, 37 to 54) were placed into three training groups: group A—one-legged endurance training (E) and the other leg sprint training (S); group B—one-legged S and the other leg no training (NT); group C—one-legged E and the other leg NT. Exercise training, performed on a bicycle ergometer with intensity adjusted to heart rate, lasted 4 weeks, with an average of 5 workouts per leg each week. The exercise intensity throughout training represented 75% for E and 150% for S of the one-legged $\dot{V}O_{2max}$ assessed pretraining and at week 3 to ensure proper training progression. Importantly, intensity and duration of each type of training produced similar total work output for each training bout. Total weekly energy output averaged 12,558 kcal (3000 J) per trained leg, with all groups achieving within 5 to 10% of this value; group A, however, performed 90 to 95% more work than group B because their training required both legs.

Pre- and posttraining measurements included needle biopsy samples from the quadriceps femoris for histochemical identification of muscle fiber type and area, glycogen concentration, and succinate dehydrogenase (SDH) and APTase enzyme activity. Subjects performed submaximal and maximal exercise for each leg and during two-legged maximal cycling (8 of 13 subjects to evaluate local metabolic adaptations to training). Measures included oxygen consumption, heart rate, arteriovenous oxygen difference ($a\text{-}\bar{v}\ O_2$ diff) in muscle blood flow (catheters inserted in the two femoral arteries and veins to measure each leg's blood flow), and glucose and lactate. Major findings showed that:

- Exercise training improved $\dot{V}O_{2max}$ (particularly for the E-trained leg) and lowered heart rate and blood lactate in submaximal exercise *only* when exercising with a trained leg.
- Training induced no change in muscle fiber composition but produced pronounced metabolic adaptations as reflected by enhanced SDH activity of the S- and E-trained legs, with no change in the NT leg. These changes generally paralleled increases in $\dot{V}O_{2max}$.
- Glycogen use during two-legged exercise remained lowest in the trained leg. Moreover, only the untrained leg continuously released lactate during submaximal exercise.

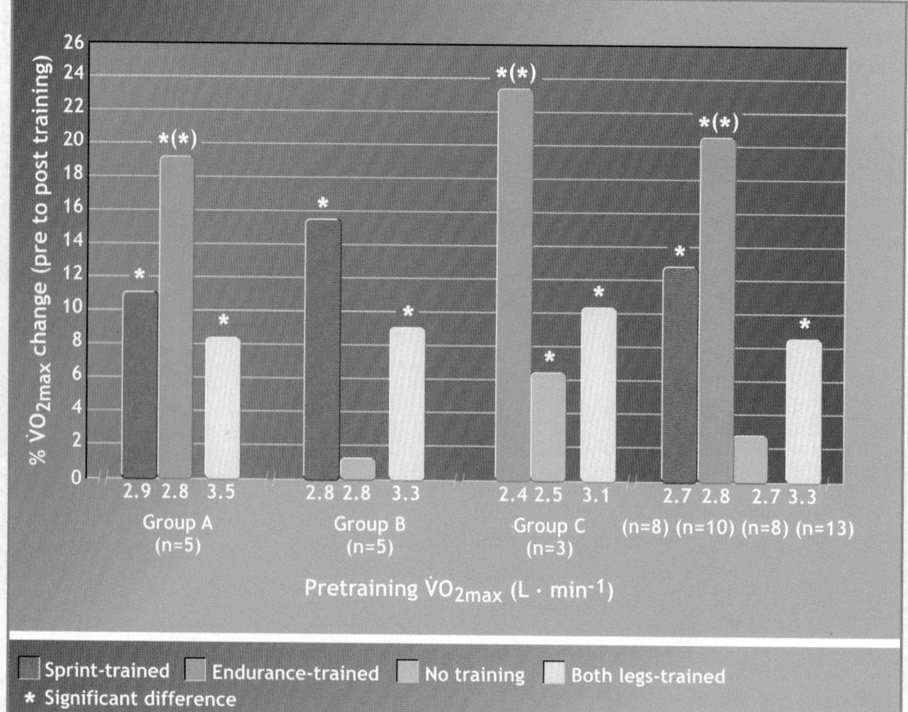

Figure 1. Mean values for percentage change in $\dot{V}O_{2max}$ in groups A, B, and C during one-legged exercise. Pretraining $\dot{V}O_{2max}$ values ($L \cdot min^{-1}$) are indicated below each bar. The *four bars on the far right* indicate average values for all untrained, sprint- or endurance-trained limbs and values for two-legged exercise regardless of training group; (*) denotes a statistically significant difference between sprint- and endurance-trained legs.

Focus on Research: Highly Specific Nature of the Training Response—*continued*

1. One-legged exercise
   Figure 1 shows that $\dot{V}O_{2max}$ increased nearly 20% with training in the E-trained leg, 11% in the S-trained leg, and 8% when exercising both legs (group A). S training of one leg only (group B) increased $\dot{V}O_{2max}$ by 15%, whereas $\dot{V}O_{2max}$ of the nontrained leg increased less than 2%. One-legged endurance training for group C increased $\dot{V}O_{2max}$ by 24% in the trained leg while $\dot{V}O_{2max}$ with the NT leg increased just 6%. These results confirmed that training only one leg exerts little effect on the nontrained leg, thus indicating considerable *training specificity.*
2. Two-legged exercise
   Analysis of pre- and posttraining two-legged $\dot{V}O_{2max}$ revealed mean increases for groups A (9%), B (10%), and C (8%). Figure 2 shows similar leg blood flow *(left panel)* in trained and untrained legs and in E-trained legs, compared with S-trained legs. In addition, similarity existed for a-$\bar{v}$ O_2 difference *(middle panel)* for S- and E-trained legs during exercise. In the four subjects with one trained and one untrained leg, the slightly higher a-$\bar{v}$ O_2 differences in the trained leg resulted from a lower oxygen content in the femoral blood draining the trained leg (greater O_2 extraction). Endurance- and sprint-trained legs showed similar calculated oxygen consumptions during exercise *(right panel);* some subjects, however, showed higher values in the trained leg than in the untrained leg.

The study's major impact demonstrated that an exercise training regimen elicits a distinct pattern of local adaptations *only* in the trained muscles. Furthermore, these specific local changes provide essential stimulation for the central cardiovascular response to exercise. Saltin and coworkers concluded that peripheral adaptations to training probably contribute as much to the training response as the well-documented improvement in central circulatory function.

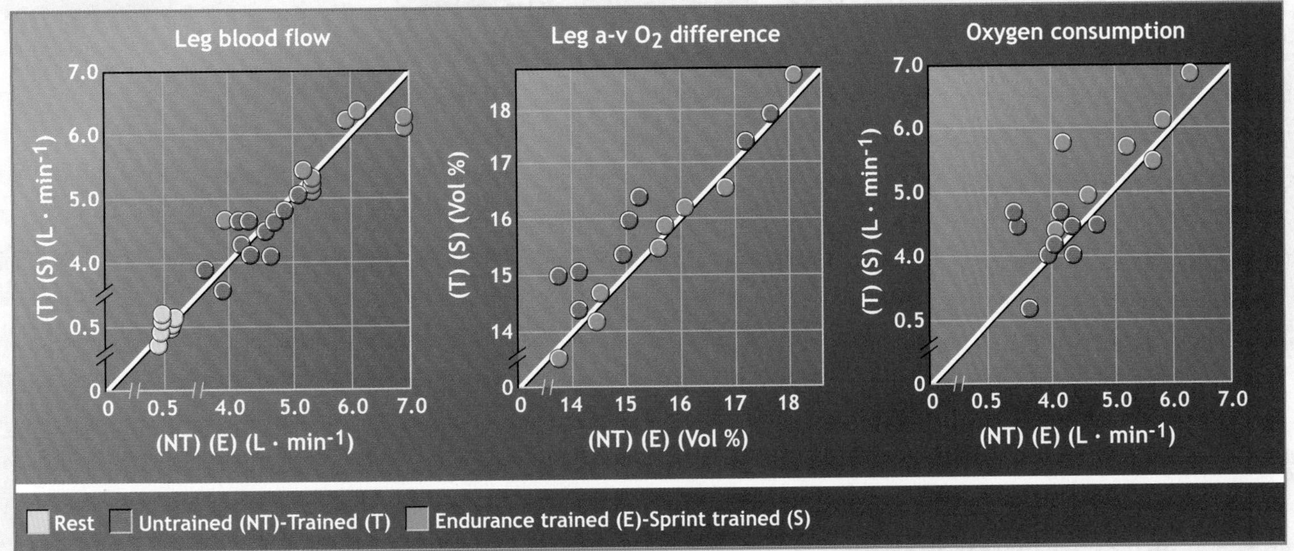

Figure 2. Leg blood flow *(left panel),* leg a-$\bar{v}$ O_2 difference *(middle panel),* and oxygen consumption *(right panel)* in each leg for subjects performing two-legged exercise for 1 hour at 70% of $\dot{V}O_{2max}$. Comparisons are made between the legs of four untrained subjects *(NT)* and four trained subjects (endurance-trained [T] or sprint-trained [S]). The panels also show trained and untrained leg comparisons for the four subjects who trained one leg with the endurance regimen and the other leg with sprint training.

Reversibility Principle

Loss of physiologic and performance adaptations (**detraining**) occurs rapidly when a person terminates participation in regular exercise.[151] Only 1 or 2 weeks of detraining significantly reduces both metabolic and exercise capacity, with many training improvements totally lost within several months. Table 21.2 shows the biologic consequences of various durations of short-term (<3 weeks) and longer-term (3 to 12 weeks) detraining in endurance-trained individuals. The data represent average responses reported in the literature. One research group provides particularly interesting findings.[192] In five subjects confined to bed for 20 consecutive days, $\dot{V}O_{2max}$ decreased by 25%. This decrease accompanied a similar decrement in maximal stroke volume and cardiac output, which decreased aerobic capacity an average of 1% each day. Additionally, the number of capillaries within trained muscle decreases between 14 and 25% within 3 weeks after training ceases.[191] For elderly subjects, 4 months of detraining results in the complete loss of endurance training adaptations on the cardiovascular system and the distribution of body water.[163]

Even among highly trained athletes, the beneficial effects of many years of prior exercise training remain transient and reversible. For this reason, most athletes begin a reconditioning program several months prior to the start of the competitive season or maintain some moderate level of off-season, sport-specific exercise to blunt the decline in physiologic functions from deconditioning.

PHYSIOLOGIC CONSEQUENCES OF TRAINING

We present many of the biologic changes that accompany training in other sections throughout this text. The following sections present a more detailed listing of the diverse adaptations to anaerobic and aerobic exercise training outlined in Table 21.3.

ANAEROBIC SYSTEM CHANGES WITH TRAINING

Figure 21.3 summarizes the metabolic adaptations in anaerobic function that accompany strenuous physical training that requires significant overload of the anaerobic systems of energy transfer. Consistent with the concept of training specificity, activities that demand a high level of anaerobic metabolism bring about specific changes in the immediate and short-term energy systems, without concomitant increases in aerobic functions. The changes that occur with sprint–power training include:

- *Increased levels of anaerobic substrates.* Muscle biopsy specimens taken before and after resistance

TABLE 21.2 ➤ CHANGES IN MEASURES OF PHYSIOLOGIC AND METABOLIC FUNCTION WITH VARIOUS DURATIONS OF DETRAINING[a]

VARIABLE	TRAINED	DETRAINED	CHANGE, % SHORT TERM DETRAINING[b]	CHANGE, % LONGER TERM DETRAINING[c]
$\dot{V}O_{2max}$, mL · kg^{-1} · min^{-1}	62.2	57.3	−8	
	62.1	50.8		−18
$\dot{V}O_{2max}$, L · min^{-1}	4.45	4.16	−7	
Cardiac output, L · min^{-1}	27.8	25.5	−8	
	27.8	25.2		−10
Stroke volume, mL	155	139	−10	
	148	129		−13
Heart rate, b · min^{-1}	186	193	4	
	187	197		5
Oxygen pulse, mL · b^{-1}	12.7	10.9		−14
Sum 3-min recovery HR	190	237		25
Plasma volume, L	2.91	2.56	−12	
a-$\bar{v}$ O_2 diff, mL · 100 mL^{-1}	15.1	15.4	−2 (NS)	
	15.1	14.1		−7
PCr, mM · (g wet wt)$^{-1}$	17.9	13.0		−27
ATP, mM · (g wet wt)$^{-1}$	5.97	5.08		−15
Glycogen, mM · (g wet wt)$^{-1}$	113.9	57.4		−50
Capillary density, cap · mm^{-2}	511	476	−7	
	464	476		−2 (NS)
Oxidative enzyme capacity			−29	−32
Myoglobin, mg · (g protein)$^{-1}$	43.3	41.0	−5 (NS)	
	43.3	40.7		−6
Insulin (rest)			17–120	
Norepinephrine/epinephrine (rest)			No change	
Norepinephrine/epinephrine (exercise)				65–100
Blood lactate			88	
Lactate threshold			−7	−18
Exercise lipolysis			−52	
Muscle glycogen synthesis			−29	−40
Time to fatigue, min			−10	
Swim power, W				−14
Elbow extension strength, ft-lb	39.0	25.5		−35

[a]Data represent an average computed from individual studies as cited in the following sources: McArdle WD, et al. Essentials of exercise physiology. Philadelphia: Lea & Febiger, 1993 (Table 12.2, 5 citations) and Wilber RL, Moffatt RJ. Physiological and biochemical consequences of detraining in aerobically trained individuals. J Strength Cond Res 1994;8:110 (101 citations). Note that a + change for heart rate represents a decline in functional capacity. Omitted values for trained and detrained excluded in original sources.

[b]Short term, 3 weeks or less in primarily aerobically trained individuals.

[c]Longer term, 3 to 12 weeks in primarily aerobically trained individuals

NS = not statistically significant

TABLE 21.3 ➤ **TYPICAL METABOLIC AND PHYSIOLOGIC VALUES FOR HEALTHY, TRAINED AND UNTRAINED MEN**[a]

VARIABLE	UNTRAINED	TRAINED	PERCENT DIFFERENCE[b]
Glycogen, mM · (g wet muscle)$^{-1}$	85.0	120	41
Number of mitochondria, mmol^3	0.59	1.20	103
Mitochondrial volume, % muscle cell	2.15	8.00	272
Resting ATP, mM · (g wet muscle)$^{-1}$	3.0	6.0	100
Resting PCr, mM · (g wet muscle)$^{-1}$	11.0	18.0	64
Resting creatine, mM · (g wet muscle)$^{-1}$	10.7	14.5	35
Glycolytic enzymes			
Phosphofructokinase, mM · (g wet muscle)$^{-1}$	50.0	50.0	0
Phosphorylase, mM · (g wet muscle)$^{-1}$	4–6	6–9	60
Aerobic enzymes			
Succinate dehydrogenase, mM · (kg wet muscle)$^{-1}$	5–10	15–20	133
Max lactate, mM · (kg wet muscle)$^{-1}$	110	150	36
Muscle fibers			
Fast twitch, %	50	20–30	−50
Slow twitch, %	50	60	20
Max stroke volume, mL	120	180	50
Max cardiac output, L · min^{-1}	20	30–40	75
Resting heart rate, b · min^{-1}	70	40	−43
Max heart rate, b · min^{-1}	190	180	−5
Max a-$\bar{v}$ O_2 diff, mL · dL^{-1}	14.5	16.0	10
$\dot{V}O_{2max}$, mL · kg^{-1} · min^{-1}	30–40	65–80	107
Heart volume, L	7.5	9.5	27
Blood volume, L	4.7	6.0	28
$\dot{V}_{Emax}$, L · min^{-1}	110	190	73
Percent body fat	15	11	−27

[a]In some cases, approximate values are used. In all cases, the trained values represent data from endurance athletes. Caution advised in assuming that the percentage differences between trained and untrained necessarily results from training, because genetic differences between individuals probably exert a strong influence on many of these factors.

[b]Percentage by which the value for the trained differs from the corresponding value for the untrained.

training (Table 21.4) show significant increases in the trained muscle's resting levels of ATP, PCr, free creatine, and glycogen accompanied by a 28% improvement in muscular strength. Other studies have shown higher levels of ATP and total creatine content in the trained muscles of sprint runners and track speed cyclists compared with distance runners and road racers.[153] Speed–power training also increases PCr content of trained skeletal muscle.[190]

- *Increased quantity and activity of key enzymes that control the anaerobic phase of glucose catabolism.* These changes do not reach the magnitude observed for oxidative enzymes with aerobic training. The most dramatic increases in anaerobic enzyme function and fiber size occur in fast-twitch muscle fibers.[93]
- *Increased capacity to generate high levels of blood lactate during all-out exercise.* An enhanced lactate-producing capacity probably results from (1) increased levels of glycogen and glycolytic enzymes and (2) improved motivation and "pain" tolerance to fatiguing exercise.[69,93]

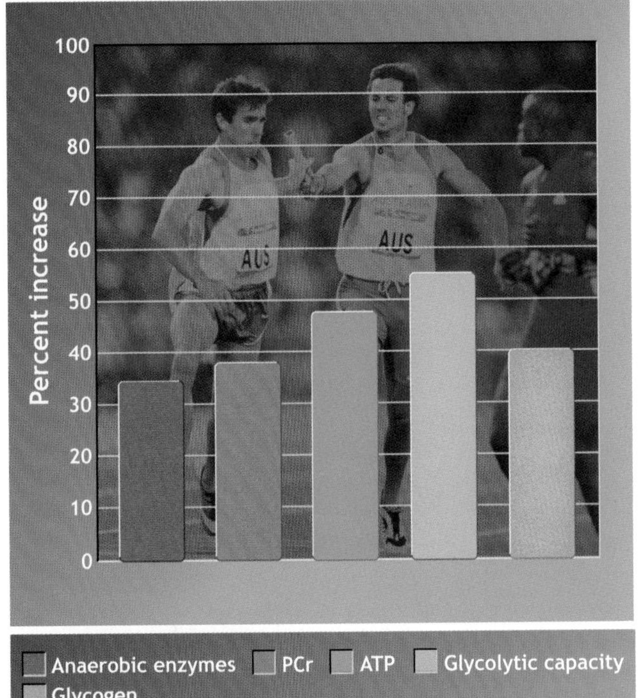

FIGURE 21.3 • Generalized potential for increases in anaerobic energy metabolism of skeletal muscle with heavy training.

TABLE 21.4 ➤ CHANGES IN RESTING CONCENTRATIONS OF PCr, CREATINE, ATP, AND GLYCOGEN FOLLOWING 5 MONTHS OF HEAVY-RESISTANCE TRAINING IN 9 MALE SUBJECTS

VARIABLE[a]	CONTROL	POSTTRAINING	PERCENT DIFFERENCE[b]
PCr	17.07	17.94	+5.1
Creatine	10.74	14.52	+35.2
ATP	5.07	5.97	+17.8
Glycogen	86.28	113.90	+32.0

[a]All values are averages expressed in mM per gram of wet muscle.
[b]All percentage differences are statistically significant.
From MacDougall JD, et al. Biochemical adaptation of human skeletal muscle to heavy resistance training and immobilization. J Appl Physiol, 1977; 43:700.

AEROBIC SYSTEM CHANGES WITH TRAINING

Figure 21. 4 shows that aerobic overload training induces significant adaptations in a variety of functional capacities related to oxygen transport and use. *With an adequate training stimulus, most of these responses are independent of race, gender and age.*[36,101,201,234,240] Many of the training-induced aerobic adaptations also occur in coronary heart disease patients undergoing high-intensity aerobic training.[71]

Metabolic Adaptations

Aerobic training significantly improves the capacity for respiratory control in skeletal muscle.

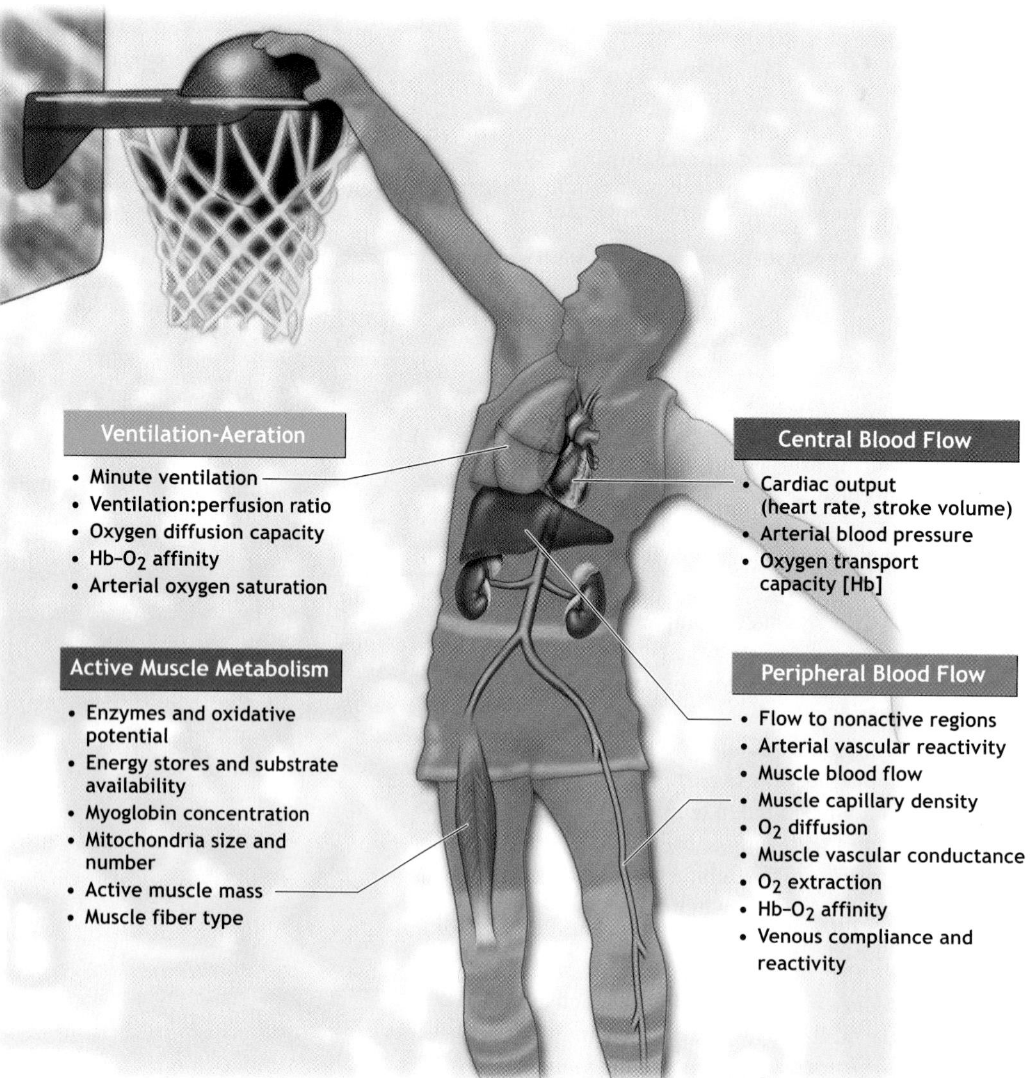

FIGURE 21.4 • Physiologic factors that can limit $\dot{V}O_{2max}$.

Metabolic Machinery

Endurance-trained skeletal muscle contains *larger* and *more numerous* mitochondria than less active muscle fibers. The enlarged mitochondrial structural machinery with training greatly *increases* capacity of subsarcolemmal and intermyofibrillar muscle mitochondria to generate ATP aerobically.[15] A nearly twofold increase in aerobic system enzymes (within 5 to 10 d of training) coincides with the increased mitochondrial capacity to generate ATP aerobically.[70,82,87]

Enzyme changes result from an increase in total mitochondrial material rather than increased enzymatic activity per unit of mitochondrial protein. Interestingly, the increase in mitochondrial protein by a factor of two greatly exceeds the typical 10 to 20% increases in $\dot{V}O_{2max}$ with endurance training. More than likely, enzymatic changes increase a person's ability to sustain a high percentage of aerobic capacity during prolonged exercise without significant blood lactate accumulation.[48,197]

FAT METABOLISM. Figure 21.5 shows that endurance training *increases* an individual's capacity to mobilize, deliver, and oxidize fatty acids for energy during submaximal exercise.[37,61,90] Enhanced fat catabolism with aerobic training becomes particularly apparent at the same absolute submaximal exercise workload, whether under fed or fasted conditions.[8,13,38] Impressive increases also occur in the trained muscle's capacity to use intramuscular triglycerides as the primary source for fatty acid oxidation.[136] A more lively, training-induced lipolysis results from:

- Greater blood flow within trained muscle.
- More fat-mobilizing and fat-metabolizing enzymes.
- Enhanced muscle mitochondrial respiratory capacity.
- Blunted catecholamine release for the same absolute power output.

Enhanced fat catabolism benefits endurance athletes because it conserves the glycogen stores so important during high-intensity prolonged exercise. Furthermore, improvement in fatty acid β-oxidation and respiratory ATP production contributes to maintaining a cell's integrity and high level of function. This would enhance endurance capacity, independent of increases in glycogen reserves or aerobic capacity.

CARBOHYDRATE METABOLISM. *Trained muscle exhibits a greater capacity to oxidize carbohydrate during maximal exercise.* Consequently, large quantities of pyruvate flow through the aerobic energy pathways, an effect consistent with increased mitochondrial oxidative capacity and enhanced glycogen storage within muscles. During submaximal exercise, however, endurance training *reduces* muscle glycogen turnover in favor of increased fatty acid combustion, as discussed previously.

Reduced total carbohydrate use as fuel in submaximal exercise with endurance training results from the combined effects of (1) decreased muscle glycogen use and (2) reduced production of (decreased hepatic glycogenolysis and gluconeogenesis) and use of plasma-borne glucose.[35] Fatty acid oxidation combined with reduced carbohydrate metabolism contributes to blood glucose homeostasis and improved endurance capacity following aerobic training. Training-enhanced hepatic gluconeogenic capacity further provides resistance to hypoglycemia during prolonged exercise.[49]

Muscle Fiber Type and Size

Aerobic training elicits metabolic adaptations in each type of muscle fiber. The basic fiber type probably does not "change" to any great extent; rather, all fibers maximize their already-existing aerobic potential.

Selective hypertrophy occurs in the different muscle fiber types in response to specific overload training. Highly trained endurance athletes have larger slow-twitch fibers than fast-twitch fibers in the same muscle. Conversely, the fast-twitch fibers of athletes trained in anaerobic power activities occupy a much greater portion of the muscle's cross-sectional area.

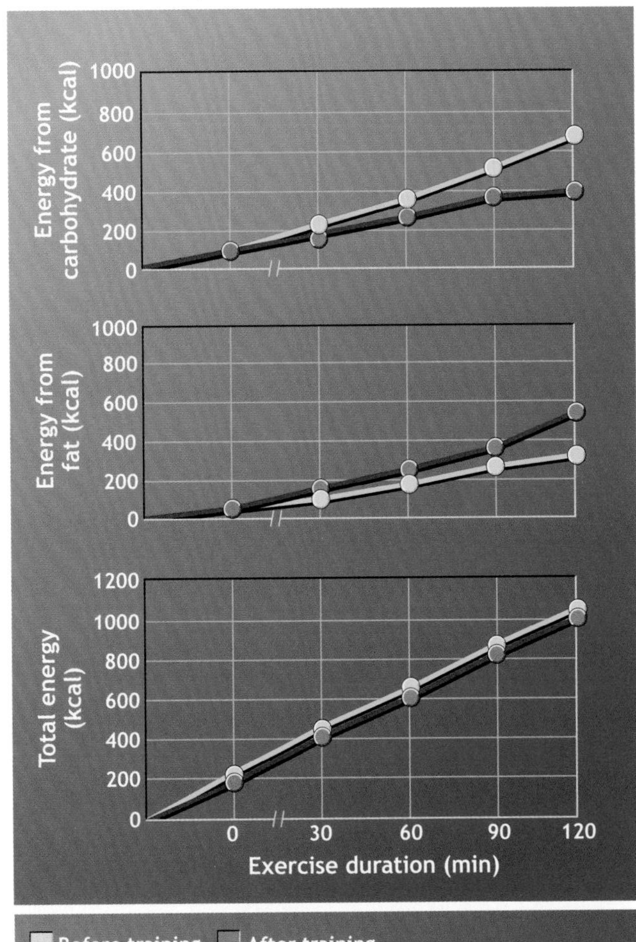

FIGURE 21.5 • Aerobic exercise training enhances capacity to catabolize fat in exercise. During constant-load, prolonged exercise, total energy derived from fat oxidation increases significantly following training. This carbohydrate-sparing adaptation may result from facilitated release of fatty acids from adipose tissue depots (augmented by a reduced blood lactate level) and an increased amount of triglyceride within the endurance-trained muscle fibers. (From Hurley BF, et al. Muscle triglyceride utilization during exercise: effect of training. J Appl Physiol 1986;5:62.)

Myoglobin

As might be expected, slow-twitch muscle fibers with high capacity to generate ATP aerobically contain relatively large quantities of myoglobin. Among animals, a muscle's myoglobin content relates to their level of physical activity.[117,159] The leg muscles of hunting dogs, for example, contain more myoglobin than the muscles of sedentary house pets;[237] similar findings exist for grazing cattle compared with penned animals.[200] Whether regular exercise exerts any effect on myoglobin levels in humans is unclear.[40,93]

Cardiovascular Adaptations

Figure 21.6 summarizes important adaptations in cardiovascular function with aerobic exercise training, which increase the delivery of oxygen to active muscle. Because of the intimate linkage of the cardiovascular system to aerobic processes, endurance training produces significant dimensional and functional cardiovascular adaptations.

Cardiac Hypertrophy: The "Athlete's Heart"

The heart's mass and volume generally *increase* with long-term aerobic training, with greater left ventricular end-diastolic volumes noted during rest and exercise. Moderate cardiac hypertrophy secondary to longitudinal myocardial cell enlargement reflects a fundamental and normal training adaptation of muscle to an increased workload, regardless of age.[148,149] This enlargement, characterized by an increase in the size of the left ventricular cavity (**eccentric hypertrophy**) and modest thickening of its walls (**concentric hypertrophy**), returns to control levels with detraining.[85]

Myocardial overload stimulates greater cellular protein synthesis, with concomitant reductions in protein breakdown.

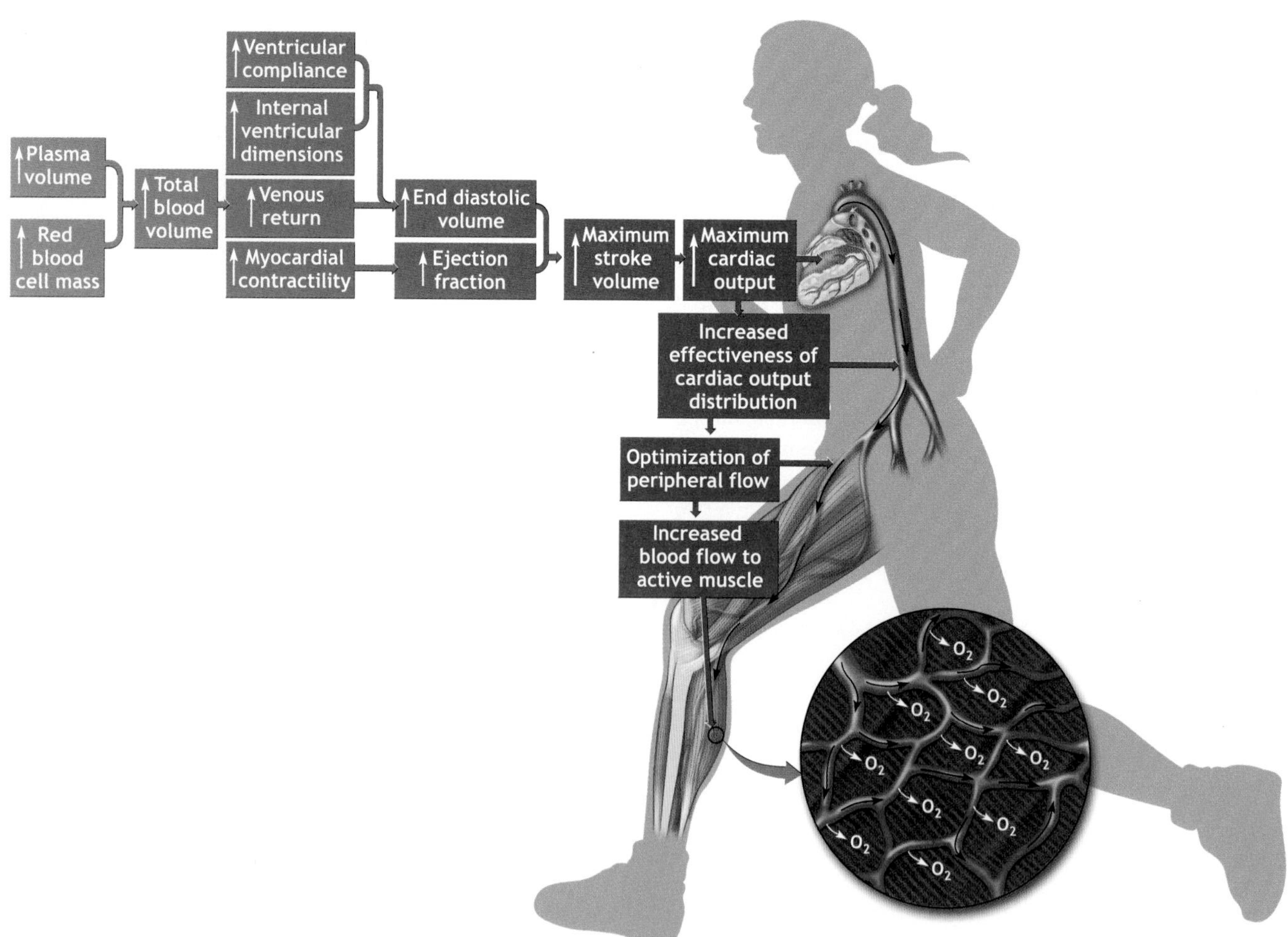

FIGURE 21.6 • Adaptations in cardiovascular function with aerobic exercise training that increases oxygen delivery to active muscles.

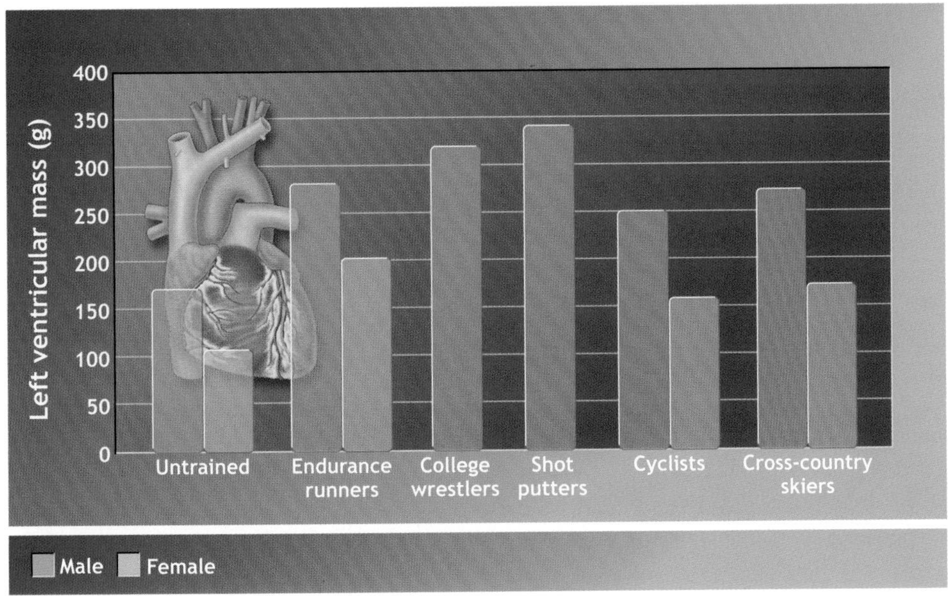

FIGURE 21.7 • General trend toward cardiac enlargement (left ventricular mass) among the untrained and various groups of male and (where applicable) female athletes.

Accelerated protein synthesis results largely from an increase in the trained muscle's RNA content. Individual myofibrils thicken, while at the same time the number of these contractile filaments increases. The heart volume of sedentary men averages 800 mL. In athletes, increases in heart volume relate to the aerobic nature of the sport—endurance athletes average 25% larger heart volume than their sedentary counterparts. Research has not yet explained to what degree the large heart volumes of endurance athletes reflect genetic endowment, training adaptations, or the combined effect of both factors. Training duration probably affects cardiac size and structure. Several studies report no changes in cardiac dimensions with short-term training, despite significant improvements in $\dot{V}O_{2max}$ and submaximal-exercise heart response.[178,223] When endurance training increases left ventricular size, the enlargement does not reflect a permanent adaptation. Instead, heart size decreases to pretraining levels—with apparently no deleterious effects—as training intensity decreases.[45,85] Figure 21.7 depicts the general trend for cardiac enlargement (reflected by left ventricular mass) in the untrained and various athletic groups.

Disease can also induce considerable cardiac enlargement. In hypertension, for example, the heart *chronically* works against an excessive resistance to blood flow (afterload). This stretches the heart muscle, which, in accordance with the Frank-Starling mechanism, generates compensatory force to overcome the added resistance to systolic ejection. In addition to ventricular dilation, individual muscle cells hypertrophy to adjust to the increased myocardial work imposed by the hypertensive state.[12] In untreated hypertension, myocardial fibers stretch beyond their optimal length, and the dilated heart weakens and eventually fails. To the pathologist, this "hypertrophied" heart represents an enlarged, distended, and functionally inadequate organ unable to deliver enough blood to satisfy minimal resting requirements.

SPECIFIC NATURE OF CARDIAC HYPERTROPHY. The ultrasonic technique of echocardiography incorporates sound waves that "map" myocardial dimensions and the volume of the heart's chambers (see Chapter 32). Echocardiography has evaluated the structural characteristics of the hearts of male and female athletes (and other species of mammals) to determine how various modes of exercise training might differentially affect cardiac enlargement.[161,214]

Research has compared male competitive swimmers, long-distance runners, wrestlers, and shot putters during their competitive seasons with untrained college men. The swimmers and runners represented athletes participating in "isotonic" or endurance events; the wrestlers and shot putters represented "isometric" or resistance-trained, power athletes. Table 21.5 shows clear distinctions in the structural characteristics of the hearts of apparently healthy athletes compared with those of healthy, untrained individuals. Also, heart structure differences among athletes relate to the nature of exercise training. For example, in the swimmers, left ventricular volume averaged 181 mL and mass equaled 308 g. In the wrestlers, left ventricular volume averaged 110 mL and mass averaged 330 g; the nonathletic controls averaged 101 mL for ventricular volume and 211 g for ventricular mass. The resistance-trained athletes had thicker ventricular walls, while those of endurance athletes remained within the normal range. Cardiac morphologic and functional adaptations, in-

TABLE 21.5 ➤ COMPARATIVE AVERAGE CARDIAC DIMENSIONS IN COLLEGE ATHLETES, WORLD-CLASS ATHLETES, AND NORMAL SUBJECTS

DIMENSION[a]	COLLEGE RUNNERS (N = 15)	COLLEGE SWIMMERS (N = 15)	WORLD CLASS RUNNERS (N = 10)	COLLEGE WRESTLERS (N = 12)	WORLD CLASS SHOT PUTTERS (N = 4)	NORMALS (N = 16)
LVID	54	51	48–59[b]	48	43–52[b]	46
LVV, mL	160	181	154	110	122	101
SV, mL	116	—[c]	113	75	68	—[c]
LV wall, mm	11.3	10.6	10.8	13.7	13.8	10.3
Septum, mm	10.9	10.7	10.9	13.0	13.5	10.3
LV mass, g	302	308	283	330	348	211

[a]LVID, left ventricular internal dimension at end diastole; LVV, left ventricular volume; SV, stroke volume; LV wall, posterobasal left ventricular wall thickness; Septum, ventricular septal thickness; LV mass, left ventricular mass.
[b]Range.
[c]Values not reported.
From Morganroth J, et al. Comparative left ventricular dimensions in trained athletes. Ann Intern Med 1975;82:521.

cluding resting bradycardia, increased stroke volume, and enlarged ventricular internal dimensions, also occur in prepubertal children who undergo intense endurance training.[155]

Figure 21.8 shows the distribution of left ventricular end-diastolic dimensions in 1309 elite Italian athletes aged 13 to 59 years.[162] End-diastolic left ventricular cavity dimension ranged from 38 to 66 mm (average, 48.4 mm) in women and 43 to 70 mm (average, 55.5 mm) in men. Ventricular cavity size of the vast majority of athletes remained within the normal range, but 14% showed substantially enlarged dimensions. A large body surface area and participation in endurance cycling, cross-country skiing, and canoeing represented the major determinants of enlarged cavity dimension. Over the 12-year study, the subjects remained free of heart problems.

Other groups also show an enlarged ventricular cavity (increased end-diastolic volume) with normal wall thickness,[143,180] although the effect appears to be less pronounced among females.[161]

Possible Explanation. *Myocardial structural and dimensional adaptations to regular exercise generally reflect specific training demands.*[52,167] As discussed in the subsequent section titled "Plasma Volume," a plasma volume increase within a day or two of the onset of endurance training probably produces intra-

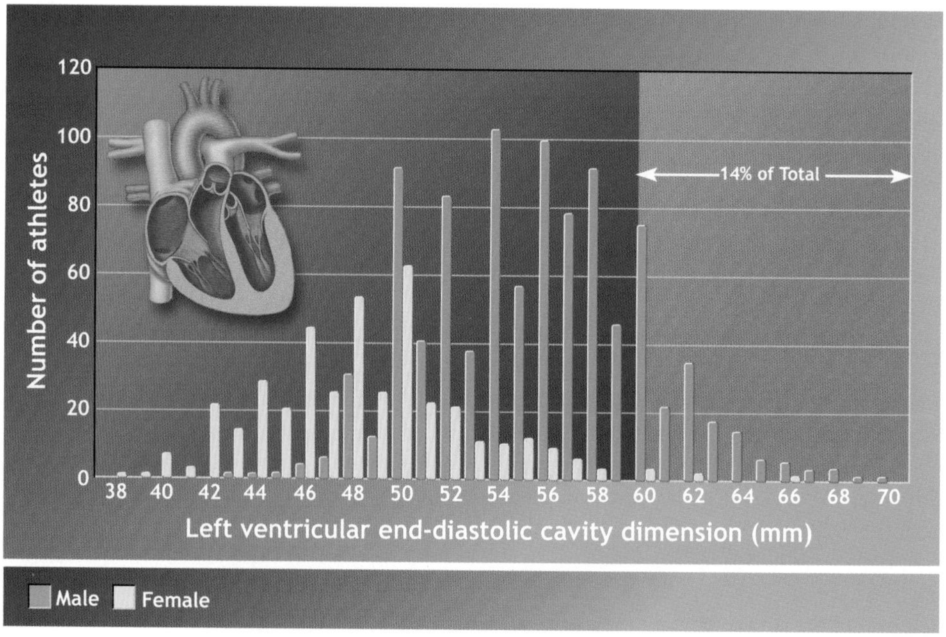

FIGURE 21.8 • Distribution of left ventricular end-diastolic cavity dimensions in 1309 highly trained athletes without evidence of structural cardiovascular disease. Fourteen percent of all athletes had markedly enlarged left ventricular cavities, ranging in size from 60 to 70 mm. (From Pelliccia A, et al. Physiologic left ventricular cavity dilation in elite athletes. Ann Intern Med 1999;130:23.)

ventricular enlargement or eccentric hypertrophy.[205,243] Increased plasma volume, coupled with a decreased heart rate and increased myocardial compliance, dilates the left ventricular cavity similar to the way added water stretches a rubber balloon.

In contrast, male and female resistance-trained athletes possess the largest intraventricular septum, ventricular wall thickness, and ventricular mass, with little enlargement in the left ventricle's internal cavity.[65,120] These athletes do not experience volume overload with training. Instead, they encounter acute episodes of significantly elevated arterial blood pressure (see Chapter 15) from high forces generated by a limited mass of skeletal muscle. An increase in ventricular wall thickness (which generally falls within the normal range when expressed as ventricular mass per unit body size, particularly fat-free body mass)[56,161,162] compensates for the additional afterload on the left ventricle without affecting ventricular cavity size. More than likely, considerable intraindividual variability exists for the heart's structural response to different forms of training. When changes do occur, the implications for myocardial blood supply and long-term cardiovascular health remain unknown. *No compelling scientific evidence indicates that specific forms of arduous exercise training can damage a normal heart.*

FUNCTIONAL VERSUS PATHOLOGIC HYPERTROPHY. Cardiac hypertrophy in response to such chronic pathologic states as hypertension is sometimes confused with moderate compensatory myocardial growth and left ventricular cavity enlargement with endurance training. Exercise stress requires that myocardial fibers generate increased tension, a critical requirement for initiating compensatory hypertrophy. However, overload application differs considerably from the chronic pressure overload from vascular disease. Exercise training imposes only a temporary myocardial stress, so nonexercise periods provide time for "recuperation." Also, dilation and weakening of the left ventricle, a frequent response to chronic hypertension, does not accompany the compensatory myocardial adaptations with exercise training. The heart size of elite athletes usually exceeds that of untrained individuals, but it generally falls within the upper range of normal limits for either body size or increase in end-diastolic volume. *The "athlete's heart" does not represent a dysfunctional organ. Rather, it demonstrates normal systolic and diastolic functions and superior functional capacity for stroke volume and cardiac output.*[145,167]

INTEGRATIVE QUESTION

In what way might cardiac hypertrophy with pressure overload (e.g., resistance training) training affect oxygenation of myocardial tissues?

Plasma Volume

A 12 to 20% *increase* in plasma volume, in the absence of changes in red blood cell mass, occurs after three to six aerobic training sessions. In fact, a significant change takes place within 24 hours of the first exercise bout, with expansion of the extracellular fluid volume requiring several weeks.[193] Intravascular volume expansion directly relates to increased synthesis and retention of plasma albumin.[152,243] A plasma volume increase enhances circulatory reserve and contributes to increased end-diastolic volume, stroke volume, oxygen transport, and temperature regulation during exercise.[72] The expanded plasma volume returns to pretraining levels within 1 week after training ceases.[205]

Heart Rate

Exercise training creates an imbalance between the tonic activity of sympathetic accelerator and parasympathetic depressor neurons in favor of greater vagal dominance—a response mediated primarily by increased parasympathetic activity and a small decrease in sympathetic discharge.[68,204] Training also decreases the intrinsic firing rate of sinoatrial (SA) nodal pacemaker tissue.[194] These training adaptations explain the resting and submaximal exercise bradycardia in highly conditioned endurance athletes or sedentary individuals who train aerobically. The reduction in submaximal heart rate indicates the magnitude of training improvement, because it generally reflects an increased maximum stroke volume and cardiac output.

EXERCISE HEART RATE: TRAINING EFFECTS. Submaximal heart rate for a standard exercise task frequently decreases by 12 to 15 $b \cdot min^{-1}$ with training, while a much smaller decrease occurs for resting heart rate.[196,239] Figure 21.9 illustrates the relationship between heart rate and oxygen consumption during graded exercise for athletes and sedentary students. The group of six endurance athletes had trained for several years; the other group consisted of three sedentary college students. The researchers evaluated the students' exercise responses before and after a 55-day training program designed to improve aerobic fitness. The lines relating heart rate and oxygen consumption remain essentially linear for both groups throughout the major portion of the exercise range. Whereas the untrained students' heart rates accelerate rapidly as exercise intensity (oxygen consumption) increases, the athletes' heart rates rise much less, that is, the slope or rate of change of the HR–$\dot{V}O_2$ lines differs considerably. Consequently, an athlete (or trained student) performs more intense exercise and achieves a higher oxygen consumption before reaching a specific submaximal heart rate than does a sedentary student. At an oxygen consumption of 2.0 $L \cdot min^{-1}$, the athletes' heart rate averaged 70 $b \cdot min^{-1}$ less than that of the sedentary students. After 55 days of training, this difference in submaximal heart rate decreased to about 40 $b \cdot min^{-1}$. In each instance, cardiac output remained about the same—the lower heart rate being compensated for by an increase in stroke volume.

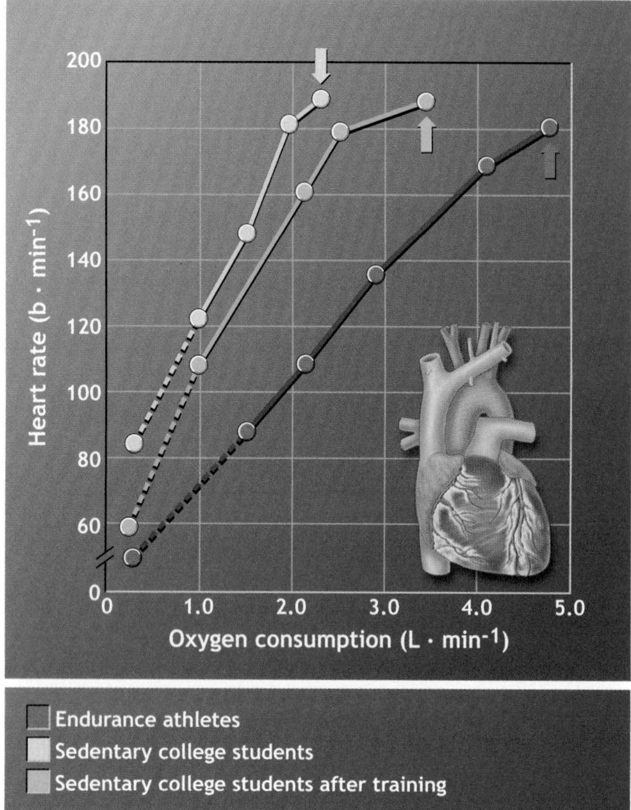

FIGURE 21.9 • Heart rate and oxygen consumption during upright exercise in endurance athletes (■) and sedentary college students before (■) and after (■) 55 days of aerobic training (⇑ = maximal values). (From Saltin B. Physiological effects of physical conditioning. Med Sci Sports 1969;1:50.)

Stroke Volume

Training causes the heart's stroke volume to *increase* during rest and exercise. This change can result from four factors: (1) an increase in internal left ventricular volume (consequent to the training-induced plasma volume expansion) and mass, (2) reduced cardiac stiffness, (3) increased diastolic filling time (owing to a training-induced bradycardia), and, possibly, (4) improved intrinsic cardiac contractile function.[108,141,241] Regardless of age, enhanced left ventricular systolic performance accompanies endurance training in healthy individuals.[53]

EXERCISE STROKE VOLUME: TRAINED VERSUS UNTRAINED. Figure 21.10 shows the stroke volume response during exercise for the men depicted in Figure 21.9.

Several important training-related observations emerge from these data:

- The heart of an endurance athlete exhibits a considerably larger stroke volume during rest and exercise than that of an untrained person of similar age.
- The greatest stroke volume increase during upright exercise for trained and untrained occurs in the transition from rest to moderate exercise. Only small increases in stroke volume accompany further increases in exercise intensity.
- Maximum stroke volume generally occurs at 40 to 50% of $\dot{V}O_{2max}$ (particularly for untrained persons); this occurs at a heart rate of 110 to 120 b · min^{-1} in young adults. Debate currently focuses on whether the stroke volume of endurance athletes actually plateaus during graded exercise (as it does for the untrained) or continues to gradually increase owing to a significantly enlarged plasma volume.[108] More than likely, endurance training blunts the small decrease in stroke volume often observed during intense exercise. This indicates that even at near-maximal heart rates, sufficient time exists for the trained heart's ventricles to fill during diastole without diminution in stroke volume.[67,211]
- A small increase in stroke volume occurs during the transition from rest to exercise for untrained persons. Consequently, the major increase in their cardiac output comes from acceleration in heart rate. For endurance athletes, *both* heart rate and stroke volume increase cardiac output; the athlete's stroke volume generally increases 60% above resting values. Relatively large stroke volume increases in transition from rest to exercise also take place in endurance-trained children and older men compared to those of healthy, untrained counterparts.[72,187]
- Eight weeks of aerobic training by previously sedentary individuals substantially increases stroke volume, but these values remain well below values for elite athletes. How much this difference reflects prolonged training, genetics, or a combination of both remains undetermined.

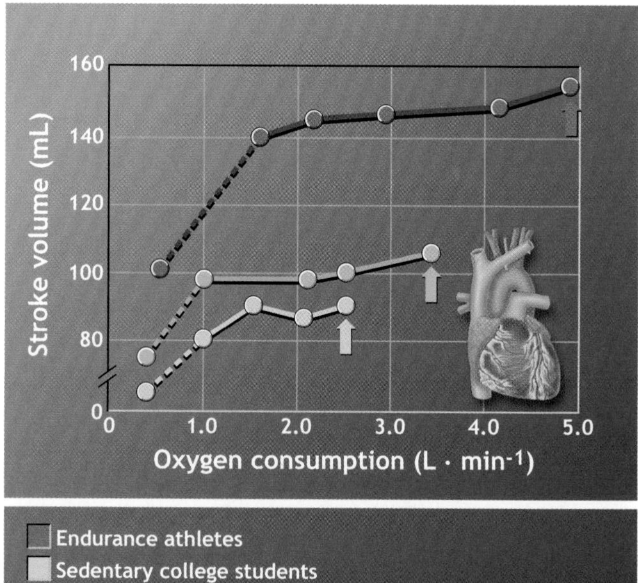

FIGURE 21.10 • Stroke volume and oxygen consumption during upright exercise in endurance athletes (■) and sedentary college students before (■) and after (■) 55 days of aerobic training (⇑ = maximal values). (From Saltin B. Physiological effects of physical conditioning. Med Sci Sports 1969;1:50.)

TABLE 21.6 ➤ MAXIMAL VALUES FOR OXYGEN CONSUMPTION, HEART RATE, STROKE VOLUME, AND CARDIAC OUTPUT IN THREE GROUPS WITH LOW, NORMAL, AND HIGH AEROBIC CAPACITIES

GROUP	$\dot{V}O_{2MAX}$ (L · MIN^{-1})	MAX HEART RATE (B · MIN^{-1})	MAX STROKE VOLUME (ML)	MAX CARDIAC OUTPUT (L · MIN^{-1})
Mitral stenosis	1.6	190	50	9.5
Sedentary	3.2	200	100	20.0
Athlete	5.2	190	160	30.4

Modified from Rowell LB. Circulation. Med Sci Sports 1969;1:15.

STROKE VOLUME AND $\dot{V}O_{2MAX}$. The data in Table 21.6 amplify the importance of stroke volume in differentiating people with high and low $\dot{V}O_{2max}$. These data represent three groups: (1) athletes, (2) healthy but sedentary men, and (3) patients with mitral stenosis, a valvular heart disease that causes inadequate emptying of the left ventricle. The differences in $\dot{V}O_{2max}$ among groups relate closely to differences in maximal stroke volume. Patients with mitral stenosis achieved an aerobic capacity and maximum stroke volume one-half that of the sedentary subjects. The importance of stroke volume also emerges in comparisons among healthy groups. Athletes achieved an average 62% larger $\dot{V}O_{2max}$ than sedentary subjects, almost entirely because of the athletes' 60% larger stroke volume (and cardiac output).

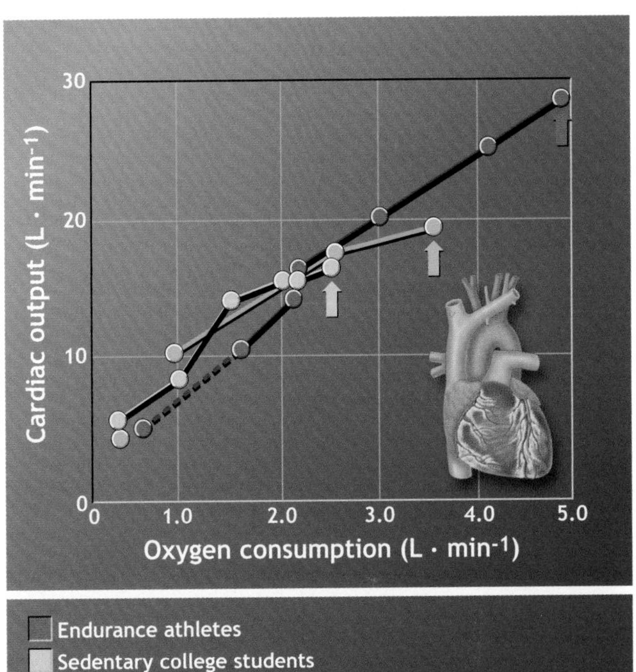

FIGURE 21.11 • Cardiac output and oxygen consumption during upright exercise in endurance athletes (■) and sedentary college students before (■) and after (■) 55 days of aerobic training (⇑ = maximal values). (From Saltin B. Physiological effects of physical conditioning. Med Sci Sports 1969;1:50.)

Cardiac Output

An increase in maximum cardiac output represents the most significant adaptation in cardiovascular function with aerobic training. Because maximal heart rate decreases slightly with training, the increased cardiac output capacity results directly from an improved stroke volume. A large maximum cardiac output (stroke volume) distinguishes champion endurance athletes from other well-trained athletes and from their untrained counterparts.

Figure 21.11 further illustrates the important role of cardiac output in sustaining aerobic metabolism. In trained athletes and students, cardiac output increases *linearly* with oxygen consumption throughout the major portion of the exercise intensity range. The linear relationship between cardiac output and oxygen consumption in graded exercise also occurs in children and adolescents. For these young people, an increase in the heart's stroke volume (and proportionate increase in cardiac output) closely matches the added cost of exercise as body mass increases with growth.[41]

TRAINING AND SUBMAXIMAL CARDIAC OUTPUT. Early reports showed that training, while improving the maximal cardiac output, reduced the heart's minute volume during moderate exercise.[7] In one study, average cardiac output of young men after 16 weeks of aerobic training decreased by 1.1 and 1.5 L · min^{-1} at a specific submaximal oxygen consumption.[54] As expected, maximal cardiac output increased 8% from 22.4 to 24.2 L · min^{-1}. With a reduced submaximal cardiac output, a corresponding increase in oxygen extraction in the active muscles matches the exercise oxygen requirement. A training-induced reduction in submaximal cardiac output presumably reflects two factors: (1) more effective distribution of blood flow and (2) enhanced ability of trained muscles to generate ATP aerobically at a lower tissue Po_2.

Oxygen Extraction (a-$\bar{v}$ O_2 Difference)

Aerobic training significantly *increases* the quantity of oxygen extracted from circulating blood.[186] An increase in arteriovenous oxygen (a-$\bar{v}$ O_2) difference results from more-effective cardiac output distribution to active muscles combined with an enhanced capacity of trained muscle fibers to extract and process the available oxygen. The a-$\bar{v}$ O_2 difference takes

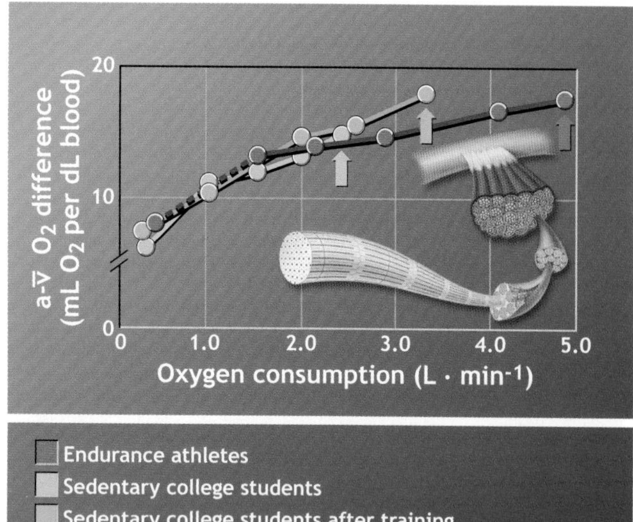

FIGURE 21.12 • The a-$\bar{v}$ O_2 difference and oxygen consumption during upright exercise in endurance athletes (■) and sedentary college students before (■) and after (■) 55 days of aerobic training (⇑ = maximal values). (From Saltin B. Physiological effects of physical conditioning. Med Sci Sports 1969;1:50.)

on even greater importance in contributing to improved aerobic capacity with training in older men and women.[112,198]

Figure 21.12 compares the relationship between oxygen extraction (a-$\bar{v}$ O_2 difference) and exercise intensity for trained athletes and untrained students. For the students, the a-$\bar{v}$ O_2 difference increases steadily during light and moderate exercise to a maximum of 15 mL of oxygen per deciliter of blood. Following 55 days of training, the students' maximum oxygen extraction increased 13% to 17 mL of oxygen. This means that during intense exercise, arterial blood released approximately 85% of its oxygen content. Actually, the active muscles extract even more oxygen, because the a-$\bar{v}$ O_2 difference reflects an *average* based on sampling of mixed-venous blood. This sample contains blood returning from tissues that use much less oxygen during exercise than active muscle. The posttraining value for maximal a-$\bar{v}$ O_2 difference for the students equals the value of the endurance athletes. Obviously, the students' lower cardiac output capacity explains the rather large difference in $\dot{V}O_{2max}$ that still characterizes athletes and students.

Blood Flow and Distribution

Trained persons perform *submaximal* exercise with a *lower* cardiac output (and unchanged or slightly lower muscle blood flow) than untrained persons. Aerobic training causes distribution of a relatively larger portion of the submaximal cardiac output to the high-oxidative skeletal muscles (composed primarily of type I fibers) at the expense of blood flow to muscles with a large percentage of type IIB fibers with low oxidative capacity.[42] Altered muscle blood flow probably results from (1) relatively rapid training-induced changes in the vasoactive properties of large arteries and local resistance vessels within skeletal and cardiac muscle, mediated by the dilation effects of endothelium-derived nitric oxide[24,43] and (2) changes within the muscle cells, related to the specific nature of the exercise training. Both adaptations support the principle of training specificity. As the muscle's ability to deliver, extract, and use oxygen increases, the active tissue's oxygen needs require proportionally less regional blood flow.

Training-induced *decreases* in splanchnic and renal blood flow in exercise result from a reduction in sympathetic nervous system outflow to these tissues.[137,150] This frees a significant quantity of blood for distribution to active muscles. Concurrently, exercise training and the accompanying frequent exposure to elevated core temperatures produces heat loss adaptations via enhanced endothelium-dependent increases in blood flow to the skin for a given internal temperature in older and younger subjects.[99,111] Augmented cutaneous blood flow facilitates the trained person's capacity to dissipate the metabolic heat generated in exercise.

SKELETAL MUSCLE BLOOD FLOW. Aerobic training *increases* total skeletal muscle blood flow during *maximal* exercise because of three factors:

1. Larger maximal cardiac output
2. Distribution of blood to muscle from nonactive areas that temporarily compromise blood flow in all-out effort
3. Enlargement of the cross-sectional areas of the large and small arteries and veins, and about a 10% increase in capillarization per gram of muscle[78,114]

The observation that oxygen extraction in skeletal muscle remains near maximal in heavy exercise supports the hypothesis that oxygen supply (blood flow), not oxygen use (extraction), limits the maximal respiratory rate of muscle tissue.[11,179]

MYOCARDIAL BLOOD FLOW. Structural and functional changes in the heart's vasculature, including modifications in mechanisms that regulate myocardial perfusion, parallel a modest training-induced myocardial hypertrophy.[74,116,149,238] Structural modifications include an increase in the cross-sectional area of the proximal coronary arteries, possible arteriolar proliferation and longitudinal growth, recruitment of collateral vessels, and an increase in capillary density. These adaptations provide adequate perfusion to support the blood flow and energy demands of the functionally improved myocardium.

Specifically, aerobic exercise training increases coronary blood flow and capillary exchange capacity by two mechanisms:

1. Ordered progression of structural remodeling that improves myocardial vascularization when new capillaries form and develop into small arterioles[115,238]
2. More effective control of vascular resistance and blood distribution within the heart muscle[228,233]

Mitochondrial mass and cellular concentration of respiratory enzymes also increase in the hearts of endurance-trained animals. The significance of vascular and cellular adaptations to the heart's functional capacity during exercise remains unclear—mainly because the healthy, untrained heart does not suffer from oxygen lack during maximum exercise. Training adaptations may provide some cardioprotection by making myocardial tissue better able to tolerate and recover from transient episodes of ischemia (more resistant to ischemic injury). The trained tissue also functions at a lower percentage of its total oxidative capacity during exercise.[149,218] In addition, myocardial training adaptations probably confer some protection from coronary artery disease. Vascular adaptations do not accompany the myocardial hypertrophy that occurs with chronic resistance training.[149]

Blood Pressure

Regular aerobic training *reduces* systolic and diastolic blood pressures during rest and submaximal exercise. The largest reduction occurs in systolic pressure, particularly in hypertensive subjects (see Chapter 32 for a more complete discussion).

Pulmonary Adaptations with Training

Aerobic training stimulates adaptations in pulmonary ventilation during submaximal and maximal exercise. Such adaptations generally reflect a breathing strategy that minimizes respiratory work at a given exercise intensity. This theoretically frees oxygen for use by the nonrespiratory active musculature.[139,222]

Maximal Exercise

Maximal exercise ventilation *increases* (increased tidal volume and breathing rate) as maximal oxygen consumption increases. This makes sense physiologically, because any increase in $\dot{V}O_{2max}$ raises both the oxygen requirement and the corresponding need to eliminate additional carbon dioxide via alveolar ventilation.

Submaximal Exercise

Several weeks of aerobic training considerably *reduces* the ventilatory equivalent for oxygen ($\dot{V}_E/\dot{V}O_2$) during submaximal exercise and lowers the percentage of the total exercise oxygen cost attributable to breathing.[29] Reduced ventilatory musculature oxygen consumption may enhance endurance for two reasons: (1) it reduces the fatiguing effects of exercise on the ventilatory musculature and (2) any oxygen freed from use by the respiratory musculature now becomes available to the active locomotor muscles.[75,97]

Studies of adolescents and young and older adults have consistently observed positive training adaptations in pulmonary ventilation during submaximal exercise.[95,227] In general, tidal volume increases and breathing frequency decreases. Consequently, air remains in the lungs for a longer time between breaths, increasing the extraction of oxygen from inspired air. For example, the exhaled air of trained individuals during submaximal exercise contains only 14 to 15% oxygen, whereas the expired air of untrained persons averages 18% at the same exercise intensity. This translates to the well-known observation that untrained persons ventilate proportionately more air to achieve the same submaximal oxygen consumption.

Significant specificity exists for ventilatory responses, not only for the type of exercise, but also in training adaptations. When subjects performed arm-only and leg-only exercise, consistently higher ventilatory equivalents occurred with the arms (Fig. 21.13).[177] As expected, the ventilatory equivalent decreased with each mode of exercise training. However, the reduction occurred *only* with exercise that used the specifically trained muscles. For the group trained by arm-crank ergometry, the ventilation equivalent showed a decrease only during arm exercise and vice versa for the leg-trained group. The ventilatory training adaptation linked closely to a less pronounced rise in blood lactate and heart rate during the specific training exercise. This suggests that the ventilatory adjustment to training results partly from local adaptations in

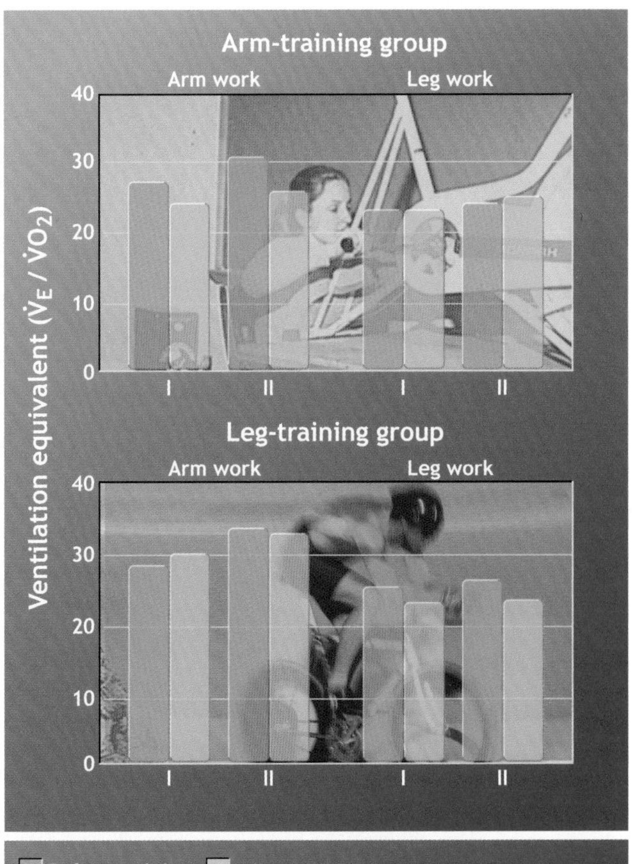

FIGURE 21.13 • Ventilation equivalents during light (I) and heavy (II) submaximal arm and leg exercise before and after arm training *(top)* and leg training *(bottom)*. (From Rasmussen B, et al. Pulmonary ventilation, blood gases, and blood pH after training of the arms and the legs. J Appl Physiol 1975;38:250.)

the specifically trained muscles. Lower lactate levels with training would remove the drive to ventilation from the additional carbon dioxide produced in lactate buffering.

Training May Benefit Ventilatory Endurance

Inspiratory muscle fatigue occurs during prolonged, high-intensity exercise.[9,91,97] Such exercise also reduces the abdominal muscles' capacity to generate maximal expiratory pressure.[62]

Exercise training enhances ability to sustain exceptionally high levels of submaximum ventilation, but exerts little effect on maximum static and dynamic lung function.[23,98,208] Endurance training also stabilizes the body's internal milieu during submaximal exercise. Consequently, exercise causes less disruption in whole-body hormonal and acid–base balance that could negatively affect inspiratory muscle function.[96] The ventilatory muscles also benefit directly from exercise training. For example, 20 weeks of run training by healthy men and women improved ventilatory muscle endurance by approximately 16% (less lactate accumulation during standard breathing exercise). The documented training-induced increase in aerobic enzyme levels and oxidative capacity of the respiratory musculature probably enhance ventilatory muscle function.[172,173,210,230] Exercise training also increases inspiratory muscle capacity to generate force and sustain a given level of inspiratory pressure.[30] These training adaptations benefit exercise performance in the following three ways:

1. Reduces overall exercise energy demands because of less respiratory work
2. Reduces lactate production by the ventilatory muscles during high-intensity, prolonged exercise
3. Enhances how ventilatory muscles' metabolize circulating lactate as metabolic fuel

Improved respiratory capacity of the ventilatory musculature would also reduce local pulmonary discomfort and breathlessness (**dyspnea**) prevalent among untrained persons during prolonged exercise. Improved ventilatory muscle endurance and reduced submaximal exercise ventilation with training delays the onset of diaphragmatic fatigue during short- and longer-term strenuous exercise.[97,133]

Blood Lactate Concentration

Figure 21.14 illustrates the generalized effect of endurance training in lowering blood lactate levels and extending the level of exercise intensity before the onset of blood lactate accumulation (OBLA) during exercise of progressively increasing intensity. The explanation underlying this effect centers on three possibilities related to the central and peripheral adaptations to training discussed in this chapter: (1) decreased rate of lactate formation during exercise, (2) increased rate of lactate clearance (removal) during exercise, and (3) combined effects of increased lactate clearance and increased lactate removal. More than likely, the combination of both factors exerts the influence.[48,104]

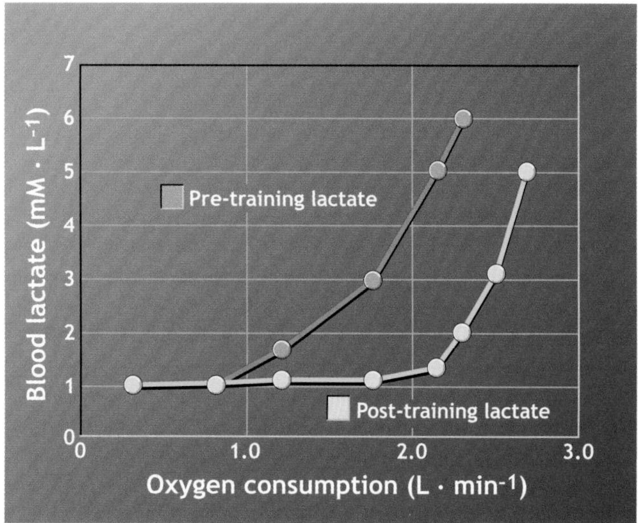

FIGURE 21.14 • Generalized response for pre- and posttraining lactate accumulation during graded exercise. (Plots based on data from the Applied Physiology Laboratory, University of Michigan, Ann Arbor.)

Does Training Improve Buffering Capacity?

Individuals who engage in vigorous anaerobic training tolerate higher blood lactate levels (and lower pH values) than untrained counterparts. This raises speculation that anaerobic training improves the body's capacity for acid–base regulation, perhaps by enhancing chemical buffers or alkaline reserve. No research has demonstrated, however, that exercise training augments buffering capacity. Motivational factors probably improve training-induced tolerance to elevated plasma acidity.

Other Aerobic Training Adaptations

- *Body composition changes:* For the obese or borderline obese person, regular aerobic exercise reduces body mass and body fat. Increases in fat-free body mass also accompany resistance training. Exercise only or combined with calorie restriction reduces body fat more than weight lost with dieting only because exercise promotes conservation of the body's lean tissue.[21,221]
- *Body heat transfer:* Well-hydrated, trained individuals exercise more comfortably in hot environments because of a larger plasma volume and more-responsive thermoregulatory mechanisms.[147] These men and women dissipate heat faster and more economically than sedentary individuals. As a result, metabolic heat generated by exercise poses less potential detriment to exercise performance and overall safety.
- *Performance changes:* Enhanced endurance performance accompanies the physiologic adaptations with training. Figure 21.15 depicts the results of cycling exercise following training performed for 40 to 60 minutes, 4 days per week for 10 weeks at an inten-

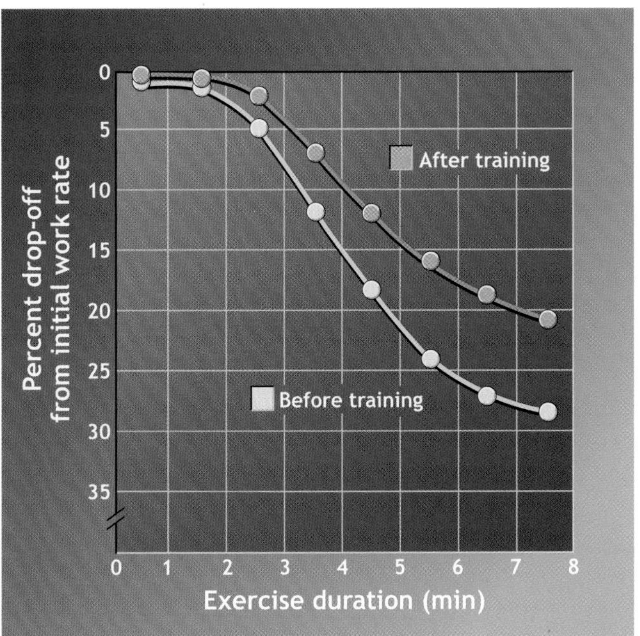

FIGURE 21.15 • Percentage drop-off from initial exercise intensity before and after 10 weeks of endurance cycling training. (From the Applied Physiology Laboratory, University of Michigan, Ann Arbor.)

sity of 85% $\dot{V}O_{2max}$ The performance test consisted of attempting to maintain a constant work rate of 265 watts for 8 minutes. Training produced significantly less drop-off in power output during the prescribed 8-minute exercise test.

- *Psychologic benefits:* Significant potential benefits on psychologic state result from regular exercise (either aerobic or resistance training), regardless of age.[57,113,224] Adaptations often occur to a degree equal to that achieved with other therapeutic interventions including pharmacologic therapy.

POTENTIAL PSYCHOLOGIC BENEFITS FROM REGULAR EXERCISE

- Reduction in state of anxiety (i.e., the level of anxiety at the time of measurement)
- Decrease in mild-to-moderate depression
- Reduction in neuroticism (long-term exercise)
- Adjunct to professional treatment of severe depression
- Improvement in mood, self-esteem, and self-concept
- Reduction in the various indices of stress

Summary View

Figure 21.16 summarizes adaptive changes in active muscle that accompany $\dot{V}O_{2max}$ improvements with endurance training. Aerobic capacity generally increases 15 to 25% over the first 3 months of intensive training and may improve by 50% over a 2-year period. When training stops, $\dot{V}O_{2max}$ decreases toward the pretraining level. Even more impressive training effects occur for aerobic enzymes of the citric acid cycle and the electron-transport chain within the mitochondria of the trained muscles. These enzymes, which facilitate carbohydrate and fat breakdown, increase rapidly and substantially

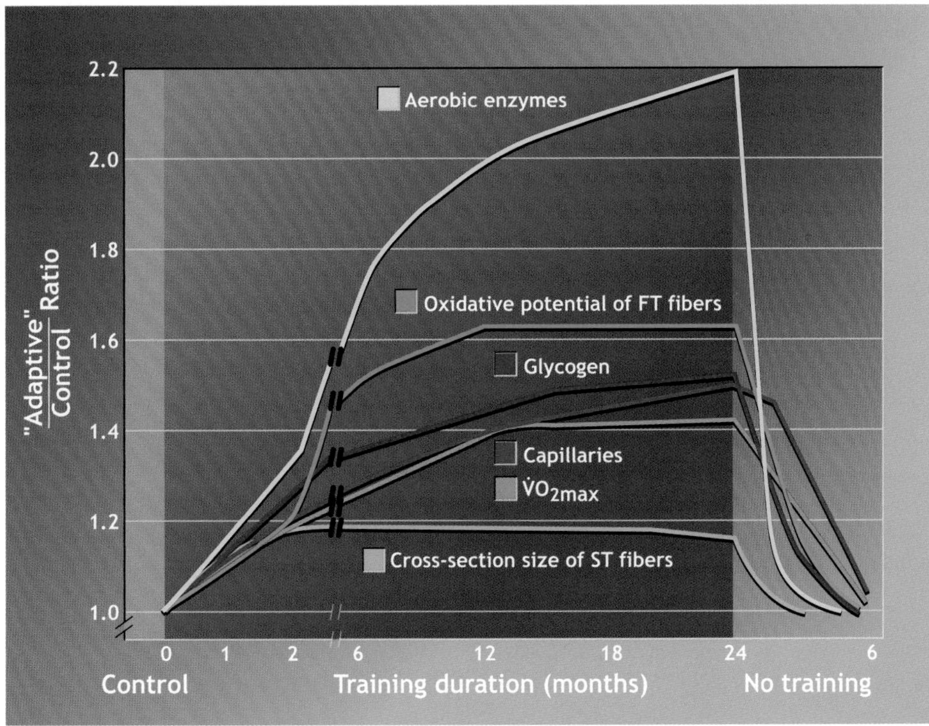

FIGURE 21.16 • Generalized summary of increase in aerobic capacity and muscle adaptations with endurance training. (Modified from Saltin B, et al. Fiber types and metabolic potentials of skeletal muscles in sedentary man and endurance runners. Ann NY Acad Sci 1977;301:3.)

throughout training in both fiber types and subdivisions. Conversely, a few weeks of detraining cause loss of a large portion of enzymatic adaptations.[40,105] The number of muscle capillaries increases throughout training.[186] When training stops, this adaptation in blood supply probably decreases relatively slowly.

Local metabolic improvement greatly exceeds improvements in the capacity to circulate, deliver, and use oxygen (reflected by $\dot{V}O_{2max}$ and cardiac output) during intense exercise. With these training adaptations, a muscle's lactate generally reaches lower levels (lower production and/or greater removal rate) than during similar submaximal exercise before training. *These cellular adjustments probably account for a trained person's ability to perform steady-rate exercise at a greater percentage of $\dot{V}O_{2max}$.*

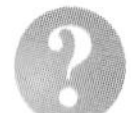

INTEGRATIVE QUESTION

Respond to the question "How long must I exercise to get in shape?"

FACTORS THAT AFFECT THE AEROBIC TRAINING RESPONSE

Four factors significantly influence the aerobic training response:

1. Initial level of aerobic fitness
2. Training intensity
3. Training frequency
4. Training duration

Initial Level of Aerobic Fitness

The magnitude of the training response depends upon initial fitness level. Someone who rates low at the start has considerable room for improvement. If capacity already rates high, the magnitude of improvement remains relatively small. Studies of sedentary, middle-aged men with heart disease showed that $\dot{V}O_{2max}$ improved by 50%, while similar training in normally active, healthy adults elicited a 10 to 15% improvement.[168] Of course, a 5% improvement in aerobic capacity represents as crucial a change for an elite athlete as a 40% increase for the sedentary person. *As a general guideline, aerobic fitness improvements generally range between 5 and 25% with endurance training.* Some of this improvement occurs within the first week of training.[83]

Training Intensity

Training-induced physiologic adaptations depend primarily on the intensity of overload. At least seven different ways can express exercise intensity:

1. Energy expended per unit time (e.g., 9 kcal · min^{-1}, or 37.8 kJ · min^{-1})
2. Absolute exercise level or power output (e.g., cycle at 900 kg-m · min^{-1}, or 147 W)
3. Relative metabolic level expressed as percentage of $\dot{V}O_{2max}$ (e.g., 85% $\dot{V}O_{2max}$)
4. Exercise below, at, or above the lactate threshold or OBLA (e.g., 4 mM lactate)
5. Exercise heart rate or percentage of maximum heart rate (e.g., 180 b · min^{-1}, or 80% HR_{max})
6. Multiples of resting metabolic rate (e.g., 6 METs)
7. Rating of perceived exertion (e.g., RPE = 14)

An example of absolute training intensity involves having all individuals exercise at the same power output or energy expenditure (e.g., 9.0 kcal · min^{-1}) for 30-minutes. When everyone performs at the same intensity, however, the task may pose a considerable stress for one person yet fall short of the training threshold for another, more fit person. For this reason, the *relative stress* on a person's physiologic systems is used to establish exercise intensity. Consequently, the assigned exercise intensity usually relates to some break point for steady-rate exercise (e.g., lactate threshold, OBLA) or some percentage of maximum physiologic capacity (e.g., %$\dot{V}O_{2max}$, %HR_{max}) or maximum exercise capacity. General practice establishes aerobic training intensity via direct measurement (or estimation) of $\dot{V}O_{2max}$ (or HR_{max}), and then assigns an exercise level to correspond to some percentage of these maximums.

Although establishing training intensity from measures of oxygen consumption provides a high degree of accuracy, its use requires sophisticated equipment and thus is impractical for the general population. An effective alternative uses *heart rate* to classify exercise for relative intensity when establishing the training protocol. Exercise heart rate is convenient because %$\dot{V}O_{2max}$ and %HR_{max} relate in a predictable way regardless of gender, fitness level, exercise mode, or age. Table 21.7 presents selected values for %$\dot{V}O_{2max}$ and the corresponding %HR_{max} obtained from several sources.[4,124] The error in estimating %$\dot{V}O_{2max}$ from %HR_{max}, or vice versa, equals about ±8%. Thus, one need only monitor heart rate to estimate the relative exercise stress or %$\dot{V}O_{2max}$ within the given error range. The relationship between %HR_{max} and %$\dot{V}O_{2max}$ remains essentially the same for arm or leg exercises among healthy subjects, normal-weight and obese groups, cardiac patients, and persons with spinal cord injuries.[60,89,142] *Importantly, however, arm (upper-body) exercise produces significantly lower HR_{max} than leg exercises. One must consider this difference when formulating the exercise prescription for different exercise modes* (see page 480).

TABLE 21.7 ➤ **RELATIONSHIP BETWEEN PERCENTAGE MAXIMUM HEART RATE AND PERCENTAGE $\dot{V}O_{2MAX}$**

PERCENT HR_{MAX}	PERCENT $\dot{V}O_{2MAX}$
50	28
60	40
70	58
80	70
90	83
100	100

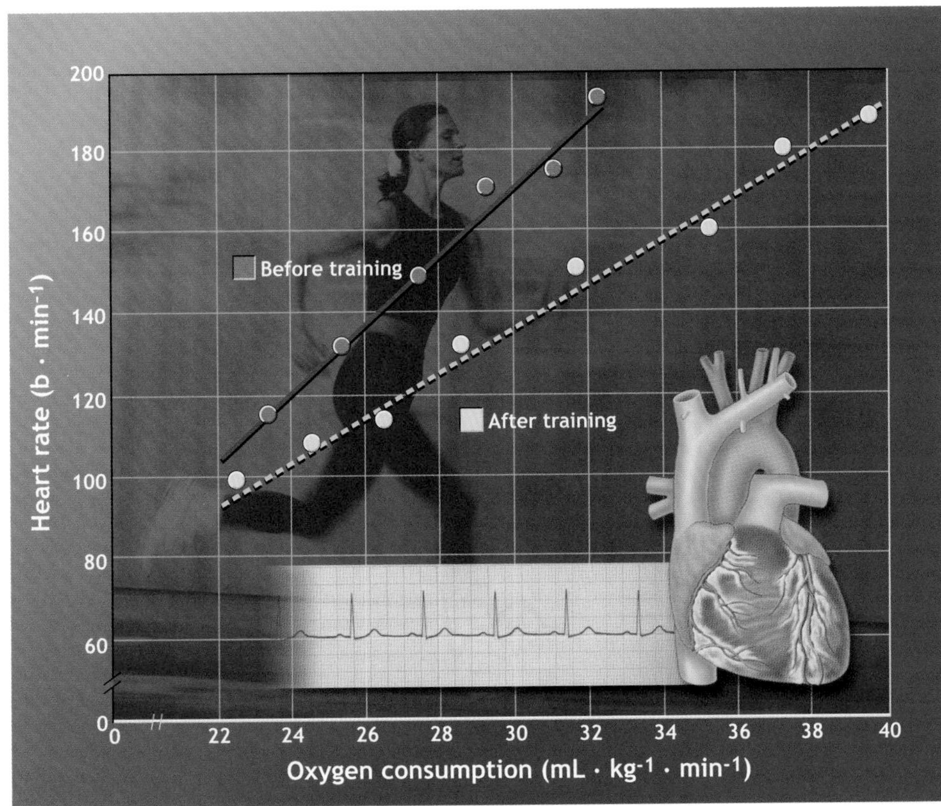

FIGURE 21.17 • Improvements in heart rate response with aerobic training in relation to oxygen consumption. A significant reduction in exercise heart rate with training usually reflects an enhanced stroke volume.

Train at a Percentage of HR_{max}

As a general rule, aerobic capacity improves if exercise intensity regularly increases heart rate to at least 55 to 70% of maximum. During lower-body exercise such as cycling, walking, or running, this heart rate increase equals about 45 to 55% of the $\dot{V}O_{2max}$, or, for college-aged men and women, a heart rate of 120 to 140 b · min^{-1}.

An alternative and equally effective method of establishing the training threshold, termed the **Karvonen method**, has subjects exercise at a heart rate equal to 60% of the difference between resting and maximum.[103] With the Karvonen method, one computes the training heart rate as follows:

$$HR_{threshold} = HR_{rest} + 0.60\,(HR_{max} - HR_{rest})$$

This approach to determining heart rate training threshold gives a somewhat *higher* value than computing the threshold heart rate simply as 70% of HR_{max}.

Clearly, positive training adaptations do not require strenuous exercise. For most healthy people, an exercise heart rate of 70% maximum represents moderate exercise with little or no discomfort. This training level, frequently referred to as "**conversational exercise**," reaches sufficient intensity to stimulate a training effect yet does not produce a level of discomfort (e.g., lactate accumulation and associated hyperpnea) that prevents a person from talking easily during the workout. *A previously sedentary person need not exercise above this heart rate to improve physiologic capacity.*

Figure 21.17 shows that as aerobic fitness improves, submaximal exercise heart rate decreases 10 to 20 b · min^{-1} for a given level of oxygen consumption. To keep pace with physiologic improvement, the exercise level then increases periodically to attain the desired exercise heart rate. A person who begins training by walking then walks more briskly; jogging then replaces walking for periods of the workout, and eventually continuous running elicits the desired exercise heart rate. In each progression, exercise remains at the same relative intensity or strenuousness. If exercise intensity progession does not adjust to training improvements, the exercise program becomes a maintenance program for aerobic fitness without further improvements.[84,85]

Is Strenuous Training More Effective?

Generally, the higher the training intensity above threshold, the greater the training improvement, particularly for $\dot{V}O_{2max}$.[50] Although a minimal threshold intensity exists below which no training effect occurs, a "ceiling" may also exist above which no further gains accrue. More-fit men and women generally require higher threshold levels to stimulate a training response than less fit persons. The ceiling for training intensity remains unknown, although 85% $\dot{V}O_{2max}$ (corresponding to 90% HR_{max}) probably represents an upper limit. Importantly, regardless of the exercise level selected, more does not necessarily produce greater results. Excessive training intensity and abrupt increases in training volume increase the risk for injury to bones, joints, and muscles.[2,100]

The "Training-Sensitive Zone"

One can determine maximum exercise heart rate immediately after several minutes of all-out effort in a specific form of exercise. This exercise intensity requires considerable motivation and stress—a requirement certainly inadvisable for adults without medical clearance, particularly individuals predisposed to coronary heart disease. Consequently, people should consider themselves average and use the **age-predicted maximum heart rates** rates presented in Figure 21.19.

Although individuals of a specific age possess varying HR_{max} values, the inaccuracy resulting from individual variation (± 10 b · min^{-1} standard deviation for any age-predicted HR_{max}) has little influence in establishing effective training for healthy people. *Maximum heart rate computes as 220 minus the person's age in years, with values independent of race or gender in children and adults.*[94,123,124]

$$HR_{max} = 220 - \text{age (y)}$$

The decrease in maximum heart rate with age probably results from reduced sympathetic output from the medulla and age-related changes in the inherent characteristics of the SA node.[186] Although this formula represents a convenient rule of thumb, it does not determine a specific person's maximum heart rate. Within normal variation, the maximum heart rate of 95% (± 2 standard deviations) of 40-year-old men and women ranges between 160 and 200 b · min^{-1}. Figure 21.18 also depicts the "training-sensitive zone" in relation to age. Aerobic system conditioning occurs as long as exercise heart rate remains within this zone.

A 40-year-old woman or man who wants to train at moderate intensity but still achieve the threshold level would select a training heart rate equal to 70% of age-predicted HR_{max}, or a target exercise heart rate of 126 b · min^{-1} (0.70×180). Then, using progressive increments of light-to-moderate exercise, the person achieves a walking, jogging, or cycling intensity that produces this heart rate. To increase training to 85% of maximum, exercise intensity must increase to produce a heart rate of 153 b · min^{-1} (0.85×180).

RUNNING VERSUS SWIMMING AND OTHER FORMS OF UPPER-BODY EXERCISE. *Estimation of HR_{max} requires an adjustment when using swimming or other upper-body exercises for training.*[60] Maximum heart rate during these exercise modes averages about 13 b · min^{-1} lower than in running for trained and untrained men and women.[66,135,138] This difference probably results from less feed-forward stimulation from the motor cortex to the medulla, in addition to less feedback stimulation from the smaller, active upper-body muscle mass. In swimming, the horizontal body position and cooling effect of the water may also contribute to a lower HR_{max}.

Establishing the appropriate exercise intensity for swimming and upper-body exercise requires subtracting 13 b · min^{-1} from the age-predicted HR_{max} in Figure 21.19. Consequently, a 30-year-old person who swims at 70% HR_{max} should select a swimming speed that produces a heart rate of

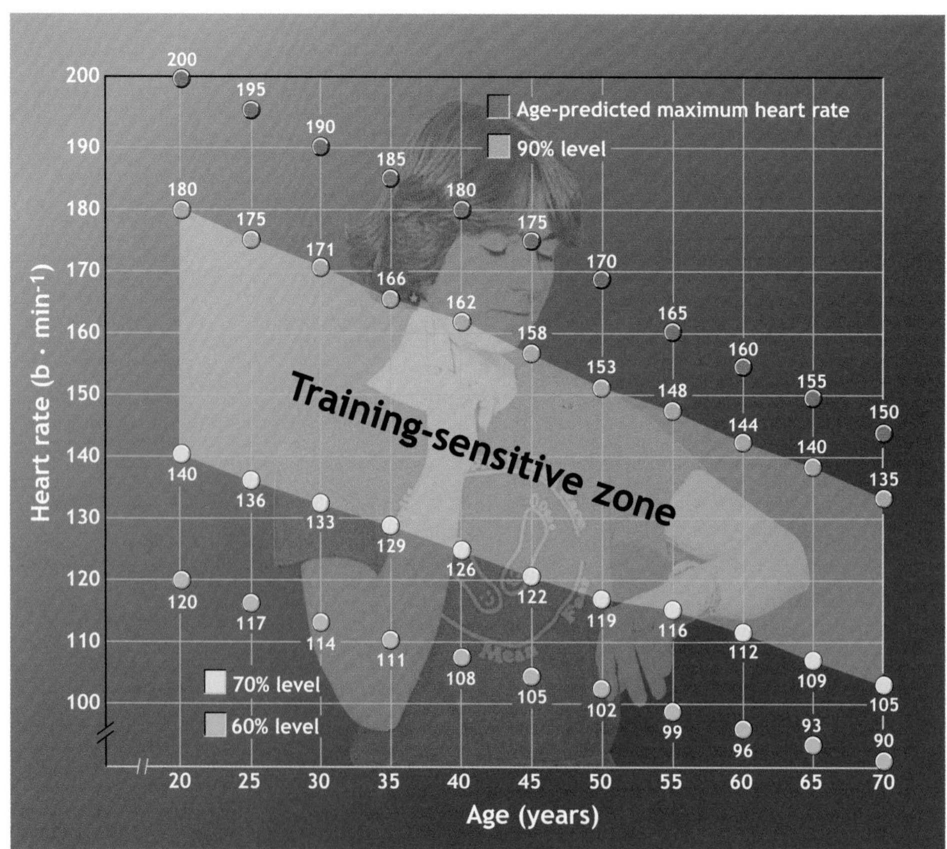

FIGURE 21.18 • Maximal heart rates and the training-sensitive zone for use in aerobic training of men and women of different ages.

124 b · min^{-1} (0.70 × [190 − 13]). This more accurately represents the appropriate threshold training heart rate for swimming. Without the appropriate heart rate adjustment, a prescription of upper-body exercise based on %HR_{max} in leg exercise results in *overestimation* of the appropriate threshold training heart rate.

Is Less-Intense Training Effective?

The often-cited recommendation of 70% HR_{max} as a training threshold for aerobic improvement represents a *general guideline* for effective yet comfortable exercise. The actual lower limit may depend on the participant's initial exercise capacity and current state of training. In addition, older and less fit, and sedentary, overweight men and women show training thresholds closer to 60% HR_{max}, which corresponds to about 45% $\dot{V}O_{2max}$.[64] Twenty to 30 minutes of continuous exercise at the 70% HR_{max} level stimulates a training effect; exercise at the lower intensity of 60% for 45 minutes also proves beneficial. *Generally, a longer exercise duration offsets a lower exercise intensity.*

Train at a Perception of Effort

In addition to oxygen consumption, heart rate, and blood lactate as indicators of exercise intensity, one also can use the **rating of perceived exertion (RPE)**.[19,183] With this psychophysiologic approach, the exerciser rates on a numerical scale (**Borg scale**, after researcher Gunnar Borg who developed this scaling system) perceived feelings in relation to the exertion level. Monitoring and adjusting RPE during exercise is a relatively easy and effective means to prescribe exercise on the basis of an individual's perception of effort that coincides nicely with objective measures of physiologic/metabolic strain (%HR_{max}, %$\dot{V}O_{2max}$, blood lactate concentration). Exercise levels corresponding to higher levels of energy expenditure and physiologic strain produce higher RPE ratings. For example, an RPE of 13 or 14 (exercise that feels "somewhat hard;" Fig. 21.19) coincides with about 70% HR_{max} during cycle ergometer and treadmill exercise; an RPE between 11 and 12 corresponds to exercise at the lactate threshold for trained and untrained individuals.[199] The RPE effectively establishes and regulates an exercise prescription for exercise intensities corresponding to blood lactate concentrations of 2.5 mM (RPE ≈ 15) and 4.0 mM (RPE ≈ 18) during a 30-minute treadmill run in which subjects self-regulated exercise intensity.[217] Individuals learn quickly to exercise at a specific RPE. In this sense, the axiom "listen to your body" becomes apropos.

RPE Scale	Equivalent % HR_{max}	Exercise Intensity % VO_{2max}
6		
7 Very, very light		
8		
9 Very light		
10		
11 Fairly light	52-66	31-50
12	61-85	51-75
13 Somewhat hard		
14	86-91	76-85
15 Hard		
16	92	85
17 Very hard		
18		
19 Very, very hard		

FIGURE 21.19 • The Borg scale (and accompanying estimates of relative exercise intensity) for obtaining the RPE during exercise. (Modified from Borg GA. Psychological basis of physical exertion. Med Sci Sports Exerc 1982;14:377.)

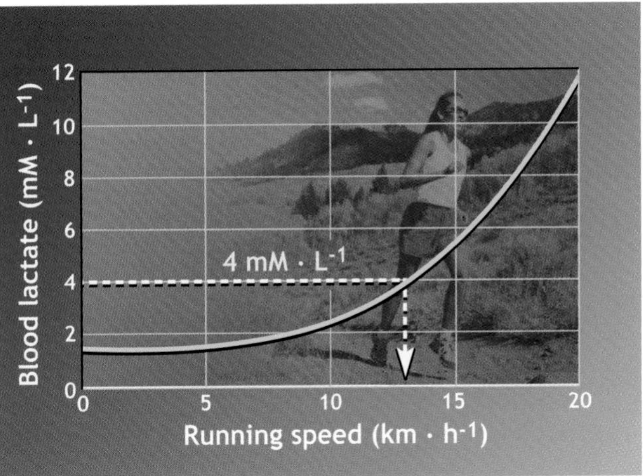

FIGURE 21.20 • Blood lactate concentration in relation to running speed for one subject. At a lactate level of 4.0 mM · L^{-1}, the corresponding running speed was approximately 13 km · h^{-1}. This speed establishes the subject's initial training intensity.

Train at the Lactate Threshold

Exercising at or slightly above the lactate threshold provides effective aerobic training, with the higher exercise levels producing the greatest benefits, particularly for fit individuals.[122,235] Figure 21.20 illustrates determination of the appropriate exercise level by plotting exercise intensity (e.g., running speed) in relation to blood lactate level. In this example, the running speed that produced a blood lactate concentration at the 4-mM level (OBLA) represented the recommended training intensity. While many coaches use the 4-mM blood lactate level as the optimal aerobic training intensity, no convincing evidence yet exists to justify this particular blood lactate level as "ideal." Regardless of the specific blood lactate level chosen for endurance training, the blood lactate–exercise intensity relationship should be evaluated periodically and the exercise intensity adjusted as aerobic fitness improves. If regular blood lactate measurement proves impractical, the exercise heart rate at the initial lactate determination remains a convenient and relatively stable marker for setting the appropriate predetermined exercise intensity. This is because no systematic training-induced change occurs in the heart rate–blood lactate relationship during incremental exercise.[58]

We endorse using RPE as an effective tool to estimate the blood lactate threshold when establishing an appropriate training intensity for continuous exercise.[217] However, recent observations indicate a change in the blood lactate concentration–RPE relationship with repeated bouts of exercise. The relationship remains altered from a single exercise bout, even after 3.5 hours of recovery.[236] This limits the use of RPE to gauge exercise intensity for a specific blood lactate concentration if repeated bouts of exercise occur during the same training session (e.g., during interval training; see page 487).

One important distinction between $\%HR_{max}$ and lactate threshold for setting training intensity lies in the physiologic dynamics each method reflects. More than likely, the $\%HR_{max}$ method establishes a level of exercise stress for overloading the central circulation (e.g., stroke volume, cardiac output), whereas the capability of the peripheral vasculature and active muscles to sustain steady-rate aerobic metabolism dictates exercise intensity adjustments based on lactate threshold.

Training Duration

No threshold duration per workout has been identified for optimal aerobic improvement. If a threshold exists, it probably depends on the interaction of many factors including total work accomplished (duration or training volume), exercise intensity, training frequency, and initial fitness level. Whereas 3- to 5-minute daily exercise periods produce training effects in some poorly conditioned people, 20- to 30-minute sessions achieve more-optimal results (within practicality for time) if intensity reaches at least 70% HR_{max}. With higher-intensity training, significant improvement occurs with only a 10-minute workout. Conversely, it requires at least 60 minutes of continuous exercise to produce a training effect when exercise intensity falls below 70% HR_{max}.

As for training volume, more does not necessarily produce greater results. In a study of collegiate swimmers, for example, one group trained for 1.5 hours daily, while another group performed two 1.5-hour exercise sessions each day.[39] Despite one group exercising at twice the daily exercise volume, *no differences* in swimming power, endurance, or performance time improvement emerged between groups.

Training Frequency

Does 2- or 5-day-a-week training produce differing effects if exercise duration and intensity remain constant for each training session? Unfortunately, the precise answer remains elusive. Some investigators report that training frequency significantly influences cardiovascular improvements while others maintain that this factor contributes considerably less than either exercise intensity or duration.[169] Studies using interval training show that training 2 days per week produced $\dot{V}O_{2max}$ changes similar in magnitude to those obtained when training 5 days per week.[59] In other studies that held total exercise volume constant, no differences emerged in $\dot{V}O_{2max}$ improvements between training frequencies of 2 and 4 or of 3 and 5 days per week.[206] As with training duration, more-frequent training becomes beneficial when training at a lower intensity.

While the extra time invested to increase training frequency may not prove profitable for improving physiologic function, the extra quantity of exercise (e.g., 3 vs. 6 d per wk) often represents a considerable caloric expenditure. *To affect meaningful weight loss through exercise, each exercise session should last at least 60 minutes at a sufficient intensity to expend 300 kcal or more.* Training only 1 day per week generally does not produce meaningful changes in anaerobic or aerobic capacity, body composition, or weight loss.[4]

Typical aerobic exercise training programs take place 3 days per week, usually with a rest day spaced between workout days. One could reasonably ask whether training on consecutive days would produce equally effective results. In an experiment concerned with this question, nearly identical improvements in $\dot{V}O_{2max}$ occurred regardless of sequencing of the 3-days-per-week training schedule.[146] This finding suggests that the stimulus for aerobic training links closely to exercise intensity and total work accomplished, *not* to the sequencing of training days.

Exercise Mode

Holding exercise intensity, duration, and frequency constant produces a similar training response, regardless of training mode—as long as the exercise involves relatively large muscle groups. Bicycling, walking, running, rowing, swimming, in-line skating, rope skipping, bench-stepping, stair climbing, and simulated arm–leg climbing all provide excellent overload for the aerobic system.[25,128,232] Based on the specificity concept, the magnitude of training improvement varies considerably depending on testing mode. Individuals trained on a bicycle show greater improvement when tested on a bicycle than treadmill.[160] Likewise, individuals who train by swimming or arm-cranking show the greatest improvement when measured during upper-body exercise.[66,135]

AMERICAN COLLEGE OF SPORTS MEDICINE'S UPDATED FITNESS GUIDELINES AND RECOMMENDATIONS

See the LWW connection site at (connection.lww.com/go/mcardle) for a full description of the latest recommendations by the American College of Sports Medicine (ACSM) concerning the recommended quantity and quality of exercise for developing and maintaining cardiorespiratory and muscular fitness and flexibility in healthy adults.[5] The guidelines for a "well-rounded training program" include flexibility exercises and modifications in previous recommendations for both aerobic and resistance training in light of the current exercise research literature. For example, a combined program of aerobic training and resistance training induces a significant increase in muscular strength and aerobic power, a decrease in body fat, and an increase in basal metabolic rate, while singular-focus programs of either resistance *only* or aerobic training *only* produced singularly larger but more-limited overall effects.[47]

- *Cardiovascular*. Recommended changes focus on helping the average person—more gradual approach with older and unfit individuals—adhere to a diverse fitness program that stimulates improvement in the full range of physical fitness components. Professionals now view exercise as exerting an additive effect; cardiovascular and health benefits derived from three 10-minute daily exercise bouts throughout the day almost equal the effects of one continuous 30-minute session. This enables many individuals to benefit from daily lifestyle exercise without the necessity of formally exercising for a distinct period in a more-structured gymnasium setting.[6,51] Clarifications have also delimited the dose of exercise required for aerobic fitness improvement. Persons should exercise at an intensity of 40–50 to 85% of $\dot{V}O_{2max}$ or 55–65 to 90% HR_{max} (lower number for unfit or sedentary persons) for at least 20 to 60 minutes more than 2 days a week. Previously sedentary or unfit individuals should exercise more than 2 days a week for at least 10 minutes. From a health perspective, further good news indicates that just moderate exercise (e.g., gardening or walking >60 min per wk) performed regularly reduces the risk of a first heart attack to the same extent as higher-intensity workouts.[119] These findings support current exercise recommendations of the American Heart Association, the Centers for Disease Control and Prevention, and the ACSM to strive for at least 30 minutes of moderate-intensity physical activity on most days.
- *Muscular strength*. The guidelines acknowledge the positive contributions of resistance training to fat-free body mass, particularly muscle and bone mass. Because single-set exercise produces only slightly less strength improvement than multiple-set exercise, men and women under 50 years of age should work major muscle groups with one set of 8 to 10 different exercises 2 to 3 days a week; weight loads should allow completion of 8 to 12 repetitions. Older and previously sedentary people perform one set of 10 to 15 repetitions. Also recognized are the potential cardiovascular benefits of regular, moderate resistance exercise—specifically, training-induced reductions in heart rate and blood pressure after training when lifting at a given resistance load.[170]
- *Joint flexibility*. A balanced fitness program should incorporate static and dynamic range-of-motion (flexibility) exercises of the body's major muscle/tendon groups (four repetitions per group) performed 2 to 3 days a week.

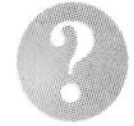

INTEGRATIVE QUESTION

What factors might account for individual differences in responsiveness of a group of individuals to the same exercise training program?

HOW LONG BEFORE IMPROVEMENTS OCCUR?

Aerobic fitness adaptations occur rapidly, with significant improvement noted within several weeks.[81] Figure 21.21 shows absolute and percentage improvements in $\dot{V}O_{2max}$ for subjects who trained 6 days per week for 10 weeks. Training consisted of stationary cycling for 30 minutes 3 days per week combined with running for up to 40 minutes on alternate days. The continuous week-to-week improvement in aerobic capacity indicates that training improvement in previously sedentary people occurs rapidly and progresses in relatively steady

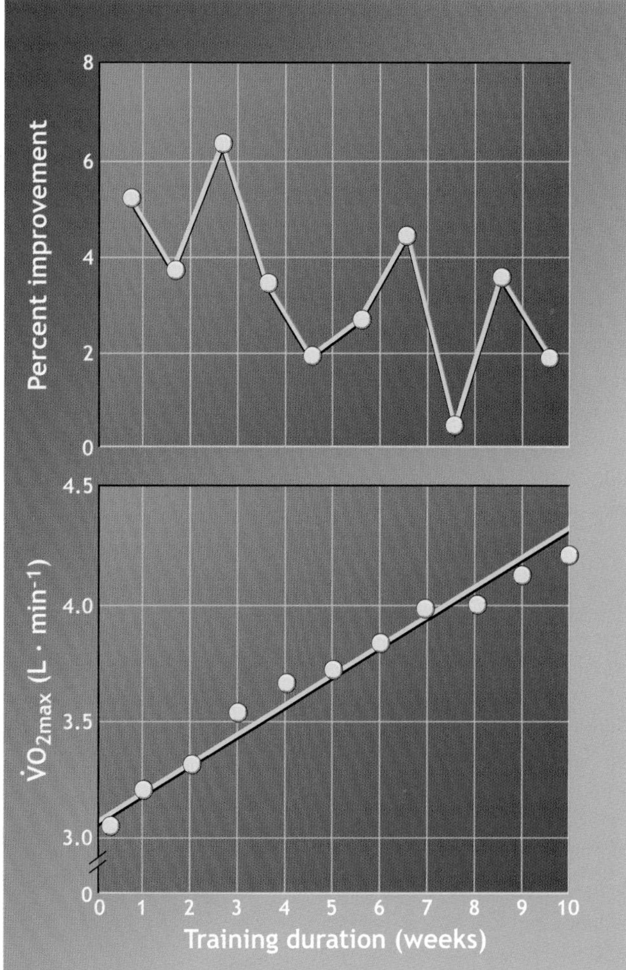

FIGURE 21.21 • Continuous improvements in $\dot{V}O_{2max}$ during 10 weeks of high-intensity aerobic training. (From Hickson RC, et al. Linear increases in aerobic power induced by a program of endurance exercise. J Appl Physiol 1977;42:373.)

TABLE 21.8 ➤ PHYSIOLOGIC RESPONSES DURING PEAK CYCLE ERGOMETER EXERCISE BEFORE AND AFTER 10 CONSECUTIVE DAYS OF AEROBIC EXERCISE TRAINING

VARIABLE	PRETRAINING	POSTTRAINING
$\dot{V}O_{2peak}$, L · min^{-1}	2.54 ± 0.29	2.80 ± 0.32*
Cardiac output, L · min^{-1}	18.3 ± 1.3	20.5 ± 1.7*
Heart rate, b · min^{-1}	189 ± 2	184 ± 2*
Stroke volume, mL	97 ± 7	112 ± 9*
a-$\bar{v}$ O_2 diff mL · dL^{-1}	13.6 ± 0.8	13.4 ± 0.6
Plasma volume (rest), mL	2896 ± 175	3152 ± 220*

*Statistically significant from pretraining valve at the .05 level.
From Mier CM, et al. Cardiovascular adaptations to 10 days of cycle exercise. J Appl Physiol 1997; 83:1900.

fashion. Of course, adaptive responses eventually level off as subjects approach their "genetically predisposed" maximums. The exact time for this leveling off remains unknown, particularly for high-intensity training. The data presented in Figure 21.17 indicate that each physiologic and metabolic system responds differently.

The data in Table 21.8 complement those in Figure 21.22 showing the rapidity of cardiovascular adaptations to aerobic exercise training.[141] Five young adult men and five women trained daily for 10 consecutive days. Exercise consisted of 1 hour of cycling—10 minutes at 65% $\dot{V}O_{2peak}$, 25 minutes at 75% $\dot{V}O_{2peak}$, and the last 25 minutes of repeat 5, 3-minute intervals at 95% $\dot{V}O_{2peak}$, followed by a 2-minute recovery. This relatively brief 10-day training period induced a 10% increase in $\dot{V}O_{2peak}$ accompanied by a 12% increase in cardiac output, 15% increase in stroke volume, and a slight decrease in heart rate during peak exercise. Resting plasma volume increased nearly 9% during the 10 days of training and correlated with the increases in exercise cardiac output and stroke volume. In addition, exercise training augmented the contractile (inotropic) response to β-adrenergic stimulation. These results indicate that significant cardiac adaptations occur with short-term exercise training in young men and women. Training-induced enhancement in inotropic response to β-adrenergic stimulation and greater blood volume at rest accompany improvements in cardiac output and stroke volume. Stroke volume increases during exercise reflected the *combined effects* of an increased left ventricular end-diastolic dimension (preload in accordance with the Frank-Starling mechanism) and increased systolic ejection.

Excessive exercise does not necessarily enhance aerobic fitness improvements. Furthermore, running injuries increase dramatically with large increases in training volume.[212] For men and women, the number of miles run per week was the only variable consistently associated with running injuries. In preadolescent children, running excessive distances may place undue strain on the articular cartilage. This type of strain could injure the bone's growth plate (epiphysis) and adversely affect normal growth.

Trainability and Genes

While a vigorous exercise-training program enhances a person's level of fitness regardless of genetic background, the limits for developing fitness capacity link closely to natural endowment. Of two individuals in the same exercise program, one might show 10 times more improvement than the other. Research in genetics indicates a genotype dependency for much of one's sensitivity in responding to maximal aerobic and anaerobic power training, including adaptations of most muscle enzymes.[20,22,46,174] In other words, both identical twins in a pair generally show a training response of similar magnitude. Figure 21.22 (A and B) indicates a clear similarity in the response of $\dot{V}O_{2max}$ (both mL · kg^{-1} · min^{-1} and %improvement) among ten pairs of male identical twins undergoing the same 20-week aerobic exercise training program. If one twin showed high responsiveness to training, a high likelihood existed that the other twin would also be a **responder**; similarly, the brother of a **nonresponder** to exercise training generally showed little improvement. Presence of the muscle-specific creatine kinase gene provides one example of the possible contribution of genetic makeup to individual differences in the responsiveness of $\dot{V}O_{2max}$ to endurance training.[181,182] Genetic makeup plays such a predominant role in

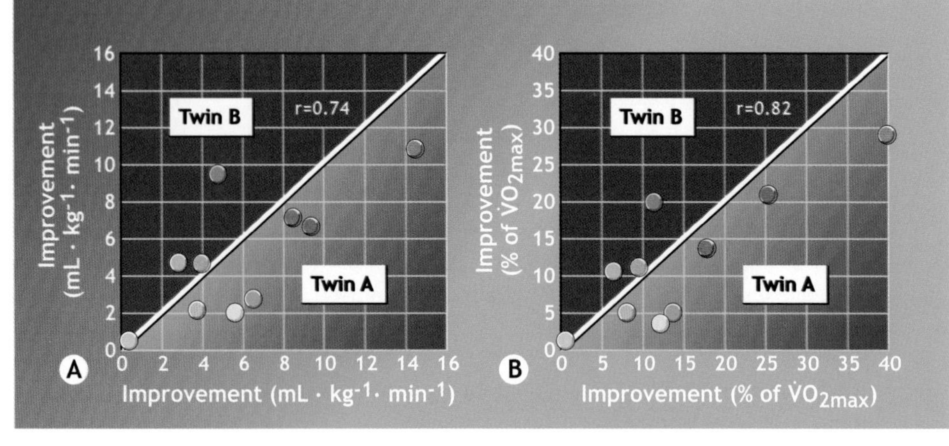

FIGURE 21.22 • Responsiveness of $\dot{V}O_{2max}$ (**A**, mL · kg^{-1} · min^{-1}; **B**, % improvement) of ten pairs of identical twins to a 20-week program of aerobic exercise training. *r*, Pearson product-moment correlation coefficient. Each of the 10 colored data points represents a twin pair. (From Bouchard C. Heredity, fitness, and health. In: Bouchard C, et al., eds. Physical activity, fitness, and health, Champaign, IL: Human Kinetics, 1990.)

training responsiveness that it makes it almost impossible to predict a specific individual's response to a given training stimulus.

MAINTENANCE OF AEROBIC FITNESS GAINS

An important question concerns the optimal exercise frequency, duration, and intensity to maintain aerobic improvements with training. In one study, healthy young adults increased $\dot{V}O_{2max}$ 25% with 10 weeks of interval training by bicycling and running for 40 minutes, 6 days a week.[80] They then joined one of two groups that continued to exercise an additional 15 weeks at the same intensity and duration but at a reduced *frequency* of either 4 or 2 days a week. Both groups maintained their gains in aerobic capacity despite up to two-thirds reduction in training frequency.

A similar study evaluated the effect of reduced training duration on the maintenance of improved aerobic fitness.[84] Upon completion of the same protocol outlined previously for the initial 10 weeks of training, subjects continued to maintain intensity and frequency of training for an additional 15 weeks, but reduced training *duration* from the original 40-minute sessions to either 26 or 13 minutes per day. They maintained almost all $\dot{V}O_{2max}$ and performance increases despite a two-thirds reduction in training duration. However, if *intensity* of training decreased and frequency and duration remained constant, even a one-third exercise intensity reduction produced a significant decline in $\dot{V}O_{2max}$.[85]

It appears that aerobic capacity improvement involves somewhat different training requirements than its maintenance. *With intensity held constant, the frequency and duration of exercise required to maintain a certain level of aerobic fitness remain considerably lower than that required for its improvement.* A small drop-off in exercise intensity, on the other hand, reduces $\dot{V}O_{2max}$. This indicates that exercise intensity plays a principal role in maintaining the increase in maximal aerobic power achieved through training.

Fitness components other than $\dot{V}O_{2max}$ more readily suffer adverse effects of reduced exercise training volume. Well-trained endurance athletes who normally trained 6 to 10 hours a week reduced weekly training to one 35-minute session and did not decrease $\dot{V}O_{2max}$ over a 4-week period.[134] However, their endurance capacity at 75% $\dot{V}O_{2max}$ significantly *decreased*, which related to reduced preexercise glycogen stores and a diminished level of fat oxidation during exercise. *These findings indicate that a single measure such as $\dot{V}O_{2max}$ cannot adequately evaluate all factors that affect training and detraining adaptations.*

Tapering for Peak Performance

In most instances, little improvement occurs in the aerobic systems during the competitive season. At best, athletes strive to prevent physiologic and performance decrements as the season progresses. Before major competition, however, athletes often reduce or **taper** training intensity and/or volume in the belief that such adjustments produce peak performance.[226] The taper period and exact alterations in training vary by sport.

Research presents no clear answers about optimum taper duration or training modification. From a physiologic perspective, probably 4 to 7 days provides sufficient time for maximum muscle and liver glycogen replenishment, optimal nutritional support and restoration, alleviation of residual muscle soreness, and healing of minor injuries. In one study of competitive runners, a 1-week taper period applied either no training (rest), low-intensity running (2 to 10 km daily at 60% $\dot{V}O_{2max}$), or high-intensity running (five 500-m repeats on day 1, decreasing one repeat each day).[203] Measurements during the taper period included blood volume, red blood cell mass, muscle glycogen content, muscle mitochondrial activity, and 1500-m race performance. Compared with the rest and low-intensity exercise taper conditions, high-intensity exercise taper produced the most benefit. This finding suggests that an optimal taper should include progressive reductions in training volume while maintaining a high level of training intensity. Further research must substantiate these findings and determine whether different sports require their unique tapering protocol.

METHODS OF TRAINING

Each year, performance improvements occur in almost all athletic competitions. These advances generally relate to increased opportunities for participation: individuals with "natural endowment" more likely become exposed to particular sports. Also, improved nutrition and health care, better equipment, and more systematic and scientific approaches to athletic training contribute to superior performance. In the following sections we present general guidelines for anaerobic and aerobic training.

Anaerobic Training

Figure 21.1 showed that the capacity to perform all-out exercise for up to 60 seconds largely depends on ATP generated by the immediate and short-term anaerobic systems for energy transfer.

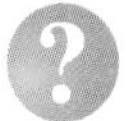

INTEGRATIVE QUESTION

In what specific ways would anaerobic exercise training improve performance in all-out physical activity?

The Intramuscular High-Energy Phosphates

Football, weightlifting, and other brief, sprint–power sport activities rely almost exclusively on energy derived from ATP and PCr, the muscles' high-energy phosphates. Engaging specific muscles in repeated 5- to 10-second maximum bursts of effort overloads this phosphagen pool. Because the intramuscular high-energy phosphates supply energy for brief, intense exercise, only small amounts of lactate accumulate and recovery progresses rapidly. Thus, exercise can begin again after about a 30-second rest period. The use of brief, all-out exercise interspersed with recovery represents a specific application of interval training to anaerobic conditioning (see page 487).

The activities selected in training to enhance ATP–PCr energy transfer capacity must engage the specific muscles at the movement speed and power output for which the athlete desires improved anaerobic power. Not only does this enhance the metabolic capacity of the specifically trained muscle fibers, but it also facilitates recruitment and modulation of firing sequence of the appropriate motor units activated in the actual movement.

Lactate-Generating Capacity

As duration of all-out effort extends beyond 10 seconds, dependence on anaerobic energy from the intramuscular high-energy phosphates decreases, with a proportionate increase in anaerobic energy transfer from glycolysis. To improve energy transfer capacity by the short-term lactic acid energy system, training must overload this aspect of energy metabolism.

Anaerobic training requires extreme physiologic and psychologic demands and considerable motivation. Repeated bouts of up to 1-minute maximum exercise stopped 30 seconds before subjective feelings of exhaustion cause blood lactate to increase to near-maximum levels. The individual repeats each exercise bout after 3 to 5 minutes of recovery. Repetition of exercise causes "lactate stacking," which results in a higher blood lactate level than with just one bout of all-out exhaustive effort.[79] Of course, as with all training, one must exercise the specific muscle groups that require enhanced anaerobic capacity. A backstroke swimmer trains by swimming the backstroke, a cyclist should bicycle, and basketball, hockey, or soccer players rapidly perform various movements and direction changes similar to those required by their sport.

As discussed in Chapter 7, recovery requires considerable time when exercise involves a significant anaerobic component. For this reason, anaerobic power training should occur at the end of the conditioning session. Otherwise, fatigue can hinder one's ability to perform subsequent aerobic training.

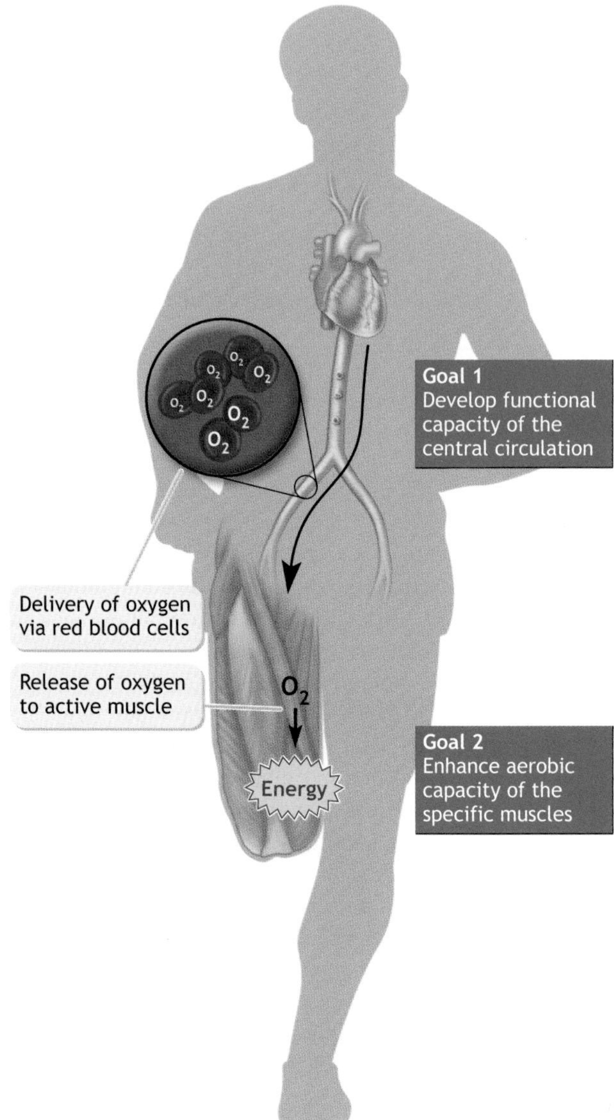

FIGURE 21.23 • The two major goals of aerobic training: *Goal 1,* develop the capacity of the central circulation to deliver oxygen; *Goal 2,* enhance the capacity of the active musculature to supply and process oxygen.

Aerobic Training

Figure 21.23 indicates two important factors in formulating an aerobic training program: (1) training must provide sufficient cardiovascular overload to stimulate increased stroke volume and cardiac output and (2) the central circulatory overload must result from exercising the sport-specific muscle groups to enhance their local circulation and "metabolic machinery." *In essence, proper endurance training overloads all components of oxygen transport and use.*[231] This consideration embodies the specificity principle as applied to aerobic training. Simply stated, runners should run, cyclists should bicycle, rowers should row, and swimmers should swim.

Relatively brief bouts of repeated exercise, as well as continuous, long-duration efforts, enhance aerobic capacity, provided exercise reaches sufficient intensity to overload the aerobic system. **Interval training**, **continuous training**, and **fartlek training** represent three common methods to improve aerobic fitness.

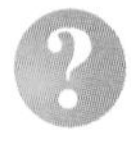

INTEGRATIVE QUESTION

What information would you need to develop a program to most effectively improve aerobic capacity for the specific physical job performance requirements for (1) firefighters, (2) police officers, and (3) oil field workers.

Interval Training

With correct spacing of exercise and rest, one can perform extraordinary amounts of high-intensity exercise, normally not possible if the exercise progressed continuously. The repeated exercise bouts (with rest periods or relief intervals) vary from a few seconds to several minutes or longer depending on the desired training outcome.[59,215,220,216] The interval training prescription evolves from the following considerations:

- Intensity of exercise interval
- Duration of exercise interval
- Length of recovery (relief) interval
- Number of repetitions of the exercise–relief interval

Consider the following example of performing a large volume of high-intensity exercise during an interval-training workout. Few people can maintain a 4-minute-mile pace for longer than 1 minute, let alone complete a mile within 4 minutes. Suppose we limited running intervals to only 10 seconds, followed by 30 seconds recovery. This scenario makes it reasonably easy to maintain these exercise–relief intervals and complete the mile in 4 minutes of actual running. Although this does not parallel a world-class performance, the example does indicate that a person can accomplish a significant quantity of normally exhausting exercise given proper spacing of rest and exercise intervals.

RATIONALE FOR INTERVAL TRAINING. Interval training has a sound basis in physiology and energy metabolism. In the example of a continuous run at a 4-minute-mile pace, anaerobic glycolysis provides a large portion of energy. Within a minute or two, the lactate level rises precipitously and the runner fatigues. During interval training, on the other hand, repeated 10-second exercise bouts permit completion of intense exercise without appreciable lactate buildup because the intramuscular high-energy phosphates provide the primary exercise energy source. Minimal fatigue results during the predominantly "alactic" exercise interval, and recovery progresses rapidly. The exercise interval can then begin after only a brief rest.

In interval training, as with other forms of physiologic conditioning, exercise intensity must activate the particular energy systems that require improvement. Table 21.9 provides practical guidelines for determining the appropriate exercise and recovery intervals.

- *Exercise interval*: Generally *add* 1.5 to 5.0 seconds to the exerciser's "best time" for training distances between 55 and 220 yards for running and 15 and 55 yards for swimming.[59] If a person can run 60 yards from a running start in 8 seconds, the training time for each repeat therefore equals 8 + 1.5, or 9.5 seconds. For an interval-training distance of 110 yards add 3 seconds, and for a distance of 220 yards add 5 seconds to the best running times. This particular type of interval training applies to training the intramuscular ATP-PCr energy system.
- Training distances of 440 yards running or 110 yards swimming: determine the exercise rate by *subtracting* 1 to 4 seconds from the best 440-yard part of a mile run or 110-yard part of a 440-yard swim. If a person runs a mile in 7 minutes (averaging 105 s per 440 yd), the interval time for each 440-yard repeat range is 104 seconds (105 − 1) to 101 seconds (105 − 4). For training intervals beyond 440 yards, *add* 3 to 4 seconds for each 440-yard portion of the interval distance. In running an interval of 880 yards, the 7-minute miler thus runs each interval at about 216 seconds [(105 + 3) × (2) = 216].
- *Relief interval*: The relief interval is either passive (rest–relief) or active (work–relief). A ratio of exercise duration to recovery duration usually formulates the duration of the relief interval. *The ratio of 1:3 generally applies to training the immediate energy system.* Thus, for a sprinter who runs 10-second intervals, the relief interval usually equals about 30 seconds (3 × 10 s). *For training the short-term energy system of glycolysis, the relief interval averages twice as long as the exercise interval, or a ratio of 1:2.* These specific work–relief ratios for anaerobic

TABLE 21.9 ➤ **GUIDELINES FOR DETERMINING INTERVAL-TRAINING EXERCISE RATES FOR RUNNING AND SWIMMING DIFFERENT DISTANCES**

Interval Training Distances (yards): Run	Swim	Work Rate for Each Exercise Interval or Repeat
55	15	1.5 } seconds *slower* than best
110	25	3.0 } times from a running (or swimming) start
220	55	5.0 } for each distance
440	110	1 to 4 seconds *faster* than the average 440-yard run or 110-yard swim times recorded during a mile run or 440-yard swim
660–1320	165–320	3 to 4 seconds *slower* than the average 440-yard run or 100-yard swim times recorded during a mile run or 440-yard swim

From Fox EL, Mathews DK. Interval training. Philadelphia: WB Saunders, 1974.

training supposedly ensure sufficient restoration of intramuscular phosphates and/or sufficient lactate removal to allow the next exercise bout to continue with minimal or no fatigue.

- *For training the long-term aerobic energy system, the exercise–relief interval ratio usually is 1:1 or 1:1.5.* During a 60- to 90-second high-intensity exercise interval, for example, oxygen consumption increases rapidly to a high level but remains insufficient to meet the exercise energy requirements. The recommended relief interval causes the succeeding exercise interval to begin before complete recovery (before return to baseline oxygen consumption). This ensures that cardiovascular and aerobic metabolic stress reach near-peak levels with repeated but relatively short exercise intervals. The duration of the rest interval takes on less importance with longer periods of intermittent exercise because sufficient time exists for adjustments in metabolic and circulatory parameters during exercise.

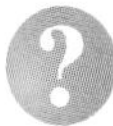

INTEGRATIVE QUESTION

A coach insists that a single exercise mode improves aerobic fitness for all physical activities requiring a high level of aerobic fitness. Give your opinion regarding the potential effectiveness of single-mode exercise to produce generalized cross-training effects?

SPRINT-TYPE INTERVAL TRAINING AFFECTS BOTH ANAEROBIC AND AEROBIC PHYSIOLOGIC SYSTEMS. Figure 21.24 shows that relatively brief but intense sprint interval training increases parameters of *both* anaerobic and aerobic metabolic capacity.[130] The 7-week training program for 12 young, adult men consisted of 30 seconds of maximum sprint effort (Wingate protocol) interspersed with 2 to 4 minutes of recovery, performed three times a week. Week 1 began with four exercise intervals with 4 minutes recovery per interval and progressed to ten exercise intervals with a 2.5-minute recovery per exercise bout by week 7. Despite this relatively brief training stimulus in

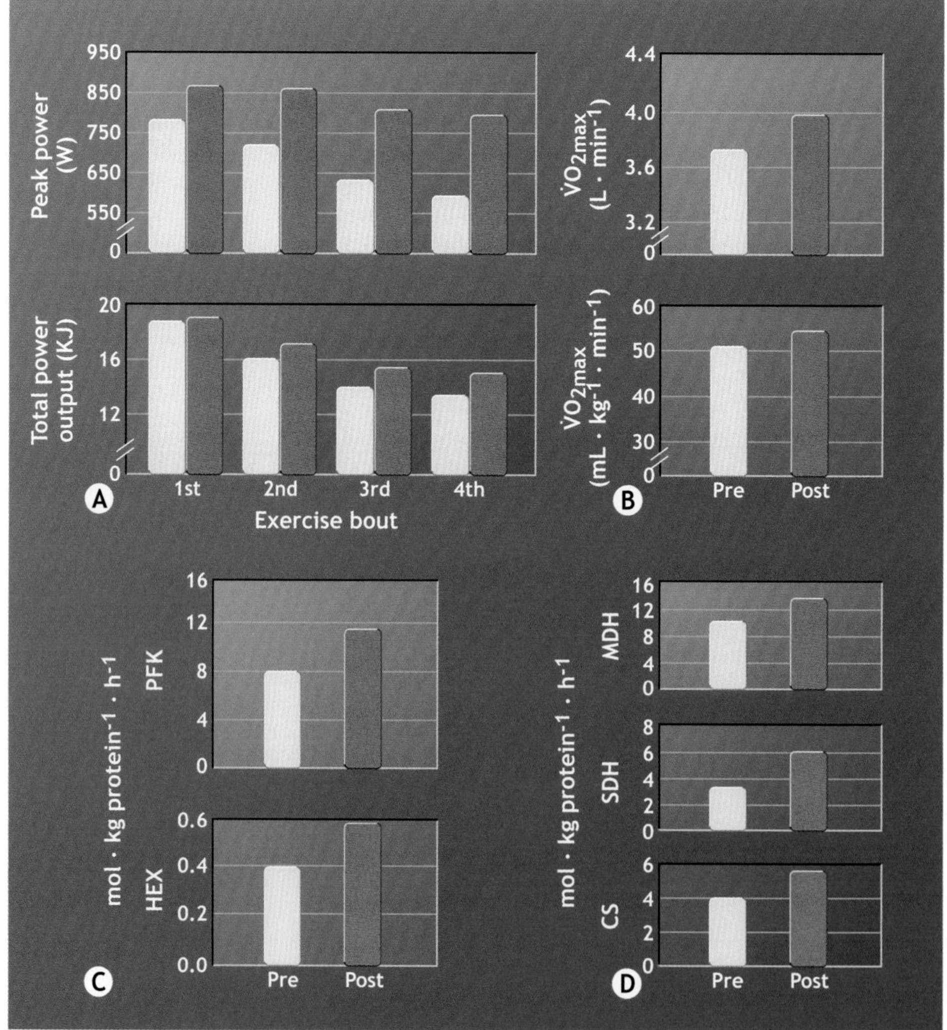

FIGURE 21.24 • Peak power output and total power output during four successive maximum 30-second efforts (**A**), $\dot{V}O_{2max}$ (**B**), maximal enzyme activity for phosphofructokinase *(PFK)* and hexokinase *(HEX)* (**C**), and maximal enzyme activity for malate dehydrogenase *(MDH)*, succinate dehydrogenase *(SDH)*, and citrate synthase *(CS)* *(D)* before *(yellow bars)* and after *(red bars)* 7 weeks of sprint interval training. (From MacDougall JD, et al. Muscle performance and enzymate adaptations to sprint interval training. J Appl Physiol 1998;84:2138.)

which exercise duration reached only 5 minutes per session during week 7, significant improvements occurred in $\dot{V}O_{2max}$, short-term power output, and maximal activity of key marker enzymes in the aerobic and anaerobic energy pathways. Positive clinical and cardiovascular adaptations to interval training also emerge among healthy elderly persons.[1]

Continuous Training

Continuous or long, slow distance (LSD) training involves steady-paced, prolonged exercise at either moderate or high aerobic intensity, usually 60 to 80% $\dot{V}O_{2max}$. The exact pace can vary, but it must at least meet a threshold intensity to ensure aerobic physiologic adaptations. Previously, we outlined the method to establish the training-sensitive zone (page 480). Continuous training for an hour or longer has become popular among joggers and other fitness enthusiasts, including competitive endurance athletes such as triathletes and cross-country skiers. For example, some elite distance runners train twice a day and run between 100 and 150 miles each week while preparing for competition. In one report (personal communication with authors), a man training for the 52.5 mile ultramarathon ran twice daily, 20 miles in the morning and 13 miles in the evening; he interspersed these runs with occasional 30- to 60-mile nonstop runs at a 7- to 8-minute per mile pace. Within this schedule, he ran more than 800 miles each month and totaled 9600 miles for the year! The precise benefits of such considerable training remain unknown.

Because of its submaximal nature, continuous exercise training progresses in relative comfort. This contrasts with the potential hazards of high-intensity interval training for coronary-prone individuals and the high level of motivation required for such strenuous exercise. Continuous training ideally suits those beginning an exercise program or wishing to accumulate a large caloric expenditure for weight loss. When applied in athletic training, continuous training actually represents "overdistance" training, with most athletes training two to five times the actual distances of competitive events.

An advantage of continuous training for endurance athletes permits exercising at nearly the same intensity as actual competition. Because specific motor unit recruitment depends on exercise intensity, continuous training may best apply to endurance athletes in terms of adaptations at the cellular level. This contrasts to interval training, which often places disproportionate stress on the fast-twitch motor units, *not* the slow-twitch units predominantly recruited in endurance competition.

Fartlek Training

Fartlek, a Swedish word meaning "speed play," represents a training method introduced to the United States in the 1940s. This relatively unscientific blending of interval and continuous training has particular application to exercise out-of-doors over natural terrain. The system uses alternate running at fast and slow speeds over both level and hilly terrain.

In contrast to the precise exercise-interval training prescription, fartlek training does not require systematic manipulation of exercise and relief intervals. Instead, the performer determines the training schema based on "how it feels" at the time, in a way similar to gauging exercise intensity based on one's rating of perceived exertion. If used properly, this method can overload one or all of the energy systems. Although lacking the systematic and quantified approaches of interval and continuous training, fartlek training provides an ideal means of general conditioning and off-season training. It also adds freedom and variety in workouts.

Insufficient evidence prevents proclaiming superiority of any specific training method for improving aerobic capacity. Each form of training produces success. One can probably use the various methods interchangeably, particularly to modify training and achieve a more psychologically pleasing exercise program.

OVERTRAINING: TOO MUCH OF A GOOD THING

Ten to 20% of athletes experience the syndrome of **overtraining**, or "staleness." As a result of complex interactions among biologic and psychologic influences, an athlete can fail to endure and adapt to training, so that normal exercise performance deteriorates, and the individual encounters increasing difficulty fully recovering from a workout.[26,107,109,176,229] This takes on crucial importance for elite athletes for whom performance decrements of 1 to 3% might cause a gold medalist to fail to qualify for competition.

Two clinical forms of overtraining have been described:

1. The less common **sympathetic form** (*basedowian* for thyroid hyperfunction patterns), characterized by increased sympathetic activity during rest; generally typified by hyperexcitability, restlessness, and impaired exercise performance. This form of overtraining may reflect excessive psychologic/emotional stress that accompanies the interaction among training, competition, and responsibilities of normal living.[118]
2. The more common **parasympathetic form** (*addisonoid* for adrenal insufficiency patterns) characterized by predominance of vagal activity during rest and exercise. More properly termed **overreaching** in the early stages (within as few as 10 d), the syndrome is qualitatively similar in symptoms to the full-blown parasympathetic overtraining syndrome but of shorter duration. Overreaching generally results from excessive and protracted overload with inadequate recovery and rest. Initially, maintenance of exercise performance requires greater effort, which eventually leads to performance deterioration in training and competition. Short-term rest intervention of a few days up to several weeks usually restores full function. Untreated overreaching eventually leads to the overtraining syndrome.

Parasympathetic overtraining syndrome represents more than just short-term inability to train as

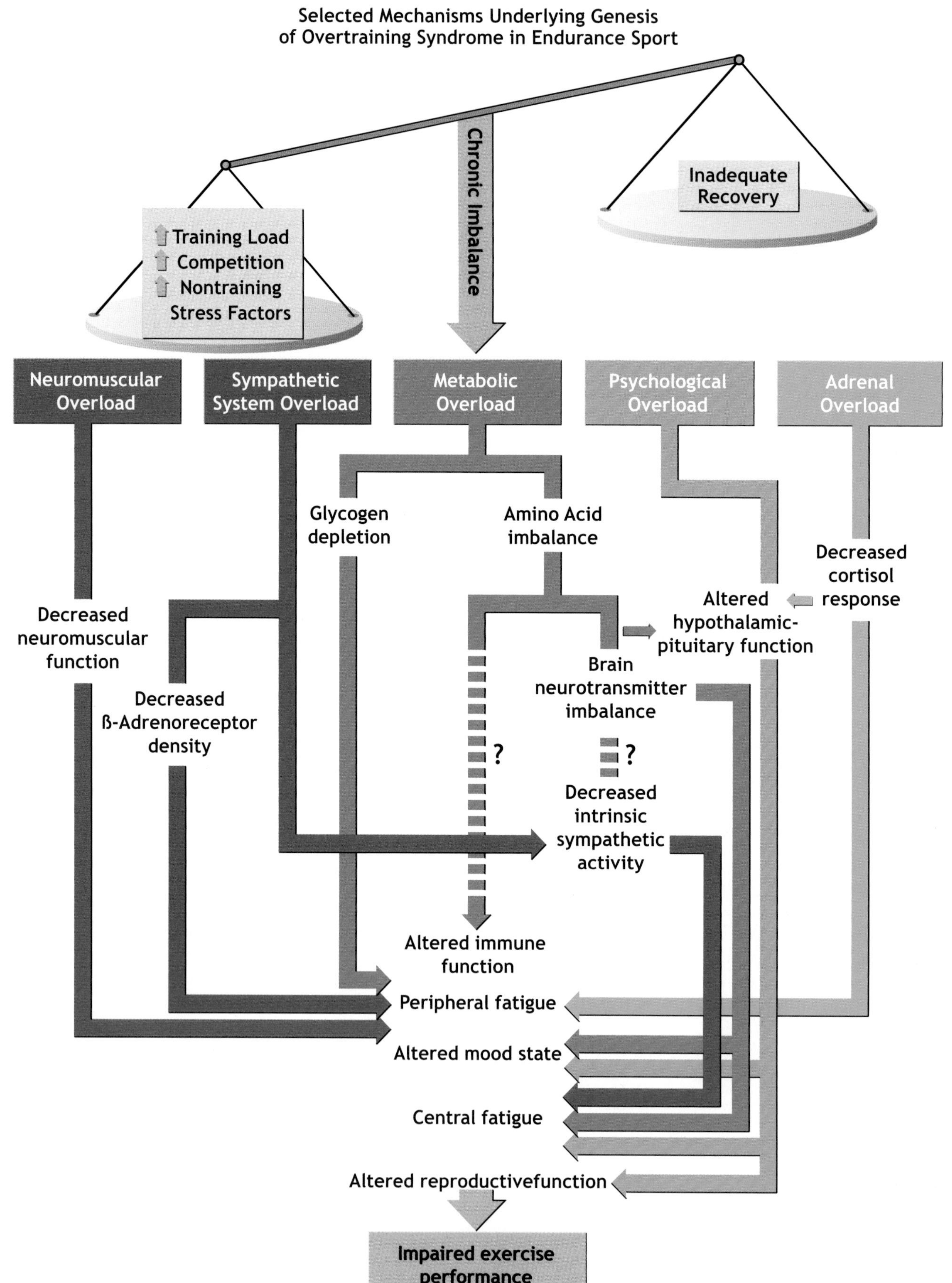

FIGURE 21.25 • Schematic overview of the genesis of the overtraining syndrome in endurance sports requiring prolonged, high-volume training. (Modified from Lehmann M, et al. Autonomic imbalance hypothesis and overtraining syndrome. Med Sci Sports Exerc 1998;30:1140.)

hard as usual or a slight dip in competition-level performance. Rather, it involves chronic fatigue experienced during exercise workouts and subsequent recovery periods. Associated symptoms include sustained poor exercise performance, altered sleep patterns and appetite, frequent infections, persistently high fatigue ratings, altered immune and reproductive function, acute and chronic alterations in systemic inflammatory responses, mood disturbances (anger, depression, anxiety), and a general malaise and loss of interest in high-level training. Injuries occur more frequently in the overtrained state. The syndrome may also result from complex interactions and subsequent effects of short- and long-term alterations in systemic inflammatory responses.[209]

DEFINITIONS OF TERMS RELATED TO THE OVERTRAINING SYNDROME[175]

- Overload: A planned, systematic, and progressive increase in training with the goal of improving performance.
- Overreaching: Unplanned, excessive overload with inadequate rest. Poor performance is observed in training and competition. Successful recovery should result from short-term (i.e., a few days up to 1 or 2 wk) interventions.
- Overtraining syndrome: Untreated overreaching that results in long-term decreased performance and impaired ability to train. Other problems may require medical attention.

Figure 21.25 gives an overview of possible factors that interact to initiate the parasympathetic-type overtraining syndrome in endurance-sports training. Interactions among chronic neuromuscular, neuroendocrine, psychologic, immunologic, and metabolic overload during long-term, high-volume training (with insufficient time for recuperation) eventually alter physiologic function and stress response to produce the overtrained state.[131,185] Preexisting medical conditions, poor diet (e.g., inadequate carbohydrate or dehydration), environmental stress (e.g., heat, humidity, altitude), and psychosocial pressures (e.g., monotonous training, frequent competition, personal conflicts) often interact to exacerbate the demands of training and increase the risk of developing overtraining syndrome.

Significant effects of overtraining include (1) functional impairments in the hypothalamo-pituitary-gonadal and adrenal axes and sympathetic neuroendocrine system as reflected by depressed urinary excretion of norepinephrine[118,225] and (2) exercise-induced increases in adrenocorticotropic hormone and growth hormone and decreases in cortisol and insulin levels.[229] In some ways the syndrome reflects the body's attempt to enforce upon the athlete an appropriate recuperative period from the sustained levels of arousal caused by prolonged heavy training and competition. Despite the highly individualized specific symptoms of the overtraining syndrome, those outlined in Table 21.10 are generally the most common. No simple, reliable method exists to diagnose overtraining in its earliest stages,[63,76,110] although deterioration in physical performance and alterations in mood rather than immune function changes provide the best indications.[156,202] Conditions that cause some athletes to thrive in training initiate overtraining in others. Generally, when symptoms emerge they persist unless the athlete rests, with complete recovery requiring weeks or even months. Currently, no reliable method exists to determine the point of complete recovery from the overtraining syndrome.

TABLE 21.10 ➤ THE OVERTRAINING SYNDROME: SYMPTOMS OF STALENESS

- Unexplained and persistently poor performance and high fatigue ratings
- Prolonged recovery from typical training sessions or competitive events
- Disturbed mood states characterized by general fatigue, apathy, depression, irritability, and loss of competitive drive
- Persistent feelings of muscle soreness and stiffness in muscles and joints
- Elevated resting pulse, painful muscles, and increased susceptibility to upper respiratory infections (altered immune function) and gastrointestinal disturbances
- Insomnia
- Loss of appetite, weight loss, and inability to maintain proper body weight for competition
- Overuse injuries

Proper periodization of training contributes significantly to preventing the overtraining syndrome. Specifically, coaches must provide for adequate recuperation during the most intense training cycles or when an athlete attempts to regain peak form following a layoff. Nutrition becomes particularly important during heavy training, with special emphasis placed on glycogen replenishment (sufficient recovery time plus high levels of dietary carbohydrate) and rehydration.

EXERCISING DURING PREGNANCY

Estimates indicate that 40% or more of women in the United States exercise during pregnancy.[77,244] Figure 21.26 illustrates the prevalence and pattern of exercise during pregnancy among 9,953 randomly selected pregnant women in 48 states, including the District of Columbia and New York City, who gave birth to live infants in 1988. Forty-two percent of all women reported exercising, one-half of whom exercised longer than 6 months. Walking was the leading activity (43% of all reported), followed by swimming (12%) and aerobics (12%). Older mothers and women who had multiple gestations, previous children, or an unfavorable reproductive history were less likely to exercise during pregnancy.

Heading Exercise Effects on the Mother

Maternal cardiovascular dynamics follow normal response patterns; moderate exercise offers no greater physiologic stress to the mother other than the additional weight gain and

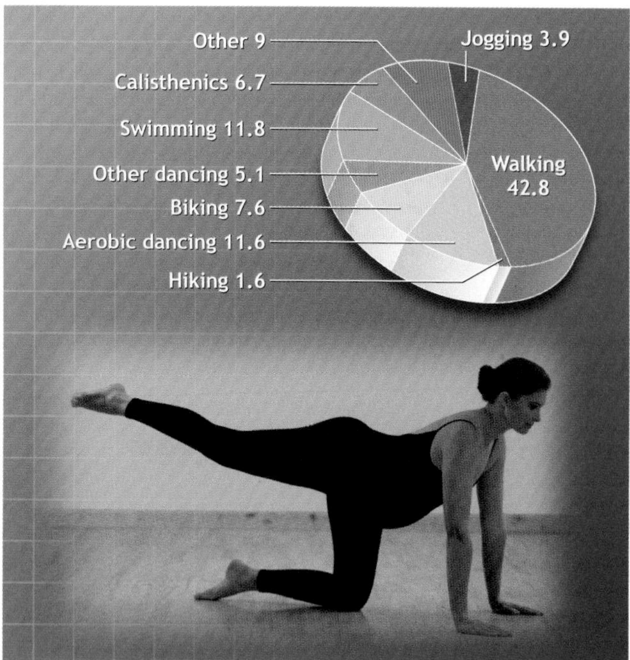

FIGURE 21.26 • Pattern of exercising (% of total) during pregnancy. (From Zhang J, Savitz DA. Exercise during pregnancy among US women. Ann Epidemiol 1996;6:53.)

possible encumbrance of fetal tissue. Pregnant women showed the same capacity as postpartum women to perform 40 minutes of cycling exercise at 70 to 75% $\dot{V}O_{2max}$. The physiologic responses to this weight-supported endurance exercise remained largely independent of gestation.[125] Furthermore, pregnancy does not compromise the absolute value for aerobic capacity ($L \cdot min^{-1}$).[127,189] As pregnancy progresses, the increase in maternal body mass and changes in coordination and balance add significantly to exercise effort with weight-bearing exercise because of an adverse effect on exercise economy.[164] Pregnancy, particularly in the last trimester, also increases pulmonary ventilation at a given submaximal exercise level.[125] Maternal exercise "hyperventilation" has been attributed to the direct stimulating effects of the hormone progesterone and an increased chemoreceptor sensitivity to carbon dioxide.[164,242] Recent evidence indicates that regular, moderate exercise during the second and third trimesters significantly reduces the ventilatory demands and rating of perceived exertion in submaximal exercise.[157] This training adaptation increases the mother's ventilatory reserve and possibly blunts exertional dyspnea during pregnancy. Table 21.11 summarizes the important maternal metabolic and cardiorespiratory adaptations to pregnancy.

Exercise Effects on the Fetus

With an increased number of women involved in physically demanding exercise, sports, and occupations, including those in the military and public safety, prudent recommendations must provide guidelines for exercise during pregnancy.[3,207] Epidemiologic evidence indicates that exercise during pregnancy does not relate to increased risk of fetal deaths or low birth weights.[195] In fact, beginning a moderate program of weight-bearing exercise early in pregnancy and continuing to exercise until term enhances fetoplacental growth.[34] In addition, a study of 577 middle-class women evaluated the effects of low–moderate exercise (<1000 kcal $\cdot$ wk^{-1}), heavier exercise (>1000 kcal $\cdot$ wk^{-1}), or no daily exercise on timely delivery and the safety and potential benefits of regular exercise during pregnancy.[77] No association emerged between low–moderate exercise and the length of gestation. A positive finding indicated that the higher volume of weekly exercise lowered rather than raised the risk of preterm birth; among births after the projected term, women who exercised more heavily delivered faster than nonexercisers.

The proposed potential exercise risks of intense maternal exercise for which repeated exposures could alter fetal growth and development include:

- Reduced placental blood flow and accompanying fetal hypoxia
- Fetal hyperthermia
- Reduced fetal glucose supply

Any factor that might temporarily compromise fetal blood supply raises concern in counseling pregnant women about exercise. Although research on humans in this area remains sparse, other species of mammals have been studied. In one investigation, treadmill exercise to exhaustion caused a fall in both uterine blood flow and arterial oxygen pressure in near-term pregnant ewes.[31] Despite this potentially negative response, a facilitated unloading of oxygen from the available blood supply maintained oxygen consumption by the utero-placental tissues and fetus. However, animals with one umbilical artery tied off to restrict placental circulation displayed a significant reduction in fetal oxygen supply during exer-

TABLE 21.11 ➤ IMPORTANT METABOLIC AND CARDIORESPIRATORY ADAPTATIONS DURING PREGNANCY

- Blood volume increases 40 to 50%; hemodilution causes reduced hemoglobin concentration
- Increase in blood volume causes dilation of left ventricle
- Slight increase in oxygen consumption at rest and during submaximal, weight-supported exercise such as stationary cycling
- Substantial increase in oxygen consumption during weight-bearing exercise such as walking and running
- Increased heart rate during rest and submaximal exercise
- Essentially no change in $\dot{V}O_{2max}$ ($L \cdot min^{-1}$)
- Increased ventilatory response—largely progesterone induced—during rest and submaximal exercise
- Possible magnified hypoglycemic response during exercise, especially late in pregnancy
- Possible blunted sympathetic nervous system responses to exercise in late gestation

Modified from Wolfe LA, et al. Maternal exercise, fetal well-being and pregnancy outcome. Exerc Sport Sci Rev 1994;22:145.

cise.[55] The researchers concluded that the fetus tolerated vigorous maternal exercise without adverse effects under normal conditions. In contrast, intense exercise posed a potential harmful reduction in oxygen supply to a fetus with some limitation in umbilical circulation.

Neonates born to exercising mothers exhibit a neurobehavioral profile as early as the fifth day after birth, which differs from that of neonates from more sedentary counterparts.[33] Exercising mothers either ran, performed aerobics, swam, or used stair-climbing exercise at least three times each week for more than 20 minutes at 55% of aerobic capacity or higher. The women in the control group led active lives that did not include regular, sustained bouts of exercise. Figure 21.27 shows data for five behavioral clusters of the Brazelton Neonatal Assessment Scales for the offspring of 34 women who exercised regularly and of 31 sedentary counterparts. No significant differences emerged between the neonates born to exercising women and those born to the sedentary controls for clusters assessing motor organization, autonomic stability, and range of state behaviors. However, the neonates born to exercising women scored significantly higher in orientation behavior and ability to regulate state (i.e., more alert and interested in the surroundings and less demanding of their mothers). The inset table indicates that axial length and head circumference remained similar between groups. However, the offspring of the exercising women were lighter and leaner than control group offspring. Although the mechanism for these differences remains unknown, the findings support the concept that continuing regular exercise throughout pregnancy modifies neonatal behavior by positively affecting early neurodevelopmental behaviors.

INTEGRATIVE QUESTION

What weight control advantage would derive during pregnancy from a daily walking program compared with a program of stationary cycling if each program remained at the same initial exercise level (i.e., constant walking speed or cycling power output), frequency, and duration?

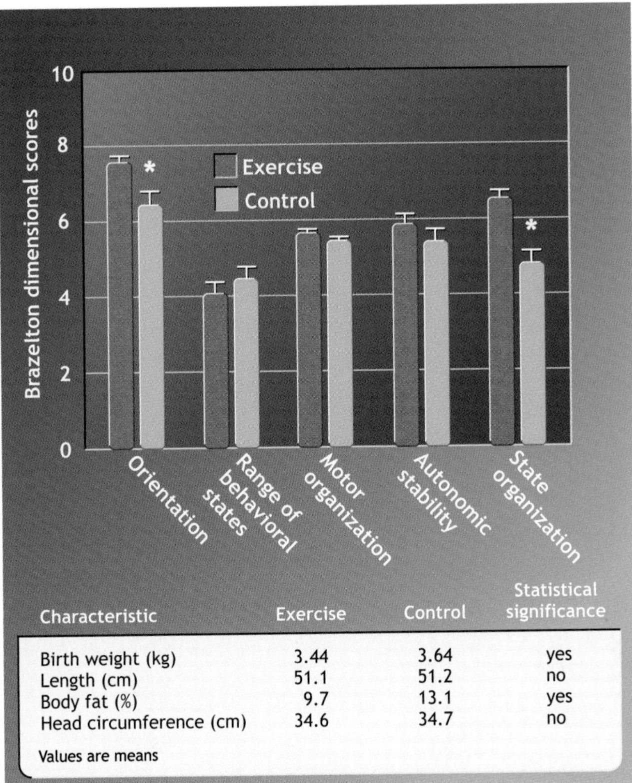

Characteristic	Exercise	Control	Statistical significance
Birth weight (kg)	3.44	3.64	yes
Length (cm)	51.1	51.2	no
Body fat (%)	9.7	13.1	yes
Head circumference (cm)	34.6	34.7	no

Values are means

FIGURE 21.27 • Behavioral constellation scores of neonates in exercise and nonexercise control groups on Brazelton Neonatal Behavioral Assessment Scales. Numbers in front of each set of vertical bars represent optimum score for each constellation; *asterisks* indicate statistical significance at the .01 level. *Insert table* presents neonatal morphometric values. (From Clapp JF III, et al. Neonatal behavioral profile of the offspring of women who continue to exercise regularly throughout pregnancy. Am J Obstet Gynecol 1999;180:91.)

Current Opinion

Reports document extreme levels of physical activity nearly to term for highly conditioned pregnant women, with no adverse effects on mother or fetus. Exercise protocols for these athletes included resistance training, endurance training, and interval training 6 days a week up to within 4 days of labor.[102] For an elite marathoner pregnant with twins, regular exercise consisted of training an average of 107 km (66.5 mi) weekly up to 3 days before birth of the twins.[10] In other research with active women with uncomplicated pregnancies, maximal exercise testing produced no untoward responses in fetal heart rate (minimal changes) or abnormal neonatal outcomes.[132] Despite these examples of extreme physical activity for well-trained women, with no apparent negative affect on maternal or fetal health, more conservative, prudent recommendations apply to most healthy, pregnant women. *Thirty to 40 minutes of moderate aerobic exercise for a previously active, healthy, low-risk woman during an uncomplicated pregnancy does not compromise fetal oxygen supply or acid–base status, induce heart rate signs of fetal distress, or produce other adverse effects to mother or fetus.*[125] Performed on a regular basis, such exercise not only maintains cardiovascular fitness, but also generates a training effect.[165,171] Hormonal action via the sympathetic nervous system during strenuous exercise probably diverts some blood from the uterus and visceral organs for preferential distribution to active muscles. This could pose a hazard to a fetus with restricted placental blood flow. The accompanying "In a Practical Sense" outlines guidelines for formulating the exercise prescription in pregnancy. The prudent approach dictates that a pregnant woman should exercise in moderation, especially if the pregnancy is at all compromised. In addition, exercise late in pregnancy may magnify the normal maternal hypoglycemic response by increasing glucose consumption by maternal skeletal muscle;

IN A PRACTICAL SENSE

➤➤ THE EXERCISE PRESCRIPTION DURING PREGNANCY

Pregnancy places unique demands on a women's physiology, necessitating some modification in exercise prescription. Pregnant women should consult a physician before initiating an exercise program (or modifying an existing program) to rule out possible complications. This pertains particularly to women of low fitness status and little exercise experience before pregnancy. The table below lists 14 common contraindications to exercising during pregnancy.

Exercise during pregnancy should heighten awareness about heat dissipation, adequate calorie and nutrient intake, and knowing when to reduce exercise intensity. For a normal, uncomplicated pregnancy, light-to-moderate exercise does not negatively affect fetal development; the benefits of a properly prescribed regular exercise during pregnancy generally outweigh potential risks.

Exercise Guidelines

Exercise mode: Avoid exercise in the supine position, particularly after the first trimester. Supine exercise can impair venous return (mass of the fetus compresses inferior vena cava), which could ultimately affect cardiac output and uterine blood flow. Non–weight-bearing exercise (e.g., cycling, swimming) minimizes the effect of gravity and the added weight associated with fetal development. Low-impact, weight-bearing exercise in moderation should not pose a risk.

Exercise frequency: Exercise 3 days a week, emphasizing continuous, steady-rate effort. With more frequent exercise, reduce the intensity.

Exercise duration: Exercise 30 to 40 minutes, depending on how the person feels.

Exercise intensity: Pregnancy alters the relationship between heart rate and oxygen consumption, making it difficult to establish guidelines from heart rate. An effective alternative establishes exercise intensity on the basis of the rating of perceived exertion (RPE), which should range between 11 ("fairly light") to 13 ("somewhat hard").

Rate of progression: Perform exercise on a regular basis; moderate aerobic exercise maintains cardiovascular fitness and often produces a small training effect. For most women the goal should not be exercise progression to induce training effects, but maintenance of cardiorespiratory fitness, muscle mass, and physician-recommended weight gain. The combined effects of pregnancy per se and regular exercise often produce improved fitness after delivery.

When to Stop Exercise and Seek Medical Advice

Discontinue exercise immediately under the following conditions:

- Any signs of vaginal bleeding
- Any gush of fluid from the vagina (premature rupture of membranes)
- Sudden swelling of ankles, hands, or face
- Persistent, severe headaches and/or disturbances in vision; unexplained lightheadedness or dizziness
- Elevated pulse rate or blood pressure that does not rapidly return to normal following exercise
- Excessive fatigue, palpitations, or chest pain
- Persistent uterine contractions (more than 6 to 8 per h)
- Unexplained or unusual abdominal pain
- Insufficient weight gain (< 1.0 kg per mo during the last two trimesters)

CONTRAINDICATIONS TO EXERCISE DURING PREGNANCY

- Pregnancy-induced hypertension
- Preterm rupture of membranes
- Preterm labor during the prior or current pregnancy
- Incompetent cervix
- Persistent second to third trimester bleeding
- Intrauterine growth retardation
- Type 1 diabetes
- History of two or more spontaneous abortions
- Multiple pregnancy
- Smoking
- Excessive alcohol intake
- History of premature labor
- Anemia
- Significant obesity

in the extreme, this response could adversely affect glucose supply to the fetus.[18,32,226]

Pregnant women should avoid supine exercise, contact sports, high-altitude exertion, hot tub immersion, and scuba diving. A decrease in uterine blood flow or elevation in maternal core temperature with extended duration exercise during environmental heat stress could compromise heat dissipation from the fetus through the placenta.[140] Because hyperthermia negatively affects fetal development (e.g., increased risk of neural tube defect), particularly in the first trimester,[144] pregnant women should exercise during warm weather in the cool part of the day for shorter intervals while maintaining regular fluid intake. Within this framework, aquatic exercise serves as an ideal form of maternal exercise.

Current fitness level and previous physical activity patterns should guide a woman's exercise behavior throughout an uncomplicated pregnancy and postpartum. Regular aerobic exercise can play an important role in maintaining functional capacity and general well-being during pregnancy. It also contributes to optimizing overall weight gain during the later stages of pregnancy,[32] and may reduce the risk for cesarean delivery in women having never born children.[27] Controversy remains about (1) whether extremes of maternal exercise benefit either mother or fetus or (2) if exercise during pregnancy benefits labor, delivery, birthweight, and general outcome.[17,166] Beginning regular exercise 6 to 8 weeks postpartum causes no deleterious effect on the volume or composition of lactation, and significantly improves the mother's aerobic fitness.[44,126]

Summary

1. Physical activities generally classify by the specific energy transfer system they predominantly activate. An effective training program commits to training the appropriate energy system(s) to improve a desired physiologic function or performance goal.
2. Physical conditioning based on sound principles produces optimum improvements. Overload, specificity, individual differences, and reversibility represent the primary training principles.
3. Exercise training initiates cellular adaptations and gross physiologic changes.
4. Anaerobic training increases resting levels of intramuscular anaerobic substrates and key glycolytic enzymes. Adaptations usually accompany concomitant increases in all-out exercise performance.
5. Aerobic training adaptations include increases in mitochondrial size and number, the quantity of aerobic enzymes, muscle capillarization, and fat and carbohydrate oxidation, all of which enhance aerobic production of ATP.
6. A linear relationship exists between heart rate and oxygen consumption from light to moderately intense exercise in trained and untrained individuals. Improved stroke volume with endurance training shifts this line significantly to the right, decreasing heart rate at any submaximal exercise level.
7. Aerobic training induces functional and dimensional changes in the cardiovascular system. These changes include decreases in resting and submaximal exercise heart rate, enhanced stroke volume and cardiac output, and an expanded a-$\bar{v}$ O_2 difference.
8. Cardiac hypertrophy represents a fundamental biologic adaptation to an increased myocardial workload imposed by exercise training. Cardiac enlargement with endurance training increases left ventricular volume and enhances stroke volume.
9. The pattern of structural and dimensional changes in the left ventricle varies with specific exercise training modes. No scientific evidence shows that regular exercise harms normal heart function.
10. Major factors that affect exercise training improvements include initial fitness level; frequency, intensity, and duration of exercise; and type (mode) of training. Of these, exercise intensity is the most crucial.
11. One can apply training intensity on either an absolute basis for exercise load or relative to a person's physiologic responses. The most practical approach sets exercise intensity to a percentage of HR_{max}. Training levels that correspond to between 60–70 and 90% of HR_{max} effectively induce aerobic fitness changes.
12. Training duration and intensity interact in their effects on the training response. Generally, 30-minute exercise sessions are practical and effective. Extending the duration compensates for reduced exercise intensity.
13. Two to 3 days a week is probably the minimum frequency for aerobic training. Optimal training frequency remains undetermined.
14. With intensity, duration, and frequency held constant, similar training improvements occur regardless of training mode when training involves large muscle groups and training evaluation remains task specific.
15. The frequency and duration of training required to maintain improved aerobic fitness are lower than those required to improve it. However, even small decreases in exercise intensity significantly reduce $\dot{V}O_{2max}$.
16. Interval, continuous, and fartlek training effectively improve the capacity of the different energy transfer systems. Interval training seems most desirable for improving the immediate and short-term anaerobic energy systems.
17. Aerobic training must consider overloading both cardiovascular function and metabolic capacity of the specific muscles. Peripheral adaptations in muscle profoundly enhance endurance performance.
18. Prolonged and intense endurance training can lead to the syndrome of overtraining, or staleness, with associated alterations in neuroendocrine and immune functions. The syndrome includes chronic fatigue, poor exercise performance, frequent infections, and general loss of interest in training. Symptoms generally persist until the athlete takes adequate time off from training, possibly several days to months.
19. At least 40% of American women exercise during pregnancy. Walking is the most common form of exercise (42%), followed by swimming (12%) and aerobics (12%).
20. Reduced placental blood flow and accompanying fetal hypoxia, fetal hyperthermia, and reduced fetal glucose supply pose the most serious potential exercise risks during pregnancy.
21. For previously active, healthy women, moderate aerobic exercise does not compromise fetal oxygen supply. It remains unclear whether extremes of maternal exercise benefit the course of pregnancy or the child in the early period after birth.

References

1. Ahmaidi S, et al. Effects of interval training at the ventilatory threshold on clinical and cardiorespiratory responses in elderly humans. Eur J Appl Physiol 1998;78:170.
2. Almeida SA, et al. Epidemiological patterns of musculoskeletal injuries and physical training. Med. Sci Sports Exerc 1999;31:1176.
3. American College of Obstetricians and Gynecologists (ACOG). Technical bulletin. Exercise during pregnancy and the postnatal period. Washington, DC: ACOG, 1985.
4. American College of Sports Medicine. Guidelines for exercise, testing and prescription. 4th ed. Philadelphia: Lea & Febiger, 1991.
5. American College of Sports Medicine. Position stand on the recommended quantity and quality of exercise for developing and maintaining cardiorespiratory and muscular fitness, and flexibility in healthy adults. Med Sci Sports Exerc 1998;30:975.
6. Anderson RE, et al. Effects of lifestyle activity vs structured aerobic exercise in obese women. JAMA 1999;281:335.
7. Andrew GM, et al. Effect of athletic training on exercise cardiac output. J Appl Physiol 1966;21:503.
8. Azevedo JL, et al. Training decreases muscle glycogen turnover during exercise. Eur J Appl Physiol 1998;78:479.
9. Babcock MA, et al. High frequency diaphragmatic fatigue detected with paired stimuli in humans. Med Sci Sports Exerc 1998;30:506.
10. Baily DM, et al. Endurance training during a twin pregnancy in a marathon runner. Lancet 1998;351:1182.
11. Bassett DR Jr, Howley ET. Maximal oxygen uptake: "classical" versus "contemporary" viewpoints. Med Sci Sports Exerc 1997;29:591.
12. Bennet DH, et al. Echocardiographic left ventricular dimensions in pressure and volume overload. Their use in assessing aortic stenosis. Br Heart J 1975;37:971.
13. Bergman BC, Brooks GA. Respiratory gas-exchange ratios during graded exercise in fed and fasted trained and untrained men. J Appl Physiol 1999;86:479.
14. Bilodeau B, et al. Upper-body testing of cross-country skiers. Med Sci Sports Exerc 1995;27:1557.
15. Bizeau ME, et al. Differential responses to endurance training in subsarcolemmal and interfyofibrillar mitochondria. J Appl Physiol 1988;85:1279.
16. Blair SN, et al. Physical fitness and all-cause mortality: a prospective study of healthy men and women. JAMA 1989;262:2395.
17. Bloom SL, et al. Lack of effect of walking on labor and delivery. N Engl J Med 1998;339:76.
18. Bonnen A, et al. Substrate and endocrine responses during exercise at selected stages of pregnancy. J Appl Physiol 1992;73:134.
19. Borg GA. Psychological basis of physical exertion. Med Sci Sports Exerc 1982;14:377.
20. Bouchard C, et al. Aerobic performance in brothers, dizygotic and monozygotic twins. Med Sci Sports Exerc 1986;18:639.
21. Bouchard C, et al. Long-term exercise training with constant energy intake. I: effect on body composition and selected metabolic variables. Int J Obes 1990;14:57.
22. Bouchard C, et al. Genetics of aerobic and anaerobic performance. Exerc Sport Sci Rev 1992;20:27.
23. Boutellier U. Respiratory muscle fitness and exercise endurance in healthy humans. Med Sci Sports Exerc 1998;30:1169.
24. Bowles DK, et al. Coronary smooth muscle and endothelial adaptations to exercise training. Exerc Sport Sci Rev 2000;28:57.
25. Brahler CJ, Blank SE. VersaClimbing elicits higher $\dot{V}O_{2MAX}$ than does treadmill running or rowing ergometry. Med Sci Sports Exerc 1995;27:249.
26. Budgett R, et al. Redefining the overtraining syndrome as the unexplained underperformance syndrome. Br J Sports Med 2000;34:67.
27. Bungum T et al. Exercise during pregnancy and type of delivery in Nullipare. J Obstet Gynecol Neonatal Nurs 2000;29:258.
28. Carroll JF, et al. Effect of training on blood volume and plasma hormone concentrations in the elderly. Med Sci Sports Exerc 1995;27:79.
29. Casaburi R, et al. Effect of endurance training on possible determinants of $\dot{V}O_2$ during heavy exercise. J Appl Physiol 1987;62:199.
30. Clanton TL, et al. Effects of swim training on lung volumes and inspiratory muscle conditioning. J Appl Physiol 1987;62:39.
31. Clapp JF III. Acute exercise stress in the pregnant ewe. Am J Obstet Gynecol 1980;136:489.
32. Clapp JF III, Little KD. Effect of recreational exercise on pregnancy weight gain and subcutaneous fat deposition. Med Sci Sports Exerc 1995;27:170.
33. Clapp JF III, et al. Neonatal behavioral profile of the offspring of women who continue to exercise regularly throughout pregnancy. Am J Obstet Gynecol 1999;180:91.
34. Clapp JF III et al.: Beginning regular exercise in early pregnancy: effect on fetoplacental growth. Am J Obstet Gynecol 2000;183:1484.
35. Coggan AR. Plasma glucose metabolism during exercise: effect of endurance training in humans. Med Sci Sports Exerc 1997;29:620.
36. Coggan AR, et al. Skeletal muscle adaptations to endurance training in 60- to 70-yr-old men and women. J Appl Physiol 1992;72:1780.
37. Coggan AR, et al. Isotopic estimation of CO_2 production during exercise before and after endurance training. J Appl Physiol 1993;75:70.
38. Coggan AR, et al. Glucose kinetics during high-intensity exercise in endurance-trained and untrained humans. J Appl Physiol 1995;78:1203.
39. Costill DL, et al. Adaptations to swimming training: influence of training volume. Med Sci Sports Exerc 1991;23:371.
40. Coyle EF, et al. Time course of loss of adaptations after stopping prolonged intense endurance training. J Appl Physiol 1984;57:1857.
41. Cunningham DA, et al. Development of cardiorespiratory function in circumpubertal boys: a longitudinal study. J Appl Physiol 1984;56:302.
42. Delp MD. Differential effects of training on the control of skeletal muscle perfusion. Med Sci Sports Exerc 1998;30:361.
43. Delp MD, Laughlin MH. Time course of enhanced endothelium-mediated dilation in aorta of trained rats. Med Sci Sports Exerc 1997;29:1454.
44. Dewey KG, et al. A randomized study of the effects of aerobic exercise by lactating women on breast-milk volume and composition. N Engl J Med 1994;330:449.
45. Dickhuth HH, et al. The long-term involution of physiological cardiomegaly and cardiac hypertrophy. Med Sci Sports Exerc 1989;21:244.
46. Dionne FT, et al. Mitochondrial DNA sequence polymorphism, $\dot{V}O_{2max}$ and response to endurance training. Med Sci Sports Exerc 1991;23:177.
47. Dolezal BA, Potteiger JA. Concurrent resistance and endurance training influence basal metabolic rate in nondieting individuals. J Appl Physiol 1998;85:695.
48. Donovan CM, et al. Enhanced efficiency of lactate removal after endurance training. J Appl Physiol 1990;68:1053.
49. Donovan CM, Sumida DD. Training enhanced hepatic gluconeogenesis: the importance for glucose homeostasis during exercise. Med Sci Sports Exerc 1997;29:628.
50. Duncan JJ, et al. Women walking for health and fitness: how much is enough? JAMA 1992;266:3295.
51. Dunn AL, et al. Comparison of lifestyle and structured interventions to increase physical activity and cardiorespiratory fitness. JAMA 1999;281:327.
52. Effron MB. Effects of resistive training on left ventricular function. Med Sci Sports Exerc 1989;21:694.
53. Ehsani AA, et al. Exercise training improves left ventricular systolic function in older men. Circulation 1991;83:96.
54. Ekblom B, et al. Effect of training on circulatory response to exercise. J Appl Physiol 1968;24:518.
55. Emmanouilides GC, et al. Fetal responses to maternal exercise in sheep. Am J Obstet Gynecol 1982;112:130.
56. Fleck SJ, et al. Magnetic resonance imaging determination of left ventricular mass: junior Olympic weightlifters. Med Sci Sports Exerc 1993;25:522.
57. Focht BC, Koltyn KL. Influence of resistance exercise of different intensities on state anxiety and blood pressure. Med Sci Sports Exerc 1999;31:456.
58. Foster C, et al. Stability of the blood lactate-heart rate relationship in competitive athletes. Med Sci Sports Exerc 1999;31:578.
59. Fox EL, et al. Frequency and duration of interval training programs and changes in aerobic power. J Appl Physiol 1975;38:481.
60. Franklin BA. Aerobic exercise training programs for the upper body. Med Sci Sports Exerc 1989;21:S141.
61. Friedlander AL, et al. Training-induced alterations of carbohydrate metabolism in women: women respond differently than men. J Appl Physiol 1998;85:1175.
62. Fuller D, et al. Expiratory muscle endurance performance after exhaustive submaximal exercise. J Appl Physiol 1996;80:1495.
63. Gabriel HHW, et al. Overtraining and immune system: a prospective longitudinal study in endurance athletes. Med Sci Sports Exerc 1998;30:1151.
64. Gaesser GA, Rich GA. Effects of high- and low-intensity exercises on aerobic capacity and blood lipids. Med Sci Sports Exerc 1984;16:269.

65. George KP, et al. Echocardiographic evidence of concentric left ventricular enlargement in female weight lifters. Eur J Appl Physiol 1998;79:88.
66. Gergley TJ, et al. Specificity of arm training on aerobic power during swimming and running. Med Sci Sports Exerc 1984;16:349.
67. Gledhill N, et al. Endurance athletes' stroke volume does not plateau: major advantage is diastolic function. Med Sci Sports Exerc 1994;26:1116.
68. Goldsmith RL, et al. Physical fitness as a determinant of vagal modulation. Med Sci Sports Exerc 1997;29:812.
69. Gollnick P, Hermansen L. Biochemical adaptation to exercise: anaerobic metabolism. Exerc Sport Sci Rev 1973;1.
70. Gollnick P, et al. Effects of training on enzyme activity and fiber composition of human skeletal muscle. J Appl Physiol 1973;34:107.
71. Hagberg JM. Physiologic adaptations to prolonged high-intensity exercise training in patients with coronary artery disease. Med Sci Sports Exerc 1991;23:661.
72. Hagberg JM, et al. Expanded blood volumes contribute to increased cardiovascular performance of endurance-trained older men. J Appl Physiol 1998;85:484.
73. Hagberg JM, et al. Specific genetic markers of endurance performance and $\dot{V}O_{2max}$. Exer Sport Sci Revs 2001;29:15.
74. Hambrecht R, et al. Effect of exercise on coronary endothelial function in patients with coronary artery disease. N Engl J Med 2000;342:454.
75. Harms CA, et al. Respiratory muscle work compromises leg blood flow during maximal exercise. J Appl Physiol 1997;82:1573.
76. Hartmann U, Mester J. Training and overtraining markers in selected sport events. Med Sci Sports Exerc 2000;32:209.
77. Hatch M, et al. Maternal leisure-time exercise and timely delivery. Am J Public Health 1998;88:1528.
78. Hepple RT. Skeletal muscle: microcirculatory adaptation to metabolic demand. Med Sci Sports Exerc 2000;32;117.
79. Hermansen L. Lactate production during exercise. In: B Pernow, B Saltin, eds. Muscle metabolism during exercise. New York: Plenum, 1971.
80. Hickson RC, Rosenkoetter MA. Reduced training frequencies and maintenance of aerobic power. Med Sci Sports Exerc 1981;13:13.
81. Hickson RC, et al. Linear increases in aerobic power induced by a strenuous program of endurance exercise. J Appl Physiol 1977;42:373.
82. Hickson RC. Skeletal muscle cytochrome c and myoglobin, endurance, and frequency of training. J Appl Physiol 1981;51:746.
83. Hickson RC, et al. Time course of the adaptive responses of aerobic power and heart rate to training. Med Sci Sports Exerc 1981;13:17.
84. Hickson RC, et al. Reduced training duration effects on aerobic power, endurance, and cardiac growth. J Appl Physiol 1985;53:255.
85. Hickson RC, et al. Reduced training intensities and loss of aerobic power, endurance, and cardiac growth. J Appl Physiol 1985;58:492.
86. Hill DW, et al. Temporal specificity in adaptations to high-intensity exercise training. Med Sci Sports Exerc 1998;30:450.
87. Holloszy JO. Metabolic consequences of endurance exercise training. In: Horton ES, Terjung RL, eds. Exercise, nutrition, and energy metabolism. New York: Macmillan, 1988.
88. Holloszy JO, Coyle EF. Adaptations of skeletal muscle to endurance exercise and their metabolic consequences. J Appl Physiol 1984;56:831.
89. Hooker SP, et al. Oxygen uptake and heart rate relationship in persons with spinal cord injury. Med Sci Sports Exerc 1993;25:1115.
90. Horowitz JF. Regulation of lipid mobilization and oxidation during exercise in obesity. Exer Sport Sci Revs 2001;29:42.
91. Hue O, et al. Ventilatory responses during experimental cycle-run transition in triathletes. Med Sci Sports Exerc 1999;31:1422.
92. Hurley BF, et al. Effects of high intensity strength training on cardiovascular function. Med Sci Sports Exerc 1984;16:483.
93. Jacobs I. Sprint training effects on muscle myoglobin, enzymes, fiber types, and blood lactate. Med Sci Sports Exerc 1987;19:368.
94. James F, et al. Responses of normal children and young adults to controlled bicycle exercise. Circulation 1980;61:902.
95. Jirka Z, Adamus M. Changes of ventilation equivalents in young people in the course of three years of training. J Sports Med 1965;5:1.
96. Johnson BD, et al. Mechanical constraints on exercise hyperpnea in endurance athletes. J Appl Physiol 1992;73:874.
97. Johnson BD, et al. Exercise induced diaphragmatic fatigue in healthy humans. J Physiol (Lond) 1993;460:385.
98. Johnson BD, et al. Respiratory muscle fatigue during exercise: implications for performance. Med Sci Sports Exerc 1996;28:1129.
99. Johnson JM. Physical training and the control of skin blood flow. Med Sci Sports Exerc 1998;30:382.
100. Jones BH, et al. Epidemiology of injuries associated with physical training among young men in the army. Med Sci Sports Exerc 1993;25:197.
101. Joyner MJ. Physiological limiting factors and distance running: influence of gender and age on record performances. Exerc Sport Sci Rev 1993;21:103.
102. Kardel KR, Kase T. Training in pregnant women: effects on fetal development and birth. Am J Obstet Gynecol 1998;178:280.
103. Karvonen MJ, et al. The effects of training on heart rate. A longitudinal study. Ann Med Exp Biol Fenn 1957;35:305.
104. Katz A, Sahlin K. Role of oxygen in regulation of glycolysis and lactate production in human skeletal muscle. Exerc Sport Sci Rev 1990;18:1.
105. Klausen K, et al. Adaptive changes in work capacity, skeletal muscle capillarization, and enzyme levels during training and detraining. Acta Physiol Scand 1981;113:9.
106. Koplan JP, et al. The natural history of exercise: a 10-yr follow-up of a cohort of runners. Med Sci Sports Exerc 1995;27:1180.
107. Krieder RB, et al. Overtraining in sport. Champaign, IL: Human Kinetics, 1998.
108. Krip B, et al. Effect of alterations in blood volume on cardiac function during maximal exercise. Med Sci Sports Exerc 1997;29:1469.
109. Kuipers M. How much is too much? Performance aspects of overtraining. Res Q Exerc Sport 1996;67:S65.
110. Kuipers H. Training and overtraining: an introduction. Med Sci Sports Exerc 1998;30:1137.
111. Kvernmo HD, et al. Enhanced endothelium dependent vasodilation in human skin vasculature induced by physical conditioning. Eur J Appl Physiol 1998;79:30.
112. Lakatta EG. Cardiovascular regulatory mechanisms in advanced age. Physiol Rev 1993;73:413.
113. Landers DM, Petruzzewllo SJ. Physical activity, fitness, and anxiety. In: Bouchard C, et al., eds. Physical activity, fitness, and health. Champaign, IL: Human Kinetics, 1994.
114. Lash JM, et al. Exercise training effects on collateral and microvascular resistance in rat model of arterial insufficiency. Am J Physiol 1995;28:H125.
115. Laughlin MH, McAllister RM. Exercise training-induced coronary vascular adaptation. J Appl Physiol 1992;73:2209.
116. Laughlin MH, et al. Control of blood flow to cardiac and skeletal muscle during exercise, In: Rowell LB, Sheperd JT, eds. Handbook of physiology, exercise: regulation and integration of multiple systems. Bethesda, MD: American Physiological Society, 1996.
117. Lawrie RA. Effect of enforced exercise on myoglobin in muscle. Nature 1953;171:1069.
118. Lehmann M, et al. Autonomic imbalance hypothesis and overtraining syndrome. Med Sci Sports Exerc 1998;30:1140.
119. Lemaitre RN, et al. Leisure-time physical activity and the risk of primary cardiac arrest. Arch Intern Med 1999;159:686.
120. Levine BD, et al. Left ventricular pressure-volume and Frank-Starling relations in endurance athletes: implications for orthostatic tolerance and exercise performance. Circulation 1991;84:1016.
121. Loftin M, et al. Effect of arm training on central and peripheral circulatory function. Med Sci Sports Exerc 1988;20:136.
122. Londeree BR. Effect of training on lactate/ventilatory thresholds: a meta-analysis. Med Sci Sports Exerc 1997;29:837.
123. Londeree BR, Moeschberger ML. Effect of age and other factors on maximal heart rate. Res Q Exerc Sport 1982;53:297.
124. Londeree BR, et al. $\%\dot{V}O_{2max}$ regressions for six modes of exercise. Med Sci Sports Exerc 1995;27:458.
125. Lotgering FK, et al. Respiratory and metabolic responses to endurance cycle exercise in pregnant and postpartum women. Int J Sports Med 1998;19:193.
126. Lotgering FK, et al. Maximal aerobic exercise in pregnant women: heart rate, O_2 consumption, CO_2 production, and ventilation. J Appl Physiol 1991;70:1016.
127. Lovelady CA, et al. Effects of exercise on plasma lipids and metabolism of lactating women. Med Sci Sports Exerc 1995;27:22.
128. Loy SF, et al. Effects of stairclimbing on $\dot{V}O_{2max}$ and quadriceps strength in middle-aged females. Med Sci Sports Exerc 1994;26:241.
129. MacDonald, MJ et al. Peripheral circulatory factors limit rate of increase in muscle O_2 uptake at onset of heavy exercise. J Appl Physiol 2001;90:83.
130. MacDougall JD, et al. Muscle performance and enzymate adaptations to sprint interval training. J Appl Physiol 1998;84:2138.

131. Mackinnon LT. Effects of overtraining and overreaching on immune function. In: Kreider R, et al., eds. Overtraining and overreaching in sport. Champaign, IL: Human Kinetics, 1997.
132. MacPhail, A et al. Maximal exercise testing in late gestation: Fetal responses. Obstet Gynecol 2000;96:565.
133. Mador M, et al. Diaphragmatic fatigue after exercise in healthy subjects. Am Rev Respir Dis 1993;148:1571.
134. Madsen K, et al. Effects of detraining on endurance capacity and metabolic changes during prolonged endurance exercise. J Appl Physiol 1993;75:1444.
135. Magel JR, et al. Metabolic and cardiovascular adjustment to arm training. J Appl Physiol 1978;45:75.
136. Martin WH III. Effect of endurance training on fatty acid metabolism during whole body exercise. Med Sci Sports Exerc 1997;29:635.
137. McAllister RM. Adaptations in control of blood flow with training: splanchnic and renal blood flows. Med Sci Sports Exerc 1998;30:375.
138. McArdle WD, et al. Specificity of run training on $\dot{V}o_{2max}$ and heart rate changes during running and swimming. Med Sci Sports 1978;10:16.
139. McConnell AK, Semple ESG. Ventilatory sensitivity to carbon dioxide: the influence of exercise and athleticism. Med Sci Sports Exerc 1996;28:685, 1996.
140. McMurray RG, Katz VL. Thermoregulation in pregnancy. Sports Med 1990;10:146.
141. Mier CM, et al. Cardiovascular adaptations to 10 days of cycle exercise. J Appl Physiol 1997;83:1900.
142. Miller WC, et al. Predicting max HR and HR-$\dot{V}O_2$ relationship for exercise prescription in obesity. Med Sci Sports Exerc 1993;25:1077.
143. Milliken MC, et al. Left ventricular mass by magnetic resonance imaging in male endurance athletes. Am J Cardiol 1988;62:301.
144. Milunsky A, et al. Maternal heat exposure and neural tube defects. JAMA 1992;268:882.
145. Mitchell JH, et al. How to recognize "athletes heart." Phys Sportsmed 1992;20(8):87.
146. Moffatt R. Placement of tri-weekly training sessions: importance regarding enhancement of aerobic capacity. Res Q 1977;48:583.
147. Montain SJ, Coyle EF. Fluid ingestion during exercise increases skin blood flow independent of increases in blood volume. J Appl Physiol 1992;73:903.
148. Moore RL, Korzick D. Cellular adaptations of the myocardium to chronic exercise. Prog Cardiovasc Dis 1996;37:371.
149. Moore RL, Palmer BM. Exercise training and cellular adaptations of normal and diseased hearts. Exerc Sport Sci Rev 1999;27:285.
150. Mueller P, et al. Renal hemodynamic responses to dynamic exercise in rabbits. J Appl Physiol 1998;85:1605.
151. Mujika I, Padilla S. Cardiorespiratory and metabolic characteristics of detraining in humans. Med Sci Sports Exerc 2001;33:413.
152. Nagashima K, et al. Mechanism for the posture-specific plasma volume increase after a single intense exercise protocol. J Appl Physiol 1999;86:867.
153. Neumann G. Anrass ungen des Stoffwech sels unter dem Einfluβ des sportlichen Trainings. In: Strauzenberg SE, Gürtler HH, et al., eds. Sportmedizin. Leipzig: Johann Ambrosius Baarth, 1990.
154. Nieuwland P, et al. Training effects on peak $\dot{V}O_2$, specific of the mode of movement, in rehabilitation of patients with coronary artery disease. !nt J Sports Med 1998;19:358.
155. Obert P, et al. Effect of long-term intensive endurance training on left ventricular structure and diastolic function in prepubertal children. Int J Sports Med 1998;19:149.
156. O'Connor PJ. Overtraining and staleness. In: Morgan WP, ed. Physical activity and mental health. Washington, DC: Taylor and Francis, 1997.
157. Ohtake PJ, Wolfe LA. Physical conditioning attenuates respiratory responses to steady-state exercise in late gestation. Med Sci Sports Exerc 1998;30:17.
158. Olson MS, et al. The cardiovascular and metabolic effects of bench stepping exercise in females. Med Sci Sports Exerc 1991;23:1311.
159. Pattengale PK, Holloszy JO. Augmentation of skeletal muscle myoglobin by a program of treadmill running. Am J Physiol 1967;213:783.
160. Pechar GS, et al. Specificity of cardiorespiratory adaptation to bicycle and treadmill training. J Appl Physiol 1974;36:753.
161. Pelliccia A, et al. Athletes heart in women. Echocardiographic characterization of highly trained elite female athletes. JAMA 1996;276:211.
162. Pelliccia A, et al. Physiologic left ventricular cavity dilation in elite athletes. Ann Intern Med 1999;130:23.
163. Pickering GP, et al. Effects of endurance training on the cardiovascular system and water compartments in elderly subjects. J Appl Physiol 1997;83:1300.
164. Pivarnik JM, et al. Physiological and perceptual responses to cycle and treadmill exercise during pregnancy. Med Sci Sports Exerc 1991;23:470.
165. Pivarnik JM, et al. Effects of maternal aerobic fitness on cardiorespiratory responses to exercise. Med Sci Sports Exerc 1993;25:993.
166. Pivarnik JM. Potential effects of maternal physical activity on birth weight: brief review. Med Sci Sports Exerc 1998;30:400.
167. Plumm BM, et al. The athlete's heart: a meta-analysis of cardiac structure. Circulation 2000;101:336.
168. Pollock ML, et al. Effects of mode of training on cardiovascular function and body composition of adult men. Med Sci Sports 1975;7:139.
169. Pollock ML, et al. Effects of frequency and duration of training on attrition and incidence of injury. Med Sci Sports 1977;9:31.
170. Pollock ML, et al. Resistance exercise in individuals with and without cardiovascular disease. Circulation 2000;101:828.
171. Potteiger JA, et al. From parturition to a marathon: a 16-week study of an elite runner. Med Sci Sports Exerc 1993;25:673.
172. Powers SK, Criswell D. Adaptive strategies of respiratory muscles in response to endurance exercise. Med Sci Sports Exerc 1996;28:1115.
173. Powers SK, et al. Myosin phenotype and bioenergetic characteristics of rat respiratory muscles. Med Sci Sports Exerc 1997;29:1573.
174. Prud'homme D, et al. Sensitivity of maximal aerobic power to training is genotype-dependent. Med Sci Sports Exerc 1984;16:489.
175. Raglin J, Bardukas A. Overtraining in athletes: the challenge of prevention. A consensus statement. ACSM's Health Fitness J 1999;3(2):27.
176. Raglin JS, Wilson GS. Overtraining in athletes. In: Hanin YL, ed. Emotion in sports. Champaign, IL: Human Kinetics, 1999:.
177. Rasmussen R, et al. Pulmonary ventilation, blood gases and blood pH after training of the arms and the legs. J Appl Physiol 1975;38:250.
178. Ricci G, et al. Left ventricular size following endurance, sprint, and strength training. Med Sci Sports Exerc 1982;14:344.
179. Richardson RS. Oxygen transport: air to muscle cell. Med Sci Sports Exerc 1998;30:53.
180. Riley-Hagen M, et al. Left ventricular dimensions and mass using magnetic resonance imaging in female endurance athletes. Am J Cardiol 1992;69:1067.
181. Rivera MA, et al. Muscle-specific creatine kinase gene polymorphism and $\dot{V}O_{2max}$ in the HERITAGE Family Study. Med Sci Sports Exerc 1997;29:1311.
182. Rivera MA, et al. Linkage between a muscle-specific CK gene marker and $\dot{V}O_{2max}$ in the HERITAGE Family Study. Med Sci Sports Exerc 1999;31:698.
183. Robertson RJ, Noble BJ. Perception of physical exertion: methods, mediators, and applications. Exerc Sport Sci. Rev 1997;25:407.
184. Roca J, et al. Evidence for tissue diffusion limitation of $\dot{V}O_{2max}$ in normal humans. J Appl Physiol 1989;67:291.
185. Rowbottom DG, et al. The hematological, biochemical and immunological profile of athletes suffering from the overtraining syndrome. Eur J Appl Physiol 1995;70:502.
186. Rowell LB. Human cardiovascular control. Cary, NC: Oxford University Press, 1994.
187. Rowland T, et al. Cardiac responses to exercise in child distance runners. Int J Sports Med 1998;19:385.
188. Rundell KW. Treadmill roller ski test predicts biathlon roller ski race results of elite U.S. biathlon women. Med Sci Sports Exerc 1995;27:1677.
189. Sady MA, et al. Cardiovascular response to maximal cycle exercise during pregnancy and at two and seven months postpartum. Am J Obstet Gynecol 1990;162:1181.
190. Saltin B, et al. Phosphagen and carbohydrate metabolism during exercise in trained middle-aged men. Scand J Clin Invest 1974;33:71.
191. Saltin B, Rowell LB. Functional adaptations to physical activity and inactivity. Fed Proc 1980;39:1506.
192. Saltin B, et al. Response to exercise after bed rest and after training. Circulation 1968;38(Suppl 7).
193. Sawka MN, et al. Blood volume: importance and adaptations to exercise training, environmental stresses, and trauma/sickness. Med Sci Sports Exerc 2000;32:332.
194. Schaefer ME, et al. Adrenergic responsiveness and intrinsic sinoatrial automaticity of exercise-trained rats. Med Sci Sports Exerc 1992;24:887.
195. Schramm WF, et al. Exercise, employment, other daily activities, and adverse pregnancy outcomes. Am J Epidemiol 1996;143:211.

196. Seals DR, Chase PB. Influence of physical training on heart rate variability and baroreflex circulatory control. J Appl Physiol 1989;66:1886.
197. Seals DR, et al. Endurance training in older men and women. II. Blood lactate responses to submaximal exercise. J Appl Physiol 1984;57:1030.
198. Seals DR, et al. Exercise and aging: autonomic control of the circulation. Med Sci Sports Exerc 1994;26:568.
199. Seip RL, et al. Perceptual responses and blood lactate concentration: effect of training state. Med Sci Sports Exerc 1991;23:80.
200. Shenk JH, et al. Spectrophotometric characteristics of hemoglobins. J Biol Chem 1934;105:741.
201. Shephard RJ. Exercise and training in women, part I: influence of gender on exercise and training responses. Can J Appl Physiol 2000;5:19.
202. Shephard RJ, Shek PN. Acute and chronic over-exertion: do depressed immune responses provide useful markers? Int J Sports Med 1998;19:159.
203. Shepley B, et al. Physiological effects of tapering in highly trained athletes. J Appl Physiol 1992;72:706.
204. Shin K, et al. Autonomic differences between athletes and nonathletes: spectral analysis approach. Med Sci Sports Exerc 1997;29:1482.
205. Shoemaker JD, et al. Relationships between fluid and electrolyte hormones and plasma volume during exercise with training and detraining. Med Sci Sports Exerc 1998;30:497.
206. Sidney KH, et al. In: Taylor AW, ed. Training: scientific basis and application. Springfield, IL: Charles C Thomas, 1972.
207. Simpson JL. Are physical activity and employment related to preterm birth and low birth weight? Am J Obstet Gynecol 1993;168:1231.
208. Sliwinski P, et al. Influence of global inspiratory muscle fatigue on breathing during exercise. J Appl Physiol 1996;80:1270.
209. Smith LL. Cytokine hypothesis of overtraining: a physiological adaptation to excessive stress? Med Sci Sports Exerc 2000;32:317.
210. Spengler CM, et al. Decreased exercise blood lactate concentrations after respiratory endurance training in humans. Eur J Appl Physiol 1999;79:299.
211. Spina RJ, et al. Exercise training prevents decline in stroke volume during exercise in young healthy subjects. J Appl Physiol 1992;72:2458.
212. Stanish WD. Overuse injuries in athletes; a perspective. Med Sci Sports Exerc 1984;16:1.
213. Starritt EC, et al. Effect of short-term training on mitochondrial ATP production rate in human skeletal muscle. J Appl Physiol 1999;86:450.
214. Stepien RL, et al. Effect of endurance training on cardiac morphology in Alaskan sled dogs. J Appl Physiol 1998;85:1368.
215. Stepto NK, et al. Effects of different interval-training programs on cycling time-trial performance. Med Sci Sports Exerc 1999;31:736.
216. Stepto NK, et al. Metabolic demands of intense aerobic interval training in competitive cyclists. Med Sci Sports Exerc, 2001;33:303.
217. Stoudemire NM, et al. The validity of regulating blood lactate concentration during running by rating perceived exertion. Med Sci Sports Exerc 1996;28:490.
218. Stranes JW, Bowles DK. Role of exercise in the cause and prevention of cardiac dysfunction. Exerc Sport Sci Rev 1995;23:349.
219. Tabata I, et al. Effects of moderate-intensity endurance and high-intensity intermittent training on anaerobic capacity and $\dot{V}O_{2max}$. Med Sci Sports Exerc 1996;28:1327.
220. Tabata I, et al. Metabolic profile of high intensity intermittent exercises. Med Sci Sports Exerc 1997;29:390.
221. Tanaka K, et al. Assessment of exercise-induced alterations in body composition of patients with coronary heart disease. Eur J Appl Physiol 1993;66:323.
222. Taylor R, Jones N. The reduction by training of CO_2 output during exercise. Eur J Cardiol 1979;9:53.
223. Thompson PD, et al. Cardiac dimensions and performance after either arm or leg endurance training. Med Sci Sports Exerc 1981;13:303.
224. Tkachuk GA, Martin GL. Exercise therapy for patients with psychiatric disorders: research and clinical implications. Prof Psychol Res Pract 1999;30:275.
225. Traeger LT, et al. Hormonal, immunological, and hematological responses to intensified training in elite swimmers. Med Sci Sports Exerc 1997;29:1637.
226. Trappe S, et al. Effect of swim taper on whole muscle and single muscle fiber contractile properties. Med Sci Sports Exerc 32:48.
227. Tzankoff SP, et al. Physiological adjustments to work in older men as affected by physical training. J Appl Physiol 1972;33:346.
228. Underwood FB, et al. Altered control of calcium in coronary smooth muscle cells by exercise training. Med Sci Sports Exerc 1994;26:1230.
229. Urhausen A, et al. Impaired pituitary hormonal response to exhaustive exercise in overtrained endurance athletes. Med Sci Sports Exerc 1998;30:407.
230. Vrabas IS, et al. Endurance training reduces the rate of diaphragm fatigue in vitro. Med Sci Sports Exerc 1999;31:1605.
231. Wagner PD. Determinants of maximal oxygen transport and utilization. Annu Rev Physiol 1996;58:21.
232. Wallick ME, et al. Physiological responses to in-line skating compared to treadmill running. Med Sci Sports Exerc 1995;27:242.
233. Wang J, et al. Chronic exercise enhances endothelium-mediated dilation of epicardial coronary artery in conscious dogs. Circ Res 1993;73:829.
234. Wanger PD. Muscle O_2 transport and O_2 dependent control of metabolism. Med Sci Sports Exerc 1995;27:47.
235. Weltman A, et al. Exercise training at and above lactate threshold in previously untrained women. Int J Sports Med 1992;13:257.
236. Weltman A, et al. Repeated bouts of exercise alter the blood lactate-RPE relation. Med Sci Sports Exerc 1998;30:1113.
237. Whipple GH. The hemoglobin of striated muscle. 1. Variations due to age and exercise. Am J Physiol 1926;76:693.
238. White FC, et al. Exercise training in swine promotes growth of arteriolar bed and capillary angiogenesis in heart. J Appl Physiol 1998;85:1160.
239. Wilmore JH, et al. Endurance exercise training has a minimal effect on resting heart rate: the HERITAGE Study. Med Sci Sports Exerc 1996;28:829.
240. Wilmore JH, et al. Cardiac output and stroke volume changes with endurance training: The HERITAGE family Study. Med Sci Sports Exerc 2001;33:99.
241. Woodiwiss AJ, et al. Reduced cardiac stiffness following exercise is associated with preserved myocardial collagen characteristics in the rat. Eur J Appl Physiol 1998;78:148.
242. Wolfe LA, et al. Maternal exercise, fetal well-being and pregnancy outcome. Exerc Sport Sci Rev 1994;22:145.
243. Yang RC, et al. Albumin synthesis after intense intermittent exercise in human subjects. J Appl Physiol 1998;84:584.
244. Zhang J, Savitz DA. Exercise during pregnancy among US women. Ann Epidemiol 1996;6:53.

CHAPTER 22

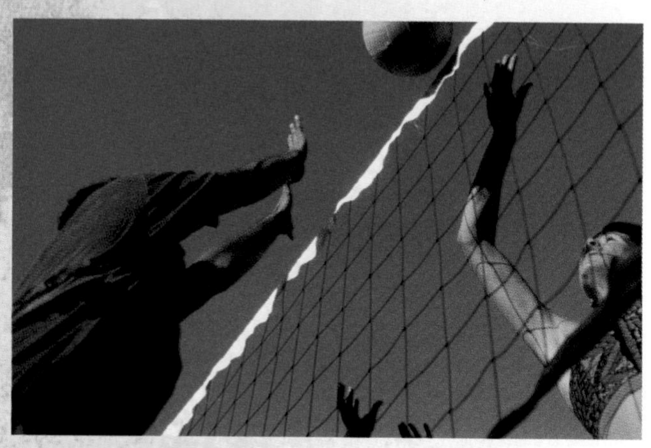

Muscular Strength: Training Muscles to Become Stronger

Chapter Objectives

- Describe the four methods to assess muscular strength: (1) cable tensiometry, (2) dynamometry, (3) one-repetition maximum (I-RM), and (4) computer-assisted isokinetic dynamometry
- Outline a procedure to assess the 1-RM for trained and untrained individuals
- Describe how to ensure test standardization and fairness when evaluating muscular strength
- Compare absolute and relative upper- and lower-body muscular strength in men and women
- Describe allometric scaling to "equalize" individuals when comparing physical and exercise performance characteristics
- Define concentric, eccentric, and isometric muscle actions, and give examples of each
- Discuss the advisability of resistance training for children and adolescents
- Summarize the main research findings on optimal number of sets and repetitions, and frequency and relative intensity of progressive-resistance exercise training
- Outline the model for strength-training periodization
- Discuss specificity of the strength-training response related to enhanced performance in sports and occupational tasks
- Differentiate between resistance training goals of competitive athletes and the untrained middle-aged and elderly
- Respond to the question: "Which is better for strength improvement: progressive resistance weight training, isometric training, or isokinetic training?"
- Describe advantages and disadvantages of plyometric training for power athletes
- Describe how "psychologic" and "muscular" factors influence maximum strength capacity and training responsiveness
- List physiologic adaptations associated with chronic resistance exercise training
- Summarize current opinion concerning resistance training's effect on muscle fiber type and number
- Develop a circuit resistance training program for middle-aged men and women to improve muscular strength and aerobic fitness
- Discuss whether specific resistance training can "shape" a muscle's appearance
- Review (1) the type of exercise most frequently associated with delayed-onset muscle soreness (DOMS), (2) the best way to minimize DOMS when initiating training, and (3) significant cellular alterations related to DOMS

PART 1 • Strength Measurement and Resistance Training

Weightlifting began in America in the early 1840s as a spectator sport practiced by "strongmen" who showcased their prowess in traveling carnivals and sideshows. By the mid-1880s, measuring muscular strength became more commonplace. As pointed out in the text's Introduction: A View of the Past, the military evaluated the strength of conscripts during the Civil War; strength measurements also provided the basis for routine fitness assessments in college and university physical education programs. In fact, an 1897 meeting of College Gymnasium Directors (Dr. D. A. Sargent, committee chair from Harvard University) established strength contests in which college undergraduates competed to determine overall body strength and the group's "strongest man." Measures included back, leg, arm, and chest strength evaluated with several of the devices depicted in Figure 9 of the "Introduction." Harvard, Columbia, Amherst, University of Minnesota, and Dickinson were the first five colleges to rank in the 1898–1899 competition.

Strength assessment became commonplace after the turn of the century, and by the mid-1900s, physical culture specialists, circus performers, body builders, competitive weight lifters, field event athletes, and wrestlers trained predominantly using "weightlifting" exercises. Most other athletes, however, refrained from lifting weights for fear such training would slow them down and increase muscle size to the point where they would lose joint flexibility and become *musclebound.* Subsequent research in the late 1950s and early 1960s dispelled this myth with experiments showing that muscle-strengthening exercises did not reduce speed or range of joint motion. Instead, the opposite usually occurred; elite weight lifters, body builders, and "muscle men" were shown to have exceptional joint flexibility without limitations in general limb movement speed. For untrained healthy individuals, heavy-resistance exercises increased both speed and power of muscular effort. Certainly, these effects would not impair subsequent sports performance.

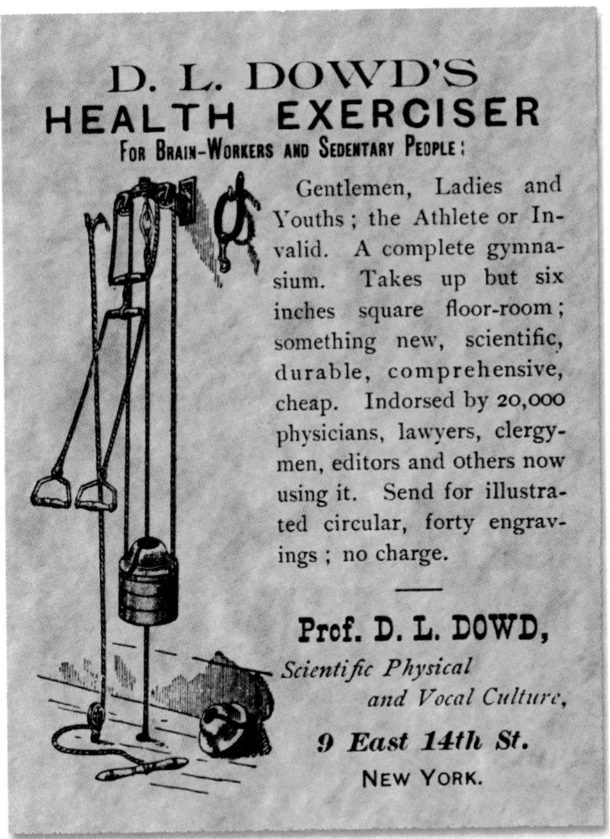

Late 1890s strength equipment advertised for home gym use. By the mid-1850s, rowing machines and strengthening devices became commonplace, eventually leading to studies of their effectiveness in American colleges (Harvard and Amherst) in the 1890s.

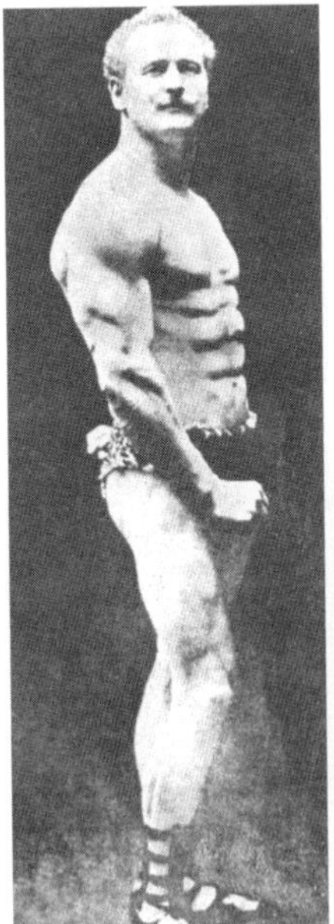
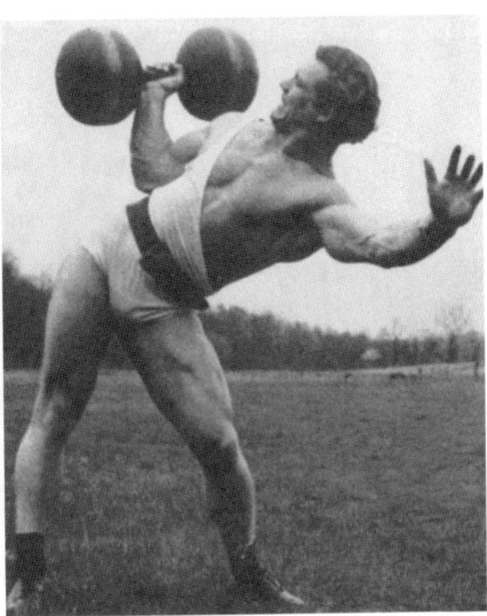

Left, Early 1890s pose of strongman Eugene Sandow (Frederick Mueller), billed by showman Florenz Ziegfeld as "The Most Perfect Man." Sandow helped to design a physical fitness training program for the British military, inspiring a future generation of body builders. *Right,* John Grimek, member of the United States 1936 Olympic weight lifting team, the only two-time Mr. America (1940, 1941), 1948 Mr. Universe, and undefeated in body-building competition. Recognized as the "best-built human" of the first half of the 20th century.

In the sections that follow, we explore the rationale underlying resistance training and physiologic adaptations when training muscles to become stronger. The discussion centers on different methods of measuring muscular strength, gender differences in strength, and resistance-training programs to increase maximum muscle strength and power.

MEASUREMENT OF MUSCLE STRENGTH

One of the following four methods commonly measures **muscle strength** or, more precisely, the maximum force or tension generated by a single muscle or related muscle groups:

- Tensiometry
- Dynamometry
- One-repetition maximum
- Computer-assisted force and power output determinations

Cable Tensiometry

Figure 22.1A shows a **cable tensiometer** and its use for measuring knee extension muscle force. Increasing the force on the cable depresses the riser over which the cable passes. This deflects the pointer and indicates the subject's strength score. The instrument measures muscle force in a static (isometric) muscle action, which produces little or no change in the muscle's external length. This application of the tensiometer differs considerably from its original use in the early 1900s for measuring the tension on the steel cables linking the upper and lower wings of a biplane aircraft. The tensiometer (lightweight, portable, and easy to use) provides the advantage of versatility for recording force measurements at virtually all angles about a specific joint's range of motion (ROM). Standardized cable-tension strength-test batteries assess the static force capacity of all the major muscle groups.[34] The tests can document strength impairment in muscles weakened from disease or injury. Muscle evaluation takes place at a specific joint angle, and repeated measurements determine strength status prior to and following resistance training. Because a particular movement activates more than one muscle group, the clinician or researcher applies the tensiometer at multiple angles in the full ROM. This approach often gives a clearer picture of muscular strength (or weakness) than relying solely on standard weightlifting tests.

Dynamometry

Figures 22.1B and C illustrate hand-grip and leg and back-lift **dynamometers** for static strength measurement based on the compression principle. An external force applied to the dynamometer compresses a steel spring and moves a pointer. The force required to move the pointer a given distance determines the external force applied to the dynamometer.

One-Repetition Maximum (1-RM)

A dynamic procedure for measuring muscular strength applies the **1-RM method**. 1-RM refers to the maximum amount of weight lifted *one time* using proper form during a standard weightlifting exercise. To test 1-RM for any muscle group, make a reasonable guess at an initial weight close to, but below, the person's maximum lifting capacity. Add weight progressively to the exercise device on subsequent attempts until the person reaches maximum lift capacity. The weight increments usually range between 1 and 5 kg, depending on the muscle group evaluated. Rest intervals of 1 to 5 minutes usually provide sufficient recuperation before attempting a lift at the next heavier weight.

ESTIMATE THE 1-RM. Impracticality and/or potential risk in performing 1-RM with preadolescents, the elderly, hypertensives,

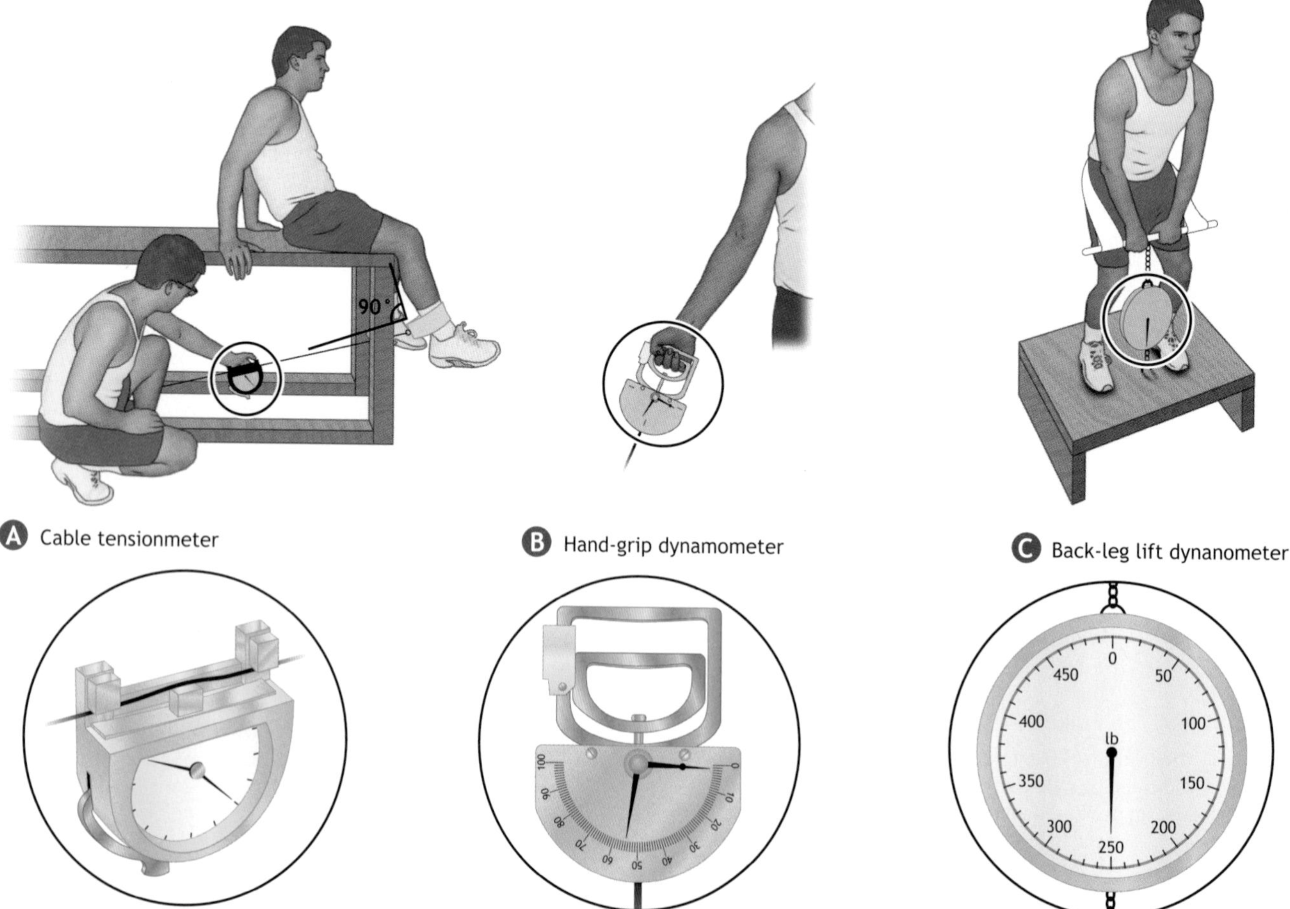

FIGURE 22.1 • Measurement of static strength with (**A**) a cable tensiometer, (**B**) a hand-grip dynamometer, and (**C**) a back-leg lift dynamometer.

cardiac patients, and other special populations requires estimating 1-RM with submaximal effort by use of the equations shown below. We present equations for untrained and resistance-trained young adults because resistance training alters the relationship between a submaximal performance (7- to 10-RM) and a maximal lift (1-RM). Generally, the weight that one lifts for 7- to 10-RM represents about 68% of the 1-RM score for the untrained person and 79% of the new 1-RM after training.[20]

Untrained:

1-RM (kg) = 1.554 × 7- to 10-RM weight (kg) − 5.181

Trained:

1-RM (kg) = 1.172 × 7- to 10-RM weight (kg) + 7.704

For example, estimate I-RM bench press score for a trained person whose 10-RM bench press equals 70 kg, as follows:

1-RM (kg) = 1.172 × 70 kg + 7.704 = 89.7 kg

Computer-Assisted, Electromechanical, and Isokinetic Methods

Microprocessor technology can rapidly quantify forces, torques, accelerations, and velocities of body segments in numerous movement patterns. Force platforms measure the external application of muscle force by a limb, as in jumping. Other electromechanical devices assess forces generated during all phases of an exercise movement (e.g., cycling) or during movements that primarily use the arms (supine bench press) or legs (leg press).

An electromechanical accommodating resistance instrument, termed an **isokinetic dynamometer**, contains a speed-controlling mechanism that accelerates to a preset, constant velocity with the application of force. Once attaining this speed, the isokinetic loading mechanism adjusts automatically to provide a counterforce to variations in force generated by the muscle as movement continues throughout the "strength curve." *Thus, one can generate maximum force (or any percentage of maximum effort) throughout the full ROM at a preestablished velocity of limb movement.* This allows training under either high-velocity (low-force) or low-velocity (high-force) conditions. A microprocessor within the dynamometer continuously monitors the immediate level of applied force. An electronic integrator in series with a recorder (or monitor) provides a readout of the average or peak force generated during any period. The voltage output from the integrator can interface directly with a computer for almost instantaneous feedback about performance (e.g., force, torque, work).

The interface of microprocessor technology with mechanical devices provides the exercise scientist with valuable data to evaluate, test, and train muscles. This technology, however, lacks universal acceptance because many still consider a maximum lift (1-RM) the best criterion of overall muscular strength. The argument for isokinetic strength measurement maintains that muscle strength dynamics involve considerably more than *just* the final outcome of a 1-RM. For example, two individuals with identical 1-RM scores could exhibit dissimilar force curves throughout the movement. Individual differences in force dynamics (e.g., time to peak tension) throughout the full ROM may reflect an entirely different underlying neuromuscular physiology that 1-RM does not assess. Figure 22.2 illustrates the differences between results from conventional 1-RM testing of knee extension (*top;* highest force score during five lifts represents *only* total weight lifted) and testing with a microprocessor-controlled, isokinetic resistance device that produces a force curve throughout the ROM (*bottom;* force related to movement duration). Note that peak torque occurred in the early phase of movement at the most advantageous angle in the ROM; the lowest torque occurred at full knee extension. Table 22.1 lists measurement units for various expressions of muscular performance during linear and angular movements.

INTEGRATIVE QUESTION

Explain why many resistance-trained athletes have their spotters during a free-weight bench press apply external force (to make the lift more difficult) in the early phase of the lift and provide assistance toward its completion.

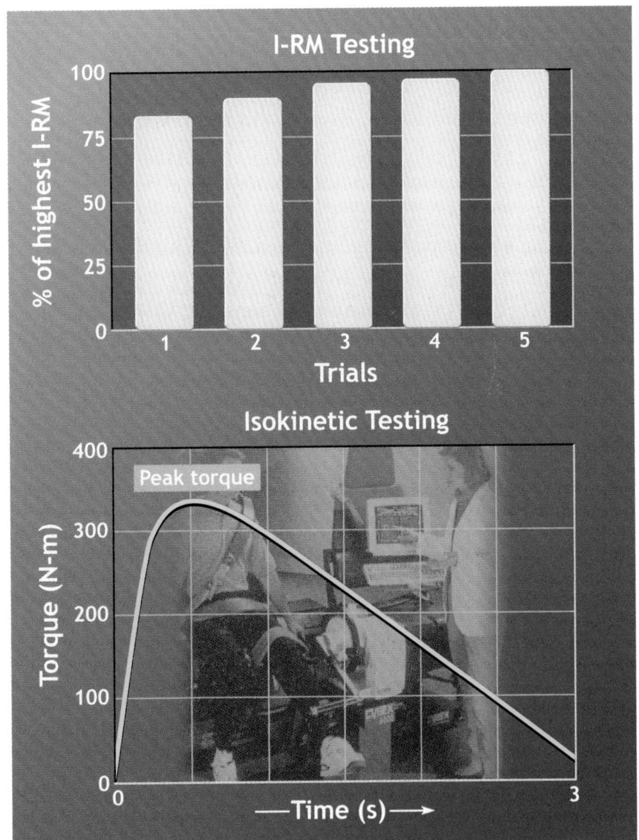

FIGURE 22.2 • *Top,* Conventional 1-RM testing. The heaviest weight lifted constitutes the 1-RM. If 150 kg is the maximum lifted, then 150 kg equals the 1-RM. *Bottom,* Force curve obtained during an isokinetic test performed at an angular velocity of 30° · s^{-1} over a 3-second interval. Peak torque in this example equals 342 N-m. Average torque is the force-time integral, or impulse divided by time. Impulse equals 602 N-m · s^{-1}, and average torque equals 200.7 N-m. Work equals the product of average torque × distance moved (90°, or 1.57 radians). Using the data for average torque and distance, work equals 174 N-m × 157 radians = 273 N-m, or 273 joules (J). Power is work per unit time, or 273 J ÷ 3.0 s = 91 W.

TABLE 22.1 ➤ INTERNATIONAL SYSTEM OF UNITS (SI) FOR VARIOUS EXPRESSIONS OF MUSCULAR STRENGTH AND POWER DURING LINEAR AND ANGULAR MOTIONS[a]

Linear Motion		Angular Motion	
Quantity	**Unit**	**Quantity**	**Unit**
Force	Newton, N	Torque, *T*	Newton meter, N · m
Velocity, *v*	Meters per second, $m \cdot s^{-1}$	Velocity, w	Radians per second, $rad \cdot s^{-1}$
Mass	Kilogram, kg	Moment of inertia, *I* or *J*	Kilogram meters squared, $kg \cdot m^2$
Acceleration, *a*	Meters per second squared, $m \cdot s^{-2}$	Acceleration, *a*	Radians per second squared, $rad \cdot s^{-2}$
Displacement, *d*	Meter, m	Displacement, θ	Radian, rad
Time, *t*	Second, s	Time, *t*	Second, s

[a]Appendix A provides additional information about SI units, including interconversions.

Resistance-Training Equipment Categories

Resistance training generally makes use of one of three categories of exercise equipment that allows for manipulation of movement speed and/or resistance on the muscle throughout the ROM. The first category includes common weightlifting equipment such as free weights and barbells. This equipment does not control for (or measure) speed of movement or resistance through a full ROM. Two subdivisions exist within the second category. One subdivision provides constant speed—controlled by true isokinetic equipment—and variable resistance. The other subdivision also provides constant speed and variable resistance with a hydraulic device, but the individual controls movement speed. In the third category, movement speed varies and resistance remains constant; this category includes some cam devices and concentric-eccentric apparatus. No machine currently allows muscles to exert force under conditions of true constant speed and true constant resistance.

Strength-Testing Considerations

The list that follows presents important considerations for muscle strength testing, regardless of measurement method:

- Standardize instructions prior to testing.
- If giving a warm-up, ensure uniformity in its duration and intensity.
- Provide the subject with adequate practice prior to testing to minimize "learning" that could compromise initial results (see next section).
- During assessment procedures, ensure consistency among subjects in the angle of limb measurement or body position on the test device.
- Predetermine a minimum number of trials (repetitions) to establish a criterion strength score. For example, if administering five repetitions of a test, what score represents the individual's strength score? Is the highest score best, or should one use the average? In most cases, an average of several trials provides a more representative (reliable) strength or power score than a single trial. Researchers report high test–retest reliability for repeated measurements of maximal-effort muscle actions when administering multiple repetitions of bench press and squat 1-RM and bidirectional hydraulic exercise on the same and different days.[117]
- Select test measures with high test score reproducibility. This crucial but often overlooked aspect of testing evaluates the variability of the subject's responses on repeated efforts. Lack of test score consistency (unreliability) often masks an individual's representative performance on the measure (or change in performance when evaluating strength improvement).

EXERCISE EQUIPMENT TO OVERLOAD SKELETAL MUSCLE

Category	*Speed*	*Resistance*	*Equipment Example*
(I)	Variable	Variable	Barbells (resistance varies through ROM even though absolute weight remains constant)
(II)	Constant	Variable	Hydraulic (person controls speed)
	Constant	Variable	Computer-regulated (movement speed controlled by computer)
(III)	Variable	Constant	CAM-adjusted equipment and concentrate-eccentric apparatus
(IV)	Constant	Constant	None available

- Recognize individual differences in body size and composition when evaluating strength scores among individuals and groups. For example, consider the "fairness" of comparing absolute muscular strength of a 120-kg football lineman with the strength of a 62-kg distance runner. Unfortunately, no clear-cut answer resolves this dilemma, but on page 507, Allometric Scaling, we present alternatives for comparing strength scores relative to body size.

Learning Factors That Affect Strength Measurements

In Chapter 19, we emphasized that the initial gains in muscular strength with resistance training result largely from neural factors instead of actual structural changes within muscle fibers. Figure 22.3 presents data from one of our laboratories for repetition-by-repetition performance improvements in maximal effort movement at an angular velocity of $5° \cdot s^{-1}$ during a supine bench press with a 5-second interval between maximal effort repetitions. The dynamometer also assessed static 1-RM at 100° angle in the ROM. This measurement differs from the conventional 1-RM determination that adds small increments of free weights on repeated lifts. The amount of improvement averaged 11.4% between maximal force on attempt 1 and attempt 5 and 2.1% between the last two attempts. Group performance improvement between the last two trials did not reach statistical significance. Strength "improvement" with repeated testing indicates the necessity for *at least* three attempts before maximum force scores begin to stabilize or plateau. The scores remained unchanged with 3-, 4-, or 5-minute rest intervals between maximal attempts. Actually, only 1-minute intervals between trials prove satisfactory for achieving the maximum lift.[216] Importantly, use of only one or two 1-RM attempts would underestimate the "true" 1-RM by as much as 11%. If a single 1-RM trial preceded a 15-week strength training program, then any strength gains attributable to training would include the 11% "learning" improvement simply from exercise familiarization, regardless of the training effect!

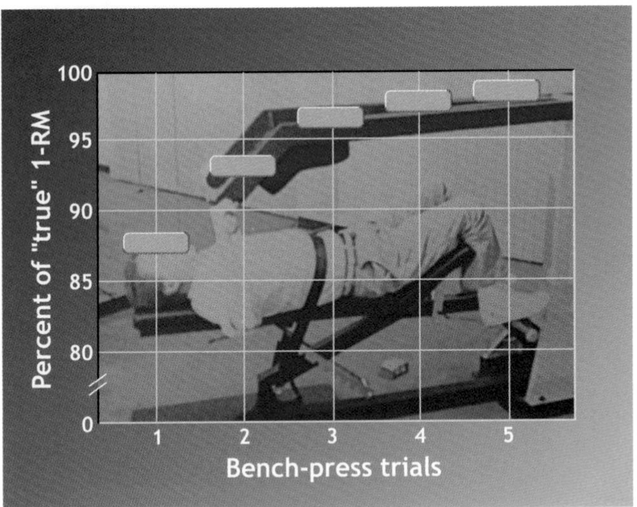

FIGURE 22.3 • Five repeated determinations of 1-RM for the supine bench press with an electromechanical dynamometer. Strong verbal encouragement was provided on each attempt. A rest interval of 5 seconds occurred between maximal-effort trials. (From Human Performance Laboratory, University of Massachusetts, Amherst.)

GENDER DIFFERENCES IN MUSCLE STRENGTH

Researchers have applied several approaches to determine if a true gender difference exists in muscle strength. These include evaluation (1) related to the muscle's cross-sectional area, (2) on an absolute basis as total force exerted, (3) related to architectural characteristics (e.g., fiber pennation angle), and (4) as relative strength related to body mass or fat-free body mass (FFM).

Strength Related to Muscle Cross-Sectional Area

Human skeletal muscle, regardless of gender, generates a maximum of between 16 and 30 newtons (N) of force per square centimeter of muscle cross section. *In the body, however, force-output capacity varies, depending on the arrangement of the bony levers and muscle architecture* (see Chapter 18). Applying the value of 30 N as a representative force capacity per cm^2 of muscle tissue indicates that a muscle with a cross-sectional area of 5.0 cm^2 can develop a maximal force of approximately 150 N. If all of the body's muscles became maximally activated simultaneously (with force applied in the same direction), the resulting force would equal 168 kN. This estimation assumes a muscle total cross section of 0.56 m^2.[53]

Figure 22.4A compares the absolute arm flexor strength of men and women in relation to muscle total cross-sectional area. Clearly, individuals with the largest muscle cross-sections generate the greatest absolute force. The near-linear relation between strength and muscle size, however, indicates little difference in arm flexor strength for the same size muscle in men and women. Figure 22.4B further demonstrates this point when expressing the strength of the men and women per unit area of muscle cross section.

One can compute muscle plus bone cross-sectional area (MCSA) and limb volume from anthropometric measures. The MCSA for the upper arm at the level of the biceps (MCSA-Bi) equals $\pi (r - [\text{BiSF} + \text{TrSF}]/4)^2$, where r is the radius of the upper arm calculated from biceps girth, BiSF is biceps skinfold, and TrSF is triceps skinfold. MCSA for the lower limb at the thigh (MCSA-Thi) is $\pi (r - [\text{ThSF}]/2)^2$, where r is the radius of the thigh and ThSF is the thigh skinfold. The following equation estimates the volume of a limb from girth measurements: volume $= \pi h/3\ (R^2/2\pi + r^2/2\pi + Rr)$, where h is the length of the upper arm or thigh in cm, R is upper arm or thigh girth, and r is elbow or knee girth. One can also predict MCSA (mm^2) from a regression equation validated by magnetic resonance imaging.[88] MCSA at the midthigh for the quadriceps in men equals $1.99\ (X_1) - 0.24\ (X_2) - 34.4$, where X_1 is midthigh girth (cm) and X_2 is thigh skinfold at the girth level.

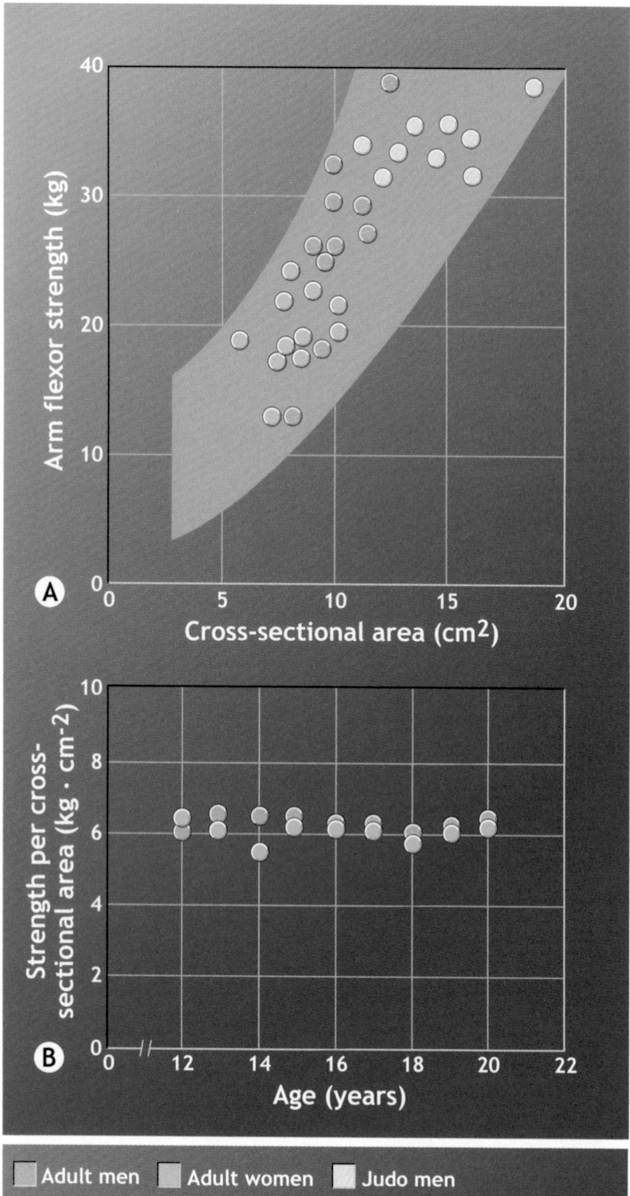

FIGURE 22.4 • **A.** Variability of upper-arm flexion strength of men and women related to the flexor muscle's total cross-sectional area. **B.** Strength per unit muscle cross-sectional area in males and females aged 12 to 20 years. (From Ikai M, Fukunaga T. Calculation of muscle strength per unit cross-sectional area of human muscle by means of ultrasonic measurements. Arbeitsphysiologie 1968;26:26.)

Absolute Muscle Strength

Comparisons of muscular strength on an absolute score basis (i.e., total force in lb or kg) indicate that men possess considerably greater strength than women for all muscle groups tested. Women score about 50% lower than men for upper-body strength and about 30% less for leg strength.[83] This gender disparity is independent of the measuring device and generally coincides with gender-related difference in muscle mass distribution.[29] Exceptions usually emerge for strength-trained female track-and-field athletes and body builders who have trained for years with progressive resistance exercise to develop the strength of specific muscle groups.

Gender Differences in Weight-Lifting Championships

A unique set of data exists on gender differences in weight-lifting competitions in which men and women participate in the same weight-lifting categories on the basis of identical body mass. Figure 22.5 displays the percentage differences in maximum weight lifted in the combined snatch and clean-and-jerk lifts during national championship competitions. Importantly, these comparisons do not "equate" or "adjust" performance scores on the basis of the well-documented gender difference in body composition. The six body weight categories range from 52 to 82.5 kg. The lighter-weight categories usually produce the smallest gender difference, with the effect most pronounced in the heavier lifters. Women of 75- and 82.5-kg body mass lift only about 60% of the maximal weight lifted by their male counterparts. This represents a more pronounced gender difference than those of other comparisons that initially matched competitors for body composition, not just body mass.

INTEGRATIVE QUESTION

What performance would you expect in maximum weight-lifting tests comparing (1) an average-size man and average-size woman and (2) a man and woman of equivalent training history and identical body mass?

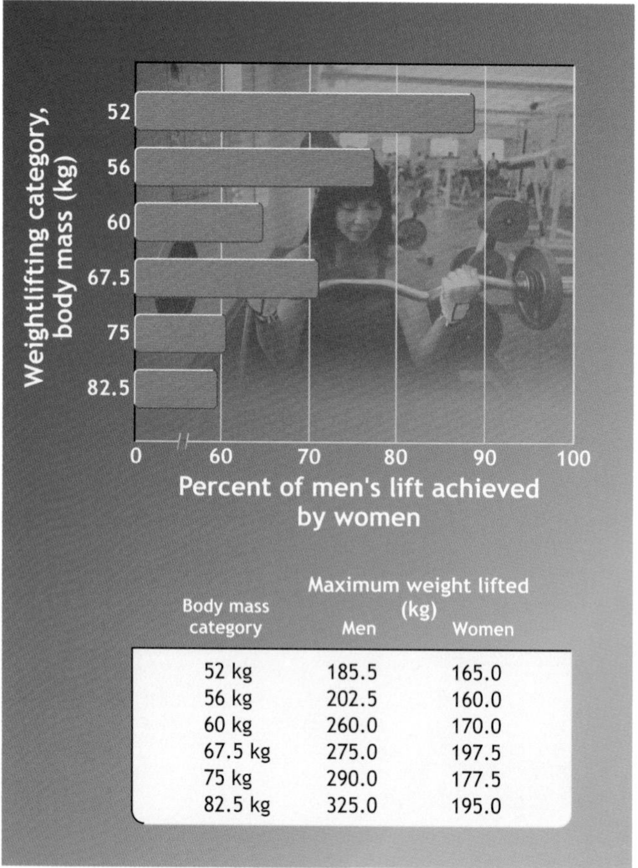

Body mass category	Maximum weight lifted (kg) Men	Women
52 kg	185.5	165.0
56 kg	202.5	160.0
60 kg	260.0	170.0
67.5 kg	275.0	197.5
75 kg	290.0	177.5
82.5 kg	325.0	195.0

FIGURE 22.5 • Difference in maximum weight lifted between men and women in the same body mass categories during a national weight lifting competition. The *inset* shows the absolute weight lifted by the men and women for each body mass category.

Relative Muscle Strength

Traditionally, comparing strength performance among individuals required creating a ratio by dividing the strength score by a reference measurement such as body mass, FFM, muscle cross section, or limb volume or girth. For example, comparing men and women for strength using a ratio score based on body mass or FFM considerably reduces (if not eliminates) the large absolute strength differences between genders.[29]

Consider the following example. A male who weighs 95 kg bench presses 114 kg; a 60-kg woman presses only 62% of the man's lift, or 70 kg. Who is "stronger?" In absolute terms, the male is clearly stronger. However, the bench press score divided by body mass creates a different situation. For the man, strength divided by body mass equals 1.20; the ratio for the woman is 1.17. In the first comparison, the male was "stronger" by 61.3%. Using the ratio score reduced the percentage difference in bench press strength to only 2.5%! Such findings support the argument that no differences exist in muscle "quality" of men and women; the observed gender difference in absolute muscle strength merely reflects differences in muscle quantity (cross-sectional area) rather than muscle fiber architectural characteristics (e.g., fiber-pennation angle) or metabolic functions. Men and women generally do not differ significantly in either upper- or lower-body strength when comparisons are made using ratio scores with lean body mass as the divisor.[83]

We must point out, however, that this traditional ratio adjustment of considering gender differences in body size may not equalize women and men on the basis of the underlying physiology. As with aerobic capacity (discussed in Chapter 11), a fair way to evaluate a potential gender difference in a criterion trait such as muscular strength or aerobic capacity either (1) compares men and women who do not differ in body size variables such as body mass or FFM and who exhibit similar training status or (2) adjusts for these variables through appropriate statistical controls. These methods preclude the need to create a ratio score because the men and women become equalized for body size and/or body composition. Using this approach, researchers assessed five measures of muscular strength for men and women using 1-RM concentric (shortening) muscle actions for the bench press and squat and isokinetic dynamometry to assess maximum force during knee flexion and extension and seated shoulder press. Figure 22.6 shows that matching men and women for body mass produced larger gender differences in the sedentary group (44.0% for the shoulders and 25.1% for knee flexion) than in the trained group (33.0% for the bench press and 10.7% for knee flexion). The percentage differences decreased (but were not at all eliminated) for both groups by matching subjects for FFM. The shoulder press (39.4%) and bench press (31.2%) produced the largest gender differences in the sedentary group, while the corresponding differences for the trained group were 30.6% (shoulder press) and 35.4% (bench press).

These results differ significantly from those of prior studies that used the traditional ratio score approach to express the strength of women and men. Without doubt, ratio scoring supports the argument that few gender differences exist in muscle quality, at least as reflected by force output capacity. In contrast, matching men and women for body size, body composition, and training status before testing yields higher upper- and lower-body strength scores for men.[151] In a latter study of military personnel (2061 men, 1301 women), mean lift capacity averaged 51% greater in men, despite a regression, ratio, or exponential mathematical adjustment in the strength score based on interindividual differences in FFM.

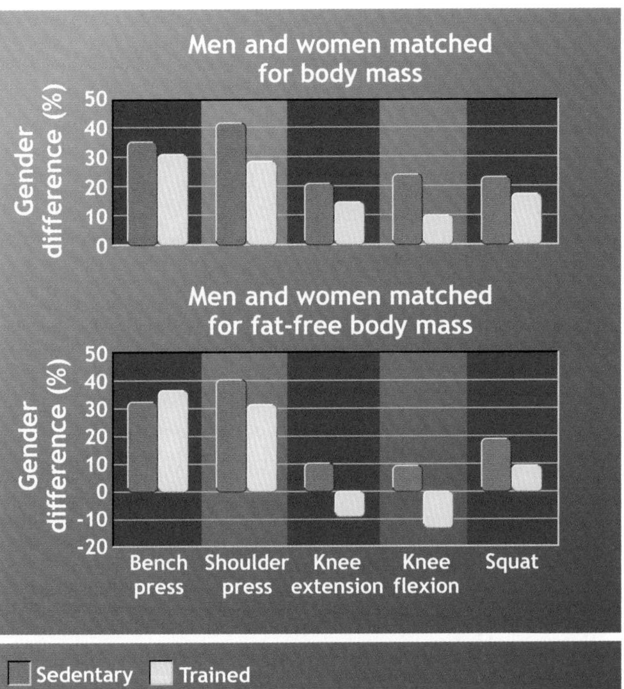

FIGURE 22.6 • Men and women matched for body mass *(top)* and fat-free body mass *(bottom)* for five measures of muscle strength. Above the zero line indicates the percentage by which the values for men exceed the values for women. (Data courtesy of Keller B. The influence of body size variables on gender differences in strength and maximum aerobic capacity. Unpublished doctoral dissertation, University of Massachusetts, Amherst, 1989.)

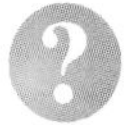

INTEGRATIVE QUESTION

Based on your knowledge of gender-related differences in physical fitness components, devise a physical test that (1) minimizes and (2) maximizes performance differences between men and women.

Allometric Scaling

Allometric scaling is a mathematical procedure to establish a proper relationship between a body size variable (usually stature, body mass, or FFM) and some other factor of interest such as muscular strength, aerobic capacity, jumping height, or running speed.[99,208] The technique provides proper statistical adjustment to evaluate the relative contribution of diverse independent variables (e.g., gender, maturation, habitual physical activity) on the dependent measure of interest (e.g., muscular strength, $\dot{V}O_{2max}$, pulmonary function).

Allometric scaling requires three assumptions: (1) a curvilinear relationship exists between the two variables in question (e.g., body mass and muscular strength), (2) the slope of the relationship passes through the origin (i.e., someone with zero body mass exhibits no muscular strength), and (3) the equation $Y = bX^a$ best describes the form of the relationship, where Y represents the outcome variable (muscular strength); X, the scaling variable (body mass); b is a constant multiplier representing the line's slope, and a is a constant exponent. Solving the scaling equation for the exponent a eliminates the influence of individual differences in the scaling factor (in this case, body mass) on the outcome variable muscular strength. Stated another way, allometric scaling permits a variable of interest to remain free of confounding effects that inherently relate to it. Transforming the basic allometric scaling equation in assumption (3) above into a log–linear model enables one to solve for exponent a. This is done by taking the log of both sides of the equation in (3) and substituting values for the outcome variable (muscular strength) and the scaling variable (body mass). The equation becomes log strength = a log body mass + log b. Linear regression then solves for a by entering the log of strength and the log of body mass into the regression. For muscular strength, slope b usually equals 0.67, but the value may vary somewhat depending on the particular data set. Data for grip strength of college-age men and women reported a body mass exponent of 0.51 to be the appropriate scaling factor, but this study did not scale to FFM, which might have given a scaling value closer to a body mass exponent to the 0.67 power. *If a linear relationship existed between muscular strength and body mass,* b *would equal 1.0, which would justify expressing strength per unit body mass without a correction.* Since this does not occur, one must express muscular strength per unit body mass raised to an appropriate power determined for the particular data set.

IS SCALING FAIR? Applying allometry to an outcome variable such as muscular strength permits comparison of individuals who exhibit large individual differences in a body-size variable. The comparison becomes free of confounding effects that inherently relate in a nonlinear manner to the variable in question. For example, how can one best compare the maximum strengths of two individuals who vary widely in body size? If one competitor weighs 100 kg (190 cm tall) and the other 70 kg (178 cm tall)— with strength scores of 125 kg for the taller, heavier person and 110 kg for the shorter, lighter person—how can we "equate" both individuals for their "expected" muscular strength? Because body mass relates to muscular strength, the traditional approach simply divides the strength score by body mass to produce a proportionate ratio score of 1.250 for the heavier person (125 kg lifted ÷ 100 kg body mass) and 1.571 for the lighter competitor. This system deems the lighter person "stronger." In effect, the approach actually penalizes the heavier person because of the disproportionately large divisor in the ratio. But is this procedure fair? The answer becomes complicated because of failure to consider differences in stature (stature also relates strongly to body mass) or total muscle mass (as reflected by FFM or lean body mass) related to body mass. To identify the strongest person (considering factors that normally affect muscular strength), one must properly scale the muscular strength outcome variable to remove the confounding influence of the body size variable(s).

Because the absolute strength of a muscle relates strongly to its cross-sectional area and because many muscles contribute to maximum force in a particular movement, should one express strength per unit cross-sectional area of the active muscles? Unfortunately, no simple answer emerges to this question or to questions raised previously. Additional complications arise when physical size characteristics between males and females and between individuals of different ages (particularly during growth and aging) potentially affect exercise performance scores. Anthropologists, biologists, and other scientists since the mid-1600s have raised and debated questions of body size scaling and outcome variables.[194,202] Thus, it is not surprising that significant discussion exists among exercise scientists about the proper scaling of variables commonly measured in exercise physiology.[103,207]

STRENGTH AND ALLOMETRIC SCALING USING BODY MASS. Figure 22.7 illustrates the relationship between body mass and several different expressions of muscular strength. The top left graph (A) plots the total weight lifted versus body mass for Olympic weight lifters. Each point represents body mass of the top weight lifters in each body mass category. Importantly, total weight lifted and body mass do not relate linearly but curvilinearly, thus supporting the belief that weight-lifting strength relates proportionally to body mass raised to the exponent 0.7 (slope of line). The *bottom six curves* (B) depict the relationship between maximal grip strength and body mass in college-age men (purple) and women (green). The *top graphs* illustrate the simple relationship between body mass and grip strength without adjustment for body size. As expected, a positive relationship emerges ($r = 0.51$ for males and $r = 0.33$ for females). The *middle graphs* depict the relationship with grip strength indexed to body mass (i.e., strength divided by body mass in kg). In this case, dividing strength by body mass penalized heavier males and females ($r = -0.43$ for males and -0.38 for females). If body mass does not represent a confounding variable, the ratio score should have approximately zero correlation ($r = 0.00$) with muscular strength. This represents an ideal situation that levies no penalty on heavier people (who may also possess a higher percentage of body fat). The *bottom graphs* illustrate the relationship between strength and allometric scaling of body mass. The body mass exponent is $a = 0.54$ for males and 0.475 for females; the resulting correlations between strength and strength raised to the appropriate exponent fall essentially to zero ($r = 0.013$ for males and 0.030 for females). This satisfies one of the basic tenets of allometry—the correlation between the scaled variable (muscular strength) and the scaling factor (body mass) must equal zero.

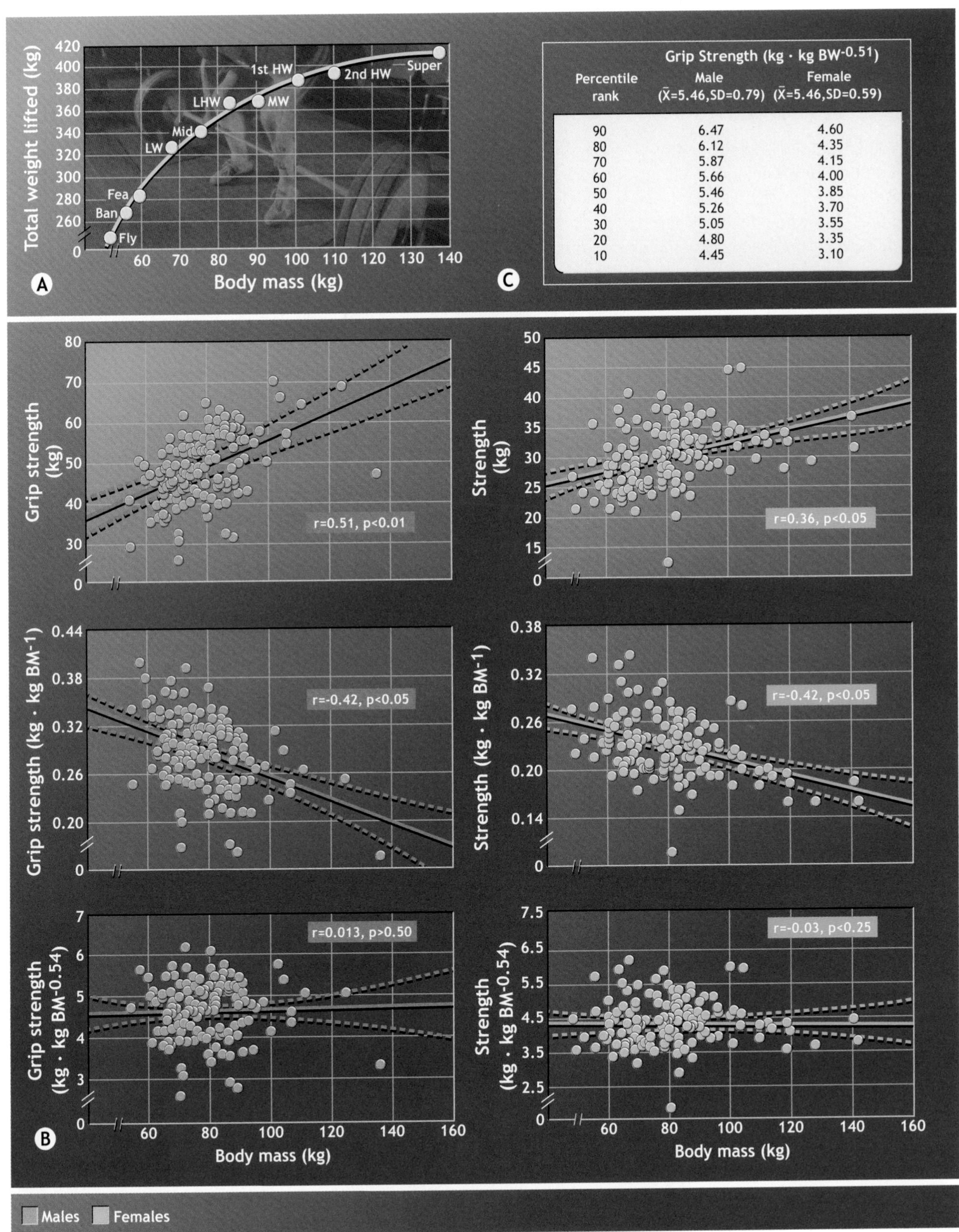

Percentile rank	Grip Strength (kg · kg BW$^{-0.51}$) Male ($\bar{X}$=5.46,SD=0.79)	Female ($\bar{X}$=5.46,SD=0.59)
90	6.47	4.60
80	6.12	4.35
70	5.87	4.15
60	5.66	4.00
50	5.46	3.85
40	5.26	3.70
30	5.05	3.55
20	4.80	3.35
10	4.45	3.10

FIGURE 22.7 • Relationship between body mass and different expressions of muscular strength. **A**. Total weight lifted in two events as a function of body mass of Olympic weight lifters (1980 Olympic games). Each point represents the body mass of the top six male weight lifters in each of the following weight categories: *Fly,* flyweight; *Ban,* bantamweight; *Fea,* featherweight; *LW,* lightweight; *Mid,* middleweight; *LHW,* light-heavyweight; *MW,* middle-heavyweight; *1st HW,* 1st heavyweight; 2nd *HW,* 2nd heavyweight; and *Super,* superheavyweight. (Modified from data of Lathan and cited by Titel K, Wutscherk H. In: Komi PV, ed. Strength and power in sport. Oxford: Blackwell Scientific Publications, 1993.) **B**. Maximal absolute grip strength, relative grip strength, and strength scaled allometrically in relation to body mass of 100 men and 105 women of college age. **C**. Percentile norms for grip strength scaled to body mass. (Data courtesy of Dr. Paul Vanderburgh.)

The inset table (C) presents percentile norms for grip strength adjusted to body mass exponent 0.51 (grip strength per $kg^{0.51}$) for college-age men and women.

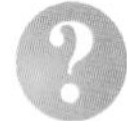

INTEGRATIVE QUESTION

You have a list of the names of young adults with the body weight of each. Justify your selection of two people: one must push a vehicle stuck in the mud while the other must move hand-over-hand on a rope strung across a ravine. *Hint:* Consider absolute and relative strength requirements of each task and the association between body mass and absolute and relative muscular strength.

TRAINING MUSCLES TO BECOME STRONGER

As a general rule, a muscle increases in strength when trained close to its current force-generating capacity. Standard weight-lifting equipment, pulleys or springs, immovable bars, or a variety of isokinetic and hydraulic devices provide effective muscle overload. Importantly, overload intensity (level of tension placed on muscle), not the type of exercise that applies the overload, generally governs strength improvements. Certain exercise methods do, however, lend themselves to precise and systematic overload applications. **Progressive-resistance weight training**, **isometric training**, and **isokinetic training** are three common exercise systems to train muscles to become stronger.[60] These systems rely on the types of muscle actions illustrated in Figure 22.8, A–C.

Different Muscle Action Forms

Neural stimulation of a muscle causes the contractile elements of its fibers to attempt to shorten along the longitudinal axis. The terms *isometric* or *static* describe muscle activation in which no observable change occurs in muscle fiber length. A **dynamic** muscle action produces movement of the skeleton. Concentric and eccentric actions represent the two types of dynamic muscle actions.

- **Concentric action** occurs when the muscle shortens, and joint movement occurs as tension develops. Figure 22.8A illustrates a concentric action when raising a dumbbell from the extended to the flexed elbow position. Similarly, lifting a fork to deliver food from the plate to the mouth requires a concentric biceps muscle action.
- **Eccentric action** occurs when external resistance exceeds muscle force and the muscle lengthens while developing tension (Fig. 22.8B). The weight slowly lowers against the force of gravity. As with the food analogy for a concentric muscle action, returning the fork to the plate involves an eccentric biceps muscle action. The muscle fibers (more specifically the sarcomeres) of the upper-arm muscles lengthen in an eccentric action to prevent the weight (or fork) from crashing to the surface. In weight lifting, muscles frequently act eccentrically as the weight slowly returns to the starting position to begin the next concentric (shortening) action. Eccentric muscle action during this "recovery" phase adds significantly to the total work of the exercise repetition. *Combined concentric and eccentric muscle actions augment the effectiveness of resistance training to enhance muscle strength and fiber size.*[78,154] Overload training that includes eccentric muscle actions also preserves strength gains better during a maintenance phase than concentric-only training.[37]
- **Isometric action** occurs when a muscle generates force and attempts to shorten but cannot overcome the external resistance (Fig. 22.8C). From a physics standpoint, this type of muscle action does not produce ex-

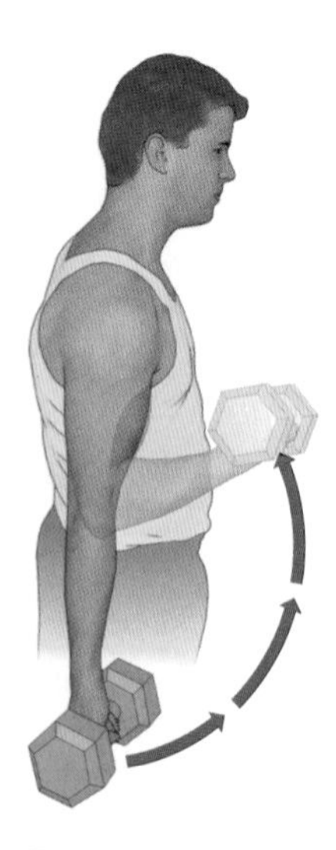

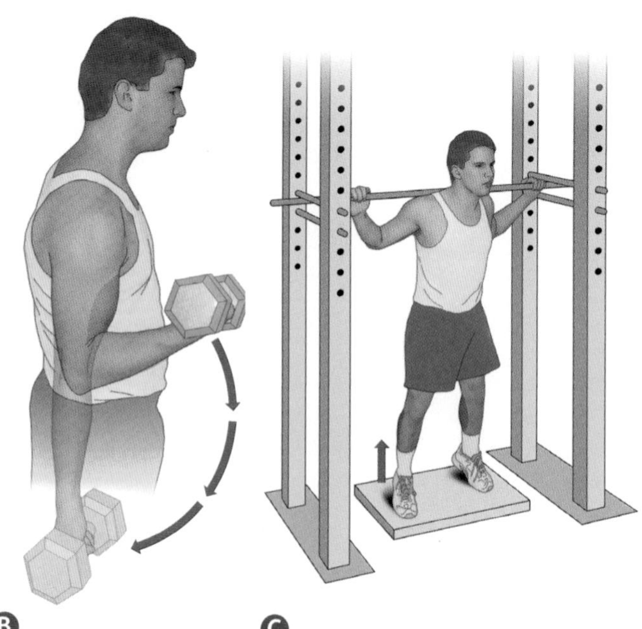

FIGURE 22.8 • Muscle force generated during (**A**) concentric (shortening), (**B**) eccentric (lengthening), and (**C**) isometric (static) muscle actions.

ternal work. However, an isometric (static) action can generate considerable force despite the lack of noticeable lengthening or shortening of muscle sarcomeres and subsequent joint movement.

The term *isotonic*, derived from the Greek word *isotonos* (*iso* meaning the same or equal, *tonos* meaning tension or strain), commonly refers to concentric and eccentric muscle actions, because in both cases movement occurs. This term lacks precision when applied to most dynamic muscle actions that involve movement, because the muscle's effective force-generating capacity continually varies as the joint angle changes throughout the ROM.

Resistance Training for Children

Exercise physiologists know relatively little concerning the benefits and possible risks of resistance training for preadolescents. Because of the formative nature of the skeletal system of growing children, obvious concern arises regarding the potential for injury from excessive musculoskeletal loading (epiphyseal fractures, ruptured intervertebral disks, lower-back bony disruptions, acute low-back trauma).[193] In addition, a child's hormonal profile lacks full development—particularly the tissue-building hormone testosterone. Thus, one might question whether resistance training in children can even induce significant strength improvements.

Closely supervised resistance training using concentric-only muscle actions with relatively high repetitions and low resistance significantly improves muscular strength with no adverse effect on bone, muscle, or connective tissue.[55,158,218] More than likely, children's strength gains result primarily from learning and enhanced neuromuscular activation rather than substantial increases in muscle size.[155] More studies must determine the benefit-to-risk ratio and long-term effects on growth and development of regular and more stressful muscle overload on children. At this time, the guidelines presented in Table 22.2 provide prudent recommendations for initiating resistance exercise training for children and adolescents.

TABLE 22.2 ➤ GUIDELINES FOR RESISTANCE-EXERCISE TRAINING AND PROGRESSION IN CHILDREN AND ADOLESCENTS

AGE (Y)	CONSIDERATIONS
7 or younger	Introduce child to basic exercises with little or no weight; develop the concept of a training session; teach exercise techniques; progress from body weight calisthenics, partner exercises, and lightly resisted exercises; keep volume low
8–10	Gradually increase the number of exercises; practice exercise technique in all lifts; start gradual progressive loading of exercises; keep exercises simple; gradually increase training volume; carefully monitor toleration to the exercise stress
11–13	Teach all basic exercise techniques; continue progressive loading of each exercise; emphasize exercise techniques; introduce more advanced exercises with little or no resistance
14–15	Progress to more-advanced youth programs in resistance exercise; add sport-specific components; emphasize exercise techniques; increase volume
16 or older	Move child to entry-level adult programs after all background knowledge has been mastered and a basic level of training experience has been gained

Note: If a child of any age begins a program with no previous experience, start the child at previous levels and move him or her to more-advanced levels as exercise toleration, skill, amount of training time, and understanding permit.
From Kraemer WJ, Fleck SJ. Strength training for young athletes. Champaign, IL: Human Kinetics, 1993.

Resistance Training

The most popular form of resistance training involves weight lifting. This method selectively strengthens specific muscles by causing them to overcome a fixed initial resistance, usually with a barbell, dumbbell, or weight plates on a pulley- or cam-type machine. For some individuals, intensive resistance training can produce a two- to three-fold increase in muscle size.

Progressive Resistance Exercise

Progressive resistance exercise (PRE) provides a practical application of the overload principle and forms the basis of most resistance-training programs. In a rehabilitation setting after World War II, researchers devised weight-training regimens to improve the strength of previously injured limbs (see "Focus on Research").[45] The procedure involved three sets of exercises, each set consisting of 10 repetitions done consecutively, without resting. The first set required one-half of the maximum weight that could be lifted 10 times, or 1⁄2 10-RM; the second set used 3⁄4 10-RM, and the final 10-RM required maximum weight. As patients trained, the exercised limbs became stronger, so the 10-RM resistance increased periodically to maintain continued strength improvements. Similar improvements occurred even when reversing the exercise intensity progression so patients performed the 10-RM as the first set.

VARIATIONS OF PRE. Studies have attempted to determine the optimal number of sets and repetitions, including frequency and relative intensity of PRE training for optimal strength improvement. The findings are generally as follows:

- Performing between 3-RM and 12-RM provides the most effective number of repetitions to improve strength.
- PRE training once weekly with 1-RM for one set increases strength significantly after week 1 of training and continues to increase strength each week thereafter up to at least week 6.

Focus on Research

Develop Strength By Increasing Load, Not Repetitions

DeLorme TL. Restoration of muscle power by heavy-resistance exercises. J Bone Joint Surg 1945;27:645.

➤ The accepted principle for muscle rehabilitation from injury prior to DeLorme's classic research involved low-resistance, high-repetition exercises—so-called endurance-building exercises. Examples include stationary cycling, stair climbing, and repetitively lifting light sandbags or weights with the aid of pulleys. The prevailing approach to restoring atrophied, weak, or "neglected" muscles relied on developing muscular endurance, not muscular strength and power. DeLorme challenged the conventional wisdom by advocating heavy-resistance exercise. He reasoned that proportionality existed between the load resisting the muscle action and the rate and extent of hypertrophy. DeLorme predicted that an inactive or injured person's strength would return to normal levels faster with heavier resistance exercise than with lighter resistance exercise.

On the basis of observations of 300 patients, most of whom required lower-extremity rehabilitation, DeLorme developed a new training system he named *progressive resistance exercise* (*PRE*). Within the PRE system, DeLorme introduced the concepts of one-repetition maximum (1-RM) strength and 10-RM strength for (1) setting the initial overload and adjusting the increasing resistance, (2) establishing maximal sets and repetitions, and (3) applying the concept of muscle-training specificity. For muscle rehabilitation, DeLorme recommended that patients accumulate 70 to 100 repetitions of an exercise using 7 to 10 sets, with a *maximum* of 10 repetitions per set. Initially, workouts began with a weight considerably less than the maximum weight lifted for 10 repetitions (10-RM) so subjects could complete 10-RM in the final set. When the person achieved 10-RM, total repetitions equaled 70 to 100. For example, if 10-RM for the first week equaled 20 pounds, then beginning the first set with 2.5 pounds and increasing 1.5 pounds after each 10-repetition set accumulated 80 repetitions when performing the final 20-pound 10-RM.

DeLorme advocated exercising once daily, 5 days per week, with workouts not exceeding 30 minutes. The patient performed one maximal lift (1-RM) only once each week. DeLorme believed that a person should exercise "smoothly, rhythmically, and without haste, but not so slowly that the mere holding of the weight would tire the patient. Sudden motions should be avoided, and a momentary pause at the end of each repetition was advocated." Weekly 1-RM measurement provided the basis for progressively adjusting the load to maintain the 10-RM training level. The figure illustrates strength improvement in one patient undergoing rehabilitation from a femur fracture. After 36 days, note the 8% gain in thigh girth (1.8 in) and the 40-pound (200%) increase in quadriceps muscle strength.

The DeLorme paper represented the first in the modern strength-training literature advocating the concept of *training specificity*. DeLorme argued that power-building and endurance exercises "were two entirely different types, each one producing its own results, and each being wholly incapable of producing the results obtained by the other." More than 55 years of subsequent research has validated the specificity concept for strength improvement, including almost every claim made by DeLorme about PRE's beneficial effects.

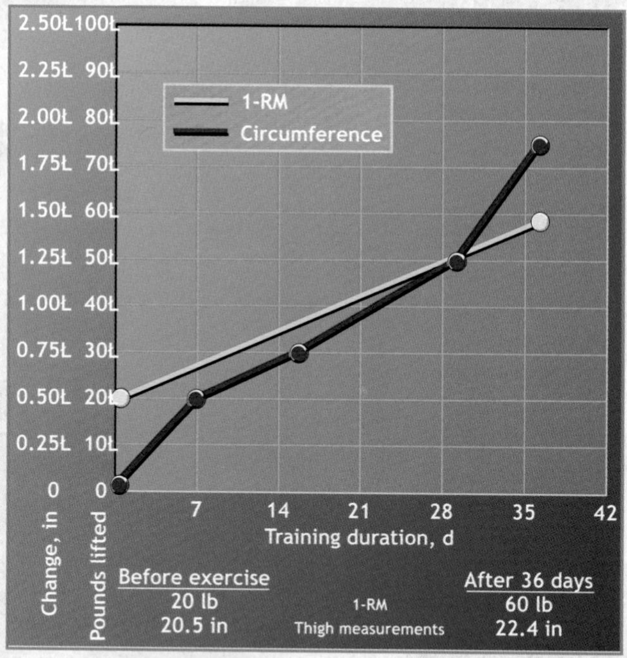

Time course of 1-RM *(yellow line)* and changes in thigh girth *(red line)* for a representative subject during 35 days of progressive-resistance exercise.

- No particular sequence of PRE training with different percentages of 10-RM proves more effective for strength improvement, as long as one 10-RM set takes place each training session.
- Performing one exercise set in both initial and longer-term training periods induces only slightly less strength improvement in recreational weight lifters than performing two or three sets.[27,77] For the serious trainer who desires to maximize muscle strength and size gains, multiple-set paradigms prove most effective.
- Single-set programs, although less effective for optimal strength improvement, generally produce most of the health and fitness benefits of multiple-set programs for healthy adults and some individuals with chronic disease. These "lower-volume" programs

also produce greater compliance and reduce financial cost and time commitment.

- The optimum number of training days per week for PRE remains unknown. Significant strength increases occur for beginners with as little as 1 day weekly.
- If PRE training includes multiple exercises, training 4 or 5 days per week may cause less improvement than training 2 or 3 times per week, because near-daily training of the same muscles may impair time for muscle recuperation between training sessions. Inadequate recovery retards progress in neuromuscular and structural adaptations and strength development.
- A fast rate of movement for a given resistance generates more strength improvement than movement at a slower rate. Neither free weights (barbells, weight plates, dumbbells) nor a diverse array of resistance exercise machines shows inherent superiority for developing muscle strength.

PERIODIZATION. In 1972, Russian scientist Leonid Mateyeev first introduced the concept of strength-training **periodization** (or periodized training);[133] it has since become incorporated into the training regimens of both novice and champion athletes.[64,132,176] Conceptually, periodization subdivides (at regular time intervals) a specific resistance-training period such as 1 year (macrocycle) into smaller periods or phases (mesocycles), with each mesocycle again separated into weekly microcycles. In essence, the training model decreases training volume and increases intensity as the duration of the program progresses. Fractionating the macrocycle into components allows manipulation of training intensity, volume, frequency, sets, repetitions, and rest periods (to prevent overtraining). It also provides a way to alter workout variety. The variation in periodization supposedly reduces any negative overtraining or "staleness" effects so the competitive athlete achieves peak performance at competition. Figure 22.9 *(top)* depicts the generalized design for periodization and a typical macrocy-

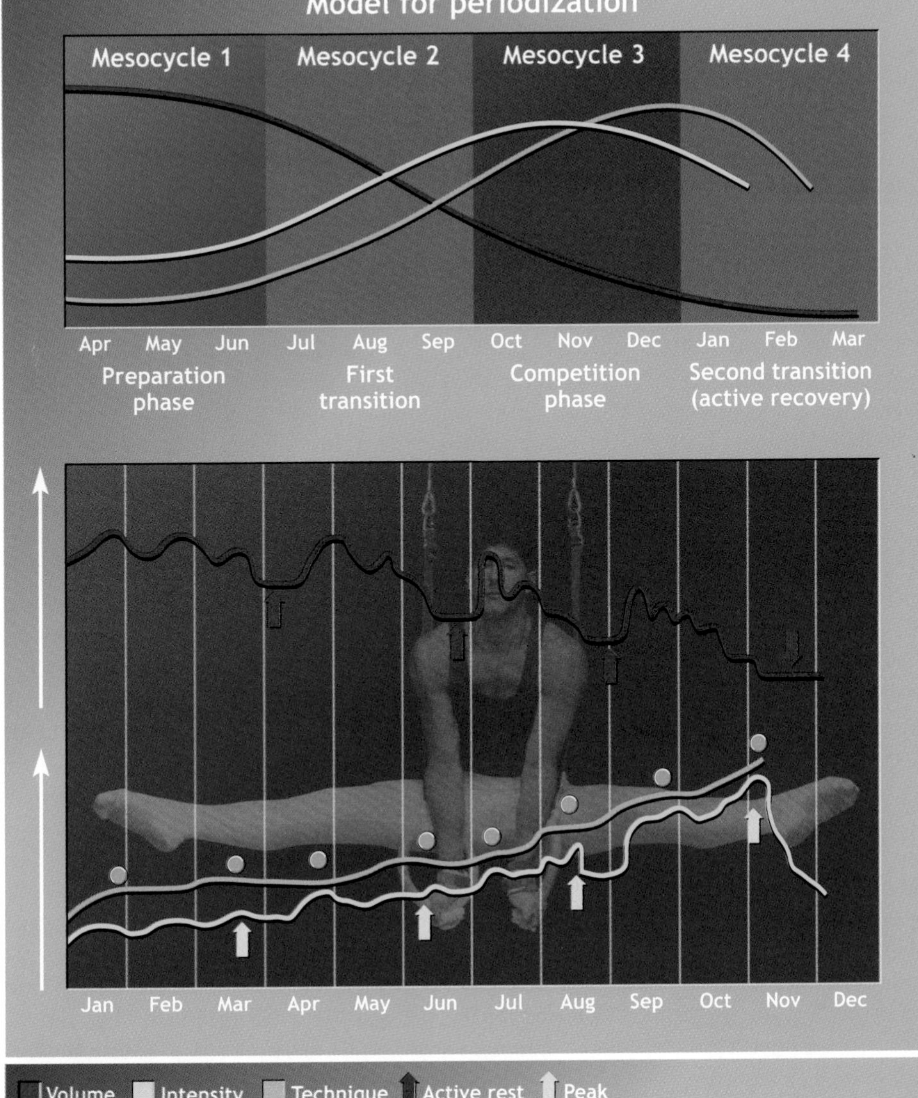

FIGURE 22.9 • *Top,* The periodization concept subdivides a macrocycle into distinct phases or mesocycles. These, in turn, usually separate into weekly microcycles. While the general plan provides modifications, the mesocycles usually include a preparation phase, a first transition phase, a competition phase, and a second transition, or active recovery phase. *Bottom,* Example of periodization for an elite athlete (gymnast) preparing for competition. Competitions took place throughout the yearly training program, so periodization focused on achieving peak performance at the end of each macrocycle. Periodization structures the intensity, duration, and frequency of strength–power workouts, attempting to avoid overtraining (staleness), minimize injury potential, and reduce training monotony, while progressing towards peak performance during competitions *(filled circles).*

cle's four distinct phases. As competition approaches, training volume gradually decreases while training intensity concurrently increases.

- **Preparation phase** emphasizes modest strength development with *high-volume* (3 to 5 sets, 8 to 12 reps), *low-intensity* workouts (50 to 80% 1-RM plus flexibility and aerobic and anaerobic training).
- **First transition phase** emphasizes strength development with workouts of *moderate volume* (3 to 5 sets, 5 to 6 reps) and *moderate intensity* (80 to 90% 1-RM plus flexibility and interval aerobic training).
- **Competition phase** lets the participant peak for competition. Selective strength development is emphasized with *low-volume, high-intensity* workouts (3 to 5 sets, 2 to 4 reps at 90 to 95% 1-RM) plus short periods of interval training that emphasize sport-specific exercises.
- **Second transition phase** (**active recovery**) emphasizes recreational activities and low-intensity workouts incorporating different exercise modes. For the next competition, the athlete repeats the periodization cycle.

Periodization structures an inverse relation between training volume and training intensity through the competition phase, and then decreases both aspects during the second transition, or recuperation, period. Note the increase in the time devoted to technique training as competition approaches, with training volume at the cycle's lowest point. The *bottom part* of Figure 22.9 shows how training volume and intensity interact within a mesocycle for an athlete in a specific sport.

Sport-specific training principles usually apply in periodization when the coach designs the athlete's training on the basis of the sport's distinct strength, power, and endurance requirements. A detailed analysis of the metabolic and technical requirements of the sport also frames the training paradigm. The concept of periodization makes intuitive sense, yet, to our knowledge, no studies have presented conclusive evidence for the superiority of this training approach, owing to difficulties controlling training intensity, training volume, the participants' general fitness level, and the composite integration of strength and rate of force development.[110,132]

To overcome such limitations, researchers have studied shorter mesocycles to determine the best combination of factors to optimize performance improvements. One study that equated training volume and intensity among three approaches to periodization (linear periodization, undulating periodization, and a nonperiodized time interval) found each training method to be equally effective.[11] The training groups made similar gains in muscular strength (25% squat, 13.1% bench press) and muscular power (7.6% vertical jump). Without equating training volume and intensity, it becomes impossible to evaluate differences in training effects reported previously.[220] A critical review of the relatively few studies of periodized strength training concluded that this approach produced greater improvements in muscular strength, body mass, lean body mass, and percentage body fat than nonperiodized multi-set and single-set training programs.[59] Considerably more research must evaluate how periodization interacts with fitness status, age, gender, and specific sports (motor) performance. Studies must equate participants on various fitness parameters and then manipulate different training protocols, accounting for factors known to affect the training response. Program evaluation must consider the following four factors: (1) biomechanics and motor control in the actual sport skill, (2) changes in segmental and whole-body composition, (3) biochemical and ultrastructural tissue adaptations, and (4) transfer of newly acquired strength to subsequent sport performance measures.

COMBINING RESISTANCE TRAINING AND PERIODIZATION: APPLICATION IN HIV-INFECTED MEN. Weight loss during HIV infection adversely affects disease outcome and increases mortality. Testosterone therapy and exercise offer relatively inexpensive and safe therapeutic modalities. In HIV-infected men, weight loss accompanies low testosterone levels[39] and deficits in muscle mass.[71,178] Therefore, combining resistance exercise with pharmacologic therapy potentially offers alternative methods to improve health outcomes by increasing muscle mass (via either resistance training, resistance training with testosterone treatments, or either separately).

To test these possibilities, a placebo-controlled, double-blind, randomized clinical trial evaluated the effects of testosterone replacement with and without resistance-exercise training on muscle strength and body composition in HIV-infected men with low testosterone levels and existing weight loss.[18] Resistance-exercise training for 16 weeks included five standard free-weight exercises (leg, bench, and overhead press, and leg curls and latissimus pulls) employing periodization procedures and testing using the same equipment and exercises as in training in accordance with the specificity-of-training principle. Each subject's initial 1-RM on the five exercises established the workout intensity. The first 4 weeks consisted of high-volume (three sets of 12–15 reps), low-intensity (60% of initial 1-RM) exercises performed thrice weekly. For the next 6 weeks, subjects trained thrice weekly using a progressive, periodized, high-intensity regimen (90% of 1-RM on heavy days, 80% of 1-RM on medium days, and 70% of 1-RM on light days) using a low volume of four sets of 4–6 repetitions of each exercise. For the 6 remaining training weeks, workout loads increased by 7% for upper-body and 12% for lower-body exercises, with set number increased from three to five. Changes in strength, thigh muscle volume, and lean body mass were compared among the four treatment modalities (placebo, no exercise; intramuscular testosterone injections, [100 mg per wk], no exercise; placebo and exercise; testosterone and exercise).

Men treated with testosterone alone, exercise alone, or both significantly increased muscular strength in the leg press (+ 22 to 30%), leg curls (+ 18 to 36%), and latissimus pulls (+ 17 to 33%). Body mass, strength, and MRI-measured thigh muscle volume improved significantly more in men in the testosterone-exercise group or exercise-alone group than in the placebo-alone group. Also, average lean mass increased by 2.3 kg in the testosterone-alone group and 2.6 kg in the testosterone-plus-exercise group but remained essentially unchanged in the placebo-alone group. The results convincingly demonstrate that progressive resistance exercise training incorporating periodization plus testosterone treatments promoted significant gains in body mass, muscle strength, and lean body mass in HIV-infected men with weight loss and low testosterone levels. Interestingly, muscle strength per unit of muscle mass increased more in men who resistance trained than in men who only received testosterone, implying that without resistance training, testosterone-only treatments failed to improve the contractile quality of skeletal muscle. Incorporating resistance-exercise training to evaluate clinical outcomes during disease progression offers great promise as a clinical intervention for HIV-infected patients.[126,192]

Practical Recommendations for Initiating a Weight-Training Program

- Avoid maximum lifts in the beginning stages of a weight-training program. Excessive resistance contributes little to strength development and greatly increases risk of muscle or joint injury (see discussion of the lower back; In a Practical Sense). *A load equal to 60 to 80% of a muscle's force-generating capacity provides sufficient stimulus to increase muscular strength.* This load generally allows completion of about 10 repetitions of a particular exercise.
- Use a lighter resistance to perform more repetitions at the start of training. Novices should initially attempt to complete 12 to 15 repetitions. This regimen does not place excessive strain on the musculoskeletal system during the early phase of the program. Use a heavier weight if 12 repetitions feel too easy. The weight is too heavy if the exerciser cannot complete 12 repetitions. This trial-and-error process may take several exercise sessions to establish the proper starting weight.
- After a week or two of training, when the muscles adapt and the exerciser learns the correct movements, the number of repetitions can decrease to between 6 and 8.
- Add more weight each time after reaching the target number of repetitions. This regimen represents progressive resistance training; as muscles become stronger, the weight increases with the lifting of a heavier load.
- The exercise sequence should proceed from larger to smaller muscle groups to avoid premature fatigue of the small group required for the movement.

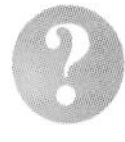

INTEGRATIVE QUESTION

Discuss the statement "There is no one *best* system of resistance training."

IN A PRACTICAL SENSE

THE LOWER BACK

Lower-back pain disability costs the Unites States more than $36 billion each year in lost workdays and employee compensation. Back injuries account for one-fourth of all work-related injuries and one-third of all compensation costs. Most cases result from on-the-job injuries, particularly in men in lumber and building retailing (*highest risk*) and construction (*most cases*); major-risk industries for women include nursing and personal care centers (*highest risk*) and hospitals (*most cases*). Grocery stores and agricultural production of crops rank among the top 10 occupations for lower-back injury for both men and women. Estimates indicate that more than 32 million adult Americans frequently experience lower-back pain, which represents the primary cause for workplace disability.[120] Workplace disability from lower back injuries also occurs in common tasks like refuse collection and other manual handling and lifting tasks.[44,48,107]

Muscular weakness, particularly in the abdominal and lower lumbar back regions, lumbar spine instability, and poor joint flexibility in the back and legs represent primary external factors related to **low-back pain syndrome.** Prevention of, and rehabilitation from, chronic low back strain commonly use muscle-strengthening and joint-flexibility exercises.[17,140,173,210] Continuing normal activities of daily living (within limits dictated by pain tolerance) yields a more rapid recovery from acute back pain than bed rest. Maintaining normal physical activity may facilitate greater recovery than specific back-mobilizing exercises performed after pain onset.[130] Prudent use of resistance training isolates and strengthens the abdomen and lower lumbar extensor muscles that support and protect the spine through its full range of motion.[163] Patients with low back pain who strengthen the lumbar extensors with the pelvis stabilized experience less pain and fewer chronic symptoms and improved muscular strength, endurance, and range of motion.[26]

Improper performance of a resistance-exercise movement (with a relatively heavy load and hips thrust forward with arched back) creates considerable compressive force on the lower spine. For example, pressing and curling exercises with back hyperextension create unusually high shearing stress on the lumbar vertebrae, often triggering low back pain. Compressive forces with heavy lifting also can trigger a range of physiologic changes that hasten damage to the disks that cushion the vertebrae. Performing half squats with barbell loads ranging from 0.8 to 1.6 times body

Continued

IN A PRACTICAL SENSE

➤➤ THE LOWER BACK—cont'd

mass produces compressive loads on the L3-L4 segment of the spine equivalent to 6 to 10 times body mass.[25,33] Thus, a person who weighs 90 kg and squats with 144 kg can create peak compressive forces in excess of 1367 kg (13,334 N)! A sudden amplification of compressive force can produce anterior disk prolapse; a lower-intensity but sustained compressive force that produces fatigue can increase posterior bulging of the lamellas in the posterior annulus.[3] In national-level male and female powerlifters, average compressive loads on L4–L5 reached 1757 kg (17,192 N).

Experiments with mice indicate that chronic disk compression in their tails—an extension of its spine, with disks similar to those in the human back—killed disk cells, eventually causing them to dehydrate outward and bulge. *One should not sacrifice proper execution of an exercise to lift a heavier load or "squeeze out" additional repetition.* The extra weight lifted through improper technique does not facilitate muscle strengthening; instead, improper body alignment or unwarranted muscle substitution during force production can precipitate injury.

Wearing a weight-lifting belt during *heavy* lifts (squats, dead lifts, clean-and-jerk maneuvers) significantly reduces intraabdominal pressure, compared with lifting without a belt.[75] The belt reduces the potentially injurious compressive forces on spinal disks during near-maximal heavy lifting, including most Olympic and power-lifting events and associated training. A person who normally trains wearing a belt should generally refrain from lifting without one. Further recommendations include performing at least some submaximal resistance training without a belt to strengthen the deep abdominal muscles. This also develops the proper pattern of muscle recruitment to generate high intra-abdominal pressures when not wearing a belt. Wearing a back belt to increase intra-abdominal pressure to ameliorate low back injuries in the workplace does not provide a clear-cut biomechanical advantage.[159] A 2-year prospective study of nearly 14,000 material-handling employees in 30 states evaluated the effectiveness of using back belts in reducing back injury worker's compensation claims and reports of low back pain.[214] Findings indicated that neither frequent back belt use (usually once a day and once or twice a week) nor a store policy that required the use of these belts related to reduced injury or reports of low back pain. Researchers continue to probe for answers about the etiology of low-back pain syndrome and how to minimize its severity and reduce its occurrence. Studies have focused on numerous contributing factors including intradisk pressure;[141] facet loads and disk fiber strains;[179] lumbar disk height and cross-sectional area;[147] compressive follower loads;[156] spinal joint force distribution;[31] ligament strain, disk shear, and facet impingement;[80] and prediction models to estimate spinal compression and shear forces.[72,104]

The following 12 exercises are ideal for general strengthening of the abdomen and lower back and improving hamstring and lower-back flexibility for individuals with no apparent lower back and spinal injuries. Symptomatic individuals require specific back exercises prescribed by a health care professional.

I. **Lower-back stretches** (hold each exercise for 30 to 60 s)

1. *Knees-to-chest stretch*: Lie supine and pull knees into chest while keeping lower back flat on the surface.

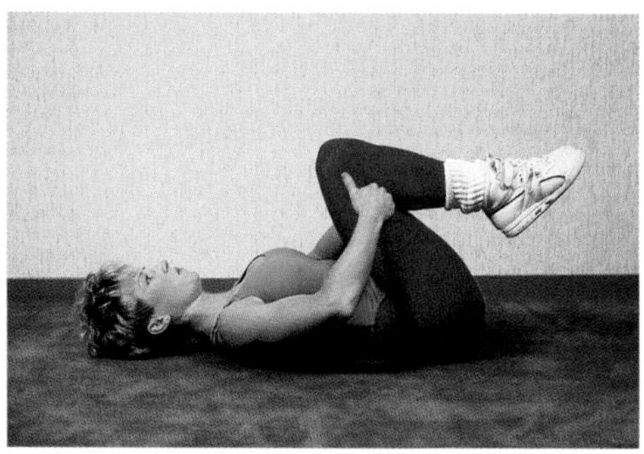

2. *Cross-leg stretch*: Cross legs like sitting male. Cross legs and pull 90°-flexed knee toward chest.

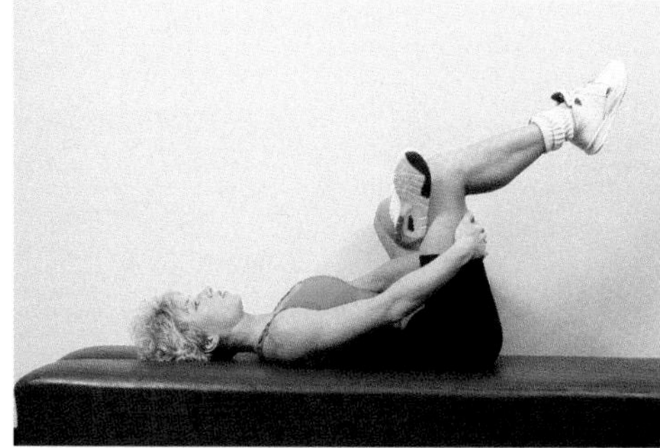

3. *Hamstring stretch*: Wrap strap over foot, keeping lower back flat; pull leg upward toward head.

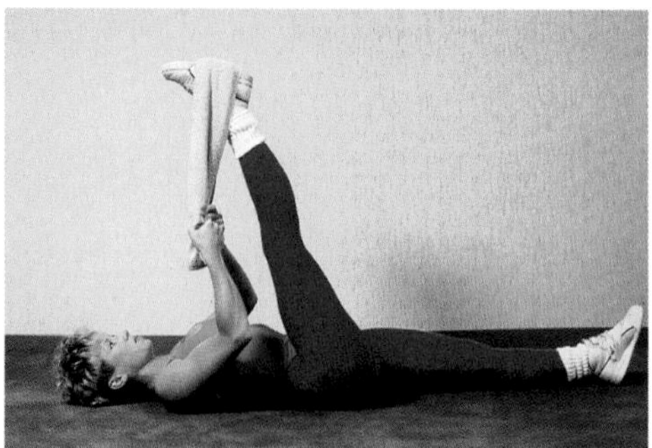

In a Practical Sense

➤➤ The Lower Back—cont'd

4. *Allah stretch*: Sit, buttocks on bilateral heels; move hands as far forward along the surface as possible.

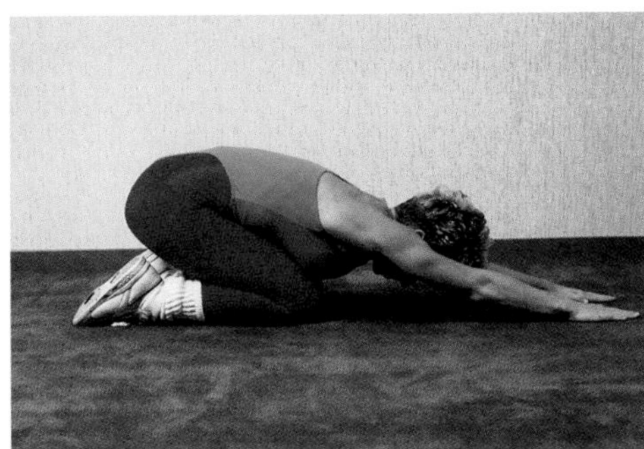

II. **Abdominal exercises**

5. *Bent-knee sit-up*: Keep hands low on neck (or across chest) with head positioned over the shoulders. Roll up slowly, engaging one row of the abdominals at a time. Raise the shoulders 4 to 6 inches off the surface.

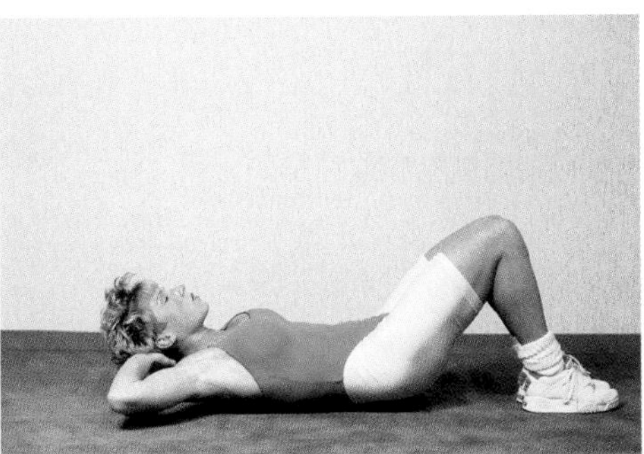

6. *Dying bug*: Flex the pelvis to flatten the lower back against the surface. Over one side bring an extended arm and flexed knee together. The opposing side should extend a straight arm overhead and straight leg backward. Maintain pelvis flexion while exchanging opposing arms and legs in this position.

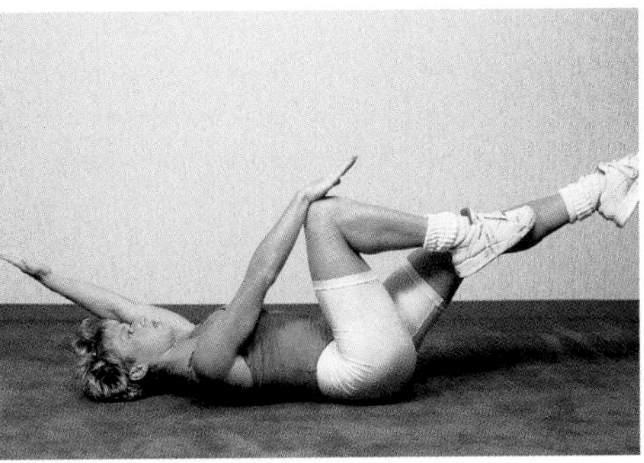

III. **Prone lumbar extension exercises**

7. *Dry-land swimming*: Lying prone with pelvic flexion, alternate lifting opposite arm and legs.

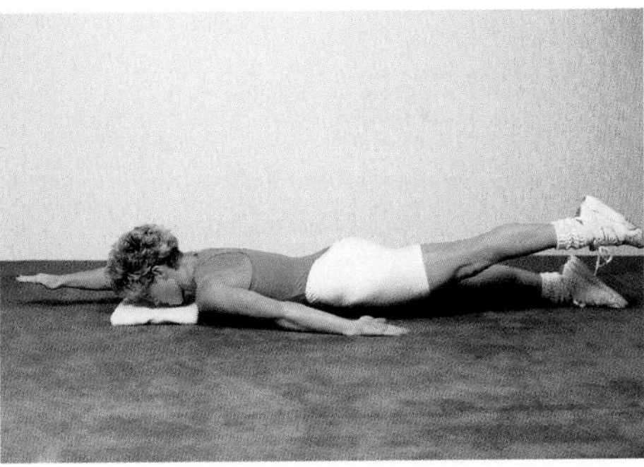

8. *Both legs up*: Lying prone with pelvic flexion, lift both legs simultaneously while keeping the head on the floor.

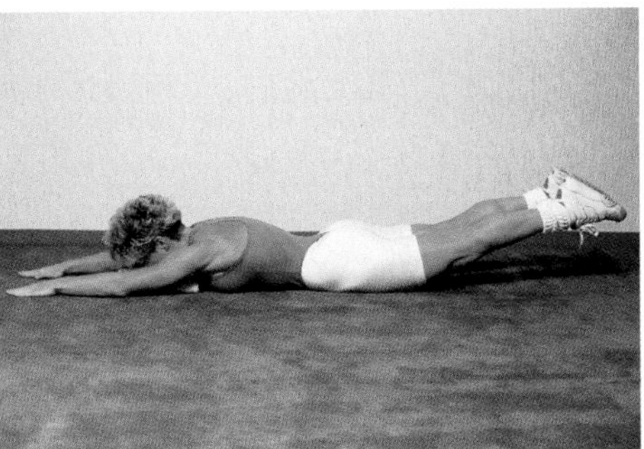

Continued

IN A PRACTICAL SENSE

➤➤ THE LOWER BACK—cont'd

9. *Upper body up*: Lying prone with pelvic flexion and arms outstretched or behind the back, lift the upper torso while keeping the legs on the floor.

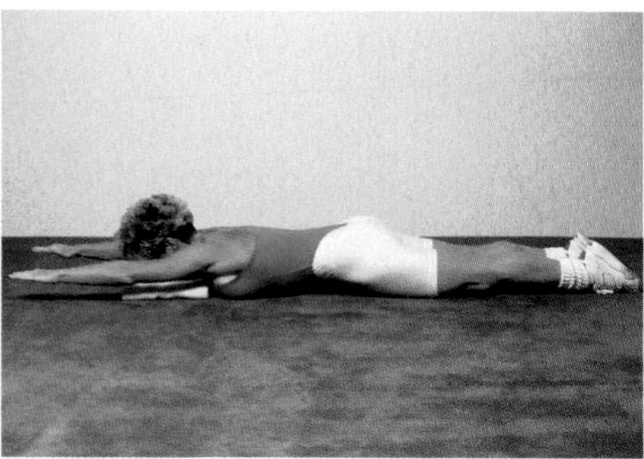

10. *Pointer (bird dog)*: Start with hands and knees on the floor. Flex pelvis into counter position. Exchange pointing opposite arm and leg while keeping the torso level.

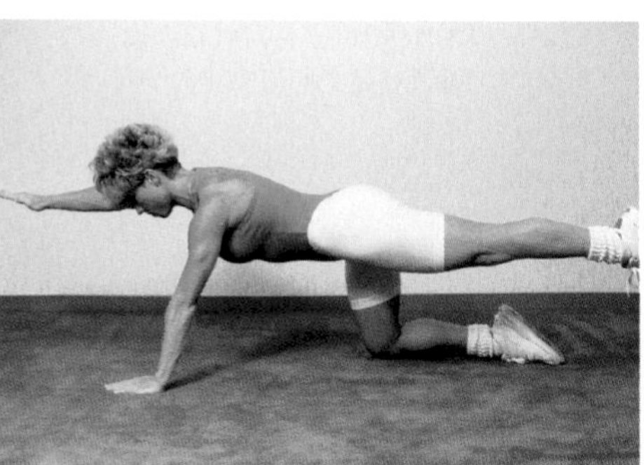

IV. **Supine pelvic-flexion exercises**

11. *Leg pointer*: Lie supine on the floor and flex the pelvis with the lower abdominals to flatten the lower back into the surface. Extend one arm upward and one leg outward while keeping the quadriceps level.

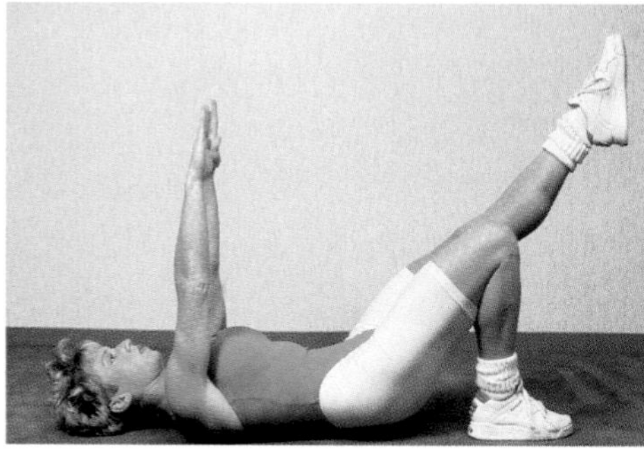

12. *Prone cobra push-up*: Keep the pelvis on the floor while pressing up with the arms, causing lower back extension.

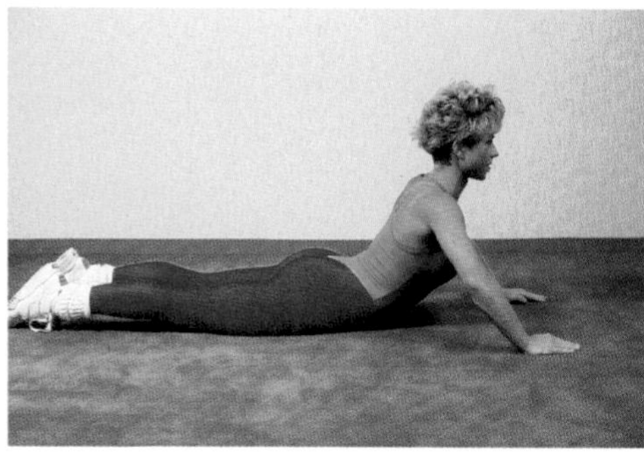

(Photos courtesy of Dr. Bob Swanson, Santa Barbara Back and Neck Care Center. Santa Barbara, CA 93108.)

Resistance Training Guidelines for Sedentary Adults, the Elderly, and Cardiac Patients: Benefits in Health and Disease

Currently, the American College of Sports Medicine, American Heart Association, Centers for Disease Control and Prevention, American Association of Cardiovascular and Pulmonary Rehabilitation, and the U.S. Surgeon General's Office consider regular resistance exercise to be an important component of a comprehensive, health-related physical fitness program.[1,6,7,61,164,204] Resistance training goals for competitive athletes focus on optimizing muscular strength, power, and hypertrophy ("high-intensity" with 1-RM to 6-RM training loads). *In contrast, goals for most middle-aged and older adults focus on maintenance (and possible increase) of muscle and bone mass and muscular strength and muscular endurance to enhance the overall health and physical-fitness profile.*[54,89,119,120,219] Adequate muscular strength in midlife maintains a margin of safety above the necessary threshold required to prevent injury in later life. For example, among 45- to 68-year-old men, hand-grip strength accurately predicted functional limitations and disability 25 years later (Fig. 22.10).[167] Men in the lowest one-third for grip strength showed the greatest risk; those in the middle one-third showed intermediate risk, and men in the top one-third experienced the least disability risk at the 25-year follow-up.

The resistance training program recommended for middle-aged and older men and women classifies as "moderate intensity." In contrast to the multiple-set, heavy-resis-

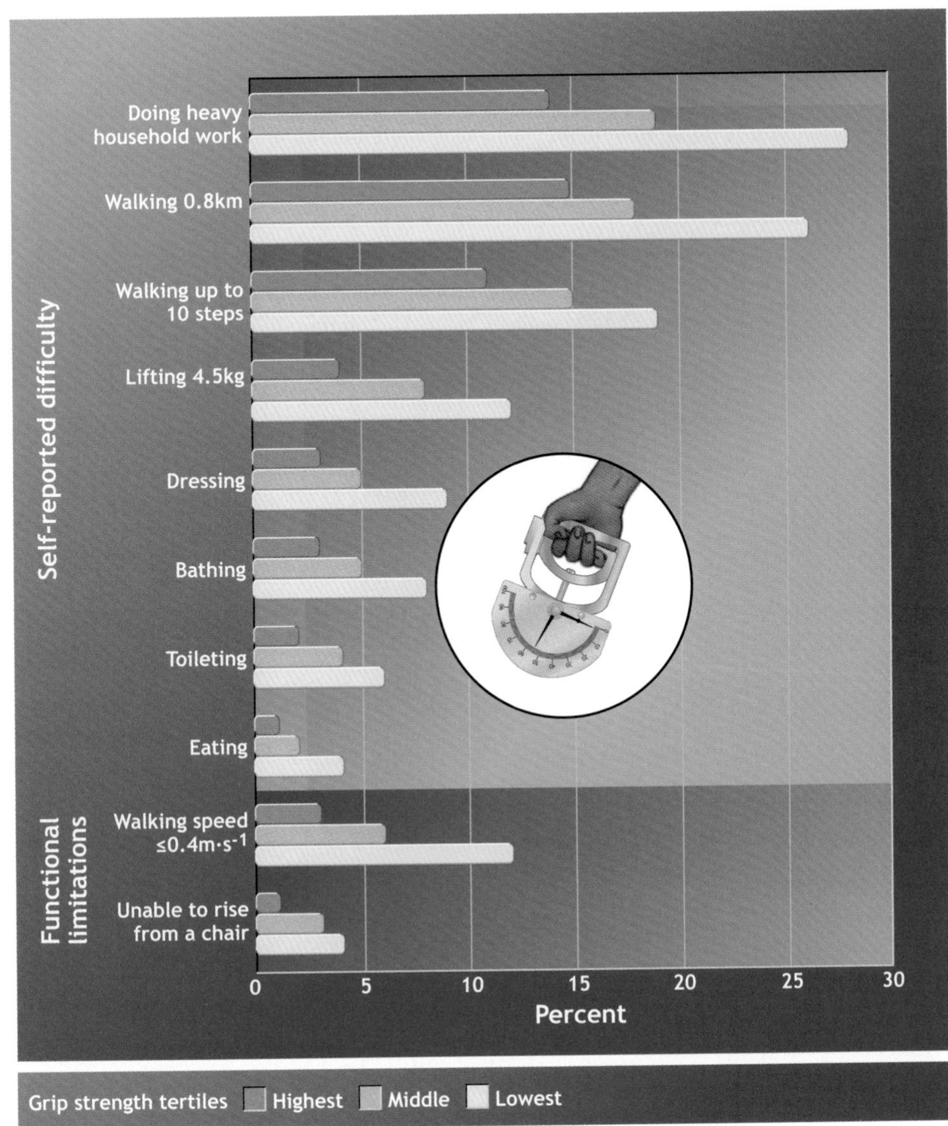

FIGURE 22.10 • Relationship between grip strength assessed in 3,218 healthy middle-aged 45 to 68–year-old men and functional limitations and difficulties 25 years later. (From Rantanen T, et al. Midlife hand grip strength as a predictor of old age disability. JAMA 1999;281:558.)

tance approach used by younger athletes, the program uses single sets of diverse exercises performed between 8- and 15-RM a minimum of twice a week. Table 22.3 presents guidelines from different groups and health organizations for prudent resistance training of older men and women and cardiac patients.[56,57]

Resistance Training Plus Aerobic Training Equals Less Strength Improvement

Concurrent resistance and aerobic training programs yield less muscular strength and power improvement than training for strength only.[81,113] This partly explains why power athletes and body builders refrain from endurance activities while participating in resistance training. More than likely, the added energy (and perhaps protein) demands of heavy endurance training impose a limit on a muscle's growth and metabolic responsiveness to resistance training. Also, a short-term bout of high-intensity endurance exercise inhibits performance in subsequent muscular strength activities.[121] Further research must determine whether this effect on maximal force output limits one's ability to overload skeletal muscle optimally to a degree that impairs strength development with concurrent strength and endurance training. If it does, then a 20- to 30-minute recovery between aerobic and strength training components might enhance the quality of the subsequent strength workout. These considerations, however, should not deter those who desire a well-rounded conditioning program offering the specific fitness and health benefits available from *both* exercise training modes.[49,89]

Isometric Strength Training

Research in Germany during the mid-1950s showed that a person could increase isometric strength about 5% weekly by performing a daily single, maximum isometric muscle action

TABLE 22.3 ➤ STRENGTH TRAINING GUIDELINES FOR SEDENTARY ADULTS, ELDERLY PERSONS, AND CARDIAC PATIENTS

GUIDELINE	SETS	REPETITIONS[a]	NUMBER OF EXERCISES	FREQUENCY (DAYS/WEEK)
Healthy sedentary adults				
1990 ACSM Position Stand[b]	1	8–12	8–10[c]	2
1995 ACSM Guidelines[d]	1	8–12	8–10	2
1996 Surgeon General's Report[e]	1–2	8–12	8–10	2
Elderly persons				
Pollock et al,[f] 1994	1	10–15	8–10	2
Cardiac patients				
1995 AHA Exercise Standards[g]	1	10–15	8–10	2–3
1995 AACVPR Guidelines[h]	1	10–15	8–10	2–3

[a]For healthy persons under age 50, weight should be sufficient to induce volitional fatigue with the number of repetitions listed. For older persons, lighter loads may be used.
[b]American College of Sports Medicine. The recommended quantity and quality of exercise for developing and maintaining cardiorespiratory and muscular fitness in healthy adults. Med Sci Sports Exerc. 1990;22:265.
[c]Minimum one exercise per major muscle group (e.g., chest press, shoulder press, triceps extension, biceps curl, pull-down [upper back], lower back extension, abdominal crunch/curl-up, quadriceps extension, leg curls [hamstrings], calf-raise).
[d]American College of Sports Medicine. Guidelines for exercise testing and prescription 5th ed. Baltimore: Williams & Wilkins, 1995; also included low-risk diseased populations.
[e]U.S. Department of Health and Human Services. Physical activity and health: a report of the surgeon general. Atlanta: US Dept. of Health and Human Services, Centers for Disease Control and Prevention, National Center for Chronic Disease Prevention and Health Promotion, 1996.
[f]Pollock ML, et al. Exercise training and prescription for the elderly. South Med J 1994;87:S88.
[g]Fletcher GF, et al. Exercise standards: a statement for health care professionals from the American Heart Association. Circulation 1995;91:580.
[h]American Association of Cardiovascular and Pulmonary Rehabilitation. Guidelines for cardiac rehabilitation programs. 2nd ed. Champaign, IL: Human Kinetics, 1995.
ACSM, American College of Sports Medicine; AHA, American Heart Association; AACVPR, American Association of Cardiovascular and Pulmonary Rehabilitation.

of only 1-second duration, or a 6-second action at two-thirds maximum.[82] Repeating this action 5 to 10 times daily produced greater gains in isometric strength.

Isometric Exercise Limitations

Isometric exercise provides muscle overload and improves strength yet offers only limited benefits for sports training. Because no movement occurs, one cannot readily evaluate the overload level and/or training progress. Also, a high degree of *specificity* affects isometric strength development. Thus, a muscle trained isometrically demonstrates improved strength primarily when the trained muscle acts isometrically, particularly at the training joint angle and body position.[108]

Isometric training to develop "strengths" for a particular movement probably necessitates training at many points through the ROM. This becomes time consuming, particularly given the availability of conventional dynamic weight training and isokinetic and other resistance activities.

Isometric Exercise Benefits

The isometric method benefits muscle testing and rehabilitation. Isometric techniques can detect specific muscle weakness, thus forming a basis for optimizing muscle overload at the appropriate joint angle.

Which Are Better, Static or Dynamic Methods?

Static and dynamic resistance training methods each significantly increase muscle "strengths." An individual's specific needs determine the optimal resistance training method (governed by the specificity of the training response).[144]

Specificity of the Training Response

An isometrically trained muscle shows greatest strength improvement when measured isometrically, whereas a dynamically trained muscle tests best when evaluated in resistance activities requiring movement. Furthermore, isometric strength developed at or near one joint angle does not readily transfer to other angles or body positions that demand use of the same muscles.[108,215] In dynamic exercise, muscles trained through movement over a limited ROM show the greatest strength improvement when measured in that ROM.[70] Even a body-position specificity exists; muscular strength of ankle plantar and dorsiflexors developed in the standing position with concentric and eccentric muscle actions showed no transfer when evaluating the same muscles' strength in the supine position.[165] Resistance training specificity makes sense because strength improvement blends adaptations in two factors: (1) the muscle fiber itself and (2) the neural organization and excitability of motor units that power discrete patterns of voluntary movement.[146,166,189] Likewise, a muscle's maximal force output depends on neural factors that effectively recruit and synchronize firing of motor units, not just local factors such as muscle fiber type and cross-sectional area.[38,106,154,183]

A 3-month study of young adult men and women emphasized the highly specific nature of resistance-training adaptations.[51] One group trained the adductor pollicis muscle isometrically with 10 daily muscle actions of 5-seconds duration at a frequency of 1 per minute. The other group trained the same muscle dynamically with 10 daily 10-repetition bouts of weight movement at one-third maximal strength. The untrained muscle served as the control. To eliminate any training influence from psychologic factors and central nervous system adaptations, a supermaximal electrical stimulation applied to the motor nerve evaluated the force capacity of the trained muscle. The results were clear—both training groups improved maximal force capacity and peak rate of force development. The improvement in maximal force for the isometrically trained group, however, nearly doubled the improvement for the dynamically trained group. Conversely, improvement in speed of force development averaged about 70% greater in the group trained with dynamic muscle actions. Such findings provide strong evidence that resistance training per se does not induce all-inclusive (general) adaptations in muscle structure and function. Rather, a muscle's contractile properties (maximal force, velocity of shortening, rate of tension development) improve in a manner highly specific to the muscle action used in training. Although both static and dynamic training methods produce significant strength increases, no one system is consistently superior to the other in diverse evaluations of muscle function. The crucial consideration concerns the intended purpose of the newly acquired strength.

PRACTICAL IMPLICATIONS. The complex interaction between the nervous and muscular systems helps explain why leg muscles strengthened in squats or deep knee bends fail to show equivalent improved force capability in other leg movements such as jumping or leg extension.[149] Low relationships emerge between dynamic measures of leg extension force at any speed and vertical jumping height.[87] Also, a muscle group strengthened and enlarged by dynamic resistance training does not demonstrate equal improvement in force capacity when measured isometrically or isokinetically.[183] Consequently, strengthening muscles for a specific athletic or occupational activity (e.g., golf, tennis, rowing, swimming, football, firefighting, package handling) demands more than just identifying and overloading the muscles used in the movement. It requires training specifically in the important movements that necessitate improved strength. Increasing leg muscle "strength" through general weight lifting probably will *not* improve performance in a variety of subsequent leg movements.[137] *Newly acquired strength seldom transfers fully to other types of movements, even those activating the same trained muscles.* For example, a standard program of weight training for leg extension increased leg extension strength by 227%. However, evaluating leg extension peak torque of the same leg with an isokinetic dynamometer detected only a 10 to 17% improvement![63] *To improve a specific physical performance through resistance training, one must train the muscle(s) in movements that mimic the movement requiring force-capacity improvement, with specific consideration for force, velocity, and power requirements.*

Specificity Not Always Observed

Most training studies support the concept of specificity, yet exceptions exist.[100,157] In one study, subjects in a free-weight (FW) training group trained three times weekly for 12 weeks using eccentric and concentric muscle actions; a second group trained by using concentric actions only with hydraulic resistance (HY); a control group did not train.[86] Training with FW and HY included five sets of supine bench presses and upright squats at an intensity of 1- to 6-RM plus five supplementary exercises at 5- to 10-RM, for a total of 20 sets per session for approximately 50 minutes. Testing before and after training included the 1-RM bench press and squat measured concentrically and eccentrically without prestretch (concentric only).

Figure 22.11 *(top)* shows that the FW group greatly increased concentric squat strength (135%), but these increases did not differ significantly from those of the group that trained using only concentric muscle actions (139%). Both groups improved about 30% when eccentric and concentric actions assessed squat strength *(bottom)*. Although the specificity principle in resistance training may encompass joint-angle or muscle-length specificity, velocity specificity, and task or movement-pattern specificity,[101,196] the principle may not fully apply to test mode.[157,160] Perhaps resistance training with free weights or hydraulic devices does not differ enough in muscle action and neuromuscular patterning to elicit highly specific training adaptations between exercise modes. Unlike isokinetic and HY routines, FW exercise includes both eccentric and concentric actions. The limiting factor in overcoming resistance in FW exercise becomes the concentric, not the eccentric muscle force. Thus, despite differences between the muscle actions in FW and HY exercise, FW- and HY-trained subjects may still experience the same training stimulus via the concentric load. A distinct possibility exists that *any* form of concentric or combined concentric–eccentric resistance training produces comparable muscle strength gains, provided that training and testing use similar movement patterns and velocities.[131]

Isokinetic Resistance Training

Isokinetic resistance training attempts to combine the positive features of both isometric exercise and dynamic weight lifting. It provides muscle overload at a preset constant speed while the muscle mobilizes its force-generating capacity *throughout* the full ROM. Any effort during the exercise movement encounters an opposing force relative to that applied to the me-

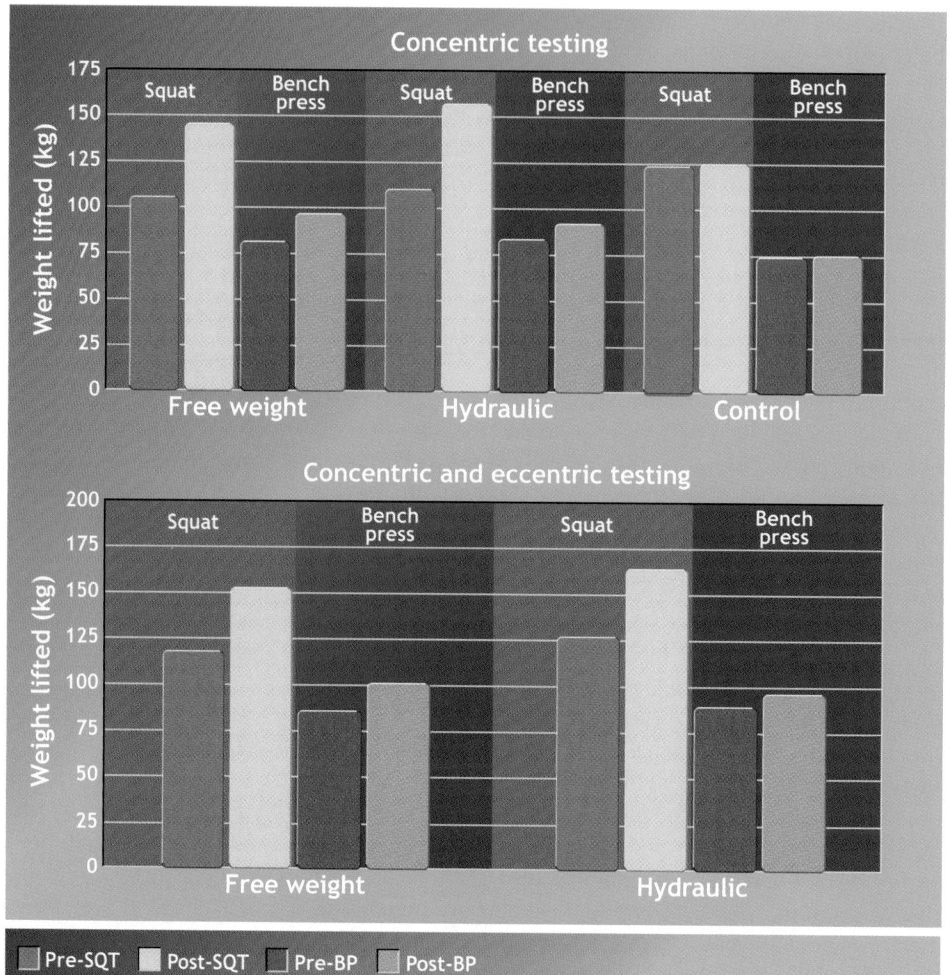

FIGURE 22.11 • Effects of 12 weeks of resistance training with concentric resistance *(top)* and combined concentric–eccentric resistance *(bottom)* on pre- and posttest squat *(SQT)* and bench press *(BP)* muscle actions. (From Hortobágyi T, Katch FI. Role of concentric force in limiting improvement in muscular strength. J Appl Physiol 1990;68:650.)

chanical device; this represents **accommodating-resistance exercise**. Theoretically, isokinetic-type training activates the largest number of motor units to overload muscles consistently—even at the relatively "weaker" joint angles—as the bone-muscle-lever mechanics produce variations in force capacity throughout the ROM.

Isokinetics Versus Standard Weight Lifting

An important distinction exists between a muscle overloaded isokinetically and one overloaded with a standard weight-lifting exercise. Figure 22.12 shows that the force capacity of a muscle (or muscle group) varies with the bony lever configuration (joint angle) as the joint moves through its ROM. During weight training, the external weight lifted usually remains fixed at the greatest load that allows completion of the movement for the desired number of repetitions. *Consequently, the resistance cannot exceed the maximum force generated at the weakest point in the ROM. Otherwise, one could not complete the movement.* The term *sticking point* describes this point in the ROM.

The fact that muscles do not generate the same maximum force through all movement phases represents a major limitation of weight lifting. To help alleviate this problem, manufacturers have devised **variable-resistance training equipment** that uses an irregularly shaped metal cam or other device to adjust resistance in accordance with the lever characteristics of a particular joint movement. This equipment still represents a classic mode of weight lifting, except that the *relative resistance* offered to the muscle theoretically remains fairly constant throughout the ROM. The machine, however, does not control the speed of movement, and the design of the mechanical device uses the average physical dimensions of a population to achieve a variable resistance. Consequently, one cannot adjust for individual variations in body structure. Furthermore, cam devices do not compensate fully for differences in mechanics and force application at all phases of the particular movement on a given piece of exercise equipment. With an isokinetically loaded muscle, on the other hand, the desired movement speed occurs almost instantaneously with force application, and the muscle generates peak power output throughout the ROM at a controlled shortening velocity.

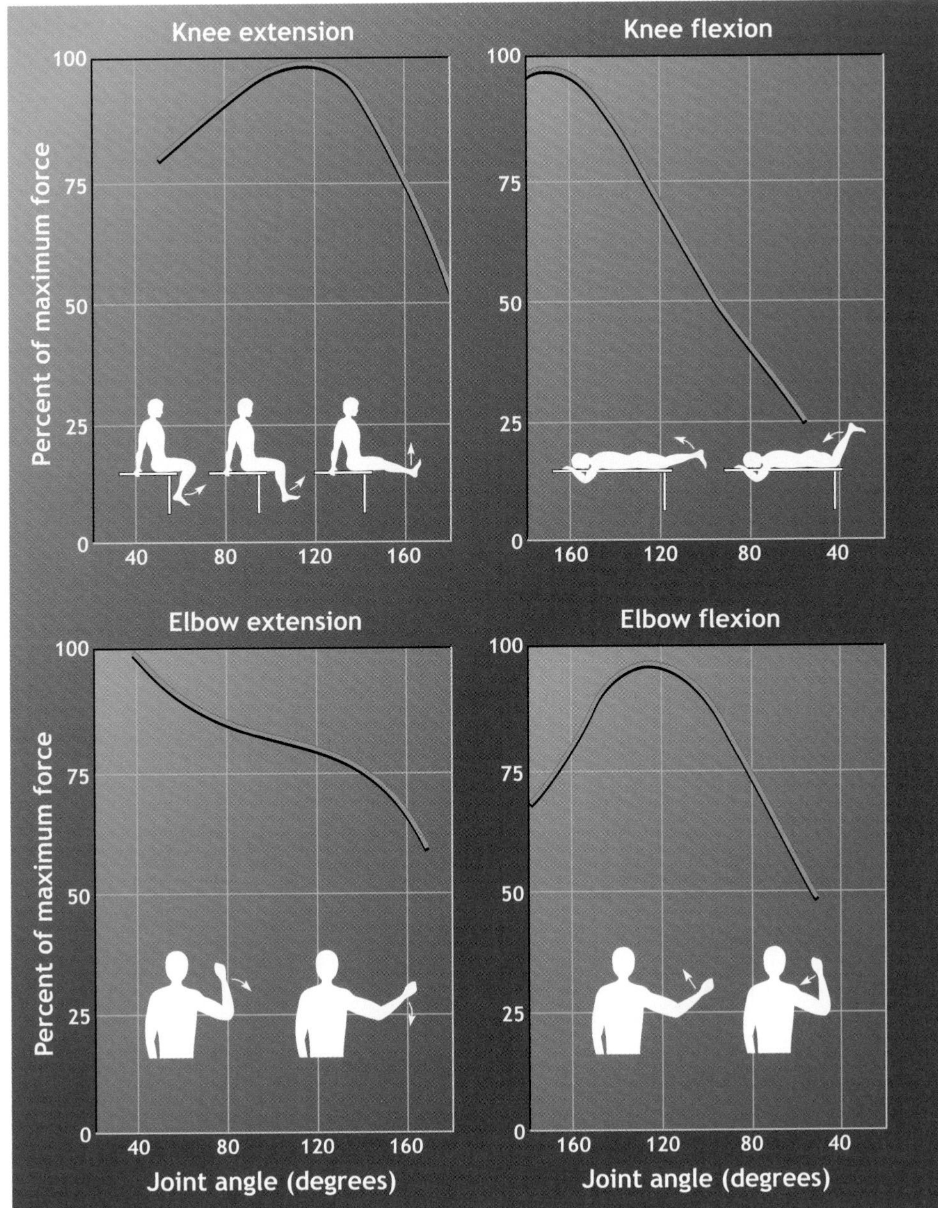

FIGURE 22.12 • Force-generating capacity of a muscle or muscle group varies with joint angle in flexion and extension throughout the ROM. Performing such dynamic movements permits computation of work and power. For rotational work, the mathematical equation is work = torque × angular displacement, where torque is the product of a force acting on the object and the perpendicular distance from the line of action of the force to the point about which the object rotates. Angular displacement is the angle through which the object rotates. To compute rotational power: power = work ÷ time = (torque × angular displacement) ÷ time. Rewriting the equation, power = torque × (angular displacement ÷ time), and power = torque × angular velocity. SI units express torque in newton-meters and angular displacement in radians (convert degrees to radians by dividing by 57.3 deg/rad). A joule is the SI unit for work accomplished in rotating an object, with power expressed in watts (joules ÷ seconds). Work and power relate as follows: work = force × distance, and power = work ÷ time = (force × distance) ÷ time. Rewriting the last expression, power = force × distance ÷ time, and power = force × velocity. (Equations from Harmon E. The measurement of human mechanical power. In Maud PJ, Foster C, eds. Physiological assessment of human fitness. Champaign, IL: Human Kinetics, 1995:88–89.)

Figure 22.13 presents a generalized two-dimensional view of torque development related to angular velocity at two specific joint angles during eccentric and concentric muscle actions. This analysis permits more-comprehensive evaluation of muscular force-generating capability than measurement at only one joint angle or with a standard 1-RM measure.

Isokinetic Exercise and Training Experiments

Experiments with isokinetic exercise have explored the force–velocity patterns in various movements related to the muscle's fiber-type composition. Figure 22.14 shows the progressive decline in peak torque output with increasing angular velocity of the knee extensor muscles in two groups who differed in sports training and predominant muscle fiber type. In movement at $180° \cdot s^{-1}$, maximal torque decrement averaged about 55% of maximal isometric ($0° \cdot s^{-1}$) force. However, the two curves in Figure 22.14 differ in peak torque, depending on the group's muscle fiber composition. Peak force at zero velocity (isometric force) remained similar for athletes with relatively high (power athletes) or low (endurance athletes) percentages of fast-twitch muscle fibers; this indicated activation of *both* fast- and slow-twitch motor units in maximal isometric knee extension. As movement velocity increased, individuals with higher percentages of fast-twitch fibers exerted greater torque per unit body mass. This indicates the desirability of a high percentage of fast-twitch fibers for power activities in which success largely depends on one's capacity to generate torque at rapid movement velocities.

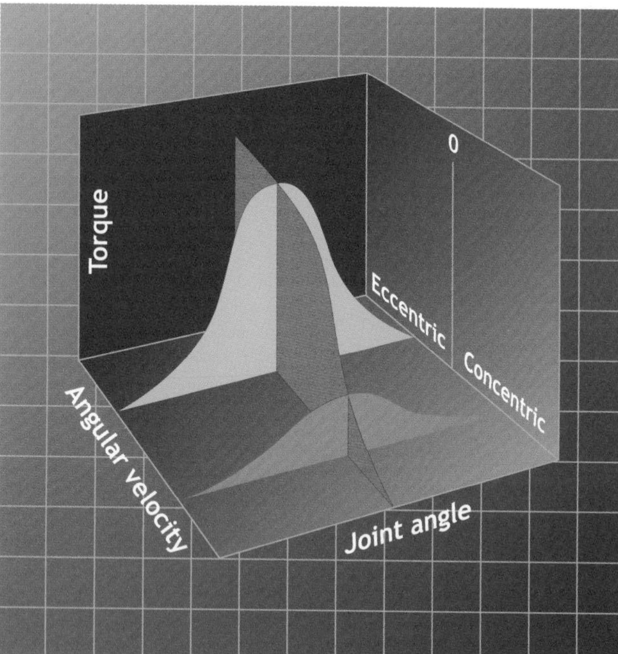

FIGURE 22.13 • Two-dimensional curve of maximal torque versus joint angle, derived from measurement at two angular velocities. The height of the line of intersection of the *red* (torque) and *blue* (angular velocity) curves represents the maximal torque at this particular combination of angular velocity and joint angle. The height of the intersection of the red and green curves also reflects maximal torque at the other angular velocity *(green curve)* and joint angle. (Two-dimensional curve analysis courtesy of Dr. E. Harmon, research physiologist and director of Biomechanics Research, U.S. Army Research Institute of Environmental Medicine, Natick, MA.)

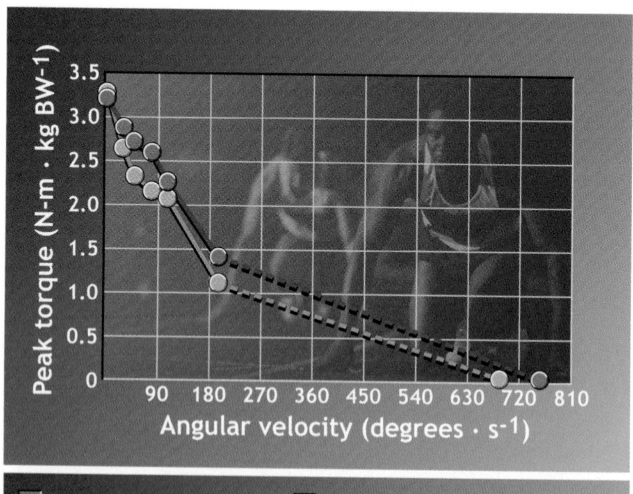

FIGURE 22.14 • Peak torque (per unit body mass) related to angular velocity of joint movement in two groups of athletes with different predominance of muscle-fiber type. The torque–velocity curves were extrapolated *(dashed line)* to the approximated maximal velocity for knee extension. (From Thorstensson A. Muscle strength, fiber types, and enzyme activities in man. Acta Physiol Scand Suppl 1976:443.)

Fast- Versus Slow-Speed Isokinetic Training

Studies of strength and power improvement with isokinetic training at slow and fast limb speeds further support the specificity of exercise performance and training response. For example, several studies show that strength and power gains from slow-speed isokinetic training relate specifically to the angular velocity of the movement used in training. In contrast, exercising at fast speeds facilitates more-general improvement; power output increased at fast *and* slow movement speeds, although measurement at the fast angular velocity used in training improved the most.[161] Muscle hypertrophy generally results only from fast-speed training and only in the fast-contracting type II muscle fibers.[40] Muscle fiber hypertrophy may account for the more-general strength improvement with fast-speed training. Furthermore, concentric muscle actions produce greater power increases and type II fiber hypertrophy from training than eccentric training at equivalent relative power levels.[134]

The attractiveness of isokinetic training allows muscular overload through a full ROM at many shortening velocities. However, applications remain limited because the most rapid speed of movement of the current isokinetic dynamometers is $400° \cdot s^{-1}$. Even this relatively "fast" movement speed does not approach limb speeds during most sports activities. In baseball pitching, for example, where upper-limb extension velocity exceeds $2000° \cdot s^{-1}$ in professional pitchers even the relatively "slow" hip rotators move at $600° \cdot s^{-1}$ during a pitch.[24] Also, the present generation of isokinetic dynamometers cannot overload eccentric muscle actions that serve important limb deceleration and "braking" control functions in normal movements.

Plyometric Training

For sports that require powerful, propulsive movements—football, volleyball, sprinting, high jump, long jump, and basketball—athletes often apply a special form of exercise training termed **plyometrics**, or explosive jump training. Plyometric exercise requires various jumps in place or rebound jumping (drop jumping from a height) to mobilize the inherent stretch–recoil characteristics of skeletal muscle and its modulation via the stretch (myotatic) reflex.

Plyometric maneuvers avoid the disadvantage of having to decelerate a mass in the latter part of the joint ROM during a fast movement to achieve maximal power production. Figure 22.15 compares the traditional bench press movement to achieve maximal power output with a ballistic bench throw that attempts to maximize power output by projecting the barbell from the hands. The results were unequivocal. During the traditional bench press, deceleration begins at about 60% of the bar position relative to the total concentric movement distance *(purple line)*. In contrast, velocity during the bench throw *(yellow line)* continues to increase throughout the ROM and remains significantly higher at all bar positions after the movement begins. This translated into significantly greater average force, average power, and peak power outputs. Simultaneous monitoring of electromyographic (EMG) activity

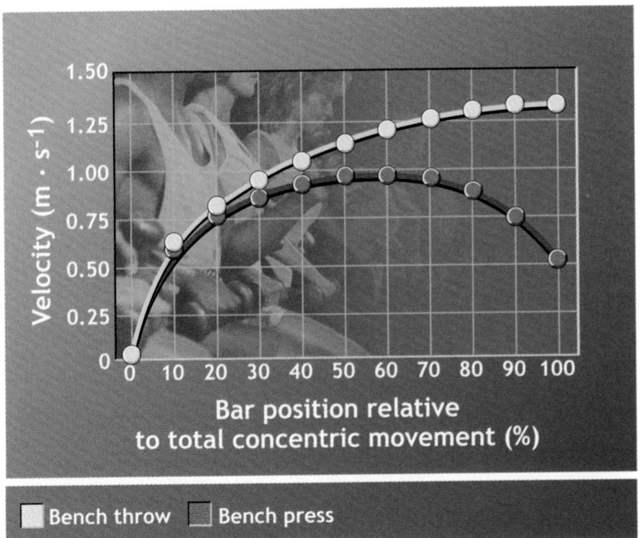

FIGURE 22.15 • Mean bar velocity in relation to total concentric bar movement for bench throw and traditional bench press performed as rapidly as possible. (Data from Newton RU, et al. Kinematics, kinetics, and muscle activation during explosive upper body movements. J Appl Biomech 1996;12:31.)

during the two conditions also showed greater muscle activity for the pectoralis major (+ 19%), anterior deltoid (+ 34%), triceps brachii (+ 44%), and biceps brachii (+ 27%) during the throw condition. Thus, achieving a faster average and peak velocity throughout the ROM produces greater power output and muscle activation (assessed by EMG) than the traditional weight-lifting exercise.

Allowing the athlete to develop greater power at the end of the movement more closely simulates the projection phase of throwing an object (ball or implement), maximal effort jumping movements, or impact in striking movements. In this form of training, called **ballistic resistance training**,[110] the athlete moves the weight or projectile as fast as possible while trying to produce maximal force before releasing it at the end of the movement. Sports performance examples include the shot put, overhead soccer throw, javelin and discuss throws, push off in the pole vault, takeoff jump for a volleyball spike, jumping for a basketball rebound, punching in boxing, and takeoff in the high jump.

Plyometric exercise overloads a muscle to provide forcible and rapid stretch (eccentric, or stretch, phase) immediately before the concentric or shortening phase of action. Like many sports situations, the rapid lengthening phase in the **stretch-shortening cycle** produces a more powerful subsequent movement largely because of two main factors:[41,203]

- Attainment of a higher active muscle state (greater potential energy) before the concentric, shortening action
- Stretch-induced evoking of segmental reflexes that potentiate subsequent muscle activation

These two effects form the basis for the alleged speed–power benefits of this training mode.[149,213,222,226] Figure 22.16 shows use of the sledge ergometer to (1) quantify force-generating capacity when affected by the stretch-shortening cycle, (2) train under such conditions, and (3) evaluate stretch reflex sensitivity and muscle stiffness under fatiguing exercise.

Practical Application of Plyometrics

A plyometric drill uses body mass and the force of gravity to provide the all-important rapid prestretch, or "cocking," phase to activate the muscle's natural elastic recoil elements. Prior stretch augments the subsequent concentric muscle action in the opposite direction. Forcibly dropping the arms to the side before vertical jumping produces an eccentric prestretch of the quadriceps muscle group and exemplifies a natural plyometric movement. Lower-body plyometric drills include a standing jump, multiple jumps, repetitive jumping in place, depth jumps or drop jumping from a height of about 1 m, single- and double-leg jumps, and various modifications. Proponents believe that repetitive plyometric actions provide neuromuscular training to enhance the power output of specific muscles and sport-specific power performances such as jumping.[79,116,149,225]

Testimonials abound about the benefits of plyometric training, but such pronouncements cannot substitute for the lack of carefully controlled evaluation of both benefits and possible orthopaedic risks of such workouts. Concern for musculoskeletal injury stems partly from the estimation that

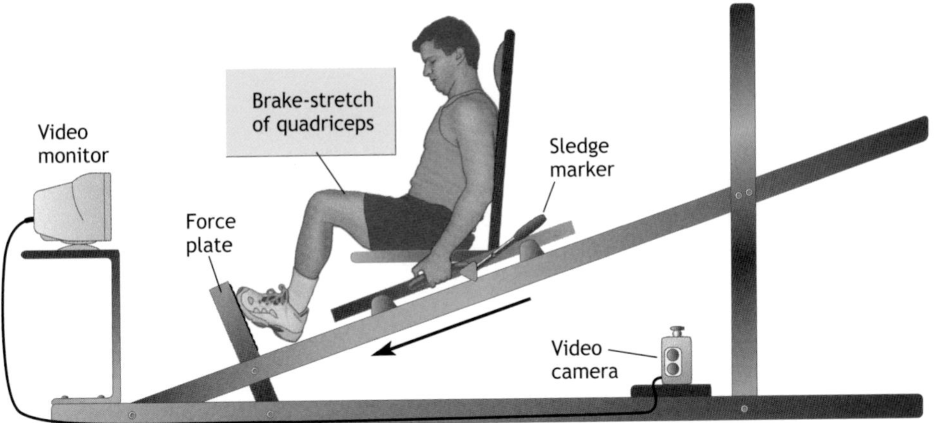

FIGURE 22.16 • The sledge ergometer for plyometric (stretch-shortening cycle) exercise and research protocols. Illustration shows braking phase (and subsequent muscle stretch) just prior to maximal activation of leg and foot extensor muscles. (Modified from Strojnik V, Komi PV. Fatigue after submaximal intensive stretch-shortening cycle exercise. Med Sci Sports Exerc 2000;32:1314.)

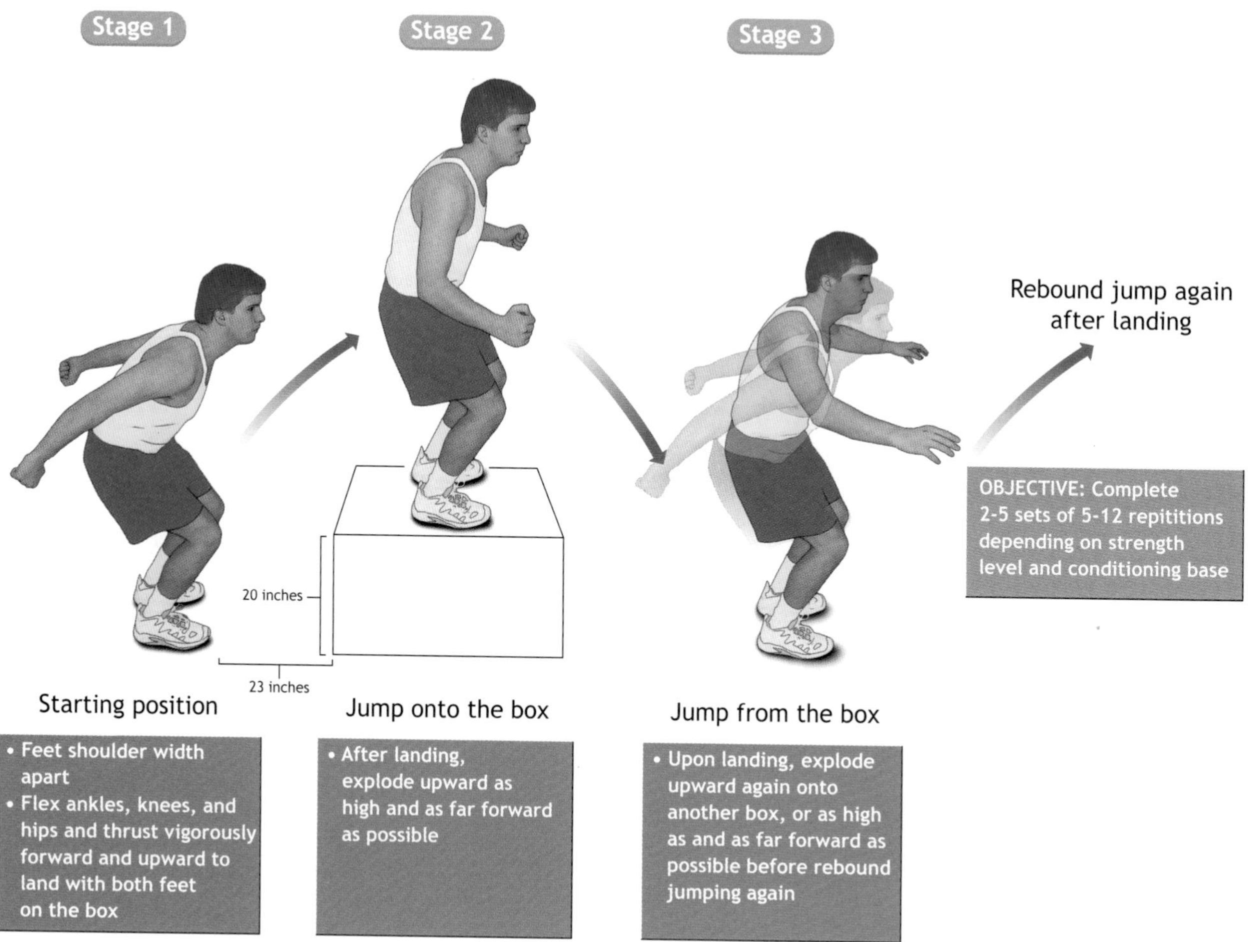

drop jumping generates external skeletal loads equal to up to 10 times body mass.[5] Research must quantify the appropriate role, if any, of plyometric drills in a complete strength–power training program. A position paper from the National Strength and Conditioning Association suggests that athletes achieve lifts of 1.5 times body weight in the squat exercise before initiating high-intensity plyometric training.[221] This practical guideline requires validation.

Figure 22.17 lists five components that contribute to the **window of explosive power development**. In this model, each component plays an important role in the contributions of the neuromuscular system to maximal power training. The window of adaptation opportunity shrinks for an athlete with already well-developed components, and expands for components in need of considerable improvement. For example, as an athlete approaches his or her high-velocity strength potential, that component's contribution to overall maximal power development diminishes. Thus, athletes should focus on training their least-developed components. Stated somewhat differently, maximal power performance improves more readily when the athlete targets specific training routines to improve the weakest links, because these have the largest adaptation window for augmenting explosive power development.

FIGURE 22.17 • Five components that contribute to explosive power development. Adapted with permission from Dr. William J. Kraemer, Human Performance Laboratory, Ball State University, Muncie, IN. (From Kraemer WJ, Newton RU. Training for muscular power. Phys Med Rehabil Clin 2000;11:341.)

PHYSICAL TESTING IN THE OCCUPATIONAL SETTING: THE ROLE OF SPECIFICITY

A comprehensive review outlines the development of physical tests and professionally and legally defensible validation strategies for preemployment occupational testing requiring diverse physical abilities or specific fitness characteristics.[94] The high specificity of components of physical performance and physiologic function (e.g., muscular strength and power, joint flexibility, aerobic fitness) combined with the specific nature of the training response casts serious doubt that broad *constructs* of physical fitness exist to any important extent. Clearly, no single measure of overall muscular strength or aerobic fitness exists. *Instead, an individual expresses an array of muscular strengths and powers and aerobic "fitnesses."* Often, these expressions of muscle function and performance relate poorly to each other, if at all. Likewise, testing a person for aerobic fitness can produce different fitness scores, depending on the activity. For example, it would not be desirable to administer the 12-minute run test in the occupational setting to infer aerobic capacity for firefighting or lumbering (both requiring significant upper-body aerobic function) or measuring static-grip or leg-strength tests to evaluate diverse dynamic strengths and powers required in these occupations.

Measurements applied in the occupational setting should most closely resemble the actual requirements of the job, not only for specific tasks but also in a manner that faithfully reflects the intensity, duration, and pace (i.e., physiologic demands) of the job. If such "content testing" remains impractical, one must substantiate alternative testing on the basis of carefully conducted validation studies.

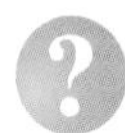

INTEGRATIVE QUESTION

Advise a candidate for a fire fighter's job about the most effective way to train for a physical test requiring 7 minutes of a series of job-related tasks (e.g., stair climb with equipment, hose drag, ladder raise, forcible entry with sledge hammer, simulated rescue dummy drag).

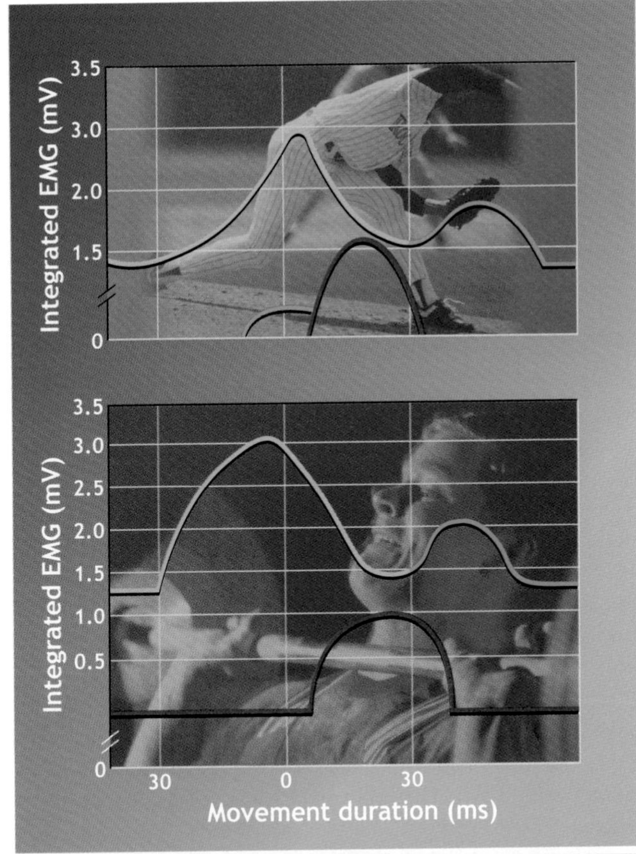

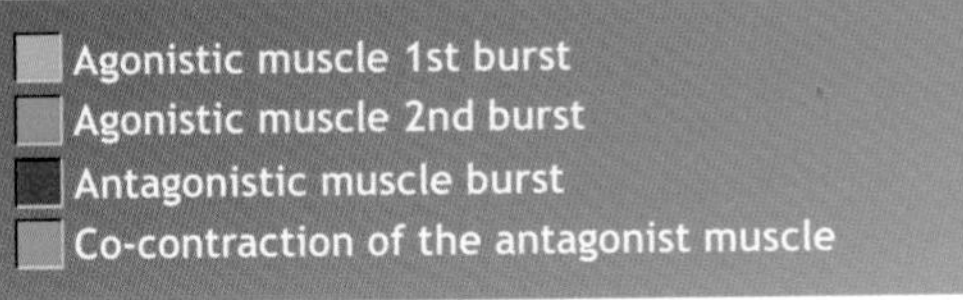

FIGURE 22.18 • Comparison of the triphasic EMG pattern during rapid elbow flexion in professional baseball pitchers and champion body builders. (Data courtesy of Dr. Pierre Lagasse, Human Motor Performance Research Laboratory, Laval University, Quebec City, Quebec, Canada.)

ELECTROMYOGRAPHY DURING MAXIMAL BALLISTIC MUSCLE ACTIONS

The electromyography (EMG) signal provides a convenient means to study intricacies of neuromuscular physiology during different muscle actions. EMG reflects both the quality and the quantity of electrical activity generated by muscle. In isometric actions, for example, the EMG signal changes in proportion to the muscle force generated. Dynamic actions reflect greater complexity because of the changing force–torque characteristics during the ROM. Rapid, ballistic movements produce an EMG characterized by alternating bursts of electrical activity in agonistic and antagonistic muscles. This produces a triphasic EMG pattern: the first burst of electrical activity occurs in the agonist, followed by signals from the antagonist (when the agonist remains electrically silent) and then another burst of agonist activity. Each phase of EMG activity relates to certain aspects of the movement pattern. The first agonist burst creates the propulsive force that initiates limb motion; the antagonist's first burst stops the limb, and the agonist's second burst produces the final limb positioning.

Our studies of professional baseball pitchers (Boston Red Sox) and champion body builders (Mr. Universe contestants) showed striking between-group differences in triphasic EMG patterns during maximal-speed, unloaded arm flexion. Figure 22.18 compares the integrated EMG signal in baseball pitchers and body builders during rapid arm flexion. For the 19 pitchers, the second burst of muscle electrical activity occurs sooner (probably a protective mechanism to slow the extremely fast limb speed), with less amplitude than for the body builders. For the 11 body builders, the first agonistic burst occurs rapidly, followed by a distinct delay before the antagonist fires. The difference in timing of electrical activity probably relates to training adaptations to distinct differences in limb acceleration patterns (baseball pitching vs. weight lifting) over many years of specific limb movement training.

EMG During Concentric Bidirectional Muscle Work

A series of experiments demonstrates the advantages of bidirectional (reciprocal) concentric muscle actions over conventional, unidirectional concentric actions. The research involved two exercise conditions with subjects seated in a device that permitted concentric-only muscle action: (1) maximal knee extension from a fully flexed right knee position or (2) maximal knee flexion from a fully extended knee position followed by extension to the original starting position. Subjects performed all actions at maximal speed. Figure 22.19 indicates maximal tension output (determined by strain gauge with simultaneous recordings of joint displacement) and integrated EMG from the vastus lateralis and vastus medialis during the two treatment conditions. Tension output increased significantly (11.4%) when maximal flexion preceded extension, as did quadriceps EMG activity (vastus medialis, 31.2%; vastus lateralis, 42.9%). Augmentation of tension output and greater EMG activity during concentric reciprocal work than with unidirectional, concentric-only work resulted from recruitment of more motor units. Facilitatory neuromuscular input from the muscle proprioceptors during the flexion phase of the reciprocal trial probably enhanced motor unit recruitment. If right and left limbs flex and then extend in alternating fashion, tension output and EMG activity of both limbs reaches higher levels than with single-limb activation, because of the facilitative influence of the double reciprocal muscle actions. **Quadruple neuromuscular facilitation** (**QNF**; a term suggested by Professor Pierre Lagasse, Human Motor Performance Research Laboratory, Laval University, Quebec City, Canada) describes such facilitatory effects during bidirectional, double concentric actions.[169]

Summary

1. Tensiometry, dynamometry, 1-RM testing with weights, and computer-assisted force and work-output determinations including isokinetic-type measurements are the most common methods of measuring muscular strength.
2. Human skeletal muscle generates a maximum force of about 30 N per cm^2 of muscle cross section, regardless of gender. On an absolute basis, men generally exert significantly greater maximal force than women.
3. The traditional method of evaluating gender differences in muscle strength creates a ratio score for strength (i.e., strength per unit body size [body mass, FFM, limb volume, girth]). When considering body size and/or composition in this manner, the large strength differences between men and women often decrease considerably. In some cases, women score higher than men.
4. Allometric scaling mathematically establishes a "proper" relationship between a body size variable (e.g., stature, body mass, FFM) and some other variable of interest, such as muscular strength or aerobic capacity. Allometry eliminates the confounding effects of factors inherently related to the variable in question. This often permits more meaningful comparisons among individuals who exhibit large differences in body size variables.
5. Optimal overload training to strengthen muscles involves three factors: (1) increasing resistance (load) to muscle action, (2) increasing the speed of muscle action, or (3) combining increased load and speed.

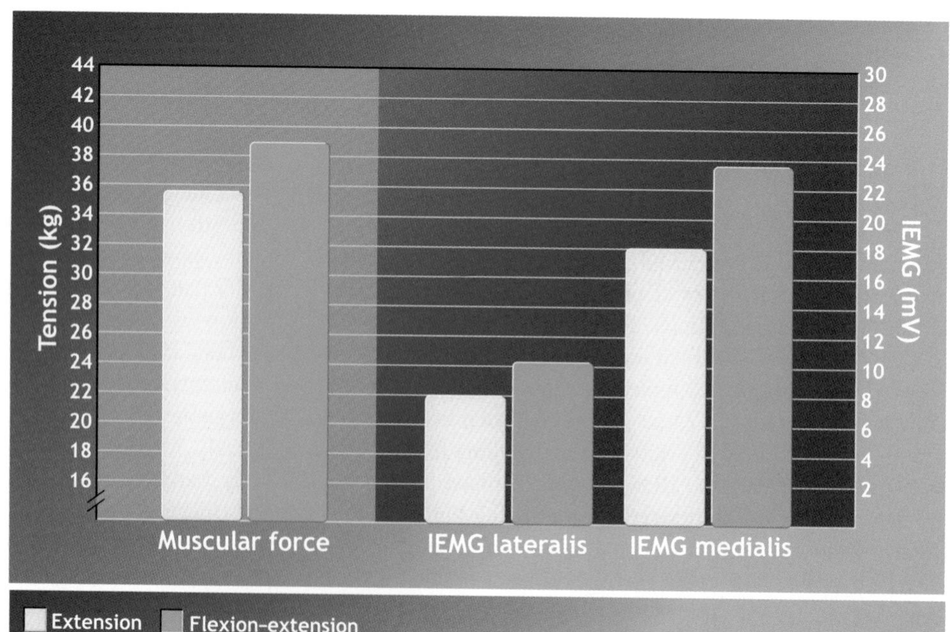

FIGURE 22.19 • Maximal knee extension force (kg) and integrated EMG (IEMG) activity in millivolts (mV) during (a) knee extension and (b) knee extension preceded by knee flexion. (From Lagasse P, et al. Neuromuscular facilitation of muscle tension output by reciprocal muscle work. Ann French-Can Assoc Adv Sci 1983;50:222.)

6. An overload between 60 and 80% of a muscle's force-generating capacity produces strength gains.
7. Progressive resistance weight training, isometrics, and isokinetic-type training are the three major strength-training systems. Each produces strength gains highly specific to the type of training. Isokinetic training offers a unique method for resistance training because of its potential to generate maximum force throughout the full ROM at different angular velocities of limb movement.
8. Closely supervised resistance training programs using relatively moderate concentric muscle actions significantly improve children's strength without adverse effects on bone, muscle, or connective tissue.
9. Periodization divides a distinct period of resistance training (macrocycle) into smaller training cycles called mesocycles; these, in turn, subdivide into weekly microcycles. Compartmentalization of training (emphasizing varied overload and sport/skill-specific neuromuscular requirements) attempts to minimize staleness and overtraining effects. It also varies the long-term training focus so that peak performance coincides with competition.
10. Resistance training for competitive athletes focuses on optimizing muscular strength, power, and hypertrophy. Training goals for middle-aged and older adults aim to modestly improve muscular strength and endurance, and maintain muscle and bone mass and enhance the overall health and fitness profile.
11. Concurrent training for muscular strength and aerobic capacity blunts the magnitude of strength improvement compared with training only for muscular strength.
12. Plyometric training drills use the inherent stretch–recoil characteristics of the neuromuscular system to facilitate muscle power development. Potential risks and benefits of such training await further research.
13. Specificity of physiologic and performance measures and their response to training casts doubt on the efficacy of general fitness measures to predict ability to perform specific tasks or occupations.
14. A triphasic EMG activity pattern characterizes rapid, ballistic limb movements. EMG patterns often differ among individuals, depending on prior athletic training and methods of strength acquisition.
15. Concentric, bidirectional muscle actions augment muscle force output and EMG activity compared with unilateral actions. This results from neuromuscular facilitation and subsequent recruitment of additional motor units with bidirectional actions.

PART 2 • Structural and Functional Adaptations to Resistance Training

Figure 22.20 lists six factors that affect the development and maintenance of muscle mass. Without a doubt, genetic factors provide the governing frame of reference that modulates each of the other factors for increasing muscle mass and strength. Muscular activity contributes little to tissue growth without appropriate nutrition to provide essential building blocks. Similarly, specific hormones and nervous system innervation provide crucial input for patterning the appropriate training response. Without tension overload, each of the other factors cannot effectively produce the desired training response.

FACTORS THAT MODIFY THE EXPRESSION OF HUMAN STRENGTH

Figure 22.21 shows that factors broadly characterized as psychologic (neural) and muscular influence the expression of human strength. A resistance-training program modifies many components of these factors, while others remain training resistant, probably determined by natural endowment or established early in life.

Psychologic–Neural Factors

Enhanced neural facilitation largely accounts for rapid and significant strength increases early in training, which often occur without an increase in muscle size and cross-

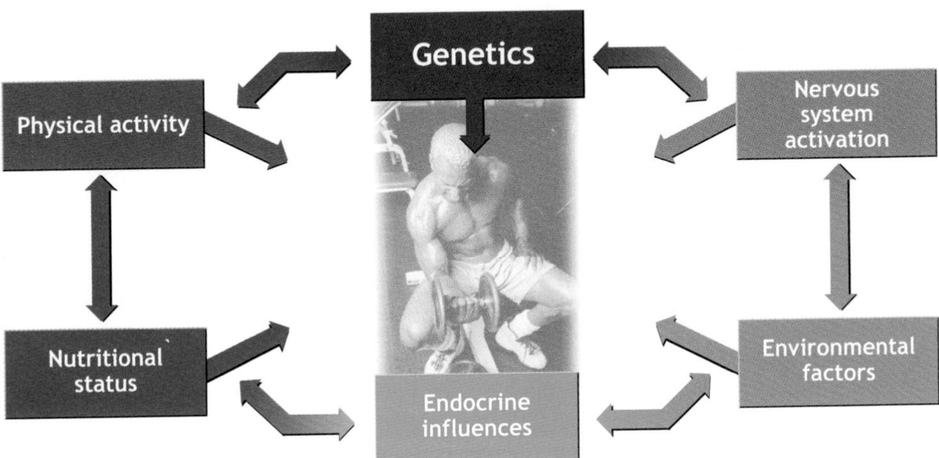

FIGURE 22.20 • Six factors that act and interact to affect development and maintenance of muscle mass.

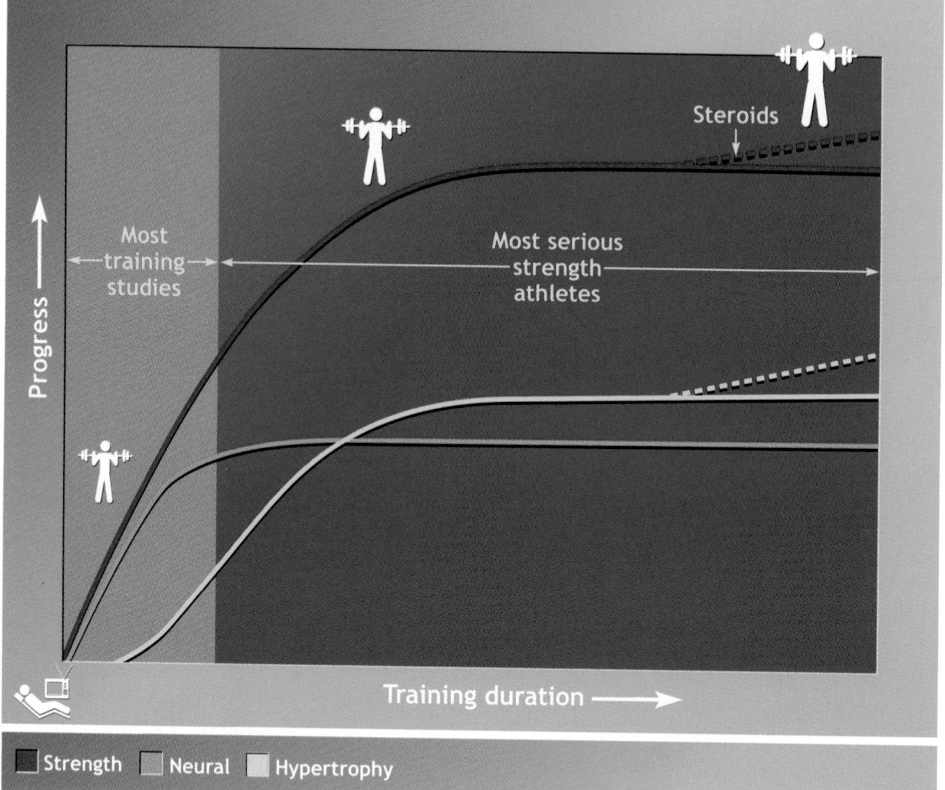

FIGURE 22.21 • Relative roles of neural and muscular adaptations in strength improvement with resistance training. Note that neural adaptations predominate in the early phase of training (this phase also encompasses most training studies). Hypertrophy-induced adaptations place the upper limit on longer-term training improvements. This tempts many athletes to use anabolic steroids and/or human growth hormone (dashed line) to induce continual hypertrophy if training alone fails. (From Sale DG. Neural adaptation to resistance training. Med Sci Sports Exerc 1988;20:135.)

sectional area.[115,146,166,189] Neural adaptations probably play a particularly important role in the rather dramatic muscular strength and power improvements of the elderly with resistance training compared with training-induced alterations in muscular hypertrophy.[74]

Figure 22.22 shows the general response curve for neural facilitation and muscle size increases during resistance training. Almost all of the relatively large strength improvements in the early phase of the program result from neural adaptations rather than from changes inherent to the muscle.

Neural adaptations with resistance training may result from influencing effects of the following:

- Greater efficiency in neural recruitment patterns
- Increased central nervous system activation
- Improved motor unit synchronization
- Lowering of neural inhibitory reflexes
- Inhibition of Golgi tendon organs

Research has considered the effects of exercise training on structural changes associated with the neuromuscular junction (NMJ). In one study with rats, endurance training improved the ratio of nerve terminal area to muscle fiber size by reducing fiber diameter without altering nerve terminal size.[211] In humans, high- and low-intensity training differentially affected the size of the NMJ.[47] Less-intense, prolonged workouts produced a more expansive NMJ area, whereas intense exercise produced greater dispersion of synapses. Further research must clarify the compensatory effects of exercise training on the structure and function of the NMJ.

A unique series of classic experiments illustrates the importance of psychologic factors in expressing human muscular strength.[92] The researchers measured arm strength in college-age men under normal conditions; immediately after a loud noise; while the subject screamed loudly at the time of exertion; under the influence of alcohol and amphetamines, or "pep pills"; and under hypnosis (told they possessed considerable strength and should not fear injury). Each of the alterations generally increased strength above normal levels; hypnosis, the most "mental" of all treatments, produced the greatest increments.

The investigators theorized that strength improvements under the various experimental treatments resulted from temporary modifications in central nervous system function. They argued that most people normally operate at a level of neural inhibition, perhaps via protective reflex mechanisms that prevent them from expressing their true strength capacity. This capacity results to a large degree from muscle cross section and fiber type and the mechanical arrangement of bone and muscle. Neuromuscular inhibition may derive from unpleasant past experiences with exercise, an overly protective home environment, or fear of injury. Regardless of the reason, the person usually cannot express maximum strength capacity. The excitement of intense competition or the influence of disinhibitory drugs or hypnotic suggestion often induces a "supermaximal" performance because of greatly reduced neural inhibition and optimal motoneuron recruitment.

Highly trained athletes often create an almost self-hypnotic state by concentrating intensely, or "psyching," before

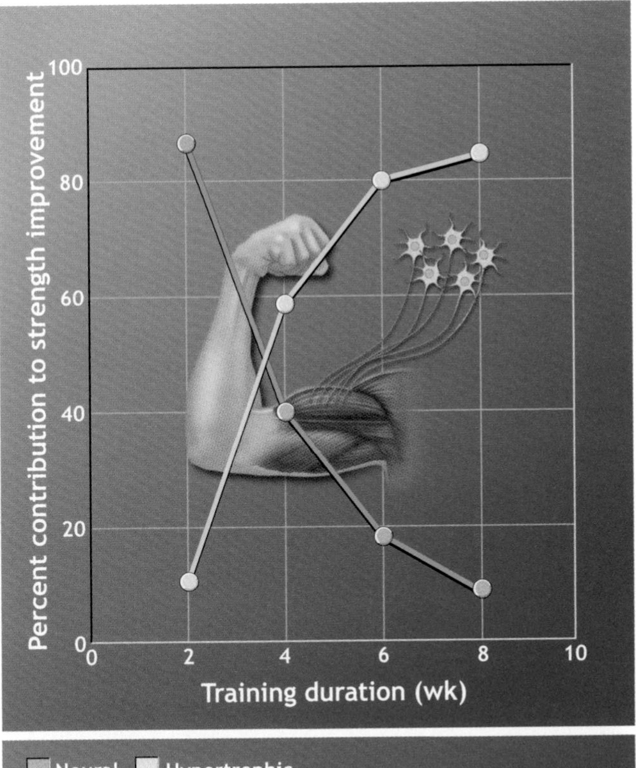

FIGURE 22.22 • Generalized response curve for showing gains in muscle strength with resistance training owing to neural (orange) versus muscular (yellow) factors. During a typical 8-week training period, approximately 90% of the strength gained over the first 2 weeks results from neural factors. In the subsequent 2 weeks, between 40 and 50% of the strength improvement still relates to nervous system adaptation. Thereafter, adaptations within the muscle fibers become progressively more important to strength improvement. Experiments of this type generally evaluate neural factors from integrated EMG recordings of the muscle groups trained.

competition. It sometimes takes years of training to perfect the "block out" of extraneous stimuli (e.g., crowd noise), so that the muscle action relates directly to the performance. This occurs particularly in power lifting competition, which demands precise, coordinated movements *with* maximal muscle tension output. Enhanced arousal level and accompanying neural disinhibition (or facilitation) could fully activate muscle groups. Increased neurologic arousal also may account for the so-called "unexplainable" feats of strength and power achieved during highly charged emergency situations.

Muscular Factors

Psychologic disinhibition and learning factors greatly modify muscle strength in the early phase of training, but ultimate strength capacity depends upon anatomic and physiologic factors within the joint–muscle unit. Table 22.4 lists physiologic and exercise performance changes associated with long-term resistance training. Most of these components show significant adaptations to training, with some modifications occurring within a few weeks.[189] Resistance training's effects on muscle fibers generally relate to adaptations in the contractile structures, which usually accompany substantial increases in muscular force and power through a given ROM. An inherent relationship exists between a muscle's power production and contraction speed. Figure 22.23 reveals that the knee extensor muscles generate approximately 60% of their maximum power at a movement speed of $100° \cdot s^{-1}$, with further power increases accompanying faster movement

TABLE 22.4 ➤ **PHYSIOLOGIC ADAPTATIONS TO RESISTANCE TRAINING**

SYSTEM/VARIABLE	RESPONSE
Muscle fibers	
Number	Equivocal
Size	Increase
Type	Unknown
Strength	Increase
Capillary density	
In body builders	No change
In power lifters	Decrease
Mitochondria	
Volume	Decrease
Density	Decrease
Twitch contraction time	Decrease
Enzymes	
Creatine phosphokinase	Increase
Myokinase	Increase
Enzymes of glycolysis	
Phosphofructokinase	Increase
Lactate dehydrogenase	No change
Aerobic metabolism enzymes	
Carbohydrate	Increase
Triglyceride	Not known
Basal metabolism	Increase
Intramuscular fuel stores	
Adenosine triphosphate	Increase
Phosphocreatine	Increase
Glycogen	Increase
Triglycerides	Not known
$\dot{V}O_{2max}$	
Circuit resistance training	Increase
Heavy resistance training	No change
Connective tissue	
Ligament strength	Increase
Tendon strength	Increase
Collagen content of muscle	No change
Body composition	
% fat	Decrease
Lean body mass	Increase
Bone	
Mineral content and density	Increase
Cross-sectional area	No change

Modified from Fleck SJ, Kramer WJ. Resistance training: physiological responses and adaptations (part 2 of 4). Phys Sportsmed, 1988;16:108.

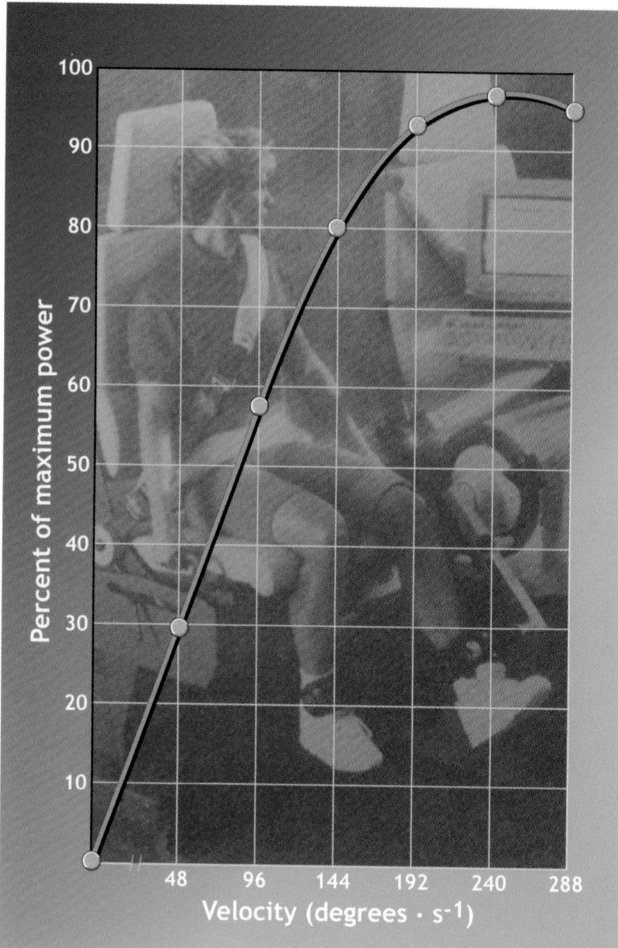

FIGURE 22.23 • Muscle power of knee extensors related to muscle contraction speed. (Data from Perrine JJ, Edgerton VR. Muscle force–velocity and power–velocity relationships under isokinetic loading. Med Sci Sports 1978;10:159.)

velocities. Work output (force × distance), in contrast to power output (force × distance ÷ time), declines as movement velocity (speed of contraction) increases.

Muscle Hypertrophy

*An increase in muscular tension (force) provides the primary stimulus to initiate skeletal muscle growth (**hypertrophy**) with exercise training*. Mechanical stress on the components of the muscular system triggers signaling proteins to activate the genes that stimulate protein synthesis. Accelerated protein synthesis that produces increases in muscle size during resistance training reflects a fundamental biologic adaptation to an increased workload regardless of gender and age.[28,30] As mentioned previously, improving muscular strength and power does not necessarily require muscle fiber hypertrophy because important neurologic factors significantly affect the expression of human strength. The later, slower-occurring strength improvements generally coincide with noticeable alterations in a muscle's subcellular molecular architecture.

Muscle growth with overload training results primarily when individual muscle fibers enlarge. The fast-twitch fibers of weight lifters, for example, average about 45% larger than those of healthy sedentary people and endurance athletes. The hypertrophic process couples directly to increased mononuclear number and synthesis of cellular components, particularly protein filaments that constitute the contractile elements.[138] Resistance exercise creates more efficient translation of mRNA that mediates the stimulation of myofibrillar protein synthesis.[217] Muscle growth can result from repeated muscle fiber injury (particularly with eccentric actions) followed by an overcompensation of protein synthesis to produce a net anabolic effect.[9] The cell's myofibrils thicken and increase in number, and accelerated protein synthesis and corresponding decreased protein breakdown forms additional sarcomeres. Intramuscular adenosine triphosphate (ATP), phosphocreatine (PCr), and glycogen also increase significantly.[127] Undoubtedly, these anaerobic energy stores contribute to the rapid rate of energy transfer required in resistance training. Body build characteristics also may explain individual differences in responsiveness to resistance training. The greatest increases in muscle mass occur for individuals with the largest relative FFM corrected for stature and body fat before training begins.[206]

Figure 22.24 shows the change in muscle fiber size that accompanies exercise-induced hypertrophy. Figure 22.24A compares exercised and nonexercised rat soleus muscle. The

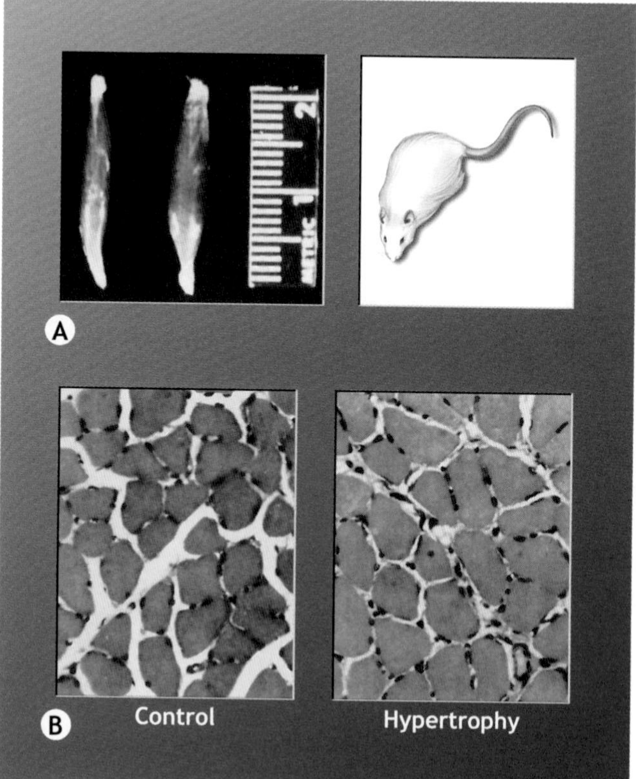

FIGURE 22.24 • **A.** Control (left) and hypertrophied (right) rat soleus muscle. **B.** Cross sections of control and hypertrophied muscles shown in A. The average diameter for 50 fibers of the hypertrophied muscle was 24 to 34% greater than that of controls; the average number of nuclei in the hypertrophied muscle was 40 to 52% greater than that of controls. (From Goldberg AL, et al. Mechanism of work-induced hypertrophy of skeletal muscle. Med Sci Sports 1975;3:185.)

hypertrophied exercised muscle appears on the *right*. Figure 22.24B represent typical cross sections of untrained and hypertrophied muscles. Hypertrophied muscle diameter averages 30% larger and the fibers contain 45% more nuclei, which increase relative to fiber size. These compensatory changes relate to marked increases in DNA synthesis and proliferation of connective tissue cells and small, mononucleated satellite cells located beneath the basement membrane adjacent to the muscle fibers.[66] Connective tissue cellular proliferation thickens and strengthens the muscle's connective tissue harness, improving the structural and functional integrity of tendons and ligaments (cartilage lacks sufficient circulation to stimulate growth).[205] Such adaptations protect joints and muscles from injury and justify resistance exercise in preventive and rehabilitative orthopaedic programs (see Focus on Research; Chapter 18).

Resistance-trained muscle fibers have increased total contractile protein and energy-generating compounds without parallel increases in capillarization, total volume of mitochondria, or mitochondrial enzymes.[175,197,200] Thus, the ratio of mitochondrial volume and/or enzyme concentration to myofibrillar (contractile protein) volume actually decreases. This training response would not hinder performance in strength and power activities because of the anaerobic nature of such efforts. It probably does, however, impede endurance in prolonged exercise by reducing the fiber's aerobic capacity per unit of muscle mass.

Significant Metabolic Adaptations Occur

Undoubtedly, success at elite levels of sport performance requires a particular muscle fiber distribution. The relatively fixed nature of muscle fiber type suggests an obvious genetic predisposition for exceptional performance. However, significant plasticity exists for metabolic potential, as specific training enhances the anaerobic and aerobic energy transfer capacity of both fiber types in men and women.[16] The heightened oxidative capacity of fast-twitch fibers with endurance training brings them to a level nearly equal to the aerobic capacity of the slow-twitch fibers of untrained counterparts.[97,98] *Age presents no barrier to training adaptations of muscle fibers.* With adequate training stimulus, skeletal muscles of older men and women adapt (fiber size, capillarization, glycolytic and respiratory enzymes) to both endurance and resistance training similar to younger persons.[36]

Endurance training induces some conversion of type IIb fibers to the more aerobic type IIa fibers.[36,223] The well-documented increase in mitochondrial size and number and a corresponding increase in total quantity of citric acid cycle and electron transport enzymes accompany these fiber subdivision changes.[84] Only specifically trained muscle fibers adapt to regular exercise; this explains why well-trained athletes who change to a sport requiring different muscle groups (or different portions of the same muscle) often feel untrained for the new activity. Within this framework, swimmers or canoeists (with well-developed upper-body musculature) do not necessarily transfer their upper body fitness to a running sport that relies predominantly on a highly conditioned lower-body musculature.

Table 22.5 summarizes changes in skeletal muscle with specific training modalities. Generally, physical activity recruits both fiber types; however, certain activities require activation of a much greater proportion of one fiber type than another.

Muscle Cell Remodeling: Current Thinking

Skeletal muscle represents dynamic tissue whose cells do not remain as fixed populations throughout life. Rather, muscle fibers undergo regeneration and remodeling in response to diverse functional demands (e.g., resistance or endurance training) to alter their phenotypic profile.[223] Activation of muscle via specific types and intensities of long-term use stimulates otherwise dormant myogenic stem cells (satellite cells) under a muscle fiber's basement membrane to proliferate and differentiate to form new fibers. Fusion of satellite cell nuclei and their incorporation into existing muscle fibers probably enables the fiber to synthesize more proteins to form additional myofibrils. This most likely contributes directly to muscular hypertrophy with chronic overload and may stimulate transformation of existing fibers from one type to another.

TABLE 22.5 ➤ EFFECTS OF SPECIFIC FORMS OF TRAINING ON SKELETAL MUSCLE

	SLOW-TWITCH FIBERS		FAST-TWITCH FIBERS	
	TYPE OF TRAINING			
MUSCLE FACTOR	STRENGTH	ENDURANCE	STRENGTH	ENDURANCE
Percentage composition	0 or ?	0 or ?	0 or ?	0 or ?
Size	+	0 or +	++	0
Contractile property	0	0	0	0
Oxidative capacity	0	++	0	+
Anaerobic capacity	? or +	0	? or +	0
Glycogen content	0	++	0	++
Fat oxidation	0	++	0	+
Capillary density	?	+	?	? or +
Blood flow during exercise	?	? or +	?	?

0, no change; ?, unknown; +, moderate increase; ++, large increase.

A variety of extracellular signal molecules, primarily peptide growth factors (e.g., insulin-like growth factor [IGF], fibroblast growth factors, transforming growth factors, and hepatocyte growth factor) govern satellite cell activity and possibly exercise-induced muscle fiber proliferation and differentiation. Figure 22.25 proposes a model for muscle cell remodeling involving satellite cell incorporation into an existing muscle fiber. A specific set of genes (gene A in the figure) is expressed in the fiber's preexisting nuclei. Chronic activation from physical activity, for example, stimulates satellite cell proliferation, with some cells differentiating and fusing (combining) with preexisting muscle fibers. These new muscle nuclei may alter gene expression (gene B in the figure) in the adapting muscle.

Studies with humans and animals support the concept that skeletal muscle adapts to altered functional demands. For example, arduous training can induce transformation in fiber type.[4,12] In one study, four athletes trained anaerobically for 11 weeks followed by 18 weeks of aerobic training. Anaerobic training increased the percentage of type IIc fibers and decreased the percentage of type I fibers; the opposite occurred during the aerobic training phase.[98] Similarly, 4 to 6 weeks of sprint training significantly increased the percentage of fast-twitch fibers, with a commensurate decrease in slow-twitch fiber percentage.[43,95] Increasing daily training duration also increases the fast- to slow-twitch shift in myosin heavy-chain phenotype in rat hindlimb muscles.[46] Such findings suggest that specific training (and perhaps inactivity) may convert type I to type II fibers (or vice versa).[180,198] Available evidence does not permit definitive statements concerning the fixed nature of a muscle's fiber composition. *More than likely, the genetic code exerts the greatest influence on fiber-type distribution.* The major direction of a muscle's fiber composition probably

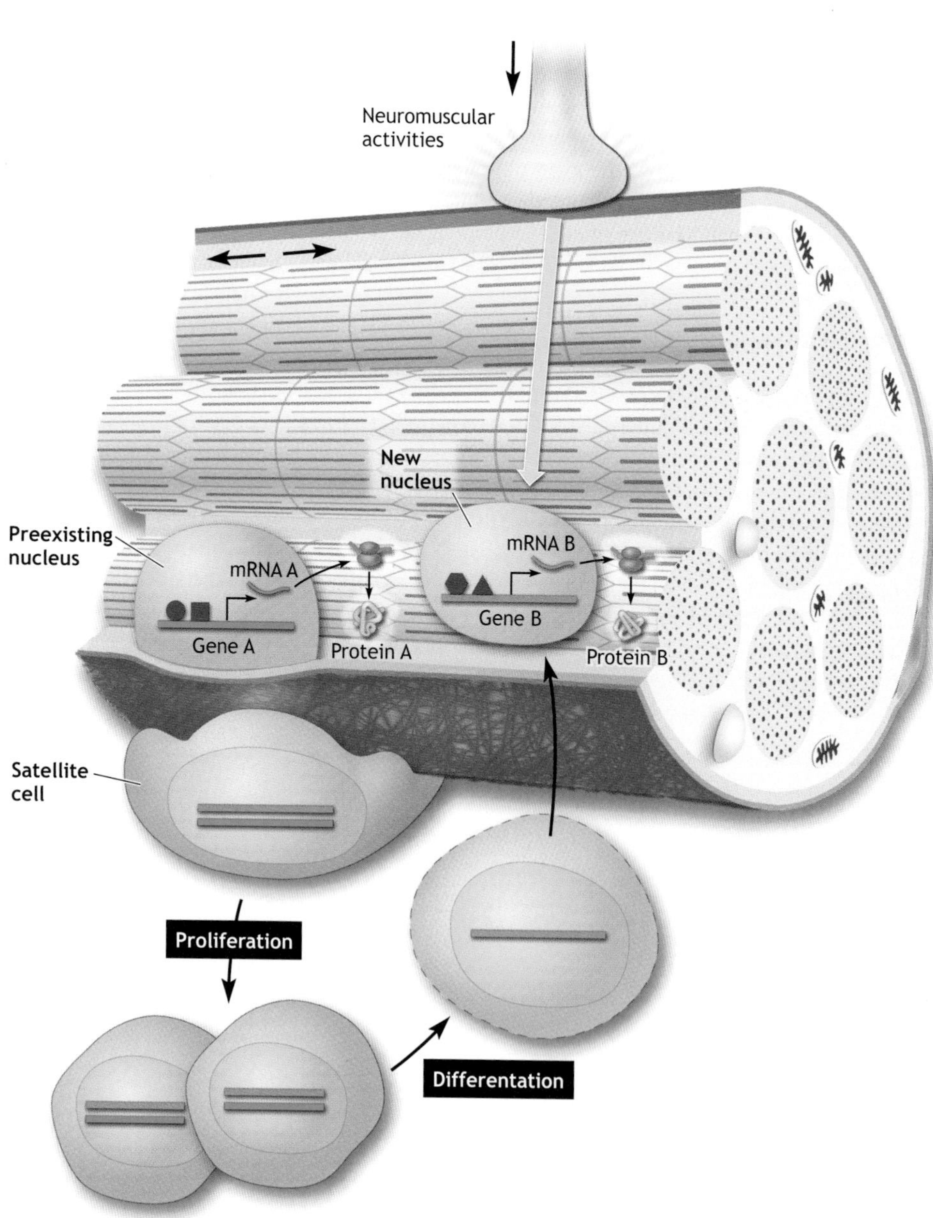

FIGURE 22.25 • A model for skeletal muscle adaptation involving satellite cells. A specific set of genes *(Gene A)* is expressed in the preexisting myonuclei. Upon stimulation from increased neuromuscular activity, for example, the satellite cells proliferate, and some of them differentiate and fuse with the preexisting myofibers. These myonuclei may alter gene expression *(Gene B)* in the adapting muscle because they have gone through an altered differentiation program under the influence of increased neuromuscular activities. (From Yan Z. Skeletal muscle adaptation and cell cycle regulation. Exerc Sport Sci Rev 2000;1:24.)

becomes fixed before birth or during the first few years of life. *The possibility does exist for some fiber-type transformation with specific chronic exercise training.*

The Elderly Respond

Women and men experience significant physiologic and performance adaptations to resistance training, independent of aging effects.[36,168,181,224] A study of five older healthy men (average, 68 y) clearly demonstrates the remarkable plasticity of human skeletal muscle among the elderly (Fig. 22.26). The men trained for 12 weeks using heavy-resistance, isokinetic, and free-weight exercises. Training increased muscle volume and cross-sectional area of the biceps brachii (13.9%) and brachialis (26.0%), while hypertrophy increased by 37.2% in the type II muscle fibers. Increases of 46.0% in peak torque and 28.6% in total work output accompanied these cellular adaptations.

Equally impressive training responses occur for older elderly persons. One hundred nursing home residents (average age 87.1 y) trained for 10 weeks with high-intensity resistance training.[58] For the 63 women and 37 men who participated, muscle strength increased an average of 113%. Strength increases also paralleled improved function, reflected by an 11.8% increase in normal gait velocity and 28.4% increase in stair-climbing speed; thigh muscle cross-sectional area increased by 2.7%.

Muscle Hyperplasia: Are New Muscle Fibers Made?

A common question concerns whether training increases the number of muscle cells (**hyperplasia**). If this does occur, to what extent does it contribute to muscle enlargement in humans? Chronic overload of skeletal muscle in various animal species develops new muscle fibers from **satellite cells** (cells between the basement layer and plasma membrane)[172] or by **longitudinal splitting**.[8,68] Under conditions of stress, neuromuscular disease, and muscle injury, the normally dormant satellite cells develop into new muscle fibers (see Fig. 22.25). With longitudinal splitting, a relatively large muscle fiber splits into two or more smaller, individual daughter cells through lateral budding. These fibers function more efficiently than the large single fiber from which they originated.[10]

Generalizing findings from research on animals to humans poses a problem. The massive cellular hypertrophy observed in humans with resistance training does not occur in many animal species. In cats, for example, muscle fiber proliferation (hyperplasia) often reflects the primary compensatory adjustment to overload. Some evidence supporting hyperplasia in humans does exist. For example, autopsy data from young, healthy men who died accidentally show that muscle fiber counts of the larger and stronger leg (leg opposite the dominant hand) contained 10% more muscle fibers than the smaller leg.[182] Cross-sectional studies of body builders with relatively large limb circumferences and muscle masses failed to show that they possessed above-normal-size individual muscle fibers.[128,129,199] The possibility exists

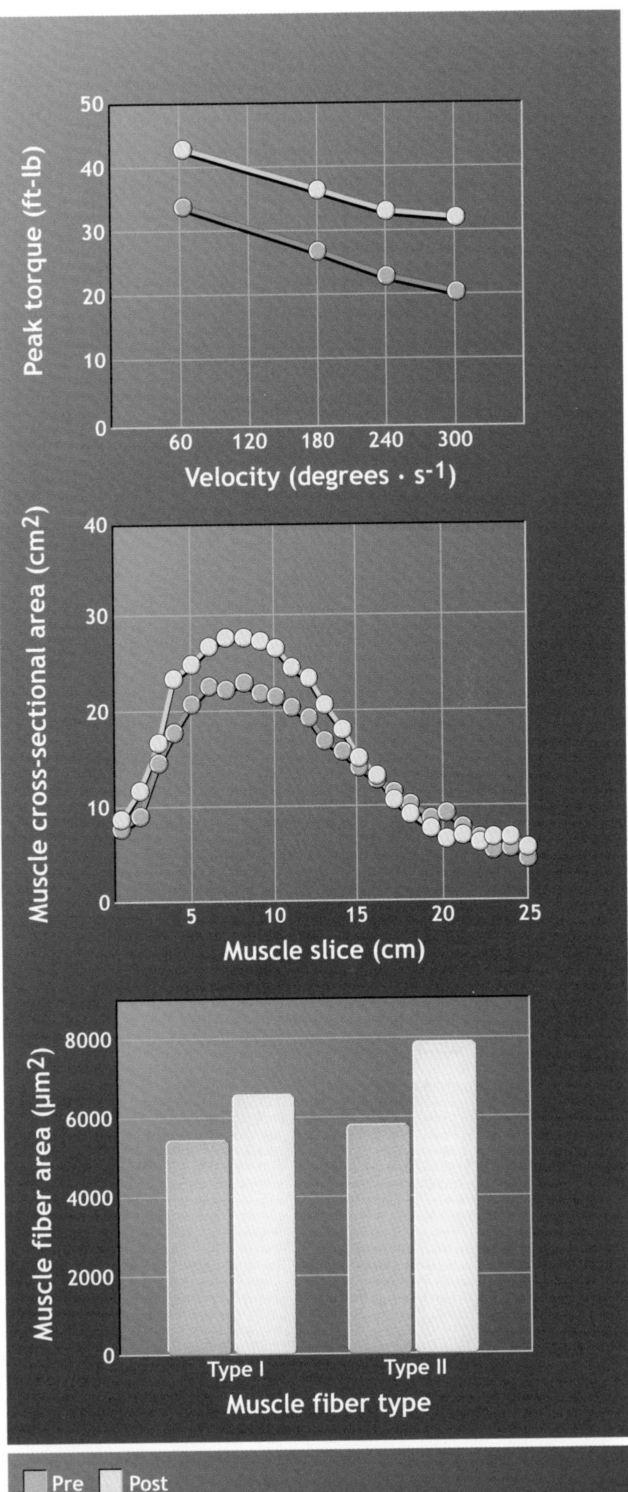

FIGURE 22.26 • The plasticity of aging muscle. Data from five men, approximately 68 years of age, before (orange) and after (yellow) 12 weeks of heavy-resistance training. *Top,* Peak torque of elbow flexors. *Middle,* Plot of flexor cross-sectional area computed from MRI scans from proximal *(right)* to distal *(left)* end of muscle. *Bottom,* Average for type I and type II fiber areas. (From Roman WJ, et al. Adaptations in the elbow flexors of elderly males after heavy-resistance training. J Appl Physiol 1993;74:750.)

that some of these body builders inherited an initially large number of small muscle fibers (that then "hypertrophy" to normal size with resistance training), yet the findings suggest the likelihood of hyperplasia with certain forms of resistance training. Muscle fibers may adapt differently to the high-volume, high-intensity training used by body builders than to the typical low-repetition, heavy-load system favored by strength and power athletes. *Even if other human studies replicate a training-induced hyperplasia (and even if the response reflects a positive adjustment), enlargement of existing individual muscle fibers represents the greatest contribution to increases in muscle size from overload training.*

Changes in Muscle Fiber-Type Composition

Research has evaluated the effects of 8 weeks of resistance exercise on muscle fiber size and fiber composition for the leg extensor muscles of 14 men who performed three sets of 6-RM leg squats three times weekly.[201] Biopsy specimens from the vastus lateralis muscle before and after training showed *no change* in percentage distribution of fast- and slow-twitch muscle fibers (indicated by the activity level of myofibrillar ATPase) with resistance training. This finding agreed with previous short-term studies using both resistance and endurance-type training; perhaps several months of resistance training in adults does not alter the basic fiber composition of skeletal muscle.[67] It remains unclear whether specific training early in life or for the prolonged periods engaged in by Olympic-caliber athletes alters a muscle fiber's inherent twitch (speed of shortening) characteristics. Some progressive fiber-type transformation may occur with prolonged, specific training (see Chapter 18). However, the current belief is that genetic factors largely determine one's predominant muscle fiber distribution.

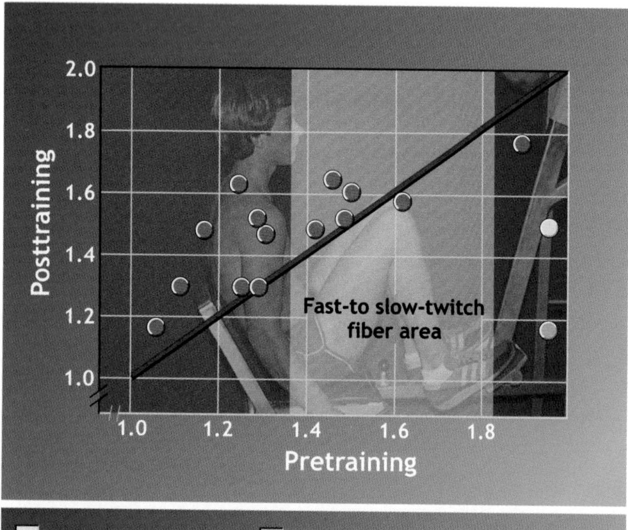

FIGURE 22.27 • Individual changes for 14 men in the ratio of fast- to slow-twitch muscle fiber area after 8 weeks of resistance training. *Orange circle on right* indicates average pretraining FT:ST area ratio; *yellow circle* represents the posttraining average. (From Thorstensson A. Muscle strength, fiber types, and enzyme activities in man. Acta Physiol Scand Suppl 1976:443.)

Metabolic characteristics of specific fibers and fiber subdivisions undergo modification within 4 to 8 weeks of resistance training. This occurs despite the lack of dramatic changes in inherent muscle fiber type with chronic exercise. A decrease in the percentage of type IIb and a corresponding increase in type IIa fibers denotes one of the more prominent and rapid training adaptations.[2,78,189] Furthermore, in the resistance training experiment described in the beginning of this section, the volume of fast-twitch fibers in the leg extensor muscles increased significantly.[201] Figure 22.27 clearly illustrates this increase for the relative areas of the fast- and slow-twitch muscle fibers before and after training. Significant hypertrophy, predominantly of the fast-twitch fibers, occurs mainly in power and Olympic-type lifters who have trained diligently over many years using progressive resistance training.[198,200] This makes sense within the framework of exercise specificity because near-maximal, high-resistance exercise requiring high levels of anaerobic power primarily recruits fast-twitch motor units.

Neuromuscular Factors

Previous sections have presented evidence that neural factors contribute importantly to muscular strength expression. The mechanism for changes in neuromuscular control with resistance training remains unclear. One study focused on strength training's effects on neuromuscular patterning. Sedentary men and women engaged in slow-speed, isokinetic training to determine its effect on the latencies and amplitudes of the muscle (M) response and patellar tendon (T) reflex as torque output improved. Percussion of the patellar tendon elicited the T reflex assessed by EMG surface electrodes over the vastus medialis. Stimulating the femoral nerve with 1-ms pulses at 0.2-Hz evaluated the M response. Subjects trained at an angular velocity of $90° \cdot s^{-1}$ with two sets of 15 concentric knee extensions 5 days per week for 10 weeks. Figure 22.28A displays improvements in peak torque output at three movement velocities (90°, 120°, and $180° \cdot s^{-1}$). Improvement ranged from 48 to 54% for men and 67 to 70% for women; values remained unchanged for a nontraining control group. Figure 22.28B shows that training did not alter T-reflex latencies for men and women. However, M-response latencies decreased significantly for all subjects, while M-response amplitude increased approximately twofold. The researchers attributed the neural and muscular changes with increased maximal torque to (1) enhanced α-motoneuron excitability (which facilitated motor unit recruitment) and (2) improved elastic properties of the specifically trained muscles.

The complexity of the exercise task also determines the time course of neural adaptation. Relatively simple muscle actions, (e.g., biceps curl) compared with more-complex maneuvers (e.g., leg press), show the most rapid neural adaptations in the early portion of training followed by strength increases that parallel muscle hypertrophy as training progresses. The more-complex multiple-joint, multiple-muscle actions require more time for neuromuscular adaptations.[32]

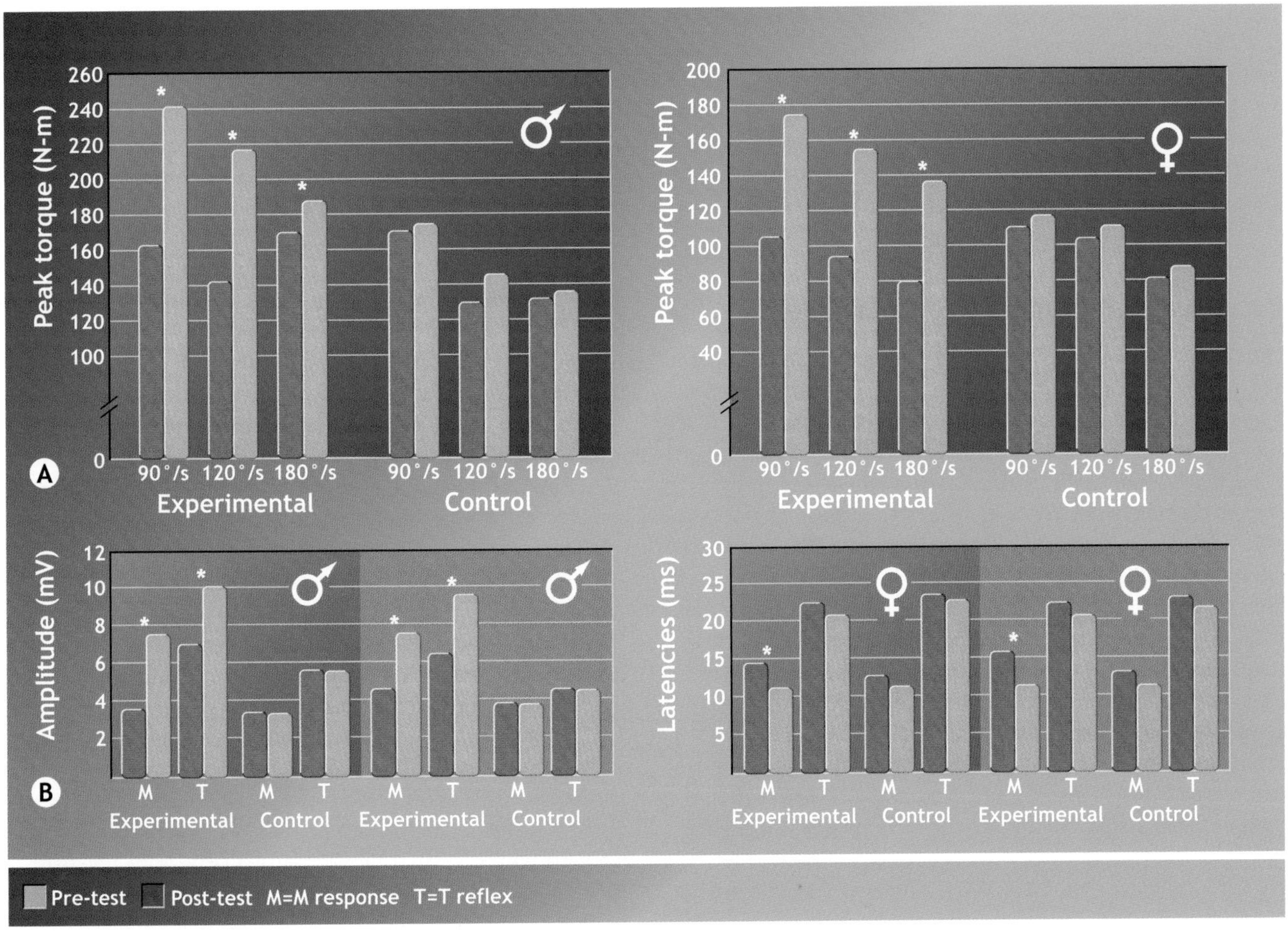

FIGURE 22.28 • Effects of slow-speed resistance training on neuromuscular factors in men and women. **A.** Changes in peak torque *(N-m)* measured concentrically at three movement velocities. **B.** Changes in vastus medialis *(M)* amplitude and latency response and patellar tendon *(T)* reflex. The *stars* indicate significant differences between pre- and posttraining values. (From Roy MA, et al. Changes in alphamotoneuron excitability following isokinetic training in sedentary males and females. Can J Appl Sport Sci 1984;9:20P.)

COMPARATIVE TRAINING RESPONSES IN MEN AND WOMEN

In today's society, women participate successfully in all sports and physical activities. Women had generally not used resistance training so as to avoid developing overly enlarged muscles similar to those of men. This hesitation was unfortunate because performance in activities like tennis, golf, skiing, dance, and gymnastics, including physically demanding occupations such as firefighting and heavy construction work, benefit from specific strength acquisition. The question often arises whether muscular strength acquisition differs between men and women, and if it does, what factors might be responsible?

INTEGRATIVE QUESTION

If women respond to resistance training essentially the same way as men, why doesn't the upper-arm girth of female body builders equal that of male body builders?

Muscular Strength and Hypertrophy

The amount of absolute muscle hypertrophy with resistance training represents a primary gender difference. Variation in hypertrophic response probably results from gender-specific differences in hormonal levels that exert strong anabolic effects, particularly the average 20- to 30-times higher testosterone levels in men.[111] Importantly, testosterone levels exist along a continuum; some women normally possess concentrations as high or higher than in men.[114]

Computed axial tomograph (CAT) scans for direct evaluation of muscle cross-sectional area show that men and women respond similarly in hypertrophic response to resistance training. Without doubt, men experience a greater absolute change in muscle size because of their larger initial muscle mass, but muscular enlargement on a percentage basis remains similar between genders.[42,155] Comparisons between elite male and female body builders also indicate substantial muscular hypertrophy in females with many years of resistance training.[187,188]

The limited data from relatively short-duration training studies suggest that women can use conventional resistance training exercise without developing overly large muscles. Gender-related differences in hormonal response to resistance exercise (e.g., increased testosterone and decreased cortisol for men) may determine any ultimate gender differences in muscle size and strength adaptations with prolonged training.[112,224] This intriguing area requires longitudinal research for a fuller description of gender differences in skeletal muscle's response to resistance training.

Does Muscle Strength Relate to Bone Density?

Laboratory experiments document differences in maximum flexion and extension dynamic strength in postmenopausal women with and without osteoporosis, defined as bone mineral density (BMD) greater than 1 standard deviation below age-adjusted norms.[96,191] Muscle strength assessed by hydraulic dynamometry represented a 5-RM bench press, a lat pull, and knee and shoulder flexion and extension concentric muscle actions at three velocities. Figure 22.29 shows chest flexion and extension strength in normal and osteoporotic women. Unequivocal results emerged; women with normal BMD (measured by dual-photon absorptiometry in the lumbar spine and femur neck) exhibited 20% greater strength in 11 of 12 test comparisons for flexion; 4 of 12 comparisons for extension showed 13% higher strength values for women with normal bone density. Quite possibly, differences in maximum dynamic strength among postmenopausal women may

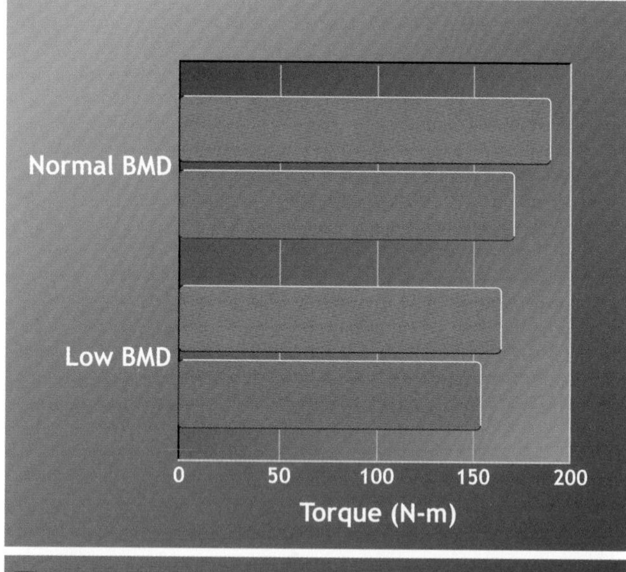

FIGURE 22.29 • Comparison of chest press extension and flexion strength in age- and weight-matched postmenopausal women with normal and low bone mineral density (BMD). Women with low BMD scored significantly lower on each measure of muscular strength than the reference group. (From Stock JL, et al. Dynamic muscle strength is decreased in postmenopausal women with low bone density. J Bone Miner Res 1987;2:338; Janey C, et al. Maximum muscular strength differs in postmenopausal women with and without osteoporosis. Med Sci Sports Exerc 1987;19:S61.)

serve a clinically useful role in screening for osteoporosis. Subsequent data complement these findings; they indicate that regional lean tissue mass (often an indication of muscular strength) also accurately predicts bone mineral density.[150]

Women with a higher risk for osteoporosis or those with existing osteoporosis can attenuate their *factor of risk* (ratio of the load on the spine to the bone's failure load) for fracture by (1) strengthening the bone by maintaining or increasing bone density and (2) lowering the magnitude of spinal forces by avoiding risky activities that increase spinal compression (e.g., lifting activities).[145] Postmenopausal women who performed 50 heel drops (rising up on the toes and then letting their body weight drop to the floor, with knees and hips extended) daily for 1 year did not increase BMD at three sites on the proximal femur, the lateral spine (L2-3), and two sites on the radius. In women more than 6 years postmenopausal, the drop exercise maintained BMD.[15]

DETRAINING

Limited data document muscle strength decrements and associated factors with cessation of resistance training. Discontinuing training for 2 weeks caused male power lifters to lose 12% of their isokinetic eccentric muscle strength and 6.4% of their type II muscle fiber area. No type I fiber area was lost.[87] Discontinuing a short period of resistance training in previously sedentary men caused loss of improved muscular strength within several weeks, most likely from reversal of training-induced neuromuscular and hormonal adaptations.[37] Encouraging news indicates that reducing training frequency to only one or two weekly sessions provides sufficient stimulus to maintain training-induced strength gains.[69]

METABOLIC STRESS OF RESISTANCE TRAINING

Traditional resistance training methods provide only minimal stimulus to improve cardiovascular fitness or reduce body fat and exert little effect on the blood-lipid profile and other heart disease risk factors.[109] For example, a program of high-intensity, variable-resistance (Nautilus) strength training produces no improvement in $\dot{V}O_{2max}$ or submaximal exercise heart rate and stroke volume,[90] although intense resistance-exercise training may cause a small blood volume increase.[139] Lack of cardiovascular improvement probably results from the relatively low "whole body" metabolic and circulatory demands of standard resistance training. Data from young men during maximal isometric and 8- to 10-RM weight-lifting exercises indicate that such activity elicits only light-to-moderate heart rate response (generally less than 130 $b \cdot min^{-1}$) and oxygen consumption (3 to 4 METs).[135]

Undoubtedly, resistance training places considerable localized stress on specific muscles. The brief activation period and relatively small muscle mass usually engaged creates lower heart rate and aerobic metabolic demands than dynamic big-muscle activities (e.g., running, hiking, climbing, swimming, cycling). A person may spend an hour or more completing a strength-training workout, yet the total time devoted to exercising does not usually exceed 8 minutes per hour! Clearly, traditional resistance-training workouts should not constitute the major portion of a program designed for cardiovascular improvement and weight control.

CIRCUIT RESISTANCE TRAINING

Modifying the traditional approach to resistance training increases the caloric cost of exercise to improve several important fitness aspects. The approach, **circuit resistance training (CRT)**, deemphasizes the brief intervals of heavy, local-muscle overload in standard resistance training. It provides a more general conditioning that improves body composition, muscular strength and endurance, and cardiovascular fitness.[13,73,102] With CRT, a person lifts a weight between 40 and 55% of 1-RM as many times as possible with good form for 30 seconds. After a 15-second rest, the participant moves to the next resistance exercise station and so on to complete the circuit, usually composed of 8 to 15 different exercises. A modification that produces similar CRT energy expenditure uses exercise:rest ratios of 1:1, with either 15- or 30-second exercise periods.[14] The circuit, repeated several times, allows for 30 to 50 minutes of continuous exercise, not just the 6 to 8 minutes of the traditional workout. As strength increases, a new 1-RM determined for each exercise provides the basis for increasing resistance.

The CRT modification of standard resistance training offers an attractive alternative for those desiring a more general conditioning program. Medically supervised CRT programs effectively train coronary-prone, cardiac, and spinal-cord-injured patients who desire a well-rounded fitness program.[105,185] CRT also provides supplemental off-season conditioning for sports requiring high levels of strength, power, and muscular endurance.

Specificity of Aerobic Improvement

Some research indicates that CRT produces nearly 50% less aerobic fitness improvement than bicycle or run training.[65] Importantly, CRT usually involves substantial upper-body exercise, but assessment of aerobic benefits from this training used treadmill or bicycle tests that predominantly activate lower-body musculature. To remove this limitation, one study assessed CRT effects on aerobic capacity with both treadmill running and arm-crank ergometry tests.[76] Aerobic capacity increased 7.8% with treadmill testing *and* 21.1% with arm-crank testing, confirming the training specificity principle. These findings take on added significance because they occurred without negative effects in a group of borderline hypertensives. The program also significantly increased muscular strength, decreased blood pressure, and modestly improved body composition.

Specificity of Hypertrophic Response

During the course of resistance training, one should not assume that a single exercise creates uniform strength improvement or hypertrophic response in the muscle(s) activated.[8] Biceps curls performed at close to 1-RM do *not* produce equal strength gains from the muscle's origin to its insertion. If they did, then the maximal force-generating capacity of the muscle would show similar percentage improvements throughout its ROM. This, however, does not occur. Similarly, electrical activity measured by surface or needle EMG or MRI to assess a muscle's cross-sectional area does not show a homogeneous response within the entire muscle during maximal activation.[21,142,174] Furthermore, the fact that a single muscle compartmentalizes into distinct regions[123] indicates that the muscle's different areas can respond differentially to the imposed stress.[52] In essence, this means that skeletal muscle remodels its internal architecture, potentially reconfiguring external orientation and hence its shape with specific resistance exercises. The overall lack of homogeneity in skeletal muscle's response to overload, coupled with intramuscular differences in fiber type and composition, probably governs the training adaptation to specific resistance exercise. The nonuniformity in response of skeletal muscle to overload training also occurs in animal models with considerable molecular differentiation.[85,170,186]

Energy Cost of Different Resistance-Exercise Methods

Table 22.6 displays energy expenditures for exercise performed using free weights, Nautilus (eccentric), Universal Gym (concentric/eccentric), Cybex (isokinetic), and Hydra-Fitness (hydraulic-concentric). Energy expenditure for hydraulic exercises averaged 9.0 kcal · min^{-1} (37.7 kJ); this averaged 35% higher than exercise with free weights, 29.4% higher than Nautilus exercise, and 11.5% more than CRT using Universal Gym equipment. The energy expenditure values for hydraulic exercise averaged about 6.4% less than slow- and fast-speed isokinetic circuit exercise. For comparison, the table gives the energy expenditure for walking at a normal pace on a level surface.

TABLE 22.6 ➤ ENERGY EXPENDITURE FOR DIFFERENT MODES OF RESISTANCE EXERCISE COMPARED TO WALKING[a]

Mode	Sex	kJ · min^{-1}	kcal · min^{-1}
Nautilus, circuit	M	29.7	7.1
	F	24.3	5.8
Nautilus, circuit	M	22.6	5.4
Universal, circuit	M	33.1	7.9
	F	28.5	6.8
Isokinetic, slow	M	40.2	9.6
Isokinetic, fast	M	41.4	9.9
Isometric and free-weight	M	25.1	6.0
Hydra-Fitness, circuit	M	37.7	9.0
Walking on level	M	22.6	5.4

[a]Based on a body weight of 68 kg.
Data from Katch FI, et al. Evaluation of acute cardiorespiratory responses to hydraulic resistance exercise. Med Sci Sports Exerc, 1985;17:168.

MUSCLE SORENESS AND STIFFNESS

Following an extended layoff from exercise, most people experience soreness and stiffness in the exercised joints and muscles. Temporary soreness may persist for several hours immediately after unaccustomed exercise, whereas a residual **delayed-onset muscle soreness (DOMS)** appears later and can last for 3 or 4 days. Any one of the following factors may produce DOMS:

- Minute tears in muscle tissue or damage to its contractile components with accompanying release of creatine kinase (CK), myoglobin (Mb), and troponin I, the muscle-specific marker of muscle fiber damage
- Osmotic pressure changes that cause fluid retention in the surrounding tissues
- Muscle spasms
- Overstretching and perhaps tearing of portions of the muscle's connective tissue harness
- Acute inflammation
- Alteration in the cell's mechanism for calcium regulation
- Combination of the above factors

Eccentric Actions Produce Muscle Soreness

The precise cause of muscle soreness remains unknown, although the degree of discomfort and muscle disturbance depends largely on the intensity and duration of effort and type of exercise performed.[50,91,162] The magnitude of active strain imposed on a muscle fiber (rather than absolute force) precipitates muscle damage and resulting soreness.[122] *Eccentric, and to some extent isometric, muscle actions generally trigger the greatest postexercise discomfort, magnified among older individuals.*[184,190,195,212] Existing muscle damage or soreness from previous exercise does not exacerbate subsequent muscle damage or impair the repair process.[152]

In one study, subjects rated muscle soreness immediately after exercise and 24, 48, and 72 hours later. Greater soreness resulted from exercise involving repeated intense strain during active lengthening in eccentric actions than from concentric and isometric actions. Soreness did not relate to lactate buildup because high-intensity, level running (concentric actions) produced no residual soreness despite significant elevations in blood lactate. In contrast, downhill running (eccentric actions) caused moderate-to-severe DOMS without lactate elevation during exercise.

Table 22.7 highlights muscle soreness and CK activity following an exercise circuit of either concentric-only or concentric and eccentric muscle actions. Group 1 performed three sets of eight exercises (concentric–eccentric) at 60% of 1-RM on Universal Gym equipment: one set equaled 20 seconds of exercise followed by 40 seconds of rest; total exercise time was 24 minutes. Group 2 followed the same exercise protocol, but they exercised maximally for each repetition on hydraulic resistance devices (Hydra-Fitness) that used concentric-only actions. Blood samples and ratings of perceived muscle soreness took place before exercise and 5, 10, and 25 hours after exercise.

TABLE 22.7 ➤ ACUTE EFFECTS OF CONCENTRIC-ONLY AND CONCENTRIC–ECCENTRIC EXERCISE ON DOMS 25 HOURS AFTER EXERCISE[a]

	Soreness Ratings			Soreness Ratings	
Site	Concentric $\bar{X}$	Concentric–Eccentric $\bar{X}$	Site	Concentric $\bar{X}$	Concentric–Eccentric $\bar{X}$
Chest	2.3	5.1	Forearm (front)	1.7	3.4
Back (upper)	2.6	2.8	Forearm (back)	1.7	2.9
Shoulders (front)	2.2	3.6	Back (lower)	1.7	2.9
Shoulders (back)	1.9	3.6	Buttocks	1.8	2.5
Biceps (mid)	1.9	4.3	Quads (mid)	2.0	4.1
Biceps (lower)	1.8	3.5	Quads (lower)	2.1	3.8
Triceps (mid)	1.9	3.4	Hamstrings (mid)	2.1	3.5
Triceps (lower)	1.9	3.0	Hamstrings (lower)	2.1	3.0

		CK Activity ($mU \cdot mL^{-1}$)	
Sample Time		Concentric $\bar{X}$	Concentric–Eccentric $\bar{X}$
Pre		86.7	126.9
5 h post		344.8	232.0
10 h post		394.3	368.5
25 h post		288.0	482.2
	Absolute increase	319.3	399.9
	Relative increase	435.6	355.4

[a]All differences between groups were statistically significant.
From Byrnes WC. Muscle soreness following resistance exercise with and without eccentric muscle actions. Res Q Exer Sport 1985;56:283.

The major difference in soreness ratings between exercise groups occurred 25 hours postexercise; the concentric–eccentric workout produced significantly higher perceived ratings of soreness for the major muscle groups exercised. The magnitude of the increase in serum CK remained the same between groups from 5 to 25 hours postexercise. Both modes of exercise elevated serum CK, but the concentric-only muscle actions did not cause DOMS.

Cell Damage

Running downhill at a 10° slope for 30 minutes produced significant DOMS 42 hours after exercise.[23] Corresponding increases also occurred in serum levels of Mb and the muscle-specific enzyme CK, both common markers of muscle injury. Acute inflammation also causes greater mobilization of leukocytes and neutrophils.[162] Subject testing also took place after 3, 6, and 9 weeks. Figure 22.30 shows the perceived soreness rating for the leg muscles in relation to elapsed post-exercise time for the three study durations. For the 3- and 6-week comparisons, differences between exercise bouts reached statistical significance, with diminished DOMS noted in the second trial *(orange)*. Similar patterns emerged for perception of muscle soreness and CK and Mb levels. Interestingly, peak soreness ratings at 48 hours did not relate to absolute or relative changes in CK or Mb. Thus, individuals reporting the greatest DOMS did not necessarily have the highest CK and Mb values. More than likely, the first bout of repetitive, high-force exercise disrupts the integrity of the sarcolemma to produce mitochondrial swelling and temporary ultrastructural muscle damage in a pool of stress-susceptible or degenerating muscle fibers.[124] The early mechanical damage to the myocytes (reflected by increased CK release) 24 hours postexercise probably is independent of an acute inflammatory cell infiltration within the muscle.[19] The subsequent decrease in muscle performance for several days after eccentric injury primarily stems from a failure in excitation–contraction coupling.[93] The fast-twitch fibers with low oxidative capacities show particular vulnerability[62], with more-extensive damage several days after exercise than in the immediate post-exercise period. Changes in plasma CK activity, soreness ratings, and skeletal muscle injury with eccentric exercise do not differ between young adult Caucasians and African American men.[177]

A single exercise bout offers significant protection against muscle soreness in subsequent exercise, with the effect lasting as long as 6 weeks.[23,148] Resistance to muscle damage in succeeding exercise may result from an eccentric exercise–induced increase in muscle fiber sarcomeres connected in series.[125] Such adaptations support the wisdom of initiating a training program with light exercise to protect against the muscle soreness that almost always follows an initial heavy-exercise bout containing an eccentric component. Actually, intense concentric exercise performed just before strenuous eccentric exercise does not magnify muscle damage. It may actually prepare the muscle to respond more effectively to the

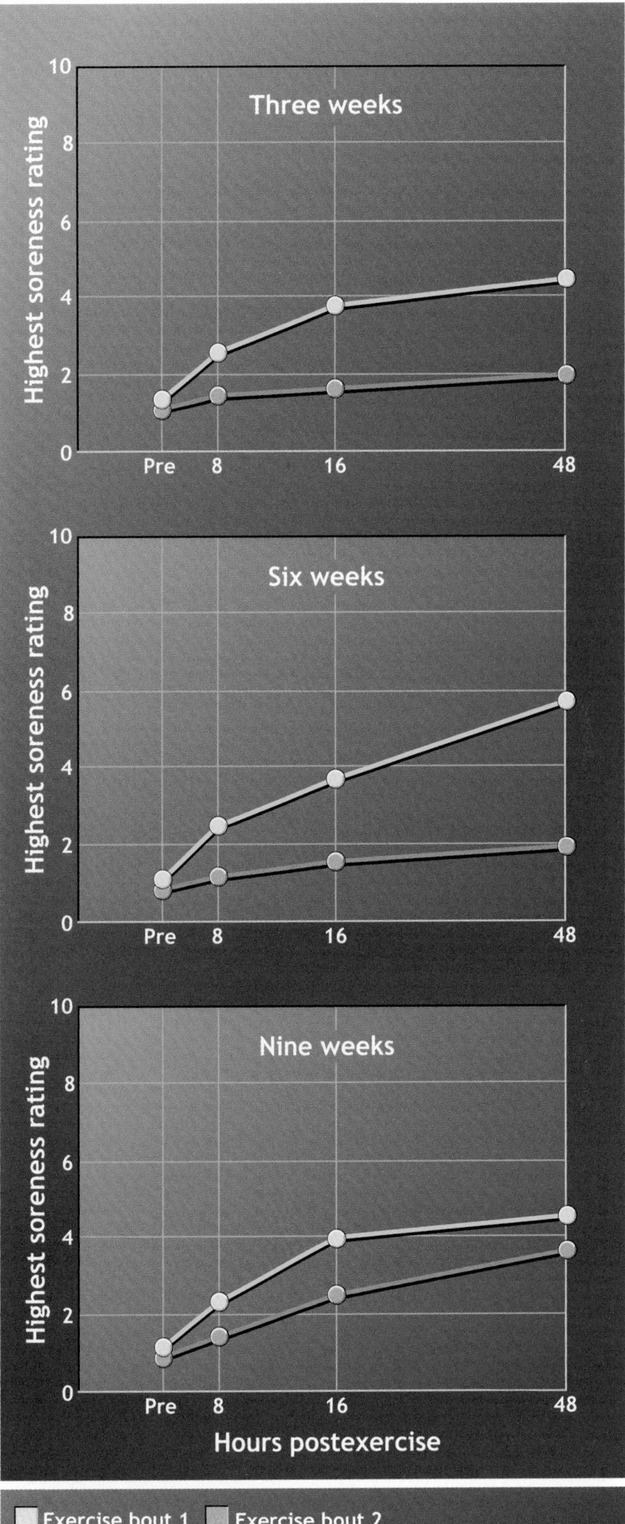

FIGURE 22.30 • Highest soreness rating before and 6, 18, and 48 hours after exercise bout 1 (*yellow*) and a subsequent exercise bout (bout 2, *orange*) performed either 3, 6, or 9 weeks later. CK and Mb showed similar results. (From Byrnes WC, et al. Delayed onset muscle soreness following repeated bouts of downhill running. J Appl Physiol 1985;59:710.)

next eccentric exercise stress.[153] However, even prior lower-intensity exercise of specific muscles does *not* provide complete protection from DOMS with more-intense exercise.[35]

Altered Sarcoplasmic Reticulum

Changes in pH, intramuscular high-energy phosphates, ionic balance, or temperature with unaccustomed exercise produce major alterations in sarcoplasmic reticulum structure and function. These effects depress the rates of Ca^{2+} uptake and release and increase free Ca^{2+} concentration as the mineral rapidly moves into the cytosol of the damaged fibers. An overload of intracellular Ca^{2+} may contribute to the autolytic process within damaged muscle fibers that degrades both contractile and noncontractile structures,[22,124] leading to reduced force capacity and eventual muscle soreness. Vitamin E supplementation protects against cellular membrane disruption and enzyme loss after muscle damage from heavy resistance exercise (see Chapter 2).[136,209]

Current DOMS Model

Figure 22.31 diagrams the probable steps in the development of DOMS and subsequent recuperation. An area of current controversy concerns whether the liberal use of nonsteroidal anti-inflammatory agents (e.g., flurbiprofen) to treat soft-tissue injury or acute pain from DOMS provides any benefit (or harm) to short- and long-term recuperation.[143]

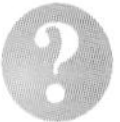

INTEGRATIVE QUESTION

How would you respond to a friend who comments: "I run and work out with free weights regularly, yet every spring my muscles are sore a day or two after a few hours of yard work."

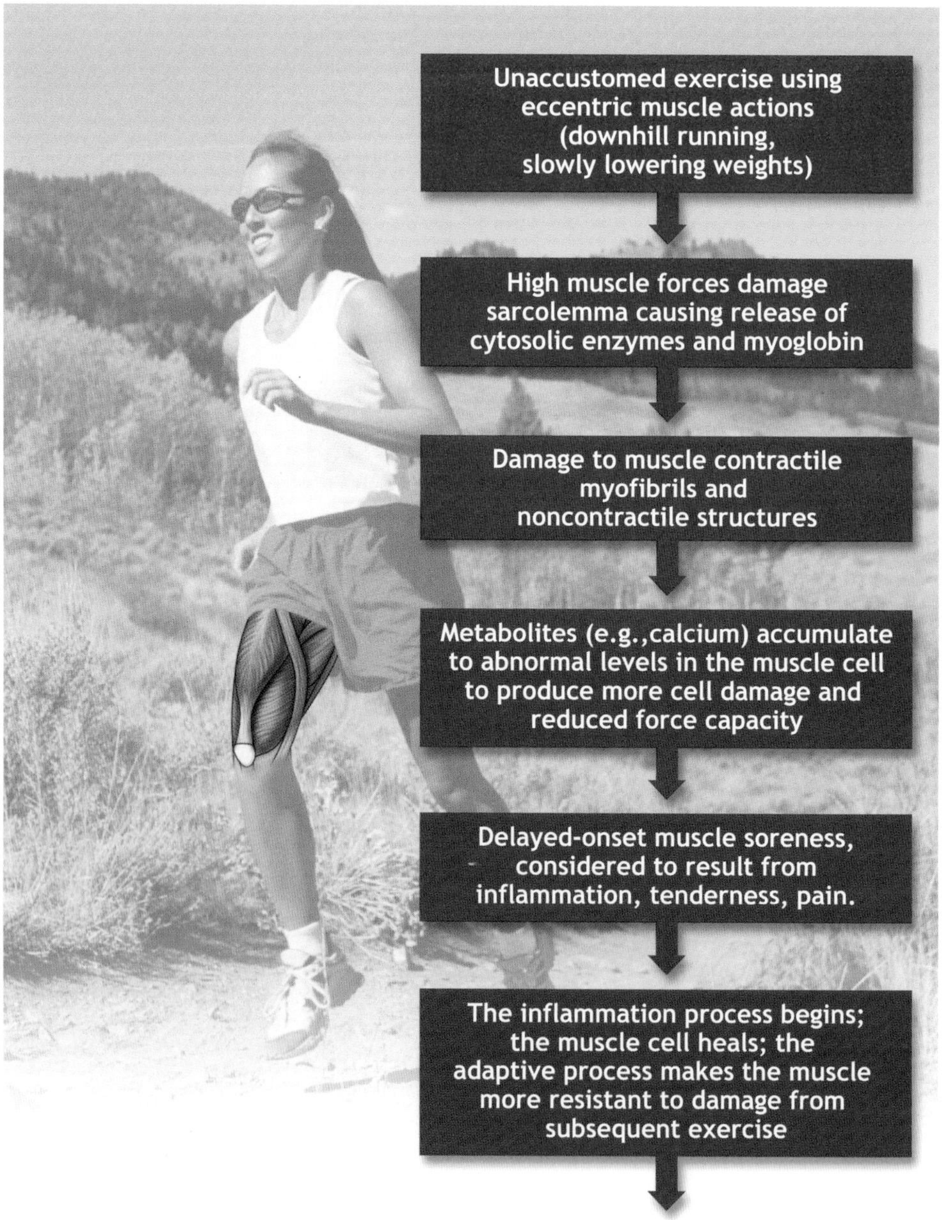

Unaccustomed exercise using eccentric muscle actions (downhill running, slowly lowering weights)

High muscle forces damage sarcolemma causing release of cytosolic enzymes and myoglobin

Damage to muscle contractile myofibrils and noncontractile structures

Metabolites (e.g.,calcium) accumulate to abnormal levels in the muscle cell to produce more cell damage and reduced force capacity

Delayed-onset muscle soreness, considered to result from inflammation, tenderness, pain.

The inflammation process begins; the muscle cell heals; the adaptive process makes the muscle more resistant to damage from subsequent exercise

FIGURE 22.31 • Proposed sequence for delayed-onset muscle soreness after unaccustomed exercise. Cellular adaptations to short-term exercise provide enhanced resistance to subsequent damage and pain.

Summary

1. Physiologic factors (size and type of muscle fibers and the anatomic-lever arrangement of bone and muscle) largely govern the upper limit of muscular strength.
2. Central nervous system influences activate the prime movers in a specific action and also exert a significant effect on maximal force capacity.
3. Genetic, exercise, nutritional, hormonal, environmental, and neural factors interact to regulate skeletal muscle mass and corresponding strength development with resistance training.
4. Three factors contribute to increased muscle strength with resistance training: (1) improved capacity for motor unit recruitment, (2) changes in motoneuron firing pattern efficiency, and (3) significant alterations within the muscle fibers' contractile elements.
5. Muscular overload of specific muscles increases strength and selectively stimulates muscle fiber hypertrophy. Muscle hypertrophy includes increased protein synthesis with myofibril thickening, proliferation of connective tissue cells, and increased number of satellite cells around each fiber.
6. Muscle hypertrophy entails structural changes within the contractile apparatus of individual fibers, particularly fast-twitch fibers, and increased anaerobic energy stores. The relative contribution of new fiber development to muscle enlargement remains undetermined.
7. The genetic code exerts the greatest influence on muscle fiber-type distribution; a muscle's fiber composition is largely fixed before birth or in the first few years of life.
8. Human muscle fibers adapt to increased functional demands via action of myogenic stem cells (satellite cells) that proliferate and differentiate to remodel the muscle.
9. Relatively short-duration resistance training for women and men generates similar strength improvements (on a percentage basis). Resistance training significantly increases a woman's muscle mass.
10. Muscle weakness in the abdominal and lower lumbar back regions and poor flexibility in back and legs represent the primary factors related to low-back syndrome. Muscle-strengthening and flexibility exercises effectively protect against and rehabilitate this condition.
11. Women at higher risk for osteoporosis (or who have the disease) can reduce their factor of risk for fracture by increasing bone density and avoiding activities that increase spinal compression.
12. Conventional resistance training contributes little to improving aerobic fitness. These exercises do not serve effectively as major activities for weight loss because of their relatively low caloric cost.
13. Circuit resistance training, by employing lower resistance and higher repetitions, effectively combines the muscle-training benefits of resistance exercise with the cardiovascular, calorie-burning benefits of continuous dynamic exercise.
14. Eccentric muscle actions induce significantly greater DOMS than concentric-only or isometric actions. Serum markers of muscle damage (e.g., CK and Mb) increase with each form of muscle action.
15. A single exercise bout provides significant protection against DOMS and damage from subsequent exercise. The protection mechanism supports the wisdom of progressing gradually (lower intensity; minimize eccentric actions) when beginning an exercise program with significant muscular force development.

References

1. ACSM position stand on exercise and physical activity for older adults. Med Sci Sports Exerc 1998;30:992.
2. Adams GR, et al. Skeletal muscle myosin heavy chain composition and resistance training. J Appl Physiol 1993;74:911.
3. Adams MA, et al. The lumbar spine in backward bending. Spine 1988;13:1019.
4. Aitken JC, et al. The effects of high intensity training upon respiratory gas exchanges during fixed term maximal incremental exercise in man. Eur J Appl Physiol 1989;58:717.
5. Allerheiligen WB. Speed development and plyometric training. In: Baechle TR, ed. Essentials of strength training and conditioning. Champaign, IL: Human Kinetics, 1994.
6. American Association of Cardiovascular and Pulmonary Rehabilitation. Guidelines for cardiac rehabilitation programs. 2nd ed. Champaign, IL: Human Kinetics, 1995.
7. American College of Sports Medicine. Position paper on the recommended quantity and quality of exercise for developing and maintaining cardiorespiratory and muscular fitness in healthy adults. Med Sci Sports Exerc 1990;22:265.
8. Antonio J. Nonuniform response of skeletal muscle to heavy resistance training: can bodybuilders induce regional muscle hypertrophy? J Strength Cond Res 2000;14:102.
9. Antonio J, Gonyea WJ. Skeletal muscle fiber hyperplasia. Med Sci Sports Exerc 1993;25:1333.
10. Antoino J, Gonyea WJ. Muscle fiber splitting in stretch-enlarged avian muscle. Med Sci Sports Exerc 1994;26:973.
11. Baker D, et al. Periodization: the effect on strength of manipulating volume and intensity. J Strength Cond Res 1994;8:235.
12. Baldwin KM, et al. Biochemical properties of overloaded fast-twitch skeletal muscle. J Appl Physiol 1982;52:457.
13. Ballor DL, et al. Metabolic response during hydraulic resistance exercise. Med Sci Sports Exerc 1987;19:363.
14. Ballor DL, et al. Physiological response to nine different exercise: rest protocols. Med Sci Sports Exerc 1989;21:90.
15. Bassey EJ, Ramsdale SJ. Weight-bearing exercise and ground reaction forces: a 12-month randomized controlled trial of effects on bone mineral density in healthy postmenopausal women. Bone 1995;16:469.
16. Baumann H, et al. Exercise training induces transitions of myosin isoform subunits within histochemically typed human muscle fibers. Pflugers Arch 1987;409:349.
17. Bentsen H, et al. The effect of dynamic strength back exercise and/or home training program in 57-year-old women with chronic low back pain: results of a prospective randomized study with a 3-year follow-up period. Spine 1997;2:1494.
18. Bhasin S, et al. Testosterone replacement and resistance exercise in HIV-infected men with weight loss and low testosterone levels. JAMA 2000;283:763.
19. Bourgeois J, et al. Naproxen does not alter indices of muscle damage in resistance-exercise trained men. Med Sci Sports Exerc 1999;31:4.

20. Braith RW, et al. Effect of training on the relationship between maximal and submaximal strength. Med Sci Sports Exerc 1993;25:132.
21. Brown JM, et al. Further evidence of functional differentiation within biceps brachii. Electromyogr Clin Neurophysiol 1993;33:301.
22. Byrd SK. Alterations in the sarcoplasmic reticulum: a possible link to exercise-induced muscle damage. Med Sci Sports Exerc 1992;24:531.
23. Byrnes WC, et al. Delayed onset muscle soreness following repeated bouts of downhill running. J Appl Physiol 1985;59:710.
24. Campbell K. Biomechanics of pitching. In: Proceedings of the 11th symposium of the International Society of Sport Biomechanics: biomechanics XI. University of Massachusetts, Amherst, 1993.
25. Cappozzo A, et al. Lumber-spine loading during half-squat exercises. Med Sci Sports Exerc 1985;17:613.
26. Carpenter DM, Nelson BW. Low back strengthening for the prevention and treatment of low back pain. Med Sci Sports Exerc 1999;31:18.
27. Carpinelli RN, Otto RM. Strength training: single vs. multiple sets (Review). Sports Med 1998;26:73.
28. Carson JA. The regulation of gene expression in hypertrophying skeletal muscle. Exerc Sport Sci Rev 1997;25:301.
29. Castro MJ, et al. Peak torque per unit cross-sectional area differs between strength-trained and untrained young adults. Med Sci Sports Exerc 1995;27:397.
30. Charette SL, et al. Muscle hypertrophy response to resistance training in older women. J Appl Physiol 1991;70:912.
31. Cheng CK, et al. Influences of walking speed change on the lumbosacral joint force distribution. Biomed Mater Eng 1998;8:155.
32. Chilibeck PD, et al. A comparison of strength and muscle mass increases during resistance training in young women. Eur J Appl Physiol 1998;77:170.
33. Cholewicki J, et al., Lumbar spine loads during the lifting of extremely heavy weights. Med Sci Sports Exerc 1991;23:1179.
34. Clarke DH, Clarke HH. Research processes in physical education, recreation, and health. Englewood Cliffs, NJ: Prentice-Hall, 1984.
35. Clarkson PM, Tremblay I. Exercise induced muscle damage, repair, and adaptation in humans. J Appl Physiol 1988;65:1.
36. Coggan AR, et al. Skeletal muscle adaptations to endurance training in 60- to 70-yr old men and women. J Appl Physiol 1992;72:1780.
37. Colliander EB, Tesch PA. Effects of detraining following short term resistance training on eccentric and concentric muscle strength. Acta Physiol Scand 1992;144:23.
38. Conley MS, et al. Resistance training and human cervical muscle recruitment plasticity. J Appl Physiol 1997;83:2105.
39. Coodley GO, et al. Endocrine function in HIV wasting syndrome. J Acquir Defic Syndr Retrovirol 1994;7:46.
40. Coyle EF, et al. Specificity of power improvements through slow and fast isokinetic training. J Appl Physiol 1981;51:1437.
41. Cronin, J.B., et al.: The role of maximal strength and load on initial power production. Med. Sci. Sports Exerc., 32:1763, 2000.
42. Cureton KJ, et al. Muscle hypertrophy in men and women. Med Sci Sports Exerc 1988;20:338.
43. Dawson B, et al. Changes in performance, muscle metabolites, enzymes and fibre types after short sprint training. Eur J Appl Physiol 1998;78:163.
44. deLooze MP, et al. Mechanical loading on the low back in three methods of refuse collecting. Ergonomics 1995;38:1993.
45. DeLorme TL, Watkins AL. Progressive resistance exercise. New York: Appleton-Century-Crofts, 1951.
46. Demirel HA, et al. Exercise induced alterations in skeletal muscle myosin heavy chain phenotype: dose-response relationship. J Appl Physiol 1999;86:1002.
47. Deschenes MR, et al. The neuromuscular junction: muscle fibre type differences, plasticity, and adaptability to increased and decreased activity. Sports Med. 1994;17:358.
48. Dolan P, et al. Bending and compressive stresses acting on the lumbar-spine during lifting activities. J Biomech 1994;27:1237.
49. Dolezal BA, Potteiger JA. Concurrent resistance and endurance training influence basal metabolic rate in nondieting individuals. J Appl Physiol 1998;85:695.
50. Duarte JA, et al. Exercise-induced signs of muscle overuse in children. Int J Sports Med 1999;20:103.
51. Duchateau J, Hainaut K. Isometric or dynamic training: differentiated effects on mechanical properties of human muscle. J Appl Physiol 1984;56:296.
52. English AW, et al. Compartmentalization of muscles and their motor nuclei: The partitioning hypothesis. Phys Ther 1993;73:857.
53. Enoka R. Neuromechanical basis of kinesiology. Champaign, IL: Human Kinetics, 1988.
54. Exercise training guidelines for the elderly. Med Sci Sports Exerc 1999;31:12.
55. Faigenbaum A, et al. The effects of different resistance training protocols on muscular strength and endurance development in children. Pediatrics 1999;104L e4(electronic issue).
56. Feigenbaum MS, Pollock ML. Strength training: rationale for current guidelines for adult fitness programs. Phys Sportsmed 1997;25(2):44.
57. Feigenbaum MS, Pollock ML. Prescription of resistance training for health and disease. Med Sci Sports Exerc 1999;31:38.
58. Fiatarone MA, et al. Exercise training and nutritional supplementation for physical frailty in very elderly people. N Engl J Med 1994;330:1769.
59. Fleck SJ. Periodized strength training: a critical review. J Strength Cond Res 1999;13:82.
60. Fleck SJ, Kraemer WJ. Designing resistance training programs. 2nd ed. Champaign, IL: Human Kinetics, 1997.
61. Fletcher GF, et al. Statement on exercise: benefits and recommendations for physical activity programs for all Americans: a statement for health professionals by the Committee on Exercise and Cardiac Rehabilitation of the Council on Clinical Cardiology. American Heart Association. Circulation 1996;94:857.
62. Frieden J, Lieber RL. Structural and mechanical basis of exercise-induced muscle injury. Med Sci Sports Exerc 1992;24:521.
63. Frontera WR, et al. Strength conditioning in older men: skeletal muscle hypertrophy and improved function. J Appl Physiol 1988;64:1038.
64. Garhammer J, Takano B. Training for weightlifting. In: Komi PV, ed. Strength and power in sport. Oxford: Blackwell Scientific Publications, 1993.
65. Gettman LR. Physiologic effects on adult men of circuit strength training and jogging. Arch Phys Med Rehabil 1979;60:115.
66. Goldberg AL, et al. Mechanism of work-induced hypertrophy of skeletal muscle. Med Sci Sports 1975;7:185.
67. Gollnick PD, et al. Effect of training on enzyme activity and fiber composition of human skeletal muscle. J Appl Physiol 1973;34:107.
68. Gonyea WJ, et al. Exercise induced increases in muscle fiber number. Eur J Appl Physiol 1986;55:137.
69. Graves JE, et al. Effect of reduced training frequency on muscular strength. Int J Sports Med 1988;9:316.
70. Graves JE, et al. Specificity of limited range of motion variable resistance training. Med Sci Sports Exerc 1989;21:84.
71. Grinspoon S, et al. Loss of lean body and muscle mass correlates with androgen levels in hypogonadal men with acquired immunodeficiency syndrome and wasting. J Clin Endocrinol Metab 1996;81:4051.
72. Guzik DC, et al. A biomechanical model of the lumbar spine during upright isometric flexion, extension, and lateral bending. Spine 1996;21:427.
73. Haennel R, et al. Effects of hydraulic circuit training on cardiovascular function. Med Sci Sports Exerc 1989;21:605.
74. Häkkinen K, et al. Changes in agonist-antagonist EMG, muscle CSA, and force during strength training in middle-aged and older people. J Appl Physiol 1998;84:1341.
75. Harmon EA, et al. Effect of a belt on intra-abdominal pressure during weight lifting. Med Sci Sports Exerc 1989;21:186.
76. Harris KA, Holly RG. Physiological response to circuit weight training in borderline hypertensive subjects. Med Sci Sports Exerc 1987;19:246.
77. Hass CJ, et al. Single versus multiple sets in long-term recreational weightlifters. Med Sci Sports Exerc 2000;32:235.
78. Hather BM, et al. Influence of eccentric actions on skeletal muscle adaptations to resistance training. Acta Physiol Scand 1991;143:177.
79. Hay JG, et al. Changes in muscle-tendon length during the take-off of a running long jump. J Sports Sci 1999;17:159.
80. Hedman TP, Fernie GR. Mechanical response of the lumbar spine to seated postural loads. Spine 1997;1:734.
81. Hennessy LC, Watson AWS. The interference effects of training for strength and endurance simultaneously. J Strength Cond Res 1994;8:12.
82. Hettinger TL, Muller EA. Muskelleistung und Muskeltraining. Int Z Angew Physiol 1953;15:111.
83. Heyward VH, et al. Gender differences in strength. Res Q Exerc Sport 1986;57:154.
84. Holloszy JO, Coyle EF. Adaptations of skeletal muscle to endurance training and their metabolic consequences. J Appl Physiol 1984;56:831.
85. Hood DA, et al. Assembly of the cellular powerhouse: current issues in muscle mitochondrial biogenesis. Exerc Sport Sci Rev 2000;28:68.

86. Hortobágyi T, et al. Interrelationships among various measures of upper body strength assessed by different contraction modes. Eur J Appl Physiol 1989;58:749.
87. Hortobágyi T, et al. The effects of detraining on power athletes. Med Sci Sports Exerc 1993;25:929.
88. Housh T, et al. Anthropometric estimation of muscle group cross-sectional area. J Strength Cond Res 1993;7:250.
89. Hurley BF, Hagberg JM. Optimizing health in older persons: aerobic or strength training? Exerc Sport Sci Rev 1998;26:61.
90. Hurley BF, et al. Effects of high intensity strength training on cardiovascular function. Med Sci Sports Exerc 1984;16:483.
91. Hyatt J-PK, Clarkson PM. Creatine kinase release and clearance using MM variants following repeated bouts of eccentric exercise. Med Sci Sports Exerc 1998;30:1059.
92. Ikai M, Steinhaus AH. Some factors modifying the expression of human strength. J Appl Physiol 1961;16:157.
93. Ingalls CP, et al. E-C coupling failure in mouse EDL muscle after in vivo eccentric contractions. J Appl Physiol 1998;85:58.
94. Jackson AS. Preemployment physical evaluation. Exerc Sport Sci Rev 1994;22:55.
95. Jacobs I. Sprint training effects on muscle myoglobin, enzymes, fiber types, and blood lactate. Med Sci Sports Exerc 1987;19:368.
96. Janney C, et al. Maximum muscular strength differs in postmenopausal women with and without osteoporosis (abstract). Med Sci Sports Exerc 1987;19:561.
97. Jansson E, Kaijser L. Muscle adaptation to extreme endurance training in man. Acta Physiol Scand 1977;100:315.
98. Jansson E, et al. Changes in muscle fiber type distribution in man after physical training. Acta Physiol Scand 1978;104:235.
99. Janz KF, et al. Longitudinal analysis of scaling $\dot{V}O_2$ for differences in body size during puberty: the Muscatine Study. Med Sci Sports Exerc 1998;30:1436.
100. Jones DA, Rutherford OM. Human muscle strength training: the effects of three different regimens and the nature of the resultant changes. J Physiol 1987;391:1.
101. Kanehisa H, Miyashita M. Specificity of velocity in strength training. Eur J Appl Physiol 1983;52:104.
102. Katch FI, et al. Evaluation of acute cardiorespiratory responses to hydraulic resistance exercise. Med Sci Sports Exerc 1985;17:168.
103. Katch VL, Katch FI. Use of weight-adjusted oxygen uptake scores that avoid spurious correlations. Res Q 1974;45:447.
104. Kee D, Chung MK. Comparison of prediction models for the compression force on the lumbosacral disc. Ergonomics 1996;39:1419.
105. Kelemen MH. Resistance training safety and assessment guidelines for cardiac and coronary prone patients. Med Sci Sports Exerc 1989;21:675.
106. Kellis E, Blatzopoulos V. Muscle activation differences between eccentric and concentric isokinetic exercise. Med Sci Sports Exerc 1998;30:1616.
107. Kingma DP, et al. Dynamic forces acting on the lumbar spine during manual handling. Can they be estimated using electromyographic techniques alone? Spine 1999;24:698.
108. Kitai TA, et al. Specificity of joint angle in isometric training. Eur J Appl Physiol 1989;58:744.
109. Kokkinos PF, et al. Strength training does not improve lipoprotein-lipid profiles in men at risk for CHD. Med Sci Sports Exerc 1991;23:1134.
110. Kraemer WJ, Newton RU. Training for muscular power. Phys Med Rehabil Clin 2000;11:341.
111. Kraemer WJ, et al. Endogenous anabolic hormonal and growth factor responses to heavy resistance exercises in males and females. Int J Sports Med 1991;12:228.
112. Kraemer WJ, et al. Changes in hormonal concentrations after different heavy-resistance exercise protocols in women. J Appl Physiol 1993;75:594.
113. Kraemer WJ, et al. Compatibility of high-intensity strength and endurance training on hormonal and skeletal muscle adaptations. J Appl Physiol 1995;78:976.
114. Kraemer WJ, et al. Acute hormonal responses to heavy resistance training in younger and older men. Eur J Appl Physiol 1998;77:206.
115. Kraus WE, et al. Skeletal muscle adaptation to chronic low-frequency motor nerve stimulation. Exerc Sport Sci Rev 1994;22:313.
116. Kubo K, et al. Influence of elastic properties of tendon structures on jump performance in humans. J Appl Physiol 1999;87:2090.
117. LaChance PF, et al. Day-to-day reliability during high and low resistance bi-directional hydraulic exercise. J Appl Sport Sci Res 1988;2:57.
118. Lawrence RC, et al. Estimates of the prevalence of arthritis and selected musculoskeletal disorders in the United States. Arthritis Rheum 1998;41:778.
119. Layne JE, Nelson ME. The effects of progressive resistance training on bone density: a review. Med Sci Sports Exerc 1999;31:25.
120. Lemmer JT, et al. Effect of strength training on resting metabolic rate and physical activity: age and gender comparisons. Med Sci Sports Exerc 2001;33:532.
121. Leveritt M, Abernethy PJ. Acute effects of high-intensity endurance exercise on subsequent resistance activity. J Strength Cond Res 1999;13:47.
122. Lieber RL, Fridén J. Muscle damage is not a function of muscle force but active muscle strain. J Appl Physiol 1993;74:520.
123. Lindman R, et al. Fiber type composition of the human female trapezius muscle: enzyme-histochemical characteristics. Am J Anat 1991;190:385.
124. Lowe DA, et al. Eccentric contraction-induced injury of mouse soleus muscle: effect of varying [Ca^{++}]. J Appl Physiol 1994;76:1445.
125. Lynn R, et al. Differences in rat skeletal muscle after incline and decline running. J Appl Physiol 1998;85:98.
126. MacArthur RD, et al. Supervised exercise training improves cardiovascular fitness in HIV-infected persons. Med Sci Sports Exerc 1993;25:684.
127. MacDougall JD. Morphological changes in human skeletal muscle following strength training and immobilization. In: Jones NL, et al. eds. Human muscle power. Champaign, IL: Human Kinetics, 1986.
128. MacDougall JD, et al. Muscle ultrastructural characteristics of the elite powerlifters and bodybuilders. Med Sci Sports 1980;2:131.
129. MacDougall JD, et al. Muscle fiber number in biceps brachii in bodybuilders and control subjects. J Appl Physiol 1984;57:1399.
130. Malmivaara A, et al. The treatment of acute low back pain—bed rest, exercises, or ordinary activity. N Engl J Med 1995;332:351.
131. Manning RM., et al. Constant vs variable resistance knee extension training. Med Sci Sports Exerc 1990;22:397.
132. Marx JO, et al. Low-volume circuit versus high-volume periodized resistance training in women. Med Sci Sports Exerc 2001;33:635.
133. Mateyeev L. Periodisierang des sportlichen training. Berlin: Berles & Wernitz, 1972.
134. Mayhew TP, et al. Muscular adaptation to concentric and eccentric exercise at equal power levels. Med Sci Sports Exerc 1995;27:868.
135. McArdle WD, Foglia GF. Energy cost and cardiorespiratory stress of isometric and weight training exercises. J Sports Med Phys Fitness 1969;9:23.
136. McBride JM, et al. Effect of resistance exercise on free radical production. Med Sci Sports Exerc 1998;30:67.
137. McBride JM, et al. A comparison of strength and power characteristics between power lifters, Olympic lifters, and sprinters. J Strength Cond Res 1999;13:58.
138. McCall GE, et al. Maintenance of mononuclear domain size in rat soleus after overload and growth hormone/IGF-I treatment. J Appl Physiol 1998;84:1407.
139. McCarthy JP, et al. Resistance exercise training and the orthostatic response. Eur J Appl Physiol 1997;76:32.
140. McGill SM. Low back stability: From frontal description to issues for performance and rehabilitation. Exerc Sport Sci Rev 2001;29:26.
141. McMillan DW, et al. Stress distributions inside intervertebral discs: the validity of experimental "stress profilometry." Proc Inst Mech Eng 1996;210:81.
142. Meyer RA, Prior BM. Functional magnetic resonance imaging of muscle. Exerc Sport Sci Rev 2000;28:898.
143. Mishra DK, et al. Anti-inflammatory medication after muscle injury. J Bone Joint Surg Am 1995;77:1510.
144. Morrissey MC, et al. Resistance training modes: specificity and effectiveness. Med Sci Sports Exerc 1995;27:648.
145. Myers ER, Wilson SE. Biomechanics of osteoporosis and vertebral fracture. Spine 1997;22:25S.
146. Narici M, et al. Human quadriceps cross-sectional area, torque, and neural activation during 6 months strength training. Acta Physiol Scand 1996;1547:175.
147. Natarajan RN, Andersson GB. The influence of lumbar disc height and cross-sectional area on the mechanical response of the disc to physiologic loading. Spine 1999;24:1873.
148. Newham DJ, et al. Repeated high force eccentric exercise; effects on muscle pain and damage. J Appl Physiol 1987;63:1381.

149. Newton RU, et al. Effects of ballistic training on preseason preparation of elite volleyball players. Med Sci Sports Exerc 1999;31:323.
150. Nichols DL, et al. Relationship of regional body composition to bone mineral density in college females. Med Sci Sports Exerc 1995;27:178.
151. Nindl BC, et al. The validity of using strength scores divided by fat-free body mass to compare lifting capacities of men and women. J Strength Cond Res 1993;7:183.
152. Nosaka K, Clarkson PM. Muscle damage following repeated bouts of high force eccentric exercise. Med Sci Sports Exerc 1995;27:1263.
153. Nosaka K, Clarkson P. Influence of previous concentric exercise on eccentric exercise-induced muscle damage. J Sports Sci 1997;15:477.
154. O'Hagan FT, et al. Comparative effectiveness of accommodating and weight resistance training modes. Med Sci Sports Exerc 1995;27:1210.
155. Ozmun JC, et al. Neuromuscular adaptations following prepubescent strength training. Med Sci Sports Exerc 1994;26:510.
156. Patwardhan AG, et al. A follower load increases the load-carrying capacity of the lumbar spine in compression. Spine 1999;24:1003.
157. Pavone E, Moffat M. Isometric torque of the quadriceps femoris after concentric, eccentric and isometric training. Arch Phys Med Rehabil 1985;66:168.
158. Payne VG, et al. Endurance training in children and youth: a meta-analysis. Res Q Exerc Sport 1997;68:80.
159. Perkins MS, Bloswick DS. The use of back belts to increase intra-abdominal pressure as a means of preventing low back injuries: a survey of the literature. Int J Environ Health 1995;1:326.
160. Petersen SR, et al. The influence of isokinetic concentric resistance training on concentric and eccentric torque outputs and cross-sectional area of the quadriceps femoris. Can J Sport Sci 1988;13:76.
161. Pipes TV, Wilmore JH. Isokinetic vs. isotonic strength training in adult men. Med Sci Sports 1976;7:262.
162. Pizza FX, et al. Exercise-induced muscle damage: effect on circulating leukocyte and lymphocyte subsets. Med Sci Sports Exerc 1995;27:363.
163. Pollock ML, et al. Effect of resistance training on lumbar extension strength. Am J Sports Med 1989;17:624.
164. Pollock ML, et al. The recommended quantity and quality of exercise for developing and maintaining cardiorespiratory fitness, strength, and flexibility in healthy adults. Med Sci Sports Exerc 1998;30:975.
165. Porter MM, Vandervoort AA. Standing strength training of the ankle plantar and dorsiflexors in older women, using concentric and eccentric contractions. Eur J Appl Physiol 1997;76:62.
166. Prevost MC, et al. The effect of two days of velocity-specific isokinetic training on torque production. J Strength Cond Res 1999;13:35.
167. Rantanen T, et al. Midlife hand grip strength as a predictor of old age disability. JAMA 1999;281:558.
168. Roman WJ, et al. Adaptations in the elbow flexors of elderly males after heavy-resistance training. J Appl Physiol 1993;74:750.
169. Roy RR, et al. The plasticity of skeletal muscle: effects of neuromuscular activity. Exerc Sport Sci Rev 1991;19:269.
170. Sakuma K, et al. Are region specific changes in fibre types attributable to nonuniform muscle hypertrophy by overloading. Eur J Appl Physiol 1995;71:499.
171. Sale DG. Influence of exercise and training on motor unit activation. Exerc Sport Sci Rev 1987;15:237.
172. Salleo A, et al. New muscle fiber production during compensatory hypertrophy. Med Sci Sports 1980;12:268.
173. Salminen JJ, et al. Leisure time physical activity in the young. Correlation with low-back pain, spinal mobility and trunk muscle strength in 15-year-old schoolchildren. Int J Sports Med 1993;14:406.
174. Sarti MA, et al. Muscle activity in upper and lower rectus abdominus during abdominal exercises. Arch Phys Med Rehabil 1996;77:1293.
175. Schantz PG, Källman M. NADH shuttle enzymes and cytochrome b_5 reductase in human skeletal muscle: effect of strength training. J Appl Physiol 1989;67:123.
176. Schmidtbleicher D. Training for power events. In: Komi PV, ed. Strength and power in sport. Oxford: Blackwell Scientific Publications, 1993.
177. Schwane JA, et al. Plasma creatine kinase responses of 18- to 30-yr-old African-American men to eccentric exercise. Med Sci Sports Exerc 2000;32:370.
178. Sellmeyer DE, et al. Endocrine and metabolic disturbances in human immunodeficiency virus infection and the acquired immune deficiency syndrome. Endocr Rev 1996;17:518.
179. Shirazi-Adl A, Parnianpour M. Effect of changes in lordosis on mechanics of the lumbar spine-lumbar curvature in lifting. J Spinal Discord 1999;12:436.
180. Simoneau J-A, et al. Human skeletal muscle fiber type alteration with high-intensity intermittent training. Eur J Appl Physiol 1985;54:240.
181. Sipalä S, Suominen H. Effects of strength and endurance training on thigh and leg muscle mass and composition in elderly women. J Appl Physiol 1995;78:334.
182. Sjöström M, et al. Evidence of fiber hyperplasia in human skeletal muscles from healthy young men. Eur J Appl Physiol 1992;62:301.
183. Sleivert GG, et al. The influence of a strength-sprint training sequence on multi-joint power output. Med Sci Sports Exerc 1995;27:1655.
184. Sorichter S, et al. Skeletal troponin I as a marker of exercise-induced muscle damage. J Appl Physiol 1998;83:1076.
185. Sparling PS, Cantwell JA. Strength training guidelines for cardiac patients. Phys Sportsmed 1989;17:191.
186. Staron RS, Hohnson P. Myosin polymorphism and differential expression in adult human skeletal muscle. Comp Biochem Physiol 1993;106B:463.
187. Staron RS, et al. Muscle hypertrophy and fast fiber type conversions in heavy resistance-trained women. Eur J Appl Physiol 1990;60:71.
188. Staron RS, et al. Strength and skeletal muscle adaptations in heavy-resistance-trained women after detraining and retraining. J Appl Physiol 1991;70:631.
189. Staron RS, et al. Skeletal muscle adaptations during the early phase of heavy-resistance training in men and women. J Appl Physiol 1994;76:1247.
190. Stauber WT. Eccentric action of muscles: physiology, injury, and adaptation. Exerc Sport Sci Rev 1989;17:157.
191. Stock JL, et al. Dynamic muscle strength is decreased in post-menopausal women with low bone density. J Bone Miner Res 1987;2:338.
192. Stringer WE, et al. The effect of exercise training on aerobic fitness, immune indices, and quality of life in HIV+ patients. Med Sci Sports Exerc. 1998;30:11.
193. Sward L. The thoracolumbar spine in young elite athletes. Current concepts on the effects of physical training. Sports Med 1992;13:357.
194. Taylor CR, et al. Scaling and energetic cost of running to body size in mammals. Am J Physiol 1970;219:1104.
195. Teague BN, Schwane JA. Effect of intermittent eccentric contractions on symptoms of muscle microinjury. Med Sci Sports Exerc 1995;27:1378.
196. Ter Haar Romeny BM, et al. Relation between location of a motor unit in the human biceps brachii and its critical firing levels for different tasks. Exp Neurol 1984;85:631.
197. Tesch PA. Enzyme activities of FT and ST muscle fibers in heavy-resistance trained athletes. J Appl Physiol 1989;83:67.
198. Tesch PA, Karlsson J. Muscle fiber types and size in trained and untrained muscles of elite athletes. J Appl Physiol 1985;59:1716.
199. Tesch PA, Larsson L. Muscle hypertrophy in body builders. Eur J Appl Physiol 1982;49:301.
200. Tesch PA, et al. Muscle capillary supply and fiber type characteristics in weight and power lifters. J Appl Physiol 1984;56:35.
201. Thorstensson A. Muscle strength, fiber types and enzyme activities in man. Acta Physiol Scand Suppl 1976:443.
202. Tittel K, Wutscherk H. Anthropometric factors. In: Komi PV, ed. Strength and power in sport. Oxford: Blackwell Scientific Publications, 1993.
203. Trimble MH, et al. Reflex facilitation during the stretch-shortening cycle. J Electromyogr Kinesiol 2000;1:179.
204. U.S. Department of Health and Human Services, Centers for Disease Control and Prevention, National Center for Chronic Disease Prevention and Health Promotion, Washington, DC, 1996.
205. Vailas AC, Vailas JC. Physical activity and connective tissue. In: Bouchard C, et al., eds. Physical activity, fitness, and health. Champaign, IL: Human Kinetics, 1994.
206. Van Etten LMLA, et al. Effect of body build on weight-training-induced adaptations in body composition and muscular strength. Med Sci Sports Exerc 1994;26:515.
207. Vanderburgh PM, Dooman C. Considering body mass differences, who are the world's strongest women? Med Sci Sports Exerc 2000;32:197.
208. Vanderburgh PM, et al. Multivariate allometric scaling of men's world indoor rowing championship performance. Med Sci Sports Exerc 1996;28:626.
209. Van der Meulen JH, et al. Contraction induced injury to the extensor digitorum longus muscles of rats: the role of vitamin E. J Appl Physiol 1997;83:817.
210. Videman T, et al. Lumbar spinal pathology in cadaveric material in relation to history of back pain, occupation and physical loading. Spine 1990;15:728.

211. Waerhaug, O, et al. Different effects of physical training on the morphology of motor nerve terminals in the rat extensor digitorum longus and soleus muscles. Anat Embryol 1992;186:125.
212. Walsh B, et al. Effect of eccentric exercise on muscle oxidative metabolism in humans. Med Sci Sports Exerc 2001;33:436.
213. Walshe JP, et al. Stretch-shorten cycle compared with isometric preload: contributions to enhanced muscular performance. J Appl Physiol 1998;84:97.
214. Wassell, J.T., et al. A prospective study of back belts for prevention of back pain and injury. JAMA 2000; 284:2727.
215. Weir JP, et al. Electromyographic evaluation of joint angle specificity and cross-training after isometric training. J Appl Physiol 1994;77:1927.
216. Weir JP, et al. The effect of rest interval length on repeated maximal bench press. J Strength Cond Res 1994;8:58.
217. Welle S, et al. Stimulation of myofibrillar synthesis by exercise I mediated by more efficient translation of mRNA. J Appl Physiol 1999;86:1220.
218. Weltman A, et al. The effects of hydraulic resistance strength training in pre-pubertal males. Med Sci Sports Exerc 1986;18:629.
219. Wescott WL, Baechle TR. Strength training past 50. Champaign, IL: Human Kinetics, 1998.
220. Willoughby D. The effects of mesocycle-length weight training programs involving periodization and partially equated volumes on upper and lower body strength. J Strength Cond Res 1993;7:2.
221. Wilson GJ, et al. Performance benefits from weight and plyometric training: effects of initial strength level. Coach Sport Sci J 1997;2:3.
222. Takarada Y, et al. Stretch-induced enhancement of mechanical power output in human multijoint exercise with countermovement. J Appl Physiol 1997;83:1749.
223. Yan Z. Skeletal muscle adaptation and cell cycle regulation. Exerc Sport Sci Rev 2000;1:24.
224. Yarasheski KE, et al. Acute effects of resistance exercise on muscle protein synthesis in young and elderly adults. Am J Physiol 1993;265:E210.
225. Young W, et al. Relationship between strength qualities and performance in standing and run-up vertical jumps. J Sports Med Phys Fitness 1999;39:285.
226. Young WB, et al. Comparison of drop jump training methods: effects on leg extensor strength qualities and jumping performance. Int J Sports Med 1999;20:295.

CHAPTER 23

Special Aids to Exercise Training and Performance

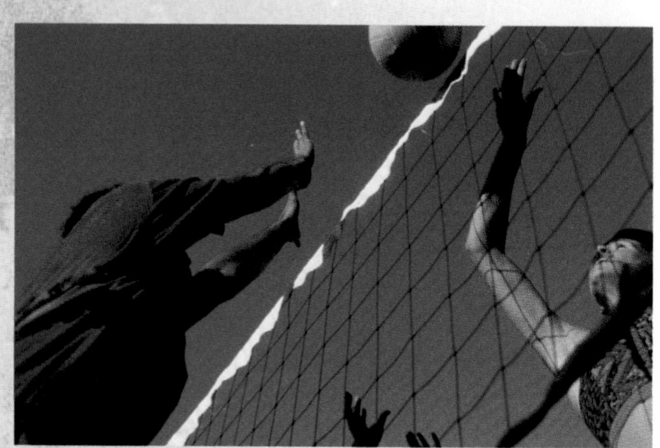

Chapter Objectives

- Define the term *ergogenic aids* and outline possible mechanisms for their purported effects
- List the categories of substances currently banned by the International Olympic Committee (IOC)
- Give examples of substances and procedures alleged to provide ergogenic benefits
- Discuss the mode of action of anabolic steroids, their effectiveness, and risks when used by males and females
- Outline a typical protocol of anabolic steroid use by athletes
- Summarize the American College of Sports Medicine's "Position Stand on Use of Anabolic Steroids"
- Discuss the medical use of human growth hormone and its potential dangers for healthy athletes
- Outline the general trend for endogenous dehydroepiandrosterone (DHEA) production during a lifetime
- Discuss the rationale for DHEA use as an ergogenic aid and potential risks from supplementing
- Summarize the controversy about whether androstenedione represents a benign nutritional supplement or a potentially harmful drug
- Discuss evidence for ergogenic effects of oral supplements of amino acids, carbohydrate–protein, or carbohydrate on hormone secretion, training responsiveness, and exercise performance
- Summarize the general research findings about ergogenic benefits and risks of taking amphetamines, caffeine, pangamic acid, buffering solutions, chromium picolinate, L-carnitine, and β-hydroxy-β-methylbutyrate
- Describe the typical time course for red blood cell reinfusion, and the mechanism for its ergogenic effect on endurance performance and $\dot{V}O_{2max}$
- Discuss the medical use of erythropoietin and its potential dangers for healthy athletes
- Define *general warm-up* and *specific warm-up,* and the potential benefits of each
- Describe possible cardiovascular benefits of moderate warm-up prior to extreme physical effort
- Provide a rationale for breathing hyperoxic gas mixtures to enhance exercise performance, and quantify its potential to increase tissue oxygen availability
- Outline the classic carbohydrate loading procedure and modified loading procedure to augment glycogen storage prior to a bout of high-intensity endurance exercise
- Describe the theoretical role for an ergogenic effect of creatine supplements, and indicate physical activities likely to benefit from supplementation
- Summarize current research and rationale for consuming medium-chain triglycerides to enhance endurance exercise performance

Considerable literature exists on the topic of **ergogenic aids** and athletic performance (*ergogenic* referring to the application of a nutritional, physical, mechanical, psychologic, or pharmacologic procedure or aid to improve physical work capacity or athletic performance). This literature includes studies of potential performance benefits of alcohol, amphetamines, hormones, carbohydrates, amino acids, fatty acids, additional red blood cells, caffeine, carnitine, creatine, phosphates, oxygen-rich breathing mixtures, massage, wheatgerm oil, vitamins, minerals, ionized air, music, hypnosis, and even marijuana and cocaine! Athletes routinely use only a few of these alleged aids, however, and only a few evoke real controversy. Specific concern focuses on the use of anabolic steroids and other exogenous hormones, nutritional components, amphetamines, and the unique procedure of "blood doping." Because warm-up and oxygen inhalation are common procedures, we include these in our discussion of the effectiveness and practicality of ergogenic aids for human physiology and exercise performance. We discuss nutritional requirements for the macro- and micronutrients for active individuals in the specific chapters dealing with these nutrients. The increasing use of herbs of undocumented benefit and quality by fitness enthusiasts and athletes to improve health, reduce stress, elevate emotional and cognitive response, enhance muscular development and exercise performance, and speed recovery raises concern about efficacy and possible toxicity ("In a Practical Sense" summarizes purported benefits, ingredients, and possible side effects of commonly used herbal compounds).

Several explanations account for heightened interest in factors that might enhance the capacity for exercise and training responsiveness in addition to one's innate physical ability and commitment to training. First, more people participate in high-level amateur and professional athletics. Second, success in competition brings significant personal recognition and approval but also more tangible rewards, ranging from valuable college scholarships to lucrative professional contracts and commercial endorsements. For many individuals, athletic success paves the way to riches, a route that sometimes results in personal misfortune.

On July 16, 1998, the international governing body of bicycle racing suspended the coach of the top-ranked Festina team of France in a drug scandal that threatened to overwhelm the 85th Tour de France, bicycle racing's most prestigious and financially rewarding competition. The suspension resulted after large quantities of illicit drugs were found in the team car. These included amphetamines, steroids, masking drugs (usually diuretics to prevent steroid detection or chemicals such as probenecid, which inhibit substances from reaching the urine), and the blood-boosting epoetin, a genetically engineered copy of the kidney hormone erythropoietin, linked to more than a dozen heart attacks among competitive cyclists. The following day, after the sixth stage of the Tour, the governing body suspended all nine members of Festina after its coach admitted supplying illegal drugs to his riders. One week later during its world championships, the International Swimming Federation, the swimming world's governing body, suspended four Chinese swimmers from all meets for 2 years for using triamterene, a banned diuretic that masks anabolic steroid use. On August 6, 1998, the organization banned from competition for 4 years the Irish swimmer who won three gold medals at the 1996 Summer Olympics, accusing her of manipulating a drug test by spiking her urine sample with alcohol to mask forbidden performance-enhancing drugs.

In this chapter, we discuss the possible ergogenic role of the more common pharmacologic and nutritional agents and physiologic procedures purported to enhance exercise performance, increase the quality and quantity of training, and augment the body's adaptation to regular exercise. The following chart presents six mechanisms by which diverse agents might induce ergogenic effects:[122]

POSSIBLE MECHANISMS OF ACTION FOR PURPORTED ERGOGENIC AIDS

- Act as a central or peripheral stimulant of the nervous system (e.g., caffeine, choline, amphetamines, alcohol)
- Increase the storage and/or availability of a limiting substrate (e.g., carbohydrate, creatine, carnitine, chromium)
- Act as a supplemental fuel source (e.g., glucose, medium-chain triglycerides)
- Reduce or neutralize performance-inhibiting metabolic by-products (e.g., pre-exercise use of sodium bicarbonate, citrate, pangamic acid, phosphate)
- Facilitate recovery (e.g., high-glycemic carbohydrates, water)
- Alter the internal environment to optimize muscle dynamics (e.g., warm-up, hyperoxic breathing)

PHARMACOLOGIC AGENTS

Many athletes use a variety of pharmacologic agents, believing that a specific drug improves skill, strength, power, or endurance. In our drug-oriented, competitive culture, drug use for ergogenic purposes continues on the upswing among high school and even junior high school athletes. When winning becomes all important, one can do little to prevent the use *and* abuse of drugs, even if little hard scientific evidence indicates performance-enhancing effects.[194] Athletes go to great lengths to promote all aspects of their health; they train hard, they eat well-balanced meals, they seek and receive medical advice for various injuries (no matter how minor), yet ironically, they ingest synthetic agents, many of which precipitate adverse effects ranging from nausea, hair loss, itching, and nervous irritability to severe consequences such as sterility, liver disease, drug addiction, and even death caused by liver and blood cancer.

The International Olympic Committee (IOC) initiated drug testing for stimulants in Olympic competition in 1968, following the death of a famed Tour de France British cyclist from

In a Practical Sense

➤➤ Commonly Used Herbal Compounds for Exercise and Training: User Beware

Aside from the influence of genetics and proper training, nutrition often exerts an important influence on athletic performance. However, in seeking the competitive edge, exercise enthusiasts and athletes fall prey to fad diets and unnecessary supplements whose potency, quality, and effectiveness lack scientific validation. Athletes often eat a suboptimal diet, particularly when they attempt to reduce body weight while training strenuously. This leads many of these men and women to use a diverse array of "nutritional" supplements, including herbal compounds (used by 23% of U.S. adults), in the hope of covering nutritional inadequacies and ensuring optimal performance and training responsiveness.

Intake of a broad range of herbal compounds as supplements for ergogenic purposes has expanded considerably during the last decade. Aside from the lack of documentation concerning the efficacy of these chemicals, many carry the potential for significant health risk. The prudent coach and exercise specialist should possess at least basic knowledge of the common herbs used by athletes, their purported effects, contraindications, and possible adverse side effects. The table lists the more popular herbs with their uses, active ingredients, common dosage, and precautionary information.

References

Fetrow C, Avila JR. Professionals handbook of complementary & alternative medicines. Springhouse, PA: Springhouse Corporation, 1999.

Schuyler W, et al. The natural pharmacy. 2nd ed. Rocklin, CA: Healthnotes, 1999.

Herbs Frequently Used by Athletes to Improve Health, Reduce Stress, Elevate Emotional and Cognitive Responses, Enhance Muscular Development and Exercise Performance, and Speed Recovery

Herb	*Other Name*	*Purported Use/Benefit*	*Active Ingredients*	*Dosage*	*Side Effects/ Interactions/Comments*
Astragalus	Huang qi	Supports immune system; benefits cardiovascular system; increases energy level; promotes tissue repair	Flavonoids, polysaccharides, triterpene glycosides, amino acids and trace minerals	9–15 g · d^{-1}	None
Bilberry	*Vaccinium myrtillus*	Diabetes; macular degeneration; retinopathy	Anthocyanosides (bioflavonoid)	240–600 mg · d^{-1} as herbal extract or 20–60 g · d^{-1} fruit	None
Bee pollen	Buckwheat pollen; puhuang	Allergies; asthma; cholesterol and triglyceride lowering	Protein, carbohydrates, minerals and essential fatty acids	500–1000 mg · d^{-1}	Allergic reactions; avoid with hypoglycemic agents
Chamomile	Camomile, roman camomile	Stress reduction; supports immune function; assists sleep; promotes tissue repair	α-Bisabol; bioflavonoids	Taken as tea 3 to 4 times per day	Avoid if you have allergies to plants
Echinacea	*Echinacea purpurea; echinacea angustifolia*	Common cold/sore throat; immune function; infection; influenza	Alkylamides, polyacetylenes; increases production of interferon	At onset of cold or flu—3–4 mL · $2h^{-1}$; or 300 mg powder · d^{-1}	Avoid if allergic to sunflower plant family
Ephedra	*Ephedra sinica; Ephedra equisetina*	Asthma; cough; weight loss; increase energy level	Alkaloids ephedrine and pseudoephedrine	1.5–6 g · d^{-1} in tea form; 12.5–25 mg · $4h^{-1}$ as over-the-counter drug	Banned substance; amphetamine-like side effects; avoid with hypertension or pregnancy
Garlic	*Allium sativum*	High blood pressure; high triglycerides; intermittent claudication	Sulfer compound allicin	600–900 mg · d^{-1}	Avoid with stomach problems; heartburn, gastritis, or ulcers
Ginseng, Asian	Pannax	Mental alertness; memory; physical endurance; type 2 diabetes; hyperlipidemia; congestive heart failure	Eleutherosides	200–600 mg · d^{-1}	Avoid with hypertension, heart disease; pregnancy and lactation; nervousness; fever or sleep disorders

IN A PRACTICAL SENSE

➤➤ COMMONLY USED HERBAL COMPOUNDS FOR EXERCISE AND TRAINING—cont'd

HERB	OTHER NAME	PURPORTED USE/BENEFIT	ACTIVE INGREDIENTS	DOSAGE	SIDE EFFECTS/ INTERACTIONS/COMMENTS
Ginseng, Siberian	Eleuthero root	Physical endurance; fatigue prevention; immune function; motion sickness	Eleutherosides	200–600 mg · d^{-1}	Avoid with hypertension, heart disease, pregnancy, and lactation; nervousness; fever or sleep disorders
Ginkgo biloba	Maidenhair tree	Age-related cognitive decline; Alzheimer's disease; intermittent claudication; depression; atheroscleroisis; impotence (of vascular origin)	Gingko flavone glycosides (bioflavonoid), terpene lactones)	120–240 mg · d^{-1}	Mild headaches lasting 1 or 2 days; mild upset stomach
Guarana	*Paullinia: cupana*	Fatigue prevention; weight loss	Guaranine (identical to caffeine)	200–800 mg · d^{-1}	Avoid with pregnancy, glucoma, heart disease, high blood pressure, history of stroke
Kava Kava	*Piper methysticum*	Anxiety; restlessness; stress, muscle relaxing; improves sleep	Kava-lactones	200–250 mg · d^{-1}	Avoid with pregnancy or if lactating; can cause drowsiness
Milk thistle	*Silybum marianum*	Alcohol-related liver disease; hepatitis; liver support	Bioflavonoid complex-silymarin	200–400 mg · d^{-1}	None
Glucosamine sulfate[a]		Osteoarthritis; joint inflammation; joint stiffness		1500 mg · d^{-1}	Avoid with diabetes
Grape seed extract		Circulatory disorders; varicose veins; atherosclerosis		75–300 mg · d^{-1}	None
Saw palmetto	*Serenoa repens, sabal serrulata*	Benign prostatic hyperplasia; urination problems in males	Liposterolic extract of saw palmetto provides fatty acids, sterols, and esters	200–300 mg · d^{-1}	None
St. John's Wort	*Hypericum perforatum*	Depression; anxiety or nervous unrest; mood disturbance of menopause	Hypericin, flavonoids	900 mg · d^{-1}	Heightens sun sensitivity; interferes with iron absorption
Witch hazel	*Hamamelis virginiana*	Eczema; hemorrhoids; varicose veins	Tannins and volatile oils	As ointment or cream 3–4 times · d^{-1}	Not for internal use; causes stomach irritation
Yohimbe	*Pausinystalia ohimbe*	Impotence; depression	Yohimbine (alkaloid)	15–30 mg · d^{-1}	Use only under medical supervision
Valerian	Heliotrope; setwall; vandal root	Stress reduction; improves sleep; benefits cardiovascular system	Essential oils	300–500 mg before sleep	None

[a]Not truly listed as an herb; usually listed as a supplement

amphetamine overdose a year earlier.[42] Since then, testing has consistently expanded, with initiation of random unannounced drug testing in track and field in 1989. The IOC currently bans the following seven categories of substances:

- Stimulants
- Narcotic analgesics
- Androgenic–anabolic steroids
- β-Blockers
- Diuretics
- Peptide hormones and analogues
- Substances that alter urine sample integrity

Lists of banned substances can be found at the following LWW connection website: http://connection.lww.com/go/mcardle. The competitive athlete should consult with the IOC Medical Commission, national governing bodies (NGBs), and international federations (IFs) for the most up-to-date list of banned substances. The United States Olympic Committee (USOC) provides background information about prohibited substances and methods on their website http://test.olympicusa.org/inside/in_1_1_4_6_5.html#TOC, with links to different sport organization Websites (NGBs and IFs). Contact the USOC Drug Control Program in Colorado Springs to obtain the most recent "Guide to Prohibited Substances and Methods."

Anabolic Steroids

Anabolic steroids gained prominence in the early 1950s for medical use in treating patients deficient in natural androgens or with muscle-wasting diseases. Other legitimate steroid uses include treatment of osteoporosis and severe breast cancer in women and countering the excessive decline in lean body mass and increase in body fat often observed in elderly men, HIV patients, and individuals undergoing kidney dialysis.

The prescription use of steroids is legal in the United States. However, the Anabolic Steroid Control Act of 1990 criminalizes the sale and possession of any anabolic steroid intended for nonmedical use. It also is a felony to buy a known counterfeit steroid or one not approved by the Food and Drug Administration (FDA). Screening for exogenous anabolic steroid use among competitive athletes includes measuring the ratio of testosterone to luteinizing hormone (T:LH) in urine or that of testosterone to epitestosterone (T:E), normally no greater than 2.0. Recent findings indicate that a urinary T:LH ratio ≥30 is a more sensitive marker of anabolic steroid use than the urinary T:E ratio ≥6.0, currently the prohibited level set by the IOC.[185]

INTEGRATIVE QUESTION

A student swears that a chemical compound added to his diet produced profound improvements in weight-lifting performance. Your review of the research literature indicates no ergogenic benefits for this compound. How would you reconcile the discrepancy?

Anabolic steroids have become an integral part of the high-technology scene of competitive American sports, beginning with the United States weight-lifting team (1955), who used Dianabol (modified, synthetic testosterone molecule methandrostenolone). The formulation of other anabolic steroids ushered in a new era in the "drugging" of competitive athletes. An estimated 1 to 3 million athletes (90% of male and 80% of female professional bodybuilders) currently use androgens, often combined with stimulants and diuretics, believing that their use augments training effectiveness.[66] Even in the sport of baseball, *estimates* based on interviews of strength trainers and current players indicate that up to 30% of professional players use anabolic steroids in the hope of performance enhancement.

Structure and Action

Anabolic steroids function in a manner similar to testosterone, the chief male hormone. By binding with special receptor sites on muscle and other tissues, testosterone contributes to male secondary sex characteristics, including gender differences in muscle mass and strength that develop at the onset of puberty. Testosterone production takes place mainly in the testes (95%), with the adrenal glands producing the remainder. Synthetically manipulating the steroid's chemical structure to increase muscle growth (from anabolic tissue building and nitrogen retention) reduces the hormone's androgenic, or masculinizing, effects. Nevertheless, a masculinizing effect of synthetically derived steroids still exists despite chemical alteration, particularly in females.

Athletes typically combine multiple steroid preparations in oral and injectable form, a practice called **stacking**, because they believe that the various androgens differ in physiologic action. They also progressively increase drug dosage—a practice called **pyramiding**—usually in 6- to 12-week cycles. The drug quantity far exceeds the recommended medical dose, often by 40-fold. The athlete then progressively reduces drug dosage in the months before competition to lower the chance of detection during drug testing. The difference between dosages used in research studies and the excess typically used by athletes has greatly contributed to the credibility gap between scientific findings (often, no effect of steroids) and what most in the athletic community believe to be true.

Table 23.1 lists examples of oral and injectable anabolic steroids, including typical retail cost and black market prices (Boston, MA). Black market prices vary considerably in different domestic regions and internationally: conservative estimates suggest at least twice the retail cost up to 100 times retail! In 1989, the FDA published a list of foreign anabolic–androgenic steroids commonly found in the domestic black market: Anabolicum, Andriol, Anadrol, Anatrofin, Asellacrin, Bolasterone, Bolfortan, Crescormin, Curablon, Cyclofenil, Deca-Durabolin, Dianabol, Dihydrolone, Durateston, Dymethyzine, Esiclene, Equipoise, Exoboline, Finaject, Furazabol, Halostein, Hombreol, Iontanyl, Laurabolin, Lipiodex, Metanabol, Methandrostenolone, Nerobol, Nilevar, Nolvadex, Nondrabolin, Nor-Diethylin, Omnifin, Oxandrolone, Oxitosona, Parabolan, Primobolan/Primobolan depot, Primotestin/Primotestin depot, Proviron, Quinalone, Retabolil, Stromba, Sustanon, Testoviron Depot, Thiomucase, Triacana, Trophobolene, Uni-Test Suspension, Undestor. Numerous other synthetic anabolic steroid drugs exist, including the popular European steroid Turinabol.

PRACTICAL EXAMPLE OF STEROID ABUSE. The cycling of steroids coincides with competition. Many athletes use the exercise training model called *periodization* (see Chapter 22, page 513) to structure their drug use. Steroid use coincides with the goal of achieving maximum muscle strength and size at competition. The off-season steroid cycle differs considerably from precompetition conditions for drugs taken and dosages. For example, an 18-week off-season cycle for bodybuilding might include four steroids (Dianabol, Plenastril, Sustanon 250, Dynabolon) taken in higher dosages during week 1 (e.g., Dianabol 120 mg; Plenastril 150 mg) to progressively reduced dosages during week 18 (e.g., Dianabol 10 mg; Plenastril 18 mg during wk 18, but 25 mg in wk 17). In this example, the total dose during week 1 was approximately 1.3 mg per kg body mass for Dianabol and 1.7 mg per kg body mass for Plenastril. The bodybuilder then follows a 6- to 8-week cycle of human chorionic gonadotropin (HCG) and Clomid (brand name for clomiphene citrate, a synthetic hormone usually given to treat female infertility) to increase testosterone concentrations. Tak-

TABLE 23.1 ➤ **EXAMPLES OF ORAL AND INJECTABLE ANABOLIC STEROIDS, INCLUDING TYPICAL RETAIL COST AND BLACK MARKET PRICES**

Generic Name	Commercial Name	Form[a]	Retail Cost[b]	Black Market[b] Cost
Oxymetholone	Anadrol-50	Oral; 50 mg	\$115/100 tabs	\$200–500
Oxandrolone	Oxandrin	Oral; 2.5 mg	\$420/100 tabs	\$600–1600
Stanazolol	Winstrol V	Oral; 2 mg	\$100/100 tabs	\$200–500
Nandrolone Phenpropionate	Durabolin Nandrobolic	Injectable; 25 mg · mL^{-1}	\$27/5 mL vial	\$200–500
Nadrolone Deconate Androlone-D 200	Deca-Durabolin Neo-durabolic	Injectable; 50 mg · mL^{-1}	\$12/2 mL vial	\$400–750

[a]Anabolic steroids are taken by mouth or injected into a muscle. Tablets or capsules taken by mouth are often called "orals." Oral androgens do not metabolize into testosterone but act directly on androgen receptors. The injectable forms, known as "oils" or "waters," usually have longer-lasting effects than orals. Injectables release slowly into the body once the injection enters a muscle (usually the buttocks). One injection (at normal concentrations prescribed medically) can maintain normal serum testosterone levels for 10–14 days. Oral androgens are not as biologically active as the injectable forms.

[b]2001 typical retail prices in the Amherst/Boston area. Prices vary depending on country and local conditions. The black market price reflects a range of prices from various sources, 2001.

ing these hormones in conjunction with exercise training supposedly increases lean body mass above the off-season level. The athlete then cycles to another 20-week regimen of steroids (e.g., Oxandrolone, Masterone, Primobolan, Stromba), using different dosages of each throughout the cycle (going from daily dose of 90 mg of Oxandrolone in wk 1 to 60 mg in wk 12 before competition; 100 mg of Masterone in wk 1 to 500 mg in wk 12; 300 mg Primobolon in wk 1 to 200 mg in wk 12; 350 mg of Stromba in wk 1 to 250 mg in wk 12). Other synthetic hormones often are added to the mix, coupled with high intakes of protein, dietary supplements, and perhaps various herbal preparations designed to further augment an anabolic effect.

A Drug with a Considerable Following

One often pictures steroid abusers as extremely muscular bodybuilders; however, abuse is also frequent in competitive athletes in road cycling, tennis, track and field, and swimming. Surveys of United States Powerlifting Team members indicate that up to two-thirds used androgenic–anabolic steroids.[58,254] In the United States, more than 300,000 men and women took anabolic steroids between 1992 and 1993.[274] Federal authorities conservatively estimate that the emerging business of illegal trafficking in steroids exceeds \$100 million yearly—a figure likely to increase significantly during the next decade. Because many competitive and recreational athletes obtain steroids on the black market, misinformed individuals may take massive and prolonged dosages without medical monitoring and suffer harmful alterations in physiologic function.

Steroid abuse among young boys and girls and its accompanying risks, including extreme virilization and premature cessation of bone growth, remains particularly worrisome.[3,95] Boys and girls as young as 11 years of age use anabolic–androgenic steroids.[81] Approximately 1 of 15 high school students or about one-half million adolescents (250,000 high school seniors) use steroids—youngsters also likely to abuse other illicit drugs and share needles.[31,71] Data from the National Institutes of Drug Abuse indicate that about 175,000 teenage girls in the United States report taking an anabolic steroid at least once within a year of the time surveyed; for teenage boys, the number rises to 325,000. Teenagers cite improved athletic performance as the most common reason for taking steroids, although 25% acknowledged enhanced appearance as a main reason.[31] In this regard, a body image disturbance may contribute to anabolic steroid abuse among teenagers and young men.[267]

Effectiveness Questioned

For more than four decades, researchers and athletes have debated the true effect of anabolic steroids on human body composition and exercise performance. Much of the confusion about anabolic steroids' ergogenic effectiveness stems from variations in experimental design, control group, specific drugs and dosages (athletes use higher dosages than those typically prescribed in clinical treatment and human research), treatment duration, accompanying nutritional supplementation, training intensity, evaluation techniques, previous experience of subjects, and individual differences in responsiveness to a drug's effect.[39] Also, the relatively small residual androgenic effect of the steroid may facilitate central nervous system activation to make the athlete more aggressive (so-called *roid rage*), competitive, and fatigue resistant. Such facilitatory effects allow the athlete to train harder for a longer time or to believe that augmented training effects have actually occurred.[154] Abnormal mood alterations and psychiatric dysfunction sometimes accompany androgen use.[228]

Research with animals suggests that anabolic steroid treatment combined with exercise and adequate protein intake stimulates protein synthesis an increases muscle protein content (myosin, myofibrillar, sarcoplasmic factors).[208] In contrast, other research found that steroid treatment did not benefit leg muscle weight of rats subjected to functional overload by surgical removal of the synergistic muscle.[162] The researchers concluded that treatment with anabolic steroids did not complement functional overload to stimulate additional muscular development.

The situation with humans often becomes difficult to interpret. Some studies show that steroid use by men who train augments body mass gains and reduces body fat, while other studies show no effect on strength and power or body composition, even with sufficient energy and protein intake to support an anabolic effect.[84,144,264] When steroid use produces body mass gains, the compositional nature of the gains (water, muscle, fat) remains unclear. Patients receiving dialysis and those infected with the HIV virus commonly experience malnutrition, reduced muscle mass, and chronic fatigue. Dialysis patients given 6 months of supplementation with the anabolic steroid nandrolone decanoate exhibited significantly increased lean body mass and level of daily function.[131] Similarly, in men with HIV, a moderately supraphysiologic androgen regimen that included the anabolic steroid oxandrolone increased lean tissue accrual and muscular strength gains from resistance exercise training substantially more than physiologic testosterone replacement alone.[226]

Dosage Is an Important Factor

In many instances, dosage variations contribute to the confusion and credibility gap between scientist and steroid user regarding the ergogenic effectiveness of anabolic steroids. One study focused on 43 healthy men with some resistance-training experience.[84] Experimental controls accounted for diet (energy and protein intake) and exercise (standard weight lifting, 3 times weekly), with steroid dosage (600 mg of testosterone enanthate injected weekly or placebo) exceeding values in previous studies with humans. Figure 23.1 shows changes from baseline average values for fat-free body mass (FFM; hydrostatic weighing), triceps and quadriceps cross-sectional muscle areas (magnetic resonance imaging), and muscle strength (1-RM) after 10 weeks of treatment. The men who received the hormone while continuing to weight train gained about 0.5 kg of lean tissue weekly, with no increase in body fat over the treatment period. Even the group receiving the drug and not training exhibited significantly increased muscle mass and strength, compared with men receiving the placebo, but their increases averaged less than those of men who trained while taking testosterone. The researchers emphasized that that they did not design their study to justify or endorse steroid use for athletic purposes, because of the health risks (see below). These data, however, did indicate that medically supervised anabolic steroid treatment could potentially restore and enhance muscle mass in those suffering from tissue-wasting diseases.

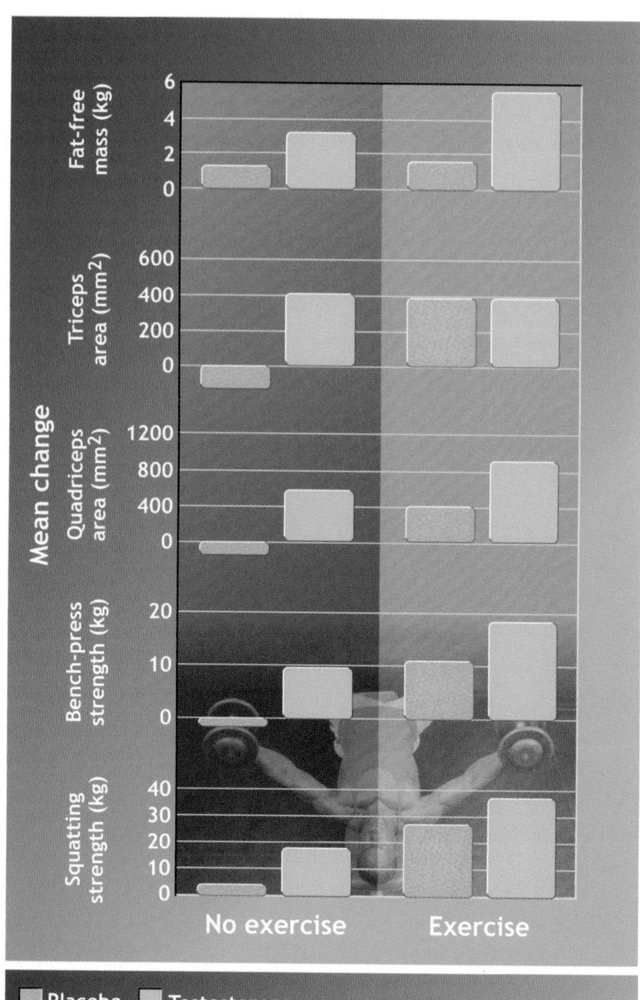

FIGURE 23.1 • Changes from baseline in average fat-free body mass, triceps and quadriceps cross-sectional areas, and muscle strength in bench press and squatting exercises over 10 weeks of testosterone treatment. (From Bhasin S, et al. The effects of supraphysiological doses of testosterone on muscle size and strength in normal men. N Engl J Med 1996;335:1.)

Do Risks Exist?

Whether anabolic steroid use by athletes carries health risks remains controversial, because research on risk involves medical observations of hospitalized patients treated for anemia, renal insufficiency, impotence, or pituitary gland dysfunction.[227] *In our opinion, the infrequent but distinct possibility of harmful side effects from anabolic steroids, particularly orally administered steroids, greatly outweighs any potential ergogenic effect.* Prolonged high dosages of steroids (often at levels 10 to 200 times therapeutic recommendations[34]) can lead to long-lasting impairment of normal testosterone endocrine function. In five male power athletes, for example, 26 weeks of steroid administration reduced serum testosterone to less than one-half the level when the study began, with the effect lasting throughout a 12- to 16-week follow-up.[84] Infertility, reduced sperm concentrations (azoospermia), and decreased testicular volume pose additional problems for the steroid user.[90] Gonadal function usually returns to normal within several months. Other hormonal alterations during steroid use by males include a sevenfold increase in estradiol concentration, the major female hormone. The higher estradiol level represented the average value for normal females, which possibly explains the **gyneco-**

mastia (usually irreversible, excessive development of the male mammary glands, sometimes secreting milk) often reported among males who take anabolic steroids.

Steroid use with exercise training may produce connective tissue damage that decreases tendon tensile strength and elastic compliance.[150,231,249] Furthermore, steroids cause (1) chronic stimulation of the prostate gland (with possible size increase), (2) injury and functional alterations in cardiovascular function and myocardial cell cultures, (3) possible pathologic ventricular growth and decreased diastolic relaxation (when combined with resistance training), and (4) increased blood platelet aggregation.[1,68,69,168] The latter could easily compromise cardiovascular system health and function and possibly increase risk of stroke and myocardial infarction.

Dramatic life-shortening resulted for adult rats exposed for 6 months to the type and relative levels of steroids used by athletes.[28] One year after termination of steroid exposure, 52% of mice given a high steroid dose had died, compared with 35% of those given a low steroid dosage and only 12% of the control animals given no exogenous hormones (Fig. 23.2). Autopsy of steroid-treated mice revealed a broad array of pathologic effects that did not appear until long after cessation of steroid use. Those most prevalent included liver and kidney tumors, lymphosarcomas, and heart damage, frequently in combination. A 6-month exposure represents about one-fifth of a male mouse's life expectancy, a relative duration considerably longer than the exposure of most humans to steroid use. However, several of the pathologic effects, particularly liver damage, represent typical effects seen in athletes taking steroids. If such findings prove applicable to humans, several decades may elapse before the true negative effects of anabolic steroid use emerge.

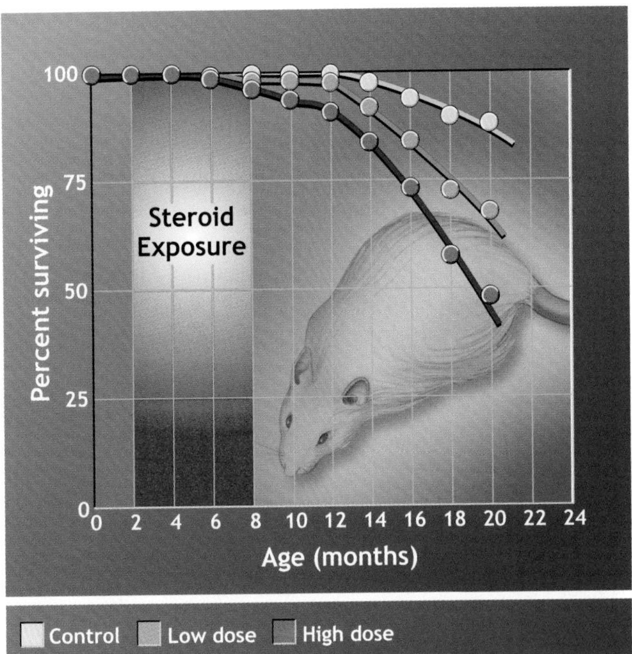

FIGURE 23.2 • Life-shortening effects of exogenous anabolic steroid use in mice. (Modified from Bronson FH, Matherne CM. Exposure to anabolic–androgenic steroids shortens life span of male mice. Med Sci Sports Exerc 1997;29:615.)

STEROID USE AND LIFE-THREATENING DISEASE. Table 23.2 lists the adverse effects and medical risks of anabolic steroid use. Concern centers on possible links between androgen abuse and abnormal liver function.[172] Because the liver almost exclusively metabolizes androgens, it becomes susceptible to damage from long-term steroid use and toxic excess, particularly steroids containing a 17-alkyl group. The development of localized blood-filled lesions, a condition called **peliosis hepatis**, is one of the serious effects of androgens on the liver.[35] In the extreme case, the liver eventually fails and the patient dies. We present these data not as a scare tactic but to emphasize the potentially serious adverse effects, even when a physician prescribes the drug in the recommended dosage. Although patients often take steroids for a longer duration than athletes, some athletes take steroids on and off for years, at dosages exceeding typical therapeutic levels (50–200 mg · d^{-1} versus the usual therapeutic dosage of 5–20 mg · d^{-1}). Preliminary data also suggest that anabolic

TABLE 23.2 ➤ SIDE EFFECTS AND MEDICAL RISKS OF ANABOLIC STEROID USE

Males: Increase	Males: Decrease	Females: Increase	Females: Decrease
Testicular atrophy	Sperm count	Voice change (deepening)	Breast tissue
Gynecomastia	Testosterone levels	Facial hair	
		Menstrual irregularities	
		Clitoral enlargement	

Males and Females: Increase	Decrease	Possible
LDL-C	HDL-C	Hypertension
LDL-C/HDL-C		Connective tissue damage
Potential for neoplastic liver disease		Myocardial damage
Aggressiveness, hyperactivity, irritability		Myocardial infarction
Withdrawal and depression when steroid use stops		Impaired thyroid function
Acne		Altered myocardial structure
Peliosis hepatitis		

steroids interfere with the responsiveness of the body's immune system.[36] The clinical significance of these findings awaits further research.

STEROID USE AND PLASMA LIPOPROTEINS. Anabolic steroid use (particularly the orally active 17-alkylated androgens) by healthy men and women rapidly reduces high-density-lipoprotein cholesterol (HDL-C) levels, elevates both low-density-lipoprotein cholesterol (LDL-C) and total cholesterol levels,[257] and reduces the HDL-C:LDL-C ratio.[49] Weight lifters who used anabolic steroids averaged an HDL-C level of 26 mg · dL^{-1} compared with 50 mg · dL^{-1} for weight lifters not taking this drug![136] Reducing HDL-C to this level significantly increases a steroid user's risk of coronary artery disease. The significantly low HDL-C levels among weight lifters remain low, even after they abstain for at least 8 weeks between consecutive steroid cycles.[212] The long-term effects of steroid use on cardiovascular morbidity and mortality are unknown.

ACSM POSITION STATEMENT ON ANABOLIC STEROIDS . As part of their long-range educational program, the **American College of Sports Medicine (ACSM)** has taken a stand on the use and abuse of anabolic–androgenic steroids. We endorse their position, which follows[4]:

AMERICAN COLLEGE OF SPORTS MEDICINE: POSITION STAND ON USE OF ANABOLIC STEROIDS

Based on a comprehensive survey of the world literature and a careful analysis of the claims made for and against the efficacy of anabolic–androgenic steroids in improving human physical performance, it is the position of the American College of Sports Medicine that:

- Anabolic–androgenic steroids in the presence of an adequate diet and training can contribute to increases in body weight, often in the lean mass compartment.
- The gains in muscular strength achieved through high-intensity exercise and proper diet can occur by the increased use of anabolic–androgenic steroids in some individuals.
- Anabolic–androgenic steroids do not increase aerobic power or capacity for muscular exercise.
- Anabolic–androgenic steroids have been associated with adverse effects on the liver, cardiovascular system, reproductive system, and psychologic status in therapeutic trials and in limited research on athletes. Until further research is completed, the potential hazards of the use of the anabolic–androgenic steroids in athletes must include those found in therapeutic trials.
- The use of anabolic–androgenic steroids by athletes is contrary to the rules and ethical principles of athletic competition as set forth by many of the sports governing bodies. The American College of Sports Medicine supports these ethical principles and deplores the use of anabolic–androgenic steroids by athletes.

ADDITIONAL RISKS FOR FEMALES . Besides the broad range of potential adverse effects discussed previously, females have additional concerns about dangers from anabolic steroid use. These include virilization (more apparent than in men), disruption of normal growth pattern by premature closure of the plates for bone growth (also for boys), altered menstrual function, dramatic increase in sebaceous gland size, acne, hirsutism (excessive body and facial hair), and generally irreversible deepening of the voice, decreased breast size, enlarged clitoris, and hair loss. Serum levels of LH, FSH, progesterone, and estrogens also decline, which may negatively affect follicle formation, ovulation, and menstrual function. The long-term effects of steroid use on reproductive function, including possible sterility, require further clarification.

Growth Hormone: Genetic Engineering Comes to Sports

Human growth hormone (**GH** or hGH), also known as **somatotropin**, currently competes with anabolic steroids in the illicit market of alleged tissue-building, performance-enhancing drugs (the Atlanta Olympics were dubbed by many the "Growth Hormone Games"). The adenohypophysis of the pituitary gland produces GH, which serves as a potent anabolic and lipolytic agent intimately involved in tissue-building processes and growth. Specifically, GH stimulates bone and cartilage growth, enhances fatty acid oxidation, and reduces glucose and amino acid breakdown.[270] Reduced GH secretion accounts for some of the decrease in FFM and increase in fat mass that accompanies aging, a condition that reverses somewhat with exogenous recombinant GH supplements produced by genetically engineered bacteria.[211] Healthy elderly men who received GH supplements exhibited significantly increased FFM (4.3%) and decreased fat mass (13.1%).[182] *Supplementation, however, did not reverse the negative effects of aging on functional measures of muscular strength and aerobic capacity.* Furthermore, men receiving the supplement experienced hand stiffness, malaise, arthralgias, and lower-extremity edema.

Excessive GH production during skeletal growth produces **gigantism**, an endocrine and metabolic disorder that causes abnormal size or overgrowth of the entire body or any of its parts. Excessive hormone production following growth cessation produces the irreversible disorder **acromegaly**, characterized by enlarged hands, feet, and facial features. Medically, children who suffer from kidney failure or who produce insufficient GH receive thrice-weekly biosynthetic GH injections until adolescence to help them achieve near-normal size.[117] In young adults with hypopituitarism, GH replacement therapy improves muscle volume, isometric strength, and exercise capacity.[132,214]

No Unanimity Among Researchers

At first glance, GH use seems appealing to strength and power athletes because at physiologic levels, this hormone stimulates amino acid uptake and muscle protein synthesis, while enhancing fat breakdown and conserving glycogen reserves.[164] However, few well-controlled studies have examined how GH supplements affect healthy subjects undergoing exercise training. In one study, six well-trained men maintained a high-protein diet while taking either biosynthetic GH or a placebo.[57] During 6 weeks of standard resistance training with GH, percentage body fat decreased and FFM increased significantly. No changes in body composition occurred for the group training with the placebo. However, subsequent investigations have not replicated these findings.[67,272] For example, 16 previously sedentary young men participating in a 12-week resistance-training program received recombinant human GH supplements ($40\ \mu g \cdot kg^{-1} \cdot d^{-1}$) or a placebo.[271] Table 23.3 shows that FFM, total body water, and whole-body protein synthesis increased more in the GH recipients, with no significant differences between groups in (1) fractional rate of protein synthesis in skeletal muscle, (2) torso and limb circumferences, or (3) muscle function in dynamic and static strength measures. The authors attributed the greater increase in whole-body protein synthesis in the GH group to a possible increase in nitrogen retention in lean tissue other than skeletal muscle—for example, connective tissue, fluid, and noncontractile protein.

Because GH occurs naturally in the body, ready detection of its use as an ergogenic substance is difficult. However, blood markers are currently available for use in screening. Such testing requires a change in current Olympic policy that permits only urine testing.[22,60] Non-prescription GH can only be obtained on the black market and often in an adulterated form. The use of human cadaver–derived GH (used until May, 1985 by U.S. physicians to treat children of short stature) greatly increases the risk for contracting Creutzfeldt-Jakob disease, an infectious, incurable, and fatal brain-deteriorating disorder. A synthetic form of GH (Protoropin and Humantrope), produced by genetic engineering, currently treats GH-deficient children (cost $20,000 to $40,000 per year). Undoubtedly, child athletes who receive GH in the belief that they will gain a competitive edge will suffer increased incidence of gigantism, while adults will develop acromegalic syndrome. Additional, less obvious side effects include insulin resistance leading to type 2 diabetes, water retention, and carpal tunnel compression syndrome.

DHEA: A Worrisome Trend

Dehydroepiandersterone (**DHEA** and its sulfated ester, DHEA sulfate, or DHEAS) is a relatively weak steroid hormone synthesized primarily from cholesterol by the adrenal cortex of primates. More DHEA (commonly referred to as "mother hormone") is produced by the body than all other known steroids. Its chemical structure closely resembles the sex hormones testosterone and estrogen, and a small amount of DHEA serves as precursor for these hormones in men and women. News reports and advertisements tout DHEA as a "superhormone," a Holy Grail that increases testosterone production, bolsters the immune system, preserves youth, invigorates sex life, decreases joint pain and fatigue, and counters the debilitating effects of aging. Sites on the World Wide Web regularly extol its benefits.

Because DHEA occurs naturally, the FDA exerts no control over its distribution or claims for its action and effectiveness. The Drug Enforcement Administration does not consider DHEA an anabolic steroid as defined in section 102(6) of the Controlled Substances Act. Instead, DHEA fits the definition of a dietary supplement. According to regulations, *dietary supplement* refers to a product (other than tobacco) intended to supplement the diet that bears or contains one or more of the following dietary ingredients: (1) vitamin, (2) mineral, (3) herb or other botanical, (4) amino acid, (5) dietary substance for use by humans to supplement the diet by increasing the total diet intake, (6) a concentrate, metabolite, constituent, extract, or combination of any ingredient described in (1) to (5). Section 201(g) of the Federal Food, Drug and Cosmetic Act defines a *drug* (in contrast to *dietary supplement*) as an article intended for use in diagnosis, cure, mitigation, treatment, or disease prevention in man or other animals. Thus, if labels on DHEA-containing products recommend DHEA for disease treatment or prevention, the FDA could regulate the product as a drug.

The lay press, mail order, and health food industry describe DHEA as a pill (even available as a chewing gum, each piece containing 25 mg) to cure just about any bodily dysfunction—protect against cancer, heart disease, diabetes, and osteoporosis; enhance sexual drive; facilitate lean tissue gain

TABLE 23.3 ➤ MAXIMAL FORCE PRODUCTION OF KNEE EXTENSOR AND FLEXOR MUSCLE GROUPS BEFORE AND AFTER TRAINING WITH OR WITHOUT GROWTH HORMONE SUPPLEMENTS

	Exercise plus Placebo			Exercise plus GH		
	Initial	Final	% Change	Initial	Final	% Change
Concentric						
Knee extensors	212 ±13[a]	248 ±10	+17	191 ±11	214 ±9	+12
Knee flexors	137 ±11[a]	158 ±7	+15	122 ±12	143 ±6	+17
Isometric						
Knee extensors	220 ±13[a]	252 ±13	+14	198 ±15	207 ±7	+5
Knee flexors	131 ±8[a]	158 ±8	+20	127 ±13	140 ±16	+10

[a]Values are mean ±SE. Maximum force (N · m) determined using a Cybex dynamometer. Concentric force measured at $60° \cdot s^{-1}$ angular velocity. Isometric force measured at 135° of knee extension. The maximum concentric force production of the knee flexor and extensor muscles increased significantly in both groups ($P < 0.05$), but these increments and the increments in maximum isometric force production were not greater in the exercise plus GH group.
From Yarasheski KF: et al. Effect of growth hormone and resistance exercise on muscle growth in young men. Am J Physiol 1992;262:E261.

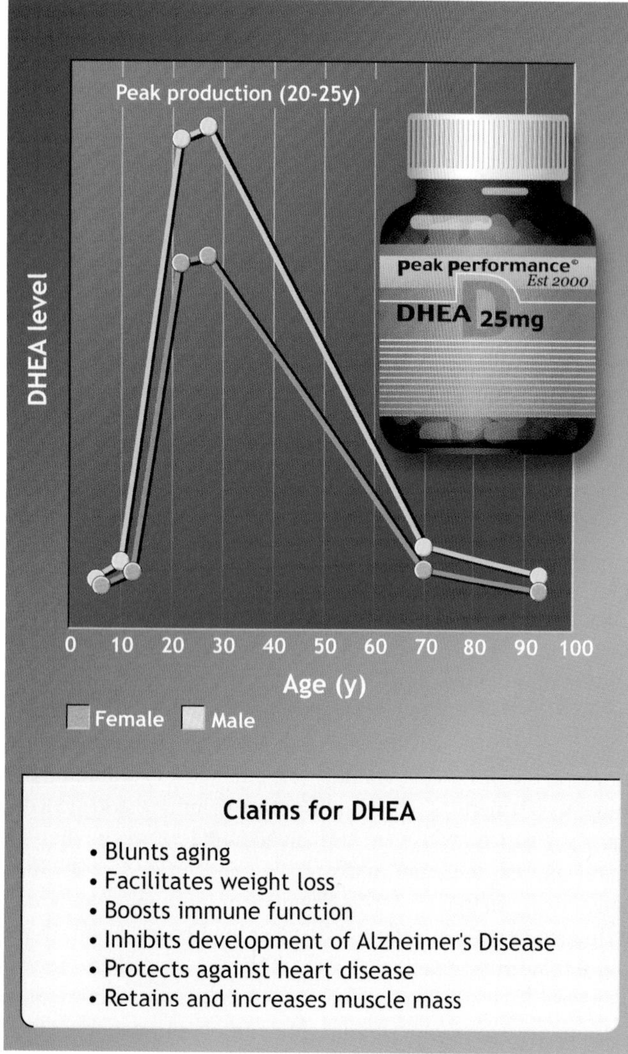

FIGURE 23.3 • Generalized trend for plasma levels of DHEA for men and women over a lifetime.

and body fat loss; enhance mood and memory; boost immunity to diverse infectious diseases including AIDS; and extend life. The hormone's detractors consider it the "snake oil" of the 21st century. The IOC and USOC have placed DHEA on their banned substance lists at zero-tolerance levels.

Figure 23.3 illustrates the generalized trend for plasma DHEA levels during a lifetime, with six common claims made by manufacturers of DHEA supplements.[118,248] Boys and girls have substantial levels of DHEA at birth, which then decline sharply. DHEA production increases steadily from age 6 to 10 years (which may contribute to the beginning of puberty and sexuality), with peak production (higher in males than females) between ages 20 and 25 years. In contrast to the glucocorticoid and mineralocorticoid adrenal steroids, whose plasma levels remain relatively high with aging, DHEA levels undergo a long, slow decline after age 30. By age 75, the plasma level is only about 20% of that in young adults. This has led to speculation that plasma DHEA levels might serve as a biochemical marker of biologic aging and disease susceptibility.[17] Popular reasoning concludes that supplementing with DHEA blunts the negative effects of aging by raising plasma levels to more "youthful" concentrations. In fact, people supplement with this "natural" hormone just in case it proves beneficial—without considering the potential for biologic harm.

An Unregulated Compound with Uncertain Safety

In 1994, the FDA reclassified DHEA (along with many other "natural" chemicals under the Dietary Supplement and Education Act) from the category of unapproved new drug (prescription required) to a dietary supplement for over-the-counter sale without prescription. Pharmaceutical companies synthesize DHEA from chemical ingredients or extract it from wild yams. Many consider the current unregulated and unmonitored use of DHEA among healthy men and women (daily dosage varies from 5 to 10 mg to as much as 2000 mg) a disaster waiting to happen. Despite its quantitative significance as a hormone, researchers know little about DHEA, particularly with respect to the following:

- Health and aging
- Cellular or molecular mechanism(s) of action
- Possible receptor site interaction (although its sulfate interacts with brain receptors for the neurotransmitter γ-aminobutyric acid [GABA])
- Potential for adverse effects from exogenous dosage, particularly among young adults with normal DHEA levels

Furthermore, appropriate DHEA dosage for humans remains uncertain. Concern exists about possible harmful effects on blood lipids, glucose tolerance, and prostate gland health, particularly because medical problems associated with hormone supplementation often do not appear until years after initiation of drug use. The National Institute on Aging mounted a media blitz to warn Americans to remain cautious about taking such "miracle" compounds (including DHEA) readily purchased through mainstream grocery chains, drug and nutrition stores, health clubs, mail-order catalogs, and the Internet.

Early support for DHEA comes from studies of rodents fed daily supplements.[61,73,97] Treatment indicated beneficial effects in preventing cancer, atherosclerosis, viral infections, obesity, and diabetes; enhancing immune function; and even extending life span. Scientists have argued, however, that research findings using rats and mice—who produce little if any DHEA—do not necessarily apply to healthy humans. Cross-sectional observations relating DHEA levels to risk of death from heart disease provided early indirect evidence for a beneficial effect in humans. A high DHEA level conferred protection in men, while for women, an elevated DHEA level represented an increased heart disease risk. Subsequent research showed only a moderate protective association for men and no association for women. Studies also suggest that DHEA supplements may provide cardioprotection during aging (more beneficial in men than women),[124] boost immune function in disease,[245] and perhaps provide antioxidant protection.[10]

In other research on humans, eight men and eight women (ages 50 to 65 y) received either 100 mg of DHEA or a placebo daily for 3 months, and the other treatment for the next 3 months.[173] Both men and women exhibited a slight 1.2% increase in lean body mass during DHEA supplementation, compared with placebo. Fat mass decreased in the men but increased slightly in the women. Chemical markers also indicated improved immune function. These findings suggest some positive effects of exogenous DHEA on muscle mass and immune function in middle-aged men and women, but no data exist for young adults. Subsequent research evaluated the effect of short-term ingestion of 50 mg DHEA daily on serum steroid hormones and the effect of 8 weeks of supplementation (150 mg daily) on resistance-training adaptations in young men.[28] Although short-term supplementation rapidly increased serum androstenedione (see next section) concentrations, it exerted *no effect* on serum testosterone and estrogen concentrations. Furthermore, long-term DHEA supplementation elevated serum androstenedione levels, but had *no effect* on anabolic hormones, serum lipids, liver enzymes, muscular strength, and lean body mass, compared with placebo given to men undergoing similar training.

Concern exists about the effect of unregulated long-term DHEA supplementation (particularly ≥50 mg daily) on bodily function and overall health. Converting DHEA into potent androgens such as testosterone promotes facial hair growth in females and alters normal menstrual function. Like exogenous anabolic steroids, DHEA appears to lower HDL-C levels, which increases heart disease risk. Limited, conflicting data exist concerning its effects on breast cancer risk. Clinicians have expressed fear that elevating plasma DHEA by supplementation might stimulate the growth of otherwise dormant prostate gland tumors or cause benign hypertrophy of the prostate gland itself. If cancer exists, DHEA may accelerate its growth. *Despite its popularity among exercise enthusiasts, no data support an ergogenic effect of exogenous DHEA on young adult men and women.*

Androstenedione: Nutritional Supplement or Potentially Harmful Drug?

Many athletes use the over-the-counter "nutritional" supplement, **androstenedione** (in addition to norandrostenediol and norandrostenedione, which convert to the steroid nandrolone), believing that it stimulates production of endogenous testosterone, enables them to train harder, builds muscle mass, and repairs injury more rapidly. Found naturally in meat and extracts of some plants, the World Wide Web touts androstenedione as "a prohormone, a metabolite only one step away from the biosynthesis of testosterone." The National Football League, the National Collegiate Athletic Association, the Men's Tennis Association, and the IOC ban its use because they feel it provides unfair competitive advantage and may endanger health, like anabolic steroids. The IOC banned the1996 Olympic shot-put gold medalist for life because he used androstenedione. Presently, Major League Baseball, the National Basketball Association, and the National Hockey League do not forbid its use.

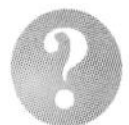

INTEGRATIVE QUESTION

Respond to the question: "If hormones such as testosterone, growth hormone, and DHEA occur naturally in the body, what harm could exist in supplementing with these 'natural' compounds?"

Originally developed by East Germany in the 1970s to enhance performance of their elite athletes, androstenedione was first commercially manufactured and sold in the United States in 1996. By calling the substance a supplement and avoiding any claims of medical benefit, the 1994 FDA rules enable marketing of androstenedione as a food ($800 million in sales yearly on the Internet and over the counter). Because many countries consider androstenedione a controlled substance, international athletes travel to the United States to purchase the compound, further contributing to the supplement industry's greater than $15 billion total yearly sales. Currently available are an androstenedione-containing chewing gum and a steroid lozenge that dissolves under the tongue.

Androstenedione is an intermediate (precursor) hormone between DHEA and testosterone, which aids the liver in synthesizing other biologically active steroid hormones. It is normally produced by the adrenal glands and gonads and converted to testosterone enzymatically by 17β-hydroxysteroid dehydrogenase found in diverse tissues of the body. Androstenedione is also an estrogen precursor.

Little scientific evidence supports claims of androstenedione's effectiveness or anabolic qualities.[65] To date, only one study has systematically evaluated whether short- and long-term oral androstenedione supplementation elevates blood testosterone concentrations or enhances muscle size and strength gains during resistance training.[139] In one phase of the investigation, 10 young-adult men received either a single 100-mg dose of androstenedione or a placebo containing 250 mg of rice flour. Figure 23.4A shows that serum androstenedione rose 175% during the first 60 minutes following ingestion and then rose further to about 350% above baseline values between minutes 90 and 270. However, short-term androstenedione supplementation did *not* affect serum concentrations of either free or total testosterone. In the experiment's second phase, 20 young, untrained men received either 300 mg of androstenedione daily ($n = 10$) or 250 mg of a rice flour placebo daily during weeks 1, 2, 4, 5, 7, and 8 of an 8-week total-body resistance-training program.

Serum androstenedione levels increased 100% in the androstenedione-supplemented group and remained elevated throughout training. Although serum testosterone levels (Fig. 23.4B) remained significantly higher in the androstenedione-supplemented group than in the placebo group before and following supplementation, free and total testosterone levels in serum remained unaltered for both groups as a result of the supplementation–training period. However, serum estradiol and estrone concentrations only increased significantly during

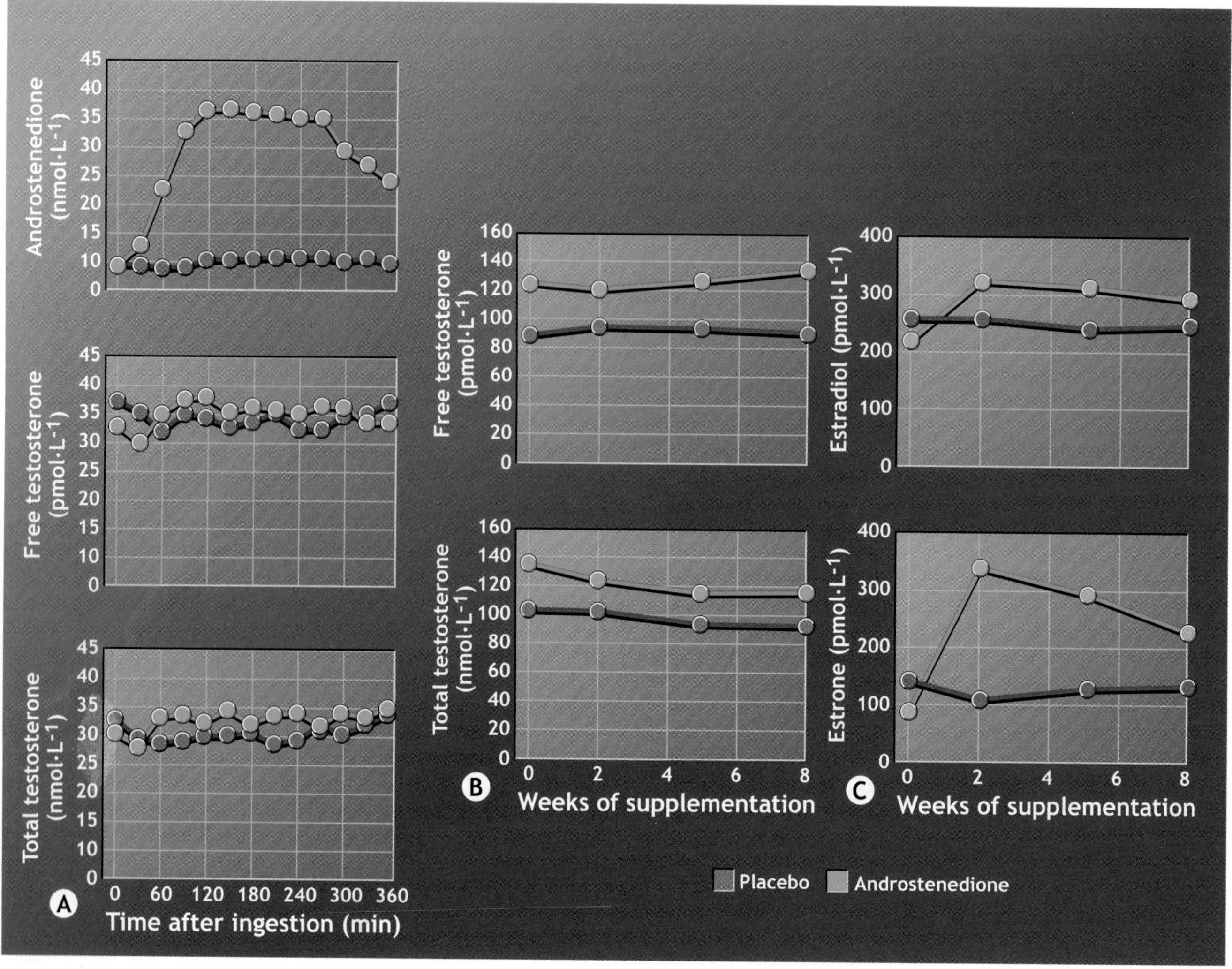

FIGURE 23.4 • **A**. Effect of acute (single dose) exogenous supplementation with 100 mg of androstenedione or placebo on serum concentrations of androstenedione and free and total testosterone. **B**. Serum free and total testosterone, and (**C**) serum estradiol and estrone with 300-mg daily supplementation of androstenedione (n = 9) and placebo (n = 10) during 8 weeks of resistance training. (From King DS, et al. Effect of oral androstenedione on serum testosterone and adaptations to resistance training in young men. JAMA 1999;281:2020.)

training for the group receiving the supplement, suggesting increased aromatization of the ingested androstenedione to estrogens (Fig. 23.4C). Furthermore, while resistance training significantly increased muscle strength and lean body mass and reduced body fat for both groups, no synergistic effect emerged for the group supplemented with androstenedione. The supplement did, however, cause a 12% (significant) HDL-C *reduction* after only 2 weeks, which remained lower for the 8 weeks of training and supplementation. Serum liver enzyme concentrations remained within normal limits for both groups throughout the experimental period.

Taken together, these findings indicate *no effect* of androstenedione supplementation on (1) basal serum concentrations of testosterone or (2) training response in terms of muscle size and strength and body composition. The potentially significant negative effects of the HDL-C reduction on overall heart disease risk and the elevated serum estrogen levels on risk of gynecomastia and possibly pancreatic and other cancers are worrisome. These findings must be viewed within the context of this specific study, because test subjects took far smaller dosages of androstenedione than are routinely taken by bodybuilders and other athletes.

Questions have concerned the legal use of androstenedione by professional baseball players during the 1998 season in their attempt to break the home run records of Babe Ruth and Roger Maris. The sport-related issues focus on (1) whether supplementation causes significant increases in muscular strength and power and (2) whether any fitness increases actually transfer to improved performance in the diverse, precise motor skills required in baseball, basketball, ice and field hockey, soccer, and golf. If positive effects occur, then scientists can objectively assess any improvements in such tasks. As far as we know, no reliable evidence demonstrates such sport-specific benefits. Further studies in larger groups of men and women for longer periods must determine what dosage, if any, raises testosterone to high enough levels for a long enough time to provide ergogenic effects and whether such use causes harm. Currently, some athletes supplement with a daily dose of androstenedione in the range of 500 to 1200 mg.

Competitive Athletes Beware

Recent research raises concern among elite athletes that androstenedione use can cause failure of a urine test for the banned anabolic steroid nandrolone.[43] This occurs because the supplement often contains contamination with trace amounts of the metabolite 19-norandrosterone, the standard marker that signals nandrolone use. Many brands of androstenedione preparations are grossly mislabeled. Analysis of nine different brands of 100-mg doses also indicate wide fluctuations in overall content ranging from zero to 103 mg of androstenedione, with one brand also containing testosterone.

INTEGRATIVE QUESTION

Outline the points you would make in a talk to a high school football team concerning whether or not they should consider using performance-enhancing chemicals and hormones.

Amino Acid Supplements for an Anabolic Effect

An emerging trend involves using nutrition as a legal alternative for "activating" the body's normal anabolic mechanisms. Highly specific dietary changes supposedly create a hormonal milieu that facilitates protein synthesis in skeletal muscle. More than 100 companies in the United States promote such alleged ergogenic stimulants. Weight lifters, bodybuilders, and fitness enthusiasts use amino acid supplements, believing that they boost the body's natural production of the anabolic hormones testosterone, GH, insulin, or insulin-like growth factor I (IGF-I) and so improve muscle size and strength and decrease body fat.[74,109] The rationale for trying nutritional ergogenic stimulants comes from the clinical use of amino acid infusion or ingestion to regulate anabolic hormones in deficient patients.

Research on healthy subjects does not provide convincing evidence for an ergogenic effect of oral amino acid supplements on hormone secretion, training responsiveness, or exercise performance. For example, in studies with appropriate design and statistical analysis, supplements of arginine, lysine, ornithine, tyrosine, and other amino acids, either singly or in combination, produced no effect on GH levels,[83,145] insulin secretion,[30,83] diverse measures of anaerobic power,[82] or all-out running performance at $\dot{V}O_{2max}$.[225] Furthermore, elite junior weight-lifters who supplemented with all 20 amino acids showed no improvement in physical performance or changes in resting or exercise levels of testosterone, cortisol, or GH.[87] Such findings support the position that taking amino acids in the quantities recommended in commercial supplements does not benefit the hormonal profile, body composition and muscle size, and exercise performance. Additionally, the indiscriminate use of amino acid supplements at dosages considered pharmacologic rather than nutritional raises the possibility of direct toxic effects or the creation of an amino acid imbalance.[156]

Stimulating an Anabolic Effect

Resistance training generally stimulates both protein synthesis and protein degradation in exercised muscle fibers. Muscle hypertrophy occurs when a net increase in protein synthesis results from a shift in the body's normal dynamic state of protein synthesis and degradation. The normal hormonal milieu (e.g., insulin and GH levels) in the period following resistance exercise stimulates the muscle fiber's anabolic processes while blunting muscle protein degradation. Dietary modifications that increase amino acid transport into muscles raise energy availability or increase anabolic hormones should theoretically augment the training effects by increasing the rate of muscle anabolism and/or depressing catabolism. Either effect should create a positive body protein balance for improved muscular growth and strength.

CARBOHYDRATE–PROTEIN SUPPLEMENTATION IN RECOVERY MAY AUGMENT HORMONAL RESPONSE TO RESISTANCE EXERCISE. A study of hormone dynamics indicates potential ergogenic effects from carbohydrate and/or protein supplements *immediately following* resistance training.[44] Nine drug-free male weight lifters with at least 2 years of resistance-training experience consumed carbohydrate and protein supplements immediately after a standard resistance-training workout. Treatment included either (1) placebo of pure water or a supplement of (2) carbohydrate (1.5 g per kg body mass), (3) protein (1.38 g per kg body mass), or (4) carbohydrate/protein (1.06 g carbohydrate plus 0.41 g protein per kg body mass) consumed immediately following and then 2 hours after the training session. Compared with the placebo condition, each nutritive supplement produced a hormonal environment (elevated plasma insulin and GH concentrations) during recovery that was conducive to protein synthesis and muscle tissue growth. Subsequent research from the same laboratory showed that protein–carbohydrate supplementation before and after resistance training altered the metabolic and hormonal responses to 3 consecutive days of heavy resistance training.[142] Changes in the immediate recovery period included increases in the concentration of glucose, insulin, GH, and IGF-I and decreased blood lactate concentration. Such data provide indirect evidence for a possible training benefit (e.g., enhanced glycogen and protein synthesis in recovery) of increasing carbohydrate or protein intake immediately after a resistance-training workout. However, data must still document actual augmented protein synthesis, muscle growth, and muscle strength from these dietary manipulations in resistance training.

POSTEXERCISE GLUCOSE AUGMENTS PROTEIN BALANCE AFTER RESISTANCE-TRAINING WORKOUTS. Research with postexercise glucose ingestion complements the previously described studies of carbohydrate/protein supplementation following resis-

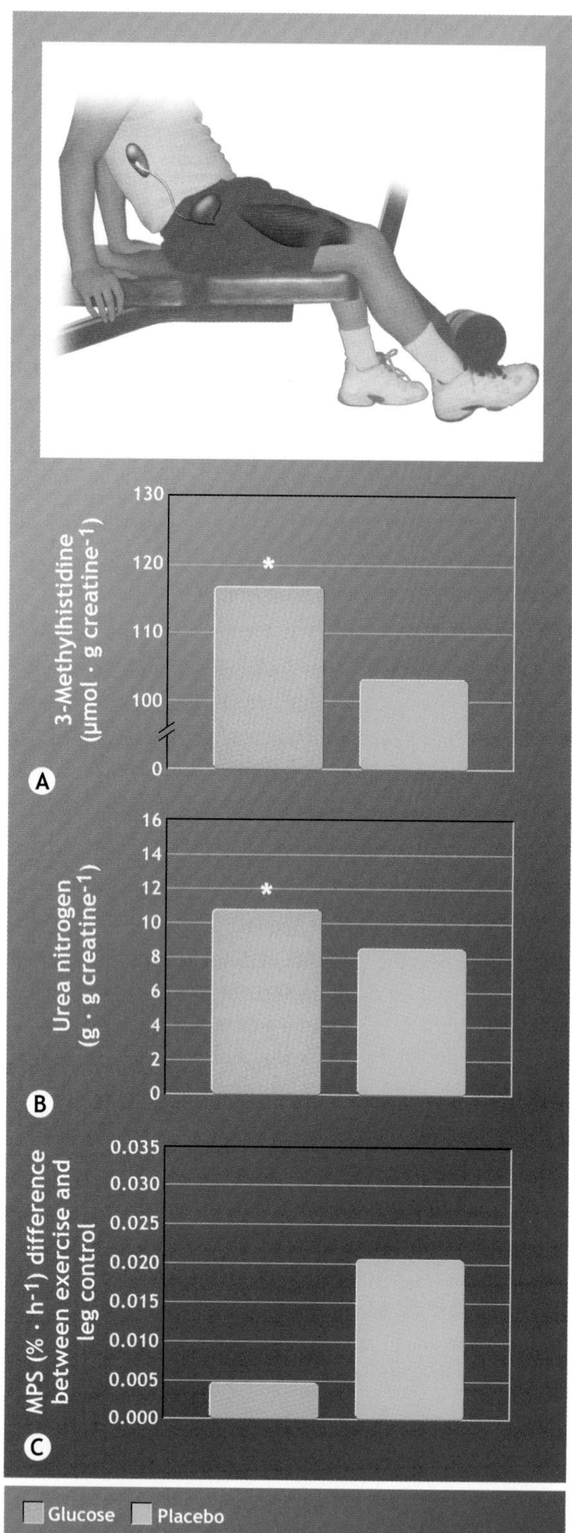

FIGURE 23.5 • Effects of glucose (1.0 g per kg body mass) versus Nutrasweet placebo, ingested immediately after exercise and 1 hour later, on protein degradation reflected by 24-hour urinary output of (**A**) 3-methylhistidine, (**B**) urinary urea nitrogen, and (**C**) rate of muscle protein synthesis (MPS) measured by vastus lateralis muscle incorporation of leucine (L-[l-^{13}C]). *Bars* for MPS indicate difference between exercise and control leg for glucose and placebo conditions. *Significantly different from placebo condition. (From Roy BD, et al. Effect of glucose supplement timing on protein metabolism after resistance training. J Appl Physiol 1997;82:1882.)

tance-training workouts.[210] Eight healthy men familiar with resistance training performed eight sets of 10 repetitions or unilateral knee extensor exercise at 85% of maximum strength (1-RM) in a placebo-controlled, randomized, double-blind trial. Immediately after the exercise session and 1 hour later, subjects received either a glucose supplement (1.0 g per kg body mass) or a placebo (Nutrasweet). Measurements consisted of (1) urinary 3-methylhistidine excretion (3-MH) as a marker of muscle protein degradation, (2) vastus lateralis muscle incorporation rate for the amino acid leucine (L-[l-^{13}C]leucine) to indicate protein synthesis, and (3) urinary nitrogen excretion to reflect protein breakdown. Figure 23.5 A and B shows that glucose supplementation significantly reduced myofibrillar protein breakdown, as reflected by decreased excretion of 3-MH and urinary nitrogen. Although not statistically significant, glucose supplementation also produced an increase in the rate of leucine incorporation into the vastus lateralis over the 10-hour postexercise period (Fig. 23.5 C). All of these alterations indicated a more positive body protein balance after exercise in the supplemented condition. The researchers speculated that the beneficial effect of glucose supplementation immediately following resistance exercise resulted from increased insulin release with intake of the high-glycemic carbohydrate (glucose). Higher plasma insulin concentrations should enhance muscle protein balance in recovery.

Although of possible significance as a natural means to stimulate anabolic processes and augment a positive protein balance in response to a bout of heavy exercise, one should view the effects of carbohydrate and/or protein supplementation in perspective. Further research must determine whether transient alterations in hormonal milieu and protein balance in recovery in the supplemented condition actually induce anabolic effects (increase lean body mass and muscular strength) compared with training without supplements. Researchers have yet to present such data.

DIETARY LIPID MAY AFFECT HORMONAL MILIEU. The diet's lipid content may modulate resting neuroendocrine homeostasis in a direction to modify tissue synthesis and training responsiveness. Research evaluated the effects of an intense resistance-exercise bout on postexercise plasma testosterone.[251] In agreement with prior research, testosterone levels significantly increased 5 minutes postexercise. However, a more impressive finding was a close association between the macronutrient composition of the individual's regular diet and baseline (resting) plasma testosterone levels. Table 23.4 shows that the quantity and percentage of dietary macronutrients correlated significantly with preexercise testosterone concentrations. More specifically, dietary lipid and saturated and monounsaturated fatty acid levels best predicted testosterone concentrations at rest—lower levels of each of these dietary components accompanied lower resting levels of testosterone. These findings support prior studies, which showed that a low-fat diet (~ 20% fat) produced lower testosterone levels than a diet with higher lipid content (~ 40% fat).[196,200,230] Interestingly, the data in Table 24.4 also show that the diet's protein percentage correlated *inversely* with testosterone levels at

TABLE 23.4 ➤ **RELATIONSHIPS BETWEEN PREEXERCISE TESTOSTERONE CONCENTRATION AND SELECTED NUTRITIONAL VARIABLES**

NUTRIENT	CORRELATION WITH TESTOSTERONE[a]
Energy, kJ	−0.18
Protein, %[b]	−0.71*
CHO, %[b]	−0.30
Lipid, %[b]	0.72*
SFA, g · 1000 $kcal^{-1} \cdot d^{-1}$	0.77†
MUFA, g · 1000 $kcal^{-1} \cdot d^{-1}$	0.79‡
PUFA, g · 1000 $kcal^{-1} \cdot d^{-1}$	0.25
Cholesterol, g · 1000 $kcal^{-1} \cdot d^{-1}$	0.53
PUFA/SFA	−0.63‡
Dietary fiber, g · 1000 $kcal^{-1} \cdot d^{-1}$	−0.19
Protein/CHO	−0.59‡
Protein/lipid	0.16
CHO/lipid	0.16

[a]Correlation coefficients are Pearson product-moment correlations.
[b]Nutrient percentage values expressed as percentage of total energy per day.
*P ≤ .01. †P ≤ .005. ‡P ≤ .05.
SFA, saturated fatty acids; MUFA, monounsaturated fatty acids; PUFA, polyunsaturated fatty acids; CHO, carbohydrate
From Volek JS, et al. Testosterone and cortisol in relationship to dietary nutrients and resistance exercise. J Appl Physiol 1997;82:49.

rest—higher dietary protein related to *lower* testosterone levels. Because many resistance-trained athletes consume considerable dietary protein, the implications of this association for the training response remain unresolved. Also, if low dietary lipid intake decreases resting testosterone levels, then individuals consuming low-fat diets (e.g., vegetarians, dancers, gymnasts, wrestlers) may experience a blunted training response. Furthermore, athletes who show low plasma testosterone levels because of overtraining might benefit from changing their diet's macronutrient composition. Whether or not this proves correct awaits further prospective trials that evaluate the effects of manipulating diet composition on hormonal balance and training responsiveness.

Amphetamines

***Amphetamines**, or "pep pills," are a group of pharmacologic compounds that exert powerful stimulating effects on central nervous system function.* Amphetamine (Benzedrine) and dextroamphetamine sulfate (Dexedrine) are used most frequently by athletes. Amphetamines exert sympathomimetic effects—their action mimics epinephrine and norepinephrine. These sympathetic hormones increase blood pressure, heart rate, cardiac output, breathing rate, metabolism, and blood glucose. Five to 20 mg of amphetamine usually exerts its effect for 30 to 90 minutes after ingestion, although its influence often persists for much longer. Amphetamines allegedly increase alertness, wakefulness, and the capacity to perform work by depressing the sensation of muscle fatigue. The deaths of two famed cyclists in the 1960s during competitive road racing were attributed to amphetamine use for just such purposes. In one of these deaths, in 1967, British Tour de France rider Tom Simpson overheated and suffered a fatal heart attack during the ascent of Mont Ventoux. Soldiers in World War II commonly used amphetamines to increase alertness and reduce feelings of fatigue. Athletes frequently use amphetamines, believing that they gain an ergogenic edge; ironically, little or no advantage exists.

Dangers of Amphetamines

Amphetamine use in athletics makes little sense for the following reasons:

- Regular use can lead to either physiologic or emotional drug dependency. This often causes a cyclical reliance on "uppers" (amphetamines) or "downers" (barbiturates)—the barbiturates reduce or tranquilize the "hyper" state brought on by amphetamines.
- General side effects include headache, tremulousness, agitation, fever, dizziness, and confusion—all of which negatively affect sports performance requiring rapid reaction and judgment and a high level of steadiness and mental concentration.
- Use eventually requires larger doses to achieve the same effect because drug tolerance increases with prolonged use; this can aggravate and even precipitate cardiovascular disorders.
- Inhibition or suppression of the body's normal mechanisms for perceiving and responding to pain, fatigue, or heat stress by amphetamines severely jeopardizes health and safety.
- The effects of prolonged intake of high doses of amphetamines remain unknown.

Amphetamine Use and Athletic Performance

Table 23.5 summarizes the results of seven experiments concerning the effects of amphetamines on physical performance. In almost all instances, amphetamines did not affect exercise capacity or performance of simple psychomotor skills.

Athletes take amphetamines to "get up" for the event and keep psychologically ready to compete. The day or evening before a contest, however, competitors often become nervous and irritable and have difficulty relaxing. Under these circumstances, a barbiturate serves to induce sleep. The athlete then regains the hyper condition by popping an upper prior to competition. Individuals knowledgeable about these drugs urge banning them from sport competition. The IOC, American Medical Association, and most sport-governing groups have rules that disqualify athletes for amphetamine use. Ironically, most research indicates that amphetamines do *not* enhance physical performance. Perhaps their greatest influence lies in the psychologic realm; athletes are easily convinced that any supplement augments performance. A placebo containing an inert substance often produces similar results!

TABLE 23.5 ➤ SUMMARY OF RESULTS ON THE EFFECTS OF AMPHETAMINES ON ATHLETIC PERFORMANCE

Study	Dose (mg)	Experiment	Effect of Amphetamines
(1)	10–20	Two all-out treadmill runs with 10-min rest between runs	None
		Consecutive 100-yd swims with 10-min rest intervals	None
		220–440-yd swims for time	None
		220-yd track runs for time	None
		100-yd to 2-mile track runs for time	None
(2)	10	Bench stepping to fatigue carrying weights equal to one-third body mass, 3 times with 3-min rest intervals	None
(3)	5	100-yd swim for speed	None
(4)	15	All-out treadmill runs	None
(5)	10	Stationary cycling at work rates of 275–2215 kg · min^{-1} for 25–35 min followed by treadmill run to exhaustion	None on submaximal or maximal $\dot{V}O_2$, heart rate, ventilation volume, or blood lactate; work time on the bicycle and treadmill increased significantly
(6)	20	Reaction and movement time to a visual stimulus	None; subjective feelings of alertness or lethargy unrelated to reaction or movement time
(7)	5	Psychomotor performance during a simulated airplane flight	Enhanced performance and lessened fatigue; if preceded by secobarbital (barbiturate), decreased performance

1. Karpovich PV. Effect of amphetamine sulfate on athletic performance. JAMA 1959;170:558.
2. Foltz EE, et al. The influence of amphetamine (Benzedrine) sulfate and caffeine on the performance of rapidly exhausting work by untrained subjects. J Lab Clin Med, 1943;28:601.
3. Haldi J, Wynn, W. Action of drugs on efficiency of swimmers. Res Q 1959;17:96.
4. Golding LA, Barnard RJ. The effects of d-amphetamine sulfate on physical performance. J Sports Med Phys Fitness 1963;3:221.
5. Wyndham CH, et al. Physiological effects of the amphetamines during exercise. S Afr Med J 1971;45:247.
6. Pierson WR, et al. Some psychological effects of the administration of amphetamine sulfate and meprobamate on speed of movement and reaction time. Med Sci Sports 1961;12:61.
7. McKenzie RE, Elliot LL. Effects of secobarbital and D-amphetamine on performance during a simulated air mission. Aerospace Med 1965;36:774.

Caffeine

Caffeine, a possible exception to the general rule against taking stimulants, remains a controlled drug in athletic competition.[53,100,155,236] Caffeine, the most widely consumed behaviorally active substance in the world, belongs to a group of lipid-soluble compounds called *purines* (proper chemical name, 1,3,7-trimethylxanthine), found naturally in coffee beans, tea leaves, chocolate, cocoa beans, and cola nuts and often added to carbonated beverages and nonprescription medicines (see Table 23.6). Sixty-three plant species contain caffeine in their leaves, seeds, or fruits. In the United States, 75% (14 million kg) of caffeine intake (per capita, 150 mg · d^{-1}) comes from coffee (3.5 kg per person per year), 15% from tea, and the remainder from the items listed in Table 23.6. Depending on preparation, one cup of brewed coffee contains between 60 and 150 mg of caffeine, instant coffee about 100 mg, brewed tea between 20 and 50 mg, and caffeinated soft drinks about 50 mg. For comparison, 2.5 cups of percolated coffee contain 250 to 400 mg or generally between 3 and 6 mg per kg of body mass. This amount of coffee produces urinary caffeine concentrations below the IOC-acceptable limit of 12 μg · mL^{-1} and National Collegiate Athletic Association limit of 15 μg · mL^{-1}. The intestinal tract absorbs caffeine rapidly, and peak plasma concentration is reached within 1 hour. It also clears from the body fairly rapidly, taking about 3 to 6 hours for blood caffeine concentrations to decrease by one half, compared with about 10 hours for other stimulants like methamphetamine.

Ergogenic Effects

Drinking 2.5 cups of regularly percolated coffee up to 1 hour before exercising significantly extends endurance in moderately strenuous aerobic exercise under laboratory conditions; it also improves performance in higher-intensity, shorter-duration physical effort. Elite distance runners who consumed 10 mg of caffeine per kg of body mass immediately before a treadmill run to exhaustion significantly improved their performance time by 1.9% compared with placebo or control conditions.[85] Data presented in "Focus on Research," page 567, show that subjects performed 90.2 minutes of exercise with caffeine and 75.5 minutes without it.[53] Consuming caffeine before exercise increased fat catabolism and reduced carbohydrate oxidation. Larger caffeine doses also induce an ergogenic effect on endurance, although this causes some individuals to exceed the IOC doping limit for urinary caffeine concentrations.[223] Interestingly, caffeine is the only substance for which the IOC has set urinary limits. The ergogenic effect of caffeine on endurance performance also applies to aerobic exercise performed at high ambient temperatures.[48]

Caffeine provides an ergogenic benefit during maximal swimming performances completed in less than 25 minutes. In a double-blind, cross-over research design, seven male and four female competent distance swimmers (<25 min for 1500 m) consumed caffeine (6 mg · kg body mass^{-1}) 2.5 hours before swimming 1500 m.[155] Figure 23.6 shows that the split times improved significantly with caffeine for each 500-m of the

TABLE 23.6 ➤ **CAFFEINE CONTENT OF COMMOM FOODS, BEVERAGES, AND OVER-THE-COUNTER MEDICATIONS**

BEVERAGES AND FOOD		OVER-THE-COUNTER PRODUCTS	
SUBSTANCE	CAFFEINE CONTENT (MG)	SUBSTANCE	CAFFEINE CONTENT (MG)
Coffee[a]		**Cold remedies**	
Coffee, Starbucks, grande, 16 oz	550	Dristan Coryban-D, Triaminicin, Sinarest	30–31
Coffee, Starbucks, tall, 12 oz	375	Excedrin	65
Coffee, Starbucks, short, 8 oz	250	Actifed, Contac, Comtrex, Sudafed	0
Coffee, Starbucks, Americano, tall, 12 oz	70		
Coffee, Starbucks, Latte or Cappuccino, grande, 16 oz	70	**Diuretics**	
		Aqua-ban	200
Brewed, drip method	110–150	Pre-Mens Forte	100
Brewed, percolator	64–124		
Instant	40–108	**Pain remedies**	
Expresso	100	Vanquish	33
Decaffeinated, brewed or instant; Sanka	2–5	Anacin; Midol	32
		Aspirin, any brand; Bufferin, Tylenol, Excedrin P.M.	0
Tea, 5 oz cup[a]			
Brewed, 1 min	9–33	**Stimulants**	
Brewed, 3 min	20–46	Vivarin tablet, NoDoz maximum-strength caplet, Caffedrine	200
Brewed, 5 min	20–50		
Iced tea, 12 oz; instant tea	12–36	NoDoz tablet	100
		Energets Lozenges	75
Chocolate			
Baker's semi-sweet, 1 oz; Baker's chocolate chips, 1/4 cup	13	**Weight control aids**	
		Dexatrim, Dietac	200
Cocoa, 5 oz cup, made from mix	6–10	Prolamine	140
Milk chocolate candy, 1 oz	6		
Sweet/dark chocolate, 1 oz	20	**Pain drugs**[b]	
Baking chocolate, 1 oz	35	Cafergot	100
Chocolate bar, 3.5 oz	12–15	Migrol	50
Jello chocolate fudge mousse	12	Fiornal	40
Ovaltine	0	Darvon compound	32
Soft drinks			
Jolt	100		
Sugar Free Mr. Pibb	59		
Mellow Yellow, Mountain Dew	53–54		
Tab	47		
Coca Cola, Diet Coke, 7-Up Gold	46		
Shasta-Cola, Cherry Cola, Diet Cola	44		
Dr. Pepper, Mr. Pibb	40–41		
Dr. Pepper, sugar free	40		
Pepsi Cola	38		
Diet Pepsi, Pepsi Light, Diet RC, RC Cola, Diet Rite	36		

[a]Brewing tea or coffee for longer periods slightly increases the caffeine content.
[b]Prescription, 1 oz ~ 30 mL.
Data from product labels and manufacturers and National Soft Drink Association, 1997. *Caffeinism* refers to caffeine intoxication characterized by restlessness, tremulousness, nervousness, excitement, insomnia, flushed face, dieresis, gastrointestinal complaints, rambling flow of thought and speech, tachycardia or cardiac arrhythmia, periods of inexhaustibility, and/or psychomotor agitation.

swim. The swim time averaged 1.9% faster with caffeine than without it (20:58.6 vs. 21:21.8). Enhanced performance with caffeine associated with a lower plasma potassium concentration before exercise and higher blood glucose levels at the end of the trial. These responses suggest a possible caffeine effect on electrolyte balance and glucose availability. Caffeine also alters the cardiovascular response to dynamic exercise in a manner that depresses regional blood flow and vascular conductance.[59]

NO DOSE-RESPONSE RELATIONSHIP. Figure 23.7 illustrates the effects of preexercise caffeine administration on endurance time of nine well-trained male cyclists. Subjects received a placebo or a capsule containing 5, 9, or 13 mg of caffeine per kg of body mass 1 hour before cycling at 80% of their maximal power output on a $\dot{V}O_{2max}$ test. All caffeine trials showed a 24% improvement in performance. However, no greater benefit occurred with caffeine quantities above 5 mg · kg body mass^{-1}. For all subjects, only the lowest caffeine dose

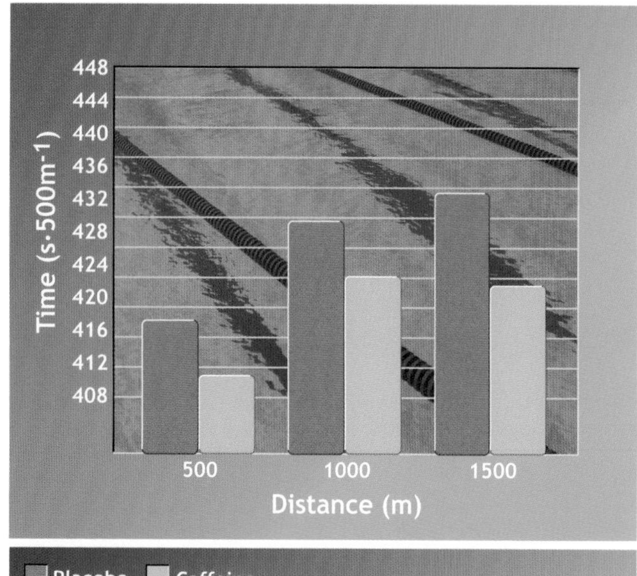

FIGURE 23.6 • Split times for each 500 m of a 1500-m time trial with caffeine and placebo. Caffeine produced significantly faster split times. (From MacIntosh BR, Wright BM. Caffeine ingestion and performance of a 1,500-metre swim. Can J Appl Physiol 1995;20:168.)

produced urinary caffeine concentrations below the doping limit set by the IOC, a finding of importance to the elite competitive athlete.

Proposed Mechanism for Ergogenic Action

A precise explanation for the ergogenic boost from caffeine remains elusive. *In all likelihood, the ergogenic effect of caffeine (or related methylxanthine compounds) in high-intensity endurance exercise results from facilitated use of fat as an exercise fuel, thus sparing the body's limited carbohydrate reserves.*[6,99,147] However, some investigators have found the ergogenic effect to be unrelated to hormonal or metabolic changes with caffeine.[236] This suggests a possible action of caffeine on specific tissues, including the central nervous system. In the quantities usually administered to humans, caffeine probably acts in either of two ways: (1) directly on adipose and peripheral vascular tissues[100,244] or (2) indirectly by stimulating epinephrine release from the adrenal medulla; epinephrine then acts as an antagonist of the adenosine receptors on adipocyte cells.[98] Adenosine receptors normally repress lipolysis. Caffeine's inhibition of adenosine receptors increases cellular levels of the second messenger cyclic 3′,5′-adenosine monophosphate (cyclic AMP). Cyclic AMP, in turn, activates hormone-sensitive lipases to promote lipolysis, which releases free fatty acids (FFAs) into the plasma. Elevated plasma FFA levels increase fat oxidation, thus conserving liver and muscle glycogen to benefit high-intensity endurance exercise.

Caffeine and its metabolites readily cross the blood–brain barrier to produce analgesic effects on the central nervous system. Caffeine also enhances motoneuronal excitability, thus facilitating motor unit recruitment. The stimulating effects of caffeine do not result from its direct action on the central nervous system. Rather, caffeine provides indirect nervous system stimulation by blocking the receptors for adenosine (discussed previously), which also serve a neuromodulator function that exerts a calming effect on brain and spinal cord neurons. Four factors probably interact to produce caffeine's facilitating effect on neuromuscular activity: (1) lowered threshold for motor unit recruitment, (2) altered excitation/contraction coupling, (3) facilitated nerve transmission, and (4) increased ion transport within the muscle. Conflicting evidence exists concerning the effect of preexercise caffeine on $\dot{V}O_{2max}$.[70,233]

INCONSISTENT EFFECTS. Prior nutrition may partly account for the variation frequently observed among individuals in response to exercise after consuming caffeine. While caffeine generally elicits group improvement in endurance, individuals who normally consume a high-carbohydrate diet show a blunted effect for caffeine on FFA mobilization.[40,258] Individual differences in caffeine sensitivity, tolerance, and hormonal response from short- and long-term patterns of caffeine consumption also affect this drug's ergogenic qualities. Interestingly, the ergogenic effects of caffeine are lower for caffeine in coffee than for an equivalent dose in a caffeine capsule in water.[101] This suggests that components in coffee actually antagonize caffeine's actions. Beneficial effects do not occur consistently in habitual caffeine users,[243] indicating that an athlete must consider "caffeine tolerance" rather than assume

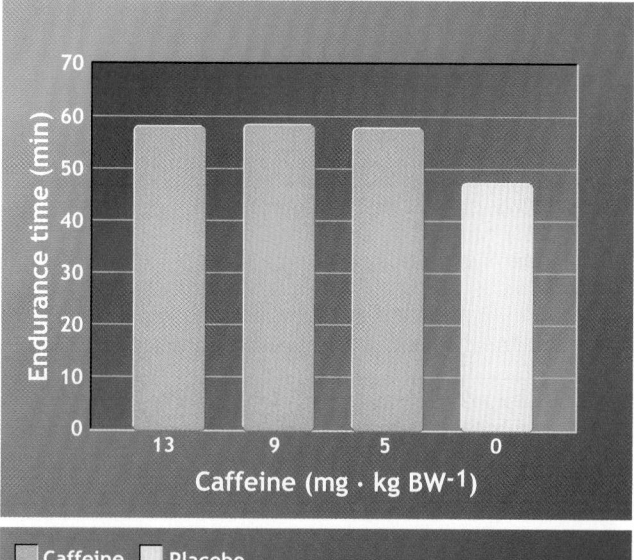

FIGURE 23.7 • Endurance performance (time to fatigue) following preexercise doses of caffeine in different concentrations. Cycling time (min) represents the average for nine male cyclists. All caffeine trials produced significantly better performance than the placebo condition. No dose-response relationship emerged between caffeine concentration and endurance performance; however, the 5-mg per kg body mass dose was the *only* treatment that passed the IOC's doping standards for urinary caffeine concentrations. (From Pasman WJ, et al. The effect of different dosages of caffeine on endurance performance time. Int J Sports Med 1995;16:225.)

Focus on Research — Ergogenic Benefits of Caffeine

Costill DL, et al. Effects of caffeine ingestion on metabolism and exercise performance. Med Sci Sports Exerc 1978;10:155.

➤ The potential ergogenic benefits of various substances and procedures have always interested sports competitors and exercise physiologists. Costill and colleagues tested the hypothesis that ingesting caffeine stimulated free fatty acid (FFA) mobilization, retarded depletion of muscle glycogen, and consequently enhanced endurance exercise performance. Previous research with animals and humans demonstrated that elevating plasma FFA spared muscle glycogen and extended exercise capacity. FFA concentration typically rose after injection of heparin, a substance that stimulates increased FFA mobilization and subsequent oxidation. Because caffeine also mobilizes FFA, Costill tested its effects on muscle glycogen levels, the metabolic mixture in exercise, and endurance performance in humans.

Two female and seven male competitive cyclists (average $\dot{V}O_{2max}$ = 60 mL · kg^{-1} · min^{-1}), consuming the same diet, performed a cycle ergometer $\dot{V}O_{2max}$ test and two additional endurance exercise trials separated by 3 days. In one trial, they consumed 200 mL of hot water containing 5 g decaffeinated coffee (D), 60 minutes before the exercise trial. The cycling test continued as long as possible at a work intensity of 80% $\dot{V}O_{2max}$. In the second trial, subjects consumed a hot drink containing 5 g D plus 330 mg of caffeine (C) 60 minutes before the exercise test. Subjects remained unaware of the experiment's purpose, with test order randomized for C and D trials. Blood samples, taken before and during each trial, provided information on plasma lactate, FFA, glycerol, glucose, and triglycerides. In addition, respiratory gas exchange throughout exercise allowed computation of RQ and estimation of the nonprotein metabolic mixture.

The figure shows that total exercise time to exhaustion increased 19.5% during trial C (90.2 min) compared with trial D (75.5 min). Although FFAs did not differ significantly between conditions, (although consistently higher in C trial) the caffeinated drink produced significantly higher plasma glycerol levels and significantly lower RQ values. The RQ allowed the researchers to estimate carbohydrate oxidation during exercise (about 240 g in both trials). In contrast, fat oxidation with caffeine (118 g) exceeded oxidation without caffeine (57 g). Subjects also perceived the exercise as easier in the C condition.

This study demonstrated that caffeine ingestion before exercise increased the rate of lipolysis during sustained exercise. Increased lipolysis could spare liver and skeletal muscle glycogen early in exercise for later use. Subsequent research has confirmed caffeine's ergogenic role in endurance exercise performance.

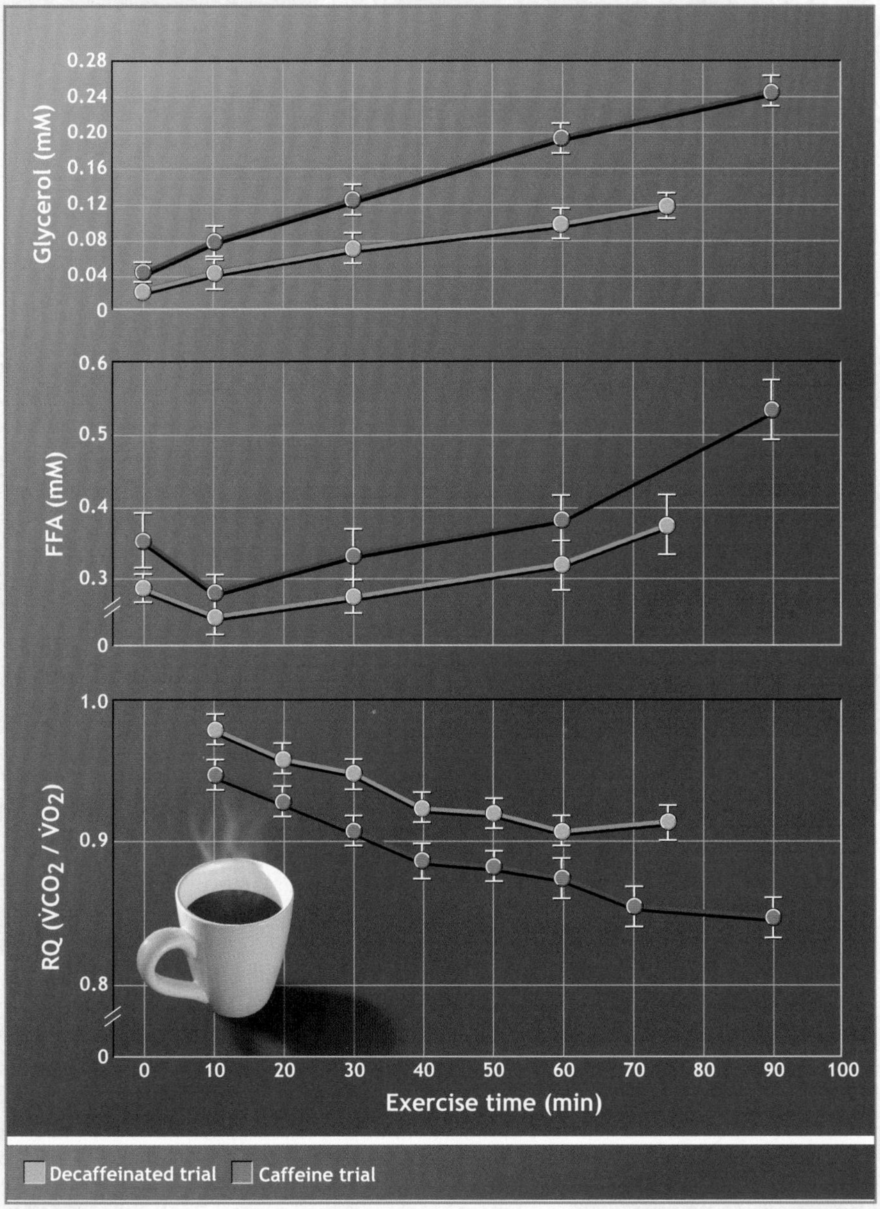

Average values for plasma glycerol, free fatty acid (FFA), and respiratory quotient (RQ) during endurance exercise after consuming either a caffeinated or decaffeinated liquid. Vertical bars (I) represent standard error of the mean.

that caffeine provides a consistent benefit to all people. *From a practical standpoint, the athlete should omit caffeine-containing foods and beverages 4 to 6 days before competition, to optimize caffeine's potential for ergogenic benefits.*[242]

Effects on Muscle

Caffeine may act directly on muscle to enhance exercise capacity.[171] A double-blind research design evaluated voluntary and electrically stimulated muscle actions under "caffeine-free" conditions and following oral administration of 500 mg of caffeine.[151] Electrically stimulating the motor nerve allowed the researchers to remove central nervous system control and quantify caffeine's direct effects on skeletal muscle. Caffeine produced no effect on maximal muscle force during voluntary or electrically stimulated muscle actions. For submaximal effort, however, caffeine increased force output for low-frequency electrical stimulation before and after muscle fatigue. These findings suggest that caffeine exerts direct, specific ergogenic effects on skeletal muscle during repetitive low-frequency stimulation. Perhaps caffeine increases the sarcoplasmic reticulum's permeability to Ca^{2+}, thus making the ion readily available for contraction. Caffeine could also influence the myofibril's sensitivity to Ca^{2+} and facilitate excitation–contraction coupling. Caffeine does not exert ergogenic effects on anaerobic metabolic capacity (glycolysis) as measured during repeated high-intensity Wingate exercise tests.[108] On page 587 of this chapter we discuss research concerning how caffeine dramatically blunts the ergogenic effect of creatine supplementation on short-term muscular power.

Warning About Caffeine

Individuals who normally avoid caffeine may experience adverse effects when they consume it. Caffeine stimulates the central nervous system; it can produce restlessness, headaches, insomnia, nervous irritability, muscle twitching, tremulousness, psychomotor agitation, and elevated heart rate and blood pressure and trigger premature left ventricular contractions. From the standpoint of temperature regulation, caffeine acts as a potent diuretic. This could cause an unnecessary preexercise loss of fluid, negatively affecting thermal balance and exercise performance in hot environments. Caffeine's effect on fluid loss is lessened when consumed during exercise because (1) catecholamine release in exercise greatly reduces renal blood flow and (2) exercise enhances renal solute reabsorption and consequently water conservation (osmotic effect).[261]

While the effects of excess caffeine generally pose no significant health risk, death from caffeine overdose can occur. The LD-50 (lethal oral dose required to kill 50% of the population) for caffeine is about 10 g (150 $mg \cdot kg$ body $mass^{-1}$) for a 70-kg person. A 50-kg woman has significant acute health risk with a caffeine intake of 7.5 g. Moderate caffeine toxicity has been reported in small children consuming 35 mg per kg of body mass. Such observations provide clear indication of the inverted U-shaped relationship between certain exogenous chemicals and health and safety (and probably exercise performance). With caffeine, ingesting small quantities produces desirable effects, but consuming a significant excess can wreak havoc.

IOC LIMIT FOR DISQUALIFICATION. The IOC permits athletes to consume some caffeine as long as its concentration in urine does not exceed 12 $\mu g \cdot mL^{-1}$. Only between 0.5 and 3.0% of ingested caffeine appears in the urine; most is metabolized by the liver (with relatively large individual variation). Athletes should know that 600 to 800 mg (4 to 7 cups of coffee) consumed over a 30-minute period significantly raises urine caffeine concentrations to levels that would cause disqualification from competition.[263] A person who degrades caffeine slowly or who excretes large nonmetabolized amounts in the urine has increased risk of a positive urine test and disqualification. Also, ingesting caffeine tablets or using caffeine suppositories or injections can trigger a positive doping test.

Pangamic Acid

Some athletes tout **pangamic acid**, commonly known as "vitamin" B_{15}, for its alleged ergogenic benefits in aerobic exercise. Proponents of pangamic acid use argue that studies in Russia showed that this compound increased the cell's ability to use oxygen, reduced lactate build-up, and enhanced endurance. As with many proposed ergogenic aids, testimonials from athletes abound regarding its effectiveness as a training aid and performance enhancer. Significant limitations in research design of the early studies of pangamic acid make interpretation of the findings difficult. Research conducted in this country has failed to show any benefit of this compound on aerobic capacity, endurance performance, or circulating levels of blood glucose and lactate.[92] From a nutritional perspective, pangamic acid has no vitamin or provitamin properties and appears to serve no particular need for the body. Concern exists that synthetic mixtures sold as B_{15} may prove harmful.[116] FDA guidelines make it illegal to sell this compound as a dietary supplement or drug.

Buffering Solutions

Maximal exercise for 30 to 120 seconds causes dramatic alterations in the chemical balance between intra- and extracellular fluids, because the muscle fibers rely predominantly on anaerobic energy transfer. As a result, significant quantities of lactate accumulate with a concurrent fall in intracellular pH. Increased acidity ultimately inhibits energy transfer and contractile dynamics in the active muscle fibers, and exercise performance declines.[133]

The bicarbonate aspect of the body's buffering system (see Chapter 14) provides a rapid first line of defense against intracellular increases in H^+ concentration. Maintaining extracellular bicarbonate at a high level facilitates H^+ efflux from the cell, which reduces intracellular acidosis.[157] This effect has led to speculation that increasing the body's bicarbonate reserve before short-term anaerobic exercise might enhance per-

TABLE 23.7 ➤ PERFORMANCE TIME AND ACID-BASE PROFILES FOR SUBJECTS UNDER CONTROL (PLACEBO) AND INDUCED PREEXERCISE ALKALOSIS CONDITIONS BEFORE AND AFTER AN 800-M RACE

VARIABLE	CONDITION	PRETREATMENT	PREEXERCISE	POSTEXERCISE
pH	Control	7.40	7.39	7.07
	Placebo	7.39	7.40	7.09
	Alkalosis	7.40	7.49[a]	7.18[b]
Lactate ($mmol \cdot L^{-1}$)	Control	1.21	1.15	12.62
	Placebo	1.38	1.23	13.62
	Alkalosis	1.29	1.31	14.29[b]
Standard HCO_3^{-1} ($mEq \cdot L^{-1}$)	Control	25.8	24.5	9.90
	Placebo	25.6	26.2	11.00
	Alkalosis	25.2	33.5[a]	14.30[b]
Performance time (min:s)		Control 2:05.8	Placebo 2:05.1	Alkalosis 2:02.9[c]

From Wilkes D. et al. Effects of induced metabolic alkalosis on 800-m racing time. Med Sci Sports Exerc 1983;15:277.
[a]Pre-exercise values significantly higher than pre-treatment values.
[b]Alkalosis values significantly higher than placebo and control values after exercise.
[c]Alkalosis time significantly faster than control and placebo times.

formance by delaying the fall in intracellular pH associated with exhaustive effort. Research in this area has produced conflicting results, perhaps owing to variations in the preexercise dose of sodium bicarbonate and the type of exercise used to evaluate preexercise alkalosis.[103,193,247]

To improve experimental design, one study investigated the effects of acute metabolic alkalosis on exhaustive, short-term exercise that produced a significant increase in anaerobic metabolites.[262] Six trained middle-distance runners ran an 880-m race (1) under control conditions and (2) following alkalosis induced by ingesting a sodium bicarbonate solution (300 mg per kg body mass) or a calcium carbonate placebo of similar concentration. Table 23.7 shows that ingesting the alkaline drink raised the subjects' pH and standard bicarbonate level before exercise. In addition, subjects ran on average 2.9 seconds faster under alkalosis and exhibited higher postexercise values for blood lactate, pH, and extracellular H^+ concentration than in the placebo condition.

The ergogenic effect of **preexercise alkalosis** also occurs for women (Fig. 23.8).[166] Ten moderately trained women

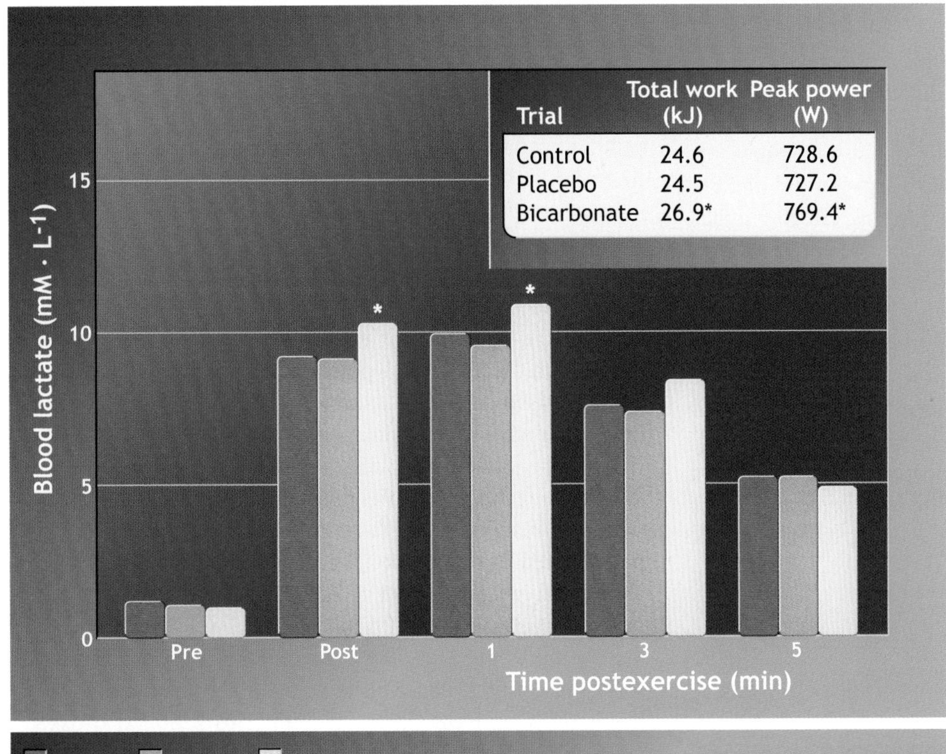

FIGURE 23.8 • Bicarbonate loading and its effects on total work, peak power output, and postexercise blood lactate levels in moderately trained women. *Significantly higher than either control or placebo. (From McNaughton LR, et al. Effect of sodium bicarbonate ingestion on high intensity exercise in moderately trained women. J Strength Cond Res 1997;11:98.)

performed one bout of maximal cycle ergometer exercise for 60 seconds on separate days under three conditions in a double-blind research design: (1) control, no treatment; (2) dose of sodium bicarbonate of 300 mg · kg body mass^{-1} in 400 mL of low-calorie flavored water 90 minutes before testing; and (3) placebo of equimolar dose of sodium chloride (to maintain intravascular fluid status similar to bicarbonate condition) administered like the bicarbonate treatment. Exercise capacity was the total work accomplished in the 60-second ride. The figure's *inset box* shows that total work performed and peak power output reached significantly higher levels with preexercise bicarbonate treatment than under either control or placebo conditions. The bicarbonate treatment produced a significantly higher blood lactate level in the immediate and 1-minute postexercise period, which explains the greater work capacity attained in this short-term, predominantly anaerobic exercise trial. Similar ergogenic benefits of induced alkalosis occur in anaerobic performances, with exogenous sodium citrate as the alkalinizing agent.[114,165]

Augmented anaerobic energy transfer during exercise probably explains the ergogenic effect of preexercise alkalosis. More than likely, increased extracellular buffering from preexercise sodium bicarbonate ingestion facilitates H^+ efflux from the working muscle fibers. This delays the fall in intracellular pH and its subsequent negative effects on muscle function. An improvement of 2.9 seconds in 800-m race time represents a dramatic performance improvement—a distance of 19 meters at race pace, which in most 800-m races brings a last-place finisher to first place!

Effect Related to Dosage and Degree of Anaerobiosis

Bicarbonate dosage and the cumulative anaerobic nature of the exercise interact to influence the potential ergogenic effect of preexercise bicarbonate loading.[119] Doses of at least 0.3 g per kg body mass facilitate H^+ efflux from the cell and significantly enhance a single 1- to 2-minute maximal effort,[96,160,166] as well as longer-term arm or leg exercise that exhausts within 6 to 8 minutes.[206] No ergogenic effect emerges for performance typical of heavy resistance training, perhaps because the absolute anaerobic metabolic load is generally lower than that in continuous, supramaximal whole-body activities.[191] Bicarbonate loading with all-out effort of less than 1 minute only exerts an ergogenic effect with repetitive (intermittent) exercise.[54] Intermittent anaerobic exercise produces high intracellular H^+ concentrations whose buffering benefits from a higher extracellular bicarbonate level. Species differences also appear to influence the ergogenic effects of bicarbonate loading; improvements occur for racehorses but not for racing greyhounds.[138,146]

INTEGRATIVE QUESTION

Advise a competitor in an Olympic weight-lifting contest who plans to bicarbonate load because each competitive event requires all-out effort of an anaerobic nature.

High-Intensity Endurance Performance

Although preexercise-induced alkalosis does not benefit low-intensity, aerobic exercise because pH and lactate remain at near-resting levels, it may enhance aerobic exercise of higher intensity. This is because high-intensity endurance exercise, while predominantly aerobic, does cause blood lactate accumulation and a decrease in pH that can negatively affect performance. A double-blind, placebo-controlled experiment determined whether ingesting a preexercise alkalinizing agent improved high-intensity endurance performance.[192] Eight trained male cyclists consumed sodium citrate (0.5 g per kg body mass) before a 30-km time trial. Race times were faster and plasma pH and lactate concentrations higher after sodium citrate ingestion than with the placebo. Despite the relatively small anaerobic component in high-intensity aerobic exercise (compared with short-term, maximal exercise), ingesting a buffer before exercising facilitates lactate and hydrogen ion efflux and improves muscle function

Although the IOC does not ban alkalinizing agents, more research must clarify the ergogenic benefits (and possible dangers) of short-term induced alkalosis. Individuals who bicarbonate load often experience abdominal cramps and diarrhea about 1 hour after ingestion. This adverse effect would surely minimize any potential ergogenic benefit. Substituting sodium citrate (0.4 to 0.5 g per kg body mass) for sodium bicarbonate can reduce or eliminate adverse gastrointestinal effects.[149,165]

β-Hydroxy-β-methylbutyrate

β-Hydroxy-β-methylbutyrate (HMB), a bioactive metabolite generated in the breakdown of the essential branched-chain amino acid leucine, may decrease protein loss during stress by inhibiting protein catabolism.[241] In rats and chicks, significantly less protein breakdown and a slight increase in protein synthesis occurred in muscle tissue (*in vitro*) exposed to HMB.[181] Data also suggest an HMB-induced increase in cellular fatty acid oxidation *in vitro* in mammalian muscle cells exposed to HMB.[45] Depending on the quantity of HMB in food (relatively rich sources include catfish, grapefruit, and breast milk), humans synthesize between 0.3 and 1.0 g of HMB daily, about 5% of which comes from dietary leucine catabolism. Because of its potential nitrogen-retaining effects, many resistance-trained athletes use HMB supplements to prevent or slow muscle damage and blunt muscle breakdown (proteolysis) associated with intense physical effort.

To determine the effect of exogenous HMB on skeletal muscles' response to resistance training, young-adult men participated in two randomized trials.[176] In study 1, 41 subjects received either 0, 1.5, or 3.0 g of HMB daily at two protein levels, either 117 g or 175 g daily, for 3 weeks. The men weight trained during this time for 1.5 hours, 3 days a week. In study 2, 28 subjects consumed either 0 or 3.0 g of HMB daily and weight trained for 2 to 3 hours, 6 days a week, for 7 weeks. In the first study, HMB supplementation significantly depressed the exercise-induced rise in muscle proteolysis (reflected by urinary 3-methylhistidine and plasma creatine phosphokinase [CPK] levels) during the first 2 weeks of exercise training. These biochemical indices of muscle damage were 20 to 60% lower in the HMB-supplemented group. In addition, the supplemented group lifted significantly more total weight during each training week (Fig. 23.9A), with the greatest effect in the group receiving the largest HMB supplement. Muscular strength increased 8% in the unsupplemented group and more in the HMB-supplemented groups (13% for the 1.5-g group and 18.4% for the 3.0-g group). Added protein (not indicated in graph) did not affect any of the measurements, but one should view this lack of effect in proper context—the "lower" protein quantity (115 g · d^{-1}) was equivalent to twice the RDA.

In the second study, those who received HMB supplementation had significantly higher FFM (measured by total body electrical conductivity) than the unsupplemented group at 2 and 4–6 weeks of training (Fig. 23.9B). However, at the last measurement during training, the difference between groups decreased and did not differ significantly from the difference between pretraining baseline values.

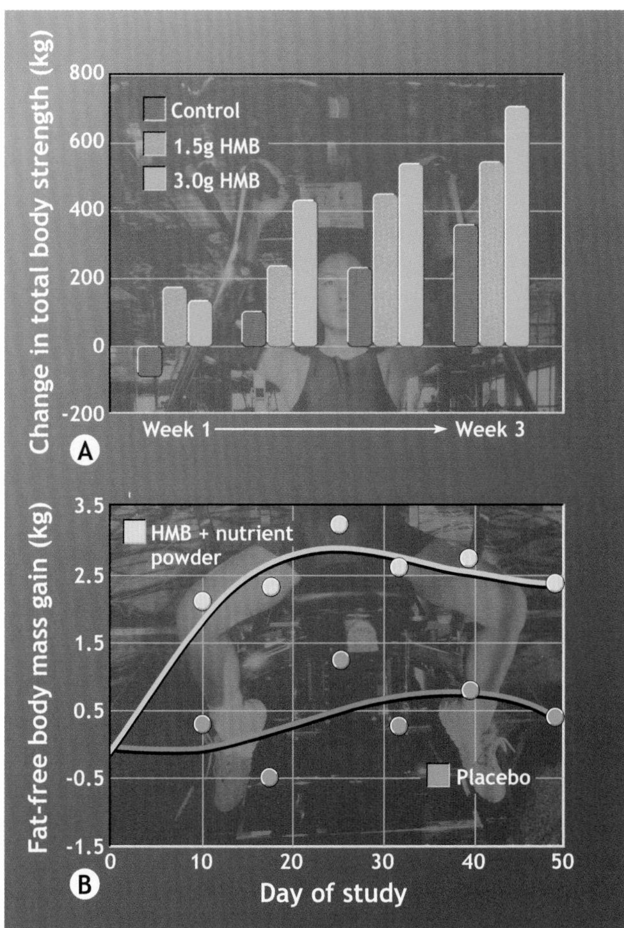

FIGURE 23.9 • **A**. Change in muscle strength (total weight lifted in upper- and lower-body exercises) during study 1 (week 1 to week 3) in subjects who supplemented with HMB. Each *group of bars* represents one complete set of upper- and lower-body workouts. **B**. Total body electrical conductivity–assessed change in FFM during study 2 for a control group that received a carbohydrate drink *(placebo)* and a group that received 3 g of Ca-HMB each day mixed in a nutrient powder *(HMB + nutrient powder)*. (From Nissen S, et al. Effect of leucine metabolite β-hydroxy-β-methylbutyrate on muscle metabolism during resistance-exercise training. J Appl Physiol 1996;81:2095.)

Although the mechanism for HMB's action on muscle metabolism, strength improvement, and body composition remains unknown, the researchers speculated that taking this metabolite during resistance training inhibits normal proteolytic processes that accompany intense muscular overload. While the results demonstrate an ergogenic effect for HMB supplementation, it remains unclear just what component of the FFM (protein, bone, water) HMB actually affects. Furthermore, the data in Figure 23.9B indicate potentially transient body-composition benefits of supplementation that tend to revert toward the unsupplemented state as training progresses.

Recent research has studied the effects of variations in HMB supplementation (approximately 3 versus 6 g · d^{-1}) on muscular strength during 8 weeks of whole body resistance training in untrained, young adult men.[88] The study's primary finding indicated that HMB supplementation, regardless of dosage, produced no difference in the majority of the strength data (including 1-RM strength) compared with the placebo group. In contrast to the findings presented in Figure 23.9A, increases in training volume remained similar among groups. In both HMB-supplemented groups in recovery, significantly lower levels of CPK indicate some potential effect of HMB in inhibiting muscle breakdown in response to resistance training. The group that consumed the lower dosage of HMB showed a greater increase in FFM than the other two groups, but inferences from these findings are limited owing to the use of skinfolds to assess body composition. HMB supplementation with a dosage as high as 6 g · d^{-1} during 8 weeks of resistance training appears to have no adverse effects on hepatic enzyme function, blood lipid profile, renal function, or immune function.[89] Additional studies by other laboratories must assess the long-term effects of HMB supplements on body composition, training response, and overall health and safety.

NONPHARMACOLOGIC APPROACHES

Besides pharmacologic procedures, athletes often use diverse physical, mechanical, physiologic, and nutritional means hoping to achieve ergogenic effects.

Temporomandibular Joint Repositioning

A number of reports in the popular and dental literature over the past 30 years have claimed either real or potential benefits to exercise performance for **temporomandibular joint (TMJ) repositioning** with a specially designed, custom-fitted bite splint that optimizes alignment of the upper and lower jaw. At the same time, elite athletes in a variety of sports (e.g., football, tennis, baseball, boxing, luge, field events, and sprint and distance running) have extolled the sports performance benefits of jaw appliances. Proponents of this form of "sports dentistry" argue that improper TMJ alignment negatively affects the skeletal frame in general and the relatively large neural and vascular component in the jaw region in particular. Consequently, correct positioning and proper stability of the mandible align the cervical vertebrae and alleviate negative neural and vascular input from the orofacial area to the brain. Advocates argue that TMJ adjustment ultimately translates into optimal exercise performance.

Little experimentation exists concerning the ergogenic effects of TMJ repositioning. Most claims for improved exercise performance emerge from case studies, anecdotal "success stories," and subjective evaluation. Even when objective measurement was made, the research design often was flawed and poorly controlled. In one of our laboratories, we evaluated the effects of a mandibular orthopedic repositioning appliance (MORA) on maximum and submaximum physiologic and performance measures in young-adult men and women with documented TMJ malalignment.[163] The subjects were randomly assigned to one of four conditions: (1) without a MORA, (2) with a placebo MORA with no bite surface to maintain usual jaw position, (3) with a MORA that optimized jaw position, and (4) with a MORA that magnified the subject's abnormal occlusion. To ensure a double-blind study, the researchers coded each of the subject's three bite splints with the code maintained by the dentists. Because the dentists did not take part in the laboratory measurements, neither the subjects nor the staff knew which bite splint was used during testing. Data analysis revealed that the MORA device produced *no effect* on measures of visual reaction and movement times; muscular strength of the grip, elbow flexors, and leg extensors; submaximal and maximal oxygen consumption; perception of effort; running economy; and all-out anaerobic exercise capacity of the arms and legs. In fact, placing the jaw in a less-than-optimal position (more than the subject's regular malocclusion) caused no deleterious effect on any performance measure. Clearly, these findings run counter to the opinion of advocates of mandibular-repositioning appliances and agree with several studies showing no effect of TMJ repositioning on isometric and isokinetic measures of muscular strength and power.[273] Such findings support the contention that the benefits of short-term TMJ repositioning on exercise performance noted in previous articles probably result from inadequacies in research design rather than any real ergogenic effects.

Red Blood Cell Reinfusion—Blood Doping

Red blood cell reinfusion, often called *induced erythrocythemia, blood boosting,* or *blood doping,* gained public prominence as a possible ergogenic technique during the 1972 Munich Olympics when an athlete allegedly used this procedure prior to his two gold medal–winning endurance runs.

How It Works

Red blood cell reinfusion involves withdrawing 1 to 4 units (1 unit = 450 mL of whole blood) of a person's blood (**autologous transfusion**), immediately reinfusing the plasma, and placing the packed red cells in frozen storage. **Homologous transfusion** infuses a type-matched donor's blood. To prevent dramatic reductions in blood-cell concentration, each unit of blood withdrawal takes place at 3- to 8-week intervals, because it takes this long to reestablish normal red blood cell levels. Stored blood cells are then infused 1 to 7 days before an endurance event; this increases red blood cell count and hemoglobin levels by as much as 8 to 20%. Hemoconcentration translates to an average hemoglobin increase for men from a normal 15 g per dL of blood to 19 g per dL (hematocrit increases 40 to 60%). Hematologic parameters remain elevated for at least 14 days.[93] Theoretically, the added blood volume contributes to a larger maximal cardiac output, while red blood cell packing increases the blood's oxygen-carrying capacity. Enhanced oxygen transport and delivery to active tissues provides significant performance benefits to endurance athletes.[25,256]

An ergogenic effect usually results from infusion of 900 to 1800 mL of freeze-preserved autologous blood. Each 500-mL infusion of whole blood (equivalent to 275 mL of packed red cells) adds about 100 mL of oxygen to the blood's total oxygen-carrying capacity—each 100 mL of whole blood carries about 20 mL of oxygen. Because an elite endurance athlete's total blood volume circulates 5 to 6 times each minute in heavy exercise, the potential "extra" oxygen available to the tissues from red cell reinfusion averages 500 mL (0.5 L).

Blood doping might also produce effects opposite to those intended. For example, a large red blood cell infusion (and increase in blood cell concentration) could increase blood viscosity, or "thickness," and thus *decrease* cardiac output, blood flow velocity, and peripheral oxygen supply—all important factors that can reduce aerobic capacity and endurance performance. Any increase in blood viscosity might also compromise blood flow through the narrowed, atherosclerotic vessels of individuals with coronary artery disease and so increase the risk for heart attack or stroke.

Does It Work?

A theoretical basis for blood doping exists, and experimental evidence justifies its use for physiologic reasons.[215] Much of the early conflict concerning ergogenic benefits resulted from poor experimental design, inconsistent criteria for exercise performance, diverse blood storage techniques, and variations in the timing and quantity of blood withdrawn and replaced. Early research in this area noted a significant, rapid increase in $\dot{V}O_{2max}$ following infusion of whole blood.[75] One study reported a 23% overnight increase in performance and a 9% increase in $\dot{V}O_{2max}$ with blood doping.[77] Although many of these early studies contained flaws in research design, subsequent investigations (including a study by a past critic of the technique) support previous findings and show physio-

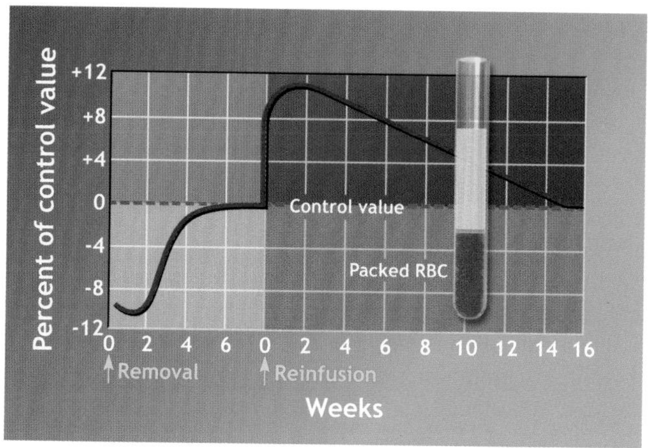

FIGURE 23.10 • Time course of hematologic changes after removal and reinfusion of 900 mL of freeze-preserved blood. (From Gledhill N. Blood doping and related issues: a brief review. Med Sci Sports Exerc 1982;14:183.)

logic and performance improvements with red blood cell reinfusion.[205,222]

Differences in results among the various studies of exercise performance following red blood cell reinfusion largely result from variations in blood storage methods. Freezing red blood cells permits storage in excess of 6 weeks without significant loss of cells. With storage at 4°C (used in some earlier studies), substantial hemolysis occurs after only 3 weeks. This represents an important difference because it usually takes a person 5 to 6 weeks to reestablish blood cells lost after withdrawal of two units of whole blood (Fig. 23.10).[93]

With appropriate blood storage methods, red blood cell reinfusion significantly elevates hematologic parameters of men and women. This in turn translates to a 5 to 13% increase in aerobic capacity, decreased heart rate and blood lactate during submaximal exercise, and augmented endurance at both sea level and altitude. In addition, significant thermoregulatory benefits during exercise in the heat (reduced body heat storage and improved sweating response) result from red blood cell reinfusion.[215,216] Increased oxygen content in arterial blood in the infused state likely "frees" blood for delivery to the skin for heat dissipation during exercise heat stress.

Table 23.8 illustrates hematologic, physiologic, and performance responses for five adult men during submaximal and maximal exercise before and 24 hours after infusion of 750 mL of packed red blood cells. These response patterns generally represent the more recent research in this area.

A New Twist: Hormonal Blood Boosting

To eliminate the cumbersome and lengthy process of blood doping, endurance athletes now use epoetin, a synthetic form of **erythropoietin (EPO)**, a hormone produced by the kidneys that regulates red blood cell production within the marrow of the long bones.[190] Medically, exogenous recombinant human EPO, commercially available since 1988, has proved useful in combating anemia in patients with severe renal disease. Normally, a decrease in red blood cell concentration or decline in the pressure of oxygen in arterial blood—as in severe pulmonary disease or on ascent to high altitude—releases this hormone to stimulate erythrocyte production. The 12% increase in hemoglobin and hematocrit that typically follows a 6-week EPO treatment significantly improves endurance exercise performance.[76] Unfortunately, if self-administration in an unregulated and unmonitored manner—simply injecting the hormone requires much less sophistication than procedures for blood doping—can increase the hematocrit more than 60%. This dangerously high hemoconcentration (and corresponding increase in blood viscosity), greatly increases the likelihood for stroke, heart attack, heart failure, and pulmonary edema.

EPO use has become particularly prevalent in cycling competition and allegedly contributed to at least 18 deaths (attributed to heart attacks) among competitive bicyclists. Because EPO cannot be detected in urine, the blood hematocrit serves as a surrogate marker. During the 1997 and 1998 competitive seasons, Tour de France officials made spot checks of hematocrits, suspending for 2 weeks any rider with an abnormally high level. This resulted in suspension of 12 riders during 1997 and six midway through the 1998 competitive season. The International Cycling Union has set a hematocrit threshold of 50% for males and 47% for females, and the International Skiing Federation uses a hemoglobin concentration

TABLE 23.8 ➤ **PHYSIOLOGIC, PERFORMANCE, AND HEMATOLOGIC CHARACTERISTICS BEFORE AND 24 HOURS AFTER REINFUSION OF 750 mL OF PACKED RED BLOOD CELLS**

VARIABLE	PREINFUSION	POSTINFUSION	DIFFERENCE	DIFFERENCE, %
Hemoglobin, g · dL blood^{-1}	13.8	17.6	3.8[b]	+27.5[b]
Hematocrit[a], %	43.3	54.8	11.5[b]	+26.5[b]
Submaximal $\dot{V}O_2$, L · min^{-1}	1.60	1.59	−0.01	−0.6
Submaximal HR, b · min^{-1}	127.4	109.2	18.2	−14.3[b]
$\dot{V}O_{2max}$, L · min^{-1}	3.28	3.70	0.42[b]	+12.8[b]
HR_{max}, b · min^{-1}	181.6	180.0	−1.6	−0.9
Treadmill run time, s	793	918	125[b]	+15.8

[a]Hematocrit presented as the percentage (%) of 100 mL (dL) of whole blood occupied by red blood cells.
[b]Difference statistically significant.
From Roberston RJ, et al. Effect of induced erythrocythemia on hypoxia tolerance during exercise. J Appl Physiol 1982;53:490.

of 18.5 g · dL^{-1} as the threshold for disqualification. Recent data suggest that hematocrit cutoff values of 52% for men and 48% for women (roughly 3 standard deviations above the mean) represent "abnormally high" or extreme values in triathletes.[180] Of course, the 50% hematocrit level cutoff raises the unanswered question of the number of disqualified "clean" cyclists. Estimates place this number between 3 and 5% because of factors that affect normal variation in hematocrit such as genetics, posture, altitude training, and hydration level.[11,29]

Current concern centers on an anomaly in iron metabolism frequently observed among high-level international cyclists. Apparently, many of these athletes show serum iron levels above 500 ng · L^{-1} (normal, 100 ng · L^{-1}), with some values as high as 1000 ng · L^{-1}. The elevated iron level results from their regular injections of supplemental iron to support increased synthesis of red blood cells induced by repeated EPO use. Chronic iron overload increases the risk of liver dysfunction among these athletes.

Warm-Up (Preliminary Exercise)

Coaches, trainers, and athletes at all levels of competition generally recommend engaging in some type of physical activity or warm-up before vigorous exercise. Conventional wisdom maintains that preliminary exercise helps the performer prepare either physiologically or psychologically and reduces the likelihood of joint and muscle injury. With animals, injuring a "warmed-up" muscle requires more force and greater muscle length than injuring a muscle in the "cold" condition.[213] The warming-up process stretches the muscle–tendon unit and possibly allows greater length and less tension on exposure to a given external load.

Warm-up generally fits into one of two categories, although overlap often exists:

- **General warm-up** uses body movements or "loosening-up" exercises unrelated to the specific neuromuscular actions of the anticipated performance. Examples include calisthenics and stretching.
- **Specific warm-up** applies big-muscle, rhythmic movements that provide skill rehearsal in the actual activity. Examples include swinging a golf club, throwing a baseball or football, tennis practice, basketball shooting and movements, and preliminary lead-up in the high jump or pole vault.

Psychologic Considerations

Competitors at all levels generally believe that performing some prior skill-related activity prepares them mentally for their event, so they can clearly focus on the upcoming performance.[209] A specific warm-up related to the activity itself also may improve the necessary skill and coordination requirements. Consequently, sports that require accuracy, timing, and precise movements generally benefit from some type of specific or "formal" preliminary practice.

The notion also exists that prior exercise, particularly before strenuous effort, gradually prepares a person to go "all out" without fear of injury. The ritual warm-up of baseball pitchers provides a good example of this belief. Is it conceivable that a pitcher would enter a game, throwing at competitive speeds, without previously warming up? Would any athlete begin competition without first stretching and engaging in a particular form, intensity, or duration of warm-up? Although most performers would respond with a definite no, objective support for this response remains elusive. One reason is the difficulty designing a well-controlled experiment with topflight athletes to determine the necessity of warming up and whether it actually improves subsequent performance with reduced risk of injury. In terms of preexercise stretching, recent research with army recruits indicates that a typical muscle-stretching protocol in the preexercise warm-up produces *no* clinically meaningful reductions in risk of exercise-related injury compared with subsequent exercise without warm-up.[189]

Certain sport-related situations require peak performance with little time for warming up. For example, a reserve player entering the last few minutes of a game has no time for stretching, vigorous calisthenics, or taking practice shots; the player must go all out and achieve optimal performance without warm-up, except that done before the game or at intermission. Do more injuries occur in such cases? Does physical performance (e.g., shooting, rebounding, or basketball defense) deteriorate during the first few minutes of this "unwarmed" condition from that preceded by a warm-up? Future research must address such questions.

Psychologic factors, including an athlete's ingrained belief in the importance of warming up, establish a definite bias in comparing maximum performance with and without warm-up. It is difficult if not impossible to obtain a maximum effort with no warm-up if a subject believes in the importance of preliminary exercise. In this regard, some researchers have hypnotized their subjects to neutralize preconceived notions about warm-up.

Physiologic Considerations

One study evaluated the effect of warm-up on 2-minute sprint-cycling performance at 120% of the power output at $\dot{V}O_{2max}$. Warm-up produced a higher muscle temperature, lower blood lactate level, and higher oxygen consumption during the first minute of exercise than the no-warm-up condition.[204] This suggests that warm-up augments local blood flow at the onset of exercise, thus increasing the aerobic contribution to muscle energy metabolism early in exercise. However, an increased muscle temperature per se does not contribute significantly to the slow component (after several minutes) of oxygen-consumption kinetics during heavy exercise.[141] Thus, any oxygen delivery–use benefits early in exercise from increased muscle temperature with warm-up may not carry over as exercise progresses.

Five mechanisms explain why warm-up should improve physical performance and exercise capacity, owing to subsequent increases in blood flow and muscle and core temperature:[19]

1. Faster muscle contraction and relaxation
2. Greater economy of movement because of lowered viscous resistance within active muscles

3. Facilitated oxygen delivery and use by muscles, because hemoglobin releases oxygen more readily at higher temperatures (Bohr effect)
4. Facilitated nerve transmission and muscle metabolism, because increased temperature accelerates the rate of bodily processes; a specific warm-up may also facilitate recruitment of motor units required in physical activity
5. Increased blood flow through active tissues as the local vascular bed dilates with higher levels of metabolism and muscle temperature

Effects on Performance

Little research has objectified the ergogenic effect of warming-up, yet more than likely, it is beneficial. Because of the strong psychologic component and possible physiologic benefits of warming-up, whether passive (massage, heat applications, and diathermy), general (calisthenics, jogging), or specific (practicing the actual movements), many exercise physiologists recommend continuing such procedures until substantial evidence justifies its elimination. A warm-up provides a comfortable way to lead up to more-vigorous exercise. *The warm-up should progress gradually and provide sufficient intensity to increase muscle and core temperatures without causing fatigue or reducing energy stores.* These considerations become highly individualized; a warm-up for an Olympic swimmer would exhaust the recreational swimmer. To gain the possible benefits from increased body temperature, the actual competition or activity should begin within several minutes after the end of the warm-up. When possible, the warm-up should activate specific muscles in a way that mimics the anticipated activity and brings about a full range of joint motion.

Sudden Strenuous Exercise

Sudden exertion can trigger the onset of myocardial infarction, particularly in sedentary people and those with latent coronary artery disease.[33,170] With this in mind, consideration of possible benefits from warming up takes on clinical significance. Several studies have evaluated the effects of preliminary exercise on the cardiovascular response to sudden, strenuous exercise. The findings provide an essentially different physiologic framework for justifying warm-up that relates importantly to adult fitness and cardiac rehabilitation programs and occupations and sports requiring sudden bursts of physical effort.

In one study, 44 men free of overt symptoms of coronary artery disease ran on a treadmill at high intensity for 10 to 15 seconds without prior warm-up.[15] Evaluation of the postexercise ECG revealed that 70% of the subjects displayed abnormal ECG changes attributable to inadequate myocardial oxygen supply. The altered ECG did not relate to age or fitness level. To evaluate the effect of a warm-up, 22 of the men with an abnormal ECG from the treadmill run-jogged in place at moderate intensity (heart rate, 145 b $\cdot$ min^{-1}) for 2 minutes before treadmill running. With warm-up, 10 men now showed normal tracings during sudden exertion, while another 10 men displayed improved ECG responses; only two subjects still showed significant abnormalities. In a subsequent study, the exercise blood pressure response also improved with prior warm-up.[16] For seven men with no warm-up, systolic blood pressure averaged 168 mm Hg immediately after the 15-second treadmill run. This decreased to 140 mm Hg when the 2-minute jog-in-place warm-up preceded exercise.

These observations indicate that coronary blood flow does not adjust to a sudden increase in myocardial work instantaneously and that transient myocardial ischemia (poor oxygen supply) can occur in apparently healthy and fit individuals. *Prior warm-up (at least 2 min of easy jogging) benefits the subsequent ECG and blood pressure responses to vigorous exercise in a manner that indicates a more favorable relationship between myocardial oxygen supply and demand.* Although a prudent practice for all people, warming up before strenuous exercise holds particular importance for individuals with limited myocardial blood flow from coronary artery disease. A brief warm-up likely provides more-optimal blood pressure and hormonal adjustments at the onset of subsequent strenuous exercise. The warm-up would serve two beneficial purposes under these conditions: (1) reduce myocardial workload and thus the myocardial oxygen requirement and (2) augment blood flow through the coronary arteries.

Oxygen Inhalation (Hyperoxia)

Athletes often breathe oxygen-enriched or **hyperoxic gas mixtures** during time-outs, at half-time, or following strenuous exercise. They believe that this procedure significantly enhances the blood's oxygen-carrying capacity and thus facilitates oxygen transport to active or recovering muscles. The fact remains, however, that when healthy people breathe ambient air at sea level, hemoglobin in the blood leaving the lungs normally remains 95 to 98% saturated with oxygen (see Chapter 13). In physiologic terms:

- Breathing air with high oxygen concentration could increase oxygen transport by hemoglobin to only a small extent, or by about 1 mL of extra oxygen for every dL of blood (+ 10 mL O_2 per L)
- Oxygen that dissolves in plasma when one breathes a hyperoxic mixture also increases by about 0.4 mL per dL of blood (+ 4.0 mL O_2 per L), or from the normal 0.3 mL (3.0 mL per L) to about 0.7 mL per dL (7.0 mL per L) of blood

Consequently, the blood's oxygen-carrying capacity under hyperoxic conditions potentially increases by about 14 mL of oxygen for every 1000 mL of blood—10 mL "extra" attached to hemoglobin and 4 mL "extra" dissolved in plasma.

Pre-exercise Oxygen Breathing

Blood volume for a 70-kg person averages about 5000 mL (5.0 L). As discussed above, breathing hyperoxic gas adds about 70 mL of oxygen to the total blood volume (5.0 L blood

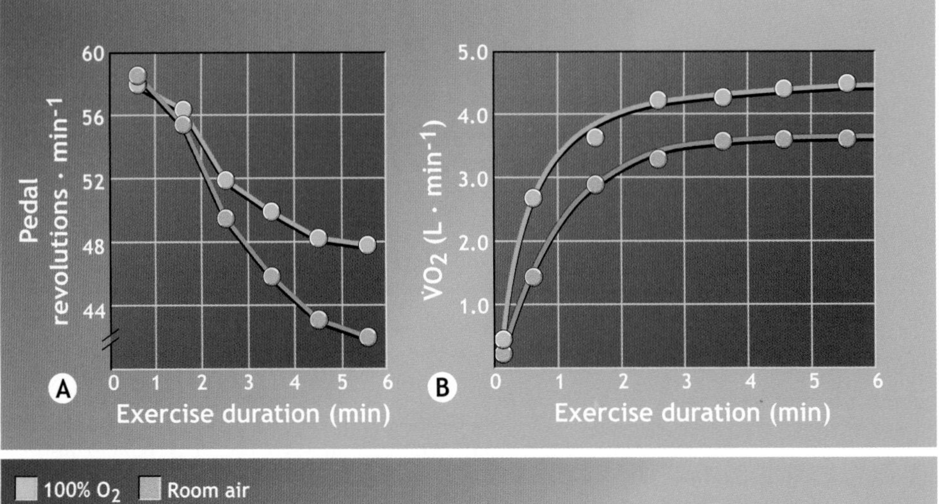

FIGURE 23.11 • **A**. Endurance (measured by pedal revolutions each minute) while breathing 100% oxygen or ambient air. **B**. Oxygen consumption curves during the endurance rides show enhanced oxygen consumption while breathing oxygen. (Data from Weltman A, et al. Effects of increasing oxygen availability on bicycle ergometer endurance performance. Ergonomics 1978;21:427.)

× 14 mL "extra" O_2 per L blood). Thus, despite any potential psychologic benefit for the athlete who believes that preexercise oxygen breathing helps subsequent performance, this procedure confers only a trivial physiologic advantage from any additional oxygen per se. Furthermore, this small benefit emerges only if subsequent exercise takes place immediately after hyperoxic breathing without breathing ambient air in the interval between hyperoxic breathing and exercise—ambient air's lower oxygen pressure causes any additional oxygen to exit the body. The football player who breathes an oxygen-rich mixture on the sideline before returning to the game or the swimmer who takes a few breaths of oxygen before moving to the blocks for the starting instructions does not gain a competitive edge because of physiologic benefits. This is particularly ironic in football, because metabolic reactions that do *not* use oxygen generate almost all of the energy to power each play.

Oxygen Breathing During Exercise

Considerable evidence indicates that breathing hyperoxic gas during submaximal and maximal aerobic exercise enhances physical performance. Oxygen breathing during vigorous exercise accelerates oxygen consumption at the onset of exercise (smaller oxygen deficit, particularly in repeated bouts of heavy effort); reduces blood lactate, heart rate, and pulmonary ventilation in submaximal exercise; and significantly increases $\dot{V}O_{2max}$.[140,153,184,202] In one study, subjects performed a 6.5-minute endurance ride on a bicycle ergometer at an exercise level equal to 115% of $\dot{V}O_{2max}$ while breathing either room air or 100% oxygen.[260] Tanks of compressed gas supplied both air and oxygen to mask a subject's knowledge of the breathing mixture. Figure 23.11A shows superior endurance (less drop-off in pedal revolutions) while breathing oxygen during exercise. Figure 23.11B shows the oxygen consumption curves during the endurance ride breathing oxygen and room air. The oxygen condition produced a higher oxygen consumption throughout exercise.

Figure 23.12 shows that the oxygen consumption of the quadriceps muscle of seven trained subjects during maximum knee-extension exercise to exhaustion varied with the level of inspired oxygen, averaging lower in hypoxia (12% O_2) than in normoxia (21% O_2) and greater in hyperoxia (100% O_2) than normoxia. The figure also includes confirmatory results (dotted yellow line) from a previous study of cycle ergometry exercise under comparable conditions.[140] Cycle ergometry produced lower muscle-specific $\dot{V}O_{2peak}$ values than

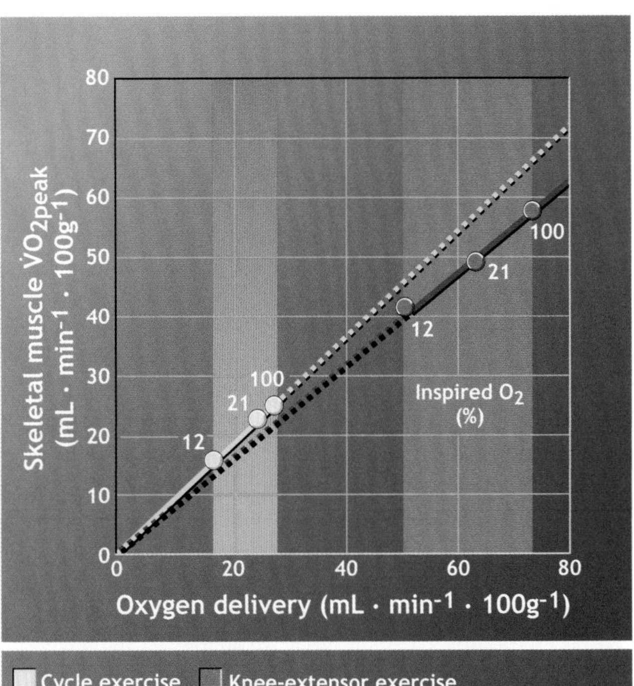

FIGURE 23.12 • Relationship between skeletal muscle $\dot{V}O_{2peak}$ and oxygen delivery per 100 g of muscle during conventional maximal cycle ergometry exercise (yellow) and knee-extension exercise (purple) under hypoxia, normoxia, and hyperoxia. (From Richardson RS, et al. Evidence of O_2 supply–dependent $\dot{V}O_{2max}$ in exercise-trained human quadriceps. J Appl Physiol 1999;86:1048.)

knee-extension exercise. However, the slopes of the lines relating oxygen delivery to peak muscle oxidative metabolism were remarkably similar for both exercise modes. For maximal knee-extension exercise, the oxygen content of the venous blood leaving the active muscles remained essentially equal among conditions and averaged approximately 4 mL · dL^{-1}. However, oxygen delivery in arterial blood increased from 17.3 to 19.5 to 21.8 mL · dL^{-1} with increasing levels of oxygen inhalation. Consequently, the hyperoxic condition during maximal exercise produced the largest a-$\bar{v}$ O_2 difference and skeletal muscle $\dot{V}O_{2peak}$. Similarly, maximal exercise intensity decreased by 25% under 12% inspired oxygen and increased by 14% under 100% inspired oxygen, compared with normoxic conditions. *Current research not only points up the ergogenic effect of breathing hyperoxic mixtures during aerobic exercise but also supports the contention that oxygen delivery to active muscles via the circulatory system, not use via mitochondrial metabolic rate, significantly limits aerobic metabolism during big-muscle exercise.*

Because breathing hyperoxic gas does not increase maximal cardiac output, the increased exercise oxygen consumption must result from an expanded a-$\bar{v}$ O_2 difference. In strenuous exercise, the small increases in arterial hemoglobin saturation and dissolved plasma oxygen with hyperoxic breathing significantly increase *total* oxygen availability as blood volume circulates 4 to 7 times each minute. More specifically, the additional 14-mL oxygen in each 1 L of blood when breathing hyperoxic gas represents considerable extra oxygen when exercising at a 20- to 30-L cardiac output. If the muscles used this added oxygen during exercise, $\dot{V}O_{2max}$ would readily increase by 5 to 10%. The increased partial pressure of oxygen in solution from breathing hyperoxic gas also facilitates its diffusion across the tissue–capillary membrane into the mitochondria. More-rapid oxygen diffusion may account for the higher oxygen consumption early in exercise under hyperoxic conditions. Reduced pulmonary ventilation under hyperoxic conditions reduces the oxygen cost of breathing. Theoretically, this liberates oxygen for use by the active, nonventilatory skeletal muscles. Hyperoxia may also increase sustained local muscle performance in intense static and dynamic movements not affected by central circulatory factors. This ergogenic effect may result from the high oxygen pressure in blood and fluids within the local active muscle environment.

Although breathing hyperoxic mixtures offers positive ergogenic benefits *during* endurance performance, limited practical application exists for sports. The "legality" of using an appropriate breathing system during actual competition seems unlikely.

Oxygen Breathing During Recovery

Research does not support the use of hyperoxic breathing mixtures as an ergogenic aid to facilitate recovery from exercise or as an adjuvant to improve subsequent performance when recovering from previous exercise. Figure 23.13 illustrates the effects of breathing hyperoxic gas in recovery from strenuous exercise on subsequent exercise performance.[259] Following 1 minute of all-out exercise on a bicycle ergometer, subjects recovered while breathing either room air or 100% oxygen for 10 or 20 minutes. They then repeated the all-out bicycle ride. No significant differences emerged in cumulative revolutions (graph A) and 6-second-by-6-second revolutions (graph B) for the 1-minute ride after breathing room air or 100% oxygen during recovery from previous all-out exercise. Also, breathing either room air or oxygen yielded similar blood lactate levels in the 10- or 20-minute recovery periods, indicating that breathing oxygen in recovery did not

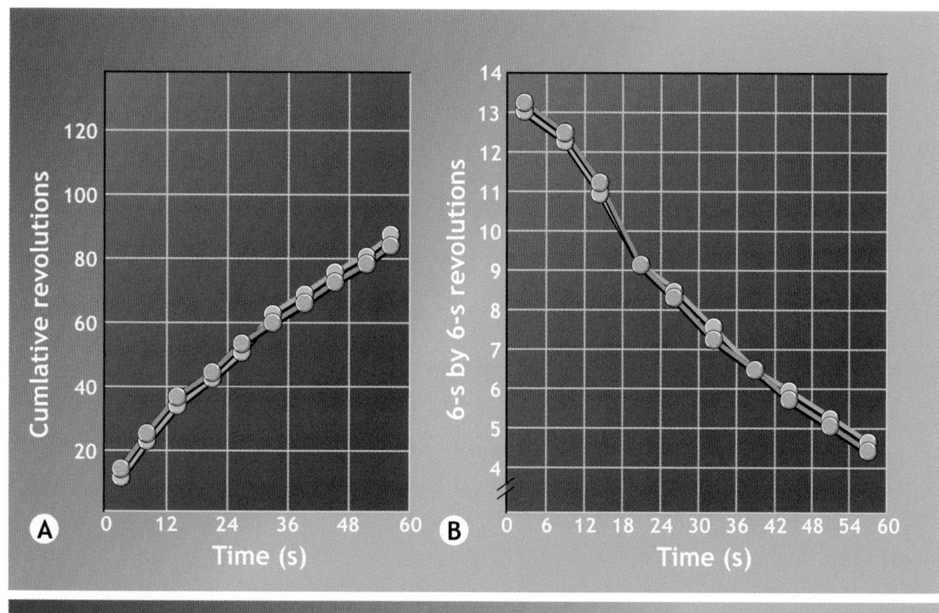

FIGURE 23.13 • Cumulative (**A**) and absolute (**B**) 6-second pedal revolutions on a bicycle ergometer during 1 minute of maximal exercise after breathing either 100% oxygen or ambient room air during recovery from a previous maximal exercise bout. (From Weltman A, et al. Exercise recovery, lactate removal, and subsequent high intensity exercise performance. Res Q 1977;48:786.)

facilitate lactate removal. Subsequent research supports these findings; it showed that breathing oxygen after short intervals of submaximal and maximal exercise did not affect recovery kinetics for minute ventilation, heart rate, or serum lactate or the level of ensuing exercise performance.[203,266]

Modification of Carbohydrate Intake

Increased carbohydrate intake before and during high-intensity aerobic exercise, including periods of heavy training, is a sound practice of macronutrient manipulation that benefits exercise performance. One of the more popular nutritional–exercise modifications used by endurance athletes to augment the body's glycogen reserves involves **carbohydrate loading**, or **glycogen supercompensation**. The procedure produces significantly higher "packing" of muscle glycogen than simply maintaining a high-carbohydrate diet. Normally, each 100 g of muscle contains about 1.7 g of glycogen; glycogen loading packs 4 to 5 g of glycogen. Although judicious adherence to this dietary technique significantly improves endurance exercise, some aspects of carbohydrate loading could prove detrimental.

Nutrient-Related Fatigue in Prolonged Exercise

Glycogen stored in the liver and active muscle supplies most of the energy for intense aerobic exercise. Prolonging such exercise reduces the body's glycogen reserves, allowing fat catabolism—from adipose tissue and liver fatty acid mobilization and intramuscular fat stores—to supply a progressively greater percentage of energy to the muscles. A significantly lowered muscle glycogen level precipitates fatigue, even though active muscles maintain sufficient oxygen and there is almost unlimited potential energy from stored fat. Ingesting a glucose and water solution near the point of fatigue allows exercise to continue, but for all practical purposes, "the muscles' fuel tank reads empty." Reliance on fat catabolism decreases power output because fat mobilization and aerobic breakdown are significantly slower than that of carbohydrate. Marathon runners use the term **hitting the wall** (endurance cyclists use *bonking*) to describe sensations of fatigue and muscle pain associated with severe glycogen depletion.

In the late 1930s, Nordic scientists reported significantly enhanced endurance performance when athletes consumed carbohydrate-rich diets. Conversely, switching to high-fat diets drastically reduced endurance capacity. Modifying the diet's macronutrient composition alters carbohydrate stores and profoundly affects subsequent prolonged, high-intensity aerobic exercise performance.[198] In a classic series of experiments, endurance capacity tripled for subjects fed a high-carbohydrate diet over that when the same subjects consumed a high-fat diet of similar energy content.[20] Because carbohydrate represents the important energy substrate during 1 to 2 hours of high-intensity exercise, researchers seek additional means of increasing the body's preexercise glycogen reserves.

Classic Loading Procedure

Table 23.9 indicates the classic procedure for achieving the supercompensation effect, which involves first reducing the muscle's glycogen content with prolonged steady-rate exercise about 6 days before competition. Because glycogen supercompensation occurs *only* in the specific muscles depleted by exercise, athletes must engage the muscles activated in their sport. Preparing for marathon running, endurance swimming, or bicycling requires 90 minutes of moderately intense submaximal exercise in the specific activity. The athlete then maintains a low-carbohydrate diet (about 60–100 $g \cdot d^{-1}$) for several days to further deplete glycogen stores. (*Note:* Glycogen depletion increases formation of intermediate forms of the glycogen-storing enzyme **glycogen synthase** within the muscle fibers.) Moderate training continues during this time. Then, at least 3 days before competing, the athlete switches to a high-carbohydrate diet (400–700 $g \cdot d^{-1}$) and maintains this intake up to the precompetition meal. The supercompensation diet should also contain adequate daily protein, minerals, and vitamins and abundant water. For athletes who follow this protocol, supercompensated muscle glycogen levels remain stable for at least 3 days during a maintenance phase (in a nonexercising individual) if the diet contains 60% of calories as carbohydrate.[94]

Athletes should learn all they can about carbohydrate loading before manipulating their dietary and exercise habits to achieve a supercompensation effect. If an athlete decides to supercompensate after weighing the pros and cons (see page 580), the new food regimen should proceed in stages during training and not for the first time before competition. For example, the athlete should start with a long run followed by a high-carbohydrate diet. A detailed log should record how the dietary manipulation affects performance. A record of subjective feelings should include exercise depletion and replenish-

TABLE 23.9 ➤ TWO-STAGE DIETARY PLAN TO INCREASE MUSCLE GLYCOGEN STORAGE

Stage 1—Depletion

Day 1: Exhausting exercise performed to deplete muscle glycogen in specific muscles

Days 2, 3, 4: Low-carbohydrate food intake (60–100 $g \cdot d^{-1}$; high percentage of protein and lipid in the daily diet)

Stage 2—Carbohydrate loading

Days 5, 6, 7: High-carbohydrate food intake (400–700 $g \cdot d^{-1}$; normal percentage of protein in the daily diet)

Competition day

High-carbohydrate precompetition meal

TABLE 23.10 ➤ **SAMPLE MEAL PLAN FOR CARBOHYDRATE-DEPLETION AND CARBOHYDRATE-LOADING PRECEDING AN ENDURANCE EVENT**

Meal	Stage 1—Depletion	Stage 2—Carbohydrate Loading
Breakfast	0.5 cup fruit juice 2 eggs 1 slice whole-wheat toast 1 glass whole milk	1 cup fruit juice 1 bowl hot or cold cereal 1 to 2 muffins 1 Tbsp butter coffee (cream/sugar)
Lunch	6 oz hamburger 2 slices bread salad (normal size) 1 Tbsp mayonnaise and salad dressing 1 glass whole milk	2–3 oz hamburger with bun 1 cup juice 1 orange 1 Tbsp mayonnaise pie or cake (one 8-in slice)
Snack	1 cup yogurt	1 cup yogurt, fruit, or cookies
Dinner	2–3 pieces of chicken, fried 1 baked potato with sour cream 0.5 cup vegetables iced tea (no sugar) 2 Tbsp butter	1–1.5 pieces of chicken, baked 1 baked potato with sour cream 1 cup vegetables 0.5 cup sweetened pineapple iced tea (sugar) 1 Tbsp butter
Snack	1 glass whole milk	1 glass chocolate milk with 4 cookies

During Stage 1, the intake of carbohydrate approaches approximately 60 g or 240 kcal; in Stage 2, the carbohydrate intake increases to 400–700 g or about 1600–2800 kcal.

ment phases. With positive results, the athlete can try the entire series—depletion, low-carbohydrate diet, and high-carbohydrate diet—but maintain the low-carbohydrate diet for only 1 day. With no adverse effects, the low-carbohydrate diet can gradually extend to a maximum of 4 days.

SAMPLE DIETS FOR ACHIEVING THE SUPERCOMPENSATION EFFECT. Table 23.10 provides a sample meal plan for carbohydrate depletion (Stage 1) and carbohydrate loading (Stage 2) preceding an endurance event.

LIMITED APPLICABILITY. Carbohydrate loading's potential benefits to exercise performance apply only to intense aerobic activities lasting more than 60 minutes, unless the athlete begins competing in a relative state of glycogen depletion. *In contrast, exercise lasting less than 60 minutes requires only normal carbohydrate intake and glycogen reserves.* Carbohydrate loading did not benefit trained runners in a 20.9-km (13-mile) run, compared with a run following a low-carbohydrate diet.[219] In addition, ingesting 40 g of carbohydrate immediately before exercise had no effect on 30-minute maximal cycling performance of well-trained cyclists.[183] Varying the carbohydrate percentage between 40 and 70% in an isocaloric diet produced no effect on intense exercise lasting either 10 or 30 minutes.[187] Furthermore, anaerobic power output of 75 seconds' duration did not improve when preexercise dietary manipulation increased muscle glycogen availability above normal levels.[111]

Endurance training increases both the rate and magnitude of glycogen replenishment.[175] For sports competition and exercise training, a daily diet containing about 60 to 70% of calories as carbohydrates provides adequate muscle and liver glycogen reserves. This diet ensures about twice as much muscle glycogen as a typical diet containing 45 to 50% carbohydrate. For well-nourished athletes, the supercompensation effect remains relatively small. During intense training, however, athletes who do not upgrade daily calorie and carbohydrate intakes to meet energy demands may experience chronic muscle fatigue and staleness.[55]

Possible Gender Difference in Glycogen Storage and Catabolism in Exercise

Research suggests that women do not increase glycogen storage when dietary carbohydrate increases from 60 to 75% of total caloric intake.[229] Other data support the notion of significant gender differences in carbohydrate metabolism in exercise before and after endurance training. During submaximal exercise at equivalent percentages of $\dot{V}O_{2max}$ (same relative workload), women derive a *smaller* proportion of the total energy from carbohydrate oxidation than men.[125] This gender difference in substrate oxidation does not persist into recovery.[120]

With similar endurance-training protocols, both women and men show a significant decrease in glucose flux for a given submaximal power output.[47,86] However, at the same relative workload after training, women show an exaggerated shift toward fat catabolism, whereas men do not.[125] This suggests that endurance training induces greater glycogen-sparing at a given relative submaximal exercise intensity for women than men. Gender differences in exercise substrate metabolism may reflect differences in sympathetic nervous system adaptation to training (i.e., more-blunted catecholamine response for women). A glycogen-sparing metabolic adaptation to training could benefit womens' performance during high-intensity endurance competition.

Negative Aspects of Carbohydrate Loading

Addition of 2.7 g of water stored with each gram of muscle glycogen makes this a heavy fuel compared with equivalent energy stored as fat. The athlete often feels "heavy" and uncomfortable with this added body mass; any extra load also directly adds to the energy cost of running, racewalking, cross-country skiing, and all other weight-bearing activities. The extra weight may negate any potential benefits from increased glycogen storage. On the positive side, water liberated during glycogen breakdown aids in temperature regulation, which benefits exercise in the heat.

The classic model for supercompensation may pose potential hazards for individuals with specific health problems. A severe, chronic carbohydrate overload, interspersed with periods of high lipid and/or high protein intake, can increase blood cholesterol and urea nitrogen levels. This could negatively affect individuals susceptible to type 2 diabetes and heart disease and those with renal disease or certain muscle enzyme deficiencies (e.g., McArdle's disease).[126] High lipid intake often causes gastrointestinal distress plus poor recovery from the exercise-depletion sequence of the loading procedure. During the low-carbohydrate phase of the loading procedure, marked ketosis can occur for individuals who exercise while carbohydrate depleted. Failure to eat a balanced diet also produces mineral and vitamin deficiencies, particularly of the water-soluble vitamins. The glycogen-depleted state reduces one's capability to train hard, possibly leading to a detraining effect during portions of the loading sequence. Adverse alterations in mood appear in individuals who train while consuming low-carbohydrate diets.[137] Dramatically reducing dietary carbohydrate for 3 or 4 days could set the stage for lean tissue loss, because muscle protein serves as gluconeogenic substrate to maintain blood-glucose levels in the glycogen-depleted state.

Modified Loading Procedure

The less-stringent **modified loading procedure** outlined in Figure 23.14 eliminates many of the potential negative outcomes of the classic glycogen-loading sequence.[219] The modified dietary protocol stimulates increases in glycogen synthase without requiring the dramatic glycogen depletion with exercise demanded by the classic loading procedure[269] and increases glycogen storage to nearly the *same* level achieved with the classic protocol.[218] The 6-day protocol does not require prior exercise to exhaustion. Rather, the athlete trains at about 75% of $\dot{V}O_{2max}$ (85% HR_{max}) for 1.5 hours and then, on successive days, gradually reduces (tapers) exercise duration. During the first 3 days, carbohydrates represent about 50% of total calories. Three days before competition, the diet's carbohydrate content increases to 70% of total energy intake.

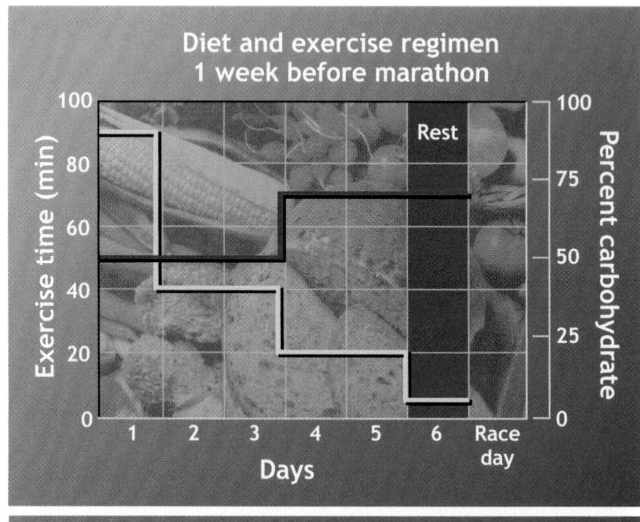

FIGURE 23.14 • A modified approach to carbohydrate loading. Recommended combination of diet and exercise for overloading muscle glycogen stores in the week before an important endurance contest. Exercise time is gradually reduced during the week, while the diet's carbohydrate content increases for the last 3 days. (From Sherman WM, et al. Effect of exercise-diet manipulation on muscle glycogen and its subsequent utilization during performance. Int J Sports Med 1981;2:114.)

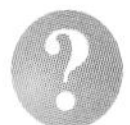

INTEGRATIVE QUESTION

What advice would you give to a sprint athlete who plans to carbohydrate load for competition?

L-Carnitine

L-Carnitine, a short-chain carboxylic acid containing nitrogen, is a vitamin-like compound found mostly in meat and dairy products. (*Note:* D,L-carnitine is toxic and should never be ingested.) The liver and kidneys synthesize L-carnitine from methionine and lysine, and about 95% of the body's carnitine is located in muscle cells. Vital to normal metabolism, carnitine facilitates the influx of long-chain fatty acids into the mitochondrial matrix (as part of the carnitine acyltransferase enzyme system) where they enter β-oxidation during energy metabolism. This carnitine-dependent process is probably an important rate-limiting step in fatty acid oxidation. Intracellular carnitine contributes to the maintenance of the acetyl-CoA:CoA ratio within the cell. Optimizing this ratio augments skeletal muscle energy metabolism by reducing inhibition of the pyruvate dehydrogenase enzyme; this facilitates conversion of pyruvate (and lactate) to acetyl-CoA, particularly in type I, slow-twitch muscle fibers.[220] Theoretically, enhanced carnitine function could inhibit lactate accumulation and enhance exercise performance.[51,234]

Rate of Fatty Acid Oxidation Affects Aerobic Exercise Intensity

During prolonged aerobic exercise, plasma FFAs often increase more than is required by the actual expenditure of energy. Speculation is that plasma FFA elevation results from inadequate mitochondrial fatty acid uptake and oxidation because of insufficient L-carnitine. Hence, increasing intracellular L-carnitine by dietary supplementation should promote fatty acid oxidation during exercise. Such an effect would increase aerobic energy transfer from fat breakdown while conserving limited glycogen reserves. Supplementation should be most beneficial under conditions of glycogen depletion, which places the greatest demands on fatty acid oxidation. Consequently, L-carnitine marketing targets endurance athletes who believe that this "metabolic stimulator" enhances fat burning and spares glycogen. Not surprisingly, the alleged fat-burning benefits of L-carnitine also appeal to the bodybuilder as a "surefire" way to reduce body fat.

While patients with progressive muscle weakness have benefited from carnitine administration, few data suggest that healthy adults require carnitine above levels in a well-balanced diet. *Research does not support ergogenic benefits, positive metabolic alterations (aerobic or anaerobic), or body fat–reducing effects from L-carnitine supplementation.*[50,115,197,253] For example, muscle carnitine levels do not differ between young and middle-aged men who consume a normal carnitine intake of about 100 to 200 mg daily. For these individuals, typical variations in muscle carnitine levels do not reflect capacity for aerobic metabolism.[224] Furthermore, no L-carnitine deficit occurs during long-term exercise or heavy training.[63] Taking up to 2000 mg of L-carnitine, either orally or intravenously during aerobic exercise, does not affect the fuel mixture metabolized, endurance performance, aerobic capacity, or the exercise level for the onset of blood lactate accumulation (OBLA).[253] Short-term administration of 2000 mg of L-carnitine to endurance athletes either 2 hours before a marathon or 20-km into an endurance run significantly increased plasma concentrations of all carnitine fractions.[50] However, plasma carnitine increases did not affect running performance, alter the metabolic mixture during the run, or enhance recovery. Even with exercise prolonged and intense enough to deplete glycogen reserves, individuals receiving L-carnitine supplements did not alter substrate metabolism to indicate enhanced fat oxidation.[64] Carnitine supplementation also exerts no effect on repetitive short-term anaerobic exercise. Lactate accumulation, acid–base balance, or performance in five 100-yard swims with 2-minute rest intervals did not differ between competitive male swimmers who consumed 2000 mg L-carnitine in a citrus drink twice daily for 7 days and those who consumed only the citrus drink.[234]

Perhaps of Some Benefit

L-carnitine acts as a vasodilator in peripheral tissues and possibly enhances regional blood flow and oxygen delivery.[115] In one study, subjects consumed either L-carnitine supplements (3000 mg · d^{-1} for 3 wk) or an inert placebo to evaluate effects on delayed-onset muscle soreness (DOMS) after eccentric muscle actions.[91] Compared with placebo conditions, subjects receiving L-carnitine experienced significantly less postexercise muscle pain and tissue damage, as reflected by lower plasma levels of the muscle enzyme creatine kinase. The vasodilation property of L-carnitine might improve oxygen supply to damaged tissue and promote clearance of muscle damage by-products, thus reducing DOMS.

Chromium

The trace mineral chromium potentiates insulin function, although its precise mechanism of action remains unclear. Insulin promotes carbohydrate transport into cells, augments fatty acid catabolism, and triggers cellular enzyme activity that facilitates protein synthesis. Chronic chromium deficiency may increase blood cholesterol and decrease the body's sensitivity to insulin, thus raising the risk for type 2 diabetes.[7] In all likelihood, some adult Americans consume less than the 50 to 200 μg of chromium considered the estimated safe and adequate daily dietary intake (ESADDI). This occurs largely because chromium-rich foods—brewer's yeast, broccoli, wheat germ, nuts, liver, prunes, egg yolks, apples with skins, asparagus, mushrooms, wine, and cheese—are not usually part of the regular daily diet. Processing also removes significant chromium from foods. In addition, strenuous exercise and associated high carbohydrate intake promote urinary chromium losses, thus increasing the potential for chromium deficiency.[8] For athletes with chromium-deficient diets, dietary modification to increase chromium intake or prudent use of chromium supplements seems appropriate.[148]

Numerous Alleged Benefits

Chromium, touted as a "fat burner" and "muscle builder," is one of the most hyped minerals in the health food/fitness literature. Supplemental intake of chromium, usually as **chromium picolinate**, often reaches 600 μg daily. This chelated picolinic acid combination supposedly yields better chromium absorption than the inorganic salt chromium chloride. Millions of Americans believe the unsubstantiated claims of health food faddists, television infomercials, and exercise zealots that additional chromium promotes muscle growth, curbs appetite, fosters body fat loss, and even lengthens life.[9] Advertising targets chromium to bodybuilders and other resistance-trained athletes as a safe alternative to anabolic steroids for favorably changing body composition. Chromium supplements supposedly potentiate insulin action, thus increasing amino acid anabolism in skeletal muscle.

Generally, studies suggesting beneficial effects of chromium supplements on body fat and muscle mass infer body composition changes from changes in body weight (or unvalidated anthropometric measurements) instead of assessing more appropriately by hydrostatic weighing. One study observed that supplementing daily with 200 μg (3.85 μmol) of chromium picolinate for 40 days produced a small increase in FFM (estimated from skinfold thickness) and decrease in body fat in young men undergoing 6 weeks of resistance training.[80] The researchers reported no data to show increased muscular strength. Another study reported increases in body mass without changes in strength or body composition in previously untrained female college students (no change in males) receiving a daily chromium supplement of 200 μg during 12 weeks of resistance training, compared with unsupplemented controls.[113]

Other research evaluated the effects of a daily 200-μg chromium supplement on muscle strength, body composition, and chromium excretion in 16 untrained males undergoing 12 weeks of resistance training.[110] Muscular strength improved significantly in both supplemented (24%) and placebo (33%) groups during training. However, no changes occurred in any of the body composition variables. The group receiving the supplement did show significantly higher chromium excretion than controls after 6 weeks of training. The researchers concluded that chromium supplements provided *no ergogenic effect* on any measured variable. Furthermore, supplementing with 800 μg of chromium picolinate (plus 6 mg of boron) proved no more effective than a maltodextrin placebo in enhancing lean tissue gain or promoting fat loss during resistance training.[2] Daily supplementation with 400 μg of chromium picolinate for 9 weeks did not promote weight loss in sedentary obese women; it actually caused significant weight gain during the treatment period.[102]

In support of chromium supplementation, significantly greater body fat loss (no increase in FFM) occurred in subjects "recruited from a variety of fitness and athletic clubs" who consumed 400 μg of chromium daily over 90 days than in subjects receiving a placebo.[135] Hydrostatic weighing and DEXA techniques assessed body composition. However, body compositional data from hydrostatic weighing do not appear in the report, and the DEXA-derived analysis indicated average body fat values of 42% for both control and experimental subjects, a seemingly extraordinary level of obesity for members of fitness clubs. Collegiate football players who received daily 200-μg supplements of chromium picolinate for 9 weeks showed no changes in body composition and muscular strength from intense weight training compared with controls receiving a placebo.[46] Similar findings of no benefit on body composition and exercise performance variables emerged from a 14-week study of NCAA Division I wrestlers in which combined chromium picolinate supplementation with a typical preseason training program was compared with identical training without supplementation.[255]

Because loss of muscle mass commonly affects older individuals, any potential ergogenic benefit to muscle from chromium supplementation should emerge readily in this group. This did not occur for older men involved in high-intensity resistance training; a high chromium picolinate dosage (924 $\mu g \cdot d^{-1}$) did not augment development of muscle size, strength, or power or FFM accretion above the unsupplemented condition.[38] Obese personnel enrolled in the United States Navy's mandatory remedial physical-conditioning program who consumed an additional 400 μg of chromium picolinate daily showed no greater loss in body weight or percentage body fat or increase in FFM than a group receiving a placebo.[235]

A comprehensive double-blind study examined the effects of a daily chromium supplement (3.3 to 3.5 μmol, either as chromium chloride or chromium picolinate) or a placebo for 8 weeks during resistance training in 36 young men.[152] For each group, dietary intakes of protein, magnesium, zinc, copper, and iron equaled or exceeded recommended levels during training; subjects also maintained adequate baseline dietary chromium intakes. Supplementation increased serum chromium concentration and urinary chromium excretion equally, regardless of its ingested form. Table 23.11 shows that compared with placebo treatment, chromium supplementation (regardless of form) did not affect training-related changes in muscular strength, physique, FFM, or muscle mass. In November 1996, the Federal Trade Commission ordered three producers of chromium supplements to cease promoting unsubstantiated weight loss and health claims (reduced body fat, increased muscle mass, increased energy level) for chromium picolinate. Under the settlement, the companies could no longer make statements of benefit unless reliable research data substantiated such claims.

Not Without a Potential Downside

Chromium competes with iron for binding to transferrin, a plasma protein that transports iron from ingested food and damaged red blood cells for delivery to tissues in need. The chromium picolinate supplement for the group whose data appear in Table 23.11 reduced serum transferrin (a measure of adequacy of current iron intake) significantly compared with chromium chloride or placebo treatments. However, other researchers observed that giving men between 56 to 69 years of age 924 μg of supplemental chromium daily as chromium picolinate for 12 weeks did not affect hematologic measures or indices of iron metabolism or status.[37] Thus, more research must determine whether chromium picolinate supplementation above recommended values adversely affects iron transport and distribution within the body. Furthermore, no studies have evaluated the safety of long-term chromium supplementation or the ergogenic efficacy of supplementation in individuals with suboptimal chromium status. Concerning the bioavailability of trace minerals in the diet, excessive dietary chromium inhibits zinc and iron absorption. At the extreme, this could induce iron-deficiency anemia, blunt the ability to train intensely, and negatively affect exercise performance requiring high-level aerobic metabolism.

Further potential bad news emerges from studies in which human tissue cultures that received extreme doses of chromium picolinate showed eventual chromosomal damage. Critics contend that such high laboratory dosages would not occur with supplement use in humans. Nonetheless, one can argue that cells continually exposed to excessive chromium (e.g., long-term supplementation) accumulate this mineral and retain it for years. Determination of the possible ill effects

TABLE 23.11 ➤ **EFFECTS OF TWO DIFFERENT FORMS OF CHROMIUM SUPPLEMENTATION ON AVERAGE VALUES FOR ANTHROPOMETRIC, BONE, AND SOFT-TISSUE COMPOSITION MEASUREMENTS BEFORE AND AFTER WEIGHT TRAINING**

	Placebo		Chromium Chloride		Chromium Picolinate	
	Pre	Post	Pre	Post	Pre	Post
Age (y)	21.1	21.5	23.3	23.5	22.3	22.5
Stature (cm)	179.3	179.2	177.3	177.3	178.0	178.2
Weight (kg)	79.9	80.5[a]	79.3	81.1[a]	79.2	80.5
Σ4 skinfold thickness (mm)[b]	42.0	41.5	42.6	42.2	43.3	43.1
Upper arm girth (cm)	30.9	31.6[a]	31.3	32.0[a]	31.1	31.4
Lower leg girth (cm)	38.2	37.9	37.4	37.5	37.1	37.0
Endomorphy	3.68	3.73	3.58	3.54	3.71	3.72
Mesomorphy	4.09	4.36[a]	4.25	4.42[a]	4.21	4.33[a]
Ectomorphy	2.09	1.94[a]	1.79	1.63[a]	2.00	1.88[a]
FFMFM (kg)[c]	62.9	64.3[a]	61.1	63.1[a]	61.3	62.7[a]
Bone mineral (g)	2952	2968	2860	2878	2918	2940
Fat-free body mass (kg)	65.9	67.3[a]	64.0	65.9[a]	64.2	66.1[a]
Fat (kg)	13.4	13.1	14.7	15.1	14.7	14.5
Body fat (%)	16.4	15.7	18.4	18.2	18.4	17.9

[a]Significantly different from pretraining value.
[b]Measured at biceps, triceps, subscapular, and suprailiac sites.
[c]Fat-free, mineral-free mass.
From Lukaski HC, et al. Chromium supplementation and resistance training: effects on body composition, strength, and trace element status of men. Am J Clin Nutr 1996;63:954.

of long-term chromium supplementation at the considerable excess ingested by some athletes requires further research.

Creatine

Meat, poultry, and fish are a rich source of creatine, providing approximately 4 to 5 g of creatine per kg of food. The body synthesizes only about 1 g of this nitrogen-containing organic compound daily from the nonessential amino acids arginine, glycine, and methionine, primarily in the kidneys, liver, and pancreas.[268] Thus, adequate dietary creatine is important. Since the animal kingdom contains the richest creatine-containing foods, vegetarians are at a distinct disadvantage for ready sources of exogenous creatine.[13,106] Skeletal muscle contains approximately 95% of the body's total 120 to 140 g of creatine.

Creatine sold in supplemental form as **creatine monohydrate (CrH_2O)** comes as a powder, tablet, capsule, and stabilized liquid. Phosphocreatine (PCr), a less frequently used form of creatine supplementation, is produced by adding phosphate salts to the CrH_2O molecule. Creatine supplements in this form produced the same training effects on body mass, muscular strength, and FFM (estimated from skinfolds) as creatine ingested in monohydrate form.[186] A person can purchase creatine over-the-counter or mail order as a nutritional supplement (but without guarantee of purity). Ingesting a liquid suspension of creatine monohydrate at the relatively high dosage of 20 to 30 g per day for 2 weeks increases intramuscular concentrations of free creatine and PCr up to 30%. These levels remain high for weeks after a few days of supplementation.[121,161] An athlete can supplement with creatine in international competition since sports' governing bodies do not consider creatine an illegal substance.

Important Component of High-Energy Phosphates

The precise physiologic mechanisms underlying the potential ergogenic effectiveness of supplemental creatine remain poorly understood. Creatine passes through the digestive tract unaltered and is absorbed into the bloodstream by the intestinal mucosa. Just about all ingested creatine is incorporated into skeletal muscle (average concentration, 125 mM [range 90 to 160 mM] per kg dry muscle). About 40% exists as free creatine; the remainder combines readily with phosphate (in the creatine kinase reaction shown below) to form PCr. Type II, fast-twitch muscle fibers store about 4 to 6 times more PCr than ATP.[41] As emphasized in Chapter 5, PCr serves as the cells' "energy reservoir" to provide rapid phosphate-bond energy to resynthesize ATP (more rapid than ATP regenerated in glycogenolysis[107]) in the reversible reaction:

$$PCr + ADP \xrightarrow{\text{creatine kinase}} C + ATP$$

PCr may also function to shuttle intramuscular high-energy phosphate between the mitochondria and muscle filament cross-bridge sites that initiate muscle action.[21] Maintaining a high sarcoplasmic ATP:ADP ratio by energy transfer from PCr becomes important in maximum effort lasting up to 10 seconds. Short-term exercise of this duration places significant demands on the rate of ATP resynthesis, which greatly exceeds energy transfer from the breakdown of intracellular macronutrients.[23,107] Improved energy transfer capacity from PCr also lessens reliance on energy from anaerobic glycolysis with its associated increase in intramuscular H^+ and decrease in pH from lactate accumulation.[14] Amounts of intramuscular PCr are limited, so it seems reasonable that any PCr increase should accomplish the following:

- Contribute to faster ATP turnover to maintain power output during short-term muscular effort
- Delay depletion of PCr
- Diminish dependence on anaerobic glycolysis and decrease subsequent lactate formation
- Facilitate muscle relaxation and recovery from repeated bouts of intense, brief effort via faster ATP and PCr resynthesis; rapid recovery allows continued higher-level power output[23,41,240]

Documented Benefits in Humans

Creatine supplementation received notoriety as an ergogenic aid from its use by British sprinters and hurdlers in the 1992 Barcelona Olympic Games. Creatine supplementation at recommended levels has been shown to exert the following three effects:

1. Improve performance in muscular strength and power activities
2. Augment short bursts of muscular endurance
3. Provide for greater muscular overload to augment training effectiveness

The literature does not report serious adverse effects from creatine supplementation for up to 4 years.[217] In fact,

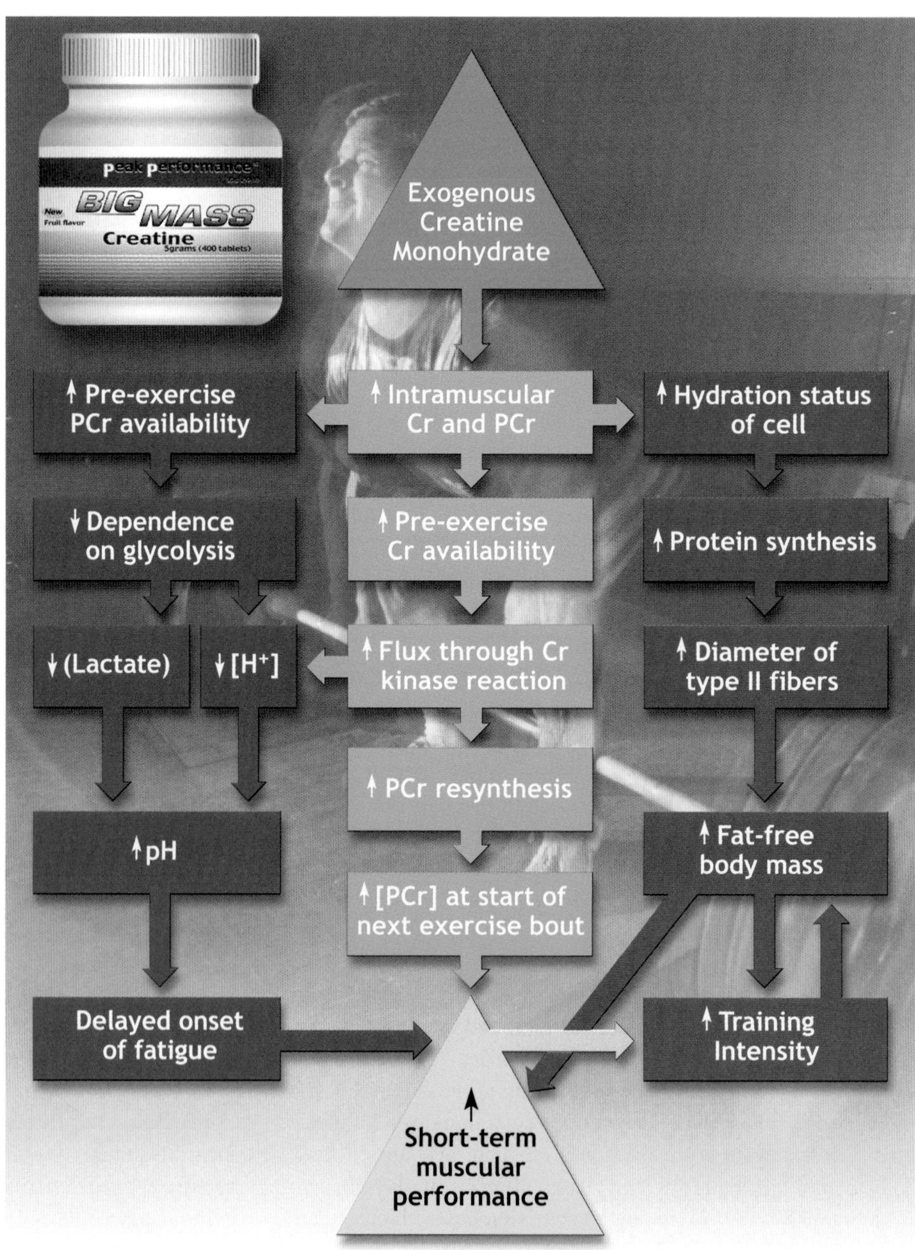

FIGURE 23.15 • Possible mechanisms to explain why increased intracellular creatine (Cr) and phosphocreatine (PCr) might enhance intense, short-term exercise performance and the exercise-training response. (Modified from Volek JS, Kraemer WJ. Creatine supplementation: its effect on human muscular performance and body composition. J Strength Cond Res 1996;10:200.)

TABLE 23.12 ➤ SELECTED STUDIES SHOWING INCREASES IN EXERCISE PERFORMANCE FOLLOWING CREATINE MONOHYDRATE SUPPLEMENTATION

REFERENCE	EXERCISE	PROTOCOL	EXERCISE PERFORMANCE
d	Isokinetic, unilat. knee extensions (180° · s^{-1})	5 bouts of 30 ext. w/1-min rest periods	Less decline in peak torque production during bouts 2, 3, and 4
e	Running	4-300 m w/4-min rest periods	Improved time for final 300- and 1000-m runs
		4-1000 m w/3-min rest periods	Improved total time for 4-1000-m runs; reduction in best time for 300- and 1000-m runs
a	Cycle ergometry (140 rev · min^{-1})	Ten 6-s bouts w/1-min rest periods	Better able to maintain pedal frequency during second 4–6 of each bout
f	Cycle ergometry (140 rev · min^{-1})	Five 6-s bouts w/30-s recovery followed by one 10-s bout	Better able to maintain pedal frequency near end of 10-s bout
b	Cycle ergometry (80 rev · min^{-1})	Three 30-s bouts w/4-min rest periods	Increase in peak power during bout 1 and increase in mean power and total work during bouts 1 and 2
c	Bench press	1-RM bench press and total reps at 70% 1-RM	Increase in 1-RM; increase in reps at 70% of 1-RM
g	Bench press	5 sets bench press w/2-min rest periods	Increase in reps completed during all 5 sets
g	Jump squat	5 sets jump squat w/2-min rest periods	Increase in peak power during all 5 sets

From Volek JS, Kraemer WJ. Creatine supplementation: its effect on human muscular performance and body composition. J Strength Cond Res. 1996;10:200.
[a]Balsom PD, et al. Creatine supplementation and dynamic high-intensity intermittent exercise. Scand J Med Sci Sports 1995;3:143.
[b]Birch R, et al. The influence of dietary creatine supplementation on performance during repeated bouts of maximal isokinetic cycling in man. Eur J Appl Physiol 1994;69:268.
[c]Earnest CP, et al. The effect of creatine monohydrate ingestion on anaerobic power indices, muscular strength and body composition. Acta Physiol Scand 1995;153:207.
[d]Greenhaff PL, et al. Influence of oral creatine supplementation on muscle torque during repeated bouts on maximal voluntary exercise in man. Clin Sci 1993;84:565.
[e]Harris RC, et al. The effect of oral creatine supplementation on running performance during maximal short-term exercise in man. J Physiol 1993;467:74P.
[f]Soderlund K, et al. Creatine supplementation and high-intensity exercise: influence on performance and muscle metabolism. Clin Sci 1994;87 (suppl):120.
[g]Volek JS, et al. Creatine supplementation enhances muscular performance during high-intensity resistance exercise. J Am Diet Assoc 1997;97:765.

studies with animals suggest that creatine or creatine analogs may exert positive effects on a number of diseases.[268] However, anecdotes indicate a possible association between creatine supplementation and cramping in multiple muscle areas during competition or lengthy practice in players of American football. This effect may result from (1) altered intracellular dynamics because of increased levels of free creatine and PCr or (2) an osmotically induced enlarged cell volume (greater cellular hydration) caused by the muscle fibers' increased creatine content. Gastrointestinal tract disturbances such as nausea, indigestion, and difficulty absorbing food have also been linked to exogenous creatine ingestion.

Figure 23.15 outlines possible mechanisms for enhancement of exercise performance and training response by creatine supplementation and elevated intramuscular free creatine and PCr. Taking a high dose of creatine helps replenish muscle creatine following intense exercise. This metabolic "reloading" should promote recovery of muscle contractile capacity, thus enabling athletes to maintain repeated efforts of high-intensity exercise. A facilitated rate of muscle relaxation may also contribute to the ergogenic action of creatine supplementation.[240] Besides benefiting weight lifting and bodybuilding, improved immediate anaerobic power output capacity also aids sprint running, swimming, kayaking, cycling, jumping, football, and volleyball. Increased intramuscular PCr concentrations should also permit increased training intensity. Ergogenic effects of creatine supplementation also occur in animals. Specifically, supplementation combined with exercise training enhanced repetitive high-intensity running performance of rats more than either training or supplementation alone.[24] From a clinical perspective, it appears that exogeneous creatine may reduce damage after traumatic head injury, although the protective mechanism remains unknown.

Oral supplements of creatine monohydrate (20 to 25 g · d^{-1}) significantly increase muscle creatine content and performance in high-intensity exercise, particularly repeated intense muscular effort (Table 23.12).[167,178,199,207,221,239,250] Even daily doses as low as 6 g daily for 5 days promote significant improvement in repeated power performance.[79] Other research evaluated a creatine dose of 30 g daily for 6 days in trained runners under two conditions: (1) four repeated 300-m runs with a 4-minute recovery and (2) four 1000-m runs with a 3-minute recovery.[112] Compared with placebo treatment, creatine supplementation significantly improved performance under both conditions, with the most impressive gains in repeated 1000-m runs. Supplementing with 20 g of creatine daily for 4 days also benefited anaerobic capacity in three 30-second Wingate tests with a 5-minute rest between trials. Creatine supplementation does not improve cardiovascular and metabolic responses during continuous incremental treadmill running[104] or performance that requires a high level of aerobic energy transfer.[12,79]

Short-term use (e.g., 20 g · d^{-1} for 5 consecutive days) produced no detrimental effect on blood pressure, plasma creatine, plasma CK activity, or the renal responses of healthy men, as measured by glomerular filtration rate and total protein and albumin excretion rates.[134,169] Only limited information exists about the effects of long-term, high-dose supplementation with creatine, particularly the effects on cardiac muscle and kidney function (creatine degrades to creatinine before excretion in urine). For healthy subjects, no differences in plasma contents and urinary excretion rates for creatinine, urea, and albumin emerged between control subjects and individuals who consumed creatine for between 10 months and 5 years.[188] In addition, glomerular filtration rate, tubular reabsorption, and glomerular membrane permeability remained normal with chronic creatine use. However, individuals with suspected renal malfunction should refrain from creatine supplementation because of the potential for exacerbating the disorder,[195] possibly via an increased production of the uraemic toxin methylguanidine.[268]

EFFECTS ON BODY COMPOSITION. Body mass increases of between 0.5 and 5.2 kg often accompany creatine supplementation,[13,72,143,252] independent of short-term changes in testosterone or cortisol concentrations.[251] In fact, short-term creatine supplementation exerts no effect on the hormonal response to resistance training.[179] It is unclear how much of the weight gain occurs from (1) the anabolic effect of creatine on muscle tissue synthesis, (2) retention of intracellular water from increased creatine stores, or (3) other factors.

Research has determined the effect of creatine supplementation plus resistance training on body composition, muscle fiber hypertrophy, and exercise performance adaptations. Creatine intake during resistance training (4-d pretraining dosage, 20 g · d^{-1}, followed by 5 g · d^{-1} during training) by young-adult females significantly increased maximal strength of trained muscles (20 to 25%), maximal intermittent exercise capacity of the arm flexors (10 to 25%), and FFM (6%) compared with the placebo condition.[238] Part of the FFM increase resulted from increased muscle water content. Data also indicate that a significant 2.42-kg body mass gain associated with creatine supplementation and resistance/agility training resulted partly from increases in fat/bone-free body mass unrelated to an increase in total body water.[143]

In more recent research, resistance-trained men, matched for physical characteristics and maximal strength, randomly received either a placebo ($n = 9$) or a creatine supplement ($n = 10$).[252] Supplementation was 25 g daily, followed by maintenance at 5 g daily. Both groups engaged in heavy resistance training for 12 weeks. Figure 23.16A shows the significantly greater training-induced increase in body mass (6.3%) and FFM (6.3%) for the creatine-supplemented group, compared with controls (3.6% increase body mass and 3.1% increase FFM). Maximum bench press (+24%) and squat (+32%) strength increases were greater in the creatine group than in controls (+16% bench press; +24% squat; Fig. 23.16B). Creatine supplementation also induced greater muscle fiber hypertrophy with resistance training, as indicated by significantly greater enlargement in types I (35 vs. 11%), IIA (36 vs. 15%), and IIAB muscle fiber cross-sectional areas (35 vs. 6%; Fig. 23.16C). The significantly larger average volume of weight lifted in the bench press during weeks 5 to 8 by the creatine supplement group suggests that higher quality of the training sessions mediated the more favorable adaptations in FFM, muscle morphology, and strength performance.

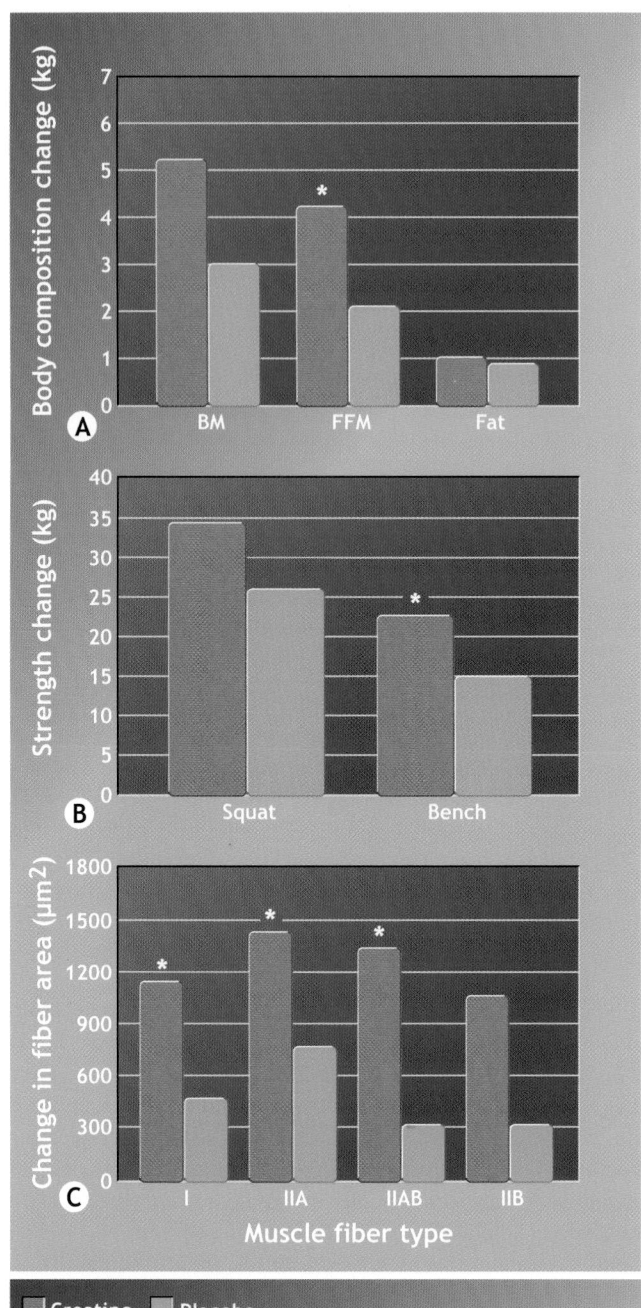

FIGURE 23.16 • Effects of 12 weeks of creatine supplementation plus heavy resistance training on changes in (**A**) body mass *(BM)* fat-free body mass *(FFM)*, and body fat, (**B**) muscular strength in the squat and bench press, and (**C**) cross-sectional areas of specific muscle fiber types. The placebo group underwent identical training and received an equivalent quantity of powdered cellulose in capsule form. * Change significantly greater than placebo group. (From Volek JS, et al. Performance and muscle fiber adaptations to creatine supplementation and heavy resistance training. Med Sci Sports Exerc 1999;31:1147.)

Creatine Loading

Many creatine users pursue a loading phase by ingesting 20 to 30 g of creatine daily (usually in tablet form or a powder added to liquid) for 5 to 7 days. Individuals who consume vegetarian-type diets show the greatest increase in muscle creatine levels because of low dietary creatine content. Large increases also characterize individuals with normally low basal levels of intramuscular creatine.[106] A maintenance phase follows the loading phase, in which the athlete supplements with as little as 2 to 5 g of creatine daily.

Practical questions for the athlete desiring to elevate intramuscular creatine levels concern (1) the magnitude and time course of intramuscular creatine increase with supplementation, (2) the dosage needed to maintain creatine increase, and (3) the rate of creatine loss, or "washout," when supplementation ceases. To provide insight into these questions, researchers studied two groups of men.[121] In one experiment, six men ingested 20 g of creatine monohydrate (approximately 0.3 g per kg of body mass) for 6 consecutive days, then stopped the supplementation. Biopsies assessed muscle creatine levels before supplement ingestion and at days 7, 21, and 35. Similarly, nine men took 20 g of creatine monohydrate daily for 6 consecutive days. Instead of discontinuing supplementation, they reduced dosage to 2-g daily (approximately 0.03 g per kg body mass) for an additional 28 days. Figure 23.17A shows that total muscle creatine concentration increased approximately 20% after 6 days. Without continued supplementation, muscle creatine content gradually declined to near baseline in 35 days. The group that continued to supplement with reduced creatine intake for an additional 28 days maintained muscle creatine content at the higher level (Fig. 23.17B).

For both groups, the increase in total muscle creatine content during the initial 6-day supplementation period averaged about 23 mmol per kg of dry muscle, which represented about 20 g (17%) of total creatine ingested. Interestingly, a similar 20% increase in total muscle creatine concentration occurred with only a 3-g daily supplement. However, this increase occurred more gradually and required 28 days rather than the 6 days with the 6-g supplement.

A rapid way to creatine-load skeletal muscle requires ingesting 20 g of creatine monohydrate daily for 6 days; switching to a reduced 2-g per day dosage keeps these levels elevated for up to 28 days. If rapidity of loading does not matter, supplementing with 3 g daily for 28 days achieves the same high levels.

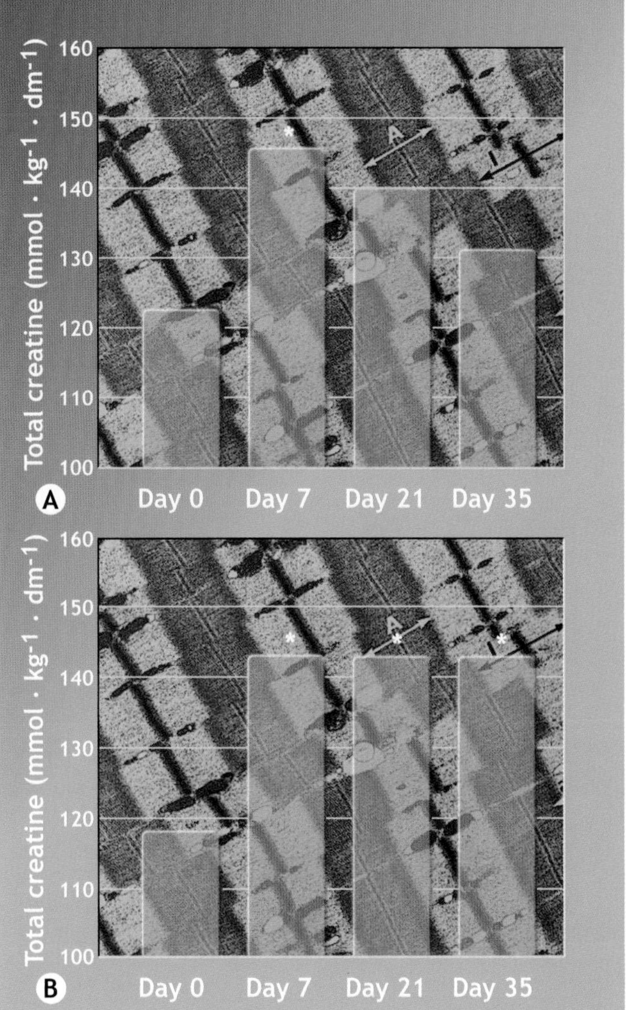

FIGURE 23.17 • **A**. Total muscle creatine concentration in six men who ingested 20 g of creatine for 6 consecutive days and then stopped the supplement. Muscle biopsies done before ingestion (day 0) and on days 7, 21, and 35. **B**. Muscle total creatine concentration in nine men who ingested 20 g of creatine for 6 consecutive days and then ingested 2 g of creatine daily for the next 28 days. Muscle biopsies done before ingestion (day 0) and on days 7, 21, and 35. Values refer to averages per dry mass (dm). *Significantly different from day 0. (From Hultman E, et al. Muscle creatine loading in men. J Appl Physiol 1996;81:232.)

CARBOHYDRATE INGESTION MAY AUGMENT CREATINE LOADING. Research now supports the common belief among athletes that consuming creatine with a sugar-containing drink increases creatine uptake and storage in skeletal muscle (Fig. 23.18).[105] For 5 days, subjects received either 5 g of creatine four times each day, or a 5-g supplement followed 30-minutes later by 93 g of a high-glycemic simple sugar four times daily. The creatine-only group significantly increased in muscle PCr (7.2%), free creatine (13.5%), and total creatine (20.7%). However, much larger increases resulted for the creatine plus sugar-supplemented group (14.7% for muscle PCr, 18.1% for free creatine, and a 33.0% for total creatine). Creatine supplementation alone did not affect insulin secretion, whereas adding sugar significantly elevated plasma insulin levels. More than likely, augmented creatine storage with a creatine plus sugar supplement resulted from insulin-mediated glucose transport into skeletal muscle, which also facilitated creatine transport into muscle fibers.

STOP CAFFEINE WHEN USING CREATINE. *Caffeine blunts the ergogenic effect of creatine supplementation.* To evaluate the effect of preexercise caffeine ingestion on both intramuscular creatine stores and high-intensity exercise performance, subjects consumed either a placebo, a daily creatine supplement ($0.5\ g \cdot kg$ body mass^{-1}), or the same daily creatine supple-

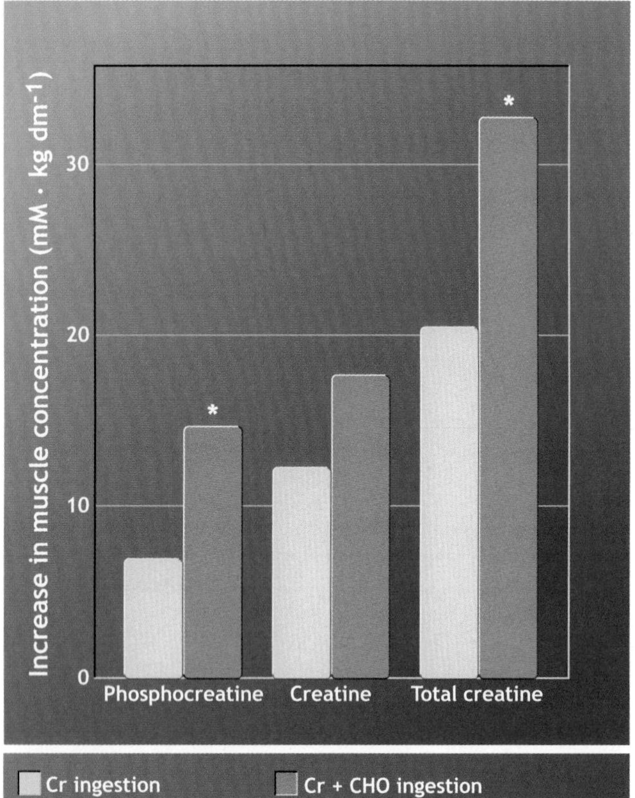

FIGURE 23.18 • Increases in dry muscle (dm) concentrations of phosphocreatine (PCr), creatine (Cr), and total creatine in one group after 5 days of Cr supplementation and in another group after 5 days of Cr and carbohydrate (CHO) supplementation. Values represent averages. * Significantly greater than creatine-only supplementation. (From Green AL, et al. Carbohydrate ingestion augments skeletal muscle creatine accumulation during creatine supplementation in humans. Am J Physiol 1996;271:E821.)

ment plus caffeine (5 mg · kg body mass^{-1}) for 6 days.[237] Under each condition, subjects performed maximal intermittent knee extension exercise to fatigue on an isokinetic dynamometer. Creatine supplementation, with or without caffeine, significantly increased intramuscular PCr (evaluated by nuclear magnetic resonance spectroscopy) between 4 and 6%. Dynamic torque production also increased 10 to 23% with creatine compared with the placebo. Consuming caffeine, however, *totally negated* creatine's ergogenic effect!

The researchers initially speculated that caffeine, through its action as a sympathomimetic agent, assists the uptake and trapping of exogenous creatine by skeletal muscle. However, no enhanced retention occurred. From a practical standpoint, caffeine supplements totally counteracted the ergogenic effect of muscle creatine loading. *Thus, athletes who load creatine should abstain from caffeine-containing foods and beverages for several days before competition.*

Some Research Shows No Benefit

While most research confirms positive effects of creatine supplementation, ergogenic effects may not emerge (1) in untrained subjects performing a single 15-second bout of sprint cycling,[52] (2) in trained subjects performing bouts of sport-specific physical activities such as swimming and running,[32,201] (3) during rapid weight loss,[177] or (4) when short-term supplementation does not increase muscle PCr.[174] The reason for these discrepancies remains unknown.

Lipid Supplementation with Medium-Chain Triglycerides

Do high-fat foods or lipid supplements elevate plasma fatty acid levels to increase energy availability from fat during prolonged aerobic exercise? Several factors affect the answer to this question. First, consuming triglycerides composed of predominantly long-chain fatty acids (12 to 18 carbons) significantly delays gastric emptying. This affects the rapidity of fat availability negatively and also slows fluid and carbohydrate replenishment, both crucial factors in high-intensity endurance exercise. Second, after digestion and intestinal absorption (normally 3 to 4 h), long-chain triglycerides reassemble with phospholipids, fatty acids, and a cholesterol shell to form fatty droplets called *chylomicrons*. Chylomicrons then travel slowly to the systemic circulation via the lymphatic system. Once in the bloodstream, tissues remove the triglycerides bound to chylomicrons. Consequently, the relatively slow rate of gastric emptying and subsequent digestion, absorption, and assimilation of long-chain triglycerides makes this energy source an undesirable supplement to augment energy metabolism in active muscle during exercise.[78]

Medium-chain triglycerides (MCTs), on the other hand, provide a more rapid source of fatty acid fuel. MCTs are processed oils, frequently produced for patients with intestinal malabsorption and tissue-wasting diseases. Marketing for the sports enthusiast hypes MCTs as "fat burners," "energy sources," "glycogen sparers," and "muscle builders." Unlike longer-chain triglycerides, MCTs contain saturated fatty acids with 8 to 10 carbon atoms along the fatty acid chain. During digestion, lipase in the mouth, stomach, and intestinal duodenum hydrolyzes MCTs to glycerol and medium-chain fatty acids (MCFAs). Their water-solubility allows MCFAs to move rapidly across the intestinal mucosa directly into the bloodstream (portal vein) without first being transported slowly as chylomicrons by the lymphatic system, as long-chain triglycerides require. Once at the tissues, MCFAs move readily through the plasma membrane, where they diffuse across the inner mitochondrial membrane for oxidation—they enter the mitochondria largely independently of the carnitine–acyl-CoA transferase system. The speed of cellular uptake and mitochondrial oxidation contrasts with the slower transfer and oxidation rate of long-chain fatty acids. Owing to their relative ease of oxidation, MCTs don't usually store as body fat. Because ingesting MCTs rapidly elevates plasma FFAs, some rersearchers speculate that these lipids might spare liver and muscle glycogen during high-intensity aerobic exercise.[158,159]

Possible Exercise Benefits Inconclusive

Although consuming MCTs does not inhibit gastric emptying, as does common fat,[18] conflicting research supports their use in exercise.[129,130,246] In early studies, subjects consumed 380 mg of MCT oil per kg of body mass 1 hour before exercising at 60 to 70% of $\dot{V}O_{2max}$ for 1 hour.[62,123] Plasma ketone levels generally increased but the exercise metabolic mixture did not change, compared with a placebo trial or a trial after subjects consumed a glucose polymer. By consuming 30 g of MCTs (estimated maximal amount tolerated in the gastrointestinal tract) before exercising, MCT catabolism contributed only 3 to 7% to the total exercise energy requirement.[127]

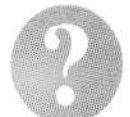

INTEGRATIVE QUESTION

Discuss the importance of the psychologic or "placebo" effect in evaluating claims for the effectiveness of particular nutrients, chemicals, or procedures as ergogenic aids.

Subsequent research investigated possible metabolic and ergogenic effects of consuming 86 g of MCT (surprisingly well tolerated by subjects). Six endurance-trained cyclists rode for 2 hours at 60% of $\dot{V}O_{2peak}$ while ingesting 2 L of either 4.3% MCT emulsion, 10% glucose plus 4.3% MCT emulsion, or a 10% glucose solution during exercise.[246] They then performed a simulated 40-km cycling time trial. Figure 23.19 shows the effects of the different beverages on average speed in the time trials. Although replacing the carbohydrate beverage with only MCTs produced an 8% decrement in performance (in agreement with another study[129]), the combined carbohydrate plus MCT solution consumed throughout exercise produced a statistically significant 2.5% improvement in cycling speed compared with the two other conditions. This ergogenic effect occurred with (1) reduced total carbohydrate oxidation at a given level of oxygen consumption, (2) higher final circulating FFA and ketone levels, and (3) lower final glucose and lactate concentrations.

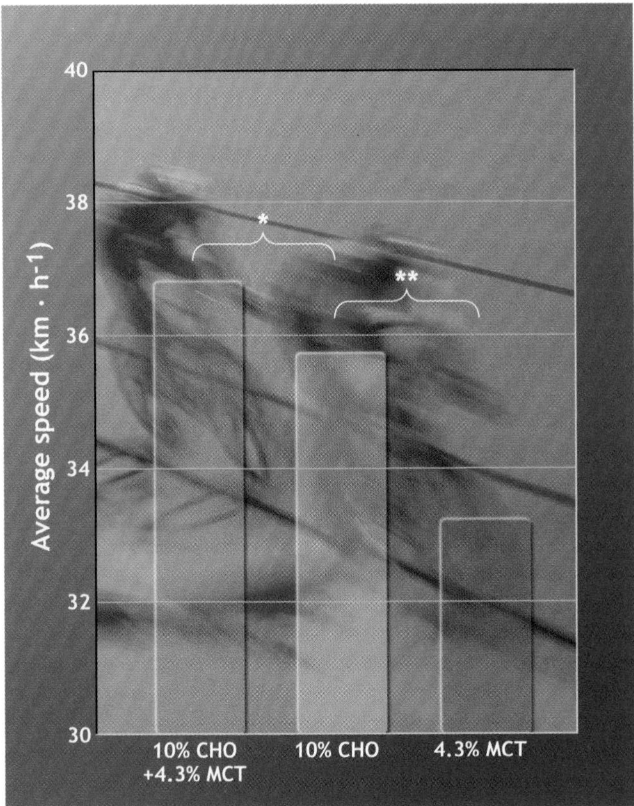

FIGURE 23.19 • Effects of carbohydrate (CHO; 10% solution), medium-chain triglyceride (MCT; 4.3% emulsion), and carbohydrate + MCT (10% CHO + 4.3% MCT) ingestion during exercise on simulated 40-km time-trial cycling speeds after 2 hours of exercise at 60% of $\dot{V}O_{2peak}$. *Significantly faster than 10% CHO trials; **Significantly faster than 4.3% MCT trials. (From Van Zyl CG, et al. Effects of medium-chain triglyceride ingestion on fuel metabolism and cycling performance. J Appl Physiol 1996;80:2217.)

The relatively small ergogenic enhancement by MCT supplementation probably occurred because this exogenous source of fatty acids contributes relatively little to the total energy expenditure (and total fat oxidation) during sustained exercise.[128] MCT ingestion does not stimulate release of bile, the fat-emulsifying agent from the gall bladder. Thus, cramping and diarrhea often accompany excess intake of this lipid. Research must validate the practical significance of the ergogenic claims for MCT, including the magnitude of any benefit and tolerance level for these lipids during exercise.

Summary

1. The term ergogenic aid describes substances or procedures that improve physical work capacity, physiologic function, or athletic performance.
2. Anabolic steroids compose a group of pharmacologic agents frequently used for ergogenic purposes. These drugs function like the hormone testosterone. Anabolic steroids may help to increase muscle size, strength, and power with resistance training in some individuals.
3. Debate exists about whether administration of growth hormone to healthy people augments muscular hypertrophy when combined with resistance training. Health risks exist for those who abuse this chemical.
4. Dehydroepiandersterone (DHEA) is a relatively weak steroid hormone synthesized from cholesterol by the adrenal cortex. DHEA levels steadily decrease throughout adulthood, prompting many individuals to supplement, hoping to counteract the effects of aging. Despite its popularity among exercise enthusiasts, available research does not indicate an ergogenic effect of DHEA.
5. No ergogenic benefits exist for healthy subjects from oral amino acid supplements on hormone secretion, training responsiveness, or exercise performance.
6. The effect on hormonal dynamics of carbohydrate and/or protein supplementation immediately following a resistance-exercise workout suggests a potential ergogenic effect on training responsiveness.

7. Little evidence supports the use of amphetamines or pep pills to aid exercise performance or psychomotor skills, other than a simple placebo effect. Adverse effects of amphetamines include drug dependency, headache, dizziness, confusion, and gastrointestinal distress.
8. Caffeine ingestion exerts an ergogenic effect in some individuals by extending endurance in aerobic exercise. This results from increased fat use for energy and conservation of the body's glycogen reserves. These effects become less apparent for individuals who maintain a high-carbohydrate diet, or who habitually use caffeine.
9. Relatively concentrated buffering solutions consumed before exercise significantly improve all-out anaerobic performance.
10. Some athletes believe supplements of the leucine metabolite β-hydroxyl-β-methylbutyrate (HMB) decrease protein loss by inhibiting protein catabolism. An objective decision about the potential benefits and risks of HMB awaits further research.
11. Red blood cell reinfusion (blood doping) involves drawing, storing, and reinfusing concentrated (packed) red blood cells several weeks later. The additional blood volume and increased red cell mass and concentration contribute to a larger maximum cardiac output and an increase in the blood's oxygen-carrying capacity and $\dot{V}O_{2max}$. Studies applying appropriate methods of blood storage and research design support the ergogenic benefits of this procedure for intense aerobic exercise and thermoregulation.
12. A physiologic rationale for why warm-up should enhance exercise performance includes possible benefits on muscle-shortening velocity and efficiency, enhanced oxygen delivery and use, and facilitated transmission of nerve impulses. Only limited research supports the benefits of warm-up beyond a positive psychologic component.
13. Moderate warm-up may prove beneficial immediately before sudden, strenuous exercise by reducing myocardial work and augmenting coronary blood flow when exercise begins. This may prevent transient myocardial ischemia and its potentially dangerous adverse effects.
14. Breathing hyperoxic gas during exercise extends endurance by increasing oxygen consumption, reducing blood lactate, and lowering pulmonary ventilation. Using this procedure before or after exercise has no ergogenic effect.
15. Carbohydrate loading generally augments endurance in prolonged submaximal exercise. Because of potential negative effects, athletes should be well informed about this procedure. A modification of the classic loading procedure provides the same high level of glycogen storage without dramatic alterations in the diet and exercise routine.
16. Athletes supplement with carnitine to possibly elevate intracellular carnitine to facilitate fat oxidation and conserve glycogen during prolonged exercise. However, research shows neither a lowering of normal intracellular carnitine levels in prolonged exercise nor any ergogenic benefits from carnitine supplementation.
17. The trace mineral chromium potentiates insulin's functions in the body. Research fails to show any beneficial effect of chromium supplements on training-related changes in muscular strength, physique, or muscle mass for individuals with adequate dietary chromium intake.
18. Creatine supplements significantly increase intramuscular creatine and PCr, enhance brief anaerobic power output capacity, and facilitate recovery from repeated bouts of intense effort. Effective creatine loading results from ingesting 20 g of creatine monohydrate for 6 consecutive days; reducing intake to 2 g daily maintains elevated levels of intramuscular creatine.
19. Owing to their relatively rapid digestion, assimilation, and catabolism for energy, some athletes believe that consuming medium-chain triglycerides (MCTs) enhances fat oxidation and conserves glycogen during endurance exercise. Ingesting about 86 g of MCTs enhances performance by an additional 2.5%.

References

1. Ajayi AAL, et al. Testosterone increases human platelet thromboxane A_2 receptor density and aggregation responses. Circulation 1995;91:2742.
2. Almada A, et al. Effects of ingesting a nutritional supplement containing chromium picolinate & boron on body composition during resistance training. FASEB J 1995;9(4):A1015.
3. American Academy of Pediatrics. Adolescents and anabolic steroids: a subject review. Pediatrics 1997;99:904
4. American College of Sports Medicine. The use of anabolic–androgenic steroids in sports. Sports Med Bull 1984;19:13.
5. American Medical Association Council on Food and Nutrition. JAMA 1973;224:1418.
6. Anderson DE, Hickey MS. Effects of caffeine on the metabolic and catecholamine response to exercise in 5 and 28°C. Med Sci Sports Exerc 1994;26:453.
7. Anderson RA, Guttman HN. Trace minerals and exercise. In: Horton ES, Terjung RL, eds. Exercise, nutrition, and energy metabolism. New York: Macmilllan, 1988.
8. Anderson RA, et al. Exercise effects on chromium excretion of trained and untrained men consuming a constant diet. J Appl Physiol 1988;64:249.
9. Anderson RA. Effects of chromium on body composition and weight loss. Nutr Rev 1998;56:266.
10. Araghiniknam M, et al. Antioxidant activity of Dioscorea and dehydroepiandrosterone (DHEA) in older humans. Life Sci 1996;59:11.
11. Audran M, et al. Effects of erythropoietin administration in training athletes and possible indirect detection in doping control. Med Sci Sports Exerc 1999;31:639.
12. Balsom PD, et al. Creatine supplementation per se does not enhance endurance exercise performance. Acta Physiol Scand 1993;149:521.
13. Balsom PD, et al. Creatine in humans with special reference to creatine supplementation. Sports Med 1994;18:268.
14. Balsom PD, et al. Skeletal muscle metabolism during short duration high-intensity exercise: influence of creatine supplementation. Acta Physiol Scand 1995;154:303.

15. Barnard RJ, et al. Cardiovascular responses to sudden strenuous exercise: heart rate, blood pressure, and ECG. J Appl Physiol 1973;34:883.
16. Barnard RJ, et al. Ischemic response to sudden strenuous exercise in healthy men. Circulation 1973;48:936.
17. Barrett-Conner E, et al. A prospective study of dehydroepiandrosterone sulfate, mortality, and cardiovascular disease. N Engl J Med 1986;315:1519.
18. Beckers EJ, et al. Gastric emptying of carbohydrate-medium chain triglyceride suspensions at rest. Int J Sports Med 1992;13:581.
19. Bergh U, Ekblom B. Physical performance and peak aerobic power at different body temperatures. J Appl Physiol 1979;46:885.
20. Bergstrom J, et al. Diet, muscle glycogen and physical performance. Acta Physiol Scand 1967;71:140.
21. Bessman SP, Savabi F. The role of the phosphocreatine energy shuttle in exercise and muscle hypertrophy. In: Biochemistry of exercise VII. Champaign, IL: Human Kinetics, 1990.
22. Birkeland KI, et al. The future of doping control in athletes. Issues related to blood sampling. Sports Med 1999;28:25.
23. Bogdanis GC, et al. Contribution of phosphocreatine and aerobic metabolism to energy supply during repeated sprint exercise. J Appl Physiol 1996;80:876.
24. Brannon TA, et al. Effects of creatine loading and training on running performance and biochemical properties of rat skeletal muscle. Med Sci Sports Exerc 1997;29:489.
25. Brechue WF, et al. Blood flow and pressure relationships which determine $\dot{V}O_{2max}$. Med Sci Sports Exerc 1995;27:37.
26. Bredle DL, et al. Phosphate supplementation, cardiovascular function, and exercise performance in humans. J Appl Physiol 1988;65:1821.
27. Bronson FH, Matherne CM. Exposure to anabolic–androgenic steroids shortens life span of male mice. Med Sci Sports Exerc 1997;29:615.
28. Brown GA, et al. Effect of oral DHEA on serum testosterone and adaptations to resistance training in young men. J Appl Physiol 1999;87:2274.
29. Browne A, et al. The ethics of blood testing as an element of doping control in sport. Med Sci Sports Exerc 1999;31:497.
30. Bucci L, et al. Ornithine supplementation and insulin release in bodybuilders. Int J Sports Nutr 1992;2:287.
31. Buckley WE, et al. Estimated prevalence of anabolic steroid use among male high school seniors. JAMA 1988;260:3441.
32. Burke LM, et al. Oral creatine supplementation does not improve sprint performance in elite swimmers. Med Sci Sports Exerc 1995;27:S146, 1995.
33. Burke AP, et al. Plaque rupture and sudden death related to exertion in men with coronary artery disease. JAMA 1999;281:921.
34. Burkett LN, Falduto MT. Steroid use by athletes in a metropolitan area. Phys Sportsmed 1984;12:69.
35. Cabasso A. Peliosis hepatitis in a young adult bodybuilder. Med Sci Sports Exerc 1994;26:2.
36. Calabrese LH, et al. The effects of anabolic steroids and strength training on the human immune response. Med Sci Sports Exerc 1989;21:386.
37. Campbell WW, et al. Chromium picolinate supplementation and resistive training by older men: effects on iron-status and hematologic indexes. Am J Clin Nutr 1997;66:944.
38. Campbell WW, et al. Effects of resistance training and chromium picolinate on body composition and skeletal muscle in older men. J Appl Physiol 1999;86:29.
39. Casaburi R, et al. Androgen effects on body composition and muscle performance. In: Bhasin S, et al, eds. Pharmacology, biology, and clinical applications of androgens: current status and future prospects. New York: Wiley-Liss, 1996.
40. Casal DC, Leon AS. Failure of caffeine to affect substrate utilization during prolonged exercise. Med Sci Sports Exerc 1985;17:174.
41. Casey A, et al. Metabolic response of type I and II muscle fibers during repeated bouts of maximal exercise in humans. Am J Physiol 1996;271:E38.
42. Catlin DH, Murray TH. Performance-enhancing drugs, fair competition, and Olympic sport. JAMA 1996;276:231.
43. Catlin DH et al. Trace contamination of over-the-counter androstenedione and positive urine test results for nandrolone metabolite. JAMA 2000;284:2618.
44. Chandler RM, et al. Dietary supplements affect the anabolic hormones after weight-training exercise. J Appl Physiol 1994;76:839.
45. Cheng W, et al. Beta-hydroxy-beta-methyl butyrate increases fatty acid oxidation by muscle cells. FASEB J 1997;11(3):A381.
46. Clancy S, et al. Effects of chromium picolinate supplementation on body composition, strength, and urinary chromium loss in football players. Int J Sports Nutr 1994;4:142.
47. Coggan AR, et al. Endurance training increases plasma glucose turnover and oxidation during moderate-intensity exercise in men. J Appl Physiol 1990;68:990.
48. Cohen BS, et al. Effects of caffeine ingestion on endurance racing in heat and humidity. Eur J Appl Physiol 1996;73:358.
49. Cohen LI, et al. Lipoprotein (a) and cholesterol in bodybuilders using anabolic androgenic steroids. Med Sci Sports Exerc 1996;28:176.
50. Colombani P, et al. Effects of L-carnitine supplementation on physical performance and energy metabolism of endurance-trained athletes—a double-blind crossover field study. Eur J Appl Physiol 1996;73:434.
51. Constantin-Teodosiu D, et al. Carnitine metabolism in human muscle fiber types during submaximal dynamic exercise. J Appl Physiol 1996;80:1061.
52. Cooke WH, et al. Effect of oral creatine supplementation on power output and fatigue during bicycle ergometry. J Appl Physiol 1995;78:670.
53. Costill DL, et al. Effects of caffeine ingestion on metabolism and exercise performance. Med Sci Sports 1978;10:155.
54. Costill DL, et al. Acid-base balance during repeated bouts of exercise: influence of HCO_3. Int J Sports Med 1984;5:228.
55. Costill DL, et al. Effects of repeated days of intensified training on muscle glycogen and swimming performance. Med Sci Sports Exerc 1988;20:249.
56. Cowart V. Steroids in sports: after four decades, time to return to the genie's bottle? JAMA 1987;257:421.
57. Crist DM, et al. Body composition response to exogenous GH during training in highly conditioned adults. J Appl Physiol 1988;65:579.
58. Curry LA, et al. Qualitative description of the prevalence and use of anabolic androgenic steroids by United States powerlifters. Percept Mot Skills 1999;88:224.
59. Daniels JW, et al. Effects of caffeine on blood pressure, heart rate, and forearm blood flow during dynamic exercise. J Appl Physiol 1998;85:154.
60. Dawson RT. Drug testing. Br J Sports Med 1999;33:219.
61. Daynes RA, Araneo BA. Prevention and reversal of some age-associated changes in immunologic responses by supplemental dehydroepiandrosterone sulfate therapy. Aging Immunol Infect Dis 1992;3:135.
62. Décombaz J, et al. Energy metabolism of medium-chained triglycerides versus carbohydrates during exercise. Eur J Appl Physiol 1983;52:9.
63. Décombaz J, et al. Muscle carnitine after strenuous endurance exercise. J Appl Physiol 1992;72:423.
64. Décombaz, J, et al. Effect of L-carnitine on submaximal exercise metabolism after depletion of muscle glycogen. Med Sci Sports Exerc 1993;25:773.
65. DeCree C. Androstenedione and dehydroepiandrosterone for athletes. Lancet 1999;354:779.
66. Delbeke FT, et al. The abuse of doping agents in competing bodybuilders in Flanders (1988–1993). Int J Sports Med 1995;16:60.
67. Deyssig R, et al. Effect of growth hormone treatment on hormonal parameters, body composition and strength in athletes. Acta Endocrinol 1993;128:313.
68. Di Bello B, et al. Effects of anabolic–androgenic steroids on weightlifters' myocardium: an ultrasonic videodensitometric study. Med Sci Sports Exerc 1999;31:514.
69. Dickerman RD, et al. Echocardiography in fraternal twin bodybuilders with one abusing anabolic steroids. Cardiology 1997;88:50.
70. Dodd S, et al. Caffeine and exercise performance. Sports Med 1993;15:14.
71. Durant RH, et al. Use of multiple drugs among adolescents who use anabolic steroids. N Engl J Med 1993;328:922.
72. Earnest CP, et al. The effect of creatine monohydrate ingestion on anaerobic power indices, muscular strength and body composition. Acta Physiol Scand 1995;153:207.
73. Eich DM, et al. Inhibition of accelerated coronary atherosclerosis with dehydroepiandrosterone in the heterotropic rabbit model of cardiac transplantation. Circulation 1993;87:261.
74. Eichner ER. Ergolytic drugs. Sports Science Exchange; Gatorade Sports Science Institute. 1989;15(2).
75. Ekblom B. Response to exercise after blood loss and reinfusion. J Appl Physiol 1972;33:175.
76. Ekblom B, Berglund B. Effect of erythropoietin administration on maximal aerobic power in man. Scand J Med Sci Sports 1991;11:88.
77. Ekblom B, et al. Central circulation during exercise after venesection and reinfusion of red blood cells. J Appl Physiol 1976;40:379.
78. Emken EA. Metabolism of dietary stearic acid relative to other fatty acids in human subjects. Am J Clin Nutr 1994;60(suppl):1023S.

79. Engelhardt M, et al. Creatine supplementation in endurance sports. Med Sci Sports Exerc 1998;30:1123.
80. Evans GW. The effect of chromium picolinate on insulin controlled parameters in humans. Int J Biosoc Med Res 1969;11:163.
81. Faigenbaum A, et al., Anabolic androgenic steroid use by 11- to 13-year old boys and girls: knowledge, attitudes, and prevalence (abstract). J Strength Cond Res 1996;10:285.
82. Fleck SJ, et al. Anaerobic power effects of an amino acid supplement containing no branched amino acids in elite competitive athletes. J Strength Cond Res 1995;9:132.
83. Fogelholm GM, et al. Low-dose amino acid supplementation: no effects on serum human growth hormone and insulin in male weight lifters. Int J Sports Nutr 1993;3:290.
84. Forbes GB, et al. Sequence of changes in body composition induced by testosterone and reversal of changes after drug is stopped. JAMA 1992;267:397.
85. French C, et al. Caffeine ingestion during exercise to exhaustion in elite distance runners. J Sports Med Phys Fitness 1991;31:425.
86. Friedlander AL, et al. Training induced alterations of carbohydrate metabolism in women: women respond differently than men. J Appl Physiol 1998;85:1175.
87. Fry A, et al. Endocrine and performance responses to high volume training and amino acid supplementation in elite junior weightlifters. Int J Sports Nutr 1993;3:306.
88. Gallagher, PM et al. β-hydroxy-β-methylbutyrate ingestion, Part I: effects on strength and fat free mass. Med Sci Sports Exerc 2000;32:2116.
89. Gallagher, PM et al. β-hydroxy-β-methylbutyrate ingestion, Part II: effects on hematyology, hepatic and renal function. Med Sci Sports Exerc 2000;32:2116.
90. Gazvani MR, et al. Conservative management of azoospermia following steroid abuse. Hum Reprod 1997;12:1706.
91. Giamberardino MA, et al. Effect of prolonged L-carnitine administration on delayed muscle pain and CK release after eccentric effort. Int J Sports Med 1996;17:320.
92. Girondola RN, et al. Effects of pangamic acid (B_{15}) ingestion on metabolic response to exercise. Biochem Med 1980;24:218.
93. Gledhill N. Blood doping and related issues: a brief review. Med Sci Sports Exerc 1982;14:183.
94. Goforth HW Jr, et al. Persistence of supercompensated muscle glycogen in trained subjects after carbohydrate loading. J Appl Physiol 1997;82:342.
95. Goldberg L, et al. Effects of a multidimensional anabolic steroid prevention intervention: the Adolescents Training and Learning to Avoid Steroids (ATLAS) program. JAMA 1996;276:1555.
96. Goldfinch J, et al. Induced metabolic alkalosis and its effects on 400-m racing time. Eur J Appl Physiol 1988;57:45.
97. Gordon GB, et al. Reduction of atherosclerosis by administration of DHEA. J Clin Invest 1988;82:712.
98. Graham TE. The possible actions of methylxanthines on various tissues. In: Riley T, Orme J, eds. The clinical pharmacology of sport and exercise. Amsterdam: Elsevier Science, 1997.
99. Graham TE, Spriet LL. Performance and metabolic responses to a high caffeine dose during exercise. J Appl Physiol 1991;71:2292.
100. Graham TE, Spirit LL. Metabolic, catecholamine, and exercise performance responses to various doses of caffeine. J Appl Physiol 1995;78:867.
101. Graham TE, et al. Metabolic and exercise endurance effects of coffee and caffeine ingestion. J Appl Physiol 1998;85:883.
102. Grant KE, et al. Chromium and exercise training: effect on obese women. Med Sci Sports Exerc 1997;29:992.
103. Granier PL, et al. Effect of $NaHCO_3$ on lactate kinetics in forearm muscles during leg exercise in man. Med Sci Sports Exerc 1996;28:692.
104. Green AL, et al. The influence of oral creatine supplementation on metabolism during sub-maximal incremental treadmill exercise. Proc Nutr Soc 1993;53:84A.
105. Green AL, et al. Carbohydrate ingestion augments skeletal muscle creatine accumulation during creatine supplementation in humans. Am J Physiol 1996;271:E821.
106. Greenhauf PL. Creatine and its application as an ergogenic aid. Int J Sports Nutr 1995;5:S100.
107. Greennauf PL, Timmons JA. Interaction between aerobic and anaerobic metabolism during intense muscle contraction. Exerc Sport Sci Revs 1998;26:1.
108. Greer F, et al. Caffeine, performance, and metabolism during repeated Wingate exercise tests. J Appl Physiol 1998;85:1502.
109. Grunewald K, Bailey R. Commercially marketed supplements for bodybuilding athletes. Sports Med 1993;15:90.
110. Hallmark MA, et al. Effects of chromium and resistive training on muscle strength and body composition. Med Sci Sports Exerc 1996;28:139.
111. Hargreaves M, et al. Effect of muscle glycogen availability on maximal exercise performance. Eur J Appl Physiol 1997;75:188.
112. Harris RC, et al. The effect of oral creatine supplementation on running performance during maximal short term exercise in man. J Physiol 1993;467:74P.
113. Hasten DL, et al. Effects of chromium picolinate on beginning weight training students. Int J Sports Nutr 1992;2:343.
114. Hausswirth C, et al. Sodium citrate ingestion and muscle performance in acute hypobaric hypoxia. Eur J Appl Physiol 1995;71:362.
115. Heinonen OJ. Carnitine and physical exercise. Sports Med 1996;22:109.
116. Herbert V. Pangamic acid ("vitamin B_{15}"). Am J Clin Nutr 1979;32: 1534.
117. Hintz RL, et al. Effect of growth hormone treatment on adult height of children with idiopathic short stature. N Engl J Med 1999;340:502.
118. Hornsby PJ. Biosynthesis of DHEAS by the human adrenal cortex and its age-related decline. Ann NY Acad Sci 1995;774:29.
119. Horswill CA, et al. Influence of sodium bicarbonate on sprint performance: relationship to dosage. Med Sci Sports Exerc 1988;20:566.
120. Horton TJ, et al. Fuel metabolism in men and women during and after long-duration exercise. J Appl Physiol 1998;85:1823.
121. Hultman E, et al. Muscle creatine loading in men. J Appl Physiol 1996;81:232.
122. Ivy JL. Food components that may optimize physical performance: an overview. In: Marriott BM, ed. Food components to enhance performance. Committee on Military Nutrition Research. Washington, DC: National Academy Press, 1994.
123. Ivy JL, et al. Contribution of medium and long chain triglyceride intake to energy metabolism during prolonged exercise. Int J Sports Med 1980;1:15.
124. Jakaubowicz D, et al. Effect of dehydroepiandrosterone on cyclic-guanosine monophosphate in men of advancing age. Ann NY Acad Sci 1995;774:312.
125. Jansson E. Sex differences in metabolic response to exercise. In: Saltin B, ed. Biochemistry of exercise VI. Champaign, IL: Human Kinetics, 1986.
126. Jetté M, et al. The nutritional and metabolic effects of a carbohydrate-rich diet in a glycogen supercompensation training regimen. Am J Clin Nutr 1978;31:2140.
127. Jeukendrup AE, et al. Metabolic availability of medium-chain triglycerides coingested with carbohydrate during prolonged exercise. J Appl Physiol 1995;79:756.
128. Jeukendrup AE, et al. Effect of endogenous carbohydrate availability on oral-medium chain triglyceride oxidation during prolonged exercise. J Appl Physiol 1996;80:949.
129. Jeukendrup AE, et al. Effect of medium-chain triacylglycerol and carbohydrate ingestion during exercise on substrate utilization and subsequent cycling performance. Am J Clin Nutr 1998;67:397.
130. Jeukendrup AE, et al. Fat metabolism in exercise: a review—part III: effects of nutritional interventions. Int J Sports Med 1998;19:371.
131. Johansen KL, et al. Anabolic effects of nandrolone decanoate in patients receiving dialysis. A randomized controlled trial. JAMA 1999;281:1275.
132. Jorgensen JA, et al. Beneficial effects of growth hormone treatment in GH-deficient adults. Lancet 1989;1:1221.
133. Juel C. Lactate-proton cotransport in skeletal muscle. Physiol Revs 1997;77:321.
134. Juhn MS, Tarnopolsky M. Potential side effects of oral creatine supplementation: a critical review. Clin J Sports Med 1998;8:298.
135. Kaats GR, et al. A randomized, double-masked, placebo-controlled study of the effects of chromium picolinate supplementation on body composition: a replication and extension of a previous study. Curr Ther Res 1998;57:747.
136. Kantor MA, et al. Androgens reduce HDL_3-cholesterol and increase hepatic triglyceride lipase activity. Med Sci Sports Exerc 1985;17:462.
137. Keith RE, et al. Alterations in dietary carbohydrate, protein, and fat intake and mood state in trained female cyclists. Med Sci Sports Exerc 1991;23:212.

138. Kesl LD, Engen RL. Effects of $NaHCO_3$ loading on acid-base balance, lactate, lactate concentration, and performance in racing greyhounds. J Appl Physiol 1998;85:1037.
139. King DS, et al. Effect of oral androstenedione on serum testosterone and adaptations to resistance training in young men. JAMA 1999;281:2020.
140. Knight DR, et al. Hyperoxia increases lung maximal oxygen uptake. J Appl Physiol 1993;75:2586.
141. Koga S, et al. Effect of increased muscle temperature on oxygen uptake kinetics during exercise. J Appl Physiol 1997;83:1333.
142. Kraemer WJ, et al. Hormonal responses to consecutive days of heavy-resistance exercise with or without nutritional supplementation. J Appl Physiol 1998;85:1544.
143. Kreider RB, et al. Effects of creatine supplementation on body composition, strength, and sprint performance. Med Sci Sports Exerc 1998;30:73.
144. Lamb DR. Anabolic steroids and athletic performance. In: Laron Z, Rogol A, eds. Hormones and sport. Rome: Serono, 1989.
145. Lambert MI, et al. Failure of commercial oral amino acid supplements to increase serum growth hormone concentrations in male bodybuilders. Int J Sports Nutr 1993;3:298.
146. Lawrence L, et al. Effect of sodium bicarbonate on racing standardbreds. J Anim Sci 1990;68:673.
147. LeBlanc J, et al. Enhanced metabolic response to caffeine in exercise-trained human subjects. J Appl Physiol 1985;59:832.
148. LeFavi RG, et al. Efficacy of chromium supplementation in athletes: emphasis on anabolism. Int J Sports Nutr 1992;2:111.
149. Linossier M-T, et al. Effect of sodium citrate on performance and metabolism of human skeletal muscle during supramaximal cycling exercise. Eur J Appl Physiol 1998;76:48.
150. Liow RYL, Tavares S. Bilateral rupture of the quadriceps tendon associated with anabolic steroids. Br J Sports Med 1995;29:77.
151. Lopes JM, et al. Effect of caffeine on skeletal muscle function before and after fatigue. J Appl Physiol 1983;54:1303.
152. Lukaski HC, et al. Chromium supplementation and resistance training effects on whole body and regional composition, strength, and trace element status of men. Am J Clin Nutr 1996;63:954.
153. MacDonald M, et al. Acceleration of $\dot{V}O_2$ kinetics in heavy submaximal exercise by hyperoxia and prior high-intensity exercise. J Appl Physiol 1997;83:1318.
154. MacDougall D. Anabolic steroids. Phys Sportsmed 1983;11:95.
155. MacIntosh BR,Wright BM. Caffeine ingestion and performance of a 1,500-metre swim. Can J Appl Physiol 1995;20:168.
156. Maher TJ. Safety concerns regarding supplemental amino acids: results of a study. In: Marrtiott BM, ed. Food components to enhance performance.. Committee on Military Nutrition Research. Washington, DC: National Academy Press, 1994.
157. Mainwood GW, Worsley-Brown P. The effects of extracellular pH and buffer concentration on the efflux of lactate from frog sartorius muscle. J Physiol (Lond) 1975;250:1.
158. Masicotte D, et al. Exogenous 13C lipids and 13C glucose oxidized during prolonged exercise in man (abstract). Med Sci Sports Exerc 1990;2:52.
159. Massicotte D, et al. Oxidation of exogenous medium-chain free fatty acids during prolonged exercise: comparison with glucose. J Appl Physiol 1992;73:1334.
160. Matson LG, Tran ZV. Effects of sodium bicarbonate ingestion on anaerobic performance: a meta-analytic review. Int J Sports Nutr 1993;3:2.
161. Maughan RJ. Creatine supplementation and exercise performance. Int J Sport Nutr 1995;5:94.
162. Max SR, Rance NE. No effect of sex steroids on compensatory muscle hypertrophy. J Appl Physiol 1984;56:1589.
163. McArdle WD, et al. Temporomandibular joint repositioning and exercise performance: a double-blind study. Med Sci Sports Exerc 1984;16:228.
164. McCall GE, et al. Maintenance of mononuclear domain size in rat soleus after overload and growth hormone/IGF-I treatment. J Appl Physiol 1998;84:1407.
165. McNaughton LR. Sodium citrate and anaerobic performance: implications of dosage. Eur J Appl Physiol 1990;61:392.
166. McNaughton LR, et al. Effect of sodium bicarbonate ingestion on high intensity exercise in moderately trained women. J Strength Cond Res 1997;11:98.
167. McNaughton LR, et al. The effects of creatine supplementation on high-intensity exercise performance in elite performers. Eur J Appl Physiol 1998;78:236.
168. Melchert RB, Lelder AA. Cardiovascular effects of androgenic-anabolic steroids. Med Sci Sports Exerc 1995;27:1252.
169. Mihic S, et al. Acute creatine loading increases fat-free mass, but does not affect blood pressure, plasma creatine, or DK activity in men and women. Med Sci Sports Exerc 2000;32:291.
170. Mittleman MA, et al. Triggering of acute myocardial infarction by heavy physical exertion. N Engl J Med 1993;329:922.
171. Mohr T, et al. Caffeine ingestion and metabolic responses of tetraplegic humans during electrical cycling. J Appl Physiol 1998;85:979.
172. Molano F, et al. Rat liver lysosomal and mitochondrial activities are modified by anabolic–androgenic steroids. Med Sci Sports Exerc 1999;31:243.
173. Mortola J, Yen SS. The effects of oral dehydroepiandrosterone on endocrine-metabolic parameters in postmenopausal women. J Clin Endocrinol Metab 1990;71:696.
174. Mujika I, et al. Creatine supplementation and sprint performance in soccer players. Med Sci Sports Exerc 2000;32:518.
175. Nakatani A, et al. Effect of endurance exercise training on muscle glycogen supercompensation in rats. J Appl Physiol 1997;82:711.
176. Nissen S, et al. Effect of leucine metabolite β-hydroxy-β-methylbutyrate on muscle metabolism during resistance-exercise training. J Appl Physiol 1996;81:2095.
177. Odland LM, et al. Effect of oral creatine supplementation on muscle [PCr] and short-term maximum power output. Med Sci Sports Exerc 1997;29:216.
178. Ööpik V, et al. Effect of creatine supplementation during rapid body mass reduction on metabolism and isokinetic muscle performance capacity. Eur J Appl Physiol 1998;78:83.
179. Op 't Eijnde B, Hespel P. Short-term creatine supplementation does not alter the hormonal response to resistance training. Med Sci Sports Exerc 2001;33:449.
180. O'Toole ML, et al. Hematocrits of triathletes: is monitoring useful? Med Sci Sports Exerc 1999;31:372.
181. Ostaszewksi P, et al. The effect of the leucine metabolite 3-hydroxy 3-methyl butyrate (HMB) on muscle protein synthesis and protein breakdown in chick and rat muscle. J Anim Sci 1996;74(suppl):138A.
182. Papadakis MA, et al. Growth hormone replacement in healthy older men improves body composition but not functional ability. Ann Intern Med 1996;124:708.
183. Palmer GS, et al. Carbohydrate ingestion immediately before exercise does not improve 20 km time trial performance in well trained cyclists. Int J Sports Med 1998;19:415.
184. Peltonen JE, et al,: Effects of oxygen fraction in inspired air on force production and electromyogram activity during ergometer rowing. Eur J Appl Physiol 1997;76:495.
185. Perry PJ, et al. Detection of anabolic steroid administration: ratio of urinary testosterone to epitestosterone vs the ratio of urinary testosterone to luteinizing hormone. Clin Chem 1997;43:731.
186. Peeters BM, et al. Effect of oral creatine monohydrate and creatine phosphate supplementation on maximal strength indices, body composition, and blood pressure. J Strength Cond Res 1999;113:3.
187. Pitsiladis YP, Maughan RJ. The effects of alterations in dietary carbohydrate intake on the performance of high-intensity exercise in trained individuals. Eur J Appl Physiol 1999;79:433.
188. Poortmans JR, Francaux M. Long-term oral creatine supplementation does not impair renal function in healthy athletes. Med Sci Sports Exerc 1999;31:1108.
189. Pope RP, et al. A randomized trial of preexercise stretching for prevention of lower-limb injury. Med Sci Sports Exerc 2000;32:271.
190. Porter DL, Goldberg MA. Physiology of erythropoietin production. Semin Hematol 1994;31:112.
191. Portington KJ, et al. Effect of induced alkalosis on exhaustive leg press performance. Med Sci Sports Exerc 1998;30:523.
192. Potteiger JA, et al. Sodium citrate ingestion enhances 30 km cycling performance. Int J Sports Med 1996;17:7.
193. Potteiger JA, et al. The effects of buffer ingestion on metabolic factors related to distance running. Eur J Appl Physiol 1996;72:365.
194. President's Council on Physical Fitness and Sports. Nutritional ergogenics and sports performance. Res Dig 1998;3(2).
195. Pritchard NR, Kalra PA. Renal dysfunction accompanying oral creatine supplements. Lancet 1998;352:234.
196. Raben AB, et al. Serum sex hormones and endurance performance after a lacto-ovo-vegetarian and mixed diet. Med Sci Sports Exerc 1992;24:1290.
197. Ransone JW, Lefavi RG. The effects of dietary L-carnitine on anaerobic exercise lactate in elite male athletes. J Strength Cond Res 1997;11:4.

198. Rauch LHG, et al. The effects of carbohydrate loading on muscle glycogen content and cycling performance. Int J Sports Nutr 1995;5:25.
199. Rawson ES, et al. Effects of 30 days of creatine ingestion in older men. Eur J Appl Physiol 1999;80:139.
200. Reed MJ, et al. Dietary lipids: an additional regulator of plasma levels of sex hormone binding globulin. J Clin Endocrinol Metab 1987;64:1083.
201. Redondo D, et al. The effect of oral creatine monohydrate supplementation on running velocity. Med Sci Sports Exerc 1994;26:S23.
202. Richardson RS, et al. Evidence of O_2 supply-dependent $\dot{V}O_{2max}$ in exercise-trained human quadriceps. J Appl Physiol 1999;86:1048.
203. Robbins MK, et al. Effect of oxygen breathing following submaximal and maximal exercise on recovery and performance. Med Sci Sports Exerc 1992;24:270.
204. Robergs RA, et al. Effects of warm-up on muscle glycogenolysis during intense exercise. Med Sci Sports Exerc 1991;23:7.
205. Robertson RJ, et al. Hemoglobin concentration and aerobic work capacity in women following induced erythrocythemia. J Appl Physiol 1984;57:568.
206. Robertson RJ, et al. Effect of induced alkalosis on physical work capacity during arm and leg exercise. Ergonomics 1987;30:19.
207. Rockwell JA, et al. Creatine supplementation affects muscle creatine during energy restriction. Med Sci Sports Exerc 2001;33:61.
208. Rogozkin V. Metabolic effects of anabolic steroids on skeletal muscle. Med Sci Sports 1979;11:160.
209. Roure R, et al. Autonomic nervous system responses correlate with mental rehearsal in volleyball training. Eur J Appl Physiol 1998;78:99.
210. Roy BD, et al. Effect of glucose supplement timing on protein metabolism after resistance training. J Appl Physiol 1997;82:1882.
211. Rudman D, et al. Effects of human growth hormone in men over 60 years old. N Engl J Med 1990;323:1.
212. Sachtleben TR, et al. Serum lipoprotein patterns in long-term anabolic steroid users. Res Q Exerc Sport 1997;68:110.
213. Safran MR, et al. The role of warm up in muscular injury prevention. Am J Sports Med 1988;16:123.
214. Salamon R, et al. The effects of treatment with recombinant human growth hormone on body composition and metabolism in adults with growth hormone deficiency. N Engl J Med 1989;321:1797.
215. Sawka MN, Young AJ. Acute polycythemia and human performance during exercise and exposure to extreme environments. Exerc Sport Sci Rev 1989;17:265.
216. Sawka MN, et al. Influence of polycythemia on blood volume and thermoregulation during exercise heat stress. J Appl Physiol 1987;62:912.
217. Schilling BK, et al. Creatine supplementation and health variables: A retrospective study. Med Sci Sports Exerc 2001;33:183.
218. Sherman WM. Carbohydrates, muscle glycogen, and muscle glycogen super-compensation. In: Williams MH, ed. Ergogenic aids in sports. Champaign, IL: Human Kinetics, 1983.
219. Sherman WM, et al. Effect of exercise-diet manipulation on muscle glycogen and its subsequent utilization during performance. Int J Sports Med 1981;2:114.
220. Siliprandi N, et al. Metabolic changes induced by maximal exercise in human subjects following L-carnitine administration. Biochim Biophys Acta 1990;1034:17.
221. Smith SA, et al. Creatine supplementation and age influence muscle metabolism during exercise. J Appl Physiol 1998;85:1349.
222. Spiret LL, et al. Effect of graded erythrocythemia on cardiovascular and metabolic responses to exercise. J Appl Physiol 1986;61:1942.
223. Spriet LL, et al. Caffeine ingestion and muscle metabolism during prolonged exercise in humans. Am J Physiol 1992;262:E891.
224. Starling RD, et al. Relationships between muscle carnitine, age and oxidative status. Eur J Appl Physiol 1995;71:143.
225. Stensrud T, et al. L-Tryptophan supplementation does not improve running performance. Int J Sports Med 1992;13:481.
226. Strawford, A, et al. Resistance exercise and supraphysiologic androgen therapy in eugonadal men with HIV-related weight loss. A randomized controlled trial. JAMA 1999;281:1282.
227. Street C, et al. Androgen use by athletes: a reevaluation of the health risks. Can J Appl Physiol 1996;21:421.
228. Su TP, et al. Neuropsychiatric effects of anabolic steroids in male normal volunteers. JAMA 1993;269:2760.
229. Tarnopolsky MA, et al. Carbohydrate loading and metabolism during exercise in men and women. J Appl Physiol 1995;78:1360.
230. Tegelman R, et al. Effects of a diet regimen on pituitary and steroid hormones in male ice hockey players. Int J Sports Med 1992;13:424.
231. Tingus SJ, Carlsen RC. Effect of continuous infusion of an anabolic steroid on murine skeletal muscle. Med Sci Sports Exerc 1993;25:485.
232. Thompson KH, et al. Studies of vanadyl sulfate as a glucose-lowering agent in STZ-diabetic rats. Biochem Biophys Res Commun 1993;197:1549.
233. Toner MM, et al. Metabolic and cardiovascular responses to exercise with caffeine. Ergonomics 1982;25:1175.
234. Trappe SW, et al. The effects of L-carnitine supplementation on performance during swimming. Int J Sports Med 1994;15:181, 1994.
235. Trent LK, Thieding-Cancel D. Effects of chromium picolinate on body composition in a remedial conditioning program. NHRC publ 94-20, 1995.
236. Trice I, Haymes EM. Effects of caffeine ingestion on exercise-induced changes during high-intensity, intermittent exercise. Int J Sports Nutr 1995;5:37.
237. Vandenberghe K, et al. Caffeine counteracts the ergogenic action of creatine loading. J Appl Physiol 1996;80:452.
238. Vandenberghe K, et al. Long-term creatine intake is beneficial to muscle performance during resistance training. J Appl Physiol 1997;83:2055.
239. Vandenberghe K, et al. Phosphocreatine resynthesis is not affected by creatine loading. Med Sci Sports Exerc 1999;31:236.
240. VanLeemputte M, et al. Shortening of muscle relaxation time after creatine loading. J Appl Physiol 1999;86:840.
241. Van Koevering M, Nissen S. Oxidation of leucine and β-ketoisocaproate to β-hydroxy-β-methylbutyrate in vivo. Am J Physiol 1992;262(Endocrinol Metabol 25):E27.
242. Van Soeren MH, Graham TE. Effect of caffeine on metabolism, exercise endurance, and catecholamine responses after withdrawal. J Appl Physiol 1998;85:1493.
243. Van Soeren MH, et al. Caffeine metabolism and epinephrine responses during exercise in users and nonusers. J Appl Physiol 1994;75:805.
244. Van Soeren MH, et al. Acute effects of caffeine ingestion at rest in humans with impaired epinephrine responses. J Appl Physiol 1996;80:999.
245. Van Vollenhoven RF, et al. An open study of dehydroepiandrosterone in systemic lupus erythematosus. Arthritis Rheum 1994;37:1305.
246. Van Zyl CG, et al. Effects of medium-chain triglyceride ingestion on fuel metabolism and cycling performance. J Appl Physiol 1996;80:2217.
247. Verbitsky O, et al. Effect of ingested sodium bicarbonate on muscle force, fatigue, and recovery. J Appl Physiol 1997;83:333.
248. Vermeulen A. Dehydroepiandrosterone sulfate and aging. Ann NY Acad Sci 1995;774:121.
249. Visuri T, Lindholm H. Bilateral distal biceps tendon avulsions with use of anabolic steroids. Med Sci Sports Exerc 1994;26:941.
250. Volek JS, et al. Creatine supplementation enhances muscular performance during high-intensity resistance exercise. J Am Diet Assoc 1997;97:765.
251. Volek JS, et al. Testosterone and cortisol in relationship to dietary nutrients and resistance training. J Appl Physiol 1997;82:49.
252. Volek JS, et al. Performance and muscle fiber adaptations to creatine supplementation and heavy resistance training. Med Sci Sports Exerc 1999;31:1147.
253. Vukovich MD, et al. Carnitine supplementation: effect on muscle carnitine and glycogen content during exercise. Med Sci Sports Exerc 1994;26:1122.
254. Wagman DF, et al. An investigation into anabolic androgenic steroid use by elite U.S. powerlifters. J Strength Cond Res 1995;9:149.
255. Walker LS, et al. Chromium picolinate effects on body composition and muscular performance in wrestlers. Med Sci Sports Exerc 1998;30:1730.
256. Wanger PD. Muscle O_2 transport and O_2 dependent control of metabolism. Med Sci Sports Exerc 1995;27:47.
257. Webb OL, et al. Severe depression of high density lipoprotein cholesterol levels in weight lifters and bodybuilders by self-administered exogenous testosterone and anabolic–androgenic steroids. Metabolism 1984;33:11.

258. Weir J, et al. A high carbohydrate diet negates the metabolic effects of caffeine during exercise. Med Sci Sports Exerc 1987;19:100.
259. Weltman AL, et al. Exercise recovery, lactate removal, and subsequent high intensity exercise performance. Res Q 1977;48:786.
260. Weltman AL, et al. Effects of increasing oxygen availability on bicycle ergometer endurance performance. Ergonomics 1978;21:427.
261. Wemple RD, et al. Caffeine vs caffeine-free sports drinks: effects on urine production at rest and during prolonged exercise. Int J Sports Med 1997;18:40.
262. Wilkes D, et al. Effect of acute induced metabolic alkalosis on 800-m racing time. Med Sci Sports Exerc 1983;15:277.
263. Williams MH. Ergogenic and ergolytic substances. Med Sci Sports Exerc 1992;24:S344.
264. Wilson JD. Androgen abuse by athletes. Endocr Rev 1988;9:181.
265. Winder WW. Effect of intravenous caffeine on liver glycogenolysis during prolonged exercise. Med Sci Sports Exerc 1986;18:192.
266. Winter FD, et al. Effects of 100% oxygen on performance of professional soccer players. JAMA 1989;262:227.
267. Wroblewska A-M. Androgenic-anabolic steroids and body dysmorphia in young men. J Psychosom Res 1997;42:225.
268. Wyss M, Kaddurak-Daouk R. Creatine and creatinine metabolism. Physiol Rev 2000;80:1007.
269. Yan Z, et al. Effect of low glycogen on glycogen synthase in human muscle during and after exercise. Acta Physiol Scand 1992;145:345.
270. Yarasheski KE. Growth hormone effects on metabolism, body composition, muscle mass, and strength. Exerc Sport Sci Rev 1994;22:285.
271. Yarasheski KE, et al. Effect of growth hormone and resistance exercise on muscle growth in young men. Am J Physiol 1992;262:E261.
272. Yarasheski KE, et al. Short-term growth hormone treatment does not increase muscle protein synthesis in experienced weight lifters. J Appl Physiol 1993;74:3073.
273. Yates JW, et al. Effect of a mandibular orthopedic repositioning appliance on muscular strength. J Am Dent Assoc 1984;108:331.
274. Yesalis CE, et al. Anabolic–androgenic steroid use in the United States. JAMA 1993;270:1217.

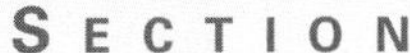

SECTION 5

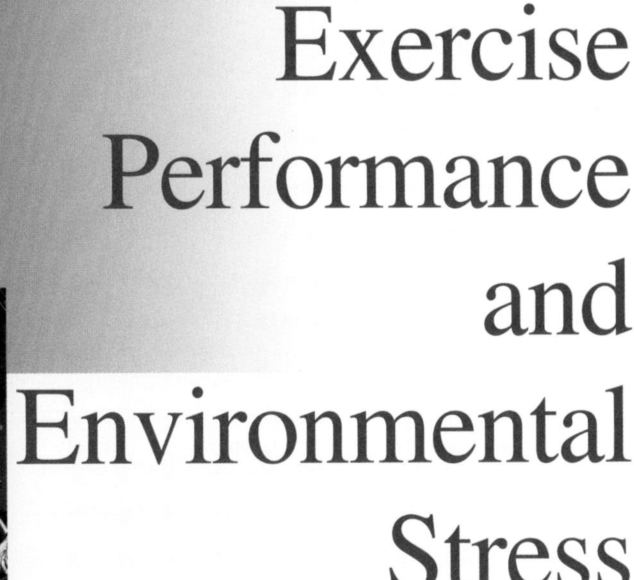

Exercise Performance and Environmental Stress

"The true explorer does his work not for any hopes of reward or honor, but because the thing he has set for himself to do is a part of his being, and must be accomplished for the sake of the accomplishment. And he counts lightly hardships, risks, obstacles, if only they do not bar him from his goal."

Admiral Robert E. Peary,
Polar Explorer

Previous chapters have focused on the physiologic and metabolic adjustments that enable humans to generate energy for exercise in "normal" environments. In this context, stress on the organism largely reflects that imposed by the specific form of exercise, such as walking, running, bicycling, or swimming (in relatively warm water). In many instances, however, the environment acts to compound the stress of exercise.

Sport activities often take place at terrestrial elevations that impair oxygenation of blood flowing through the lungs to severely limit aerobic energy metabolism for exercise. At the other extreme, exploration beneath the water's surface poses a different challenge. Divers must transport their sea-level environment in the form of a gas mixture compressed in a scuba tank carried on the back. However, some diving enthusiasts use no external assistance, and the length of an underwater excursion becomes limited by (1) the quantity of air inhaled into the lungs just before the dive and (2) the buildup of arterial carbon dioxide during the dive. In both breath-hold diving and scuba diving, the environment provides unique challenges and dangers for the participant. These dangers exist often independent of the stress of exercise. Consideration must also focus on the thermal quality of the environment. On land, exercising in a hot, humid environment or under conditions of extreme cold can impose a severe stress. These environmental demands not only impair exercise capacity but, in the extreme, pose a severe threat to the health and safety.

The Badwater 135-mile ultra-marathon vividly illustrates the acute environmental extremes to which individuals voluntarily expose themselves during exercise. The race begins during high summer at Death Valley National Monument, CA, the lowest point in the continental United States (282 ft below sea level). It stretches 41 miles across the desert at sea level and then climbs more than 8,600 vertical feet during the race's remaining 95 miles. In addition to frequent 50 mile per hour headwinds, ambient temperature varies by as much as 100° F, from 130° F at the start to below freezing at the finish at the base of Mount Whitney, CA.

Space exploration and accompanying acute and chronic exposures to near-zero gravity presents an entirely unique set of environmental stressors that impinge on physiologic function, structural mass, and exercise capacity both during flight and upon return to earth.

The extent that each environmental stressor deviates from neutral conditions, and the duration of the exposure, determine the total effect on the body. In addition, the effect of several environmental stressors operating at the same time (e.g., extreme cold exposure at high altitude) may exceed the simple additive consequence of each stressor imposed separately.

In the four chapters that follow, we explore the specific problems encountered at altitude, during exercise in hot and cold environments, and during prolonged exposure to microgravity. We also discuss the immediate physiologic adjustments and long-term adaptations as the body strives to maintain internal consistency despite an environmental challenge. The chapter on sport diving considers the unique problems associated with this increasingly popular form of sport and recreation. We recommend the following five texts (or chapters from texts) for the student interested in the specifics of human adaptation to diverse forms of environmental stress.

References

Dill DB, ed. Handbook of physiology. Serction 4: adaptation to the environment. Washington, DC: American Physiological Society, 1964.

Frisancho AR. Human adaptation: a functional interpertation. St. Louis: C.V. Mosby, 1993.

Nicogossian AE, et al. Space physiology and medicine, 3rd ed. Philadelphia: Lea & Febiger, 1994.

Pandolf K et al., eds. Performance physiology and environmental medicine at terrestrial extremes. Carmel, IN: Cooper Publishing Group, 1988.

Toner MM, McArdle WD. Human thermoregulatory responses to acute cold stress with special reference to water immersion. In Fregley MJ, Blatteis, CM, eds. Handbook of physiology, environmental physiology. Section 4, vol. 1. New York: Oxford University Press, 1996.

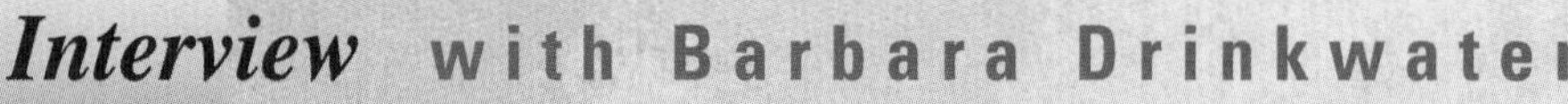

Interview with Barbara Drinkwater

Education: BS (Douglass College, Rutgers University, New Brunswick, NJ); MEd (University of North Carolina, Greensboro, NC); PhD (Purdue University, West Lafayette, IN).

Current Affiliation: Retired May 1, 2000. Previously Research Physiologist. Department of Medicine. Pacific Medical Center, Seattle, WA.

Research Focus: The response of women to exercise as mediated by environmental factors and aging. Special areas of interest have been the female athlete, her physical performance under environmental stressors such as heat and altitude, the effect of exercise-associated amenorrhea on bone health, and the role of exercise, calcium, and exercise in preventing osteoporosis.

Memorable Publication: Drinkwater, B.L.: Bone mineral content of amenorrheic and eumenorrheic athletes. *New Eng. J. Med.* 311:277, 1984.

Statement of Contributions: ACSM Honor Award

In recognition of her distinguished scientific contributions as one of the foremost investigators of exercise and physiological issues pertaining to women, particularly with, respect to the study of bone mineral content relative to menstrual function, pregnancy, physical activity, and calcium intake, and for her distinguished international leadership and professional contributions to exercise science and sports medicine.

Dr. Drinkwater began her well-known scientific work with a series of landmark studies, first on the aerobic capacity, training, and detraining characteristics of young women track athletes, and then on the influence of air pollutants and thermal stress on the working capacity of humans. She has demonstrated a continuing interest in gender differences and aging on aerobic capacity, body composition, and thermal responses. Indeed, an anthology of the woman in sport would be incomplete without reference to her data-based studies and scholarly reviews of the physiological responses of women to exercise, particularly in reference to age, fitness, and heat stress.

Dr. Drinkwater has earned the respect of the international scientific community for her primary scientific contribution, the interactions of menstrual function, estrogen and exercise on bone mineral content. Her work has clarified the importance of adequate menstrual function on bone mineral density in young athletic women, the long term consequences of bone mineral losses following athletic amenorrhea, and the role of estrogen relative to physical activity for the prevention of bone mineral loss in menopause.

Second only to her scientific contributions, Dr. Drinkwater has demonstrated an exemplary commitment to professional leadership and development of beginning scholars and clinicians. She has served or chaired many of the vital committees of ACSM, and was elected as Trustee, Vice President, and President. She remains a strong voice that brings an important message to the American College of Sports Medicine Foundation, where she serves on the Board of Directors. Dr. Drinkwater is an icon that represents unfailing support, nurturing, and challenging of beginning investigators and clinicians in exercise science and sports medicine.

Dr. Drinkwater's highly regarded contributions to the international scientific community, her professional leadership, and her commitment to the development of beginning scientists and clinicians form the basis of recognizing her with ACSM's highest distinction.

➤ What first inspired you to enter the exercise science field? What made you decide to pursue your advanced degree and/or line of research?

In 1965, I was teaching a methods course in track and field to physical education majors. One of them asked me why women weren't allowed to compete in the marathon, and were restricted to running twice around the track. I decide to investigate the scientific rationale and found instead that myths and prejudice, not science, limited women's participation in sports. Several years later I had the opportunity to join the Institute of Environmental Stress at the University of California, Santa Barbara. With the encouragement of the director, Steven M. Horvath, PhD, I began the series of studies that would demonstrate clearly that women of all ages could attain high levels of aerobic power and that cardiovascular fitness, not gender, accounted for the previous notion that women could not tolerate exercise in the heat.

➤ What influence did your undergraduate education have on your final career choice?

My undergraduate degree was in Physical Education. I had an excellent program that emphasized science as well as sports skills and teaching methods. However, none of the female faculty members had a doctorate degree, and graduate education was never mentioned. The assumption in those days was that we "majors" would go directly into teaching. However, I'm sure it was my love for sport and the excellent courses I had in physiology and kinesiology that later led me into the exercise science field.

➤ Who were the most influential people in your career, and why?

Oddly enough, the most influential individual in my career was Ben Winer, PhD, who taught the statistics courses I took in the doctoral program at Purdue. He was an outstanding teacher, and the skills and knowledge of experimental design that I gained in his classes led to my unofficial role of statistician and advisor on study designs at Institute of Environmental Stress. Obviously, I owe a great deal to Steve Horvath as well, who gave me the opportunity to work at the Institute. A career encompasses not only your research and teaching, but your professional contributions as well. Individuals such as Charles Tipton, John Sutton, Carl Gilsolfi, Peter Raven, Chris Wells, Toby Tate, and a multitude of others all enhanced that aspect of my career.

Their support and encouragement had a tremendous impact on my career and me.

➤ **What has been the most interesting/enjoyable aspect of your involvement in science? What was the least interesting/enjoyable aspect?**

The most enjoyable aspect of my scientific career has been the opportunity to encourage and "open some doors" for younger women on the road toward their own careers. That, plus the opportunity to speak to a wide variety of audiences about topics of importance to their health and well being, have given me a great deal of satisfaction. The least enjoyable aspect has been the constant need to search for funds to keep the research program going.

➤ **What is your most meaningful contribution to the field of exercise science, and why is it so important?**

I would like to think that my most meaningful contribution to the field of exercise science has been to stimulate interest of other investigators in evaluating women's response to exercise, environmental stress, and aging. In terms of a specific area of research, I would have to select the area of the Female Athlete Triad, which demonstrates that the amenorrhea experienced by many female athletes can lead to irreversible bone loss. Until our 1984 paper in the New England Journal of Medicine, *amenorrhea was assumed to be a benign—and welcome—condition by the athletes. When additional studies confirmed our results, athletes and those responsible for their health began to take the Triad seriously.*

➤ **What advice would you give to students who express an interest in pursuing a career in exercise science research?**

My advice to an undergraduate student would be to select as many science courses as possible in areas related to exercise science and work hard to get good grades. Your selection to the better graduate programs will depend largely on your grade point average and the recommendations of your professors. If you are not a serious student, you are not going to have a successful career in research. In selecting a doctoral program, investigate thoroughly before applying. Not only will you be spending 4 to 5 years of your life in that department, but you will be depending on the reputation of that program and the faculty to secure a postdoctoral position. Among the factors to consider are the publications of the faculty and graduate students, ongoing research in your area of interest, laboratory facilities and equipment, success of graduates in obtaining postdoctoral positions, and the requirements for the PhD. If possible, talk with some recent graduates of the program and get their honest appraisal of their experience.

➤ **What interests have you pursued outside of your professional career?**

Sports, aviation, and animals. I've been active in a number of sports, but am now totally involved with golf—playing several times a week and even taking my clubs over to Australia to play when not at an Olympic venue. When I was in Santa Barbara, I found time to get a commercial pilot's license, an instrument rating, and an instrument instructor's rating. I spent many hours in the air on trips throughout California and the Southwest. When I moved to Vashon in 1982, I had two dogs and one cat. Within 6 months, a puppy found at the dump and another 6 cats that had come out of the woods joined the family. At that point, I decided the island needed a humane society so I started one. Sixteen years later, the program is going strong and now includes a low-cost spay neuter program, a lost-and-found hotline, an adoption service, education programs in the schools, and medical–surgical help as well.

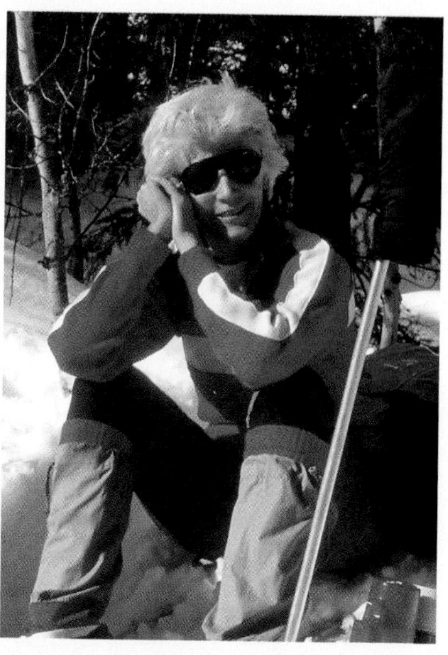

➤ **Where do you see the exercise science field (particularly your area of greatest interest) heading in the next 20 years?**

The exercise science field is so diverse that it may be impossible to make a general statement regarding future directions. I do believe there will be increasing interest in the interaction of exercise and health. As our population continues to age, the rising cost of medical care will force an emphasis on lifestyle and other preventive measures. The Surgeon General's Healthy People 2000 Report has made physical activity and fitness the number one priority for health promotion and disease prevention. The responsibility for providing data-based evidence that physical activity does indeed prevent or ameliorate disease states, as well as defining the optimum exercise program for each segment of the population, will be the responsibility of the exercise scientist who is challenged by studying integrated physiological systems.

➤ **You have the opportunity to give a "last lecture." Describe its primary focus.**

I can't even conceive of accepting an invitation to give a "last lecture"! The actual final lecture I give will be one that I probably accepted to give six months earlier, and in the interim I've decided I've said enough, I have nothing new to say, and it's time to leave the stage to younger professionals with new and exciting data and insights. I hope I have the good sense to recognize that time when it comes.

CHAPTER 24

Exercise at Medium and High Altitude

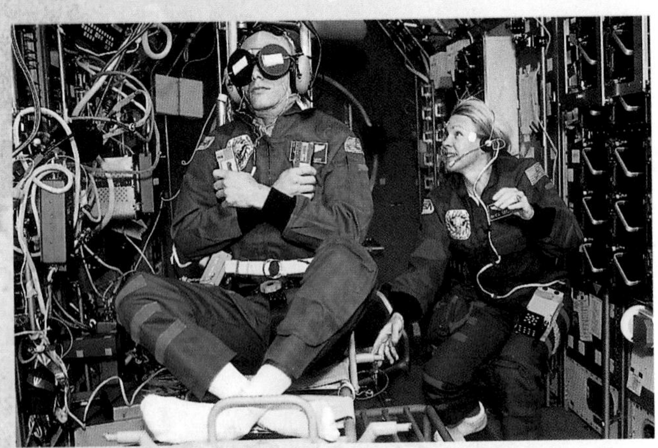

Chapter Objectives

- Outline the effects of increasingly higher altitudes on (1) partial pressure of oxygen in ambient air, (2) oxygen saturation of hemoglobin in pulmonary capillaries, and (3) $\dot{V}O_{2max}$
- Describe and quantify the oxygen transport cascade at sea level and at 4300 m
- Discuss immediate and longer-term physiologic adjustments to altitude exposure
- Give symptoms, possible causes, and treatment for acute mountain sickness, high-altitude pulmonary edema, and high-altitude cerebral edema
- Describe the "lactate paradox" and possible causes for its occurrence
- Summarize factors that affect the time course for altitude acclimatization
- Graph the relation between the decrease in $\dot{V}O_{2max}$ (% sea-level value) with increasing altitude or simulated altitude exposure
- Discuss alterations in circulatory function that offset the benefits of altitude acclimatization on oxygen transport capacity
- Discuss whether altitude training produces greater improvement than sea-level training on sea-level exercise performance
- Describe the training concept "living high, training low"

More than 40 million people live, work, and recreate at terrestrial elevations between 3048 m (10,000 ft) and 5486 m (18,000 ft) above sea level. In terms of the earth's topography, these elevations encompass the range generally considered **high altitude**. High-altitude natives inhabit permanent settlements as high as 5486 m in the Andes and Himalayas. However, prolonged exposure of an unacclimatized person to this altitude can cause death from the ambient air's subnormal oxygen pressure (**hypoxia**), even if the person remains inactive. The physiologic challenge of even medium altitude becomes readily apparent during physical activity. In the United States, close to 1 million people a year ascend Pikes Peak, Colorado (4300 m) by train, car, or railroad, and thousands of others do so by climbing, cycling, and even running. Millions more throughout the world ascend to high altitudes for mountaineering, trekking, tourism, business, and scientific and military excursions. Whatever the purpose, many newcomers to altitude do not take sufficient time to acclimatize to the physiologic challenge of the reduced partial pressure of oxygen (Po_2) in ambient air.

THE STRESS OF ALTITUDE

Altitude's challenge comes directly from the decreased ambient Po_2, not from the reduced total barometric pressure per se or any change in the relative concentrations (percentages) of gases in inspired (ambient) air. Figure 24.1 illustrates the barometric pressure, the pressures of the respired gases, and the percentage saturation of hemoglobin at various terrestrial elevations. Figure 24.2 shows changes that occur in oxygen availability (reflected by Po_2) in ambient air, alveolar air, and arterial and mixed-venous blood as one ascends from sea level to Pikes Peak. The progressive change in the environment's oxygen pressure and in various body areas is termed the **oxygen transport cascade.**

Air density decreases progressively as one ascends above sea level. For example, the barometric pressure at sea level averages 760 mm Hg, and at 3048 m the barometer reads 510 mm Hg; at an elevation of 5486 m, the pressure of a column of air at the earth's surface equals about one-half its pressure at sea level. Although dry ambient air at sea level and

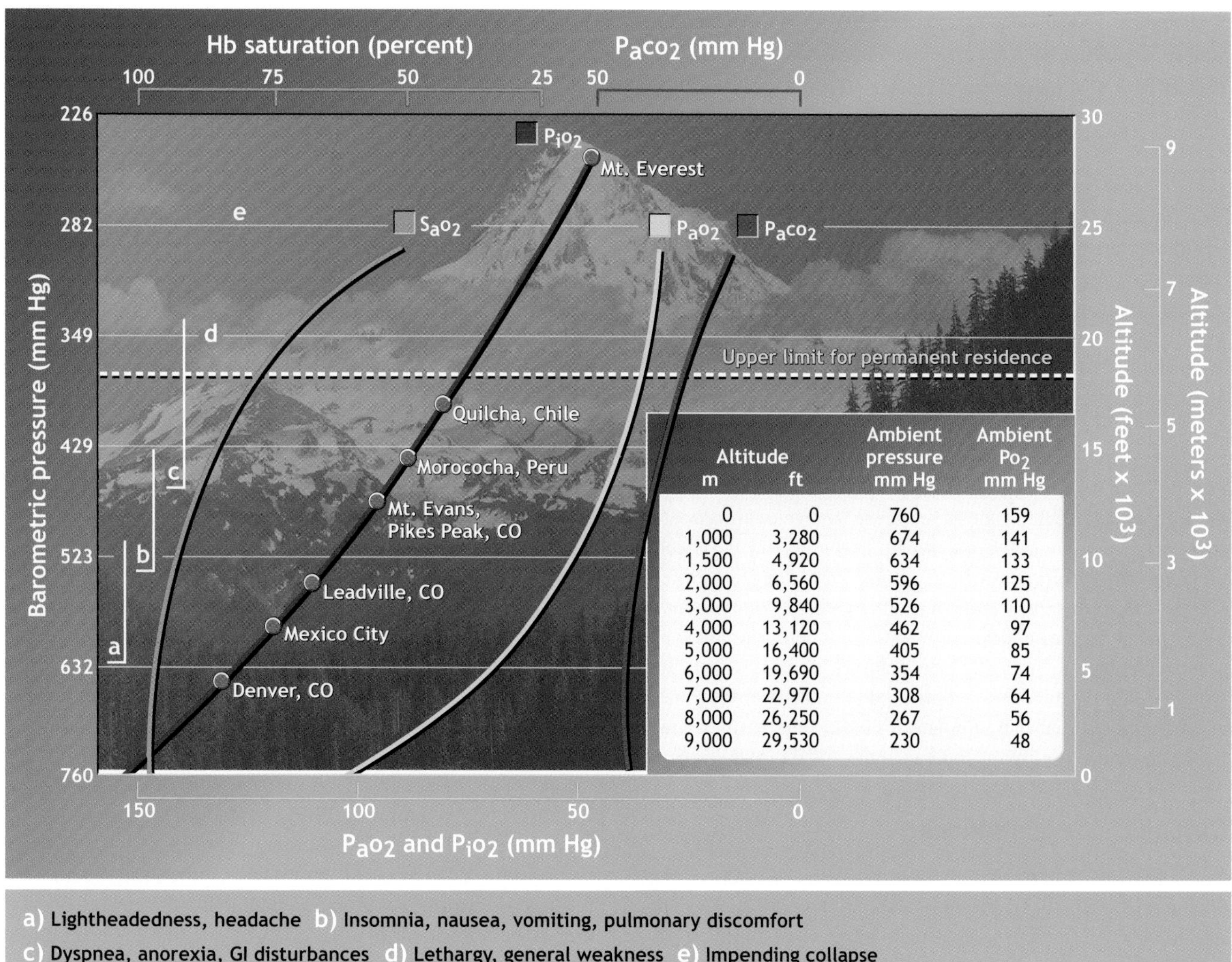

Altitude m	Altitude ft	Ambient pressure mm Hg	Ambient Po_2 mm Hg
0	0	760	159
1,000	3,280	674	141
1,500	4,920	634	133
2,000	6,560	596	125
3,000	9,840	526	110
4,000	13,120	462	97
5,000	16,400	405	85
6,000	19,690	354	74
7,000	22,970	308	64
8,000	26,250	267	56
9,000	29,530	230	48

FIGURE 24.1 • Changes in environmental and physiologic variables with progressive elevations in altitude (P_aO_2, partial pressure of arterial oxygen; P_aCO_2, partial pressure of arterial carbon dioxide; P_iO_2, partial pressure of oxygen in inspired air; S_aO_2, oxygen saturation of hemoglobin).

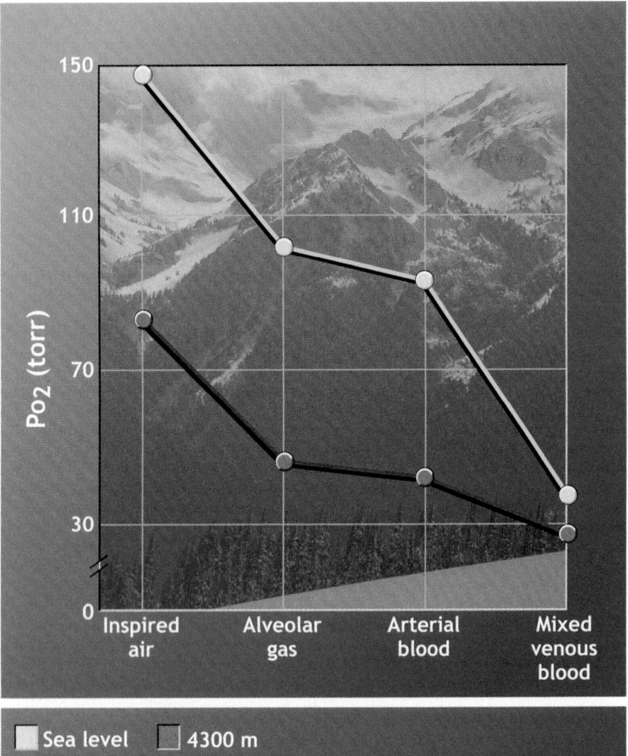

FIGURE 24.2 • Oxygen transport cascade from sea level to 4,300 m (14,108 ft).

altitude contains 20.93% oxygen, the Po_2 (density of the oxygen molecules) of air decreases directly with the fall in barometric pressure upon ascending to higher elevations (Po_2 = 0.2093 × barometric pressure). Thus, ambient Po_2 at sea level averages about 150 mm Hg, but only 107 mm Hg at 3048 m. At the summit of Mt. Everest (8848 m; 29,028 ft) ambient air pressure on a day climbers usually ascend to the summit ranges between 251 and 253 mm Hg, with a concomitant alveolar Po_2 of about 25 mm Hg (ambient air Po_2 between 42 and 43 mm Hg).[104] This equals only about 30% of the oxygen available in air at sea level. *The reduction in Po_2, and accompanying arterial hypoxia, precipitates the immediate physiologic adjustments to altitude and longer-term acclimatization.* **Acclimatization** refers to adaptations produced by a change in the natural environment, whether a change in season or place or residence. In contrast, **acclimation** refers to adaptation produced in a controlled laboratory environment as in chambers that can simulate high altitude or microgravity, hypoxic environments, and extremes of thermal stress.

Oxygen Loading at Altitude

The oxyhemoglobin dissociation curve is S-shaped (see Chapter 13, Fig. 13.3), and only a small change occurs in hemoglobin's percentage saturation with oxygen until an altitude of about 3048 m. At 1981 m (6500 ft), for example, alveolar Po_2 decreases from its sea level value of 100 mm Hg to 78 mm Hg, yet hemoglobin remains 90% saturated with oxygen. This relatively small arterial desaturation exerts little effect on a person during rest or even mild exercise, but performance in vigorous aerobic activities deteriorates. The relatively poor performances of men and women in middle-distance and distance running and swimming during the 1968 Olympics in Mexico City (altitude 2300 m; 7546 ft) resulted from the small reduction in oxygen transport at this altitude.[18] No world records emerged in events lasting longer than 2.5 minutes. Altitude does not impair the short-term anaerobic energy system at moderate altitude (e.g., glycogen storage, pathways of glycolysis and corresponding phosphorylase and phosphofructokinase enzyme activity, although maximal lactate accumulation becomes depressed at extreme elevation [see page 612]) or success in sprint–power activities such as sprint running, speed skating, track cycling, jumping, and discus.[27,30] However, impaired performance has been reported for reported for repeated interval sets of short-term power output (15-s training intervals) in elite athletes.[12] Performance in single bouts of such activities often improves because of lower air density (air resistance or drag force) at altitude than at sea level. In addition the lessened air resistance from a 24% reduction in air density at 2300 m should improve performance in the shot put (+6 cm), hammer throw (+53 cm), and javelin (+162 cm).[22] The oxygen cost for stationary cycling remains unaltered during altitude exposure.

In the transition from moderate altitude to higher elevations, values for alveolar (arterial) Po_2 are on the steep part of the oxyhemoglobin dissociation curve. This dramatically reduces hemoglobin oxygenation and oxygen transport capacity and negatively affects even mild aerobic activities. At high elevations in the Andes and Himalayas, oxygen loading of hemoglobin decreases dramatically, and physical activity becomes difficult to sustain. A small change in inspired Po_2 (i.e., barometric pressure) greatly affects aerobic capacity at the summit of Mt. Everest. For well-acclimatized mountain climbers, for example, breathing ambient air with a Po_2 of 48.5 mm Hg produces a $\dot{V}O_{2max}$ of 1450 mL · min^{-1}. This declines to 1070 mL · min^{-1} with only a 6–mm Hg decrease in inspired Po_2–a decrease of 63 mL O_2 · min^{-1} in $\dot{V}O_{2max}$ for each 1 mm Hg drop in inspired Po_2.[103,104]

Sudden exposure to 4300 m, for example, causes a 32% reduction in aerobic capacity compared with sea-level values.[110] At altitudes above 5182 m (17,000 ft), permanent living becomes nearly impossible, and mountain climbing frequently requires the aid of hyperoxic breathing mixtures.[74] At 5486 m (18,000 ft), arterial Po_2 averages 38 mm Hg and hemoglobin maintains only 73% oxygen saturation. Amazingly, however, reports describe acclimatized mountaineers who lived for weeks at 6706 m (22,000 ft) breathing only ambient air.[42] In fact, members of two Swiss expeditions to Mt. Everest remained at the summit for 2 hours without using breathing equipment![73] This represents an impressive feat considering that arterial Po_2 averages only 25 mm Hg, with a corresponding arterial blood oxygen saturation of 58%. An unacclimatized person becomes unconscious within 30 seconds under these conditions.[106] For acclimatized men at simulated extreme altitudes that approach the summit of Mt. Everest, $\dot{V}O_{2max}$ decreases by 70% from 4.13 L · min^{-1} to 1.17 L · min^{-1}, or from 49.1 mL · kg^{-1} · min^{-1} to 15.3 mL · kg^{-1} · min^{-1}.[34] These low values reflect the sea-level aerobic capacity of a sedentary 80-year-old man. Despite the significant physiologic strain imposed by high altitude, mountaineer Tom Whittaker, age 50, became the first amputee to reach Mt. Everest's summit (third attempt) on May 27, 1998. Although remarkable performances at high altitude reflect exceptions and not the rule, they demonstrate the enormous adaptive capability of humans to survive and even work without external support at extreme terrestrial elevations (see "Focus on Research").

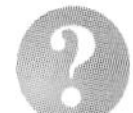

INTEGRATIVE QUESTION

Respond to this question: "If altitude has such negative effects on the body, how come certain track and field records are broken during competition at higher elevations?"

Focus on Research

High Altitude: A Hostile Environment

Pugh LGCE, et al. Muscular exercise at great altitudes. J Appl Physiol 1964;19:431.

Since the first ascent of Mt. Everest (8848 m; 29,028 ft) in 1953 by Sir Edmund Hillary and Tenzig Norgay, scientists have studied relationships between terrestrial elevation, partial pressure of oxygen in ambient air, arterial hemoglobin oxygen loading, and cardiovascular function to explain reduced exercise capacity at altitude. Early experiments at high altitude posed enormous scientific challenges owing to equipment limitations and lack of trained personnel with mountaineering experience. The experiments, carried out by the Himalayan Scientific and Mountaineering Expedition of 1960–1961 (sponsored by the publishers of *World Book Encyclopedia,* Chicago, IL, and the Medical Research Council, London, England), represent "classic" experiments in environmental physiology. Discoveries from this legendary scientific expedition provided the underpinnings to current understanding about physical work at high altitude. The research by L. G. C. E. Pugh and coworkers was part of the first series of studies to demonstrate that lung diffusion capacity, cardiac output, and the oxygen cost of extreme pulmonary ventilation limit exercise capacity at altitudes above 5800 m (19,000 ft).

The researchers used bicycle ergometer exercise to assess physical working capacity at sea level and at altitudes ranging from 4650 m to 7440 m (barometric pressure of 440 to 300 mm Hg). They established a base station at 4650 m but used a prefabricated laboratory hut at 5800 m (barometric pressure of 380 mm Hg) to conduct most of the research.

Subjects included eight men—six experienced mountaineers and one "sportsman," all acclimatized to high altitude, and one high-altitude Sherpa guide. The scientists with the Himalayan Scientific Expedition were five of the seven "lowland" subjects. The Sherpa guide carried the bicycle ergometer (20 kg) to the laboratory hut. Subjects pedaled at 50 RPM, with expired air collected by the Douglas bag method. A dry-gas meter measured expired air volumes with respiratory gas concentrations analyzed with a Lloyd-Haldane chemical analyzer. The exercise protocol (preceded by a 10-min warm-up) included 6 minutes of exercise (12 min at sea level) starting at 300 kg-m · min^{-1} with increments of 300 kg-m · min^{-1}. The test terminated when the subject would not exercise for at least 2 minutes at a given intensity. Oxygen consumption, pulmonary ventilation, heart rate, respiratory exchange ratio, and venous blood samples (not secured from all subjects) were obtained during the last 2 minutes at each exercise level.

Figure 1 presents the researchers' original plot of $\dot{V}O_{2max}$ in relation to terrestrial elevation. Clearly, $\dot{V}O_{2max}$ decreased from sea level upward and declined steeply above 6000 m, to reach an average of 1.42 L · min^{-1} at 7440 m.

(continued)

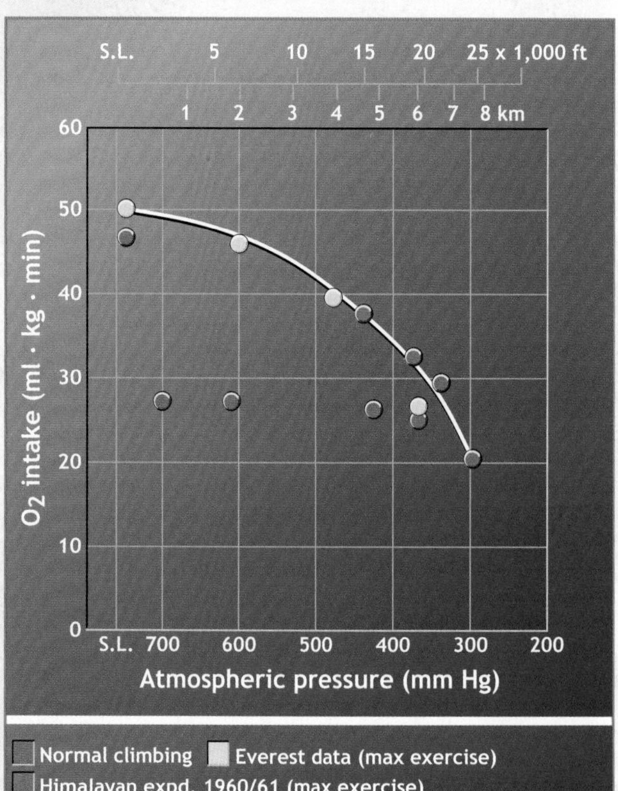

Figure 1. Oxygen consumption during submaximal (purple symbols; men climbing at their typical pace) and maximal (yellow and orange symbols) exercise in relation to ambient barometric pressure and terrestrial elevation. S.L., sea level.

Focus on Research High Altitude: A Hostile Environment

Figure 2 shows pulmonary ventilation (STPD and BTPS) and heart rate in response to $\dot{V}O_2$ during exercise at different altitudes. The curves for pulmonary ventilation shift to the left and increase in slope during exercise at higher elevations, with submaximal effort requiring the greatest ventilation at the highest altitude. This altitude-related hyperventilation reflects the experience of mountain climbers at great altitude; any slight increase in mountain slope or snow conditions brings them to a halt with breathlessness. Only the highest altitude produced apparent impairment of maximum exercise ventilation. Heart rates remained elevated during submaximal exercise at altitude.

Figure 3 shows a tendency for a higher respiratory exchange ratio (R) at all exercise levels at 5800 m than at sea level. At $\dot{V}O_2$s above 2.0 L · min^{-1}, R increased nearly vertically, a response consistent with the extreme hyperventilation at high altitude. Altitude exposure increased exercise blood lactate (not shown), which also contributed to exercise hyperventilation. Finally, comparisons of data for the Sherpa guide with those of the other subjects showed his superior work capacity, attributable to economy of ventilation with preservation of a normal blood pH and maintenance of a relatively higher arterial Po_2. The guide also maintained a high pulmonary diffusing capacity for oxygen and a high cardiac output relative to work intensity (measured in a separate experiment).

These pioneering studies demonstrated physiologic links to exercise limitations at high altitude and formed the foundation for expanding knowledge of human physical working capacity at extreme terrestrial elevations.

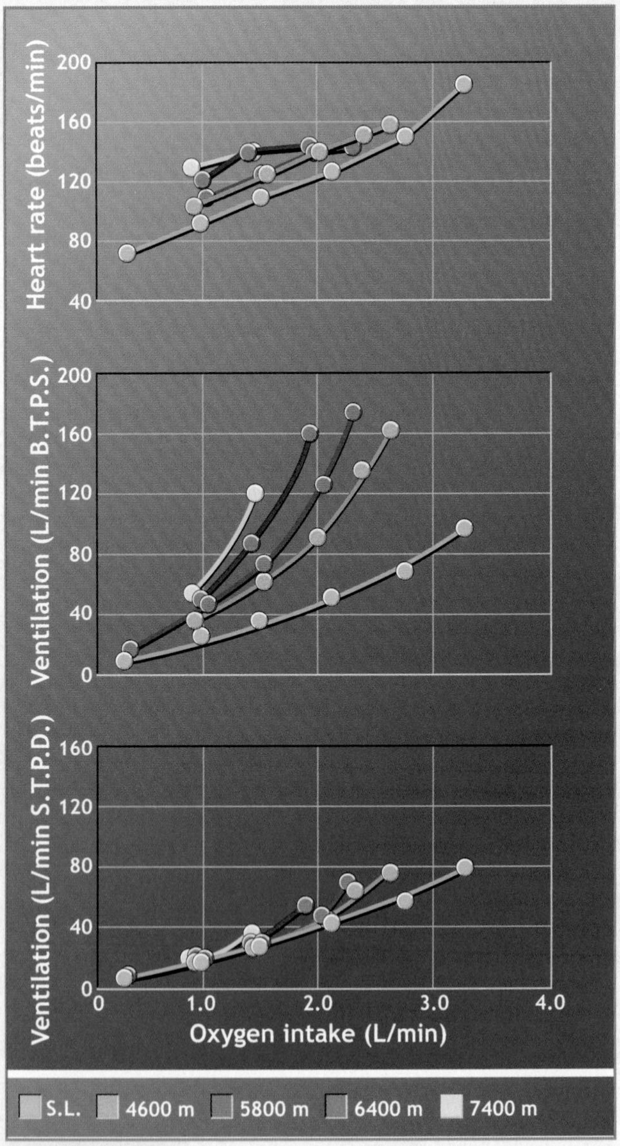

Figure 2. Pulmonary minute ventilation (BTPS, STPD) and heart rate in relation to oxygen consumption at sea level and altitudes up to 7400 m (24,440 ft). S.L., sea level.

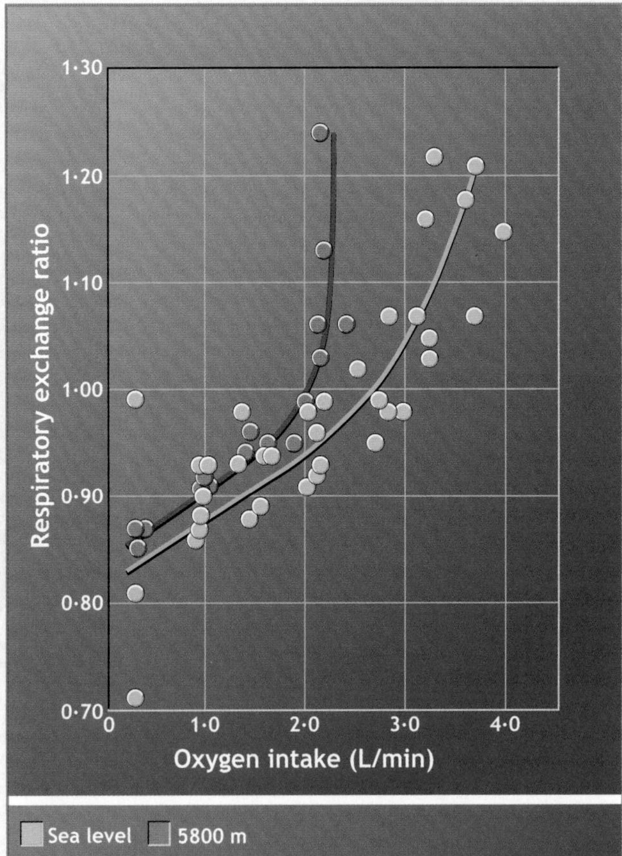

Figure 3. Respiratory exchange ratio during graded exercise at sea level and 5800 m (19,000 ft).

ACCLIMATIZATION

During the many years that mountaineers attempted to climb the world's highest peaks, they knew that it required weeks to adjust to successively higher elevations. *The term **altitude acclimatization** broadly describes adaptive responses in physiology and metabolism that improve tolerance to altitude hypoxia.* Each adjustment to a higher elevation proceeds progressively, and full acclimatization requires time. Successful adjustment to medium altitude affords only partial adjustment to a higher elevation. Residents of moderate altitudes, however, do show less decrement in physiologic capacity and exercise performance than lowlanders when both groups travel to a higher altitude.[63]

Table 24.1 indicates that compensatory responses to altitude occur almost immediately, while other adaptations take weeks or even months. The rapidity of the body's response remains largely altitude dependent, although considerable individual variability exists for both the rate and success of acclimatization.[71,75] A person can retain many of the beneficial submaximal exercise responses associated with 16 days of acclimatization at 4300 m despite intermittent sojourns to sea level for up to 8 days.[8] This suggests that certain aspects of acclimatization regress more slowly than they are acquired.

Immediate Responses to Altitude

Arrival at elevations of 2300 m and higher initiates rapid physiologic adjustments to compensate for the thinner air and accompanying reduction in alveolar Po_2. The two more important responses include:

- Increase in the respiratory drive to produce hyperventilation
- Increase in blood flow during rest and submaximal exercise

Hyperventilation

Hyperventilation from reduced arterial Po_2 is the most important and clear-cut immediate response of the native lowlander to altitude exposure.[21,44,91] Once initiated, this "hypoxic drive" increases during the first few weeks and can remain elevated for a year or longer during prolonged altitude residence.[52]

The aortic arch and branching of the carotid arteries in the neck contain peripheral chemoreceptors sensitive to reduced oxygen pressure. A significant reduction in arterial Po_2, which occurs at altitudes above 2000 m, progressively stimulates these receptors. This modifies inspiratory activity to increase alveolar ventilation and cause alveolar Po_2 to rise toward the level in ambient air. Increases in alveolar Po_2 with hyperventilation facilitate oxygen loading in the lungs and provide the rapid first line of defense against reduced ambient Po_2 at altitude. For females, variations in menstrual cycle phase do not affect ventilatory responses and exercise performance decrements during acute altitude exposure compared with those at sea level.[9] Mountaineers who respond with a strong, hypoxic ventilatory drive to sudden altitude exposure perform exercise tasks at extreme altitudes more effectively (and reach higher altitude) than climbers with a blunted hypoxic ventilatory response.[91]

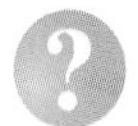

INTEGRATIVE QUESTION

From a physiologic perspective, what represents a safe altitude for flight in an airplane with a non-pressurized cabin?

Increased Cardiovascular Response

Resting systemic blood pressure increases in the early stages of altitude adaptation.[44] In addition, submaximal exercise heart rate and cardiac output rise as much as 50% above sea level values, while the heart's stroke volume remains un-

TABLE 24.1 ➤ IMMEDIATE AND LONGER-TERM ADJUSTMENTS TO ALTITUDE HYPOXIA

SYSTEM	IMMEDIATE	LONGER-TERM
Pulmonary acid–base	Hyperventilation	Hyperventilation
	Bodily fluids become more alkaline due to reduction in CO_2 (H_2CO_3) with hyperventilation	Excretion of base (HCO_3^-) via the kidneys and concomitant reduction in alkaline reserve
Cardiovascular	Increase in submaximal heart rate	Submaximal heart rate remains elevated
	Increase in submaximal cardiac output	Submaximal cardiac output falls to or below sea-level values
	Stroke volume remains the same or decreases slightly	Stroke volume decreases
	Maximum cardiac output remains the same or decreases slightly	Maximum cardiac output decreases
Hematologic		Decreased plasma volume
		Increased hematocrit
		Increased hemoglobin concentration
		Increased total number of red blood cells
Local		Possible increased capillarization of skeletal muscle
		Increased red-blood-cell 2,3-DPG
		Increased mitochondrial density
		Increased aerobic enzymes in muscle
		Loss of body weight and lean body mass

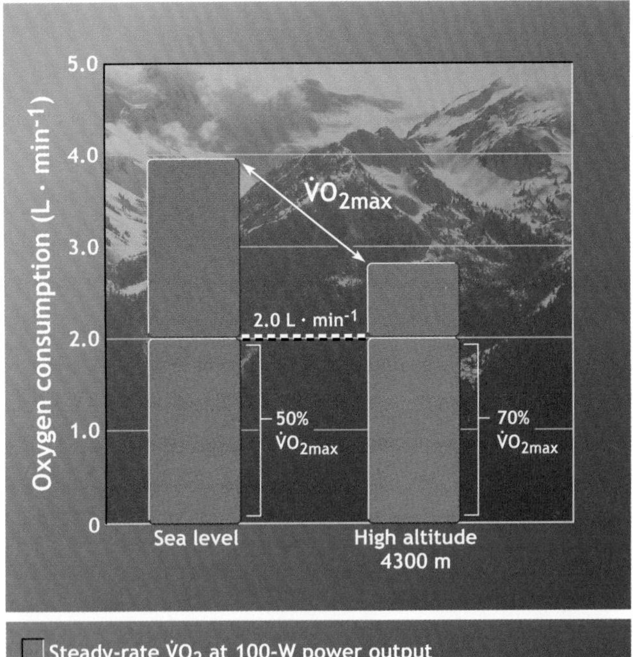

FIGURE 24.3 • Comparison of oxygen cost and relative strenuousness of submaximal exercise at sea level and high altitude.

changed.[49] The increased submaximal exercise blood flow at altitude largely compensates for arterial desaturation. For example, a 10% increase in cardiac output during rest or moderate exercise offsets a 10% reduction in arterial oxygen saturation, at least in terms of total oxygen transported through the body. Figure 24.3 shows that while the oxygen cost of submaximal exercise at 100 watts on a bicycle ergometer at sea level and high altitude remains unchanged at about 2.0 $L \cdot min^{-1}$, the relative strenuousness of the effort increases dramatically at altitude. In this example, submaximal exercise representing 50% of sea-level $\dot{V}O_{2max}$ equals 70% of $\dot{V}O_{2max}$ at 4300 m.

Catecholamine Response

Norepinephrine activity progressively increases over time during rest and exercise with altitude exposure.[67,68] Increased blood pressure and heart rate at altitude coincide with the steady rise in plasma levels and excretion rates of norepinephrine. Norepinephrine levels peak in women and men after 6 days of high-altitude exposure and then remain stable.[65,66,107] In addition to affecting heart rate and blood pressure, increased sympathoadrenal activity contributes to regulation of stroke volume, vascular resistance, and substrate use during short- and long-term hypobaric exposures. Figure 24.4 shows the 24-hour urinary excretion of norepinephrine and epinephrine during control (sea level) measurements and following exposure to 4300-m altitude for 7 days. Epinephrine showed little change, but norepinephrine excretion increased significantly by the fourth day. Urinary norepinephrine levels remain elevated for approximately 1 week following return to sea level.[96]

Table 24.2 shows metabolic and cardiorespiratory responses to moderate and maximal cycling exercise in young men at sea level and during brief exposure to simulated altitude of 4000 m.[94] Despite the increase in pulmonary ventilation during submaximal exercise at "altitude," arterial oxygen saturation decreased from 96% at sea level to 70% during all exercise intensities. In submaximal exercise, increased cardiac output entirely compensated for the blood's reduced oxygen content. Augmented blood flow resulted from the higher heart rate because the heart's stroke volume remained unchanged during short-term altitude exposure. With an increase in cardiac output, submaximal exercise oxygen consumption remained essentially identical at sea level and altitude. The greatest altitude effect on aerobic metabolism emerged during maximal exercise when $\dot{V}O_{2max}$ decreased to 72% of the sea level value.

With maximal exercise during short-term altitude exposure (≤7d), ventilatory and circulatory adjustments fail to compensate for the depressed arterial oxygen content. Figure 24.5 illustrates the relationship between pulmonary ventilation and oxygen consumption up to maximum during bicycle ergometer exercise at sea level and simulated altitudes from 1000 to 4000 m. Each 1000-m increase in altitude caused a proportionate increase in exercise ventilation volume. However, when exercise oxygen consumption exceeded 2.0 $L \cdot min^{-1}$, pulmonary ventilation increased disproportionately at progressively higher elevations.

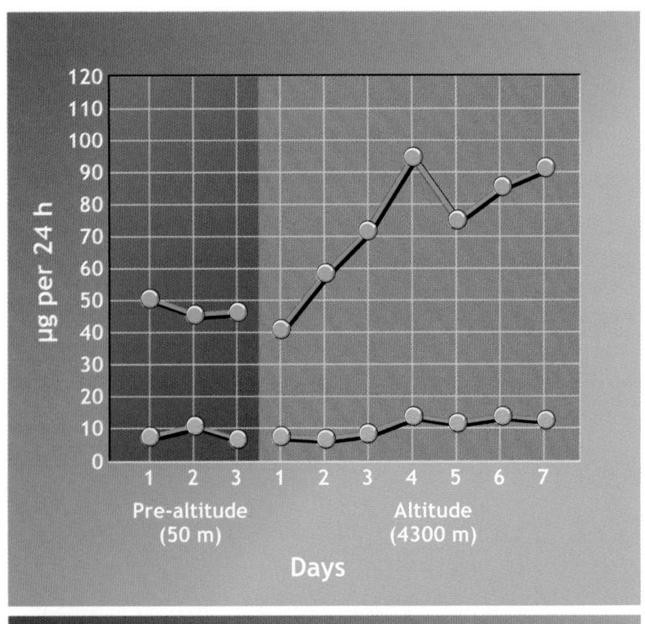

FIGURE 24.4 • Effects of a 7-day stay at 4300-m (14,108-ft) on urinary norepinephrine and epinephrine in eight male sea-level residents. (Modified from Surks MJ, et al. Changes in plasma thyroxine concentration and metabolism, catecholamine excretion and basal oxygen uptake during acute exposure to high altitude (14,100 ft). J Clin Invest 1966;45:1442.)

TABLE 24.2 ➤ **CARDIORESPIRATORY AND METABOLIC RESPONSE DURING SUBMAXIMAL AND MAXIMAL EXERCISE AT SEA LEVEL AND SIMULATED ALTITUDE OF 4000 M (13,115 FT)**

EXERCISE LEVEL	$\dot{V}O_2$ (L · MIN^{-1})		$\dot{V}$E (L · MIN^{-1} BTPS)		ARTERIAL SATURATION (%)	
Altitude, m	*0*	*4000*	*0*	*4000*	*0*	*4000*
600 kg-m · min^{-1}	1.50	1.56	39.6	53.7	96	71
900 kg-m · min^{-1}	2.17	2.23	59.0	93.7	95	69
Maximum	3.46	2.50	123.5	118.0	94	70

EXERCISE LEVEL	$\dot{Q}$ (L · MIN^{-1})		H R (B · MIN^{-1})		S V (ML)		A-$\bar{V}$ O_2 DIFF (ML O_2 · dL^{-1})	
Altitude, m	*0*	*4000*	*0*	*4000*	*0*	*4000*	*0*	*4000*
600 kg-m · min^{-1}	13.0	16.7	115	148	122	113	10.8	9.4
900 kg-m · min^{-1}	19.2	21.6	154	176	125	123	11.4	10.4
Maximum	23.7	23.2	186	184	127	126	14.6	10.8

From Sternberg J, et al. Hemodynamic response to work at simulated altitude 4000 m. J Appl Physiol 1966;21:1589.
$\dot{Q}$= cardiac output

Fluid Loss

Because ambient air in mountainous regions remains cool and dry, considerable body water evaporates as inspired air becomes warmed and moistened in the respiratory passages. This fluid loss often leads to moderate dehydration and accompanying symptoms of dryness of the lips, mouth, and throat. Fluid loss becomes pronounced for physically active people because of large daily total sweat loss and exercise pulmonary ventilation volumes (and hence water loss). Physically active individuals should have access to water at all times.

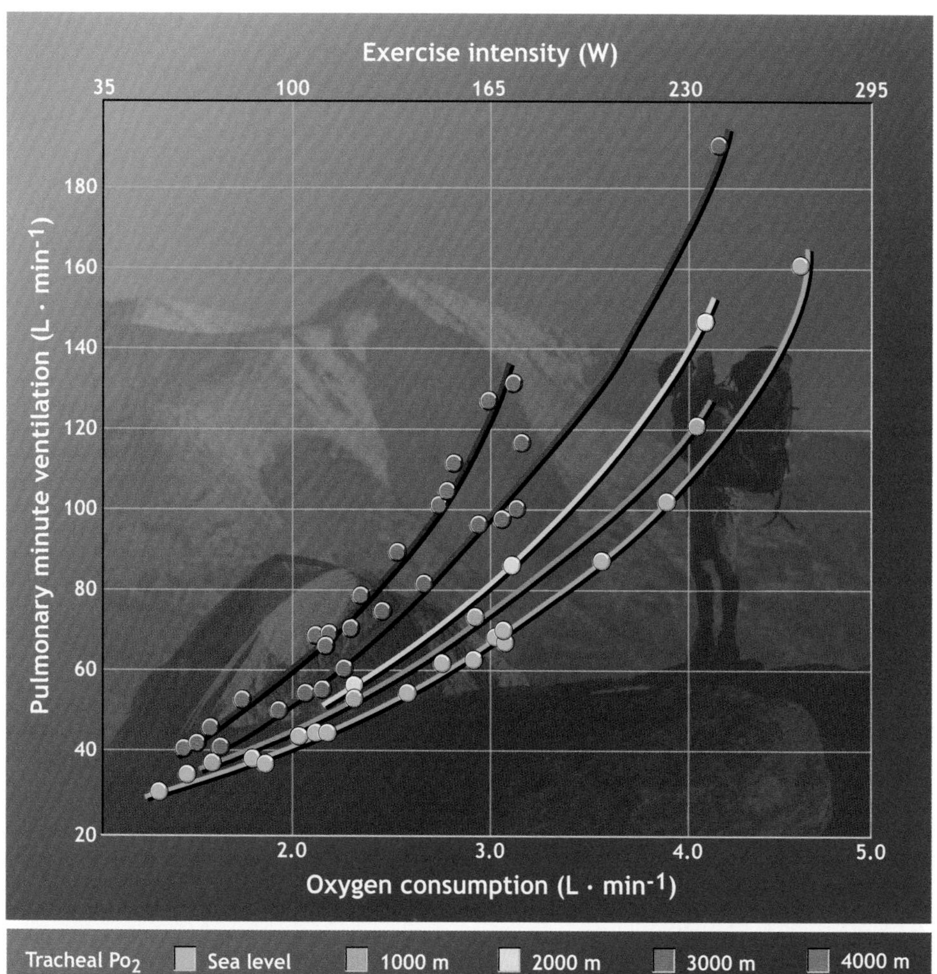

FIGURE 24.5 • Effects of a progressive increase in simulated altitude from sea level (tracheal PO_2 = 149 mm Hg) to 4000 m (tracheal PO_2 = 87 mm Hg) on the relationship between pulmonary ventilation and oxygen consumption during cycle ergometry. (Modified from Åstrand PO. The respiratory activity in man exposed to prolonged hypoxia. Acta Physiol Scand 1954;30:343.)

IN A PRACTICAL SENSE

➤➤ IDENTIFICATION AND TREATMENT OF ALTITUDE-RELATED MEDICAL PROBLEMS

Natives who live and work at high altitudes as well as newcomers risk a variety of medical problems associated with reduced arterial P_{O_2}. These problems usually remain mild and dissipate within several days, depending on the rapidity of the ascent and degree of exposure. Other medical complications significantly compromise overall health and safety. Three medical conditions threaten those who ascend to high altitude:

1. **Acute mountain sickness (AMS)**, the most common malady
2. **High-altitude pulmonary edema (HAPE)**, which reverses if the person returns quickly to a lower altitude
3. **High-altitude cerebral edema (HACE)**, a potentially fatal condition if not diagnosed and treated immediately

Acute Mountain Sickness

Most people experience the discomfort of AMS during the first few days at altitudes of 2500 m and above. This relatively benign condition, which becomes exacerbated by exercise in the first few hours of exposure,[80] possibly results from acute reduction in cerebral oxygen saturation.[85] It occurs most frequently in those who ascend rapidly to a high altitude without benefiting from gradual and progressive acclimatization to lower altitudes. Symptoms (Table 1) usually begin within 4 to 12 hours and dissipate within the first week.[35,39,54] Headache, the most frequent symptom, probably results from increased cerebral hemodynamics from short-term hyperventilation.[45] Most symptoms become prevalent above 3000 m. Rapid ascent to 4200 m almost guarantees some form of AMS.[61]

Decreased thirst sensation and severe appetite suppression can occur during the early stages, often resulting in a 40% reduction in energy intake and consequent body mass loss. Diets low in salt and high in carbohydrates are well tolerated during the early stay at high altitude. A potential benefit of maintaining carbohydrate reserves through dietary intake lies in the liberation of more energy per unit oxygen with carbohydrate oxidation than with fat (5.0 kcal vs. 4.7 kcal per L of O_2). Also, high blood lipid levels following a high-fat meal may reduce arterial oxygen saturation. Benefits of maintaining a high-carbohydrate diet include:

1. Enhanced altitude tolerance
2. Reduced severity of mountain sickness
3. Lessened physical performance decrements during the early stages of altitude exposure

Even moderate exercise becomes intolerable for persons suffering the effects of AMS. Symptoms subside and often disappear as acclimatization progresses. Acclimatizing slowly to moderate altitudes below 3048 m followed by a gradual progression to higher elevations (termed *staged ascent*) usually prevents AMS. Climbers should spend several nights at 2500 to 3000 m before going higher, and an extra night should be added for each additional 600 to 900 m climbed. Abrupt increases of more than 600 m in the altitude for sleeping should be avoided at 2500 m or higher ("climb high–sleep low"). If acclimatization proves ineffective, a 300-m descent usually alleviates symptoms; supplemental oxygen and the drug acetazolamide (Diamox) facilitate recovery.

High-Altitude Pulmonary Edema

For unknown reasons, about 2% of sojourners to altitudes above 3000 m experience HAPE. Symptoms (Table 1) usually manifest within 12 to 96 hours following rapid ascent. Major predisposing factors for HAPE include level of altitude, rate of ascent, and individual susceptibility.[6] Fluid accumulates in the brain and lungs in this life-threatening condition.[3,79] At first, symptoms do not seem severe, but the syndrome progresses to pulmonary edema and fluid retention by the kidneys. Chest examination reveals wheezy, raspy sounds known as *rales*. Even in well-acclimatized individuals, HAPE can develop with severe exertion at elevations above 5486 m (18,000 ft), probably the result of increased pulmonary artery pressure with damage to the blood-gas barrier.[105]

Table 2 lists appropriate methods to avoid and treat HAPE. Treatment to prevent severe disability or even death requires immediate descent to lower altitude on a stretcher (or flown to safety), because physical activity from walking potentiates complications. With proper treatment, symptoms decrease within hours, with complete clinical recovery within days. HAPE poses no problem for healthy individuals who journey to and recreate without acclimatization at altitudes below 1676 m.

TABLE 1. IMPORTANT ALTITUDE-RELATED MEDICAL CONDITIONS

CONDITION	SYMPTOMS
Acute mountain sickness (AMS)	Severe headache, fatigue, irritability, nausea, vomiting, loss of appetite, indigestion, flatulence, generalized weakness, constipation, decreased urine output with normal hydration, sleep disturbance
High-altitude pulmonary edema (HAPE)	Debilitating headache and severe fatigue; excessively rapid breathing and heart rate; rales;[a] cough producing pink frothy sputum; bluish skin color (from low blood P_{O_2}); disruption of vision, bladder, and bowel functions; poor reflexes; loss of coordination of trunk muscles; paralysis on one side of the body
High-altitude cerebral edema (HACE)	Staggered gait, dyspnea upon exertion, severe weakness/fatigue, persistent cough with pulmonary infection, pain or pressure in substernal area, confusion, impaired mental processing, drowsiness, ashen skin color, loss of consciousness

[a]Excess mucus in the lungs diagnosed as clicking sounds heard through a stethoscope.

IN A PRACTICAL SENSE

➤➤ IDENTIFICATION AND TREATMENT OF ALTITUDE-RELATED MEDICAL PROBLEMS—cont'd

TABLE 2. PREVENTION AND TREATMENT OF HIGH-ALTITUDE PULMONARY EDEMA

Prevention

1. Slow ascent for susceptible individuals (average increase in sleeping altitude of 300–350 m · d^{-1} above 2500 m)
2. No ascent to higher altitude with symptoms of AMS
3. Descent when AMS symptoms do not improve after a day of rest
4. Under circumstances of high risk: avoid vigorous exercise when not acclimatized
5. Nifedipine: 20 mg slow-release formulation every 6 hours (or 30–60 mg sustained-release formulation once daily) for susceptible individuals when slow ascent is impossible

Treatment

1. Descent by at least 1000 m (primary choice in mountaineering)
2. Supplemental oxygen: 2–4 L · min^{-1} (primary choice in areas with medical facilities)
3. When 1 and/or 2 not possible:
   - Administer 20 mg nifedipine slow-release formulation every 6 hours
   - Use portable hyperbaric chamber (see Fig. 26.10)
   - Descend to low altitude as soon as possible

High-Altitude Cerebral Edema

HACE is a potentially fatal neurologic syndrome that develops within hours or days in individuals with AMS. HACE occurs in about 1% of people exposed to altitudes above 2700 m; it involves increased intracranial pressure that causes coma and death if left untreated. The early symptoms (Table 1), similar to those of AMS and HAPE, progressively worsen as the altitude stay progresses. Cerebral edema probably results from cerebral vasodilation and elevations in capillary hydrostatic pressure that cause movement of fluid and protein from the vascular compartment across the blood–brain barrier.[36] An enlarged cerebral fluid volume eventually distorts brain structures, particularly the white matter, which exacerbates symptoms and increases sympathetic nervous system activity. Tissue hypoxia caused by high-altitude exposure may also initiate a series of local events that stimulate angiogenesis (new capillary vessel growth) in brain tissue.[108] Because of the difficulty in adequately diagnosing HACE at high altitude, immediate descent to a lower elevation is mandatory.

OTHER CONDITIONS

Chronic mountain sickness (CMS), prevalent in a small number of altitude natives, can develop after months and years at altitude. CMS relates to excessive polycythemia, perhaps the result of a genetically linked variation in the EPO response to hypoxic stress.[72] CMS symptoms include lethargy, weakness, sleep disturbance, bluish skin coloring (cyanosis), and change in mental status. **High-altitude retinal hemorrhage** (HARH) affects virtually all climbers at altitudes above 6700 m (21,982 ft). HARH usually progresses unnoticed with no specific treatment or means for prevention. Hemorrhage in the macula of the eye—the oval "yellow spot" region in the back of the eyeball close to the optic disc—can produce irreversible visual defects. Retinal bleeding probably results from surges in blood pressure with exercise that cause blood vessels in the eye to dilate and rupture from increased cerebral blood flow.[97]

SENSORY FUNCTIONS. Figure 24.6 shows deterioration in a variety of sensory and mental functions with the decrease in arterial oxygen saturation at altitude. Neurologic alterations range from a 5% decrease in sensitivity to light at 1524 m to a further 25% decrease in light sensitivity and 30% decrease in visual acuity when elevation doubles to 3048 m, and a 25% deterioration in coding task performance and simple reaction time at 6096 m.

MYOCARDIAL FUNCTION. Individuals with normal electrocardiograms at sea level including patients with stable chronic heart failure generally show no adverse changes to indicate myocardial ischemia (e.g., arrythmias, angina, ECG abnormalities) at simulated high altitudes, even during maximal exercise.[2,82,95] Even on Mt. Everest, contractile function of the heart remains stable despite the considerable chronic hypoxia.[77] Because little information exists about the effects of altitude on individuals with coronary artery disease and with congestive heart failure, these patients should avoid high-altitude exposure altogether.[61]

Longer-Term Adjustments to Altitude

Hyperventilation and increased submaximal exercise cardiac output provide a rapid and relatively effective counter to the acute challenge of altitude exposure. Concurrently, other slower-acting adjustments occur during a prolonged altitude stay. The most important longer-term adjustments involve:

- Regulation of acid–base balance of body fluids altered by hyperventilation
- Synthesis of hemoglobin and red blood cells and accompanying changes in local circulation and aerobic cellular function
- Elevated sympathetic neurohumoral activity as reflected by a significant increase in norepinephrine that peaks within 1 week at altitude.

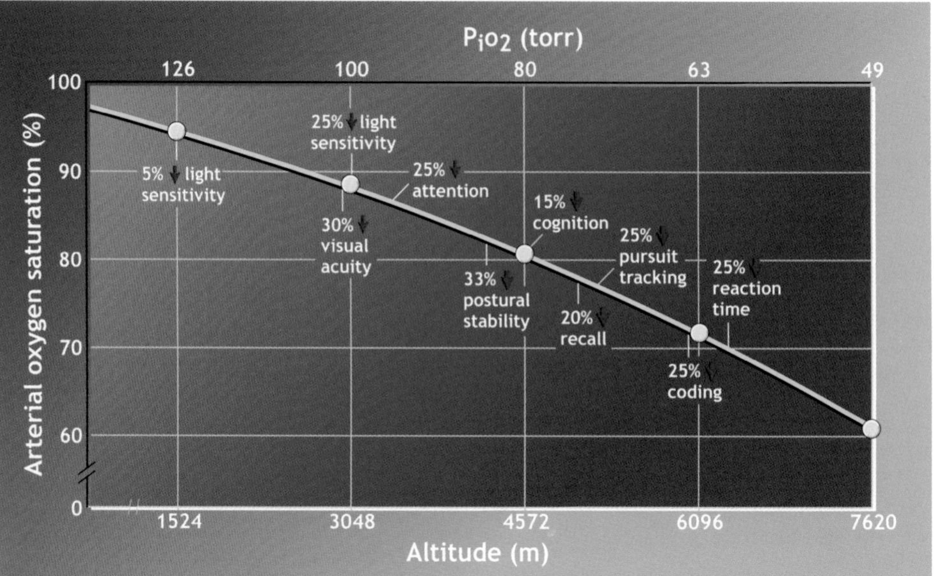

FIGURE 24.6 • Arterial saturation as a function of increasing altitude and the corresponding impairment (↓) in diverse sensory and mental functions. (Modified from Fulco CS, Cymerman A. Human performance and acute hypoxia. In: Pandolf KB, et al., eds. Human performance physiology and environmental medicine at terrestrial extremes. Carmel, IN: Cooper Publishing Group, 1988.)

Each of these acclimatization components improves tolerance to the relative hypoxia of medium and high altitudes.

Acid–Base Readjustment

The beneficial effect of hyperventilation at altitude to increase alveolar PO_2 produces the opposite effect on the body's carbon dioxide level. Because ambient air contains essentially no carbon dioxide, the increased breathing volumes at altitude dilute normal alveolar carbon dioxide concentrations. This creates a larger-than-normal gradient for diffusion ("wash out") of carbon dioxide from the blood to the lungs, causing arterial PCO_2 to decrease considerably. With exposure to 3048 m, for example, alveolar PCO_2 drops to about 24 mm Hg, in contrast to its usual 40 mm Hg value at sea level. Alveolar PCO_2 drops as low as 10 mm Hg during a prolonged stay at high altitude.

Carbon dioxide loss from the bodily fluids in a hypoxic environment creates a physiologic disequilibrium. We pointed out in Chapter 13 that carbonic acid (H_2CO_3) normally carries the largest quantity of carbon dioxide in the body. This relatively weak acid readily dissociates into H^+ and HCO_3^-, which move to the lungs in the venous circulation. H^+ and HCO_3^- recombine in the pulmonary capillaries to form H_2CO_3, which in turn forms carbon dioxide and water; carbon dioxide diffuses from the blood into the alveoli and leaves the body. A decrease in carbon dioxide level with hyperventilation increases the pH from loss of carbonic acid, and bodily fluids become more alkaline.

Because hyperventilation represents a sustained and beneficial response to altitude exposure, adjustments proceed during acclimatization to minimize the accompanying negative disruption in acid–base balance. Control of ventilatory-induced alkalosis advances slowly as the kidneys excrete base (HCO_3^-) through the renal tubules. In turn, restoration of normal pH increases the respiratory center's responsiveness, thus enabling even greater hyperventilation in response to altitude hypoxia.

REDUCED BUFFERING CAPACITY AND THE "LACTATE PARADOX." *Establishing acid–base equilibrium with acclimatization occurs at the expense of a loss of absolute alkaline reserve.* Thus, although the pathways of anaerobic metabolism remain unaffected at altitude, the blood's capacity for buffering acid gradually decreases, and the critical level lowers for acid metabolite accumulation. A general depression in maximum lactate concentrations becomes apparent in maximal exercise above 4000 m.[76]

On immediate ascent to high altitude, a given submaximal exercise load increases blood lactate concentration compared with sea level values. Presumably, increased lactate accumulation results from greater reliance on anaerobic glycolysis with altitude hypoxia. Surprisingly, the same submaximal and maximal exercise with large muscle groups after several weeks of hypoxic exposure produces *lower lactate levels*, despite a lack of increase in either $\dot{V}O_{2max}$ or regional blood flow in active tissues. The question arises concerning this apparent physiologic contradiction, termed the **lactate paradox**, "How is lactate accumulation reduced without a concomitant increase in tissue oxygenation, when the hypoxemia associated with high altitude should promote lactate accumulation?"

Research to resolve the lactate paradox points to reduced output of the glucose-mobilizing hormone epinephrine during chronic high-altitude exposure.[10] Because glucose and glycogen are the only macronutrient sources for anaerobic energy (and lactate formation), reduced glucose mobilization blunts the capacity for lactate formation. Reductions in intracellular ADP during long-term altitude exposure may also inhibit activation of the glycolytic pathway. In addition, depressed lactate formation during maximal exercise may partly reflect an overall reduced central nervous system drive, which would blunt capacity for all-out physical effort.[48,64] Reduced blood lactate accumulation at high altitude is apparently not related to the decreased buffering capacity that accompanies high-altitude acclimatization.[47]

Hematologic Changes

An increase in the blood's oxygen-carrying capacity is the most important longer-term adjustment to altitude exposure. Two factors account for this adaptation: (1) an initial decrease in plasma volume, followed by (2) increased synthesis of erythrocytes and hemoglobin.

PLASMA VOLUME DECREASE. During the first several days of altitude exposure, the body's fluid balance changes in a direction that shifts fluid from the intravascular space to the interstitial and intracellular spaces. The decrease in plasma volume that occurs within several hours of altitude exposure increases red blood cell concentration.[90] After a week at 2300 m, for example, the plasma volume decreases by about 8%, whereas the concentration of red blood cells (hematocrit) increases 4% and hemoglobin, 10%. A 1-week stay at 4300 m decreases plasma volume 16 to 25% with concomitant increases in hematocrit (6%) and hemoglobin (20%).[37] The rapid reduction in plasma volume (and accompanying hemoconcentration) increases the oxygen content of arterial blood significantly above values observed on arrival at altitude. Diuresis (increased urine output) accompanies the shift in fluid from the plasma during acclimatization, which maintains balance in the fluid compartments at a lower total body water content.

RED BLOOD CELL MASS INCREASE. Reduced arterial Po_2 at altitude stimulates an increase in the total number of red blood cells, a condition termed **polycythemia**. The erythrocyte-stimulating hormone **erythropoietin (EPO)**, synthesized and released primarily from the kidneys in response to localized arterial hypoxia, initiates red blood cell formation within 15 hours after altitude ascent. In the weeks that follow, erythrocyte production in the marrow of the long bones increases considerably and remains elevated throughout the altitude stay.[34] The blood of a typical miner in the Andes contains 38% more erythrocytes than the blood of a lowlander. In some apparently healthy high-altitude natives, red cell count may reach levels 50% above normal—8 million cells per mm^3 compared with 5.3 million for the native lowlander![62] Climbers acclimatized at 6500 m during a 1973 Mt. Everest expedition showed a 40% increase in hemoglobin concentration and a 66% increase in hematocrit.[16] This probably approaches the upper limit for a beneficial hematologic response. Any further erythrocyte packing increases blood viscosity and restricts blood flow and oxygen diffusion to the tissues.

INTEGRATIVE QUESTION

For their assault on Mt. Everest, elite mountaineers spend a total of 3 months at camps at 16,600 feet, 19,500 feet, 21,300 feet, 24,000 feet, and 26,000 feet before their final ascent. Explain the physiologic rationale for a "stage ascent" approach to mountaineering.

Polycythemia translates directly to an increase in the blood's capacity to transport oxygen. For example, the oxygen-carrying capacity of blood in high-altitude residents of Peru averages 28% above sea-level values.[43] In well-acclimatized mountaineers, the blood carries 25 to 31 mL of oxygen per dL of blood, compared with 20 mL for lowland residents.[74] Thus, despite reduced hemoglobin oxygen saturation at altitude, the *quantity* of oxygen in arterial blood may approach or even equal sea-level values.

Figure 24.7A illustrates the general trend for hemoglobin and hematocrit increases during acclimatization. For eight young women who lived and worked for 10 weeks at the 4267-m summit of Pikes Peak. Because the researchers' previous work showed significantly fewer hematologic changes during acclimatization in women than in men (possibly because of inadequate iron intake), each woman received iron supplementation prior to, during, and on return from altitude.

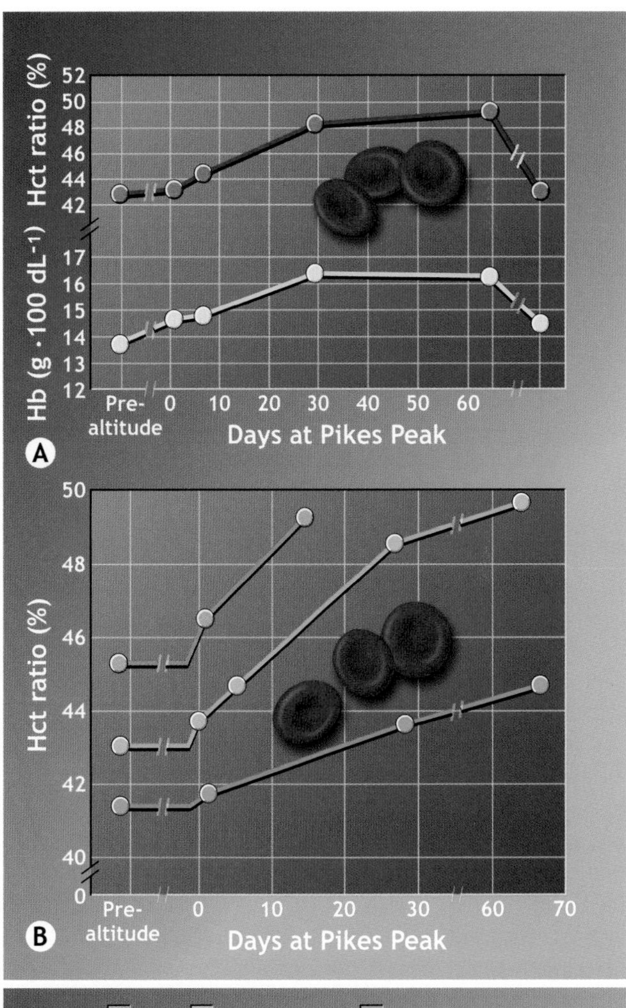

FIGURE 24.7 • **A**. Effects of altitude on hemoglobin (Hb; yellow line) and hematocrit (Hct; red line) levels of 8 young women from the University of Missouri (213 m) prior to, during, and 2 weeks after exposure to 4267 m at Pikes Peak, Colorado. (From Hannon JP, et al. Effects of altitude acclimatization on blood composition of women. J Appl Physiol 1968; 26: 540.) **B**. Hematocrit response of young women receiving supplemental iron (+Fe) prior to and during altitude exposure compared to groups of male and female subjects receiving no supplemental iron. (Courtesy of Dr. J. P. Hannon.)

Red blood cell concentration increased rapidly upon reaching Pikes Peak. Hemoconcentration resulted from a reduction in plasma volume within the first 24 hours at altitude. Hemoglobin concentration and hematocrit continued to rise in the month that followed and then stabilized for the remainder of the stay. Prealtitude values reestablished within 2 weeks after the women returned to Missouri.

Figure 24.7B shows that iron supplementation increased the prealtitude values for hematocrit and hemoglobin. One might anticipate this finding, as young women frequently suffer from mild dietary iron insufficiency with depressed iron reserves (see Chapter 2). Comparison of the acclimatization curve for the iron-supplemented women with another group of women not given additional iron showed a greater hematocrit increase in the supplemented group. Iron supplementation enhanced hematocrit increases at altitude to a level equivalent to that of men at the same location. These findings indicate that athletes with borderline iron stores may not respond to acclimatization as effectively as individuals who arrive at altitude with iron reserves adequate to sustain an increase in erythrocyte production.

Cellular Adaptations

A topic of considerable debate concerns whether extreme terrestrial hypoxia stimulates vascular and cellular adaptations in humans that improve local oxygen extraction and maximize oxidative functions.[30,40,69,99] Any improvement in the energy state of the muscle with acclimatization probably does not result from a reorginazation of metabolic pathways.[31] Animals born and raised at high altitude showed more concentrated capillarization of skeletal muscle (number per mm^2) than sea-level counterparts.[100] Chronic hypoxia may also initiate remodeling of capillary diameter and length and the formation of new capillaries to significantly increase oxygen conductance to neural tissues.

Human residents of sea level also show increased tissue capillarization during an altitude stay.[71] A more prolific microcirculation reduces the oxygen diffusion distance between the blood and tissues to optimize tissue oxygenation at altitude when arterial Po_2 decreases. Furthermore, muscle biopsy specimens from humans living at altitude indicate that myoglobin increases up to 16% after acclimatization.[78] Additional myoglobin augments oxygen "storage" in specific fibers and facilitates intracellular oxygen release and delivery at a low tissue Po_2. Whether the small increase in mitochondrial number and concentration of aerobic energy transfer enzymes with prolonged exposure[59] (or when training under normobaric hypoxic versus normoxic conditions[69]) reflects exercise training effects or the hypoxic environment remains unclear.[41,88]

High-altitude natives benefit from the slight shift to the right of the oxyhemoglobin dissociation curve at altitude. This effect decreases hemoglobin's affinity for oxygen to favor more oxygen release to tissues for a given drop in cellular Po_2. Facilitated oxygen release from hemoglobin with long-term altitude exposure occurs from an increased concentration of red blood cell 2,3-diphosphoglycerate (2,3-DPG; see Chapter 13).[55] Increased 2,3-DPG coupled with more circulating hemoglobin (and red blood cells) favorably affects the long-term resident's capacity to supply oxygen to active tissue during physical activity.

Changes in Body Mass and Body Composition

Prolonged high-altitude exposure significantly reduces lean body mass (muscle fibers atrophy up to 20%) and body fat, with the magnitude of weight loss directly related to terrestrial elevation. Six men participated in a 40-day progressive decompression to an ambient pressure of 249 mm Hg in a hyperbaric chamber to simulate an ascent of Mt. Everest.[84] Daily caloric intake from a depressed appetite decreased by 43% during the exposure period. Reduced energy intake reduced body mass 7.4 kg, predominantly from the muscle component of the fat-free body mass. In addition to depressed appetite and food intake during high-altitude exposure, intestinal absorption efficiency decreases to compound the difficulty in maintaining body weight.[13,23,101] The basal metabolic rate also increases significantly upon arrival at altitude, which further affects the tendency to lose weight. To some extent, one can override an accelerated metabolic rate and minimize weight loss by consciously increasing energy intake while at altitude.

Time Required for Acclimatization

The time required to acclimatize to altitude depends on terrestrial elevation. Acclimation to one altitude ensures only partial adjustment to a higher elevation. As a broad guideline, it takes about 2 weeks to adapt to altitudes up to 2300 m. Thereafter, each 610-m altitude increase requires an additional week to fully acclimatize, up to 4600 m. Athletes desiring to compete at altitude should begin intense training as soon as possible during acclimatization. Rapid initiation of training minimizes detraining effects brought about by the normal tendency to reduce physical activity in the first few days at altitude.[53] Acclimatization adaptations dissipate within 2 or 3 weeks after returning to sea level.

METABOLIC, PHYSIOLOGIC, AND EXERCISE CAPACITIES AT ALTITUDE

The stress of high altitude significantly restricts work capacity and physiologic function. Even at lower altitudes, the physiologic and metabolic adjustments do not fully compensate for the reduced ambient oxygen pressure, and exercise performance deteriorates. Certain circulatory parameters, particularly stroke volume and maximum heart rate, acclimatize in a direction that reduces oxygen transport capacity and $\dot{V}O_{2max}$.[26,29,87]

Maximal Oxygen Consumption

Figure 24.8A depicts the relationship between the decrease in $\dot{V}O_{2max}$ (% of sea-level value) and increasing altitude or simulated exposures (i.e., hypobaric chambers or normobaric hy-

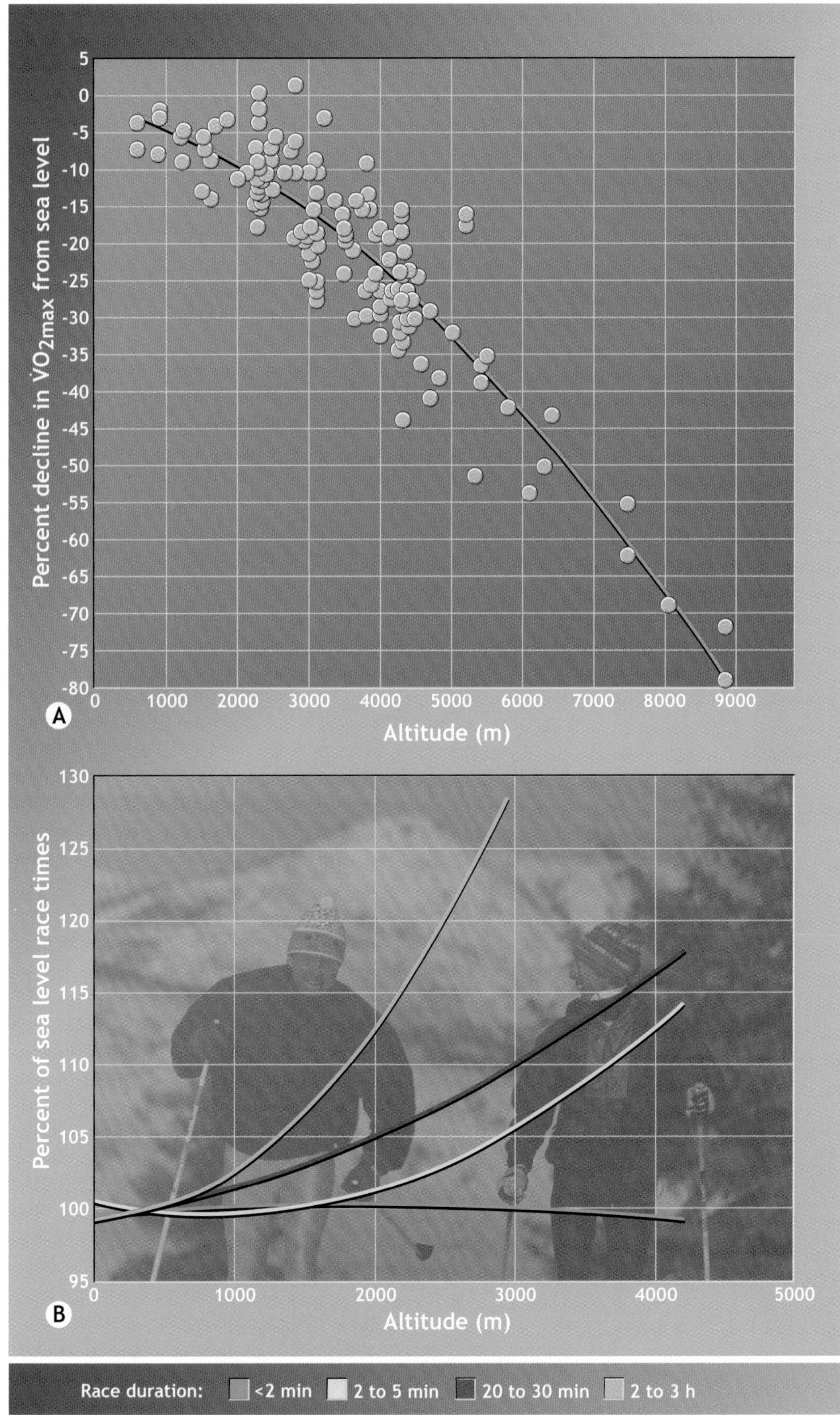

FIGURE 24.8 • A. Reduction in $\dot{V}O_{2max}$ as a percentage of the sea-level value in relation to altitude exposure, derived from 146 average data points from 67 different civilian and military investigations conducted at altitudes from 580 m (1902 ft) to 8848 m (29,021 ft). "Altitudes" represent data from actual terrestrial elevations or simulated elevations with hypoxic chambers or hypoxic gas breathing. The *orange curvilinear line* is a database regression line drawn using the 146 points. **B**. Generalized trend in performance decrements in relation to altitude exposure for runners and swimmers, primarily during competition. (Modified from Fulco CS, et al. Maximal and submaximal exercise performance at altitude. Aviat Space Environ Med 1998;69: 793.)

poxic gas breathing) as reported in diverse civilian and military studies.[27] Variation in points about the orange line depicting the relationship most likely result from disparities in experimental design and procedures and physiologic differences among subjects. The figure indicates that small declines in $\dot{V}O_{2max}$ become noticeable beginning at an altitude of 589 m. *Thereafter, arterial desaturation causes the $\dot{V}O_{2max}$ of men and women to decrease at a rate of 7 to 9% per 1000-m altitude increase up to 6300 m, where aerobic capacity declines at a more rapid, nonlinear rate.*[19,75,86] For example, aerobic capacity at 4000 m averages 75% of the sea-level value. At 7000 m, $\dot{V}O_{2max}$ averages one-half the sea-level value; the $\dot{V}O_{2max}$ of a relatively fit man atop Mt. Everest is about 1000 mL · min^{-1}, which corresponds to an exercise power output of only 50 watts on a bicycle ergometer.[73]

Physical conditioning prior to altitude exposure offers little protection because the endurance athlete experiences a slightly greater percentage reduction in $\dot{V}O_{2max}$ than does an untrained person. In addition, large variability exists among individuals in the decrement in $\dot{V}O_{2max}$ with altitude exposure. Men experience the largest decrease, particularly those with a large lean body mass, a large sea-level aerobic capacity, and a low sea-level lactate threshold.[81] To some extent, arterial desaturation and decrease in $\dot{V}O_{2max}$ are more pronounced in individuals with a blunted hyperventilation response to exercise in a hypoxic environment.[28] Despite any unique effects of altitude exposure on aerobically fit individuals, a standard exercise task at altitude still provides relatively less stress for well-conditioned women and men because they perform it at a lower percentage of $\dot{V}O_{2max}$.

Circulatory Factors

Even after several months of acclimatization to hypoxia, $\dot{V}O_{2max}$ remains significantly below sea-level values, despite relatively rapid and pronounced increases in hemoglobin concentration. This occurs because reduced circulatory capacity—combined effect of lowered maximum heart and stroke volume—offsets the hematologic benefits of acclimatization.[29,50]

Submaximal Exercise

The immediate altitude response to exercise increases submaximal cardiac output (Table 24.2), but this response diminishes as acclimatization progresses and does not improve with prolonged exposure.[49] Reduced exercise cardiac output results mainly from a progressive decrease in the heart's stroke volume (associated with diminished plasma volume) as the altitude stay progresses. Despite the reduced cardiac output, submaximal oxygen consumption remains stable through an expanded a-$\bar{v}$ O_2 difference. To some extent, an increased submaximal heart rate offsets the decrease in stroke volume during submaximal exercise.

Maximal Exercise

Maximum cardiac output decreases after about a week above 3048 m and remains lower throughout one's stay.[33,75] *Reduced blood flow during maximal exercise results from the combined effect of decreases in maximum heart rate and stroke volume, both of which continue to decrease with the length and magnitude of altitude exposure.*[49–52,86,89] This blunted cardiac response does not result from myocardial hypoxia, at least as reflected by electrocardiographic and coronary blood flow measurements during vigorous exercise at high altitudes.[38,87] Decreased plasma volume and increased total peripheral vascular resistance contribute to the reduced maximum stroke volume. Enhanced parasympathetic tone induced by prolonged altitude exposure probably reduces the maximum heart rate.[89]

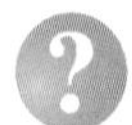

INTEGRATIVE QUESTION

If altitude acclimatization improves endurance exercise performance at altitude, why does it not improve similar performance immediately upon return to sea level?

Performance Measures

Figure 24.8B illustrates the generalized trend in exercise performance decrements, primarily during competition for athletes at different altitude exposures. Altitude exerts no adverse effect on events lasting less than 2 minutes. For longer-duration events, performance times are longer (poorer performance) at higher elevations than at sea level. The threshold for decrements occurs at about 1600 m for events with a duration of 2 to 5 minutes, while only a 600- to 700-m altitude induces poorer performance in events lasting longer than 20 minutes. For the 1- and 3-mile runs, medium altitude (2300 m) causes a 2 to 13% performance decrement for fit subjects.[25] This coincides with the 7.2% increase in 2-mile run times for highly trained middle-distance runners at the same altitude.[1] Even after 29 days of acclimatization, high-altitude exposure significantly increases 3-mile run time, compared with times for the same run near sea level.[76] The small improvement in endurance performance during acclimatization, despite lack of concomitant increase in $\dot{V}O_{2max}$, relates to three factors: (1) increased minute pulmonary ventilation (ventilatory acclimatization), (2) increased arterial oxygen saturation and cellular aerobic functions, and (3) blunting of the blood lactate response in exercise (see "lactate paradox," page 612).

AEROBIC CAPACITY ON RETURN TO SEA LEVEL

Sea-level exercise performance does not significantly improve after living at altitude when $\dot{V}O_{2max}$ serves as the improvement criterion.[46,56,70] An 18-day stay at 3100 m produced no significant change in the altitude-induced 25% reduction in aerobic capacity in young runners.[33] Furthermore, $\dot{V}O_{2max}$ was about the same as the prealtitude measure on return to sea level. Even in studies showing small improvements in either $\dot{V}O_{2max}$ or exercise performance at altitude and on return to sea level, the change often relates to an increase in physical activity (i.e., the effects of training and/or repeated testing) during altitude exposure.[20,51]

Possible Negative Effects

Several physiologic changes during prolonged altitude exposure negate adaptations that could improve exercise performance on return to sea level. For example, the residual effects of a loss of muscle mass and a reduced maximum heart rate and stroke volume would not enhance sea-level performance. Any reduction in maximum cardiac output at altitude offsets benefits from an increase in the blood's oxygen-carrying capacity. Although a blunted circulatory capacity returns to normal after a few weeks at sea level, so also do potentially positive hematologic adaptations.[37] Within a physiologic context, the controversial use of blood doping (see Chapter 23) mimics the hematologic benefits of altitude exposure without the potential negative effects on maximum cardiovascular dynamics and body composition.

ALTITUDE TRAINING AND SEA-LEVEL PERFORMANCE

Most research does not support endurance training at altitude to improve subsequent sea-level exercise performance. Altitude acclimatization improves capacity for exercise at altitude, particularly high altitude. However, the effect of altitude training on aerobic capacity and endurance performance immediately on return to sea level remains unclear. As discussed above, altitude adaptations in local circulation and cellular metabolism, combined with compensatory increases in the blood's oxygen-carrying capacity, should theoretically improve subsequent sea-level performance. Also, positive pulmonary adaptations and responses during prolonged hypoxic exposure do not regress immediately upon descent from altitude.[92] Furthermore, if tissue hypoxia provides an important training stimulus, altitude plus training should act synergistically, and the total effect should exceed similar training at sea level. Unfortunately, much of the exercise training–altitude exposure research contains experimental design flaws that limit evaluation of this possibility. Poor control over subjects' physical activity at altitude makes it difficult to discern whether any improved $\dot{V}O_{2max}$ or performance score on return to sea level represents a training effect, an altitude effect, or synergism between altitude and training.

Researchers used equivalent groups to compare the effectiveness of altitude training (2300 m) and equivalent training at sea level.[1] Six middle-distance runners trained at sea level for 3 weeks at 75% of their sea-level $\dot{V}O_{2max}$. Another group of six runners trained an equivalent distance at the same percentage $\dot{V}O_{2max}$ measured at 2300 m. The groups then exchanged training sites and continued to train for 3 weeks at the same relative intensity as the preceding group. Initially, 2-mile run times were 7.2% slower at altitude, compared with those at sea level. Run times improved 2.0% for both groups during altitude training, but postaltitude performance at sea level remained the same as the prealtitude sea-level runs. Figure 24.9 shows that short-term altitude exposure decreased $\dot{V}O_{2max}$ 17.4% for both groups; it improved only slightly after 20 days of altitude training. When the runners returned to sea level after altitude training, aerobic capacity remained 2.8% *below* prealtitude sea-level values. Clearly, for these well-conditioned middle-distance runners, no synergistic effect emerged from combining aerobic training at medium altitude compared with equivalent sea-level training.

Others have duplicated these observations for $\dot{V}O_{2max}$ and endurance performance at both moderate and higher altitudes.[24,53] Highly trained male track athletes flew to Nunoa, Peru (altitude 4000 m), where they continued to train and acclimatize for 40 to 57 days. $\dot{V}O_{2max}$ decreased 29% below sea-level values after the initial 3 days at altitude; after 48 days it still remained 26% lower. The 440-yard, 880-yard, and 1- and 2-mile runs during a "track meet" with the altitude natives measured running performance after acclimatization. The times after acclimatization remained considerably slower than prealtitude, sea-level times, particularly for the longer runs. Furthermore, when the athletes returned to sea level, $\dot{V}O_{2max}$ and running performance generally did not differ from prealtitude measures. On no occasion did a runner improve his previous prealtitude run time. In fact, running times in the longer events averaged 5% *below* prealtitude trials. In other studies, training in a hypobaric chamber provided no additional benefit to sea-level performance compared with similar training (albeit at a higher absolute exercise level) at sea

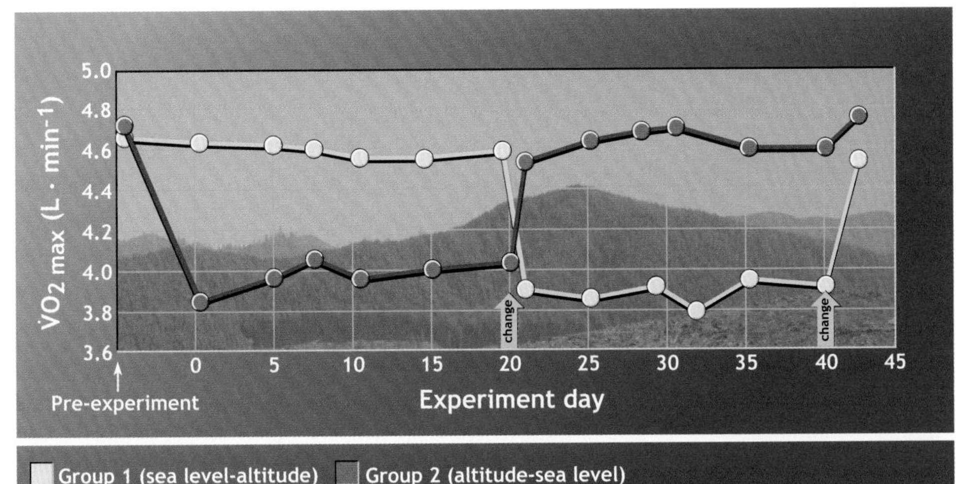

FIGURE 24.9 • Maximal oxygen consumption of two equivalent groups during training for 3 weeks at altitude and 3 weeks at sea level. Group 1 trained first at sea level and continued training for 3 weeks at altitude. For Group 2, the procedure reversed, and they trained first at altitude and then at sea level. Green arrows in figure indicate change in training site. (From Adams WC, et al. Effects of equivalent sea-level and altitude training on $\dot{V}O_{2max}$ and running performance. J Appl Physiol 1975;39:262.)

TABLE 24.3 ➤ EFFECT OF ALTITUDE ON TRAINING INTENSITY FOR SIX COLLEGIATE ATHLETES

	ALTITUDE (M)			
	300	2300	3100	4000
Intensity of workout (% $\dot{V}O_{2max}$ at 200 m)	78	60	56	39

From Kollias J, Buskirk ER. Exercise and altitude. In Science and medicine of exercise and sports. 2nd ed. Johnson WR, ER Buskirk, eds. New York: Harper & Row. 1974: .

level. As expected, the "altitude"-trained group eventually showed significantly better exercise performance at simulated altitude than sea-level residents.[98]

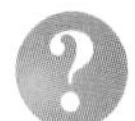

INTEGRATIVE QUESTION

Give your opinion (and rationale) about what effects a 2-week exposure to an altitude of 3000 m would have on maximal exercise performance of a 60-second duration.

Decrement in Absolute Training Level at Altitude

One must lower the absolute workload to perform aerobic exercise at the same relative intensity at altitude as at sea level. Otherwise, anaerobic metabolism provides a larger portion of the energy for exercise at altitude (see Fig. 24.3), and fatigue develops.[109] Exposure to 2300 m and higher makes it nearly impossible to train at the same absolute exercise intensity as at sea level. Table 24.3 shows the reduction in training intensity relative to sea-level standards for six college athletes. At 4000 m, for example, the runners could train only at the intensity equivalent to 39% of the sea-level $\dot{V}O_{2max}$, compared to an intensity of 78% when training at sea level. The absolute exercise training level at altitude may become so reduced that an athlete cannot maintain peak condition for sea-level competition. In this regard, elite athletes benefit from periodically returning from altitude to sea level for intense training to offset any "detraining" during a prolonged altitude stay (see next section). Intermittent returns to a lower altitude would not interfere with acclimatization and might even benefit altitude performance.[8,20] Regardless of the training model, athletes who train at altitude should include high-intensity speed work to maintain muscle power.

COMBINE ALTITUDE STAY WITH LOW-ALTITUDE TRAINING

Research has focused on the optimal combination of high-altitude stay plus low-altitude training in competitive runners. Athletes who lived at 2500 m but returned regularly to 1250 m to train at near–sea-level intensity (i.e., **live high–train low**) showed greater average increases in $\dot{V}O_{2max}$ and 5000-m run performance than athletes who lived and trained only at 2500 m or those who lived and trained only at sea level.[57] This indicates that strategies that combine (1) altitude acclimatization and (2) maintenance of sea-level training intensity provide *synergistic benefits* to endurance performance at sea level. Regular training exposure to a near–sea-level environment appears to prevent the impaired systolic function (i.e., reduced maximum stroke volume and cardiac output) typically observed during training at altitude. Debate exists concerning whether intermittent altitude exposure increases red blood cell mass and hemoglobin concentration.[4,58]

Not all individuals benefit to the same degree from a living-high, training-low strategy. Within the group showing physiologic and performance increases with this protocol, certain individuals classified as "responders," while others showed little positive adjustment.[17] These "nonresponders" displayed a significantly smaller increase in plasma concentration of the erythrocyte-producing hormone EPO after 30 hours at altitude than the responders. Such individuals would experience a blunted increase in hematocrit during acclimatization to altitude exposure. These findings suggest that three prerequisites exist for benefit from the combination of altitude living and lower-altitude training:

1. The altitude stay must take place at an elevation high enough to raise EPO concentrations to increase total red blood cell volume and $\dot{V}O_{2max}$.
2. The athlete must respond to the altitude stress with increased EPO output.
3. Training must take place at an elevation low enough to maintain training intensity and exercise oxygen consumption at near sea-level values.

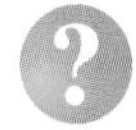

INTEGRATIVE QUESTION

Respond to a person who suggests that periodic breath holding while exercising at sea level should bring about similar physiologic adaptations as training at altitude.

At-Home Acclimatization

Inability to maintain sea-level training intensity represents a significant negative aspect of a sojourn to altitude to improve subsequent sea-level performance from hematologic changes with acclimatization. Failure to maintain the muscular power outputs of sea-level training at altitude may actually initiate a detraining effect. Application of the live high–train low training model poses significant practical and financial hurdles. For these reasons, some endurance athletes use the banned (and dangerous) practices of blood doping and EPO injections to increase hematocrit and hemoglobin concentration, without the bother and potential negative effects of an altitude stay.

A more prudent approach makes use of the observation that altitude's beneficial effects on erythropoiesis and aerobic capacity require relatively short-term exposures to hypoxia.

For example, daily intermittent exposures of 3 to 5 hours for 9 days to simulated altitudes of 4000 to 5500 m in a hypobaric chamber significantly increased endurance performance, red blood cell count, and hemoglobin concentration in elite mountain climbers.[15,83] Intermittent hypoxic training under normobaric conditions provides an added bonus with clinical and cardioprotective implications because such exercise augments training's effect on selected metabolic and cardiovascular risk factors.[5]

In the absence of a hypobaric chamber, three approaches create an "altitude" environment where an athlete, mountaineer, or hot-air balloonist living at sea level spends a large enough portion of the day to stimulate an altitude acclimatization response.

- In the **Gamow Hypobaric Chamber**, a person rests and sleeps for about 10 hours each day. The chamber's total air pressure can decrease to simulate the barometric pressure of a preselected altitude. Reductions in barometric pressure bring about proportionate reductions in the inspired air's Po_2 to simulate altitude exposure and induce physiologic adaptations.
- To eliminate the necessity of constructing an enclosure to withstand differentials between sea-level ambient air pressure and the reduced pressure in the hypobaric chamber, one can simulate altitude at sea level by increasing the nitrogen percentage of the air within an enclosure. Increased nitrogen percentage correspondingly reduces the air's oxygen percentage, thus decreasing the Po_2 of inspired air. Nordic skiers have applied this technique by living for 3 to 4 weeks in a specially constructed house that provides "air" with only 15.3% oxygen, compared with its normal concentration of 20.9%. The system requires mixing nitrogen gas and carefully monitoring the breathing mixture.
- The **Wallace Altitude Tent** (Fig. 24.10), a suitcase-sized unit developed by British Olympic cyclist Shaun Wallace, continuously supplies air with an oxygen content of approximately 15% to simulate an altitude of 2500 m. The 70-pound unit consists of a portable tent that fits over a normal bed; a "hypoxic generator" (housed in an airline suitcase) continually feeds altitude-simulating hypoxic air into the tent. The porosity of the tent's material limits the rate of diffusion of outside oxygen into the tent and maintains the 15% oxygen concentration. Equilibration of the tent's environment at the 15% oxygen level requires about 90 minutes. The manufacturer proclaims: "Easily set up at home, or in a hotel whilst on-the-road, the system provides the beneficial physiological adaptations associated with living at 9000′ altitude, without any compromise in training quality—the ultimate in high–low training." Future research must verify the effectiveness of this unique approach to endurance training.

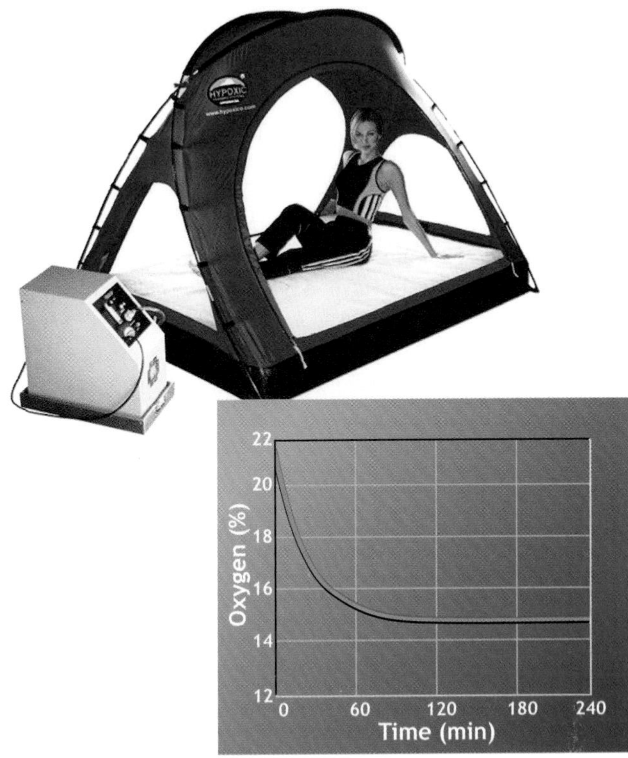

FIGURE 24.10 • The Wallace Altitude Tent fits over a double or queen-size bed or can be constructed for in-home use as a semipermanent cubicle. Patches of "breathable" nylon permit diffusion of ambient oxygen (at higher Po_2) into the tent (at lower Po_2) to maintain the percentage of oxygen within the tent at about 15%. A hypoxic generator *(left of tent)* continuously supplies air with oxygen content that equilibrates within the tent at near 15%. The *inset* shows the time course for equilibration of air within the tent to reach the 15% oxygen level. (Photo courtesy of Hypoxico Inc, Shaun Wallace, Cardiff, CA.)

Summary

1. The progressive reduction in ambient Po_2 as one ascends in altitude eventually causes inadequate hemoglobin oxygenation in arterial blood. Arterial desaturation produces noticeable performance decrements in aerobic physical activities at altitudes of 2000 m and higher. Altitude does not adversely affect short-term (anaerobic) sprint and power performances that depend on energy from intramuscular high-energy phosphates and glycolytic reactions.
2. Reduced Po_2 and accompanying hypoxia at altitude stimulate physiologic responses and adjustments that improve altitude tolerance during rest and exercise. Hyperventilation and increased submaximal cardiac output via elevated heart rate are the primary immediate responses to altitude exposure.
3. Medical problems ranging from mild to life-threatening often emerge during altitude exposure. AMS, HAPE, and HACE are the most prominent maladies. The potentially lethal conditions of

HAPE and HACE require the patient's immediate removal to a lower altitude.

4. Acclimatization entails physiologic and metabolic adjustments that greatly improve tolerance to altitude hypoxia. The main adjustments involve (1) reestablishment of acid–base balance of the bodily fluids, (2) increased synthesis of hemoglobin and red blood cells, and (3) improved local circulation and cellular metabolism. Adaptations 2 and 3 significantly facilitate oxygen transport and use.
5. The rate of altitude acclimatization depends on the terrestrial elevation. Noticeable improvements occur within several days. The major adjustments require about 2 weeks, although acclimatization to relatively high altitudes may require 4 to 6 weeks.
6. The alveolar Po_2 averages 25 mm Hg at the summit of Mt. Everest. For acclimatized men, this reduces $\dot{V}O_{2max}$ by 70%, to about 15 mL $O_2 \cdot kg^{-1} \cdot min^{-1}$. An unacclimatized individual loses consciousness within 30 seconds at this altitude.
7. Acclimatization does not fully compensate for the stress of altitude. Despite acclimatization, $\dot{V}O_{2max}$ decreases about 2% for every 300 m above 1500 m. A significant decrement in endurance-related exercise performance parallels the reduced aerobic capacity.
8. Altitude-related decrements in physiologic function (e.g., reduction in maximum heart rate and stroke volume) offset any beneficial effects of acclimatization. This partly explains the inability to achieve sea-level $\dot{V}O_{2max}$ values at altitude, even after acclimatization.
9. Despite certain altitude acclimatization adaptations that should increase aerobic capacity and endurance performance on return to sea level, research results do not support such an effect. This probably results from the altitude-related decrease in maximum heart rate and maximum stroke volume.
10. Training at altitude provides no more benefit to sea-level performance than equivalent training at sea level.
11. Athletes benefit from periodically returning from altitude to sea level for intense training to offset any "detraining" from lower levels of exercise during a prolonged altitude stay.

References

1. Adams WC, et al. Effects of equivalent sea-level and altitude training on $\dot{V}O_2$ max and running performance. J Appl Physiol 1975;39:262.
2. Agostoni P, et al. Effects of simulated altitude-induced hypoxia on exercise capacity in patients with chronic heart failure. Am J Med 2000;109:450.
3. Anholmm JD, et al. Radiographic evidence of interstitial pulmonary edema after exercise at altitude. J Appl Physiol 1999;86:503.
4. Ashenden MJ, et al. "Live high, train low" does not change the total haemoglobin mass of male endurance athletes sleeping at a simulated altitude of 3000 m for 23 nights. Eur J Appl Physiol 1999;80:479.
5. Baily DM, et al. Training hypoxia: modulation of metabolic and cardiovascular risk factors in men. Med Sci Sports Exerc 2000;32:1058.
6. Bärtsh P. High altitude pulmonary edema. Med Sci Sports Exerc 1999;31(Suppl 1):S23.
7. Basnyat B, et al. Myocardial infarction or high-altitude pulmonary edema. Wilderness Environ Med 2000; 11:196.
8. Beidleman BA, et al. Exercise responses after altitude acclimatization are retained during reintroduction to altitude. Med Sci Sports Exerc 1997;29:1588.
9. Beidleman BA, et al. Exercise VE and physical performance at altitude are not affected by menstrual cycle phases. J Appl Physiol 1999;86:1519.
10. Bender PR, et al. Decreased exercise muscle lactate release after high altitude acclimatization. J Appl Physiol 1989;67:1456.
11. Boero JA, et al. Increased brain capillaries in chronic hypoxia. J Appl Physiol 1999;86:2111.
12. Brosnan MJ, et al. Impaired interval exercise responses in elite female cyclists at moderate simulated altitude. J Appl Physiol 2000;11:196.
13. Butterfield GE. Nutrient requirements at high altitude. Clin Sports Med 1999;18:607.
14. Butterfield GE, et al. Increased energy intake minimizes weight loss in men at altitude. J Appl Physiol 1992;72:1741.
15. Casas M, et al. Effect of intermittent exposure to hypobaric hypoxia and exercise on human physical performance. J Physiol Biochem (Rev Esp Fisiol) 1997;53:160.
16. Cerretelli P. Limiting factors to oxygen transport on Mount Everest. J Appl Physiol 1976;40:658.
17. Chapman RF, et al. Individual variation in responses to altitude training. J Appl Physiol 1998;85:1448.
18. Craig AB Jr. Olympics 1968: a post-mortem. Med Sci Sports 1969;1:177.
19. Cymerman A, et al. Operation Everest II: maximal oxygen uptake at extreme altitude. J Appl Physiol 1989;66:2446.
20. Daniels J, Oldridge N. The effects of alternate exposure to altitude and sea level on world-class middle-distance runners. Med Sci Sports 1970;2:107.
21. Dempsey JA. Effects of acute through life-long hypoxic exposure on exercise pulmonary gas exchange. Respir Physiol 1971;13:62.
22. Dickinson ER, et al. Project Olympics. Schweiz Z Sportsmed 1966;14:305.
23. Dinmore AJ, et al. Intestinal carbohydrate absorption and permeability at high altitude (5,730 m). J Appl Physiol 1994;76:1903.
24. Emonson DL, et al. Training-induced increases in sea level $\dot{V}O_{2max}$ and endurance training are not enhanced by acute hypobaric exposure. Eur J Appl Physiol 1997;76:8.
25. Faulkner JA, et al. Maximum aerobic capacity and running performance at altitude. J Appl Physiol 1968;24:685.
26. Ferretti G, et al. Oxygen transport system before and after exposure to chronic hypoxia. Int J Sports Med 1990;11:S15.
27. Fulco CS, et al. Maximal and submaximal exercise performance at altitude. Aviat Space Environ Med 1998;69:793.
28. Gavin TP, et al. Ventilation's role in the decline in $\dot{V}O_{2max}$ and SaO_2 in acute hypoxic exercise. Med Sci Sports Exerc 1998;30:195.
29. Gonzalez NC, et al. Increasing maximal heart rate increases maximal O_2 uptake in rats acclimatized to simulated altitude. J Appl Physiol 1998;84:164.
30. Green HJ, et al. Operation Everest II: adaptations in human skeletal muscle. J Appl Physiol 1989;66:2454.
31. Green HJ, et al. Human skeletal muscle exercise metabolism following an expedition to Mount Denali. Am J Physiol Regul Integr Comp Physiol. 2000;279:R1872.
32. Green HJ, et al. Increase in submaximal cycling efficiency mediated by altitude acclimatization. J Appl Physiol 2000;89:1189.
33. Grover RF, Reeves JT. Exercise performance of athletes at sea level and 3,100 meters altitude. In: Goddard RF, ed. The effects of altitude on physical performance. Chicago, IL: Athletic Institute, 1967.
34. Groves BM, et al. Operation Everest II: elevated high-altitude pulmonary resistance unresponsive to oxygen. J Appl Physiol 1987;63:521.
35. Hackett PH, Roach RC. High altitude medicine. In: Auerbach PA, ed. Wilderness medicine, management of wilderness and environmental emergencies. St Louis, MO: Mosby-Year Book, 1995.
36. Hackett PH, et al. High-altitude cerebral edema evaluated with magnetic resonance imaging. Clinical correlation and pathophysiology. JAMA 1998;280:1920.
37. Hannon JP, et al. Effects of altitude acclimatization on blood composition of women. J Appl Physiol 1969;26:540.
38. Harris CW, Hansen JE. Electrocardiographic changes during exposure to high altitude. Am J Cardiol 1966;18:183.

39. Honigman B, et al. Acute mountain sickness in a general tourist population at moderate altitude. Ann Intern Med 1993;118:587.
40. Hoppeler H, Desplanches D. Muscle structural modifications in hypoxia. Int J Sports Med 1992;13:S166.
41. Hoppeler H, et al. II. Morphologic adaptations of human skeletal muscle to chronic hypoxia. Int J Sports Med 1990;11:53.
42. Hunt J, Hillary E. The conquest of Everest. New York: EP Dutton, 1954.
43. Hurtado A. Animals in high altitudes: resident man. In: Dill DB, et al., eds. Handbook of physiology. Baltimore: Williams & Wilkins, 1964.
44. Insalaco G, et al. Cardiovascular and ventilatory response to isocapnic hypoxia at sea level and at 5,050 m. J Appl Physiol 1996;80:1724.
45. Jansen GF, et al. Cerebral vasomotor reactivity at high altitude in humans. J Appl Physiol 1999;86:681.
46. Jensen K, et al. High-altitude training does not increase maximal oxygen uptake or work capacity at sea level in rowers. Scand J Sci Med Sports 1993;3:256.
47. Kayser B, et al. Maximal lactate capacity at altitude: effect of bicarbonate loading. J Appl Physiol 1993;75:1070.
48. Kayser B, et al. Fatigue and exhaustion in chronic hypobaric hypoxia: influence of exercising muscle mass. J Appl Physiol 1994;76:634.
49. Klausen K. Cardiac output in man in rest and work during and after acclimatization to 3800 m. J Appl Physiol 1969;21:609.
50. Klausen K. Exercise under hypoxic conditions. Med Sci Sports 1969;1:43.
51. Klausen K, et al. Effect of high altitude on maximal working capacity. J Appl Physiol 1966;21:1191.
52. Klausen K, et al. Exercise at ambient and high oxygen pressure at high altitude and at sea level. J Appl Physiol 1970;29:456.
53. Kollias J, Buskirk ER. Exercise at altitude. In: Johnson WR, Buskirk ER, eds. Science and medicine of exercise and sports. New York: Harper and Row, 1974.
54. Krasney JA. Brief review: a neurogenic basis for acute altitude sickness. Med Sci Sports Exerc 1994;26:195.
55. Lenfant CP, et al. Effect of chronic hypoxic hypoxia on the O_2-Hb dissociation curve and respiratory gas transport in man. Respir Physiol 1969;7:7.
56. Levine BD, et al. Altitude training does not improve running performance more than equivalent training near sea level in trained runners. Med Sci Sports Exerc 1992;24:769.
57. Levine BD, Stray-Gunderson J. "Living high–training low": effect of moderate-altitude acclimatization with low-altitude training on performance. J Appl Physiol 1997;83:102.
58. Liu Y, et al. Effect of "living high–training low" on the cardiac functions at sea level. Int J Sports Med 1998;19:380.
59. MacDougall JD, et al. Operation Everest II: structural adaptations in skeletal muscle in response to extreme simulated altitude. Acta Physiol Scand 1991;142:421.
60. Mairbaurl H. Red blood cell function in hypoxia at altitude and exercise. Int J Sports Med 1994;15:51.
61. Malconian MK, Rock PB. Medical problems related to altitude. In: Pandolf K, et al., eds. Human performance physiology and environmental medicine at terrestrial extremes. Carmel, IN: Cooper Publishing Group, 1994.
62. Manier G, et al. Pulmonary gas exchange in Andean natives with excessive polycythemia—effect of hemodilution. J Appl Physiol 1988;65:2107.
63. Maresch CM, et al. Maximal exercise during hypobaric hypoxia (447 torr) in moderate-altitude natives. Med Sci Sports Exerc 1983;15:360.
64. Mazzeo R, et al. β-Adrenergic blockade does not prevent the lactate response to exercise after acclimatization to high altitude. J Appl Physiol 1994;76:610.
65. Mazzeo RS, et al. Acclimatization to high altitude increases muscle sympathetic activity both at rest and during exercise. Am J Physiol 1995;269(Renal Fluid Electrolyte Physiol. 38):R201.
66. Mazzeo RS, et al. Catecholamine response during 12 days of high-altitude exposure (4,300 m) in women. J Appl Physiol 1998;84:1151.
67. Mazzeo RS, et al. Sympathoadrenal responses to submaximal exercise in women after acclimatization to 4,300 meters. Metabolism 2000;49:1036.
68. Mazzeo RS, et al. Catecholamine responses to alpha-adenergic blockade during exercise in women acutely exposed to altitude. J Appl Physiol 2001;90:121.
69. Melissa L, et al. Skeletal muscle adaptations to training under normobaric hypoxic versus normoxic conditions. Med Sci Sports Exerc 1997;29:238.
70. Mizuno M, et al. Limb skeletal muscle adaptation in athletes after training at altitude. J Appl Physiol 1990;68:496.
71. Mizuno M, et al. Limb skeletal muscle adaptation in athletes after training at altitude. J Appl Physiol 1990;68:496.
72. Ou LC, et al. Polycythemic responses to hypoxia: molecular and genetic mechanisms of chronic mountain sickness. J Appl Physiol 1998;1242.
73. Pugh LCGE. Muscular exercise on Mount Everest. J. Physiol (London) 1958;141:233.
74. Pugh LCGE. Physiological and medical aspects of the Himalayan Scientific and Mountaineering Expedition, 1960–61. Br Med J 1962;2:621.
75. Pugh LCGE. Animals in high altitudes: an above 5000 meters-mountain exploration. In: Dill DB, et al., eds. Handbook of physiology. Baltimore: Williams & Wilkins, 1964.
76. Pugh LCGE. Athletes at altitude. J Physiol (London) 1967;192:619.
77. Reeves JT. Operation Everest II; preservation of cardiac function at extreme altitude. J Appl Physiol 1987;63:531.
78. Reynafarje C. Myoglobin content and enzymatic activity of muscle and altitude adaptation. J Appl Physiol 1962;17:301.
79. Richalet JP. High altitude pulmonary oedema: still a place for controversy? Thorax 1995;50:923.
80. Roach RC, et al. Exercise exacerbates acute mountain sickness at stimulated high altitude. J Appl Physiol 2000;88:581.
81. Robergs RA, et al. Multiple variables explain the variability in the decrement in $\dot{V}O_{2max}$ during acute hypobaric hypoxia. Med Sci Sports Exerc 1998;30:869.
82. Rock PB, et al. Operation Everest II. Electrocardiography during maximal exercise at extreme altitude. Med Sci Sports Exerc 1986;18:S74.
83. Rodríguez FA, et al. Intermittent hypobaric hypoxia stimulates erythropoiesis and improves aerobic capacity. Med Sci Sports Exerc 1999;31:264.
84. Rose MS, et al. Operation Everest II: nutrition and body composition. J Appl Physiol 1988;65:2545.
85. Saito S, et al. Exercise-induced cerebral deoxygenation among untrained trekkers at moderate altitudes. Arch Environ Health 1999;54:271.
86. Saltin B, et al. Maximal oxygen uptake and cardiac output after 2 weeks at 4300 m. J Appl Physiol 1968;25:400.
87. Saltin B. Exercise and the environment: focus on altitude. Res Q Exerc Sport 1996;67:1.
88. Saltin B, et al. Morphology, enzyme activities and buffer capacity in leg muscles of Kenyan and Scandinavian runners. Scand J Med Sci Sports 1995;5:209.
89. Savard GK, et al. Cardiovascular response to exercise in humans following acclimatization to extreme altitude. Acta Physiol Scand 1995;154:199.
90. Sawka MN, et al. Blood volume: importance and adaptations to exercise training, environmental stresses, and trauma/sickness. Med Sci Sports Exerc 2000;32:332.
91. Schoene RB, et al. Relationship of hypoxic ventilatory response to exercise performance on Mount Everest. J Appl Physiol 1984;56:1478.
92. Schoene RB, et al. Operation Everest II: ventilatory adaptations during gradual decompression to extreme altitude. Med Sci Sports Exerc 1990;22:804.
93. Sharp C. Exercise at altitude. BR J Sports Med 2000;34:404.
94. Stenberg, J, et al. Hemodynamic response to work at simulated altitude, 4,000 m. J Appl Physiol 1966;21:1589.
95. Suarez JM, et al. Operation Everest II. Left ventricular systolic function in man at high altitude assessed by two dimensional echocardiography. Am J Cardiol 1987;60:137.
96. Surks MJ, et al. Changes in plasma thyroxine concentration and metabolism, catecholamine excretion and basal oxygen uptake during acute exposure to high altitude (14,100 ft). J Clin Invest 1966;45:1442.
97. Sutton JR. High altitude retinal hemorrhage. Semin Respir Med 1983;5:159.
98. Terrados N, et al. Effects of training at simulated altitude on performance and muscle metabolic capacity in competitive road cyclists. Eur J Appl Physiol 1988;57:203.
99. Terrados N, et al. Is hypoxia a stimulus for synthesis of oxidative enzymes and myoglobin? J Appl Physiol 1990;68:2369.
100. Valdivia E. Total capillary bed in striated muscle of guinea pigs native to Peruvian mountains. Am J Physiol 1958;194:585.
101. Westerterp-Plantenga MS, et al. Appetite at "high altitude" [Operate Everest III (Comex-'97)]: a simulated ascent on Mount Everest. J Appl Physiol 1999;87:391.

102. West JB. Do climbs to extreme altitudes cause brain damage? Lancet 1986;2:387.
103. West JB. High life: a history of high altitude physiology and medicine. New York: Oxford University Press, 1998.
104. West JB. Barometric pressure on Mt. Everest: new data and physiological significance. J Appl Physiol 1999;86:1062.
105. West JB. Invited review; pulmonary capillary stress failure. J Appl Physiol 2000;89:2483.
106. West JB, et al. Pulmonary gas exchange on the summit of Mount Everest. J Appl Physiol 1983;55:678.
107. Wolfel EE, et al. Systemic hypertension at 4,300 m is related to sympathoadrenal activity. J Appl Physiol 1994;76:1643.
108. Xu F, Severinghaus JW. Rat brain VEGF expression in alveolar hypoxia: a possible role in high-altitude cerebral edema. J Appl Physiol 1998;85:53.
109. Young AJ. Energy substrate utilization during exercise in extreme environments. Exerc Sport Sci Rev 1990;18:65.
110. Young AJ, Young PM. Human acclimatization to high terrestrial altitude. In: Pandolf KB, et al., eds. Human performance physiology and environmental medicine at terrestrial extremes. Indianapolis: Benchmark Press, 1988.

CHAPTER 25

Exercise and Thermal Stress

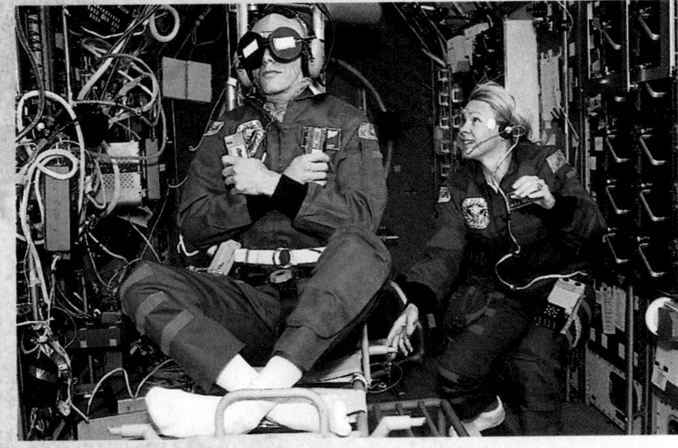

Chapter Objectives

- Discuss the role of the hypothalamus in maintaining thermal balance
- Explain the four physical factors that contribute to heat gain and heat loss
- Discuss how the circulatory system serves as a "workhorse" for thermoregulation
- List desirable clothing characteristics for exercising in cold and warm weather
- Indicate how (1) football equipment and (2) the cycling helmet affect heat dissipation and thermoregulation in exercise
- Discuss factors that maintain cutaneous and muscle blood flow and blood pressure during exercise in the heat
- Describe the responses of cardiac output, heart rate, and stroke volume during exercise in the heat versus exercise in a thermoneutral environment
- Graph the relationship between core temperature and exercise intensity expressed as a percentage of $\dot{V}O_{2max}$
- Quantify fluid loss during hot-weather exercise, and indicate the consequences of dehydration on physiology and performance
- Describe the purposes of fluid replacement and proposed benefits of (1) preexercise hyperhydration and (2) glycerol supplementation when exercising in a hot environment
- Discuss how acclimatization, training, age, gender, and body fat modify heat tolerance during exercise
- Give symptoms, possible causes, and treatment for heat cramps, heat exhaustion, and exertional heat stroke
- Describe factors that constitute the WB-GT index and the relative importance of each factor
- List six factors that reduce the insulation properties of clothing
- Summarize the American College of Sports Medicine WB-GT recommendations for endurance activities like running and cycling
- Discuss the immediate and possible longer-term physiologic adjustments to cold stress
- Indicate the purpose of the wind chill index and factors that comprise it

Humans can tolerate a drop in deep body temperature of 10°C but only an increase of 5°C. **Temperature** technically represents the mean kinetic energy of a substance's molecules. The potential for heat exchange between substances (e.g., blood to capillary walls) or objects (e.g., playing surface to participant's body) reflects a functional definition of this term. Over the past 20 years, more than 100 football players have died from excessive heat stress during practice or competition. Hyperthermia and dehydration also contributed to the deaths of three, apparently healthy collegiate wrestlers just before their 1997 competitive season.[165] Unfortunately, heat injury occurs commonly in a variety of longer-duration athletic events. A proper understanding of thermoregulation and the best ways to support these mechanisms should prevent such tragedies. A major part of this responsibility rests with the people who organize and guide athletic events and physical activity programs.[103,119]

➤ PART 1 • Mechanisms of Thermoregulation

THERMAL BALANCE

Figure 25.1 shows that body temperature or, more specifically, the temperature of the deeper tissues (**core**), represents a dynamic equilibrium between factors that add and subtract body heat. Integration of mechanisms that alter heat transfer to the periphery (**shell**) regulates evaporative cooling and varies the body's heat production to sustain thermal balance. Core temperature rises if heat gain exceeds heat loss, as readily occurs with vigorous exercise in a warm, humid environment; in contrast, core temperature falls in the cold, when heat loss exceeds heat production.

Table 25.1 presents thermal data for heat production and heat loss via sweating during rest and maximal exercise. The chemical reactions of energy metabolism produce body heat gains that can reach considerable levels during muscular activity. From shivering alone, whole body metabolism increases up to 3- to 5-fold.[69,163] Metabolism often rises 20 to 25 times above the resting level to about 20 kcal · min^{-1} during intense aerobic exercise by elite athletes; this theoretically can increase core temperature by 1°C (1.8°F) every 5 to 7 minutes. The body also absorbs heat from solar radiation and from objects warmer than the body. Heat leaves the body via the physical mechanisms of radiation, conduction, and convection, but most importantly by water vaporization from the skin and respiratory passages. Under optimal conditions, evaporative cooling with maximal sweating accounts for a heat loss of about 18 kcal · min^{-1}.

Circulatory adjustments provide the "fine tuning" for temperature regulation. Heat conservation occurs when blood shunts rapidly to the deep cranial, thoracic, and abdominal cavities and

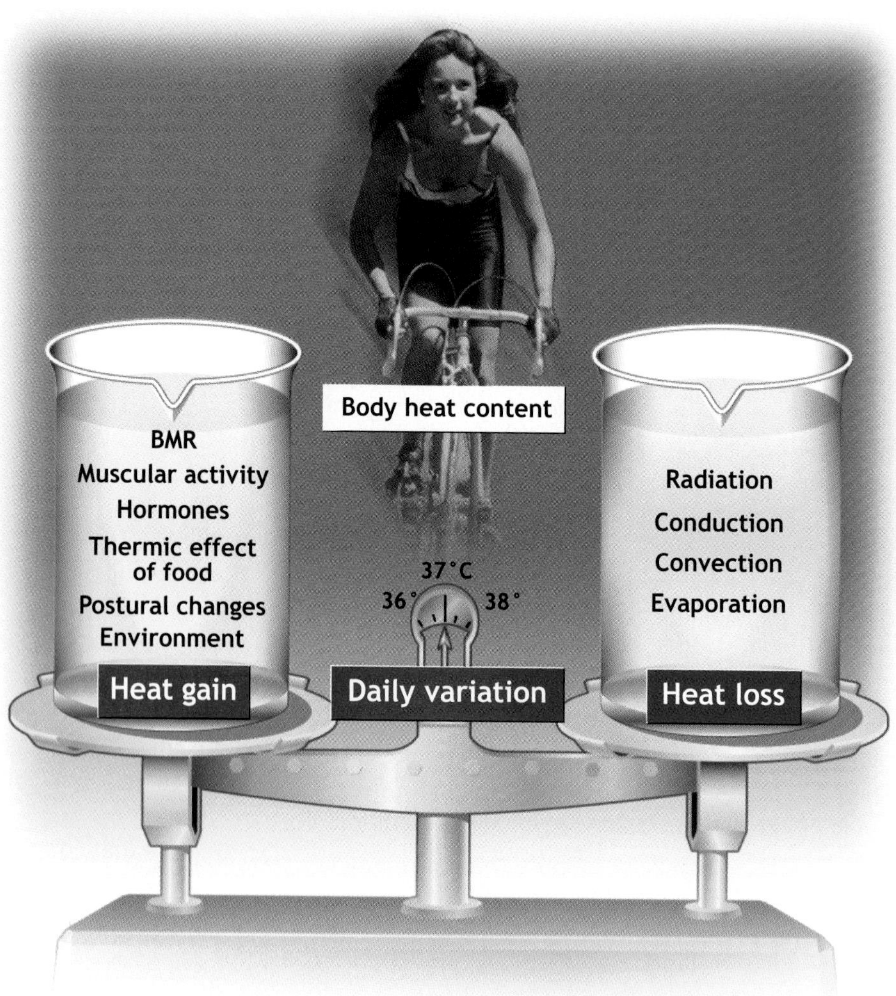

FIGURE 25.1 • Factors contributing to heat gain and heat loss to regulate core temperature at about 37°C.

TABLE 25.1 ➤ THERMODYNAMICS DURING REST AND EXERCISE

CONDITION	REST	MAXIMAL EXERCISE
Body's heat production 1 L O_2 consumption ~ 4.82 kcal	~0.25 L $O_2 \cdot min^{-1}$ ~1.2 kcal $\cdot min^{-1}$	~4.0 L $O_2 \cdot min^{-1}$ ~20.0 kcal $\cdot min^{-1}$
Body's capacity for evaporative cooling Each 1 mL sweat evaporation = ~ 0.6 kcal body heat loss	**Maximal sweating** ~30 mL $\cdot min^{-1}$ = 18 kcal $\cdot min^{-1}$	
Core temperature increase	No increase	~1°C every 5 to 7 minutes

portions of the muscle mass. This optimizes insulation from subcutaneous fat and other components of the body's shell. Conversely, when internal heat increases, peripheral vessels dilate and warm blood flows to the cooler periphery.[71] The drive to maintain thermal balance remains so strong that it readily triggers a sweat rate of 2.0 L $\cdot$ h^{-1} in exercise in the heat, or an oxygen consumption of 1200 mL $\cdot$ min^{-1} from shivering in severe cold.

HYPOTHALAMIC REGULATION OF TEMPERATURE

*The **hypothalamus** contains the central coordinating center for temperature regulation.* This group of specialized neurons at the floor of the brain acts as a "thermostat"—usually set and carefully regulated at 37°C ± 1°C—that continually makes thermoregulatory adjustments to deviations from a temperature norm. Unlike the home thermostat, however, the hypothalamus cannot "turn off" the heat; it can only initiate responses to protect the body from either a buildup or loss of heat.

Two ways activate the body's heat-regulating mechanisms:

1. Thermal receptors in the skin provide input to the central control center
2. Changes in blood temperature perfusing the hypothalamus directly stimulates this area

Figure 25.2 shows the diverse structures embedded within the skin and subcutaneous tissue. The *blowup* on the right depicts the dynamics of sweat evaporation from the skin surface.

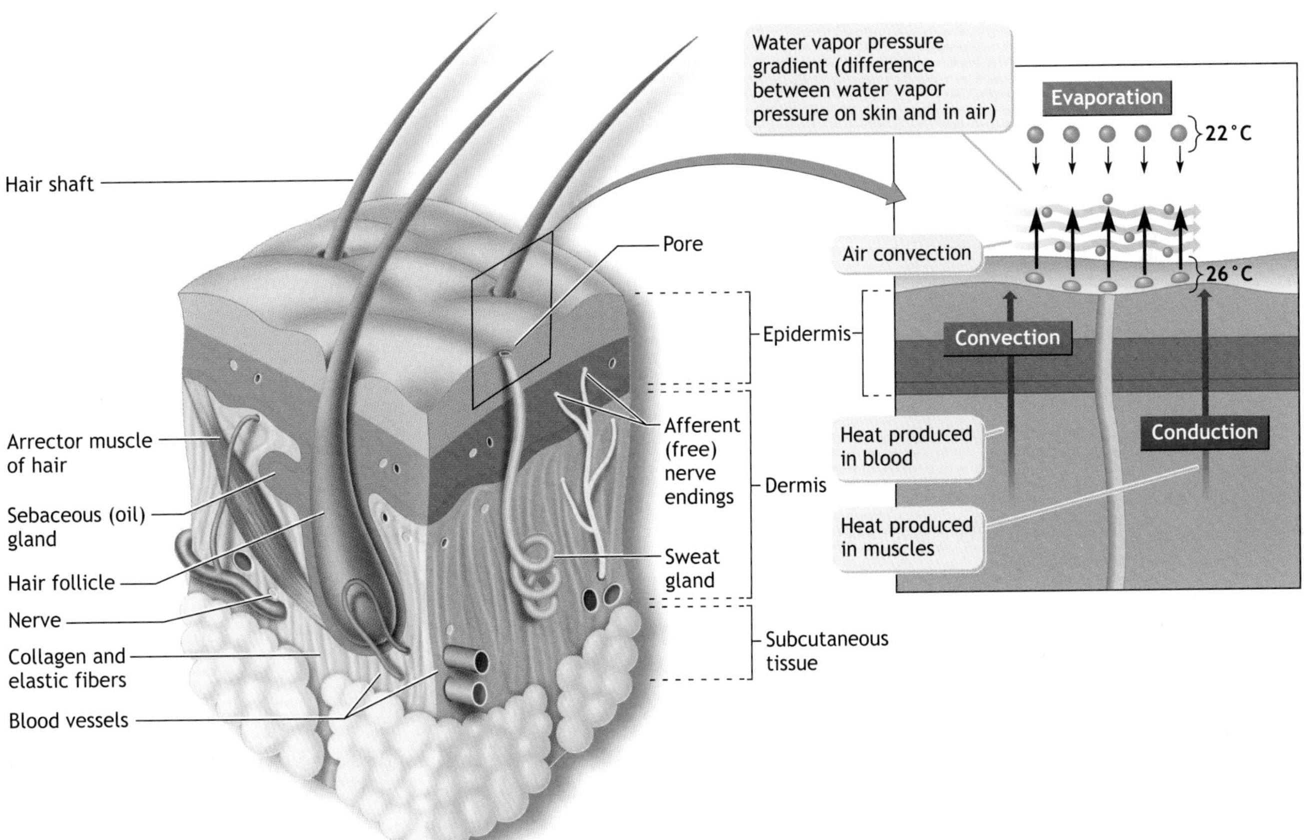

FIGURE 25.2 • Schematic illustration of the skin and underlying structures. The blowup of the skin surface shows the dynamics of conduction, convection, and sweat evaporation for heat dissipation from the body. Each 1 L of water evaporated from the skin transfers 580 kcal of heat energy to the environment.

Peripheral thermal receptors responsive to rapid changes in heat and cold exist predominantly as free nerve endings in the skin. The more-numerous cutaneous cold receptors generally exist near the skin surface. Cold receptors play an important role in initiating regulatory responses to a cold environment. The cutaneous thermal receptors act as an "early warning system" to relay sensory information to the hypothalamus and cortex. This direct input evokes appropriate heat-conserving or heat-dissipating physiologic adjustments, and the individual consciously seeks relief from a thermal challenge.

The central hypothalamic regulatory center plays the primary role in maintaining thermal balance. In addition to receiving peripheral input, cells in the anterior portion of the hypothalamus detect slight changes in blood temperature. Heightened activity of these cells stimulates other hypothalamic regions to initiate coordinated responses for heat conservation (posterior hypothalamus) or heat loss (anterior hypothalamus). In contrast to the importance of peripheral receptors in detecting cold, the temperature of the blood perfusing the hypothalamus provides the primary means to monitor body warmth.

THERMOREGULATION IN COLD STRESS: HEAT CONSERVATION AND HEAT PRODUCTION

The normal heat transfer gradient flows from the body to the environment, and generally core temperature regulation involves no physiologic strain. However, excessive heat loss can occur in extreme cold, particularly at rest. In this case, the body's heat production increases while heat loss slows to minimize any decline in core temperature.

Vascular Adjustments

Stimulation of cutaneous cold receptors constricts peripheral blood vessels, which immediately reduces the flow of warm blood to the body's cooler surface and redirects it to the warmer core. For example, cutaneous blood flow averages 250 $mL \cdot min^{-1}$ in a thermoneutral environment, yet with severe cold stress this flow approaches zero.[72] Consequently, skin temperature declines toward ambient temperature, maximizing the insulatory benefits of skin, muscle, and subcutaneous fat. A person with excessive body fat exposed to cold stress greatly benefits from this heat-conserving mechanism.[157] For a thinly clad person with a normal body fat content, cutaneous blood flow regulation generally provides effective thermoregulation at ambient temperatures between 25 and 29°C (77 to 84°F).

Muscular Activity

Shivering generates significant metabolic heat, but physical activity provides the greatest contribution in defending against cold. Exercise energy metabolism sustains a constant core temperature in air as cold as −30°C (−22°F) without reliance on a heavy, restrictive clothing barrier. Internal temperature, not the body's heat production per se, mediates the thermoregulatory response to cold.[115] Shivering still occurs during vigorous exercise if the core temperature remains low. As a result, cold stress often induces higher exercise oxygen consumption from shivering than occurs performing the same exercise in a warmer environment.

When exercise metabolism decreases (e.g., from fatigue), shivering alone may not prevent a decline in core temperature.[163] To some extent, the variability among individuals in shivering response likely dictates the diverse outcomes for those caught unprepared for accidental wet–cold exposures. General muscle fatigue induced by prior heavy exercise does not appear to blunt the shivering response.[161]

Hormonal Output

Increased heat production during cold exposure results partly from action of the two "calorigenic" adrenal medulla hormones epinephrine and norepinephrine. Prolonged cold stress probably also stimulates release of thyroxine, the thyroid hormone that initiates increased resting metabolism.

THERMOREGULATION IN HEAT STRESS: HEAT LOSS

The body's thermoregulatory mechanisms primarily protect against overheating.[96,144] Dissipating heat efficiently becomes crucial during exercise in hot weather when inherent competition exists between (1) mechanisms that maintain a large muscle blood flow and (2) thermoregulatory mechanisms. Figure 25.3 illustrates the potential avenues for heat exchange during exercise. Body heat loss occurs by four physical processes—**radiation**, **conduction**, **convection**, and **evaporation**.

Heat Loss By Radiation

Objects continually emit electromagnetic heat waves. Because our bodies usually remain warmer than the environment, the net exchange of radiant heat energy moves through the air to solid, cooler objects in the environment. This form of heat transfer does not require molecular contact between objects; it provides the means for the sun's warming effect on the earth. A person can remain warm by absorbing radiant heat energy from direct sunlight or by reflection from snow, sand, or water, even in subfreezing air temperatures. The body absorbs radiant heat energy from the surroundings when an object's temperature exceeds skin temperature, making evaporative cooling the only avenue for heat loss.

Heat Loss By Conduction

Heat exchange by conduction involves direct heat transfer from one molecule to another through a liquid, solid, or gas. The circulation transports most of the body heat to the shell, but a small amount continually moves by conduction directly through the deep tissues to the cooler surface. Heat loss by conduction then involves warming air molecules and cooler surfaces that contact the skin.

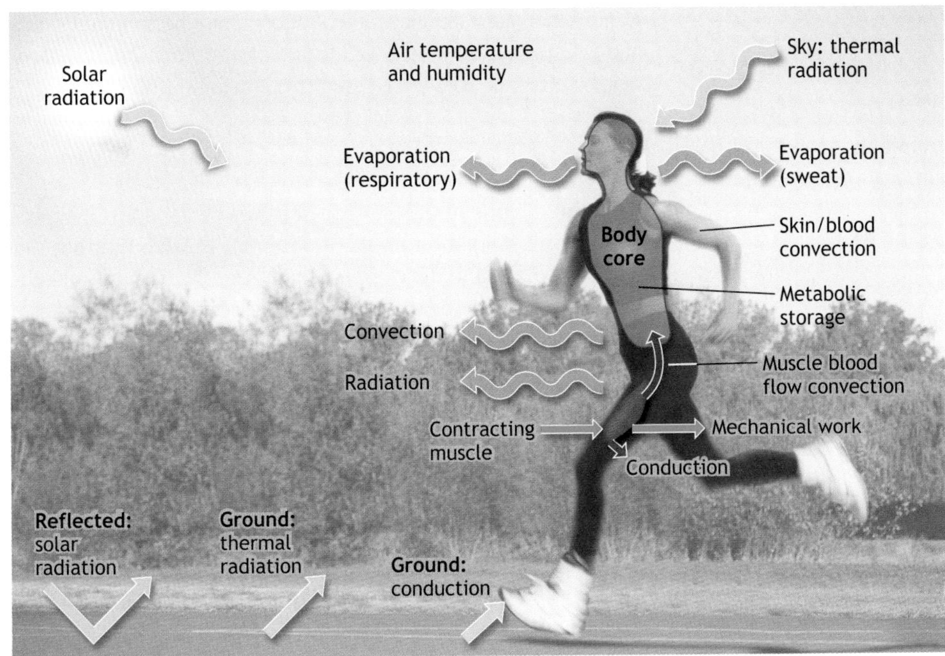

FIGURE 25.3 • Heat production within active muscle and its transfer from the core to the skin. Under appropriate environmental conditions, excess body heat dissipates to the environment, regulating core temperature within a narrow range. (From Gisolfi CV, Wenger CB. Temperature regulation during exercise: old concepts, new ideas. Exerc Sport Sci Rev 1984;12:339.)

The rate of conductive heat loss depends on two factors: (1) the temperature gradient between the skin and surrounding surfaces and (2) their thermal qualities. For example, immersing the body in water can produce considerable heat loss. Placing one hand in room-temperature water clearly illustrates this phenomenon. Why does the hand in water feel much colder than the hand in air, even though the water and air have identical temperatures? The answer is straightforward: water absorbs several thousand times more heat than air and conducts it away from the warmer body part. Sitting in an indoor swimming pool with water at 83°F provides more discomfort than sitting on the pool deck at the same temperature. Warm-weather hikers often gain considerable body heat when exercising in a warm environment. Lying on a rock shielded from the sun facilitates some body heat loss by conductance between the rock's cool surface and the hiker's warmer surface.

Heat Loss By Convection

The effectiveness of heat loss by conduction depends on how rapidly the air (or water) adjacent to the body exchanges once it warms. If air movement or convection proceeds slowly, the air next to the skin warms and acts as a "zone of insulation" that minimizes further conductive heat loss. Conversely, if cooler air continually replaces warmer air about the body on a breezy day, in a room with a fan, or when running, heat loss increases because convection continually replaces the zone of insulation. For example, air currents at 4 miles per hour are about twice as effective for body cooling as air currents at 1 mile per hour. The cooling effect of airflow forms the basis of the wind chill index (see p. 649), which indicates the equivalent still-air temperature for a particular ambient temperature at different wind velocities. Convection also exerts an important effect on thermal balance in water because the body loses heat more rapidly swimming than remaining motionless.

Heat Loss By Evaporation

Evaporation provides the major defense against overheating. Water vaporizing from the respiratory passages and skin surface continually transfers heat to the environment. Each liter of water that vaporizes extracts 580 kcal from the body and transfers it to the environment.

The body's surface contains approximately 2 to 4 million sweat glands. During heat stress, these eccrine glands—controlled by cholinergic sympathetic nerve fibers—secrete large quantities of hypotonic saline solution (0.2 to 0.4% NaCl). Evaporation of sweat from the skin exerts a cooling effect. The cooled skin in turn cools the blood diverted from interior tissues to the surface. In addition to heat loss through sweat evaporation, about 350 mL of insensible perspiration seeps through the skin each day and evaporates to the environment. Also, about 300 mL of water vaporizes daily from the moist mucous membranes of the respiratory passages. This is seen as "foggy breath" in cold weather.

Evaporative Heat Loss at High Ambient Temperatures

As ambient temperature increases, conduction, convection, and radiation decrease in their effectiveness for facilitating body heat loss. When ambient temperature exceeds body temperature, the body actually gains heat by these three thermal transfer mechanisms. In such environments (or when conduction, convection, and radiation become inadequate to dissipate a large metabolic heat load), sweat evaporation from the skin and respiratory tract provide the *only* means for heat dissipation. Generally, increases in ambient temperature induce proportionate increases in sweating rate.

Heat Loss in High Humidity

Three factors influence the total amount of sweat vaporized from the skin and/or pulmonary surfaces:

1. Surface exposed to the environment
2. Temperature and relative humidity of the ambient air
3. Convective air currents about the body

***Relative humidity** represents the most important factor determining the effectiveness of evaporative heat loss.* Relative humidity refers to the ratio of the water in ambient air at a particular temperature to the total quantity of moisture that air could contain, expressed as a percentage. For example, 40% relative humidity means that ambient air contains only 40% of the air's moisture-carrying capacity at the specific temperature. With high humidity, the ambient vapor pressure approaches that of the moist skin (about 40 mm Hg), and evaporation greatly diminishes, even though large quantities of sweat bead on the skin and eventually roll off. This form of sweating represents useless water loss that can produce dehydration and overheating. A dangerous rise in core temperature can occur in athletes who compete in moderate to high-intensity sports lasting 30 minutes or longer in environments that exceed 35°C and 60% relative humidity. "In a Practical Sense" describes how to assess the heat quality of the environment and gives recommendations concerning physical activity in relation to ambient temperature, radiant heat, and relative humidity.

Continually drying the skin while sweating also thwarts evaporative cooling. *Sweat per se does not cool the skin; evaporation cools the skin.* Individuals can tolerate relatively high environmental temperatures provided relative humidity remains low. Most people find hot, dry desert climates more comfortable than cooler but more humid tropical climates.

INTEGRATIVE QUESTION

In deciding on the starting time for an upcoming summer marathon, indicate what past meteorological information would be most valuable and why.

Integration of Heat-Dissipating Mechanisms

The mechanisms for heat loss remain the same whether the heat load originates internally (metabolic heat) or externally (environmental heat).

Circulation

The circulatory system represents the "workhorse" for maintaining thermal balance (see "Focus on Research, page 635). At rest in the heat, heart rate and cardiac output increase while superficial arterial and venous blood vessels dilate to divert warm blood to the body shell. This manifests itself as a flushed or reddened face on a hot day or during vigorous exercise. With extreme heat stress, 15 to 25% of the cardiac output passes through the skin. Enhanced cutaneous blood flow greatly increases the thermal conductance of peripheral tissues and favors radiative heat loss to the environment, particularly from the hands, forehead, forearms, ears, and tibial areas.

Evaporation

Sweating begins within several seconds of the start of vigorous exercise and, after about 30 minutes, reaches equilibrium in direct relation to the exercise load. An effective thermal defense exists when evaporative cooling combines with a large cutaneous blood flow. The cooled peripheral blood then flows to the deeper tissues to absorb additional heat on its return to the heart.

Hormonal Adjustments

Because sweating produces loss of water and electrolytes, heat stress initiates hormonal adjustments to conserve salts and fluid.[31] Fluid conservation makes urine more concentrated during heat stress. Concurrently, repeated days of exercise in the heat or just a single exercise bout stimulates adrenocortical release of the sodium-conserving hormone **aldosterone**, which acts on the renal tubules to increase sodium reabsorption. Aldosterone also reduces sweat's osmolality. Thus, sweat sodium concentration decreases during repeated heat exposure to further conserve electrolytes. At the same time, exercise and/or hypohydration stimulates **vasopressin** (also called *antidiuretic hormone*) release from the neurohypophysis of the hypothalamus. Vasopressin increases the permeability of the collecting tubules of the kidneys to facilitate fluid retention. The magnitude of aldosterone and vasopressin release depends on hypohydration severity and physical activity intensity.[110]

EFFECTS OF CLOTHING ON THERMOREGULATION

Clothing insulates the body from its surroundings. It can reduce radiant heat gain in a hot environment or retard conductive and convective heat loss in the cold.

Clothing Insulation (clo units)

Research by the military has established standards for the insulatory properties of clothing to meet environmental challenges. The **clo unit** is an index of thermal resistance. It indicates the insulatory capacity provided by any layer of trapped air between the skin and clothing, including the clothing's insulation value. Assuming an environment with negligable air movement and body movement to disturb the insulatory layer of air about the body, a clo unit of 1 maintains a sedentary person at 1 MET (a unit of resting metabolism) indefinitely in an environment of 21°C (68.8°F), and 50% relative humidity.

An individual's metabolic rate at a given environmental temperature also affects the clo unit requirement. Data in the inset table on page 630 show six conditions of metabolic intensity from sleeping to heavy work (expressed in MET units) and three environmental temperatures (0°C, −20°C, −50°C). Note that

In a Practical Sense

►►Assessing Heat Quality of the Environment: How Hot Is Too Hot?

A variety of factors determine the physiologic strain imposed by environmental heat. These include:

- Air temperature and relative humidity
- Individual differences in body size and fatness
- State of training
- Degree of acclimatization
- Environmental influences such as convective air currents and radiant heat gain
- Exercise intensity
- Amount, type, and color of clothing

Several football deaths from heat injury occurred with air temperature below 75°F (23.9°C), but with relative humidity above 95%. *Prevention is the most effective control of heat stress injuries.*[38] Most importantly, acclimatization greatly reduces the likelihood of heat injury. Another consideration requires evaluating the environment for its potential thermal challenge using the **wet bulb–globe temperature (WB-GT)** index. This index of environmental heat stress, developed by the military, provides important information to the National Collegiate Athletic Association to establish thresholds for (1) increased risk of heat injury and (2) exercise performance decrements.[103] The WB-GT index depends on ambient temperature, relative humidity, and radiant heat as related in the following equation:

$$\text{WB-GT} = 0.1 \times \text{DBT} + 0.7 \times \text{WBT} + 0.2 \times \text{GT}$$

where DBT represents the dry-bulb temperature (air temperature) recorded by an ordinary mercury thermometer, and WBT equals the wet-bulb temperature recorded by a similar thermometer except that a wet wick surrounds the mercury bulb (Fig. 1). With high relative humidity, little evaporative cooling occurs from the wetted bulb, so this thermometer's temperature remains similar to that of the dry-bulb. On a dry day, however, significant evaporation occurs from the wetted bulb, which maximizes the difference between the two thermometer readings. A small difference between thermometer readings indicates high relative humidity, whereas a large difference indicates little air moisture and rapid evaporation. GT represents the globe temperature recorded by a thermometer with a black metal sphere enclosing its bulb. The black globe absorbs radiant energy from the surroundings to measure this source of heat gain. Most industrial supply companies sell this relatively inexpensive thermometer.

The *top* portion of the inset table in Figure 1 presents WB-GT guidelines to reduce the chance of heat injury in athletic activities. These standards apply to lightly clothed humans but do *not* consider the specific heat

WB-GT Range °F	°C	Recommendations
80-84	26.5-28.8	• Use discretion, especially if unconditioned or unacclimatized
85-87	29.5-30.5	• Avoid strenuous activity in the sun
> 88	> 31.2	• Avoid exercise training

WBT Range °F	°C	Recommendations
60	15.5	• No prevention necessary
61-65	16.2-18.4	• Alert all participants to problems of heat stress and importance of adequate hydration
66-70	18.8-21.1	• Insist that appropriate quantity of fluid be ingested
71-75	21.6-23.8	• Rest periods and water breaks every 20 to 30 minutes; limits placed on intense activity
76-79	24.5 26.1	• Practice curtailed and modified considerably
> 80	> 26.5	• Practice cancelled

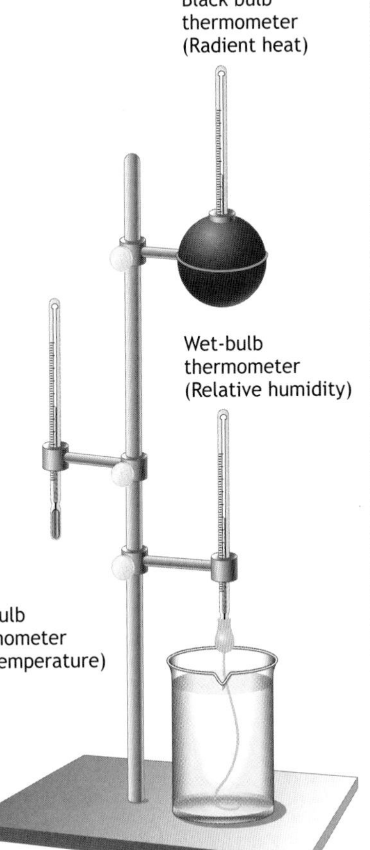

Figure 1. Apparatus to measure wet bulb–globe temperature (WB-GT). *Inset table.* Guidelines to reduce risk of heat injury for outdoor athletic activities by use of the WB-GT and wet-bulb temperature (WBT). (Modified from Murphy RJ, Ashe WF. Prevention of heat illness in football players. JAMA 1965;194:650.)

IN A PRACTICAL SENSE

➤➤ASSESSING HEAT QUALITY OF THE ENVIRONMENT: HOW HOT IS TOO HOT?—CONT'D

load imposed by uniforms or equipment. For American football, the lower end of each temperature range serves as the more prudent guide. One can also assess ambient heat load from the wet-bulb thermometer (WBT) because this reading reflects both air temperature and relative humidity. The *bottom* portion of the inset table presents heat stress recommendations based on the WBT.

The American College of Sports Medicine proposes the following recommendations concerning risk for heat injury with continuous exercise based on the WB-GT:

AMERICAN COLLEGE OF SPORTS MEDICINE WB-GT RECOMMENDATIONS FOR CONTINUOUS ACTIVITIES SUCH AS ENDURANCE RUNNING AND CYCLING[3]

- *Very high risk*: Above 28°C (82°F)—postpone race
- *High risk*: 23 to 28°C (73–82°F)—heat-sensitive individuals (e.g., obese, low physical fitness, unacclimatized, dehydrated, previous history of heat injury) should not compete
- *Moderate risk*: 18 to 23°C (65–73°F)
- *Low risk*: Below 18°C (65°F)

Without the WBT, but knowing relative humidity (local meteorologic stations or media reports), the **heat-stress index** (Fig. 2) also evaluates the relative heat stress. The index should rely on data close to the actual race site to eliminate potential error from meteorologic data some distance from the event. Data collected on the 24-hour trend for ambient temperature and relative humidity justified the change in race time for the 1996 Olympic marathon run in Atlanta from 6:30 PM to 7:00 AM to reduce heat injury risk.

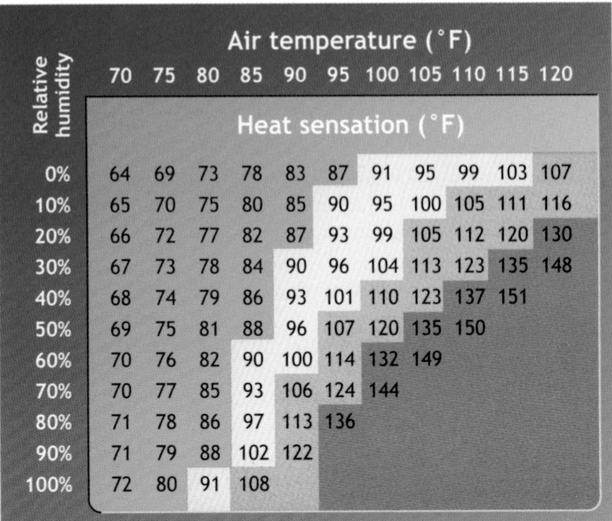

Air temperature (°F) / Heat sensation (°F)

Relative humidity	70	75	80	85	90	95	100	105	110	115	120
0%	64	69	73	78	83	87	91	95	99	103	107
10%	65	70	75	80	85	90	95	100	105	111	116
20%	66	72	77	82	87	93	99	105	112	120	130
30%	67	73	78	84	90	96	104	113	123	135	148
40%	68	74	79	86	93	101	110	123	137	151	
50%	69	75	81	88	96	107	120	135	150		
60%	70	76	82	90	100	114	132	149			
70%	70	77	85	93	106	124	144				
80%	71	78	86	97	113	136					
90%	71	79	88	102	122						
100%	72	80	91	108							

90°–105°F	Possibility of heat cramps
105°–130°F	Heat cramps or heat exhaustion likely, heat stroke possible
130°+	Heat stroke a definite risk

Figure 2. The heat-stress index.

for each activity condition, the clo unit requirement increases almost proportionally from sleeping to heavy work at the three extremes of temperature. Stated somewhat differently, a close inverse relationship exists between metabolic intensity and the insulation required (more clothing required for less work). At rest (1 MET) at 0°C, the clo requirement is 5.4, but when temperature drops to −50°C, the clo requirement increases by 130% to 12.4.

CLO VALUES REQUIRED TO MAINTAIN CORE TEMPERATURE RELATED TO PHYSICAL ACTIVITY LEVEL AND AMBIENT TEMPERATURE

ACTIVITY	TEMPERATURE, °C		
	0	−20	−50
Heavy work, 6.0 METs	1.0	1.6	2.2
Moderate work, 3.0 METs	1.6	2.8	4.2
Light work, 2.0 METs	2.6	4.0	6.2
Very light work, 1.5 METs	3.4	5.6	8.2
Rest, 1.0 MET	5.4	8.3	12.4
Sleep, 0.8 METs	6.7	10.6	15.5

Six factors affect the insulation (clo) value of clothing:

1. *Wind speed*—increased speed disturbs the zone of insulation
2. *Body movements*—pumping actions of arms and legs disturb the zone of insulation
3. *Chimney effect*—loosely hanging clothing ventilates the trapped air layers away from body
4. *Bellows effect*—vigorous body movements increase ventilation of air layers for conserving body heat
5. *Water vapor transfer*—clothing resists the passage of water vapor and thus decreases body heat loss by evaporative cooling
6. *Permeation efficiency factor*—how well clothing absorbs liquid sweat by capillary action (wicking); wicking sweat away from the body surface reduces the cooling effect of evaporation, thus improving clothing's effectiveness for conserving body heat

Table 25.2 presents clo values for common garments. To determine the total insulatory value of what a person wears, add the individual clo values for each garment. Without wind penetration or air movement around the clothing, the clo

TABLE 25.2 ➤ CLO VALUES FOR SOME COMMON GARMENTS[a]

Garment Description	Clo	Garment Description	Clo
Underwear, pants		**Jacket**	
Pantyhose	0.02	Vest	0.13
Panties	0.03	Light summer jacket	0.25
Briefs	0.04	Jacket	0.35
Pants, long legs	0.1	**Coats, jacket, and overtrousers**	
Underwear, shirts		Coat	0.6
Bra	0.01	Down jacket	0.55
Shirt, sleeveless	0.06	Parka	0.7
T-shirt	0.09	**Accessories**	
Shirt with long sleeves	0.12	Socks	0.02
Half-slip, nylon	0.14	Thick, ankle socks	0.05
Shirts		Thick, long socks	0.1
Tube top	0.06	Slippers, quilted fleece	0.03
Short sleeve	0.09	Shoes (thin soled)	0.02
Light-weight blouse, long sleeves	0.15	Shoes (thick soled)	0.04
Light-weight blouse, long sleeves	0.20	Boots, gloves	0.05
Normal, long sleeves	0.25	**Skirts, dresses**	
Flannel shirt, long sleeves	0.3	Light skirt, 15 cm above knee	0.10
Trousers		Light skirt, 15 cm below knee	0.18
Shorts	0.06	Heavy skirt, knee-length	0.25
Walking shorts	0.11	Light dress, sleeveless	0.25
Light-weight trousers	0.20	Winter dress, long sleeves	0.4
Normal trousers	0.25	**Sleepwear**	
Flannel trousers	0.28	Long-sleeve, long gown	0.3
Overalls	0.28	Thin-strap, short gown	0.15
Sweaters		Hospital gown	0.31
Sleeveless vest	0.12	Long-sleeve, long pajamas	0.50
Thin sweater	0.2	**Robes**	
Long sleeves, turtleneck (thin)	0.26	Long-sleeve, wrap, long	0.53
Sweater	0.28	Long-sleeve, wrap, short	0.41
Thick sweater	0.35	**Coveralls**	
Long sleeves, turtleneck (thick)	0.37	Daily wear, belted, work	0.49
		Highly insulating multicomponent, filling coveralls	1.03
		Fibre-pelt	1.13

[a]Higher numbers indicate greater insulatory capacity.

value for a given weight of clothes equals 0.15 times clothing weight in pounds. For example, wearing 10 pounds of clothes produces a clo value of 1.5 (0.15 × 10 lb).

Cold-Weather Clothing

In providing insulation from the cold, the mesh of the cloth fibers traps air that then becomes warm. This establishes a barrier to heat loss, because both the cloth and air conduct heat poorly; insulation becomes more effective with a thicker zone of trapped air above the skin. For this reason, several layers of light clothing, or garments lined with animal fur, feathers, or synthetic fabrics (with numerous layers of trapped air) provide better insulation than a single bulky layer. The clothing layer against the skin should also effectively wick moisture away from the body's surface to the next insulating clothing layer for subsequent evaporation. Wool or synthetics (e.g., polypropylene) that insulate well and dry quickly serve this purpose. A wool cap contributes considerably to heat conservation; nearly 30 to 40% of body heat dissipates through the highly vascularized head region that represents only about 8% of the body's total surface area. Conversely, cooling the head during exercise in hot weather reduces symptoms of thermal discomfort. When clothing becomes wet, through either external moisture or condensation from sweating, it loses almost 90% of its insulating properties. This actually facilitates heat loss from the body, because water conducts heat 25 times faster than air.

The thermoregulatory challenge when exercising in cold air arises not from inadequate insulation, but rather from metabolic heat dissipation through a thick air–clothing barrier. Cross-country skiers alleviate this problem by removing layers of clothing as the body warms. This maintains core temperature without reliance on evaporative cooling. *The ideal winter garment in cold, dry weather blocks air movement but allows water vapor to escape through the clothing if sweating occurs.*

Warm-Weather Clothing

Dry clothing, no matter how lightweight, retards heat exchange more than the same clothing fully wet. Switching to a dry tennis, basketball, or football uniform in hot weather makes little sense for temperature regulation. Evaporative heat loss occurs only when the clothing becomes wet throughout. A dry uniform simply prolongs the time lag between sweating and evaporative cooling.

Different materials absorb water at different rates. Cottons and linens readily absorb moisture. In contrast, heavy sweatshirts and rubber or plastic clothing produce high relative humidity close to the skin, retarding vaporization of moisture from its surface; this significantly blunts or even prevents evaporative cooling. Warm-weather clothing should fit loosely to permit free circulation of air between the skin and environment to promote convection and evaporation from the skin. Color also exerts an influence; dark colors absorb light rays and add to radiant heat gain, whereas lighter color clothing reflects heat rays.

Football Uniforms

Of all athletic uniforms and equipment, football gear presents the most significant barrier to heat dissipation. Even with loose-fitting porous jerseys, the wrappings, padding (with its plastic covering), helmet, and other objects of "armor" effectively seal off 50% of the body's surface from the benefits of evaporative cooling. The 6 or 7 kg of equipment, frequently transported over a relatively hot artificial playing surface, also adds significantly to the total metabolic load. The large size of many of these athletes further magnifies heat stress, particularly for offensive and defensive linemen with their relatively small surface area mass:body ratio and a higher body fat percentage than smaller teammates at the other positions.[167]

Figure 25.4 shows the metabolic and thermal stress provided by the football uniform.[91] The experiment tested nine men running for 30 minutes at 25.6°C (78°F) and 35% relative humidity. In one test, the men wore only shorts; in another, they wore the complete football uniform including helmet and plastic padding. In a third series, they wore shorts and carried a backpack containing 6.2 kg, the exact weight of the uniform and equipment.

Wearing football gear while exercising produced significantly higher rectal and skin temperatures during exercise and recovery than the other exercise conditions. Skin temperature directly beneath the padding averaged only 1°C less than rectal temperature. This indicates that subcutaneous blood in these areas cooled by only about one-fifth as much as blood near the skin surface directly exposed to the environment. Because rectal temperature remained elevated in recovery with uniforms, a rest period offers limited value in normalizing thermal status unless the athlete removes the uniform. The dark green line shows that the weight of the uniform accounts for a large portion of the heat load. Not wearing the uniform

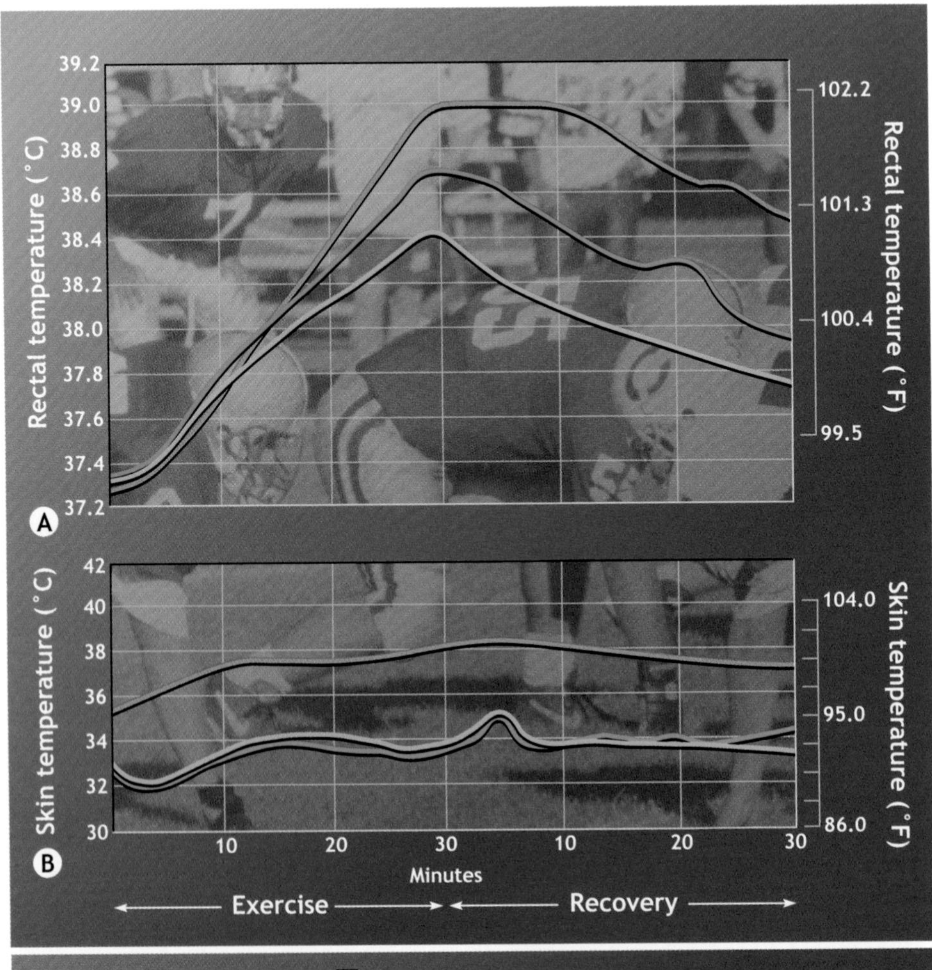

FIGURE 25.4 • Effects of full football uniform and its equivalent weight on (**A**) rectal temperature, and (**B**) skin temperature during exercise. Subjects ran at 9.6 km · h^{-1} for 30 minutes at 25.6°C and 35% relative humidity. The uniform caused the largest heat stress, because of its effect in retarding evaporative cooling. This significantly elevated rectal and skin temperatures. (From Mathews DK, et al. Physiological responses during exercise and recovery in a football uniform. J Appl Physiol 1969;26:611.)

(light green line) produced cooler skin temperatures and lower sweat rates. Without the uniform, evaporation from the skin progressed freely, whereas the uniform insulated the athlete and reduced the effective evaporative surface.

The Modern Cycling Helmet Does Not Thwart Heat Dissipation

Wearing a commercially available cycling helmet provides vital protection against possible head trauma, but does the helmet impede thermoregulatory processes in a hot–dry or hot–humid environment? Because the head provides a significant avenue for heat loss during exercise-induced hyperthermia,[126] many competitive cyclists believe riding without a helmet reduces thermal strain and physical discomfort. This belief persists even though the design of the current commercial protective helmet retains aerodynamic and lightweight features, with ventilation ports for convective and evaporative cooling. To evaluate physiologic and perceptual responses of wearing a helmet, 10 male and 4 female competitive cyclists pedaled for 90 minutes at 60% of $\dot{V}O_{2peak}$ in both hot–dry (35°C, 20% relative humidity) and hot–humid (35°C, 70% relative humidity) environments, with and without a protective helmet.[148] The results for oxygen consumption, heart rate, core, skin, and head skin temperatures, rating of perceived exertion, and perceived thermal sensations of the head and body showed that exercising in a hot–humid environment produced significantly greater thermal stress than exercising under thermoneutral conditions. Wearing the helmet, however, did *not* increase the riders' heat strain or perceived heat sensation from the head or body.

Summary

1. Humans tolerate only relatively small variations in internal (core) temperature. Exposure to heat or cold stress initiates thermoregulatory mechanisms that generate and conserve heat at low ambient temperatures and dissipate heat at high temperatures.
2. The "thermostat" for temperature regulation resides in the brain's hypothalamus. This coordinating center initiates adjustments in response to input from thermal receptors in the skin and changes in the temperature of blood perfusing the hypothalamic region.
3. Heat conservation in cold stress results from vascular adjustments that shunt blood from the cooler periphery to the warmer deep tissues of the body's core. If this mechanism proves ineffective, shivering provides a significant input of metabolic heat. Prolonged cold stress stimulates release of hormones that elevate resting metabolism.
4. Heat stress diverts warm blood from the body's core to the shell. Four factors—radiation, conduction, convection, and evaporation—contribute to heat dissipation. Evaporation provides the major physiologic defense against overheating at high ambient temperatures and during exercise.
5. The effectiveness of evaporative heat loss diminishes dramatically in warm, humid environments, making a person particularly vulnerable to dehydration and spiraling core temperature.
6. Practical heat-stress indices (e.g., wet bulb–globe temperature index, heat-stress index) use combinations of ambient temperature, radiant heat, and relative humidity to evaluate the environment's potential heat challenge.
7. Three factors influence sweat vaporization from the skin or pulmonary surfaces: surface exposure, ambient air temperature and relative humidity, and convective air currents.
8. Vigorous exercise generates significant metabolic heat to help maintain core temperature in cold air environments, even if the person wears little clothing.
9. The clo index reflects thermal resistance from clothing—the insulatory capacity of air trapped between skin and clothing including the clothing's insulation value. A clo value of 1.0 maintains a person in thermal balance indefinitely at 1 MET at 68.8°F, and 50% relative humidity in still air.
10. In the cold, wearing several layers of light clothing traps a zone of air against the skin, which provides more effective insulation from cold than a single thick layer of clothing. Wet clothing loses its insulating properties, greatly facilitating heat flow from the body.
11. Ideal warm-weather clothing is lightweight, loose fitting, and light colored. Even with these characteristics, heat loss slows until the clothing becomes wet and allows for evaporative cooling.
12. Football uniforms impose a significant barrier to heat dissipation because they effectively shield about 50% of the body's surface from the benefits of evaporative cooling.

➤ PART 2 • Thermoregulation and Environmental Stress During Exercise

EXERCISE IN THE HEAT

The refrigerating mechanism of evaporative cooling dissipates metabolic heat during exercise, particularly in hot weather. This places a demand on the body's fluid reserves and often produces relative hypohydration. Excessive sweating leads to more serious fluid loss and a reduced plasma volume. This causes circulatory failure in the extreme, and core temperature rises to lethal levels.

Circulatory Adjustments

The body faces two competitive cardiovascular demands when exercising in the heat:

1. The muscles require delivery of arterial blood (oxygen) to sustain energy metabolism.
2. Arterial blood must divert to the periphery to transport metabolic heat for cooling at the skin surface; this blood cannot deliver its oxygen to the active muscles.

Submaximal exercise produces similar cardiac outputs in hot and cold environments.[137] However, the heart's stroke volume usually remains lower in the heat in proportion to the fluid deficit created in exercise.[109] The reduced stroke volume closely associates with a reduction in blood volume.[52] This translates to *higher heart rates* at all submaximal levels of exercise in the heat. In contrast, the reflex compensatory increase in heart rate in maximal exercise cannot offset the stroke volume decrease, so maximal cardiac output decreases.

Vascular Constriction and Dilation

Maintaining adequate cutaneous and muscle blood flow during exercise under heat stress requires that other tissues temporarily compromise their blood supply. For example, during environmental heat stress compensatory constriction of the splanchnic vascular bed and renal tissues rapidly counteracts active vasodilation of the subcutaneous vessels responsible for 80 to 95% of elevated skin blood flow.[70,99,174] A significant, prolonged reduction in renal and visceral tissue blood flow probably contributes to the relatively large number of liver and renal complications during exertional heat stress.

Maintenance of Blood Pressure

Aside from redirecting blood to the skin and active tissues during exercise, vasoconstriction in the viscera increases total vascular resistance. A balance between dilation and constriction usually maintains arterial blood pressure during exercise in the heat. In heavy exercise (with accompanying dehydration), relatively less blood diverts to peripheral areas for heat dissipation.[44] Reduced peripheral blood flow reflects the body's attempt to maintain cardiac output in the face of a diminishing plasma volume caused by sweating. *Circulatory regulation and muscle blood flow take precedence over temperature regulation during exercise in the heat.* When submaximal exercise progresses without excessive physiologic strain, a greater dependence still exists on anaerobic metabolism than in cooler conditions.[176] This results in earlier accumulation of lactate, encroachment on glycogen reserves, and premature fatigue during prolonged moderate exercise.[43] Two factors increase blood lactate accumulation: (1) decreased lactate uptake by the liver because of reduced hepatic blood flow and (2) reduced muscle catabolism of circulating lactate because a large portion of the cardiac output diverts to the periphery for heat dissipation.

Core Temperature During Exercise

The heat generated by active muscles can raise core temperature to fever levels that would incapacitate a person if caused by external heat stress alone.[8] Champion runners show no ill effects from rectal temperatures as high as 41°C (105.8°F) at the end of a 3-mile race. Aerobically fit subjects perform longer in uncompensably (thermoregulatory mechanisms inadequate) hot environments and tolerate higher levels of hyperthermia than subjects with lower aerobic fitness.[20] However, an abnormally high core temperature for trained and untrained subjects impairs exercise performance. Fatigue generally coincides with core temperatures between 38 and 40°C; this temperature range likely reflects a "critical" high body temperature for fatigue during exercise.[54,121]

Temperature Regulated at a Higher Level

Within limits, the increase in core temperature with exercise does not reflect a failure of the heat-dissipating mechanisms or contribute to early fatigue. To the contrary, it represents a well-regulated response even during exercise in the cold. Figure 25.5A illustrates the relationship between esophageal (core) temperature and power output (oxygen consumption) for five men and two women of varying fitness levels during exercise of increasing severity. Core temperature increases to a higher level for all subjects as exercise intensity increases, although considerable intersubject variation exists in temper-

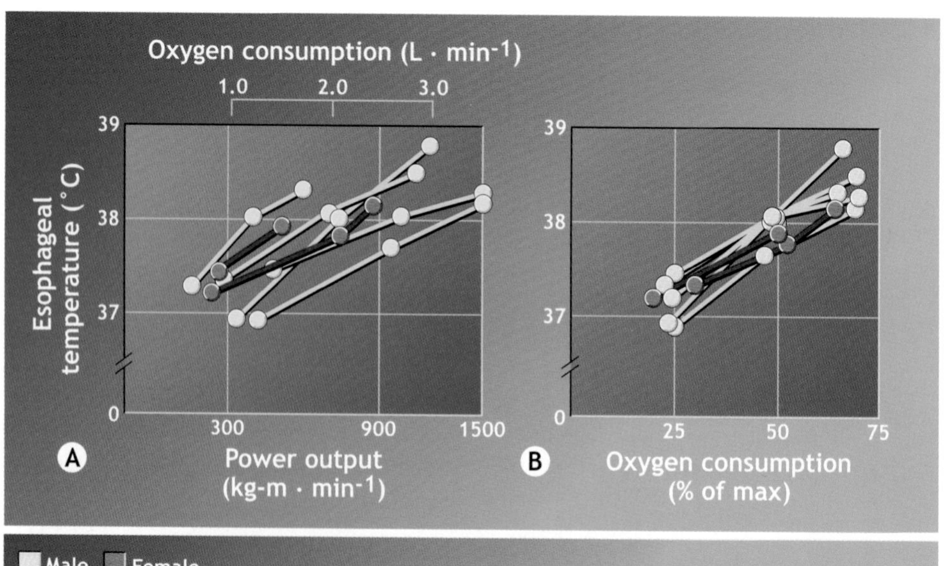

FIGURE 25.5 • Relationship between esophageal temperature and (**A**) oxygen consumption (absolute exercise intensity expressed as power output) and (**B**) oxygen consumption as a percentage of $\dot{V}O_{2max}$. (From Saltin B, Hermansen L. Esophageal, rectal, and muscle temperature during exercise. J Appl Physiol 1966;21:1757.)

Focus on Research

Heat Stress and Cardiovascular Dynamics in Exercise

Rowell LB, et al. Reductions in cardiac output, central blood volume, and stroke volume with thermal stress in normal men during exercise. J Clin Invest 1966;45:1801.

➤ Early research about heat-acclimatized men showed no increase in cardiac output (CO) during exercise in a hot, humid environment. The 1966 research by Rowell and colleagues constituted the first study of cardiac output of unacclimatized men during heat stress and exercise. The data showed reduced cardiac output at high ambient temperatures and exercise intensities and helped explain an unacclimatized man's limited exercise capacity during environmental heat stress.

The researchers tested the hypothesis that maximum blood flow decreased during strenuous exercise in the heat in unacclimatized subjects (six men; mean age, 23 y; mean body surface area, 1.97 m^2; mean $\dot{V}O_{2max}$ at 23.6°C, 3.80 L · min^{-1}) by measuring CO seven times during each of four exercise intensities at 25.6°C and 43.3°C in the same subjects (56 CO determinations per subject). The men walked for 15 minutes on a motor-driven treadmill at 3.5 mph at 7.5, 10, 12.5, and 15% grade. They rested for 15 to 20 minutes between walks.

The care given to accuracy of CO measurements represented a unique aspect of the research. Open-circuit spirometry techniques measured oxygen consumption ($\dot{V}O_2$). The indicator dilution method assessed CO by indocyanine green dye injected into the right atrium and sampled from the aortic arch. Detailed repeat measurements reduced within-subject variability. Stroke volume (SV), arteriovenous oxygen differences (a-$\bar{v}$ O_2 difference), heart rate (HR), and central blood volume (CBV) were also determined.

Figure 1 presents data for $\dot{V}O_2$, SV, a-$\bar{v}$ O_2 difference, CBV, and HR at each work load at the two different temperatures. Exercise $\dot{V}O_2$ remained unaffected by ambient temperature, while HR increased markedly at 43.3°C. At the two lowest exercise intensities, CBV at 43.4°C remained 16% below control values at 25.6°C. Decrements in CBV paralleled the percentage decrease in SV (also 16%). CVC and SV remained reduced at the two higher exercise intensities, but SV showed reductions that were more pronounced.

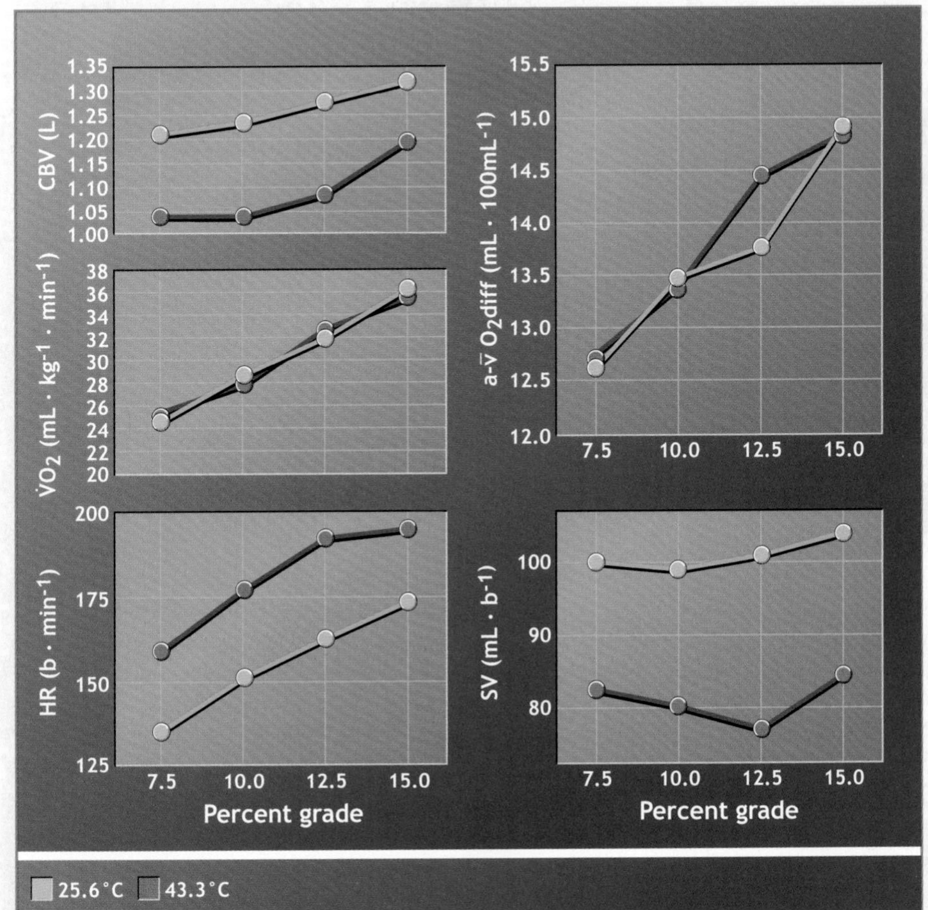

Figure 1. Central blood volume (CBV), oxygen consumption ($\dot{V}O_2$), heart rate (HR), arteriovenous oxygen difference (a-$\bar{v}$ O_2 diff), and stroke volume (SV) during exercise of increasing intensity at 25.6°C and 43.4°C.

Focus on Research Heat Stress and Cardiovascular Dynamics in Exercise—continued

Figure 2 presents the average CO responses to exercise at 25.6°C and 43.3°C at each of the four intensities (indicated as *percent grade* on the *right*). Ambient air temperature exerted only a small effect on CO during the first two exercise intensities. With further increases in intensity (12.5 and 15% grades), CO decreased more markedly during heat stress. For example, CO averaged 1.1 L · min^{-1} lower at 12.5% grade at 43.3°C than in the cooler environment. Three subjects attained near-maximal HRs at 12.5% grade. However, they failed to increase CO at the most intense exercise level, although $\dot{V}O_2$ increased the expected amount via a widened a-$\bar{v}$ O_2 difference.

This important experiment demonstrated that heat dissipation during moderate-to-severe exercise at a high ambient temperature occurs by repartitioning of CO rather than by increasing it. The decrease in CBV and SV during exercise in heat stress suggests a redistribution of blood from the core to the periphery coincident with a more rapid circulation time. The study showed for the first time that the failure of cardiac output to increase adequately during heat stress constitutes an important contributory factor limiting unacclimatized man's capacity to exercise in the heat.

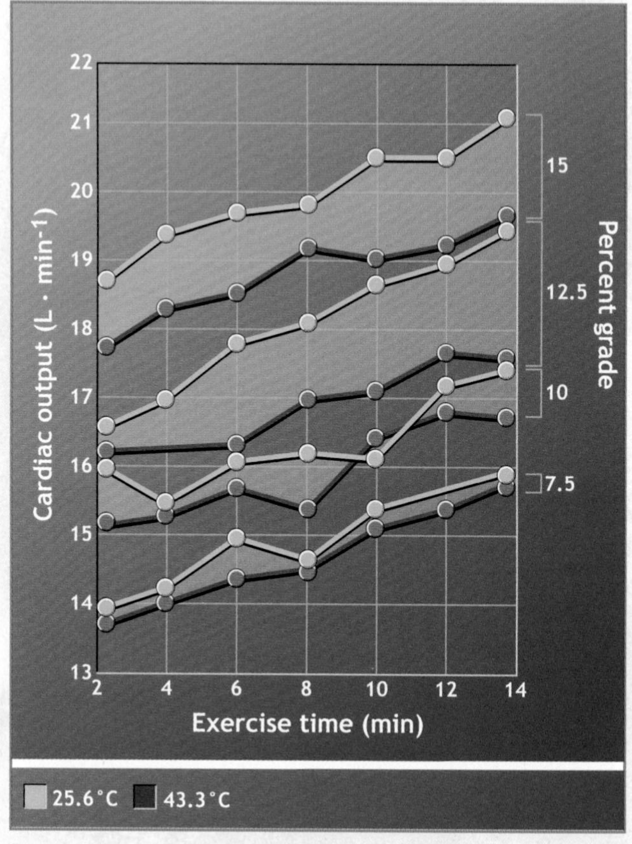

Figure 2. Average responses for cardiac output during different intensities (percent grade) of exercise at 25.6°C and 43.3°C.

ature response. However, the lines move closer together in Figure 25.5B, which plots core temperature in relation to exercise oxygen consumption expressed as a percentage of each person's $\dot{V}O_{2max}$. This indicates that relative workload (i.e., the percentage of exercise capacity) determines the change in core temperature with exercise. *More than likely, a modest rise in core temperature represents a favorable adjustment that optimizes physiologic and metabolic functions.*

In general, exercise at 50% $\dot{V}O_{2max}$ in a comfortable environment increases core temperature to a new steady level of about 37.3°C (99°F), whereas work at 75% of maximum elevates temperature to 38.5°C (101°F), regardless of the absolute exercise oxygen consumption. This means that a fit person generates more total energy (heat) in exercise at the same percentage of $\dot{V}O_{2max}$ as a less fit person, yet both maintain about the same core temperature.[141] The extra metabolic heat for the trained person dissipates via a larger sweat output. However, the trained person exercises with a lower core temperature than the untrained person at identical exercise levels.

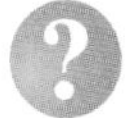

INTEGRATIVE QUESTION

What mechanisms might explain how improved aerobic fitness increases exercise tolerance in a warm, humid environment?

Water Loss in the Heat: Dehydration

Dehydration refers to body water loss from a hyperhydrated state to euhydration or from euhydration downward to hypohydration. A moderate exercise workout over 1 hour generally produces a sweat loss of 0.5 to 1.0 L. Much greater water loss occurs from several hours of heavy exercise in a hot environment. Exercise performed in less challenging thermal environments (e.g., cross-country skiing, or swimming) still produces significant sweating.[151] For swimmers and divers, water immersion stimulates fluid loss through increased urine production. Non-exercise-induced water loss also occurs when power athletes (wrestlers, boxers, weight lifters, and rowers) aggressively attempt to "make weight" through rapid weight loss induced by common dehydration techniques—external heat exposure via sauna, steam room, hot whirlpool or shower, fluid and food restriction, diuretic and laxative use, and vomiting. Athletes often combine these techniques, hoping to accelerate weight loss. *The risk of heat illness greatly increases when a person begins exercising in a dehydrated state.*

Fluid deficits (*hypovolemia*) in the intracellular and extracellular compartments with hypohydration can rapidly reach levels that reduce the body's ability to dissipate heat and increase the rate of heat storage owing to reductions in (1) sweating rate and (2) skin blood flow for a given core temperature. The reduced heat tolerance severely compromises cardiovascular function and exercise capacity, particularly with intense exercise in hot environments.[112,146] Because sweat remains hypotonic to other body fluids, the hypovolemia from sweating correspondingly increases plasma osmolality.

In terms of exercise performance, rapid weight loss through dehydration does not impair muscular strength (effects on muscular endurance remain equivocal) or a single bout of power performance up to a duration of 60 seconds.[53,111] Losing body water rapidly before exercising even improves muscular power and strength on a relative basis (per kg of body mass).[68] When high-intensity exercise lasts longer than 1 minute, dehydration profoundly impairs physiologic function and optimal ability to train and compete. For wrestlers, moderate hypohydration equivalent to 1.5% of body mass produced poorer intermittent all-out exercise performance compared with similar exercise in the euhydrated state.[98]

Magnitude of Fluid Loss

For an acclimatized person, water loss by sweating reaches a peak of about 3L · h^{-1} an hour during intense exercise in the heat and can average nearly 12 L on a daily basis. Several hours of intense sweating can produce sweat-gland fatigue that ultimately interferes with core temperature regulation. Elite marathon runners frequently experience fluid loss in excess of 5 L during competition, a loss equivalent to 6 to 10% of body mass. For a slower-paced ultramarathon, the average fluid loss rarely exceeds 500 mL per hour. Even in a temperate climate of 10°C (50°F), soccer players lose an average of 2 L during a 90-minute game.[93] *The ability of acclimatized humans to sustain their exceptional potential for evaporative cooling necessitates adequate fluid replacement.*

Sports other than distance running also induce a large sweat output and accompanying fluid loss. Football, basketball, and hockey players lose large quantities of fluid during competition. High school wrestlers often lose 9 to 13% of their preseason body mass prior to certification; the greatest portion of this weight loss results from voluntarily reducing water intake and excessive sweating just prior to the weigh-in. Collegiate wrestlers, excluding heavyweights, regain an average of 3.7 kg during the 20 hours between weigh-in and competition.[147] In their desire to "make weight," high school and collegiate wrestlers usually compete in a dehydrated state, with significantly reduced blood and plasma volumes.[173,178] Transient, reversible mood alterations and impaired short-term memory also accompany rapid weight loss in collegiate wrestlers.[19]

Significant Consequences

Almost any dehydration impairs physiologic function and thermoregulation. As dehydration progresses and plasma volume decreases, peripheral blood flow and sweating rate diminish, and thermoregulation becomes progressively more difficult. Preexercise dehydration equivalent to 5% of body mass significantly increases rectal temperature and heart rate and decreases sweating rate, $\dot{V}O_{2max}$, and exercise capacity, compared with exercise under normal hydration.[143] A reduced central blood volume lowers ventricular filling pressure and helps to explain the elevated heart rate and 25 to 30% stroke volume reduction in the dehydrated state. An increase in heart rate, however, does not offset the reduced stroke volume; consequently, cardiac output and arterial blood pressure decline.[25,50] The elevation in core temperature relates directly to a reduced sweating rate and cutaneous blood flow.[116]

Fluid loss becomes most apparent during exercise in hot, humid environments because the high vapor pressure of ambient air thwarts evaporative cooling. Figure 25.6 shows the linear dependency between sweating rate (during rest and exercise) and the air's moisture content as reflected by wet-bulb temperature (see "In a Practical Sense"). Ironically, excessive sweat output in high humidity contributes little to cooling because of minimal evaporation.

Physiologic and Performance Decrements

Reduced peripheral blood flow and increased core temperature in exercise relate closely to dehydration level. A fluid loss equivalent to only 1% of body mass significantly increases rectal tem-

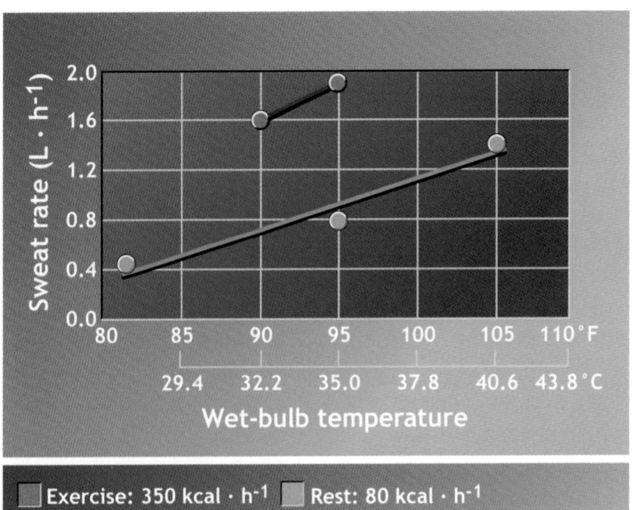

FIGURE 25.6 • The effect of humidity (wet-bulb temperature) on sweat rate at rest and during exercise in the heat. Ambient dry-bulb temperature was 43.4°C (110°F). (From Iampietro PF. Exercise in hot environments. In: Shephard RJ, ed. Frontiers of fitness. Springfield, IL: Charles C Thomas, 1971.)

perature compared with the same exercise and normal hydration.[34] For each liter of sweat-loss dehydration, exercise heart rate increases 8 b · min^{-1}, with a corresponding 1.0 L · min^{-1} decrease in cardiac output.[25] A water loss of 4 to 5% of body mass (common among high school and collegiate wrestlers) impairs physical work capacity and physiologic function.[16,21] The 5 hours between weigh-in and match time may not adequately ensure complete rehydration and electrolyte balance at the time of competition.[170] Because a large portion of water lost through sweating comes from blood plasma, circulatory capacity progressively decreases as sweat loss progresses. Bodily fluid loss manifests itself by decreased plasma volume, reduced skin blood flow for a given core temperature, reduced stroke volume, increased near-compensatory heart rate, and a general deterioration in circulatory and thermoregulatory efficiency in exercise.[142] For exercise performance, dehydration equal to 4.3% of body mass reduced walking endurance by 48%; concurrently, $\dot{V}O_{2max}$ decreased by 22%.[27] These same experiments showed that endurance performance (−22%) and $\dot{V}O_{2max}$ (−10%) decreased when dehydration averaged only 1.9% of body mass. Clearly, even modest dehydration imposes adverse thermoregulatory effects during exercise.

Diuretics

Diuretic-induced dehydration draws a greater percentage of water from the plasma than body water lost through sweating.[21] Wrestlers who use diuretic drugs to lose body water rapidly to make weight place themselves at a distinct disadvantage because of the adverse effects of reduced plasma volume on thermoregulation and cardiovascular function. In addition, drugs that induce diuresis can markedly impair neuromuscular function, which does not occur with comparable fluid loss through exercise.[17] Chemicals that induce vomiting and diarrhea for sudden weight loss not only cause dehydration but also promote excessive mineral loss with accompanying muscle weakness and impaired neuromuscular function.

MAINTAINING FLUID BALANCE: REHYDRATION AND HYPERHYDRATION

Fluid replacement must focus on maintaining plasma volume so circulation and sweating progress at optimal levels. Blunting hypohydration by ingesting fluid during exercise increases blood flow to the skin for more effective cooling, independent of any change in plasma volume.[108] Prevention of dehydration and its consequences, especially hyperthermia, occurs *only* with an adequate and strictly observed water replacement schedule.[18,92,117] Meeting this requirement often presents difficulties, because some coaches and athletes feel that ingesting water hinders performance. Left on their own, most individuals voluntarily replace only about one-half of the water lost in exercise (<500 mL · h^{-1}).[122] For wrestlers, dehydration represents a way of life. Older ballet dancers, with their continual preoccupation with maintaining a thin appearance, often demonstrate similar behaviors. Those responsible for such programs must steadfastly promote proper hydration for thermoregulation, exercise performance, and safety.

Adequate hydration provides the most effective defense against heat stress. The ideal hydration protocol balances water loss with water intake, not pouring water over the head or body. No evidence indicates that restricting fluid intake during training in some way makes an athlete better able to adjust to subsequent work in the heat. *A well-hydrated athlete always functions at a higher level than one who exercises in a dehydrated state.* Chapters 2 and 3 discuss the body's fluid compartments and specific factors that influence gastric emptying and subsequent intestinal fluid absorption. These chapters also provide practical recommendations for oral rehydration beverages and possible complications from excessive water intake in prolonged exercise (hyponatremia).

Ingesting "extra" water (**hyperhydration**) before exercising in the heat may offer a small thermoregulatory protection. Hyperhydration delays development of hypohydration with inadequate fluid replacement during exercise, increases sweating during exercise, and brings about a smaller rise in core temperature in **uncompensable heat stress**, in which evaporative cooling is inadequate to maintain thermal balance.[81,116] Acute preexercise hyperhydration effectively results from consuming (1) at least 500 mL of water before sleeping the night before exercising in the heat, (2) another 500 mL upon awakening, and (3) an additional 400 to 600 mL of cold water 20 minutes before exercise. An extended, systematic regimen of hyperhydration (4.5 L · d^{-1}) 1 week before soccer competition by elite young soccer players in Puerto Rico increased body water reserves (despite greater urine output) and improved temperature regulation during a soccer match in warm weather.[129] The structured sequence of preexercise hyperhydration produced a 1.1 L greater total body fluid volume than the volume with the athletes' normal daily 2.5-L fluid intake.

Preexercise hyperhydration does not replace the need for continual fluid replacement during exercise. In most instances, the benefits of hyperhydration subside if the individual remains euhydrated during exercise. However, in activities like distance running, matching fluid loss with fluid intake becomes virtually impossible because only 800 to 1000 mL of fluid empty from the stomach each hour. This rate of stomach emptying does not match a water loss that can average nearly 2000 mL per hour. Under these conditions, preexercise hyperhydration may prove beneficial.

A Benefit from Exogenous Glycerol?

The United States Olympic Committee (USOC) has banned the use of the diuretic glycerol—a component of the triglyceride molecule, a gluconeogenic substrate, an important constituent of the plasma membrane's phospholipids, and an osmotically active natural metabolite. The two-carbon glycerol molecule achieved clinical notoriety (along with mannitol, sorbitol, and urea) for its role in producing an osmotic diuresis. The capacity for influencing water movement within the body makes glycerol effective in reducing excess accumulation of fluid (edema) in the brain and eye. An osmotic effect occurs because concentrated extracellular glycerol enters brain tissues, cerebrospinal fluid, and the eye's aqueous humor at a slow rate, which draws fluid from these tissues.

When consumed with 1 to 2 L of water, glycerol facilitates intestinal water absorption[166] and extracellular fluid retention, mainly in the plasma and interstitial fluid compartments.[45,49,80,130] An expanded body fluid volume potentially sets the stage for fluid excretion from increased renal filtrate and urine flow. Because proximal and distal kidney tubules reabsorb large amounts of glycerol, much of the fluid portion of the increased renal filtrate is also reabsorbed; this averts marked diuresis and promotes hyperhydration.

The normal plasma glycerol concentration at rest averages 0.05 mM; it may rise to 0.5 mM during prolonged exercise with accompanying carbohydrate depletion and elevated fat catabolism. The kidneys generally reabsorb from the renal filtrate almost all of the glycerol from food and metabolism. Thus, an exaggerated increase in urine glycerol concentration most likely indicates glycerol supplementation.

Proponents of glycerol supplementation maintain that its hyperhydration effect reduces overall heat stress in exercise, as reflected by increased sweating rate; this leads to a lower exercise heart rate and body temperature and enhances endurance performance.[87] Reducing heat stress with augmented hyperhydration before exercise, using glycerol plus water supplementation, would therefore increase the safety of the exercise participant. One g of glycerol per kg of body mass (with 1 to 2 L of water) is the typical recommended preexercise glycerol dose; its hyperhydration effect lasts up to 6 hours.

Not all research demonstrates meaningful thermoregulatory benefits from glycerol hyperhydration over preexercise hyperhydration with plain water.[81] For example, exogenous glycerol diluted in 500 mL of water consumed 4 hours before exercise failed to promote fluid retention or ergogenic effects.[64] Also, no cardiovascular or thermoregulatory advantages result from consuming glycerol with small volumes of water during exercise.[113] Side effects of exogenous glycerol ingestion include headache, nausea, dizziness, bloating, and light-headedness. Those favoring glycerol supplementation argue that failure to reverse the USOC's glycerol ban only increases the exposure of elite athletes to risk of heat injury, including potentially fatal heat stroke. A definitive conclusion about thermoregulatory benefits of exogenous glycerol awaits further research.

Adequacy of Rehydration

Changes in body mass indicate water loss and adequacy of rehydration during and following exercise participation. Voiding small volumes of dark yellow urine with a strong odor also qualitatively indicates inadequate hydration. Well-hydrated individuals typically produce large volumes of light-colored urine without a strong smell. Table 25.3 presents recommendations for fluid intake with acute weight loss during exercise. These standards initially applied to a 90-minute football practice, but they easily adapt to most exercise situations.

Athletes can be weighed before and after practice. Each pound of weight lost represents 450 mL (15 fl oz) of dehydration. Periodic water breaks during activity help deter fluid depletion. Because the thirst mechanism imprecisely monitors water needs, coaches and trainers must urge athletes to rehydrate themselves routinely. If a person relied entirely on thirst for rehydration, it could take several days to reestablish fluid balance following severe dehydration.[135] Alcohol-containing beverages generally impede restoration of fluid balance, particularly if the rehydration fluid contains 4% or more alcohol.[95,153-155]

TABLE 25.3 ➤ RECOMMENDED FLUID AVAILABILITY AND INTAKE FOR A STRENUOUS 90-MINUTE ATHLETIC PRACTICE[a]

Weight Loss		Minutes between Water Breaks	Fluid per Break		Fluid Availability for an 11-Member Squad	
LB	KG		OZ	ML	GAL	L
8	3.6	No practice recommended	—		—	
7.5	3.4		—		—	
7	3.2	10	8–10	266	6.5–8	27.4
6.5	3.0	10	8–9	251	6.5–7	25.5
6	2.7	10	8–9	251	6.5–7	25.5
5.5	2.5	15	10–12	325	5.5–6.5	22.7
5	2.3	15	10–11	311	5.5–6	21.8
4.5	2.1	15	9–10	281	5–5.5	19.9
4	1.8	15	8–9	251	4.5–5	18.0
3.5	1.6	20	10–11	311	4–4.5	16.1
3	1.4	20	9–10	281	3.5–4	14.2
2.5	1.1	20	7–8	222	3	11.4
2	0.9	30	8	237	2.5	9.5
1.5	0.7	30	6	177	1.5	5.7
1	0.5	45	6	177	1	3.8
0.5	0.2	60	6	177	0.5	1.9

[a]Based on an 80% replacement of weight loss.

Electrolyte Replacement

Because sweat remains hypotonic to bodily fluids, water replacement is the immediate concern during exercise rather than mineral replenishment. For a fluid loss of less than 2.7 kg in adults, adding a slight amount of salt to food readily replenishes the sodium lost in sweat. Adding sodium and potassium chloride to the drinking water provided little benefit to men and women who became sweat-loss dehydrated by 3% of body mass on 5 successive days but received food and water *ad libitum* during each daily recovery period.[23] During prolonged exercise, the kidneys' sodium-conserving mechanisms generally balance sodium losses.[67]

Added Sodium May Benefit Rehydration

Chapter 3 discusses that electrolytes (and glucose) added to the rehydration beverage bring about a more complete rehydration than plain water.[127,149,171] Restoration of water and electrolyte balance in recovery occurs more rapidly by (1) adding moderate-to-high amounts of sodium (between 20 and 60 mmol · L^{-1}) to the rehydration drink or (2) combining solid food (with appropriate sodium content) with plain water.[94,96,138] Adding a small amount of potassium (2 to 5 mmol · L^{-1}) may enhance water retention in the intracellular space and reestablish any extra potassium excretion that accompanies sodium retention by the kidneys.[28] A beverage that tastes good to the individual also contributes to voluntary rehydration during and in recovery from exercise.[132,172]

To restore fluid balance, the volume of ingested fluid following exercise must exceed by 25 to 50% the exercise sweat loss, because the kidneys continually form some urine regardless of hydration status. Pure water absorbed from the gut rapidly dilutes plasma sodium. In turn, decreased plasma osmolality stimulates urine production and blunts the normal sodium-dependent stimulation of the thirst mechanism. These responses are counter to the goal of rehydration. Unless the beverage contains sufficient sodium, excess fluid intake merely increases urine output without fully benefiting rehydration.[156] *Maintaining a relatively high plasma sodium concentration by adding sodium to ingested fluid sustains the thirst drive, promotes retention of ingested fluids (lower urine output), and restores lost plasma volume more rapidly during rehydration.*

Figure 25.7 illustrates the effect of a rehydration beverage with added sodium on ingested fluid retention in recovery. Six healthy men exercised in a warm, humid environment until sweating produced a 1.9% weight loss. They then ingested one of four test drinks (2045 mL) containing sodium concentrations of either 2, 26, 52, or 100 mmol · L^{-1} (typical "sports drinks" contain 10 to 25 mM sodium; normal plasma sodium concentration ranges between 138 and 142 mM) over a 30-minute period beginning 30 minutes after stopping exercise. From the 1.5-hour urine sample onward, urine volume inversely related to the rehydration beverage's sodium content. At the end of the study period, a difference in total body water content of 787 mL existed between trials using drinks with the lowest and highest sodium content. The drink containing 100 mM sodium contributed to the greatest fluid retention.

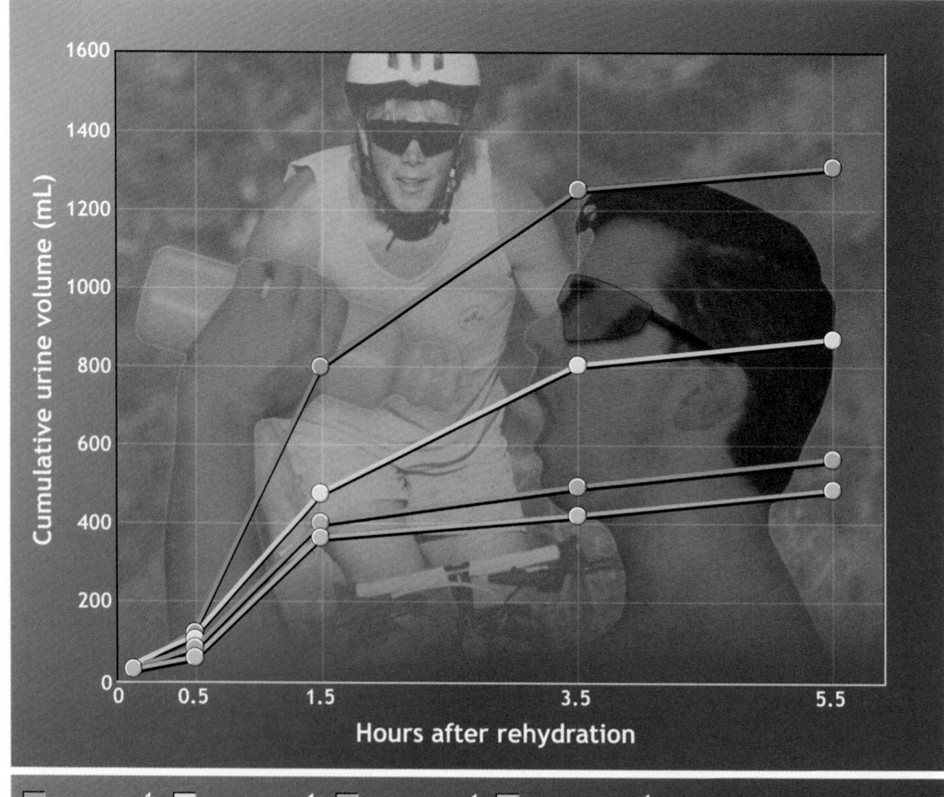

FIGURE 25.7 • Cumulative urine output during recovery from exercise-induced dehydration. The oral rehydration beverages were four test drinks (equivalent to 1.5 times body mass loss, or approximately 2045 mL) containing sodium (and matching anion) in a concentration of either 2, 26, 52, or 100 mmol · L^{-1}. (From Maughan RJ, Leiper JB. Sodium intake and post-exercise rehydration in man. Eur J Appl Physiol 1995; 71:311.)

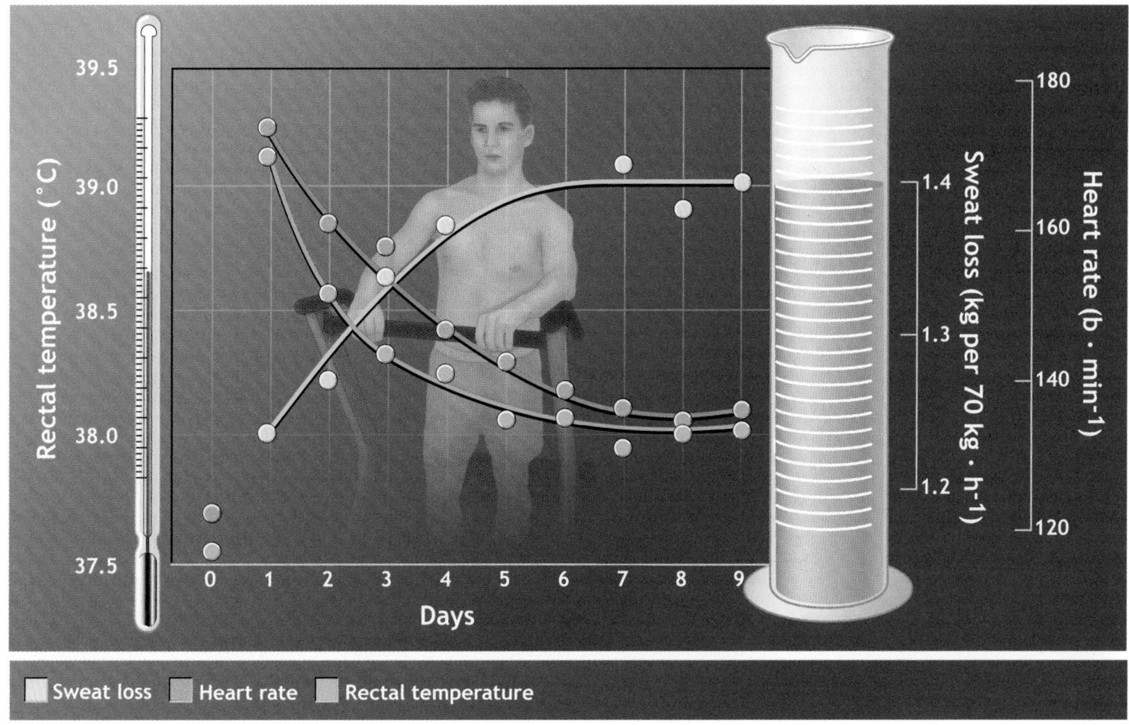

FIGURE 25.8 • Average rectal temperature, heart rate, and sweat loss during 100 minutes of daily heat-exercise exposure for 9 days. On day 0, the men walked on a treadmill at an exercise intensity of 300 kcal · h^{-1} in a cool climate. Thereafter, they performed the same daily exercise in the heat at 48.9°C (26.7°F wet bulb). (From Lind AR, Bass DE. Optimal exposure time for development of acclimatization to heat. Fed Proc 1963;22:704.)

With prolonged exercise in the heat, sweat loss can deplete the body of 13 to 17 g of salt (2.3 to 3.4 g · L^{-1} of sweat) daily, about 8 g more than is typically consumed. It seems prudent in this deficit situation to replace the lost sodium by adding about one-third teaspoon of table salt to 1 L of water. Moderate exercise generally produces a negligible potassium loss in sweat.[24,33] Even at competitive physical activity levels, potassium loss in sweat ranges between 5 and 18 mEq, which poses little or no immediate danger.[28] With heavy sweating, increasing the intake of potassium-rich foods (citrus fruits and bananas) replaces most potassium losses. *Except in unusual cases, minor adjustments in food intake and electrolyte conservation by the kidneys adequately compensate for mineral loss through sweating.*

Whole Body Precooling

"Cold treatments" that periodically apply cold towels to the forehead and abdomen during exercise or a cold shower before exercising in the heat improve heat transfer at the body's surface only slightly above that with the same exercise without skin wetting.[10] However, whole body precooling (core temperature decrease of 0.7°C) with up to 60 minutes immersion in water at 23.5°C significantly increased subsequent exercise endurance in a hot, humid environment. Time to exhaustion inversely related to initial body temperature (lowered via precooling) and directly related to the rate of heat storage.[51] Precooling with cold-water immersion enhanced the rate of heat storage and caused less thermoregulatory strain—attenuated rise in skin and rectal temperatures and heart rates—during exercise.[13] In addition, whole-body precooling of the skin by 5 to 6°C without concomitant reduction in core temperature reduced thermal strain and increased distance cycled in 30 minutes under warm, humid conditions.[73] On the other hand, whole body precooling provided no thermoregulatory benefit during a simulated triathlon,[12] or on the physiologic responses to a 90-minute soccer-specific exercise protocol under normal environmental conditions.[36]

FACTORS THAT MODIFY HEAT TOLERANCE

Major factors that interact to improve physiologic adjustments and exercise tolerance during environmental heat stress include acclimatization, training status, age, gender, and body composition.

Acclimatization

Relatively easy tasks performed in cool weather become taxing if attempted on the first hot day of spring. The early stages of preseason training for warm-weather sports often pose the greatest hazards for heat injury, because thermoregulatory mechanisms have not adjusted to the dual challenge of exercise and environmental heat. Repeated exposure to hot environments (particularly when combined with exercise), with accompanying elevated core and skin temperatures and profuse sweating, improves the capacity for exercise with less discomfort upon subsequent heat exposure.[120,143,158,168]

*The term **heat acclimatization** describes the collective physiologic adaptive changes that improve heat tolerance.* Data from a classic study in the early 1960s (Fig. 25.8) show that the major acclimatization occurs during the first week of heat exposure, with full acclimatization thereafter. The process requires only 2 to 4 hours of daily heat exposure. The first several sessions in the heat should include 15 to 20 minutes of light-intensity physical activity. Thereafter, exercise sessions should increase in duration and intensity.

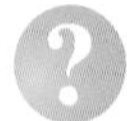

INTEGRATIVE QUESTION

Your Maine-based soccer team competes in Hawaii in early spring. Discuss how you would prepare the team to compete in this hot–humid environment (1) making all precompetition preparations at your school or (2) if time, money, and travel were not considerations.

Table 25.4 summarizes the main physiologic adjustments during heat acclimatization. *Optimal acclimatization requires adequate hydration.* During exercise, larger quantities of blood flow to cutaneous vessels to facilitate heat transfer from the core to the periphery. A more effective cardiac output distribution also helps stabilize blood pressure during exercise. A lowered threshold for sweating complements these "circulatory acclimatizations." Consequently, cooling begins before core temperature increases appreciably. Sweating capacity, the most significant factor for heat acclimatization, increases early in acclimatization and nearly doubles after 10 days of heat exposure; sweat also becomes more dilute (less salt lost) and distributes more evenly over the skin surface. Concurrently, heat acclimatization reduces sodium loss from the kidneys. Adjustments in circulation and evaporative cooling enable the heat-acclimatized person to exercise with lower skin and core temperatures and heart rates than an unacclimatized person.[1] A lower exercise core temperature requires diversion of less blood to the skin, thus freeing more of the cardiac output for active muscles. Acclimatization also reduces carbohydrate use in exercise, a response consistent with acclimatization-induced plasma epinephrine reduction.[42] The major benefits of acclimatization dissipate within 2 to 3 weeks after returning to a more temperate environment.

Training Status

Exercise-induced "internal" heat stress with training in a cool environment induces qualitatively similar adjustments in peripheral circulation and evaporative cooling as training in hot ambient temperatures. These training adaptations facilitate elimination of metabolic heat generated by exercise. They generally occur with an 8- to 12-week training period at an exercise intensity that exceeds 50% of aerobic capacity. This makes well-conditioned men and women living in a temperate climate respond more effectively to a sudden, severe heat stress than their sedentary counterparts.[5,6,34] Exercise training increases the sensitivity and capacity of the sweating response so that sweating begins at a lower core temperature, producing larger volumes of more-dilute sweat. This results partly from intrinsic adaptations in the sweat glands with training.[15] Concurrently, a training-induced adjustment in the cutaneous circulation provides greater skin blood flow at a given internal temperature or percentage of $\dot{V}O_{2max}$, independent of age.[70] Enhanced physical fitness also sustains better blood flow to the gastrointestinal tract. This maintains the normal barrier to endotoxin movement from the gut lumen into the plasma, blunting the potential for endotoxin-induced fever that could aggravate exercise hyperthermia.[140] Plasma and extravascular fluid volumes also increase during the initial stages of aerobic training.[22,85,89,97] Controversy exists as to whether an expanded plasma volume necessarily enhances the sweating response or provides added thermoregulatory benefit during during physical activity in hot weather (e.g., lower submaximal heart rate and increased stroke volume and cardiac output).[143] The thermoregulatory benefit for exercise training occurs only if the individual remains fully hydrated during exercise.[145]

As one might expect, exercise "heat conditioning" in cool weather offers fewer benefits than acclimatization from similar exercise training in the heat. *A physically active person cannot achieve full heat acclimatization without exposure to environmental heat stress.* Athletes who train and compete in hot weather have a distinct thermoregulatory advantage over athletes who train in cool climates and only periodically compete in hot weather.

TABLE 25.4 ➤ **PHYSIOLOGIC ADJUSTMENTS DURING HEAT ACCLIMATIZATION**

Acclimatization Response	Effect
• Improved cutaneous blood flow	• Transports metabolic heat from deep tissues to the body's shell
• Effective distribution of cardiac output	• Appropriate circulation to skin and muscles to meet demands of metabolism and thermoregulation; greater blood pressure stability during exercise
• Lowered threshold for start of sweating	• Evaporative cooling begins early in exercise
• A more effective distribution of sweat over skin surface	• Optimum use of effective surface for evaporative cooling
• Increased sweat output	• Maximizes evaporative cooling
• Lowered salt concentration of sweat	• Dilute sweat preserves electrolytes in extracellular fluid
• Lower skin and core temperatures and heart rate for a standard exercise	• Frees greater portion of cardiac output for distribution to active muscles
• Less reliance on carbohydrate catabolism during exercise	• Carbohydrate sparing

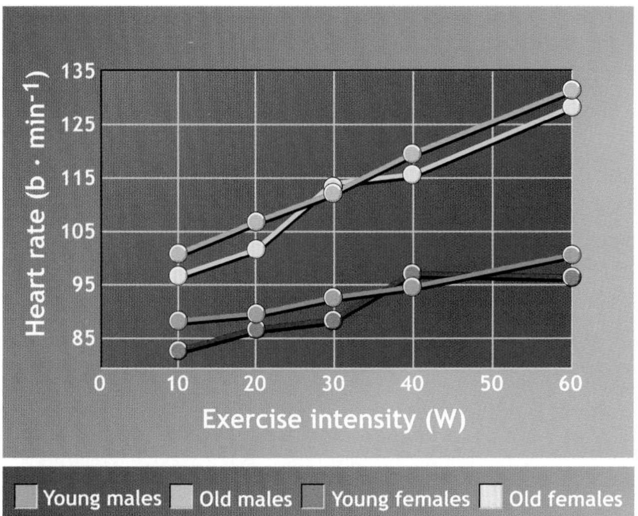

FIGURE 25.9 • Heart rate during moderate exercise in the heat by young and old men and women. Dry-bulb ambient temperature was 33.5°C, and wet-bulb was 28.5°C. (Modified from Henshel A. The environment and performance. In: Simonsen E, ed. Physiology of work capacity and fatigue. Springfield, IL: Charles C Thomas, 1971.)

Age

Debate exists about the effects of aging on the ability to tolerate and acclimatize to moderate heat stress.[4,74,134,137] An early study exposed men and women aged 60 to 93 years to 70 minutes of heat stress during exercise at intensities ranging from 2 to 5 METs.[59] Figure 25.9 shows the relationship between heart rate and exercise intensity in the heat for these older subjects and for young men and women. The less fit elderly subjects exercised at higher heart rates than young adults of the same gender. However, environmental heat imposed no greater physiologic strain for the older groups because their body temperature increased an average of only 0.3°C, compared with 0.2°C for the younger group. Testing the elderly subjects in the spring and fall evaluated their extent of natural heat acclimatization during the summer months. After the summer, all subjects showed significantly lower heart rates during the standard thermal–exercise stress.

Comparisons between young and middle-aged competitive runners indicate no age-related decrements in thermoregulation during marathon running.[133] Trained 50-year-old men showed little impairment in thermoregulatory function compared with young men.[124] Likewise, sweating capacity for men aged 58 to 84 years adequately regulated body temperature during prolonged desert walks.[32] *Research that controls for body size and composition, aerobic fitness level, level of hydration, degree of acclimatization, and chronological age shows little or no age-related decrements on thermoregulatory capacity or heat-stress acclimatization.*[75,160]

Age-Related Differences

Some age-related factors affect thermoregulatory dynamics despite equivalence between young and older adults in capacity to regulate core temperature during heat stress. Aging delays the onset of sweating and blunts the magnitude of the sweating response, by either a (1) modified sensitivity of thermoreceptors, (2) limited sweat gland output per se, or (3) dehydration-limited sweat output with insufficient fluid replacement.[66,74] Aging also alters the intrinsic structure and function of the skin itself and its vasculature.[77,90,136] Vascular changes include depressed peripheral vascular sensitivity that impairs local cutaneous vasodilation, because of two factors: (1) smaller release of vasomotor tone and (2) less-active vasodilation once sweating begins.[65] For example, older athletes show a 25 to 40% lower skin blood flow with increased core temperature compared with younger athletes.[76] Contributing factors also include the combined effects of a lower cardiac output and reduced blood distribution from the splanchnic and renal circulations with aging.[106] Furthermore, older adults do not recover from dehydration as effectively as younger counterparts, mainly from a reduced thirst drive.[75] This places these elderly in a chronic state of hypohydration (with a less than optimal plasma volume), which could impair thermoregulatory dynamics. An altered thirst mechanism and a shift in the operating point for control of body fluid volume and composition also contributes to the decrease in total blood volume.[29,88]

Children

Children show a lower sweating rate and a higher core temperature during heat stress than adolescents and adults, even though children possess a larger number of heat-activated sweat glands per unit skin area.[9,40] A reduced sweating response possibly results from underdeveloped peripheral mechanisms, including the sweat glands and their surrounding tissues, rather than from a blunted central drive related to sweating.[150] The age difference in thermoregulation lasts through puberty; it generally does not limit exercise capacity except during extreme environmental heat stress.[39] Sweat composition also differs between children and adults; sweat of children shows higher sodium and chlorine concentrations and lower concentrations of lactate, H^+, and potassium.[40,105] *From a practical standpoint, exercise intensity should decrease for children exposed to heat; children also require more time to acclimatize than more-mature competitors.*[63]

Gender

Early comparisons of thermoregulation in men and women indicated that men exhibited greater tolerance to environmental heat stress during a standard bout of exercise. However, a major flaw in this research required that women exercise at a higher percentage of their aerobic capacity than men. When researchers controlled for this factor and compared men and women of equal fitness (or exercised both at the same $\%\dot{V}O_{2max}$), thermoregulatory differences between the genders became less pronounced.[35,57,62] Most researchers now concede that women tolerate the thermal stress of exercise at least as well as men of comparable aerobic fitness and level of acclimatization; both genders also acclimatize to the same degree.[2,158]

Sweating

Sweating represents the distinct gender difference in thermoregulation. Women sweat less prolifically than men, despite possessing more heat-activated sweat glands per unit skin area.[15] Women start to sweat at higher skin and core temperatures; they also produce less sweat than men for a comparable heat-exercise load, even after equivalent acclimatization.[33]

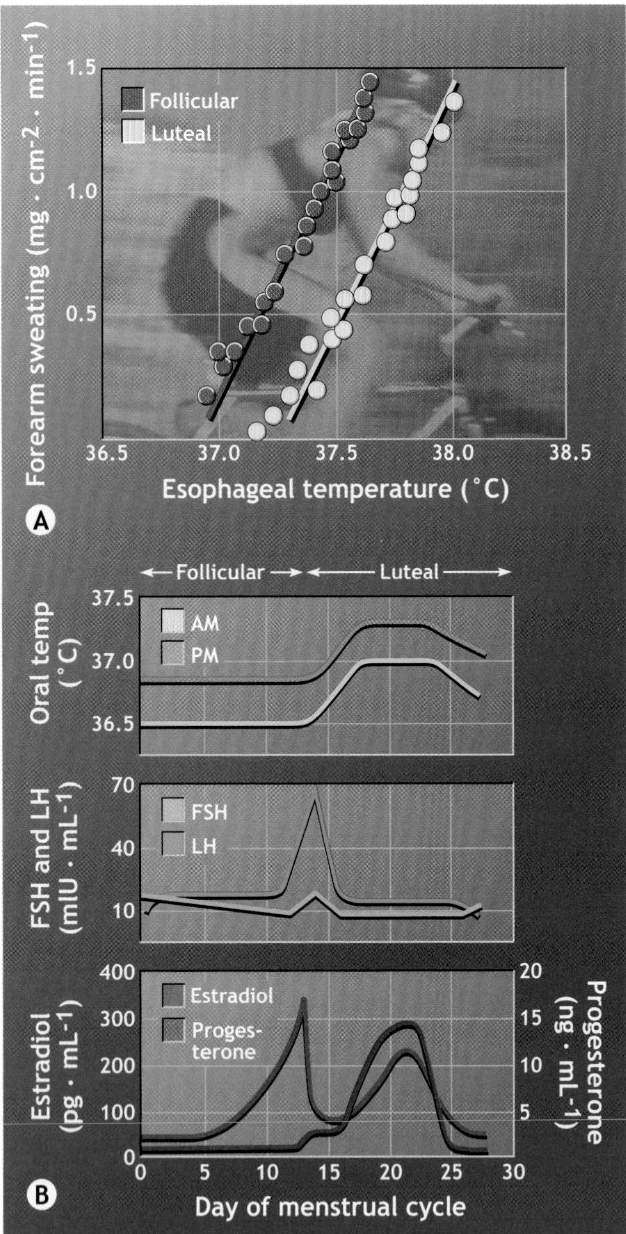

FIGURE 25.10 • A. Forearm sweating response in relation to esophageal temperature during cycle ergometer exercise performed at 60% $\dot{V}O_{2max}$ at 35°C during the follicular and luteal phases of the menstrual cycle. (Modified from Stephenson LA, Kolka MA. Menstrual cycle phase and time of day alter reference signal controlling arm blood flow and sweating. Am J Physiol 1985;249: R186.) **B**. Oral temperature and hormonal changes during the follicular and luteal phases of the menstrual cycle. Menses typically occurs during days 1 to 5. (Modified from Stephenson LA, Kolka MA. Effect of gender, circadian period and sleep loss on thermal responses during exercise. In: Pandolf KB, et al., eds. Human performance physiology and environmental medicine at terrestrial extremes. Carmel, IN: Cooper Publishing Group, 1994.)

EVAPORATIVE VERSUS CIRCULATORY COOLING. Despite a lower sweat output, women have a heat tolerance similar to men of equal aerobic fitness at the same exercise level.[158] Women probably use circulatory mechanisms for heat dissipation, whereas men make greater use of evaporative cooling. Clearly, producing less sweat to maintain thermal balance protects women from dehydration during exercise at high ambient temperatures.

Ratio of Body Surface Area to Body Mass

The typically smaller female possesses a relatively large external surface per unit of body mass exposed to the environment, offering a favorable dimensional characteristic for heat dissipation. Consequently, under identical conditions of heat exposure, women tend to cool faster than men. Children possess a similar "geometric" advantage during heat stress, because of their larger ratio of surface area-to-mass than adults.

Menstruation

Phases of the menstrual cycle influence cutaneous vascular control in women in a manner that dramatically alters skin blood flow and the sweating response during rest and physical activity.[18,159] Figure 25.10A shows sweating response at the forearm versus esophageal temperature during cycle ergometer exercise at 60% $\dot{V}O_{2max}$ at 35°C during the follicular and luteal phases of the menstrual cycle. The shift of the curve to the right during the luteal phase indicates that a significantly higher core temperature threshold initiates sweating during this phase. A similar response occurs during heavier exercise at 80% of aerobic capacity.[79] An upward resetting of the thermoregulatory set-point for sweating during the luteal phase probably reflects a unique feature of hormone dynamics throughout the cycle.[60,159] Figure 25.10B diagrams the normal hormonal responses during the follicular and luteal phases. An upward shift of approximately 0.4°C in oral temperature (equivalent to core temperature increase in part A of the figure) persists for about 6 days during the luteal phase. Note that estradiol exhibits a biphasic upward shift—once in the follicular and once in the luteal phase—but the progesterone surge coincides with the increase in oral temperature during the luteal phase. *The change in thermoregulatory sensitivity during the luteal phase does not affect ability to exercise or perform hard physical work.*[34,86] However, one must consider the menstrual cycle phase when evaluating thermoregulatory dynamics during exercise and thermal stress.

Body Fat Level

Excess body fat is a liability when exercising in the heat. Because the specific heat of fat exceeds that of muscle tissue, fat increases the insulatory quality of the body shell and retards heat conduction to the periphery. The large, overly fat person has a smaller ratio of body surface area-to-body mass for effective sweat evaporation than a leaner, smaller person.

Excess body fat also directly adds to the metabolic cost of weight-bearing activities. Compounding this effect by adding the weight of sports equipment (e.g., football or lacrosse gear), intense competition, and a hot, humid environment places the overly fat person at a distinct disadvantage for temperature regulation and exercise performance. Fatal heat stroke (see next section) occurs 3.5 times more frequently in excessively overweight young adults than in individuals of average body size.[58]

INTEGRATIVE QUESTION

Describe the ideal personal physical and physiologic characteristics that minimize heat injury risk in exercise during environmental heat stress.

COMPLICATIONS FROM EXCESSIVE HEAT STRESS

On average, 381 people died in the United States from excessive heat stress each year between 1979 and 1996, and about one-half of these were men and women 65 years of age and older. If the normal signs of heat stress—thirst, tiredness, grogginess, and visual disturbances—go unheeded, cardiovascular compensation begins to fail. This initiates a cascade of disabling complications collectively termed **heat illness**. Heat cramps, heat exhaustion, and heat stroke constitute the major heat illnesses in order of increasing severity. Heat-related disabilities are more apparent among overweight, unacclimatized, and poorly conditioned individuals, including those who exercise when dehydrated.[37,46,55] No clear-cut demarcation exists between these maladies because symptoms often overlap. When heat illness occurs, immediate action must reduce the heat stress and rehydrate the person until medical help arrives. Table 25.5 summarizes the salient features of the cardiovascular response patterns during three distinct stages of exercise hyperthermia. These stages—compensation, crisis, and failure—apply to heat exhaustion and heat stroke. The response patterns are broadly classified as either central circulatory effects, peripheral effects, or central nervous system effects.

Heat Cramps

Heat cramps (involuntary muscle spasms) occur during or after intense physical activity, usually in the specific muscles exercised. Core temperature often remains within normal range. An imbalance in the body's fluid level and electrolyte concentrations produces this form of heat illness. Sweating also causes electrolyte loss during prolonged heat exposure. Failure to replenish these minerals often leads to muscle pain and spasm, most commonly in the abdomen and extremities. Drinking copious amounts of water and increasing daily salt intake several days before heat stress generally prevents this heat-related malady.

TABLE 25.5 ➤ CARDIOVASCULAR RESPONSES DURING THE THREE STAGES OF EXERCISE HYPERTHERMIA

	Central Circulation		Peripheral	Rectal Temperature	Central Nervous System Status
Compensation	↑ CO ↑ SV, ↑ HR ↓ PV Respiratory alkalosis	↓ Low SPBF ↓ PV	↓ Low TPVR ↑ Skin BF ↑ Muscle BF	37.0°C to 39.5°C	Premonitory signs Dizziness Headache Euphoria Psychoses
Crises	↑↓ CO ↑ MABP ↓ SV ↑↑ HR Tachycardia (180 b · min^{-1}) Metabolic acidosis	↑↓ SPBF ↓ PV Moderate CVP	↓ TPVR ↑↓ Skin BF	39.5°C 41.5°C	Cerebral congestion ↴ Cerebral edema ↴ Intracranial hypertension
Failure	↓↓ CO ↓↓ MABP ↑ HR Tachycardia Metabolic acidosis	↑↑ SPBF (autoregulatory escape); high CVP but low if hypovolemic	↓ TPVR ↓ Low skin BF	41.5°C	Coma, decreased cerebral perfusion ↴ Cerebral ischemia ↴ Neurologic damage, seizures

Data from Hubbard RW, Armstrong LE. The heat illnesses: biochemical, ultrastructural, and fluid-electrolyte considerations. In: Pandolf K et al., eds. Human performance physiology and environmental medicine at terrestrial extremes. Carmel, IN: Cooper Publishing Group, 1994; original data of Kielblock AJ, et al. Cardiovascular origins of heatstroke pathophysiology: an anesthetized rat model. Aviat Space Environ Med 1982:53:171.

Abbreviations: CO, cardiac output; SV, stroke volume; HR, heart rate; SPBF, splanchnic blood flow; PV, plasma volume; TPVR, total peripheral vascular resistance; BF, blood flow; MABP, mean arterial blood pressure; CVP, central venous pressure. ↑ = moderate increase; ↑↑ = strong increase; ↓ = moderate decrease; ↓↓ = strong decrease; ↑↓ = increase then decrease; ↴ = progressing to.

Heat Exhaustion

Heat exhaustion usually develops in unacclimatized people, often during the first heat wave of the summer or with the first hard training session on a hot day. Exercise-induced heat exhaustion probably results from ineffective circulatory adjustments compounded by a depletion of extracellular fluid, principally plasma volume from excessive sweating. Blood usually pools in the dilated peripheral vessels; this drastically reduces the central blood volume necessary to maintain cardiac output. Characteristics of heat exhaustion include a weak and rapid pulse, low blood pressure in the upright position, headache, dizziness, and general weakness. Sweating may decrease somewhat, but core temperature does not rise to dangerous levels (i.e., >40°C or 104°F). A person experiencing heat exhaustion symptoms should stop exercising and move to a cooler environment. Intravenous therapy replenishes fluid most effectively.

Heat Stroke

***Heat stroke**, the most serious and complex of the heat-stress maladies, requires immediate medical attention.* Heat stroke reflects failure of the heat-regulating mechanisms from an excessively high core temperature. The *classic form* of heat stroke—core temperature >105°F, altered mental status, absence of sweating—usually occurs during heat waves. It affects the very young, the elderly, and those with chronic diseases. In classic heat stroke, environmental heat overloads the body's heat-dissipating mechanisms. Severe heat stress also produces a continuum of potentially negative alterations in the immune system and in leukocyte adhesion and activation processes (unrelated to elevated catecholamine levels).[56] One in every three individuals who survive a near-fatal case of classic heat stroke remains permanently disabled with multisystem organ dysfunction.[30]

Exertional heat stroke is a state of extreme hyperthermia from the interactive effects of two factors:

1. Significant metabolic heat load in exercise
2. Challenge for heat dissipation imposed by a hot–humid environment

When thermoregulation fails, sweating diminishes, the skin becomes dry and hot, and body temperature rises to 41.5°C and higher; this places an inordinate strain on cardiovascular function. The often-subtle symptoms compound the complexity of emergency hyperthermia. With intense exercise, usually by young, highly motivated individuals, sweating may progress, but body heat gain greatly overpowers the avenues for heat loss. Other predisposing factors for exertional heat stroke include low physical fitness, obesity, inadequate acclimatization, sweat gland dysfunction, dehydration, and infectious disease. If untreated, the disability progresses rapidly, and death ensues from circulatory collapse and damage to the central nervous system and other organ systems. While the person is awaiting medical treatment, aggressive steps must be taken to lower core temperature, because mortality relates to both the magnitude and duration of hyperthermia. Immediate treatment includes fluid replacement and body cooling through alcohol rubs, application of ice packs, and whole-body immersion in cold or even ice water.[7] Prudent treatment also includes specific drug therapy to counter possible endotoxin effects precipitated by heat stroke pathology.[55]

Oral Temperature Unreliable

Oral temperature inaccurately measures core temperature after strenuous exercise. One report indicated large, consistent differences between oral and rectal temperatures; rectal temperature following a 14-mile race in a tropical climate averaged 103.5°F, while oral temperature remained normal at 98°F![139] Part of the discrepancy lies in the effects on oral temperature of evaporative cooling of the mouth and airways during high levels of exercise pulmonary ventilation.

Summary

1. Core temperature normally increases during exercise; the relative stress of exercise determines the magnitude of the increase. A well-regulated temperature adjustment creates a more favorable environment to maintain normal physiologic and metabolic functions.
2. Excessive sweating compromises fluid reserves, creating a relative state of dehydration. Sweating without fluid replacement decreases plasma volume, which leads to circulatory dysfunction and a precipitous rise in core temperature.
3. Exercise in a hot, humid environment poses a significant thermoregulatory challenge because the large sweat loss in high humidity contributes little to evaporative cooling.
4. Fluid loss of more than 4 to 5% of body weight significantly impedes heat dissipation, compromises cardiovascular function, and diminishes exercise capacity.
5. Adequate fluid replacement maintains plasma volume so circulation and sweating progress optimally. The ideal replacement schedule during exercise matches fluid intake to fluid loss, a process effectively monitored by changes in body weight.
6. The small intestine can absorb about 1000 mL of water each hour. Factors that affect absorption rate include stomach volume and the temperature and osmolality of the oral rehydration beverage. A small amount of electrolytes in the rehydration beverage facilitates fluid replacement more than drinking plain water.
7. The diet generally replaces minerals lost through sweating. With prolonged exercise in the heat, adding a small amount of salt to the replacement fluid (1 tsp $\cdot$ L^{-1}) facilitates sodium replenishment.

8. Repeated heat stress initiates thermoregulatory adjustments that improve exercise capacity and reduce discomfort on subsequent heat exposure. Heat acclimatization triggers favorable cardiac output distribution while increasing sweating capacity. Ten days of heat exposure generally promotes full acclimatization.
9. Aging affects thermoregulatory functions but does not appreciably affect temperature regulation during exercise or acclimatization to moderate heat stress.
10. Women and men show equivalent efficiency in thermoregulation during exercise when controlled for levels of fitness and acclimatization. However, women produce less sweat than men when both exercise at the same core temperature.
11. Heat cramps, heat exhaustion, and heat stroke constitute the major heat illnesses. Heat stroke, a medical emergency, is the most serious and complex of these maladies.
12. Oral temperature after exercising inaccurately measures core temperature. This discrepancy results partly from evaporative cooling of the mouth and airways with relatively high levels of pulmonary ventilation during exercise and recovery.

EXERCISE IN THE COLD

Human exposure to extreme cold produces significant physiologic and psychologic challenges. Cold ranks high among the differing terrestrial environmental stressors for its potentially lethal consequences.[163] In addition to the effects of environmental cold stress per se, core temperature becomes further compromised (with increased susceptibility for hypothermia) during chronic exertional fatigue and sleep loss, inadequate nourishment, reduced tissue insulation, and a blunted shivering heat production.[177]

Water provides an excellent medium to study physiologic adjustment to cold because it conducts heat about 25 times faster than air at the same temperature. Consequently, immersion in cool water of only 28° to 30°C often imposes a thermal stress that rapidly initiates an array of thermoregulatory adjustments. People frequently shiver if they remain inactive in a pool or ocean environment because of a large conductive heat loss to the water. Even when exercising at moderate intensity in cold water, exercise metabolism often generates insufficient heat to counter the large thermal drain. This becomes most notable during swimming, because heat transfer by convection increases significantly with the movement of water past the skin surface.

Light and moderate exercise in cold water produce higher oxygen consumptions and lower body temperatures than identical exercise in warmer water.[26,100,162] For example, swimming at a submaximal pace in a flume at 18°C (64°F) requires 500 mL of oxygen more per minute than swimming at the same speed in 26°C (79°F) water.[114] The additional oxygen consumption directly relates to the added energy cost of shivering because the body attempts to combat heat loss in colder water. Shivering also serves an important role in recovering from hypothermia; it attenuates the typical postexercise decline in core temperature and facilitates core rewarming.[48]

Body Fat, Exercise, and Cold Stress

Differences in body fat content among individuals exert a significant influence on physiologic function in the cold during rest and exercise.[101,102,123,152] Successful ocean swimmers, for example, usually possess a relatively large amount of subcutaneous fat compared with highly trained non-ocean swimmers.[125] The additional fat increases the effective insulation in cold water when peripheral blood diverts from the body's shell to the core. With this advantage, athletes with greater thermal insulation from fat accretion swim in cool ocean water with almost no fall in core temperature. For leaner swimmers, exercise does not generate sufficient heat to offset the heat drain to the water, and the body's core cools.

To a large extent, consider the stress from "cold" as highly relative. The physiologic strain from cold-water and cold-land environments depends not only on environmental temperature, but also on one's level of metabolism and the resistance to heat flow provided by body fat.[128,164] A person with excess body fat who rests comfortably immersed to the neck in 26°C water may sweat about the forehead during vigorous exercise. For this person, 18°C provides a more favorable water temperature for high-intensity exercise. For a lean person, on the other hand, water at 18°C proves debilitating during rest and exercise. An optimum water temperature exists for each person and for each physical activity. For most persons, water temperatures between 26°C (78.8°F) and 30°C (86.0°F) allow effective heat dissipation in sustained exercise without compromising exercise capacity from large deviations in core temperature. Even colder water may optimize performance in shorter-term, near-maximal exercise, particularly for fatter people. For some as yet unexplained reason, older adults do not withstand the challenge of cold during rest and low-intensity exercise as effectively as their younger counterparts with similar aerobic capacities.[41] Perhaps age-related variations in body composition or hormonal functions provide part of the explanation.

Children and Cold Stress

Cold water provides an exceptionally stressful thermoregulatory environment for children. A child's distinctly large ratio of body surface area-to-mass, although facilitating heat loss in a warm environment, becomes a liability during cold stress, as body heat dissipates rapidly. During exercise in the less stressful cold-air environment, children rely on two mechanisms to compensate for their relatively large body surface: (1) augmented energy metabolism and (2) more effective peripheral vasoconstriction in the limbs.[157]

ACCLIMATIZATION TO COLD

Humans possess much less capacity for adaptation to long-term cold exposure than to prolonged heat exposure.[175] Indeed, the basic response of Eskimos and Lapps involves

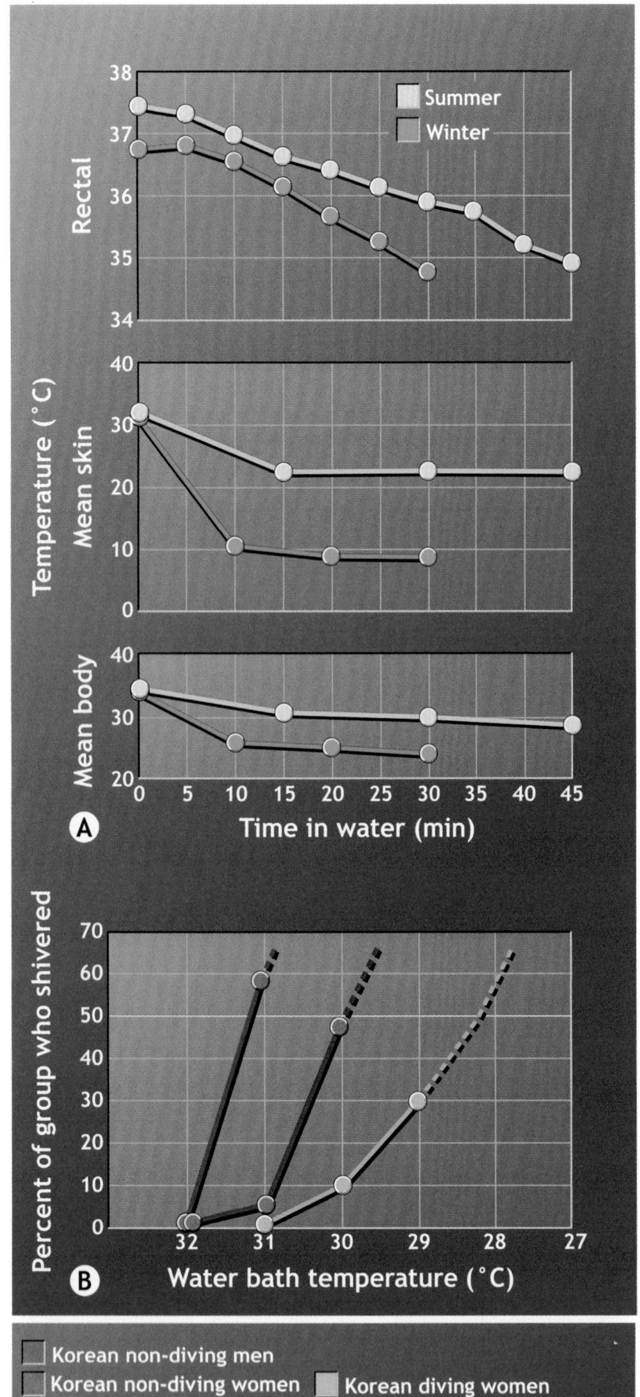

Figure 25.11 • **A**. Differences in rectal temperature, mean skin temperature, and mean body temperature in relation to water temperature during summer and winter in Ama divers upon resurfacing from a dive. (Modified from Kang DH, et al. Energy metabolism and body temperature of the Ama. J Appl Physiol 1965;18:483.) **B**. Shivering response in professional Ama divers compared with that of nondiving Korean men and women at different immersion temperatures. The point at which the lines cross the horizontal line at 50 indicates the water temperature that 50% of a group began to shiver (Modified from Hong SK. Comparison of diving and nondiving women of Korea. Fed Proc 1963;22:831.)

avoiding the cold or minimizing its effects. For example, their clothing provides a near-tropical microclimate, and the temperature inside an igloo generally averages 21°C (70°F).

The Ama

Studies of the **Ama**, the women divers of Korea and southern Japan, indicate some human cold adaptation.[61] These women tolerate daily prolonged exposure to diving for food in cold water that in winter averages 10°C (50°F). During the summer, when water temperature rises to 25°C, the Ama perform three bouts of diving, each about 45 minutes long. In winter, they perform only one 15-minute dive each day. The women generally remain in the water until oral temperature declines to about 34°C (93.2°F). Figure 25.11A shows skin and core temperature responses of the Ama relative to time in the water. Mean skin and mean body temperatures always remained lower during the winter dives. Figure 25.11B shows the relationship between water temperature and the coldest water temperatures when at least 50% of the group started shivering for the Ama and for nondiving Korean women and men. The response curve for the Ama (light blue) shifted to the right, clearly indicating a blunted thermogenic response (higher shivering threshold) until water temperature reached about 28°C. An elevated resting metabolism also may contribute to how the Ama tolerate extreme cold. In winter, resting metabolic rate increased by about 25% compared to nondiving women living in the same country. Interestingly, the Ama and nondiving female counterparts had equivalent body fat percentages. This suggests that circulatory adaptations aid these divers by retarding heat transfer from the core to the skin during cold-water immersion.

Other Examples of Cold Adaptation

A type of general cold adaptation occurs with regular and prolonged cold-air exposure. As a result, heat production does not balance heat loss, and the person regulates at a lower core temperature during cold stress.[82,98] Some peripheral circulatory adaptations also reflect a form of acclimation with severe local cold exposure.[83,84,118] Repeated cold exposure of the hands or feet increases blood flow through these tissues during cold stress. This commonly occurs in fishermen who routinely handle nets and fish in cold water. While this local adaptation actually facilitates heat loss from the periphery, it provides a self-defense because a vigorous circulation of warm blood in exposed tissue thwarts tissue damage from localized hypothermia. Chronic cold exposure may also blunt the typical depression of immune responses with acute cold stress.[78] Although not specifically a form of cold acclimatization, improved physical fitness, as reflected by a high aerobic capacity and relatively large muscle mass, enhances a person's thermoregulatory defense against cold stress. This manifests itself in a larger shivering response and earlier (more sensitive) onset of shivering with cold exposure.[11]

INTEGRATIVE QUESTION

What information contributes to predicting an individual's survival time during extreme cold exposure?

HOW COLD IS TOO COLD?

Cold injuries from overexposure continue to rise because of increased participation by the general population in such outdoor winter activities as ice skating, ice fishing, cross-country skiing, snowboarding, snowmobiling and all-season walking, hiking, jogging, and cycling. Pronounced peripheral vasoconstriction during severe cold exposure can cause the temperature of the skin and the extremities to fall to dangerous levels, particularly when compounded by marked increases in convective and conductive heat loss. Predisposing factors to frostbite include alcohol use, low physical fitness, fatigue, dehydration, and poor peripheral circulation.[131] Early warning signs of cold injury include tingling and numbness in the fingers and toes or a burning sensation in the nose and ears. Overexposure from failure to heed these warning signs can lead to tissue damage as frostbite; in the extreme, irreversible damage occurs that requires surgical removal of the tissue. From military operations and occupational perspectives, application of external heat to the torso *during* cold exposure can overcome the local effects of environmental cold and maintain fingers and toes at a comfortable temperature for up to 3 hours with exposure to −15°C.[14]

In severe cold stress (e.g., near drowning in prolonged cold-water submersion), the brain experiences significant decrements in temperature, which reduce this tissue's oxygen needs. In addition to reduced oxygen requirements from cooling, the central nervous system benefits from a redistribution of blood from tissues that can compromise their supply for relatively long periods of time. Other responses include potential benefits from the mammalian dive reflex (see Chapter 26, p. 662) and possibly cold-induced changes in neurotransmitter release.[47]

INTEGRATIVE QUESTION

Explain the greater likelihood for resuscitation and survival from cold-water drowning than from drowning in warmer water.

The Wind-Chill Index

One dilemma in evaluating the thermal quality of an environment relates to the inadequacy of ambient temperature alone to assess coldness validly. Many of us have experienced the chilling winds of a spring day, even though air temperature remained well above freezing. In contrast, a calm subfreezing day may feel comfortable. *Wind creates the difference—air currents on a windy day magnify heat loss because the warmer insulating air layer surrounding the body continually exchanges with the cooler ambient air.*

The **wind chill index**, presented in Figure 25.12 and used by the National Weather Service since 1973, illustrates the cooling effect of wind on bare skin for different temperatures and wind velocities. For example, a 30°F ambient air reading becomes equivalent to 0°F with a wind speed of 25 mph, while a 10°F reading equals −29°F at the same wind velocity. In addition, if a person runs, skis, or skates into the wind the effective cooling increases directly with the forward velocity. Thus, running at 8 mph into a 12-mph headwind cre-

Wind speed (mph)	Ambient temperature (°F)*															Wind speed (mph)
	40	35	30	25	20	15	10	5	0	-5	-10	-15	-20	-25	-30	
	Equivalent temperature (°F)															
Calm	40	35	30	25	20	15	10	5	0	-5	-10	-15	-20	-25	-30	Calm
5	37	33	27	21	16	12	6	1	-5	-11	-15	-20	-26	-31	-35	5
10	28	21	16	9	4	-2	-9	-15	-21	-27	-33	-38	-46	-52	-58	10
15	22	16	11	1	-5	-11	-18	-25	-36	-40	-45	-51	-58	-65	-70	15
20	18	12	3	-4	-10	-17	-25	-32	-39	-46	-53	-60	-67	-76	-81	20
25	16	7	0	-7	-15	-22	-29	-37	-44	-52	-59	-67	-74	-83	-89	25
30	13	5	-2	-11	-18	-26	-33	-41	-48	-56	-63	-70	-79	-87	-94	30
35	11	3	-4	-13	-20	-27	-35	-43	-49	-60	-67	-72	-82	-90	-98	35
**40	10	1	-6	-15	-21	-29	-37	-45	-53	-62	-69	-76	-85	-94	-101	40**

Little danger   Danger   Great danger

FIGURE 25.12 • The wind-chill index.

ates the equivalent of a 20-mph wind speed. Conversely, running at 8 mph with a 12-mph wind at one's back creates a relative wind speed of only 4 mph. The *yellow-shaded zone in the left of the figure* denotes relatively little danger from cold injury for a properly clothed person. In contrast, in the *orange-shaded zone,* which generally begins at about 22°F, the danger to exposed flesh increases, especially for the ears, nose, and fingers. In the *red-shaded zone,* the equivalent wind-chill temperatures pose serious risk of exposed flesh freezing within minutes.

Perhaps an Exaggeration

Recent assessments by several groups of researchers indicate that the wind-chill index—based on Antarctic expeditions in the 1940s that measured the time that cans of water froze at different temperatures and wind speeds—significantly *overestimates* cold air's effects on human skin. Recently, the National Weather Service reassessed its computer model that calculates the wind-chill index as a public health tool to reduce hypothermia, frostbite, and related cold injuries. Critics maintain that the index does not consider the significant difference between body heat loss in the sun and shade, or the diverse rates of freezing of different areas of the human body. The following is an example from a proposed modification of the wind chill index for an air temperature 10°F above zero relative to current assessments (Fig. 25.12):

PROPOSED MODIFICATION OF WIND CHILL INDEX FOR AIR TEMPERATURE OF 10°F

Wind Speed (mph)	Current Wind Chill	Proposed Wind Chill
5	6	10
10	−9	0
15	−18	−8
20	−25	−14
25	−29	−19
30	−33	−23
35	−35	−26
40	−37	−29

Respiratory Tract During Cold-Weather Exercise

Cold ambient air generally poses no special danger of damaging respiratory passages. Even in extreme cold, incoming air warms to between 26°C and 32°C as it reaches the bronchi, although values as low as 20°C have been observed with breathing large volumes of cold, dry air.[104] Warming an incoming breath of cold air greatly increases its capacity to hold moisture. Thus, humidification of inspired cold air causes a significant water and heat loss from the respiratory tract, chiefly with large ventilatory volumes during exercise. Airway moisture loss during cold-weather exercise contributes to mouth dryness, a burning sensation in the throat, irritation of the respiratory passages, and general dehydration. Wearing a scarf or cellulose mask-type baklava that covers the nose and mouth and traps the water in exhaled air (and warms and moistens the next incoming breath) helps minimize uncomfortable respiratory symptoms.

Summary

1. Water conducts heat about 25 times faster than air; immersion in water of only 28 to 30°C provides considerable thermal stress that initiates rapid thermoregulatory adjustments.
2. Heat production from shivering and physical activity offsets heat flux to a cold environment. Shivering increases the metabolic rate by 3 to 6 METs.
3. Subcutaneous fat provides excellent insulation against cold stress. It greatly enhances the effectiveness of vasomotor adjustments and enables individuals with excess body fat to retain a large percentage of metabolic heat. Enhanced insulation from body fat becomes apparent in cold water, where fatter individuals exhibit less thermal and cardiovascular strain and greater exercise tolerance than leaner counterparts.
4. Individuals exhibit much less physiologic adaptation to chronic cold stress than to prolonged heat exposure. In most instances, appropriate clothing enables humans to tolerate some of the coldest climates on earth.
5. Ambient temperature and wind influence the coldness of an environment. The wind-chill index determines the wind's cooling effect on exposed tissue.
6. Considerable water loss occurs from the respiratory passages during exercise on a cold day, but inspired ambient air temperature generally does not pose a danger to respiratory tract tissues.

References

1. Adams WC, et al. Thermoregulation during marathon running in cool, moderate, and hot environments. J Appl Physiol 1975;38:1030.
2. American College of Sports Medicine. American College of Sports Medicine position stand on prevention of thermal injuries during distance running. Sports Med Bull 1984;19:8.
3. American College of Sports Medicine. American College of Sports Medicine position stand on heat and cold illnesses during distance running. Med Sci Sports Exerc 1996;28(12):1.
4. Anderson RK, Kenney WL. Effect of age on heat-activated sweat gland density and flow during exercise in dry heat. J Appl Physiol 1987;63:1089.
5. Armstrong LE, Pandolf KB. Physical training, cardiorespiratory physical fitness and exercise-heat tolerance. In: Pandolf KB, et al., eds. Human performance physiology and environmental medicine at terrestrial extremes. Indianapolis: Benchmark Press, 1988.
6. Armstrong LE, Maresh CM. Effects of training, environment, and host factors on the sweating response to exercise. Int J Sports Med 1998;19(suppl 2):S103.
7. Armstrong LE, et al. Whole-body cooling of hyperthermic runners: comparison of two field therapies. Am J Emerg Med 1996;14:355.
8. Asmussen E, Bøje O. Body temperature in muscular work. Acta Physiol Scand 1945;10:1.
9. Bar-Or O. Temperature regulation during exercise in children and adolescents. In: Gilsolfi CV, Lamb DR, eds. Perspectives in exercise science and sports medicine, vol 2. Indiana: Benchmark Press, 1989.

10. Bassett DR Jr, et al. Thermoregulatory responses to skin wetting during prolonged treadmill running. Med Sci Sports Exerc 1987;19:28.
11. Bittel JHM, et al. Physical fitness and thermoregulatory reactions in a cold environment. J Appl Physiol 1988;65:1984.
12. Bolster DR, et al. Effects of precooling on thermoregulation during subsequent exercise. Med Sci Sports Exerc 1997;31:251.
13. Booth J, et al. Improved running performance in hot humid conditions following whole body precooling. Med Sci Sports Exerc 1997;29:943.
14. Brajkovic D, et al. Influence of localized auxiliary heating on hand comfort during cold exposure. J Appl Physiol 1998;85:2054.
15. Buono MJ, Sjoholm NT. Effect of physical training on peripheral sweat production. J Appl Physiol 1988;65:811.
16. Burge CM, et al. Rowing performance, fluid balance, and metabolic function following dehydration and rehydration. Med Sci Sports Exerc 1993;25:1358.
17. Caldwell JE, et al. Diuretic therapy, physical performance, and neuromuscular function. Phys Sportsmed 1984;12:73.
18. Charkoudian N, Hohnson JJ. Female reproductive hormones and thermoregulatory control of skin blood flow. Exerc Sport Sci Rev 2000;28:108.
19. Choma CW, et al. Impact of rapid weight loss on cognitive function of collegiate wrestlers. Med Sci Sports Exerc 1998;30:746.
20. Cheung SS, Mclellan TM. Heat acclimation, aerobic fitness, and hydration effects on tolerance during uncompensable heat stress. J Appl Physiol 1998;84:1731.
21. Claremont AD, et al. Heat tolerance following diuretic induced dehydration. Med Sci Sports 1976;8:239.
22. Convertino VA. Blood volume: its adaptation to endurance training. Med Sci Sports Exerc 1991;23:1338.
23. Costill DL, et al. Water and electrolyte replacement during repeated days of work in the heat. Aviat Space Environ Med 1975;46:795.
24. Costill DL, et al. Muscle water and electrolytes following varied levels of dehydration in man. J Appl Physiol 1976;40:6.
25. Coyle EF, Montain SJ. Benefits of fluid replacement with carbohydrate during exercise. Med Sci Sports Exerc 1992;24:S324.
26. Craig AB Jr, Dvorak M. Thermal regulation of man exercising during water immersion. J Appl Physiol 1968;25:28.
27. Craig FN, Cummings EG. Dehydration and muscular work. J Appl Physiol 1966;21:670.
28. Cunningham JJ. Is potassium needed in sports drinks for fluid replacement during exercise? Int J Sport Nutr 1997;7:154.
29. Davy KP, Seals DR. Total blood volume in healthy young and older men. J Appl Physiol 1994;76:2059.
30. Dematte JE, et al. Near-fatal heat stroke during the 1995 heat wave in Chicago. Arch Intern Med 1998;129:173.
31. DeSouza MJ, et al. Menstrual status and plasma vasopressin, renin and aldosterone exercise responses. J Appl Physiol 1989;67:736.
32. Dill DB, et al. Cardiovascular responses and temperature in relation to age. Aust J Sports Med 1975;7:99.
33. Dill DB, et al. Capacity of young males and females for running in desert heat. Med Sci Sports 1977;9:137.
34. Drinkwater BL. Women and exercise: physiological aspects. Exerc Sport Sci Rev. Collomore Press, Lexington MA. 1984.
35. Drinkwater BL, et al. Aerobic power as a factor in women's response to work in hot environments. J Appl Physiol 1976;41:815.
36. Drust B, et al. Investigation of the effects of the precooling on the physiological responses to soccer-specific intermittent exercise. Eur J Appl Physiol 2000;81:11.
37. Eichner ER. Treatment of suspected heat illness. Int J Sports Med 1998;19:S150.
38. Epstein Y, et al. Exertional heat stroke: a case series. Med Sci Sports Exerc 1999;31:224.
39. Falk B, et al. Longitudinal analysis of the sweating response of pre-, mid-, and late-pubertal boys during exercise in the heat. Am J Hum Biol 1992;4:527.
40. Falk B, et al. Thermoregulatory responses of pre-, mid-, and late pubertal boys to exercise in dry heat. Med Sci Sports Exerc 1992;24:688.
41. Falk B, et al. Response to rest and exercise in the cold: effects of age and aerobic fitness. J Appl Physiol 1994;76:72.
42. Febbraio MA, et al. Muscle metabolism during exercise and heat stress in trained men: effect of acclimatization. J Appl Physiol 1994;76:589.
43. Fink WJ, et al. Leg muscle metabolism during exercise in the heat and cold. Eur J Appl Physiol 1975;34:183.
44. Fortney SM, et al. Effect of hyperosmolarity on control of blood flow and sweating. J Appl Physiol 1984;57:1668.
45. Freund BJ, et al. Glycerol hyperhydration: hormonal, renal, and vascular fluid responses. J Appl Physiol 1995;79:2069.
46. Frye AJ, Kamon E. Responses to dry heat of men and women with similar capacities. J Appl Physiol 1981;50:65.
47. Giesbrecht GG. Cold stress, near drowning and accidental hypothermia: a review. Aviat Space Environ Med 2000;71:733.
48. Giesbrecht GG, et al. Inhibition of shivering increases core temperature afterdrop and attenuates rewarming in hypothermic humans. J Appl Physiol 1997;83:1630.
49. Gleeson MR, et al. Comparison of the effects of pre-exercise feeding of glucose, glycerol, and placebo on endurance and fuel homeostasis in man. Eur J Appl Physiol Occup Physiol 1986;55:645.
50. Gonzalez-Alonso JR, et al. Reductions in cardiac output, mean blood pressure and skin vascular conductance with dehydration are reversed when venous return is increased. Med Sci Sports Exerc 1994;26:S163.
51. Gonzalez-Alonso JR, et al. Influence of body temperature on the development of fatigue during prolonged exercise in the heat. J Appl Physiol 1999;86:1032.
52. Gonzalez-Alonso J, et al. Stroke volume during exercise: interaction of environment and hydration. Am J Physiol Heart Circ Physiol 2000;278:H321.
53. Greiwe JS, et al. Effects of dehydration on isometric muscular strength and endurance. Med Sci Sports Exerc 1998;30:284.
54. Hales JRS, et al. Limitation of heat tolerance. In: Fregly MJ, Blatteis CM, eds. Handbook of physiology—environmental physiology. American Physiological Society and Oxford University Press, NewYork, 1996.
55. Hales JRS. Hyperthermia and heat illness: pathological implications for avoidance and treatment. Ann NY Acad Sci 1997;813:534.
56. Hammami MM, et al. Lymphocyte subsets and adhesion molecules expression in heatstroke and heat stress. J Appl Physiol 1998;84:1615.
57. Haymes EM. Physiological responses of female athletes to heat stress: a review. Phys Sportsmed 1984;12:45.
58. Henshel A. Obesity as an occupational hazard. Can J Public Health 1967;58:491.
59. Henshel A. The environment and performance. In: Simonsen E, ed. Physiology of work capacity and fatigue. Springfield, IL: Charles C Thomas, 1971.
60. Hessemer V, Bruck K. Influence of menstrual cycle on thermoregulatory, metabolic, and heart rate responses to exercise at night. J Appl Physiol 1985;59:1902.
61. Hong SK, Rahn H. The diving women of Korea and Japan. Sci Am 1967;216:34.
62. Horstman DH, Christensen E. Acclimatization to dry heat: active men vs. active women. J Appl Physiol 1982;52:825.
63. Inbar O, et al. Conditioning vs. work-in-the-heat as methods for acclimatizing 8–10 year old boys to dry heat. J Appl Physiol Environ Exerc Physiol 1981;50:406.
64. Indner WJ, et al. The effect of glycerol and desmopressin on exercise performance and hydration in triathletes. Med Sci Sports Exerc 1998;30:1263.
65. Inoue Y, et al. Relationship between skin blood flow and sweating rate, and age related regional differences. Eur J Appl Physiol 1998;79:17.
66. Inoue Y, et al. Mechanisms underlying the age-related decrement in the human sweating response. Eur J Appl Physiol 1999;79:121.
67. Irving RA, et al. The immediate and delayed effects of marathon running on renal function. J Urol 1986;136:1176.
68. Jacobs I. The effects of thermal dehydration on performance of the Wingate anaerobic test. Int J Sports Med 1980;1:21.
69. Jacobs I, et al. Thermoregulatory thermogenesis in humans during cold stress. Exerc Sport Sci Rev 1994;22:221.
70. Johnson JM. Physical training and the control of skin blood flow. Med Sci Sports Exerc 1998;30:382.
71. Johnson JM, Proppe DW. Cardiovascular adjustments to heat stress. In: Fregly MJ, Blatteis CM, eds. Handbook of physiology. Sect 4: Environmental physiology, vol 1. New York: Oxford University Press, 1996.
72. Johnson JM, et al. Regulation of the cutaneous circulation. Fed Proc 1986;45:2841.
73. Kay D, et al. Whole-body pre-cooling and heat storage during self-paced cycling performance in warm humid conditions. J Sports Sci 1999;17:937.
74. Kenney WL, Anderson RK. Response of older and younger women in dry and humid heat without fluid replacement. Med Sci Sports Exerc 1988;20:155.
75. Kenney WL, Johnson JM. Control of skin blood flow during exercise. Med Sci Sports Exerc 1992;24:303.

76. Kenney WL, et al. Alpha 1-adrenergic blockage does not alter control of skin blood flow during exercise. Am J Physiol 1991;260:H855.
77. Kenney WL, et al. Decreased active vasodilator sensitivity in aged skin. Am J Physiol 1997;272(Heart Circ Physiol 41):H1605.
78. Kizaki T, et al. Relationship between cold tolerance and generation of suppressor macrophages during acute cold stress. J Appl Physiol 1997;83:1116.
79. Kolka MA, Stephenson LA. Thermoregulation during active and passive heating during the menstrual cycle. (Abstract). Physiologist 1985;28:368.
80. Koenigsberg PS, et al. Sustained hyperhydration with glycerol ingestion. Life Sci 1995;57:645.
81. Latzka WA, et al. Hyperhydration: tolerance and cardiovascular effects during uncompensable heat stress. J Appl Physiol 1998;84:1858.
82. LeBlanc J. Factors affecting cold acclimation and thermogenesis in man. Med Sci Sports Exerc 1988;20:S193.
83. LeBlanc J. Local adaptation to cold of Gaspé fisherman. J Appl Physiol 1962;17:950.
84. Leftheriotis G, et al. Finger and forearm vasodilatory changes after local acclimation. Eur J Appl Physiol 1990;60:49.
85. Luetkemeier MJ, Thomas EL. Hypervolemia and cycling time trial performance. Med Sci Sports Exerc 1994;26:503.
86. Lynch NJ, Nio MA. Effects of menstrual cycle phase and oral contraceptive use on intermittent exercise. Eur J Appl Physiol 1998;78:565.
87. Lyons TP, et al. Effects of glycerol-induced hyperhydration prior to exercise in the heat on sweating and core temperature. Med Sci Sports Exerc 1990;22:477.
88. Mack GW, et al. Body fluid balance in dehydrated healthy older men: thirst and renal osmoregulation. J Appl Physiol 1994;76:1615.
89. Mack GW, et al. Influence of exercise intensity and plasma volume on active cutaneous vasodilatation in humans. Med Sci Sports Exerc 1994;26:209.
90. Martin HL. Maximal skin vascular conductance in subjects aged 5-85 yr. J Appl Physiol 1995;79:297.
91. Mathews DK, et al. Physiological responses during exercise and recovery in a football uniform. J Appl Physiol 1969;26:611.
92. Maugham RF. Fluid and electrolyte loss and replacement in exercise. In: Williams C, Devlin JT, eds. Foods, nutrition and sports performance. London: E & F Spoon, 1992.
93. Maughan RJ, Leiper JB. Fluid replacement requirements in soccer. J Sports Sci 1994;12(special issue):S29.
94. Maughan RJ, Lieper JB. Sodium intake and post-exercise rehydration in man. Eur J Appl Physiol 1995;71:311.
95. Maughan RJ, et al. Rehydration and recovery after exercise. Sports Science Exchange, Gatorade Sports Science Institute, 1996;9(3).
96. Maughan RJ, et al. Restoration of fluid balance after exercise-induced dehydration: effect of food and fluid intake. Eur J Appl Physiol 1996;73:317.
97. Maw GJ, et al. Whole-body hyperhydration in endurance-trained males determined using radionuclide dilution. Med Sci Sports Exerc 1996;28:1038.
98. Maxwell NS, et al. Intermittent running: muscle metabolism in the heat and effect of hypohydration. Med Sci Sports Exerc 1999;31:675.
99. McAllister RM. Adaptations in control of blood flow with training: splanchnic and renal blood flows. Med Sci Sports Exerc 1998;30:375.
100. McArdle WD, et al. Thermal adjustment to cold-water exposure in exercising men and women. J Appl Physiol 1984;56:1572.
101. McArdle WD, et al. Thermal adjustment to cold-water exposure in resting men and women. J Appl Physiol 1984;56:1565.
102. McArdle WD, et al. Thermal responses of men and women during cold-water immersion: influences of exercise intensity. Eur J Appl Physiol 1992;65:265.
103. McCann DJ, Adams WC. Wet bulb globe temperature index and performance in competitive distance runners. Med Sci Sports Exerc 1997;29:955.
104. McFadden ER Jr. Respiratory heat and water exchange: physiological and clinical implications. J Appl Physiol 1984;54:331.
105. Meyer F, et al. Sweat electrolyte loss during exercise in the heat: effects of gender and maturation. Med Sci Sports Exerc 1992;24:776.
106. Minson CT, et al. Age alters the cardiovascular response to direct passive heating. J Appl Physiol 1998;84:1323.
107. Moran DS, et al. Evaluating physiological strain during cold exposure using a new cold strain index. Am J Physiol 1999; 277(2 Pt 2):R556.
108. Montain SJ, Coyle EF. Fluid ingestion during exercise increases skin blood flow independent of increases in blood volume. J Appl Physiol 1992;73:903.
109. Montain SJ, Coyle EF. The influence of graded dehydration on hyperthermia and cardiovascular drift during exercise. J Appl Physiol 1992;73:1340.
110. Montain SJ, et al. Aldosterone and vasopressin responses in the heat: hydration level and exercise intensity effects. Med Sci Sports Exerc 1997;29:661.
111. Montain SJ, et al. Hypohydration effects on skeletal muscle performance and metabolism: a ^{31}P-MRS study. J Appl Physiol 1998;84:1889.
112. Montain SJ, et al. Thermal and cardiovascular strain from hypohydration: influence of exercise intensity. Int J Sports Med 1998;19:87.
113. Murray R, et al. Physiological responses to glycerol ingestion during exercise. J Appl Physiol 1991;71:144.
114. Nadel ER. Thermal and energetic exchanges during swimming. In: Problems with temperature regulation during exercise. New York: Academic Press, 1977.
115. Nadel ER, et al. Thermoregulatory shivering during exercise. Life Sci 1973;13:983.
116. Nadel ER, et al. Effect of hydration state on circulatory and thermal regulation. J Appl Physiol 1980;49:751.
117. Nadel ER, et al. Influence of fluid replacement beverages on body fluid homeostasis during exercise and recovery. In: Gisolfi CV, Lamb DR, eds. Perspectives in exercise science and sports medicine, vol 3. Carmel, IN: Benchmark Press, 1990.
118. Nelms JD, Soper JG. Cold vasodilatation and cold acclimatization in the hands of British fish filleters. J Appl Physiol 1962;17:444.
119. Nielsen B. Olympics in Atlanta: a fight against physics. Med Sci Sports Exerc 1996;28:665.
120. Nielsen B. Heat acclimatization—mechanisms of adaptation to exercise in the heat. Int J Sports Med 1998;19(Suppl 2):S1534.
121. Nielsen B, et al. Acute and adaptive responses to exercise in a warm, humid environment. Pflügers Arch 1997;434:49.
122. Noakes TD. Fluid replacement during exercise. Exerc Sports Sci Rev 1993;21:297.
123. Noakes TD. Exercise and the cold. Ergonomics 2000;43:1461.
124. Pandolf KB, et al. Thermoregulatory responses of middle-aged and young men during dry-heat acclimatization. J Appl Physiol 1988;65:65.
125. Pugh LCGE. A physiological study of channel swimming. J Clin Invest 1960;37:538.
126. Rasch W, Cabanac M. Selective brain cooling is affected by wearing headgear during exercise. J Appl Physiol 1993;74:1229.
127. Rehrer NJ. The maintenance of fluid balance during exercise. Int J Sports Nutr 1996;15:122.
128. Rennie DW. Tissue heat transfer in water: lessons from the Korean divers. Med Sci Sports Exerc 1988;20:S177.
129. Rico-Sanz J, et al. Effects of hyperhydration on total body water, temperature regulation and performance of elite young soccer players in a warm climate. Int J Sports Med 1996;17:85.
130. Riedesel ML, et al. Hyperhydration with glycerol solutions. J Appl Physiol 1987;63:2262.
131. Rintamaki H. Predisposing factors and prevention of frostbite. Int J Circumpolar Health 2000;59:114.
132. Rivera-Brown AM, et al. Drink composition, voluntary drinking and fluid balance in exercising, trained, heat-acclimatized boys. J Appl Physiol 1999;86:78.
133. Robinson S. Training, acclimatization and heat tolerance. Can Med Assoc J 1967;96:795.
134. Robinson S, et al. Acclimatization of older men to work in the heat. J Appl Physiol 1965;20:583.
135. Rolls BJ, et al. Thirst following water deprivation in humans. Am J Physiol 1980;239(Regul Integrat Comp Physiol 8):476.
136. Rooke GA, et al. Maximal skin blood flow is decreased in elderly men. J Appl Physiol 1994;77:11.
137. Rowell LB. Human cardiovascular control. Cary, NC: Oxford University Press, 1994.
138. Roy ML, et al. Effect of sodium in a rehydration beverage when consumed as a fluid or meal. J Appl Physiol 1998;85:1329.
139. Rozycki TJ. Oral and rectal temperatures in runners. Phys Sportsmed 1984;12:105.
140. Sakurada S, Hales JR. A role for gastrointestinal endotoxins in enhancement of heat tolerance by physical fitness. J Appl Physiol 1998;84:207.
141. Saltin B, Hermansen L. Esophageal, rectal and muscle temperature during exercise. J Appl Physiol 1966;21:1757.
142. Sawka MN. Physiological consequences of hypohydration: exercise performance and thermoregulation. Med Sci Sports Exerc 1992;24:657.

143. Sawka MN, Coyle EF. Influence of body water and blood volume on thermoregulation and exercise performance in the heat. Exerc Sport Sci Rev 1999;27:167.
144. Sawka MN, Wegner CB. Physiological responses to acute-exercise heat stress. In: Pandolf KB, et al., eds. Human performance physiology and environmental medicine at terrestrial extremes. Indianapolis, IN: Benchmark Press, 1988.
145. Sawka MN, et al. Influence of hydration level and body fluids on exercise performance in the heat. JAMA 1984;252:1165.
146. Sawka MN, et al. Hydration effects on temperature regulation. Int J Sports Med 1998;19(suppl 2):S108.
147. Scott JR, et al. Acute weight gain in collegiate wrestlers following a tournament weigh-in. Med Sci Sports Exerc 1994;26:1181.
148. Sheffield-Moore M, et al. Thermoregulatory responses to cycling with and without a helmet. Med Sci Sports Exerc 1997;29:755.
149. Shi X, et al. Effects of carbohydrate type and concentration and solution osmolality on water absorption. Med Sci Sports Exerc 1995;27:1607.
150. Shibasaki M, et al. Mechanisms of underdeveloped sweating responses in prepubertal boys. Eur J Appl Physiol 1997;76:340.
151. Shimizv T, et al. Human thermoregulatory responses during prolonged walking in age at 25, 30, and 35°C. Eur J Appl Physiol 1998;78:473.
152. Shiraki K, Claybaugh JR. Effects of diving and hyperbaria on responses to exercise. Exerc Sport Sci Rev 1995;23:459.
153. Shirreffs SM, Maughan RJ. The effect on alcohol consumption on fluid retention following exercise-induced dehydration in man. J Physiol 1995;489:33P.
154. Shirreffs SM, Maughan RJ. The effect of alcohol consumption on the restoration of blood and plasma volume following exercise-induced dehydration in man. J Physiol 1996;491:64P.
155. Shirreffs SM, Maughan RJ. Restoration of fluid balance after exercise-induced dehydration: effects of alcohol consumption. J Appl Physiol 1997;83:1152.
156. Shirreffs SM, Maughan RJ. Rehydration and recovery of fluid balance after exercise. Exer Sport Sci Rev 2000;1:27.
157. Smolander J, et al. Thermoregulation during rest and exercise in the cold in pre- and early-pubescent boys and young men. J Appl Physiol 1992;72:1589.
158. Stephenson LA, Kolka MA. Thermoregulation in women. Exerc Sport Sci Rev 1993;21:231.
159. Stephenson LA, Kolka MA. Effect of gender, circadian period and sleep loss on thermal responses during exercise. In: Pandolf KB, et al., eds. Human performance physiology and environmental medicine at terrestrial extremes. Carmel, IN: Cooper Publishing, 1994.
160. Tankersley GG, et al. Sweating and skin blood flow during exercise: effects of age and maximal oxygen uptake. J Appl Physiol 1991;71:230.
161. Tikuisis P, et al. Physiological responses of exercise-fatigued individuals exposed to wet-cold conditions. J Appl Physiol 1999;86:1319.
162. Toner MM, McArdle WD. Physiological adjustments of a man to cold. In: Pandolf KB, et al., eds. Human performance physiology and environmental medicine at terrestrial extremes. Carmel, IN: Cooper Publishing, 1988.
163. Toner MM, McArdle WD. Human thermoregulatory responses to acute cold stress with special reference to water immersion. In: Fregly MJ, Blatteis CM, eds. Handbook of physiology. Sect 4: Environmental physiology, vol 1. New York: Oxford University Press, 1996.
164. Toner MM, et al. Thermal responses during arm and leg and combined arm-leg exercise in water. J Appl Physiol 1984;56:1355.
165. U.S. Department of Health and Human Services. Hyperthermia and dehydration-related deaths associated with intentional weight loss in three collegiate wrestlers—North Carolina, Wisconsin, and Michigan, November-December, 1997. MMWR 1998;47:105.
166. Wapnir PA, et al. Enhancement of intestinal water absorption and sodium transport by glycerol in rats. J Appl Physiol 1996;81:2523.
167. Wailgum TD, Palone AM. Heat tolerance of college football linemen and backs. Phys Sportsmed 1984;12:81.
168. Wegner CB. Human heat acclimatization. In: Pandolf KB, et al., eds. Human performance physiology and environmental medicine at terrestrial extremes. Indianapolis, IN: Benchmark Press, 1988.
169. Weller A, et al. Physiological responses to a cold, wet, and windy environment during prolonged intermittent walking. Am J Physiol 1997;272(Regul Integrat Comp Physiol 41):R226.
170. Widerman PM, Hagen RD. Body weight loss in a wrestler preparing for competition: a case study. Med Sci Sports Exerc 1982;14:413.
171. Wilk B, Bar-Or O. Effect of drink flavor and NaCl on voluntary drinking and hydration in boys exercising in the heat. J Appl Physiol 1996;80:1112.
172. Wilmore JH, et al. Role of taste preference on fluid intake during and after 90 min of running at 60% of $\dot{V}O_{2max}$ in the heat. Med Sci Sports Exerc 1998;30:587.
173. Yankanich J, et al. Precompetition weight loss and changes in vascular fluid volume in NCAA division I college wrestlers. J Strength Cond Res 1998;12:138.
174. Yoshida E, et al. Relationship between aerobic power, blood volume, and thermoregulatory responses to exercise-heat stress. Med Sci Sports Exerc 1997;29:867.
175. Young AJ. Human adaptation to cold. In: Pandolf KB, et al., eds. Human performance physiology and environmental medicine at terrestrial extremes. Indianapolis: Benchmark Press, 1988.
176. Young AJ. Energy substrate utilization during exercise in extreme environments. Exerc Sport Sci Rev 1990;18:65.
177. Young AJ, et al. Exertional fatigue, sleep loss, and negative energy balance increase susceptibility to hypothermia. J Appl Physiol 1998;85:1210.
178. Zambraski EJ, et al. Iowa wrestling study: weight loss and urinary profiles of collegiate wrestlers. Med Sci Sports 1976;8:105.

CHAPTER 26

Sport Diving

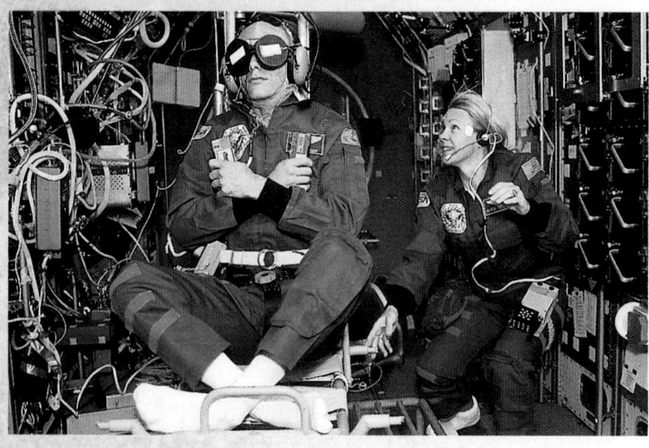

Chapter Objectives

- Outline the chronology of historical milestones in diving from antiquity to present
- Quantify, with examples, the relationship between depth under water and gas pressure and volume
- Discuss the rationale for snorkel size and the underwater depth for its use
- Describe factors that limit the depth of a breath-hold dive
- Describe the effects of hyperventilation on breath-hold duration, and potential risks of using this maneuver before diving
- Outline evidence that supports a "diving reflex" in humans
- Describe open-circuit and closed-circuit scuba systems
- List causes, symptoms, and treatment of air embolism, lung burst, pneumothorax, mask squeeze, aerotitis, nitrogen narcosis, decompression sickness, and oxygen poisoning
- Discuss the decompression schedule for diving with compressed air in terms of its purpose and factors that influence it
- Outline the rationale for saturation diving, and describe the environment where the diver lives for prolonged dives to exceptional depths
- Give reasons for using helium–oxygen breathing mixtures and the limitations to deep diving under such conditions
- Describe the closed-circuit, mixed-gas system used by the U.S. Navy in technical diving

An estimated 5 million scuba divers work and recreate in the United States, with an additional 200,000 divers trained each year. The sections below outline general principles of diving, including potential dangers as a person descends and ascends beneath the water. Unquestionably, safe diving requires thorough knowledge of diving physics and physiology. We emphasize the relationships among diving depth, pressure, and gas volume and the potentially toxic effects of various gases breathed in diving.[3,6,11,33,34]

DIVING HISTORY—ANTIQUITY TO THE PRESENT

Men and women have practiced breath-hold diving for centuries as they hunted for sponges and food, salvaged artifacts and treasures, repaired ships, observed marine life, and participated in military maneuvers. The 5th century historian Herodotus tells of the underwater exploits of the Greek patriot Scyllias against the Persians. When Scyllias, taken as prisoner aboard ship, learned that Xerxes planned to attack a Greek flotilla, he escaped by jumping overboard. The Persians presumed he had drowned. To the contrary, Scyllias used a hollow reed as a snorkel and remained undiscovered, surfacing at night to cut each enemy ship loose from its moorings, saving the Greek Navy from sure disaster. Understandably, each dive could last only a few minutes until the discovery of how to remain underwater for longer durations. Using longer "snorkels" did not work because the diver could not inhale against water pressure at depths greater than several feet. Rebreathing from an air-filled bag submerged under water also failed because the buildup of exhaled carbon dioxide caused the diver to lose consciousness.

The first solutions to these problems took place in the 1530s with the invention of diving bells supplied with surface air. The bell, positioned a few feet from the surface, had its bottom open to water with its top portion containing air compressed by water pressure. A diver in the bell with his head surrounded by air could then hold his breath, swim from the bell for a minute or two, and return for a short while, repeating the process until the air remaining in the bell became toxic.

In England and France in the16th century, diving suits made of leather allowed descent to depths up to 60 feet. Manual pumps delivered fresh air from the surface to the diver. Soon metal helmets could withstand greater water pressures, and divers could descend much further. By the 1830s, perfection of the surface-supplied air helmet allowed extensive underwater salvage work.

Starting in the 19th century, two main avenues of investigation—one scientific and the other technologic—accelerated underwater exploration. Two scientists, Paul Bert and John Scott Haldane, explained the physiologic effects of water pressure on body tissues and also defined safe limits for compressed air diving. Technological improvements with compressed air pumps, carbon dioxide scrubbers, and demand-valve regulators allowed prolonged underwater explorations.

Chronology of Selected Events in Diving History

4500 BC Archeologists unearth shells in Mesopotamia dated to this period that must have originated from the sea floor.

3200 BC Archeologists discover mother-of-pearl (abalone) shell ornaments dated to this period from the Egyptian Theban VI Dynasty.

2500 BC Greek divers make sponges widely available in commerce; *The Illiad* and *The Odyssey* mention diving and sponges.

550 BC Pearl diving documented in India and Ceylon.

500 BC Scyllias demonstrates the practical use of breath-hold diving in military exploits against the Persian Navy.

100 BC The Ama, Japan's women breath-hold divers of antiquity and modern times (see Chapter 24), gather pearl oysters, shellfish, and edible seaweed.

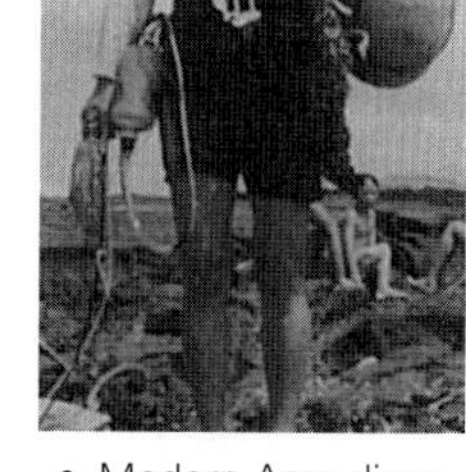

• Modern Ama diver.

1500 da Vinci designs the first "snorkel" device and dive fins for the hands and feet.

1530 Invention of the first diving bell.

1650 First effective air pump developed by Von Guericke, which Robert Boyle makes use of in compression and decompression experiments with animals.

1667 Physicist Robert Boyle makes first recorded observation of decompression sickness or "the bends" by documenting a gas bubble in the eye of a viper that had been compressed and then decompressed.

1690 Sir Edmund Halley (of comet fame) patents a practical diving bell (led-coated wood with glass at the top to allow light to enter), 60 cubic feet (1.7 m^3) in volume connected by a pipe to weighted barrels of air replenished from the surface; permits dives to 60 feet for 90 minutes.

1715 John Lethbridge's constructs his "diving engine" built from an oak cylinder and supplied with compressed surface air. The diver remained submerged for 30 minutes at 60 feet while protruding his arms (sealed by greased leather cuffs) into the water for salvage work.

1776 First confirmed submarine battle; David Bushnell's American *Turtle* against the H.M.S Eagle (British) in New York harbor.

1788 John Smeaton's popular diving bell uses a hand pump to supply fresh surface air and a one-way valve to prevent air from returning to the pump when it stops.

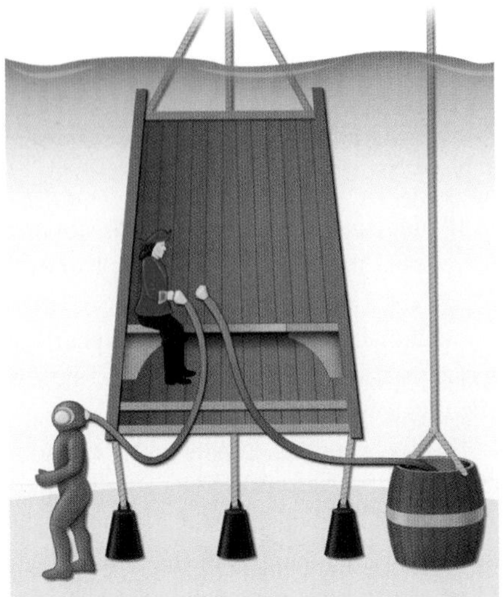

• Halley's diving bell used weighted barrels of air to replenish the bell's atmosphere (late 17th century).

1808 Freiderich von Drieberg invents a bellows-in-a-box device (named Triton) worn on the diver's back, which delivers compressed air from the surface. The device never worked successfully, but nonetheless suggested compressed air could be used in diving, an idea conceived by Halley in the late 1690s.

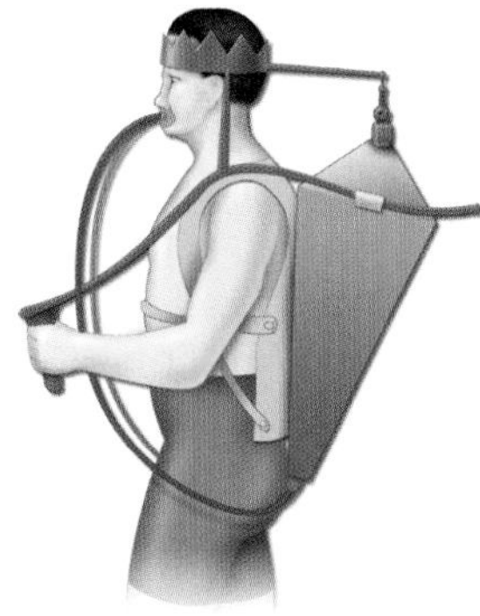

• Triton diving apparatus invented by von Drieberg

1823 "Smoke helmet" patented by Charles Anthony Deane for fighting structural fires. Later modified for diving, the helmet fastened over the head with weights and received surface air through a hose. In 1828, Charles and his brother John market the helmet with a loosely attached "diving suit" so the diver could perform salvage work but only in the full vertical position to prevent water from entering the suit.

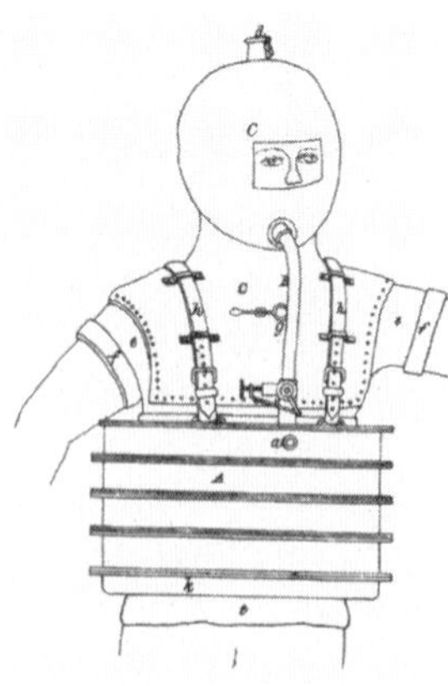

• James' first practical self-contained diving apparatus comprised of copper or leather helmet with a glass plate window attached to a waterproof tunic sealed at the waist and wrists by "elastic bandages."

1825 First prototype for scuba invented by William James incorporates a cylindrical belt (air reservoir) around the diver's trunk that supplies air at 450 psi to a helmet by a hand operated valve and rubber tube. The diver inhales through the nose and exhales through a mouthpiece connected by a short tube to an escape valve in the helmets' crown. With the reservoir charged to 30 atmospheres, James believed a diver would have enough air to last approximately 60 minutes.

1837 Augustus Siebe, the father of diving, seals the Deane brothers' diving helmet to the waist-length jacket to create a full, watertight rubber suit that received surface air. This suit served as the forerunner for modern hardhat diving gear.

1839 Seibe's diving suit used during salvage of the British warship *HMS Royal George* sunk in 1782 to a depth of 65 feet; divers reported the first symptoms of decompression sickness.

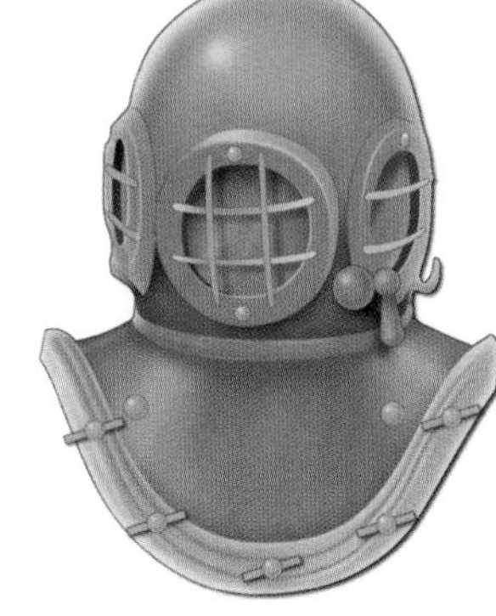

• Siebe's early diving suit

1843 From the experience salvaging the *HMS Royal George*, the British Royal Navy establishes the first diving school.

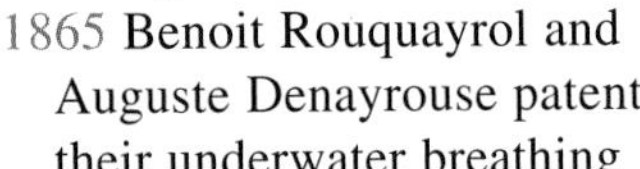

1865 Benoit Rouquayrol and Auguste Denayrouse patent their underwater breathing apparatus ("aerophore") consisting of a steel tank of compressed air (250–350 psi) worn on the back connected through an automatic demand valve to a mouthpiece. This forerunner of modern scuba enables the diver to disconnect from a tether that supplies surface air and swim freely with the tank for several minutes.

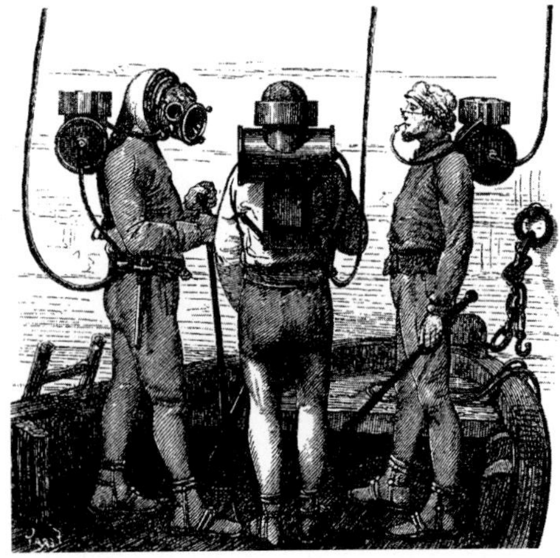

• Aerophore SCUBA apparatus patented in 1865 by Benoit Rouquayrol and Auguste Denayrouse.

1873 Dr. Andrew H. Smith, surgeon to the New York Bridge Company (builders of the Brooklyn Bridge), reports about bends in workers who leave their pressurized caisson. Smith recommends chamber recompression for future projects, but does not mention nitrogen bubbles as the cause of decompression sickness.

1878 First self-contained diving apparatus developed by Henry A. Fleus uses compressed oxygen (not compressed air). Rope soaked in caustic potash absorbs carbon dioxide so the diver can rebreathe exhaled air without bubbles entering the water. The apparatus provides divers up to three hours of "bottom time."

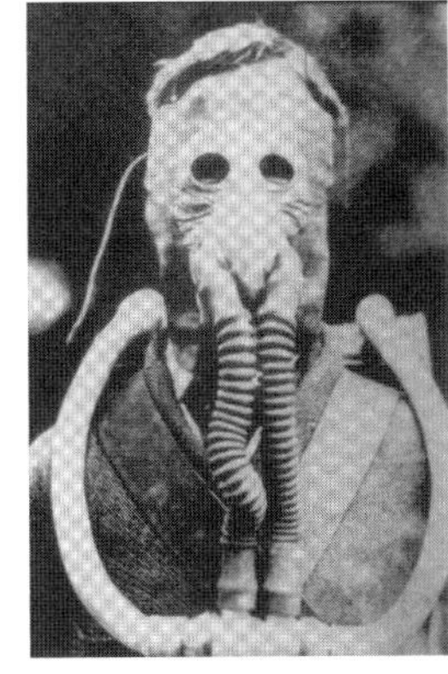

• Fleuss first practicable self-contained diving apparatus using the closed circuit principle.

1878 Paul Bert publishes *La Pression Barometrique,* which describes physiologic studies of pressure changes. Bert proves that nitrogen gas bubbles cause decompression sickness (the "bends" or caisson disease), gradual ascent prevents the problem, and recompression relieves pain.

1908. John Haldane, Arthur Boycott, and Guybon Damant publish "The Prevention of Compressed-Air Illness," a landmark paper that describes staged decompression to combat decompression sickness. Based on this work, the British Royal Navy and United States Navy develop diving tables for compressed air diving up to 200 feet deep.

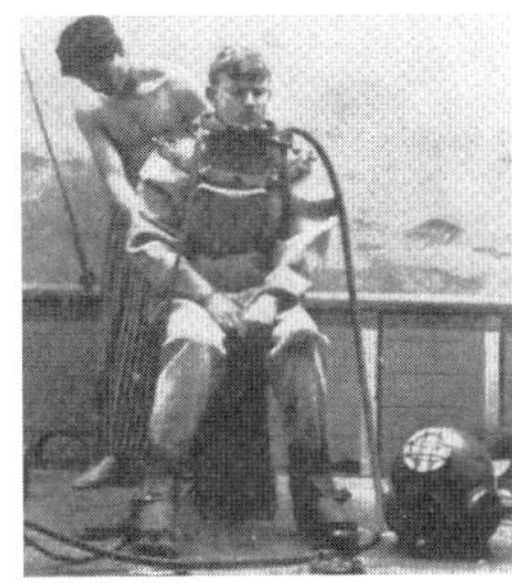

• Pearl deep sea diver (circa 1896).

1912 Sir Robert Davis designs the first pressurized submersible decompression chamber.

1917 The U.S. Bureau of Construction and Repair first introduces the Mark V diving helmet, which revolutionizes salvage operations in World War II.

1920s U.S. researchers experiment with helium–oxygen mixtures for deep dives.

1924 The U.S. Navy and Bureau of Mines conduct the first experiments with helium–oxygen mixtures.

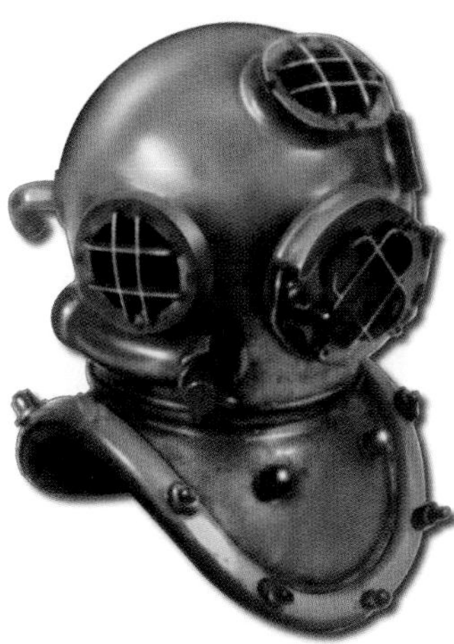

• U.S. Navy Mark V diving helmet

1930 William Beebe and Otis Barton descend 1426 feet in a 4'9" bathysphere attached to a barge by a steel cable.

1930s Guy Gilpatric pioneers use of rubber goggles with glass lenses for skin diving. By the mid-1930s, face masks, fins, and snorkels are in common use.

1933 French Navy captain Yves Le Prieur modifies the Rouquayrol-Denayrouse "aerophore" by combining a new demand valve with a 1500 psi high-pressure air tank without a regulator to eliminate restricting effect of hoses and lines. The diver breathes fresh air by opening a tap, while exhaled air escapes under the edge of the diver's mask.

1934 William Beebe and Otis Barton descend 3028 feet in a bathysphere near Bermuda, setting a depth record that remained until 1948.

1935 French navy adopts Le Prieur's scuba.

1936 Le Prieur establishes the world's first scuba diving club, called the "Club of Divers and Underwater Life."

1938 Edgar End and Max Nohl make the first intentional saturation "dive" in a Milwaukee hospital hyperbaric chamber (27 hr at a101-ft depth). Decompression takes 5 hours, and Nohl suffers the bends.

1939 A new diving bell, the McCann-Erickson Rescue Chamber, makes the first successful rescue of men aboard the submarine *USS Squalus*, a new 310-foot submarine sunk in 243 feet of water in the North Atlantic. The chamber fits over the submarine's escape hatch, which four men at a time entered under one atmosphere of pressure.

1941-1944 Italian divers, working out of midget submarines during World War II, use closed-circuit scuba to place explosives under British naval and merchant marine vessels. The British adopt this technology to sink the German battleship *Tirpitz.*

1942-43 Jacques-Yves Cousteau (French naval lieutenant) and Emile Gagnan (engineer for a Parisian natural gas company) redesign a car regulator to supply compressed air to a diver on initiation of a breathing cycle. They attach their new demand valve regulator to hoses, a mouthpiece, and a pair of compressed air tanks, which they patent as the *Aqua Lung*. Frederic Dumas descends to 210 feet in the Mediterranean Sea and experiences *l'ivresse des grandes profondeurs* —the rapture of the great depths. Cousteau achieves worldwide acclaim for

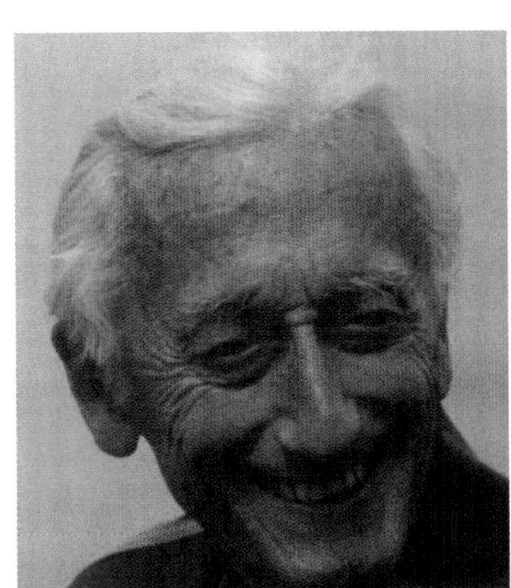

• Top left. Captain Jacques Cousteau (1910-1997); Bottom left. First AquaLung dive in the Marne River. Bottom right. 1943 Cousteau-Gagnan regulator.

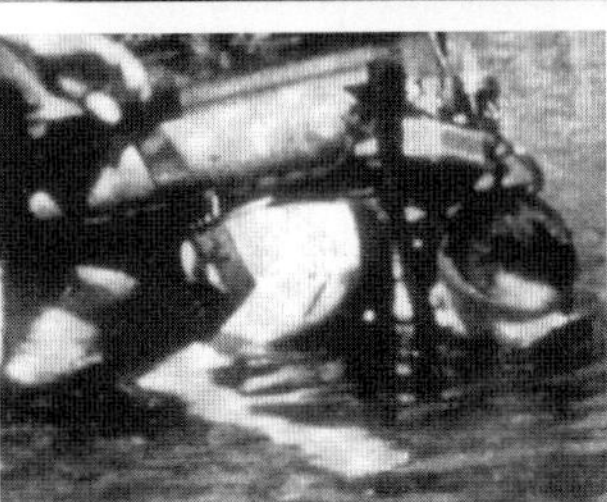

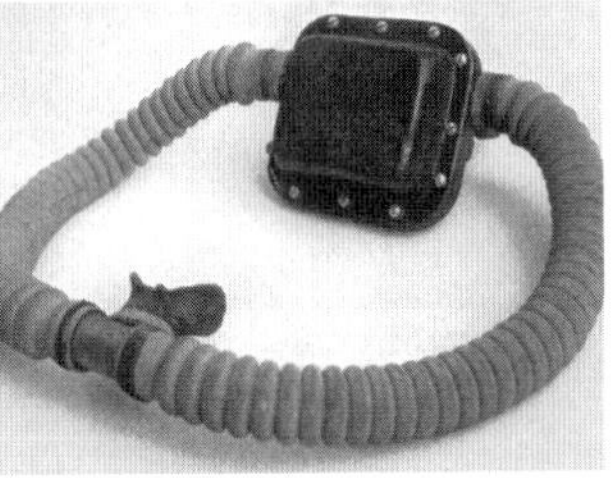

his underwater explorations, movies, books, and dedication to environmental causes <www.cousteau.org/>.

1947 Frederic Dumas uses the Aqua Lung and dives to 94 m (307 ft) in the Mediterranean Sea.

1948 Otis Barton descends in a modified bathysphere to 1370 m (4500 feet) off the coast of California.

1950s Augus and Jaquet Picard develop the bathyscaphe (deep boat), a completely self-contained vessel. In 1954, the bathyscaphe sets a diving record of 4050 m (13,287 ft).

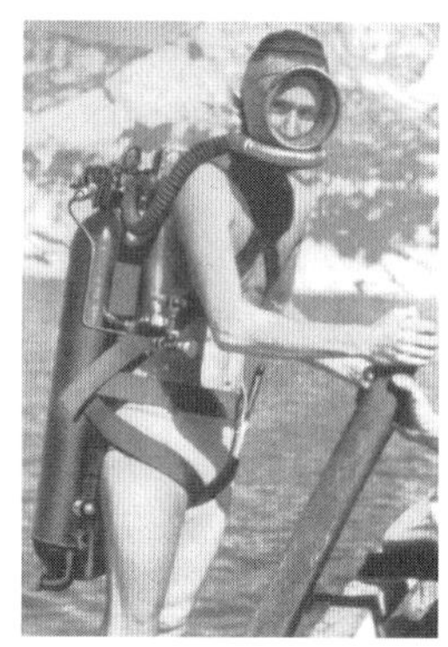

• Dumas with the 1943 AquaLung Costeau-Gagnan unit. Note the waist level control valve.

1959 The YMCA begins the first nationally organized course for scuba certification.

1960 Jacques Picard and Don Walsh descend to approximately 35,820 ft (10,916 m, 6.78 miles; water pressure 16,883 psi, temperature 37.4°F) in the August Picard-designed, Swiss-built, U.S. Navy-owned bathyscaphe *Trieste* in the Pacific Ocean to the bottom of the Mariana Trench (deepest known seafloor depression on earth)

1960s As accident rates for scuba divers climb, the first national agencies form to train and certify divers; NAUI (National Association of Underwater Instructors) forms in 1960, and PADI (Professional Association of Diving Instructors) forms in 1966.

1962 Albert Falco and Claude Wesley spend seven days under 10 m (33 ft) of water near Marseilles in an underwater-living habitat named *Diogenes*.

1963–1965 Divers live and work in underwater habitats for a month at a time at 60 m.

1968 John J. Gruener and R. Neal Watson dive to 133 m breathing compressed air.

1970s Implementation of diving safety standards including the following: certification cards to indicate a minimum training level and as a requirement for tank refills, change from J-valve reserve systems to non-reserve K valves, adoption of submersible pressure gauges, and use of the buoyancy compensator and single-hose regulators.

1980 Divers Alert Network founded at Duke University as a nonprofit organization to promote safe diving.

1981 Record 686-m (2250-ft) "dive" is made in a Duke Medical Center chamber. Stephen Porter, Len Whitlock, and Erik Kramer live in the 8-foot chamber for 43 days, breathing a nitrogen, oxygen, and helium mixture.

1983 Introduction of the first commercially available dive computer (Orca Edge).

1985 Robert Ballard (www.ife.org) and Ralph White use a remote controlled camera to explore the wreck of the *Titanic* (12,500 ft- or 3810-m depth).

1990s. Estimated 500,000 new scuba divers certified yearly in the United States as this activity's popularity increases for recreational and commercial purposes.

PRESSURE–VOLUME RELATIONSHIPS AND DIVING DEPTH

Diving Depth and Pressure

Water remains essentially noncompressible owing to its high density. Consequently, its pressure against a diver's body increases directly with the depth of the dive. Two forces produce increased external pressure (**hyperbaria**) in diving: (1) weight of the column of water directly above the diver (hydrostatic pressure) and (2) weight of the atmosphere (*ata*, or *bar*) at the water's surface. Table 26.1 shows that a column of sea water exerts a force of 1 sea-level ata (760 mm Hg, or 14.7 lb per in^2 [*psi*]) for each 33-feet (10-m) descent below the water's surface. Because fresh water is less dense than sea water, a depth of approximately 34 feet corresponds to 1 ata in fresh-water diving. Thus, a dive to 33 feet in sea water exposes the diver to a pressure of 2 ata—1 ata from the weight of ambient air at the surface and the other from the weight of the column of water itself. Diving from sea level to 66 feet (20 m) exposes a diver to an absolute external pressure of 3 ata; the pressure is 4 ata at 99 feet (30 m), and so on. Clearly,

TABLE 26.1 ➤ RELATIONSHIP OF DEPTH IN WATER TO PRESSURE AND GAS VOLUME

Depth		Pressure		Hypothetical Lung Volume	Inspired Air (mm Hg)	
FT	M	ATM	MM HG	(ML)	Po_2	PN_2
Sea level		1	760	6,000	159	600
33	10	2	1,520	3,000	318	1,201
66	20	3	2,280	2,000	477	1,802
99	30	4	3,040	1,500	636	2,402
133	40	5	3,800	1,200	795	3,003
166	50	6	4,560	1,000	954	3,604
200	60	7	5,320	857	1,113	4,204
300	90	10	7,600	600	1,590	6,006
400	120	13	9,880	461	2,068	7,808
500	150	16	12,160	375	2,545	9,610
600	180	19	14,440	316	3,022	11,412

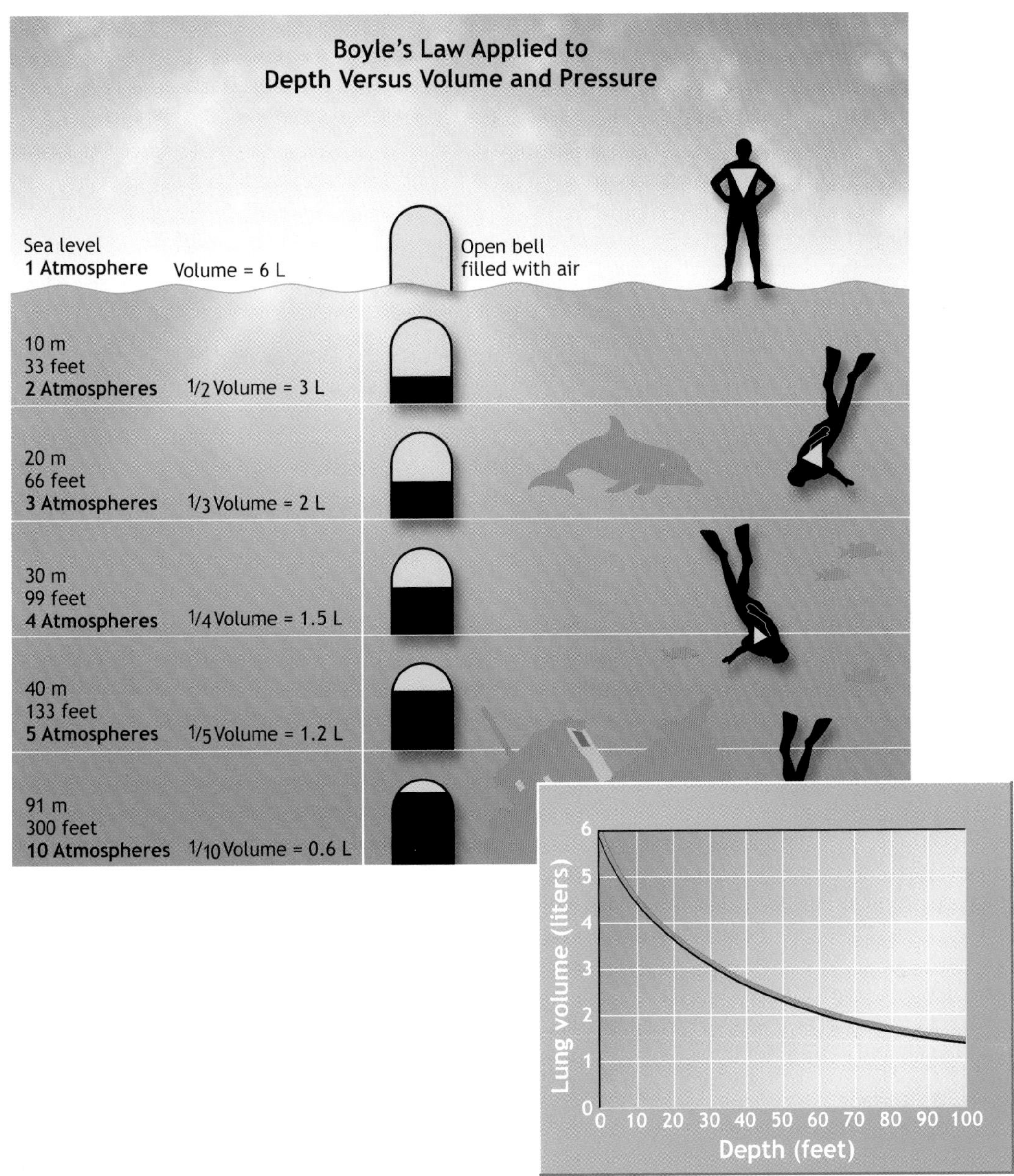

FIGURE 26.1 • Any gas volume varies inversely with the pressure acting upon it. A 6-L volume, whether in an open bell or in the flexible thoracic cavity, compresses to 3 L in 33 feet (10 m) of seawater (fsw) because of a doubling of the external water pressure. At 99 fsw, or 4 ata, the gas decreases to 25% of its original volume, or 1.5 L. The *inset figure* graphically illustrates the curvilinear relation between lung volume at the surface and depth in sea water. The volume change per unit depth change is greatest nearest the water's surface.

considerable external pressure accrues when diving relatively short distances below the surface.

Water constitutes a significant portion of the body's tissues, so they too remain incompressible and not particularly susceptible to the increased external pressure during diving. The body also contains air-filled cavities—notably the lungs, respiratory passages, and sinus and middle ear spaces. Volume and pressure in these cavities change considerably with any increase or decrease in diving depth.[5,42] *Pain, injury, and even death occur unless adjustments equalize the rapid and significant changes in pressure that occur in a hyperbaric environment.*

Diving Depth and Gas Volume

Boyle's law *states that at constant temperature, the volume of a given mass of gas varies inversely with its pressure.* When pressure doubles, the volume halves; conversely, reducing the pressure by one-half expands the volume of any gas to twice its previous size. Figure 26.1 (and Table 26.1) shows that if divers fills their lungs with 6 L of air at the surface and then descend to 10 m, the lung volume compresses to 3 L. Diving an additional 10 m to a depth of 20 m (external pressure now 3 ata) reduces the original 6-L lung volume by two-thirds, to 2 L. At 91 m (300 ft), the lung volume compresses to approximately 0.6 L simply from the compressive force of water against the air-filled thoracic cavity. For most individuals, any further increase in diving depth reduces the pulmonary air volume to an extent that seriously damages the chest wall and lung tissue. As the diver returns to the surface, the air volume reexpands to its *original* 6-L volume. For the scuba diver who breathes pressurized air beneath the water, a 6-L lung volume at a 10-m depth expands to 12 L at the water's surface; this 6-L volume at 50-m depth occupies 36 L at sea-level pressure. Failure to permit this "extra" air volume to escape through the nose or mouth during ascent ruptures lung tissue from the powerful force of expanding gases.

SNORKELING AND BREATH-HOLD DIVING

Swimming at the water's surface with fins, mask, and snorkel is a common form of recreation and sport for activities like spear fishing and exploring shallow areas of clear water. A J-shaped tube, or **snorkel**, allows the swimmer to breathe continually with the face immersed in water. The swimmer periodically takes a full breath of air and dives to explore beneath the water's surface. After about 30 seconds, the carbon dioxide level in arterial blood increases causing the diver to sense the need to breathe and surface quickly. Snorkeling is essentially an extension of swimming, limited entirely by the swimmer's breath-holding ability.

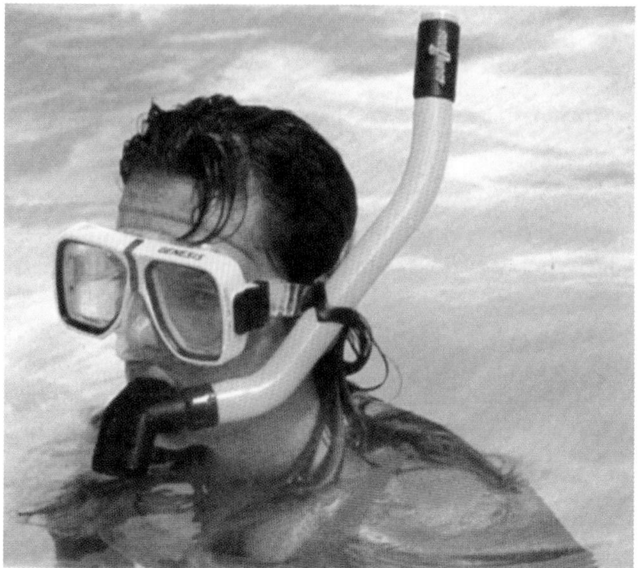
Basic tools for snorkeling and breath-hold diving.

Limits to Snorkel Size

Novice skin divers often speculate that if only the snorkel were longer they could swim deeper in the water and still breathe ambient air through the top of the snorkel. Some beginners believe they can sit at a pool bottom and breathe through a garden hose extending up to the pool deck! Although the idea of a longer snorkel seems intriguing, two factors limit snorkel length and volume:

1. Increased hydrostatic pressure on the chest cavity as one descends beneath the water
2. Increased pulmonary dead space by enlarging the snorkel's volume

Inspiratory Capacity and Diving Depth

When breathing through a snorkel, the diver inspires air at atmospheric pressure. At a depth of about 3 feet (1 m), the compressive force of water against the chest cavity becomes so large that the inspiratory muscles can no longer overcome external pressure and expand thoracic dimensions. This makes inspiration impossible without air at sufficient pressure to counter the compressive force of water at the particular depth. This forms the basis for scuba, which we discuss on page 660 of this chapter.

Snorkel Size and Pulmonary Dead Space

In Chapter 12 we discussed that not all inspired air enters the alveoli. Approximately 150 mL of each breath fills the nose, mouth, and other nondiffusible portions of the respiratory tract. The snorkel, an extension of the airways, adds to the volume of the anatomic dead space. Consequently, the ideal snorkel averages about 15 inches (38 cm) in length, with an inside diameter of five-eighths to three-quarters of an inch to minimize the effects of added dead space and resistance to breathing.[37] Any further increase in snorkel size (volume) significantly increases anatomic dead space volume, thus encroaching on alveolar ventilation.

Breath-Hold Diving

The duration of a breath-hold dive depends upon:

- Breath-hold duration until arterial carbon dioxide pressure reaches the breath-hold breakpoint
- Relationship between the diver's total lung capacity (TLC) and residual lung volume (RLV)

During a full inspiration of ambient air, approximately 1 L of oxygen moves into the respiratory passages and lungs. Upon breath-hold, 650 mL of this oxygen sustains metabolism before partial pressures of arterial oxygen (Po_2) and carbon dioxide (Pco_2) reach levels that signal the need for renewed breathing.[8] With some practice, most people can breath-hold for up to 1 minute, and 2 minutes represents a typical upper limit. During this time, arterial Po_2 drops to 60 mm Hg, whereas Pco_2 the most important factor controlling breath-holding rises to 50 mm Hg, thus signaling an urgency to breathe. Increased physical activity greatly reduces breath-holding time because oxygen consumption and carbon dioxide production increase directly with exercise intensity.

Hyperventilation and Breath-Hold Diving: Blackout

Hyperventilation before breath-hold diving significantly extends the breath-hold period; at the same time, the risk to the diver greatly increases. **Blackout**, a sudden loss of consciousness, poses a serious danger in skin diving; it usually afflicts divers who try to extend the dive's duration beyond reasonable limits. Blackout probably results from a critical reduction in arterial Po_2, which contributes to a total relaxation of respiratory muscles.

The breakpoint for breath-holding corresponds to an increase in arterial Pco_2 to 50 mm Hg. However, some people can ignore this stimulus and continue breath-holding until arterial carbon dioxide reaches levels that cause severe disorientation and even blackout.[9] When hyperventilation precedes breath-hold, arterial Pco_2 decreases from its normal value of 40 mm Hg to 15 mm Hg. Lowering the body's carbon dioxide content before the dive significantly extends the duration of breath-hold until arterial Pco_2 increases to a level that stimulates ventilation. For example, 270 seconds is the longest breath-hold recorded while breathing air without prior hyperventilation. Breath-holds of 15 to 20 minutes have been reported with hyperventilation followed by several deep breaths of pure oxygen.[25]

The combination of hyperventilation, breath-holding, and exercise in the underwater environment poses serious risks.[9,10] Consider the following scenario: A skin diver hyperventilates at the surface before a dive to reduce arterial Pco_2 and augment breath-hold duration. The diver now takes a full inhalation and descends beneath the water. Alveolar oxygen continually moves into the blood for delivery to active muscles. Owing to previous hyperventilation, arterial carbon dioxide levels remain low, freeing the diver from the urge to breathe. Concurrently, as the diver swims deeper, the external water pressure compresses the thorax, increasing gas pressure within this cavity. Increased intrathoracic pressure maintains a relatively high alveolar Po_2. Consequently, even though the absolute quantity of alveolar oxygen decreases as oxygen moves into the blood during the dive, Po_2 remains adequate to continually load hemoglobin as the dive progresses. When the diver senses the need to breathe from the eventual CO_2 buildup and begins to ascend, significant reversals occur in intrathoracic pressure. As water pressure on the thorax decreases with ascent, lung volume expands and alveolar Po_2 decreases to a level where no gradient exists for oxygen diffusion into arterial blood. This places the diver in a hypoxic state. Near the surface, alveolar Po_2 may reach such low levels that dissolved oxygen actually diffuses from the venous blood returns to the lungs and flows into the alveoli, causing the diver to suddenly lose consciousness before surfacing.

ADDITIONAL CONSIDERATIONS. Two responses provide additional risks from hyperventilation preceding a breath-hold dive.

1. A normal quantity of arterial carbon dioxide maintains the acid–base balance of the blood, mediated by H^+ release as carbonic acid forms from the union of carbon dioxide and water. By reducing the blood's carbon dioxide content through hyperventilation, H^+ concentration decreases, causing the blood pH to shift in the direction of increased alkalinity.
2. A normal arterial Pco_2 provides a continuous stimulus for dilation of the arterioles in the brain.[31] Any significant reduction in arterial carbon dioxide with hyperventilation could reduce cerebral blood flow and cause dizziness or even loss of consciousness. This obviously creates danger in the aquatic environment.

Depth Limits with Breath-Hold Diving: Thoracic Squeeze

Progressing deeper beneath the water subjects the body's air cavities to tremendous compressive forces. Generally, when the lung volume compresses below 1.5 to 1.0 L (i.e., to RLV) internal and external pressures fail to equalize, and **lung squeeze** occurs ("In a Practical Sense" provides equations for estimating RLV from measures of age, body mass, and stature). Excessive hydrostatic pressure on pulmonary air volume causes extensive damage to pulmonary tissues.

Commercial breath-hold diving generally does not exceed depths of 100 fsw, and lung squeeze generally occurs at depths between 150 and 200 fsw. However, individuals show considerable variability in the safe depth for breath-hold diving without danger of lung squeeze. The world record for breath-hold diving depth following a single breath of air is 417 fsw (127 m), a level about 20 yards above the typical cruising depth of nuclear submarines. Francisco Ferreras (height, 6 ft 3 in; weight, 220 lb) achieved this remarkable physiologic feat. Estimates indicate that the external water pressure against the diver's thoracic cavity at this depth would compress his chest girth from 50 inches to 20 inches. Wearing fins and a hooded wet suit, Ferreras was lowered down a cable anchored to the ocean floor. At the desired depth, a balloon-like bag inflated that facilitated ascent to the surface. The total round trip took about 2.5 minutes. Cuban diver Deborah Andollo set the woman's record of 363 fsw (110 m).

The ratio of the diver's TLC to RLV at the surface generally determines the critical diving depth before lung squeeze; this ratio typically averages 4:1 at the surface. For example, for a diver with a 6.0-L TLC and a 1.5-L RLV, Boyle's law predicts that TLC would compress to RLV at 30 m, or 4 ata external pressure. *No danger from lung squeeze exists if lung volume remains greater than RLV, because sufficient air remains in the lungs and rigid respiratory passages to equalize pressure and prevent damage from compression.* If TLC during a dive decreases below RLV (i.e., if TLV ÷ RLV falls below 1.00) pulmonary air pressure becomes less than the external water pressure. The unequalized pressure creates a relative vacuum within the lungs. In severe cases of lung squeeze, blood literally bursts from the pulmonary capillaries through the alveoli and into the lungs. In this situation, divers literally drown in their own blood. Further increases in depth cause compression fractures of the ribs as the chest cavity caves in from excessive external pressure.

In many instances, the ratio TLV:RLV at the surface significantly *underestimates* the actual impressive depths achieved by trained breath-hold divers. Part of the explana-

IN A PRACTICAL SENSE

ESTIMATING RESIDUAL LUNG VOLUME FROM AGE, STATURE, AND BODY MASS

In breath-hold diving, residual lung volume (RLV) plays a significant role by affecting the depth a diver can achieve without danger of lung squeeze. In fact, the diver's TLC:RLV ratio at the surface generally determines the critical diving depth before lung squeeze.

Laboratory techniques of helium dilution, nitrogen washout, or oxygen dilution routinely measure RLV (see Chapter 12). Each procedure requires complicated and expensive laboratory equipment. An alternative, although less valid, approach estimates RLV with gender-specific prediction equations based on age, stature, and body mass. The standard error of estimate for predicting RLV ranges between ± 325 to 500 mL.

RLV Prediction Equations

Variables: age (y); St, stature (cm); BM, body mass (kg).

Normal-weight males

$$\text{RLV (L)} = (0.022 \times \text{Age}) + (0.0198 \times \text{St}) - (0.015 \times \text{BM}) - 1.54$$

Normal-weight females (only age and stature used)

$$\text{RLV (L)} = (0.007 \times \text{Age}) + (0.0268 \times \text{St}) - 3.42$$

Overweight males (%fat ≥25) *and females* (%fat ≥30)

$$\text{RLV (L)} = (0.0167 \times \text{Age}) + (0.0130 \times \text{BM}) + (0.0185 \times \text{St}) - 3.3413$$

Examples

1. Male: age, 21.0 years; body mass; 80 kg; stature, 182.9 cm

$$\begin{aligned}\text{RLV (L)} &= (0.022 \times 21) + (0.0198 \times 182.9) - (0.015 \times 80) - 1.54 \\ &= 0.462 + 3.621 - 1.2 - 1.54 \\ &= 1.34 \text{ L}\end{aligned}$$

2. Female: age, 19 years; stature, 160.0 cm

$$\begin{aligned}\text{RLV (L)} &= (0.007 \times 19) + (0.0268 \times 160.0) - 3.42 \\ &= 0.133 + 4.288 - 3.42 \\ &= 1.00 \text{ L}\end{aligned}$$

3. Overweight male: age, 35 years; body mass, 104 kg; stature, 179.5 cm

$$\begin{aligned}\text{RLV (L)} &= (0.0167 \times 35) + (0.0130 \times 104) + (0.0185 \times 179.5) - 3.3413 \\ &= 0.5845 + 1.352 + 3.321 - 3.3413 \\ &= 1.39 \text{ L}\end{aligned}$$

Grimby G, Söderholm B. Spirometric studies in normal subjects, III: static lung volumes and maximum ventilatory ventilation in adults with a note on physical fitness. Acta Med Scand 1963;2:199.

Miller WCT, et al. Derivation of prediction equations for RV in overweight men and women. Med Sci Sports Exerc 1998;30:322.

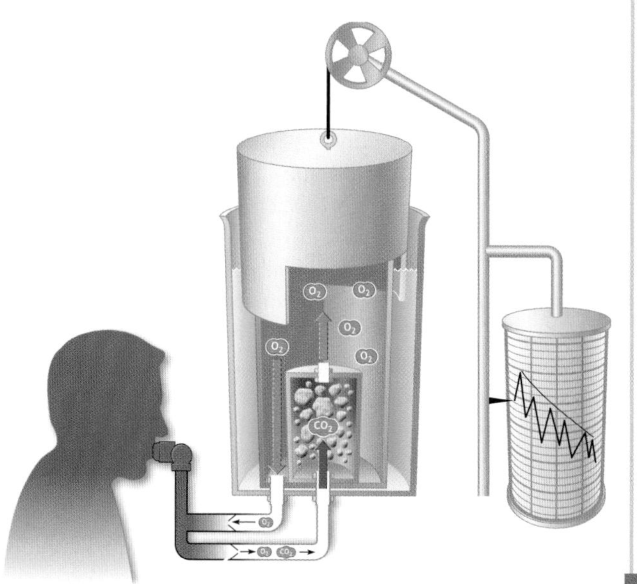

tion may relate to a reduced RLV as immersion progresses because of a shift toward greater intrathoracic blood volume. Consequently, a smaller RLV underwater increases the TLV:RLV and increases the maximal depth before reaching the critical ratio.

OTHER PROBLEMS. If pressures within the internal air spaces do not continually equalize with external hydrostatic pressures, problems other than lung squeeze limit the depth of a breath-hold dive. For example, if air at ambient pressure remains trapped within the middle ear (from inflamed tissue or a mucous plug) and cannot equilibrate with air in the lungs, the external hydrostatic pressure moves the eardrum inward and it eventually ruptures.[11] A ruptured eardrum frequently occurs at relatively shallow depths.

The sinuses also provide difficulty for skin divers. Air compressed in the lungs by the external force of water attempts to move into the paranasal sinuses. However, sinuses inflamed and irritated from infection provide extremely narrow openings that hinder sinus space equilibration with pressure changes in the respiratory tract. Failure to equilibrate creates a relative vacuum in the sinus cavities that distorts their tissues' shape, causing intense sinus pain. With severe disequilibrium, fluid and blood move into the sinuses to fill the vacuum.

A Diving Reflex in Humans?

Classic physiologic responses to immersion, collectively termed the **diving reflex**, enable diving mammals to spend considerable time underwater.[14,27] These include (1) bradycardia, (2) decreased cardiac output, (3) increased peripheral vasoconstriction, and (4) lactate accumulation in underperfused muscle. A modified diving response has also been described for humans during face immersion, breath-hold face immersion, and dives to modest depths.[16,20,27,35] The research has primarily documented increased vagal activity that induces significant bradycardia in humans during face immersion and diving, particularly in cool and cold water. Elevated blood lactate concentration during breath-hold dives to 65 m at energy expenditures only slightly above rest also suggests a diving-mediated peripheral vasoconstriction that decreases blood flow (oxygen) to muscles.[15]

Recent data have expanded the findings on blood lactate concentration to include hemodynamic aspects of breath-hold diving in thermoneutral and cool water by elite divers to depths of 40 to 55 m.[17] Figure 26.2A illustrates the responses for one diver during descent to 40 m, bottom stay, and ascent (depth indicated by *green line*) in water at 25°C and 35°C. The electrocardiographic tracing (Fig. 26.2B) shows the longest R–R interval recorded during the cool-water dive. After an initial tachycardia, bradycardia rapidly ensued and became most pronounced in cool water, where heart rate decreased to only 16 b · min^{-1} near the bottom. Because stroke volume did not change appreciably during the dive, reductions in cardiac output *(yellow line)* mainly resulted from lower heart rates. Cardiac output decreased to a low of 3 L · min^{-1} (25°C) compared with the control value of 6.4 L · min^{-1} at the surface. A large number of frequent, diverse arrhythmic beats, often more frequent than true sinus beats accompanied bradycardia, particularly in the cool-water dives. Arterial blood pressure also increased suddenly and dramatically, reaching 280/200 and 290/150 mm Hg in two divers. This hypertensive response reflected overall peripheral vasoconstriction; the significant increase in blood lactate concentrations reflected increased anaerobic metabolism.

Overall, the intense cardiovascular responses to breath-hold diving in elite divers resembles response patterns of diving mammals. The occurrence of arrythmias and large increases in blood pressure probably reflect species differences and less perfect adaptation by humans.

SCUBA DIVING

The discussion of snorkeling emphasized that at depths below 1 m, inspiratory muscle power cannot overcome the compressive force of water against the thoracic cavity. Air under pressure from an external source to promote inspiratory action counteracts the external hydrostatic force. The **self-contained underwater breathing apparatus (scuba)**, principally developed in 1943 by French oceanographer Jacques-Yves Costeau and Emile Gagnon, is the most common apparatus for supply-

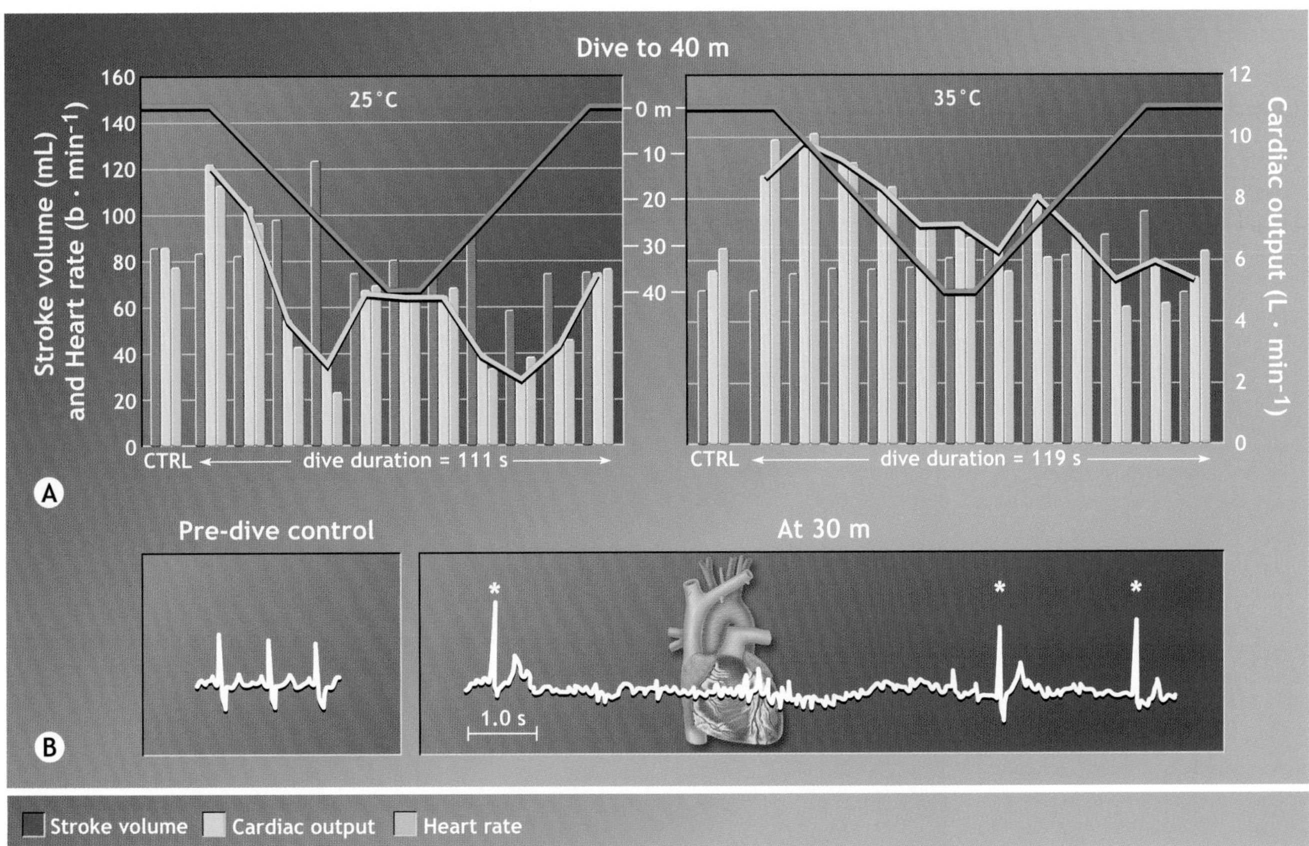

FIGURE 26.2 • A. Heart rate, stroke volume, and cardiac output for an elite breath-hold diver throughout a dive to 40 m in warm (35°C) and cool (25°C) water. *Green line,* diving depth in relation to time; *yellow line,* cardiac output throughout the dive; *CTRL,* control measures prior to dive. **B.** Electrocardiographic tracing showing longest R-R interval during the dive in 25°C water. (*), QRS complex during the dive. (From Ferrigno M, et al. Cardiovascular changes during deep breath-hold dives in a pressure chamber. J Appl Physiol 1997;83:1282.)

ing air under pressure to permit complete independence from the surface. *Sport divers should use only this form of scuba.* The scuba system, strapped to the diver's chest or back, includes a tank of compressed air and a demand regulator valve (which delivers air the diver needs at a particular depth) with hose and mouthpiece or full face mask. Two basic scuba designs exist: (1) the common **open-circuit system** and (2) the **closed-circuit system**, used primarily for clandestine military operations and special applications that require mixed gases.

Underwater commercial operations frequently apply surface-demand diving techniques in operations below 50-m depth. This approach supplies air directly from a compressor at the surface to the diver via a direct reinforced hose. German inventor Augustus Siebe (1788-1872) provided the original design for this system in 1819; it consisted of a copper helmet (hard hat) riveted to a leather jacket, with air delivered continuously from the surface. The excess supplied air and the expired air bubbled out from the bottom of the jacket. If the diver moved significantly from the vertical position, water would rush in through the bottom of the jacket and fill the headpiece. Siebe subsequently modified this design in 1840; he constructed a full waterproof diving suit bolted to a breastplate and helmet that allowed a diver to work in any position, because the suit encapsulated the entire body. Valves admitted air through the diver's helmet as needed, and expired air exited the helmet also through valves.[22] Siebe's "closed" diving helmet allowed divers to dive safely to depths previously impossible to attain.

Open-Circuit Scuba

Figure 26.3 illustrates the typical open-circuit scuba system for submerged swimming with neutral buoyancy in relatively shallow water. For most diving purposes, the steel or aluminum tanks (lightweight titanium that withstands high pressures also used) contain 2,000 L (70–80 ft^3) of air compressed to about 3,000 psi; deeper and longer exposures require 3,500 L (120 ft^3) of compressed air. One tank supplies enough air for a 0.5- to 1-hour dive to moderate depths. The compressed air flows through a **two-stage regulator** valve that (1) reduces the tank pressure to a near-breathable pressure at a particular depth and (2) releases air on demand at pressure equal to ambient, so the diver can inspire without difficulty. The start of inspiration creates a slight negative pressure. This opens the demand valve and releases air to the diver at a pressure nearly equal to the water's external pressure. The positive pressure created with exhalation closes the inspiratory valves and discharges the exhaled air into the water. The scuba gear contains gauges that continually monitor tank pressure and diving depth.

Open-circuit scuba presents several drawbacks. The air exhaled into the water generally contains approximately 17% oxygen, so the open-circuit system wastes about 75% of the total oxygen in the tank. In addition, the diver requires a significant mass of air at increased depths to provide tidal volume for adequate pulmonary ventilation. As an extreme example, inhalation of a 5-L volume at 300 fsw (90 m) requires the equivalent of 50 L of air at sea level! This dramatic effect of pressure on air volume greatly limits the time one can remain at great depth before depleting the scuba tank's air. Factors that influence the energy cost of swimming underwater (and thus pulmonary ventilation) include gender (lower in women than men), gear and number of tanks (25% greater with two tanks), fin type (flexible fin lower than rigid fin), and diver's experience (lower in advanced divers).[30] Because diving tanks contain moisture-free compressed air, each breath produces significant heat and moisture loss as the inspired air warms and humidifies on its passage down the respiratory

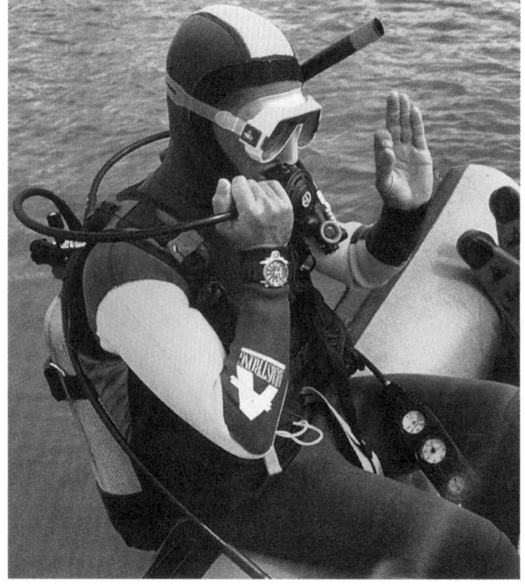

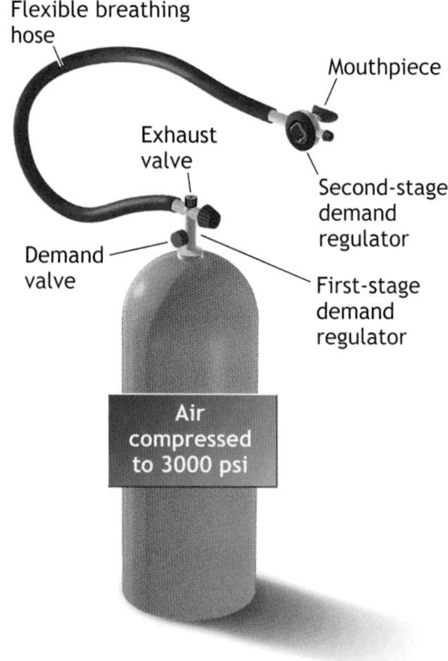

FIGURE 26.3 • General design of an open-circuit scuba unit. Compressed air flows through a two-stage regulator that (1) reduces tank pressure to a near-breathable pressure at a specific depth and (2) releases air to the diver on demand at pressure equal to "ambient" so the diver breathes without difficulty.

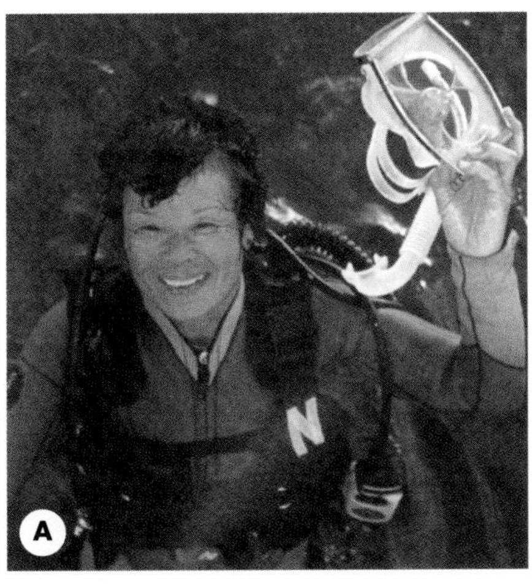

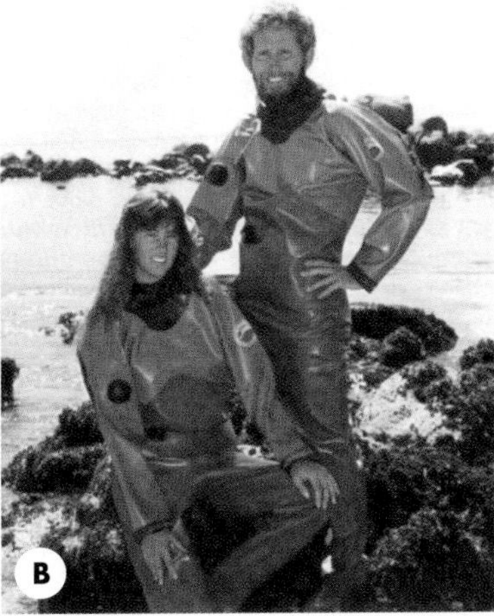

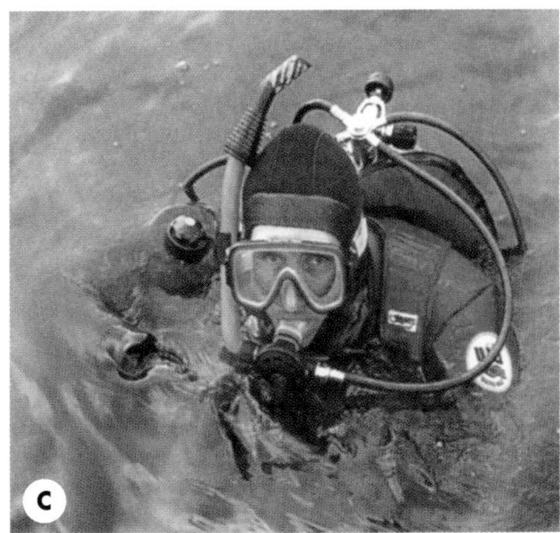

(A) Wet suits are available in 3- to 9-mm thickness and a variety of styles. **(B)** Dry suits are preferred for diving in colder water. **(C)** A hood is important for cold-water diving because up to 50% of body heat escapes through the head.

tract. This causes significant body heat loss during prolonged diving. To counter heat loss, the diver breathes a *heated* gas mixture to avoid hypothermia during deep diving with compressed helium–oxygen (see p. 670).

The **wet suit**, the most common protective garment worn by recreational scuba divers, counters cold stress during diving. This garment, constructed of air-impregnated rubber (usually foam neoprene), traps water against the diver's skin, which warms to body temperature to provide the insulatory boundary. The suit, filled with thousands of tiny gas bubbles, provides insulation. Wet suits generally furnish sufficient thermal protection for relatively short dives, even in ice water. For longer dives in moderately cold water (17 to 18.5°C), however, a full wet suit offers insufficient thermal protection.[1] Compression of the wet suit as the diver descends progressively diminishes the suit's insulating properties.

The modern **dry suit**, made from foam neoprene, crushed neoprene, vulcanized rubber, or heavy-duty nylon with laminated waterproof materials, and often worn over insulating garments, enhance protection from cold stress. This protective clothing ensemble, designed to keep the diver dry, has seals at the neck, wrists, and ankles and a waterproof zipper to prevent water from entering the suit. Dry-suit underwear traps a layer of air between the diver and the water for additional insulation. Layering of underwear adjusts insulation to water temperature.

Figure 26.4 shows the theoretical air time limits for a diver performing similar work at various underwater depths.[28,37,38] These times assume a completely filled standard compressed air tank and ascent and descent at 60 feet per minute. For example, a single aluminum tank containing 80 ft^3 of air compressed to 3000 psi normally sustains an 80-minute dive near the surface. At a depth of 10 m, this tank supplies enough air for about 40 minutes, whereas at 3 ata or 20 m, dive duration decreases by one-third to 27 minutes. These time limits vary with the diver's body size, type and intensity of physical activity, fitness level, and diving experience, all of which affect exercise energy cost and ventilatory volumes.

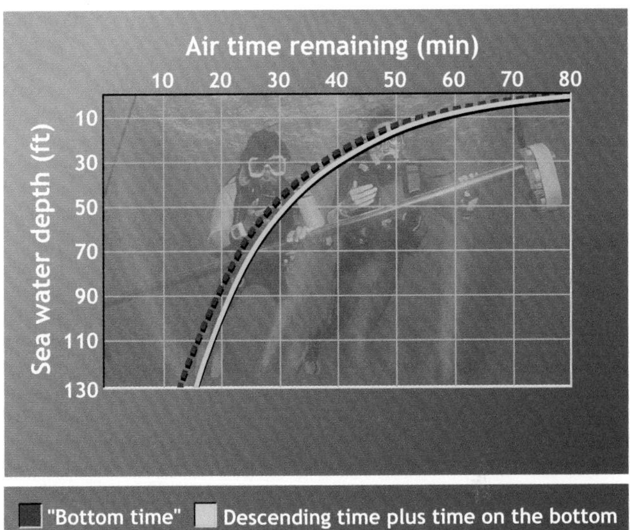

FIGURE 26.4 • Theoretical air time for a single tank containing 80 ft^3 of air. The *yellow line* includes the time spent descending (at a rate of 60 ft · min^{-1}) plus time on the bottom; *dashed line,* indicates only "bottom time."

Closed-Circuit Scuba

The need for shallow diving maneuvers during World War II produced a new diving form that used rebreathing of pure oxygen and absorption of carbon dioxide within a closed system. The closed-circuit underwater breathing apparatus operates in the same manner as the closed-circuit spirometer described in Chapter 8. A small cylinder feeds pure oxygen into a bellows or bag from which the diver breathes. The breathing bag acts as a pressure regulator. Valves in the breathing mask direct the exhaled gas through a carbon dioxide–absorbing canister containing soda lime; the carbon dioxide–free gas then passes back to the diver. The oxygen cylinder replenishes the oxygen consumed in energy metabolism, allowing the diver to continually rebreathe oxygen, the only gas removed from the tank. Thus, only a small oxygen cylinder sustains the submerged diver for 3 hours or longer. Because no expired air releases into the water, the system provides a near-silent and bubble-free operation for clandestine activities. Figure 26.5 illustrates a closed-circuit scuba design currently used by the U.S. Navy that requires only a single bottle of compressed oxygen. The other type of closed-circuit system uses mixed gas: one bottle of pure oxygen and a second bottle of a mixed gas containing either helium and oxygen (**heliox**) or nitrogen and oxygen (**nitrox**; see p. 671).

The closed-circuit system requires a high level of proficiency for safe use. Two main problems exist with closed-circuit scuba. First, a serious medical emergency occurs if carbon dioxide output exceeds its rate of absorption or if absorption fails altogether. With a faulty rebreathing system, the diver may not receive warning symptoms and can drown from becoming anesthetized by arterial carbon dioxide buildup. Second, high concentrations of inspired oxygen, particularly when breathed under high pressures beneath the water, produce a variety of adverse effects on physiologic functions, mainly those related to the central nervous system. These problems remain minimal if the depth–time limits do not exceed the recommendations in Table 26.2. Closed-circuit oxygen breathing generally should not exceed a maximum depth of 25 fsw and definitely should not exceed 50 fsw, because of high risk of central nervous system seizures from oxygen poisoning. Minimal risk usually exists in military diving, because most operations require swimming underwater in relatively shallow depths to avoid detection at night. (We discuss oxygen poisoning more fully later in this chapter.) Decompression sickness does not pose a problem because no inert gas absorption occurs when rebreathing pure oxygen. The increased resistance to breathing and the generally large dead space common with the closed-circuit system limit heavy physical work.

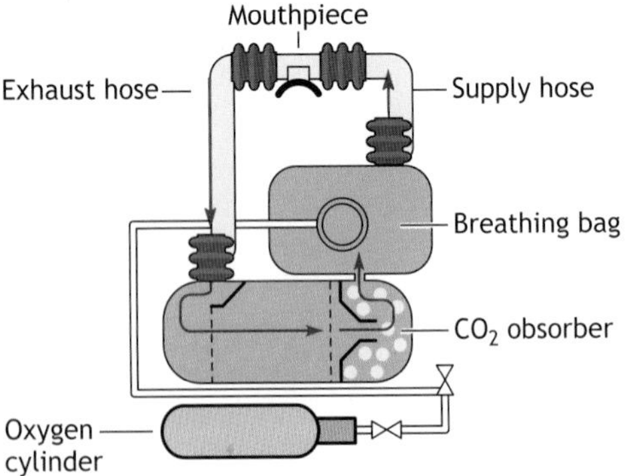

FIGURE 26.5 • General design of a closed-circuit scuba system used by the U.S. Navy. A small cylinder of pure oxygen feeds into a bellows or bag from which the diver breathes. The breathing bag acts as a pressure regulator. Appropriate valves in the breathing mask direct the exhaled gas through a CO_2-absorbing canister containing soda lime; the CO_2-free gas then passes back to the diver. The oxygen cylinder replenishes oxygen consumed in metabolism. *Arrows* indicate direction of airflow.

TABLE 26.2 ➤ U.S. NAVY–RECOMMENDED DEPTH–TIME LIMITS BREATHING PURE OXYGEN DURING WORKING DIVES[a]

Depth (ft)	Depth (m)	Time (min)
Normal Operations		
10	3.0	240
15	4.6	150
20	6.1	150
25	7.6	75
Exceptional Operations		
30	9.2	45
35	10.7	20
40	12.2	10

[a]No symptoms of oxygen poisoning were noted at these depths and durations.

SPECIAL PROBLEMS WITH BREATHING GASES AT HIGH PRESSURES

Figure 26.6 shows the primary risks from breathing compressed air and other gas mixtures in scuba diving. **Henry's law** states that the quantity of gas dissolved in a liquid at a given temperature varies directly with the (1) pressure differential between the gas and the liquid and (2) solubility of the gas in the liquid. Underwater breathing systems must supply air, oxygen, or other gas mixtures at sufficient pressure to overcome the force of water against the diver's thorax. For example, at 3 ata of pressure (20-m depth) the respired gas requires delivery at approximately 2,280 mm Hg (3 × 760 mm Hg), whereas gas delivery at 60 m requires a pressure of 5,320 mm Hg. The following sections consider the specific dynamics of breathing gases at high pressures and their effects on physiologic functions. We also examine the physical responses of a gas to abrupt changes in pressure. Figure 26.7 summarizes the main hazards of scuba diving posed by im-

Unique risks in scuba diving

- Increased resistance to breathing with increased density of compressed gas mixture at depth
- Toxicity of oxygen at high pressures
- Anesthetic effects of nitrogen at high pressures
- Excess heat loss from environmental stress and inhaled gas mixture
- Free-gas development in gas-supersaturated body tissues

FIGURE 26.6 • Important factors that contribute to risk in scuba diving.

proper equalization of pressure within the body's air spaces (and diving mask) in response to changes in external pressure.

Air Embolism

An air volume breathed underwater expands in direct proportion to the reduction in external pressure as the diver ascends to the surface. Air breathed at a depth of 10 m doubles in volume if brought to the surface. If normal breathing continues during ascent, the expanding air vents freely through the nose and mouth. However, if a diver takes a full breath at 10 m but fails to exhale while ascending, the rapidly expanding gas eventually ruptures the lungs before the diver reaches the surface. **Lung burst** becomes a real possibility in scuba diving. Many inexperienced divers react to a perceived underwater danger by filling their lungs and then holding their breath while rapidly swimming to the surface. This particular diving hazard does not necessarily require a deep dive. Accidents caused by breath-hold ascent with scuba frequently occur in shallow dives; changes in pressure exert the greatest effect on the expanding lung volume near the water surface (see *inset box* in Fig. 26.1). *Inhaling a full breath of compressed air in 6 feet of water causes serious overdistension of lung tissue if the diver fails to exhale during ascent.* Fatal **air embolism** can occur in swimming pools as shallow as 8 feet for an inexperienced diver using scuba. Air embolism from pulmonary

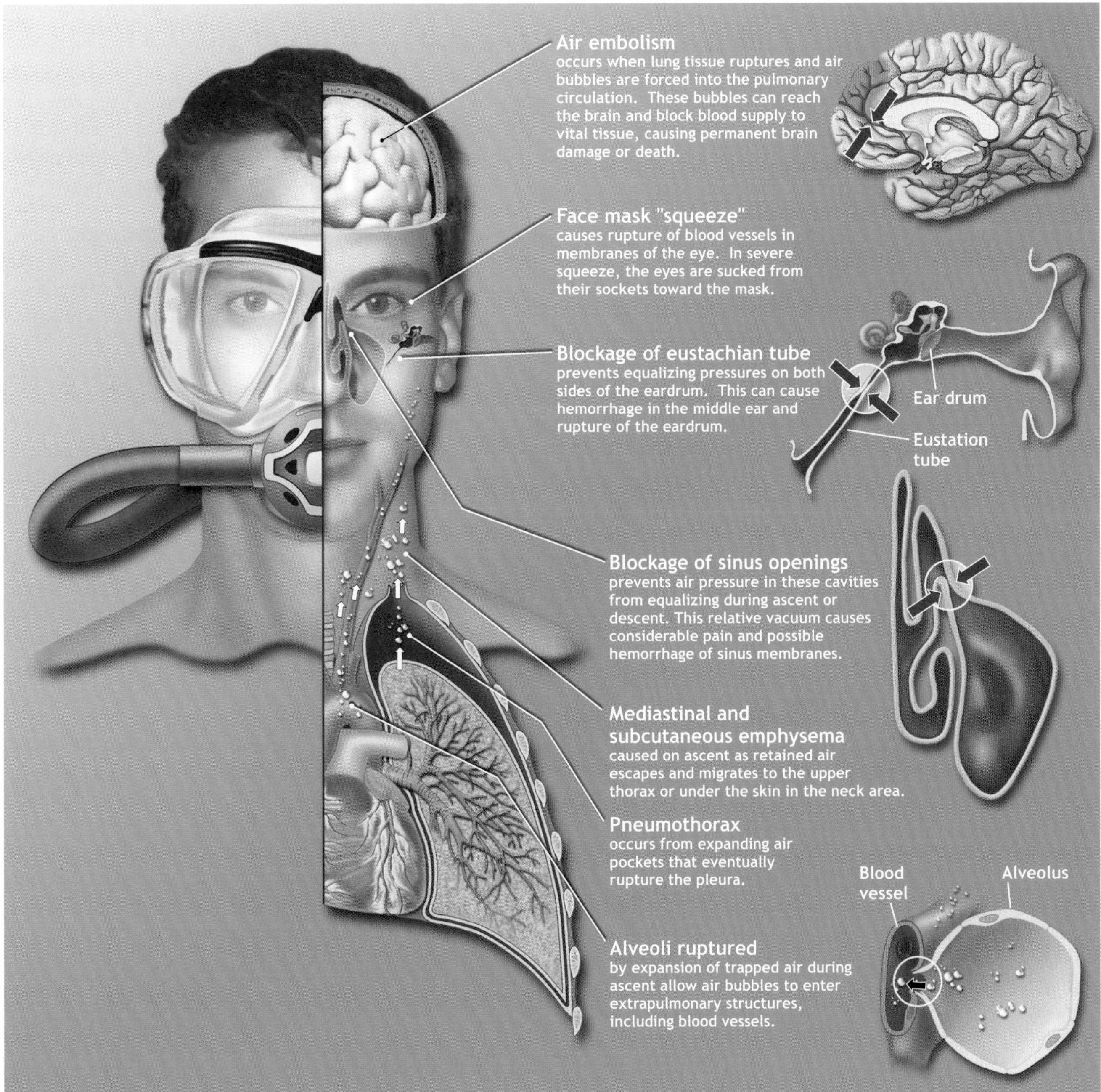

FIGURE 26.7 • Scuba diving hazards from an inability to equalize internal and external gas pressures.

barotrauma ranks second only to drowning as a cause of death among recreational scuba divers.

If expansion of air in the respiratory tract causes lung tissue to rupture during ascent from under water—because of either breath-holding or pulmonary obstruction (bronchospasm, excessive pulmonary secretions, or bronchial inflammation)—air bubbles (**emboli**) may enter the pulmonary venous system. Emboli then flow to the heart and enter the systemic circulation. Because the diver usually maintains a head-up, vertical position on ascent, the bubbles move upward in the body. Eventually, they lodge in the small arterioles or capillaries and restrict blood supply to vital tissue. General symptoms of air embolism include confusion, weakness, dizziness, and blurred vision. Severe blockage of pulmonary, coronary, and cerebral circulation causes collapse, unconsciousness, and frequently death. Effective treatment for air embolism requires rapid decompression to reduce bubble size and force them into solution to open the plugged vessels. Even with rapid, expert treatment, 16% of air embolism victims die.

Pneumothorax: Lung Collapse

Air forced through the alveoli when lung tissue ruptures sometimes migrates laterally to burst through the pleural sac covering the lungs. In about 10% of cases of this form of pulmonary barotrauma, an air pocket forms in the chest cavity outside the lungs, between the chest wall and lung itself. Continued expansion of trapped air during ascent collapses the ruptured lung (**pneumothorax**). Pneumothorax treatment often requires surgical intervention with a syringe to extract the air pocket.

To eliminate the danger of air embolism and pneumothorax, instructors teach divers to ascend slowly and breathe normally when using scuba gear. The diver's lungs must remain free from any disease that could lead to air trapping (e.g., chronic obstructive pulmonary disease), which creates difficulty equalizing alveolar pressure and external pressure during ascent.

Mask Squeeze

Air in a facemask or goggles before a dive equals ambient air pressure at the surface. However, as the diver progresses deeper, a considerable pressure differential develops between the inside and outside of the mask. This creates a relative vacuum within the mask. For example, wearing swimming goggles to improve vision and protect the eyes from irritants during a dive beneath the water can cause the eyes to bulge, or squeeze, from their sockets. This leads to capillary rupture and hemorrhage of the eyes and surrounding soft tissue. This can occur at swimming the deep end of many pools.[12] The squeeze effect occurs because most goggles are constructed from rigid materials. Consequently, displacement of the eye and surrounding soft tissue into the air space between the eye and the goggles provides the only means of equalizing the difference in air pressure between the goggle space and external water pressure during breath-hold diving. As newer pools with separate diving wells reach depths of 14 feet (4.3 m), the use of goggles poses a distinct risk to swimmers who dive to this depth.

Breath-hold diving with a face mask that covers both the eyes and nose represents a somewhat different situation than diving with only swim goggles. Air pressure within the mask that covers the eyes and nose readily equalizes to external water pressure as air flows freely between the nasal passages and the lungs' relatively large air volume. In breath-hold diving, air in the lungs compresses and passes through the nose to equalize mask pressure. With scuba, inspired air automatically adjusts to the external water pressure. Therefore, periodically exhaling through the nose into the mask balances pressures on both sides of the face mask.

Aerotitis: Middle-Ear Squeeze

Divers often encounter problems equalizing pressure within the air space of the eustachian tubes, the passages that connect the middle ear with the back of the throat.[3,39] These relatively narrow, mucus-lined channels generally resist air flow. In healthy individuals, the tubes remain clear enough that changes in external pressure against the eardrum equalize by pressure changes transmitted from the lungs through the eustachian tubes. In both skin and scuba diving (and air travel in nonpressurized aircraft), middle-ear pressure usually equalizes with external pressure by blowing gently against closed nostrils. Swallowing, yawning, or moving the jaws from side to side also helps to "pop" the ears.

In upper-respiratory tract infection, the eustachian tube membranes swell and produce mucus that often plugs cranial air passages. The greatest difficulty involves equalizing middle-ear pressure during descent, because an equal force from the ear canal does not readily match the pressure change against the outer surface of the eardrum. The magnitude of pressure changes in diving considerably exceed those experienced in air travel. Divers can suffer severe pain only a few feet under water because the eardrum stretches and moves inward toward the plugged canal. Further pressure disequilibrium creates a relative vacuum in the middle ear that hemorrhages tissues. Complete blockage of the eustachian tubes can rupture the eardrum, causing water to rush into the middle ear as pressure equalizes.

NEVER USE EARPLUGS. *Never wear earplugs while diving.* During a dive, the external water pressure pushes the earplug deep into the external ear canal. A pocket of ambient air trapped between the plug and eardrum may rupture the eardrum outward during descent. People with the following conditions should *not* dive: respiratory disease, perforated eardrum, or temporary blockage of the eustachian tubes from infection. In the latter case, diving can resume when the infection subsides, and the ear canals clear.

Aerosinusitis

Inflamed, congested sinuses prevent air pressure in these cavities from equalizing during diving.[29] Sinus air pressure that does not equalize during descent remains at atmospheric pressure while external pressure increases. This relative vacuum creates "sinus squeeze," causing sinus membranes to bleed as blood occupies the space to equalize the pressure differential.

Nitrogen Narcosis: Rapture of the Deep

The total pressure of the respired gas during diving increases in direct proportion to the diving depth. Likewise, the partial pressure of each gas in the breathing mixture increases, so that at 10 m the nitrogen partial pressure doubles the sea-level value to 1200 mm Hg. With each additional 10-m depth, nitrogen partial pressure increases by 600 mm Hg—inspired PN_2 equals 4,200 mm Hg at a 60-m depth. At each successive depth, the gradient increases for the net flow of nitrogen across the alveolar membrane into the blood and eventually into the tissue fluids for equilibration. At 20 m, for example, all tissues eventually contain three times as much nitrogen than before the dive. Tissue perfusion, solubility coefficients of tissue, body composition, and temperature all influence nitrogen uptake at the tissue level.

Some 300 fsw generally sets the limit for compressed air diving, because dissolved nitrogen accumulation in the body's fluids and tissues renders all but the most experienced divers incapable of accomplishing meaningful work. The U.S. Navy sets the maximum operating depth at 190 fsw for breathing compressed air. In 1935, Dr. Albert Behnke (see Chapter 28) and coworkers demonstrated that the increase in inspired nitrogen pressure while breathing compressed air during diving produced the narcotic effect. An increase in the pressure and quantity of dissolved nitrogen causes physical and mental changes characterized by a general state of euphoria similar to alcohol intoxication, a condition termed **rapture of the deep**. Dissolved nitrogen at a depth of 30 m produces effects similar to those felt after consuming some alcohol on an empty stomach; at 60 m, the feelings resemble the effects of two or three martinis. Eventually, high nitrogen levels produce a numbing, anesthetic effect on the central nervous system. The term **nitrogen narcosis** collectively describes these symptoms. At the extreme, mental processes deteriorate so that a diver may feel that the scuba serves little purpose and may actually remove it and swim deeper instead of toward the surface.

Because nitrogen diffuses slowly into body tissues, the narcosis effect depends on dive depth and duration. Considerable individual variation exists for nitrogen sensitivity, but a mild narcosis usually appears after an hour or more at 30 to 40 m—the maximum recommended depth for recreational scuba divers. Treatment requires that the diver ascend to a shallower depth, where complete recovery usually occurs rapidly.[37] The precise role of body fatness in nitrogen narcosis remains controversial.[23]

Decompression Sickness

With rapid ascent, the external pressure against the diver's body decreases dramatically. Excess dissolved nitrogen in the body tissues begins to separate from the dissolved state and eventually form bubbles in the tissues, an effect not unlike the appearance of carbon dioxide bubbles when removing the cap from a carbonated beverage. With the cap in place, the gas remains dissolved under pressure. Removing the cap suddenly reduces pressure above the fluid, causing bubbles to form. **Decompression sickness** *occurs when dissolved nitrogen moves out of solution and forms bubbles in body tissues and fluids.* It results from ascending to the surface too rapidly after a deep, prolonged dive, often made possible with double and triple air tanks. Because nitrogen reaches equilibrium slowly in many tissues, particularly fatty tissues, it leaves the body slowly.[21,41] This means that women (with a greater average percentage body fat than men) and obese men face greater risk for decompression sickness. Figure 26.8 compares nitrogen elimination after a simulated "dive" by two dogs who differed in fat content. The relatively fat dog eliminated considerably more nitrogen over the 4-hour decompression than the leaner dog.

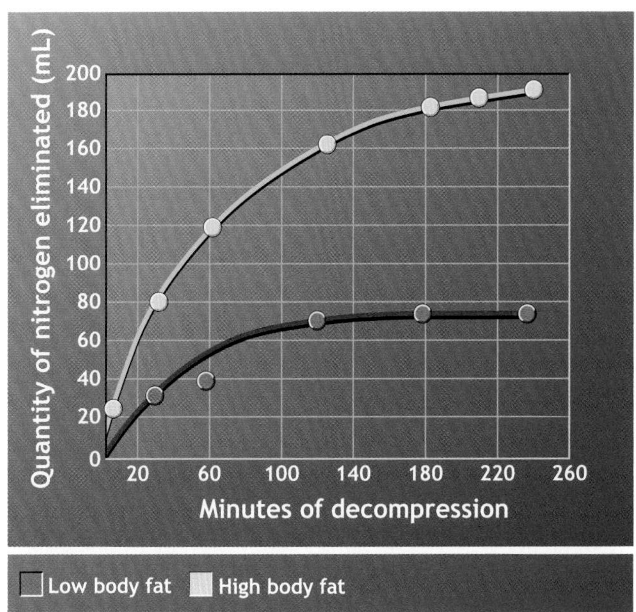

FIGURE 26.8 • Nitrogen elimination from body tissues of a relatively lean dog and one higher in body fat during decompression in a chamber. (Courtesy of Dr. A. R. Behnke.)

The term *bends,* a synonym for decompression sickness, emerged during construction of piers for the Brooklyn Bridge (1869–1883) to reflect the bent-over position of limping workers who emerged from the caisson. Vann poignantly describes the time course and horrendous consequences of decompression sickness in an early history of this malady:[40]

> In 1900, for example, a Royal Navy diver descended to 150 fsw in 40 minutes, spent 40 minutes at depth searching for a torpedo, and ascended to the surface in 20 minutes without apparent difficulty. Ten minutes later, he complained of abdominal pain and fainted. His breathing was labored, he was cyanotic, and he died after 7 min. An autopsy the next day revealed the organs to be healthy, but gas was present in the liver, spleen, heart, cardiac veins, venous, subcutaneous, and cerebral veins and ventricles.

Nitrogen Elimination: Zero Decompression Limits

Diving at a depth of 30 m for up to 30 minutes represents the time limit before sufficient nitrogen dissolves to pose danger from decompression sickness. About 18 minutes is the limit at 40 m, and one can spend almost an hour at 20 m without danger from decompression sickness. If a diver exceeds the depth–duration recommendations for compressed air diving shown in Figure 26.9, the ascent to the surface must progress in a preestablished manner. With this approach, a recreational or commercial diver ascends at a prescribed, relatively slow rate designed not to require stops. This rate of ascent enables all excess dissolved nitrogen to diffuse from the tissues into the blood and escape through the lungs without bubbles forming.[37,41] **Stage decompression** requires that the diver make one or more stops on ascent to the surface. The time required for the slowest tissue compartment to lose sufficient nitrogen to allow the ascent to the next depth determines the duration of such pauses (termed *stage-decompression stops*). For example, a dive to 30 m for 50 minutes requires one 2-minute decompression stop at 6 m (20 ft) and a 24-minute stop at 3 m (10 ft). Surface stage decompression involves transfer of the diver from the water (after several in-water stops) to a decompression chamber at the surface. The judicious use of a hyperoxic breathing mixture facilitates recompression.

A conservative approach recommends that the sport diver not exceed a 20- to 25-m depth (30-m maximum). During single or repetitive dives the diver should never approach the time limits indicated by the decompression tables.[13] The recommendations in Figure 26.9 assume a *single* dive, with a minimum of 12 hours between dives. For repeated dives within 12 hours, the diver must consult the appropriate repetitive dive decompression schedules.[36] These recommendations account for the residual nitrogen remaining in the body at the start of the next dive if it occurs within the 12-hour period. Interestingly, air travel within 24 hours of scuba diving increases risk of decompression sickness because commercial airlines usually pressurize cabins to an equivalent altitude of 7000 feet. This further reduction in ambient atmospheric pressure may suffice to initiate bubble formation from excess nitrogen dissolved in body tissues during the prior preflight dive(s).

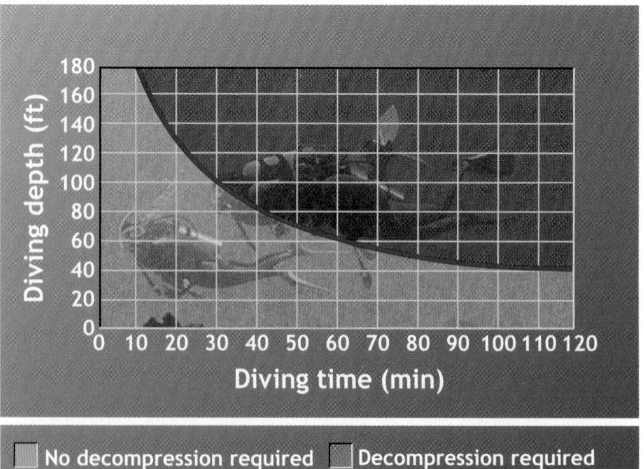

FIGURE 26.9 • Zero decompression limits. Any single dive falling on the left side of the curve requires no decompression provided the rate of ascent does not exceed 60 ft per minute (m = ft × 0.34048). Dives on the right side of the line require the decompression period specified in the Navy standard decompression tables.[35]

Consequences of Inadequate Decompression

Overwhelming evidence indicates that bubbles within the vascular circuit initiate complications from decompression injury. With the exception of bubbles in central nervous tissue that cause lesions in brain and spinal cord and damage intravertebral disks, the primary bubbles form in the venous and arterial vascular bed.[4] Symptoms of decompression sickness usually appear within 4 to 6 hours after a dive. Severe violation of decompression procedures (e.g., diver runs out of air and ascends too rapidly) initiates symptoms immediately; these progress to paralysis within minutes. Indications of inadequate decompression are dizziness, itchy skin, and aching pain in the legs and arms, particularly in tight tissues such as ligaments and tendons (the classic and most common characteristic). The degree of injury depends on the size of the bubbles and where they form. Bubbles in the lungs cause choking and asphyxia, whereas bubbles in the brain and coronary arteries block the flow of blood and deprive these vital tissues of oxygen and nutrients, producing cellular damage and death. Central nervous system bends occur with some frequency; failure to provide immediate treatment leads to permanent neural damage.

Treatment for the bends involves lengthy recompression in a **hyperbaric chamber**. This specialized device elevates external pressure to force nitrogen gas back into solution. Gradual decompression then follows to provide sufficient time for the expanding gas to leave the body as the diver returns to the "surface." Immediate recompression offers the best chance for success; any delay decreases the prognosis for complete recovery. Figure 26.10 shows a collapsible, lightweight, transportable chamber for rapid deployment in treating decompression accidents during transport of the diver to an appropriate facility. The chances are slim for a sport diver to have ready access to such a recompression chamber. This makes it imperative that divers adhere strictly to recommendations for diving depth and duration.

HIGHER PREVALENCE WITH A PATENT FORAMEN OVALE. Decompression sickness sometimes occurs after uneventful dives, without any reported errors in recommended decompression procedures. Divers with lesions localized in the high cervical spinal cord and brain areas show a significantly higher prevalence of patent foramen ovale (PFO) of the myocardium than divers with decompression sickness localized in the lower spinal cord.[18] PFO consists of an interatrial septum channel that forms a functional valve between the right and left atria. This channel could cause specific decompression sickness because nitrogen bubbles that the pulmonary vasculature nor-

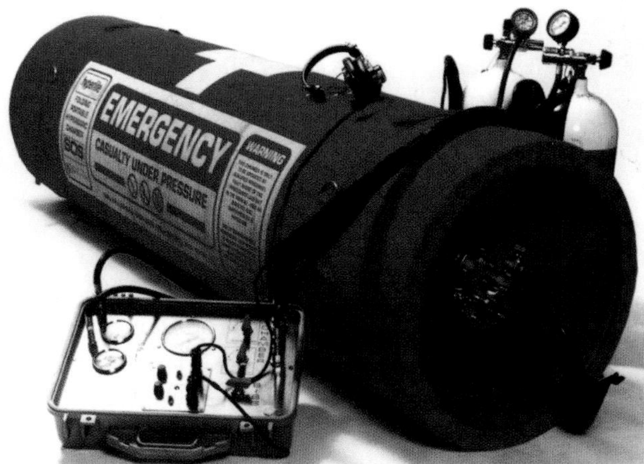

FIGURE 26.10 • Portable, collapsible recompression chamber (50 kg) for diving in remote locations. A compressed air cylinder provides a working pressure differential of 2.1 ata (bars), or 70 fsw, between the chamber environment and ambient conditions; the diver receives oxygen via a breathing mask. The tube is constructed from para-aramid fiber (like Kevlar) in a matrix of silicone rubber. This provides flexibility (can fold when not in use) and considerable strength under pressure (burst pressure approximately 14 ata differential pressure). (Manufactured by SOS Limited, London, England; photo courtesy of John Selby.)

TABLE 26.3 ➤ **REPRESENTATIVE DEPTH–TIME LIMITS FOR CLOSED-CIRCUIT DIVING WITH 100% OXYGEN**

DEPTH (FSW)	MAXIMUM TIME (MIN)
25	240
30	80
35	25
40	15
50	10

Adapted from United States Navy diving manual, vol 2 Mixed gas diving, rev 3. NAVSEA publication 0994 LP-001-9020. May 1991.

mally filters pass through the PFO into the arterial circulation. The bubbles then migrate preferentially into the carotid and/or vertebral arteries. Divers with unexplained decompression sickness but with symptoms suggesting cerebral or high spinal localization should receive evaluation for PFO.

Oxygen Poisoning

Inspiring a gas with a Po_2 above 2 ata (1,520 mm Hg) greatly increases a diver's susceptibility to **oxygen poisoning**, particularly at elevated metabolic rates during physical activity.[2,24] For this reason, closed-circuit scuba that uses pure oxygen places severe restrictions on both diving depth and duration (Table 26.3). At depths greater than 25 fsw (7.6 m), the diver should *not* rebreathe pure oxygen except in extraordinary circumstances. A decreased vital capacity strongly indicates impaired pulmonary function under hyperoxic conditions.[7]

Breathing high pressures of oxygen negatively affects bodily functions in three ways:

1. It irritates respiratory passages and eventually induces bronchopneumonia if exposure persists.
2. It constricts cerebral blood vessels at pressures above 2 ata and alters central nervous system function.
3. It blunts carbon dioxide elimination.

For carbon dioxide elimination, an elevated inspired Po_2 may force sufficient oxygen into solution in the plasma to supply the diver's metabolic needs. As such, oxygen remains combined with hemoglobin (oxyhemoglobin) as blood returns to the pulmonary capillaries. This causes carbon dioxide buildup because deoxygenated hemoglobin normally transports significant carbon dioxide as carboaminohemoglobin from the tissues (see Chapter 13). Treatment for oxygen poisoning consists of breathing air at sea-level pressure.

Carbon Monoxide Poisoning

Potentially lethal carbon monoxide gas combines some 200 times more readily with hemoglobin than oxygen. Thus, only a small quantity of carbon monoxide in the inspired mixture readily induces tissue hypoxia. Carbon monoxide poisoning becomes of concern during deep dives because the partial pressures of all gases in the breathing mixture (including impurities) increase greatly.

Contaminants from automotive and industrial exhausts, including carbon monoxide and oxides of sulfur, may reach high levels in urban areas. For this reason, one should not fill a scuba tank during air pollution alerts. Aside from the contaminants present in ambient air, operating the gasoline or diesel engine compressor contributes additional carbon monoxide and oil impurities. Placing the compressor's engine exhaust downstream from the air intake eliminates this potential source of contamination. The antidote for carbon monoxide poisoning requires breathing hyperbaric oxygen as soon as possible. High pressures of inspired oxygen hasten dissociation of carbon monoxide from the hemoglobin molecule.

Women at Risk?

Women make up about 35% of the recreational scuba divers in the United States, but they do not experience a greater risk than men of equivalent physical fitness for decompression sickness, nitrogen narcosis, oxygen toxicity, air embolism, or diving accidents. The research literature remains sparse about the risks of open-circuit scuba diving to the fetus during pregnancy. Prudent guidelines recommend that pregnant women *refrain* from scuba diving during the entire length of pregnancy to eliminate any risk of injury to the fetus from maternal breathing of compressed air at elevated pressures.[36]

DIVES TO EXCEPTIONAL DEPTHS: MIXED-GAS DIVING

Commercial, military, scientific, rescue, and technical divers often descend to depths in excess of 160 fsw. Recall that at depths greater than 60 fsw, diving with compressed air and saturation diving (see p. 670) significantly increases the risk of oxygen toxicity. This depth and lower require inhalation of compressed mixed gases (non-air) with a lower PO_2 (Fig. 26.11). Although oxygen always exists in the breathing mixture in mixed-gas diving, it represents only a small fraction of the mix in dives to extreme depths. Consequently, precise management of oxygen concentrations becomes a primary consideration in **mixed-gas diving**.

Helium–Oxygen Mixtures

Helium, the second lightest known element, is the most common inert gas substituted for nitrogen in deep diving. Helium does not induce narcosis at any inspired pressure.[32]

Helium in the breathing mixture in diving came into its own during the 1939 rescue of remaining crew members and salvage of the submarine *Squalus,* which sank in 75 m of water. For these purposes, a compressor at the water's surface continually supplied the divers with a helium-oxygen (**heliox**) mixture. Breathing colorless, odorless, tasteless, nonexplosive, and relatively nontoxic heliox mixtures significantly reduces typically increased breathing resistance imposed by nitrogen, because of helium's extremely low density. During rapid descent to depths in excess of 300 fsw up to 2280 fsw, divers have experienced potentially incapacitating nausea, muscle tremors, and other central nervous effects, a condition termed **high-pressure nervous syndrome** (**HPNS**). This condition probably results from the direct effects of the extremes of hydrostatic pressure on excitable nerve cells. Slowing the rate of descent (compression) and adding a small amount of narcotic gas (e.g., 5% N_2) to the heliox breathing mixture relieves the tremor associated with HPNS. The term **trimix** describes the helium–nitrogen–oxygen combination.

Other negative effects of breathing helium include:

- Changes in voice characteristics (high-pitched, cartoon-like quality), which interfere with voice communication among divers. Electronic voice unscramblers remedy this effect.
- Considerable heat loss for divers living in a heliox environment; this is due to helium's high thermal conductivity (6 × air). The thermal challenge contributes to weight loss, common among saturation divers.

The increased risk for central nervous system oxygen toxicity when breathing surface-supplied heliox gas makes it crucial

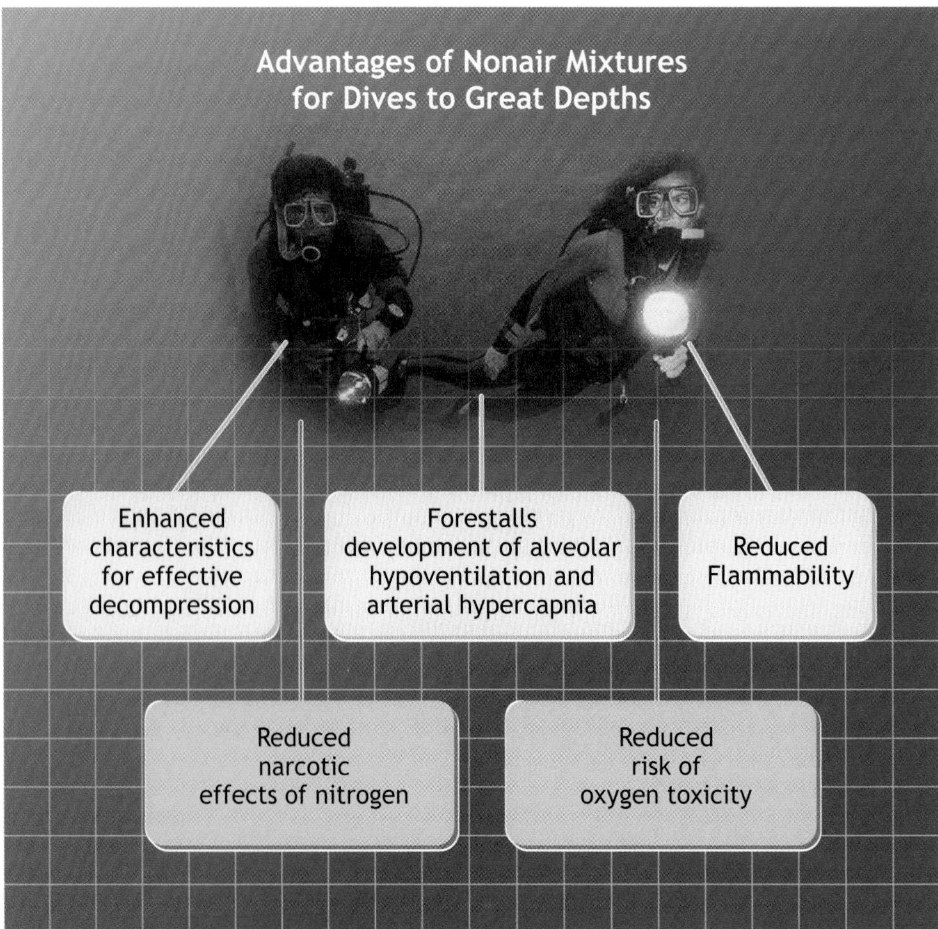

FIGURE 26.11 • Rationale for breathing gas mixtures other than compressed air when diving to great depths. Avoidance of nitrogen narcosis and oxygen poisoning are the *overwhelming* reasons for breathing non-air mixtures.

TABLE 26.4 ➤ **REPRESENTATIVE NORMAL OXYGEN PARTIAL PRESSURE LIMITS FOR SURFACE-SUPPLIED HELIOX DIVING**

EXPOSURE TIME (MIN)	MAXIMUM OXYGEN PARTIAL PRESSURE (ATA)
13	1.8
20	1.7
30	1.6
40	1.5
80	1.4
Unlimited	1.3

Adapted from United States Navy diving manual, vol 2. Mixed gas diving, rev 3. NAVSEA publication 0994 LP-001-9020. May 1991.

that the diver not exceed the oxygen exposure limits put forth in Table 26.4.

Saturation Diving

Breathing an heliox mixture supports a safe dive to depths greater than 300 fsw, but the time the diver must remain "in-water" for decompression becomes prohibitive. Thus, dives below 300 fsw generally take place with **saturation diving** in a deep-diving system using a helium–oxygen–nitrogen breathing mixture that maintains oxygen pressure between 0.4 and 0.6 ata (Po_2, 300 to 450 mm Hg). In saturation diving, each inert gas in a mixture begins to concentrate in body tissues as diving depth and duration progress. Within 24 to 30 hours, the gases equilibrate and become *saturated* in body tissues to equal the pressures of the inspired gases. Once the tissues achieve saturation, the decompression procedure remains identical, regardless of the dive's duration.

The deep-diving system consists of a chamber where the divers live under pressure for 2 to 4 weeks. The system also contains a deck decompression chamber and transfer capsule or diving bell for transport of personnel under pressure to and from the worksite. Once at the worksite, the divers exit, tethered to an umbilicus-supplied breathing apparatus. Saturation diving provides benefits in offshore oilfield work with dives for up to a month at depths of 1500 fsw. Successful dives to depths of 2300 fsw in a dry chamber apply principles of saturation diving with a breathing mixture of hydrogen, helium, and oxygen. Decompression from a saturation dive takes 8 to 24 hours per 10-m ascent.

A critical consideration in saturation diving with heliox mixtures is maintaining normoxic Po_2 in the breathing mixture. Breathing the wrong mixture or the correct mixture at the wrong pressures creates the potential for a tragic fatality. Oxygen percentages must be held within ±0.10% of the desired value to avoid either hypoxia or oxygen toxicity. Figure 26.12 shows the typical recommended percentage of oxygen in heliox for various diving depths.[19] For example, the oxygen concentration to obtain a desired Po_2 of 0.35 ata (Po_2, 270 mm Hg) at a depth of 1200 fsw requires a breathing mixture with approximately 0.7% oxygen.

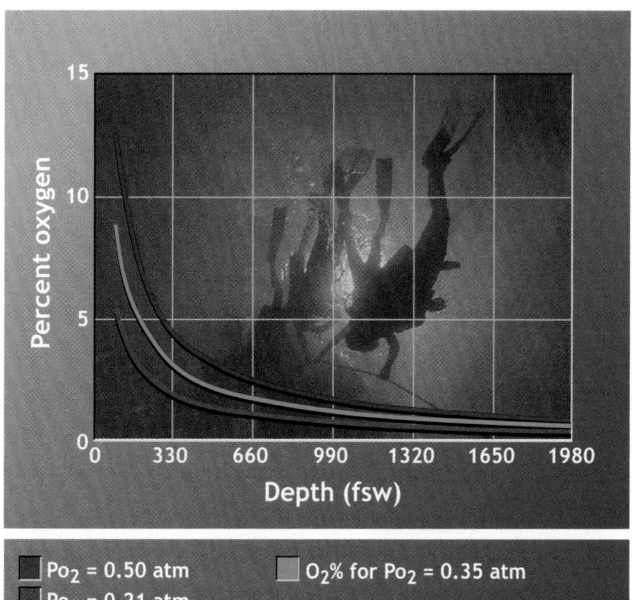

FIGURE 26.12 • Range of oxygen concentrations for deep saturation diving. The *green line* represents the oxygen concentration that maintains oxygen at 0.35 atm (Po_2 = 266 mm Hg), a common choice for Po_2. The *purple line* shows the oxygen needed to provide the normoxic level of 0.21 atm. The *red line* represents 0.5 atm (Po_2 = 380 mm Hg), the upper limit of continuous exposure to avoid whole-body oxygen toxicity. The low oxygen concentrations needed at great depths become difficult to mix and analyze within acceptable tolerance limits; thus, they are usually mixed as the diving chamber becomes pressurized. (From Hamilton RW. Mixed-gas diving. In: Diving medicine. Bove AA, ed. 3rd ed. Philadelphia: WB Saunders, 1997.)

Technical Diving

The term **technical diving** defines untethered dives (scuba or closed-circuit rebreathing) beyond the traditional compressed air range for military operations, science, salvage, and recreational pursuits. For example, many recreational scuba divers now consider the typical depth limit of 130 fsw imposed by diving with compressed air too restrictive. They wish to expand their diving depths for personal achievement, recreation, and exploration (e.g., cave diving). Technical diving requires special equipment, expertise, and management of gas mixtures. Technical divers routinely use various mixtures of trimix compressed gas to dive below 300 fsw. Blending a depth-specific gas mixture enables the diver to control both the risk of hyperoxia and the narcotic potential of the mixture's nitrogen.

Closed-circuit nitrogen-oxygen and helium-oxygen scuba, originally developed for military operations, now appear in the recreational technical diving community. These highly sophisticated systems maintain a constant partial pressure of oxygen in the inhaled mixture regardless of depth. Figure 26.13 illustrates a closed-circuit mixed-gas system used by the U.S. Navy. An oxygen sensor (#19) and microprocessor (#21) in the breathing loop continually detect and regulate falling Po_2. The sensors activate valves that add the precise quantity of 100% oxygen to regulate inspired Po_2 at 0.75 ata

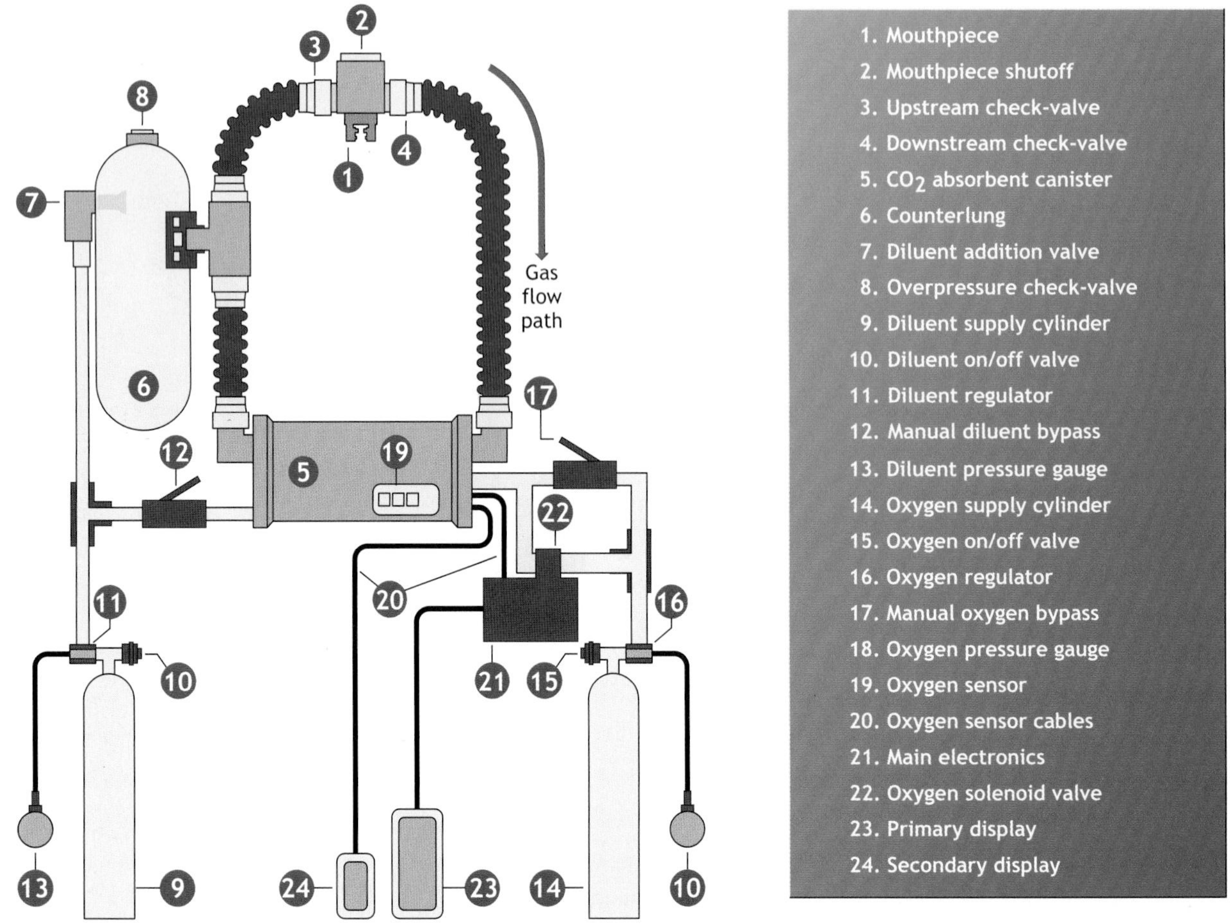

Gas
flow
path
1. Mouthpiece
2. Mouthpiece shutoff
3. Upstream check-valve
4. Downstream check-valve
5. CO2 absorbent canister
6. Counterlung
7. Diluent addition valve
8. Overpressure check-valve
9. Diluent supply cylinder
10. Diluent on/off valve
11. Diluent regulator
12. Manual diluent bypass
13. Diluent pressure gauge
14. Oxygen supply cylinder
15. Oxygen on/off valve
16. Oxygen regulator
17. Manual oxygen bypass
18. Oxygen pressure gauge
19. Oxygen sensor
20. Oxygen sensor cables
21. Main electronics
22. Oxygen solenoid valve
23. Primary display
24. Secondary display

FIGURE 26.13 • Closed-circuit mixed-gas system used by the U.S. Navy for diving to great depths. A microprocessor and oxygen sensors in the breathing loop continually detect falling Po_2 and activate valves that add the precise amount of 100% oxygen to regulate the partial pressure of inspired oxygen. One high-pressure gas bottle supplies pure oxygen, and a second provides either air or a heliox mixture as a diluent. As with the typical closed-circuit system, a chemical bed continually absorbs the carbon dioxide produced in metabolism (approximate cost, $35,000 to $45,000).

(427 mm Hg). One of two high-pressure gas bottles (#s 9 and 14) supplies pure oxygen, and the other provides either air or a heliox mixture as the diluent gas. As with the typical closed-circuit system, a chemical bed absorbs carbon dioxide produced in metabolism. Monitors within the facemask provide continual feedback about Po_2 and diving depth. A fiberglass casing worn on the diver's back contains the microprocessor, gas bottles, breathing bag, and insulated carbon dioxide absorbent canister (cold decreases the life of the CO_2 absorbent).

ENERGY COST OF UNDERWATER SWIMMING

As with swimming at the surface, drag forces impede the diver's forward movement and greatly increase the energy cost of swimming underwater. Figure 26.14 shows the curvilinear relationship between oxygen consumption and underwater swimming speed. For example, a swimmer with a $\dot{V}O_{2max}$ of 35 mL · kg^{-1} · min^{-1} could swim underwater at a speed of 1.2 knots (1.4 mph) for only several minutes. This speed creates minimal stress for a diver with a $\dot{V}O_{2max}$ of 65 mL · kg^{-1} · min^{-1}.

Oxygen consumption
(mL · kg-1 · min-1)
40.0
35.0
30.0
25.0
20.0
15.0
10.0
5.0
0.4
0.6
0.8
1.0
1.2
1.4
Swimming speed (knots)

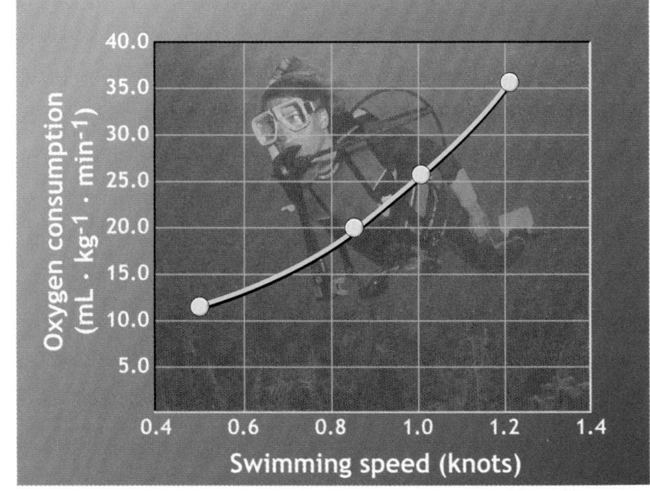

FIGURE 26.14 • Generalized curvilinear relationship between oxygen consumption (mL · kg^{-1} · min^{-1}) and underwater swimming speed (1.0 knot = 1.15 mph).

Focus on Research: The Cost of Swimming Underwater

Donald KW, Davidson WM. Oxygen uptake of 'booted' and 'fin swimming' divers. J Appl Physiol 1954;7:31.

➤ Use of scuba allows thousands of individuals to enjoy underwater diving. The duration of independence underwater depends on the depth of the dive and the physiologic/metabolic demands of physical activity before the tank empties of compressed air. Minute pulmonary ventilation increases with increasing muscular effort underwater, thus decreasing time underwater.

Early research on underwater diving, particularly with closed-circuit scuba, attempted to establish the interactions between energy expenditure, pulmonary airflow, quantity of oxygen available in the tank, and the diver's rate of return to the surface, to avoid complications such as oxygen poisoning, anoxia, and nitrogen narcosis. Fundamental data required detailed measurements of oxygen consumption ($\dot{V}O_2$) and carbon dioxide production ($\dot{V}CO_2$) to determine the amount of oxygen supplied in the tank and the total CO_2 absorbent required. The study by Donald and Davidson, completed in 1944 but not published until 1954, was among the first to quantify $\dot{V}O_2$ of divers and underwater swimmers during different forms of physical effort. This research demanded considerable technical expertise to permit accurate $\dot{V}O_2$ measurements in the underwater environment.

Subjects included 13 British military divers and 13 military "commando" frogmen, all in top physical condition. Each subject underwent multiple measurements under diverse exercise conditions. The researchers used a modified closed-circuit breathing system. Divers breathed pure oxygen under all conditions, which included work in a tank (12-ft depth) and in open seawater. Divers wore either (1) a full rubber diving suit with leather or rubber boots (5 to 7 lb in the sole) that allowed them to assume the vertical position with ease or (2) the familiar frogman well-fitting rubber suit with rubber swim fins.

Measurements were taken during rest at the surface, sitting underwater (12-ft depth), standing underwater, with minimum movement (moving along the bottom as slowly and gently as possible without stopping and avoiding any marked postural changes), and with maximum movement (moving as fast as possible to cover the greatest distance).

Additional $\dot{V}O_2$ measurements were made while subjects rode an underwater cycle ergometer (leg exercise) outfitted with paddles attached to the pedals to increase resistance. Pedal revolutions per minute (rpm) controlled exercise intensity. A metronome placed in the diver's line of vision maintained pedaling rate. Thirty rpm represented light exercise maintained easily for 15 minutes, 40 rpm provided heavy exercise for 15 minutes, and 45 rpm caused fatigue within 10 minutes. For heavy arm exercise, the diver stood underwater while alternately lifting a 21-lb weight (18-in-lift per minute) by means of a pulley system. The frogmen swam 2 to 3 feet below the surface at (1) a medium speed of 1.3 to 1.7 ft · s^{-1} for 20 minutes and (2) a fast speed of 1.7 to 2.3 · s^{-1} for 10 minutes.

Tank Series: Booted Divers

$\dot{V}O_2$ with subjects seated and standing still underwater remained low and remarkably near the divers' calculated resting values. Since these men experienced near-neutral buoyancy underwater, it is likely that lying and standing quietly required less postural effort than in air, hence the low underwater energy expenditure. While these resting data have little application to practical diving conditions, they do help to explain the prolonged periods trained divers can stay underwater with limited oxygen supply if they remain inactive.

$\dot{V}O_2$ during the minimum-movement experiments reached the same magnitude as that for walking about 2.0 mph on the level in air; the underwater maximum-movement $\dot{V}O_2$ equaled the out-of-water $\dot{V}O_2$ for walking at 4 mph. Even though the energy expenditure values during un-

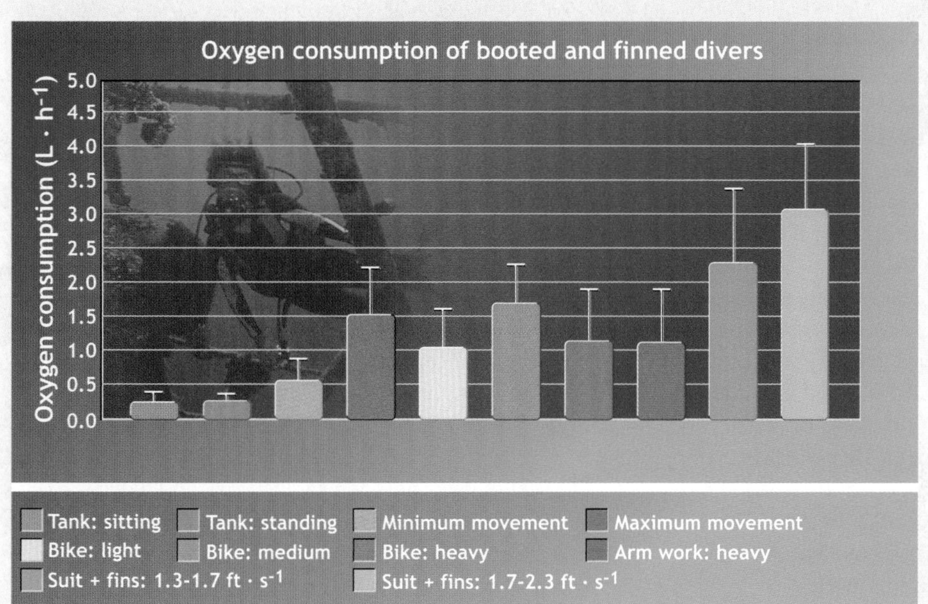

Average and minimum and maximum (shown as error bars) values for $\dot{V}O_2$ for different activities during booted and finned diving. (From Donald KW, Davidson WM. Oxygen uptake of 'booted' and 'fin swimming' divers. J Appl Physiol 1954;7:31.)

Focus on Research — The Cost of Swimming Underwater—continued

derwater effort were relatively low, the divers complained of fatigue, possibly owing to the minimal involvement of the total leg musculature during work under water.

Underwater Swimming with Fins

Eight of the 13 swimmers had $\dot{V}O_2$s of 2.3 L · min^{-1} or above during a 20-minute swim at the slower speed. At the faster speed, sustained for 10 minutes, 4 of 8 swimmers achieved $\dot{V}O_2$s over 3.0 L · min^{-1}, with one swimmer exceeding 4.0 L · min^{-1}, just slightly below his maximum level in air. These $\dot{V}O_2$s during underwater swimming are similar to those reported for athletes during different sustained sport activities out of the water and considerably higher than those previously calculated for underwater activities. The results indicated a need to reconsider the maximum size of CO_2 absorbent canisters used in most closed-circuit diving systems.

The figure shows the marked differences in $\dot{V}O_2$ under the different exercise conditions. These carefully designed experiment formed the foundation for further research on underwater energy expenditure. Such information contributed to the growing understanding of diving physiology and the construction of safer diving systems.

Summary

1. Breath-hold diving has been practiced for centuries. The advent of deep-sea diving had its origins in the 14th century with the invention of diving bells supplied with surface air.
2. The underwater environment routinely exposes divers to high pressures (hyperbaria) and the possibility of rapid pressure changes. Severe injury and even death ensue unless divers adjust to equalize pressures in the body's air-filled cavities.
3. Two factors limit snorkel size: (1) increased hydrostatic pressure on the chest cavity during descent and (2) increased pulmonary dead space from enlarging the snorkel's internal volume.
4. The duration of a breath-hold dive depends on time until arterial P_{CO_2} reaches the breath-holding breakpoint.
5. Hyperventilation significantly increases breath-holding time; it also increases the likelihood of underwater blackout. Blackout results from a critical reduction in arterial oxygen pressure, an abnormal change in arterial carbon dioxide pressure, an acid–base imbalance, or the combined effects of all three factors.
6. The point at which the diver's lung volume compresses to RLV generally determines maximum depth for breath-hold diving. Below this critical depth, internal and external pressures cannot equalize, and lung squeeze results. The TLV:RLV ratio at the surface often significantly underestimates the impressive depths achieved by trained breath-hold divers.
7. Breath-hold diving by elite divers produces intense cardiovascular changes that resemble response patterns of diving mammals, suggesting a modified diving reflex in humans. Responses include (1) bradycardia, (2) decreased cardiac output, (3) increased peripheral vasoconstriction, and (4) lactate accumulation in underperfused muscle.
8. Because scuba supplies breathing mixtures at great depths and pressures, specific hazards result from improper equalization of pressures in the lungs, sinus, and middle-ear spaces with the external water pressure. The most significant dangers include air embolism, pneumothorax, mask and middle-ear squeeze, and aerosinusitis.
9. Gases breathed at high pressures move across the alveolar membrane and eventually dissolve and equilibrate in the fluids of all tissues. High tissue oxygen and nitrogen pressures exert profound effects on physiologic function. The maximum recommended diving depth for breathing compressed air is about 30 m, before the potential for adverse effects.
10. Prolonged breathing of a gas with a P_{O_2} above 2 ata increases a diver's susceptibility to oxygen poisoning. Closed-circuit scuba systems that use pure oxygen severely restrict dive depth and duration.
11. During ascent, a gradient exists for the net flow of nitrogen from body fluids into the lungs. Bubbles form in tissues when excess nitrogen fails to exit through the lungs if ascent progresses too rapidly. Decompression sickness or bends describe this extremely painful condition.
12. Diving to depths below 60 fsw requires inhalation of compressed mixed gases. Oxygen always exists in the breathing mixture in mixed-gas diving, but it represents only a small fraction of the mix in dives to extreme depths. Thus, precisely managing oxygen concentrations becomes a primary consideration in diving with gas mixtures.
13. Breathing mixtures of helium and oxygen (heliox) enables dives to depths of 2,000 fsw. Heliox diving eliminates nitrogen narcosis risk and reduces oxygen poisoning risk.
14. Rapid descent to depths from 300 fsw to 2,800 fsw when breathing heliox mixtures often produces

nausea, muscle tremors, and other central nervous system effects (termed high-pressure nervous syndrome [HPNS]). HPNS probably results from the direct effects of extreme hydrostatic pressure on excitable nerve cells

15. Drag forces that impede a diver's forward movement greatly increase the energy cost of swimming underwater.

References

1. Arieli R, et al. Thermal status of wet-suited divers using closed circuit O_2 apparatus in sea water of 17–18.5°C. Eur J Appl Physiol 1997;76:69.
2. Arieli R. Latency of oxygen toxicity of the central nervous system in rats as a function of carbon dioxide production and partial pressures of oxygen. Eur J Appl Physiol 1998;78:454.
3. Becker GD. Barotrauma resulting from scuba diving: an otolaryngological perspective. Phys Sportsmed 1985;13:113.
4. Behnke AR. Decompression sickness: advances and interpretations. Aerosp Med 1971;42:255.
5. Bove A, Davis J. Diving medicine. Philadelphia: WB Saunders, 1990.
6. Bove AA. Medical aspects of sport diving. Med Sci Sports Exerc 1988;28:591.
7. Clark JM, et al. Effects of prolonged oxygen exposure at 1.5, 2.0, or 2.5 ATA on pulmonary function in men (predictive studies V). J Appl Physiol 1999;86:243.
8. Corteix C, et al. Chemical and nonchemical stimuli during breath holding in divers are not independent. J Appl Physiol 1993;75:2022.
9. Craig AB Jr. Causes of loss of consciousness during underwater swimming. J Appl Physiol 1961;16:583.
10. Craig AB Jr. Summary of 58 cases of loss of consciousness during underwater swimming and diving. Med Sci Sports 1976;8:171.
11. Craig AB Jr. Principles and problems of underwater diving. Phys Sportsmed 1980;8:72.
12. Craig AB Jr. Physics and physiology of swimming goggles. Phys Sportsmed 1984;12:107.
13. Davis JC. Decompression sickness in sport scuba diving. Phys Sportsmed 1988;16(2):108.
14. Elsner R, Gooden B. Metabolic conservation by cardiovascular adjustments. In: Diving and asphyxia. A comparative study of animals and man. New York: Cambridge University Press, 1983.
15. Ferretti G, et al. alveolar gas composition and exchange during deep breath-holds in elite divers. J Appl Physiol 1991;70:794.
16. Ferrigno M, et al. Simulated breath-hold diving to 20 meters: cardiac performance in humans. J Appl Physiol 1987;62:2160.
17. Ferrigno M, et al. Cardiovascular changes during deep breath-hold dives in a pressure chamber. J Appl Physiol 1997;83:1282.
18. Germonpré P, et al. Patent foramen ovale and decompression sickness in sport divers. J Appl Physiol 1998;84:1622.
19. Hamilton RW. Mixed-gas diving. In: Bove AA, ed. Diving medicine. 3rd ed. Philadelphia: WB Saunders, 1997.
20. Hayashi N, et al. Face immersion increases vagal activity as assessed by heart rate variability. Eur J Appl Physiol 1997;76:394.
21. Hierholzer J, et al. MRI in decompression illness. Neuroradiology 2000;42:368.
22. Kindwall EP. A short history of diving and diving medicine. In: Bove AA, ed. Diving medicine. 3rd ed. Philadelphia: WB Saunders, 1997.
23. Kizer KW. Women and diving. Phys Sportmed 1981;9:84.
24. Lambertsen CJ. Effects of oxygen at high partial pressure. In: Fenn WO, Rahn H, eds. Handbook of physiology. Washington, DC: American Physiological Society, 1965.
25. Lanphier EH, Rahn H. Alveolar gas exchange during breath-hold diving. J Appl Physiol 1963;18:471.
26. Lin Y-C. Breath-hold diving in terrestrial mammals. In Exercise and Sport Sciences Reviews. Vol. 10. Edited by R.L. Terjung. Philadelphia, Franklin Institute, 1982.
27. Magel JR, et al. Heart rate response to apnea and face immersion. J Sports Med Phys Fitness 1982;22:135.
28. Miller JW. NOAA diving manual. Washington, DC: U.S. Department of Commerce, U.S. Government Printing Office, 1979.
29. Parell GJ, Becker GD. Neurological consequences of scuba diving with chronic sinusitis. Laryngoscope 2000;110:1358.
30. Pendergast DR, et al. Energetics of underwater swimming with scuba. Med Sci Sports Exerc 1996;28:573.
31. Poulin MJ, et al. Fast and slow components of cerebral blood flow response to step decreases in end-tidal P_{CO_2} in humans. J Appl Physiol 1998;85:388.
32. Rostain JD, et al. EEG and sleep disturbances during dives at 450msev in helium-nitrogen-oxygen mixture. J Appl Physiol 1997;83:575.
33. Smith DJ. Diagnosis and management of diving accidents. Med Sci Sports Exerc 1998;28:587.
34. Strauss RH. Diving medicine. Am Rev Respir Dis 1979;119:1001.
35. Sterba JA, Lundgren CEG. Breath-hold duration in man and the diving response induced by face immersion. Undersea Biomed Res 1988;15:361.
36. Taylor MB. Women in diving. In: Bove AA, ed. Diving medicine. 3rd ed. Philadelphia: WB Saunders, 1997.
37. The NOAA diving manual. Washington, DC: U.S. Government Printing Office, 1991.
38. US Navy dive manual, Navsea 0994-Lp-001-9020, vol 1, rev 3. Feb 1993.
39. Uzun C, et al. Use of the nine-step inflation/deflation test as a predictor of middle ear barotrauma in sports scuba divers. Br J Audiol. 2000;34:153.
40. Vann RD. Mechanisms and risks of decompression. In: Bove AA, ed. Diving medicine. 3rd ed. Philadelphia: WB Saunders, 1997.
41. Wienke BR. Basic decompression theory and applications. Flagstaff, AZ: Best Publishing, 1991.
42. Wienke BR. Basic diving physics and applications. Flagstaff, AZ: Best Publishing, 1994.

CHAPTER 27

Microgravity: The Last Frontier

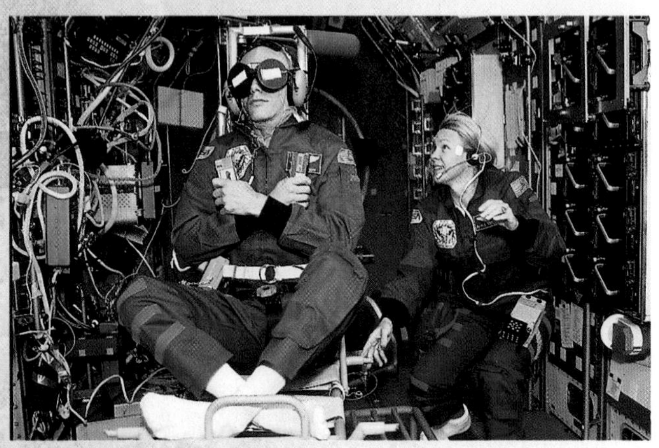

Chapter Objectives

- Define the term gravity and list factors that affect the magnitude of gravitational force
- Differentiate between zero-g and weightlessness
- Outline factors that contribute to a sense of "free fall" for an individual in a falling elevator
- Describe four strategies for simulating microgravity with nonhuman objects and animals and humans
- Describe how the KC-135 airplane creates brief periods of microgravity during astronaut training
- List five important physiologic/anatomic responses to microgravity exposure; differentiate between short-term and long-term responses
- Give reasons for denitrogenation prior to extravehicular activity (EVA), and procedures to achieve this effect
- Summarize NASA's research recommendations concerning bone loss with microgravity exposure
- Discuss the role of hindlimb unloading to study mammalian responses to microgravity
- Outline the goals of exercise countermeasures to ensure astronaut health and safety during missions and return to Earth
- Describe the rational for using lower-body negative pressure and its role as a countermeasure during space flight
- Outline interactions among energy balance, nutrition, and protein dynamics during space travel
- Describe the time course for postflight recovery from space flight for various physiologic systems
- List five high-priority, future research areas targeted by the Committee on Space Biology and Medicine of the National Research Council
- List 10 significant spin-off technologies from space biology research

THE WEIGHTLESS ENVIRONMENT

The pioneering efforts of mainly German, Russian, and American scientists and engineers advanced aerospace medicine from the early test flights of rocket-propelled jet aircraft to the technologic innovations of today's **International Space Station (ISS)** that orbits 220 nautical miles above Earth. The remarkable successes of man's escape from Earth's atmosphere and subsequent return originated in antiquity, when prophets and philosophers could only dream of contacting celestial bodies. From flying machine designs of the Renaissance to successful hot-air balloon ascents during the mid-1700s, the obsession to explore the universe has not waned. The reliability of powerful rocketry now makes space adventure possible, creating new challenges about how best to tame the short- and long-term physiologic stress imposed by escaping Earth's gravitational field.

The early jet flights could not test human's responses to changing gravitational forces because that era's test aircraft could not accommodate specialized laboratory equipment. Nevertheless, knowing how to cope with the unique environmental stressors (and health challenges) of high-altitude exposure still required new understanding unavailable from conventional medicine. The field of **aerospace medicine** emerged from a need to deal with unconventional situations not encountered in normal gravity. Few in the medical establishment could predict the response of mice, cats, dogs, monkeys, or humans to space flight. Primates and eventually humans in more powerful rocket tests followed the earliest "space-travelers," lower life forms carried aloft by test aircraft. Concurrently, research progressed by use of space cabin simulators on Earth. Scientists focused on psychophysiologic responses to changing gravitational forces and prolonged isolation while performing complex motor and mental tasks. The experience from simulations and manned flights provided new understanding about space flights' impact on human structure and function.

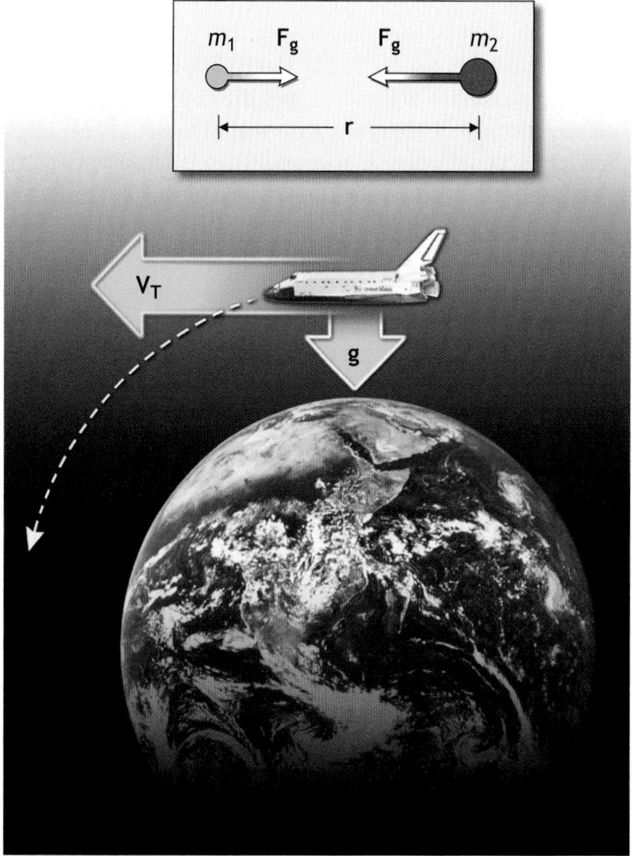

Top. Two different size masses (m_1 and m_2), depicted as the red- and green-filled ovals, and separated by a distance r exert attractive gravitational forces (Fg) on each other. The forces on each particle have equal magnitude even when their masses differ markedly. Stated more formally, the gravitational force between small masses is proportional to the product of the masses, and inversely proportional to the square of the separation between them. *Bottom.* Microgravity refers to the perceived "weightlessness" associated with free fall. The forces acting on an astronaut orbiting Earth in a spacecraft are not balanced—both astronaut and spacecraft accelerate towards the Earth's center. They do not "fall" to the Earth because its surface is curved and they are moving at a high enough tangential velocity (V_T) that "balances" gravity's downward force on the spacecraft. No perceived force (i.e., weight) exists because nothing counteracts the force of gravity.

Gravity

On the Earth's surface, **gravity** provides an invisible attraction that makes any mass exert downward force or have weight. Gravity behaves in the same fundamental way between the Earth and any object on it, or between any of the planets that revolve about the sun in our solar system, or between a planet and its moons. The universality of the gravitational law discovered in 1687 by **Sir Isaac Newton** (1642–1727) can be stated as follows and depicted in the top of the accompanying unnumbered figure on the top right:

> Every particle in matter in the universe attracts every other particle with a force directly proportional to the product of the masses of the particles and inversely proportional to the square of the distance separating them.

Law of Universal Gravitation

The mathematical equation describing Newton's law of gravity is as follows:

$$F_g = G\, m_1\, m_2 \div r^2$$

where F_g = magnitude of gravitational force on either particle, m_1 and m_2 = masses of the particles; r = distance between particles, and G = gravitational constant. Mathematically, a very small gravitational force can exist between any two objects, but it can never quite reach zero. The relative term *small* usually refers to an apparent weight of an object one millionth that on Earth's surface (i.e., 0.000001 times less than on Earth—nearly, but not quite, weightless).

A difference in definition exists between g and G. Lower-case *g* represents acceleration due to gravity; it relates the weight (w) of a body to its mass (m) so that $w = mg$. Thus, the value for *g* differs at different locations on Earth and other planetary bodies. Capital G relates the gravitational force between any two bodies to their masses and the distance between them. The G value remains the same for any two bodies, independent of their location in space. In 1798, English physicist and chemist Sir Henry Cavendish (1731–1810) performed the experiment that "weighed the earth," using a torsion balance instrument designed by John Mitchell (1724–1793, founder of the science of *seismology*) to determine G accurately. Refined instrumentation has determined the presently accepted value for the universal constant G as 6.67259(85) $\times 10^{-11}$ $Nm^2 \cdot kg^{-2}$.

When a person sits in a chair on Earth, the force of gravity pulls the person into the seat because the chair provides an equal and opposite force (Newton's third law). Every mass (m) on Earth requires support from a force (F) equal to its weight (w) such that w (or F) $= mg$. Stated somewhat differently, the constant acceleration force per second (s) of descent on a freely falling body at or near Earth's surface has a value of 1g, or the equivalent magnitude of 9.80665 or 9.91 $m \cdot s^{-2}$, 980 $cm \cdot s^{-2}$, or 32 $ft \cdot s^{-2}$. On the moon's surface, the attractive force of the moon rather than Earth causes the acceleration of gravity, where $g = 1.6\ m \cdot s^{-2}$. Near the sun's surface, the value of g increases tremendously by a factor of nearly 169 to 270 $m \cdot s^{-2}$.

Microgravity and Weightlessness

To achieve an orbit around Earth or move away from it, the velocity of a rocket must exceed the downward pull of Earth's gravity. The gravitational pull on the rocket decreases as the rocket moves further from Earth. When the rocket reaches a specified distance from Earth sufficient for orbit, a traveler experiences a weightless feeling because *nearly* all of the forces acting on the body remain in balance. To reach a point in space where the gravitational pull from Earth equals one-millionth the force at Earth's surface requires traveling 6.37 million km, or 16.6 times the distance from Earth to the moon, or 1400 times the highway distance between New York City and San Francisco. In a practical sense, a rock dropped from a window 5 m above the ground requires 1 second to touch ground. In an environment with only 1% of Earth's gravitational pull, the same drop takes 10 seconds. In a microgravity environment equal to one-millionth of the gravity on Earth, the same 5-m drop would take 1000 seconds, or approximately 17 minutes.

The issue of gravitational force also applies to **escape velocity (V_{esc})**, which depends on the mass (M) and radius (r) of the celestial body a spacecraft attempts to leave. Knowing Earth's M (5.98×10^{24} kg) and r (6378 km, or 6.378×10^6 m), computing the Earth's V_{esc} of 11.2 $km \cdot s^{-2}$ is as follows:

$$\begin{aligned} V_{esc} &= \sqrt{(2 \times G \times M \div r)} \\ &= \sqrt{2 \times (6.67 \times 10^{-11}\ Nm \cdot kg^{-2}) \times (5.98 \times 10^{24}\ kg)} \\ &\quad \div (6.378 \times 10^6\ m) \\ &= 1.12 \times 10^4\ m \cdot s^{-1} \\ &= 11.2\ km \cdot s^{-2} \\ &= 40{,}200\ km \cdot h^{-1} \\ &= 11.2\ km \cdot s^{-2}\ (25{,}039\ mi \cdot h^{-1}) \end{aligned}$$

On the moon, with significantly less gravity than Earth, a spacecraft must achieve approximately one-fifth the escape velocity (5321 mph, or 2.38 $km \cdot s^{-2}$ of the corresponding 25,039 mph required on Earth. Leaving the planet Jupiter would require an extremely large escape velocity (133,018 mph: 59.5 $km \cdot s^{-2}$) compared with the Earth or moon because of Jupiter's huge mass (1.9×10^{27} kg), radius (71,492 km), and distance (6.63×10^{10} m) from Earth.

Spacecraft orbit Earth at a relatively close distance (typically 200 to 450 km), so astronauts experience only an *apparent* sense of weightlessness. In essence, the force of gravity never truly reaches an absolute value of zero (called **zero-g**), because a gravitational force still exists. Consequently, the term **microgravity**, not weightlessness (or zero-g), correctly describes what astronauts feel during space flight in Earth orbit when the rocket's altitude exceeds approximately 160 km (100 mi) at a velocity of approximately 17,500 mph. In a microgravity environment, an object's apparent weight is small compared with its actual weight due to Earth's gravity. On the space shuttle or the ISS, the microgravity environment at 220-km altitude is qualitatively the same as in a spacecraft orbiting a thousand Earth radii away (6,370,000 km) to escape Earth's gravitational field, where g would now equal one-millionth the force of Earth's gravity.

The 121-ft space shuttle, used as an orbiting laboratory, can carry a payload of 29,479 kg into orbit, with each main engine producing a thrust of 170,068 kg at sea level while burning a liquid oxygen and hydrogen mixture. After achieving orbital velocity, the astronaut and spacecraft continually accelerate toward a single point at the Earth's center. However, they do not fall to Earth because of the planet's curved surface and because both craft and crew move at a high enough tangential velocity (V_T) to the Earth (see bottom of unnumbered figure on previous page). The spacecraft's speed creates an outward centrifugal force that "balances" the downward gravitational force on the spacecraft. When spacecraft velocity decreases (reduced V_T)—a planned maneuver during re-entry—the craft falls toward Earth under gravity's pull.

The orbit essentially creates a state of continuous **free-fall** in which the astronaut does not perceive any force (i.e., weight) because nothing counteracts gravity. Thus, the astronaut experiences a feeling of floating. During this time, astronaut and spacecraft accelerate at the same rate in orbit and no buoyancy effects exist. No pressure gradient pushes the astronaut against the vehicle's floor or walls. In fact, the vehicle and its inhabitants maintain a state of continuous free-fall around the Earth in a microgravity environment (1.0×10^{-6}), as the vehicle's falling path remains parallel to the Earth's surface. The spacecraft and any unfixed object within it fall *around* the Earth, not toward it. All objects in a state of free-fall experience the same acceleration regardless of their mass. Interestingly, springboard divers launch themselves into the air when performing dives and then experience the free-fall of microgravity (at a rate independent of the diver's mass).

Spacecraft that maintain Earth orbit at an established velocity produce high-quality microgravity. The United

States reusable launch vehicles (space shuttles) stay in orbit for no longer than 18 days (16 d planned mission plus a 2-d contingency capability); before the Russian Mir Space Station was deorbited (March 21, 2001), it remained in orbit for 15 years (launched Feb. 20, 1986), maintaining continuous free fall as it circled Earth. Currently, the 454-metric ton (356 × 290-ft wing span) ISS orbits Earth every 90 minutes.

A spacecraft sustains circular orbit because the centripetal acceleration of uniform circular motion remains approximately the same as gravity (centripetal acceleration $= v^2 \div r$, where v = object velocity; r = distance from the object's center to the center of Earth [E]). For a typical space shuttle orbit, acceleration due to gravity at a shuttle's typical 296-km altitude can be computed from the equation:

$$F = Gm_E\, m \div r_E^{\,2}$$

where F = force of Earth's gravity on a mass (m) at Earth's surface. Also, $F = mg$, where $g = Gm_E \div r_E^2$: thus, $F = Gm_E\, m \div r^2$, which represents the force of Earth's gravity on a mass (m) at distance r from Earth's center. Since $F = ma$, where $a = Gm_E \div r^2$, this means that $gr_E^{\,2} = ar^2$, and $a = gr_E^{\,2} \div r^2$. The latter represents acceleration due to Earth's gravity at a distance r from Earth's center. We know the Earth's radius (6.37×10^6 m), therefore acceleration (a) due to gravity at the space shuttle's altitude computes as follows:

$$a = 9.8\ \text{m} \cdot \text{s}^{-2}\,(6.37 \times 10^6\ \text{m})^2 \div (6.67 \times 10^6\ \text{m})^2$$
$$= 8.9\ \text{m} \cdot \text{s}^{-2}$$

In this example, $8.9\ \text{m} \cdot \text{s}^{-2}$ achieves approximately 90% of the acceleration due to gravity at Earth's surface. Using the same equation, one could predict 10^{-6} microgravity at a distance 6.37×10^9 miles from the center of Earth.

Passenger in a Falling Elevator

When an elevator descends quickly, one feels a lessening of weight because of the reduced force between the feet and the elevator floor. If the elevator cable suddenly snaps and the elevator plummets downward, the force against the feet equals zero until the elevator strikes bottom. Consider the example of a 60-kg woman. If she could lift her feet off the floor before hitting the ground, she would float within the elevator compartment. No force pushes her up because she and the elevator fall together at the same speed and acceleration. This applies equally to any other objects in the elevator. If a scale were present in the elevator, the woman's weight would not register because the scale too would be falling. **Apparent weight**, computed as $AW = m(a - g)$, depends on the person's mass (m) and acceleration (a). Substituting in the equation yields a weightless (zero-g) condition: $(60\ \text{kg})(-9.81\ \text{m} \cdot \text{s}^{-2} - 9.81\ \text{m} \cdot \text{s}^{-2}) = 0\ \text{kg}$. *During free fall, everything in the elevator remains weightless because the person and elevator car (including a scale) accelerate downward at the same rate due to gravity alone.*

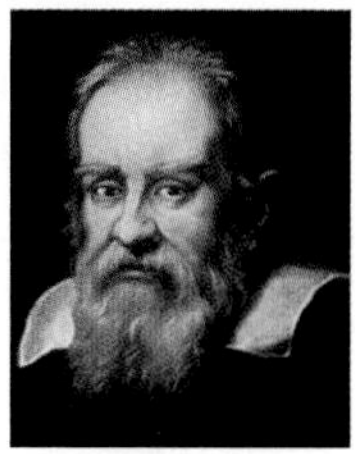

Galileo Galilei (1564–1642)

Galileo, in his classic *Two New Sciences,* makes the case of a similar "falling" experiment in which, legend has it, he simultaneously dropped a cannonball and musket ball of different masses from the Leaning Tower of Pisa. Galileo observed that both objects fell downward at approximately the same rate and consequently touched the ground at the same time. In his demonstration of the two falling masses, F and g both equaled zero, as both objects hit the ground at the same time, similar to the situation of the person and elevator striking the ground simultaneously. The term *zero-g* correctly applies to these temporary weightless conditions.

Examples of Near–Zero-g During Space Flight

Space flight provides the ubiquitous condition of near–zero-g. Liquids fail to remain in open cups or glasses, so drinks must be squeezed into the mouth from special containers. No "up" or "down" exists inside the space vehicle; to keep from floating freely, astronauts must anchor or tether themselves to a fixed object within the cabin (e.g., a wall or other

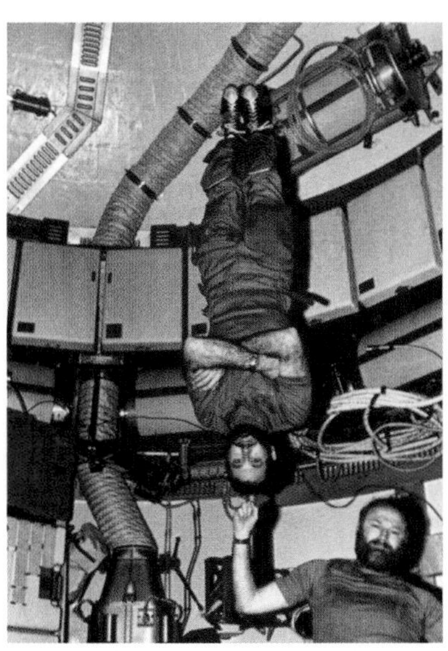

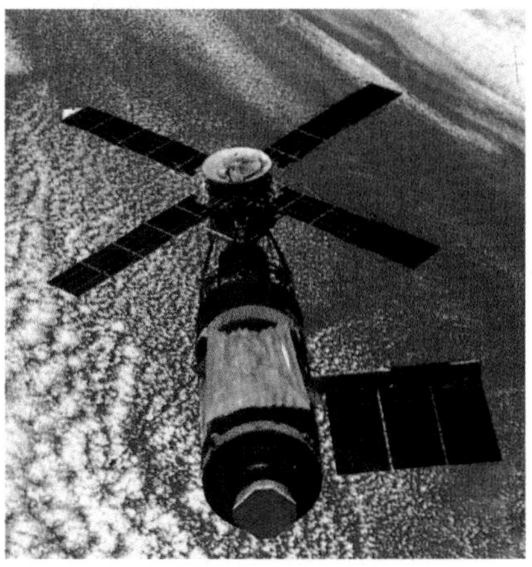

Demonstration of microgravity aboard Spacelab (photo above shows the entire vehicle in orbit; note the solar panels), where no "up" or "down" exists.

attached object). Astronauts aboard the 1973–1974 Skylab missions wore shoes with a triangular-shaped cleat on the sole. The floors, made of aluminum alloy webbing with triangular openings, provided a contact surface for the shoe, which when twisted, locked the foot in place. The cleated shoes provided a stable base to apply leverage for movement. The contact surface provides reaction forces to gravitational or inertial and accelerational forces. These enable the body's muscoloskeletal-neural internal "sensors" to achieve control over posture and locomotion.

In microgravity, blood and fluid volumes shift upward into the thoracocephalic region, causing a puffy-face appearance as fluid relocates from extracellular to intracellular spaces.[73] Correspondingly, a 2- to 5-cm decrease occurs in waist girth (a legitimate way in space to wear otherwise tight-fitting pants!). The initial net shift of fluid also produces eye redness, "bird-type" (skinny) legs, nasal congestion, headaches, and nausea. Concomitant reductions in blood volume affect cardiovascular function, manifested by decreased plasma and red blood cell volume, increased venous pooling, blunted baroreceptor reflex, and **orthostatic intolerance** (defined as compromised venous return to the heart during upright posture in a gravity environment).

On Earth, the constant downward pressure of 1g compresses intervertebral disks. In microgravity, however, the removal of gravitational force causes the disks to expand, and stature actually increases by as much as 5 cm (Fig. 27.1 top). The *bottom* of Figure 27.1 illustrates that posture also changes during microgravity exposure. Compared with preflight, joints move toward the midpoint in their range of motion, so

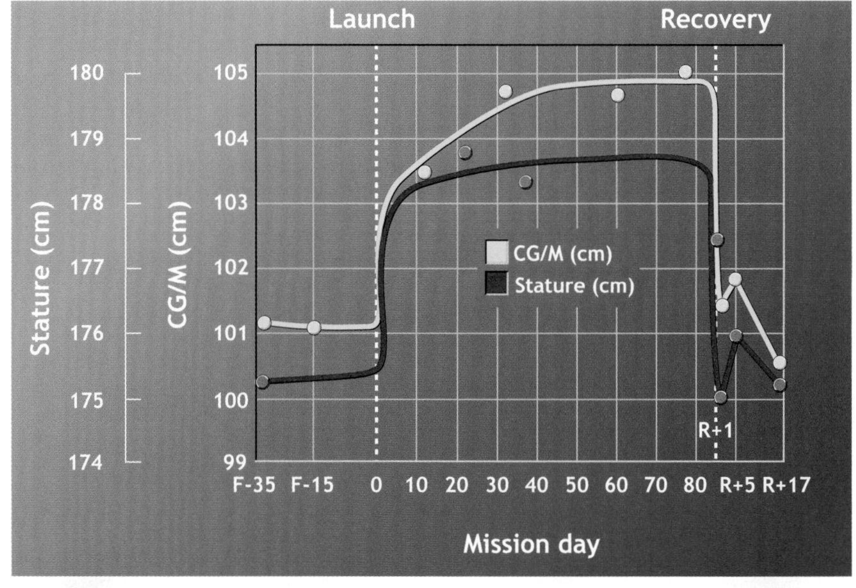

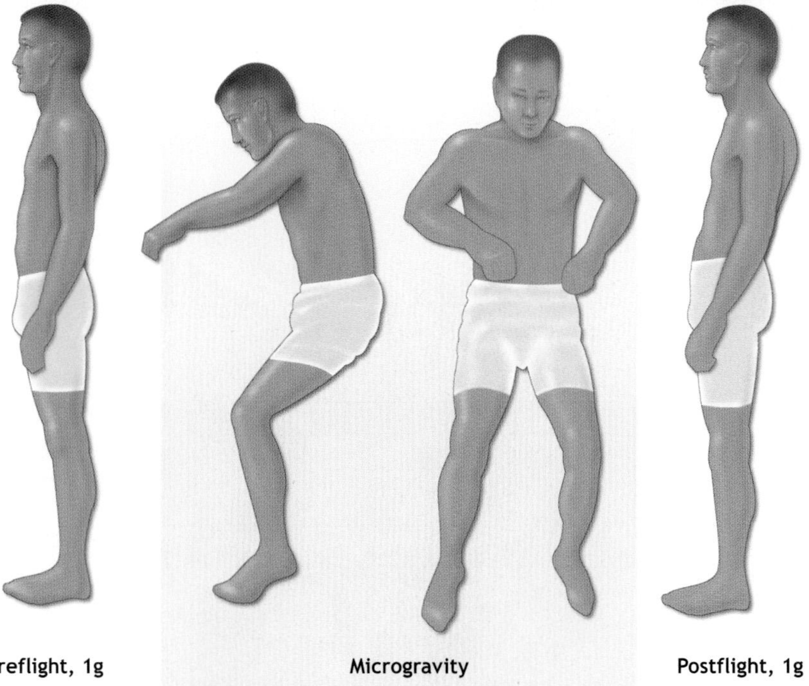

FIGURE 27.1 • *Top.* Change in center of gravity/mass (CG ÷ M) and stature before (F), during an 84-day Skylab 4 mission, and 17 days postflight (R). *Bottom.* General changes in posture under conditions of Earth's gravity (1g) and microgravity. (From Thornton WE, et al. Anthropometric changes and fluid shifts. In: Johnson RS, Dietlein LF, eds. Biomedical results from Skylab. NASA SP-377. Washington, DC: Government Printing Office, 1977.)

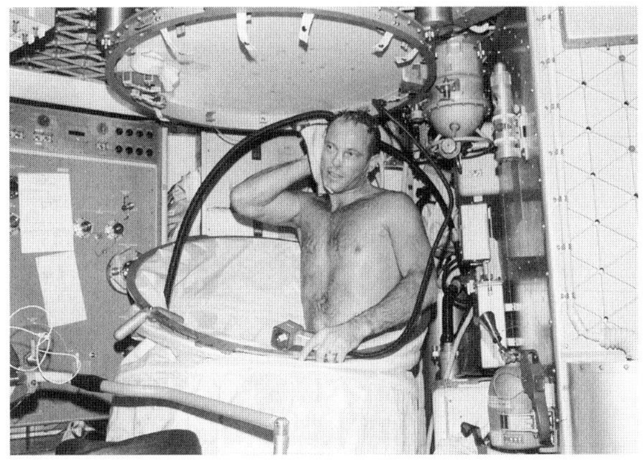

FIGURE 27.2 • Astronaut Jack Lousma, Skylab 3 pilot, takes a hot bath in the crew quarters of the Orbital Workshop (OWS). In deploying the shower facility, the shower curtain pulled up from the floor and attached to the ceiling. The water came through a push-button showerhead connected to a flexible hose, and a vacuum system drew off the water. (Photo courtesy of NASA, Lyndon B. Johnson Space Center, Houston, TX.)

that hips and knees flex slightly, causing the body to crouch. Arms tend to float in front of the body unless consciously forced downward. Note the postural sway with head protruding forward with accompanying lordosis immediately following the mission upon return to Earth.

New technology and techniques to offset the effects of microgravity often replace the most ordinary tasks on Earth. Anchoring of eating utensils becomes essential or else they float freely away. The same holds true for food; crumbs fall downward to one's plate or napkin on Earth, while in a microgravity environment, they disperse in all directions to pose a menace if inhaled or they migrate to clog a sensitive instrument. Similarly, sprinkled salt or pepper fails to reach the intended food. Spilled water does not drip downward, but drifts upward to form mostly stationary, suspended particles within the cabin. When these globules contact a solid object, they spread like pancake batter and cling to surfaces, making them difficult to remove. Without the reacting force of friction, simple chores such as showering require new strategies and unique skills. Figure 27.2 shows the shower facility aboard the 1973 Skylab 3 vehicle. Shower facilities were not included on subsequent shuttle flights because of the cumbersome nature of the equipment and the time required to shower. Instead, astronauts now use a sprayable hand washer and take a sponge bath. The sponge absorbs the sprayed water, which the astronaut then squeezes into an airflow system that carries the fluid into a waste collection tank.

Gravity on Moon and Mars

Gravity on celestial bodies is always a positive number because it represents the magnitude of a vector quantity. The attractive force on the moon's surface, for example, produces a g force of $1.6\ m \cdot s^{-2}$, or approximately one-sixth that on Earth. When astronauts land on Mars, they will experience a g force of $3.7\ m \cdot s^{-2}$, approximately 40% as large as experienced on the Earth's surface at sea level.

To reach the Martian surface, astronauts will rely on a lander vehicle (see schematic illustration below) to descend from the main launch spacecraft to the Martian surface. Suppose the Earth weight of the Mars lander (w_{lander}) equaled 39,200 N (mass remains the same on Mars or anywhere in between Earth and Mars). Mars has a radius of 3.40×10^6 m and a mass of 6.42×10^{23} kg. The distance r from the center of Mars can be computed as:

$$\begin{aligned} r &= (6.0 \times 10^6\ m) + (3.40 \times 10^6\ m) \\ &= 9.4 \times 10^6\ m \end{aligned}$$

The mass of the Mars lander (m_{lander}) equals its Earth weight divided by the factor for the acceleration of gravity on Earth:

$$\begin{aligned} m_{lander} &= w_{lander} \div g = 39{,}200\ N \div 9.9\ m \cdot s^{-2} \\ &= 4000\ kg \end{aligned}$$

From the following equation:

$$\begin{aligned} F_g &= Gm_{mars}m \div r^2 \\ &= (6.67 \times 10^{-11}\ Nm^2 \cdot kg^{-2})(6.42 \times 10^{23}\ kg)(4000\ kg) \div (9.4 \times 10^6\ m)^2 \\ &= 1940\ N \end{aligned}$$

The acceleration due to Mars gravity can be calculated as follows:

$$\begin{aligned} g_{mars} &= F_g \div m \\ &= 0.48\ m \cdot s^{-2} \end{aligned}$$

To determine F_g and g_{mars} at Mars' surface, replace $r = 9.4 \times 10^6$ m with $r_{mars} = 3.40 \times 10^6$ m. At the surface of Mars, $F_g = 15{,}000$ N and $g_{mars} = 3.7\ m \cdot s^{-2}$

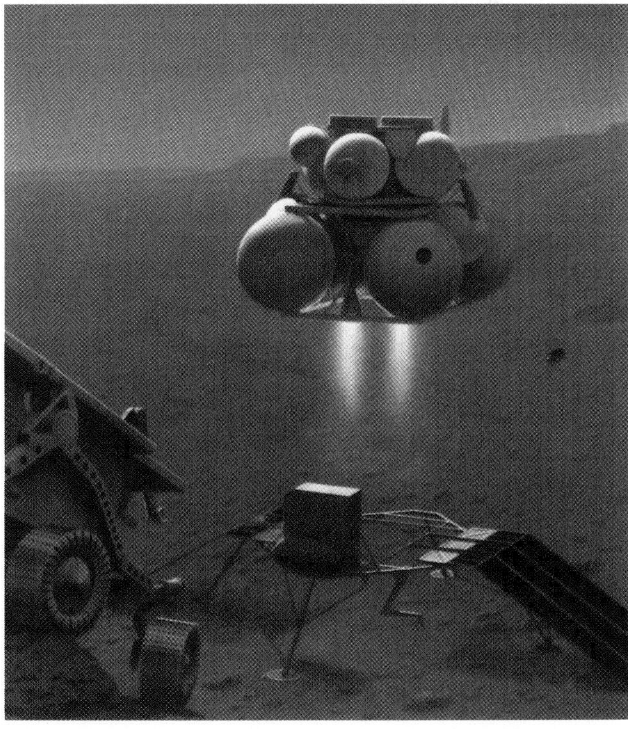

Concept drawing of a Mars lander vehicle to transport crew members between an orbiting space launch vehicle and the Martian surface.

Strategies for Simulating Microgravity

Different types of strategies have simulated space flight's microgravity environment, allowing researchers to manipulate various experimental conditions before deciding the best procedure(s) for a particular mission. One strategy uses sophisticated test equipment that creates zero-gravity conditions for relatively brief times for use with nonhuman objects dropped from towers and into tubes or within sounding rockets as they fall to Earth after achieving a maximum altitude. Another employs parabolic airplane flights with living and nonliving objects, whereas a third strategy simulates microgravity conditions with animals and humans using head-down bed rest, confinement, water immersion, or immobilization.

Nonhuman Testing

The Microgravity Research Division of the **National Aeronautics and Space Administration** (**NASA**) Office of Life and Microgravity Sciences and Applications (www.microgravity.hg.nasa.gov/) directs a basic and applied research program from the Marshall Space Flight Center that supports ground-based and flight experiments requiring microgravity conditions of varying duration and quality. In microgravity, researchers study the fundamental states of matter—solids, liquids, and gases—and the forces acting upon them. In addition to the space shuttles and ISS, NASA researchers use four other methods to achieve either zero-gravity or microgravity (3 of the 4 shown on this page and the fourth shown on page 687 [Fig. 27.4]). These include (1) two drop towers, one tower where objects fall 24 m, and one in-ground shaft 132-m deep and 6.1-m diameter, and one drop tube 105-m high for achieving 2.2 to 5.2 seconds of zero-gravity conditions; (2) sounding rockets that fly suborbital parabolic trajectories with a payload that produces several minutes of high-quality microgravity during the rocket's coast and before atmospheric re-entry; (3) bioreactor (rotating wall cylinder to randomize the gravity vector in cell culture samples, which reduces shear forces and simulates microgravity exposure (www.science.nasa.gov/newhome/br/bioreactor.htm) by perpendicular rotation to the gravity vector that intersects the center of the cell (which alters cytoplasmic viscosity and disrupts normal particle distribution, causing particle "suspension"); and (4) reduced-gravity aircraft that achieve microgravity conditions for 25 to 30 seconds.

The longest zero-gravity drop time currently available (approximately 10 s) occurs in Japan in a 490-m deep vertical mine shaft converted to a drop facility (jem.tksc.nasda.go.jp/index_e.html). The Bremen Drop Tower at Bremen University, Germany, consists of a 146-m tall concrete shaft that produces one-millionth of Earth's gravity (1.0 micro-g or 1.0×10^{-6} g). In all of the drop facilities, polystyrene pellets decelerate the payload as it hits the ground from its fall within the tube whose air has been evacuated to minimize drag. The 105-m drop tube at Marshall Space Flight Center can create a vacuum of less than a billionth of an atmosphere. Sensations similar to those from a drop in the reduced gravity facilities can be experienced on most roller coaster amusement park rides.

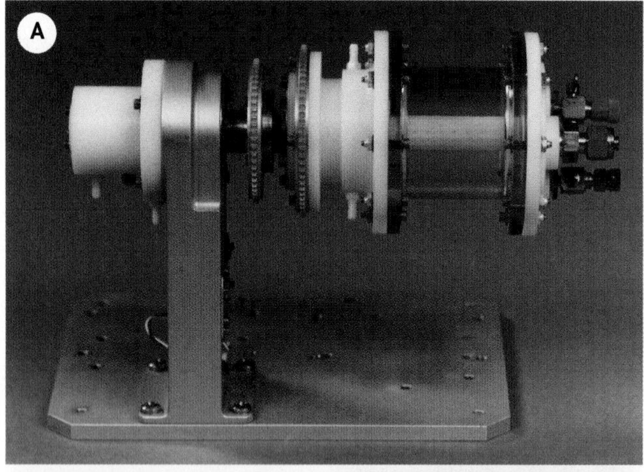

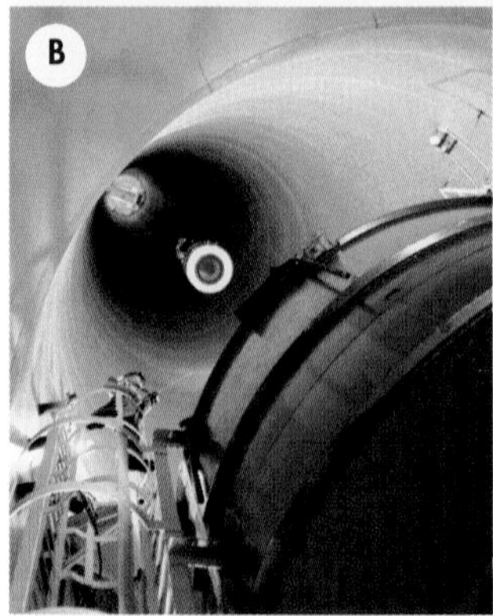

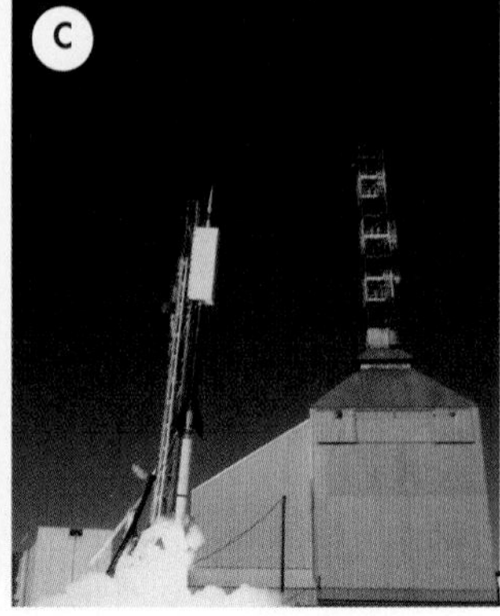

A. Bioreactor apparatus. **B**. Drop tower facility. Note object in mid-flight within the tower. **C**. Launch of sounding rocket.

Human Testing

Researchers have devised five basic strategies to simulate a microgravity environment and study its effects on humans: (1) head-down bed rest, (2) wheelchair confinement of paraplegics, (3) water immersion, (4) immobilization and confinement, and (5) parabolic flights.

HEAD-DOWN BED REST. Head-down bed rest has yielded the most information about human physiologic dynamics in simulated microgravity. Results of these studies have confirmed experimental findings in space about physiologic responses and adaptations, including psychologic stress, hormonal changes, and immune function[13,78]; this makes the head-down bed rest strategy a particularly useful space flight analogue. Subjects remain confined to bed for an extended time (weeks, months, or a year) in a horizontal or head-down tilt position (−3 to −12°), often followed by physiologic measurements in response to positive acceleration at forces up to 3g in a centrifuge.

WHEELCHAIR CONFINEMENT OF PARAPLEGICS. Prolonged wheelchair confinement produces postural hypotension, particularly in paraplegics, who seldom experience full erect posture following their disability.[25] As in longer space flight missions

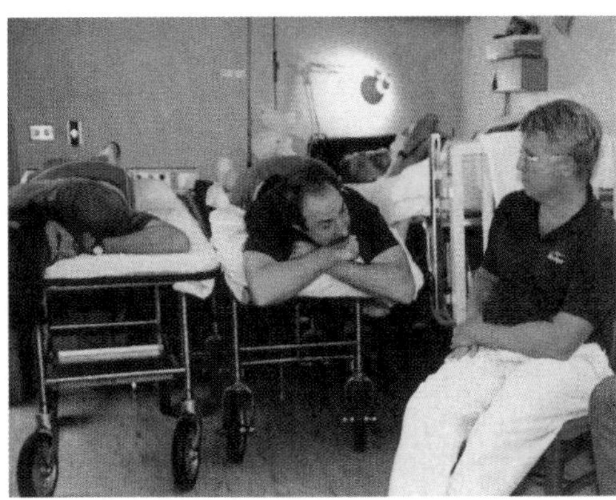

Bed rest, head-down experimental strategy to study postural hypotension and associated cardiovascular functions.

(>21 d), years of sitting constrain fluctuations in hydrostatic gradients normally experienced by nonparaplegics during routine daily activities. Short-term exercise stress (e.g., graded, arm-crank exercise to maximum[91]) has been used to study paraplegics' responses for heart rate, systolic and diastolic blood pressure, forearm vascular resistance (FVR), and vasoactive hormones.[34] In general, exercise eliminated orthostatic hypotension and increased FVR and baroreflex sensitivity independent of blood volume changes. These positive cardiovascular adjustments in paraplegics to less frequent, but relatively intense exercise, have relevance as a postflight countermeasure to the potentially debilitating effects of prolonged missions on orthostatic stability and baroreflex functions following return to Earth's gravitational environment. The intriguing possibility of immediate benefit from short-term, intense postflight exercise would maximize overall mission efficiency by reducing the time devoted to in-flight exercise and concomitant demands for additional food and water associated with daily exercise.[35]

WATER IMMERSION. Subjects lie supine in a water tank for up to 24 hours (wet immersion technique) or lie on a thin sheet to prevent the skin from touching the water (dry immersion technique). Figure 27.3 illustrates maneuvers under water in a space suit as a simulation modality of near–zero-g conditions. The astronaut performs complex hand–eye coordination tasks to mimic skills required during **extravehicular activity** (**EVA**) during orbital missions.

IMMOBILIZATION AND CONFINEMENT.

- Whole-body or segmental casts restrict limb and body movements in humans and animals. A recent approach immobilizes the nondominant arm in a sling, except during sleep and bathing, for 4 weeks.[91] This procedure produces an effective analogue for simulating the effects of "weightlessness" on human skeletal muscle loading. Changes in muscle structure and function (e.g., torque production, cross-sectional area, histochemical muscle fiber analysis, and integrated electromyography, or IEMG) produce results similar in magnitude and direction to data obtained from humans following exposure to real and simulated microgravity environments.
- Confining animals to small cages severely restricts their movement.
- A harness provides partial body support by suspending an animal in a head-down position with gravitational loading removed from the hind limbs (see the unnumbered figure on page 717).

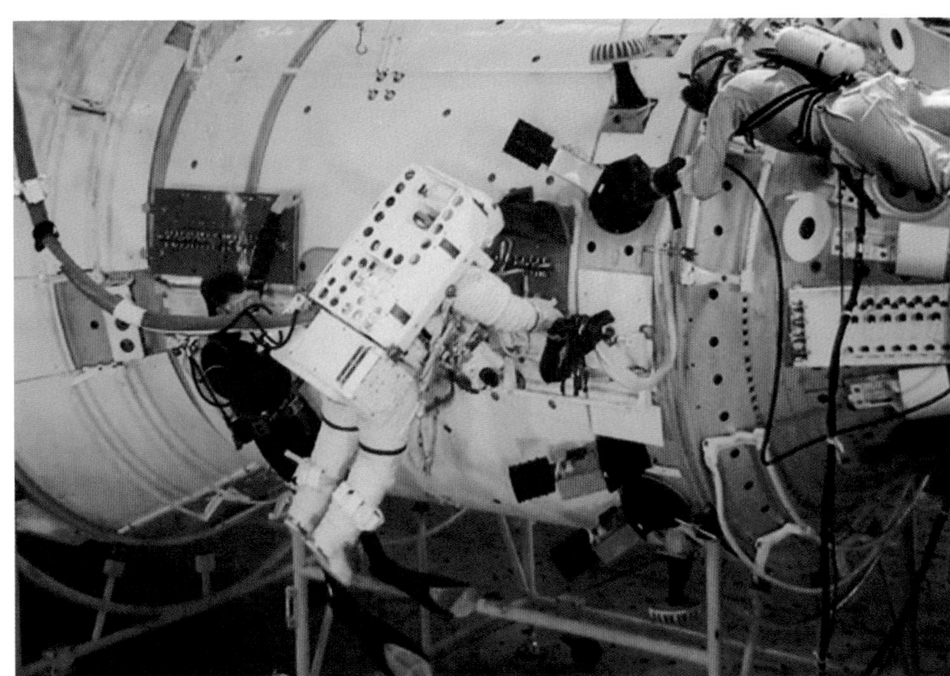

FIGURE 27.3 • An astronaut with the assistance of scuba divers performs a simulated EVA maneuver to the space shuttle in the Weightless Environment Training Facility. (Photos courtesy of NASA, Lyndon B. Johnson Space Center, Houston, TX.)

PARABOLIC FLIGHTS. Figure 27.4 *(top)* illustrates the strategy to evaluate physiologic responses to microgravity produced when NASA's KC-135 aircraft climbs rapidly at a 45° angle and then follows a path called a parabola. The aircraft produces a near–zero-g effect (1×10^{-3} g) for about 30 seconds (*center purple area* in the figure) just as the aircraft achieves 9500 m of the 10,000-m ascent (termed *pull-up*) before it slows. The plane then traces a parabola (pushover), descending rapidly at a 45° angle (termed *pull-out*) to 7300 m. The forces of acceleration and deceleration produce 2 to 2.5 times normal gravity during the pull-up and pull-out phases of the flight; the brief pushover at the apogee generates an environment with less than 1% of Earth's gravity. The gut-wrenching sensations produced during KC-135 training flights have earned the plane the nickname "vomit comet."

During repeated brief parabolic roller coaster-like maneuvers, scientists evaluate how humans and equipment function during intermittent forces ranging from 1.8g to near–zero-g, similar to those experienced during liftoff and re-entry of space vehicles. Depending on the mission, astronaut training can include up to 60 **parabolic flights** daily for a week, providing nearly 3 hours of cumulative weightlessness. Some career astronaut–researchers have accumulated 4000 and 5000 parabolas during a decade of KC-135 flight experiments, equivalent to 28 to 36 hours of simulated weightlessness.

The *bottom left* of Figure 27.4 shows scientists measuring shock-absorption parameters from vibrations during motorized treadmill exercise on KC-135 parabolic flights. Adding 245 kg to the base of the treadmill blunted the impact forces (and vibration effects) of the exercising subject. The adjacent photo shows astronauts testing both aerobic (rowing) and resistance-training equipment during the flights. Scientific information gleaned from the reduced-gravity aircraft flights has translated into on-board exercise regimens as countermeasures to gravity's effects during space shuttle and ISS missions (see page 719).

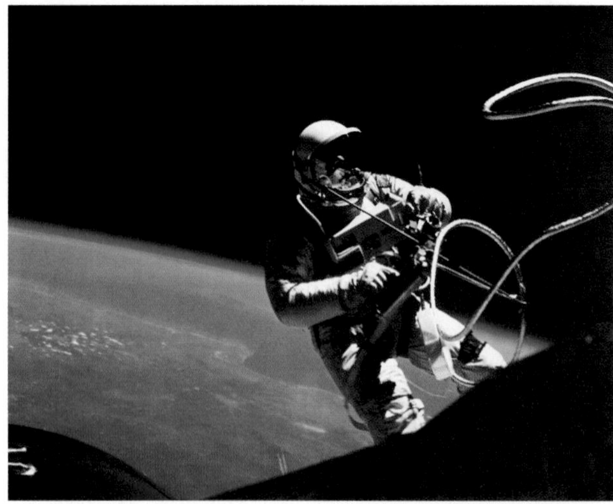

Astronaut Edward H. White II performed an EVA during the third revolution of the Gemini 4 spacecraft (June 9, 1965). White remained secured to the spacecraft by a 25-foot umbilical line and a 23-foot tether line, both wrapped in gold tape to form one cord. In his right hand, White carries a handheld, self-maneuvering unit. His gold-plated helmet visor protected him from the unfiltered rays of the sun.

Mathematical Modeling and Computer Simulations

Researchers generally consider an entire physiologic system (e.g., cardiovascular, thermoregulatory, hormonal, respiratory, muscular) or subdivide it into its component parts. For example, elements of the cardiovascular system include the heart, lungs, blood vessels, and blood. Each constituent can further subdivide into parts and factors such as wall compliance, wall thickness, and blood flow within the heart's chambers or through its valves and specific vasculature. Researchers mathematically model each component on the basis of known values for a particular function (e.g., HR_{max} in young adults averages close to 200 b · min^{-1} [standard deviation of ± 10 b · min^{-1}]).

Armed with numerous facts about the entire system, a computer-based model recreates how the system would respond to weightlessness when changes affect single or multiple components. Scientists have applied mathematical models of the thermoregulatory and cardiovascular systems to establish design criteria for the astronaut's space suit. For example, the model predicts the range of energy expenditures an astronaut might encounter with EVA (shown in unnumbered figure below; from 180 to 200 kcal · kg^{-1} · h^{-1} assessed during different space missions). On shuttle *Atlantis* STS-98 flight of 12 days and 21 hours (Feb. 7, 2001–Feb. 20, 2001), astronauts conducted 3 space walks over a period of 19 hours and 49 minutes. They used hand and power tools to bolt the U.S. Destiny Laboratory Module onto the station. By 2005, about 160 space walks will have been completed totaling 960 clock-hours or 1920 man-hours to assemble and maintain the station. Knowing the limits of sustained energy expenditure based on prior laboratory research establishes a reasonable completion time for the EVA and provides parameters for garment design for effective dissipation of the work-induced heat load above the basal requirement. Simulating different aspects of the EVA (speed of movement, intensity of effort, duration of task) and how different physiologic systems respond and adapt allows scientists the luxury of predicting outcomes under specified conditions. Well-designed mathematical models should ultimately predict physiologic response in microgravity with high accuracy.

HISTORICAL OVERVIEW OF AEROSPACE PHYSIOLOGY AND MEDICINE

This section briefly highlights the early history of aerospace medicine, paying tribute to pioneers and their accomplishments that ushered in the modern space age. Today's astronauts must overcome numerous diverse challenges as they prepare to live in space for prolonged periods. Perhaps during the middle of this century, thousands of individuals will routinely travel into space, some establishing permanent space colonies relatively near Earth orbit, while others participate in exploration-class missions to Mars and beyond. For example, the first human Mars mission will require 160 days to reach the planet. Astronauts will then spend 569 days establishing a base colony, including exploration, followed by a 154-day return voyage to Earth. This sojourn

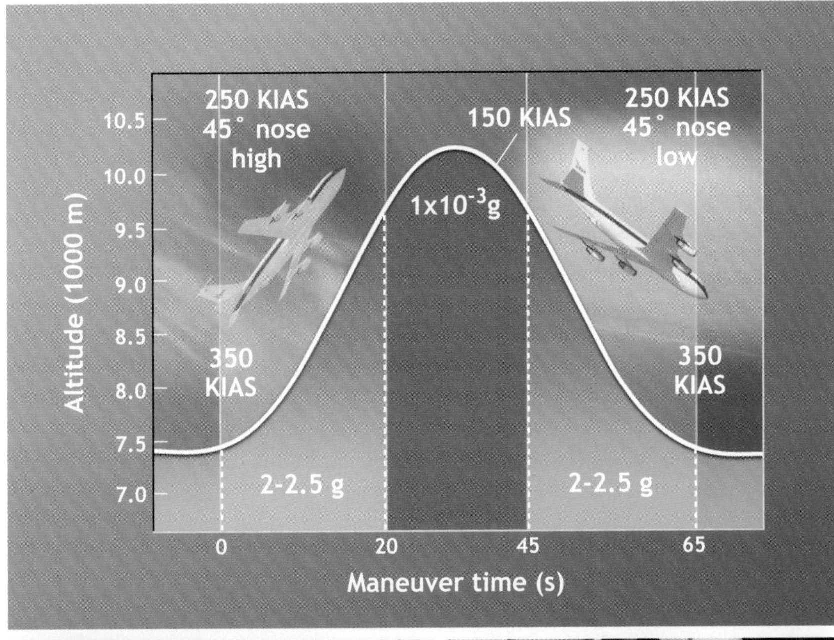

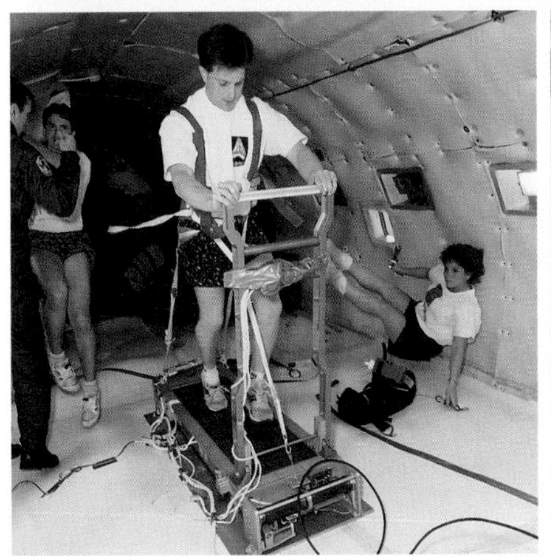

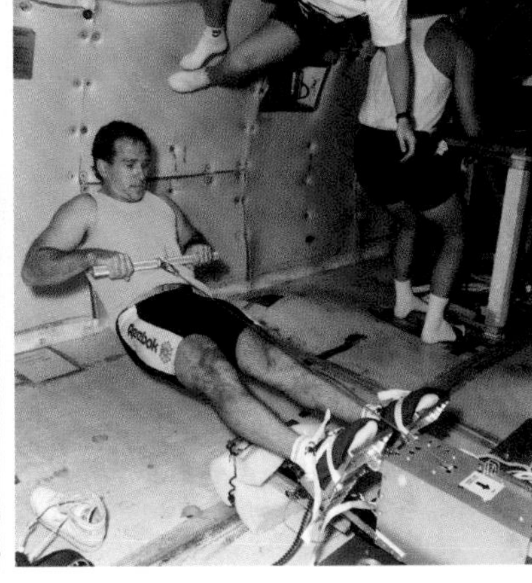

FIGURE 27.4 • *Top.* Parabolic (Keplerian trajectory) flight profile of NASA's KC-135 aircraft used to achieve brief periods of weightlessness. KIAS, knots indicating air speed. (From: Nicogossian AE, et al. Space physiology and medicine. 3rd ed. Philadelphia: Lea & Febiger, 1994.) *Bottom left.* Evaluating the shock absorption qualities caused by vibrations while running on a motorized treadmill during KC-135 flights. *Bottom right.* Evaluating exercise equipment (aerobic and strength) during KC-135 flights. (Photos courtesy of NASA, Lyndon B. Johnson Space Center, Houston, TX.)

provides three distinct travel phases: (1) rapid transition between a 1-g environment on Earth to microgravity, (2) 6 months in near–zero-g traveling to and from Mars, and (3) exposure to 0.38g while working and living on Mars. Each transition requires an integrated strategy of suitable countermeasures against physiologic deconditioning from prolonged microgravity, including radiation's potential negative effects (see page 701).[27]

In addition to experiencing varied gravitational forces, astronauts on Mars must contend with a hostile environment that includes viscous windstorms of several hundred miles per hour that can last for weeks, not to mention temperature extremes from –220°F to + 81°F. The thin atmosphere consists mostly of carbon dioxide (93.5%), so living on Mars requires a sustained presence of Earth's atmosphere. It is of interest that an astronaut's sleep cycle will probably not be adversely affected, because the Martian day lasts only 37 minutes longer than a day on Earth. However, a year on Mars lasts 687 days, with each of its four seasons twice as long as Earth's. Current research focuses on the interplay of multidisciplinary countermeasures, including exercise/fitness, nutrition/energy balance, and pharmacologic interventions to ensure astronaut health and well being and a successful mission.

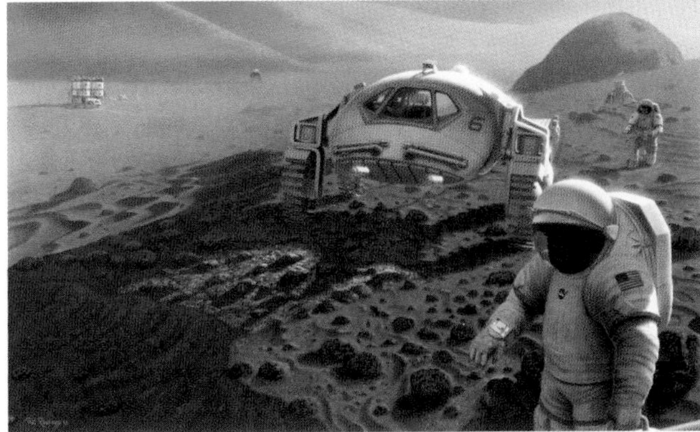

Conceptual drawing of a future exploration mission on Mars.

As humans venture into unexplored regions of space, new scientific knowledge about adaptations to microgravity affects exploration efforts. Research in exercise physiology and interrelated disciplines has significantly expanded knowledge about (1) microgravity's effects on human structure and function and adaptations and (2) countermeasure strategies to minimize undesirable outcomes. Throughout the history of aerospace exploration, achieving each new milestone fostered new challenges to improve human safety and health, while at the same time trying to match aircraft performance with the ambitious demands of flying faster and higher. A single historical event in 1957—the Russian **Sputnik-1** orbiting satellite (discussed shortly)—significantly impacted future research concerning physiologic function during high-altitude flights that accelerated man's quest to explore heavenly bodies beyond planet Earth.

Foundations

Progress in the embryonic field of aerospace physiology and medicine accelerated following World War II, primarily from impetus provided by the successful rocket-carrying bombs launched by the German Air Force against Britain in the war's late stages. German scientists who pioneered the successful V-2 rocket, the world's first operational long-range ballistic missile, immigrated to the United States and joined the rocket development program at the Army Ballistic Missile Agency of the Redstone Arsenal, Huntsville, Alabama, (named the George C. Marshall Space Flight Center in 1960 to honor the former Army Chief of Staff during World War II, Secretary of State, and Nobel Prize winner). By 1950, the U.S. military had capitalized on German rocket technology and launched new V-2 style rockets and advanced high-altitude balloons carrying primates and other animals to the fringes of space. With war no longer a major threat, research concentrated on developing more-sophisticated and powerful rocket engines capable of placing humans in Earth orbit.

Early Years

The first national civil aeronautics laboratory, now known as National Aeronautics and Space Administration Langley Research Center, was established in 1917 in Hampton, Virginia. This research facility currently focuses on aeronautics, earth science, space technology and structures, and materials research (www.larc.nasa.gov/). In 1951, the Aeromedical Association created a Space Medicine Branch for systematic evaluation of human function in a weightless environment. Two new research laboratories (U.S. Air Force School of Space Medicine [www.sam.brooks.af.mil/] and Naval Aerospace Medical Institute [www.hq.nasa.gov/office/pao/History/SP-60/cover.html]) also devoted time and resources to studying space medicine. These military research facilities partnered with universities and private sector laboratories to create a formidable team to study high-performance aircraft and unmanned guided missiles at high altitudes. Research eventually included human adaptation to high-altitude exposures. This included development in the 1930s of pressurized suits that allowed pilots to achieve higher altitudes than ever before (50,000 ft), paving the way for the 1961–1963 Mercury series of suborbital flights and eventual lunar missions.[82] From 1951 to 1957, the two new laboratories and auxiliary support facilities produced significant information, mostly about "hardware" aspects of space flight but also biomedical evaluations during suborbital flights with lower animal forms (bacteria, mice) and primates.

Suborbital Flights

In December 1946, experiments sponsored by the National Institutes of Health at Holloman's Aeromedical Field Laboratory (and later at Wright-Patterson Air Force Base and White Sands Air Force Base) studied cosmic radiation's effects on fungus spores (unsuccessful, as the cylinders carrying the microbes vanished on re-entry) and how fruit flies survived without deleterious effects at an altitude of 171 km. The Albert Project (named for the monkey sealed in the nose cone of the V-2 rocket) attempted to record respiration during space flight, but the respiration apparatus failed just before launch, and Albert perished. He would not have survived anyway because the parachute recovery apparatus also failed on the rocket's re-entry.

A second launch (Albert II) occurred 1 year later on June 14, 1949, but the primate died on impact when the recovery chute again failed. Fortunately, respiratory and electrocardiographic instruments verified that the primate functioned well during the 83-mile ascent and return. Two additional V-2 rocket flights provided supportive evidence that a primate could successfully withstand re-entry forces of 5.5g and exposure to cosmic radiation. A fifth V-2 launch substituted a mouse for the monkey, and an on-board camera photographed the mouse at fixed intervals. The mouse died on impact (once again the recovery system failed), but the mouse displayed normal muscular function and coordination during the subgravity flight. Additional flights in 1951 that monitored cardiovascular and respiration dynamics of primates showed no negative responses during these relatively brief missions.

With subsequent travel, rocketry systems improved and the on-board monkey and mice "animalnauts" survived intact during suborbital flights to altitudes of 36 miles. High-altitude balloon flights also proved successful. In September, 1950, eight white mice withstood a 97,000-ft ascent without negative physiologic consequences. The balloon experiments continued with fruit flies, mice, hamsters, cats, and dogs for up to 24 hours. Most of these experiments ended in failure, mainly from equipment malfunction. Nonetheless, the invaluable experience gained from rocket and balloon launchings, instrumentation and recovery techniques, and the growing body of scientific data related to cosmic radiation and subgravity physiologic responses would greatly benefit subsequent human endeavors. The years 1946 through 1952 marked the practical beginning of Air Force research in space biology and set the stage for the next round of experimentation with new and more powerful rockets.

High-Altitude Explorations

Between 1952 and 1957, research in high-altitude exploration matched the United States' enthusiasm for its embryonic space biology programs. Study areas included human reaction to subgravity or near–zero-g conditions, human re-entry into Earth's atmosphere, effects of abrupt and sustained acceleration and deceleration on human response to rocket flight, and equipment design for better accommodation for primate and human explorers as they pushed the envelope by ascending higher (120,000-ft balloon ascent) and for longer durations (up to 74 h). In 1952, the National Advisory Committee for Aeronautics (NACA; established in 1915 to foster aviation), proposed new research to (1) extend airplane velocity to Mach 10 (see below) at altitudes from 12 to 50 miles and (2) identify problems with space flights at speeds that required a 25,039-mph (40,200 km · h^{-1}, or 1.12×10^4 m · s^{-1}) escape velocity from Earth's gravity.

Mach numbers were named to honor Austrian physicist Ernst Mach (1838–1916) who established basic principles of supersonics and ballistics. The Mach number represents the ratio of an object's velocity to the velocity of sound, which travels at 1089 ft · s^{-1}, or 331.9 m · s^{-1}, at 0°C. For example, Mach 10 refers to 10 times the speed of sound. Interestingly, professor Mach rejected Newton's concepts of absolute time and space before Einstein, who cited Mach's inertial theories in the early 1900s in developing his relativity theory.

By 1954, characteristics for a new hypersonic research aircraft had been defined, and 1 year later, North American Aviation won the competition to build the X-15 airplane. Construction began in September 1957, ushering in a new era that featured high-performance aircraft capable of hypersonic speeds (4250 mph) at altitudes close to the fringes of the atmosphere (67 mi, or 353,760 ft). Concurrently, the United States had committed to launch an Earth-orbiting satellite as part of the International Geophysical Year (July 1, 1957, to December 31, 1958) to gather scientific information about our planet. At the same time, the early phases of developing a potential space vehicle and sophisticated satellite program were about to change in sudden and dramatic fashion.

The Rocket Launch That Shocked the World

On October 4, 1957, the Russians shocked the world when their 83.6-kg, 58-cm diameter aluminum alloy Sputnik-1, shown below, became the first Earth-orbiting satellite. One month later, on November 3, a larger 508-kg Sputnik-2 remained in orbit for almost 200 days with a dog on board. These space milestones—achieved 4 months before the Naval Research Laboratory launched its inaugural, tiny 1.6-kg Vanguard 1 orbiting, unmanned satellite—jolted the United States' scientific and government establishments into a sense of urgency to surpass Russia's apparent space technology supremacy. Two factors contributed to a "space race" to achieve dominance of this new frontier: (1) fear of losing potential military superiority in space and (2) fear of losing the "education race" to an enlightened Russian youth who possibly excelled in mathematics and science.

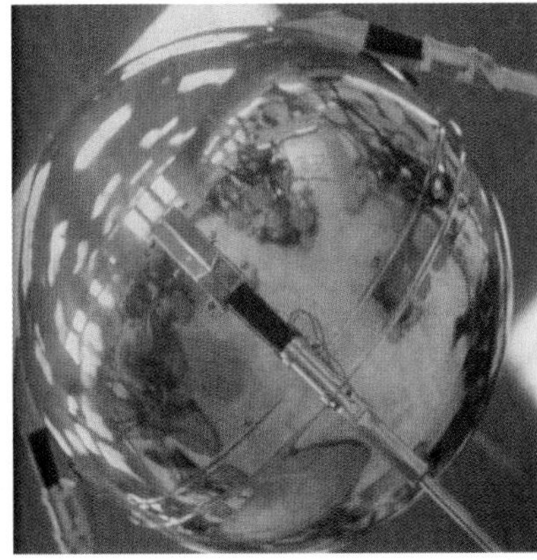

Sputnik-1 satellite

MODERN ERA

In 1958, the newly formed NASA laid the groundwork for future discoveries that would affect almost every facet of our lives. These included discoveries about rocketry and propulsion systems, physiologic requirements and adaptations to manned space flight, and more than 30,000 practical "technology-transfer" payoffs (discussed on page 742) from interdisciplinary experiments in physical chemistry, microbiology, genetics, medicine, and exercise physiology.

National Aeronautics and Space Administration

Reacting swiftly to the perceived Soviet threat of technologic superiority, the United States Congress passed the National Aeronautics and Space Act, signed into law on July 29, 1958, by President Dwight D. Eisenhower. As a new federal agency, NASA began operation on October 1, 1958, less than a year after the successful Sputnik-1 launch. For the first time in our history, a single government agency had responsibility for conquering a new frontier only dreamt about by the early aeronaut explorers. These pioneers included Wilson, who attached thermometers to kites, 1749; the Montgolfier brothers Joseph and Etienne, who in 1783 ascended in large-capacity hot air balloons that they designed; and physicist J. A. C. Charles in one of the first free ascents with a passenger and gondola in a hydrogen-filled balloon (1783); Grey, Piccard, Anderson, and Steven, who flew in high-altitude balloons (1920s–1930s); Aida de Costa, the first woman to pilot a powered gasoline air-

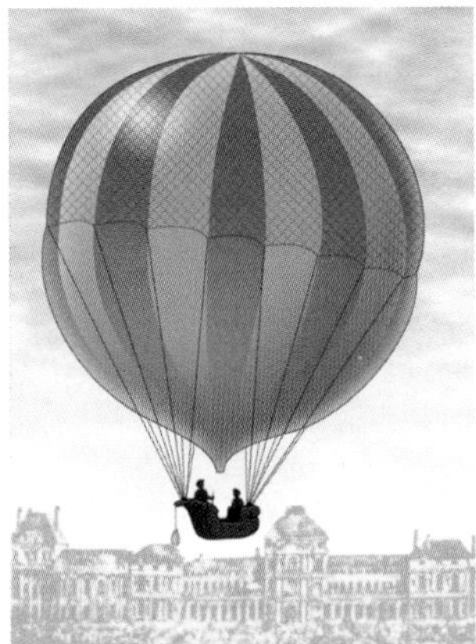

A physician (Pilâtre de Rozier) and military officer (Marquis d' Arlandes) made the first manned, sustained hydrogen balloon free ascent to 85 m that lasted 25 minutes and covered 8 km over Paris, France on November 21,1783. The two men carried a pail of water and sponge to arrest sparks that often ignited small fires that threatened the 23-m-by-15-m balloon made of painted cloth fabric and paper. The balloon weighed 725 kg (including a fire basket made of wrought iron wire) with an estimated lift (payload) of 770 kg. In 1785, de Rozier became the first fatality when his balloon exploded at about 1000 m.

craft (dirigible) solo, in Paris on June 29, 1903, months before Orville Wright's (1871–1948) flight; such scientists as Johannes Kepler (1571–1630), who penned an imaginary moon visit *(Somnium, sive Astronomia Lunaris);* and an emerging cadre of science writers (e.g., Jules Verne, 1865, *De la Terre a la Lune;* Hale, *Brick Moon*, serialized in *Atlantic Monthly* magazine in 1869–1870; Eyraud, *Voyage a Venus*, 1875).

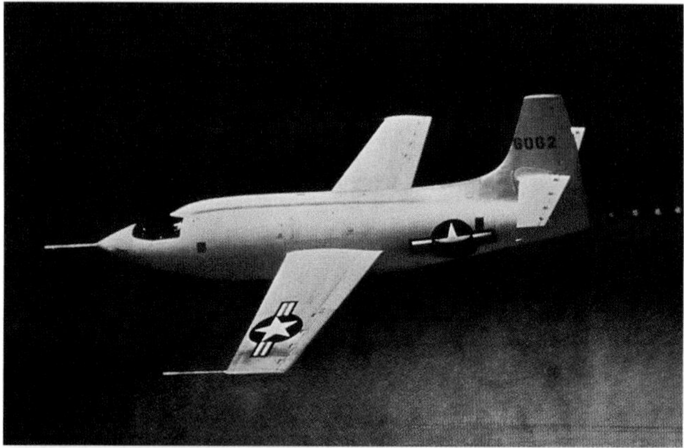

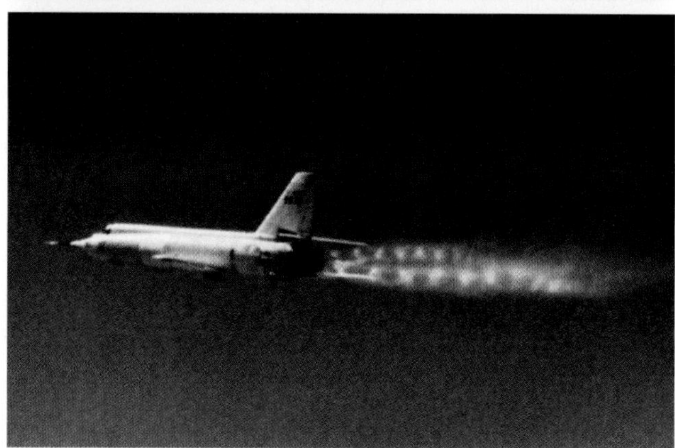

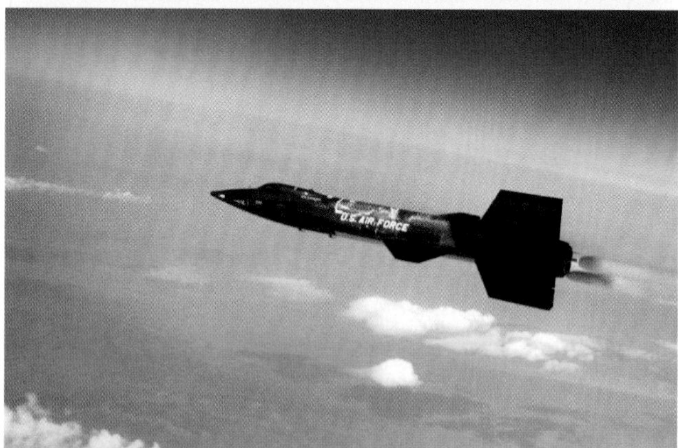

FIGURE 27.5 • *Top.* The X-1 made the world's first supersonic flight (Mach 1.45) by breaking the sound barrier on October 14, 1947. The Douglas D-558-2 skyrocket (not shown) flew to Mach 2 on November 20, 1953). *Middle.* The X-2 achieved Mach 3 on September 27, 1956. *Bottom.* Top view of the X-15 during high altitude and speed trials. Test pilot Joe Walker flew the X-15 to a world-record altitude of 354,200 feet (67.1 mi) on August 22, 1963. Three years later on October 3, 1967, Peter Knight piloted the X-15 to Mach 6.7. His vehicle's launch weight (rocket plus fuel) was approximately 33,000 pounds (landing weight, 14,700 lb). The X-15 had a fuel capacity of 1003 gallons of liquid oxygen and 1445 gallons of anhydrous ammonia. (Photos from Stillwell WH. X-15. Research results with a selected bibliography. www.hq.nasa.gov/office/pao/History/SP-60/cover.html.)

At its inception, NASA inherited 8000 employees and a $100 million budget; it supervised three major research laboratories (Langley Aeronautical Laboratory, established in 1918; Ames Aeronautical Laboratory, founded in 1940; and Lewis Flight Propulsion Laboratory, created in 1941). NASA also supervised two smaller facilities at Monroc Dry Lake in the California desert for high-speed flight research and Wallops Island, Virginia, for testing rockets. NASA absorbed the Jet Propulsion Laboratory, managed by the California Institute of Technology, and the Army Ballistic Missile Agency, whose engineers were developing the massive rocket engines required for space flight. NASA assimilated the technical resources obtained from 13 prior years of jet aircraft research with the X-1 (which achieved Mach 1) and X-2 (which achieved Mach 3) rocket airplanes, including engineering information gleaned from hundreds of other rocket and jet airplane flights. Figure 27.5 shows the X-1, X-2, and X-15 rocket aircraft, the predecessors of NASA's successful shuttle aircraft.

NASA had two main goals: (1) launching a man into space and returning him safely to Earth and (2) developing the capability of humans to endure space missions.[88] Achieving this second goal had been a Herculean task because the current knowledge of microgravity's effects remained restricted to laboratory simulations. Scientists knew little about how humans would respond to the rigors of microgravity and what might happen during extended sojourns beyond Earth's gravitational field. Experts publicly expressed concern about possible deleterious effects of space flight on human function and overall health. In 1958, the National Academy of Sciences–National Research Council Committee on Bioastronautics listed 30 potential ill effects from human exposure to the space environment during launch and re-entry (Table 27.1). Many of these concerns proved justified and are discussed in subsequent sections.

TABLE 27.1 ➤ PREDICTED DELETERIOUS EFFECTS OF WEIGHTLESSNESS DURING LAUNCH, TRAVEL, AND RE-ENTRY

• Anorexia	• Bone demineralization
• Nausea	• Renal calculi
• Disorientation	• Motion sickness
• Sleeplessness	• Pulmonary atelectasis
• Fatigue	• Tachycardia
• Restlessness	• Hypertension
• Euphoria	• Hypotension
• Hallucinations	• Cardiac arrhythmia
• Decreased g tolerance	• Postflight syncope
• Gastrointestinal disturbance	• Decreased work capacity
• Urine retention	• Reduced blood volume
• Diuresis	• Reduced plasma volume
• Muscular incoordination	• Dehydration
• Muscle atrophy	• Weight loss
• Sleepiness	• Infectious illnesses

Modified from Dietlein LF. Skylab: a beginning. In: Johnston RS, Dietlein LF, eds. Biomedical results from Skylab (NASA SP-377). Washington, DC: U.S. Government Printing Office. 1977.

In the race to become first in space, scientists could not afford the luxury of years to conduct systematic research. Instead, a test pilot's prior flight experience provided "seat-of-the pants" solutions to important aeronautical questions. Fortunately, the fully pressurized flight suits used by Navy test pilots during high-altitude reconnaissance became the first "space suits" during the early rocket missions. This allowed NASA to proceed on a fast track toward eventually putting a human into space.

United States Races Into Space

Besides initiating human space flight, NASA's other top priority centered on a plan to allow humans to work for extended periods during prolonged space missions. These two goals required advanced technologies in rocket design and effective approaches to prepare test pilots for missions never attempted previously. To put a human into Earth orbit required new ways of looking at the man–machine interface. On the human side, engineers had to design a fail-safe life-support system, provide for food and water, integrate an efficient method to remove metabolic by-products, and implement temperature control to ensure crew safety during liftoff, flight, and re-entry. Research had to determine physiologic responses to extremes of acceleration and reduced gravity, including short- and long-term adjustments to prolonged weightlessness. Could a human function competently during liftoff, propelled upward at thousands of miles per hour, and then perform flawlessly in maneuvering the space vehicle and returning it to Earth safely? Engineers needed to develop rocket engines with sufficient thrust to achieve escape velocity. The pilot's capsule required intricate communication and navigation controls. The capsule's weight and size had to dovetail with rocket design and launch requirements. In addition, a capsule recovery system required development for safe re-entry. The human and engineering requirements facing NASA provided significant challenges to say the least, and the race into space was on with no turning back.

The current human space program owes a debt of gratitude to thousands of men and women from many countries whose imaginations and careers spearheaded possibilities of space exploration. The following sections review key achievements of the United States and Russian space programs related to advances in space medicine and physiology. These superpowers played the dominant role in the space effort, but not without significant contributions from European, Japanese, and Canadian human space programs. Their remarkable successes culminated in the launches (Nov. and Dec. 1998) of Russian and United States rockets to initiate assembly of the ISS (Fig. 27.6). On October 30, 2000, the

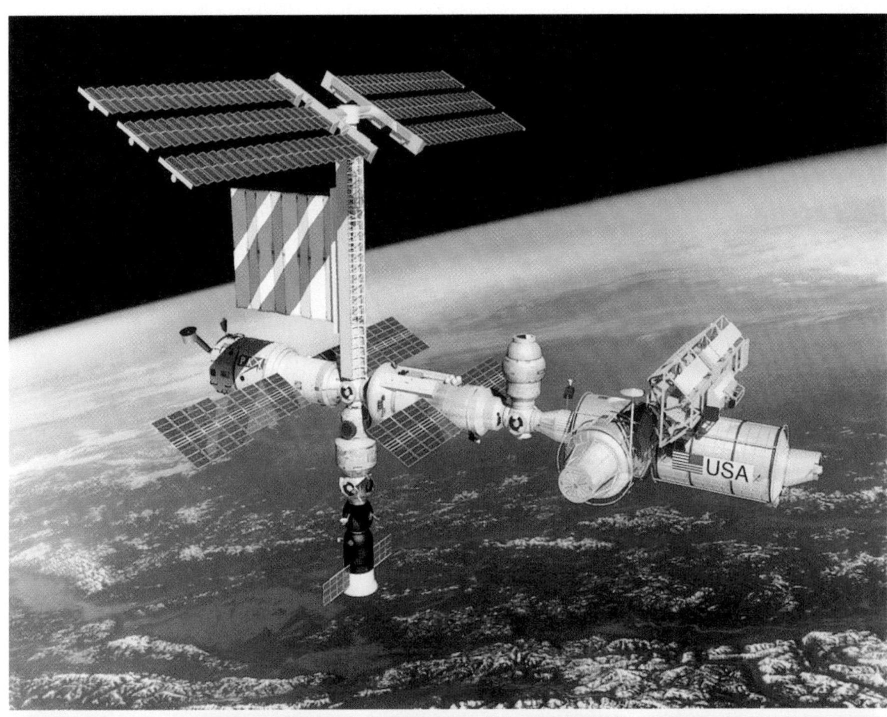

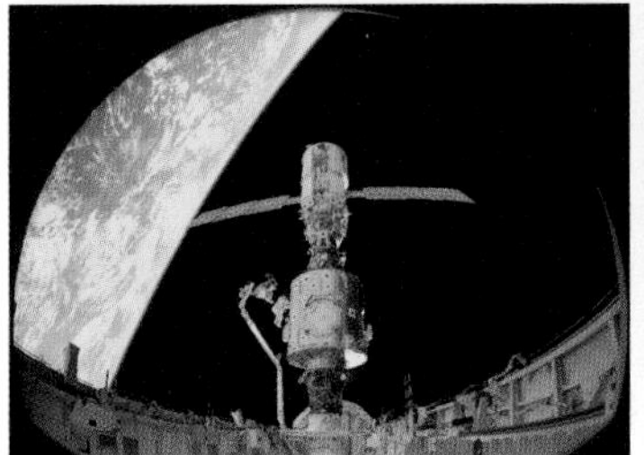

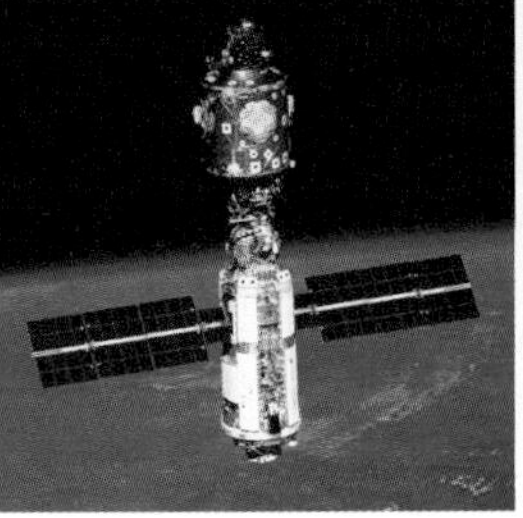

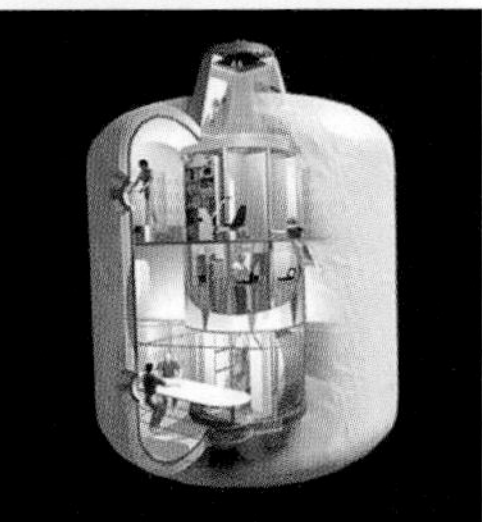

FIGURE 27.6 • *Top.* International Space Station (ISS) projected for completion in 2004. The most complex (and expensive) construction project ever undertaken involves 16 nations (United States, Canada, Belgium, France, Denmark, Germany, Italy, the Netherlands, Norway, Spain, Sweden, Switzerland, United Kingdom, Japan, Russia, Brazil). The program utilizes more than 100,000 people at space agencies and hundreds of contractors and subcontractors worldwide. The 460-ton ISS necessitates 45 United States and Russian rocket missions to launch and assemble the more than 100 major components. Constructing this giant space outpost complex, the size of almost two football fields, will require 160 space walks (approximately 1800 h) by pairs of astronauts. *Bottom left.* A robot arm from the Space Shuttle Endeavor lifts *Unity*, the first of the ISS modules, to join the Russian control module Zayra. *Bottom middle.* ISS view from STS-96 *Discovery* during a fly-around following separation of the American and Russian spacecraft. *Bottom right.* Computer-generated cutaway view of the Translab Module, the large-volume (12,000 ft^3) habitation module for ISS scheduled for flight 16A in late 2004.

Souyz Expedition 1 crew began it's rendezvous with the ISS for a four-month stay to prepare the ISS for future missions to continue the on-orbit assembly. This includes installation of solar arrays and batteries, thermal control systems, communications equipment, and the 8.5-m long, 4.3-m diameter U.S. Laboratory Module *Destiny*, the centerpiece of the ISS for conducting fundamental scientific experiments. The *Destiny* will focus on basic and applied research in biotechnology, fluid physics, combustion, and the life sciences. Completing the $60 billion ISS by 2004 draws on knowledge gained previously from scientific studies of relatively brief (hours and days) and longer (>1 y) physiologic responses and adaptations to microgravity. Living aboard the ISS, in turn, will generate new knowledge about prolonged adaptations of humans for projected sojourns to Mars and beyond.

United States Human Space Program

Table 27.2 summarizes the salient accomplishments of NASA's human space program beginning with Project Mercury and continuing with Gemini, Apollo, Skylab, Apollo-Soyuz, and Space Shuttle. Voluminous medical data exist from the initial six Mercury flights (1961–1963) to the present extended-duration flights of the United States and Soviet cooperative endeavors. NASA currently oversees 15 flight and research facilities in the United States (www.nasa.gov/nasaorgs/index.html).

TABLE 27.2 ➤ ACCOMPLISHMENTS OF THE UNITED STATES AND SOVIET HUMAN SPACE PROGRAMS: FROM PROJECT MERCURY TO THE INTERNATIONAL SPACE STATION

PROGRAM	YEARS	ACCOMPLISHMENTS
Project Mercury	May 1961 to May 1963	Twenty unmanned missions; two suborbital, four orbital manned missions. Longest flight 34 h, 19 min, 49 s; 22 Earth orbits. Alan Shepard, (1923–1998) first U.S. astronaut makes suborbital flight of 15 min, 28 s on May 5, 1961 (5 other astronauts completed successful missions).
	Feb. 12, 1962	John Glenn became the first American to orbit Earth (3 times) in his spacecraft *Friendship 7*.
	May 15 to 16, 1963	Astronaut L. Gordon Cooper piloted *Faith 7* during a 22-orbit mission, becoming the first astronaut to launch a satellite (beacon) while in orbital flight, and first American to re-entry in manual mode (maximum orbital speed achieved was 17,546.6 mph at a perigee of 100.2 and apogee of 165.9 statute mi). His flight suit temperature reached 92°F and cabin temperature109°F.
Project Gemini	May 1961 to Nov 1966	Two umanned missions; 10 human space missions; first U.S. extravehicular activity (EVA; 22 min on Gemini IV); first rendezvous and docking (Gemini VIII; 6 h, 33 min after lift-off); first use of fuel cells for electrical power; evaluation of guidance and navigation systems for future rendezvous missions; biomedical experiments successfully conducted on Gemini IV, V, VII. Longest EVA on last Gemini XII (5 h, 30 min). The Kennedy Space Center (KSC) at Cape Canaveral, FL serves as the primary launch facility for the U.S. Space Program. Over a 20-month period (March 1965 to Nov. 1966), the 10 Project Gemini human missions built a bridge between the relatively "simple" Mercury flights and the technologically challenging Apollo moon program. They accomplished rendezvous between two spacecraft in orbit, mastered space docking, and made the first controlled re-entries to Earth.
Apollo Program	Oct 1961 to Dec 1972	Six unmanned Apollo-Saturn missions; 12 manned missions achieved significant biomedical results concerning physiologic responses: • Vestibular disturbances • Suboptimal food consumption (1260–2903 kcal · d^{-1}) • Postflight dehydration and weight loss • Decreased postflight orthostatic tolerance from tilt tests • Reduced postflight orthostatic tolerance first 3 days • Cardiac arrhythmias (Apollo 15) • Decreased red cell mass (2–10%) and plasma volume (4–9%) **Moon Flights:** *Apollo 10* launched from KSC on May 18, 1969, on a 9-day mission. The spacecraft orbited the moon and the lunar module (LM) descended to an altitude of 15 km over the planned site for the first lunar landing. Color TV was transmitted to earth. The command module (CM) landed safely in the Pacific May 26, 1969. *Apollo 11* orbits the moon; Apollo astronauts Neil Armstrong and Edwin Aldrin Jr., became the first men to walk on the moon. The spacecraft returned and landed in the Pacific on July 24, 1969, fulfilling the space goal set by President Kennedy on May 25, 1961.

TABLE 27.2 ➤ ACCOMPLISHMENTS OF THE UNITED STATES AND SOVIET HUMAN SPACE PROGRAMS: FROM PROJECT MERCURY TO THE INTERNATIONAL SPACE STATION—*continued*

Program	Years	Accomplishments
Apollo Program—*continued* 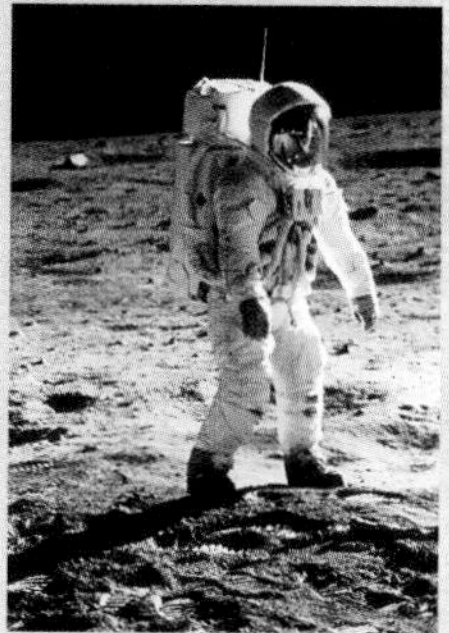 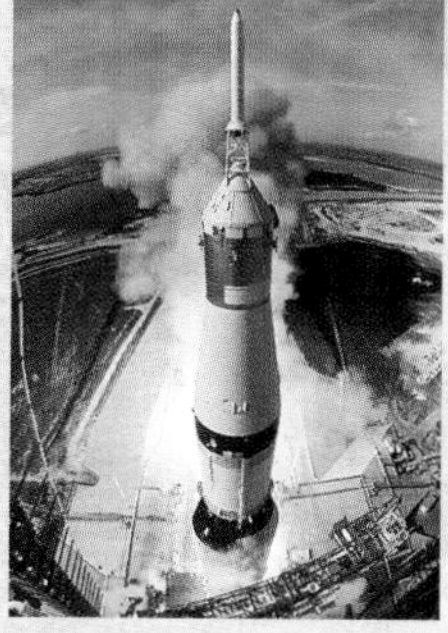 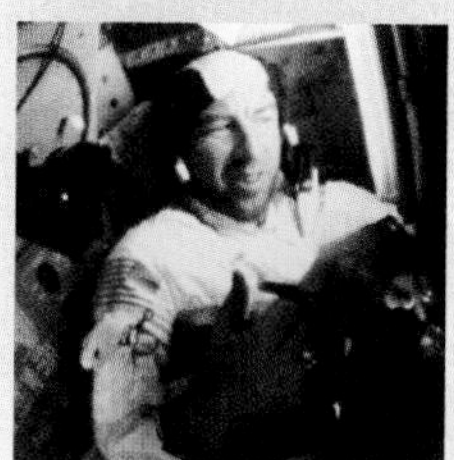 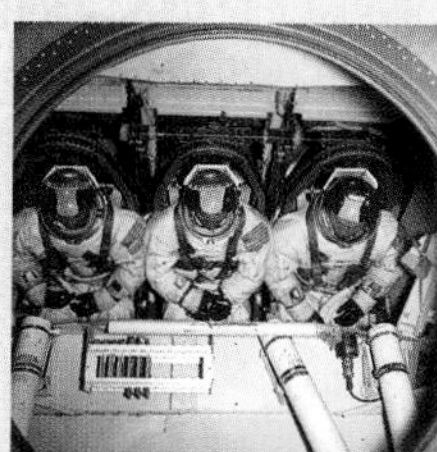		*Apollo 12* launched on Nov. 14, 1969, and landed on the moon 163 m from the Surveyor III spacecraft. The two astronauts performed two EVAs on the lunar surface; retrieved samples and pans of Surveyor III; left the lunar surface after a stay of 31 h, 31 min; redocked and landed in the Pacific on Nov. 24, 1969. *Apollo 13* launched on a lunar landing mission on April 11, 1970, but 7 h, 55 min into the flight an explosion in an oxygen tank required an abort. The astronauts powered up the LM and used the LM propellant for a free-return trajectory around the moon. They returned safely to Earth and landed in the mid-Pacific on April 17. *Apollo 14* launched from KSC on Jan. 31, 1971, and the LM landed on the Fra Mauro area of the moon on February 5. Two EVAs were performed, the second using a mobile equipment transporter to permit a longer traverse. The LM lifted off from the moon February 6 and the CM splashed down in the Pacific on Feb. 9, 1970. *Apollo 15* launched July 26, 1971, and on July 30 the LM landed in the Hadley-Apennine region of the moon. Three EVAs were completed with a total EVA time of 18 h, 35 min. The LM ascent stage lift-off on August 2 was the first televised, and the lunar roving vehicle was used for the first time. *Apollo 15's* CM landed in the Pacific on August 7, 1971. *Apollo 16* launched from KSC on April 16, 1972, and landed in the moon's Descartes region April 20. Three EVAs were completed, using the lunar roving vehicle for a distance of 26.7 km. The LM lifted off April 23 and docked with the command service module (CSM) to transfer astronauts and samples. The CM landed in the Pacific April 27. *Apollo 17,* the final manned lunar landing mission, launched from KSC on Dec. 7, 1972. The astronauts in the LM landed in the Taurus-Littrow region of the moon on Dec. 11 and explored the area on the lunar roving vehicle during three 22 h EVAs. Lift-off occurred on Dec. 14, and the CM landed in the Pacific Dec. 19.
Project Skylab Program 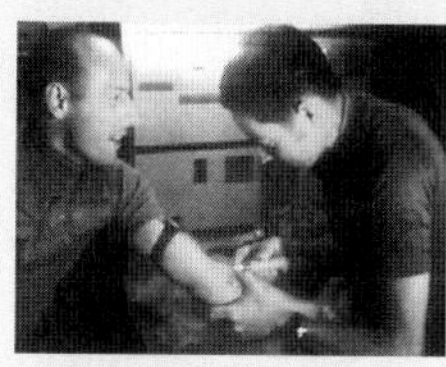 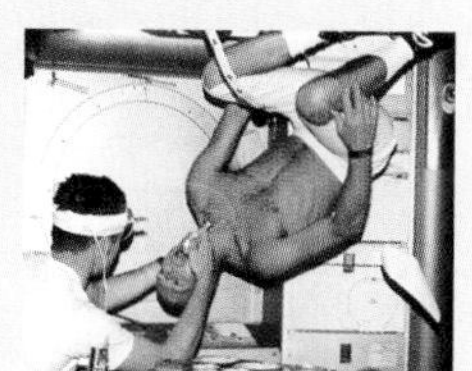 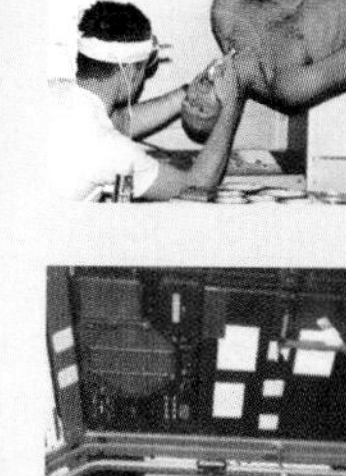 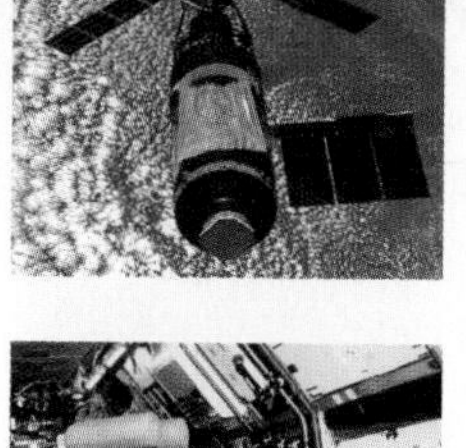 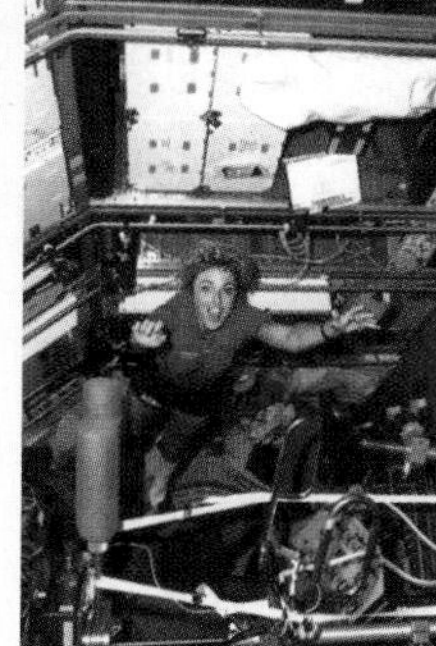	May 1973 to Feb 1974	One unmanned and three manned missions. *Skylab 1* (unmanned) launched into orbit May 14, 1973 by a Saturn V booster. Almost immediately, technical problems developed due to vibrations during lift-off. A critical meteoroid shield ripped off, taking one of the craft's two solar panels with it; a piece of the shield wrapped around the other panel, keeping it from deploying. Skylab maneuvered so its Apollo Telescope Mount (ATM) solar panels faced the sun to maximize electricity. Because of the loss of the meteoroid shield, workshop temperatures increased to 52°C (126° F). The Skylab 2 launch was postponed while NASA engineers trained (10 d) the crew to make the workshop habitable. The engineers "rolled" Skylab to lower workshop temperature. Extensive scientific studies on 28-, 59-, and 85-day missions showed humans could live and work in space for extended periods using countermeasures against deleterious adaptations. *Skylab 2,* first manned mission, launched May 25, 1973, for 28 d, 50 min. The crew rendezvoused with Skylab on the fifth orbit. After making substantial repairs, including deployment of a parasol sunshade that cooled the inside temperature to 23.8°C (75°F), by June 4 the workshop became fully operational. The crew conducted solar astronomy and Earth resources experiments, medical studies, and five student experiments; 404 orbits and 392 experiment-hours completed; three EVAs totaled 6 h, 20 min. *Skylab 3* (July 28–Sep. 25, 1973; 59 d, 11 h). Continued maintenance of the space station and extensive scientific and medical experiments completed. Completed 858 Earth orbits and 1081 hours of solar and Earth experiments; three EVAs totaled 13 h, 43 min. *Skylab 4* (Nov. 16, 1973–Feb. 8, 1974; 84 d, 1 h). Last of the Skylab missions; included observation of the *Comet Kohoutek* among numerous experiments. Completed 1214 Earth orbits and four EVAs totaling 22 h, 13 min.

TABLE 27.2 ➤ ACCOMPLISHMENTS OF THE UNITED STATES AND SOVIET HUMAN SPACE PROGRAMS: FROM PROJECT MERCURY TO THE INTERNATIONAL SPACE STATION—*continued*

Program	Years	Accomplishments
Apollo-Soyuz Test Project (ASTP) 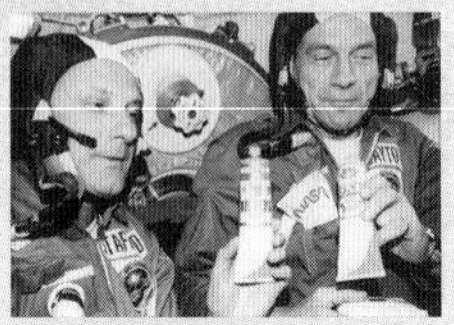	July 1975 (9 d)	First U.S. and Soviet project that successfully tested rendezvous and docking systems, and medical and technical cooperation from July 15–24, 1975 (9 d, 7 h, 28 min). The Soyuz launched just over 7 hours prior to the launch of the Apollo CSM. Apollo then maneuvered to rendezvous and docked 52 hours after the Soyuz launch. The Apollo and Soyuz crews conducted diverse experiments for 2 days. After separation, Apollo remained in space an additional 6 days. Soyuz returned to Earth approximately 43 hours after separation.
Space Shuttle Program 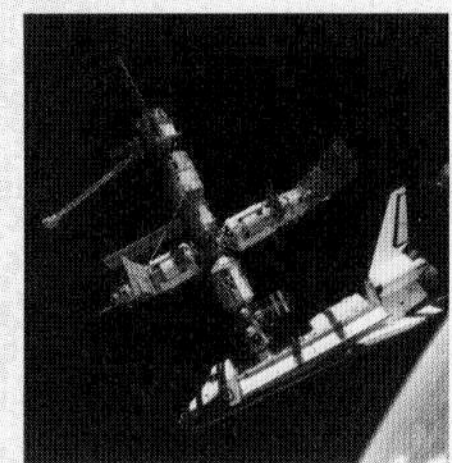 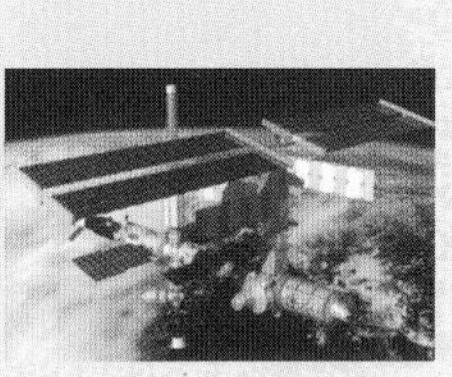	March 1979 to present	First reusable spacecraft that operated under sea-level atmospheric pressure while in orbit. The pressurized spacelab module provides a sophisticated scientific laboratory to study physiologic and medical aspects of extended flight, including extended EVA.
International Space Station 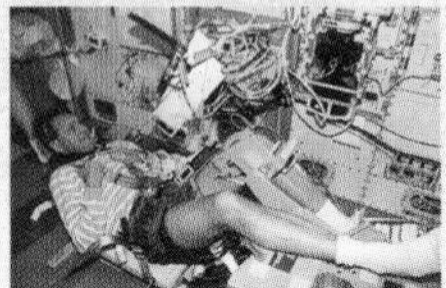 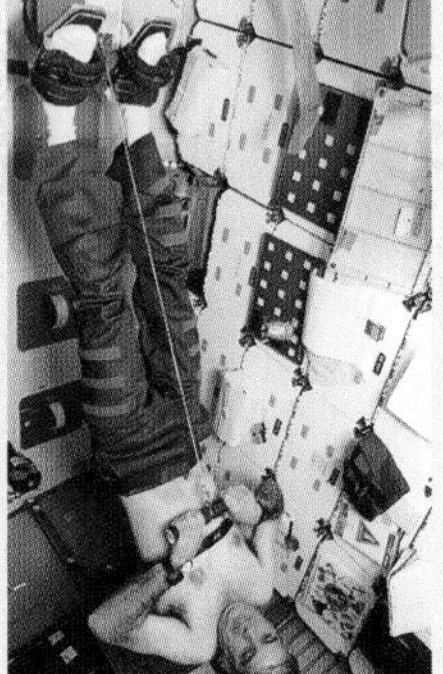 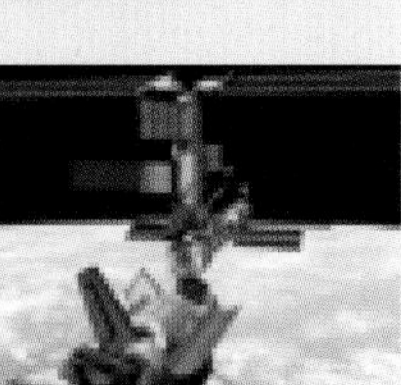 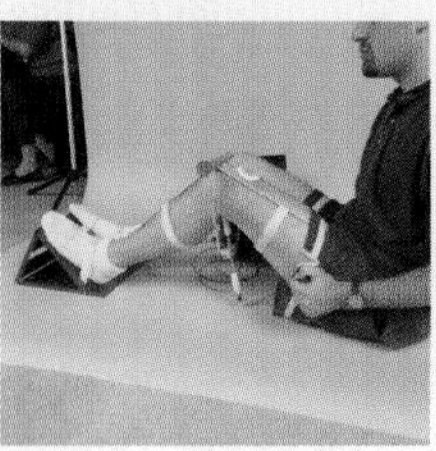 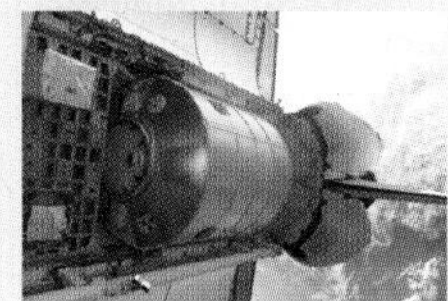		The International Space Station (ISS), an international cooperative research platform, provides a state-of-the-art research facility, studies gravity's effects on physical, chemical, and biologic systems, serves as an advanced facility for technology and human exploration, and as a commercial platform for space research and development. The ISS is designed to accomplish three main goals: (1) advance scientific knowledge, (2) to live, explore, and work productively in space, and (3) use attributes of space to improve products and processes on Earth. Major research areas include fundamental biology, physical science (materials science, biotechnology, fundamental physics, fluid physics, combustion), biomedical research and countermeasures, advanced human support technology, space science, and Earth observation.
	Nov. 1998 to Feb. 2002	Dec 7, 1998, Shuttle *Endeavor* mated *Unity* module with Russian control module *Zayra.*
	Nov. 2000 to Feb. 2001	Four modules on-orbit (*Unity* node; *Zarya* functional cargo block; *Zvezda* service module, *Destiny* U.S. Lab). Five assembly and resupply flights. Expedition I crew arrived November 2, 2000 on *Soyuz.*
	Feb. 2001 to June 2001	Six assembly and resupply flights (lab outfitting and remote manipulator); major focus on radiation research, bone and muscle studies, psychosocial studies, fluids science, protein crystallization. Expedition 2 crew arrived February 2001 on Shuttle.
	June 2001 to Oct. 2001	Studies of subregional bone and muscle structure and function; effects of prolonged space flight on human skeletal muscle (pre/post flight measurements); crystal growth, cell biology, pulmonary function, susceptibility to renal stone formation.
	Oct. 2001 to Feb. 2002	Studies of multiple plant experiments in space, biomass production, astroculture, commercial generic bioprocessing, biological habitats, centrifuge, physical sciences apparatus (fluids, laser cooling, low temperature, materials science, alpha magnetic spectrometry).
	March 8, 2001 to July 2001	Expedition 2 arrived on Space Shuttle Discovery (STS-102) March 8, 2001, with the Multi-Purpose Logistics Module (un-piloted, reusable cargo cylindrical carrier 6.4 m long and 4.5 m diameter, 4.5 tons, that provides equipment and supplies for the *Destiny* module. This new module also included components that provide life support, fire detection and suppression, electrical distribution, and computer functions. The crew will work with 18 different experiments. Shuttle Discovery flight STS-104 (July 12, 2001) will consist of five assembly and resupply flights, including the Joint Airlock. STS-105 is slated to launch August 5, 2001.

Resources

Johnston RS. Introduction. In: Biomedical results of apollo (NASA SP-368). Johnson RS, et al., eds. Washington, DC: U.S. Government Printing Office, pp. 3–7, 1975.
Link MM. Space medicine in Project Mercury (NASA SP-4003). Washington, DC: U.S. Government Printing Office, 1965.
Nicogossian AE, et al Space physiology and medicine. 3rd edition. Philadelphia: Lea & Febiger. 1994.
www.spaceflight.NASA.gov

Perhaps the most significant technologic achievement of the 20th century took place on July 20, 1969, when Apollo 11 astronauts Edwin "Buzz" Aldrin and Neil Armstrong landed on the moon's surface in the lunar module Eagle after it separated from the main spacecraft at 50,000 feet. With these words, "Houston, Tranquility Base here. The Eagle has landed," the world knew a momentous accomplishment had taken place. Seven hours later, Armstrong's hopeful words as he set foot on the lunar surface—"One small step for man, one giant leap for mankind"—resonated worldwide to demonstrate that humans could travel to the moon, explore its surface, and return safely to Earth. Aldrin joined him on the surface several minutes later, and for two hours they collected rocks, planted the American flag on lunar soil in the Sea of Tranquility, and took photographs. Thus, it had taken almost a decade and $25.4 billion to achieve the goal President John F. Kennedy first stated on May 25, 1961:

> I believe that this nation should commit itself to achieving the goal, before this decade is out, of landing a man on the Moon and returning him safely to Earth. No single space project in this period will be more impressive to mankind, or more important for the long-range exploration of space; and none will be so difficult or expensive to accomplish.

Indeed, the Apollo program achieved its three main objectives: (1) ensuring the safety and health of crew members, (2) preventing contamination of Earth by extraterrestrial organisms, and (3) studying specific effects of space exposure on the human body. During the Apollo program, 12 astronauts walked on the moon during six lunar landings. Table 27.3 summarizes this program's significant medical findings.

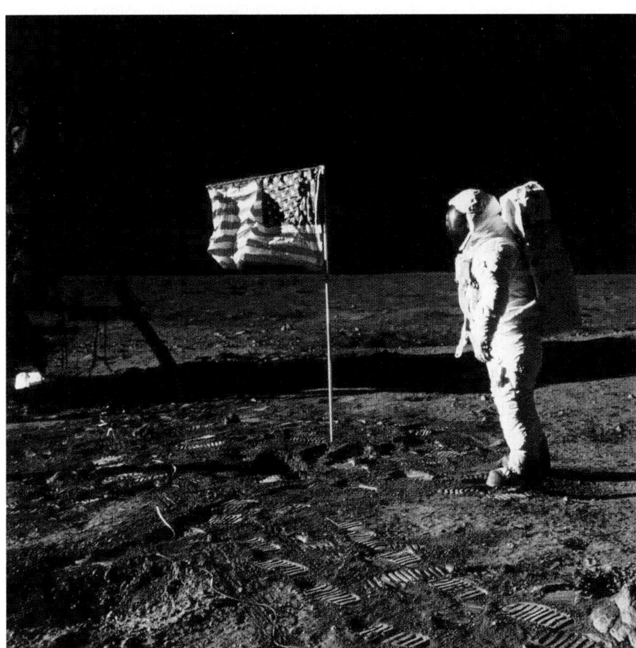

Astronaut Edwin E. Aldrin, Jr., lunar module pilot of the first lunar landing mission, poses beside the deployed United States flag (stiffened by inserts) during Apollo 11 EVA on the lunar surface (July 20, 1969). The lunar module is darkly outlined on the left, and the astronaut's footprints are visible in the soil (foreground).

TABLE 27.3 ➤ SIGNIFICANT BIOMEDICAL FINDINGS FROM APOLLO SPACE MISSIONS

- Vestibular disturbances
- Inflight cardiac arrhythmia
- Reduced postflight orthostatic tolerance
- Reduced postflight exercise tolerance
- Postflight dehydration and weight loss
- Flight diet adequate; food consumption suboptimal
- Decreased red cell mass, plasma volume
- Negative inflight balance trend for nitrogen, calcium, other electrolytes
- Increased inflight adrenal hormone secretion
- No inflight diuresis

Dietlein LF. Summary and conclusions. In: Biomedical results from Skylab (NASA SP-377). Johnston RS, Dietlein LF, eds. Washington, DC: U.S. Government Printing Office. 1977:579.

Soviet Space Program

The Soviet human space program began in 1957 when Sputnik-1 crystallized the United States' efforts to join the race into space. The first Soviet cosmonaut in space, Lt. Colonel Yuri Gagarin, prepared for manned space flight as a test pilot in the Vostok program. On April 12, 1961, Gagarin completed a single Earth orbit in 108 minutes and ejected from the Vostok spacecraft at 7000 m in a parachute landing. The Soviets withheld the news that Gagarin might have perished when the Vostok spacecraft malfunctioned on re-entry. His return unharmed scored another key space victory for the Soviet Union in their quest for supremacy in space. Longer-duration missions for up to 5 days in space followed this historic flight. The first woman in space, Valentina Tereshkova, flew in Vostok-6 in 1963, the last mission of this series. The two succeeding Soviet missions, named Voskhad, advanced space science by completing (1) the first EVA that lasted 8 minutes, by cosmonaut Aleksei Leonov (who exited the spacecraft through a canvas tube attached to the Voskhod 2) and (2) medical studies of lung function, middle-ear (vestibular) function, blood pressure, muscular strength (hand grip), and blood composition from the first

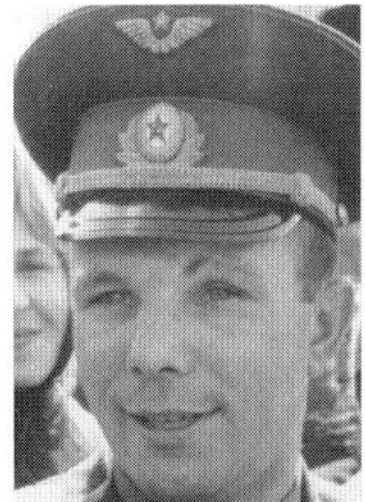

Pioneer cosmonaut Yuri A. Gagarin ("Columbus of the Cosmos"; 1934–1968), the first human to orbit the Earth in the *Vostok* I spacecraft.

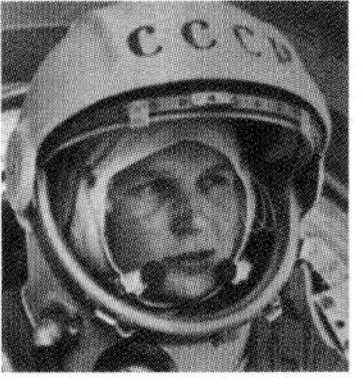

Cosmonaut Colonel-Engineer Valentina Tereshkova (1937–) the first woman in space, orbited Earth 48 times during a 3-day flight (June 17–19, 1963). Nineteen years later, Svetlana Savitskaya became the second Russian woman in space (1982, 1984).

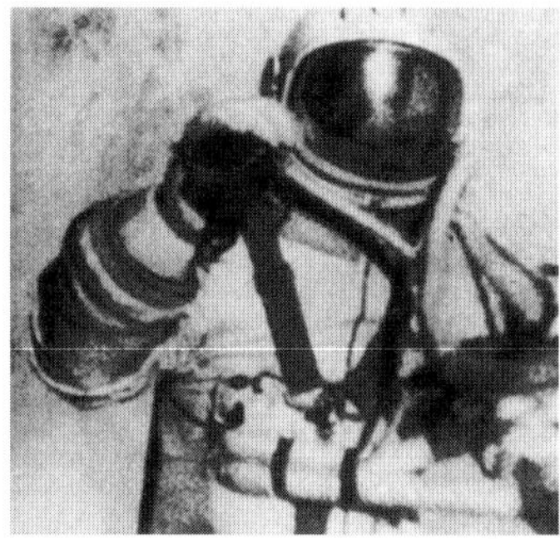

Cosmonaut Aleksei Leonov (1934–), copilot of *Voskhod* 2, performed the first EVA for 10 minutes during the second orbit of a 1-day flight before returning safely to the spacecraft through an inflatable airlock, but not without first releasing air from his spacesuit as a desperate measure when he had difficulty reentering the narrow passageway (March 18, 1964). The Soviets did not disclose this brush with disaster, so Leonov returned a hero, once again demonstrating Soviet supremacy in space. Leonov also served as command pilot for Soyuz 19 in the Apollo-Soyuz Test Project (July 15–21, 1975).

blood sample taken during weightlessness by Dr. Boris Yegorov, the first space physician.

The next period of Soviet exploration included manned flight aboard the advanced Soyuz-1 spacecraft, but a tragic accident stalled several planned rendezvous and docking missions. In January 1969, Soyuz flights 4 and 5 completed mission-critical maneuvers (rendezvous, docking, EVA transfer) for a future moon landing. Unfortunately, four unmanned spacecraft designed to test a powerful booster rocket needed to achieve moon orbit exploded on launch, canceling that phase of the program. One year later, the 18-day Soyuz mission included extensive experiments to evaluate microgravity's effects on heart function, vision, muscular strength, and hematologic variables. Unfortunately, an in-flight exercise countermeasures effort did *not* reduce problems experienced with balance (one aspect of orthostatic intolerance) and muscle weakness.

April 19, 1971, marked the launch of the world's first space station, Salyut-1 shown below. Forty-nine days later,

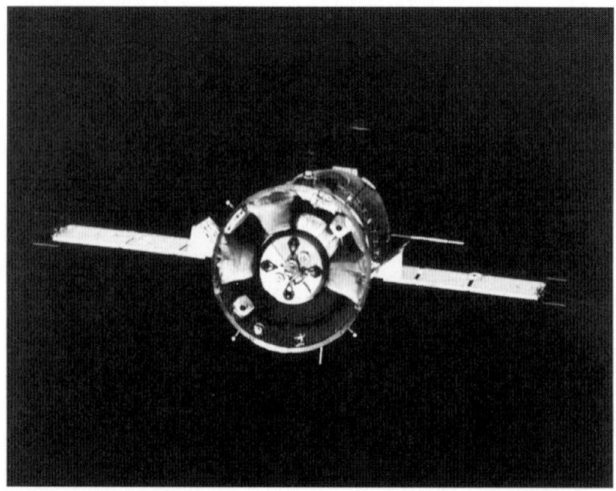

Salyut-1, the first scientific space station, launched from the Baikonur launch cosmodrome (Kazakstan, Russia) on June 6,1971 stayed in orbit for 23.8 days. The 6790-kg station included a telescope, spectrometer, electrophotometer, and television. The crew conducted medical-biological experiments.

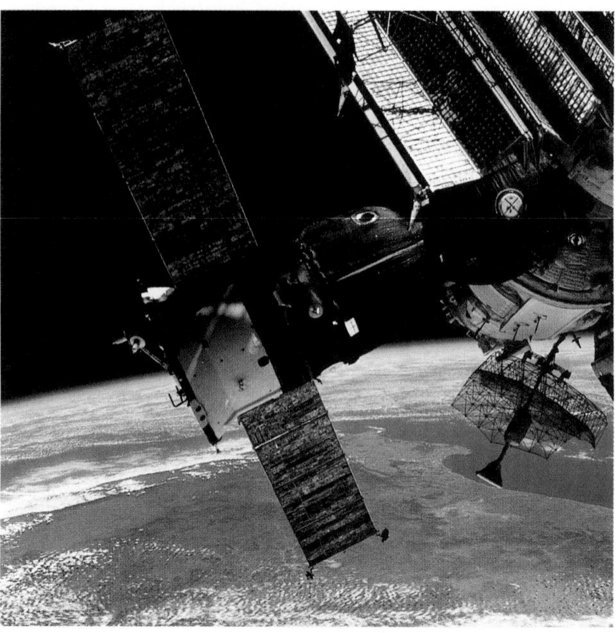

Shuttle *Atlantis* (STS-71) performs the first shuttle docking with the Russian Space station *Mir* June 27-July 7, 1995.

three cosmonauts from Soyuz-11 boarded Salyut-1 to become the space station's first crew. Over the next 6 years, the Soviets launched four additional Salyut space stations, the cosmonauts performing biomedical experiments on 24 missions, 10 of them involving humans, but only 5 experiments categorized successful. The longest mission (Soyuz-18) lasted 63 days. Subsequent missions on advanced Salyut-6 and Salyut-7 space stations lengthened flight duration and increased the number of crew members. Between 1977 and 1981, five two-man crews completed flights of 96, 140, 175, 185, and 74 days. Thirteen other crews completed shorter flights. During the Salyut-6 program, the Soviets accumulated about 3 years of flight experience and 5 hours of EVA. In 1982, two cosmonauts accumulated 211 days in orbit. American and Soviet cooperation in space commenced during July 15–24, 1975, with the first docking of an Apollo spacecraft with a Soyuz spacecraft (Apollo–Soyuz Test Project or ASTP). This mission established the basis for future American–Russian cooperation between the American Space Shuttle and Mir Space Station shown in close proximity prior to docking in the above photo. The 143-ton *Mir*, almost twice as heavy as Skylab (76 tons) and the largest manufactured object in space ($4.2 billion to build and maintain), was purposely deorbited after 15 years of unprecedented scientific achievements (46 expeditions and 23,000 experiments, including the longest continuous space mission [438 d] and 16 spacewalks totaling 77 h). *Mir* plunged in fiery descent from the Earth's atmosphere into the Pacific Ocean on March 22, 2001. Twenty-two years earlier, the U.S. first space station *Skylab*, despite three repair attempts to save this science space station from failure after only six years in orbit, also met a fiery re-entry from Earth's atmosphere in the southeastern Indian Ocean on July 11, 1979.

MEDICAL EVALUATION FOR ASTRONAUT SELECTION

Candidates for astronauts currently undergo extensive medical and psychologic evaluation.[50,93] However, little factual information existed about what to expect during space flight or the personal characteristics necessary for mission success when NASA devised the first medical evaluation in 1959. Approximately 600 active military test pilots from the Navy, Air Force, Army, and Marine Corps served as the initial candidate pool. From this group, NASA invited 110 for further testing. Thirty-two pilot finalists qualified for the next phase of testing, which included the exhaustive 23-item test battery listed in Table 27.4. The final evaluative criteria for the Mercury astronaut selection included (1) younger than age 40 years, (2) less than 71 inches tall (no weight requirement), (3) excellent physical condition, (4) college degree in engineering or equivalent, (5) minimum of 1500 hours flying time, (6) graduation from test pilot school, and (7) qualified test pilot.

First Astronauts

The test battery identified a final group of candidates believed best qualified to achieve the following goals:

- *Survive*—demonstrate ability to fly in space and return safely
- *Perform*—demonstrate ability to perform effectively under the conditions of space flight
- *Serve as a backup for automatic controls and instrumentation*—increase the reliability of flight systems
- *Serve as a scientific observer*—go beyond what the instruments and satellites can observe and report
- *Serve as an engineering observer and true test pilot*—to improve the flight system and its components

In April 1959, NASA selected its final seven astronauts (Fig. 27.7). This elite group of men, survivors of an extraordi-

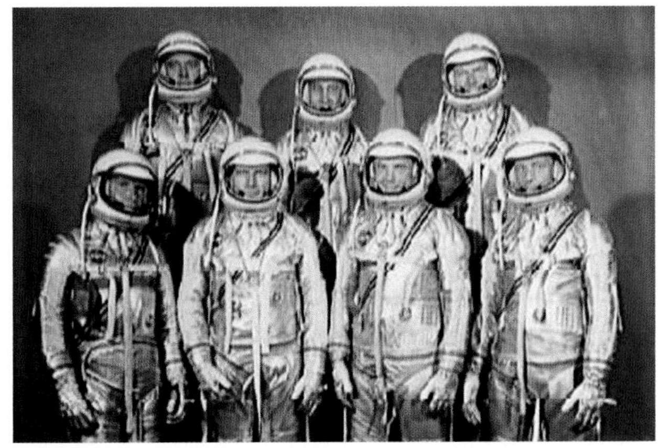

FIGURE 27.7 • Project Mercury-7 astronauts. (Photo courtesy of NASA, Lyndon B. Johnson Space Center, Houston, TX.)

TABLE 27.4 ➤ PHYSIOLOGIC AND PSYCHOLOGIC TESTING OF THE FIRST AMERICAN PROJECT MERCURY ASTRONAUTS

PHYSIOLOGIC TESTS	PSYCHOLOGIC TESTS
1. *Harvard step test:* Subject steps up 20 inches to platform and down once every 2 s for 5 min to measure physical fitness	1. Extensive interviews (psychiatrists)
2. *Treadmil maximum workload:* Subject walks at constant rate on moving platform elevated 1° each min; test continues until heart rate reaches 180 b · min^{-1}; test of physical fitness	2. Rorschach (ink blot)
3. *Cold pressor:* Subject plunges feet into tub of ice water; pulse and blood pressure measured before and during test	3. Thematic apperception (stories suggested by pictures)
4. *Complex behavior simulator:* A panel with 12 signals, each requiring a different response, measures ability to react reliably in confusing situations	4. Draw-a-person
5. *Tilt table:* Subject lies on steeply inclined table for 25 min to measure heart's ability to compensate for unusual body position for extended duration	5. Sentence completion
6. *Partial pressure suit:* Subject taken to simulated altitude of 65,000 ft for 1 h in MC-1 partial pressure suit; measure of cardiovascular efficiency and breathing at low ambient pressures	6. Self-inventory from 566-item questionnaire
7. *Isolation:* Subject enters a dark, soundproof room for 3 h to assess adaptation to unusual circumstances and coping without external stimuli	7. Officer effectiveness inventory
8. *Acceleration:* Subject placed in centrifuge with seat inclined at various angles; assesses near–multiple gravity forces	8. Personal-preference schedule from 225 pairs of self-descriptive statements
9. *Heat:* Subject spends 2 h in chamber at 130°F; measures reactions of heart and body functions to this stress	9. Preference evaluation from 52 statements
10. *Equilibrium and vibration:* Subject seated on chair that rotates simultaneously on two axes; subject required to maintain chair on even keel using control stick with and without vibration; subject tested with and without blindfold	10. Determination of authoritarian attitudes
11. *Noise:* Subject exposed to different sound frequencies to determine susceptibility to high-frequency tones	11. Peer ratings
	12. Interpretation of the question, "Who am I?"
	13. Wechsler Adult Scale
	14. Miller Analogies Test
	15. Raven Progressive Matrices
	16. Doppelt Mathematical Reasoning Scale
	17. Engineering analogies
	18. Mechanical comprehension
	19. Air Force Officer Qualification Test
	20. Aviation qualification test (USN) space memory
	21. Spatial orientation
	22. Gottschaldt Hidden Figures
	23. Guilford-Zimmerman Spatial Visualization

narily elaborate search and selection process, would train to enter an unknown environment, using a life-support system previously tested only during high-altitude balloon flights. Unknown at that time, NASA had identified, conducted, and completed similar tests with female test pilots with extensive flight experience. However, an executive decision had been made that the new astronauts would only be males with commissions in the armed services with prior fighter pilot training and experience.

Beginning in 1977, NASA adopted medical evaluation criteria for astronaut selection, relying on some test procedures gleaned from exercise physiology research experiments that assessed maximal physiologic responses during treadmill and cycle-ergometer tests. The standards, modified in 1991, reflect changes in NASA's objectives for space exploration; personnel now include pilots, mission specialists, payload specialists, and space flight participants. The strictest stan-

TABLE 27.5 ➤ MEDICAL TESTS ADMINISTERED TO U.S. ASTRONAUTS AND COSMONAUT CANDIDATES, 1977–1992

Astronaut Candidates	Cosmonaut Candidates
Medical history NASA Medical Survey Questionnaire	*Medical history* Includes surgical history and examination
Physical examination Includes rectal examination, pelvic examination, and Pap smear, proctosigmoidoscopy	*Physical examination* Includes rectal examination, pelvic examination, and uterine ultrasound
Cardiopulmonary evaluation Includes history and examination, pulmonary function tests, exercise stress test, blood pressure, resting and 24-h ECG, echocardiogram	*Cardiopulmonary evaluation* Includes history and examination, pulmonary function tests, exercise stress test, blood pressure, resting and 24-h ECG, echocardiogram, phono- and mechanocardiography, cardiac cycle analysis
Musculoskeletal evaluation Muscle mass, anthropometry	*Musculoskeletal examination* Anthropometry
Radiographic evaluation Chest films (PA and lateral), sinus films, mammography, interview with radiation safety officer, review of medical radiation exposure history	*Radiographic evaluation* Chest films (abdominal flat plate), cranium, spine, renal, and urologic x-rays, abdominal and urogenital ultrasound, radioisotope liver test, excretory urogram and urofluorometry
Laboratory examinations Complete blood workup (clinical biochemistry; hematology; immunology; serology; endocrinology) Urinalysis, including 24-h urine chemistry renal-stone profile, and urine endocrinology Stool analysis for occult blood, ova, and parasites	*Laboratory examinations* Complete blood workup (clinical biochemistry; hematology; immunology; serology) Urinalysis, including 24-h urine chemistry and renal-stone profile Stool analysis for ova and parasites Analysis of duodenal and intestinal secretions
Otorhinolaryngologic (ENT) evaluation Includes history and examination, audiometry, tympanometry	*Otorhinolaryngologic (ENT) evaluation* Includes history and examination, audiometry, tympanometry, exo- and endoscopy, vestibular function, optokinetic stimulation
Ophthalmologic evaluation Includes visual acuity, refraction, and accommodation, color and depth perception, phorias, tonometry, perimetry, funduscopic examination with retinal photographs	*Ophthalmologic evaluation* Includes visual acuity, refraction, and accommodation; color and depth perception; night vision; tonometry; extraocular muscles; slit-lamp examination and ophthalmoscopy
Dental examination Includes panorex and full dental x-rays within prior 2 years	*Dental examination* Orthopantomography, electro-odontodiagnosis, vacuum test
Neurologic evaluation Includes history and examination, EEG at rest, EEG with photic stimulation, EEG during hyperventilation, Valsalva's maneuver, and sleep	*Neurologic evaluation* Includes history and examination, Doppler study of cranial vessels, EEG with photic stimulation, autonomic reflexes, skin thermometry
Psychiatric and psychologic evaluation Includes psychiatric interview, psychologic tests	*Psychiatric and psychophysiologic evaluation* Includes psychiatric interview, psychometric testing, personality inventory, sleep monitoring
Other tests Drug screen; PPD skin test; microbiologic, fungal, and viral tests; pregnancy test; screen for sexually transmitted disease; abdominal ultrasound	*Functional testing* Decompression and hypoxia, centrifugation (Gz and Gx), postural tests, lower-body negative pressure, ergometry, thermal testing, parabolic flight

From Pool SL, et al. Medical evaluation for astronaut selection and longitudinal studies. In: Nicogossian AE, et al., eds. Space physiology and medicine. 3rd ed. Philadelphia: Lea & Febiger, 1994:375. Cosmonaut data reported by Pool et al. who cite Yazov D, Chazov E. Ordinance from the USSR Minister of Defense and the USSR Minister of Health no. 390/585. On the implementation of instructions for medical qualification and control regarding the health of cosmonaut candidates, cosmonauts, and cosmonaut instructors. Moscow, 1989.

dards for vision and hearing apply to pilots and mission specialists, with less stringent requirements in these two areas for the two other personnel categories. Soviet selection and training program standards for cosmonauts clearly resemble the United States model. Table 27.5 compares medical testing for astronaut and cosmonaut finalists. Table 27.6 lists medical events previously reported during space flight missions. The left column includes common events; the right column lists those with one or only a few reported cases.

In addition to medical screening and testing, NASA conducts retrospective and longitudinal studies of astronauts matched against a large control group of Johnson Space Center employees.

The family of curves in Figure 27.8 compares sitting pulse rate and blood pressure, hearing, maximum oxygen consumption, and the health-related Framingham Risk Score for astronauts and age- and body-size matched controls. Until about age 40, astronauts score better on health and fitness variables than controls. The comparative data provide an important baseline for future studies of the possible effects of acute and chronic microgravity exposure on parameters concerned with long-term health and aging. For example, NASA sponsors three types of studies:

1. *Data analysis from single flights*. This involves ongoing data collection about space motion sickness symptoms experienced before, during, and after flights. Such studies aim to validate ground-based predictive tests of an individual's susceptibility to this malady and to define operationally acceptable countermeasures.
2. *Longitudinal studies spanning several missions*. Such studies help to quantify any cumulative effects of repeated exposure to the space environment, particularly the effects of radiation on cancer risk and repeated weightlessness on bone mineral loss.
3. *Longitudinal studies throughout careers*. Long-term medical surveillance to provide information about occupational injuries and maladies during, or for a significant time following, space flight. The longest-duration study of physiologic responses after microgravity exposure involves studies of astronaut John Glenn, Jr., the first American to orbit Earth, who piloted the 1962 Friendship 7 capsule atop a Mercury-Atlas 6 Earth-orbital space mission. Thirty-six years later, on October 29, 1998, at age 77, Glenn served as a Payload Specialist 2 on Shuttle Discovery STS-95 for an 8-day mission. The experiments involved studies of bone and muscle loss, balance, and sleep disorders (www.spaceflight.nasa.gov/).

Exercise Physiology Laboratory

Exercise physiology research had been conducted in various laboratories at the Johnson Space Center (JSC) in Houston, Texas soon after the center had been established. However, the official NASA Exercise Physiology Laboratory at JSC (*www.jsc.nasa.gov/sa/sd/sd3/exl/index.htm*) began operations in 1994. The laboratory uses both ground-based and in-flight investigations to assess effects of microgravity exposure on cardiopulmonary and musculoskeletal changes and to develop suitable countermeasures to these changes. The laboratory assesses preflight, inflight, and postflight aerobic exercise performance and capacity using graded treadmill and cycle ergometer (sitting and recumbent) submaximal and maximal exercise tests. The laboratory also uses isokinetic and isometric testing devices to evaluate muscular strength and endurance, along with other equipment (lactate analyzer, reaction/response device, underwater weighing tank and bioelectrical impedance analyzer, interactive video system) to monitor physiologic and performance capacity and body composition. Laboratory personnel also define in-flight medical requirements for the Space

TABLE 27.6 ➤ MEDICAL EVENTS IN MANNED SPACEFLIGHT

COMMON	ONE OR FEW REPORTED CASES
Space motion sickness	Urinary tract infection
Nasal/sinus congestion	Prostatitis
Constipation	Nephrolithiasis
Headache	Cardiac dysrhythmias:
Back pain	extrasystoles, bigeminy, quadrageminy, supraventricular tachycardia, ventricular tachycardia (sustained, asymptomatic)
Skin irritation/dryness	Chemical pneumonitis
Abscess	Aspiration of foreign body
Minor abrasions/contusions	Gastroenteritis
Musculoskeletal sprain/strain	Decompression sickness (limb bends)
Corneal irritation/abrasion	Eye trauma
Upper respiratory infection	Contact dermatitis
Insomnia	Spatial disorientation
	Serous otitis

From Barratt M. Principles of diagnosis and treatment for spaceflight. In: Dietlein LF, Pestov ID. Health performance, and safety of space crews, vol 4. Space biology and medicine series. In press.

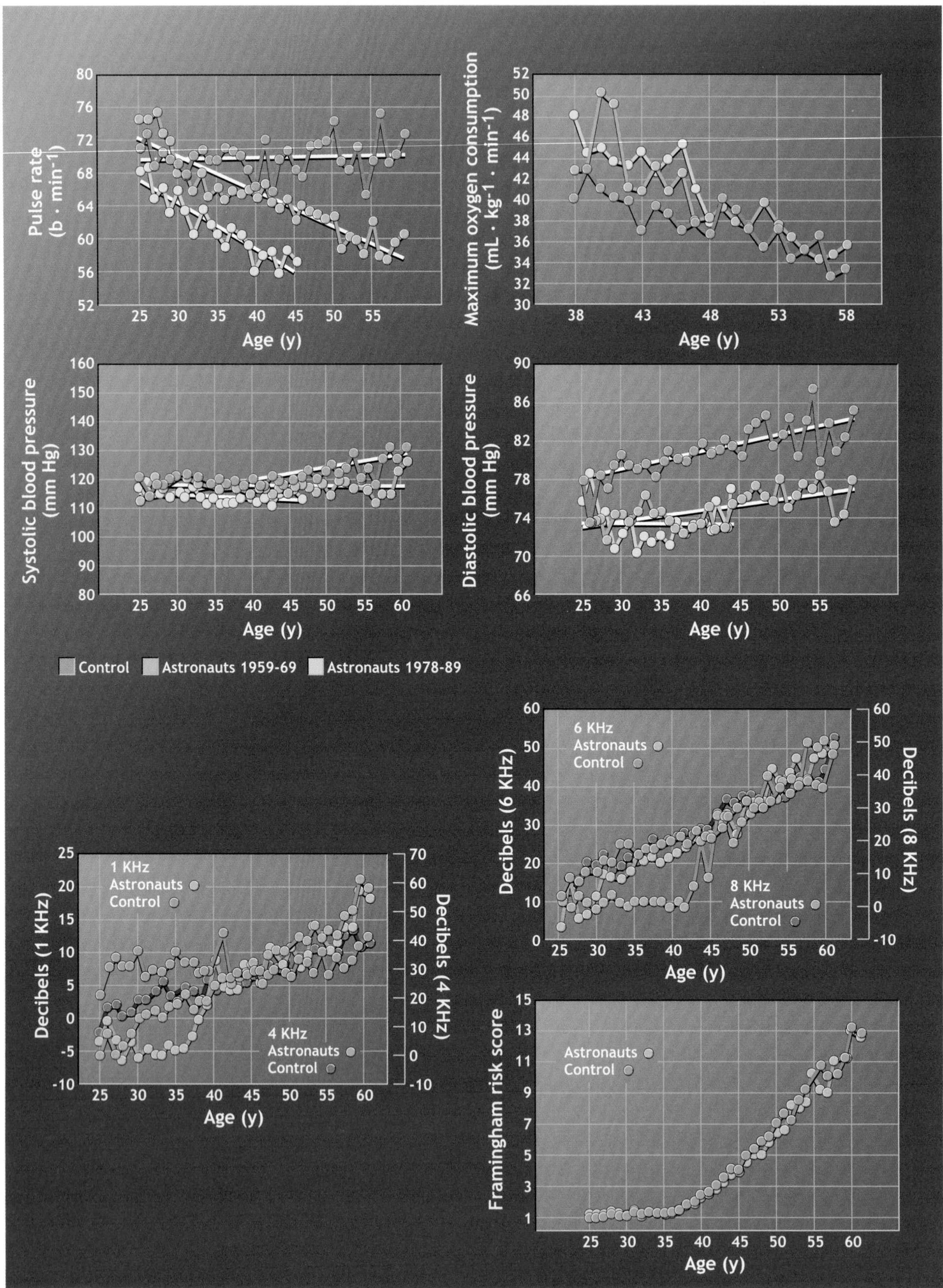

FIGURE 27.8 • Comparison of astronaut subgroups and control group on selected variables. *Top four graphs.* Sitting pulse rate, maximum oxygen consumption, and systolic and diastolic blood pressures. *Solid lines* represent regression lines indicating average trend. *Bottom Left.* Hearing acuity compared at 1, 4, 6, and 8 KHz. *Bottom right.* Framingham Risk Score (derived from six risk factors; higher score, greater risk). (From Pool SL, et al. Medical evaluation for astronaut selection and longitudinal studies. In: Nicogossian AE, et al., eds. Space physiology and medicine. 3rd ed. Philadelphia: Lea & Febiger, 1994.)

Station Crew Health Care System and the science requirements for the Extended-Duration Orbiter Medical Project (EDOMP), to address concerns about the physiologic condition of shuttle astronauts during up to 16-day missions. The laboratory collaborates with university researchers in exercise physiology and related disciplines in projects that deal with bone and muscle, cardiovascular function, endocrinology, environmental physiology, neuroscience, nutritional biochemistry, preflight adaptation training, and psychologic and behavioral dynamics.

Occupational Health Program

In addition to NASA's exercise physiology laboratory, the Occupational Health Program (OHP) (ohp.ksc.nasa.gov/welcome.html) consists of approximately 400 occupational medicine and environmental health professionals distributed across 10 primary NASA centers. This team provides comprehensive medical support to a diverse, highly technologic workforce of more than 60,000 civil servant and contractor employees involved in the human exploration and development of space, aeronautics research, and earth and space science activities. The traditional occupational health program elements include medical surveillance, industrial hygiene, health physics, emergency medical response, employee assistance programs, physical fitness programs, and overall health and wellness programs. Astronauts in training for a mission participate at the Johnson Space Center in developmental fitness regimens in modern facilities similar to most university and commercial gymnasia.

RADIATION EFFECTS. *For astronauts living in low-Earth orbit for long time periods, including exploratory Mars missions and beyond, radiation exposure poses potentially serious health concerns.*[105] Current preflight requirements include projecting a mission radiation dosage, assessing the probability of solar flares during the mission, and quantifying the radiation exposure history of flight crew members. Each crew member carries a passive dosimeter (radiation-measuring device), and highly sensitive dosimeters located throughout the spacecraft continually monitor radiation in case of solar flares or other radiation contingencies.

Future research must resolve the short- and long-term biologic impact on cellular microarchitecture of galactic cosmic ray particles (nuclei of high atomic number) with high energies (HZE) and high linear energy transfer (LET). Different kinds of radiation during liftoff and aboard the spacecraft on short-duration missions at nominal orbit generally pose an "acceptable" level of hazard to astronaut health (e.g., blood-forming organs, lenses of eyes, skin). For the Skylab 4 mission, with an average cumulated dose of 43.20 mGy (absorbed radiation dose expressed in **Gray units**, where 1 Gy = 1J ÷ kg of absorbed ionization in any material or 100 rads) over 57 days (compared with only 0.07 mGy for Mercury and 1.31 mGy on 43 shuttle missions), astronauts could fly one 84-day Skylab mission a year for 50 years before exceeding the career limits for radiation exposure.[2,86,139]

Biologic doses expressed in dose equivalents describe an amount of radiation that produces the same "health decrement" as an equal dose of low-LET radiation. Dose equivalents are expressed in Sieverts (S_v or rem; 1 S_v = 100 rem). One S_v equals the dose received in Gy or rad multiplied by a qualitative factor Q. At doses of 10 to 50 rem, no obvious radiation effects occur, except minor blood changes. For 50 to 100 rem, 5 to 10% of subjects experience fatigue, nausea, and vomiting for about 1 day but no serious disability and little or no danger of dying. Thereafter, symptoms increase progressively with increasing dose, and above 550 rem, death almost always occurs within 6 months. A single short-term dose beyond 4500 rem produces incapacitation within hours, and all persons die within 1 week.[140] We outline goals for future research about radiation effects on page 741.

PHYSIOLOGIC ADAPTATIONS TO MICROGRAVITY

Space flight has produced considerable biomedical information about human physiology in microgravity, beginning in 1961 with astronaut Alan Shepard's brief solo flight aboard *Freedom 7* (see Table 27.2 and unnumbered figure below). In the ensuing 39 years, researchers have quantified physiologic adaptations to relatively brief space missions (1 to 14 d) and flights lasting longer than 2 weeks, including postflight adaptations.

Figure 27.9 displays a generalized schema of the dynamics of physiologic functions with microgravity exposure. These include the effects of two major factors: (1) reduced hydrostatic gradients and (2) reduced loading and disuse of weight-bearing tissues. The graphic reveals how these two factors influence the following six systems: (1) cardiovascular and cardiopulmonary, (2) hematologic, (3) fluid, electrolyte, and hormonal, (4) muscle, (5) bone, and (6) neurosensory and vestibular. Each system has been color coded, with *arrows* indicating how one system might influence an-

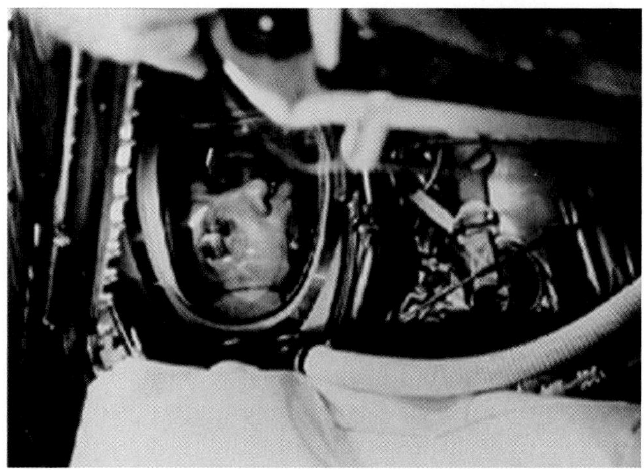

Astronaut Alan Shepard's (1923-1998) historic 15-minute, 28-second solo flight on May 5, 1961 on Mercury 3 rocket *Freedom 7* (achieved 116.5 statute mi-altitude and traveled 303 statute mi at a maximum velocity of 5134 mph). Shepard logged 216 cumulative hours of space flight, including 9 hours of cumulative EVA on Apollo 14.

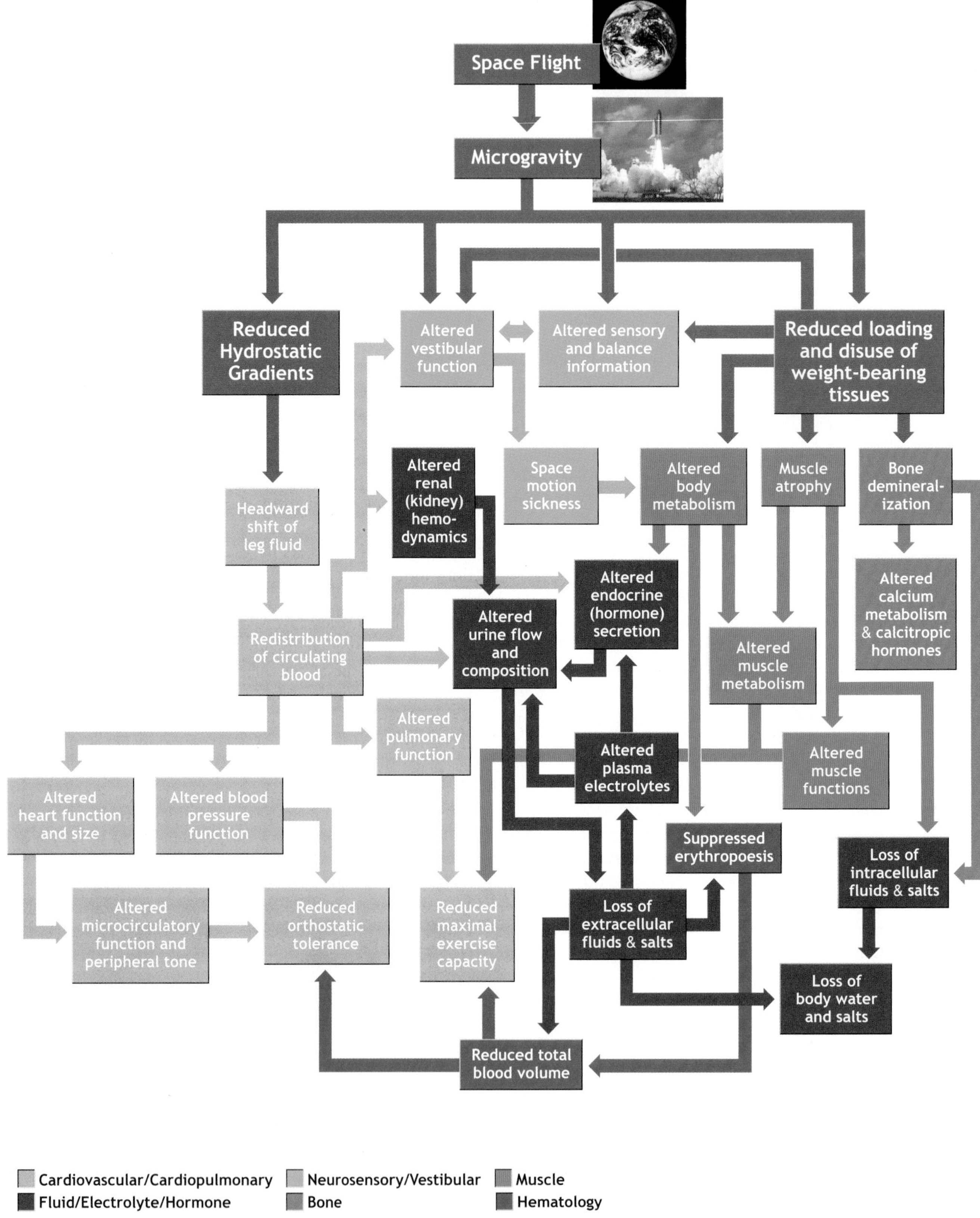

FIGURE 27.9 • General schema of microgravity's effects on physiologic alterations from (1) reduced hydrostatic gradients and (2) reduced loading and disuse of weight-bearing tissues. (Modified from Lujan BF, White RJ. Human physiology in space. [www.nsbri.org/humanphysiologyspace/].)

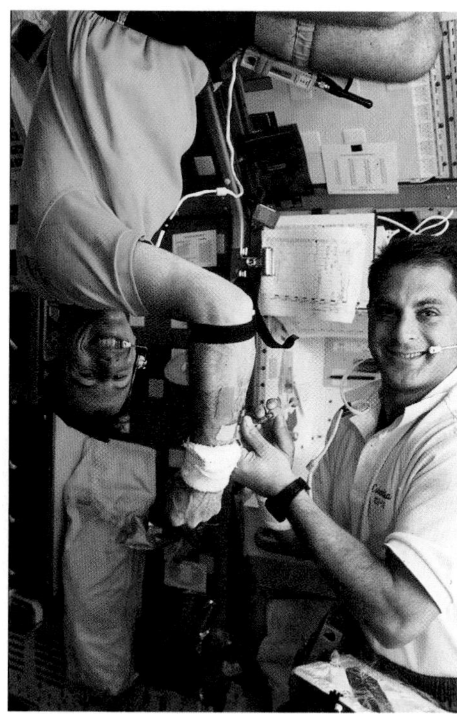

Blood sampling to assess changes in blood volume during a *Skylab* medical experiment. Note the blue thigh cuff used to monitor changes in lower limb fluid shifts.

other. For example, trace the pathways between a decrease in hydrostatic gradients (top left) and reduced total blood volume (bottom center). How many different pathways interact to reduce total blood volume? Similarly, trace how altered sensory and balance information also affect blood volume and maximal exercise capacity. Two of the current NASA research efforts focus on (1) the impact of reduced bone density on risk of bone fractures and (2) the functional impact of skeletal muscle atrophy (reduced strength) on performing mission-related tasks. These physiologic responses to microgravity, in addition to reduced stroke volume related to orthostatic hypotension and possible syncope, have implications for developing and testing effective countermeasure strategies (see page 719).

In addition to the flow chart of physiologic events, we present separate tables with detailed information about the cardiovascular, pulmonary, body fluid, sensory, and musculoskeletal responses to microgravity. The information comes from almost four decades of cumulative research from Mercury, Gemini, Apollo, ASTP, Vostok, Voskhod, Soyuz, Shuttle Spacelab, Skylab, Salyut, and Mir missions. Excellent summary resource materials exist about these responses,[4,10,18,21,26,28–32,37,40,49,52,65,87,104,106,120,125,134,136] including many of the Internet sites listed on pages 747–748.

Cardiovascular Adaptations

The decrease in total fluid volume during the first few days in microgravity reduces the heart's total work effort. With continued microgravity exposure, overall heart size decreases, mainly from reduced left ventricular volume, particularly left ventricular end-diastolic volume. Perhaps such adaptations represent an appropriate response to microgravity without compromising "normal" cardiovascular function during a mission.

Table 27.7 summarizes adaptations in 15 cardiovascular variables for space missions through 1992, while Figure 27.10 displays pre- to postflight changes in stroke volume during upright exercise, expressed as a percentage of preflight baseline. Also shown are changes in aerobic capacity (not listed in Table 27.7) as a function of intensity and frequency of 20-minute inflight cycle ergometer exercise bouts during four different missions. Maximal oxygen consumption declined significantly regardless of training regimen, except for group 1, which maintained heart rate above 130 $b \cdot min^{-1}$ and exercised

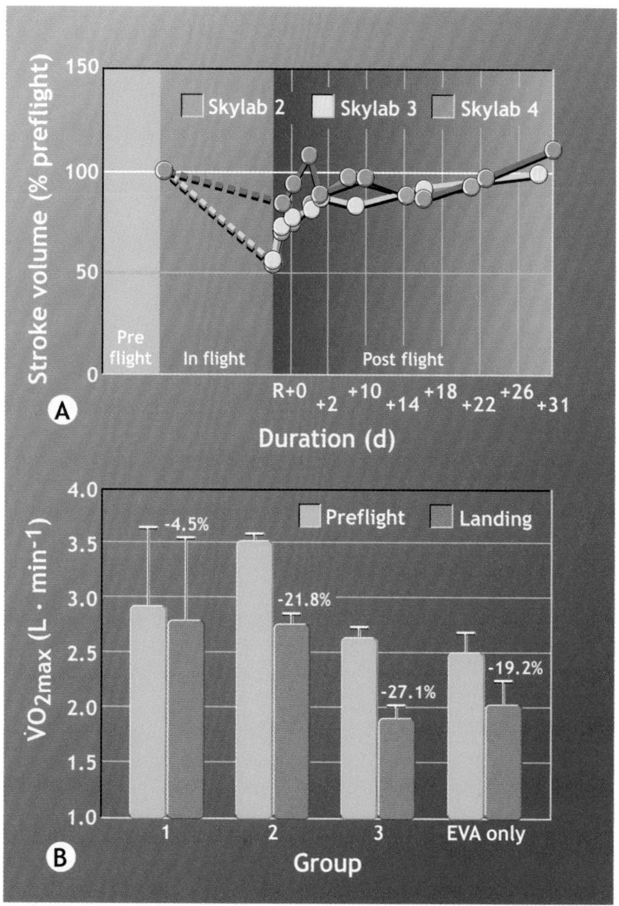

Group 1 (n=3): Ex.>3x/week, HR >130, >20min/session (regular exercise group)
Group 2 (n=5): Ex.>3x/week, HR <130, >20min/session (reduced intensity exercise group)
Group 3 (n=8): Ex.<2x/week; HR and min/session variable (minimal exercise group)
EVA Only (n=4): EVA subjects. Minimal other exercise peformed during flight (Hubble Mission)

FIGURE 27.10 • Pre- to postflight changes in (**A**) stroke volume during upright exercise (Skylab 2-4). R, return to Earth, and (**B**) aerobic capacity related to intensity and frequency of 20-minute in-flight cycle ergometry. (Data for A from Michel EL, et al. Results of Skylab medical experiment M171-metabolic activity. In: Johnson RS, Dietlein LF, eds. Biomedical results from Skylab. NASA SP-377. Washington, DC: Government Printing Office, 1977. Data for B from Sawin CF. Biomedical investigations conducted in support of the extended duration orbiter medical project. Aviat Space Environ Med 1999;70:169.)

TABLE 27.7 ➤ CHANGES IN CARDIOVASCULAR VARIABLES ASSOCIATED WITH MICROGRAVITY

		LONG SPACE FLIGHTS (>2 WK)	
PHYSIOLOGIC MEASURE	**SHORT SPACE FLIGHTS (1–14 D)**	**PREFLIGHT VS. IN-FLIGHT**	**PREFLIGHT VS. POSTFLIGHT**
Heart rate (resting)	Variable in flight; increased after flight; peaks during launch and re-entry; RPB up to 1 week	Normal or slightly increased	Increased; RPB 3 weeks
Blood pressure (resting)	Normal; decreased after flight	Diastolic blood pressure reduced or unchanged	Decreased mean arterial pressure
Orthostatic tolerance	Decreased after flights longer than 5 hours; exaggerated cardiovascular responses to tilt test, stand test, and LBNP after flight; RPB 3–14 days	Exaggerated cardiovascular responses to in-flight LBNP (especially during first 2 wk); last in-flight test comparable to recovery-day test	Exaggerated cardiovascular responses to LBNP; RPB up to 3 weeks
Total peripheral resistance	Decreased in flight; no increase at landing despite drop in stroke volume and increase in HR	Tendency toward decrease	Increased after landing
Cardiac size	Normal or slightly decreased C/T ratio after flight	C/T ratio decreased after flight	
Stroke volume	Increased in flight by as much as 60% (SLS-1); compensated by decreased HR	Increased early in flight, then decreased	12% decrease on average
Left end-diastolic volume	Same as stroke volume	Same as in short-duration missions	16% decrease on average
Cardiac output	Elevated 30 to 40% in flight (SLS-1); reduced immediately after flight	Unchanged	Variable; RPB 3–4 weeks
Central venous pressure	Elevated above resting supine level before launch; transient increase followed by levels below preflight upon attaining orbit	Not measured	Not measured
Left cardiac muscle mass thickness	Unchanged	Unchanged	11% decrease; return to normal after 3 weeks
Cardiac electrical activity (ECG/VCG)	Moderate rightward shift in QRS and T waves after flight	Increased P-R interval, QT interval, and QRS vector magnitude	Slight increase in QRS duration and magnitude; increase in P-R interval duration
Arrhythmia	Usually PABs and PVBs; isolated cases of nodal tachycardia, ectopic beats, and supraventricular bigeminy in flight	PVBs and occasional PABs; sinus or nodal arrhythmia at release of LBNP in flight	Occasional unifocal PABs and PVBs
Systolic time intervals	Not measured	Not measured; PEP/ET ratio RPB 2 weeks	Increase in resting and LBNP-stressed
Exercise capacity	No change or decreased ≤12% after flight; increased HR for same $\dot{V}O_2$; no change in efficiency; RPB 3–8 days	Submaximal exercise capacity unchanged	Decreased after flight; recovery time inversely related to amount of in-flight exercise rather than mission duration
Venous compliance in legs	Not measured	Increased: continues to increase for 10 days or more; slow decrease later in flight	Normal or slightly increased

Data from Nicogossian AE, et al. Space physiology and medicine, 3rd ed. Philadelphia: Lea & Febiger, 1994:216.
RPB, return to preflight baseline; LBNP, lower-body negative pressure; C/T, cardiothoracic; ECG, electrocardiogram; VCG, vectorcardiogram; PAB, premature atrial beat; PVB, premature ventricular beat; HR, heart rate; SLS-1, Spacelab Life Sciences-1

longer than 20 minutes more than three times weekly. In contrast to these reported studies, some in-flight ergometer and treadmill studies have reported that astronauts maintained their level of aerobic capacity during relatively brief missions.

INTEGRATIVE QUESTION

Contrast the hemodynamic responses when a person moves from the upright to the upside-down position on Earth and in a microgravity environment.

Pulmonary Adaptations

A tight linkage exists between the cardiovascular, pulmonary, and metabolic systems. The cells' demand for oxygen during rest and exercise remains invariant regardless of the environment. Any change in external work above a resting baseline triggers immediate ventilatory responses that increase breathing rate and tidal volume. Augmented alveolar ventilation maintains an adequate pressure differential for diffusion of oxygen across lung tissues for delivery by the cardiovascular system to the site of increased energy metabolism.

Table 27.8 summarizes changes in pulmonary variables during two Spacelab missions (see unnumbered photo on right). Figure 27.11 depicts changes in pulmonary diffusing capacity for carbon monoxide measured preflight on days 2, 4, and 9 during the mission and within 6 hours before or after landing and then at days 1, 2, 4, and 6 postflight. Note that diffusing capacity increases in the sitting and standing positions during 3 days in microgravity and then returns to the baseline values achieved preflight.

Denitrogenation and EVA

Before astronauts perform EVA maneuvers, they must "washout" the nitrogen from their fluids and tissues to prevent decompression sickness (DCS, or the bends) from changes in gas pressures within the cabin and EVA garment. They do this

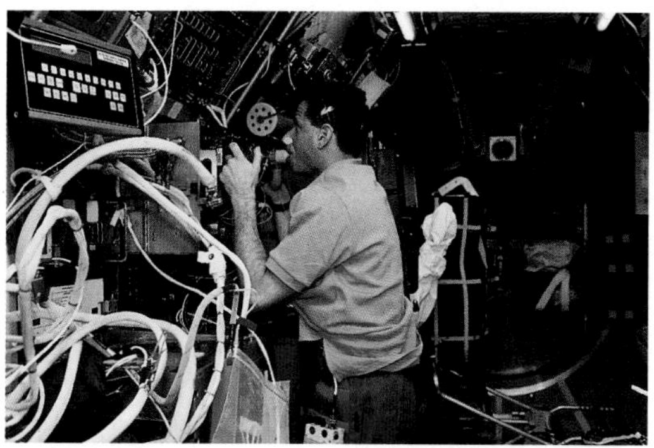

The automated ALFE (Astronaut Lung Function Experiment) hardware makes detailed measurement of lung function in microgravity. Tests include monitoring the motion in the rib cage and abdomen during rest, exercise, and following deep breathing, the patterns of gas distribution in the lungs when inhaling various gas mixtures, and breathing maneuvers to measure the concentrations and volumes of inhaled and exhaled gases before and following different durations and modes of exercise.

TABLE 27.8 ➤ CHANGES IN PULMONARY SYSTEM VARIABLES ASSOCIATED WITH MICROGRAVITY DURING SPACELAB LIFE SCIENCES-1 (FLIGHT STS 40, JUNE 5, 1991) AND GERMAN SPACELAB MISSION D-2 ABOARD STS-55 (APRIL 26, 1993)

PHYSIOLOGIC RESPONSE TO MICROGRAVITY (1–14 D)	REFERENCE LETTER	NUMBER OF SUBJECTS	CHANGES IN MICROGRAVITY (IN-FLIGHT VS. PREFLIGHT STANDING MEASUREMENTS)
Pulmonary blood flow			
Total pulmonary blood flow (cardiac output)	A	4	18% increase
Cardiac stroke volume	A	4	4% increase
Diffusing capacity (carbon monoxide)	A	4	28% increase
Pulmonary capillary blood volume	A	4	28% increase
Diffusing capacity of alveolar membrane	A	4	27% increase
Pulmonary blood flow distribution	C	7	More uniform but some inequality remained
Pulmonary ventilation			
Respiration frequency	E	8	9% increase
Tidal volume	E	8	15% decrease
Alveolar ventilation	E	8	Unchanged
Total ventilation	E	8	Small decrease
Ventilatory distribution	B	7	More uniform but some inequality remained
Maximal peak expiratory flow rate	E	7	Decreased by ≤12.5% early in flight but then returned to normal
Pulmonary gas exchange			
O_2 uptake	E	8	Unchanged
CO_2 output	E	8	Unchanged
End-tidal Po_2	E	8	Unchanged
End-tidal Pco_2	E	8	Small increase when CO_2 concentration in spacecraft increased
Lung volumes			
Functional residual capacity	D	4	15% decrease
Residual lung volume	D	4	18% decrease
Closing volume	B	7	Unchanged as measured by argon bolus

Note: Pulmonary blood flow in normal subjects equals cardiac output. The ability of carbon monoxide to diffuse into the blood is a standard clinical test of the integrity of the alveolar membrane and its surrounding capillary blood supply. The data indicate that more alveoli are expanded and ventilated in space than on Earth. Closing volume refers to the volume in the lung where the alveoli close in significant numbers.

A. Prisk OK, et al. Pulmonary diffusing capacity, capillary blood volume and cardiac output during sustained microgravity. J Appl Physiol 1993;75:15.
B. Guy HJB, et al. Inhomogeneity of pulmonary ventilation during sustained microgravity as determined by single-breath washouts. J Appl Physiol 1994;76:1719.
C. Prisk OK, et al. Inhomogeneity of pulmonary ventilation during sustained microgravity on Spacelab SLS-1. J Appl Physiol 1994;76:1730.
D. Elliott AR, et al. Lung volumes during sustained microgravity on Spacelab SLS-1. J Appl Physiol 1994;77:2005.
E. Prisk OK, et al. Pulmonary gas exchange and its determinants during sustained microgravity on Spacelab SLS-1. J Appl Physiol 1995;76:1290.
Modified from West JB, et al. Pulmonary function in space. JAMA. 1997;277:1957.

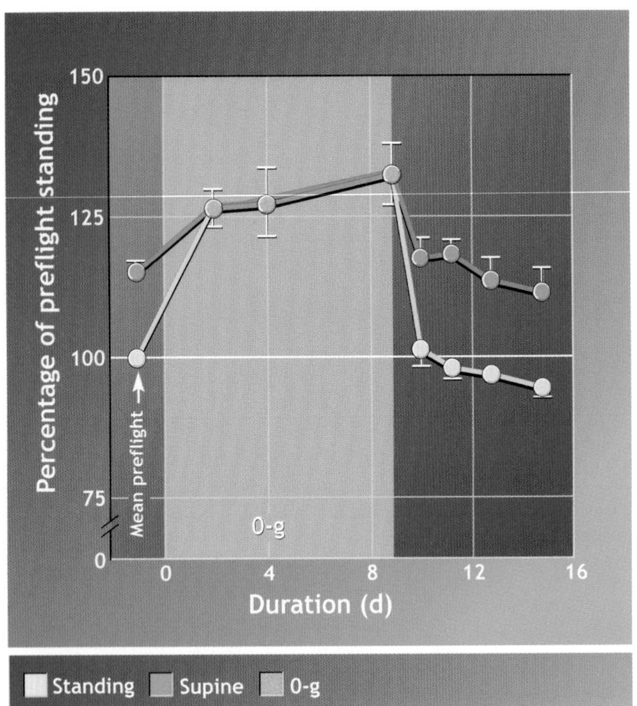

FIGURE 27.11 • Pulmonary diffusing capacity for carbon monoxide preflight, on flight days 2, 4, and 9 and 6 hours following landing and on days 1, 2, 4, and 6 postflight. Data are referenced to the preflight standing value. (From Prisk GK, et al. Pulmonary diffusing capacity, capillary blood volume, and cardiac output during sustained microgravity. J Appl Physiol 1993;75:15,1993.)

by using a 10.2 pounds per square inch atmosphere (psia) staged decompression of the shuttle for at least 12 hours. This also includes 100 minutes of **preoxygenation**, breathing 100% O_2 at 14.7 psia prior to decompression and before decompression to the suit pressure of 4.3 psia (equivalent to 9144-m altitude). Even a slight incapacitation from DCS during an EVA could hinder safe return to the spacecraft and provoke a medical emergency. Scientists have proposed several ways to induce **denitrogenation**. First, reduce the total pressure inside the spacecraft from 760 to 630 torr (approximate barometric pressure of Denver, CO) to shorten overall time for denitrogenation prior to EVA. Second, have astronauts sleep in a special low-pressure compartment prior to EVA. Thus, the several hours devoted to denitrogenation during sleep would not encroach upon valuable work time. A seemingly simple solution would increase the pressure within the space suit to keep N_2 in solution to avoid forming bubbles. This, however, would cause the suit to stiffen considerably, rendering limb maneuverability nearly impossible.

The rate of denitrogenation depends on at least two factors: (1) tissue nitrogen capacity, which increases with body fat content (N_2 elimination takes longer in fatter people) and (2) the tissues' oxygenation; this ultimately depends on cardiac output, which decreases in the supine position during flight.[94] In prolonged missions, as lower limb muscles begin to atrophy in the weightless environment, the time for denitrogenation also may change.

EXERCISE-ENHANCED PREOXYGENATION. Recent experiments using exercise-enhanced preoxygenation (10 min of upper- and lower-body exercise at 75% estimated $\dot{V}O_{2max}$ breathing 100% O_2) eliminated DCS during 36 U-2 reconnaissance flights at altitudes of 29,000 to 30,000 feet in a pilot who previously experienced 25 episodes of DCS.[48] Another experiment investigated the efficiency of either a 1-hour or a 15-minute preoxygenation period, each beginning with 10 minutes of dual-cycle ergometry performed at 75% of $\dot{V}O_{2peak}$ for enhancing preoxygenation efficiency by increasing perfusion gradients and minute ventilation.[135] Male subjects accomplished a 1-hour preoxygenation with exercise, a 15-minute preoxygenation with exercise, or a 1-hour resting preoxygenation before exposure to 4.3 psia for 4 hours while performing light-to-moderate exercise. The incidence of DCS following the 1-hour preoxygenation with exercise was significantly less (42%; $n = 26$) than following the 1-hour resting preoxygenation (77%; $n = 26$). The incidence and onset of DCS following the 15-minute preoxygenation with exercise (64%; $n = 22$) did not differ significantly from the 1-hour resting control. *Thus, 1 hour of preoxygenation with exercise significantly improves resistance to DCS, illustrating the potentially positive effect of exercise on ameliorating DCS during critical mission EVA maneuvers.*

Body Fluid Adaptations

Table 27.9 summarizes preflight to postflight adaptations in 24 body fluid variables. Figure 27.12 reports data for three variables: (1) percentage change in plasma volume and red cell mass during Spacelab 1 and three Skylab missions, (2)

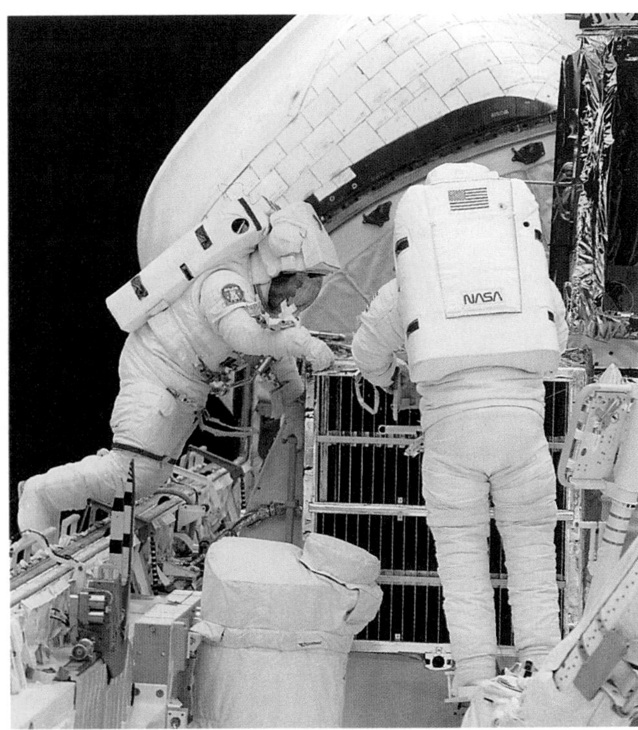

American and Russian astronauts work side-by-side for several hours during construction of the International Space Station.

TABLE 27.9 ➤ CHANGES IN BODY FLUID VARIABLES ASSOCIATED WITH MICROGRAVITY

Physiologic Measure	Short Space Flights (1–14 d)[a]	Long Space Flights (>2 wk)[b]	
		Preflight vs. In-Flight	Preflight vs. Postflight
Total body water	3% decrease by flight day 4 or 5		Decreased after flight
Plasma volume	Decreased after flight (except Gemini-7 and -8); decreased in flight (SLS-1)		Markedly decreased after flight. RPB 2 weeks increased at R + 0; decreased R + 2 (hydration effect)
Hematocrit	Slightly increased after flight		Decreased after flight; RPB 2–4 weeks after landing
Hemoglobin	Normal or slightly increased after flight	Increased in first in-flight sample; slowly declines later in flight	Decreased from near-preflight values on landing day; RPB 1–2 months
Red blood cell (RBC) mass	Decreased after flight (approx. 9% on SLS-1); RPB at least 2 weeks	Decreased ~15% during first 2–3 weeks in flight; begins to recover after about 60 days; recovery of RBC mass is independent of time spent in space	Decreased after flight; RPB 2 weeks to 3 months after landing
Red blood cell morphology	No significant changes observed after flight	Increase in percentage of echinocytes; decrease in discocytes	Rapid reversal of in-flight changes in distribution of red blood cell shapes; significantly increased potassium influx; RPB 3 days
Red blood cell half-life (^{51}Cr)	No change; verified on SLS-1		No change
Reticulocytes	Decreased after flight; RPB 1 week		Decreases at landing shift to increases over preflight values by 7 days after landing; greatest changes seen after longer flights
Iron turnover	No change		No change
Mean corpuscular volume	Increased after flight; RPB at least 2 weeks		Variable, but within normal limits
Mean corpuscular hemoglobin	Increased after flight; RPB 2 weeks		Variable, but within normal limits
White blood cells	Increased after flight, especially neutrophils; lymphocytes decreased; RPB 1–2 days; no significant change in T/B lymphocyte ratio		Increased, especially neutrophils; postflight reduction in number of T cells and T-cell function as measured by PHA responsiveness, RPB 3–7 days; transient postflight elevation in B cells, RPB 3 days
Plasma lipids	Decreased cholesterol and triglycerides in flight		
Plasma glucose	Decreased during and immediately after flight	Decreased for the first 2 months then leveled off	Postflight hyperglycemia with increased lactate and pyruvate
Plasma proteins	Occasional postflight elevations in α_2-globulin, due to increases of haptoglobin, ceruloplasmin, and α_2-macroglobulin; elevated IgA and C_3		No significant changes
Red blood cell enzymes	No consistent postflight changes	Decrease in phosphofructokinase; no evidence of lipid peroxidation or red blood cell damage	No consistent postflight changes
Serum/plasma electrolytes	Increased K and Ca in flight (SLS-1); decreased Na in flight; decreased K and Mg after flight	Decreased Na, Cl, and osmolality; slight increase in K and PO_4	Postflight decreases in Na, K, Cl, Mg; increase in PO_4 and osmolality
Serum/plasma hormones	Decreased ANF, aldosterone, and ADH in flight (SLS-1); increased cortisol and angiotensin 1 in flight (SLS-1)	Increases in cortisol; decreases in ACTH, insulin	Postflight increases in angiotensin, aldosterone, thyroxine, TSH and GH; decrease in ACTH

Continued

TABLE 27.9 ➤ CHANGES IN BODY FLUID VARIABLES ASSOCIATED WITH MICROGRAVITY—cont'd

		Long Space Flights (>2 wk)	
Physiologic Measure	Short Space Flights (1–14 d)	Preflight vs. In-Flight	Preflight vs. Postflight
Insulin		Decreased during long missions	Decreased after flight
Serum/plasma metabolites and enzymes	Postflight increases in blood urea nitrogen, creatinine, and glucose; decreases in lactic acid dehydrogenase, creatinine phosphokinase, albumin, triglycerides, cholesterol, and uric acid		Postflight decrease in cholesterol, uric acid
Urine volume	Decreased after flight	Decreased early in flight	Decreased after flight
Urine electrolytes	Postflight increases in Ca, creatinine, PO_4, and osmolality; decreases in Na, K, Cl, Mg	Increased osmolality, Na, K, Cl, Mg, Ca, PO_4; decrease in uric acid excretion	Increase in Ca excretion; initial postflight decreases in Na, K, Cl, Mg, PO_4, uric acid; Na and Cl excretion increased in second and third week after flight
Urinary hormones	In-flight decreases in 17-OH-corticosteroids, increase in aldosterone; postflight increases in cortisol, aldosterone, ADH, and pregnanediol; decreases in epinephrine, 17-OH-corticosteroids, androsterone, and etiocholanolone	In-flight increases in cortisol, aldosterone, and total 17-ketosteroids; decrease in ADH	Increases in cortisol, aldosterone, norepinephrine, decreases in total 17-OH-corticosteroids, ADH
Urinary amino acids	Postflight increases in taurine and β-alanine; decreases in glycine, alanine, and tyrosine	Increased in flight	Increased after flight

[a]Biomedical data from Mercury, Gemini, Apollo, ASTP, Vostok, Voskhod, Soyuz, Shuttle Spacelab.
[b]Biomedical data from Skylab, Salyut, Mir missions.
Data from Nicogossian AE, et al. Space physiology and medicine. 3rd ed. Philadelphia: Lea & Febiger, 1994:217.
SLS, Spacelab Life Sciences; RPB, return to preflight baseline; R, return to Earth.

percentage change in total hemoglobin during four Salyut (Russian) missions, and (3) blood volume related to orthostatically stressed heart rate response during Apollo, SMEAT (Skylab Medical Experiments Altitude Tests), and Skylab missions.

Sensory System Adaptations

Table 27.10 summarizes space flight adaptations in the sensory system categories of audition, gustation and olfaction, somatosensory, and vision for relatively short (<14 d) and longer (>14 d) space missions. The bottom of the table lists general vestibular system changes. Part A of Figure 27.13 schematically shows multisensory interactions that readjust these sensory responses disturbed by microgravity. Sensorimotor integration plays a pivotal role in posture and movement control, ambulation, and manipulating objects at 1g, which necessitate proper adjustment in body orientation. In essence, the sensory-motor control system consists of a highly complex, tightly integrated neural complex that modulates vestibular, visual, somatosensory, tactile, and proprioceptive input within a central command-processing center. Disturbance in one aspect of the system usually initiates an override, readjustment, or temporary substitution by other system components to maintain the system's functional integrity.[38,59,68,79,80,92,130] Considerable research has assessed how microgravity affects spatial orientation, postural control, vestibulo-ocular reflexes, and vestibular processing. Studies have also focused on mechanisms related to space motion sickness and perceptual motor performance.[89,90] The unnumbered figure below shows an in-flight experiment on 1993 Spacelab Life Sciences 2 shuttle flight STS-58 using a rotating chair to study vestibular function.

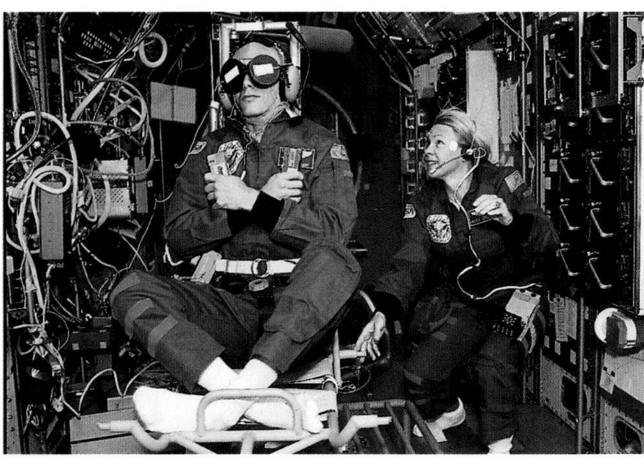

Photo courtesy of Dr. Martin Fettman, Colorado State University, Fort Collins, CO, payload specialist on STS-58, who participated in the rotating chair experiments depicted in this photo.

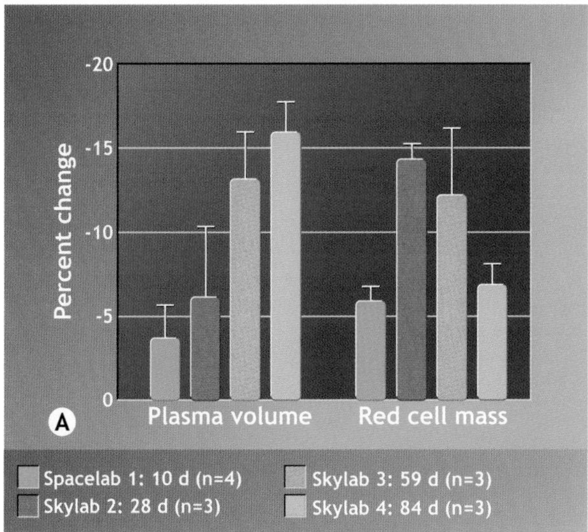

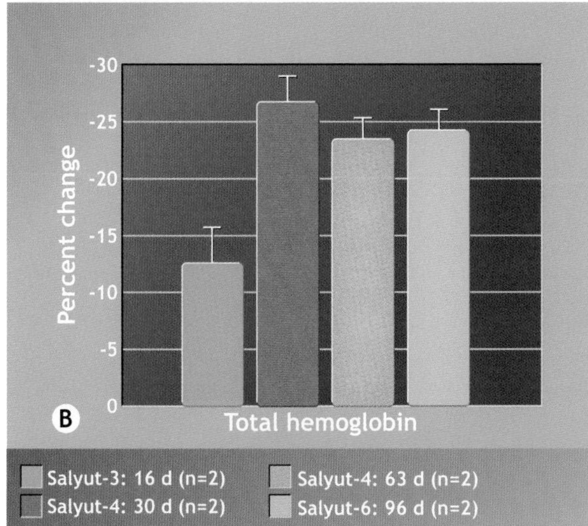

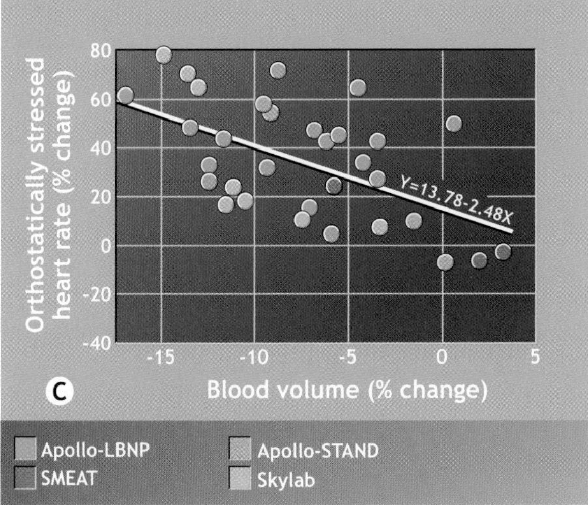

FIGURE 27.12 • Pre- to postflight changes in (**A**) plasma volume and red blood cell mass (Spacelab 1; Skylab 2-4), (**B**) total hemoglobin (Salyut 3-4; 6), and (**C**) blood volume in relation to orthostatically-stressed heart rate (Apollo, Skylab, and SMEAT [Skylab Medical Experiments Altitude Tests]). *Error bars* in A and B represent standard errors of measurement. (Data for A and B redrawn from Convertino VA. Physiological adaptations to weightlessness: effects on exercise and work performance. Exerc Sports Sci Rev 1990;18:119.)

Part B of Figure 27.13 displays the immediate effects of space flight on postural reflexes in crew members from eight missions that lasted 4 to 10 days. Immediate postflight measurements were made within 1 to 5 hours in 10 of the 13 subjects. The greatest postural instability occurred in tests requiring vestibular information. These experiments demonstrated a two-stage readaptation process following microgravity exposure. The first stage occurred quickly, within a few hours after landing; in a second, slower stage, stability returned to near normal in approximately 4 days. On longer Russian Mir missions (140 and 175 d), recovery of postural parameters to preflight levels required approximately 6 weeks. Apparently, readaptation of postural control upon return from space coincides with mission duration, with a prominent role played by visual cues.[26]

Musculoskeletal Adaptations

Table 27.11 examines musculoskeletal adaptations during exposure to microgravity. *NASA's greatest biomedical concern involves the significant 1% per month loss in weight-bearing bone mass during space missions.*

Increased Calcium Loss

Table 27.12 summarizes data from 18 male crew members aboard Russian MIR station missions lasting between 4 and 14.4 months. Bone mineral density (BMD) declined at all seven sites measured, with spine, neck of femur, trochanter, and pelvis decreasing more than 1% per month. On the shorter 4- to 14-day Gemini flights, BMD decreased 3 to 9% in the os calcis (heel bone).[132] Loss of BMD at the os calcis and radius occurred during Apollo Skylab missions and showed no recovery, even after 97 days postflight.[122,131] During the Skylab II 28-day orbital mission, crew members experienced a daily negative 50-mg calcium balance;[137] daily calcium loss averaged 140 mg on the 84-day mission. Increased bone calcium loss, if coupled with a high fluid and salt intake, could alter plasma filtrate composition and pH to favor supersaturation of kidney stone-forming salts.[138]

Figure 27.14 illustrates how reduced mechanical stress in microgravity affects calcium balance. The *top panel* shows how three skeletal loading factors—reduced gravity (microgravity), normal gravity, and above-normal gravity loading—adjust calcium distribution in the digestive (intestine), cardiovascular, renal (kidney), and skeletal (bone) systems. Under normal 1-g conditions, the small intestine absorbs approximately 250 to 500 mg of calcium for every 1000 mg consumed, with the remainder excreted in feces (▼▼). In contrast, in a microgravity environment, reduced calcium intestinal absorption exacerbates calcium fecal loss (▼▼▼). Abnormal calcium excretion from bone resorption disrupts calcium homeostasis, which in turn decreases total body calcium and bone mass. With increased gravitational loading, calcium absorption by bone increases, sparing overall calcium loss (▼). In the *bottom panel,* the flow diagram shows proposed parallel dynamics of the calcium/endocrine response and skeletal struc-

TABLE 27.10 ➤ CHANGES IN SENSORY SYSTEM VARIABLES ASSOCIATED WITH MICROGRAVITY

		Long Space Flights (>2 wk)	
Physiologic Measure	Short Space Flights (1–14 d)	Preflight vs. In-Flight	Preflight vs. Postflight
Audition	No change in thresholds after flight	One report of lowered thresholds during a 1-year flight	No change in thresholds after flight
Gustation and olfaction	Subjective and varied human experience; no impairments noted	Same as shorter missions	Same as shorter missions
Somatosensory	Subjective and varied human experience; no impairments noted	Subjective experiences (e.g., tingling in feet)	
Vision	Intraocular tension tends to increase during flight and decrease at landing; postflight decreases in visual field; retinal blood vessels constricted after flight; dark-adapted crews reported light flashes with eyes open or closed; decrease in visual motor task performance and contrast discrimination; no change in in-flight contrast discrimination or distant and near visual acuity	Light flashes reported by dark-adapted subjects; frequency related to latitude (highest in South Atlantic anomaly, lowest over poles)	No significant changes except for transient decreases in intraocular pressure
Vestibular system	40–70% of astronauts/cosmonauts exhibit in-flight neurovestibular effects including immediate reflex motor responses (postural illusions, sensations of tumbling or rotation, nystagmus, dizziness, vertigo) and space motion sickness (pallor, cold sweating, nausea, vomiting); motion sickness symptoms appear early in flight and subside or disappear in 2–7 days; postflight difficulties in postural equilibrium with eyes closed or other vestibular disturbances	In-flight vestibular disturbances are same as for shorter missions; markedly decreased susceptibility to provocative motion stimuli (cross-coupled angular acceleration) after adaptation period of 2–7 days; cosmonauts have reported occasional reappearance of illusions during long missions.	Immunity to provocative motion continues for several days after flight; marked postflight disturbances in postural equilibrium with eyes closed; some cosmonauts exhibit additional vestibular disturbances after flight, including dizziness, nausea, and vomiting

Data used by permission from Nicogossian AE, et al. Space physiology and medicine. 3rd ed. Philadelphia: Lea & Febiger, 1994:219.

ture and composition to altered gravitational loading with adequate diet and endocrine balance.

Without suitable countermeasures, progressive calcium losses during future missions of several years duration will likely compromise astronaut well-being, particularly increasing bone fracture risk upon return to Earth. On-board, multimode exercise training and lower-limb exercise has *not* prevented BMD loss, despite United States and Soviet crew members' commitment to intense workouts. Researchers hope that future research using valid animal and bed rest models will reveal the basic mechanism of bone remodeling during prolonged microgravity exposures.[85,103,119] These studies must consider hormonal and cellular factors as affected by alterations in mechanical stimulation that probably alter bone sensors to subsequently affect this organ's structural integrity.[42] Biochemical markers of bone turnover during 120 days of bed rest (skeletal unloading) demonstrated that the combined effects of accelerated bone resorption and retarded bone formation accounted for bone loss.[54] BMD measurements at the distal radius and tibia in 15 cosmonauts on the MIR space station on missions of 1, 2, and 6 months revealed the following:[128] (1) cancellous and cortical bone of the radius changed significantly at each of the time points, (2) for the weight-bearing tibial site, cancellous BMD appeared normal after 1 month and deteriorated thereafter. After 2 months, bone loss became noticeable in the tibial cortices, (3) at 6 months, cortical bone loss was less evident than cancellous bone loss and cumulative time in microgravity did not relate to BMD changes, and (4) after return to Earth for durations similar to time in space (1 to 6 mo), tibial bone loss still persisted. The scientists concluded that even with on-board, dedicated physical exercise intervention, bone loss persists and can remain pathologic for a prolonged period following the mission. Alterations in circulation to bone during microgravity exposure can alter the balance between bone resorption and bone formation. Thus, bone blood flow may play an important role in bone remodeling in microgravity.[14]

Part of the solution to the problem of bone loss in prolonged microgravity may lie in selecting crew members with the greatest resistance to bone loss, including applying targeted prevention and/or treatment strategies.[123] Individual differences in the rate of bone loss during space flight probably relate to genetic factors. Thus, identifying the genetic basis of osteoporosis may exclude susceptible individuals from prolonged missions. Hopefully, effective combinations of pharmacologic, nutritional, and exercise countermeasures together with screening procedures will combat bone loss during space missions. Studying female crew members

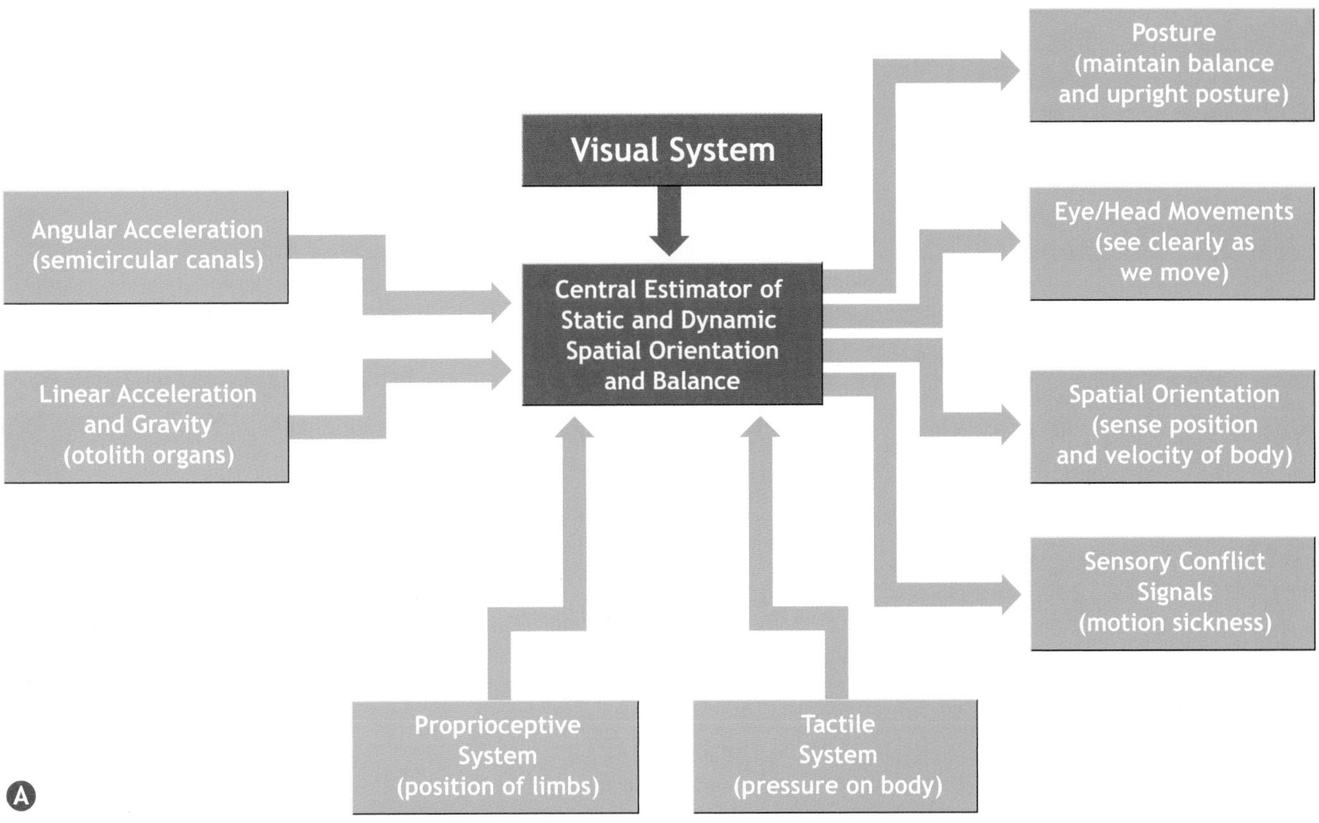

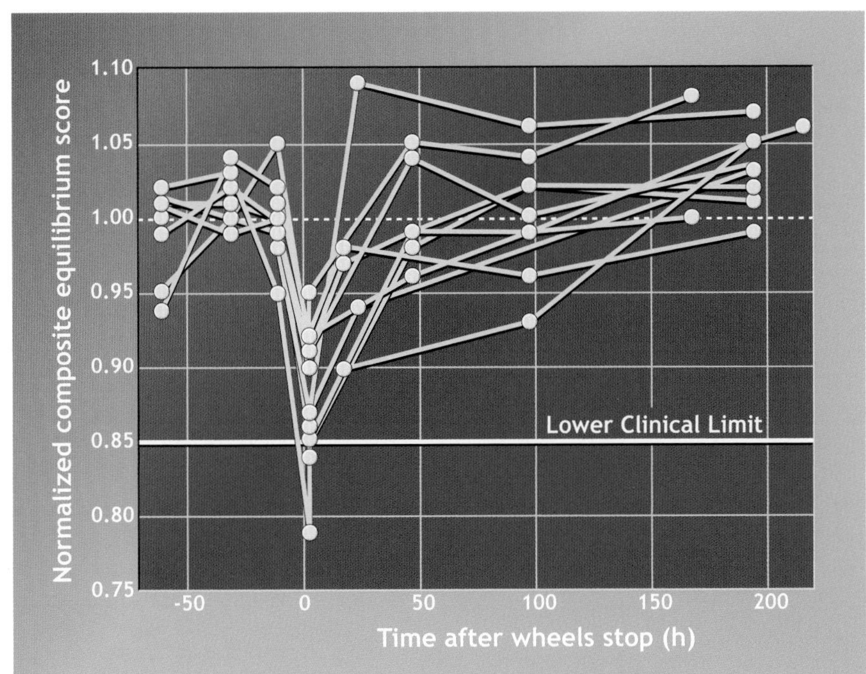

FIGURE 27.13 • **A**. Schematic representation of sensory motor system that controls eye movements and posture, and perception of orientation and motion. **B**. Changes in anterior-posterior sway (composite equilibrium score) in 10 astronauts at various times after the space shuttle returned to Earth (*wheels stop*). The tests involved perturbation of a posture platform under different conditions of visual, vestibular, and proprioceptive input. Dashed horizontal line at 1.00 represents normal response. (Data reported in Daunton NG. Adaptation of the vestibular system to microgravity. In: Fregly MJ, Blatteis CM, eds. Handbook of physiology. Section 4, Environmental physiology, vol 2. American Physiological Society. New York: Oxford University Press, 1996:765. Data for A modified from Young LR, et al. M.I.T./Canadian vestibular experiments on the Spacelab-1 mission: 2. Visual vestibular tilt interaction in weightlessness. Exp Brain Res 1986;64:299. Data for B modified from Paloski WH, et al. Recovery of postural equilibrium control following space flight. Ann NY Acad Sci 1992;656:747.)

TABLE 27.11 ➤ CHANGES IN MUSCULOSKELETAL VARIABLES ASSOCIATED WITH MICROGRAVITY

Physiologic Measure	Short Space Flights (1–14 d)	Long Space Flights (>2 wk)	
		Preflight vs. In-Flight	Preflight vs. Postflight
Stature	Slight increase during first week in flight (~1.3 cm); RPB 1 day	Increased during first 2 weeks in flight (maximum 3–6 cm); stabilizes thereafter	Height returns to normal on R + 0
Body mass	Postflight weight losses average about 3.4%; about 2/3 of the loss due to water loss, the remainder due to loss of lean body mass and fat	In-flight weight losses average 3–4% during first 5 days; thereafter, weight either declines or increases for the remainder of mission; early in-flight losses are probably due to loss of fluids; later losses are metabolic	Rapid weight gain during first 5 days after flight, mainly due to replenishment of fluids; slower weight gain from R + 5 days to R + 2 or 3 weeks; amount of postflight weight loss inversely related to in-flight caloric intake
Protein synthesis	Elevated 40% on flight day 8 (SLS-1), suggesting a "stress response"		
Body composition		Fat is probably replacing muscle tissue; muscle mass is partially preserved depending on exercise regimen	
Total body volume	Decreased after flight	Center of mass shifts headward	Decreased after flight
Limb volume	In-flight leg volume decreases exponentially during the first flight day; thereafter, rate of decrease declines and plateaus within 3–5 days; postflight decrements in leg volume up to 3%; rapid increase immediately after flight, followed by slower RPB	Same as short missions early in flight; leg volume continues to decrease slightly throughout mission; arm volume decreases slightly	Rapid increase in leg volume immediately after flight, followed by slow RPB
Muscle strength	Decreased during and after flight; RPB 1–2 weeks		Postflight decrease in leg muscle strength, particularly extensors; increased use of in-flight exercise appears to reduce postflight losses in strength, regardless of mission duration; arm strength normal or slightly decreased after flight
EMG analysis	Postflight EMGs from gastrocnemius suggest increased susceptibility to fatigue and reduced muscular efficiency; EMGs from arm muscles show no change		Postflight EMGs from gastrocnemius show shift to higher frequencies, suggesting deterioration of muscle tissue; EMGs indicate increased susceptibility to fatigue; RPB about 4 days
Reflexes (Achilles tendon)	Reflex duration decreased after flight		Reflex duration decreased after flight (by 30% or more); reflex magnitude increased; compensatory increase in reflex duration about 2 weeks after flight; RPB about 1 month
Nitrogen and phosphorus balance		Negative balances early in flight shift to less negative or slightly positive balances later	Rapid return to markedly positive balances after flight
Bone density	Os calcis density decreased after flight; radius and ulna show variable changes, depending on method		Os calcis density decreased after flight; amount of loss correlate with mission duration; little or no loss from non–weight-bearing bones; RPB is gradual; the time course has not been determined
Calcium balance	Increasing negative calcium balance in flight	Excretion of Ca in urine increases during first month in flight, then plateaus; fecal Ca excretion declines until day 10, then increases continually throughout flight; Ca balances becomes increasingly negative throughout flight	Urine Ca content drops below preflight baselines by day 10; fecal Ca content declines, but does not reach preflight baseline by day 20; markedly negative Ca balance after flight, becoming much less negative by day 10; Ca balance still slightly negative on day 20; RPB at least several weeks

RPB, return to preflight baseline; SLS, Spacelab Life Sciences; R, return to Earth; EMG, electromyography.
Data used by permission from Nicogossian AE, et al. Space physiology and medicine. 3rd ed. Philadelphia: Lea & Febiger, 1994:220.

TABLE 27.12 ➤ **BONE LOSS ON MIR SPACE STATION (DATA EXPRESSED AS PERCENTAGE BONE MINERAL DENSITY LOST PER MONTH)**

Variable	Crew Members (n)	Mean Loss (%)	SD*
Spine	18	1.07**	0.63
Neck of femur	18	1.16**	0.85
Trochanter	18	1.58**	0.98
Total body	17	0.35**	0.25
Pelvis	17	1.35**	0.54
Arm	17	0.04	0.88
Leg	16	0.34**	0.33

*Standard deviation
** $p < .01$.
From LeBlanc A, et al. Bone mineral and lean tissue loss after long duration spaceflight. Am Soc Bone Miner Res 1996;11:S323.

should offer a wealth of new information for comparison with terrestrial research on gender-related bone loss including how reduced gravity affects hormone status. Carefully controlled, longitudinal studies in an microgravity environment (i.e., long-term studies on the ISS) become crucial to better understand skeletal biology.[123]

Skeletal Muscle Adaptations

Bone loss during prolonged microgravity exposure coincides with significant decrements in muscle mass and strength. Deterioration in muscle structure and function (see "Focus on Research," next page) could compromise crew health and safety during an exploration-class mission, including performance of critical EVA tasks, landing maneuvers, and procedures for leaving orbit on return to Earth. The absence of

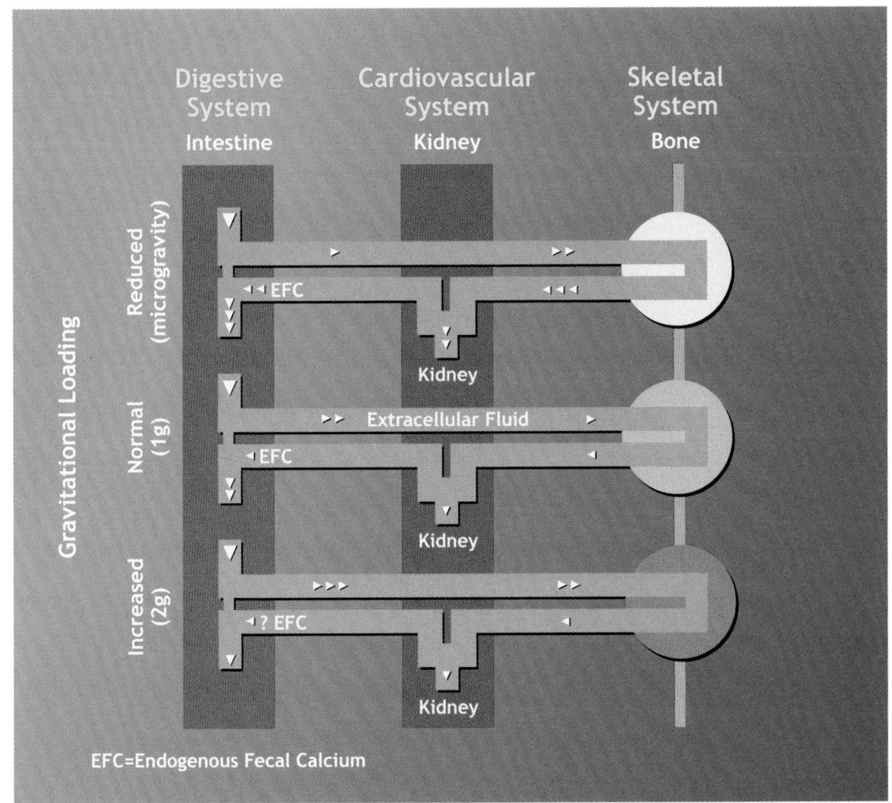

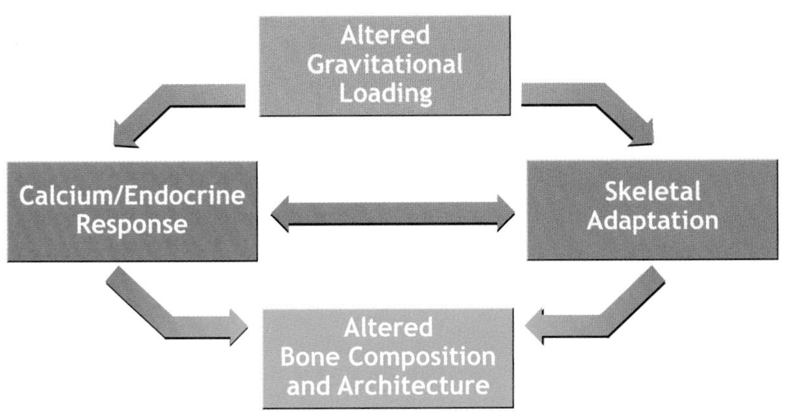

FIGURE 27.14 • Influence of gravitational loading on calcium balance. *Top.* How the digestive system (intestine), cardiovascular system (kidney), and skeletal system (bone) adjust calcium distribution in response to (1) reduced (microgravity), (2) normal (1g), and (3) increased (2g) gravitational skeletal loading. The *shading within the circle in the right panel* represents the adaptation in whole-body bone mineral (darker-shading greater Ca accretion) to the different loading conditions. *Bottom.* Flow diagram proposing parallel calcium/endocrine and skeletal adaptive responses to changing gravitational loading, assuming adequate diet and endocrine balance. (Adapted from Morey-Holton ER, et al. The skeleton and its adaptation to gravity. In: Fregly MJ, Blatteis CM, eds. Handbook of physiology. Section 4, Environmental physiology, vol 2. American Physiological Society. New York: Oxford University Press, 1996.)

Focus on Research: Microgravity's Affects on Muscle Fibers

Edgerton VR, et al. Human fiber size and enzymatic properties after 5 and 11 days of space flight. J Appl Physiol 1995;78:1733.

➤ From the beginning of manned space flight, it has been assumed that prolonged exposure to near–zero-gravity would negatively affect neuromuscular function. Early experiments by the Soviet Union showed that space flight impaired a number of neuromotor components. Some neural adaptations persisted for days and weeks after space flight. A principal issue not addressed by the Soviets was the degree to which neuromotor changes related to muscular components. This study by Edgerton and colleagues was the first to objectify space flight's effects on human muscle fibers. The researchers measured size and capillarization of single muscle fibers and activities of myofibrillar adenosinetriphosphatase (ATPase), succinate dehydrogenase (SDH), and α-glycerophosphate dehydrogenase (GPD) of astronauts who flew either one 11-day or one of two 5-day missions.

Five male (age 40 y; range 33 to 46 y) and three female (age 38 y, range 36 to 40 y) astronauts served as subjects. Five of the subjects participated in a 261–hour flight; two subjects flew for 120 hours; and one subject flew for 128 hours. Preflight (3 to 16 wk before the mission) and postflight (2 to 3 h after landing), a 6-mm needle was used to obtain muscle biopsies from the midportion of the vastus lateralis muscle. For postflight measures, all subjects minimized their walking and standing between landing and the biopsy. Tissue was quick-frozen in liquid nitrogen for subsequent analyses according to standard procedures.

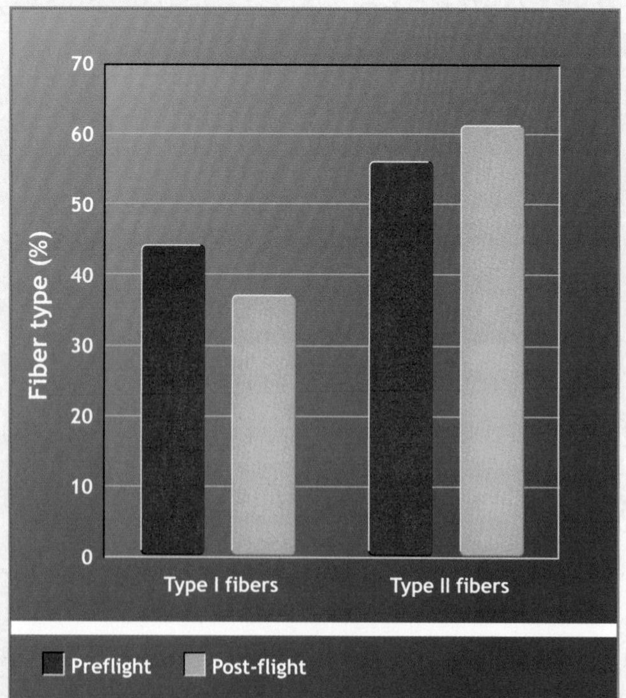

Figure 1. Muscle fiber–type percentage before and immediately after 11 days of space flight.

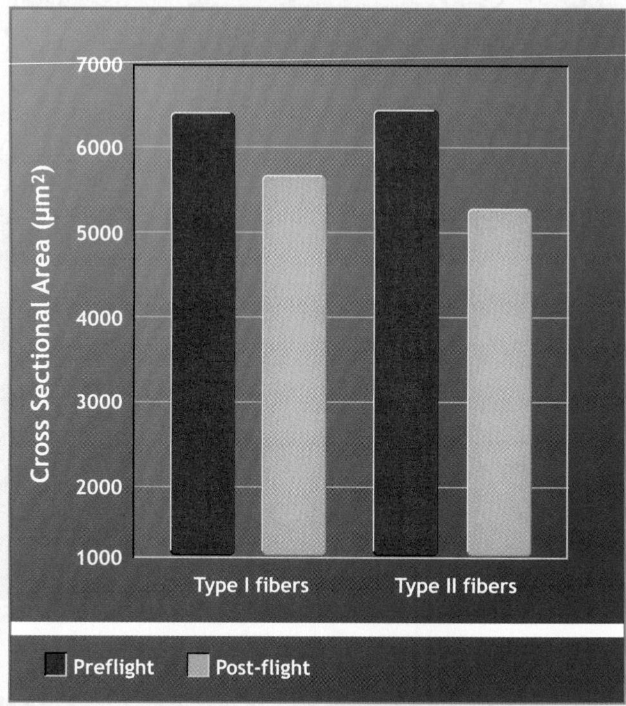

Figure 2. Cross-sectional area of type I and type II muscle fibers before and immediately after 11 days of space flight.

Figures 1 and 2 present the results for muscle fiber type and cross-sectional area (CSA), respectively, for type I and type II muscle fibers. The percentage of fibers classified as type I averaged 6 to 8% less after the mission. This reduction seemed to be compensated for by an increase in the percentage of type IIA fibers with no change in type IIB fibers. A similar pre- to postflight difference was noted for the three subjects who flew for 5 days, but this difference was not statistically significant.

After the 11-day flight, CSA averaged 16 to 36% smaller than preflight values. Although relative atrophy among fiber types was greatest for type IIB and least for type I fibers, mean fiber size decreased significantly for all fibers. Crew members of 5-day missions also exhibited some evidence of muscle atrophy .

The table presents results for fiber enzyme activities, enzyme ratios, total enzyme activities per fiber, and number of capillaries per fiber for all subjects on 5- and 11-day missions. A 32% decrease in total SDH activity in type II fibers was the only significant difference in enzyme activity during space flight. SDH activity per unit mass of the fibers did not change for either type I or type II fibers, but SDH activity per fiber decreased from muscle atrophy. No loss of total activity occurred for ATPase or GPD, because the increase in activity per unit mass countered any atrophy effect.

The absolute number of capillaries supplying each type of muscle fiber decreased significantly from space flight. However, since mean fiber size also decreased (Fig. 2), capillary number per unit muscle CSA remained unchanged.

Focus on Research: Microgravity's Affects on Muscle Fibers

EFFECTS OF 5 TO 11 DAYS OF SPACE FLIGHT ON MUSCLE FIBER CAPILLARIZATION AND SELECTED ENZYME LEVELS

	Type I Fibers			Type II Fibers		
Variable	Preflight	Postflight	%Diff	Preflight	Postflight	%Diff
ATPase activity	383.0	376.0	−2	471.0	513.0	−9*
SDH activity	232.0	203.0	−13	184.0	158.0	−14
ATP/SDH	1.8	2.1	17*	2.9	4.0	38*
GPD activity	5.9	10.6	80	25.0	23.0	−8
Total ATPase	212.0	177.0	−17	258.0	211.0	−18
Total SDH	133.0	97.0	−27	105.0	71.0	−32*
Capillaries per fiber	4.7	3.8	−19*	4.8	3.6	26*

*Significantly different at the 0.05 level.

Because of the close association between the CSA of single fibers, motor units, and whole muscle and the muscle's force-generating capacity, the present results suggest a loss in strength of the vastus lateralis within 11 days of space flight. The loss in CSA within 11 (and perhaps even 5 d) of microgravity exposure agrees with previous data on small mammals (rats) and supports the usefulness of animal models to study human responses to space travel. Astronauts showed considerable variation in preflight and inflight physical activity levels. More than likely, some of the between-subject variation in muscle atrophy related to physical activities during flight. For example, two of the three subjects who exercised four or more times during the flight showed little or no atrophy, while an astronaut with a high level of preflight physical fitness exhibited the greatest atrophy.

The work of Edgerton and colleagues showed that skeletal muscle adapts relatively rapidly to microgravity exposure, with a significant loss in CSA, selected enzyme activity, and fiber capillarization. These highly variable responses may partly relate to physical fitness level before launch and extent of in-flight exercise.

gravity virtually eliminates the load-bearing effects on antigravity muscles, rendering them particularly susceptible to impaired performance in emergencies.

Such exigencies would also apply to low-orbit missions. For example, egress from an orbiting spacecraft, even under normal conditions, taxes the major muscle groups of the arms, legs, and torso. The current launch and entry suit (LES) that must be worn during all landing and exiting procedures weighs 23 kg, including a parachute pack weighing an additional 12 kg in the event of an emergency bailout. The additional weight could potentially impair operational performance during an emergency requiring lifting, pushing and pulling, climbing, and jumping. In an expedited contingency landing, a crew member deploys a 20-kg flight package that includes an inflatable slide that must be lifted up against the side hatch and locked into designated slots before inflation. Another scenario involves escape through the top window of the flight deck. This would require climbing out of the spacecraft's top window using a ground descent device to rappel to the surface.

Concentric and Eccentric Strength

The important role of concentric and eccentric muscle actions in space missions[1,8,12,15,16,19,23,24,31,44] has focused experiments on pre- and postflight assessment of submaximal and maximal muscle functions. For example, concentric strength of Skylab crews was tested isokinetically before and after flights.[116] Tests conducted 5 days after the 28-day flight showed decrements of approximately 25% in leg extensor strength. Even greater losses would probably have occurred had testing been conducted immediately upon landing. Subsequently, longer Skylab missions (59 and 84 d) and (59 d) provided preflight fitness and conditioning that emphasized strengthening exercises for the lower extremities. This emphasis on preflight fitness produced smaller strength decrements during flight than during Skylab II. On longer (110 to 237 d) and short (7 d) Russian missions, isokinetic concentric strength declined up to 28%.[46] The 7-day Salyut-6 mission caused significant decrements in torque/velocity relationships in the gastrocnemius/soleus, anterior tibialis, and ankle extensor musculature. On the longer 110- to 237-day missions, cosmonauts' average triceps strength loss ranged between 20 and 50%. Significant losses in peak torque also occurred for isokinetic measures of ankle flexion and extension at all measured angular velocities of movement (Fig. 27.15). Current studies of cosmonauts are investigating the utility of functional electrostimulation (FES) to minimize atrophy, morphologic changes, and neuromuscular coordination patterns of skeletal muscles during prolonged space missions.[81] FES trains lower-extremity muscle groups using 1-second tetanic muscle actions followed by 2 seconds of relaxation continuously at 20 to 30% of maximum tetanic muscle force for up to 6 hours daily.

EXTENDED-DURATION ORBITER MEDICAL PROJECT. Table 27.13 displays changes between 17 astronauts' preflight and landing (postflight) concentric and eccentric abdominal strength, ec-

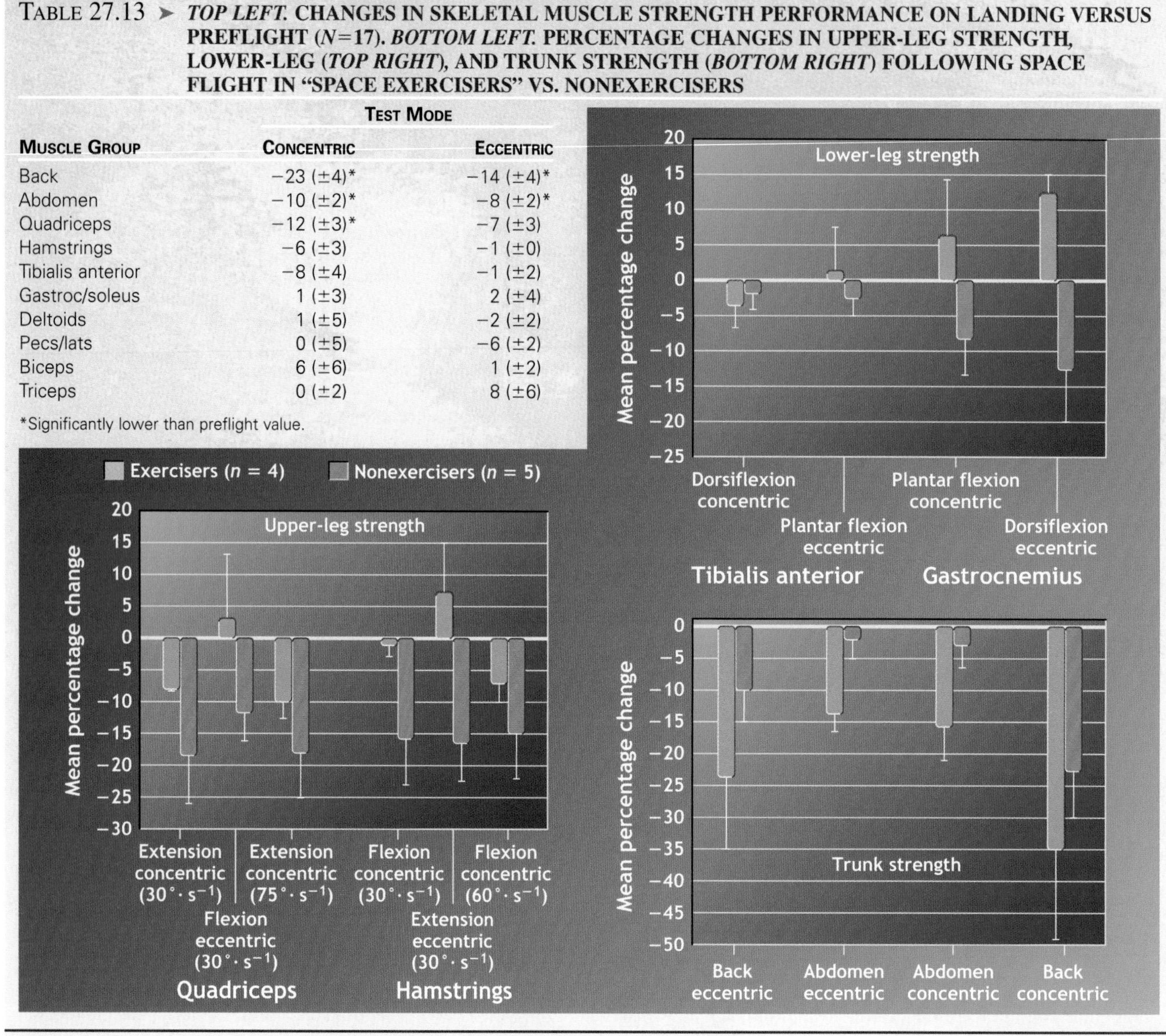

TABLE 27.13 ➤ *TOP LEFT.* CHANGES IN SKELETAL MUSCLE STRENGTH PERFORMANCE ON LANDING VERSUS PREFLIGHT ($N = 17$). *BOTTOM LEFT.* PERCENTAGE CHANGES IN UPPER-LEG STRENGTH, LOWER-LEG (*TOP RIGHT*), AND TRUNK STRENGTH (*BOTTOM RIGHT*) FOLLOWING SPACE FLIGHT IN "SPACE EXERCISERS" VS. NONEXERCISERS

	Test Mode	
Muscle Group	**Concentric**	**Eccentric**
Back	−23 (±4)*	−14 (±4)*
Abdomen	−10 (±2)*	−8 (±2)*
Quadriceps	−12 (±3)*	−7 (±3)
Hamstrings	−6 (±3)	−1 (±0)
Tibialis anterior	−8 (±4)	−1 (±2)
Gastroc/soleus	1 (±3)	2 (±4)
Deltoids	1 (±5)	−2 (±2)
Pecs/lats	0 (±5)	−6 (±2)
Biceps	6 (±6)	1 (±2)
Triceps	0 (±2)	8 (±6)

*Significantly lower than preflight value.

Data from Extended Duration Orbiter Medical Project. 1989–1995. Final report NASA/SP-1999-534. NASA. Lyndon B. Johnson Space Center. Houston, TX, 1999.

centric strength of the quadriceps/soleus, and concentric quadriceps strength assessed at $30° \cdot s^{-1}$. Note that for each muscle group tested, greater strength loss occurred in concentric than in eccentric modes, with the greatest losses in the back (−23%) and quadriceps (−12%) muscles within 5 hours after landing. The three *inset figures* display the percentage strength changes in upper- and lower-leg and trunk flexor muscles. The unique aspect of these data compares space "exercisers" with "nonexercisers." The exercisers trained by running on the treadmill (see page 721) at intensities from 60 to 85% of preflight $\dot{V}O_{2peak}$ estimated from heart rate. Interestingly, testing conducted 7 days postflight revealed that onboard treadmill exercise did *not* ameliorate strength loss in all muscle groups. Preservation of muscle integrity even after only 9 to 11 days of space flight may be limited to those muscles exercised—in accord with the principle of specificity of exercise training.

Muscle Ultrastructural Changes

Permanent neuromuscular dysfunction has not yet been demonstrated during prolonged space missions. Nevertheless, in-flight and postflight changes during missions of nearly 1 year reveal altered muscular coordination patterns, some delayed-onset muscle soreness (DOMS), and generalized muscular fatigue and weakness. Many unanswered questions remain about human muscle physiology and biochemistry adaptations related to microgravity exposure in humans.

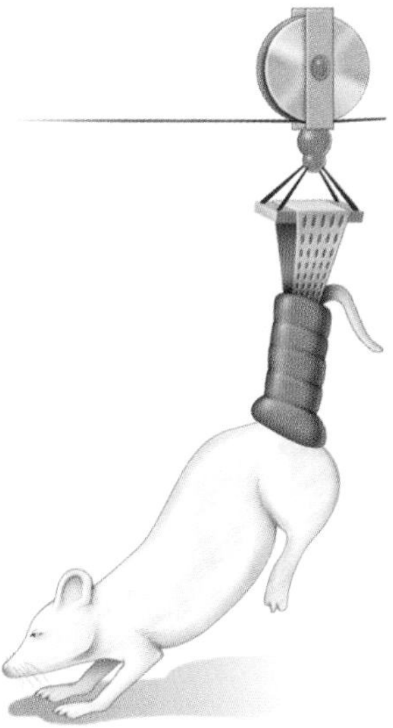

Hind limb suspension (unloading)

Animal models using head-down, tail-suspended, non–weight-bearing rodents (see above illustration) rely on reduced gravity's effects on skeletal muscle-contractile morphology and physiology. Placing rodents in a harness that elevates the hindquarters eliminates the normal loading of the weight-bearing hindlimb muscles. The model mimics the fluid shifts of microgravity; it produces reduced sensory input to the motor centers and less mechanical stimulation of connective, muscular, and osseous tissues. Specifically, both spaceflight and non–weight-bearing confinement atrophies rat skeletal muscles, mainly the slow twitch (type 1) leg-extensor fibers.[3,5,31,57,97,99] Also, non–weight bearing in microgravity reduces contractile activity (assessed by EMG) of male rat hindlimb soleus muscle by 75%.[21,34]

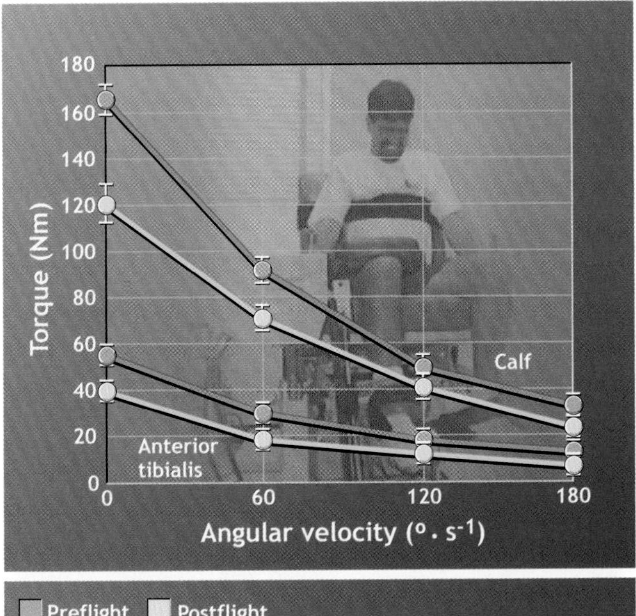

FIGURE 27.15 • Force–velocity relationship of ankle flexors (anterior tibialis) and extensor calf muscles measured by isokinetic dynamometry at four angular velocities in six cosmonauts before and after 110 to 237 days in microgravity on Salyut-7. (Data summarized from Convertino VA. Effects of microgravity on exercise performance. In: Garrett WE, Kirkendall DT, eds. Exercise and sport science. Philadelphia: Lippincott Williams & Wilkins, 2000.)

Maximal Explosive Leg Power Before and After Space Missions

Figure 27.16 shows different duration space flight effects on maximal explosive power (MEP) and maximal cycling power (MCP) assessed preflight and 26 days postflight for astronauts exposed to microgravity for up to 180 days. The *inset illustration at the bottom left* shows the ergometer–dynamometer to assess MEP. Subjects made six maximal pushes with both feet against the force platform for approximately 250 milliseconds at a knee angle of 110° with a 2-minute rest between pushes. MCP involved five to seven "all-out" pedal revolutions for 5 to 6 seconds on a bicycle ergometer following either 5 to 7 minutes of mild aerobic exercise or free-wheel pedaling. The *top figure* shows the percentage of premission scores for MEP and MCP for four astronauts at four periods after mission completion. Astronaut 1, who spent 31 days in orbit, recovered nearly all MEP by 11 days postflight. For the other three astronauts, whose missions lasted 169 to 180 days, MEP recovery approached only 77% of the preflight value. For the two astronauts tested 26 days postflight, MEP for astronaut 3 was 80% of his premission score, while astronaut 4 achieved only 57%. In contrast, each astronaut's MCP, a measure of more-sustained power output, recovered more rapidly throughout the postflight measurement period, with final scores within 10% of premission values.

The *bottom figure (right)* compares all values for MCP plotted relative to corresponding MEP scores, expressed as a percentage of premission values. On average, MCP deterioration exceeded loss of MEP. The researchers attributed the differential deterioration in the two forms of maximal exercise to muscular and neurologic factors involved in each form of effort. In essence, the absence of gravity appears to rearrange postural muscle tone and locomotor coordination substantially. More than likely, this adversely affects the motor control system, and in one astronaut it negatively affected the normal motor unit recruitment pattern. Changes in neural drive during long-term missions (90 to 180 d) could impact the contractile and elastic characteristics of lower limb musculature.[61]

NASA's Research Recommendations Concerning Muscle Structure and Function

NASA has provided a series of recommendations for research in muscle physiology with prolonged microgravity exposure.[106]

1. Determine cellular and molecular mechanisms of muscle fatigue, impaired neuromuscular coordination, and delayed-onset muscle soreness (DOMS). Evaluate whether these deficits relate to muscle fiber atrophy and increased susceptibility to damage and compromised microcirculation.
2. Use human bed rest and animal non–weight-bearing experiments to determine how musculoskeletal weight-bearing and non–weight-bearing transduces into molecular signals that regulate muscle mass and protein isoform expression.
3. Use neonatal rodents as the research model to study myogenesis (muscle cell growth), fiber-type

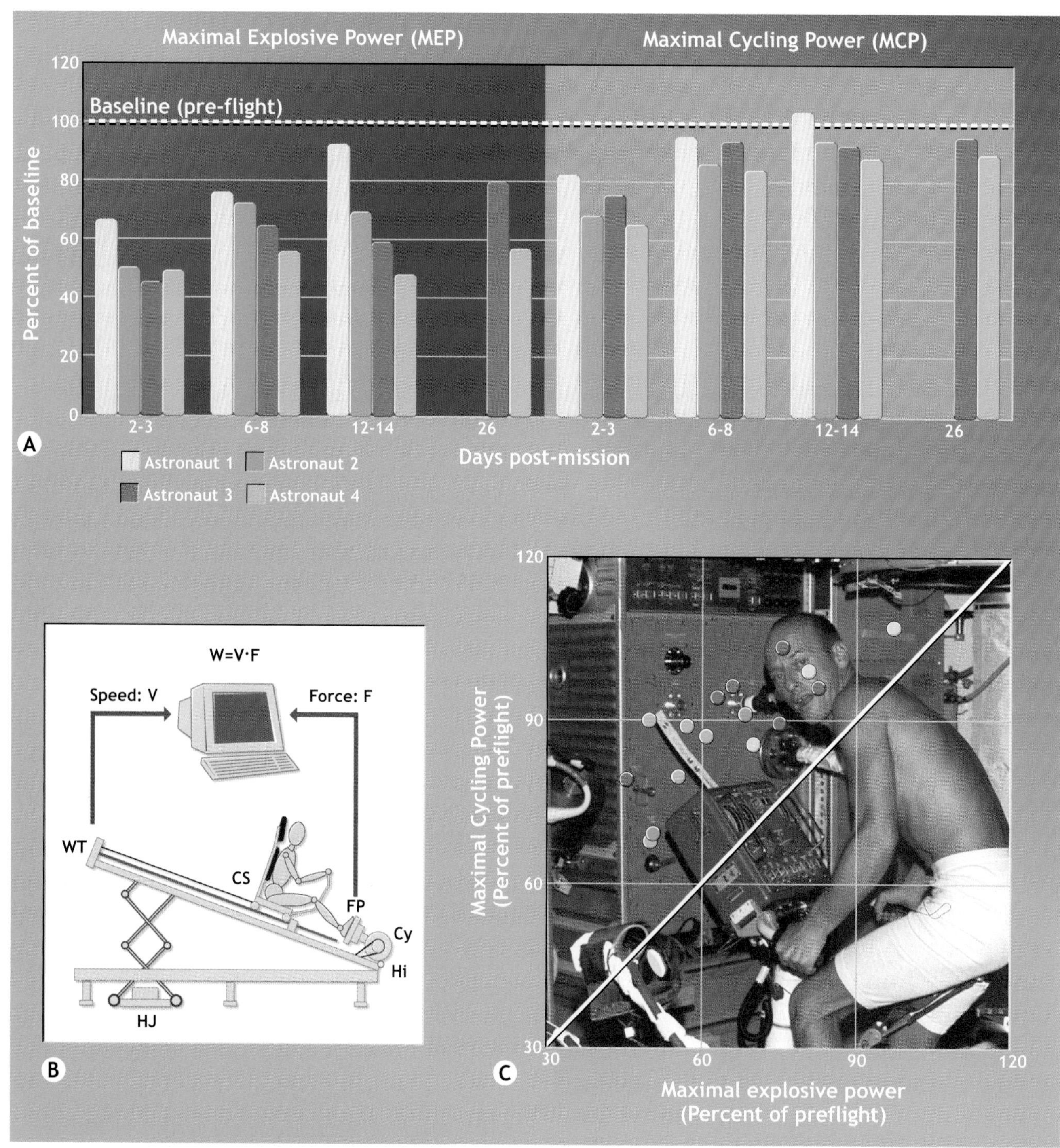

FIGURE 27.16 • **A**. Effects of up to 180 days in microgravity on changes in maximal explosive power (MEP) and maximal cycling power (MCP). **B**. The ergometer–dynamometer assessed MEP of the lower limbs by varying either force or velocity. HJ, hydraulic jack; WT, wire tachometer; CS, carriage seat; FP, force platform; Cy, isokinetic cycle ergometer; Hi, hinge. MEP was assessed within less than 0.3 s, and MCP determined during all-out pedaling on a cycle ergometer for 5 to 6 s. **C**. Plot of MCP versus MEP scores expressed as a percentage of premission values. (Data modified from Antonutto G, et al. Effects of microgravity on maximal power of lower limbs during very short efforts in humans. J Appl Physiol 1999;86:85.)

differentiation, and muscular and spinal development. Emphasize mechanisms related to how muscle cells sense working length and gravity's mechanical stress.

4. Investigate key receptor functions of proteins, including growth and hormone factors, to probe the neuromuscular system's basic adaptation mechanisms to microgravity.

COUNTERMEASURE STRATEGIES

Countermeasures *systematically attempt to neutralize (or minimize) space flight's potentially harmful deconditioning effects on crew physiologic function, performance, and overall health during mission-critical maneuvers, particularly re-entry and landing.* In the absence of gravity, no linear, downward head-to-foot acceleration forces (referred to as +Gz) act on the body. This makes normal biologic functions more susceptible to short- and longer-term maladaptations such as **space motion sickness (SMS)**, a syndrome characterized by headache and dizziness, drowsiness, malaise, poor concentration, disorientation, nausea, pallor, and sudden vomiting without dry heaves. Some symptoms resemble those of terrestrial motion sickness. SMS symptoms often dissipate on their own or with medication during the first few days of space flight. On re-entry after short-duration missions, SMS can manifest as a **general re-entry syndrome (GRS)** imposing potentially deleterious effects on astronaut performance. GRS symptoms include vertigo, nausea, instability, and fatigue induced by reimposition of increased +Gz during re-entry and landing. In contrast to the relatively acute emergence of SMS, weeks and months of prolonged absence of normal gravitational loading adversely affect bone and muscular structure and function. Concurrently, fluid shifts within the vascular system produce significant loss of electrolytes and bone minerals. Cumulative negative effects during sustained missions could trigger more-severe medical complications such as increased risk of developing renal stones, orthostatic intolerance, neurosensory and motor dysfunctions, and musculoskeletal injuries (including bone fracture) in the weeks and months following return to Earth.

Without an appropriate countermeasures program, microgravity's deleterious effects mimic adverse changes with prolonged bed rest. For example, 30 days of bed rest dramatically impairs skeletal muscle function; knee extensor strength declines nearly 23%, while knee flexor strength and leg volume decrease 10 to 12%. Limb volume reductions result from decreased muscular cross-sectional area due to fiber-protein loss. The 28-day Skylab 2 mission decreased muscular function and leg volume to an extent comparable to that with bed rest (see unnumbered illustration below of method used to assess changes in leg volume).[21] The protein loss has been attributed in part to a normal adaptive response to decreased workload on weight-bearing muscles.[107] Decrements in cardiovascular function generally parallel losses in muscle strength and size.[117,118]

Projected travel time for an exploration-class mission to Mars requires approximately 6 months of isolation in microgravity, more than a year of planetary habitation at 0.38g, followed by a 6-month return trip (in microgravity) to Earth. Thus,

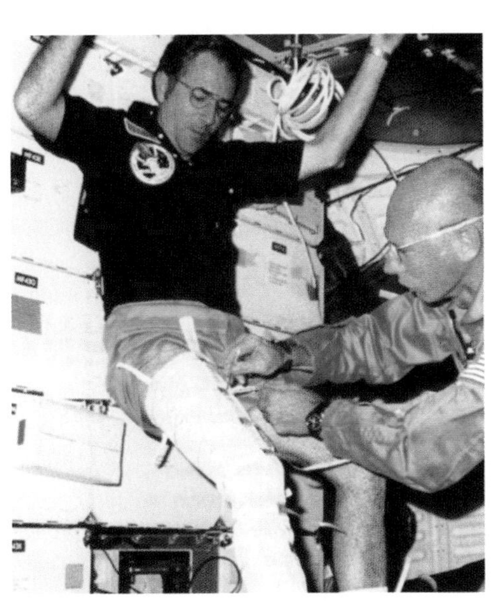

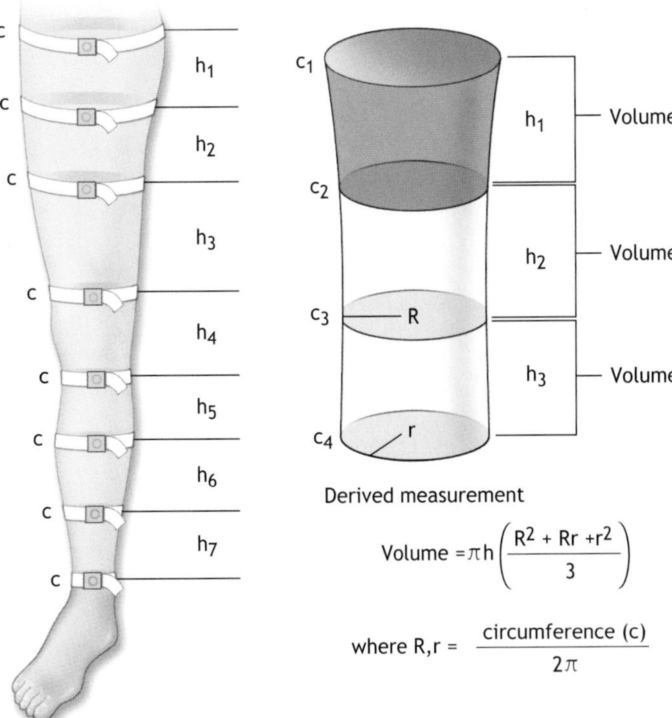

The leg volume measuring system assesses changes in leg segmental volume from fluid shifts in the lower body during short and longer duration missions. Determining the truncated cone, segmental volume (e.g., h_1) requires two circumferences (c_1 and c_2) and the distance between them.

TABLE 27.14 ➤ ADVERSE EFFECTS OF SPACE FLIGHT AND PROPOSED COUNTERMEASURES

Area	Major Findings	Clinical/Operational Consequences	Countermeasures under Evaluation
Cardiovascular	Fluid loss Electrolyte changes Electrical activity disturbances Neuroreflex readjustments	Orthostatic intolerance	Fluid/electrolyte replenishment Exercise
Neurovestibular	Motion sickness Gait disturbances Motor performance degradation	Decreased productivity	Palliative treatments (intramuscular promethazine) Adaptation trainers
Musculoskeletal	Bone mass loss Muscle mass loss	Renal stone formation Muscle/joint injuries Bone fractures	Diet Exercise, lower-body negative pressure Drugs (biphosphonates, etc.)
Immunologic, endocrinologic	Changes in immune response *in vitro* Inappropriate hormonal secretion or metabolism	Susceptibility to infection (?) Synergistic radiation effects Allergic reactions and disorders	Growth factors (?)

Note: Third column lists factors (renal stone formation, muscle/joint injuries, bone fractures) undocumented in NASA reports.
From Nicogossian AE, et al. Countermeasures to space deconditioning. In: Nicogossian AE, et al., eds. Space physiology and medicine. 3rd ed. Philadelphia: Lea & Febiger. 1994: 447.

on-board countermeasures play a critical role in minimizing pathology or impaired motor task performance to preserve crew health and safety. More than likely, gender-related factors affect these health and performance goals.[39] In-flight resistance and endurance exercises show the greatest overall potential as exercise countermeasures to combat deleterious effects of sustained microgravity. Table 27.14 lists examples of adverse effects and clinical consequences of prolonged microgravity exposure in four functional body areas and the possible countermeasure strategies.

In-Flight Exercise

Four exercise modes have played predominant roles during in-flight workouts aboard space missions: (1) treadmill walking and running, (2) cycle ergometry, including maximal exerecise performed 24 h before landing,[84] (3) leg rowing, and (4) upper- and lower-body multijoint dynamic resistance exercise. Figure 27.17 shows different exercise modes during KC-135 flights and space missions. At the end of this section, we discuss the latest exercise mode—the human-powered centrifuge.

Lunar–Mars Life Support Test Experiment

NASA conducts research to examine the efficacy of exercise testing and prescription protocols for onboard countermeasures on future space flights. The experiments provide insights into potentially useful training methodologies for application to space missions, particularly targeted resistance exercise for lower-extremity muscles, those most likely to suffer impairment. The 60-day trial studied men and women before, during, and after a 60-day confined-chamber experiment at 1g in the Life Support Systems Integration Unit, a component scheduled for a future ISS mission. A combined exercise countermeasure protocol quantified the following:

- Training effects from exercise countermeasures
- Subjects' tolerance to combined aerobic and resistance training countermeasures
- Methods to quantify the performance of exercise countermeasures for valid monitoring of exercise compliance

Measurements included:

1. $\dot{V}O_{2peak}$. Subjects pedaled an electronically braked cycle ergometer in the upright position at 75 rpm at increasing workloads of 50, 100, and 150 W for men and 50, 75, and 100 W for women. Exercise then continued in 25-W increments to volitional termination.
2. *Submaximal and maximal sustained aerobic exercise.* Subjects cycled for three 5-minute periods at 75 rpm at exercise intensities representing 25, 50, 75, and 100% of $\dot{V}O_{2peak}$.
3. *Resistance exercise.* Subjects performed maximal-effort bench press, seated shoulder press, latissimus dorsi pull, squat, and heel raise on a multifunction exercise station preprogrammed for fast- and slow-speed movement velocities.

In the chamber, subjects exercised 6 days per week, alternating between preprogrammed 32-minute cycle ergometer aerobic workouts at 40 to 80% of $\dot{V}O_{2peak}$ and the five resistance exercises used in the pretest assessment. They performed three sets of 6- to 12-RM of each exercise beginning with a warm-up at 50% 1-RM. Movement speed varied from $10° \cdot s^{-1}$ at the slow speed to $20° \cdot s^{-1}$ at the fastest speed. Submaximal ergometer tests were administered on days 15, 30, and 58 in lieu of the aerobic workout. Subject compliance with the exercise program averaged 91%.

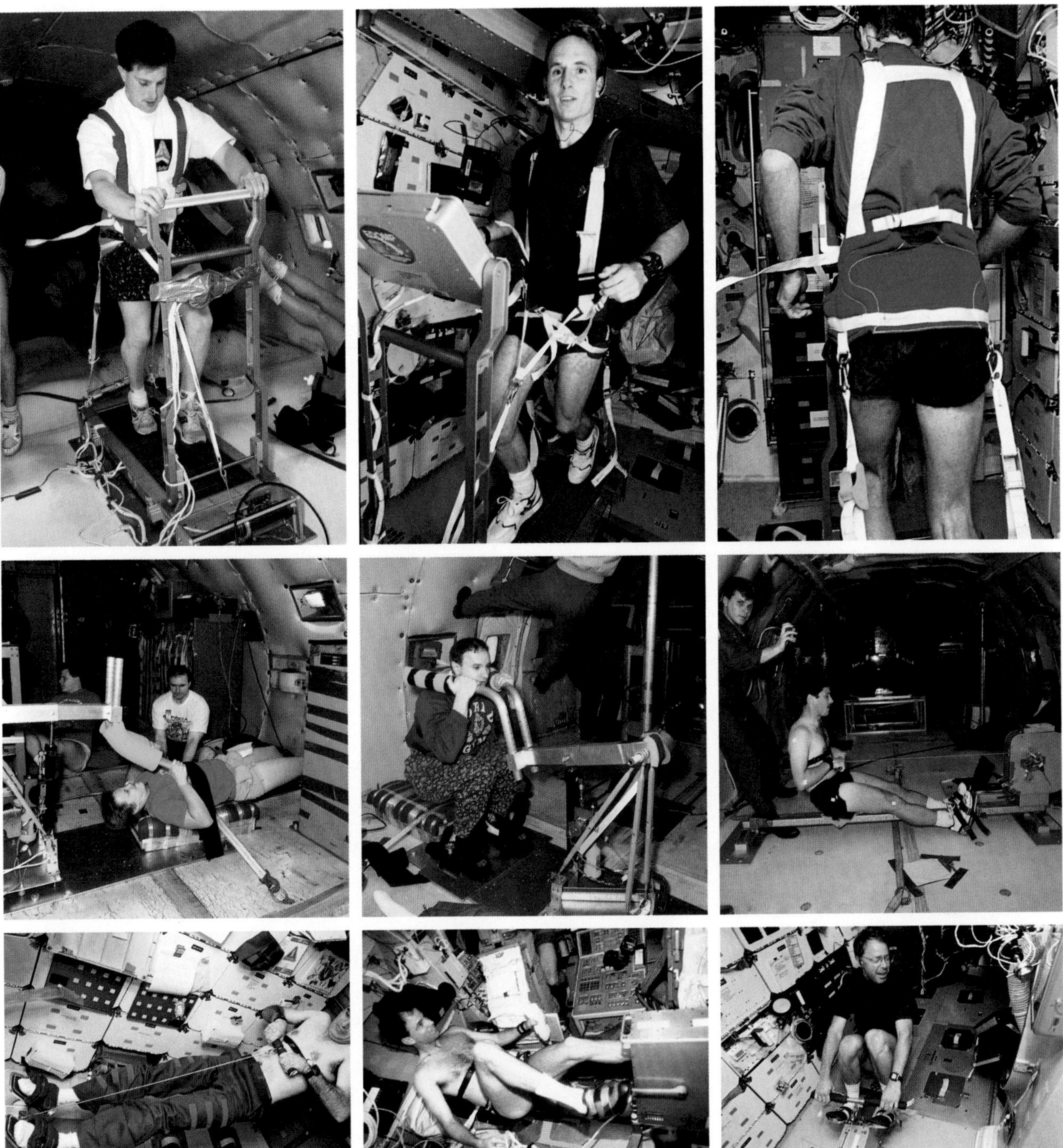

FIGURE 27.17 • Examples of exercise training and measurement using different exercise modes during microgravity conditions. *Top*. Tethered treadmill exercise during KC-135 training (*left*) and space shuttle mission (*middle and right*). Note the strap arrangement around the upper body and straps anchored to the hips to keep the astronaut tethered to the treadmill. *Middle*. KC-135 training for upper-arm bench press exercise (*left*), squat exercise (*middle*), and upper-arm rowing exercise (*right*). *Bottom*. Exercise training aboard different space shuttle missions showing upper-arm, cycling, and rowing modes. (Photos courtesy of NASA, Lyndon B. Johnson Space Center, Houston, TX.)

Figure 27.18 shows peak torque developed at low, medium, and high movement speeds with resistance exercises during training weeks 2, 5, and 8. Within-subject evaluation revealed that all subjects improved in "strength" measures (peak torque, average peak torque, total work) at each speed over the 8-week period. The pre- to postchamber exercise oxygen consumptions shown in the *top left panel* of Figure 27.19 reveal that average $\dot{V}O_{2peak}$ increased 7% during chamber confinement, ranging between 1 and 20%, with the initially high-fit subjects improving the least. Peak posttraining workload also increased (13%), as did exercise duration (7%). Submaximal exercise heart rate (*bottom left panel*) declined 6% during the last test session ("submax 3") compared with pretraining values. Ratings of perceived exertion and systolic

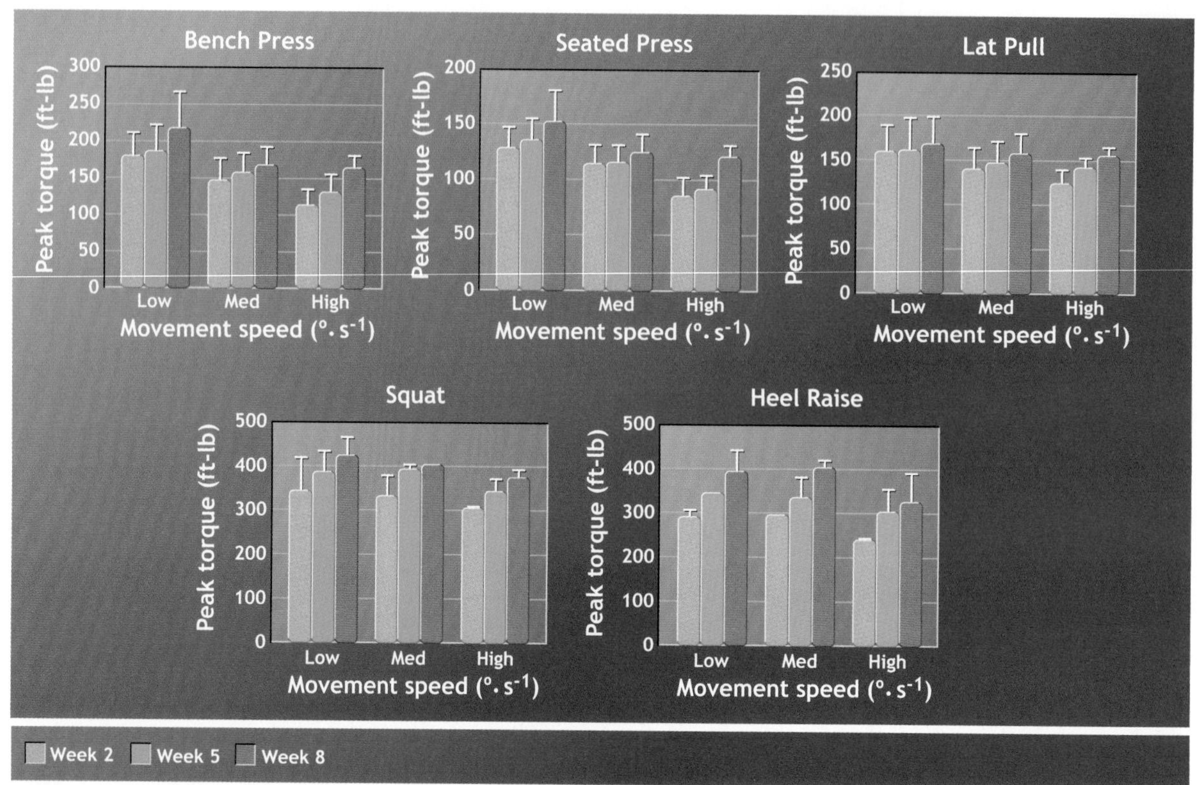

FIGURE 27.18 • Peak torque developed at low, medium, and high movement training speeds during bench press, seated press, lat pull, squat, and heel raise during weeks 2, 5, and 8. (Adapted from Lee SL, et al. Exercise Countermeasures Demonstration Project during the Lunar-Mars Life Support Test Project. Phase IIA. NASA. NASA/TP-98-206537. Lyndon B. Johnson Space Center, Houston, TX. 1998.)

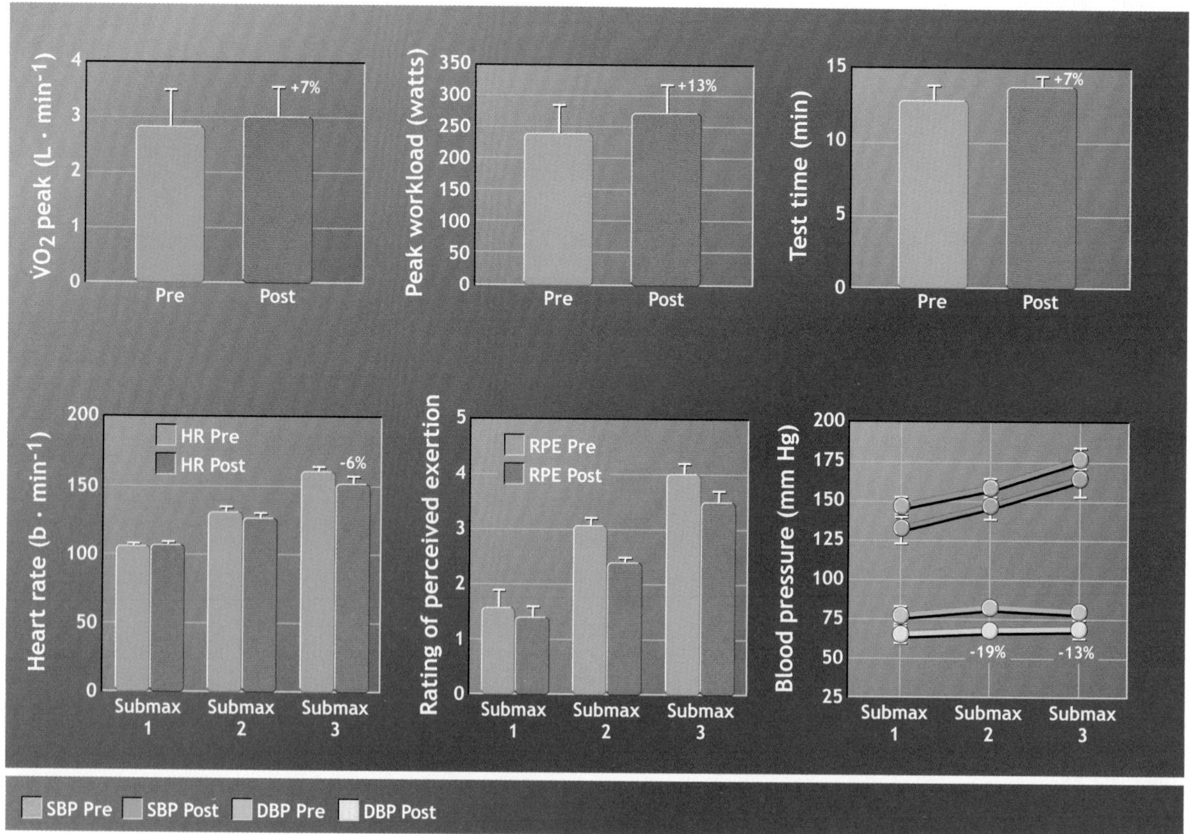

FIGURE 27.19 • The 60-day lunar-Mars countermeasures experiment. *Top.* Comparison of pre- versus post-$\dot{V}O_{2peak}$, peak workload, and test duration on the bicycle ergometer. *Bottom.* Heart rate, rating of perceived exertion (RPE), and blood pressure during three submaximal test sessions. (Adapted from Lee SL, et al. Exercise Countermeasures Demonstration Project during the Lunar-Mars Life Support Test Project. Phase IIA. NASA. NASA/TP-98-206537. Lyndon B. Johnson Space Center, Houston, TX. 1998.)

blood pressure during the three training sessions did not change. In contrast, diastolic blood pressure declined significantly by 19% after 30 days ("submax 2") and 13% at 58 days ("submax 3").

Countermeasures on Long-Duration Missions

The prolonged Russian Mir missions made extensive use of exercise countermeasures based on considerable prior experience with extended space missions. Like their American counterparts, cosmonauts did not exercise during the flight's first 48 to 72 hours to provide sufficient recovery from SMS that affects nearly 70% of astronauts and cosmonauts on their first flight. The Soviet cosmonaut Titov deserves credit as the first person to experience SMS—refractory dizziness when making head movements and subsequent nausea and illness after 6 hours during the 1961 Vostok-2 mission.[43] On current space shuttle missions, an intramuscular injection of Phenergan relieves SMS, replacing Dexedrine and other drug combinations that evoke strong negative central nervous system responses.

Toward the end of the flight's first week and over the next 24 days, cosmonauts exercise twice daily, progressing to 1 hour of continuous ergometer cycling at an initial workload of 900 kg-m · min^{-1}. Exercise intensity progressively increases to maintain heart rate between 80 to 90% of age-predicted maximum. They add 5 to 15 minutes of daily strengthening exercise (hamstrings, trunk extensors) using bungee-cord devices. On missions exceeding 1 month, cosmonauts exercise twice daily for 1 hour on a passive (subject-driven) treadmill with a restraint system similar to that used by space shuttle astronauts (see schematic on right of U.S. space shuttle passive treadmill in which a rapid-onset centrifugal brake provides seven braking levels to control drag forces on the running track). To simulate gravitational forces, straps from their side—called subject load devices—secure the cosmonaut to the treadmill. Treadmill exercise, using a harness and bungee tether system, generates the effects of 0.5 to 0.7g, while exercise on Salyut and Mir treadmills generated a "gravitational" pull of 0.62g. The nonmotorized treadmill requires running at a positive percentage grade to overcome frictional resistance. At present, the treadmill provides the only mode of on-board exercise. Astronauts wear a monitor (ear oximeter) secured to the ear to record heart rate continuously by an infrared sensor that detects pulsating blood flow in the earlobe. A mechanical sensor wire on the side of the treadmill displays distance run from number of treadmill revolutions completed.

Figure 27.20 compares heart rate response during continuous *(top)* and intermittent *(bottom)* treadmill exercise during two shuttle missions. Astronauts did not attain assigned target heart rates (representing 60, 70, or 80% $\dot{V}O_{2max}$) when exercising continuously for 30 minutes during an 11-day mission. More than likely, altered running mechanics while wearing the bungee apparatus affected ability to attain target heart rates.

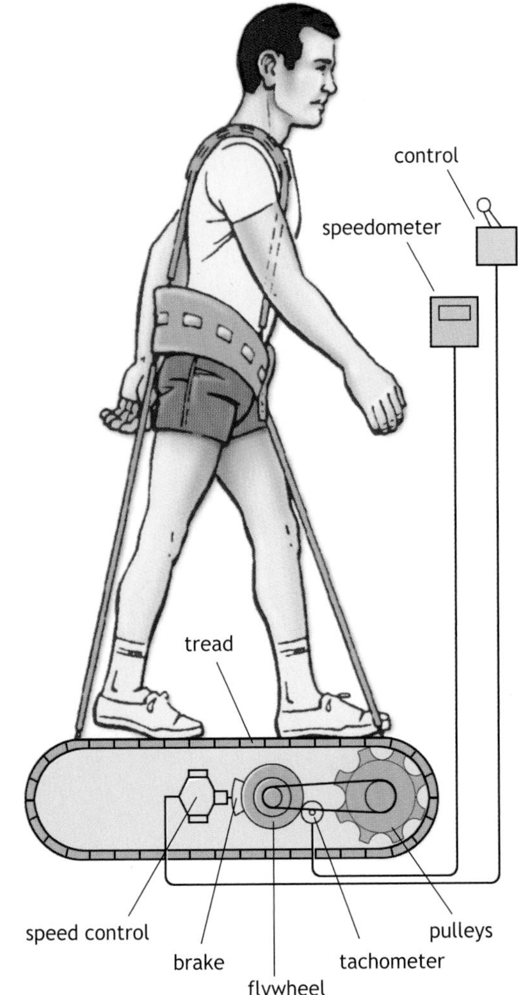

Schematic details of subject-driven U.S. Space Shuttle treadmill.

INTEGRATIVE QUESTION

What type of exercise training program would you advise an astronaut to undertake (1) 6 months prior to a Mars mission and (2) during the mission?

New Approach: Human-Powered Centrifuges Simulate Gravitational Loading

NASA currently supports new countermeasures that use unique exercise devices to combat the deleterious effects of space flight deconditioning.

SELF-POWERED HUMAN CENTRIFUGE. Because force and acceleration represent two distinct entities ($F = m \times a$), simply applying force to an object (e.g., bungee cord or lower-body negative-pressure device) in microgravity does not mean that it regulates a beneficial "loading" of the skeleton similar to that with exercise on Earth. An animal or human placed in a rotating centrifuge does experience the force benefits produced by a sustained-acceleration "gravity" field. In this regard, a self-powered human centrifuge, dis-

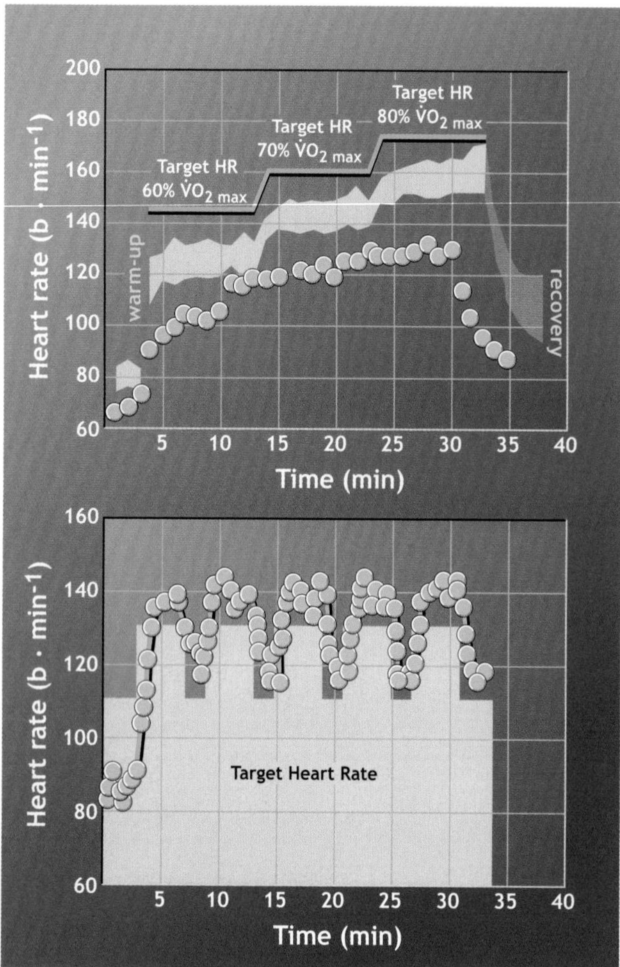

FIGURE 27.20 • *Top.* Heart rate during continuous treadmill exercise at 60, 70, and 80% of $\dot{V}O_{2max}$ on an 11-day shuttle mission. The *light green shaded area* shows the exercise heart rate range during workout days 3 to 11. *Green circles* represent heart rate during a familiarization run on flight day 2. The intense workouts helped to minimize orthostatic dysfunction upon landing. *Bottom.* Heart rate during five intervals of a treadmill exercise routine using the shuttle treadmill. (Adapted from Lee SL, et al. Exercise Countermeasures Demonstration Project during the Lunar-Mars Life Support Test Project. Phase IIA. NASA. NASA/TP-98-206537. Lyndon B. Johnson Space Center, Houston, TX. 1998.)

played schematically in Figure 27.21, offers promise for counteracting adverse physiologic effects of extended-duration space missions.[58]

Pedaling the **Space Cycle™** propels the centrifuge in a curvilinear motion about a fixed central shaft rigidly fixed within the spacecraft. A centrifuge effect produces artificial gravity as the rider rotates about the shaft while pedaling. Irregularly shaped cams fixed to the foot crankshaft allow an adjustable spring-loaded device to trace a path around the cam and provide resistance to pedaling. Altering cam configuration generates foot force profiles to simulate walking, jogging, and cycling. Combining artificial gravity with impact-loading exercise offers the potential for an effective countermeasures strategy against orthostatic intolerance, macro- and microscopic skeletal muscle deterioration, and loss of bone mass.

The Space Cycle™, designed for the ISS, would simulate gravitational acceleration (+Gz) experienced while standing on Earth and provide axial loading on the rider's long bones. The added "stress" in microgravity should also provide similar 1g stress on the musculoskeletal system. Thus, missions lasting a year or more should benefit from artificially induced gravity produced by human powered, in-flight centrifugation.

In addition to the Space Cycle™, NASA's Ames Research Center has developed its own self-powered human centrifuge to evaluate the countermeasure potential of this exercise mode with and without the effect of +Gz acceleration (Fig. 27.22).[45] The **Ames centrifuge** consists of a short-arm, dual-couch device powered by a chain-linked cycle foot drive. Approximately two pedal revolutions produce a 360° rotation of the centrifuge, which could generate a maximum of 5g. Research with this device required subjects to perform exercise under two conditions: (1) pedaling the centrifuge for 2 minutes at 25, 50, and 75% of maximum cycling rpm, defined as all-out until volitional fatigue and (2) exercising at the same

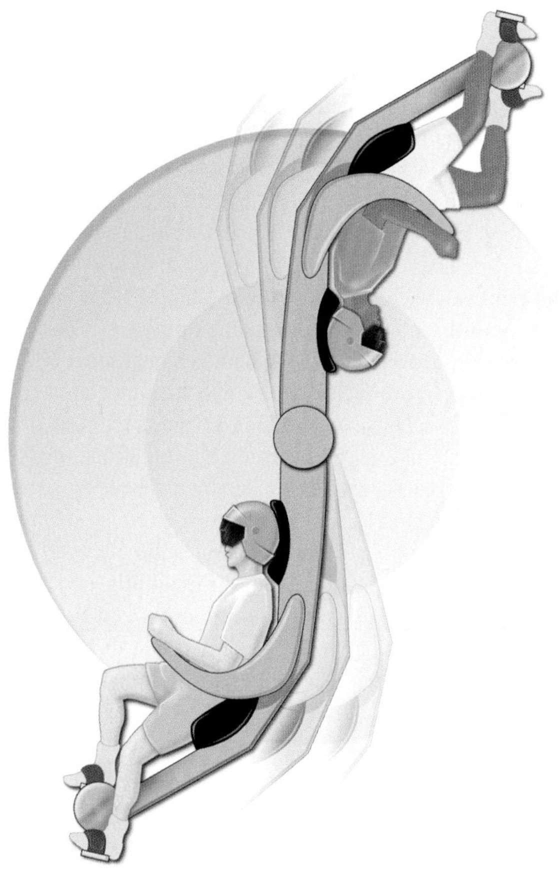

FIGURE 27.21 • Pedaling the self-powered human centrifuge (Space Cycle™) creates artificial gravity by producing head-to-foot acceleration (+Gz). Added instrumentation can monitor extremity strength, power output, body mass, and other parameters for on-going functional and medical research. Restricting head movements by wearing a harness attached to the frame combined with virtual reality headgear to maintain a horizontal visual experience could minimize sensory input conflict during cycling, dramatically reducing space motion sickness. (From Kreitenberg A, et al. The "Space Cycle"™ self powered human centrifuge: a proposed countermeasure for prolonged human space flight. Aviat Space Environ Med. 1998;69:66.

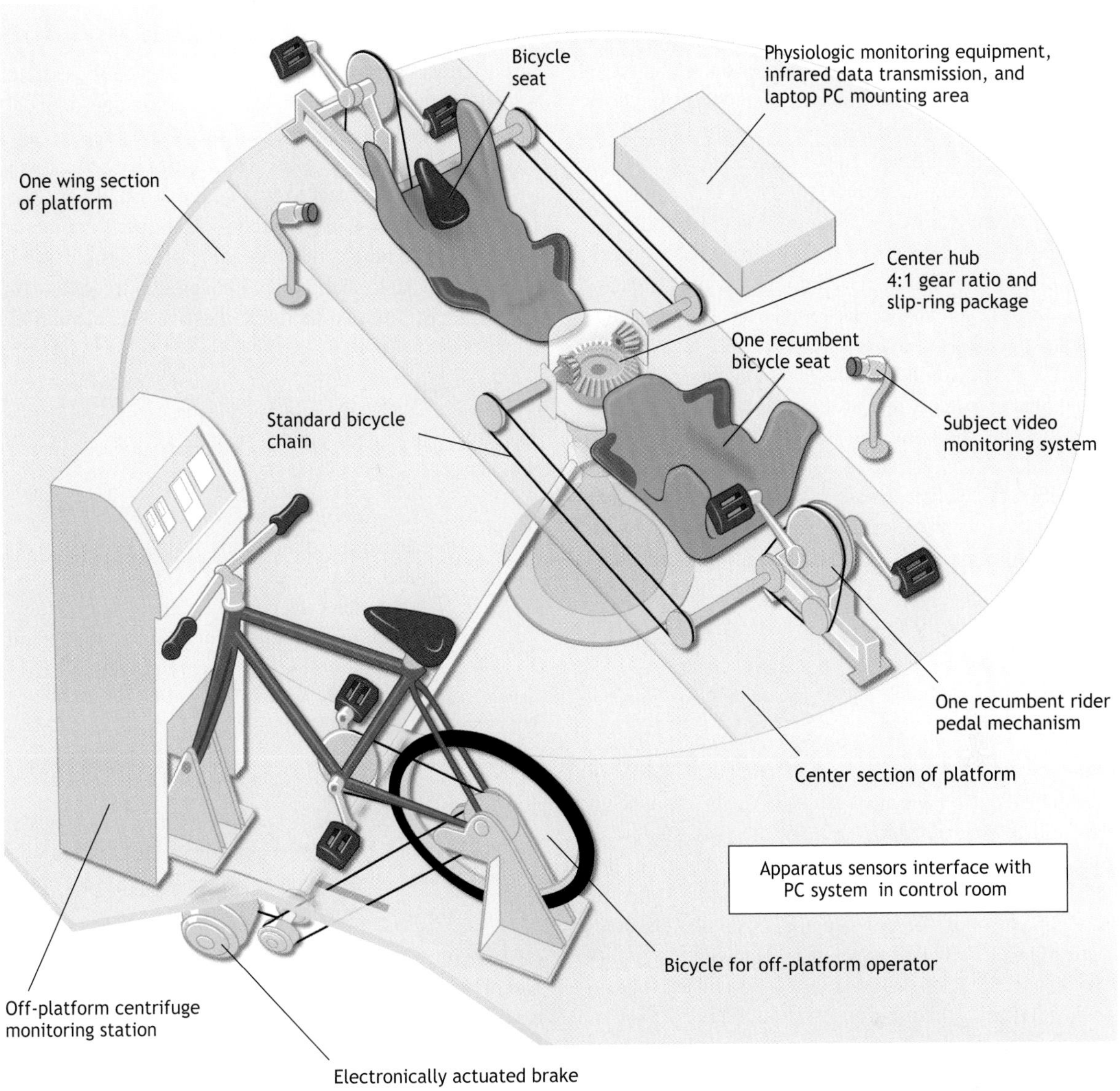

Bicycle seat
Physiologic monitoring equipment, infrared data transmission, and laptop PC mounting area
One wing section of platform
Center hub 4:1 gear ratio and slip-ring package
One recumbent bicycle seat
Standard bicycle chain
Subject video monitoring system
One recumbent rider pedal mechanism
Center section of platform
Apparatus sensors interface with PC system in control room
Bicycle for off-platform operator
Off-platform centrifuge monitoring station
Electronically actuated brake

Exercise Acceleration
Passive Acceleration
Heart rate (b•min-1)
Time (s)
86
80
34
6
90
41
3
-6
100%
75% max
50% max
25% max

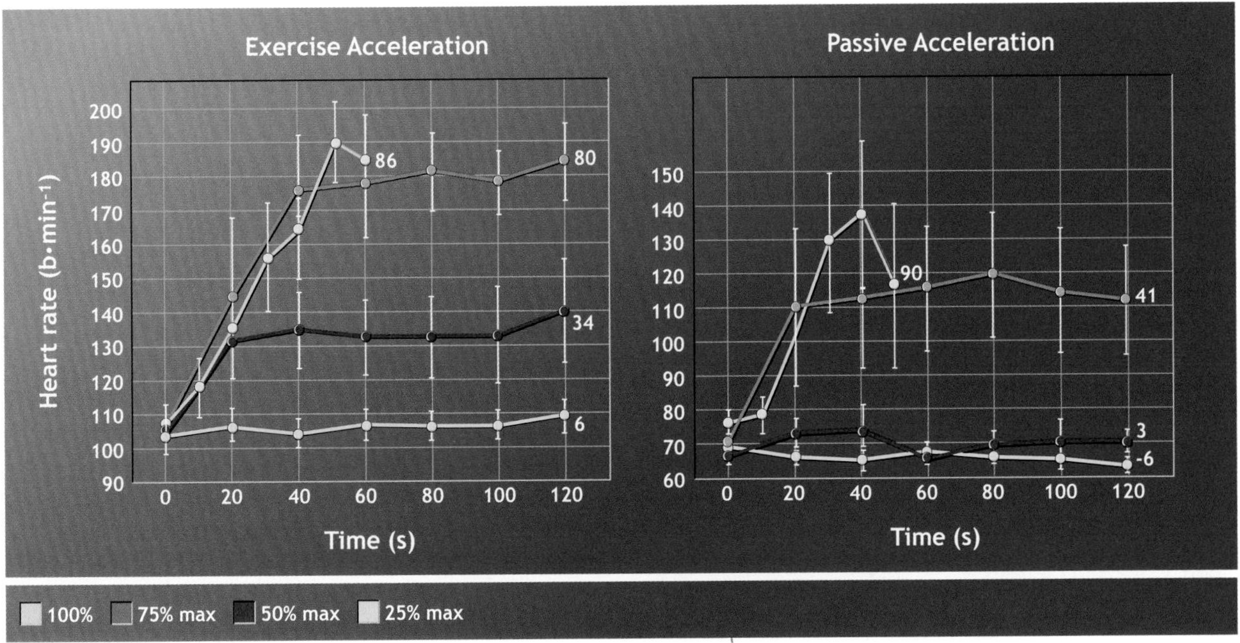

FIGURE 27.22 • *Top*. The Ames centrifuge. *Bottom*. Comparison of the effects of two conditions (exercise acceleration and passive acceleration) on heart rate response at different percentages of maximal acceleration. Numbers at the end of lines represent final HR increase above rest. (Modified from Greenleaf JE, et al. Cycle-powered short radius (1.9 m) centrifuge: effect of exercise versus passive acceleration on heart rate in humans. NASA technical memorandum 110433. 1997. NASA. Ames Research Center. Moffett Field, CA, 1997.)

three intensities without centrifuge acceleration. Changes in heart rate under the two conditions assessed the effects of only exercise and exercise coupled with +Gz acceleration. Subjects remained blindfolded during exercise to prevent nausea or vertigo. They achieved 3.9 Gz (43.7 rpm) for maximal-acceleration exercise, 0.2 Gz at 25% (11.0 rpm), 1.0 Gz at 50% (21.8 rpm), and 2.2 Gz (32.8 rpm) at 75% maximum Gz. The *bottom* of Figure 27.22 compares the effects of the two conditions (exercise acceleration and passive acceleration) on heart rate response at different percentages of maximal acceleration. The numbers at the end of each trial (shown at the *right*) represent heart rate at the end of exercise minus heart rate at the start. Pedaling the Ames centrifuge produced its intended effect—it augmented heart rate response to exercise, especially at 75% maximum Gz. Additional research must quantify how much exercise and artificial gravity exposure (optimal magnitude, frequency, and duration) is most effective during space missions for full adaptation of head, arm, and leg movement equilibrium.[60]

Space Pharmacology

SMS remains the most persistent short-term problem during space flight. Approximately 50% of cosmonauts, 60% of Apollo astronauts, and 71% of first-time shuttle astronauts encountered mild-to-severe SMS. Table 27.15 lists the incidence and severity of SMS during 36 space shuttle flights through 1991. Note the decline in prevalence from 77 episodes to 34 episodes for crew members on their second shuttle flight. On the 1993 Space Shuttle Life Sciences mission (SLS-2), only one astronaut experienced nausea (but no actual sickness) during the mission's first few days.[111]

SMS is not confined to orbital flight; nearly 10% of astronauts experience it during re-entry or immediately upon landing, including training during parabolic flights.[101] Ninety-two percent of cosmonauts report SMS upon return from missions lasting several months or longer.[56] To date, no single pharmacologic treatment prevents or cures SMS. On shuttle missions, the disorder shows no preference for commanders, pilots, or mission specialists, gender or age, career versus noncareer astronauts, or first-time versus repeat flyers. Incomplete understanding of the cause(s) of SMS hampers its treatment, but pharmacologic treatment usually provides most individuals relief within 3 days. Additional countermeasure strategies, including mechanical and electrical stimulation and biofeedback techniques, have attempted to minimize SMS effects, but medication still proves the most effective.

TABLE 27.15 ➤ INCIDENCE AND SEVERITY OF SPACE MOTION SICKNESS DURING 36 SPACE SHUTTLE FLIGHTS

	Number of Crewmembers		
Motion Sickness Rating	First Shuttle Flight	Later Shuttle Flight	Totals
None	32 (29%)	28 (45%)	60 (35%)
Mild	36 (33%)	24 (39%)	60 (35%)
Moderate	29 (27%)	10 (16%)	39 (23%)
Severe	12 (11%)	0 (0%)	12 (7%)
Totals	109 (64%)	62 (36%)	171 (100%)

From Nicogossian AE, et al. Countermeasures to space deconditioning. In: Nicogossian AE, et al. eds. Space physiology and medicine. 3rd ed. Philadelphia: Lea & Febiger, 1994: 230.

Medications

The following medications provide pharmacologic therapy for SMS:

1. *Anticholinergics (parasympatholytics)* blunt parasympathetic nervous system effects. Scopolamine in a dose of 0.6 to 1.0 mg proves most effective to eradicate approximately 90% of symptoms.
2. *Antihistamines* (action antagonistic to histamine) offer some protection but are not as effective as scopolamine.
3. *Sympathomimetics* mimic sympathetic nervous system effects. Amphetamine with scopolamine confers beneficial effects.
4. *Sympatholytics* inhibit sympathetic nervous system effects. Some of these drugs (e.g., trimethobenzamine, chlorpromazine, prochlorperazine) provide only marginal relief.

"**Scope-dex**," a combination of scopolamine (parasympatholytic) and amphetamine (sympathomimetic) exhibits the best overall success in minimizing SMS.

Lower-Body Negative Pressure

Figure 27.23 shows the in-flight **lower-body negative pressure (LBNP) apparatus** aboard Skylab (A, B) and shuttle (C) missions. This device serves two functions:

1. Assesses the status of orthostatic deconditioning during space flight and postlanding.
2. Functions as a countermeasure against adverse orthostatic changes with short- and long-term missions.

The LBNP device applies negative pressure to the lower limbs. This forces fluid in the vascular system to migrate downward from the upper torso to the lower body, thereby redistributing the blood volume in a manner resembling the early in-flight response to microgravity. During three, 6-month MIR missions, cosmonauts wore thigh cuffs (rather than rely on an LBNP device) at 1, 3 to 4, 5 to 5.5 months and used echocardiography to assess cardiovascular parameters (see unnumbered figure on next page). Data were contrasted with control sessions 30 days preflight and 3 and 7 days postflight.[51] In all cosmonauts, a significantly reduced vasoconstrictive response and a less efficient blood flow redistribution toward the brain coincided with ortho-

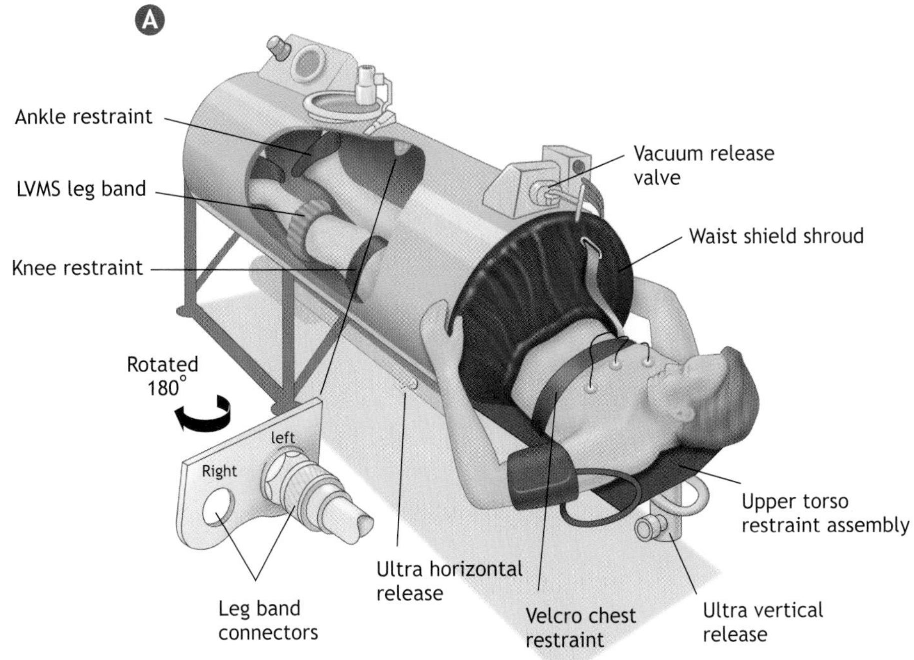

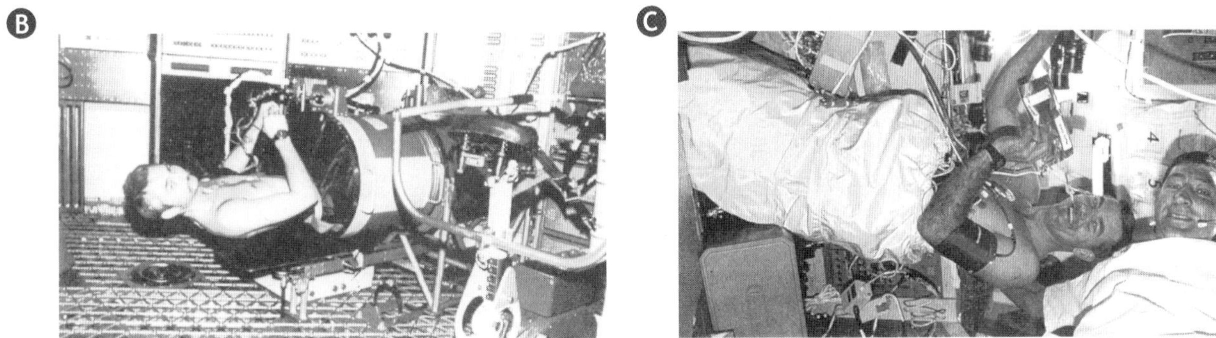

FIGURE 27.23 • **A**. Schematic diagram of the lower-body negative pressure (LBNP) apparatus (used aboard Skylab) illustrating the upper- and lower-body restraint assembly, including the leg volume measuring system (LVMS) leg band. The waist seal shroud maintains controlled and regulated negative pressure from 0 to 50 mm Hg below ambient pressure. During ground tests, a vacuum provides negative pressure; during flight, negative pressure occurs from the space vacuum. **B**. LBNP device beginning with the 28-day Skylab 2 mission (1973). The 20-inch diameter, 48-inch long cylindrical chamber separates longitudinally to provide access to the legs, beginning at the subject's waist at the iliac crests, and ease of securing leg bands to measure change in lower-limb (calf) volume. Lower-leg volume changes on exposure to negative pressure because of caudal displacement of blood and other fluids. **C**. LBNP assessment aboard an early shuttle mission. (From Nicogossian AE, et al., eds. Space physiology and medicine, 3rd ed. Philadelphia: Lea & Febiger, 1994.)

static intolerance during postflight stand tests. In addition, the vascular response to LBNP tests remained depressed during the flights. Thus, the thigh cuffs compensated partially for the cardiovascular changes induced by microgravity but not for microgravity deconditioning. Upregulation of nitric oxide (NO; a potent vasodilator and natriuretic) may explain orthostatic intolerance in microgravity.[126] If this mechanism proves correct, administration of an inducible nitric oxide synthase inhibitor (iNOS) may help to attenuate orthostatic intolerance when astronauts return to Earth following a mission; it also may benefit patients following extended bed rest.

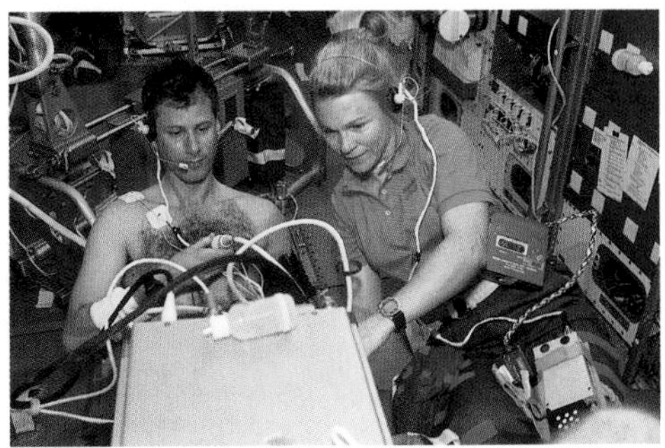

Echocardiography to assess cardiovascular parameters during space flight.

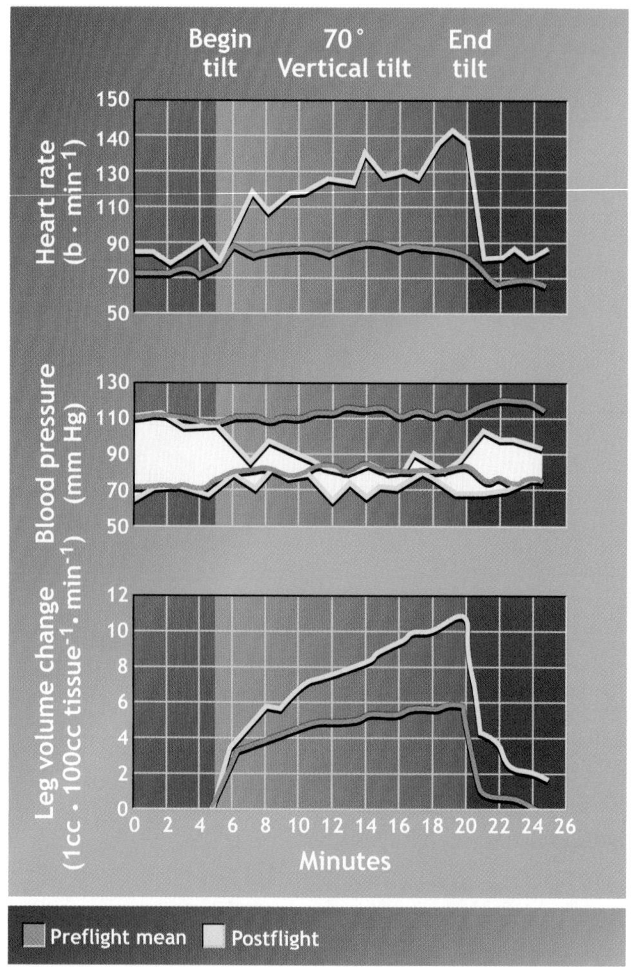

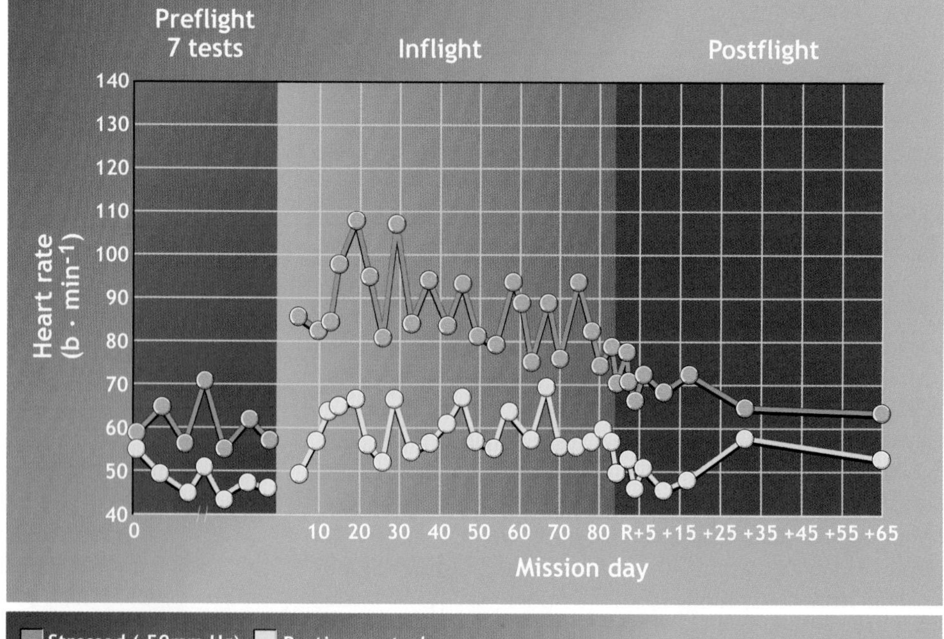

FIGURE 27.24 • LBNP evaluation of cardiovascular dynamics during space missions: *Top.* Gemini 14-day pre–postflight changes in heart rate, blood pressure, and leg volume. *Bottom.* Resting heart rate in a −50 mm Hg LBNP test in one crew member during an 80-day Skylab mission. (From Charles JB, et al. Cardiopulmonary function. In Nicogossian AE, et al., eds. Space physiology and medicine, 3rd ed. Philadelphia: Lea & Febiger, 1994.)

Assessing Orthostatic Deconditioning Effects

Disruptions in cardiovascular dynamics, particularly heart rate, blood pressure, and leg volume changes during space missions could compromise crew performance and mission success.[7,22] For example, orthostatic testing conducted after Gemini (14 d) and during Skylab (80 d) missions documented the degree of orthostatic deconditioning effects. The Gemini vehicles (including Mercury and Apollo) had barely enough room for the astronauts, so they could not accommodate an on-board LBNP chamber. Thus, testing on Gemini took place only before and after flights. Also, Gemini flights used a tilt table rather than LBNP (Fig. 27.24, *top panel*). A 15-minute, 70° vertical LBNP tilt test produced dramatic changes in heart rate, systolic and diastolic blood pressure, and leg volume during the prolonged Skylab mission, compared with the same variables assessed 3 weeks prior to liftoff. Heart rate increased 100%, from 70 b · min^{-1} at rest at the start of the LBNP tilt test to 140 b · min^{-1} at the end of the procedure. Systolic blood pressure declined more (30%) than diastolic blood pressure (<10%) during the tilt, whereas leg volume increased 10-fold during the test.

The *bottom* of Figure 27.24 shows the pattern of resting heart rate in a −50 mm Hg LBNP test in one crew member during the 80-day Skylab 4 mission and 2 months postflight. While not as dramatic as the shorter-duration Gemini experiments, the resting heart rate increase in response to LBNP during Skylab confirmed the relative instability (and variability) of heart rate, particularly during the first month of space flight, compared with that at the end of the mission.

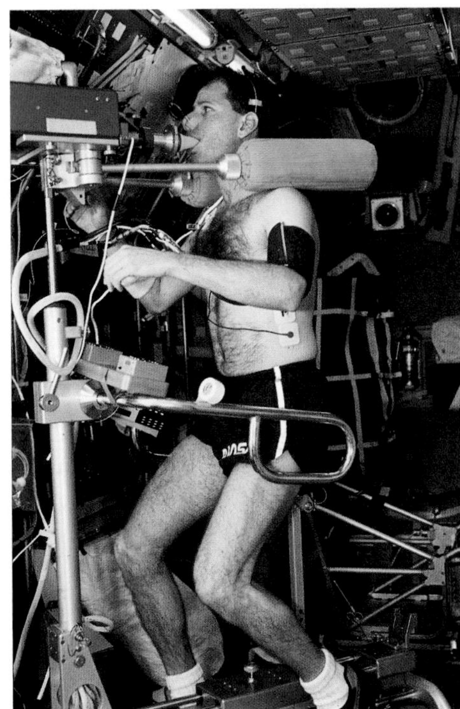

Measuring oxygen consumption on the space treadmill during a shuttle mission. Note the shoulder supports and handrails. Biosensors continuously monitor physiologic functions.

Heart rate with LBNP during preflight never exceeded 75 b · min^{-1}, but it always exceeded this value throughout the mission. On Skylab missions 2 and 3, resting heart rate averaged approximately 109 b · min^{-1}, a 55% increase over preflight values.

LBNP Combined Countermeasures

A countermeasure combination of LBNP and increased fluid ingestion during space flight improves performance on a postflight upright standing posture test.[9,127] For example, two groups of 26 male astronauts consumed either no fluid or a loading volume of 32 oz of water or juice plus eight salt tablets (to facilitate fluid retention) 1 hour before leaving Earth orbit during shuttle missions 1 through 8.[11] Figure 27.25 shows the fluid-loading countermeasure effects on postflight heart rate responses in the supine and standing positions. All crew members showed similar preflight heart rates. Crew members who used the liquid countermeasures did not experience syncope after landing mainly because approximately 40% of the ingested fluid increased plasma volume for nearly 4 hours. Astronauts who loaded fluid before re-entry also had

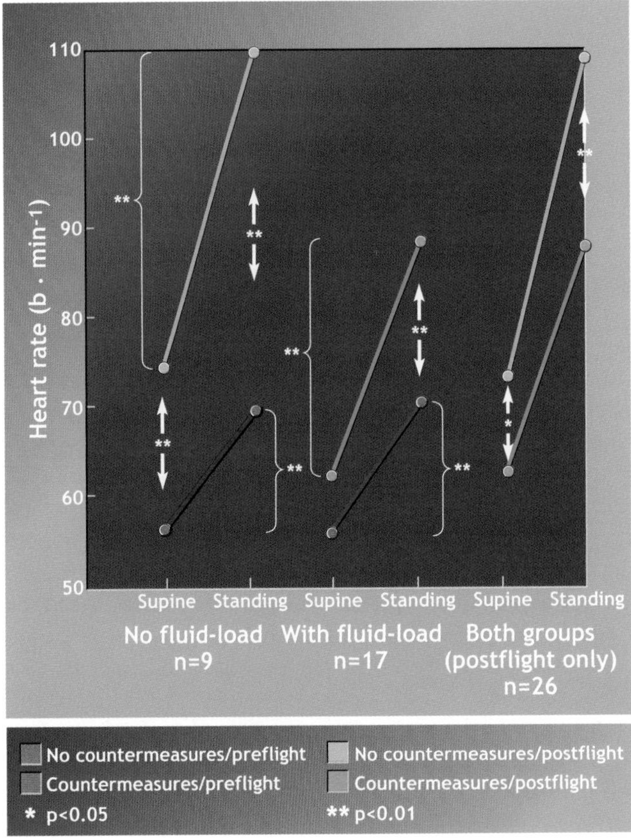

FIGURE 27.25 • Effect of forced–liquid-loading countermeasures on heart rate response to moving from supine to standing before (preflight) and after (postflight) space flight. Postflight refers to period of space mission 1 hour before leaving Earth orbit. (Modified from Bungo MW, et al. Cardiovascular deconditioning during space flight and the use of saline as a countermeasure to orthostatic intolerance. Aviat Space Environ Med 1985;5:985.)

lower heart rates and maintained a more stable mean blood pressure. Overall, the hyperhydration countermeasures were more effective during short (3 to 7 d) missions than during longer (10 d) ones.

The protective benefits of *combined* countermeasures significantly reduce the incidence of orthostatic intolerance assessed by postural tests postflight to only 5%.[100] In contrast, fluid loading alone prior to re-entry loses its effectiveness after 7 days in microgravity[20] or during a 7-day, 6° head-down bed rest[17], because the vascular space cannot maintain enough fluid to restore plasma volume to a level that exerts significant benefits. Another countermeasure tactic, in addition to combined countermeasures, reduces air temperature inside the space cabin the night before landing. Keeping the cabin "as cold as tolerable" helps to dissipate heat in the cabin (and ultimately in the space garments) during re-entry and postlanding when the cabin's air temperature can reach 26.7 to 32°C. The astronaut's liquid cooling garment uses a thermoelectric cooler to keep the precirculated water cool before it circulates through the full-torso garment. Reducing an astronaut's sweating response during re-entry and landing minimizes fluid loss.

NASA GUIDELINES. The flight rule requiring astronauts to **isotonic fluid load** (hyperhydrate) prior to re-entry with 8 g of NaCl in 1 L of water (referred to as the "soak") sometimes produced nausea and vomiting, causing some astronauts to ignore the rule. Adding natural sugars to sweeten the fluid and increase palatability also triggered undesirable fluid loss through copious urine flow (diuresis). More than likely, this discontinued fluid countermeasure application may itself have contributed negatively to postflight evaluation of physiologic parameters.

Current NASA guidelines concerning combined countermeasures for re-entry now require (1) preinflation of anti-g suits, (2) use of a liquid cooling garment that circulates chilled water through tubes in the flight suit, and (3) consumption 2 hours before landing of 15 mL per kg of preflight body mass of an isotonic fluid, consommé or potassium citrate (Astroade). Determining the efficacy of these combined procedures requires additional research using appropriate control conditions during re-entry and landing. Nevertheless, incorporation of the liquid cooling garment has decreased the frequency of orthostatic symptoms to approximately 5%, with a corresponding 50% decrease in postflight nausea.[100]

Nutrition

An optimal diet for space flight should theoretically satisfy the energy balance equation to provide energy (calorie) intake equal to the energy required for the mission. Dietary management may also counter the diverse adverse effects of physiologic adaptation to microgravity.[35] This goal, although seemingly straightforward, has not been accomplished successfully on most missions. *Almost every space journey produces weight loss compared with similar-duration ground-based activities on Earth.*[95,96,111,129] Disruption in energy balance results from combined effects of (1) increased energy demands of the physical requirements of space flight and (2) decreased food intake during microgravity exposure. Both factors negatively affect the space traveler's energy balance, similar to the early monkeys in flight. The effects of a negative energy balance became manifested not only in weight loss but also in impaired fluid, electrolyte, and mineral balance. Each of these factors in turn influences cardiovascular, musculoskeletal, immunologic, and endocrinologic functions. Cosmonauts in the Russian space program have also reported weight loss during extended missions.

Adequacy of Food Intake

During the relatively brief 1961–1963 Mercury missions of up to 34 hours, astronauts ate pureed foods and bite-sized cubes through their helmet faceplates. John Glenn, the first American space diner, consumed 270 kcal of pureed applesauce and beef and gravy with vegetables during the flight. On the longer Gemini flights, astronauts were supposed to consume 2800 kcal daily, but actually ate only 30 to 50% of this amount. Their rations consisted of bite-sized cubes of meat, dessert, and bread, in addition to rehydratable fruits, salads, meats, soups, desserts, and beverages, designed to supply a macronutrient mixture of 16% protein, 31% lipid, and 53% carbohydrate.

To improve taste, the meals on Apollo flights contained greater variety—astronauts could preselect from 70 foods—with the foods thermostablized to withstand temperature extremes and with relatively normal moisture content to improve taste. Bread made from irradiated flour could be preserved for at least 1 month, enabling astronauts to consume sandwiches throughout their mission. They were supposed to consume their individualized diets for 21 days preflight, throughout the flight, and for 18 days postflight. The spacecraft's galley area contained a freezer, food chiller, and hot and cold outlets to provide drinking water and to rehydrate foods. During EVA and moon missions, astronauts consumed calorie-dense fruit bars and fruit-flavored beverages from a delivery system within their space suit. Crew members were encouraged to consume an additional 800 to 1000 kcal as food bars every third day. Protein intake varied between 52 and 126 g daily, averaging 76 g.

Physiology experiments on subsequent Skylab missions required more-stringent guidelines and control of food intake to maintain validity of on-board studies of mineral balance, body fluid characteristics, bone mineral composition, body mass, and other biomedical parameters. The Skylab contains freezers and refrigerators to give astronauts and cosmonauts more varied food choices. Experience in planning nutritious meals in space has carryover to human health, particularly because the tools for space-based nutrition research must meet stringent design criteria for flight. New technologies developed in space have potential in studies of both normal and abnormal nutritional states on Earth, such as malnutrition in special populations from infants to the elderly.[67]

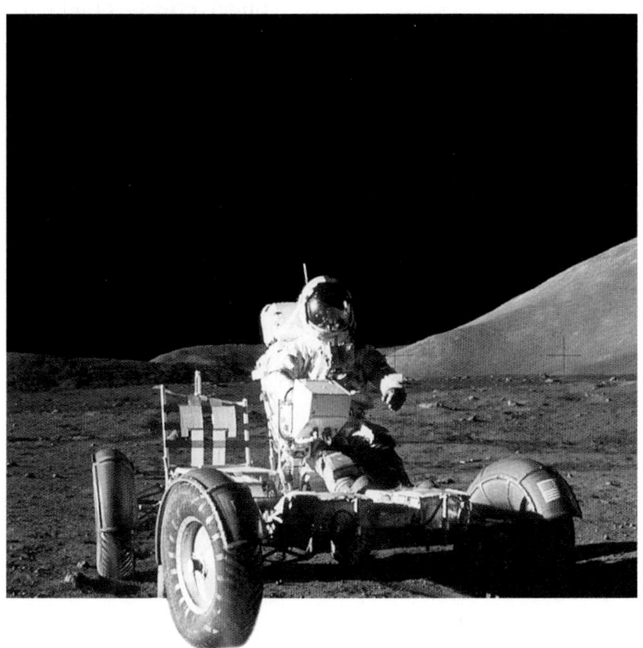

Astronaut Eugene A. Cernan, Apollo 17 mission commander, makes a short checkout of the Lunar Roving Vehicle during the early part of the first Apollo 17 EVA at the Taurus-Littrow landing site of NASA's sixth and final Apollo lunar landing mission (Dec. 10, 1972). Improved access to between-meal snacks during EVA maneuvers helped astronauts more closely balance energy intake and energy expenditures.

Effects on Body Weight

The graphs in Figure 27.26 summarize the large individual variation in body weight changes for the commander, scientist–pilot, and pilot crew members during three Skylab missions lasting 24, 56, and 84 days. On each mission, all crew members lost weight and did not regain it, except the commander (Skylab 4), whose weight returned to prelaunch values by mission's end. The most dramatic weight loss (3 to 4%) generally occurred over the first 10 days of each mission, mainly from fluid loss. Weight loss reversed within 5 days after the crew returned to Earth. This same weight loss pattern during space flight and weight regain postflight occurred during the 1996 Life Sciences and Microgravity (LSM) mission (liftoff.msfc.nasa.gov/Shuttle/msl/main.html).[113]

INTEGRATIVE QUESTION

How would you measure an astronaut's body weight in microgravity?

Food Intake on Skylab

The relatively large Skylab vehicle with its own food galley changed the way astronauts dined in space. The crew preselected commercially available foods, which were then preassembled into complete meals. Flexible aluminum and plastic pouches contained beverages and natural food items, and cans contained the thermostabilized foods. Estimated basal energy expenditure (using the Harris-Benedict equation to predict BMR) multiplied by 1.7 for men and 1.6 for women, established the total energy content of daily meals. Thus, a basal requirement of 1752 kcal for a male allowed an additional 1226 kcal for nonbasal activities (1752 kcal × 1.7 = 2978 kcal [1752 + 1226]). Even with these conservative computations, astronauts fail to balance energy intake with energy expenditure and thus lose weight. For example, on Columbia shuttle flight STS-40 (June 5 to 14, 1991), the fifth dedicated SLS-1 mission, four payload crew members weighed and recorded all food consumed before, during, and after flight. Figure 27.27 shows clearly that the astronauts underconsumed recommended energy intake by 33% during the 9-day mission, with considerable individual variation in macronutrient intake. Daily protein intake varied between 34 and 149 g; lipid intake ranged between 11 and 42% of total calories ingested, and carbohydrate ranged between 37 and 72%.

Comparison of Energy and Macronutrient Intake for Apollo, Skylab, and Space Shuttle Missions

Table 27.16 *(top)* summarizes the dietary intakes for Apollo, Skylab, and space shuttle astronauts during space flight; the *bottom* of the table lists macronutrient proportions, expressed as a percentage of total energy intake.[113] For comparison, the space flight intakes are contrasted with World Health Organization equations that predict daily requirements. Three salient findings emerge. First, for each mission, energy intake never achieved the predicted optimum. It came closest on Skylab (99.1% predicted), but reached only 64.2% of predicted on Apollo and 67.5% on the space shuttle. Second, astronauts consumed a relatively higher percentage of carbohydrate (58%) and lower percentage of lipid (28%) during flight than in preflight; preflight calories from carbohydrate averaged 52%; those from lipid averaged 33%. Third, considerable individual variation exists in energy expenditure during space flight, ranging from 28 to 47 kcal · kg^{-1} · d^{-1}. Perhaps the relative ease of preparing foods of high carbohydrate content explains the shift in macronutrient preference during space flight.[62,63] Of nutritional significance, daily calcium intake averaged approximately 25% lower than values recommended by the National Research Council (see connection/lww.com/go/mcardle). The reduced total water consumption during flight[63] results in part from food intake but also from reduced fluid consumption, possibly from reduced sensitivity of the thirst mechanism.[70]

DAILY NUTRITIONAL RECOMMENDATIONS FOR 90- TO 360-DAY SPACE MISSIONS. Table 27.17 lists daily recommended macro- and micronutrient intake proposed by the Biomedical Operations Research Branch of NASA, charged with nutritional optimization of space missions. The reference values for space travelers frequently exceed the Dietary Reference Intakes for an average American man and woman. Nevertheless, because of large variations among individuals in energy expenditure, it will not be possible for a single recommended nutrient intake to apply to all astronauts on their missions. Instead, astronauts will probably receive individually customized meal plans to meet nutrient and energy requirements of the mission. The astronauts' total energy expenditure consists of their

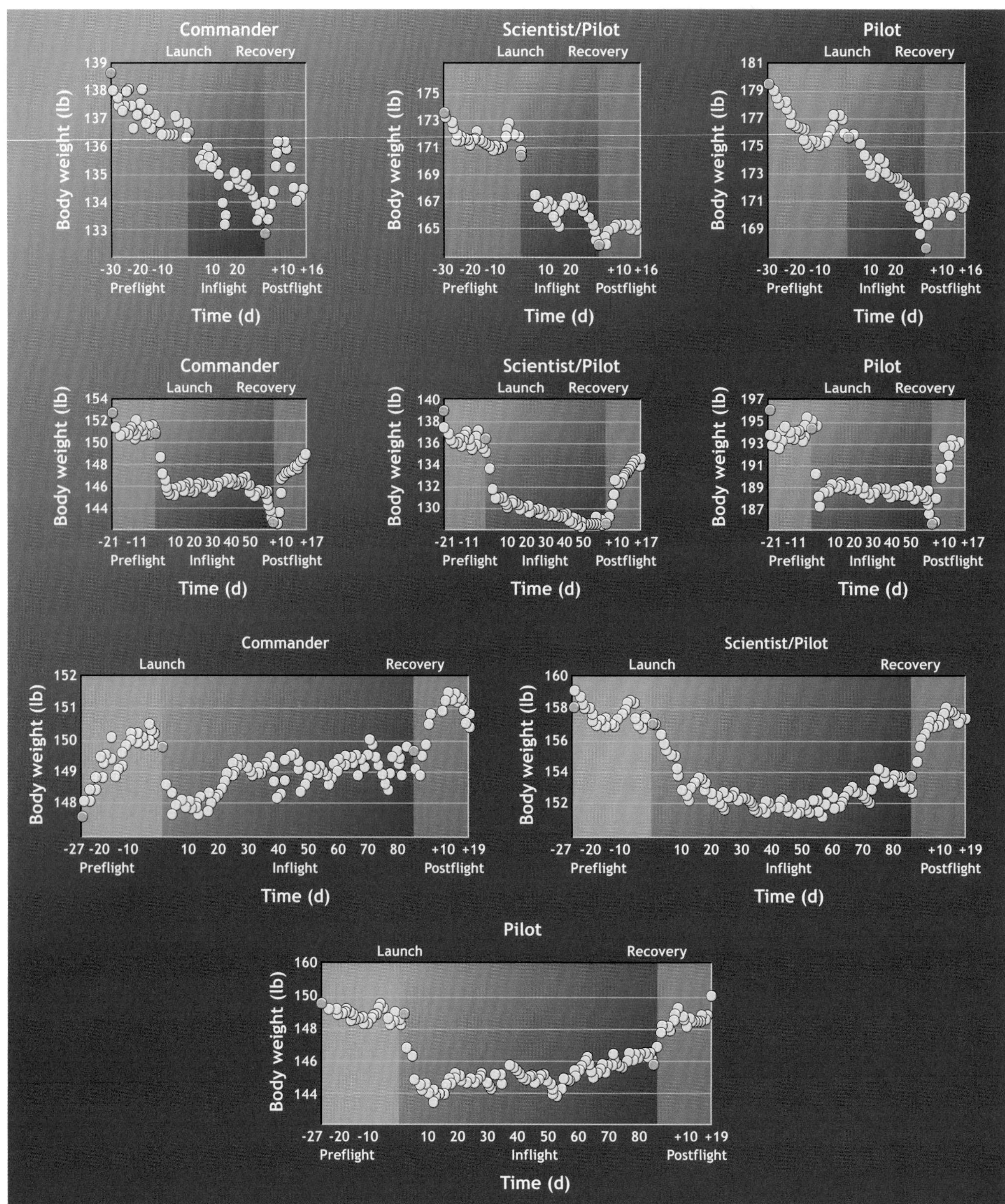

FIGURE 27.26 • Changes in body weight of crew personnel during three Skylab missions *Top*. Skylab 2, 24 days. *Middle*. Skylab 3, 56 days. *Bottom three*. Skylab 4, 84 days. *Orange circles* denote body weight at transitions at various phases in mission sequence. Note that for each astronaut body weight decreases dramatically during microgravity exposure. (From Thornton WE, Ord J. Physiological mass measurements in Skylab. In: Johnson RS, Dietlein LF, eds. Biomedical results from Skylab. NASA SP-377. Washington, DC: Government Printing Office, 1977.)

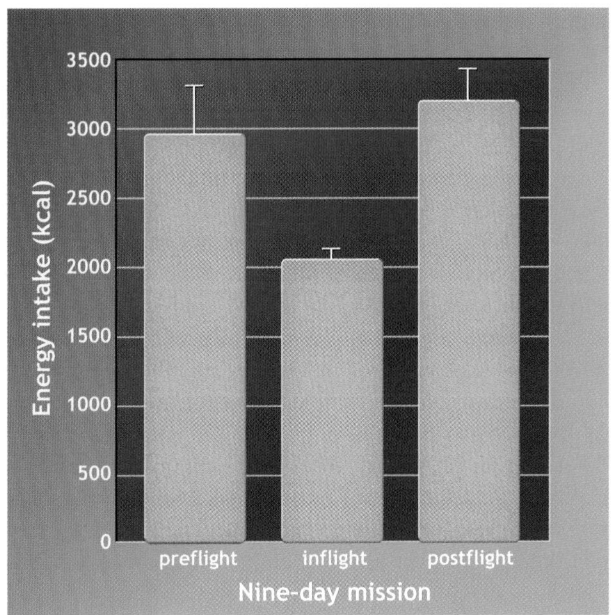

FIGURE 27.27 • Daily energy intake during the shuttle STS-40 flight before, during, and postflight. (From Lane HW, Rambaut PC. Nutrition. In Nicogossian AE, et al., eds. Space physiology and medicine, 3rd ed. Philadelphia: Lea & Febiger, 1994.)

BMR, the energy cost of planned in-flight exercise, and any EVA activity.

During future stays on Space Station Freedom, the iron requirement (see Table 27.17) changes from the current daily standard of 15 mg · d^{-1} for women to 10 mg · d^{-1}, because of decreased red blood cell mass and turnover and altered iron metabolism in space.[71,124] The challenge to researchers becomes identifying ways to ensure that astronauts have a total food intake adequate to balance energy requirements and achieve optimal macro- and micronutrient intake to sustain "good" health throughout a mission, regardless of duration. This will pose a challenge for future interplanetary travel, particularly with respect to whether pregnancy and birth can be sustained successfully without gravity.[98] Considerably more ground-based and space-mission research with animals and humans should provide additional insights.

ALTERED PROTEIN DYNAMICS. *Atrophy of skeletal muscles that support posture and locomotion represents a characteristic maladaptation to microgravity during short- and long-duration exposures.*[36] Decreases in lean body mass, muscle volume, and muscle strength, and changes in muscle fiber microarchitecture[141] accompany space-induced muscle atrophy.

TABLE 27.16 ➤ ***TOP.* DIETARY INTAKES FOR APOLLO, SKYLAB, AND SPACE SHUTTLE ASTRONAUTS DURING SPACE FLIGHT. *BOTTOM.* MACRONUTRIENT PROPORTIONS AS A PERCENTAGE OF ENERGY INTAKE (%kJ) IN APOLLO, SKYLAB, AND SPACE SHUTTLE DIETS BEFORE AND DURING SPACE FLIGHT**

	APOLLO	SKYLAB	SPACE SHUTTLE
Energy			
kJ · d^{-1}	7864 ± 1734[a]	11,906 ± 1300	8346 ± 1364
WHO predicted requirements (%)	64.2 ± 13.6	99.1 ± 8.2	67.5 ± 19.3
Protein			
g · d^{-1}	76.1 ± 18.7	111.0 ± 18.4	75.7 ± 20.2
% of kJ intake	16.2 ± 2.1	15.5 ± 1.2	15.0 ± 2.8
Carbohydrate intake			
g · d^{-1}	268.8 ± 49.1	413.3 ± 59.3	282.9 ± 49.5
% of kJ intake	58.1 ± 7.1	58.1 ± 4.4	57.0 ± 5.1
Lipid			
g · d^{-1}	61.4 ± 21.4	83.2 ± 13.8	62.7 ± 13.8
% of kJ intake	28.8 ± 5.4	26.4 ± 3.8	28.2 ± 4.1
Water (mL · d^{-1})	1647 ± 188[b]	2829 ± 529	1923 ± 376
Calcium (mg · d^{-1})	774 ± 212	902 ± 152	853 ± 226
Before flight			
Carbohydrate	NA[c]	50.5 ± 3.5	53.1 ± 6.2
Lipid	NA	33.4 ± 3.2	31.7 ± 5.0
Protein	NA	16.1 ± 0.9	14.7 ± 2.1
During flight			
Carbohydrate	58.1 ± 7.1	58.1 ± 4.4	57.0 ± 5.1
Lipid	28.8 ± 5.4	26.4 ± 3.8	28.2 ± 4.1
Protein	16.2 ± 2.1	15.5 ± 4.1	15.0 ± 2.8

To convert kJ to kcal divide by 4.186
[a]Values are means ± standard deviations.
[b]n=3.
[c]Not available.
Modified from Lane HW, et al. Nutrition in space: lessons from the past applied to the future. Am J Clin Nutr 1994; 60:801S–805S.

TABLE 27.17 ➤ DAILY MACRO AND MICRONUTRIENT NASA RECOMMENDATIONS FOR 90- TO 360-DAY SPACE MISSIONS

NUTRIENT	RECOMMENDATIONS[a]
Energy	WHO (moderate activity level)
Protein	12–15% of total energy consumed
Carbohydrate	50% of total energy consumed
Lipid	30-35% of total energy consumed
Fluid	238-357 mL per MJ consumed
Fiber	10-25 g
Vitamin A	1000 μg retinol equiv
Vitamin D	10 μg
Vitamin E	20 mg α-tocopherol equiv
Vitamin K	80 μg for men; 65 μg for women
Vitamin C	100 mg
Vitamin B_{12}	2.0 μg
Vitamin B_6	2.0 mg
Thiamin	1.5 mg
Riboflavin	2.0 mg
Folate	400 μg
Niacin	20 mg
Biotin	100 μg
Pantothenic acid	5.0 mg
Calcium	1000-1200 mg
Phosphorus	1000-1200 mg
Magnesium	350 mg for men; 280 mg for women
Sodium	<3500 mg
Potassium	3500 mg
Iron	10 mg
Copper	1.5-3.0 mg
Manganese	2.0-5.0 mg
Fluoride	4.0 mg
Zinc	15 mg
Selenium	70 μg
Iodine	150 μg
Chromium	100-200 μg

[a]Recommendations generated by two nutritional advisory committees to NASA. Courtesy of Dr. Helen Lane, NASA Chief Nutritionist. Biomedical Research Branch at the NASA Houston Space Center, Houston, TX. WHO, World Health Organization

Such changes suggest poor adaptation in whole-body protein (nitrogen) balance.[75,110,111] Isotopic methods that assess tissue protein turnover show that astronauts increase their protein breakdown rate by approximately 30% on mission days 2 to 8, thereby resulting in negative nitrogen balance. In addition, elevations occur in urinary cortisol, fibrinogen, and interleukin-2 (IL-2). These changes suggest that space flight triggers a stress response similar to the response pattern from physical injury.[111] In both stressful situations, tissue protein becomes a substrate for energy metabolism, which fosters a negative nitrogen balance (protein catabolism). This supports the recommendation of a daily protein intake of 1.5 g per kg body mass during space travel.[66] In addition, long space missions (4 to 9 mo on the Russian Mir Space Station) and shorter-duration space shuttle flights (up to 15 d) are associated with decreased oxidative damage from decreased oxygen radical production (in the electron transport chain) from reduced in-flight energy intake. However, increased oxidative damage occurs postflight from combined increases in metabolic rate and possible loss of in-flight host antioxidant defenses.[109] The potential beneficial effects of postflight antioxidant supplementation remain unknown.

Figure 27.28 plots daily energy intake and urine-based nitrogen balance assessment during three Skylab missions and two SLS missions. Note the in-flight negative nitrogen balance on Skylab compared with a preflight baseline despite near-normal energy intake. On the two shuttle missions, both daily calorie intake and nitrogen balance were negatively affected compared with preflight values. Based on Russian data aboard the Salyut-7 space mission, the estimated energy cost of twice-daily in-flight exercise sessions was approximately 20 kcal per kg body mass. Adding this energy requirement to an already inadequate daily energy intake would provoke further protein loss to absorb the energy deficit.[55] Future research must determine effective combinations of exercise and nutritional supplementation to stabilize energy and protein balance during space missions.

INTEGRATIVE QUESTION

Explain if consuming additional protein during a space mission can help to restore fat-free body mass.

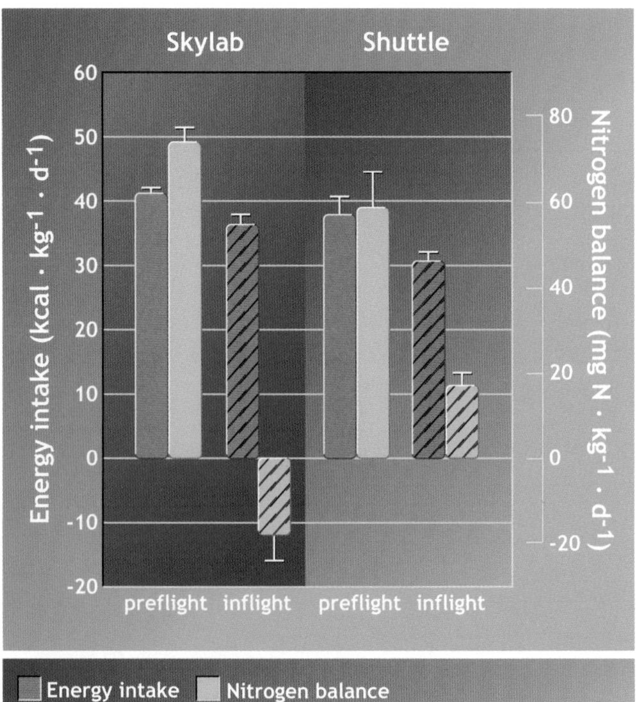

FIGURE 27.28 • Daily energy intake (*left axis*) and daily urine-based nitrogen balance (*right axis*) during space flight on three Skylab missions and two Life Sciences Space Shuttle missions (SLS-1 and SLS-2). Values are means ±SE; (Modified from Stein TP, et al. Diet and nitrogen metabolism during space flight on the shuttle. J Appl Physiol 1996;81:82).

Energy Expenditure and Balance Dynamics on the Space Shuttle

The 1996 LMS shuttle mission measured energy expenditure and energy balance in four crew members for 12 days before liftoff, during the 17-day flight, and for 15 days postflight.[113] In addition, a complementary bed-rest study with 6° head-down tilt to simulate microgravity evaluated energy expenditure and energy balance in eight subjects. The bed-rest study had three phases: (1) 15-day pre–bed rest ambulatory period, (2) 17 days of bed rest (except when subjects exercised to match the in-flight exercise routines), and (3) a 15-day recovery period. Subjects in both experiments performed submaximal and maximal bicycle ergometer exercise tests on days 13 and 8 before launch and on days 4 and 8 postflight. During space flight days 2, 8, and 13, crew members performed an additional ergometer test to assess cardiorespiratory responses to exercise at 85% $\dot{V}O_{2max}$.

Measurements included doubly labeled water (DLW; $^2H_2{}^{18}O$) and body composition by DXA before and after space flight/bed rest to quantify either positive energy balance (fat stored) or negative energy balance (fat catabolized). Nutrient intake assessment required that subjects quantify each food item consumed and not consumed with a bar code reader and a verbal description (using a cassette recorder) to estimate the contents remaining in the individual food package. During pre- and postflight periods, subjects consumed prepared meals of known nutrient content. The Spacelab contained a system to collect, measure, and save a 20-mL daily urine sample to estimate nitrogen balance from nitrogen and creatinine excretion.

The top of Figure 27.29 displays three energy intake periods expressed as kcal · kg^{-1} · d^{-1} during preflight, flight, and postflight. Note that within each period, a relative stabilization (adaptation) takes place for energy intake, probably from resetting of setpoint mechanisms that regulate energy balance. The *histogram inset* expresses average energy intake in kilocalories per day to highlight the dramatic 45% lower in-flight energy intake (1708 kcal · d^{-1}) compared with the remarkably similar values preflight (3025 kcal · d^{-1}) and postflight (3151 kcal · d^{-1}).

The bottom graphic compares the energy intake during the first 2 weeks of space flight for Skylab missions 2, 3, and 4 and the two shuttle LMS missions. Astronauts on the shuttle LMS *(bottom red curve)* remained in substantial negative energy balance throughout the flight. Astronauts on the previous three Skylab missions participated in a metabolic balance study so daily energy intakes remained fairly stable during the different-duration missions. In contrast, astronauts on shuttle LMS consumed food ad libitum, while at the same time undertaking vigorous daily exercise that contributed to their relatively high average total daily energy expenditure of 40.8 kcal · kg^{-1} · d^{-1} (3238 kcal). Interestingly, no differences occurred among the three methods to estimate energy balance, which supported the validity of the methodology and the following main research conclusions:

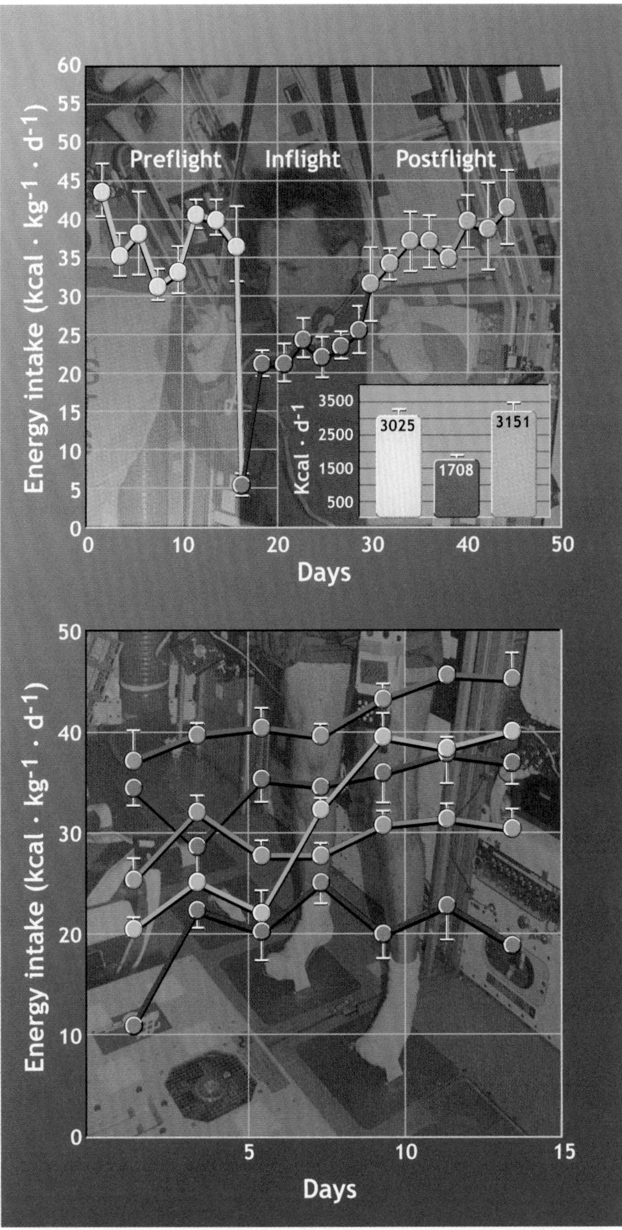

FIGURE 27.29 • *Top.* Energy intake before, during and after space flight on shuttle LMS. The *histogram inset* expresses the data as average kcal · d^{-1} during each mission phase. *Bottom.* Energy intake during the first 2 weeks of space flight for Skylab missions 2 (28 d), 3 (56 d), and 4 (84 d); two shuttle missions (SLS-1 and SLS-2 combined); and shuttle LMS. (Data modified from Stein TP, et al. Energy expenditure and balance during space flight on the space shuttle. Am J Physiol 1999;45:R1739.)

- Severe negative energy balance and corresponding loss of body mass, body fat, and protein could compromise a mission and adversely affect an astronaut's health in a manner resembling prolonged malnutrition
- High levels of physical activity during space flight may disrupt mechanisms that maintain energy balance

Persistent, severe 1400-kcal negative daily energy balance on future extended-duration flights would ultimately mobilize an astronaut's entire fat energy reserves (approximately 160,000 kcal) within 120 days and produce terminal starvation. Obviously, researchers must determine how best to ensure that astronauts consume adequate daily nutrition to counterbalance the energy requirements of space flight, including the demands of exercise countermeasures and normal work tasks, and decreased efficiency to remove the metabolic byproducts of exercise (e.g., CO_2, heat).[108] Cosmonauts on the Mir mission partially resolved their in-flight energy deficits by curtailing physical activity. Theoretically, they could remain in orbit for 660 days before severe undernutrition compromised physiology and performance.

Nutritionally Related Effects of Space Flight on Physiologic Functions

Since the first space missions, researchers have tracked adaptations in physiologic function during microgravity exposure. A prevailing theory about such changes concerns the interactions among nutritional variables and endocrine functions and their combined effects on cardiopulmonary, hormonal, skeletal, and body fluid functions and body mass and composition.[41,47,71,76,114,115] Figure 27.30 shows the triad of nutritionally related effects of space flight on physiologic systems. The interrelated triad components—fluid shifts, physical unloading of weight-bearing structures, and metabolic changes—in many ways link to shifts in endocrine function. The *inset table* shows endocrine changes during stress, simulated microgravity (bed rest), and space flight. Note that the responses to bed rest do not generally mirror endocrine changes in space flight, but they do mimic the stress-mediated responses. An attractive hypothesis, therefore, posits that the endocrine effects of space flight relate more to nutritional changes characterized best by stress-related models, not a model that incorporates bed rest.[64] The similarity between the catabolic effects of the increased demands on energy metabolism (and resulting negative energy balance) and catabolic effects of resultant space flight "stress" would help to explain space-induced decreases in body mass and lean body mass and bone density, in addition to shifts in extracellular and intracellular water compartments.

Body Composition Changes. Figure 27.31 shows percentage changes in body composition variables of 10 astronauts assessed by densitometry and multifrequency bioelectrical impedance analysis before and 2 days following 7- to 16-day missions. No significant changes occurred in body fat or extracellular water, with the 2.3% decline in body mass attributable to a loss in fat-free body mass (FFM). Note that all three

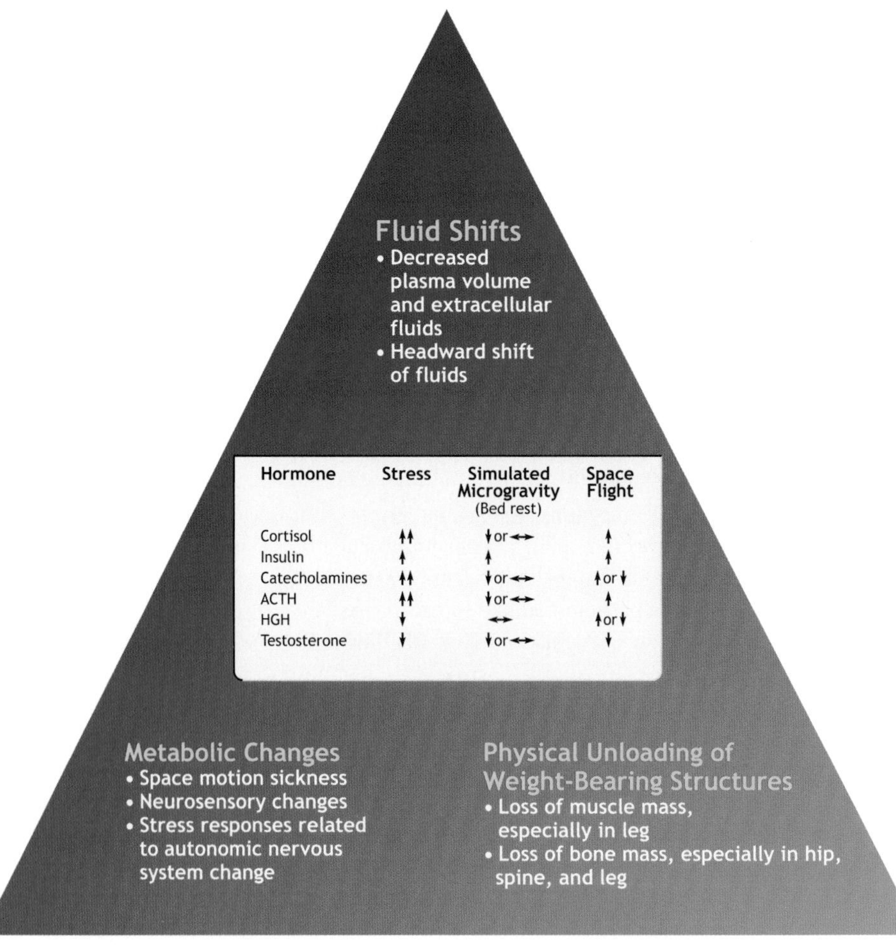

Hormone	Stress	Simulated Microgravity (Bed rest)	Space Flight
Cortisol	↑↑	↓ or ↔	↑
Insulin	↑	↑	↑
Catecholamines	↑↑	↓ or ↔	↑ or ↓
ACTH	↑↑	↓ or ↔	↑
HGH	↓	↔	↑ or ↓
Testosterone	↓	↓ or ↔	↓

Figure 27.30 • Triad of nutritionally related effects of space flight on physiologic systems. The *inset* shows endocrine changes during stress, simulated microgravity (bed rest studies), and space flight. ↑, increase; ↑↑, large increase; ↓, decrease; ↔, no change. (Modified from Lane HW, Gretebeck RJ. Nutrition, endocrinology, and body composition during space flight. Nutr Res 1998;18:1923.

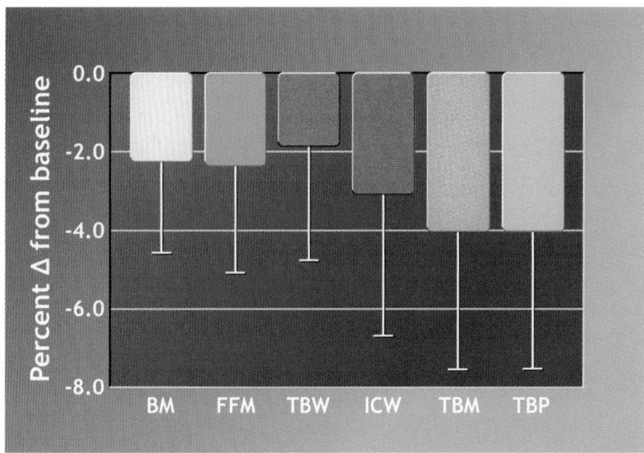

FIGURE 27.31 • Percentage changes (Δ) in body composition variables of 10 astronauts assessed by densitometry and multifrequency bioelectrical impedance analysis before and 2 days after 7- to 16-day missions. BM, body mass; FFM, fat-free body mass; TBW, total body water; ICW, intracellular water; TBM, total body mineral; TBP, total body protein. (Data from Greenisen MC, et al. Functional performance evaluation. In: Extended Duration Orbiter Medical Project. NASA Johnson Space Center final report. 1989–1995. [NASA/SP-1999-534] NASA. Lyndon B. Johnson Space Center. Houston, TX. 1999.)

components of FFM (water, protein, and mineral) declined from 3 to 4% in the postflight measures. The 3% loss of intracellular water—attributable to decreased protein and mineral levels within other tissues including muscle—explains the decrease in total-body water. Whether such alterations in body composition parameters affect in-flight performance awaits further study. However, body composition variables did not help to explain the 12% postflight reduction in $\dot{V}O_{2max}$. An integrative approach assesses regional body composition (calf muscle volume) and MRI-derived characteristics of muscle (transverse relaxation of calf muscles) following multiple shuttle/*Mir* missions lasting 16 to 28 weeks.[74]

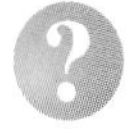

INTEGRATIVE QUESTION

What role should diet and exercise play in prolonged-duration space missions?

OVERVIEW OF PHYSIOLOGIC RESPONSES TO SPACE FLIGHT

Numerous research reports discuss short- and long-term consequences of space flight on human physiology.[6,9,17,21,49,72] From the first single-pilot flights of Project Mercury in the early 1960s to the extended Soviet Soyez missions of the 1990s, scientists have pondered how best to minimize the deleterious effects of microgravity during flight and upon return to Earth. Figure 27.32 diagrams the two main physical stressors from space travel: (1) decreased hydrostatic pressure gradients within the cardiovascular system (displayed on the *left*) and (2) decreased weight loading on muscles (displayed on the *right*), both of which ultimately increase physiologic strain *(orange box at the bottom)* and negatively affect an astronaut's physical performance (red box at the bottom).[21] Note that the three effects (decreased $\dot{V}O_{2max}$ and muscular strength and increased fatigability), combined with an increased thermal load, add significantly to the total physiologic strain. Exercise countermeasures, specifically site-specific lower-body eccentric and concentric resistance exercise, coupled with relatively intense cardiovascular workouts on a cycle ergometer and treadmill can mitigate deleterious effects from prolonged microgravity sojourns, particularly when astronauts return to a 1-g Earth environment.

Short- and Long-Term Responses

Two categories, short- and long-term, describe the time course of physiologic response and adaptation in the transitions from Earth's 1-g environment to microgravity in low-Earth orbit and then return to 1g following a mission. Short-term responses occur within 24 hours or the first few days of a mission. The second category describes longer-term changes following a mission. Figure 27.33 shows a generalized flow diagram of the immediate or short-term (<24 h) and delayed or long-term (>24 h) responses. Both the immediate and delayed responses eventually contribute to orthostatic hypotension (bottom purple box), the most common malady following space flight.

In space, body fluids no longer move "downward" from gravity's pull so fluids redistribute toward the chest and upper body (note facial puffiness from cranial edema). Lower-body fluid loss gives the legs a birdlike appearance. Excess fluid buildup in the torso triggers fluid elimination by the kidneys. Mean arterial pressure increases in the cranial region from a preflight normal of 70 mm Hg to 100 mm Hg in space (Fig. 27.33, *top*), while mean pressure at the feet declines 50% from its normal 200 mm Hg; heart volume also decreases slightly. The immediate change in body fluid distribution activates a plethora of additional responses and lower sympathetic nervous system activity. Restricted stimulation environments such as space flight and other stress-inducing situations from prolonged confinement and isolation share many of the same responses and adaptations.[77]

Time Course of In-Flight Adaptations

Figure 27.34 shows the time course for shifts in four main categories of physiologic function during 1 year of sustained microgravity. The *green horizontal line* represents baseline function on Earth (denoted as 0% change). Within the first 3 weeks, up to a 10% change in cardiovascular function reflects a deconditioning response; within 14 days, a 10% change occurs in body fluid redistribution, and within 3 months, bone mass declines by 5%. Bone mass declines further to 15% between months 5 and 6, when it appears to stabilize for several months before decreasing further to 17% after 1 year in microgravity. Like bone mass, muscle structure and function deteriorate at a slower rate than cardiac deconditioning and fluid redistribution, but the magnitude of the decrement reaches higher values.

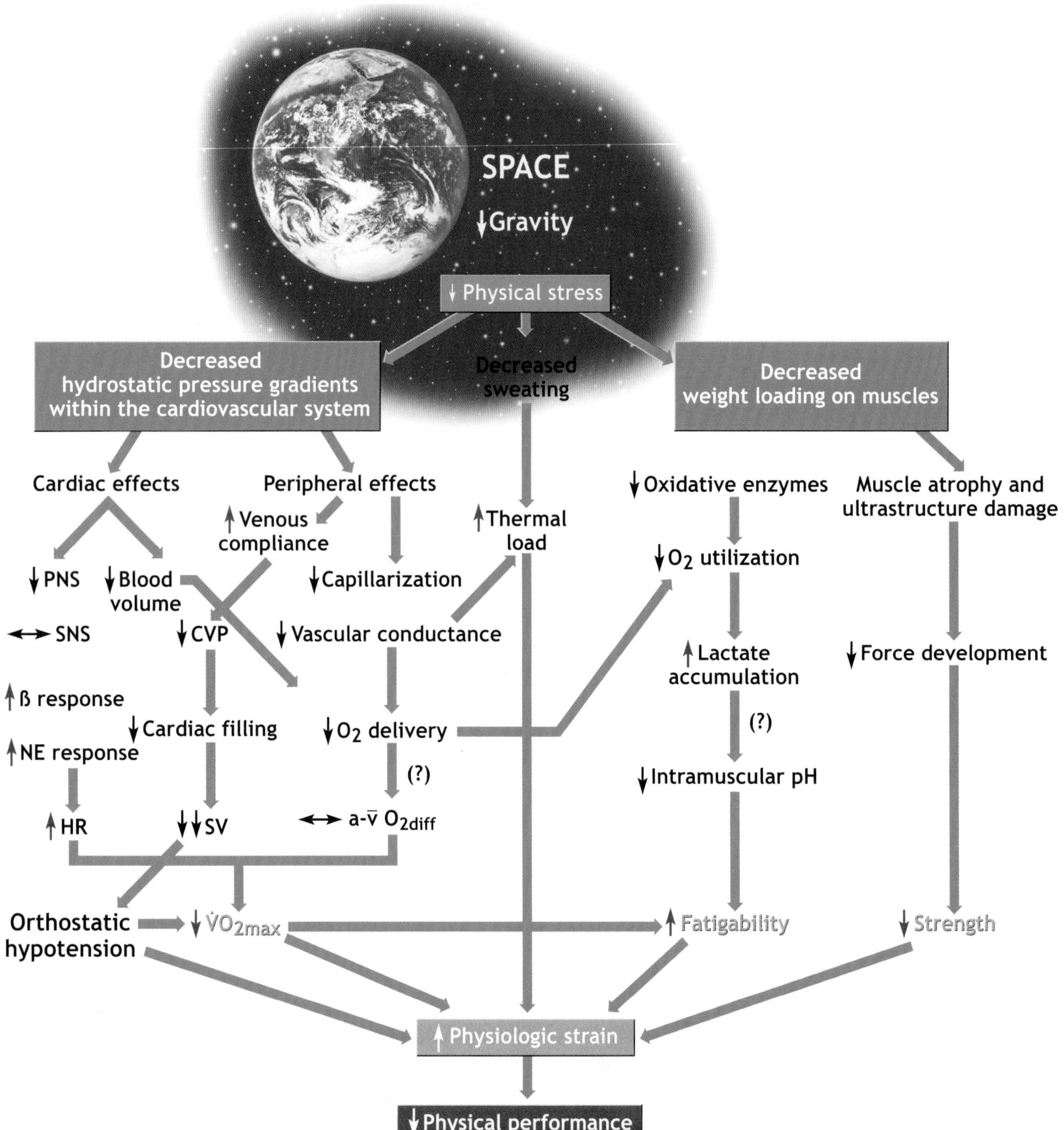

FIGURE 27.32 • Model of the relationship between physical stress of the space environment and adaptation of cardiovascular and muscular systems with resulting increased physiologic strain and decreased physical performance. SNS, sympathetic nervous system; CVP, central venous pressure; β, beta adrenegric; NE, norepinephrine; HR, heart rate; SV, stroke volume; a-$\bar{v}$ O_{2diff}, arteriovenous oxygen difference; ,↑ increase; ↓, decrease; ↓↓, large decrease; ↔, no change. (From Convertino VA. Effects of microgravity on exercise performance. In: Garrett WE, Kirkendall DT, eds. Exercise and sport science. Philadelphia: Lippincott Williams & Wilkins, 2000.

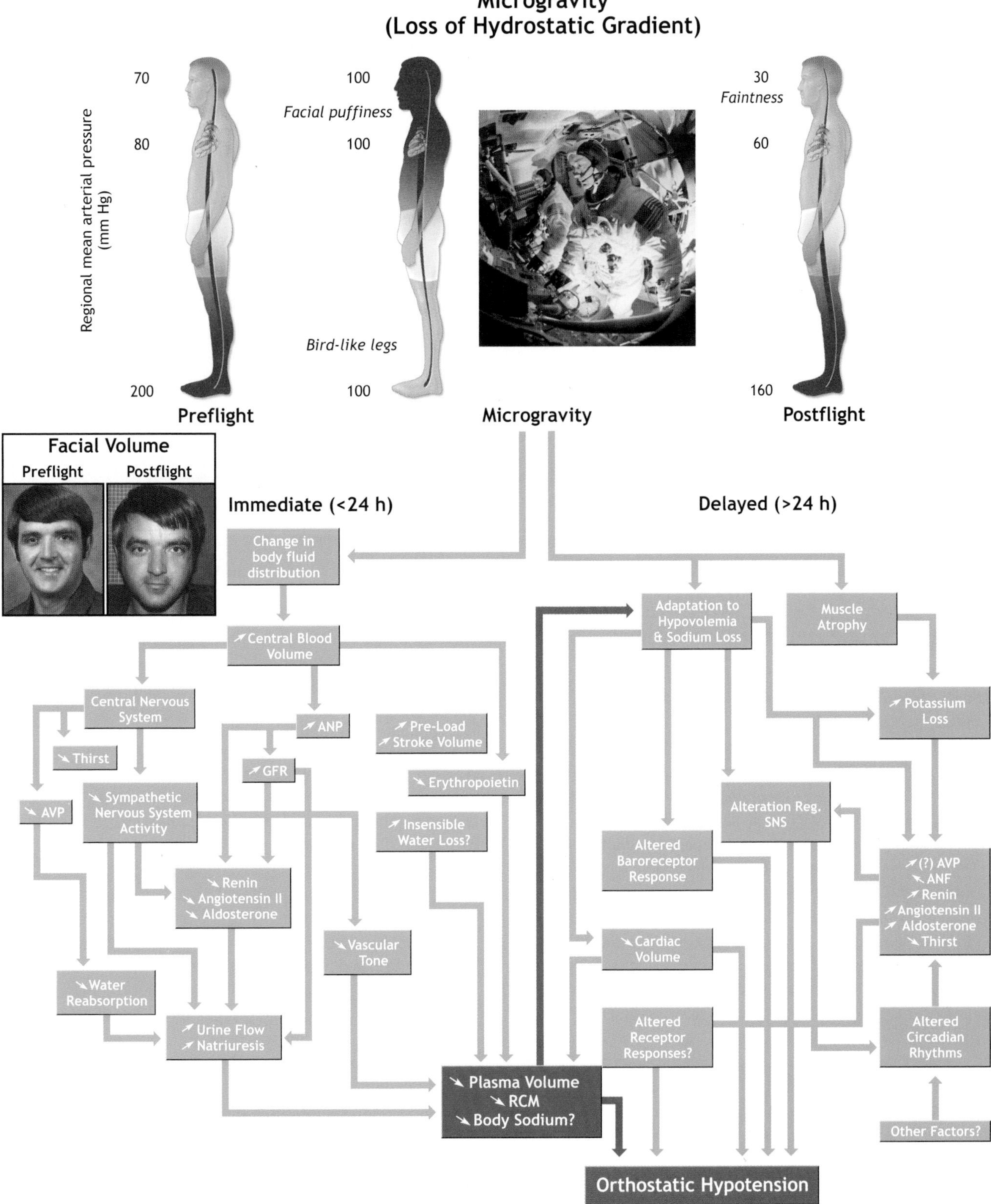

FIGURE 27.33 • Proposed immediate (<24 h) and delayed (>24 h) responses to microgravity compared with those under preflight (1g) and postflight (1g) conditions. AVP, arginine vasopressin; ANP, atrial natriuretic peptide; GFR, glomerular filtration rate; RCM, red cell mass; SNS, sympathetic nervous system; ↗, increase; ↘, decrease, ?, possible. (Photos courtesy of NASA, Lyndon B. Johnson Space Center, Houston, TX. Figures denoting changes in mean arterial pressure are modified from Hargens AR, et al. Control of circulatory function in altered gravitational fields. Physiologist 1992;35:S80. Additional graphic information modified from Maillet A, et al. Cardiovascular and hormonal changes induced by isolation and confinement. Med Sci. Sports Exerc 1996;28:S53.)

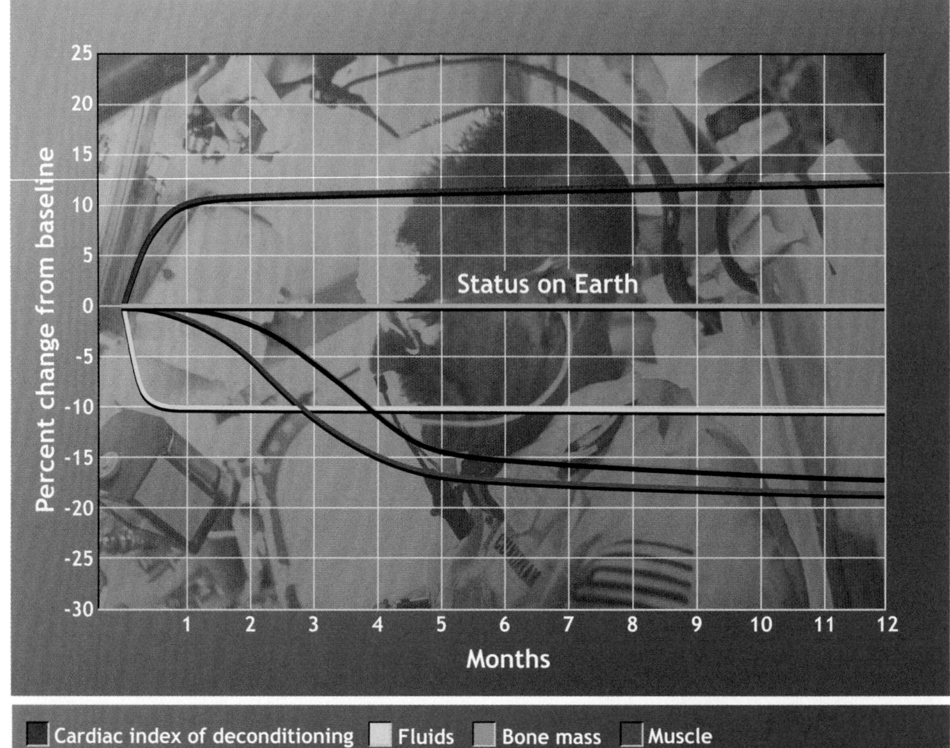

FIGURE 27.34 • Time course of four main shifts in physiologic function during 1 year in microgravity. The *horizontal green line* represents baseline function on Earth at 1g (denoted as zero percentage change). The cardiac index of deconditioning (*red line*) reflects severity of orthostatic intolerance to gravitational stress. (Modified from: Nicogossian A, et al. Overall physiologic response to space flight. In Nicogossian AE, et al., eds. Space physiology and medicine, 3rd ed. Philadelphia: Lea & Febiger, 1994.)

Time Course of Postflight Readaptations

Figure 27.35 shows how 3 months of recovery affects the neurovestibular and cardiovascular systems, fluid and electrolyte balance, red blood cell mass, and lean body mass. For reference, the *lower horizontal line* indicated by the arrow at the bottom left (*1-g set point*) represents baseline measures expected under normal 1-g conditions. The *colored lines* for each variable indicate average trends, but considerable inter- and intraindividual differences exist in recovery (readaptation) rate.

Analysis of the "recovery" curves reveals two characteristics: (1) the response rate is nonlinear, with some processes appearing bimodal with relatively high rate constants and (2) recovery time varies depending on the variable evaluated. For example, the rapid change in fluid distribution during the first few weeks of microgravity exposure shown previously in Figure 27.34 recovers to baseline within the first week of return to 1g *(yellow curve)*. In contrast, the *light green curve* for lean body mass and *purple curve* for cardiovascular deconditioning require approximately 6 weeks to approach baseline. Insufficient data exist about readaptation rate for other biomedical variables such as bone mass and nutritional status (e.g., calcium, iron).

FUTURE RESEARCH PRIORITIES

Before NASA attempts an interplanetary Mars mission sometime after 2014, a host of questions remain concerning astronaut health and safety, including priorities for the most-productive research strategies in gravitational biology.[33,83] The Committee on Space Biology and Medicine of the National Research Council[106] has targeted high-priority research areas concerning astronauts' health, safety, and performance during and following long-duration missions. The committee identified the following five broad topic areas for continued research:

1. Loss of weight-bearing bone and muscle
   - Emphasize studies that provide mechanistic insights into effective countermeasures to prevent bone and muscle deterioration during and after space flight.
   - Investigate mechanisms of changes that reproduce in-flight and postflight effects from ground-based models such as hindlimb unloading in rodents.
   - Develop a database on the course of microgravity-related bone loss and its reversibility in humans via preflight, in-flight, and postflight recording of BMD.
   - Obtain hormone profiles on humans before, during, and after space flight.
   - Investigate the relationship between exercise levels and protein energy balance in flight.
2. Vestibular function, the vestibular ocular reflex, and sensorimotor integration
   - Determine whether the same mechanisms control posture and movement on Earth and in space.
   - Determine how microgravity exposure affects central and peripheral vestibular function and development from recordings of signal processing following otolith afferent stimulation.
   - Determine if microgravity affects vestibulo-oculomotor system mechanisms in learning new motor patterns to sensory perturbations.

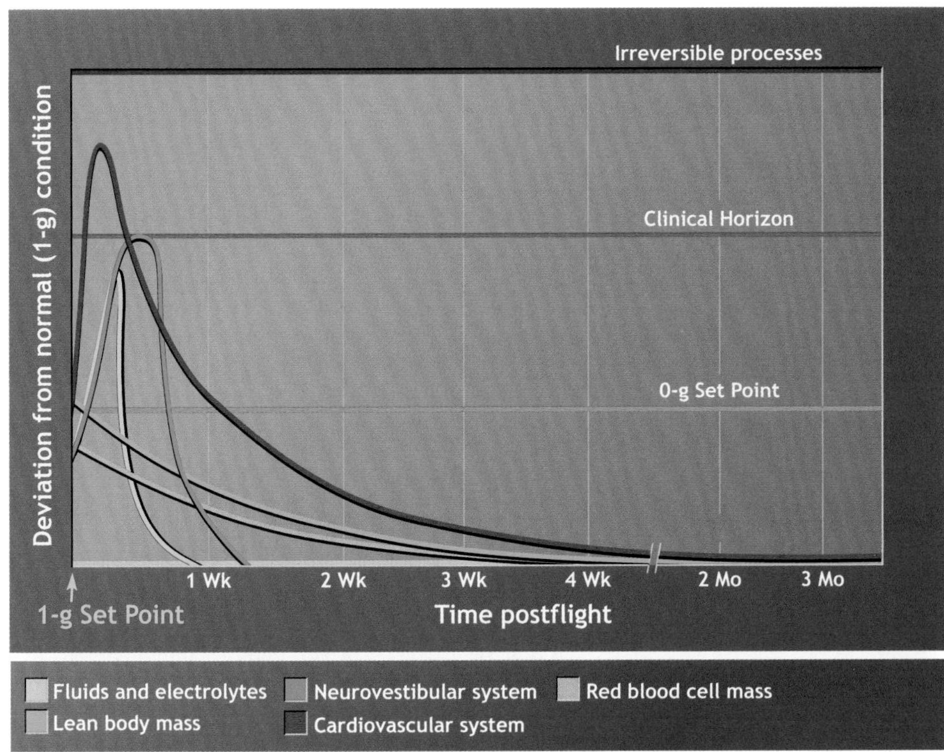

Figure 27.35 • Time course of physiologic shifts during readaptation to 1g, in which flight duration only minimally affects the readaptations. (Modified from Nicogossian AE, et al., eds. Space physiology and medicine, 3rd ed. Philadelphia: Lea & Febiger, 1994.)

3. Orthostatic intolerance upon return to Earth's gravity
   - Study effects of long-duration exposure to microgravity on the magnitude, time course, and mechanisms of cardiovascular adjustments.
   - Determine the specific mechanisms underlying inadequate total peripheral resistance during postflight orthostatic stress.
   - Reevaluate current antiorthostatic countermeasures to refine those that offer protection and eliminate those that do not. Studies should control factors carefully to avoid confounding effects of multiple, simultaneous interventions. Studies about simultaneous bone and/or muscle protection should receive priority.
   - Identify and validate methods for referencing intrathoracic vascular pressures to systemic pressures related to cardiac and pulmonary volume and compliance.
4. Radiation hazards
   - Determine the carcinogenic risks following irradiation by protons and HZE particles.
   - Determine if exposure to heavy ions at the level occurring during prolonged deep-space missions poses a risk to central nervous system integrity and function.
   - Determine how selection and design of the space vehicle affect its radiation environment and crew exposure.
   - Determine whether the combined effects of radiation and stress on the immune system in space flight could produce additive or synergistic effects on host defenses.
5. Physiologic effects of stress
   - Analyze the interactions between the hypothalamic-pituitary-adrenal axis and the immune system during space flight to determine the role played by host response to stressors in altering host defenses.

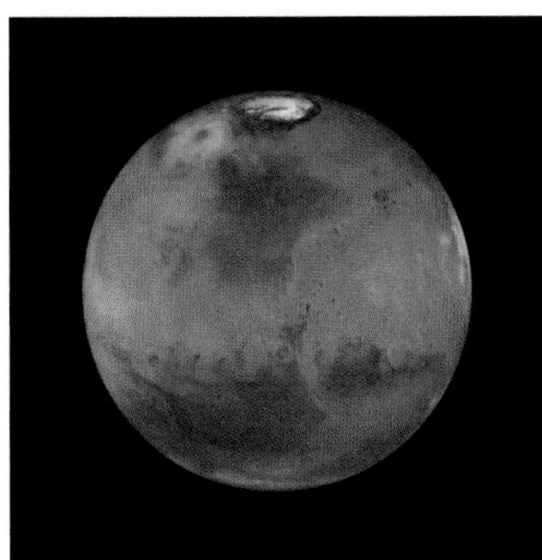

NASA has developed a long-term Mars exploration program that charts a course for the next two decades. In 2005, NASA plans to launch the Mars Reconnaissance Orbiter. NASA proposes to develop and launch a roving long-range, long-duration science laboratory as a major leap in surface measurements and pave the way for a future sample return mission as early as 2007. In the second decade of the century, NASA plans additional science orbiters, rovers and landers, and the first mission to return samples of Martian rock and soil to Earth. Current plans call for the first sample return mission in 2014, and a second in 2016 using miniaturized surface science instruments and deep drilling to hundreds of meters.

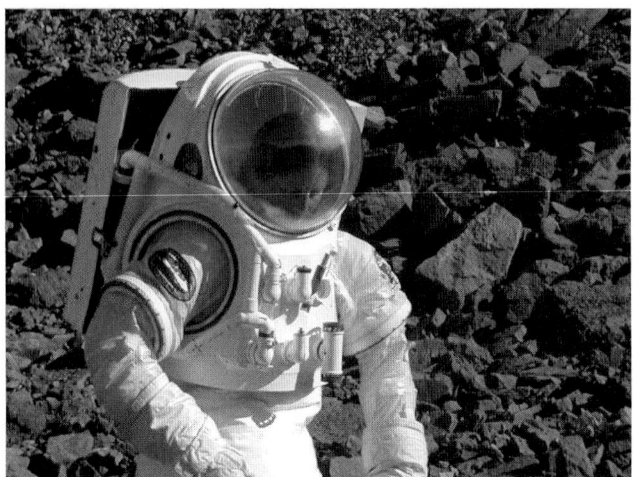

Dr. Kelly Snook tests the Mars prototype suit as part of The Haughton-Mars Project (HMP), a NASA-led international field research program centered on the scientific study of the Haughton impact crater and its surroundings on Devon Island (the largest uninhabited island on Earth), Nunavut, Canadian high arctic, considered a Mars analog.

In addition to the above five specific areas concerning astronauts' health, safety, and performance, cell biology in space research can provide information about the following central themes:[106]

- How do cells replicate and maintain their genomes, including regulation of their proliferative capacity and survival?
- How do individual cells carry out genetically defined programs of differentiation and development into specialized tissue and multicellular organisms?
- How do cells generate and maintain their complicated internal cytoarchitecture, including the cytoskeleton and the host of specialized membrane-bound organelles and membrane domains, to regulate both growth and form?
- How do cells synthesize and maintain organelle substructure?
- How do organisms respond at the cellular level to changes in their extracellular environments?

NASA's cooperative efforts with the scientific and industrial sector continue to develop advanced instrumentation and methodologies for space-based studies at the cellular level. The new generation of space vehicles now under development for interplanetary-class explorations will integrate cutting-edge research in the physical sciences to make endeavors to tame the space environment a success.

DERIVING PRACTICAL BENEFITS FROM SPACE BIOLOGY RESEARCH

NASA maintains a database of all its programs and technologies with commercial potential and benefits (technology.nasa.gov/techfinder/). Technologies developed over the past 30 years from NASA's current 15 centers to meet the challenges of space exploration have also produced more than 30,000 secondary commercial applications. Notable spin-off technologies include improved pacemakers and implantable heart pumps, cell-culturing devices, synthetic soil mixtures, new composite materials, quartz timing crystals, radiation-blocking lenses for sunglasses, excimer laser angioplasty, robotic surgery, smoke-detection equipment, cordless tools, microbe autoanalysis, equipment to diagnose balance disorders, advanced x-ray imaging, skin-damage assessment, and ocular screening. Consider the following nine examples from different decades that have directly benefited the medical, fitness, and wellness industries:

- *1999*. The Space Station In-Flight Cytometry Project pioneered a new triangular flow cell technology that improves resolution and provides three times more uniformity on a day-to-day basis than older systems. With flow cytometry, photodetectors evaluate tissue cells in a suspension as they flow through a sensing region where light signals indicate their important biologic properties. The original research emerged from NASA's need to know how microgravity affected the immune system. Preliminary evidence from space shuttle flights suggested a depressive effect on immunity. To help decipher this medical mystery, NASA sought hardware development of a machine that could rapidly separate and examine cells. The cancer-fighting benefits of flow cytometry include evaluating mutant cells in their early developmental state. The technique also determines cellular sensitivity to different chemotherapy drugs, cellular growth patterns, and the capacity of cancer cells to spread. The equipment permits a better understanding of a patient's tumor, which translates into more-rapid and effective treatment and more-positive confirmation of tumor status. Other potential clinical uses of flow cytometry involve early detection of leukemia, chemosensitivity studies before undertaking chemotherapy, antibody analysis, and detection of pathogenic organisms.

  Other technologies included the Parking Garage Automation System (PGAS), a state-of-the-art network sensor system that can be installed around and within public parking garages to guide a motorist to an open facility and eventual parking space; a new imaging sensor based on technology that greatly reduces power consumption and lowers the number of parts required in imaging systems (thus reducing cost). Applications include PC video conferencing, camcorders, digital still cameras, portable video cell phones, broadcast television, and medical applications (e.g., x-ray products including DXA technology to assess BMD with 1/100th the dosage of a dental x-ray); a chemical/mechanical heat pump that uses an environmentally safe fluid with zero ozone-depletion potential to improve performance by up to 20% in vapor-compression heat pumps, air conditioners, and

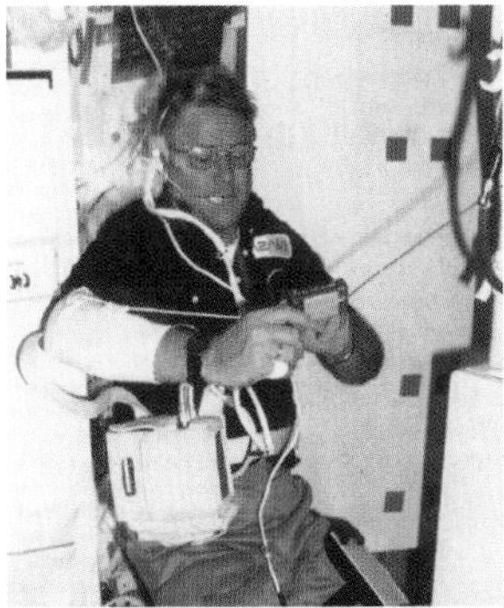
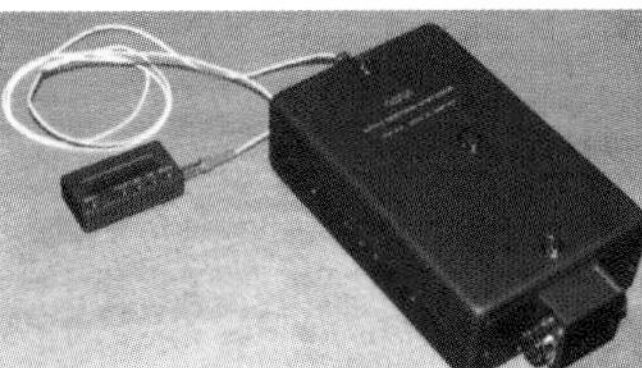

Telemetry Patient Monitoring System (PMS) transmits vital signs from single or multiple individuals to a computer for processing.

refrigeration systems; a 9-oz portable device (PocketScience) approximately the size of a pocket calculator, which uses two AA batteries and sends and receives e-mail and faxes from anywhere in the world without incompatibility concerns. The device operates by holding it against a phone handset and pushing a button. Internally, the device functions by incorporating special modulation schemes and error-correction, data-compression, and data-communication protocols.

- *1998.* NASA designed an improved telemetry system for ground monitoring of astronauts' vital signs in space. An outgrowth of this research, the Patient Monitoring System (see above unnumbered figure), monitors hospital patients with a small transmitter that allows the individual to move freely, unencumbered by wires. The electrocardiogram is transmitted to a recorder and central control station, where medical personnel can simultaneously monitor multiple patients at different building locations.
- *1997.* NASA-sponsored research developed a new insulated capacitive electrode for astronaut use on longer-duration missions; it uses a thin dielectric film electrode. NASA licensed the electrode technology to a manufacturer of personal heart rate monitors and exercise machines in the physical fitness, medical, and home markets. To assess heart rate, the exerciser grasps a handle fitted with the electrode. While the person exercises, readout of the heart rate score appears within 10 seconds via a light-emitting diode (LED).
- *1997.* A scalp-cooling system based on NASA space suit technology helps patients undergoing cancer chemotherapy retard hair loss. The system cools the head before, during, and after drug administration, with application time depending on the drug and its dosage. With scalp cooling, 63% of patients lost almost no hair, and 9% suffered only moderate hair loss.
- *1996.* NASA–Ames Research Center devised methods to improve neurosurgical techniques. On prolonged space missions, robotic telepresence surgery allows a surgeon on Earth to control a procedure during space flight by issuing commands. Robotics also has significant surgical potential on Earth. For example, brain tumors typically have a different density than normal brain tissue, allowing neurosurgeons to locate tumor edges by tactile differences. Potentially, the robotic telepresence procedure may feel differentiations in brain structures with greater precision, allowing more-exact movements and greater instrument control during an operation. The robot's probes, smaller than standard probes, still provide speed and maximum pressure under control of a computer program that "learns" as it gains experience. The neural-net software learns to distinguish tumors from normal brain tissue by remembering the pressure signatures of the different tissues. A biopsy needle then extracts a tissue sample through the probe. The robot would execute each command within safe limits and then await further instructions. With robotic computer control and miniaturized probes (approximately one-third the size of a 0.2-in probe), surgeons reduce the likelihood of injuring brain tissue or penetrating an artery. A modified form of the brain surgery robot could be used for other kinds of surgery requiring pressure, temperature, or chemical sensors.
- *1994.* Research at Dreyden Research Center created a device that prevents needle pricks of patient and surgeon during postoperative suturing.
- *1987.* "Cool suits," originally developed for NASA, protect wearers from fatigue, dehydration, and possible physical collapse from an elevated body temperature. The device consists of helmet liners and/or body vests through which a fluid circulates; a refrigeration unit cools the fluid as it passes through tubes to the garments. Auto racers now use this equipment to counter the excruciatingly high temperatures in their vehicle cockpits.
- *1986.* A microminiaturized fluid control system initially designed to search for microorganisms during the Viking Lander Mars exploration delivers preprogrammed amounts of insulin via a Programmable Implantable Medication System (PIMS) to diabetics over extended periods.

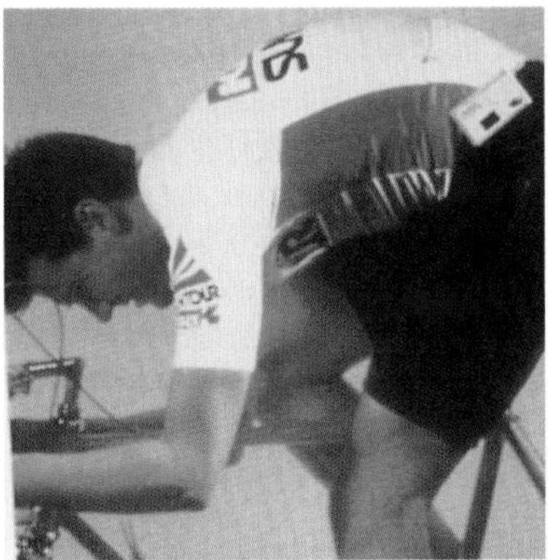

Programmable Implantable Medication System (PIMS) delivers preprogrammed amounts of insulin to diabetics.

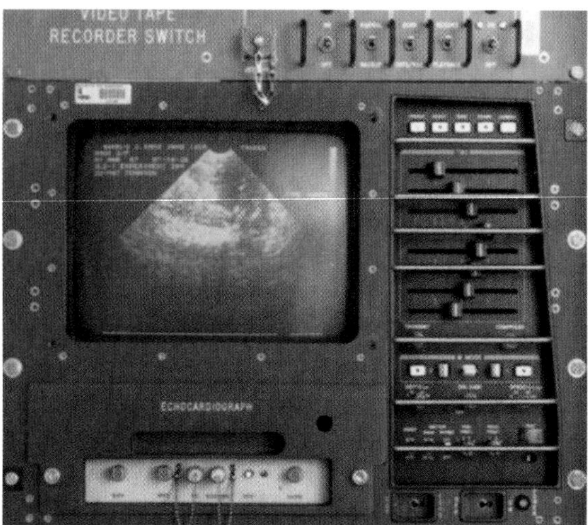

Ultrasound instrument monitors heart function during space missions.

- *1976.* Ames Research Center teamed with Stanford Children's Hospital, Palo Alto, CA, to analyze crippled children's gait patterns. To eliminate the typical long bundle of wires leading to recording equipment, NASA scientists adapted their biotelemetry technique that uses radio transmission to monitor astronauts' bodily functions in space. The modified instrumentation uses tiny electrical sensors placed on the legs to collect information about how each muscle group contributes to a child's walking. Small radio transmitters send signals to a receiver. Exercise physiology laboratories have used the same technique extensively to collect physiologic data during different modes of exercise under a variety of environmental conditions.

  Ames Research Center engineers also developed an ultrasound instrument to monitor heart function during space missions (above unnumbered figure). The device formed images of internal structures similar to the way submarines use sonar to detect underwater objects. Ultrasound has proven safer and easier than catheterization, which requires injecting a dye into the circulation and taking x-ray pictures of the structures. The technique initially tested acutely ill infants. Twenty-five years later, ultrasound testing remains routine technology in diverse medical specialties.

INTEGRATIVE QUESTION

Counter the argument that "spending money and resources on space missions is a waste of time and taxpayers' money."

Summary

1. On Earth's surface, gravity provides an invisible attraction force that makes any mass exert downward force or have weight. Sir Isaac Newton (1642–1727) discovered the universality of the gravitational law.
2. The escape velocity of an object from celestial body depends on the mass and radius of that body. Escape velocity from Earth equals 25,039 $\text{mi} \cdot \text{h}^{-1}$.
3. The force of gravity never reaches an absolute zero value (called zero-g) because a gravitational force still exists. The term *microgravity,* not *weightlessness* (or *zero-g*), describes what an astronaut perceives during space flight.
4. When an elevator descends quickly, one perceives a lessening of weight because of reduced force between the feet and elevator floor. If the elevator cable suddenly snaps and the elevator plummets downward, the force against the feet equals zero until the elevator strikes bottom. If persons could lift their feet off the floor before hitting the ground, they would experience free-fall similar to space flight.
5. Two different strategies have simulated space flights' microgravity environment: (1) test equipment to create gravity conditions for brief periods using sounding rockets and objects dropped from towers and into tubes and (2) simulated microgravity conditions using humans in head-down bed rest, wheelchair-bound individuals, water immersion, immobilization and confinement, and parabolic flights plus in vitro centrifugation, mathematical modeling, and computer simulations.
6. On October 4, 1957, the Russian's Sputnik-1 became the first Earth-orbiting satellite. One month later, Sputnik-2 remained in orbit for almost 200 days with a dog on board.
7. NASA had two main early goals: (1) launch a man into space and return him safely to Earth and (2) develop the capability of humans to endure space missions.
8. The most significant technologic achievement of the 20th century took place when Apollo 11 astronauts Aldrin and Armstrong landed on the moon's surface.
9. During the first few days in microgravity, fluid shifts from the lower body to the upper body. Total fluid volume also decreases, which reduces the heart's work effort. Continued microgravity exposure decreases overall heart size, mainly from reduced left ventricular volume, particularly left ventricular end-diastolic volume.
10. In microgravity, the greatest postural instability occurs in tests requiring vestibular information. Readaptation begins quickly within a few hours after landing and returns to near normal in approximately 4 days.
11. NASA's greatest biomedical concern during space missions involves the significant 1% per month loss in weight-bearing bone mass. This effect could compromise crew health and safety during an exploration-class mission to Mars, including performance of critical EVA tasks, landing maneuvers, and procedures for leaving orbit on return to Earth.

12. Permanent neuromuscular dysfunction has not occurred during prolonged space missions. However, in-flight and postflight changes during missions of nearly 1 year reveal altered muscular coordination patterns, delayed-onset muscle soreness and generalized muscular fatigue and weakness.
13. Countermeasures systematically attempt to minimize space flight's potentially harmful deconditioning effects on crew physiologic function, performance, and overall health during mission-critical maneuvers during re-entry and landing.
14. Without gravity, normal biologic functions become more susceptible to short- and longer-term maladaptations such as SMS—a syndrome characterized by headache and dizziness, drowsiness, malaise, poor concentration, disorientation, nausea, pallor, and sudden vomiting without dry heaves.
15. The energy balance equation has not been satisfied successfully on most space missions for two reasons: (1) increased energy demands of space flight and (2) decreased food intake.
16. Decreases in lean body mass, muscle volume, and muscle strength; altered muscle fiber microarchitecture; and atrophy of skeletal muscles that support posture and locomotion characterize maladaptations to microgravity.
17. Astronaut health, safety, and performance during and following long-duration missions require additional research about (1) loss of weight-bearing bone and muscle; (2) vestibular function, the vestibular ocular reflex, and sensorimotor integration; (3) orthostatic intolerance upon return to Earth's gravity; (4) radiation hazards; and (5) stress-related physiologic effects.
18. Technologies developed by NASA over the past 30 years have produced more than 30,000 secondary commercial spinoff applications, many providing new breakthroughs in the medical, health, and physical sciences.

References

1. Akima H, et al. Leg-press resistance training during 20 days of 60 head-down-tilt bed rest prevents muscle deconditioning. Eur J Appl Physiol 2000;82:30.
2. Bailey JV, et al. Radiological protection and medical dosimetry for the Skylab crewman. In: Johnston RS, Dietlein LF, eds. Biomedical results from Skylab (NASA SP-377). Washington, DC: U.S. Government Printing Office, 1977.
3. Baldwin KM. Effect of spaceflight on the functional, biochemical, and metabolic properties of skeletal muscle. Med Sci Sports Exerc 1996;28:983.
4. Berry CA. Summary of medical experience in the Apollo 7 through Apollo 11 manned space flights. Aerosp Med 1970;41:500.
5. Blewett C, et al. Quantitative EMG analysis in soleus and plantaris during hindlimb suspension and recovery. J Appl Physiol 1993;74:2057.
6. Blomqvist GR. Regulation of the systemic circulation at microgravity and during readaptation to 1G. Med Sci Sports Exerc 1996;28(10 suppl):S9.
7. Buckey JC, et al. Orthostatic intolerance after spaceflight. J Appl Physiol 1996;81:7.
8. Bulbulian R, et al. The effects of strength training and centrifuge exposure on 1 Gz tolerance. Aviat Space Environ Med 1994;65:1097.
9. Bungo MW, et al. Cardiovascular deconditioning during space flight and the use of saline as a countermeasures to orthostatic intolerance. Aviat Space Environ Med 1985;5:985.
10. Burton RE, Smith AH. Adaptation to acceleration environments. In: Fregly MJ, Blatteis CM, eds. Handbook of physiology. Section 4, Environmental physiology, vol 2. American Physiological Society. New York: Oxford University Press, 1996:943.
11. Charles JB, Lathers CM. Cardiovascular adaptation to spaceflight. J Clin Pharmacol 1991;31:1010.
12. Chou JL, et al. Acceleration tolerance: effect of exercise, acceleration training; bed rest and weightlessness deconditioning. A compendium of research (1950–1996). NASA TM-112214. Washington, DC: National Aeronautics and Space Administration, 1997.
13. Chouker AM, et al. Simulated microgravity, psychic stress, and immune cells in men: observations during 120-day 6° HDT. J Appl Physiol 2001;90:1736.
14. Collaeran PN, et al. Alterations in skeletal perfusion with simulated microgravity: a possible mechanism for bone remodeling. J Appl Physiol 2000;89:1046.
15. Convertino VA. Aerobic fitness, endurance training and orthostatic intolerance. Exerc Sport Sci Rev 1987;15:223.
16. Convertino VA. Potential benefits of maximal exercise just prior to return from weightlessness. Aviat Space Environ Med 1987;58:568.
17. Convertino VA. Physiological adaptations to weightlessness: effects on exercise and work performance. Exerc Sports Sci Rev 1990;18:119.
18. Convertino VA. Exercise and adaptation to microgravity environments. In: Fregly MJ, Blatteis CM, eds. Handbook of physiology. Section 4, Environmental physiology, vol 2. American Physiological Society. New York: Oxford University Press, 1996:815.
19. Convertino VA. Exercise as a countermeasure for physiological adaptation to prolonged spaceflight. Med Sci Sports Exerc 1996;28:999.
20. Convertino VA. G-factor as a tool in basic research: mechanisms of orthostatic tolerance. J Grav Physiol 1999;6:P-73.
21. Convertino VA. Effects of microgravity on exercise performance. In: Garrett WE, Kirkendall DT, eds. Exercise and sport science. Philadelphia: Lippincott Williams & Wilkins, 2000.
22. Convertino VA. Mechanisms of blood pressure regulation that differ in men repeatedly exposed to high-G acceleration. Am J Physiol Regul Integr Comp Physiol 2001;280:R947.
23. Convertino VA, et al. Changes in size and compliance of the calf after 30 days of simulated microgravity. J Appl Physiol 1989;66:1509.
24. Convertino VA, et al. Changes in volume, muscle compartment, and compliance of the lower extremities in man following 30 days of exposure to simulated microgravity. Aviat Space Environ Med 1989;60:653.
25. Convertino VA, et al. Impairment of carotid-cardiac vagal baroreflex in wheelchair-dependent quadriplegics. Am J Physiol 1991;260:R576.
26. Daunton NG. Adaptation of the vestibular system to microgravity. In: Fregly MJ, Blatteis CM, eds. Handbook of physiology. Section 4, Environmental physiology, vol 2. American Physiological Society. New York: Oxford University Press, 1996:765.
27. Davis JR. Medical issues for a mission to Mars. Aviat Space Environ Med 1999;70:162.
28. DeHart RL. Fundamentals of aerospace medicine. 2nd ed. Baltimore: Williams & Wilkins, 1996.
29. Dietlein LF. Skylab: a beginning. In: Johnston RS, Dietlein LF, eds. Biomedical results from Skylab (NASA SP-377). Washington, DC: U.S. Government Printing Office, 1977.
30. Dietlein LF, Johnson RS. U.S. manned space flight: the first twenty years. A biomedical status report. Acta Astronaut 1981;8(9):893.
31. Edgerton VR, Roy RR. Regulation of skeletal muscle fiber size, shape and function. J Biomech 1991;24(suppl 1):123.
32. Edgerton VR, Roy RR. Neuromuscular adaptations to actual and simulated spaceflight. In: Fregly MJ, Blatteis CM, eds. Handbook of physiology. Section 4, Environmental physiology, vol 1. American Physiological Society. New York: Oxford University Press, 1996:721.
33. Edgerton VR, Roy RR. Physiology of a microgravity environment. Invited review: gravitational biology of the neuromotor systems: a perspective to the next era. J Appl Physiol 2000;89:1224.
34. Engelke KA, et al. Autonomic functions and orthostatic responses 24 h after acute intense exercise in paraplegic subjects. Am J Physiol 1994;26:R1189.
35. Fettman MJ. Dietary instead of pharmacological management to counter the adverse effects of physiological adaptations to space flight. Pflugers Arch 2000;441:R15.
36. Fitts RH, et al. Physiology of a microgravity environment. Invited review: microgravity and skeletal muscle. J Appl Physiol 2000;89:823.

37. Fortney SM, et al. The physiology of bed rest. In: Fregly MJ, Blatteis CM, eds. Handbook of physiology. Section 4, Environmental physiology, vol 2. American Physiological Society. New York: Oxford University Press, 1996:889.
38. Fowler B, et al. A review of cognitive and perceptual-motor performance in space. Aviat Space Environ Med. 2000;71:A66.
39. Frabjem K, et al. Effects of gender on the autonomic modulation of the cardiovascular responses to lower body negative pressure. Aviat Space Environ Med 2000;71:626.
40. Fregly MJ, Blatteis CM, eds. Handbook of physiology. Section 4, Environmental physiology, vol 1. American Physiological Society. New York: Oxford University Press, 1996.
41. Fritsch-Yelle JM, et al. Subnormal norepinephrine release relates to presyncope in astronauts after spaceflight. J Appl Physiol 1996;81:2134.
42. Frost HM. Perspectives: a proposed general model of the "Mechanostat." Anat Rec 1996;244:139.
43. Graybiel A, et al. Equipment M131. Human vestibular function. In: Johnson RS, Dietlein LF, eds. Biomedical results from Skylab. NASA SP-377. Washington, DC: Government Printing Office, 1977.
44. Greenleaf JE, et al. Handgrip and general muscular strength and endurance during prolonged bedrest with isometric and isotonic leg exercise training. Aviat Space Environ Med 1983;54:696.
45. Greenleaf JE, et al. Cycle-powered short radius (1.9 m) centrifuge: effect of exercise versus passive acceleration on heart rate in humans. NASA technical memorandum 110433. Ames Research Center. Moffett Field, CA: NASA, 1997.
46. Grigoriev AI, Koslovskaya IB. Effect of weightlessness and hypokinesia on velocity and strength properties of human muscles. Kosm Biol Aviakosm Med 1987;21:27.
47. Grigoriev AI, et al. Metabolic and hormonal status of crewmembers in short-term spaceflight. Aviat Space Environ Med 1987;58:A121.
48. Hankins TC, et al. Test and evaluation of exercise-enhanced preoxygenation in U-2 operations. Aviat Space Environ Med 2000;71:822.
49. Hargens AR, Watenpaugh DE. Cardiovascular adaptation to spaceflight. Med Sci Sports Exerc 1996;28(8):977.
50. Harris BA, et al. Physical examination during space flight. Mayo Clinic Proc 1997;72:301.
51. Herault S, et al. Cardiac, arterial and venous adaptation to weightlessness during 6-month MIR spaceflights with and without thigh cuffs (bracelets). Eur J Appl Physiol 2000;81:384.
52. Hoffler GW. Cardiovascular studies of U.S. space crews: an overview and perspective. In: Hwang NHC, Normann NA, eds. Cardiovascular flow dynamics and measurements. Baltimore: University Park Press, 1977:335.
53. Huntoon Cl, et al. Endocrine and biochemical functions. In: Nicogossian AE, et al. Space physiology and medicine. 3rd ed. Philadelphia: Lea & Febiger. 1994:305.
54. Inoue M, et al. Altered biochemical markers of bone turnover in humans during 120 days of bed rest. Bone 2000;26:281.
55. Iyengar A, Rao BS. Effect of varying energy and protein intake on nitrogen balance in adults engaged in heavy manual labor. Br J Nutr 1979;41:19.
56. Jennings RT. Managing space motion sickness. J Vestib Res 1997;8:67.
57. Kraemer WJ, et al. The effects of 10 days of spaceflight on the shuttle Endeavor on predominantly fast-twitch muscles in the rat. Histochem Cell Biol 2000;114:349.
58. Kreitenberg A, et al. The "Space Cycle"™ self-powered human centrifuge: a proposed countermeasure for prolonged human spaceflight. Aviat Space Environ Med 1998;69:66.
59. Lackner JR, DiZio P. Multisensory, cognitive and motor influences on human spatial orientation in weightlessness. J Vestib Res 1993;3:361.
60. Lackner JR, DiZio P. Artificial gravity as a countermeasure in long-duration space flight. J Neurosci Res 2000 15;62:169.
61. Lambertz D, et al. Effects of long-term spaceflight on mechanical properties of muscles in humans. J Appl Physiol 2001;90:179.
62. Lane HW. Energy requirements for space flight. J Nutr 1992;122:13.
63. Lane HW, Gretebeck RJ. Metabolic energy required for flight. Adv Space Res 1994;14:147.
64. Lane HW, Gretebeck RJ. Nutrition, endocrinology, and body composition during space flight. Nutr Res 1998;18:1923.
65. Lane H, Schoeller DA. Nutrition in space flight and weightlessness. Boca Raton, FL: CRC Press, 1999.
66. Lane HW, Smith SM. Physiological adaptations to space flight. Life Support Biosphere Sci 1999;6:13.
67. Lane HW, et al. Nutrition in space: lessons from the past applied to the future. Am J Clin Nutr 1994;60:801S.
68. Layne CS, et al. Neuromuscular activation patterns during treadmill walking after space flight. Exp Brain Res 1997;113:104.
69. Layne CS, et al. Effect of long-duration spaceflight on postural control during self-generated perturbations. J Appl Physiol 2001;90:997.
70. Leach CS, Johnson PC. Influence of spaceflight on erythrokinetics in man. Science. 1984;225:216.
71. Leach CS, et al. The endocrine and metabolic responses to space flight. Med Sci Sports Exerc 1982;15:432.
72. Leach CS, et al. Changes in total body water during space flight. J Clin Pharmacol 1991;31:1001.
73. Leach CS, et al. Regulation of body fluid compartments during short-term spaceflight. J Appl Physiol 1996;81:105.
74. LeBlanc A, et al. Muscle volume, MRI relaxation times (T2), and body composition after spaceflight. J Appl Physiol 2000;89:2158.
75. Leonard JI, et al. Quantitation of tissue loss during prolonged space flight. Am J Clin Nutr 1983;38:667.
76. Lovejoy JC, et al. A paradigm of experimentally induced mild hyperthyroidism: effects on nitrogen balance, body composition, and energy expenditure in healthy young men. J Clin Endocrinol Metab 1997;82:765.
77. Maillet A, et al. Cardiovascular and hormonal changes induced by isolation and confinement. Med Sci Sports Exerc 1996;28(10 Suppl):S53.
78. Maillet A, et al. Orthostatic tolerance and hormonal changes in women during 120 days of head-down bed rest. Aviat Space Environ Med 2000;71:706.
79. Massion L. Movement, posture and equilibrium: interaction and coordination. Prog Neurobiol 1992;38:35.
80. Massion L, et al. Axial synergies under microgravity conditions. J Vestib Res 1993;3:275.
81. Mayr W, et al. MYOSTIM-FES to prevent muscle atrophy in microgravity and bed rest: preliminary report. Artif Organs 1999;23:428.
82. Mohler S. The world's first practical flight pressure suit. Aviat Space Environ Med 1998;69:802.
83. Moody SA, Golden C. Developmental biology research in space: issues and directions in the era of the international space station. Dev Biol 2000 1;228:1.
84. Moore AD, et al. Maximal exercise as a countermeasure to orthostatic intolerance after spaceflight. Med Sci Sports Exerc 2000;33:75.
85. Navidi M, et al. Effect of excess dietary salt on calcium metabolism and bone mineral in a spaceflight rat model. J Appl Physiol 1995;78:70.
86. Nelson GA. Radiation in microgravity. In: Fregly MJ, Blatteis CM, eds. Handbook of physiology. Section 4, Environmental physiology, vol 2. American Physiological Society. New York: Oxford University Press, 1996:785.
87. Nicogossian AE, Gaiser K. Biomedical challenges of spaceflight. In: DeHart RL, ed. Fundamentals of aerospace medicine. 2nd ed. Baltimore: Williams & Wilkins, 1996:953.
88. Nicogossian AE, et al. Space physiology and medicine. 3rd ed. Philadelphia: Lea & Febiger, 1994.
89. Oman CM. Motional sickness. A synthesis and evaluation of the sensory conflict theory. Can J Physiol Pharmacol 1990;68:294.
90. Oman CM. Sensory conflict theory and space sickness: our changing perspective. J Vestib Res 1997;8:51.
91. Parcell AC, et al. An upper arm model for simulated weightlessness. Acta Physiol Scand 2000;169:47.
92. Peusner KD. Development of the gravity sensing system. J Neurosci Res 2001 15;63:103.
93. Pool SL, et al. Medical evaluation for astronaut selection and longitudinal studies. In: Nicogossian AE, et al. Space physiology and medicine. 3rd ed. Philadelphia: Lea & Febiger, 1994.
94. Prisk GK, et al. Pulmonary diffusing capacity, capillary blood volume, and cardiac output during sustained microgravity. J Appl Physiol 1993;81:2134.
95. Rambaut PC, et al. Observations on energy balance in man during space flight. Am J Physiol 1977;233:R208.
96. Rice BL, Lane HW. Dietary studies in the joint US–Russian space program. J Am Diet Assoc 1997;97(10 suppl 2):S127.
97. Riley DA, et al. Rat hindlimb unloading: soleus histochemistry, ultrastructure, and electromyography. J Appl Physiol 1990;69:58.
98. Ronca AE, et al. Physiology of a microgravity environment. Selected contribution: effects of spaceflight during pregnancy on labor and birth at 1 G. J Appl Physiol 2000;89:849.
99. Roy RR, et al. The plasticity of skeletal muscle: effects of neuromuscular activity. Exerc Sport Sci Rev 1991;19:269.

100. Sawin CF. Biomedical investigations conducted in support of the extended duration orbiter medical project. Aviat Space Environ Med 1999;70:169.
101. Schlegel TT, et al. Orthostatic intolerance and motion sickness after parabolic flight. J Appl Physiol. 2001;90:67-82.
102. Serrador JM, et al. Cerebral vasoconstriction precedes orthostatic intolerance after parabolic flight. Brain Res Bull. 2000 1;53:113.
103. Smith SM, et al. Calcium metabolism before, during and after a 3-mo spaceflight: kinetic and biochemical changes. Am J Physiol 1999;277:1.
104. Space Science Board. National Research Council. A strategy for space biology and medical sciences for the 1980s and 1990s. Washington, DC: National Academy Press, 1987.
105. Space Studies Board. National Research Council. Radiation hazards to crews of interplanetary missions: biological issues and research strategies. Washington, DC: National Academy Press, 1996.
106. Space Science Board. National Research Council. A strategy for research in space biology and medicine in the new century. Washington, DC: National Academy Press, 1998.
107. Stein TP. Nutrition and muscle loss in humans during spaceflight. Adv Space Biol Med 1999;7:49.
108. Stein TP. The relationship between dietary intake, exercise, energy balance and the space craft environment. Pflugers Arch. 2000;441:R21.
109. Stein TP, Leskiw MJ. Oxidant damage during and after spaceflight. Am J Physiol Endocrinol Metab 2000;278:375.
110. Stein TP, et al. The effect of spaceflight on human protein metabolism. Am J Physiol 1993;264:E824.
111. Stein TP, et al. Diet and nitrogen metabolism during spaceflight on the shuttle. J Appl Physiol 1996;81:82.
112. Stein TP, et al. Measurement of energy expenditure in rhesus monkeys during spaceflight using doubly labeled water ($^{2}H_2{}^{18}O$). J Appl Physiol 1996;81:201.
113. Stein TP, et al. Energy expenditure and balance during spaceflight on the space shuttle. Am J Physiol 1999;45:R1739.
114. Strollo F. Hormonal changes in humans during spaceflight. Adv Space Biol Med. 1999;7:99.
115. Strollo F. Adaptation of the human endocrine system to microgravity in the context of integrative physiology and ageing. Pflugers Arch. 2000;441:R85.
116. Thornton WE, Rummel JA. Muscular deconditioning and its prevention in space flight. In: Johnson RS, Dietlein LF, eds. Biomedical results from Skylab. Chapter 32. NASA SP-377. Washington, DC: Scientific and Technical Information Office. National Aeronautics and Space Administration, 1977.
117. Thornton WE, et al. Anthropometric changes and fluid shifts. In: Johnson RS, Dietlein LF, eds. Biomedical results from Skylab. NASA SP-377. Washington, DC: Scientific and Technical Information Office. National Aeronautics and Space Administration, 1977.
118. Thornton WE, et al. Changes in leg volume during microgravity simulation. Aviat Space Environ Med 1992;63:789.
119. Tipton CM. Animal models and their importance to human physiological responses in microgravity. Med Sci Sports Exerc 1996:S94.
120. Tipton CM, Hargens A. Physiological adaptations and countermeasures associated with long-duration spaceflights. Med Sci Sports Exerc 1996;28:974.
121. Turner RT. Invited review: what do we know about the effects of spaceflight on bone? J Appl Physiol. 2000;89:840.
122. Tilton FE, et al. Long-term follow-up of Skylab bone demineralization. Aviat Space Environ Med 1980;11:1209.
123. Turner RT. Physiology of a microgravity environment. Invited review: what do we know about the effects of spaceflight on bone? J Appl Physiol 2000;89:840.
124. Udden MM, et al. Human erythropoiesis during spaceflight. Blood 1991;78(suppl 1):367A.
125. Van Huss WD, Heusner WW. Space flight research relevant to health, physical education, and recreation. With particular reference to Skylab's life science experiments. NAS 1979;19:148.
126. Vaziri ND, et al. Upregulation of NOS by simulated microgravity, potential cause of orthostatic intolerance. J Appl Physiol 2000;89:338.
127. Vernikos J, Convertino VA. Advantages and disadvantages of fludrocortisone or saline load in preventing post-spaceflight orthostatic hypotension. Acta Astronaut 1994;33:259.
128. Vico L, et al. Effects of long-term microgravity exposure on cancellous and cortical weight-bearing bones of cosmonauts. Lancet 2000;355:1607.
129. Vodovotz T, et al. Food and nutrition in space. Nutrition 2000;16:534.
130. Vogel H, Kass JR. European vestibular experiments on Spacelab-1 mission: 7. Ocular counter rolling measurements pre- and post-flight. Exp Brain Res 1986;64:284.
131. Vogel JM, Whittle MW. Bone mineral changes: the second manned Skylab mission. Aviat Space Environ Med 1976;47:396.
132. Vose GP. Review of roentgenographic bone demineralization studies of the Gemini spaceflights. Am J Roentgenol Radium Ther Nucl Med 1974;121:1.
133. Watenpaugh DE, et al. Effects of spaceflight on human calf hemodynamics. J Appl Physiol. 2001;90:1552.
134. Wautenpaugh DE, Hargens AR. The cardiovascular system in microgravity. In: Fregly MJ, Blatteis CM, eds. Handbook of physiology. Section 4, Environmental physiology, vol 1. American Physiological Society. New York: Oxford University Press, 1996:631.
135. Webb JT, et al. Exercise-enhanced preoxygenation increases protection from decompression sickness. Aviat Space Environ Med 1996;67:618.
136. West JB, et al. Respiratory system in microgravity. In: Fregly MJ, Blatteis CM, eds. Handbook of physiology. Section 4, Environmental physiology, vol 1. American Physiological Society. New York: Oxford University Press, 1996:675.
137. Whedon GD, et al. Mineral and nitrogen balance study, results of metabolic observations on Skylab II 28-day orbital mission. Acta Astronom 1975;2:297.
138. Whitson PA, et al. Alterations in renal stone risk factors after space flight. J Urol 1993;150:803.
139. Yasuda H, et al. Effective dose equivalent on the ninth Shuttle–Mir mission (STS-91). Radiat Res. 2000;154:705.
140. Young RW. Acute radiation syndrome. In: Conklin JJ, Walker RI, eds. Military radiobiology. New York: Academic Press, 1987.
141. Zhou MY, et al. Myosin heavy chain isoforms of human muscle after short term spaceflight. J Appl Physiol 1995;78:1740.

Microgravity-Related Internet Sites

Ask the Microgravity Scientist
zeta.lerc.nasa.gov/science/comments.htm
Astronaut Biographies
www.jsc.nasa.gov/Bios/
Aviation, Space, and Environmental Medicine
www.asma.org/html/journal.htm
California Institute of Technology Space Radiation laboratory
www.srl.caltech.edu/
California Institute of Technology Jet Propulsion laboratory
www.jpl.nasa.gov/
California Space Institute
calspace.ucsd.edu/
Centennial of Flight
centennialofflight.gov/
Directorate of Manned Spaceflight and Microgravity
www.estec.esa.nl/spaceflight/index.htm
Discovery Channel
www.discovery.com/stories/science/iss/iss.html
Dryden Flight Research Center
www.dfrc.nasa.gov/
Emotion of Space
www.hq.nasa.gov/osf/station/sp_emotion.html
Encyclopedia Astronautica
www.friends-partners.org/~mwade/spaceflt.htm
Euro Space Center Web Cam
www.ping.be/eurospace/cam.htm
Exercise Physiology Laboratory at NASA-Johnson Space Center
www.jsc.nasa.gov/sa/sd/sd3/exl/index.htm
Glenn Public Affairs Image Gallery
www.grc.nasa.gov/WWW/PAO/html/paogalry.htm
Goleta Air & Space Museum
www.air-and-space.com/%7ebrianl/museums.htm
History of Astronomy and Space Science
www-hpcc.astro.washington.edu/scied/astro/astrohistory.html
Human Physiology in Space
www.nsbri.org/HumanPhysSpace/index.html
ImageNet
zeno.grc.nasa.gov/

International Space Station Challenge
voyager.cet.edu/iss/
J-Track Satellite Tracking
liftoff.msfc.nasa.gov/RealTime/jtrack/
Johnson Space Center
www.jsc.nasa.gov/
Keck Observatory
www2.keck.hawaii.edu:3636/
Kennedy Space Center
www.ksc.nasa.gov/
Lewis Center for Educational Research
www.avstc.org/
Malin Space Science Systems
www.mass.com
Marshall Space Flight Center
www.msfc.nasa.gov/
Microgravity News and Research
www.microgravity.com/
Microgravity News
mgnews.msfc.nasa.gov/site/
Microgravity Science Division
microgravity.grc.nasa.gov/
Moonlink
www.moonlink.com/
Mullard Space Science Laboratory
www.mssl.ucl.ac.uk
NASA Ames Center for Bioinformatics
biocomp.arc.nasa.gov/
NASA Astronaut Biographies
www.jsc.nasa.gov/Bios/
NASA Basics of Space Flight Learners' Workbook
www.jpl.nasa.gov/basics/bsf.htm
NASA Centers' Homepages
www.nasa.gov/hqpao/nasa_centers.html
NASA Education Program
education.nasa.gov/
NASA Facts
www.jsc.nasa.gov/pao/factsheets/factsheets/spinoffs/
NASA Historical Archive
science.ksc.nasa.gov/history/history.html
NASA History Office
www.hq.nasa.gov/office/pao/History/history.html
NASA Human Spaceflight
spaceflight.nasa.gov
NASA Image Exchange
nix.nasa.gov/
NASA International Space Station
spaceflight.nasa.gov/station/
NASA Langley Research Center
www.larc.nasa.gov/
NASA Life & Microgravity
www.hq.nasa.gov/office/olmsa/
NASA Life Sciences Research laboratories
www.jsc.nasa.gov/sa/sd/sd3/sd3.htm
NASA Medical Sciences Division
www.jsc.nasa.gov/sa/sd/default.html
NASA Microgravity
microgravity.grc.nasa.gov/
NASA Observatorium
observe.ivv.nasa.gov/nasa/core.shtml.html
NASA Office of Space Flight
www.hq.nasa.gov/osf
NASA Photo Gallery
www.nasa.gov/gallery/photo/index.html
NASA Realtime Data
spaceflight.nasa.gov/realdata/tracking/index.html
NASA Search
www.nasa.gov/search/
NASA Space Shuttle
www.spaceflight.nasa.gov/shuttle/
NASA Space Shuttle Launches
science.ksc.nasa.gov/shuttle/missions/missions.html
NASA Spacelink
spacelink.nasa.gov
NASA Technology
nasatechnology.nasa.gov/
National Space Biomedical Institute
www.nsbri.org/
National Space Development Agency of Japan (NASDA)
www.nasda.go.jp/index_e.html
National Space Science Data Center
nssdc.gsfc.nasa.gov/
On-line Educational materals
spacelink.nasa.gov/Instructional.Materials/On-line.Educational.Activities/
Physics Classroom
www.glenbrook.k12.il.us/gbssci/phys/Class/BBoard.html
Rover Ranch
prime.jsc.nasa.gov/ROV/
Russian Space Agency
liftoff.msfc.nasa.gov/rsa/rsa.html
Russian Space Research Institute
arc.iki.rssi.ru/Welcome.html
San Diego Aerospace Museum
www.aerospacemuseum.org/
Science at NASA
science.nasa.gov/default.stm
Science Joy Wagon (The Physics Zone)
www.sciencejoywagon.com/physciszone/
Smithsonian National Air and Space Museum
www.nasm.edu/
Space.com
www.space.com/
Space Grant Web Sites
calspace.ucsd.edu/spacegrant/webmap/sg_homepages.html
SpaceNews.com
www.spacenews.com/
SpaceZone
www.spacezone.com/audsch.htm
Space Science
spacescience.nasa.gov
Space Team Online
quest.arc.nasa.gov/space/team/index.html
Space Telescope Science Institute
oposite.stsci.edu/pubinfo/
Space Weather.com
spaceweather.com
Spacedaily
www.spacedaily.com/
Universe Today
www.universetoday.com/
Vanderbilt Center for Space Physiology and Medicine
www.mc.vanderbilt.edu/gcrc/space/
Visible Earth
visibleearth.nasa.gov/
Women of NASA
quest.arc.nasa.gov/women/intro.html

SECTION 6

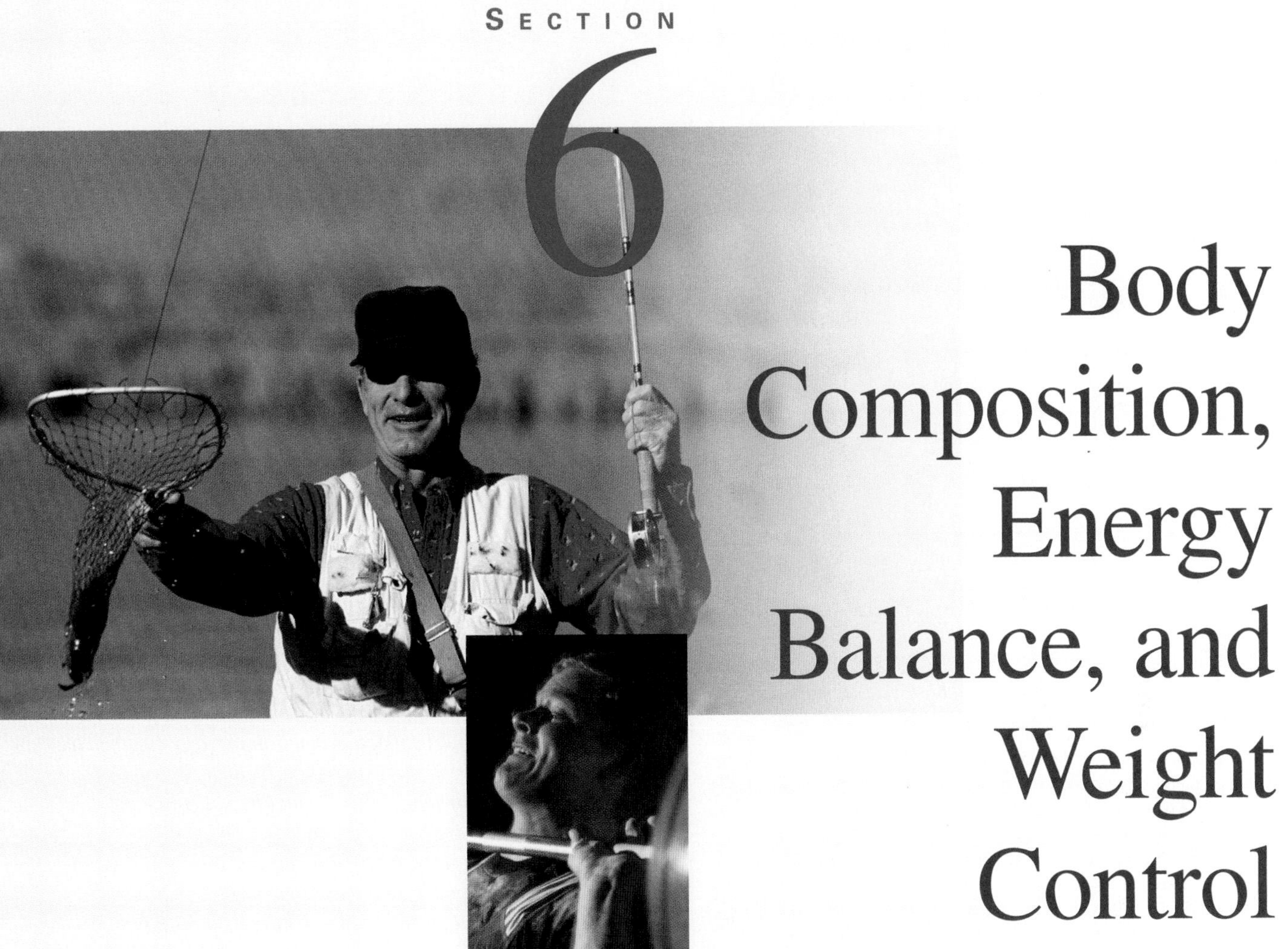

Body Composition, Energy Balance, and Weight Control

Overview

The accurate appraisal of body composition provides an important component in a comprehensive program of total physical fitness. In this regard, height–weight tables—a frequently used standard—serve only limited value in evaluating physique because "overweight" and "overfat" do not necessarily coincide. Athletes clearly illustrate this point in that many exceed some average weight for height and gender but otherwise possess relatively little body fat. Such individuals do not require weight loss, which might adversely affect their sports performance. In contrast, a prudent weight loss program would surely benefit the more than 97 million overweight men and women in the United States. This group spends nearly $50 billion each year, purchasing 54 million diet books, products, and services at more than 1500 weight-control clinics in the hope of permanently reducing excess fat. To this end, regular physical activity plays a crucial role in maintaining a healthful body composition and a high level of physiologic function.

In this section, we discuss body composition, its components and assessment, and the differences between sedentary and physically active men and women. We also deal with topics relevant to obesity and discuss the use of diet and exercise for weight loss and weight maintenance.

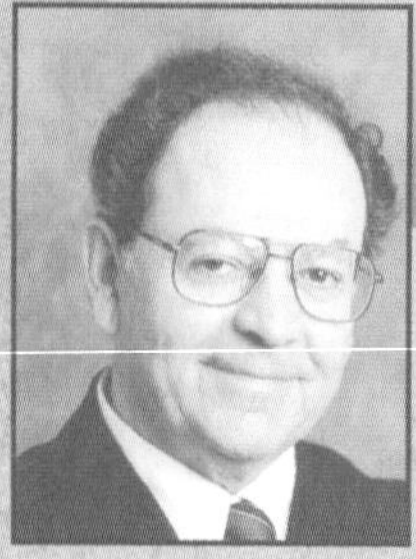

Interview with Dr. Claude Bouchard

Education: B Ped (Laval University, Quebec City, Canada); MSc (University of Oregon, Eugene, OR); PhD (Population genetics, University of Texas, Austin, TX); Postgraduate Training (Deutsche Sporthochschule, Institute for Research on Circulation and Sport Medicine, Cologne; Growth Research Center, Université de Montreal)

Current Affiliation: Professor and Executive Director, George A. Bray Chair in Nutrition. Louisiana State University. Pennington Biomedical Research Center. Baton Rouge, LA.

Honors and Awards: See Appendix E.

Research Focus: Genetics of adaptation to exercise and nutritional interventions, and genetics of obesity and its co-morbidities.

Memorable Publication: Bouchard C, et al. Genomic scan for maximal oxygen uptake and its response to training in the HERITAGE Family Study J Appl Physiol 2000;88:551.

Statement of Contributions: ACSM Citation Award
In recognition of his impressive research accomplishments in exercise science, genetics, child growth and maturation, diet and exercise clinical trials, and public health.

Dr. Bouchard has made important contributions to many areas of human performance research, and has been a leader in synthesizing current knowledge to produce consensus statements in exercise science. Among other things, he has conducted innovative research on the effects of experimental manipulation of diet and exercise in monozygotic twins. He has collected more data on energy balance from carefully controlled studies in this unique population than anyone in the world. This research has led to a better understanding of the variability of responses to dietary manipulation and exercise training and to the genetics of these complex processes.

His career is characterized by high scientific standards, immense productivity, breadth of interests, creative study designs, and a willingness to collaborate with others. He serves as an ideal role model for us all.

➤ What first inspired you to enter the exercise science field? What made you decide to pursue your advanced degree and/or line of research?

As a student in what was known as College Classic (the equivalent of high school, but it takes nine years and emphasizes the humanities), I became fascinated with human movement and performance. At that time, it was a very diffuse interest. That is, I was curious about the biomechanics, the exertion and the physiology, or the medical aspect, and the aesthetic of human movement. I had several career options, but came rapidly to the conclusion that I would move on to the local university, Université Laval, to learn about exercise and sports with the goal of approaching them from a scientific point of view. As you can see, even before I became a student in physical education, I was fascinated by science and human movement.

During my undergraduate studies, I was very frustrated by the poor science to which I was exposed, so I decided to go on to graduate studies. For 2 years during the summer, I traveled with friends on the East Coast of the USA and in the Midwest for the purpose of visiting universities and meeting faculty to select one for a Master's degree program. I visited at least 15 such institutions, and finally ended up at the University of Oregon, an institution that had been highly recommended to me. There, I was exposed to the teachings of Sigerseth, Clarke, Brumbach, Poley, and others.

After earning my Master's degree in Oregon, I felt that I was not quite ready to benefit from a PhD program. Following the advice of a few of my friends, I decided to go to the Sporthochschule in Cologne to work with Professor Wildor Hollmann. He was the Director of the Institute fur Kreislaufforschung und Sportmedizin, or the Institute for Research on Circulation and Sport Medicine. I knew that I could not obtain a degree there, but wanted to get more hands-on research experience. By then, my interests included not only performance but the health implications of exercise. I stayed there for 18 months and learned much.

Then, I was offered a position at my alma mater, Laval University, in Quebec. I decided to accept the position with the expectation to leave after three years or so to obtain my PhD. If I had done so immediately, I would have entered an endocrinology PhD program, as I had made contact to be admitted in the lab of Professor Hans Selye at the Université de Montreal. But I became so involved in the development of the programs and the facilities at Laval University that it was eight years before I left for my doctoral studies. By then, I had decided that genetics and biological individuality would be the focus of my research for the last decades of my career.

I opted to work with Professor Robert Malina, a colleague who had training in both physical education and biological anthropology, at the University of Texas. I spent 3 productive years there, which I completed with 10 months of postgraduate work at the Université de Montreal in the Human Growth and Development Center.

Obviously, mine has not been a linear career path. But I always felt that I was sharpening the focus of my research interest all along. Every phase in my career has been a useful one in the sense that it took me closer to what I am doing today—investigating the genetic and molecular basis of the response to exercise, and of obesity and its comorbidities. It would have been impossible to select this line of research 35 years ago, since the field did not exist. The study of individual differences could not be even contemplated at the molecular level then.

➤ Who were the most influential people in your career, and why?

Three scientists have played key roles at different times of my career. The first was Professor Fernand Landry. He was a fac-

ulty member at the University of Ottawa, but he was from the same city where I was born and went to the same colleges and community organizations that I later attended. He stimulated my interest in the biological sciences in general and the marvels of the human body's adaptation to exercise and training. He had a lasting impact on my career choices.

The second was Professor Wildor Hollmann. I got to know him very well during my stay in Cologne at his Institute. He stimulated my interest in the general topic of physical activity and health, particularly cardiovascular health. He was a very kind and patient mentor.

The last one was Professor Robert Malina. We became good friends during my doctoral studies at the University of Texas. Bob is a scholar with a strong interest in human diversity. We shared this research focus and many of the small pleasures of life.

➤ What has been the most interesting/enjoyable aspect of your involvement in science? What was the least interesting/enjoyable aspect?

The most enjoyable aspect is that you always think out of the commonly accepted paradigm and look toward the future. You verify one fact only to refocus on the new questions generated by the previous experience. You also constantly meet people who are of the same mind, colleagues who are always trying to be innovative and creative in the presence of the same set of facts as you. The life of a scientist is never dull if you have the chance to interact with the best in your field.

The least enjoyable aspect is the fact that you have to hunt for research funds all the time, particularly if you run a large laboratory operation. At one point, there were 55 people working on my research projects, and I was spending at least one-third of my time writing grant applications or renewals to maintain all of these positions.

➤ What is your most meaningful contribution to the field of exercise science, and why is it so important?

If I have contributed anything, it is evidence for the magnitude of the individual differences in fitness and performance in the sedentary state and in the response to regular exercise. My group has also demonstrated over a period of 20 years that these individual differences were not random. They are characterized by familial clustering and are accounted for by a substantial genetic effect. We have identified some of the areas responsible for the heterogeneity in fitness and performance levels, and in trainability.

I have also spent considerable research resources investigating the genetic and molecular basis of obesity and the metabolic disturbances seen in some obese individuals, but not in others. To this end, we have used a combination of twin and family studies as well as intervention protocols to begin the dissection of the complex genotypes that predispose individuals to become overweight and then obese.

I am also proud of my contributions to the efforts undertaken over the past 15 years to arrive at evidence-based consensus concerning the role of physical activity in health and disease.

➤ What advice would you give to students who express an interested in pursuing a career in exercise science research?

You will eventually need to become highly specialized in your own research pursuit, but try to acquire a broad-based understanding of the parent discipline. If you elect to become an exercise molecular biologist, you will find it useful to become an excellent biologist first. Maintaining a reasonable understanding of the changes occurring in biology in general will be a strong asset throughout your career. First, you will derive more satisfaction from your own research because you will be able to see the general implications of your work. Second, you are likely to find that a career in exercise science is more interesting if you understand what is going in the broader field of science to which you are related.

➤ What interests have you pursued outside of you professional career?

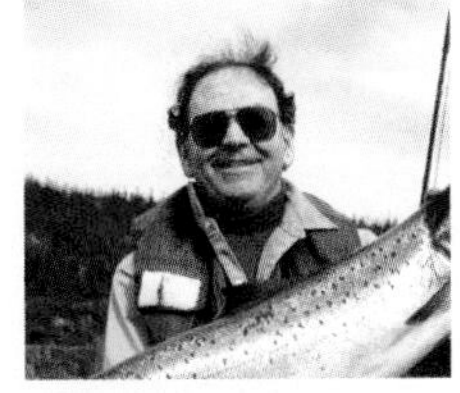

At age 20, I learned to ski and enjoyed it tremendously for many years. I shifted progressively from downhill to cross-country skiing, which I still like to do. At present, my preferred activities are hiking, fly fishing for trout and salmon, working out at the gym, reading, classical music, and wine tasting. I also enjoy traveling, but these days most of my travel is for business purposes.

➤ Where do you see the exercise science field (particularly your area of greatest interest) heading in the next 20 years?

In the next 20 years, the field of exercise science will incorporate the advances in molecular biology and genetics, something that it has failed to do in the past 10 years. The techniques of genomics and proteomics will become common technologies in our field. The benefits should be enormous, as exercise science can offer a wealth of opportunities to verify the functional consequences of DNA sequence variations in people who are not symptomatic for any disease. Such advances in the field of exercise science should make it possible for the exercise science discipline to become a significant player in preventive medicine and public health, as it will be able to develop the probes to identify those who are likely to benefit most from a physically active lifestyle. It will also change the way exercise science contributes to sports performance, as it will have the tools to identify the talented individuals at an early age.

➤ You have the opportunity to give a "last lecture." Describe its primary focus.

It would be on the extent and the causes of biological individuality and its implications for human health in a Darwinian evolutionary perspective.

CHAPTER 28

Body Composition Assessment

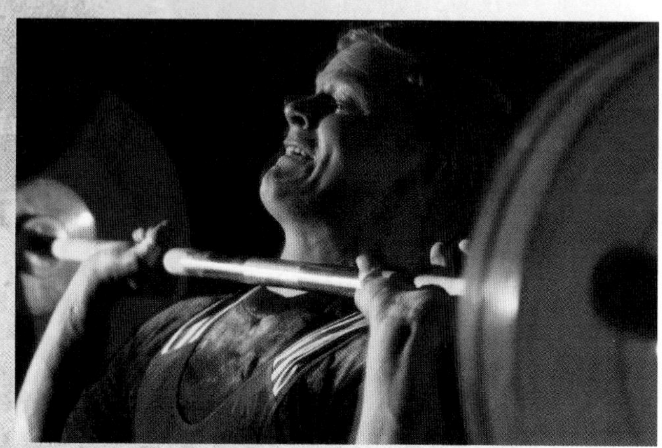

Chapter Objectives

- Summarize the early research on inadequacies of "height–weight" tables
- Outline current systems for classifying overweight and obese conditions
- Delineate characteristics of the "reference man" and "reference woman," including specific values for storage fat, essential fat, and sex-specific essential fat
- Discuss the prevalence of menstrual irregularities within the general population and specific athletic groups, and factors associated with its occurrence
- Describe Archimedes' principle applied to human body volume measurement
- Discuss limitations in the assumptions for computing percentage body fat from whole body density
- Give the anatomic locations for six frequently measured skinfolds and girths
- Describe how skinfolds and girths provide meaningful information about body fat and its distribution
- Discuss the rationale underlying use of bioelectrical impedance analysis, and factors that affect body composition estimates with this technique
- Summarize the rationale, strengths, and weaknesses of near-infrared interactance, ultrasound, x-ray, computed tomography, magnetic resonance imaging, dual-energy x-ray absorptiometry, and air-displacement plethysmography
- Give representative average values with variation limits for percentage body fat of typical young and older men and women

Body composition evaluation quantifies the major structural components of the body—muscle, bone, and fat. The life insurance actuarially based **height–weight tables** provide the most popular means of assessing the extent of "overweightness" based on gender and bony frame size (see "In a Practical Sense"). Stature (in cm) and mass (in kg) are the proper scientific terms in SI units for height and weight, respectively. We acknowledge this distinction and have changed body weight to body mass and height to stature when it preserves readability.

Height–weight tables give unreliable information about the relative composition (quality) of an individual's body and instead provide statistical landmarks based on the average ranges of body mass related to stature associated with the lowest mortality rate for people aged 25 to 59 years. They do not consider specific causes of death or quality of health (morbidity) before death.

LIMITATIONS OF HEIGHT–WEIGHT TABLES

- Use unvalidated estimates of body frame size
- Developed from data derived primarily from white populations
- Focus specifically on mortality data that may not reflect obesity-related comorbidities
- Provide no assessment of body composition

A person may weigh considerably more than the average weight-for-height standard yet still rate "underfat" for body composition. "Extra" weight for this person exists as muscle mass. According to the tables, the desirable body weight (assuming a large frame size) for a professional football player 188-cm tall and weighing 116 kg is 78 to 88 kg. Similarly, body weight without regard for frame size for young adult men 188-cm tall averages 85 kg. Using either criterion, conventional standards would classify this player as overweight, implying that he should lose at least 28 kg just to achieve the upper limit of the desirable body weight range. He must lose an additional 3 kg to match his "average" American male counterpart. If the player followed these guidelines, he most likely would no longer play football and might even jeopardize his overall health. Body fat for the football player (even though he weighed 31 kg more than the average) was only 12.7% of his body mass, compared with about 15.0% body fat for untrained young men.

Navy physician Dr. Albert Behnke first observed body composition variations between elite athletes and untrained individuals in studies of football players in the early 1940s (see "Focus on Research," page 755).[10] Careful evaluation of each player's body composition revealed that extreme muscular development primarily contributed to their excess weight. These observations clearly pointed out that the term **overweight** refers only to a body mass in excess of some standard, usually the average for a given stature. Being above an average, ideal, or desirable body mass based on height–weight tables should not necessarily dictate whether someone begins a reducing regimen. A better alternative determines body composition by one of the laboratory or field techniques reviewed in this chapter. Table 28.1 lists examples of terms and definitions common to the area of body composition.

TABLE 28-1 ➤ TERMS FREQUENTLY USED IN DESCRIBING AND MEASURING BODY COMPOSITION

TERM	DEFINITION
Abdominal fat	Subcutaneous and visceral fat in the abdominal region
Adipose tissue mass (ATM)	Fat (about 83%) plus its supporting structures (about 2% protein and 15% water); consists predominantly of white adipocytes (cells with a single fat droplet, mainly as triglyceride)
Anthropometry	Standardized techniques (e.g., calipers, tapes) to quantify (or predict) body size, proportion, and shape (*anthropo*, human; *metry*, measure)
Body density (Db)	Body mass (BM) expressed per unit body volume (body mass ÷ body volume)
Body mass index (BMI)	Ratio of BM to stature squared (body mass ÷ stature^2)
Densitometry	Archimedes' principle of water displacement to estimate whole body density; other terms include *hydrostatic weighting, hydrodensitometry, underwater weighing*
Essential lipids	Compound lipids (phospholipids) needed for cell membrane formation—about 10% of total body fat
Fat mass (FM)	All extractable lipids from adipose and other body tissues
Fat-free body mass (FFM)	All residual lipid-free chemicals and tissues, including water, muscle, bone, connective tissue, and internal organs
Intra-abdominal fat	Visceral fat in the abdominal cavity
Lean body mass (LBM)	FFM plus essential body fat
Minimal body mass	BM plus essential fat (includes sex-specific essential fat); 48.5 kg for the reference woman; computed from bone diameters, stature, and constants
Nonessential lipids	Triglycerides found mainly in adipose tissue—about 90% of total body fat
Reference man and reference woman	Behnke's reference standards for men and women that partition body mass into lean body mass, muscle, and bone, with fat subdivided into storage and essential fat; standards for body dimensions developed from military and anthropometric surveys
Relative body fat (%BF)	FM expressed as a percentage of total body mass
Specific gravity	Body mass in air divided by loss of weight in water (body mass ÷ [body mass − body weight in water])
Stature	Height expressed in metric units
Subcutaneous fat	Adipose tissue beneath the skin
Visceral adipose tissue (VAT)	Adipose tissue within and surrounding thoracic (e.g., heart, liver, lungs) and abdominal (e.g., liver, kidneys, intestines) cavities

IN A PRACTICAL SENSE

➤➤ DETERMINING BODY FRAME-SIZE FROM STATURE AND TWO BONE DIAMETERS

Body frame-size (BFS) becomes a useful measure for evaluating "normalcy" of body weight with standardized charts that categorize weight by frame size (bony structure). A combination of stature and bony widths (bone diameter measurements) adequately defines BFS, because BFS relates to the fat-free body mass (bone and muscle) and not to body fat.

MEASUREMENTS

1. Stature (height [Ht]) measured in cm
2. Biacromial diameter (cm) measured as the distance between the most lateral projections of the acromial processes (see figure)
3. Bitrochanteric diameter (cm) measured as the distance between the most lateral projection of the greater trochanters (see figure)

CALCULATIONS

Regression analyses determines BFS values for women and men from Ht and the sum of the biacromial and bitrochanteric bone diameters (ΣBia + Bitroc) with the following equations:

$$\text{Female: BFS} = \text{Ht} \times 10.357 + (\Sigma\text{Bia} + \text{Bitroc})$$
$$\text{Male: BFS} = \text{Ht} \times 8.239 + (\Sigma\text{Bia} + \text{Bitroc})$$

Steps

1. Measure stature and biacromial and bitrochanteric diameters; take two measurements and use the average.
2. Compute the sum of the average biacromial and bitrochanteric diameter measurements.
3. Compute BFS by substituting in the appropriate gender-specific formulas (example illustrated in Table 1).
4. Determine frame-size category by referring to Table 2.

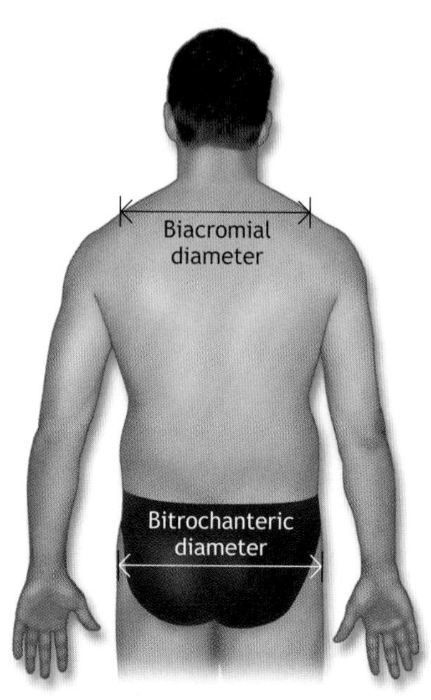

Example

Table 1 shows calculations of BFS for a male and female of different heights and bony diameters. The male's height corresponds to a value below the 10th percentile for height-by-age for men in the U.S. population. This height, combined with large breadth measurements, results in a medium frame-size ranking (Table 2). In contrast, the female's height of 173.4 cm ranks above the 90th percentile for the U.S. population. However, her small breadth measurements also result in a medium frame-size ranking (Table 2).

Katch VL, Freedson PS. Body size and shape: derivation of the "HAT" frame size model. Am J Clin Nutr 1982;36:669.

TABLE 1. EXAMPLE OF BFS CALCULATIONS FOR A MALE AND FEMALE OF DIFFERENT HEIGHTS AND BONY MEASUREMENTS

VARIABLE	SUBJECT A (MALE)	SUBJECT B (FEMALE)
Ht	167.3 cm	173.4 cm
Biacromial diameter	48.0 cm	29.8 cm
Bitrochanter diameter	35.0 cm	22.2 cm
ΣBia + Bitroc	83.0 cm	52.0 cm
BFS value	1461.4	1847.9 cm
	[BFS = Ht × 8.239 + ΣBia + Bitroc]	[BFS = Ht × 10.357 + ΣBia + Bitroc]
	[BSF = 167.3 × 8.239 + 83.0]	[BSF = 173.4 × 10.357 + 52.0]
	[BSF = 1461.4]	[BSF = 1847.9]
Frame size category from Table 2	Medium	Medium

TABLE 2. BFS CATEGORIES

	FRAME-SIZE CATEGORY		
Sex	**Small**	**Medium**	**Large**
Male	<1459.3	1459.4–1591.9	>1592.0
Female	<1661.9	1662.0–1850.7	>1850.8

Focus on Research: Overweight But Not Overfat

Welham WC, Behnke AR. The specific gravity of healthy men; body weight/volume and other physical characteristics of exceptional athletes and of naval personnel. JAMA 1942;18:498.

➤ The Welham and Behnke research is one of the most frequently cited studies in the body composition and exercise physiology literature. These investigators tested the hypothesis that differences in body fat among men relate chiefly to the body's specific gravity and not body mass per se. The hypothesis predicted that heavy but lean men would have higher body specific gravity values than counterparts of similar body mass, but with high body fat levels. If correct, a relatively large body mass may not always provide an appropriate measure of excessive fatness.

In 1942, the relation between the body density and estimates of body fatness remained undetermined, although scientists knew the specific gravity of the body's fat and nonfat (fat-free) components. Twenty-five professional football players, most of whom had been designated All-Americans, classified unfit for military service because of excessive body weight according to standard height–weight tables. Measurements included stature, body mass, and whole-body density determined by hydrostatic weighing. A unique aspect of the body density assessment corrected body volume from estimates of residual lung volume.

The *inset figure* shows the relationship between body density and "weight by height" for the athletes. The *vertical line* at a weight:height ratio of 2.65 represents the upper limit for classification as fit for military service. Men of this age who fell to the right of the vertical line did not qualify for life insurance because of their excessive body weight; 17 of the players classified as overweight. However, the high body densities of 11 of these men indicated a low percentage body fat. Body mass of all the players averaged 90.9 kg (200 lb), and body density averaged 1.080 g · cm^{-3}. For the 6 heaviest men, body mass averaged 104.5 kg (230 lb), with body density at 1.059 g · cm^{-3}.

Welham and Behnke's research was the first to show that variations in body density related mainly to individual differences in the body's fat content. The research also pointed up the inadequacies of height–weight tables to infer body fatness or determine a desirable body weight, particularly among highly trained large athletes. The researchers suggested that a body density of 1.060 g · cm^{-3} should serve as the demarcation for excessive fatness for men. With this criterion, 23 of the 25 lean but heavy football payers qualified as fit (and not overly fat) for military service.

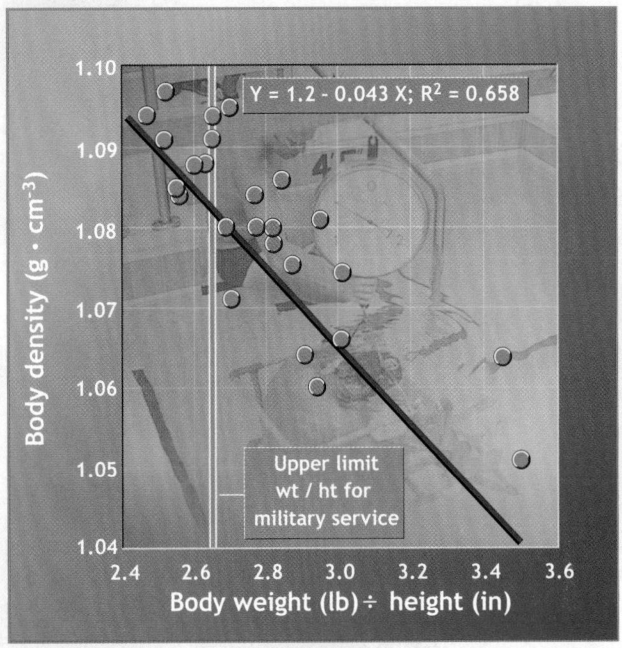

Relationship between body density and weight-to-height ratio for 25 All-American football players.

THE BODY MASS INDEX: A SOMEWHAT BETTER ALTERNATIVE

Clinicians and researchers frequently use the **body mass index (BMI)**, derived from body mass and stature, to assess the "normalcy" for a person's body weight. This measure exhibits a somewhat higher association with body fat and disease risk than do estimates based simply on stature and mass although independent effects of ethnicity should be considered.[36,54] BMI computes as follows:

$$\text{BMI} = \text{Body mass (kg)} \div \text{stature (m}^2\text{)}$$

The importance of this easily obtained index lies in its curvilinear relationship with the all-cause mortality ratio. As BMI increases throughout the range of moderate and severe overweight, so also does the risk increase for cardiovascular complications (including hypertension and stroke), certain cancers, diabetes, gallstones, osteoarthritis, and renal disease.[21,137]

The largest ever prospective study of more than 1 million United States adults (457,785 men and 588,369 women) during 14 years of follow-up provided the data that revealed the relationships between BMI and mortality risk. Figure 28.1A shows that smoking status and presence or absence of disease at time of enrollment in the study substantially modified the association between BMI and risk of premature death from all causes. Men and women who never smoked and remained disease free at the study's start (light green lines) experienced the greatest health risk from excess weight. In contrast, excessive leanness related to increased death risk among current and former smokers with a history of disease. In healthy people, the nadir of the curve for BMI and mortality occurred between a

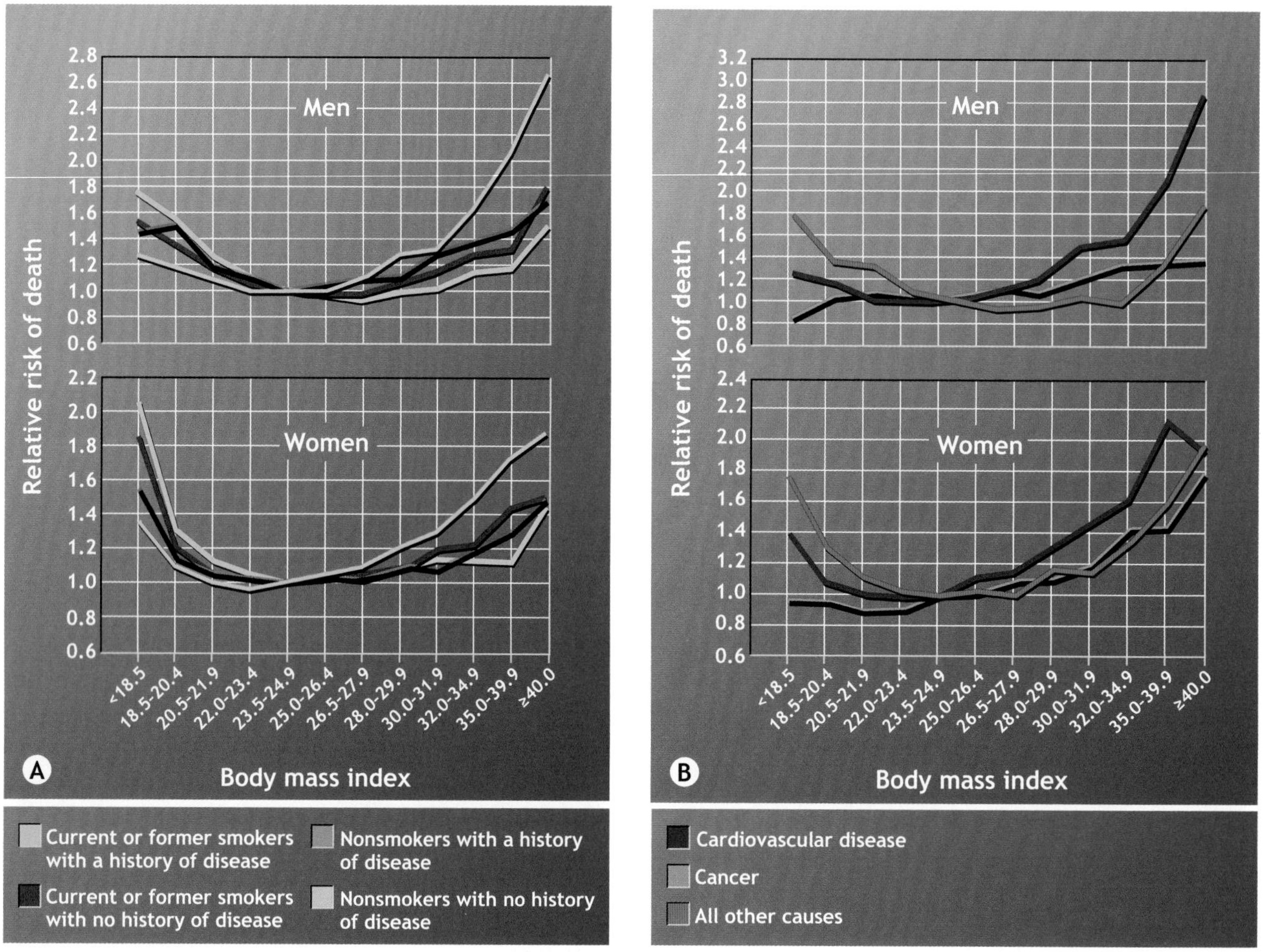

FIGURE 28.1 • **A**. Multivariate relative risk of death from *all causes* among men and women according to body mass index (BMI), smoking status, and disease status. Data from four mutually exclusive subgroups. Nonsmokers had never smoked. **B**. Multivariate relative risk of death from cardiovascular disease, cancer, and all other causes according to BMI among men and women who had never smoked and had no history of disease at enrollment. Subjects with BMIs of 23.5 to 24.9 composed the reference category in both figures. (From Calle EE, et al. Body-mass index and mortality in a prospective cohort of U.S. adults. N Engl J Med 1999;341:1097.)

BMI of 23.5 and 24.9 for men (e.g., 5′10″ at 174 lb) and 22.0 and 23.4 for women (e.g., 5′5″ at 150 lb), with a gradient of increasing risk associated with moderate overweight. Among white men and women with the highest BMI, relative death risk equaled 2.58 (men) and 2.00 (women), compared with counterparts with a BMI of 23.5 to 24.9 (relative risk 1.0).

Figure 28.1B shows the clear association in men and women between excess weight and a greater death risk from

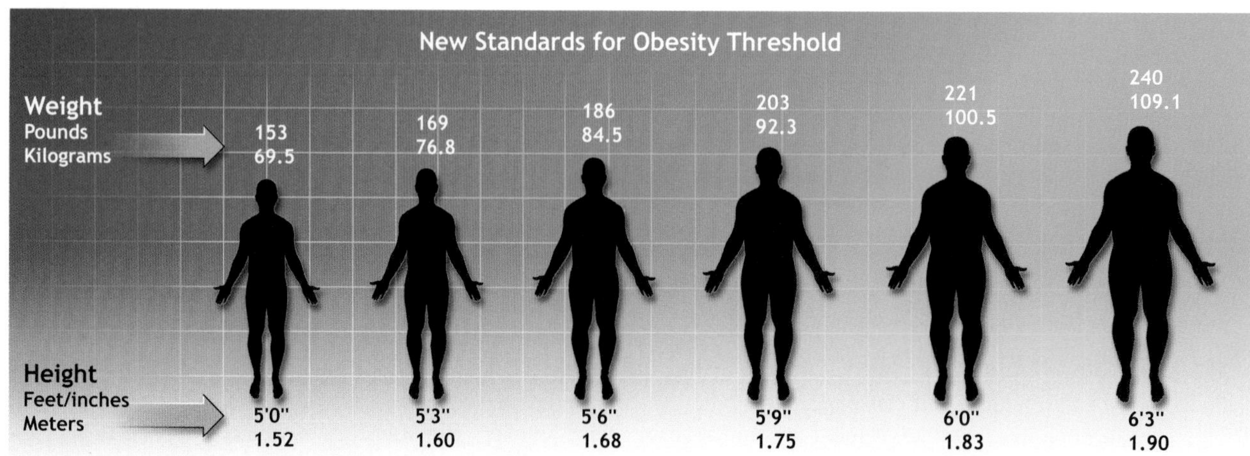

heart disease or cancer. A positive relationship emerged between BMI and cancer risk, with no elevation in risk among the leanest men and women. A J-shaped curve described BMI and cardiovascular disease risk, while a U-shaped curve predicted risk of death for all other causes. The authors attribute the increased death risk among the lean men and women depicted in the J- and U-shaped curves to the presence of disease at the time of death.

New Standards for Overweight and Obesity

On June 18, 1998, the 24-member expert panel convened by the National Heart, Lung and Blood Institute lowered the BMI demarcation point for "overweight" to 25 from 27. Based on the association between obesity and disease, individuals with a BMI of 30 or more were categorized as obese. The *unnumbered figure* on previous page shows the current standards for identifying the obesity threshold (defined by BMI ≥30.0) for six heights from 5′0″ to 6′3″. People with a BMI of 30 average approximately 30 pounds overweight. For example, a man 6′0″ weighing 221 pounds and a woman weighing 186 pounds at 5′6″ both have a BMI of 30, and both are approximately 30 pounds overweight. These revised standards place 97 million Americans in the overweight and obese categories—up from 72 million under the previous standard. For the first time in the United States, overweight people (BMI above 25) outnumber people of desirable weight; shockingly, 59% of American men and 49% of women have BMIs exceeding 24! Analysis of available data by ethnicity and gender shows that significantly more black, Mexican, Cuban, and Puerto Rican males and females classify as overweight than their white counterparts.[136]

Figure 28.2 A and B present the revised growth charts for the United States for boys and girls age 2 to 20 years. These charts represent data combined from five national health examination surveys collected from 1963 to 1994 and five supplementary data sources. As yet, no absolute BMI standard has been set to classify children and adolescents as overweight and obese.[99,120] However, expert panels recommend the use of BMI-for-age to identify the ever increasing number of children and adolescents at the upper end of the distribution who are either overweight (≥95th percentile) or at risk for overweight (≥85th percentile and ≤95th percentile (see Chapter 30). Less specific recommendations exist for the lower end of the distributions, but BMIs in this range may indicate underweight or at risk for underweight.

Example BMI Computation

Male: stature, 175.3 cm, 1.753 m (69 in); body mass, 97.1 kg (214.1 lb)

$$\text{BMI} = 97.1 \div (1.753)^2 = 31.6 \text{ kg} \cdot \text{m}^{-2}$$

This man's BMI falls considerably above the threshold for the upper-range BMI for men.

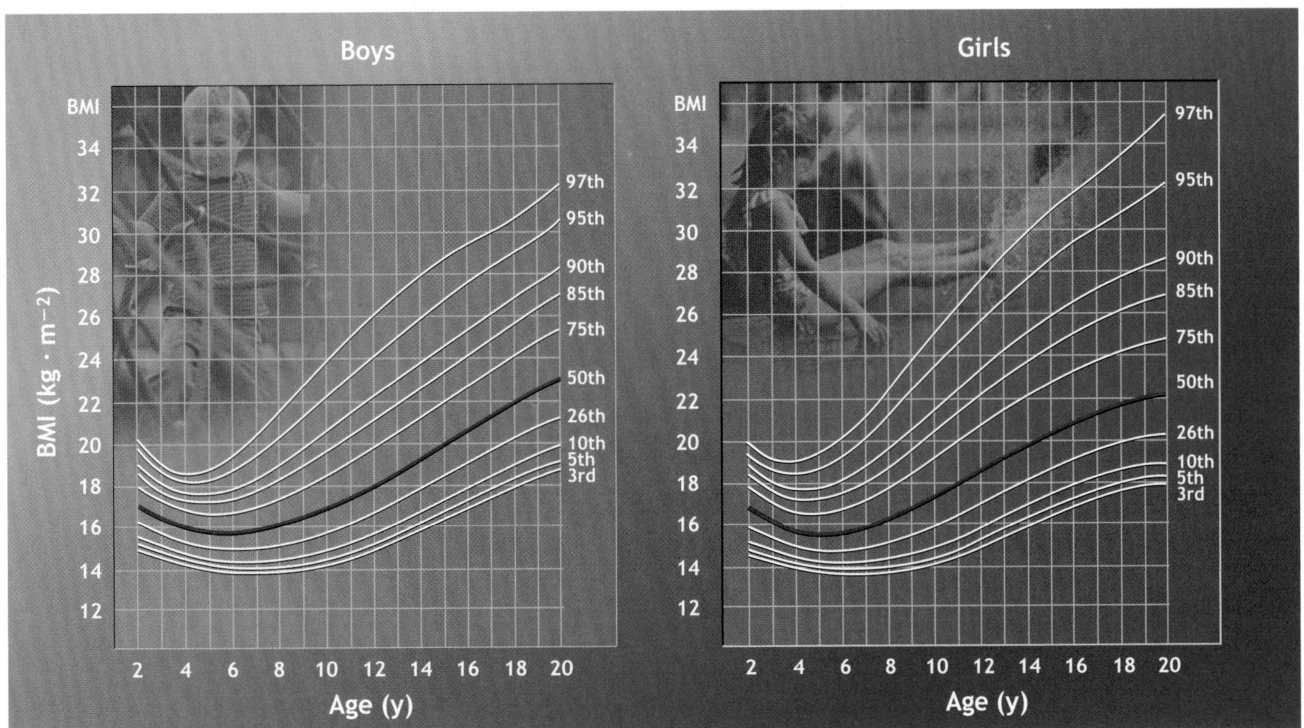

FIGURE 28.2 • Body mass index-for-age percentiles for boys and girls ages 2 to 20 years. Developed by the National Center for Health Statistics in collaboration with the National Center for Chronic Disease Prevention and Health Promotion (2000) (From Kuczmarski, RJ, et al.: CDC growth charts: United States. Advance Data 2000; 314. From Vital and Health Statistics of the Centers for Disease Control and Prevention/ National Center for Health Statistics.)

BMI Limitations

The BMI, like the height–weight tables, fails to consider the body's proportional composition or the all-important component of body fat distribution, referred to as fat patterning. Specifically, factors other than excess body fat—bone, muscle mass, and even increased plasma volume induced by exercise training—affect the numerator of the BMI equation. A high BMI could lead to an incorrect interpretation of overfatness in lean individuals with excessive muscle mass because of genetic makeup or exercise training.

The possibility of misclassifying someone as overweight using BMI standards applies particularly to large-size field athletes, bodybuilders, weight lifters, heavier wrestlers, and most professional football players. For example, the BMI for seven defensive linemen from a former NFL Super Bowl team averaged 31.9 $kg \cdot m^{-2}$ (team BMI averaged 28.7), clearly signaling these athletes as overweight and placing many of them in the moderate category for mortality risk. However, the players' body fat content, 18.0% for the linemen and 12.1% for the team, indicated that they were not overfat.

The pattern of misclassification of body weight relative to body fat content also applies to the typical NFL player from 1920 to 1996. Figure 28.3 plots the average BMI for all NFL roster players at each fifth-year interval between 1920 and 1996, based on 53,333 players. Average body fat content of players measured during the late 1970s through the 1990s fell below the range typically associated with population data for men. Those with body fat determinations, evaluated with densitometry during this era, included roster players of the New York Jets, Washington Redskins, New Orleans Saints, and Dallas Cowboys (Table 28.2). Almost all players from 1960 onward classify as overweight based on standard height–weight tables. For the BMI data up to 1989, values for linebackers, skill players, and defensive backs represent the low category for disease risk, while the BMIs for offensive and defensive linemen place them at "moderate" risk. After 1989, risk for linebackers increased from the low to the moderate category. The BMIs for offensive and defensive linemen, the largest NFL players, quickly approached high risk and remained in that category. This certainly does not bode well from a health perspective for these large-size players, at least based on BMI risk predictions for the general population.

In contrast to professional football players, the BMI for National Basketball Association players for the 1993–1994 season averaged only 24.5 $kg \cdot m^{-2}$. This relatively low BMI places them in the very low risk category and below the overweight category, yet height–weight standards would classify them as overweight.

Another category of world-class athletes—racing cyclists who participated in the Tour de France—had remarkably low BMIs. In the 1997 race, the BMI for 170 competitors averaged 21.5 $kg \cdot m^{-2}$ (1.79 m stature, 68.75 kg body mass). Three

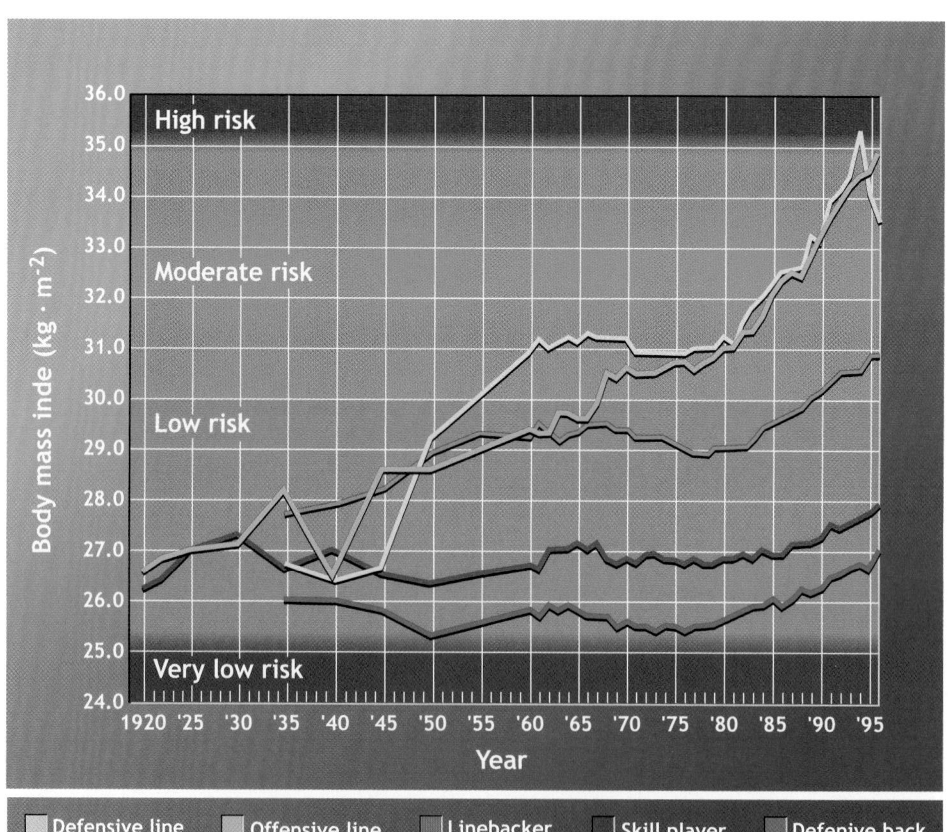

FIGURE 28.3 • BMIs for all players in the National Football League between 1920 and 1996 (n = 53,333). Categories include offensive and defensive linemen, linebackers, skill players (quarterbacks, receivers, backfield), and defensive backs. (Data compiled by K. Monahan and F. Katch, Exercise Science Department, University of Massachusetts, Amherst, 1996).

TABLE 28.2 ➤ PHYSIQUE AND BODY COMPOSITION OF "UNDERFAT" PROFESSIONAL FOOTBALL PLAYERS AND "OVERWEIGHT" OFFENSIVE AND DEFENSIVE PROFESSIONAL LINEMEN AND SHOT PUTTERS

VARIABLE	ALL-PRO DEFENSIVE BACKS 1	2	3	4	ALL-PRO OFFENSIVE BACK (N = 1)	DALLAS DEFENSIVE LINEMEN 1977 (N = 10)	DALLAS LINEMEN 1977 (N = 5)	OLYMPIC SHOT-PUTTERS (N = 13)
Age (y)	27.1	30.2	29.4	24.0	32	31	29	24
Stature (cm)	184.7	181.9	187.2	181.5	184.7	193.8	197.6	187.0
Mass (kg)	87.9	87.1	88.4	88.9	90.6	116.0	116.5	112.3
Relative fat (%)	3.9	3.8	3.8	2.5	1.4	18.6	13.2	14.8
Absolute fat (kg)	3.4	3.3	3.4	2.2	1.3	21.6	15.4	16.6
Fat-free body mass (kg)	84.5	83.8	85.0	86.7	89.3	94.4	101.1	95.7
Lean:fat ratio	24.85	25.39	25.00	39.41	68.69	4.37	6.57	5.77
Girth (cm)								
Shoulders	122.1	119.0	120.5	117.2	121.8	129.5	122.5	133.3
Chest	101.6	101.0	99.5	107.5	102.0	116.5	109.9	118.5
Abdomen, avg	81.8	85.5	81.0	82.6	81.7	102.0	97.0	100.3
Buttocks	98.0	99.0	101.9	102.0	96.5	112.8	111.5	112.3
Thigh	61.0	61.0	58.5	64.0	63.2	66.2	69.3	69.4
Knee	39.5	41.3	41.1	38.0	41.0	44.8	45.8	42.9
Calf	37.6	38.8	38.8	37.8	41.3	43.5	42.4	43.6
Ankle	21.8	23.1	23.5	22.4	22.7	25.8	25.7	24.7
Forearm	31.8	29.1	31.1	31.8	33.5	33.5	34.8	33.7
Biceps	38.0	35.8	37.1	37.7	40.4	41.5	41.7	42.2
Wrist	18.5	17.2	17.4	17.5	18.0	19.3	19.3	18.9

From Katch FI, Katch VL. The body composition profile: techniques of measurement and applications. Clin Sports Med 1984;3:30.

years later in the 2000 race, the BMI for 162 competitors remained essentially unchanged (21.5 kg · m^{-2}; 1.79 m stature, 69.1 kg body mass). The BMI among cyclists from Switzerland (N = 5), France (N = 36), Spain (N = 22), Italy (N = 30), Belgium (N = 14), Netherlands (N = 12), Germany (N = 9), and USA (N = 8) remained within narrow limits (20.8 kg · m^{-2} for Swiss cyclists to 22.3 kg · m^{-2} for USA cyclists). On average, stature among teams was within 0.2 m (1.78 to 1.80 m) and body mass ranged from 66.8 kg (Swiss) to 72.1 kg (USA). Because of the homogeneity in body size variables among these top-level performers, it seems unlikely that body composition variables *per se* will help to explain individual differences in cycling performance. Instead, experiments have focused on physiological and nutritional variables during extended-duration endurance cycling performance.[20,44,123]

Miss America and BMI—Undernourished Role Models?

Many consider Miss America beauty pageant contestants to possess the ideal combination of beauty, grace, and talent. Each competitor survives the rigors of local and state contests, thus satisfying judges that finalists have "ideal qualities" worthy of role-model status. The consummate image of the Miss America physique to some extent shapes society's generalized "ideal" for female size and shape. The contest, televised worldwide to millions of viewers, reinforces this notion. However, do such images reinforce an unhealthful message to those who attempt to emulate such physiques?[45]

Figure 28.4 shows the BMIs of Miss America contestants from available data between 1922 to 1999 (excluding 1927–1933, when the pageant was not held). Also included for comparison about body size is Behnke's standard for the reference woman (see page 761). The *bottom horizontal dashed line* in the figure designates the World Health Organization (WHO) cutoff for undernutrition established at a BMI of 18.5 kg · m^{-2}.[202] The *top horizontal dashed line* represents the BMI for the reference woman (Fig. 28.5; stature, 1.638 m; body mass, 56.7 kg; BMI, 21.1 kg · m^{-2}). The downward slope of the regression line from 1922 to 1999 shows a clear tendency for relative undernutrition from the mid-1960s to approximately 1990. Using the WHO cutoff, the BMIs of 30% (n = 14) of the 47 Miss America winners fell below 18.5. Raising the BMI cutoff to 19.0 kg · m^{-2} adds another 18 women, or a total of 48% of the winners, with undesirable values. Approximately 24% of contest winners had BMIs between 20.0 and 21.0 kg · m^{-2}, and no winner after 1924 had a BMI equaling that of the reference woman!

Interestingly, 1965 was the last year for which we could locate girth measurements from official press releases or newspaper coverage of the contest. We compared the percentage difference between the Miss America girth averages with the corresponding measurements for the reference woman (bottom row of right inset table). For the average bust, waist, and hip values (35.1, 24.0, 35.4), Miss America's measurement exceeded the reference woman's bust measurement by 2.6 inches (8%) but fell 7% below for

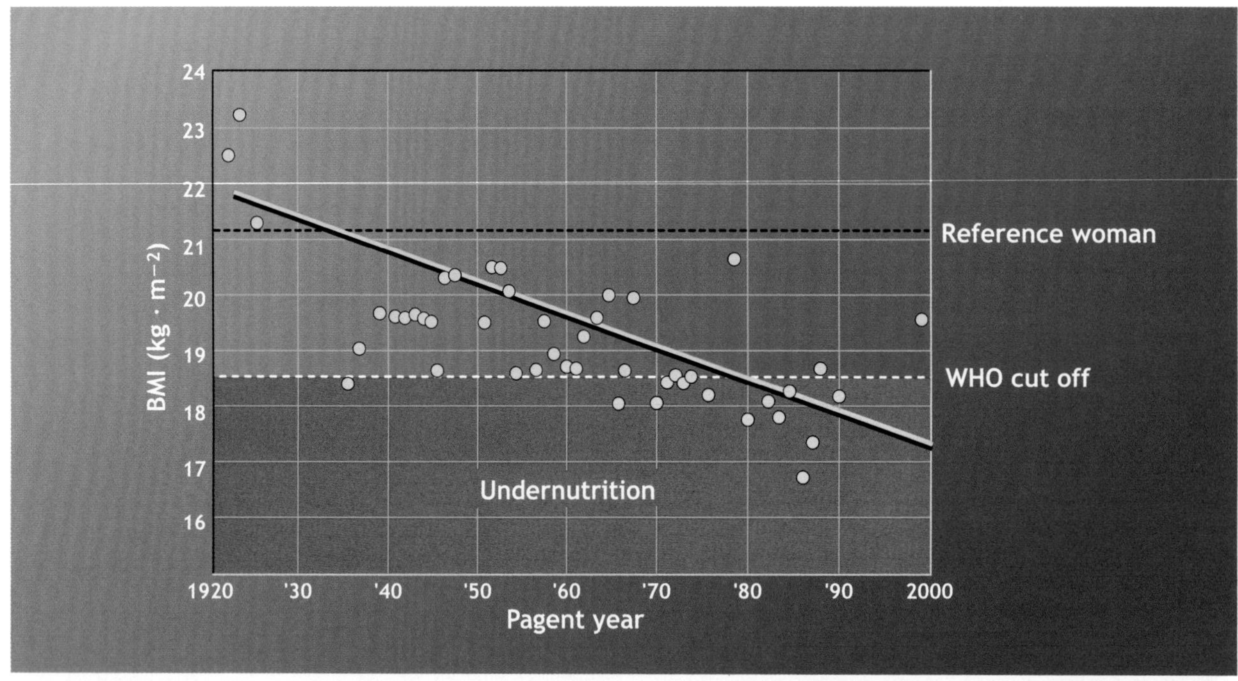

1922-1948	Age	Ht	Wt	1951-1968	Age	Ht	Wt	1970-1999	Age	Ht	Wt
1922	18	65	135	1951	20	65.5	119	1970	21	65.5	110
1923	19	65	140	1952	25	70	143	1971	21	68	121
1924	18	66	132	1953	19	66.5	128	1972	22	67	118
1926	18	52.5	118	1954	20	68	132	1973	23	68	120
1936	22	66	114	1955	19	68.5	124	1974	23	69	125
1937	17	66.5	120	1957	19	67	120	1976	18	70.5	128
1939	19	67	126	1958	20	68.5	130	1979	22	64	121
1941	19	65.5	120	1959	21	65	114	1980	22	67	114
1942	21	65	118	1960	21	67	120	1983	25	67	115
1943	21	68	130	1961	18	66	116	1984	20	66	110
1944	21	67	125	1962	19	65.5	118	1985	20	68	120
1945	18	70	136	1964	21	66.5	124	1986	21	69	114
1946	21	68	123	1965	22	124	124	1987	21	68.5	116
1947	21	67	130	1966	19	115	115	1988	24	70	131
1948	18	69	138	1967	19	116	116	1990	24	67.5	118
				1968	19	135	135	1999	24	69	133

Girths (inches)

	Bust	Waist	Hips	Calf	Thigh	Ankle	Biceps	Wrist
1926	33	24.5	33.5	12.5	19.5	7	–	–
1935	33	23	35.5	–	–	–	–	–
1926	34	23.5	34.5	13	19	8.5	9.5	5.5
1941	34	24	36	14	23	8	11	6
1942	34	24	34.5	–	–	–	–	–
1943	36	23	35	–	–	–	–	–
1944	36.5	25	37.5	13	19.5	8	–	–
1945	35.5	25	35	14.5	20	8.5	–	–
1946	35.5	25.5	36	13.5	22	8.5	–	–
1947	35	25	–	–	–	–	–	–
1948	37	25	–	–	–	–	–	–
1951	35	25	–	–	–	–	–	–
1952	36	24	36	–	–	–	–	–
1953	35	23	35	–	–	–	–	–
1954	37	24	36	–	–	–	–	–
1955	34.5	22	35	–	–	–	–	–
1957	35	23	35	–	–	–	–	–
1958	35	25	36	–	–	–	–	–
1959	34	22	35	–	–	–	–	–
1960	36	24	36	–	–	–	–	–
1961	35	22	35	–	–	–	–	–
1962	35	24	35	–	–	–	–	–
1964	35	23	35	–	–	–	–	–
1965	36	24	36	–	–	–	–	–
Ref W*	36.1	30.3	36.8	14.1	21.6	8.9	12.5	6.8

Ref W* = Behnke's reference woman; stature = 163.8 cm, body mass = 56.7 kg

FIGURE 28.4 • Body mass index (BMI) of 47 Miss America pageant contestants from 1922 to 1999. The *top horizontal black line* represents the BMI for Behnke's reference woman (21.1 kg · m^{-2}). The *bottom horizontal white line* designates the World Health Organization's (WHO) BMI demarcation for undernutrition (18.5 kg · m^{-2}). The *left inset table* shows the available data for age, height (in), and weight (lb) for the contest winners. The *right inset table* shows selected girths for 24 Miss America winners from 1926 to 1965.

the waist value (−1.8 in) and 5% (−1.7 in) for the hips. Unfortunately, no contemporary data exist from 1966 to 2000, so we cannot compare the modern Miss America's physique with historical data.

COMPOSITION OF THE HUMAN BODY

Current evaluation of body composition partitions body mass into different compartments whose sum equals the body mass. In 1921, Czech anthropologist J. Matiega described a four-component model consisting of the weight of the skeleton (S), skin plus subcutaneous tissue (Sk + St), skeletal muscle (M), and a remainder (R).[119] The sum of the four components equaled the body mass:

$$\text{Total body mass} = S + [Sk + St] + M + R$$

Matiega's early attempt to describe human physique analytically used anthropometric measurements to approximate the first three anatomic entities of his four-component model. The thickness of four bony structures (wrists, ankles, and humeral and femoral condyles) plus stature estimated S. Six skinfolds (upper arm, forearm, thigh, calf, thorax, and abdomen) plus body surface area determined the mass of Sk + St. Upper-arm, thigh, and calf girths (subtracting a skinfold and determining the radius of each area to compute cross-sectional area) ascertained M. In essence, the body's major structural components included the mass of muscle, fat, and bone.

Over the past 65 years, numerous studies have focused on body composition and how best to measure its various components. Most methodologies partition the body into two distinct compartments: (1) fat-free body mass and (2) fat mass. The density of homogenized samples of fat-free body tissues in small mammals is approximately 1.100 g · cm^{-3} at 37°C.[152] Fat-free tissue maintains a water content of 73.2%,[133] with potassium at 60 to 70 mmol · kg^{-1} in men and 50 to 60 mmol · kg^{-1} in women.[14] Fat stored in adipose tissue has a density of 0.900 g · cm^{-3} at 37°C.[128] Subsequent body composition studies expanded the two-component model to account for biologic variability in three (water, protein, fat) or four (water, protein, bone mineral, fat) distinct components.[80,200] Women and men differ significantly in relative quantities of specific body composition components. Consequently, gender-specific reference standards provide a framework for evaluating "normal" body composition. Behnke's proposed model for the reference man and reference woman proves useful for such purposes.[9]

Reference Man and Reference Woman

Figure 28.5 shows the different body composition compartments for the **reference man** and **reference woman**. The schema partitions body mass into lean body mass, muscle, and bone, with total body fat subdivided into storage and essential fat components. This model integrates the average physical dimensions from thousands of individuals measured in large-scale civilian and military anthropometric surveys

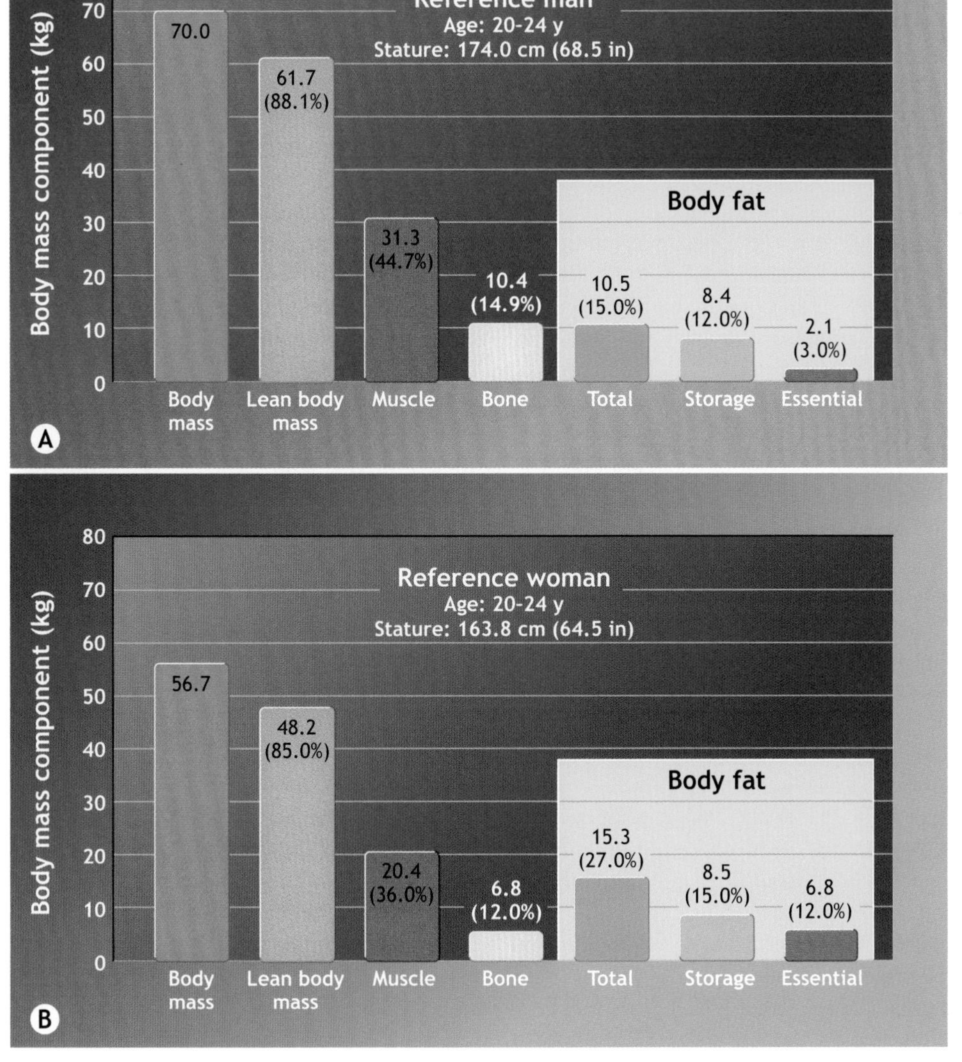

FIGURE 28.5 • Behnke's theoretical model for the body composition of the reference man (**A**) and reference woman (**B**). Values in parenthesis indicate percentage of total body mass.

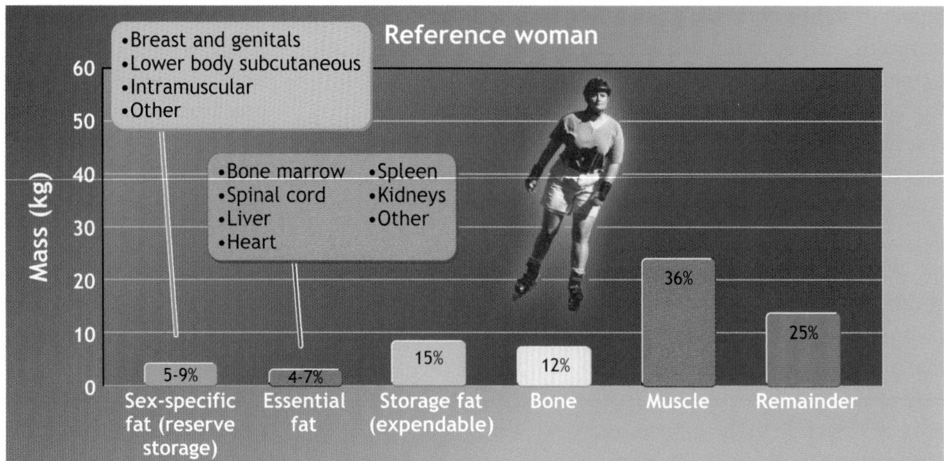

FIGURE 28.6 • Theoretical model for body fat distribution for the reference woman with body mass of 56.7 kg, stature, 163.8 cm, and 27% body fat. (From Katch VL, et al. Contribution of breast volume and weight to body fat distribution in females. Am J Phys Anthropol 1980;53:93.)

with data from laboratory studies of tissue composition and structure.

The reference man is taller and heavier, his skeleton weighs more, and he possesses a larger muscle mass and lower body fat content than the reference woman. These differences exist even when one expresses fat, muscle, and bone as a percentage of body mass. Just how much of the gender difference in body fat relates to biologic and behavioral factors, perhaps from lifestyle differences, is unclear. More than likely, hormonal differences play an important role. The concept of reference standards does not mean that men and women should strive to achieve this body composition or that the reference man and woman reflect some "average." Instead, the reference model proves useful for statistical comparisons and interpretations of data from other studies of elite athletes, individuals involved in exercise training, different racial and ethnic groups, and the underweight and obese.

Essential and Storage Fat

In the reference model, total body fat exists in two storage sites or depots: essential fat and storage fat. **Essential fat** consists of the fat in heart, lungs, liver, spleen, kidneys, intestines, muscles, and lipid-rich tissues of the central nervous system and bone marrow. *Normal physiologic functioning requires this fat.* In the heart, for example, dissectible fat from cadavers represents approximately 18.4 g or 5.3% of an average heart weighing 349 g in males and 22.7 g or 8.6% of a heart weighing 256 g in females.[201] In the female, essential fat includes additional **sex-specific essential fat**. Whether any of this fat provides reserve storage for metabolic fuel is unclear.

The **storage fat** depot includes fat primarily in adipose tissue. The adipose tissue energy reserve contains approximately 83% pure fat, 2% protein, and 15% water within its supporting structures. Storage fat includes the visceral fatty tissues that protect the various internal organs within the thoracic and abdominal cavities from trauma, and the larger adipose tissue volume deposited beneath the skin's surface. Although a similar proportional distribution of storage fat exists in men and women (12% of body mass in men, 15% in women), the total percentage of essential fat in women, which includes the sex-specific fat, averages four times that in men. *More than likely, the additional essential fat serves biologically important functions for child bearing and other hormone-related functions.* Considering the reference body's total quantity of storage fat (approximately 8.5 kg), this depot represents, at least theoretically, 63,500 kcal of available energy, or the energy equivalent of running nonstop at a 9-minute-per-mile pace for 114 hours!

Figure 28.6 partitions the distribution of body fat for the reference woman. As part of the 5 to 9% sex-specific fat reserves, breast fat probably contributes no more than 4% of body mass for women whose total fat content ranges between 14 and 35%.[90] We interpret this to mean that other substantial sex-specific fat depots exist (e.g., pelvic, buttock, and thigh regions) that contribute to the female's body-fat stores.[155]

FAT-FREE BODY MASS AND LEAN BODY MASS. The terms **fat-free body mass (FFM)** and **lean body mass** refer to specific entities. Lean body mass (a theoretical entity) contains the small percentage of non–sex-specific essential fat equivalent to approximately 3% of body mass (located chiefly within the central nervous system, bone marrow, and internal organs). In contrast, FFM represents the body mass devoid of *all* extractable fat (FFM = body mass − fat mass). Behnke points out that FFM refers to an *in vitro* entity appropriate to carcass analysis.[9] Behnke considered the lean body mass an *in vivo* entity relatively constant in water, organic matter, and mineral content throughout the active adult's life span. *In normally hydrated, healthy adults, the FFM and lean body mass differ only in the essential fat component.*

Figure 28.5 showed that the lean body mass in men and the **minimal body mass** in women consist chiefly of essential fat (plus sex-specific fat for females), muscle, water, and bone. The whole-body density of the reference man with 12% storage fat and 3% essential fat is 1.070 g · cm^{-3}; the density of his FFM is 1.094 g · cm^{-3}. If the reference man's total body fat percentage equals 15.0% (storage fat plus essential fat), the density of a hypothetical fat-free body attains the upper limit of 1.100 g · cm^{-3}.

In the reference woman, the average whole body density of 1.040 g · cm^{-3} represents a body fat percentage of 27%; of this, approximately 12% consists of essential body fat. A density of 1.072 g · cm^{-3} represents the minimal body mass of 48.5 kg. In actual practice, density values exceeding 1.068 for women (14.8% body fat) and 1.088 g · cm^{-3} for men (5% body fat) rarely occur except in young, lean athletes.

Minimal Leanness Standards

A biologic lower limit seems to exist beyond which a person's body mass cannot decrease without impairing health status or altering normal physiologic functions.

Men

To estimate the lower body-fat limit in men (i.e., lean body mass), subtract storage fat from body mass. For the reference man, the lean body mass (61.7 kg) includes approximately 3% (2.1 kg) essential body fat. Encroachment into this reserve may impair optimal health and capacity for vigorous exercise.

Low body fat values exist for male world-class endurance athletes and some conscientious objectors to military service who voluntarily reduced body fat stores during a prolonged experiment with semistarvation.[93] The low fat levels of marathon runners, ranging from 1 to 8% of body mass, probably reflect an adaptation to the severe training for distance running. A low body fat level reduces the energy cost of weight-bearing exercise; it also provides a more effective gradient to dissipate metabolic heat generated during prolonged, high-intensity exercise.

Considerable variation exists in the FFM of different athletes, with values ranging from a low of 48.1 kg in some jockeys to over 160 kg in football offensive linemen and 100 kg in shot putters.[9] Seven elite sumo wrestlers *(seki-tori)* possessed an average FFM of 109 kg.[97] Table 28.2 (page 759) presents data on the physique status and body compositions of selected professional football players we have measured, many of whom classify as both underfat and overweight. Striking differences emerge among these athletes in body size, relative body fat, FFM, lean:fat ratio, and a matrix of girth measures. The defensive and offensive backs in football rated underfat compared with the reference man (or any other nonathletic standard). In contrast, linemen and shot putters were clearly overweight for their statures; body mass relative to stature (mass per unit size) represented the 90th percentile for nonathletic males.

Women

In contrast to the lower limit of body mass for the reference man (with 3% essential fat), the lower limit for the reference woman includes approximately 12% essential fat. This theoretical limit developed by Dr. Behnke, termed **minimal body mass**, is 48.5 kg for the reference woman. Generally, the leanest women in the population do not fall below 10 to 12% body fat, a narrow range probably at the lower limit for most women in good health.[82] *Behnke's theoretical concept of minimal body mass in women, incorporating approximately 12% essential fat, corresponds to the lean body mass in men that includes 3% essential fat.*

Calculation of Minimal Body Mass

A relatively simple method can estimate a woman's minimal body mass based on bone diameter measurements.[9] Body mass below the computed minimal body mass indicates an underweight condition that requires medical supervision. The following equation determines minimal body mass, where D is the sum of eight bone diameters, H (dm) is stature in decimeters, and 33.5 and 0.111 are constants:

$$\text{Minimal body mass} = (D/33.5)^2 \times H\ (\text{dm}) \times 0.111$$

Table 28.3 describes how to compute minimal body mass of a young, thin-appearing woman with a body mass of 38.7 kg and stature of 166.7 cm, or 16.67 dm. Standard methods were used to assess the eight bone diameters. Clearly, by Behnke's standards, this woman is underweight, because her scale-determined 38.7-kg body mass remains 8% below her recommended predicted minimal body mass of 41.9 kg.

Five-Level Model of Body Composition

Figure 28.7 shows a proposed five-level model for examining the human body.[189] Each level of the model becomes more elaborate—atoms, molecules, cells, tissue systems, whole body—as the body's complexity of biologic organization in-

TABLE 28.3 ➤ **HOW TO COMPUTE MINIMAL BODY MASS**[a]

DIAMETER	MEASUREMENT (CM)
Biacromial	34.4
Chest	23.8
Biiliac	22.7
Bitrochanteric	29.8
Knees[b]	16.1
Ankles[b]	11.5
Elbows[b]	11.1
Wrists[b]	10.0
Sum	159.4

[a]Data for a woman with stature of 166.7 cm (16.67 dm); body mass of 38.7 kg.
[b]Sum of right and left sides.
Step 1. Compute D, which is the sum of the eight diameters. Note that the last four measurements represent the sum of the right and left sides.
Step 2. Substitute in the equation for minimal body mass:
Minimal body mass = $(D/33.5)^2 \times H \times 0.111$
= $(159.4/33.5)^2 \times 16.67 \times 0.111$
= 41.9 kg

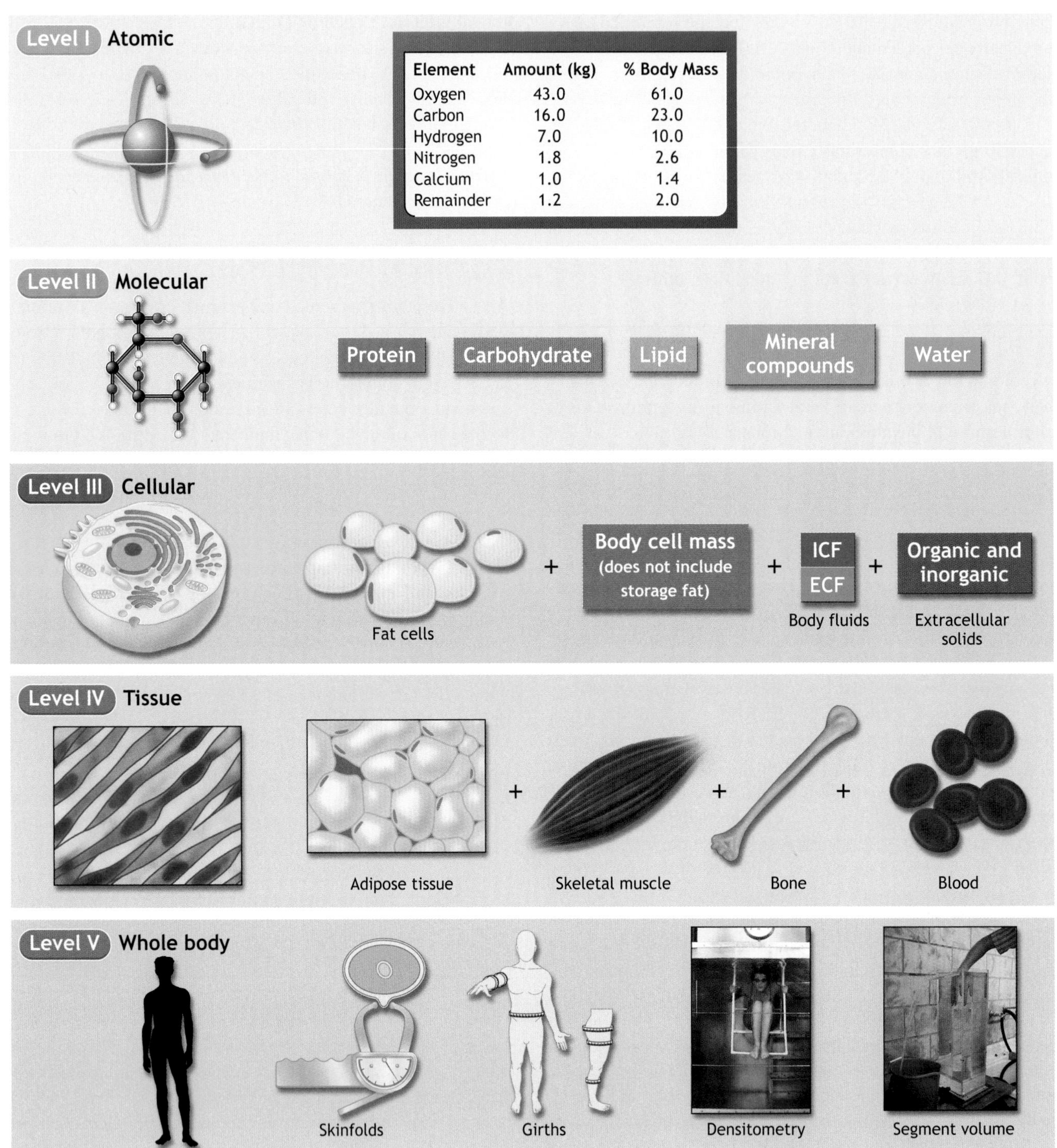

FIGURE 28.7 • Five-level multicomponent model to assess and interpret body composition. Each level progresses in complexity of biologic organization. Use of appropriate measurement techniques to assess the components within a particular organization level is the model's key feature. This allows researchers to focus on a particular body composition aspect in relation to specific and/or general biologic effects. Measurements could include changes in tissue composition from weight gain or loss or more theoretical aspects related to cellular and tissue functions. ICF, intracellular fluid; ECF, extracellular fluid. (Modified from Wang ZM, et al. The five-level model: a new approach to organizing body composition research. Am J Clin Nutr 1992;56:19.)

creases in accord with advances in physics and chemistry assessment techniques. Note that subdivisions exist within each of the five levels. The model primarily attempts to identify and then quantify each level's various components. An essential feature provides separate and distinct levels, each with directly or indirectly measurable characteristics. Examples of measurement include the following for a reference body weighing 70 kg:

- **Atomic level**. Body mass equals the sum of all the body's atoms (O + C + H + N + Ca + remainder). For a typical 70-kg man, this is generally 60% oxygen, 23% carbon, 10% hydrogen, 2.6% nitrogen, 1.4% calcium, and less than 1% for the remaining atoms. Cadaver or tissue biopsy samples determine the elemental composition. Whole-body ^{40}K counting assesses total body potassium,[135] with total body sodium, chlorine, phosphorus, and calcium determined by delayed-γ neutron activation,[27] total body nitrogen by prompt-γ neutron activation,[28] and total body carbon by inelastic neutron scattering.[91]

- **Molecular level**. The body's elements form molecules that constitute more than 100,000 different chemical compounds. Water, fat (essential and storage), glycogen, protein (nitrogen-containing compounds), and minerals (metallic and nonmetallic elements) are the major constituents. Certain elements can be sampled from body fluids and estimated by isotopic dilution,[48] and single[147] and dual-energy x-ray absorptiometry quantify osseous (bone containing 99% of the body's Ca and 86% of its P) and nonosseous mineral-containing compounds.[146]
- **Cellular level**. Three main compartments make up the body mass: (1) cells (cell mass = cells from muscles + connective [including fat cells], epithelial, and nervous tissues); (2) extracellular fluids (plasma + interstitial fluid); (3) extracellular solids (organic and inorganic extracellular solids). Isotopic dilution procedures measure extracellular fluid and plasma volumes. Determination of the naturally occurring radioactive isotope of potassium (^{40}K) assesses body cell mass because more than 95% of the body's potassium remains in the intracellular fluid compartment.
- **Tissue and organ level**. The body contains 11 subsystems—circulatory, respiratory, nervous, integumentary, muscular, endocrine, respiratory, lymphatic, digestive, skeletal, and reproductive. This level of body composition evaluation groups four tissue systems to represent total body mass (adipose tissue + skeletal muscle + bone + blood). Computed tomography, magnetic resonance imaging, and ultrasound procedures estimate the volumes of subcutaneous fat, visceral adipose tissue, and segmental muscle mass.
- **Whole-body level**. Common anthropometric procedures include measurement of skinfolds, girths, bone diameters, body mass, stature, BMI, surface area, segment lengths, segmental and total body volume, and body density (hydrodensitometry).

Underweight and Thin

The terms *underweight* and *thin* at times describe considerably different physical conditions. Measurements in our laboratories have focused on the structural characteristics of apparently thin females.[88] We initially screened subjects subjectively as thin or "skinny." Each of 26 women were measured for skinfolds, circumferences, and bone diameters, and percentage body fat and FFM from hydrodensitometry.

Unexpectedly, the women's percentage body fat averaged 18.2%, only 7 percentage points below values of 25 to 27% body fat typically reported for young adult women. Another striking finding included equivalence in four trunk and four extremity bone diameter measurements for the thin-appearing women compared to 174 women who averaged 25.6% fat and 31 women who averaged 31.4% body fat. *Thus, appearing thin or skinny did not necessarily correspond to a diminutive frame size or low body fat content proposed in the Behnke model for the lower limits of minimal body mass and essential body fat.*

We recommend three criteria to designate an underweight adult female:

1. Body mass lower than minimal body mass calculated from skeletal measurements outlined in Table 28.3
2. Body mass lower than the 20th percentile by stature
3. Percentage body fat lower than 17% assessed by a criterion method

Leanness, Regular Exercise, and Menstrual Irregularity

Physically active women, particularly participants in the "low weight" or "appearance" sports (e.g., distance running, body building, figure skating, diving, ballet, and gymnastics), increase their likelihood for one of three maladies: (1) delayed onset of menstruation, (2) irregular menstrual cycle (**oligomenorrhea**), or (3) complete cessation of menses (**amenorrhea**).[61,113] Menstrual and ovarian dysfunction results largely from changes in the pituitary gland's normal pulsatile secretion of luteinizing hormone, regulated by gonadotropin-releasing hormone from the hypothalamus.[114]

Amenorrhea occurs in 2 to 5% of women of reproductive age in the general population, but it can reach 40% in some athletic groups. As a group, ballet dancers remain lean and exhibit a greater incidence of menstrual dysfunction, eating disorders, and a higher mean age at menarche than age-matched, nondance counterparts.[51,191] One-third to one-half of female endurance athletes exhibit some menstrual irregularity. In premenopausal women, irregularity or absence of menstrual function accelerates bone loss and increases the risk of musculoskeletal injury during exercise and longer interruption of training (see Chapter 2).[7,61,138]

A high level of chronic physical stress (**exercise stress hypothesis**) may disrupt the hypothalamic-pituitary-adrenal axis and modify the output of gonadotropin-releasing hormone, which results in irregular menstruation. A concurrent hypothesis maintains that an energy reserve inadequate to sustain pregnancy (**energy availability hypothesis**) induces cessation of ovulation. Some researchers argue that 17% body fat represents a critical level for onset of menstruation, with 22% fat needed to sustain a normal cycle.[51,52] They reason that body fat below these levels triggers hormonal and metabolic disturbances that affect the menses. Research with animals has identified leptin, a hormone intimately linked to body fat levels and appetite control (see Chapter 30), as a principal chemical that initiates puberty.[24,176] Thus, a linkage may exist between hormonal regulation of sexual maturity onset (and perhaps continued optimal sexual function) and the level of stored energy reflected by accumulated body fat.

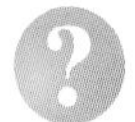

INTEGRATIVE QUESTION

What arguments counter the following position? No true sex difference exists in body fat, but only a difference caused by gender-related patterns of regular physical activity and caloric intake.

Lean:Fat Ratio

The **lean:fat ratio** may play a key role in normal menstrual function (perhaps through peripheral fat's role in converting androgens to estrogens or through leptin production in adipose tissue), but other factors may as well. *Many physically active females who are below the supposedly critical 17% body fat level have normal menstrual cycles with a high level of physiologic and exercise capacity.*[50] Conversely, some amenorrheic athletes maintain body fat levels considered average for the population. In one of our laboratories, we compared 30 athletes and 30 nonathletes, all having less than 20% body fat, for menstrual cycle regularity.[86] Four athletes and three nonathletes, ranging from 11 to 15% body fat, maintained regular cycles, whereas seven athletes and two nonathletes had irregular cycles or were amenorrheic. For the total sample, 14 athletes and 21 nonathletes maintained regular menstrual cycles. These data provide clear evidence that normal menstrual function *does not require* a critical body fat level of 17 to 22%.

Potential causes of menstrual dysfunction include the complex interplay of physical, nutritional, genetic, hormonal, regional fat distribution, psychologic, and environmental factors.[179,204] An intense exercise bout triggers release of an array of hormones, some of which may disrupt normal reproductive function.[59,197] Intense and/or prolonged exercise that releases cortisol and other stress-related hormones may alter ovarian function via the hypothalamic-pituitary-adrenal axis.[31,113]

Further research must determine whether regular intense exercise produces a cumulative hormonal effect sufficient to disrupt normal menses. In this regard, when injuries to young amenorrheic ballet dancers prevent them from exercising regularly, normal menstruation resumes even though body weight remains low.[191] Additional predisposing factors for reproductive endocrine dysfunction among athletes include nutritional inadequacy and an exercise-induced energy deficit with heavy training.[74,205] Prolonged exercise per se causes no disruption in the pulsatile release of luteinizing hormone, independent of the hormonal disturbance caused by exercise on energy and/or glucose availability.[114] Consuming well-balanced, nutritious meals may prevent or reverse athletic amenorrhea without requiring that the athlete reduce exercise training volume or intensity.[112]

In all likelihood, 13 to 17% body fat probably represents the minimum associated with regular menstrual function. The effects and risks of sustained amenorrhea on the reproductive system remain unknown. A gynecologist/endocrinologist should evaluate failure to menstruate or cessation of the normal cycle because it may reflect a significant medical condition (e.g., pituitary or thyroid gland malfunction or premature menopause).[6,111,164] As we point out in Chapter 2, prolonged menstrual dysfunction affects bone mass profoundly and negatively.

Delayed Onset of Menstruation and Cancer Risk

The delayed onset of menarche in chronically active young females may offer positive health benefits.[52,53,170] Female athletes who start training in high school or earlier show a lower lifetime occurrence of cancers of the breast and reproductive organs, in addition to non–reproductive-system cancers than their less-active counterparts. Even among older women, regular exercise appears to protect against reproductive cancers. Swedish researchers studied the country's entire female population aged 50–74 years in 1994–1995.[132] Compared to 3368 controls without endometrial cancer, higher levels of occupational and leisure-time physical activity in nonsmokers of normal body mass during ages 18 to 30 years related to significantly lower postmenopausal endometrial cancer risk. Women who exercise an average of 4 hours a week after menarche reduce their risk of breast cancer by 50% compared with age-matched inactive women.[12] One proposed mechanism for reduced cancer risk links less total estrogen production (or a less potent estrogen form) over the athlete's lifetime with fewer ovulatory cycles because of the delayed onset of menstruation.[180,193] Lower body fat levels in athletes also may contribute to lowered risk because peripheral fatty tissues convert androgens to estrogen.

COMMON TECHNIQUES TO ASSESS BODY COMPOSITION

Procedures to evaluate body composition involve:

1. Direct measurement by chemical analysis of the animal carcass or human cadaver
2. Indirect estimation by hydrostatic weighing, simple anthropometric measurements, or other procedures

Direct Assessment

Two approaches directly assess body composition. One technique uses a chemical solution to literally dissolve the body to determine its mixture of fat and fat-free components. The other technique involves physical dissection of fat, fat-free adipose tissue, muscle, and bone. Considerable research has chemically assessed body composition in various animal species, but few studies have directly determined human fat content.[26,48] These analyses are labor intensive and tedious, require specialized laboratory equipment, and involve ethical questions and legal hurdles in obtaining cadavers for research purposes.

Direct body composition assessment suggests that while considerable individual differences exist in total body fatness, the compositions of skeletal mass and the fat-free and fat tissues remain relatively stable. Based on these assumptions, researchers have developed mathematical equations to predict the body's fat percentage on the basis of the assumed constancy of these tissues.

Indirect Assessment

Diverse indirect procedures assess body composition.[153] One involves Archimedes' principle applied to hydrostatic weighing (also referred to as *densitometry* or *underwater weighing*). This method computes percentage body fat from body density, the ratio of body mass to body volume. Other procedures predict body fat from skinfold thickness and girth measurements, x-ray, total body electrical conductivity or impedance, near-infrared interactance, ultrasound, computed tomography, air plethysmography, and magnetic resonance imaging.

Hydrostatic Weighing: Archimedes' Principle

The Greek mathematician and inventor **Archimedes** (287–212 BC) discovered a fundamental principle currently applied to evaluate human body composition. An itinerant scholar of that time described the circumstances surrounding the event:

> King Hieron of Syracuse suspected that his pure gold crown had been altered by substitution of silver for gold. The King directed Archimedes to devise a method for testing the crown for its gold content without dismantling it. Archimedes pondered over this problem for many weeks without succeeding, until one day, he stepped into a bath filled to the top with water and observed the overflow. He thought about this for a moment, and then, wild with joy, jumped from the bath and ran naked through the streets of Syracuse shouting, "Eureka, Eureka! I have discovered a way to solve the mystery of the King's crown."

Archimedes reasoned that a substance such as gold must have a volume proportional to its mass, and measuring the volume of an irregularly shaped object would require submersion in water, with collection of the overflow. To apply his reasoning, Archimedes took lumps of gold and silver of the same mass as the crown, and submerged each in a container full of water. He discovered the crown displaced more water than the lump of gold and less than the lump of silver. This could only mean that the crown consisted of *both* silver and gold as the king suspected.

Essentially, Archimedes compared the **specific gravity** of the crown with the specific gravities for gold and silver. He probably also reasoned that an object submerged or floating in water becomes buoyed up by a counterforce that equals the weight of the volume of water it displaces. This buoyant force supports an immersed object against gravity's downward pull. Thus, an object loses weight in water. *Because the object's loss of weight in water equals the weight of the volume of water it displaces, its specific gravity refers to the mass of an object in air divided by its loss of weight in water.* The loss equals the weight in air minus the weight in water.

$$\text{Specific gravity} = \text{Mass in air} \div \text{Loss of weight in water}$$

In practical terms, suppose a crown weighed 2.27 kg in air and 0.13 kg less, or 2.14 kg, when weighed underwater (Fig. 28.8). Dividing the crown's mass (2.27 kg) by its weight loss in water (0.13 kg) yields a specific gravity of 17.5. Be-

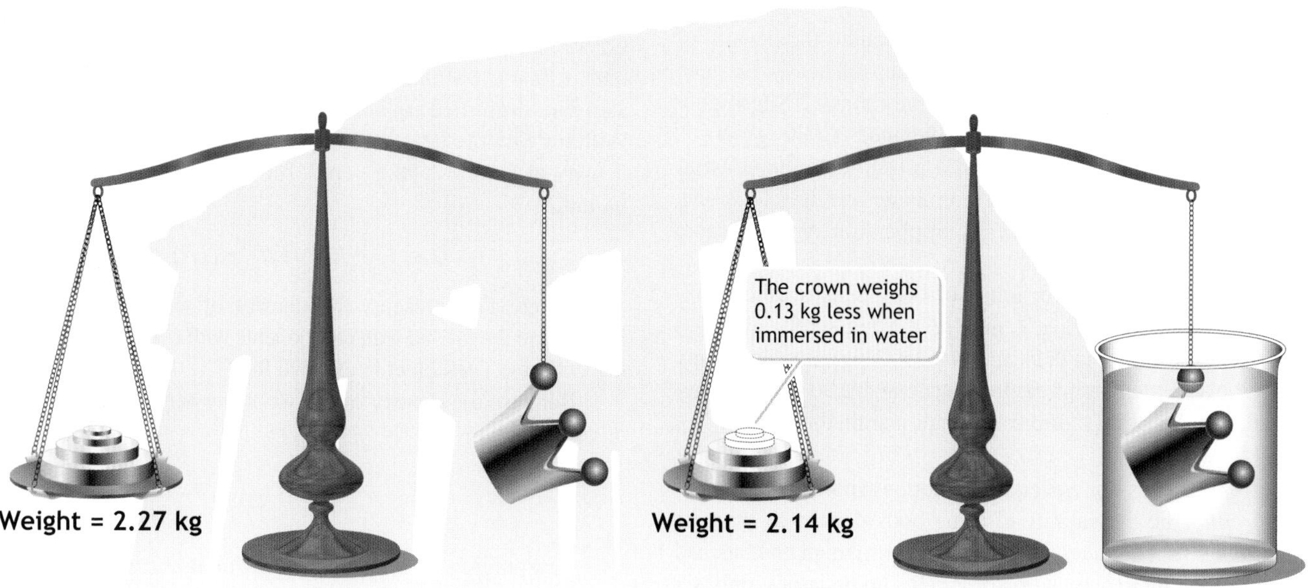

FIGURE 28.8 • Archimedes' principle of buoyant force to determine the volume and, subsequently, specific gravity of the king's crown.

cause this ratio differs considerably from the specific gravity of gold, 19.3, we too can conclude "Eureka, the crown is a fraud!" The physical principle Archimedes discovered allows us to use water submersion to determine the body's volume. Dividing a person's body mass by body volume yields body density (density = mass ÷ volume), and from this an estimate of percentage body fat.

One can think of specific gravity as an object's "heaviness" related to its volume. Objects of the same volume may vary considerably in density, defined as mass per unit volume. One gram of water occupies exactly 1 cm^{-3} at a temperature of 39.2°F (4°C); the density would equal 1 $g \cdot cm^{-3}$. Water achieves its greatest density at 4°C; thus, increasing water temperature increases the volume of 1 g of water and decreases its density. Therefore, one must correct the volume of an object weighed in water for water density at the weighing temperature (see Appendix A). The temperature effect distinguishes density from specific gravity.

INTEGRATIVE QUESTION

Why does a piece of steel or concrete sink rapidly when placed in water while a boat made of either substance floats readily?

Validity of Hydrostatic Weighing to Estimate Body Fat. Experimental evidence supports the validity of hydrostatic weighing to estimate the body's fat content. Behnke's early studies of Navy divers placed 64 subjects into two groups based on their body density. The mean difference between the groups in body mass (12.4 kg) and body volume (13.3 L) allowed Behnke to easily discern body composition differences between the groups. The ratio of the average differences (Δ mass÷ Δ volume) equaled 0.933 $g \cdot cm^{-3}$, a value within the density range of 0.92 to 0.96 $g \cdot cm^{-3}$ for human adipose tissue. Thus, the difference in body mass between the high- and low-density groups represented the density of adipose tissue. Body density for a group of heavy but lean professional football players (lean body mass 20 kg higher than that of the Navy divers) averaged 1.080 $g \cdot cm^{-3}$. Behnke stated, "Here indeed was a presumptive demonstration that fat could be separated from bone and muscle *in vivo* or 'the silver from the gold' by application of a principle renowned in antiquity."[9]

The lower and upper limits of body density among humans range from 0.93 $g \cdot cm^{-1}$ in the massively obese to nearly 1.10 $g \cdot cm^{-3}$ in the leanest males. This coincides nicely with the 1.10 density of fat-free tissue and 0.90 for homogenized samples of fat tissue from small mammals at 37°C.[94]

Possible Limitations. Several assumptions (not verified in humans) underlie the validity of using body density to estimate total body fat. Although 19th-century German anatomists had studied the gross composition of various body tissues, only six adult human bodies had been analyzed for skin, muscle, adipose tissue, bone, and organ components. Anatomic studies in 1984 presented data from 12 embalmed (6 male, 6 female) and 13 nonembalmed (6 male, 7 female) cadavers ranging in age from 55 to 94 years (see "Focus on Research," Chapter 29).[26]

The time-consuming and meticulous cadaver analyses indicate possible limitations in the two-compartment fat and fat-free model for body composition assessment. The data could not affirm that the densities of the fat-free components (bone, mineral, muscle, and water) remained constant among individuals. Also, muscle as a percentage of the FFM ranged between 41.9% (female) and 59.4% (male); similarly, bone ranged between 17.4% (male) and 25.7% (female). Other experiments also demonstrate large individual variation in bone density in living humans. Interindividual variation in the density and percentage contribution of the fat-free tissue components indicates limitations in using whole body density as the "gold standard" for estimating percentage body fat and FFM. One hopes that additional cadaver studies over a broad age range of "healthy" men and women will improve the theoretical model for estimating components of human body composition.

Computing Body Density. For illustrative purposes, suppose that a 50-kg person weighs 2 kg submerged in water. According to Archimedes' principle, loss of weight in water of 48 kg equals the weight of the displaced water. One can easily compute the volume of water displaced by correcting for the density of water at the weighing temperature. In this example, 48 kg of water equals 48 L, or 48,000 cm^{-3} (1 g of water = 1 cm^{-3} by volume at 39.2°F). Measuring the person at a water temperature of 39.2°F requires no density correction for water temperature. In practice, researchers use warmer water and apply the appropriate density value for water at the weighing temperature. The density of this person, computed as mass ÷ volume, equals 50,000 g (50 kg) ÷ 48,000 cm^3, or 1.0417 $g \cdot cm^{-3}$. The next step estimates percentage body fat and the mass of fat and fat-free tissues.

Computing Percentage Body Fat. An equation that incorporates whole-body density can estimate the body's fat percentage. The simplified equation derived by UC Berkley scientist William Siri (1919–1998) substitutes 0.90 $g \cdot cm^{-3}$ for the density of fat and 1.10 $g \cdot cm^{-3}$ for the density of the fat-free tissues.[167,168]

$$D = F + L \div (F/f) + (L/l)$$

Where D represents the density of the whole system; F and L are the fat and lean components with densities of f and l, respectively. The object is to solve for F.

Because the density of the whole system equals the sum of its parts,

$$F + L = 1.00$$
$$D = 1.00 \div (F/f) + (L/l)$$

Rearranging terms, the proportional contribution of F becomes,

$$F = 1.00 \div D \times f \times l \div (l - f) - f \div (l - f)$$

The final derivation, referred to as the **Siri equation**, computes percentage body fat as:

$$\text{Percentage body fat} = (495 \div \text{body density}) - 450$$

This equation assumes the two-component model of body composition. The density of fat extracted from adipose tissue is 0.90 g · cm^{-3} at 36°C, and 1.10 g · cm^{-3} for fat-free tissue. The pioneer researchers in this area maintained that each of these densities remains relatively constant among individuals despite large individual variations in total fat and FFM. They also assumed that the densities of the lean tissue components of bone and muscle remained the same among individuals.

In the previous example (body mass, 50 kg and body volume, 48 L), the resulting whole body density of 1.0417 g · cm^{-3} converted to percentage fat by the Siri equation equaled 25.2%.

$$\text{Percentage body fat} = (495 \div 1.0417) - 450 = 25.2\%$$

Several formulas other than Siri's equation also estimate percentage body fat from body density.[17,92] The basic difference among the formulas in calculating body fat generally averages less than 1% body fat units for body fat levels between 4 and 30%.

LIMITATIONS OF DENSITY ASSUMPTIONS. The generalized density values for the fat-free (1.10 g · cm^{-3}) and fat (0.90 g · cm^{-3}) tissue compartments represent averages for young and middle-aged adults. These "constants" vary among individuals and groups, particularly the density and chemical composition of the FFM. Such variation places some limitation in partitioning body mass into fat and fat-free components and predicting percentage body fat from whole-body density.[54,118] More specifically, the average density of the FFM is higher for blacks and Hispanics than for whites (1.113 g · cm^{-3} blacks, 1.105 g · cm^{-3} Hispanics, and 1.100 g · cm^{-3} whites).[142,161,171] A racial difference also exists among adolescents.[178,203] Consequently, using the existing equations formulated from assumptions for whites to calculate body composition from body density in blacks or Hispanics *overestimates* FFM and *underestimates* percentage body fat.[33] The following proposed modification of the Siri equation computes percentage body fat from body density for blacks:

$$\text{Percentage body fat} = (437.4 \div \text{body density}) - 392.8$$

Applying constant density values for the different tissues in growing children or aging adults also introduces errors in predicting body composition.[108] For example, the water and mineral contents of the FFM continually change during the growth period and the well-documented demineralization of osteoporosis with aging.[192] Reduced bone density makes the actual density of the fat-free tissue of young children and the elderly lower than the assumed 1.10 g · cm^{-3} constant. This invalidates the underlying assumptions of the two-compartment model (i.e., assumed constant densities of the fat and fat-free masses) and *overestimates* relative body fat calculated from densitometry. For this reason, many researchers do not convert body density to percentage body fat in children and aging adults. Others apply a multicompartment model to adjust for such factors in computing percentage body fat from body density in prepubertal children.[108,169,195] Table 28.4 presents equations adjusted to maturation level to predict body fat from whole-body density of boys and girls ages 7 to 17.

In professional American football players and competitive bodybuilders, exercise training-related increases in bone mineral mass, muscle mass, and extracellular fluid volume could affect the density of the fat-free component (thus affecting body fat estimates with hydrostatic weighing). The density of the fat-free component in such athletes could theoretically exceed 1.10 g · cm^{-3}. This would *underestimate* relative fat (when assuming a density of 1.10 g · cm^{-3}) and account for negative percentage body fat in exceptionally lean individuals.[3] On the other hand, water, protein, and minerals (and ratios of total body potassium and total body water) contribute similarly to FFM in white, male long-distance runners and their untrained counterparts,[145] even though FFM constitutes a larger proportion of the runner's body mass. Such data support use of the classic two-compartment model to evaluate an athlete's body composition, at least for trained white male runners.

Adjust for Large Musculoskeletal Development. Chronic resistance training affects the density of the FFM, altering body fat estimation from whole-body density determinations.[131] Fourteen white male weight lifters with significant muscular development and 14 nontrained controls were measured for body density (hydrostatic weighing), total body wa-

TABLE 28.4 ➤ **PERCENTAGE BODY FAT ESTIMATED FROM BODY DENSITY (BD) USING AGE- AND GENDER-SPECIFIC CONVERSION CONSTANTS TO ACCOUNT FOR CHANGES IN THE DENSITY OF THE FAT-FREE BODY MASS AS A CHILD MATURES**

AGE (YEARS)	BOYS	GIRLS
7–9	% Fat = (5.38/BD − 4.97) × 100	% Fat = (5.43/BD − 5.03) × 100
9–11	% Fat = (5.30/BD − 4.89) × 100	% Fat = (5.35/BD − 4.95) × 100
11–13	% Fat = (5.23/BD − 4.81) × 100	% Fat = (5.25/BD − 4.84) × 100
13–15	% Fat = (5.08/BD − 4.64) × 100	% Fat = (5.12/BD − 4.69) × 100
15–17	% Fat = (5.03/BD − 4.59) × 100	% Fat = (5.07/BD − 4.64) × 100

From Lohman T. Applicability of body composition techniques and constants for children and youth. Exerc Sports Sci Rev 1986;14:325.

ter (deuterium dilution), and bone mineral content (dual-energy x-ray absorptiometry). Comparisons included estimations of percentage body fat using both the two-compartment model applied in the Siri equation and a four-compartment model using the body's fat, water, mineral, and protein content and corresponding densities. Percentage body fat estimated from body density (Siri equation) produced significantly higher values than percentage body fat estimated from the four-compartment model for the weight trainers but not for untrained controls. A *lower FFM density* in weight trainers than in controls (1.089 vs. 1.099 g · cm^{-3}) explained this discrepancy; it resulted from larger water and smaller mineral and protein fractions of the FFM in the resistance-trained men. For them, incorrect assumptions underlying the Siri equation *overestimated* percentage body fat.

For the weight lifters, muscularity increased disproportionately to changes in bone mass. A lower FFM density occurred because the density of their fat-free muscle (1.066 g · cm^{-3} at 37°C) was below the 1.1 g · cm^{-3} value assumed in the Siri equation. Disproportionate increases in muscle mass relative to increases in bone mass accounted for the reduced density of the FFM below 1.1 g ·cm^{-3}, thus overpredicting percentage body fat based on the two-compartment model. If resistance training does indeed progressively alter FFM density, then applying the Siri equation would not accurately reflect true body composition changes from this mode of training.

Based on revised densities of the FFM (1.089 g · cm^{-3}) and fat mass (0.9007 g · cm^{-3}), the researchers recommend modifying Siri's equation as follows for more accurate appraisal resistance-trained white males:

$$\text{Percentage body fat} = (521 \div \text{body density}) - 478$$

Computing Fat Mass. Using data from the example on page 768, fat mass is computed by multiplying body mass by percentage fat.

$$\begin{aligned} \text{Fat mass} &= \text{body mass} \times (\%\ \text{fat}/100) \\ &= 50\ \text{kg} \times 0.252 \\ &= 12.5\ \text{kg} \end{aligned}$$

Further computations could subdivide this person's fat mass into essential and storage fat. A female with 25.2% body fat has approximately 12% essential fat, or 6.0 kg (0.12 × 50 kg); the remaining 13.2% (6.6 kg) exists as storage fat (0.132 × 50 kg). For a male with 3% essential fat and 22.2% storage fat (based on 25.2% body fat), the corresponding values equal 1.5 kg for essential fat and 11.1 kg for storage fat. Clearly, for a man and a woman with identical percentage body fat, the man rates "fatter," because storage fat represents a larger percentage of total body fat. Each gram of body fat (83% pure fat) contains approximately 7.5 kcal (7500 kcal per kg). Thus, one can compute the approximate potential energy stored in each fat depot. For storage fat in this example, the values are 49,500 kcal for the woman and 83,260 kcal for the man; for essential fat, including a female's sex-specific fat, the values are 45,000 kcal for the woman and 11,250 kcal for the man.

Computing Fat-Free Body Mass. Compute FFM by subtracting the absolute fat mass from body mass.

$$\begin{aligned} \text{Fat-free body mass} &= \text{body mass} - \text{fat mass} \\ &= 50\ \text{kg} - 12.5\ \text{kg} \\ &= 37.5\ \text{kg} \end{aligned}$$

Body Volume Measurement

The principle discovered by Archimedes applies body volume measurement in one of two ways: (1) water displacement or (2) hydrostatic weighing. Body volume requires accurate measurement, because small volume variations substantially affect the density calculation and, hence, computed percentage body fat and FFM.

Water Displacement

One can measure the volume of an object submerged in water by the corresponding rise in the level of water within a container. With this technique, a finely calibrated tube secured to the side of the container that measures the rise of water permits accurate volume measurements. When measuring body volume in this manner, one must account for the volume of air remaining in the subject's lungs during submersion. The usual protocol assesses this lung volume before the subject enters the tank and subtracts it from the total body volume determined by water displacement. **Water displacement** has proved effective in assessing arm and leg volumes and their corresponding changes with exercise training, weight gain or loss, or physical inactivity.

Hydrostatic Weighing

Hydrostatic weighing is the most common application of Archimedes' principle to determine body volume. It computes body volume as the difference between body mass measured in air (M_a) and body weight measured during water submersion (W_w; *weight* is the correct term, since the body's mass remains unchanged under water). *Body volume equals loss of weight in water with the appropriate temperature correction for water's density.*

Figure 28.9 illustrates the measurement of body volume by hydrostatic weighing under four different conditions. The first step accurately assesses the subject's body mass in air, usually ±50 g. The subject, who wears a thin nylon swimsuit, sits in a lightweight, plastic tubular chair suspended from the scale and submerged beneath the water's surface. A swimming pool serves the same purpose as the tank, with the scale and chair assembly suspended from a support at the side of the pool or diving board. The tank maintains a comfortable water temperature at approximately 95°F, similar to skin temperature. Recording water temperature provides the correction factor to determine water density at the weighing temperature (see Appendix A). A diver's belt secured around the waist (or placed across the lap) prevents the subject from floating toward the surface during submersion. The underwater weight of

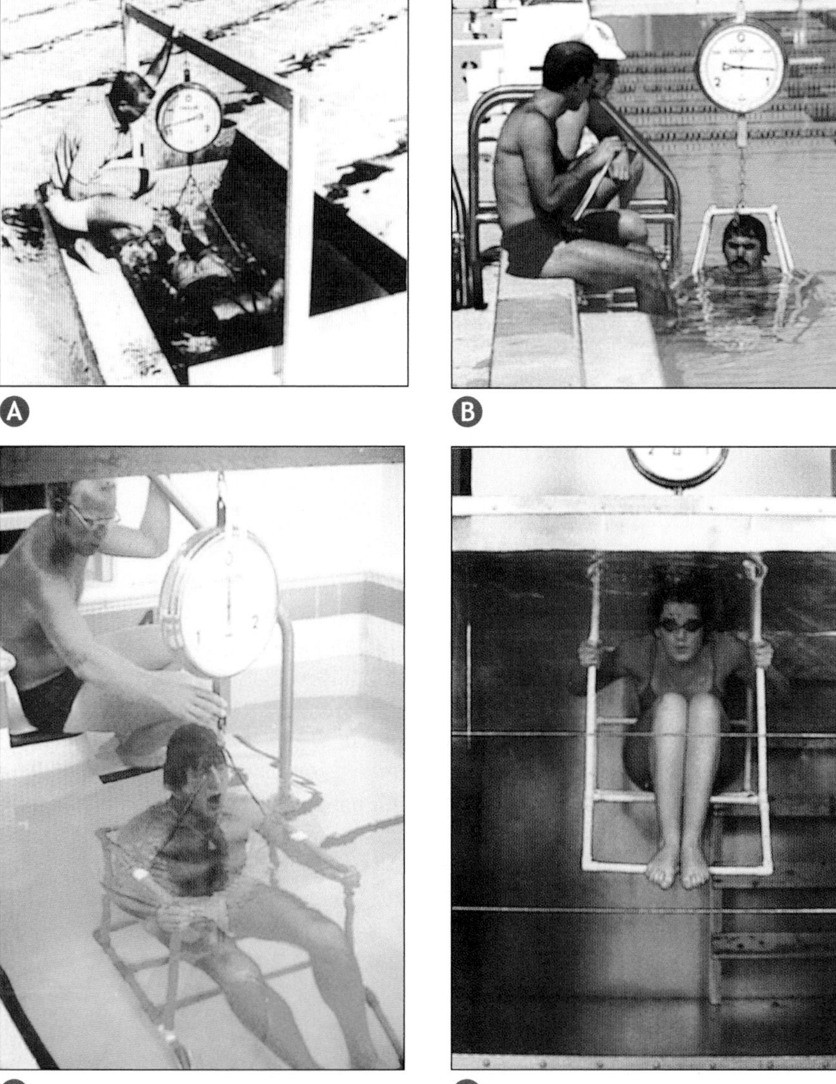

FIGURE 28.9 • Measuring body volume by underwater weighing. Prone and supine underwater weighing methods provide the same values, with residual lung volume measured before, during, or after the underwater weighing. Measurements taken (**A**) prone in a swimming pool, (**B**) seated in a swimming pool, (**C**) seated in a therapy pool, and (**D**) seated in a stainless steel tank with Plexiglas front in the laboratory. For any of the methods, subjects can use a snorkel with nose clip if they express apprehension about submersion. The final calculation of underwater weight must account for these objects.

this belt and chair (tare weight) is subtracted from the subject's total weight under water.

Seated with the head above water, the subject makes a forced maximal exhalation while slowly lowering the head under the water. The breath is held for 5 to 8 seconds to allow the scale pointer to stabilize before recording the reading at the midpoint of the oscillations. The subject repeats the procedure 8 to 12 times to obtain a dependable underwater weight score. This practice accounts for the "learning curve" in making forced exhalations during submersion.[75] Even when achieving a full exhalation, a small volume of air, the residual lung volume, remains in the lungs. Body volume calculation requires subtracting the buoyant effect of the residual lung volume, measured immediately before, during, or following the underwater weighing.[134] Reproducibility of body volumes measured several times on the same day or on consecutive days remains high, with test–retest reliability coefficients usually exceeding $r = 0.94$.[87] Failure to account for residual lung volume *underestimates* whole body density because the lungs' air volume contributes to buoyancy. This omission would create a "fatter" person on conversion of body density to percentage body fat. One can substitute a modified underwater weighing procedure that does not require full head submersion for subjects who exhibit anxiety in making a forced maximal exhalation while submerged (or younger or older subjects, the infirm, handicapped, or other special populations). The modification where the subject sits with water level just below the chin yields body density values that are nearly identical to the standard procedure with full head immersion.[37]

VARIATIONS WITH MENSTRUATION. Normal fluctuations in body mass (chiefly body water) related to the menstrual cycle generally do not affect body density and body fat assessed by hydrostatic weighing. However, some females can experience noticeable changes in body water (>1.0 kg) during menstruation. Water retention of this magnitude does affect body density and introduces a small error in computing percentage body fat.[18]

CALCULATING BODY COMPOSITION FROM BODY MASS, BODY VOLUME, AND RESIDUAL LUNG VOLUME. Data for two professional football players, an offensive guard and a quarterback, illustrate the sequence of steps in computing body density, percentage fat, fat mass, and FFM (Table 28.5). Mass ÷ volume is the conventional formula for density, with density expressed in grams per cubic centimeter, mass in kilograms, and volume in liters. The difference between M_a and W_w equals body volume, after applying the appropriate water temperature correction (D_w). Air remaining in the lungs and other "spaces" of the body (abdominal viscera, sinuses) contributes some buoyancy at the time of underwater weighing. In the extreme, consuming 800 mL of a carbonated beverage increases gastric gas volume by approximately 600 mL. This underestimates body density by hydrostatic weighing by 0.7% and overestimates percentage body fat by 11% compared with measures made before drinking the beverage.[148] However, in most subjects, abdominal gas and sinus air volume remain small (<100 mL) and can be ignored. *This contrasts with the relatively large and variable residual lung volume, which requires measurement and subsequent subtraction from the total body volume.*

Whereas the residual lung volume tends to decrease slightly in a person immersed in water compared to the volume in air (probably owing to water's compressive force against the thoracic cavity), the difference exerts only a small effect on computed percentage body fat.[68] Consequently, most laboratories measure residual lung volume in air just before underwater weighing.

The following formula computes body density (D_b) from underwater weighing variables:

$$D_b = \text{mass} \div \text{volume}$$
$$= M_a \div [(M_a - W_w) \div D_w] - RLV$$

For ease in computation, the following formula can be used:

$$D_b = M_a \times D_w / (M_a - W_w - RLV \times D_w)$$

TABLE 28.5 ➤ MEASUREMENTS OF TWO PROFESSIONAL FOOTBALL PLAYERS FROM UNDERWATER WEIGHING

VARIABLE	SYMBOL	DEFENSIVE LINEMAN	RUNNING BACK
Body mass (kg)	M_a	121.73	97.37
Net underwater weight (kg)	M_w	7.30	6.52
Water temperature correction	D_w	0.99336	0.99336
Residual lung volume (L)	RLV	1.213	1.374
Total body volume (L)	TBV	113.89	90.08
Body density (g · cm⁻³)	D_b	1.0688	1.0809
BODY COMPOSITION			
Relative percentage body fat (%)	%Fat	13.1	8.0
Absolute body fat (kg)	FM	15.9	7.2
Fat-free body mass (kg)	FFM	105.8	90.2

[a]Siri equation; %fat = (495/density) − 450.

The lower part of Table 28.5 presents body composition results for the two football players based on body density.

Skinfold and Girth Measurements

In field situations, two relatively simple procedures that measure either subcutaneous fat (**skinfolds**) or circumferences (**girths**) predict body fatness with reasonable accuracy.

Subcutaneous Fat Measurement

The rationale for using skinfolds to estimate body fat comes from the interrelationships among three factors: (1) adipose tissue depot fat directly beneath the skin (subcutaneous fat), (2) internal fat, and (3) whole body density.

THE CALIPER. By 1930, a pincer-type caliper accurately measured subcutaneous fat at selected anatomic sites. The three calipers shown in Figure 28.10 operate on a principle similar to that of a micrometer that measures distance between two points. Measuring skinfold thickness requires grasping a fold of skin and subcutaneous fat firmly with the thumb and forefingers, pulling it away from the underlying muscle tissue following the natural contour of the skinfold. When calibrated, the pincer jaws exert a relatively constant tension ($10\ g \cdot mm^{-2}$) at the point of contact with the double layer of skin plus subcutaneous tissue. The caliper dial indicates skinfold thickness in millimeters, recorded within 2 seconds after applying the full force of the caliper. This time limitation avoids skinfold

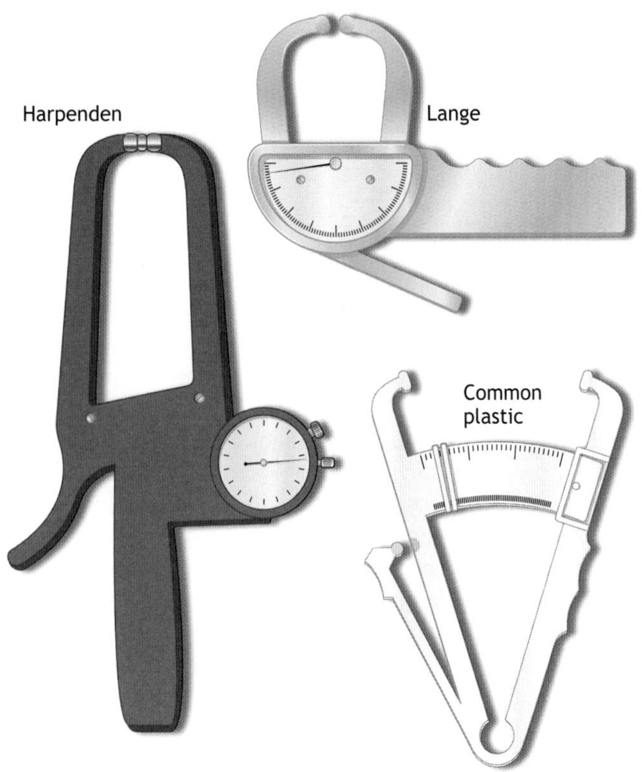

FIGURE 28.10 • Common calipers for skinfold measurements. The Harpenden and Lange calipers provide constant tension at all jaw openings.

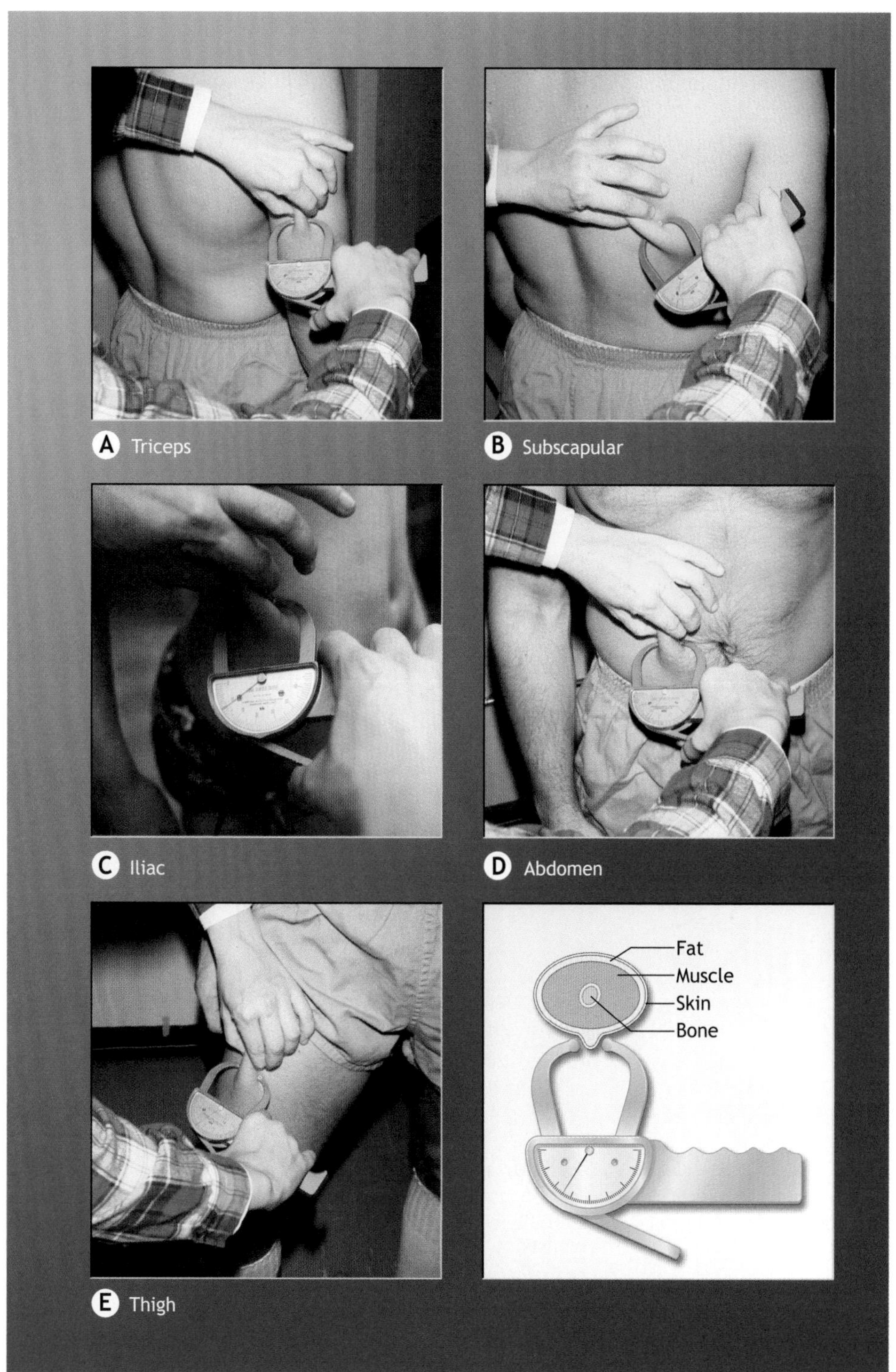

FIGURE 28.11 • Anatomic location of five common skinfold sites: **A**. Triceps. **B**. Subscapular. **C**. Iliac. **D**. Abdominal. **E**. Thigh. Measurements are taken on the right side of the body in the vertical plane, except diagonally at subscapular and suprailiac sites.

compression when taking the measurement.[8] For research purposes, the investigator should have considerable experience in taking measurements and demonstrate consistency in duplicating values for the same subjects on the same day, consecutive days, or even weeks apart. A good rule of thumb to achieve consistency requires duplicate or triplicate practice measurements on approximately 50 individuals who vary in body fat. This amount of careful attention to detail usually ensures high reproducibility of measurement (test–retest reliability at all sites, $r > 0.90$).

MEASUREMENT SITES. The most common anatomic sites for skinfold measurements include triceps, subscapular, suprailiac, abdominal, and upper thigh sites. The investigator should take a minimum of two or three measurements in rotational order at each site on the right side of the body with the subject standing. The average value represents the skinfold score. Figure 28.11 shows the anatomic location of the most frequently measured skinfold sites:

- Triceps: Vertical fold at the posterior midline of the right upper arm, halfway between the tip of the

shoulder and tip of the elbow; elbow remains in an extended, relaxed position
- Subscapular: Oblique fold, just below the bottom tip of the right scapula
- Suprailiac (iliac crest): Slightly oblique fold, just above the right hipbone (crest of ileum); the fold follows the natural diagonal line
- Abdominal: Vertical fold 1 inch to the right of the umbilicus
- Thigh: Vertical fold at the midline of the right thigh, two-thirds of the distance from the middle of the patella (kneecap) to the hip

Other sites include:

- Chest: Diagonal fold with its long axis directed toward the right nipple; on the anterior axillary fold as high as possible
- Biceps: Vertical fold at the posterior midline of the right upper arm

Usefulness of Skinfold Scores

Skinfold measurements provide fairly consistent and meaningful information about body fat and its distribution. We recommend two ways to use skinfolds. The first sums the skinfold scores to indicate *relative* fatness among individuals. The sum-of-skinfolds and individual values reflect either absolute or percentage body fat changes before and after an intervention program.

One can draw the following conclusions from the skinfold data in Table 28.6, obtained from a 22-year-old female college student before and after a 16-week aerobic exercise program:

- The largest changes in skinfold thickness occurred at the suprailiac and abdominal sites
- The triceps showed the largest percentage decrease and the subscapular the smallest percentage decrease
- Total reduction in subcutaneous skinfolds at the five sites was 16.6 mm, or 12.6% below the "before" condition

A second use of skinfolds incorporates population-specific mathematical equations to predict body density or percentage body fat. The equations prove accurate for subjects similar in age, gender, training status, fatness, and race to the group on which they were derived.[15,42,80,140] *When meeting these criteria, predicted body fat for an individual usually ranges between 3 and 5% body fat units computed from body density with hydrostatic weighing.*

From experiments in our laboratories, we developed equations to predict body fat from triceps and subscapular skinfolds in young women and men:[83–85]

Young women, ages 17 to 26 years

$$\% \text{ Body fat} = 0.55A + 0.31B + 6.13$$

Young men, ages 17 to 26 years

$$\% \text{ Body fat} = 0.43A + 0.58B + 1.47$$

In both equations, A is triceps skinfold (mm), and B is subscapular skinfold (mm).

We computed the "before" and "after" percentage body fat of the woman who participated in the 16-week physical-conditioning program (Table 28.6). Percentage body fat equals 24.4% by substituting the pretraining values for triceps (22.5 mm) and subscapular (19.0 mm) skinfolds into the equation.

$$\begin{aligned} \% \text{ Body fat} &= 0.55A + 0.31B + 6.13 \\ &= 0.55\,(22.5) + 0.31(19.0) + 6.13 \\ &= 12.38 + 5.89 + 6.13 \\ &= 24.4\% \end{aligned}$$

Substituting the posttraining values for triceps (19.4 mm) and subscapular (17.0 mm) skinfolds produced a body fat value of 21.1%.

$$\begin{aligned} \% \text{ Body fat} &= 0.55(19.4) + 0.31(17.0) + 6.13 \\ &= 10.67 + 5.27 + 6.13 \\ &= 22.1\% \end{aligned}$$

Percentage body fat determined before and after a physical conditioning or weight-loss program provides a convenient means of evaluating alterations in body composition, often independent of body weight changes.

Skinfolds and Age

In young adults, approximately one-half of the body's total fat consists of subcutaneous fat, with the remainder visceral and organ fat. With advancing age, proportionately more fat deposits internally than subcutaneously. Thus, the same skinfold score reflects a *greater* total percentage of body fat as one gets older. *For this reason, use age-adjusted* ***generalized equations*** *to predict body fat from skinfolds or girths in older men and women.*[71,72,149,181]

User Beware

The person taking skinfold measurements must develop expertise with the proper techniques. Also, with extremely obese people, the thickness of the skinfold often exceeds the width of the caliper's jaws. The particular caliper used may also contribute to errors of measurement.[57] It often becomes difficult to determine which sets of skinfold data provide the

TABLE 28.6 ➤ CHANGES IN SELECTED SKINFOLDS OF A YOUNG WOMAN DURING A 16-WEEK EXERCISE PROGRAM

Skinfolds (mm)	Before	After	Absolute Change	Percentage Change
Triceps	22.5	19.4	−3.1	−13.8
Subscapular	19.0	17.0	−2.0	−10.5
Suprailiac	34.5	30.2	−4.3	−12.8
Abdomen	33.7	29.4	−4.3	−12.8
Thigh	21.6	18.7	−2.9	−13.4
Sum	131.3	114.7	−16.6	−12.6

best comparisons because of the lack of standards for judging the results of different investigators. Thus, a prediction equation developed by one researcher (which may show high validity for the sample measured) may produce large prediction errors when another person applies the equation to skinfolds from a dissimilar group. The error in predicting body fat could approach plus or minus 200% or more![80]

INTEGRATIVE QUESTION

A friend complains that three different fitness centers determined her percentage body fat from skinfolds as follows: 25%, 29%, and 21%. How can you reconcile the differences?

Application of the Surface Area Formula

The surface area formula method described below may improve the validity of body fat estimates for diverse populations, although limitations still exist. The basic equation is as follows:

$$\% \text{ Fat} = \Sigma \text{ skinfolds} \div 3F \times k(sf)$$

where Σ skinfolds is the sum of values at two or more skinfold sites, depending on availability; $3F = 3\sqrt{\text{mass/stature}}$ (with body mass in kg and stature in dm); and k(sf) is skinfolds/3F × %fat. The %fat derives from a criterion method such as underwater weighing, and represents the observed average for the group or population of a particular age, gender, training status, or sport for which the equation applies. Thus, diverse populations require different k(sf) constants. For example, consider the mean values for a population of sedentary young men: stature, 18.42 dm; mass, 72.16 kg; Σ 3 skinfolds, 67.3 mm; % fat, 15.3. Compute the specific k(sf) constant for this group as:

$$k(sf) = \frac{67.3}{3\sqrt{3.9175} \times 15.3} = 0.741$$

By first calculating the specific k(sf) constant based on group data, one computes the percentage body fat for any similar individual with the basic equation. For example, if body mass for a young man is 74.0 kg, stature is 17.52 dm, and Σ3 skinfolds is 57.5 mm, then one computes percentage fat as follows:

$$\begin{aligned}\%\text{fat} &= \Sigma \text{ skinfolds} \div 3F \times k(sf)\\ &= 57.5 \div 6.166 \times 0.741\\ &= 12.6\%\end{aligned}$$

This method estimated the body fat content of the two champion body builders in Table 29.10, Chapter 29. For the reference group of male body builders, 3F is 6.666, %fat is 6.4, Σ 3 skinfolds is 30.4 mm, and k (sf) is 0.71818.

Measurement of Girths

Apply a linen or plastic measuring tape (not a metal tape) lightly to the skin surface so the tape remains taut but not tight. This avoids skin compression, which produces below-normal scores. Take duplicate measurements at each site and average the scores. Figure 28.12 shows six common anatomic landmarks for anthropometric measurement:

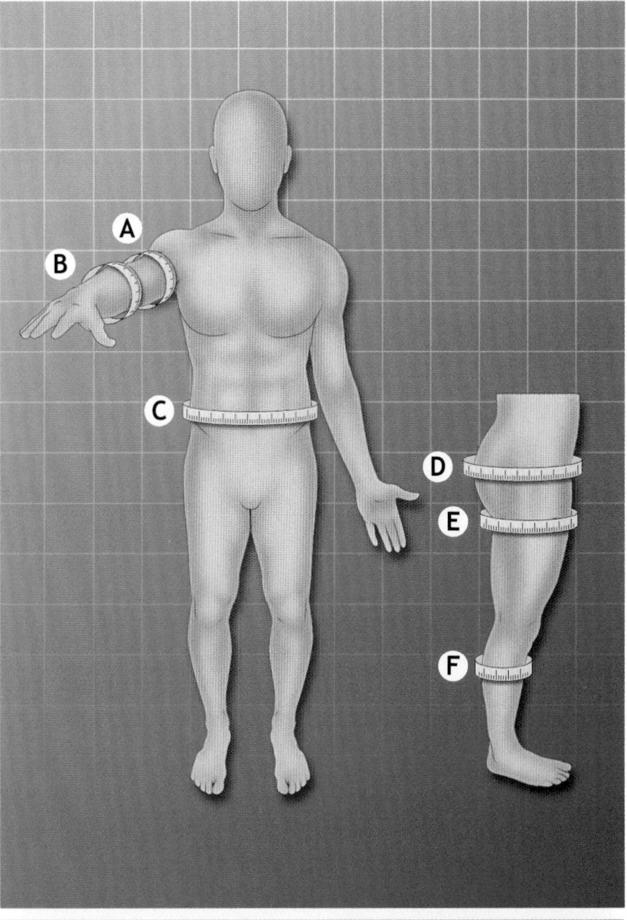

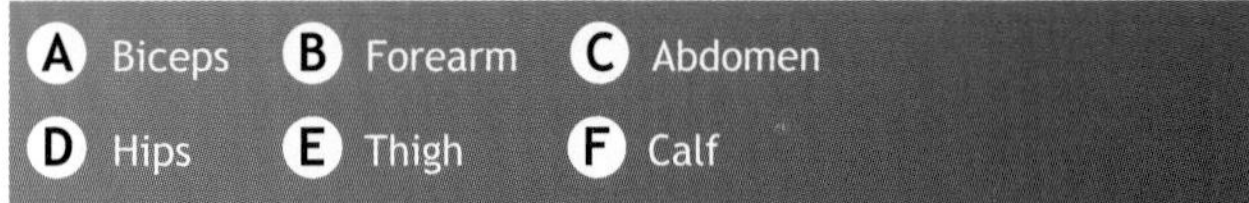

FIGURE 28.12 • Landmarks for measuring various girths at six common anatomical sites (see text for description).

- Right upper arm (biceps): Arm straight and extended in front of the body; measurement taken at the midpoint between the shoulder and the elbow
- Right forearm: Maximum girth with arm extended in front of the body
- Abdomen: 1 inch above the umbilicus
- Buttocks: Maximum protrusion with heels together
- Right thigh: Upper thigh, just below the buttocks
- Right calf: Widest girth midway between ankle and knee

Different prediction equations based on girths exist for each gender and various age groups.[83,181,182] The equations for these subgroups, although cross-validated on different samples with moderate validity, nevertheless show significant population specificity. The equations do not apply to individuals who (1) appear overly thin or excessively fat, (2) train regularly in strenuous endurance sports or activities with a substantial resistance-training component, and (3) differ in race from the specific group used to derive the original equations.[15,84,140]

Usefulness of Girth Scores

Girths prove most useful in ranking individuals within a group according to relative fatness. As with skinfolds, girth-based equations can predict body density and/or percentage body fat. The equations and constants presented in "Body Composition," on the LWW connection website: connection.lww.com/go/mcardle for young and older men and women predict an individual's body fat to within ± 2.5 to 4.0% body fat units of the actual value, provided the individual portrays the similar physical characteristics as the original validation group. Such relatively small prediction errors make girth predictions particularly useful in nonlaboratory settings. Specific equations based on girths also accurately estimate body composition of obese adult men and women.[181,194] Along with predicting percentage body fat, girths can analyze patterns of body fat distribution, including changes in fat patterning during weight loss.[60,186]

Body Fat Predictions From Girths

From the appropriate tables in "Body Composition," on the LWW connection website: connection.lww.com/go/mcardle, substitute the corresponding constants *A, B,* and *C* in the formula shown at the bottom of each table. This requires one addition and two subtraction steps. The following four-step example shows how to compute percentage fat, fat mass, and FFM for a 21-year-old man who weighs 79.1 kg:

Step 1. Measure the upper arm, abdomen, and right forearm girths with a cloth tape to the nearest 0.25 inch (0.6 cm): upper arm = 11.5 inch (29.21 cm); abdomen = 31.0 inch (78.74 cm); right forearm = 10.75 inch (27.30 cm)

Step 2. Determine the three constants *A, B,* and *C* corresponding to the three girths from the table: *A*, corresponding to 11.5 inch, is 42.56; *B*, corresponding to 31.0 inch = 40.68; and *C*, corresponding to 10.75 inch = 58.37.

Step 3. Compute percentage body fat by substituting the constants from step 2 in the formula for young men (which is shown in "Body Fat Prediction From Girths," on the LWW connection website: connection.lww.com/go/mcardle) as follows:

$$\begin{aligned}\text{Percentage fat} &= A + B - C - 10.2\\ &= 42.56 + 40.68 - 58.37 - 10.2\\ &= 83.24 - 58.37 - 10.2\\ &= 24.87 - 10.2\\ &= 14.7\%\end{aligned}$$

$$\begin{aligned}\text{Fat mass} &= \text{Body mass} \times [\%\text{fat} \div 100]\\ &= 79.1\ \text{kg} \times [14.7 \div 100]\\ &= 79.1\ \text{kg} \times 0.147\\ &= 11.63\ \text{kg}\end{aligned}$$

Step 4. Determine FFM

$$\begin{aligned}\text{FFM} &= \text{Body mass} - \text{fat mass}\\ &= 79.1\ \text{kg} - 11.63\ \text{kg}\\ &= 67.5\ \text{kg}\end{aligned}$$

Application of Surface Anthropometry: The Body Profile

A matrix of 11 girths illustrated in the top of Figure 28.13 constructs a muscular and nonmuscular body profile for college versus professional baseball players to provide a quantitative assessment of body shape.[82] If the anthropometric proportions of the individual conform to group symmetry, all of the deviation values on the body profile would fall within ±2% units of the vertical (zero deviation) reference line.

Practical application of the **body profile** allows quantification of the relative proportions of the body's girth dimensions and charts any *changes* in physical dimensions due to chronic exercise training, dietary intervention, or aging.[81] The body profile method also can quantify differences (or similarities) in physique status among athletes in diverse sports (e.g., gymnasts vs. distance swimmers) or within the same sport (e.g., football defensive lineman vs. quarterbacks; soccer goalies vs. forwards; small vs. large bodybuilders; basketball centers vs. guards). The *lower part* of Figure 28.13 shows age trends in girth patterns for females aged 4 to 64 years. Note that the waist (designated a nonmuscular region) increases progressively from age 30 to age 64 years. If all of the girths remained in relative proportion with aging, no positive (or negative) deviations would occur in the body profile; all measurements would plot as a vertical line as they do for the reference woman at ages 20 to 24 years.

Bioelectrical Impedance Analysis

A small alternating current flowing between two electrodes passes more rapidly through hydrated fat-free body tissues and extracellular water than through fat or bone tissues because of the greater electrolyte content (lower electrical resistance) of the fat-free component. *Impedance to electric current flow relates to the quantity of total body water; this in turn relates to FFM, body density, and percentage body fat.*

A person lies on a flat, nonconducting surface, with injector (source) electrodes attached on the dorsal surfaces of the foot and wrist and detector (sink) electrodes attached between the radius and ulna (styloid process) and at the ankle between the medial and lateral malleoli (Fig. 28.14). A painless, localized electrical current (approximately 800 μA at a frequency of 50 kHz) is introduced, and the impedance (resistance) to current flow between the source and detector electrodes is determined.[49] Conversion of the impedance value to body density—adding body mass and stature; gender, age, and sometimes race; level of fatness; and several girths to the equation—computes percentage body fat from the Siri equation or other similar density conversion equations.

Influence of Hydration Level and Ambient Temperature

Hydration level, even small fluid changes that occur with endurance exercise, affects the accuracy of **bioelectrical impedance analysis (BIA)** and may give incorrect information

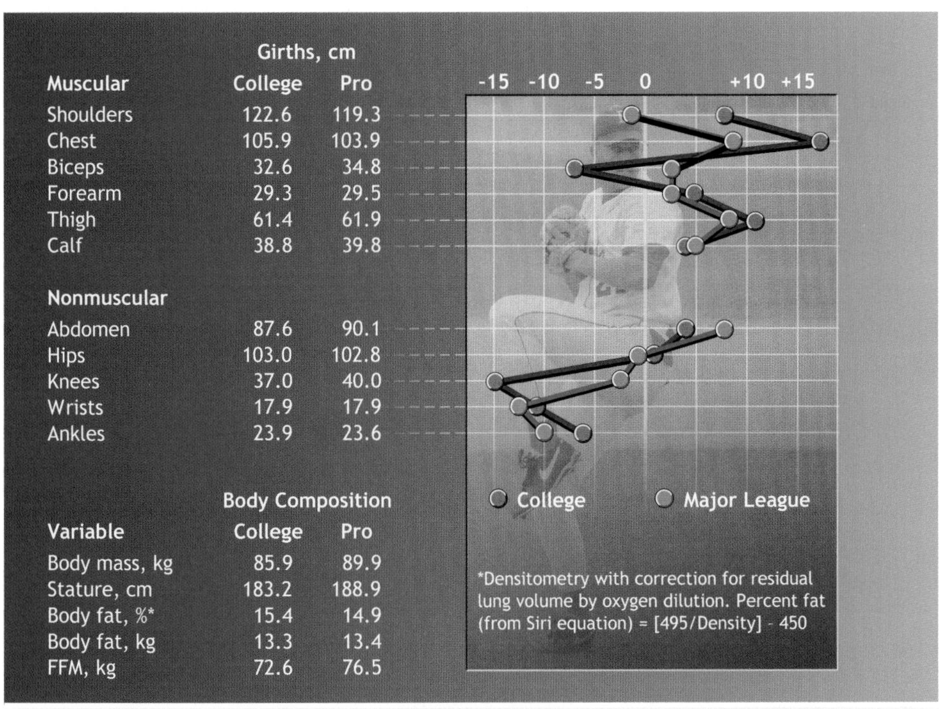

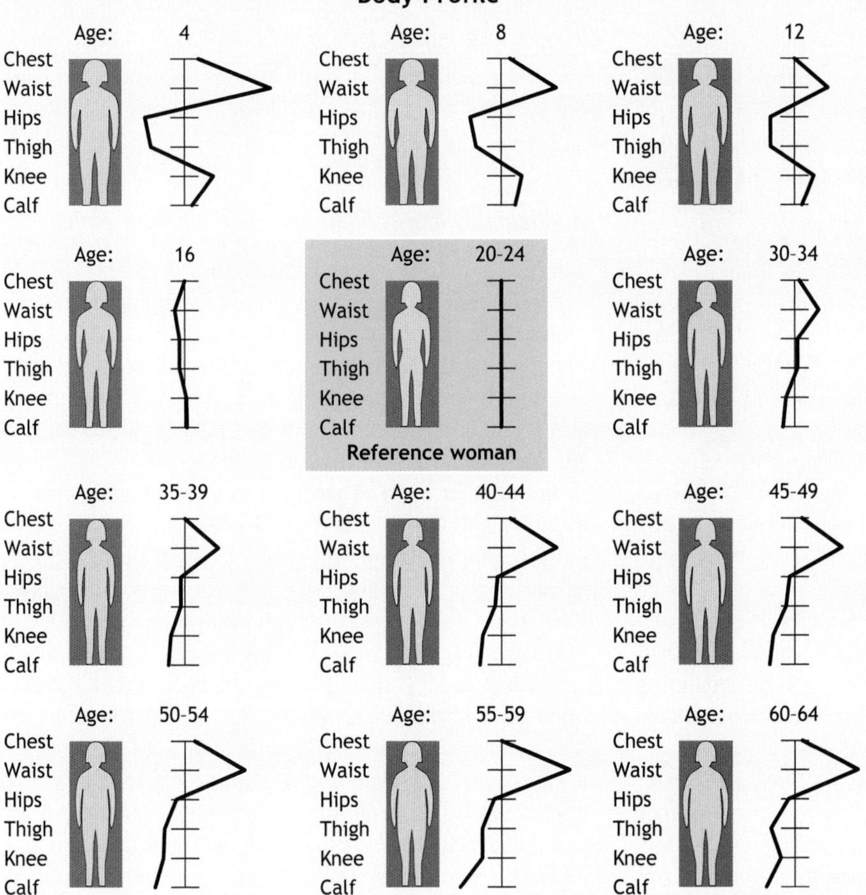

FIGURE 28.13 • *Top.* Body profile analysis using the girth technique to display muscular and nonmuscular areas relative to values established for the reference man (indicated by the *vertical yellow zero line*). The college data represent Division I university baseball pitchers ($n = 9$; University of Massachusetts, Amherst) and the pro data are from major league baseball pitchers ($n = 23$; Boston Red Sox). *Bottom.* Age trends in girth patterns for females aged 4 to 64 years. Details about constructing the body profile are contained in Katch FI, Katch VL. The body composition profile: techniques of measurement and applications. Clin Sports Med 1984;3:31 and Katch FI, et al. The ponderal somatogram: evaluation of body size and shape from anthropometric girths and stature. Hum Biol 1987;59:439.

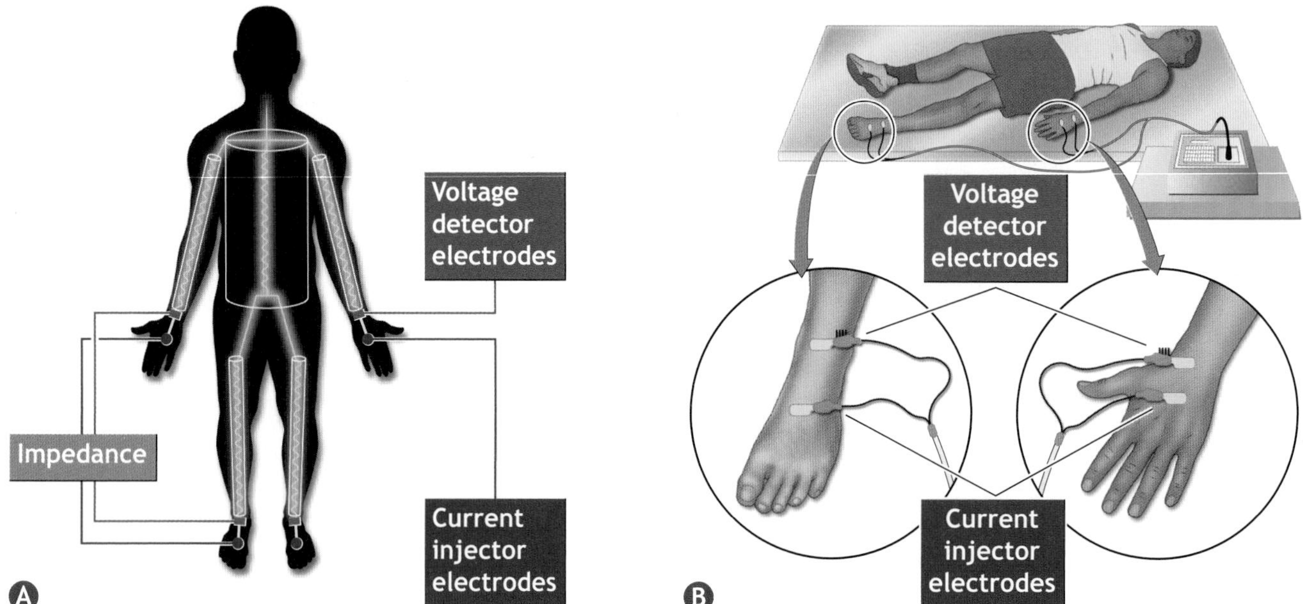

FIGURE 28.14 • Method to assess body composition by bioelectrical impedance analysis. **A**. Four-surface electrode technique applies current via one pair of distal (injector) electrodes, while the proximal (detector) electrode pair measures electrical potential across the conducting segment. (**B**) Standard placement of electrodes, and body position during whole-body impedance measurement.

about an individual's body fat content.[98,160] Hypohydration or hyperhydration alters the body's normal electrolyte concentrations, which in turn affects current flow, independent of real body composition changes. For example, losing body water through prior exercise sweat loss or voluntary fluid restriction decreases the impedance measure. This lowers the percentage body fat estimate; hyperhydration produces the opposite effect (higher body fat estimate).

Skin temperature (influenced by ambient conditions) also affects whole-body resistance, and thus the BIA prediction of body fat. Predicted body fat is significantly lower in a warm environment (moist skin produces less impedance to electrical flow) than in a cold one.[5,23]

Even with normal hydration and environmental temperature, body fat predictions with BIA prove less satisfactory than hydrostatic weighing. BIA tends to overpredict body fat in lean and athletic subjects and underpredict body fat in obese subjects.[115,162] The tendency to overestimate true percentage body fat may be more pronounced among black athletes.[65,162] BIA predicts body fat less accurately than girths and skinfolds.[16,41,89,172] Whether BIA detects small changes in body composition during weight loss is also unclear.[40,101,139,154,159] Conventional BIA technology cannot determine regional fat distribution.

At best, BIA represents another noninvasive, safe, relatively easy, and reliable means to assess total body water. The BIA technique requires that experienced personnel make measurements under strictly standardized conditions, particularly electrode placement and the subject's body position, hydration status, plasma osmolality and sodium concentration, previous food and beverage intake, skin temperature, and recent physical activity.[13,100,190] Level of body fatness and racial characteristics probably also influence BIA's predictive accuracy.[4,143,187,203] Fatness-specific BIA equations exist that predict body fat for obese and nonobese American Indian, Hispanic, and white men and women.[172] With proper measurement standardization, the menstrual cycle does not affect body composition assessment by BIA.[125]

Applicability of BIA in Sports and Exercise Training

Coaches and athletes need a safe, easily administered, rapid, and valid tool to assess body composition and detect changes with caloric restriction or exercise training. A major limitation in achieving these goals concerns BIA's lack of sensitivity to small body-compositional changes.[139,162] This presents a problem without appropriate control over factors that affect measurement accuracy and reliability.[40] For example, sweat-loss dehydration or reduced glycogen reserves (and associated loss of glycogen-bound water) from a prior training session reduce body resistance (impedance) to electrical current flow. This overestimates FFM and underestimates percentage body fat. Research using adequate sample sizes also must establish the validity and reliability for BIA among female athletes.

Chapter 29 ("In a Practical Sense") includes BIA equations (in addition to skinfolds and girths) to estimate body density and percentage body fat for athletes in general as well as athletes in specific sports. Without sport-specific equations, population-based generalized equations (accounting for age and gender) usually provide an acceptable alternative for body fat estimation.[25,71,165,177]

Near-Infrared Interactance

Near-infrared interactance (NIR) applies technology developed by the U.S. Department of Agriculture to assess body composition of livestock and the lipid content of various grains. The commercial versions to assess body composition in humans (Futrex-5000 and 1000 models for adults and model 5000A for children and adolescents) use principles of light absorption and reflection. A fiber optic probe, or light wand, emits a low-energy beam of near-infrared light into the single measuring site at the anterior midline surface of the dominant biceps. A detector within the same probe measures the intensity of the reemitted light, expressed as optical density. Shifts in the wavelength of the reflected beam as it interacts with organic material in the arm, added to the manufacturer's prediction equation (including subject's body mass and stature, estimated frame size, gender, and physical activity level) computes percentage body fat and FFM. The safe, portable, lightweight equipment requires minimal training to use and necessitates little physical contact with the subject during measurement. These test administration aspects make NIR popular for body composition assessment in health clubs, hospitals, and weight-loss centers.

Questionable Validity

Early research indicated a significant relationship between spectrophotometric measures of light interactance at various body sites and body composition assessed by total body water.[32] Subsequent research with humans has not confirmed NIR's validity compared to hydrostatic weighing and skinfold measurements. NIR does *not* accurately predict body fat across a broad range of body fat levels; NIR provides less accuracy than skinfolds.[16,25,64,173,174,184] It overestimates body fat in lean men and women and underestimates it in fatter subjects.[126] Figure 28.15 shows the inadequacy of NIR, compared with skinfold measurements, to predict body fat determined by hydrostatic weighing. In more than 47% of the subjects, an error greater than 4% body fat units occurred with NIR, with the largest errors at the extremes of body fatness. Furthermore, NIR produced large errors—standard error of estimate and total prediction error—when estimating percentage body fat for children[22] and youth wrestlers[67] and significantly underestimated body fat in collegiate football players.[66] NIR does not accurately assess body compositional changes from resistance training.[16] *Well-controlled studies do not find NIR to be a valid method for assessing human body composition.*

Ultrasound Assessment of Fat

Ultrasound technology can (1) assess the thickness of different tissues (fat and muscle) and (2) obtain an image of the deeper tissues such as a muscle's cross-sectional area. The method converts electrical energy through a probe into high-frequency (pulsed) sound waves that penetrate the skin surface into the underlying tissues. The sound waves pass through adipose tissue and penetrate the muscle layer. They then reflect from the fat–muscle interface (after reflection from a bony surface) to produce an echo, which returns to a receiver within the probe. The simplest type of ultrasound (A-mode) does not produce an image of the underlying tissues. Rather, the time required for sound wave transmission through the tissues and back to the transducer converts to a distance score to indicate fat or muscle thickness. In the more expensive and technically demanding B-mode ultrasound, a two-dimensional image provides considerable detail and tissue differentiation.[69]

Ultrasound exhibits high reliability for repeat measurements of subcutaneous fat thickness at multiple sites in the lying and standing positions on the same day and different days.[70,76] The technique has application for determining total and segmental subcutaneous adipose tissue volume.[2] It may prove particularly useful with the obese, who show considerable variation and compression of subcutaneous body fat with skinfold measures. Ultrasound used to map muscle and fat thickness at different body regions and quantify changes in the topographic fat patterns serves as a valuable adjunct to body composition assessment. In hospitalized patients, ultrasonic fat and muscle thickness determinations aid in nutritional assessment during weight loss and weight gain. Ultrasonic imaging also serves a clinical role in assessing tissue growth and development, including fetal development and structure and function of the heart and other organs.

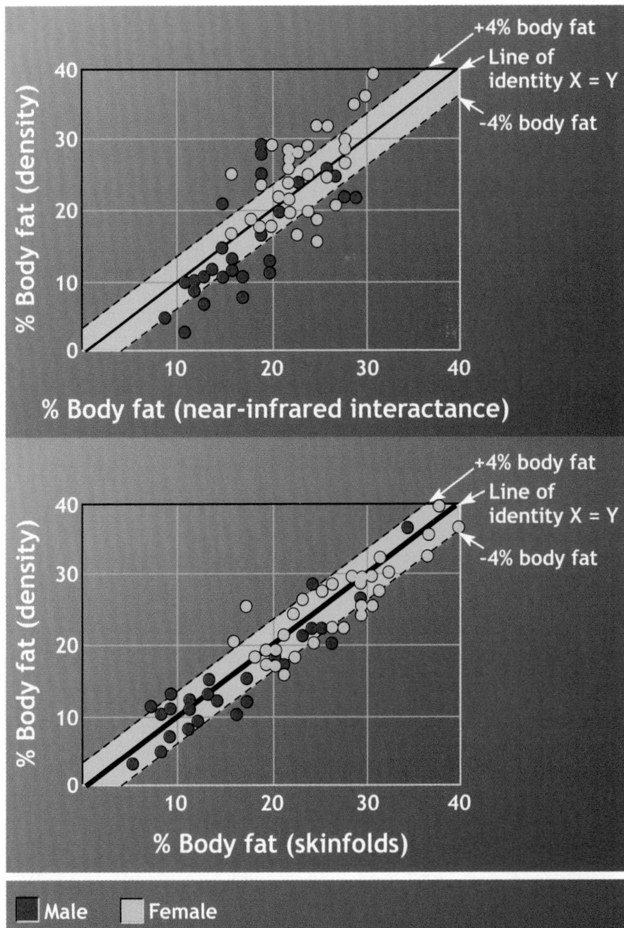

FIGURE 28.15 • Comparison of near-infrared interactance (Futrex-5000) (*top*) and skinfolds (*bottom*) for assessing percentage body fat. Shaded area about line incoprporates ±4% body fat units (From McLean K, Skinner JS. Validity of Futrex-5000 for body composition determination. Med Sci Sports Exerc 1992;24:253.)

With imaging devices, the reflected sound waves from the soft tissues convert to a real-time image for convenient visualization or for computer digitization (area, volume, and diameter) directly from the image. Color and multiple-frequency imaging allows clinicians to trace blood flow through organs and tissues or use miniaturized probes to clearly identify internal tissues, vessels, and organs. In consumer-oriented research, ultrasonic imaging of thigh fat depth provided evidence that advertised treatments using two topical cream applications to the thighs and buttocks to reduce "cellulite" (dimpled fat) failed to reduce local fat thickness compared to control conditions.[30]

Arm X-Ray Assessment of Fat

X-ray technology can analyze regional body fat deposition.[77,78] The thickness of fat layers at points *A, B,* and *C* in Figure 28.16 transforms the fat widths into a body fat value with the skinfold-surface area equation on page 775. Fat thickness from the roentgenogram substitutes in the equation for the skinfold values. The k constant derives in the same manner and differs among individuals depending on age, level of fitness, and race.[77,78] Comparing percentage body fat from roentgenograms with body fat by hydrostatic weighing established the validity of the x-ray procedure ($r = 0.90$ in young and older white and black men and women). For an individual, conversion of the x-ray widths of fat to total body fat percentage generally falls within ±3% units of body fat determined by underwater weighing. This represents accuracy similar to the percentage body fat estimated from skinfolds or girths. The x-ray procedure also includes assessment of muscle size, which contributes useful information to studies of body composition with training, aging, and changes in body mass.[38]

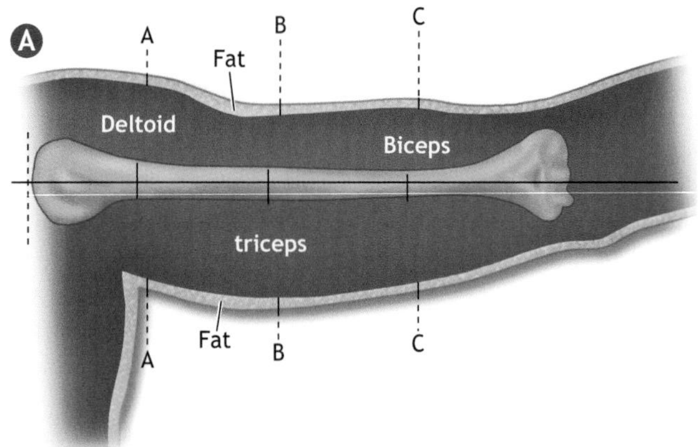

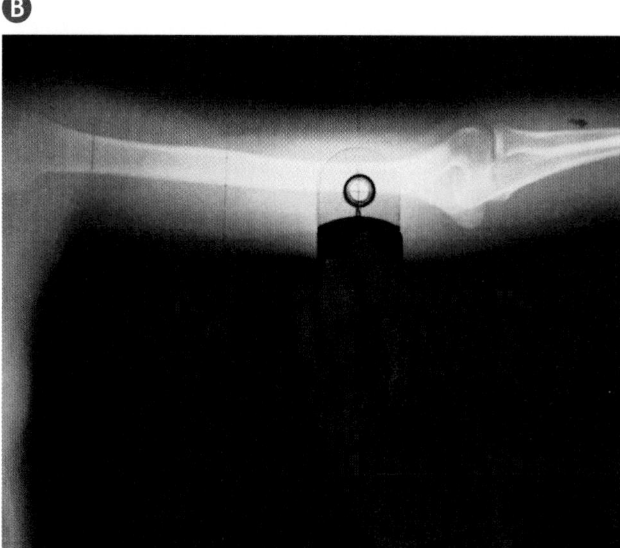

FIGURE 28.16 • **A**. Schematic diagram of an arm radiograph of a 24-year-old female. *Vertical lines* perpendicular to the long axis of the humerus at points *A, B,* and *C* represent the six fat widths. Total body fat computed from the radiograph equaled 23.6%; body fat by underwater weighing equaled 23.3%. **B**. Technician uses a digitizer to calculate fat width on the radiograph. A clear demarcation between fat, muscle, and bone appears on the radiograph, which permits accurate assessment of radiographic widths. A computer processes the information from the digitizer and transmits it to a printer and graphics plotter. (Line art and photo courtesy of Dr. A. R. Behnke.)

Computed Tomography, Magnetic Resonance Imaging, and Dual-Energy X-Ray Absorptiometry

Computed Tomography

Computed tomography (**CT**) generates detailed cross-sectional, two-dimensional radiographic images of different body segments when an x-ray beam (ionizing radiation) passes through tissues of different densities. The CT scan produces pictorial and quantitative information about total tissue area, total fat and muscle area, and thickness and volume of tissues within an organ.[56,130]

Figure 28.17, A–C, shows CT scans of the upper legs and a cross section at the midthigh of a professional walker who walked 11,200 miles through the 50 United States in 50 weeks. Total cross section and muscle increased significantly, and subcutaneous fat decreased correspondingly in the midthigh region in the "after" scans (not shown). Studies have demonstrated the efficacy of CT scans to establish the relationship between simple anthropometric measures (skinfolds and girths) at the abdomen and total adipose tissue volume measured from single or multiple pictorial "slices" through this region.[163] CT scans determined deep and total abdominal adipose tissue accumulation at the L4–L5 region in a Canadian cohort of 110 men; measures also included skinfold thickness and waist girth.[35] The single cut through the L4–L5 region minimizes radiation dose and provides the best view of visceral and subcutaneous fat. Figure 28.18 illustrates the high correlation ($r = 0.82$) between waist girth and deep **visceral adipose tissue** (**VAT**) area; men with larger waist girth also possessed greater VAT. The relationship exceeded the association between subcutaneous fat thickness (skinfolds) and VAT. An increased amount of deep abdominal

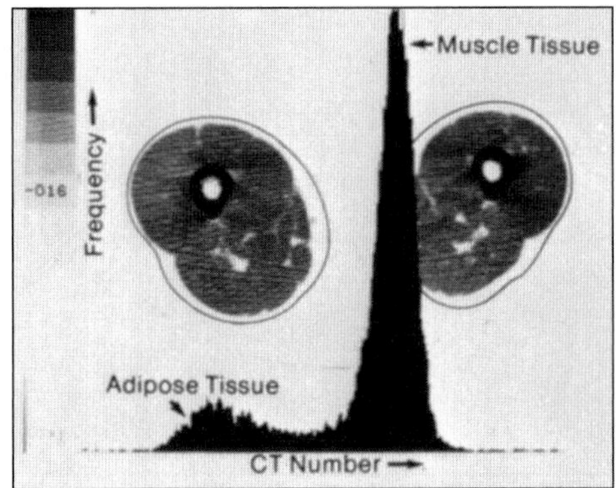

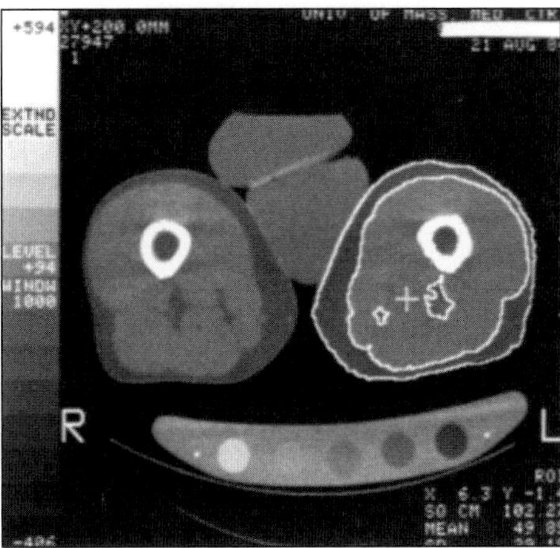

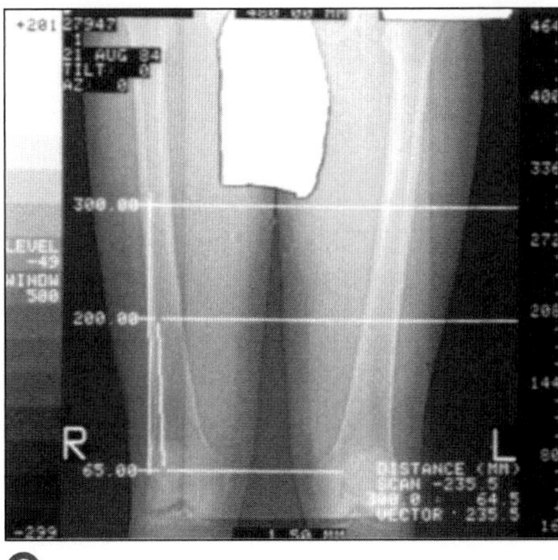

C

FIGURE 28.17 • CT scans. **A**. Plot of pixel elements (CT scan) illustrating the extent of adipose and muscle tissue in a cross section of the thigh. The two other views show a cross section of the midthigh (**B**) and an anterior view of the upper legs (**C**), prior to a 1-year walk across the United States by a champion walker. (CT scans courtesy of Dr. Steven Heymsfeld, Obesity Research Center, St. Luke's-Roosevelt Hospital, Columbia University, College of Physicians and Surgeons, New York, NY.)

adipose tissue relates to increased risk for type 2 diabetes, blood lipid profile disorders, hypertension, and cardiovascular disease. Chapter 30 discusses health risks from abdominal obesity of the deep type.

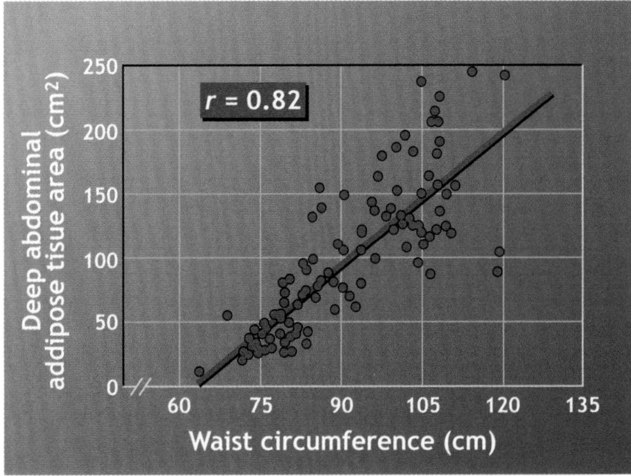

FIGURE 28.18 • Relationship between deep visceral adipose tissue (VAT) determined by CT scanning and waist girth in 110 men, ages 18 to 42 years, who varied considerably in percentage body fat by densitometry ($\bar{X}$ = 22.9%; range, 2.2 to 39.9%). The best predictors of VAT included *(a)* abdominal skinfold thickness in mm, *(b)* waist girth in cm, and *(c)* waist:hip ratio. VAT (cm^2) = −363.12 + [−1.113*a*] + [3.478*b*] + [186.7*c*]. For example, if abdominal skinfold is 23.0 mm, waist girth is 92.0 cm, and waist:hip ratio is 0.929, then by substitution in the equation, VAT = 104.7 cm^2. (Modified from Dépres J-P, et al. Estimation of deep abdominal adipose-tissue accumulation from simple anthropometric measurements in men. Am J Clin Nutr 1991;54:471.)

Magnetic Resonance Imaging

Magnetic resonance imaging (**MRI**) is a valuable, noninvasive means of gaining information about the body's tissue compartments.[1,103,130,175,196] Figure 28.19 shows a color-enhanced MRI transaxial image of the midthigh of a 30-year-old male middle-distance runner. Computer software subtracts fat and bony tissues *(lighter-colored areas)* to compute thigh muscle cross-sectional area *(red area)*. With MRI, electromagnetic radiation (not ionizing radiation as in CT scans) in a strong magnetic field excites the hydrogen nuclei of the body's water and

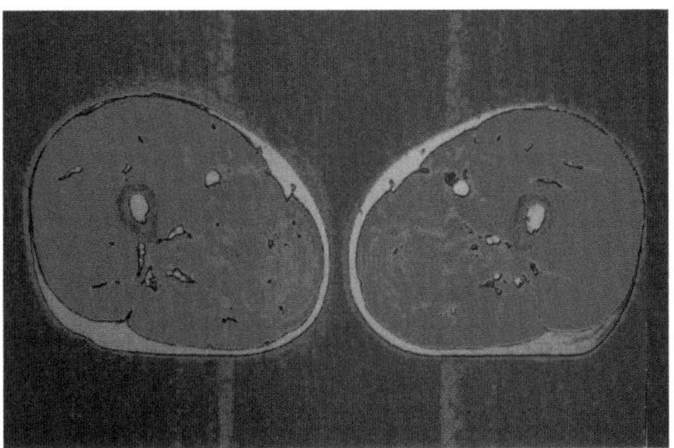

FIGURE 28.19 • MRI scans of the midthigh of a 30-year-old male middle-distance runner. (MRI scans courtesy of J. Staab, Department of the Army, USARIEM, Natick, MA.)

lipid molecules. The nuclei then project a detectable signal that rearranges under computer control to visually represent the various body tissues. MRI effectively quantifies total and subcutaneous adipose tissue in individuals of varying degrees of body fatness. Combined with muscle mass analysis, MRI can assess changes in a muscle's lean and fat components following resistance-exercise training or during different stages of growth and aging,[73] as well as postflight changes in muscle volume after a 17-day space mission and 16- to 28-week duration shuttle/MIR missions.[102] MRI has wide acceptance for medical diagnosis such as muscular dystrophy,[55] but one might ask: "How does MRI imaging for quantifying muscle mass or body fat compare with standard criterion methods that evaluate body composition?"

Figure 28.20 *(top)* shows a plot of percentage body fat determined by MRI scanning of 30 transaxial images along the length of the body and underwater weighing of 20 Swedish women, ages 23 to 40 years. Total fat from scans of the calves, thighs, lower and upper trunk, and lower and upper arms provided the basis for computing MRI percentage body fat. Good agreement emerged between the two independent body fat estimates ($r = 0.84$), thus validating MRI to assess body fat. Similar relationships emerged between MRI-determined total body fat and hydrostatic weighing and total body water estimates of the body's fat content.[127]

The *bottom* of Figure 28.20 shows the distribution of total adipose tissue, subcutaneous adipose tissue, and non subcutaneous adipose tissue measures from different body regions. The *bar graphs* show the smallest to the largest adipose tissue depots. Of all body regions, adipose tissue in the lower trunk (both subcutaneous and nonsubcutaneous) contained the greatest percentage total body fat (38.5%); the lower arm region included 2.7%, the smallest amount. The *pie chart* at *lower right* of the figure shows the relative amounts of adipose tissue in each body compartment expressed as a percentage of the total volume of MRI-determined body fat. Subcutaneous fat accounted for 75.2% of the total 21.8 L of body fat. Because nonsubcutaneous fat accounts for the remaining 24.8% of the total, it seems reasonable to conclude that "excess" fat probably deposits to the greatest extent in the subcutaneous tissues.

COMPARISON OF LEAN AND OBESE. Seventeen MRI-derived tissue slices from groups of lean and obese females provided comparative data for total and VAT volume at four anatomic sites between the top of the patella and the sternal notch. Body fat determined by densitometry for the light women (BMI, 20.6 $kg \cdot m^{-2}$) averaged 25.4%; the heavy women's BMI averaged 42.4 $kg \cdot m^{-2}$, with about 42% body fat. The three graphs in Figure 28.21 display differences between the relatively light and heavy groups in total body tissue (sum of fat and nonfat tissues), total adipose tissue, and subcutaneous adipose tissue at the 17 sites. The results show a fairly consistent pattern in the assessment of MRI-derived adipose tissue volumes. The overfat subjects possessed 165% more subcutaneous adipose tissue and 155% more total adipose tissue. Abdominal and upper-thigh regions showed the largest fat accretion. Interestingly, the light women had a greater amount of nonfat tissue (not shown) at the upper-thorax and lower-thigh regions. The *inset graph* shows the strong relationship between MRI-determined percentage of body adipose tissue (using 4 instead of 17 sites) and percentage body fat determined by densitometry. MRI yields a wealth of useful information for accurately assessing total and regional body composition. Future MRI studies should evaluate athletic groups and determine the singular and combined short- and long-term effects of dietary manipulation and exercise training on regional (trunk and extremities) and total body composition during weight gain and weight loss.

EXERCISE TRAINING. MRI and dual-energy x-ray absorptiometry (DXA, discussed in next section) assessed changes in regional (trunk and extremities) and whole-body fat mass, lean mass, and bone mineral content at 3 and 6 months after 31 women began periodized resistance training.[141] To determine the magnitude of change, results were compared with women (controls) who did not train and 18 men tested only once. MRI measured changes in thigh muscle morphology in a subset of 11 women exercisers. Periodized training combined aerobic and resistance exercise 5 days a week for 24 weeks. The training group decreased fat mass by 10% and body mass and soft tissue lean mass by 2.2%, but bone mineral content did not change. Soft tissue lean mass was distributed less in women's arms than men's both before and after training. The most striking training-induced differences occurred in the tissue composition of the women's arms (31% loss in fat mass without change in lean mass) compared with the legs (5.5% gain in lean mass without change in fat mass). Fat decreased in the trunk by 12% with no change in soft tissue lean mass. The changes reported for fat mass by MRI and DXA showed close relationships ($r = 0.72$ to 0.92). Both techniques also assessed increases in lean leg tissue mass similarly. This experiment reinforced the importance of apprising changes in regional tissue morphology (including total body changes) with an experimental treatment, in this case the effects of periodized resistance training.

Dual-Energy X-Ray Absorptiometry

Dual-energy x-ray absorptiometry (DXA), another high-technology procedure, quantifies fat and nonbone regional lean body mass, including the mineral content of the body's deeper bony structures.[96,110,116,150,156,196] It has become the accepted clinical tool for assessing spinal osteoporosis and related bone disorders.[43,147] DXA does not require the assumptions about the biologic constancy of the fat and fat-free components inherent with hydrostatic weighing.[95]

With DXA, two distinct low-energy x-ray beams (short exposure with low radiation dosage) penetrate bone and soft tissue areas to a depth of approximately 30 cm. The subject lies supine on a table so that the source and detector probes pass across the body at a slow speed of 1 $cm \cdot s^{-1}$. An entire DXA scan takes approximately 12 minutes. Computer software reconstructs the attenuated x-ray beams to produce an image of the underlying tissues and quantify

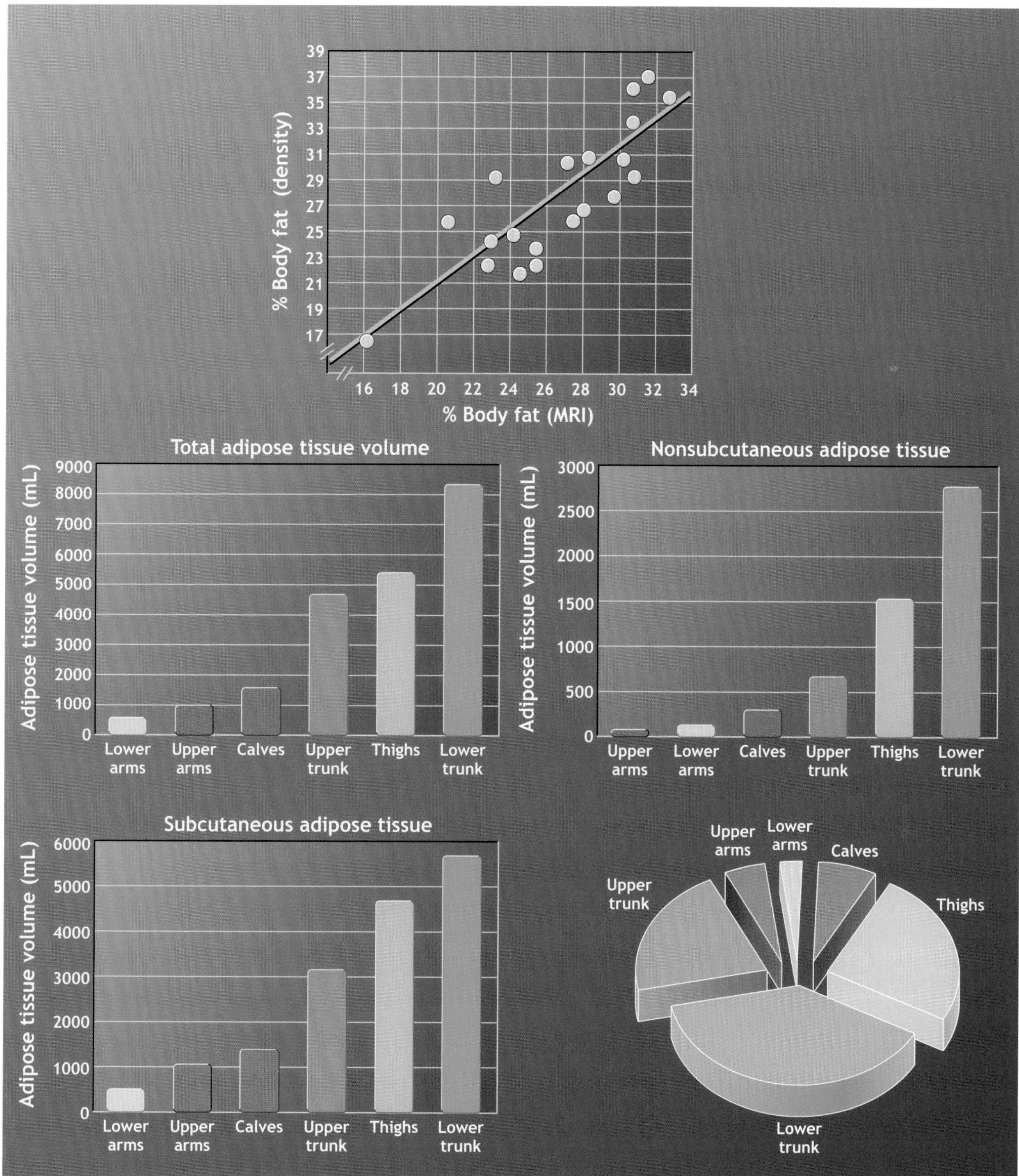

FIGURE 28.20 • *Top.* Percentage body fat determined by hydrostatic weighing (density) and MRI scanning (graph created from individual data points presented in the original article). *Bottom bar graphs.* Distribution of adipose tissue (total, subcutaneous, and nonsubcutaneous) within the various body compartments; arrangement progresses from smallest to largest. The *right pie chart* displays the percentage of total adipose tissue distributed in the different body regions. (Modified from Sohlstrom A, et al. Adipose tissue distribution as assessed by magnetic resonance imaging and total body fat by magnetic resonance imaging, underwater weighing, and body-water dilution in healthy women. Am J Clin Nutr 1993;58:830.)

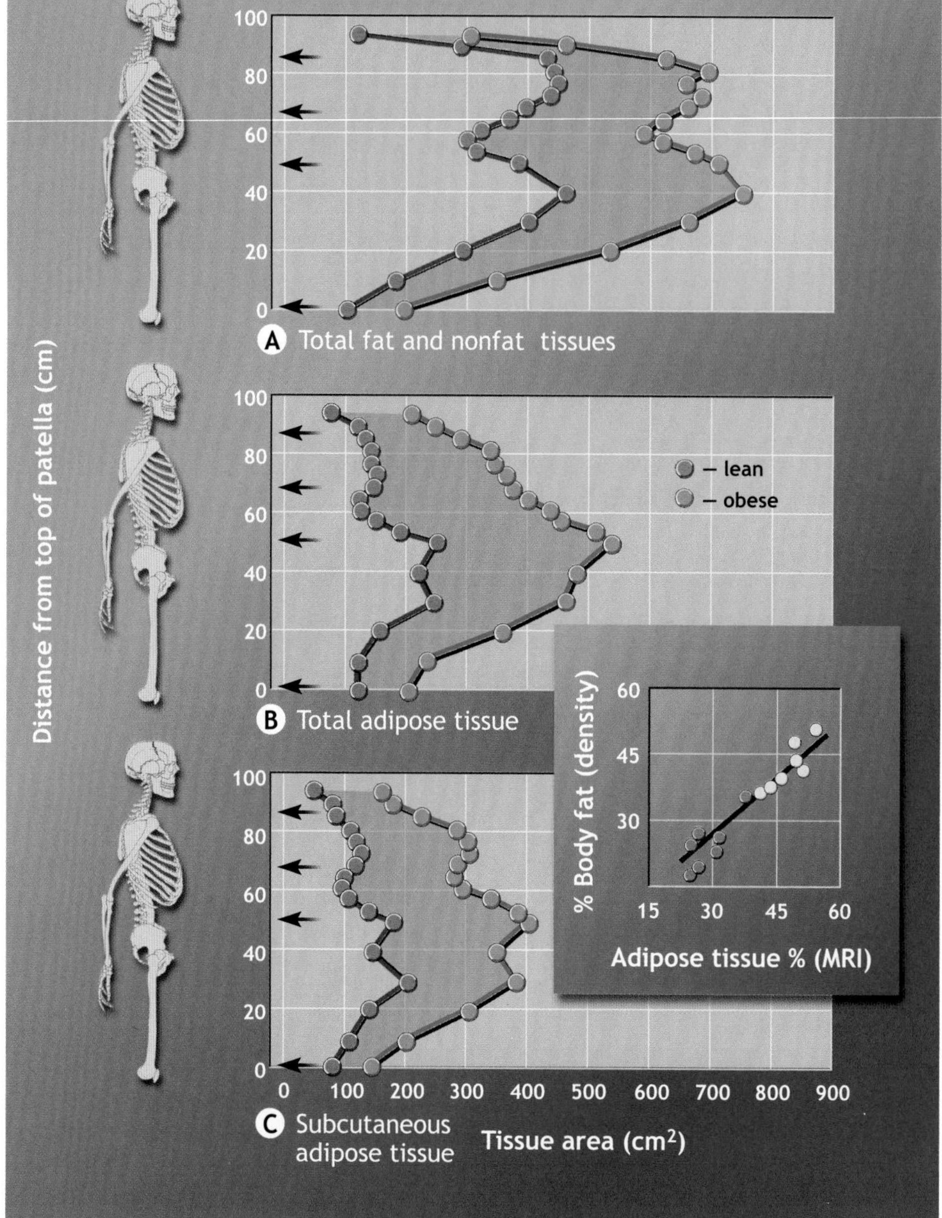

FIGURE 28.21 • MRI-determined distribution of body tissues. **A**. Total body tissues (sum of fat and nonfat tissues). **B**. Total adipose tissue. **C**. Subcutaneous adipose tissue in seven lean (*red*) and seven obese (*blue*) females. *Arrows to the right of the* y *axis* indicate the four anatomic markers in relation to position on the skeleton. The *inset graph* displays the relationship between percentage body adipose tissue (using 4 instead of 17 MRI sites) and percentage body fat determined by hydrostatic weighing in obese and lean subjects. (Modified from Fowler PA, et al. Total and subcutaneous adipose tissue in women: the measurement of distribution and accurate prediction of quantity by using magnetic resonance imaging. Am J Clin Nutr 1991;54:18.)

bone mineral content, total fat mass, and FFM. Analysis also includes selected trunk and limb regions for detailed study of tissue composition and possible relation to disease risk, including the effects of exercise training and detraining.[11,105,117,199]

DXA shows excellent agreement with other independent estimates of bone mineral content (within 1% of each other).[147] Strong relationships also exist between DXA-determined total body fat and body fat by either densitometry,[62,121] segmental body composition (upper- and lower-extremity mass), total body potassium, or total body nitrogen.[122] Figure 28.22 shows the strong association between percentage body fat estimates by DXA and underwater weighing over a broad age range in men and women. The strength of the prediction decreases for older and fatter subjects but remains within the typical range for comparisons between discrete methodologies. Using a more robust model of body composition assessment, the error is less than 2% body fat units between DXA and densitometry in the heterogeneous age group of adults shown in the figure.[63]

DXA AND BODY COMPOSITION IN ANOREXIA NERVOSA. DXA has evaluated the skeletal and regional body composition characteristics in anorexia nervosa. In one study, body mass averaged 44.4 kg (97.9 lb) for the 10 anorectic women. Figure 28.23 shows an anorectic female *(left two images)* and a typical female whose body fat percentage averaged 25% of her 56.7-kg (125-lb) body mass. Although lean body mass of the anorectic women approached the normal average of 43.0 kg, body fat equaled only 7.5%, a value more than three times less than that of comparison groups of typical young women. All of the women had been anorectic for at least 1 year, and the duration of amenorrhea averaged 3.1 years (range, 1 to 8 y). The *inset table* compares regional bone mineral densities (BMD, g · cm^{-2}) in the anorectic females with a group of 287 normal-fat females aged 20 to 40 years. The values in the *right column* represent the percentage for BMD of the anorectic group relative to the comparison group. Total body BMD averaged 10% lower, the L2–L4 region of the lumbar spine averaged 27% less, and the femoral neck BMD fell 13% below that of the normals. Spine BMD in the anorectics reached the identical average for 70-year-old women. Diminished BMD in anorexia nervosa, in addition to reducing skeletal size significantly, may make these young women particularly vulnerable to osteoporotic fractures at a relatively young age.

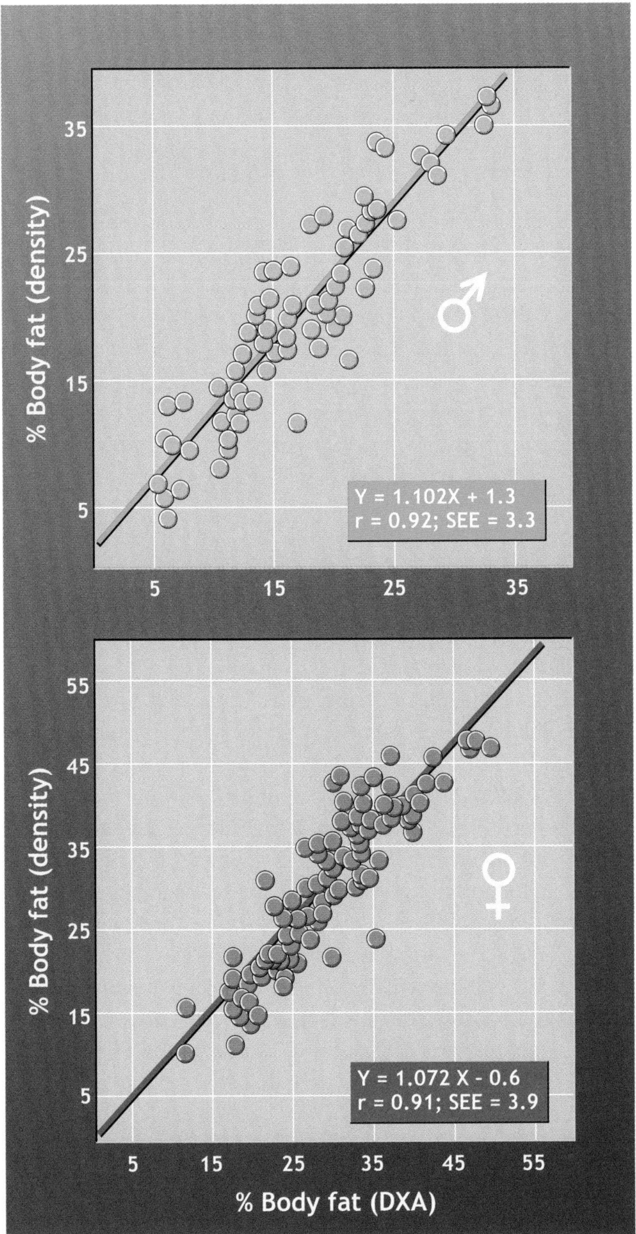

FIGURE 28.22 • Comparison of total body fat determined by densitometry and DXA in men (*top*) and women (*bottom*). (Modified from Snead DB, et al. Age-related differences in body composition by hydrodensitometry and dual-energy absorptiometry. J Appl Physiol 1993;74:770.)

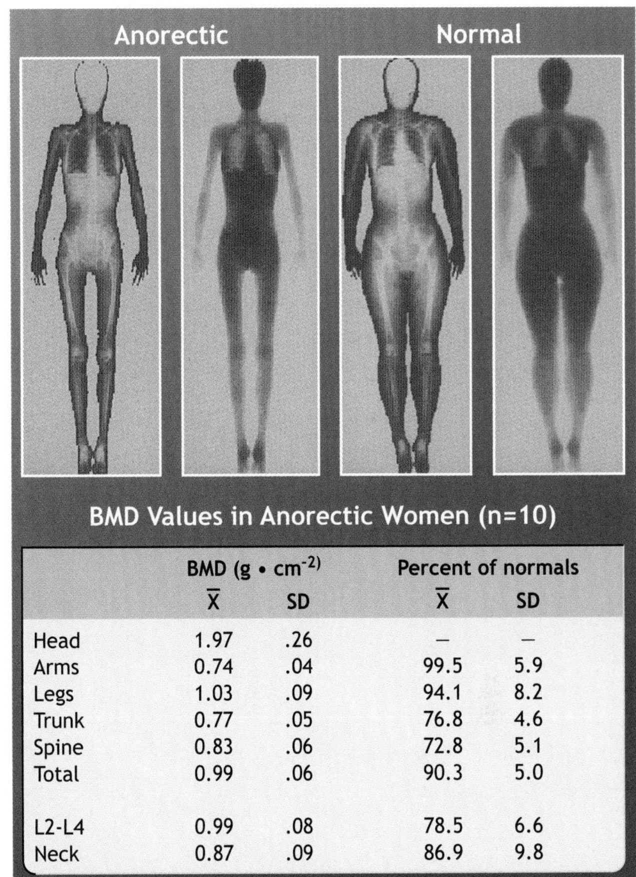

BMD Values in Anorectic Women (n=10)

	BMD (g • cm^{-2}) X̄	SD	Percent of normals X̄	SD
Head	1.97	.26	–	–
Arms	0.74	.04	99.5	5.9
Legs	1.03	.09	94.1	8.2
Trunk	0.77	.05	76.8	4.6
Spine	0.83	.06	72.8	5.1
Total	0.99	.06	90.3	5.0
L2-L4	0.99	.08	78.5	6.6
Neck	0.87	.09	86.9	9.8

FIGURE 28.23 • Example of an anorectic female (*left*) and a typical female (*right*) whose body fat percentage averaged 25% with a body mass of 56.7 kg (125 lb). The average anorectic subject weighed 44.4 kg (97.9 lb) with 7.5% body fat estimated by DXA. The *inset table* compares the regional bone mineral densities (BMDs, g · cm^{-2}) in the anorectic females with those of a group of 287 females aged 20 to 40 years with average body fat. The values in the *right columns* represent the percentage for BMD of the anorectic group relative to the comparison group. (Photo courtesy of R. B. Mazess, Department of Medical Physics, University of Wisconsin, Madison, WI, and the Lunar Radiation Corporation, Madison, WI. Data from Mazess RB, et al. Skeletal and body composition effects of anorexia nervosa. Paper presented at the international symposium on in vivo body composition studies. June 20–23, Toronto, Ontario, Canada, 1989.)

DENSITOMETRY AND SKINFOLDS IN ANOREXIA NERVOSA. A recent study[151] assessed body composition by densitometry and skinfolds in two groups of anorectic patients (97 of the restricting type [AN-RT] who lost weight only through fasting and rigorous physical exercise, and 33 binging-purging type [AN-BPT] who used binge eating, self-induced vomiting, or laxatives). During a 6-month inpatient treatment program,

TABLE 28.7 ➤ CHANGES IN BODY COMPOSITION FOLLOWING WEIGHT REGAIN IN ANOREXIA NERVOSA PATIENTS OF RESTRICTING TYPE (AN-RT) AND BINGING-PURGING (AN-BPT) TYPE

COMPOSITION[1]	BEFORE WEIGHT GAIN	AFTER WEIGHT GAIN
AN-RT (*n* = 97)		
Weight (kg)	39.5 ± 4.6[2]	52.2 ± 4.0
Density (kg · L^{-1})	1.071 ± 0.009	1.047 ± 0.007
Fat-free mass (kg)	34.5 ± 3.5[2]	40.3 ± 3.2
Fat mass (kg)	5.02 ± 1.8[3]	11.9 ± 4.6
Percentage body fat (%)	12.5 ± 3.5[4]	22.8 ± 3.0
AN-BPT (*n* = 33)		
Weight (kg)	44.0 ± 5.1	53.4 ± 4.0
Density (kg · L^{-1})	1.067 ± 0.008	1.049 ± 0.007
Fat-free mass (kg)	37.9 ± 3.7	12.5 ± 3.5
Fat mass (kg)	6.2 ± 2.0	11.8 ± 2.1
Percentage body fat (%)	13.8 ± 3.4	22.2 ± 3.0

[1]±SD
[2-4]Significantly different from AN-BPT by underwater weighing:[2] $P < 0.001$,[3] $P < 0.005$,[4] $P < 0.01$.

COMPOSITION[1]	BEFORE WEIGHT GAIN	AFTER WEIGHT GAIN
Biceps	3.68 ± 1.47[2]	6.79 ± 2.10
Triceps	5.64 ± 2.32	12.25 ± 3.51
Subscapular	5.47 ± 1.56	10.52 ± 277
Suprailiac	4.11 ± 1.39	8.93 ± 2.88
Side	4.54 ± 1.55	10.69 ± 3.39
Waist	6.66 ± 3.39	15.96 ± 5.23
Abdomen	5.59 ± 2.13	11.33 ± 4.24
Chin	4.75 ± 1.93	9.28 ± 2.27
Thigh anterior	9.01 ± 4.69	21.93 ± 7.45
Thigh posterior	9.83 ± 4.93	25.16 ± 6.58
Calf lateral	6.30 ± 3.19	10.85 ± 3.72
Calf medial	5.88 ± 3.05	10.43 ± 3.80
Upper body[3]	26.37 ± 8.9	57.44 ± 15.4
Total body	71.48 ± 26.02	154.2 ± 31.5

From Probst M, et al. Body composition of anorexia nervosa patients assessed by underwater weighing and skinfold-thickness measurements before and after weight gain. Am J Clin Nutr 2001;73:190.
[1]±Significantly different from skinfold thickness before wight gain, $P < 0.001$.
[2]±SD; *n* = 130.
[3]Upper body: subscapula, suprailiac, side, waist, and abdomen.

subjects consumed 10,460-12,552 = kJ (2500-3000 kcal) daily. Table 28.7 displays the values in both groups for body composition and skinfolds before and following weight gain. On admission, 33 subjects had body fat lower than 10% (BMI, 13.7 kg · m^{-2}), 68 subjects ranged in fatness between 10 to 15% (BMI, 14.8 kg · m^{-2}), and 39 subjects exceeded 15% (BMI, 16.0 kg · m^{-2}). Following treatment and weight gain, BMI improved considerably for each subgroup to above the normal range for typical female cohorts.

Positive adaptations in body composition occurred following the treatment program. In addition to gradually increasing body mass by 12.7 kg in AN-RT and 9.4 kg in AN-BPT, fat mass increased 137% for AN-RT and 90.3% for AN-BPT. These gains in adipose tissue mass were accompanied by more modest gains in FFM (5.8 kg or 16.8% in AN-RT and 3.7 kg or 9.8% for AN-BPT). Essentially, the differences in whole body composition and regional adipose tissue thickness assessed by skinfolds on admission between the two anorectic types disappeared with weight regain. For the sum of 12 skinfolds, tissue mass at each anatomic site approximately doubled from a total 71.5 mm to 154.2 mm, with similar percentages in the upper and lower body regions. Of added importance to changes in body composition with weight regain in anorectics is the need to provide support therapies about the "fear of fat" syndrome, which initially contributes to this growing health malady. Two aspects of recovery should include the following: (1) carefully supervised physical reconditioning program, and (2) educational programs about the effects of low body mass (and low body fat) on normal growth and bone health.

BOD POD As a Criterion Method?

A relatively new procedure to estimate body volume holds promise to possibly replace densitometry for assessing the body volume of individuals ranging in size from infants to large athletes.[124,157] The new method has adapted air displacement plethysmography first reported in the late 1800s[106] and using helium in the 1950s as the gas displaced.[167,168] The subject sits inside a small chamber (marketed commercially as **BOD POD**; Life Measurement Instruments, Concord, CA).[34] Measurement requires only 3 to 5 minutes, and high reproducibility of test scores (r >0.90) exists within and across days. Figure 28.24A shows the BOD POD. After being weighed to the nearest 5 g on an electronic scale (*bottom left* of BOD POD illustration), the subject sits comfortably in the 750-L volume, dual-chamber fiberglass shell. The molded front seat separates the unit into front and rear chambers. The electronics, housed in the rear chamber, contain the pressure transducers, breathing circuit, and air circulation system.

The BOD POD determines body volume by measuring the initial volume of the empty chamber and then the volume with the person inside. To ensure measurement accuracy, the person should wear a tight-fitting swimsuit.[47] The person's volume is the initial volume minus the reduced chamber volume with the subject inside. The subject breathes several breaths into an air circuit to assess pulmonary gas volume, which when subtracted from measured body volume yields body volume. Body density computes as body mass (measured in air) ÷ body volume (measured in BOD POD, including a correction for a small negative volume caused by isothermal effects related to skin surface area). The Siri equation converts body density to percentage body fat. Figure 28.24B shows the regression of percentage body fat assessed by hydrostatic weighing versus percentage body fat assessed by BOD POD in 42 men and 26 women ages 21 to 56 years who differed in ethnicity (47 non-Hispanic white, 10 Hispanic, 7 African American, 4 Asian American), body mass (52–129 kg), and stature (145–191 cm). A difference of only 0.3% (0.2% fat units) occurred between body fat determined

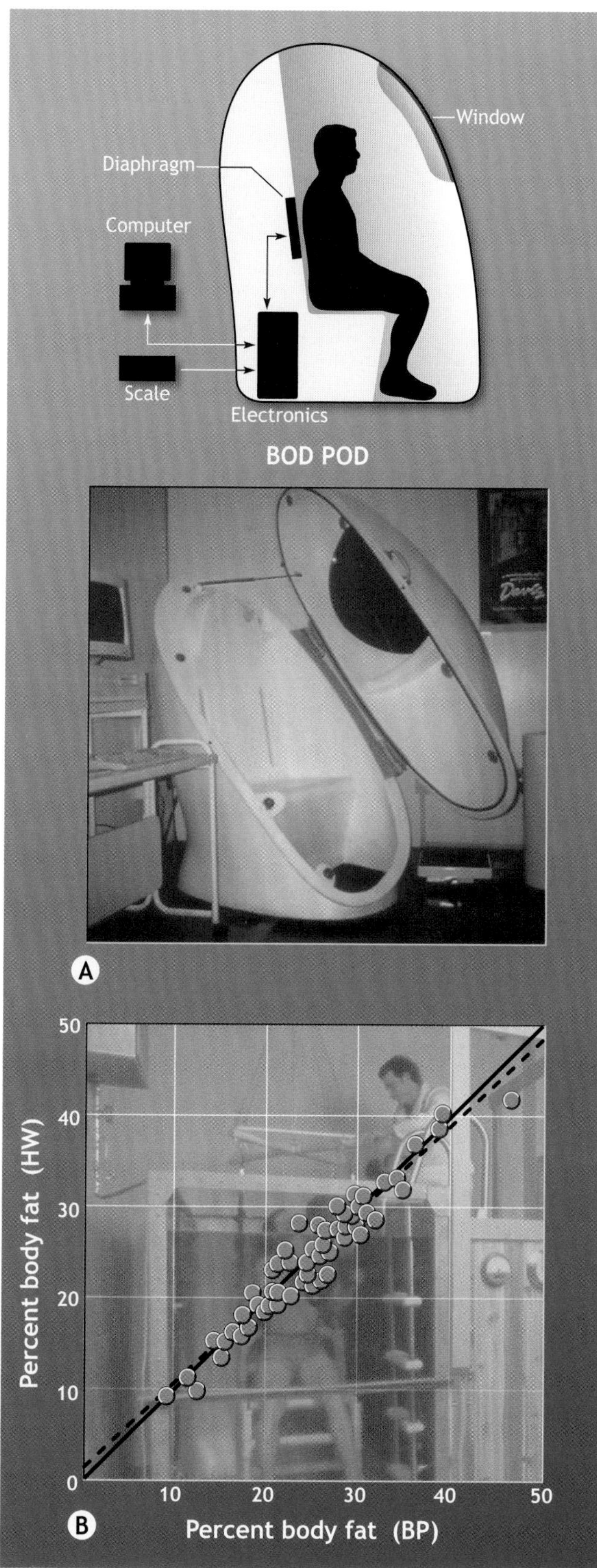

FIGURE 28.24 • A. BOD POD for measuring human body volume. (Photo courtesy of Dr. Megan McCrory, Tufts University, Boston.) **B**. Regression of percentage body fat by hydrostatic weighing (HW) versus percentage body fat by BOD POD (BP). (Data from McCrory MA, et al. Evaluation of a new air displacement plethysmograph for measuring human body composition. Med Sci Sports Exerc 1995;27:1686.)

by hydrostatic weighing and by BOD POD; the validity correlation was $r = 0.96$ between the two methods.

Future studies must determine BOD POD validity for more-homogeneous groups that represent the typical body fat range for young men and women (i.e., 10 to 20% body fat for men and 20 to 30% for women). Assessments in children, adolescents, and older subjects, including various athletic populations, also require quantification of test score reliability and validity. Recent data indicate that assessments of collegiate football players with BOD POD, although producing reliable scores, underpredicted percentage body fat compared with hydrostatic weighing and DXA values.[29]

Underprediction of %body fat also occurred in a heterogeneous sample of black men who varied considerably in age, stature, body mass, %body fat, and self-reported physical activity level and socioeconomic status.[188] BOD POD significantly underestimated body density (hence, %body fat) compared to densitometry (−1.9% fat units) and DXA(−1.6% fat units). Similar underpredictions of %body fat compared to DXA-devived %body fat (−2.9% fat units) occurred in 54 boys and girls 10 to 18 years of age.[107] In contrast, a BOD POD validation study in 25 young children ages 9 to 14 concluded that compared to DXA, total body water, and densitometry, BOD POD precisely and accurately estimated fat mass without introducing bias estimates.[46]

INTEGRATIVE QUESTION

Outline your response to a student who asks: "Why by some criteria for obesity am I considered overfat, while my body fat assessment with other methods falls within normal limits?"

AVERAGE PERCENTAGE BODY FAT

Table 28.8 lists average values for percentage body fat in samples of men and women throughout the United States. Values representing ±1 standard deviation provide some indication of the variation or spread from the average: the column headed "68% Variation Limits" indicates the range of percentage body fat that includes one standard deviation, or approximately 68 of every 100 persons measured. As an example, the average percentage body fat of 15.0% for young men from the New York sample includes the 68% variation limits from 8.9 to 21.1% body fat. Interpreting this statistically, for 68 of every 100 young men measured, percentage fat ranges between 8.9 and 21.1%. Of the remaining 32 young men, 16 possess more than 21.1% body fat, while 16 other men have a body fat percentage below 8.9. *In general, percentage body fat for young adult men averages between 12 and 15%; the average fat value for women falls between 25 and 28%.*[108,109]

Representative Samples Are Lacking

Considerable data describe average body composition for many groups of men and women of different ages and fitness levels and athletic specialties (see Chapter 29). However, no

TABLE 28.8 ➤ AVERAGE VALUES OF BODY FAT FOR YOUNGER AND OLDER WOMEN AND MEN FROM SELECTED STUDIES

STUDY	AGE RANGE	STATURE (CM)	MASS (KG)	% FAT	68% VARIATION LIMITS
Younger women					
North Carolina, 1962	17–25	165.0	55.5	22.9	17.5–28.5
New York, 1962	16–30	167.5	59.0	28.7	24.6–32.9
California, 1968	19–23	165.9	58.4	21.9	17.0–26.9
California, 1970	17–29	164.9	58.6	25.5	21.0–30.1
Air Force, 1972	17–22	164.1	55.8	28.7	22.3–35.3
New York, 1973	17–26	160.4	59.0	26.2	23.4–33.3
North Carolina, 1975	—	166.1	57.5	24.6	—
Army Recruits, 1986	17–25	162.0	58.6	28.4	23.9–32.9
Massachusetts, 1998	17–31	165.2	57.8	21.8	16.7–27.9
Older women					
Minnesota, 1953	31–45	163.3	60.7	28.9	25.1–32.8
	43–68	160.0	60.9	34.2	28.0–40.5
New York, 1963	30–40	164.9	59.6	28.6	22.1–35.3
	40–50	163.1	56.4	34.4	29.5–39.5
North Carolina, 1975	33–50	—	—	29.7	23.1–36.5
Massachusetts, 1993	31–50	165.2	58.9	25.2	19.2–31.2
Younger men					
Minnesota, 1951	17–26	177.8	69.1	11.8	5.9–11.8
Colorado, 1956	17–25	172.4	68.3	13.5	8.3–18.8
Indiana, 1966	18–23	180.1	75.5	12.6	8.7–16.5
California, 1968	16–31	175.7	74.1	15.2	6.3–24.2
New York, 1973	17–26	176.4	71.4	15.0	8.9–21.1
Texas, 1977	18–24	179.9	74.6	13.4	7.4–19.4
Army Recruits, 1986	17–25	174.7	70.5	15.6	10.0–21.2
Massachusetts, 1998	17–31	178.1	76.4	12.9	7.8–19.0
Older men					
Indiana, 1966	24–38	179.0	76.6	17.8	11.3–24.3
	40–48	177.0	80.5	22.3	16.3–28.3
North Carolina, 1976	27–50	—	—	23.7	17.9–30.1
Texas, 1977	27–59	180.0	85.3	27.1	23.7–30.5
Massachusetts, 1993	31–50	177.1	77.5	19.9	13.2–26.5

systematic evaluation exists for the body composition of a representative sample of the general population to warrant establishing norms or precise recommended values for body composition. At this time, it seems appropriate only to present average values from various studies of different age groups.

The general trend of these data indicates a distinct tendency for percentage body fat to steadily increase with advancing age. The mechanisms leading to an increase in body fat with age are poorly understood. It also remains unanswered the extent to which the additional fat in older age poses an increased health risk. The trend does not necessarily imply a desirable or normal aging process, because participation in vigorous physical activity throughout life frequently blunts body fat accretion with age.[183] Body composition could change with age because the aging skeleton becomes demineralized and porous; osteoporosis reduces body density because of significant decreases in bone density. Regular physical activity, on the other hand, maintains or increases bone mass while preserving muscle mass. Reduced daily physical activity provides another reason for the relative increase in body fat with age. A sedentary lifestyle tends to increase storage fat and reduce muscle mass. This would occur even if the daily caloric intake remained unchanged.

DETERMINING GOAL BODY WEIGHT

Average values for percentage body fat approximate 15% for young men and 25% for young women. In contact sports and activities that require muscular power (e.g., football, sprint swimming, and running), successful performance usually requires a large body mass with average or below-average body fat. In contrast, successful athletes in weight-bearing endurance activities generally possess a relatively light body mass and low body fat. One hopes that attaining a low body mass does not compromise lean tissue mass and energy reserves. *Proper assessment of body composition, not body weight, determines a person's ideal body weight. For athletes,* ***goal body weight*** *must coincide with optimizing sport-specific measures of physiologic functional capacity and exercise performance.* The following equation computes a goal body weight based on a desired body fat level:

$$\text{Goal body weight} = \text{fat-free body mass} \div 1.00 - \text{desired \%fat}$$

Suppose a 91-kg (200-lb) man, currently with 20% body fat, wants to know how much fat weight to lose to attain a body fat composition of 15%. The computations progress as follows:

$$\text{Fat mass} = 91 \text{ kg} \times 0.20 = 18.2 \text{ kg}$$
$$\text{Fat-free body mass} = 91 \text{ kg} - 18.2 \text{ kg} = 72.8 \text{ kg}$$

$$\text{Goal body weight} = 72.8 \text{ kg} \div (1.00 - 0.10) = 72.8 \text{ kg} \div 0.90 = 80.9 \text{ kg (178 lb)}$$

$$\text{Goal fat loss} = \text{Current body weight} - \text{Goal body weight} = 91 \text{ kg} - 80.9 \text{ kg} = 10.1 \text{ kg (22.2 lb)}$$

If this man lost 10.1 kg of body fat, his new body mass of 80.9 kg would contain fat equal to 10% of body mass. These calculations assume no change in FFM during weight loss. Moderate caloric restriction plus increased daily energy expenditure through exercise induce fat loss and conserve the FFM. Chapter 30 discusses prudent yet effective approaches to fat loss.

Summary

1. Standard height–weight tables reveal little about an individual's body composition. Studies of athletes clearly show that overweight does not necessarily coincide with excessive body fat.
2. BMI relates more closely to body fat and health risk than simply body mass and stature. However, BMI fails to consider the body's proportional composition.
3. Total body fat consists of essential fat and storage fat. Essential fat contains fat present in bone marrow, nerve tissue, and organs; it is not a labile energy reserve, but instead an important component for normal biologic function. Storage fat represents the energy reserve that accumulates mainly as adipose tissue beneath the skin and visceral depots.
4. Storage fat averages 12% of body mass for men and 15% for women. Essential fat averages 3% of body mass for men and 12% for women. The greater essential fat in females probably relates to childbearing and hormonal functions.
5. A person probably cannot reduce body fat below the essential fat level and still maintain good health.
6. Menstrual dysfunction occurs in athletes who train hard and maintain low body fat levels. The precise interaction between the physiologic and psychologic stress of intense, regular training and competition, hormonal balance, energy and nutrient intake, and body fat requires further study.
7. Delayed onset of menarche in chronically active young females may confer health benefits, because such individuals show a lower lifetime occurrence of reproductive organ and other cancers.
8. The most popular indirect methods of body composition assessment include hydrostatic weighing and prediction methods that incorporate skinfold and girth measurements. Hydrostatic weighing determines body density, with subsequent estimation of percentage body fat. The computation assumes a constant density for the body's fat and fat-free tissue compartments.
9. Part of the error inherent in predicting body fat from whole-body density lies in the correctness of assumptions concerning the densities of the body's fat and fat-free components. These densities, especially fat-free body mass, differ from assumed constants because of race, age, and athletic experience.
10. Common body composition assessments use prediction equations from relationships among selected skinfolds and girths and body density and percentage fat. The equations show population specificity because they are most accurate with subjects similar to those who participated in the equations' original derivation.
11. The body profile provides a practical method to (1) subdivide anthropometric dimensions into muscular and nonmuscular components and (2) monitor dimensional changes from training, diet, growth, and aging.
12. The concept of BIA states that hydrated fat-free body tissues and extracellular water facilitate electrical flow, compared with fat tissue, because of the greater electrolyte content of the fat-free component. Impedance to electric current flow relates to the body's fat quantity.
13. Near-infrared interactance should be used with caution when assessing body composition in the exercise sciences; this methodology currently lacks verification of adequate validity.
14. Ultrasound, x-ray, CT, MRI, and DXA indirectly assesses body composition. Each has a unique application and special limitations for expanding knowledge of the compositional components of the live human body.
15. An air displacement method (BOD POD) offers promise for body compositional assessment.
16. Based on data from healthy young adults, average males possess a body fat content of approximately 15% and women, 25%. These values often provide a frame of reference for evaluating the body fat of individual athletes and specific athletic groups.
17. Goal body weight computes as fat-free body mass ÷ 1.00 − desired %fat.

References

1. Abate N, et al. Prediction of total subcutaneous abdominal, intraperitoneal, and retroperitoneal adipose tissue masses in men by a single axial magnetic imaging slice. Am J Clin Nutr 1997;65:403.
2. Abe T, et al. Total and segmental subcutaneous adipose tissue volume measured by ultrasound. Med Sci Sports Exerc 1996;28:908.
3. Adams J, et al. Total body fat content in a group of professional football players. Can J Appl Sport Sci 1982;7:36.
4. Ainsworth BE, et al. Predictive accuracy of bioimpedance in estimating fat-free mass of African-American women. Med Sci Sports Exerc 1997;29:781.
5. Baumgartner RN, et al. Bioelectric impedence for body composition. Exerc Sport Sci Rev 1990;18:193.
6. Beals KA, Manore MM. Behavioral, psychological, and physical characteristics of female athletes with subclinical eating disorders. Int J Sport Nutr Exerc Metab 2000;10:128.

7. Beckvid Henriksson G et al. Women endurance runners with menstrual dysfunction have prolonged interruption of training due to injury. Gynecol Obstet Invest 2000:49:41.
8. Becque MD, et al. Time course of skin-plus-fat compression in males and females. Hum Biol 1984;58:33.
9. Behnke AR, Wilmore JH. Evaluation and regulation of body build and composition. Englewood Cliffs, NJ: Prentice-Hall, 1974.
10. Behnke AR, et al. The specific gravity of healthy men. JAMA 1942;118:495.
11. Bemben DA, et al. Musculoskeletal responses to high- and low-intensity resistance training in early postmenopausal women. Med Sci Sports Exerc 2000:32:1949.
12. Bernstein L, et al. Physical exercise and a reduced risk of breast cancer in young women. J Natl Cancer Inst 1994;86:1403.
13. Bioelectrical impedance analysis in body composition measurement: National Institutes of Health technology assessment conference statement. Am J Clin Nutr 1996;64(suppl):524S.
14. Boddy K, et al. Body potassium and fat free mass. Clin Sci 1973;44:622.
15. Brandon LJ. Comparison of existing skinfold equations for estimating body fat in African American and white women. Am J Clin Nutr 1998;67:1115.
16. Broeder CE, et al. Assessing body composition before and after resistance or endurance training. Med Sci Sports Exerc 1997;29:705.
17. Brožek, J, et al. Densitometric analysis of body composition: revision of some quantitative assumptions. Ann NY Acad Sci 1963;110:113.
18. Bunt JC, et al. Impact of total body water fluctuations on estimation of body fat from body density. Med Sci Sports Exerc 1989;21:96.
19. Burke LM, et al. Carbohydrate loading failed to improve 100-km cycling performance in a placebo-controlled trial. J Appl Physiol 2000:88:1284.
20. Burke LM, et al. Effect of fat adaptation and carbohydrate restoration on metabolism and performance during prolonged cycling. J Appl Physiol 2000;89:2413.
21. Calle EE, et al. Body-mass index and mortality in a prospective cohort of U.S. adults. N Engl J Med 1999;341:1097.
22. Cassady SL, et al. Validity of near infrared body composition analysis in children and adolescents. Med Sci Sports Exerc 1993;25:1185.
23. Caton JR, et al. Body composition by bioelectrical impedance: effect of skin temperature. Med Sci Sports Exerc 1988;20:489.
24. Chehab FF, et al. Early onset of reproductive function in normal female mice treated with leptin. Science 1997;275:88.
25. Clark RR, et al. A comparison of methods to predict minimal weight in high school wrestlers. Med Sci Sports Exerc 1993;25:1541.
26. Clarys JP, et al. Gross tissue weights in the human body by cadaver dissection. Hum Biol 1984;56:459.
27. Cohn SH, Dombrowski CS. Measurement of total body calcium, sodium, chlorine, nitrogen, and phosphorus in man by in-vivo neutron activation. J Nucl Med 1971;12:499.
28. Cohn SN, et al. Indexes of body cell mass: nitrogen versus potassium. Am J Physiol 1983;244:E305.
29. Collins MA, et al. Evaluation of the BOD POD for assessing body fat in collegiate football players. Med Sci Sports Exerc 1999;31:1350.
30. Collis N, et al. Cellulite treatment: a myth or reality—a prospective randomized, controlled trial of two therapies, endermologie and aminophylline cream. Plast Reconstr Surg 1999;104:1110.
31. Constantine NW, Warren MP. Physical activity, fitness, and reproductive health in women: clinical observations. In: Bouchard C, et al., eds. Physical activity, fitness, and health. Champaign, IL: Human Kinetics, 1994.
32. Conway JM, et al. A new approach for the estimation of body composition: infrared interactance. Am J Clin Nutr 1984;40:1123.
33. Côté KD, Adams WC. Effect of bone density on body composition estimates in young adult black and white women. Med Sci Sports Exerc 1993;25:290.
34. Dempster P, Aitkens S. A new air displacement method for the determination of human body composition. Med Sci Sports Exerc 1995;27:1692.
35. Déspres J-P, et al. Estimation of deep abdominal adipose-tissue accumulation from simple anthropometric measurements in men. Am J Clin Nutr 1991;54:471.
36. Deurenberg-Yap M, et al. The paradox of low body mass index and high body fat percentage among Chinese, Malays and Indians in Singapore. Int J Obes Relat Metab Disord 2000;24:1011.
37. Donnelly JE, et al. Hydrostatic weighing without head submersion. Description of a method. Med Sci Sports Exerc 1988;20:66.
38. Drumm S, et al. Changes in body composition, anthropometry, and arm radiography following 10 weeks of hydraulic resistive circuit exercise. Med Sci Sports Exerc 1984;16:184.
39. Dulloo AG, et al. Normal caffeine consumption: influences on thermogenesis and daily energy expenditure in lean and postobese human volunteers. Am J Clin Nutr 1989;49:44.
40. Durenberg P, et al. Changes in fat-free mass during weight loss measured by bioelectrical impedance and by densitometry. Am J Clin Nutr 1989;49:33.
41. Eliakim A, et al. Assessment of body composition in ballet dancers: correlation among anthropometric measurements, bio-electrical impedance analysis, and dual-energy X-ray absorpitometry. Int J Sports Med 2000;21:598.
42. Ellis KJ, et al. Body composition of a young, multiethnic female population. Am J Clin Nutr 1997;65:724.
43. Engelen MP, et al. Dual-energy x-ray absorptiometry in the clinical evaluation of body composition and bone mineral density in patients with chronic obstructive pulmonary disease. Am J Clin Nutr 1998;68:1298.
44. Febbraio MA, et al. Effects of carbohydrate ingestion before and during exercise on glucose kinetics and performance. J Appl Physiol 2000:89:2220.
45. Field AE, et al. Exposure to mass media and weight concerns among girls. Pediatrics 1999;103:E36.
46. Fields DA, Goran MI. Body composition techniques and the four-compartment model in children. J Appl Physiol 2000;89:613.
47. Fields DA, et al. Validation of the BOD POD with hydrostatic weighing: influence of body clothing. Int J Obes Relat Metab Disord 2000;24:200.
48. Forbes GB. Human body composition. New York: Springer-Verlag, 1987.
49. Foster KR, Lukaski HC. Whole-body impedance—what does it measure? Am J Clin Nutr 1996;64(suppl):388S.
50. Freedson PS, et al. Physique, body composition, and psychological characteristics of competitive female body builders. Phys Sportsmed 1983;11:85.
51. Frisch RE, et al. Delayed menarche and amenorrhea in ballet dancers. N Engl J Med 1980;303:17.
52. Frisch RE, et al. Lower lifetime occurrence of breast cancer and cancers of the reproductive system among former college athletes. Am J Clin Nutr 1987;45:328.
53. Frisch RE, et al. Lower prevalence of non-reproductive cancers among female former college athletes. Med Sci Sports Exerc 1989;21:250.
54. Gallagher D, et al. Healthy percentage body fat ranegs: an approach for developing guidelines based on body mass index. Am J Clin Nutr 2000;72:694.
55. Gong QY, et al. Estimation of body composition in muscular dystrophy by MRI and stereology. J Magn Reson Imaging 2000;12:467.
56. Goodpaster BH, et al. Composition of skeletal muscle evaluated with computed tomography. Ann N Y Acad Sci 2000;904:18.
57. Gore CJ, et al. Skinfold thickness varies directly with spring coefficient and inversely with jaw pressure. Med Sci Sports Exerc 2000;32:540.
58. Hagerman FC, et al. Effects of high-intensity resistance training on untrained older men. I. Strength, cardiovascular, and metabolic responses. J Gerontol A Biol Sci 2000;55:B336.
59. Harber VJ. Menstrual dysfunction in athletes: a energetic challenge. Exerc Sport Sci Rev 2000;1:19.
60. Harris TB, et al. Waist circumference and sagittal diameter reflect total body fat better than visceral fat in older men and women. The Health, Aging and Body Composition Study. Ann N Y Acad Sci 2000;904:462.
61. Hetland ML, et al. Running induces menstrual irregularities but bone mass is unaffected, except in amenorrheic women. Am J Med 1993;95:53.
62. Heymsfield SB, et al. Appendicular skeletal muscle mass: measurement by dual-photon absorptiometry. Am J Clin Nutr 1990;52:214.
63. Heymsfield SB, et al. Body composition of humans: comparison of two improved four-compartment models that differ in expense, technical complexity, and radiation exposure. Am J Clin Nutr 1991;52:52.
64. Hicks VL, et al. Validation of near-infrared interactance and skinfold methods for estimating body composition of American Indian women. Med Sci Sports Exerc 2000;32:531.
65. Hortobagyi T, et al. Comparison of four methods to assess body composition in black and white athletes. Int J Sports Nutr 1992;2:60.
66. Houmard JA, et al. Validity of a near-infrared device for estimating body composition in a college football team. J Appl Sport Sci Res 1991;5:53.

67. Housh TJ, et al. Validity of near-infrared interactance instruments for estimating percent body fat in youth wrestlers. Pediatr Exerc Sci 1996;8:69.
68. Hsieh S, et al. Measurement of residual volume sitting and lying in air and water (and during underwater weighing) and its effects on computed body density. Med Sci Sports Exerc 1985;17:204.
69. Ishida Y, et al. Reliability of B-mode ultrasound for the measurement of body fat and muscle thickness. Am J Hum Biol 1992;4:511.
70. Ishida Y, et al. Body fat and muscle thickness distributions in untrained young females. Med Sci Sports Exerc 1995;27:270.
71. Jackson AS, Pollock ML. Generalized equations for predicting body density of men. Br J Nutr 1978;40:497.
72. Jackson AS, et al. Generalized equations for predicting body density of women. Med Sci Sports 1980;12:175.
73. Janssen, et al. Skeletal muscle mass and distribution in 468 men and women aged 18–88 yr. J Appl Physiol 2000;89:81.
74. Kaiserauer S, et al. Nutritional, physiological, and menstrual status of distance runners. Med Sci Sports Exerc 1989;21:120.
75. Katch FI. Practice curves and errors of measurement in estimating underwater weight by hydrostatic weighing. Med Sci Sports 1969;1:212.
76. Katch FI. Reliability and individual differences in ultrasound assessment of subcutaneous fat: effects of body position. Hum Biol 1983;55:789.
77. Katch FI. Assessment of lean body tissues by radiography and bioelectrical impedance. In: Body composition in youth and adults. Columbus, OH: Ross Laboratories, 1985.
78. Katch FI, Behnke AR. Arm x-ray assessment of body fat in men and women. Med Sci Sports Exerc 1984;16:316.
79. Katch FI, Hortobagyi T. Validity of surface anthropometry to estimate upper-arm muscularity, including changes with body mass loss. Am J Clin Nutr 1990;52:591.
80. Katch FI, Katch VL. Measurement and prediction errors in body composition assessment and the search for the perfect prediction equation. Res Q Exerc Sport 1980;51:249.
81. Katch FI, Katch VL. Computer technology to evaluate body composition, nutrition, and exercise. Prev Med 1983;12:619.
82. Katch FI, Katch VL. The body composition profile: techniques of measurement and applications. Clin Sports Med 1984;3:31.
83. Katch FI, McArdle WD. Prediction of body density from simple anthropometric measurements in college-age men and women. Hum Biol 1973;45:445.
84. Katch FI, McArdle WD. Validity of body composition prediction equations for college men and women. Am J Clin Nutr 1975;28:105.
85. Katch FI, Michael ED. Prediction of body density from skinfold and girth measurements of college females. J Appl Physiol 1968;25:92.
86. Katch FI, Spiak DL. Validity of the Mellits and Cheek method for body-fat estimation in relation to menstrual cycle status in athletes and non-athletes below 22 percent fat. Ann Hum Biol 1984;11:389.
87. Katch FI, et al. Estimation of body volume by underwater weighing: description of a simple method. J Appl Physiol 1967;23:811.
88. Katch FI, et al. The underweight female. Phys Sportsmed 1980;8:55.
89. Katch FI, et al. Validity of bioelectrical impedance to estimate body composition in cardiac and pulmonary patients. Am J Clin Nutr 1986;43:972.
90. Katch VL, et al. Contribution of breast volume and weight to body fat distribution in females. Am J Phys Anthropol 1980;53:93.
91. Kehayias JJ, et al. Measurement of body fat by neutron inelastic scattering: comments on installation, operation, and error analysis. In: Yasumura S, et al., eds. In vivo body composition studies. New York: Plenum Press, 1990.
92. Keys A, Brožek, J. Body fat in adult men. Physiol Rev 1960;33:245.
93. Keys A, et al. The biology of human starvation. Minneapolis: University of Minnesota Press, 1950.
94. Kodama AA. In vivo and in vitro determinations of body fat and body water in the hamster. J Appl Physiol 1971;31:218.
95. Kohrt WM. Body composition by DXA: tried and true? Med Sci Sports Exerc 1995;27:1359.
96. Kohrt WM. Preliminary evidence that DEXA provides an accurate assessment of body composition. J Appl Physiol 1998;84:372.
97. Kondo M, et al. Upper limit of fat-free mass in humans: a study of Japanese sumo wrestlers. Am J Hum Biol 1994;6:613.
98. Koulmann N, et al. Use of bioelectrical impedance analysis to estimate body fluid compartments after acute variations of the body hydration level. Med Sci Sports Exerc 2000;32:857.
99. Kuczmarski RJ, et al. CDC growth charts: United States. Advance data, number 314: June 8, 2000. From Vital and Health Statistics of the Centers for Disease Control and Prevention/National Center for Health Statistics.
100. Kushner RF, et al. Clinical characteristics influencing bioelectrical impedance analysis measurements. Am J Clin Nutr 1996;64(suppl):423S.
101. Kyle UG, et al. Physical activity and fat-free and fat mass by bioelectrical impedance in 3853 adults. Med Sci Sports Exerc 2001;33:576.
102. LeBlanc A, et al. Muscle volume, MRI relaxation times (T2), and body composition after spaceflight. J Appl Physiol 2000;89:2158.
103. Lee RC, et al. Total-body skeletal muscle mass: development and cross-validation of anthropometric prediction models. Am J Clin Nutr 2000;72:796.
104. Legro RS, et al. Rapid maturation of the reproductive axis during perimenarche independent of body composition. J Clin Endocrinol Metab 2000;85:1021.
105. Lehtonen-Veromaa M, et al. Influence of physical activity on ultrasound and dual-energy X-ray absorptiometry bone measurements in peripubertal girls: a cross-sectional study. Calcif Tissue Int 2000;66:248.
106. Lim TPK. Critical evaluation of the pneumatic method for determining body volume: Its history and technique. Ann NY Acad Sci 1963;110;72.
107. Lockner DW, et al. Comparison of air-displacement plethysmography, hydrodensitometry, and dual X-ray absorptiometry for assessing body composition of children 10 to 18 years of age. Ann N Y Acad Sci 2000;904:72.
108. Lohman TG, Going SB. Multicomponent models in body composition research: opportunities and pitfalls. Basic Life Sci 1993;60:53.
109. Lohman TG, et al. Body fat measurement goes high-tech: not all are created equal. ACSM Health Fitness J 1997;1:30.
110. Lohman TG, et al. Assessing body composition and changes in body composition. Another look at dual-energy X-ray absorptiometry. Ann N Y Acad Sci 2000;904:45.
111. Long TD, et al. Lack of menstrual cycle effects on hypothalamic-pituatary-adrenal axis response to insulin-induced hypoglycaemia. Clin Endocrinol (Oxf) 2000;52:781.
112. Loucks AB, Callister R. Induction and prevention of low-T3 syndrome in exercising women. Am J Physiol 1993;264:R924.
113. Loucks AB, et al. Hypothalamic-pituitary-thyroidal function in eumenorrheic and amenorrheic athletes. J Clin Endocrinol Metab 1992;75:514.
114. Loucks AB, et al. Low energy availability, not stress of exercise, alters LH pulsatility in exercising women. J Appl Physiol 1998;84:37.
115. Lukaski HC. Methods for the assessment of human body composition: traditional and new. Am J Clin Nutr 1987;46:537.
116. Lukaski HC. Soft tissue composition and bone mineral status: evaluation by dual-energy x-ray absorptiometry. J Nutr 1993;123:438.
117. Maddalozzo GF, Snow CM. High intensity resistance training: effects on bone in older men and women. Calcif Tissue Int 2000;66:399.
118. Martin AD, Drinkwater DT. Variability in the measures of body fat assumptions or techniques? Sports Med 1991;11:277.
119. Matiega J. The testing of physical efficiency. Am J Phys Anthropol 1921;4:223.
120. Maynard LM et al. Childhood body composition in relation to body mass index. Pediatrics 2001;107:344.
121. Mazes RAB, et al. Total body composition by dual photon (^{153}Gd) absorptiometry. Am J Clin Nutr 1984;40:834.
122. Mazes RAB, et al. Dual energy x-ray absorptiometry for total-body regional bone-mineral and soft-tissue composition. Am J Clin Nutr 1990;51:1106.
123. McConell GK, et al. Effect of carbohydrate ingestion on glucose kinetics and muscle metabolism during intense endurance exercise. J Appl Physiol 2000;89:1690.
124. McCrory MA, et al. Evaluation of a new air displacement plethysmograph for measuring human body composition. Med Sci Sports Exerc 1995;27:1686.
125. McKee JE, Cameron N. Bioelectrical impedance changes during the menstrual cycle. Am J Hum Biol 1997;9:155.
126. McLean K, Skinner JS. Validity of the Futrex-5000 for body composition determination. Med Sci Sports Exerc 1992;24:253.
127. McNeill G, et al. Body fat in lean and overweight women estimated by six methods. Br J Nutr 1991;65:95.
128. Mendez J, et al. Density of fat and bone mineral of mammalian body. Metabolism 1960;9:472.

129. Mikat RP. Chest, waist, and hip circumference estimations from stereo photographic digital topography. J Sports Med Phys Fitness 2000;40:58.
130. Mitsiopoulos N, et al. Cadaver validation of skeletal muscle measurement by magnetic resonance imaging and computerized tomography. J Appl Physiol 1998;85:115.
131. Modlesky CM, et al. Density of the fat-free mass and estimates of body composition in male weight trainees. J Appl Physiol 1996;80:2085.
132. Moradi T, et al. Physical activity and postmenopausal endometrial cancer risk (Sweden). Cancer Causes Control 2000;11:829.
133. Morales MF, et al. Studies on body composition. J Biol Chem 1945;158:677.
134. Morrow JR Jr. Accuracy of measured and predicted residual lung volume on body density measurement. Med Sci Sports Exerc 1986;18:647.
135. Myhre LG, Kessler WV. Body density and potassium 40 measurements of body composition as related to age. J Appl Physiol 1966;21:1251.
136. National Center for Health Statistics. Health, United States. Hyattsville, MD: Public Health Service, 1990.
137. National Task Force on the Prevention and Treatment of Obesity. Obesity, overweight and health risk. Arch Intern Med 2000;160:898.
138. Nattiv A. Stress fractures and bone health in track and field athletes J Sci Med Sport 2000;3:268.
139. Nelson ME, et al. Analysis of body composition techniques and models for detecting change in soft tissue with strength training. Am J Clin Nutr 1996;63:678.
140. Nindl BC, et al. Comparison of body composition assessment among lean black and white male collegiate athletes. Med Sci Sports Exerc 1998;30:769.
141. Nindl BC, et al. Regional body composition changes in women after 6 months of periodized physical training. J Appl Physiol 2000;88:2251.
142. Ortiz O, et al. Differences in skeletal muscle and bone mineral mass between black and white females and their relevance to estimates of body composition. Am J Clin Nutr 1992;55:8.
143. Panotopoulos G, et al. Dual x-ray absorptiometry, bioelectrical impedance, and near infrared interactance in obese women. Med Sci Sports Exerc 2001;33:665.
144. Patel R, et al. Long-term precision of DXA scanning assessed over seven years in forty postmenopausal women. Osteoporos Int 2000:11:68.
145. Penn I-W, et al. Body composition and two-compartment model assumptions in male long distance runners. Med Sci Sports Exerc 1994;26:392.
146. Peppler WW, Mazes RB. Total body bone mineral and lean body mass by dual photon absorptiometry. Theory and measurement procedure. Calcif Tissue Int 1981;33:353.
147. Pierson RN Jr, et al. High precision in-vivo neutron activation analysis: a new era for compartmental analysis in body composition. In: Yasumura S, et al., eds. In vivo body composition studies. New York: Plenum Press, 1990.
148. Ploutz-Snyder L, et al. Gastric gas and fluid emptying assessed by magnetic resonance imaging. Eur J Appl Physiol 1999;79:212.
149. Pollock ML, Jackson AS. Measurement of cardiorespiratory fitness and body composition in the clinical setting. Compr Ther 1980;6:12.
150. Prior BM, et al. In vivo validation of whole body composition estimates from dual-energy X-ray absorptiometry. J Appl Physiol 1997;83:623.
151. Probst M, et al. Body composition of anorexia nervosa patients assessed by underwater weighing and skinfold-thickness measurements before and after weight gain. Am J Clin Nutr 2001;73:190.
152. Rathbun EN, Pace N. Studies on body composition. J Biol Chem 1945;158:667.
153. Roche LF, et al., eds. Human body composition. Champaign, IL: Human Kinetics, 1996.
154. Ross R, et al. Sensitivity of bioelectrical impedance to detect changes in body composition. J Appl Physiol 1989;67:1643.
155. Rubeffe-Scrive ML, et al. Fat cell metabolism in different regions in women: effect on menstrual cycle, pregnancy, and lactation. J Clin Invest 1985;75:1973.
156. Salamone LM, et al. Measurement of fat mass using DEXA: a validation study in elderly adults. J Appl Physiol 2000;89:345.
157. Sardinha LB, et al. Comparison of air displacement plethysmography with dual-energy absorptiometry and 3 field methods for estimating body composition in middle-aged men. Am J Clin Nutr 1998;68:786.
158. Sargent LA, et al. Family history of diabetes identifies a group at increased risk for the metabolic consequences of obesity and physical inactivity in EPIC-Norfolk: a population-based study. The European Prospective Investigation into Cancer. Int J Obes Relat Metab Disord 2000;24:1333.
159. Sartorio A, et al. Changes of bioelectrical impedance after a body weight reduction program in highly obese subjects. Diabetes Nutr Metab 2000;13:186.
160. Saunders MJ, et al. Effects of hydration changes on bioelectrical impedance in endurance trained individuals. Med Sci Sports Exerc 1998;30:885.
161. Schutte JE, et al. Density of lean body mass is greater in blacks than whites. J Appl Physiol 1984;56:1647.
162. Segal K, et al. Use of bioelectrical impedance analysis measurements as an evaluation for participating in sports. Am J Clin Nutr 1996;64(suppl):469S.
163. Seidell JC, et al. Abdominal fat depots measured with computed tomography: effects of degree of obesity, sex, and age. Eur J Clin Nutr 1988;42:805.
164. Shangold MM, et al. Evaluation and management of menstrual dysfunction in athletes. JAMA 1990;262:1665.
165. Sinning WE, et al. Validity of "generalized" equations for body composition analysis in male athletes. Med Sci Sports Exerc 1985;17:124.
166. Slaughter MH, et al. Skinfold equations for estimation of body fatness in children and youths. Hum Biol 1988;60:709.
167. Siri WE. Apparatus for measuring human body volume. Rev Sci Instrum 1956;27:729.
168. Siri WE. Body volume measurement by gas dilution. In: Brožek J, Henschel A, eds. Techniques for measuring body composition. Washington, DC: National Academy of Sciences–National Research Council, 1961.
169. Slaughter MH, et al. Skinfold equations for estimation of body fatness in children and youths. Hum Biol 1988;60:709.
170. Stager JM, Hatler LK. Menarche in athletes: the influence of genetics and prepubertal training. Med Sci Sports Exerc 1988;20:369.
171. Stolarczyk LM, et al. Predictive accuracy of bioelectrical impedance in estimating fat-free mass of Hispanic women. Med Sci Sports Exerc 1995;27:1450.
172. Stolarczyk LM, et al. The fatness-specific bioelectrical impedance analysis equations of Segal et al: are they generalizable and practical? Am J Clin Nutr 1997;66:8.
173. Stout JR, et al. Validity of percent body fat estimations in males. Med Sci Sports Exerc 1994;26:632.
174. Stout JR, et al. Validity of methods for estimating percent body fat in young women. J Strength Cond Res 1996;10:25.
175. Thomas EL, et al. Magnetic resonance imaging of total body fat. J Appl Physiol 1998;85:1778.
176. Thong FS, et al. Plasma leptin in female athletes: relationship with body fat, reproductive, nutritional, and endocrine factors. J Appl Physiol 2000;88:2037.
177. Thorland WG, et al. Midwest wrestling study: prediction of minimal weight for high school wrestlers. Med Sci Sports Exerc 1991;23:1102.
178. Thorland WG, et al. Estimation of body composition in black adolescent male athletes. Pediatr Exerc Sci 1993;5:116.
179. To WW, et al. Hormonal predisposition to menstrual dysfunction in collegiate dance students. Acta Obstet Gynecol Scand 2000;79:1117.
180. Toniolo PG, et al. A prospective study of endogenous estrogens and breast cancer in postmenopausal women. J Natl Cancer Inst 1995;87:190.
181. Tran ZV, Weltman A. Predicting body composition of men from girth measurements. Hum Biol 1988;60:167.
182. Tran ZV, Weltman A. Generalized equation for predicting body density of women from girth measurements. Med Sci Sports Exerc 1989;21:101.
183. Vaccaro P, et al. Body composition and physiological responses of Masters female swimmers 20 to 70 years of age. Res Q Exerc Sport 1984;55:278.
184. Vehrs P, et al. Reliability and concurrent validity of Futrex and bioelectrical impedance. Int J Sports Med 1998;19:560.
185. Visscher TL, et al. Underweight and overweight in relation to mortality among men aged 40-59 and 50-69 years: the Seven countries Study. Am J Epidemiol 2000;151:600.
186. Wadden TA, et al. Body fat deposition in adult obese women. II. Changes in fat distribution accompanying weight reduction. Am J Clin Nutr 1988;47:229.

187. Wagner DR, et al. Predictive accuracy of BIA equations for estimating fat-free mass of black men. Med Sci Sports Exerc 1997;29:969.
188. Wagner DR, et al. Validation of air displacement plethysmography for assessing body composition. Med Sci Sports Exerc 2000;32:1339.
189. Wang ZM, et al. The five-level model: a new approach to organizing body composition research. Am J Clin Nutr 1992;56:19.
190. Ward IC, et al. Reliability of multiple frequency bioelectrical impedance analysis: an intermachine comparison. Am J Hum Biol 1997;9:63.
191. Warren MP. The effects of exercise on pubertal progression and reproductive function. J Clin Endocrinol Metab 1980;51:1150.
192. Webster BL, Barr SI. Body composition analysis of female adolescent athletes. Med Sci Sports Exerc 1993;25:648.
193. Wells CL. Physical activity and cancer prevention. Focus on breast cancer. ACSM Health Fitness J 1999;3(1):13.
194. Weltman A, et al. Accurate assessment of body composition in obese females. Am J Clin Nutr 1988;48:1179.
195. Weststrate JA, Duerenberg P. Body composition in children: proposal for a method for calculating body fat percentage from total body density or skinfold-thickness measurements. Am J Clin Nutr 1989;50:1104.
196. Williams MJ, et al. Regional fat distribution in women and risk of cardiovascular disease. Am J Clin Nutr 1997;65:855.
197. Williams NI, et al. Effects of short-term strenuous endurance exercise upon corpus luteum function. Med Sci Sports Exerc 1999;31:949.
198. Williamson DA, et al. Body image assessment for obesity (BIA-O): development of a new procedure. Int J Obes Relat Metab Disord 2000;24:1326.
199. Winters KM, Snow CM. Detraining reverses positive effects of exercise on the musculoskeletal system in premenopausal women. J Bone Miner Res 2000;15:2495.
200. Withers RT, et al. Comparisons of two-, three-, and four-component models of body composition analysis in men and women. J Appl Physiol 1998;85:238.
201. Womack HC. The relationship between human body weight, subcutaneous fat, heart weight, and epicardial fat. Hum Biol 1983;55:667.
202. World Health Organization. Obesity: preventing and managing the global epidemic. Report of a WHO consultation presented at the World Health Organization; June 3–5, 1997; Geneva, Switzerland. Publication WHO/NUT/NCD/98.1.
203. Yanovski JA, et al. Differences in body composition of black and white girls. Am J Clin Nutr 1996;64:833.
204. Yeager KK, et al. The female athlete triad: disordered eating, amenorrhea, osteoporosis. Med Sci Sports Exerc 1993;25:775.
205. Zanker CL, Swaine IL. The relationship between serum oestradiol concentration and energy balance in young women distance runners. Int J Sports Med 1998;19:104.

CHAPTER 29

Physique, Performance, and Physical Activity

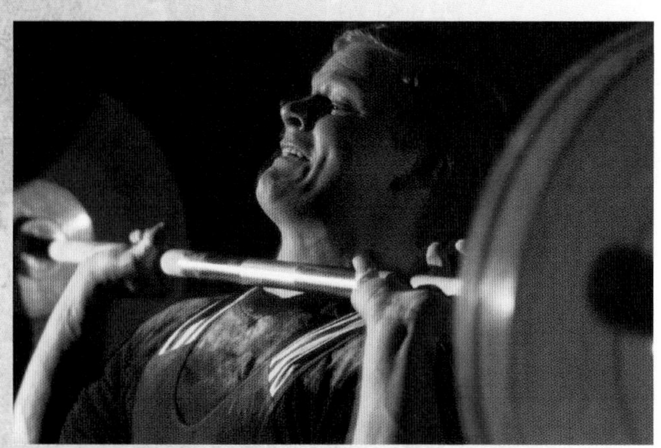

Chapter Objectives

- Compare body composition characteristics of average young men and women with elite competitors in endurance running, wrestling, triathlon, and weight lifting and bodybuilding
- Give examples of gender differences in world record performances for track and field, weight lifting, and cycling, speed skating, and swimming
- Contrast body fat values for male and female competitive swimmers with runners and give possible reasons for the differences
- Summarize body composition characteristics, including body mass index of early American professional football players and their modern-day counterparts, and compare the modern professionals with current collegiate players
- Describe procedures commonly used by high school wrestlers to "make weight" before competition
- Contrast body composition characteristics of elite high-school wrestlers with less successful counterparts
- Contrast body composition, girths, and excess muscle mass of male and female bodybuilders
- Compare ratios of fat-free body mass (FFM) to fat mass of competitive female bodybuilders to those of other elite female athletes
- Discuss the unique characteristics of the body profiles of champion male and female bodybuilders, male and female collegiate gymnasts, and National Basketball Association professional basketball players
- Discuss the upper limit of FFM in "large-size" athletes

Body composition evaluation partitions the gross size of a person into two major structural components—body fat and fat-free body mass (FFM). In Chapter 28, we emphasize that physique differs considerably between adult men and women. Pronounced physique differences also emerge among sports participants of the same gender such as Olympic competitors, track and field specialists, wrestlers, and football players; differences also exist among highly proficient adolescent competitors. In this chapter, we take a closer look at the physiques of champion athletes in different sports categories and competition levels.

Different anthropometric methodologies have quantified physique status. Visual appraisal often describes individuals as small, medium, or large, or thin (**ectomorphic**), muscular (**mesomorphic**), or fat (**endomorphic**). This approach, termed **somatotyping**, describes body shape by placing a person into a category such as thin or muscular. Visual appraisal quantifies neither body dimensions (e.g., size of the chest or shoulders nor how biceps development compares with thigh or calf development). While somatotyping offers a valuable adjunct in analyzing physique status of world-class athletes,[6–8,12] and familial heritabilities,[34,44] we focus on the body fat and FFM components of body composition. Our review quantifies aspects of physique for Olympic competitors, endurance runners, collegiate and professional football players, triathletes, high school wrestlers, champion male and female bodybuilders, collegiate gymnasts, and NBA professional basketball players.

PHYSIQUES OF CHAMPION ATHLETES

Early studies of Olympic competitors linked physique to a high level of sports achievement.[12,35] Table 29.1 and Table 29.2 list the anthropometric characteristics of male and female competitors in the 1964 Tokyo and 1968 Mexico City Olympics.[14,21] Bone diameters and stature provided estimates of lean body mass and percentage body fat. Table 29.3 lists anthropometric data for body mass, stature, and eight skinfolds for male and female swimmers, divers, and water polo athletes at the Sixth World Championships in Perth, Australia, 1992.

Also of interest are the body size differences among different groups of athletes within a particular sport. Figure 29.1 *(top)* compares the body mass, stature, chest girth, upper- and lower-limb girths, and leg length for 12 male swimmers rated "best" in the 200- and 400-m free-style with those of less successful counterparts. The bottom figure also compares selected body size variables between the 12 "best" 50-, 100-, and 200-m female breaststroke swimmers with other com-

TABLE 29.1 ➤ AGE, BODY SIZE, AND BODY COMPOSITION OF MALE ATHLETES WHO COMPETED IN SELECTED EVENTS IN THE TOKYO AND MEXICO CITY OLYMPICS

SPECIALTY	EVENT	OLYMPICS	N	AGE (Y)	STATURE (CM)	MASS (KG)	LBM[a] (KG)	BODY FAT[b] (%)
Sprint	100–200 m; 4 × 100 m; 110-m hurdles	Tokyo	172	24.9	178.4	72.2	64.9	10.1
		Mexico City	79	23.9	175.4	68.4	62.8	8.2
Long-distance running	3000, 5000, 10,000 m	Tokyo	99	27.3	173.6	62.4	61.5	1.4
		Mexico City	34	25.3	171.9	59.8	60.1	−0.5[c]
Marathon	42.2 km	Tokyo	74	28.3	170.3	60.8	59.2	2.7
		Mexico City	20	26.4	168.7	56.6	58.1	2.7
Decathlon		Tokyo	26	26.3	183.2	83.5	68.5	18.0
		Mexico City	8	25.1	181.3	77.5	67.1	13.4
Jump	High, long, triple jump	Tokyo	89	25.3	181.5	73.2	67.2	8.2
		Mexico City	14	23.5	182.8	73.2	68.2	6.8
Weight throwing	Shot, discus, hammer	Tokyo	79	27.6	187.3	101.4	71.6	29.4
		Mexico City	9	27.3	186.1	102.3	70.7	30.9
Swimming	Free, breast, back, butterfly, medley	Tokyo	450	20.4	178.7	74.1	65.1	12.1
		Mexico City	66	19.2	179.3	72.1	65.6	9.0
Basketball		Tokyo	186	25.3	189.4	84.3	73.2	13.2
		Mexico City	63	24.0	189.1	79.7	73.0	8.4
Gymnastics	All events	Tokyo	122	26.0	167.2	63.3	57.0	9.9
		Mexico City	28	23.6	167.4	61.5	57.2	7.0
Wrestling	Bantam and featherweight	Tokyo	29	27.3	163.3	62.3	54.4	12.7
		Mexico City	32	22.5	166.1	57.0	56.3	1.2
Rowing	Single and double skulls; pairs, fours, eights	Tokyo	357	25.0	186.0	82.2	70.6	14.1
		Mexico City	85	24.3	185.1	82.6	69.9	15.4

[a]Calculated by Behnke's method: LBM = $h^2 \times 0.204$, where h = stature, dm (see reference 3).
[b]Body fat (%) = (Body mass − LBM)/Body mass × 100.
[c]Error resulting from specific prediction equation as percentage body fat cannot reach a zero or negative value.
Adapted from De Garay, et al. Genetic and anthropological studies of olympic athletes. New York: Academic Press, 1974, and Hirata K. Physique and age of Tokyo Olympic champions. J Sports Med Phys Fitness 1966;6:207.

TABLE 29.2 ➤ AGE, BODY SIZE, AND BODY COMPOSITION OF FEMALE ATHLETES WHO COMPETED IN SELECTED EVENTS IN THE TOKYO AND MEXICO CITY OLYMPICS

SPECIALTY	EVENT	OLYMPICS	N	AGE (Y)	STATURE (CM)	MASS (KG)	LBM[a] (KG)	BODY FAT[b] (%)
Sprint	100–200 m;	Tokyo	85	22.7	166.0	56.6	49.6	12.4
	100-m hurdles	Mexico City	28	20.7	165.0	56.8	49.0	13.7
Jump	High, long,	Tokyo	56	23.6	169.5	60.2	51.7	14.1
	triple jump	Mexico City	12	21.5	169.4	56.4	51.7	8.4
Weight	Shot, discus,	Tokyo	37	26.2	170.4	79.0	52.3	33.8
throwing	hammer	Mexico City	9	19.9	170.9	73.5	52.6	28.5
Swimming	Free, breast, back,	Tokyo	272	18.6	166.3	59.7	49.8	16.6
	butterfly, medley	Mexico City	28	16.3	164.4	56.9	48.6	14.5
Diving	Spring, high	Tokyo	65	18.5	160.9	54.1	46.6	13.9
		Mexico City	7	21.1	160.4	52.3	46.3	11.5
Gymnastics	All events	Tokyo	102	22.7	157.0	52.0	44.4	14.7
		Mexico City	21	17.8	156.9	49.8	44.3	11.0

[a]Calculated by Behnke's method: LBM (lean body mass) = $h^2 \times 0.18$, where h = stature, dm (see reference 3).
[b]Body fat (%) = (Body mass − LBM)/Body mass × 100.
Adapted from De Garay, et al. Genetic and anthropological studies of olympic athletes. New York: Academic Press, 1974, and Hirata K. Physique and age of Tokyo Olympic champions. J Sports Med Phys Fitness 1966;6:207.

TABLE 29.3 ➤ COMPARISON OF BODY MASS, STATURE, AND EIGHT SKINFOLDS IN MALE AND FEMALE SWIMMERS, DIVERS, AND WATER POLO ATHLETES AT THE SIXTH WORLD CHAMPIONSHIPS HELD IN PERTH, AUSTRALIA, 1992

MALES	MASS (KG)	STATURE (CM)	TRI[a]	SCAP	SUPRA	ABD	THI	CALF	BIC	ILIAC
Swimming	78.4	183.8	7.0	7.9	6.3	9.4	9.6	6.5	3.7	9.2
Diving	66.7	170.9	6.8	7.9	6.0	9.6	9.6	6.0	3.8	8.5
Water polo	86.1	186.5	9.2	9.9	8.2	14.9	12.6	7.9	4.3	13.4
FEMALES										
Swimming	63.1	171.5	12.1	8.8	7.3	12.1	19.1	11.4	5.9	9.8
Diving	53.7	161.2	11.4	8.5	6.8	11.1	18.2	9.7	4.9	7.9
Water polo	64.8	171.3	15.3	10.5	9.6	17.6	23.4	13.5	7.1	12.1

[a]Abbreviations for fatfolds (mm): Tri, triceps; Scap, subscapular; Supra, supraspinale; Abd, abdomen; Calf, mid-calf; Bic, biceps; Iliac, iliac crest.
Modified from Mazza JC, et al. Absolute body size. In: Carter JE, Ackland TR, eds. Kinanthropometry in aquatic sports. A study of world class athletes. Human Kinetics Sport Science Monograph Series, vol 5. Champaign, IL: Human Kinetics, 1994.

petitors. Little doubt exists that the best male swimmers are heavier and taller and have larger chest, upper-arm, and thigh girths and upper- and lower-limb lengths than counterparts not ranking among the top 12. The best female breaststroke swimmers, also taller and heavier, possessed larger arm span, foot and arm lengths, and hand and wrist breadths than less successful competitors.

Gender

Table 29.1 indicates that for the men, basketball players, rowers, and weight throwers were tallest and heaviest; they also possessed the largest FFM and percentage body fat. For example, weight throwers in both Olympiads averaged 30% body fat, whereas 94 marathon and 133 long-distance runners averaged an exceptionally low 1.6% body fat. The largest body composition discrepancy within a sports category emerged in comparisons of the Tokyo wrestlers (12.7% body fat) and wrestlers in Mexico City (1.2% body fat). Age, stature, and FFM were similar in both groups, making this difference even more remarkable.

For female Olympians, a relatively low body fat percentage is the most striking physique characteristic. Except for weight throwers (31% body fat), competitors in the other sports groups approximated the 13.1% average body fat for all 676 female participants in both Olympiads.

For aquatic athletes (Table 29.3), skinfolds at most sites were larger in females than in males. As noted in Chapter 10, a swimmer's morphology significantly alters the horizontal components of lift and drag. Selected anthropometric variables influence the magnitude of propulsive and resistive forces that affect the swimmer's forward movement.[9,10] In well-trained freestyle swimmers, arm length, leg length, and hand and foot size—factors governed largely by genetics—significantly in-

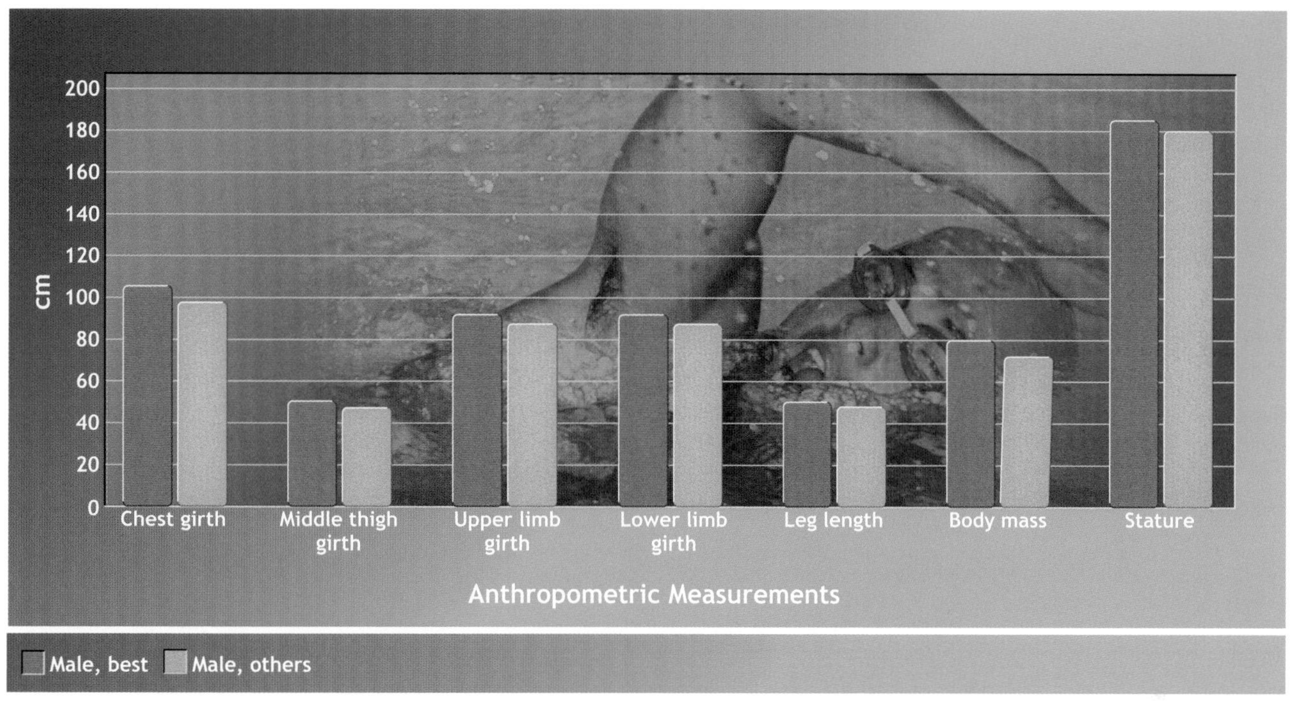

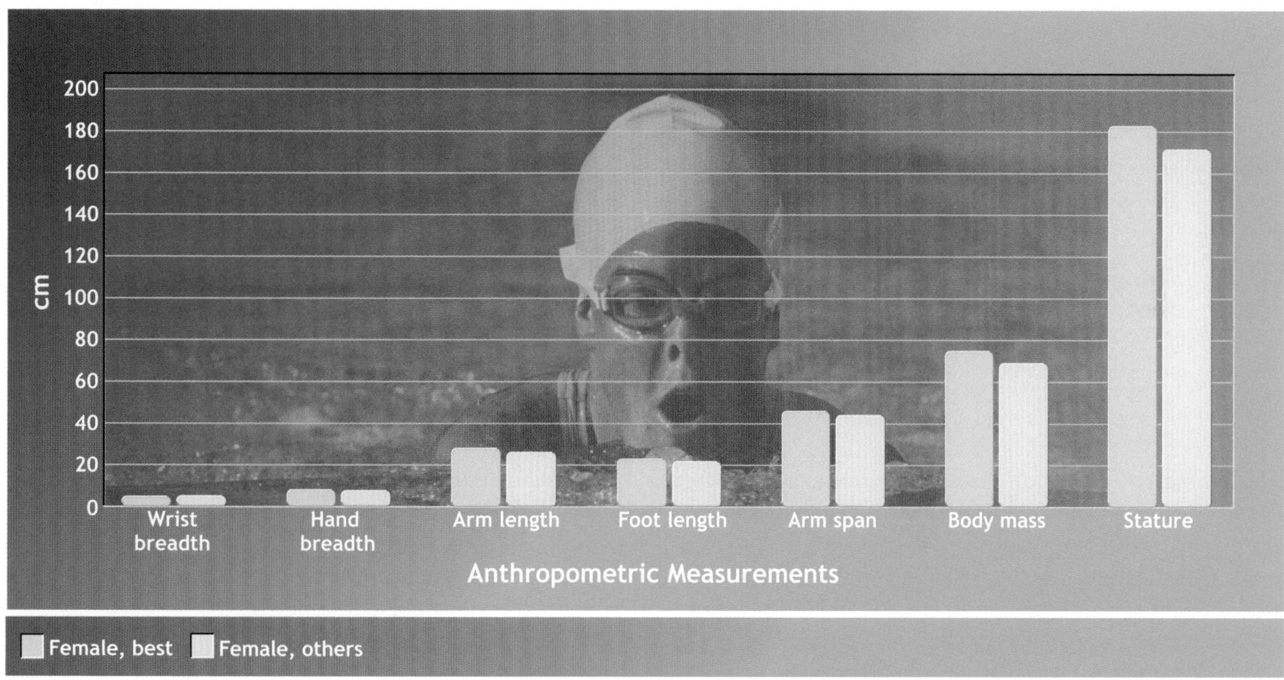

FIGURE 29.1 • *Top.* Comparison of the body mass, stature, chest and limb girths, and leg length of the best (top 12 ranks) 200- and 400-m freestyle male swimmers with those of the remaining competitors. *Bottom.* Comparison of differences in body size variables including arm span (actual values divided by 4) between the best 50-, 100-, and 200-m female breaststroke swimmers (top 12 ranks) and the rest of the competitors. Y-axis in cm for all variables except body mass, which is in kg. (Modified from Mazza JC, et al. Absolute body size. In: Carter JE, Ackland TR, eds. Kinanthropometry in aquatic sports. A study of world- class athletes. Human Kinetics Sport Science Monograph Series, vol 5. Champaign, IL: Human Kinetics, 1994.)

fluence stroke length and stroke frequency.[19] Table 29.4 presents additional anthropometric comparisons between male and female Olympians in five different sports (including swimming) at the 1976 Montreal Summer Olympics.

Fat-Free-to-Fat Ratio

Figure 29.2 compares the ratio of FFM to fat mass (FM), derived from data in the world literature for the specific sport, among male and female competitors. The *inset tables* present

TABLE 29.4 ➤ SELECTED ANTHROPOMETRIC MEASUREMENTS IN MALES AND FEMALES WHO COMPETED IN FIVE DIFFERENT SPORTS AT THE MONTREAL OLYMPIC GAMES

	CANOE		GYMNASTICS		ROWING		SWIMMING		TRACK	
MEASUREMENT[a]	M	F	M	F	M	F	M	F	M	F
Stature	185.4	170.7	169.3	161.5	191.3	174.3	178.6	166.9	179.1	168.5
Upper extremity L	82.4	76.0	76.0	72.2	85.2	76.0	80.2	74.7	80.9	74.8
Lower extremity L	88.0	81.8	78.9	76.5	91.7	82.3	84.1	78.1	86.9	80.3
Biacromial D	41.4	36.8	39.0	35.9	42.5	37.4	40.8	37.1	40.2	36.3
Biiliac D	28.1	27.3	25.8	25.0	30.2	28.2	27.9	26.7	27.1	27.2
Arm relaxed G	32.2	27.6	30.7	24.3	31.7	27.6	30.6	27.3	29.1	24.5
Arm flexed G	35.3	29.6	33.9	25.9	34.9	29.3	33.3	28.2	32.2	26.4
Forearm G	29.3	25.4	27.5	23.2	30.3	25.5	27.4	23.9	27.9	23.3
Chest G	102.6	88.9	95.1	83.5	103.7	89.6	98.6	88.0	94.3	83.8
Waist G	80.6	69.8	72.8	63.2	84.0	70.8	79.3	69.4	77.7	67.4
Thigh G	54.6	54.0	51.0	49.9	60.2	57.5	55.4	52.8	56.0	53.9
Calf G	37.5	34.9	34.7	33.3	39.3	37.0	36.9	34.0	37.6	34.9

[a]L, length; D, diameter; G, girth; all values are in centimeters.
Adapted from Carter JE, et al. Anthropometry of Montreal Olympic athletes. In: Carter JEL, ed. Physical structure of Olympic athletes. Part 1: The Montreal Olympic Games Anthropological Project. Basal: Karger, 1982.

data for average body mass, percentage body fat, and FFM. Male marathon runners and gymnasts have the largest FFM:FM, while American football offensive and defensive linemen and shot putters show the smallest ratios. Among females, bodybuilders have the largest FFM:FM values (equal to those of males), while the smallest FFM:FMs emerge for field-event participants. Surprisingly, female gymnasts and ballet dancers rank intermediate compared with other female sport participants.

World Records

Figure 29.3 compares world records for males and females through 1991 and comparative data for 2000 for maximum running speed at distances between 100 m and 10,000 m. Essentially, the percentage difference in performance between genders remained invariate over the 9-year interval. The percentage gender difference averages about 10% for all running events, including the 400-m hurdles and 400-m to 3200-m relay races (*top right inset figure*). The *lower left inset figure* shows that gender differences in world record times (expressed as maximum running speed [$m \cdot s^{-1}$]) remain remarkably similar for 100-m through 10,000-m events. Males achieve identical running speeds for 100 and 200 m; speed then declines steadily for both genders as distance increases. For example, the percentage decline between 100 m and 800 m equals 29% for men and 35% for women. A lesser rate of decline in running speed occurs over the longer distances, with the cumulative decrement in maximum speed between 800 and 10,000 m averaging 28% for men and women.

Among weight lifters (*top left inset figure*) in the same body-weight category, women in the 56-kg weight class achieve 82.0% of the men's best performance; thereafter, the percentage difference increases at the higher body-weight categories. In field events (not listed), the percentage of the men's best performance achieved by the women is as follows: long jump, 84.0%; high jump, 83.3%; javelin throw, 82.5%; and triple jump, 83.2%.

Figure 29.4 shows further comparisons in world record performances between males and females for swimming, speed skating, and cycling. In the 400-, 800-, and 1500-m freestyle swims, females achieve times closer to those of males (94% of best male times) than in the shorter distances (90.7%). The percentage differences remain about the same in speed skating and middle-distance swimming events in 400- through 1500-m distances; in cycling from 1 km to 100 km, females achieve only 87% of males' best times.

A reasonable question is whether continued improvement in training methods and performance techniques can overcome the apparent gender limits to maximal performance, particularly in events that require exceptional muscular strength/power and anaerobic capacity. *If gender equality in sports performance does emerge, it may occur first in a middle-distance swimming event.*

GEOGRAPHIC REGION. Figure 29.5 shows gender differences in six running and two field events from five world geographic regions, including comparisons with world and Olympic records through March 2000. As in Figure 29.3, the percentage difference reflects the woman's record relative to the record for men. This remarkable data set reveals that existing gender differences in world and Olympic competition persist fairly uniformly across geographic regions. Notable deviation from all other contrasts occurs in the 800-m run for the Nordic region (84.7%). In general, more-pronounced sex differences exist in South American records than in world and Olympic records.

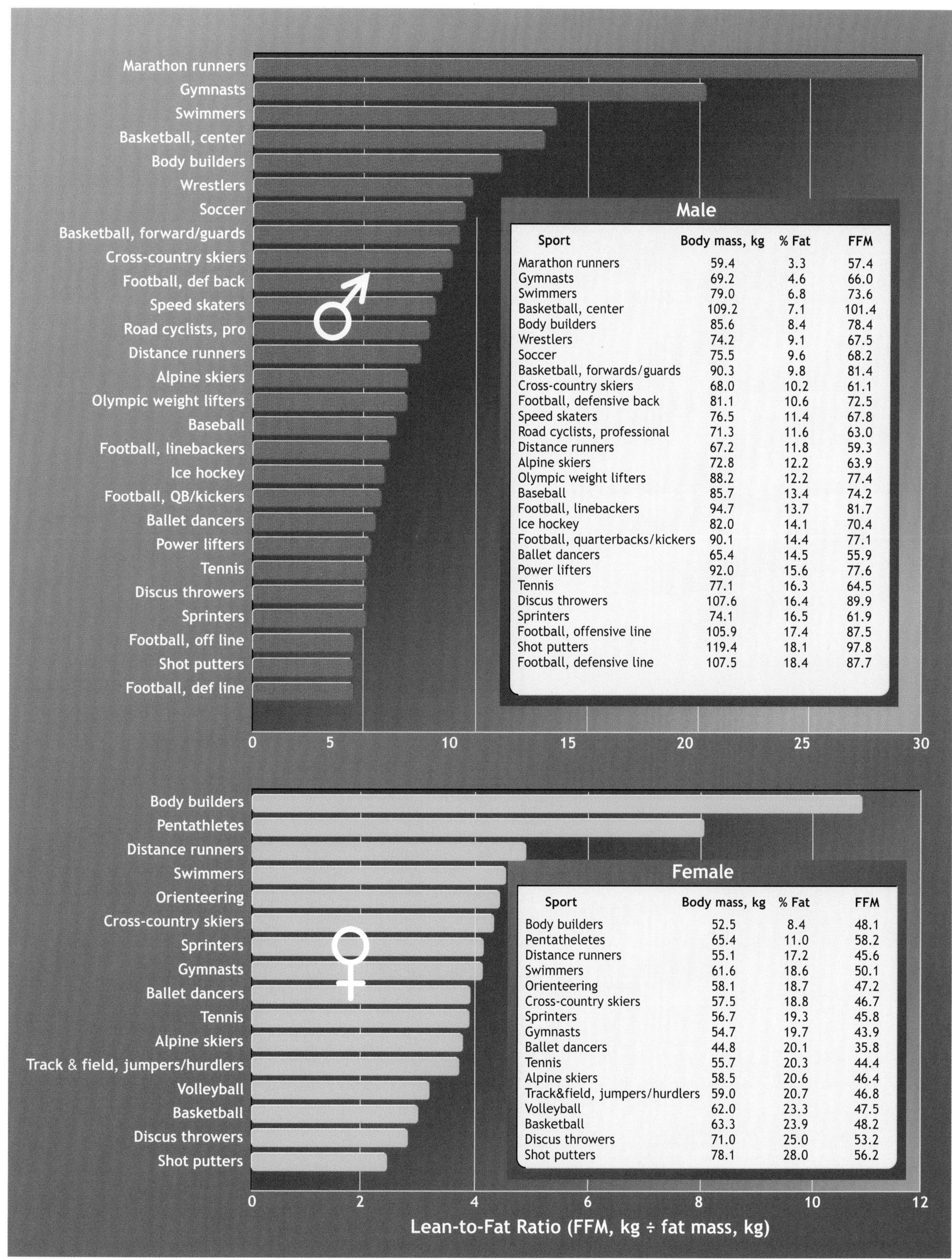

Male

Sport	Body mass, kg	% Fat	FFM
Marathon runners	59.4	3.3	57.4
Gymnasts	69.2	4.6	66.0
Swimmers	79.0	6.8	73.6
Basketball, center	109.2	7.1	101.4
Body builders	85.6	8.4	78.4
Wrestlers	74.2	9.1	67.5
Soccer	75.5	9.6	68.2
Basketball, forwards/guards	90.3	9.8	81.4
Cross-country skiers	68.0	10.2	61.1
Football, defensive back	81.1	10.6	72.5
Speed skaters	76.5	11.4	67.8
Road cyclists, professional	71.3	11.6	63.0
Distance runners	67.2	11.8	59.3
Alpine skiers	72.8	12.2	63.9
Olympic weight lifters	88.2	12.2	77.4
Baseball	85.7	13.4	74.2
Football, linebackers	94.7	13.7	81.7
Ice hockey	82.0	14.1	70.4
Football, quarterbacks/kickers	90.1	14.4	77.1
Ballet dancers	65.4	14.5	55.9
Power lifters	92.0	15.6	77.6
Tennis	77.1	16.3	64.5
Discus throwers	107.6	16.4	89.9
Sprinters	74.1	16.5	61.9
Football, offensive line	105.9	17.4	87.5
Shot putters	119.4	18.1	97.8
Football, defensive line	107.5	18.4	87.7

Female

Sport	Body mass, kg	% Fat	FFM
Body builders	52.5	8.4	48.1
Pentatheletes	65.4	11.0	58.2
Distance runners	55.1	17.2	45.6
Swimmers	61.6	18.6	50.1
Orienteering	58.1	18.7	47.2
Cross-country skiers	57.5	18.8	46.7
Sprinters	56.7	19.3	45.8
Gymnasts	54.7	19.7	43.9
Ballet dancers	44.8	20.1	35.8
Tennis	55.7	20.3	44.4
Alpine skiers	58.5	20.6	46.4
Track&field, jumpers/hurdlers	59.0	20.7	46.8
Volleyball	62.0	23.3	47.5
Basketball	63.3	23.9	48.2
Discus throwers	71.0	25.0	53.2
Shot putters	78.1	28.0	56.2

FIGURE 29.2 • Comparison of the lean:fat ratios among male and female competitors in diverse sports. Values are based on the average body mass and percentage body fat for each sport from various studies in the literature. The lean:fat ratio is FFM (kg) ÷ fat mass (kg). The values in the *inset tables* represent averages for body composition if the literature contained two or more citations about a specific sport. The equation of Siri (Chapter 28) converted body density to percentage body fat.

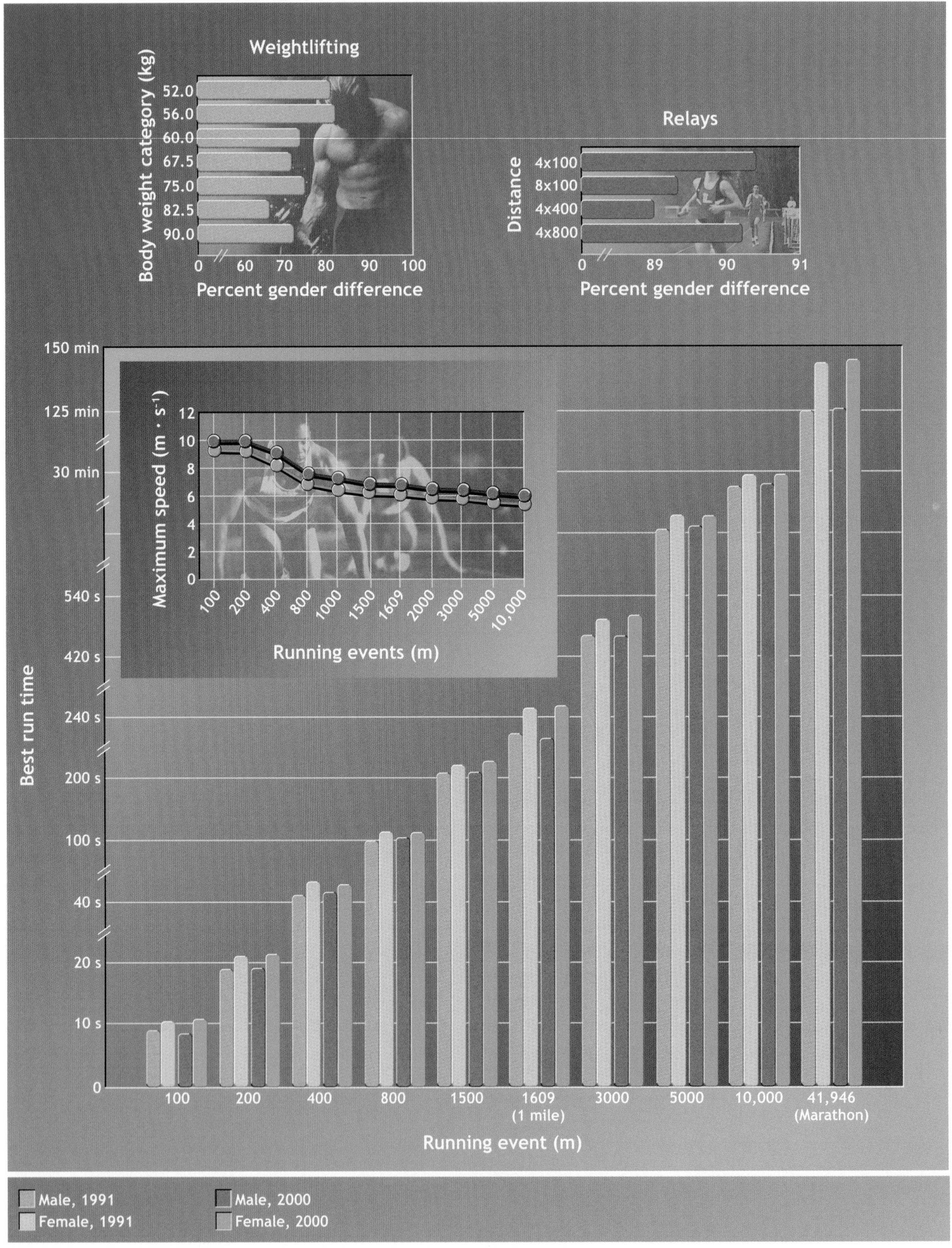

FIGURE 29.3 • *Main figure.* World records at 1991 and 9 years later in 2000 in various running events for males and females, from 100 m to the marathon. Considering all events in the 1991 and 2000 data sets, women achieved between 88 and 94% of the performance of men. The *top left inset* shows percentage differences between genders (% of male values achieved by females) for total weight lifted in the snatch and clean and jerk for six weight classifications. The *top right inset* displays percentage differences in four common relay events. The *lower inset* expresses the gender differences in world record times as maximum running speed ($m \cdot s^{-1}$) for 100 m through 10,000 m. (Weight-lifting data from the International Powerlifting Federation [www.ipf.com]).

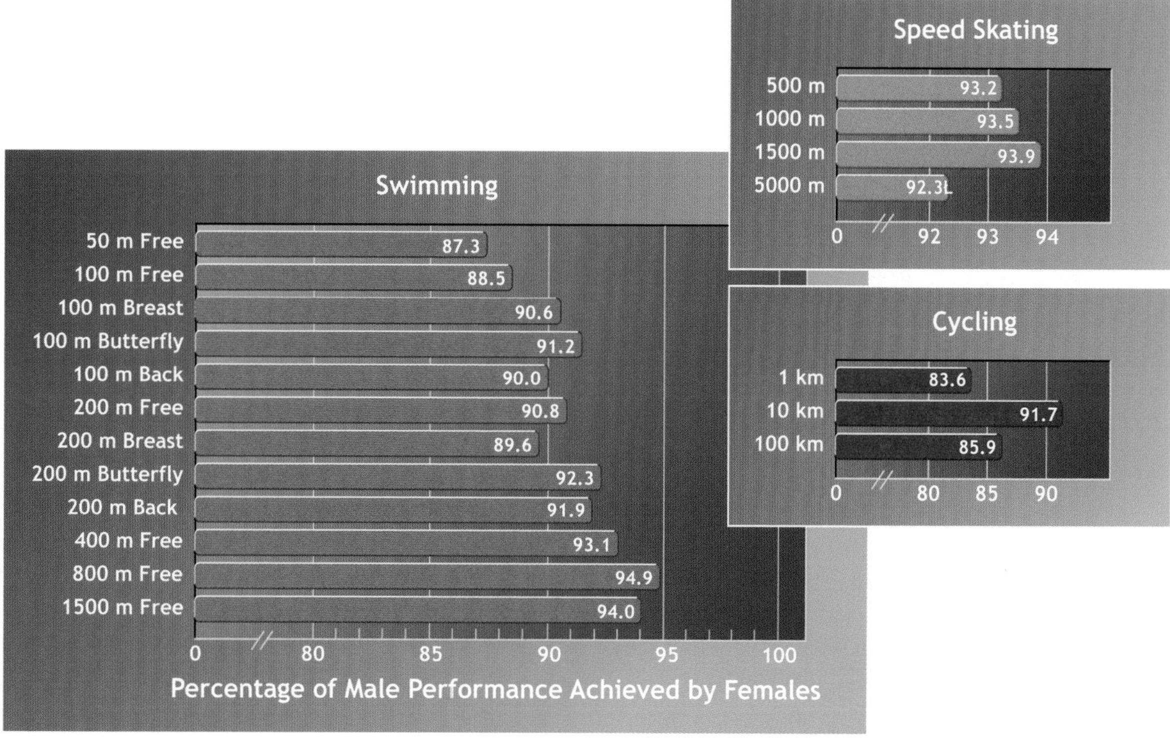

FIGURE 29.4 • Gender differences in swimming, speed skating, and cycling world record performances through June 1, 2000.

Racial Differences

Racial differences in physique may significantly affect athletic performance.[51] Black sprinters and high jumpers, for example, have longer limbs and narrower hips than white counterparts. From a mechanical perspective, a black sprinter with leg and arm size identical to that of a white sprinter would have a lighter, shorter, and slimmer body to propel. This might confer a more favorable power:body mass ratio at any given body size. Greater power output provides an advantage in jumping and sprint running events, in which generating rapid energy

Gender Differences (%) in "Best" Performance by World Geographic Region

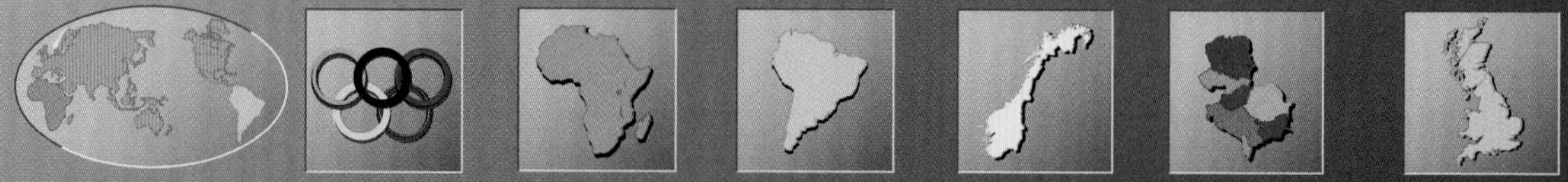

Event	World record	Olympic record	African record	SouthAmerican record	Nordic record	Balkan record	Commonwealth record
100 m	93.3	92.7	89.9	89.2	90.6	93.4	91.6
200 m	90.5	90.5	88.2	87.9	90.1	91.8	90.9
400 m	90.7	90.1	90.0	90.6	90.5	90.1	90.8
800 m	89.3	90.0	88.8	87.2	84.7	91.0	87.5
1500 m	89.4	90.8	88.1	87.4	87.8	91.5	87.4
5000 m	88.3	84.3	85.9	86.7	90.8	91.0	86.5
High jump	85.3	85.8	85.5	84.1	83.1	87.1	83.2
Long jump	84.0	83.1	86.1	81.2	84.8	87.9	81.7

FIGURE 29.5 • Gender differences (% of male values achieved by females) in eight outdoor track performance grouped by five world regions, including world records and Olympic performances through June 1, 2000.

for short durations is crucial to success. The advantage diminishes somewhat in the various throwing events. Compared with whites and blacks, Asian athletes have short legs relative to upper torso components, a dimensional characteristic beneficial in short and longer distance races and in weight lifting. In fact, successful weight lifters of all races (compared with other athletic groups) have relatively short arms and legs for their stature.

Percentage Body Fat of Elite Athletes

Considerable literature describes body fat levels of male and female competitive athletes in diverse sports.

By Category

Figure 29.6 presents six classifications of sports activities based on common characteristics and performance requirements, with percentage body fat rankings within each category for male and female competitors (where applicable). This provides an overview of percentage body fat of athletes within a broad grouping of relatively similar sports.

Field Event Athletes

Figure 29.7 shows body composition obtained by hydrostatic weighing and anthropometry—percentage body fat, fat weight, FFM, and lean:fat ratio—for the 10 top American athletes in the discus, shot put, javelin, and hammer throw 2 years before the 1980 Moscow Olympics. For comparison, data describe international elite middle- and long-distance runners (average treadmill $\dot{V}O_{2max} = 76.9$ mL · kg^{-1} · min^{-1}) and Behnke's reference man. Table 29.5 lists the corresponding data for girth and skinfold anthropometry. Shot-putters clearly possessed the largest overall body size (body mass and girths), followed by athletes in the discus, hammer, and javelin throw.

Female Endurance Athletes

Table 29.6 presents data for body mass, stature, and body composition of 11 female long-distance runners of national and international caliber.[59] The runners averaged 15.2% body fat (hydrostatic weighing), similar to reported data for high school cross-country runners[3] but considerably lower than the 26% body fat reported for sedentary females of the same age, stature, and body mass.[30] Compared with other athletic groups, the runners have relatively less fat than collegiate basketball players (20.9%),[49] gymnasts (15.5%),[50] younger distance runners (18%),[35] swimmers (20.1%),[32] or tennis players (22.8%).[32]

Interestingly, the runners' average body fat equaled the 15% value generally reported for nonathletic males. The 6 to 9% body fat of several apparently healthy runners in Table 29.6 falls within the range reported for topflight male endurance athletes. The leanest women in the population, based on Behnke's reference standards, have essential fat equal to 12 to 14% of body mass. This apparent discrepancy between

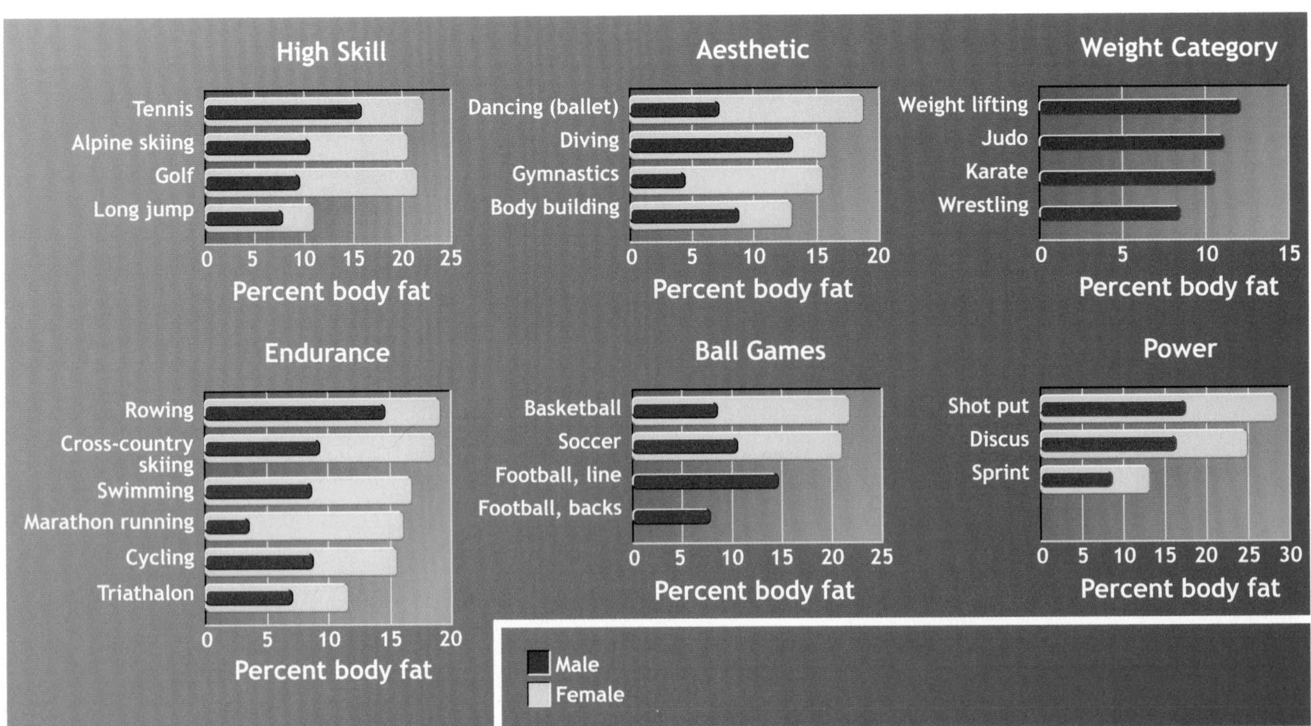

FIGURE 29.6 • Percentage body fat in athletes grouped by sport category. The value for males is displayed within the *bar* (*in red*) when a corresponding value exists for females (*yellow*). The values for percentage body fat (from body density by the Siri equation) represent averages from the literature.

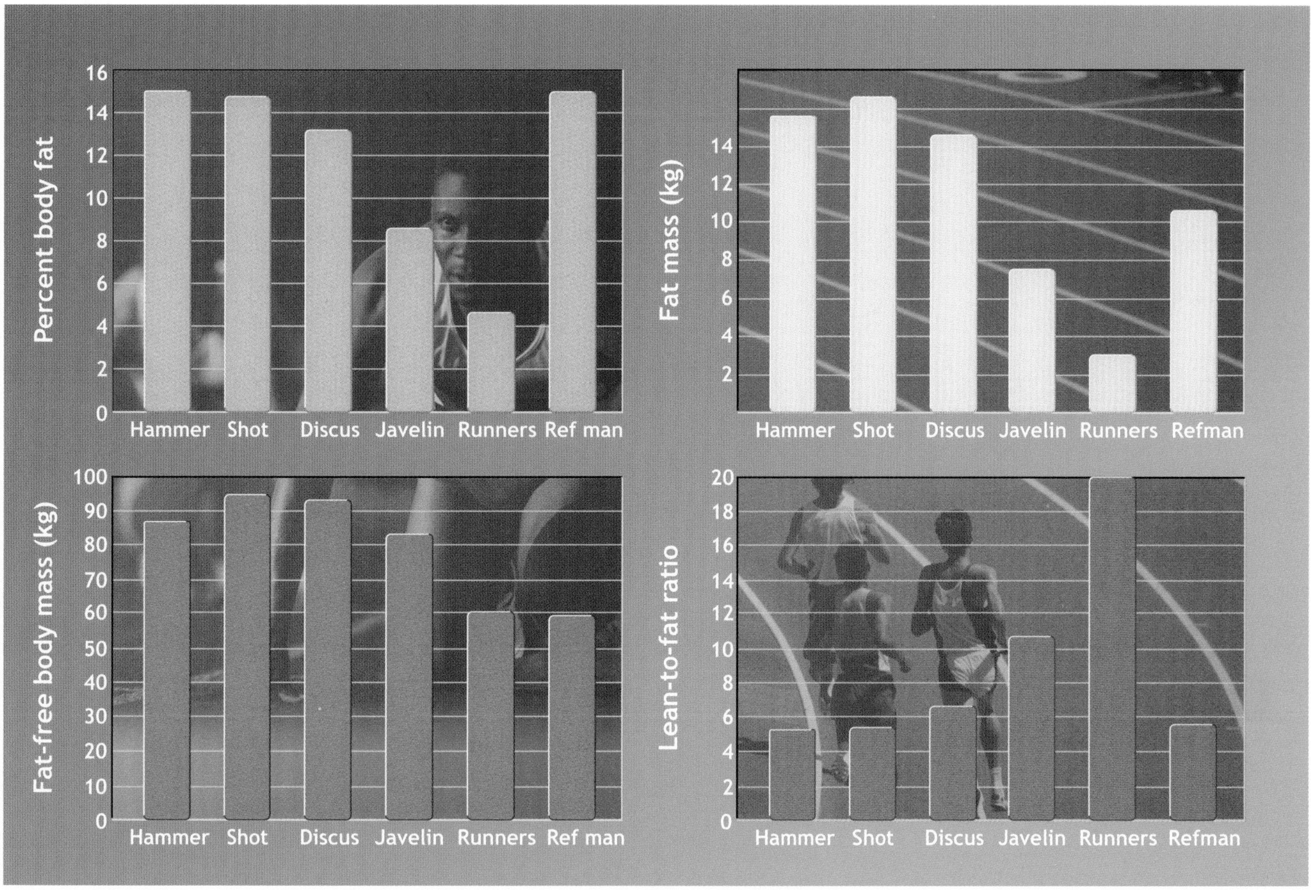

FIGURE 29.7 • Body composition (determined by hydrostatic weighing) of the 10 top American male athletes in the discus, shot put, javelin, and hammer throw. Data collected by two of the authors (FK and VK) at a 1978 U.S. Olympic minicamp at the University of Houston, Houston, TX. Athletes include former gold medalist Wilkins (discus) and world record holder Powell (discus). Data for the international elite middle- and long-distance runners from Pollock ML, et al. Body composition of elite class distance runners. Ann NY Acad Sci 1977;301:361. Reference man *(Ref. man)* data from Behnke's model in Chapter 28.

estimated fat content of distance runners and the theoretical lower limit for body fat in women requires further study. Note the relatively high body fat (35.4%) of one of the best runners; clearly, other factors must override limitations to distance running imposed by excess fat.

Male Endurance Athletes

Table 29.7 presents body composition data for 11 male elite middle- and long-distance runners and 8 elite marathoners. The group included Steve Prefontaine, former American record holder in the 800- and 1500-m runs, and Frank Shorter, the 1976 Olympic gold medalist in the marathon. A representative sample of 95 untrained college-aged men provides comparison data.

Both groups of runners maintain extremely low body fat values, considering that essential fat theoretically constitutes about 3% of body mass. Clearly, these competitors represent the lower end of the lean-to-fat continuum for topflight athletes. This physique characteristic most likely influences success in distance running. This makes sense for several reasons. First, effective heat dissipation during running maintains thermal balance—excess fat thwarts heat dissipation. Second, excess body fat is "dead weight"; it adds directly to exercise energy cost without providing propulsive energy.

For body dimensions and structure, male distance runners generally have smaller girths and bone diameters than untrained males.[12] Structural differences, particularly bone diameters, reflect a genetic influence similar to the distinct anthropometric characteristics of aquatic athletes (see Fig. 29.1). The best long-distance runners inherit a slight build, not only in stature but also in skeletal dimensions. Blending a genetically optimal physique profile with a lean body composition, a highly developed aerobic system, and proper psychologic attitude for prolonged, intensive training, provides the prime ingredients for a champion.

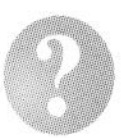

INTEGRATIVE QUESTION

Discuss the physiologic and anthropometric characteristics necessary for successful endurance running performance.

TABLE 29.5 ➤ SKINFOLD AND GIRTH ANTHROPOMETRY OF THE TOP 10 AMERICAN ATHLETES IN THE DISCUS, SHOT PUT, JAVELIN, AND HAMMER THROW

MEASUREMENT[a]	DISCUS	SHOT PUT	JAVELIN	HAMMER	RUNNERS	REF MAN
Body mass, kg	108.2	112.3	90.6	104.2	63.1	70.0
Stature, cm	191.7	187.0	186.0	187.3	177.0	174.0
Skinfolds, mm						
Triceps	13.0	15.0	11.9	12.7	5.0	—
Scapular	18.0	23.8	12.5	21.5	6.4	—
Iliac	24.5	29.6	17.0	27.4	4.6	—
Abdomen	25.6	31.4	18.4	29.1	7.1	—
Thigh	16.4	15.7	13.3	17.3	6.1	—
Girths, cm						
Shoulders	129.8	133.3	121.5	127.4	106.1	110.8
Chest	113.5	118.5	104.6	111.3	91.1	91.8
Waist	94.1	99.1	86.6	94.8	74.6	77.0
Abdomen	97.5	101.5	87.8	98.0	74.2	79.8
Hips	110.4	112.3	102.0	108.7	87.8	93.4
Thighs	66.3	69.4	61.5	67.3	51.9	54.8
Knees	41.5	42.9	40.0	41.0	36.2[b]	36.6
Calves	42.6	43.6	39.5	41.5	35.4	35.8
Ankles	25.4	24.9	24.1	24.3	21.0	22.5
Biceps	41.8	42.2	37.7	39.9	28.2	31.7
Forearms	33.1	33.7	30.8	32.4	26.4	26.4
Wrists	18.7	18.9	18.2	18.4	16.0	17.3
Diameters, cm						
Biacromial	44.5	43.8	43.2	44.8	39.5	40.6
Chest	33.1	33.7	30.8	32.6	31.3	30.0
Bi-iliac	31.3	31.2	29.6	30.4	28.0	28.6
Bitrochanter	35.5	34.9	33.7	34.8	32.2	32.8
Knee	10.2	10.5	10.0	10.2	9.5	9.3
Wrist	6.3	6.2	6.0	6.2	5.6	5.6
Ankle	7.6	7.6	7.5	7.4	—	7.0
Elbow	7.6	7.6	7.6	7.2	—	7.0

[a]Details about measurement procedures from Katch FI, Katch VL. The body composition profile: techniques of measurement and applications. Clin Sports Med, 1984;3:31. Data correspond to the athletic groups presented in Fig. 29.7.
[b]Not measured; value computed from the ratio for the reference man calf to knee.

TABLE 29.6 ➤ BODY COMPOSITION OF FEMALE ENDURANCE RUNNERS

SUBJECTS	AGE (Y)	STATURE (CM)	MASS (KG)	FFM (KG)	BODY FAT (KG)	BODY FAT (%)
1[a]	24	172.7	52.6	49.5	3.1	5.9
2[b]	26	159.8	71.5	46.2	25.3	35.4
3[c]	28	162.6	50.7	47.6	3.1	6.1
4	31	171.5	52.0	47.3	4.7	9.0
5	33	176.5	61.2	50.8	10.4	17.0
6	34	166.4	52.9	44.8	8.1	15.2
7	35	168.4	55.0	48.7	6.3	11.6
8	36	164.5	53.1	44.3	8.8	16.6
9	36	182.9	61.5	50.4	11.1	18.1
10	36	182.9	65.4	55.7	9.7	14.8
11	37	154.9	53.6	44.0	9.6	18.0
Average	32.4	169.4	57.2	48.1	9.1	15.2

[a]World's best time in marathon (2:49:40) as of 1974.
[b]World's best time in 50-mile run (7:04:31); established 18 months after the body composition evaluation.
[c]Noted U.S. distance runner. Five consecutive national and international cross-country championships.
From Wilmore JH, Brown CH. Physiological profiles of women distance runners. Med Sci Sports 1974;6:178.

Triathletes

The triathlon combines continuous endurance performance in swimming, bicycling, and running. The extreme of triathlon requirements, the ultraendurance Ironman competition, requires competitors to swim 3.9 km (2.4 mi), bicycle 180.2 km (112 mi), and run a standard 42.2-km (26.2-mi) marathon. The course records for the Ironman triathlon in Kailuja-Kona, Hawaii, stand at 8:04:08 for men (1996) and only a 10.6% slower time of 8:55:28 (1992) for women. The serious triathlete's training averages nearly 4 hours daily, covering a total of 280 miles per week by swimming 7.2 miles (30:00 min per mi pace), bicycling 227 miles (18.6 mph), and running 45 miles (7:42 min per mi pace).[22] Percentage body fat of six male and three female participants in the 1982 Ironman triathlon ranged between 5.0 and 11.3% for men and 7.4 and 17.2% for women. Body fat averaged 7.1% for the top 15 male finishers, with corresponding $\dot{V}O_{2max}$ values of 72.0 mL $\cdot$ kg^{-1} $\cdot$ min^{-1}. Triathletes have body fat content and aerobic capacity comparable to those of other athletes in single endurance sports,[43] with an overall physique most closely resembling that of elite cyclists[42] or swimmers[38] rather than elite

TABLE 29.7 ➤ **BODY COMPOSITION CHARACTERISTICS OF ELITE MALE MIDDLE- AND LONG-DISTANCE RUNNERS AND ELITE MARATHONERS**

Group	Stature (cm)	Mass (kg)	Density ($g \cdot cm^{-3}$)	Body Fat (%)	FFM (kg)	Fat Mass (kg)	Sum 7 Skinfolds (mm)
Distance runners							
Brown	187.3	72.10	1.07428	10.8	64.31	7.79	53.0
Castaneda	178.6	63.34	1.09102	3.7	61.00	2.34	32.5
Crawford	171.8	58.01	1.09702	1.2	57.31	0.70	32.5
Geis	179.1	66.28	1.07551	10.2	59.52	6.76	49.0
Johnson	174.6	61.79	1.08963	4.3	59.13	2.66	35.5
Manley	177.8	69.10	1.09642	1.5	68.06	1.04	32.0
Ndoo	169.3	53.97	1.08379	6.7	50.35	3.62	33.5
Prefontaine	174.2	68.00	1.08842	4.8	64.74	3.26	38.0
Rose	175.6	59.15	1.08248	7.3	54.83	4.32	31.5
Tuttle	176.8	61.44	1.09960	0.2	61.32	0.12	31.5
Mean	170.5	60.92	1.08916	4.5	58.18	2.74	34.5
(standard deviation)	(5.0)	(5.30)	(0.00832)	(3.5)	(4.90)	(2.38)	(7.4)
Marathon runners							
Cusack	174.6	64.19	1.08096	7.9	59.12	5.07	45.5
Galloway	180.9	65.76	1.08419	6.6	61.42	4.34	43.0
Kennedy	167.0	56.52	1.09348	2.7	54.99	1.53	37.0
Moore	184.1	64.24	1.09193	3.3	62.12	2.12	37.0
Pate[a]	179.6	57.28	1.09676	1.3	56.54	0.74	32.5
Shorter	178.4	61.17	1.09475	2.2	59.82	1.35	45.0
Wayne	172.1	61.61	1.07859	8.9	56.13	5.48	42.5
Williams	177.2	66.07	1.09569	1.8	64.88	1.19	41.5
Mean	176.8	62.11	1.08954	4.3	59.38	2.73	40.5
(standard deviation)	(5.6)	(3.66)	(0.00718)	(3.0)	(3.38)	(1.92)	(4.6)

[a]Dr. Russel Pate is an exercise physiologist, Department of Exercise Science, University of South Carolina, Columbia, SC.
Data from Pollock ML, et al. Body composition of elite class distance runners. Ann NY Acad Sci 1977;301:361.

runners. Male triathletes possess aerobic capacities similar to those of trained swimmers; $\dot{V}O_{2max}$ values for females cluster at the upper range for endurance runners. Aerobic capacity of these athletes during swimming consistently averages below values during treadmill running or stationary cycling.[36]

Swimmers Versus Runners

Male and female competitive swimmers generally have higher body fat levels than distance runners. Speculation suggests that the cool water of the training environment produces lower core temperatures than with equivalent land exercise. A lower core temperature may prevent the decreased appetite that often accompanies heavy training on land, despite swim training's significant energy requirement.

Limited evidence indicates similar daily energy intake for male collegiate swimmers (3380 kcal) and distance runners (3460 kcal), which balances training energy expenditure. In contrast, female swimmers averaged a higher daily energy intake of 2490 kcal, compared with 2040 kcal for their running counterparts.[29] However, the swimmers had a higher estimated daily energy expenditure than the runners. The swimmers' energy expenditure even surpassed energy intake, placing them in a slightly *negative* energy balance. Thus, a positive energy balance (intake greater than output) does not explain typically higher body fat levels in male (12%) and female (20%) swimmers than in male (7%) and female (15%) runners. Subsequent research from the same laboratory evaluated energy expenditure and fuel use for swimmers and runners during each form of training (45 min at 75–80% $\dot{V}O_{2max}$) and 2 hours recovery.[16] The hypothesis was that differences in hormonal response and substrate catabolism between the two exercise modes accounted for body fat differences between groups. However, the results indicated that the small between-group differences in energy expenditure, substrate use, and hormone levels could *not* account for body fat differences.

Future research must determine whether real differences in physiologic response to land and water training account for body composition differences between swimmers and runners. An alternative explanation suggests that self-selection causes individuals with higher body fat levels to compete in swimming. Excess body fat presents a liability to energy cost and thermoregulation during weight-bearing exercise on land, yet it contributes importantly to buoyancy and perhaps hydrodynamic economy to forward swimming movement from reduced drag forces.

American Football Players

The first detailed body composition analyses of American professional football players in the early 1940s clearly demonstrated the inadequacy of determining a person's optimal body mass from height–weight standards (see "Focus on Research," Chapter 28)[57] The players as a group had a body fat content that averaged only 10.4% of body mass, while FFM averaged

Focus on Research

Body Composition Analysis By Dissection

Clarys JP, et al. Gross tissue weights in the human body by cadaver dissection. Hum Biol 1984;56:459.

➤ Chemical and anatomic dissection procedures provide two *direct* methods to study human body composition. The chemical method quantifies body water, lipid, protein, and various mineral elements in different tissues and the whole body. Anatomic dissection partitions the body into components, including skin, muscle, adipose tissue, bone, and whole organs. Since 1940, the body composition literature reveals only eight complete analyses of adult humans, with only three done by chemical methods.

Until the research of Clarys and colleagues, no comparisons existed between indirect (body density assessment) and direct dissection assessment of body composition. These researchers used anthropometry, radiography, photogrammetry, densitometry, and complete anatomic dissection of 25 cadavers to determine the gross tissue mass of skin, adipose tissue, muscle, bone, and vital organs (see figure). The cadavers ranged in age from 55 to 94 years and included 12 embalmed (6 male, 6 female) and 13 nonembalmed (6 male, 7 female) whites. For each cadaver, analysis included removing skeletal muscle and other major organs (brain, heart, lungs, liver, kidneys, and spleen). Bones were then separated at their articulations and scraped to leave surfaces free of muscle and adipose tissue. Muscle included the ligaments, and bone retained the cartilage of any articular surface. Airtight plastic buckets stored all dissected tissues, including scrapings. The tissues were weighed to within 0.1 g and their densities determined. Complete cadaver dissection took approximately 15 hours and required a team of 10 to 12 anatomists and kinesiologists.

The figure shows an average adipose tissue mass of 40.5% of total body mass in females and 28.1% in males. The researchers introduced the concept of adipose tissue-free weight (ATFW)—the whole-body mass minus the mass of all dissectible adipose tissue (adipose tissue contains about 83% pure fat). Muscle accounted for 52% of the ATFW in males and 48.1% in females, while bone constituted 19.9% of ATFW in males and 21.3% in females. Combining the data for males and females, the average proportion of the ATFW included 8.5% skin, 50.0% muscle, and 20.6% bone.

Densitometry to estimate the fat and fat-free mass (FFM) assumes a constant density for the FFM. This in turn requires that the proportions of the FFM components—fat-free muscle, fat-free adipose tissue, fat-free bone, and other fat-free tissues—remain unchanged from one person to another, including the densities for each tissue. Although Clarys' research did not include measures of whole-body fat, considerable variation existed in the ATFW. The extent of the variation challenges the important assumption of a constant density for the body's FFM when using hydrostatic weighing to assess body fat.

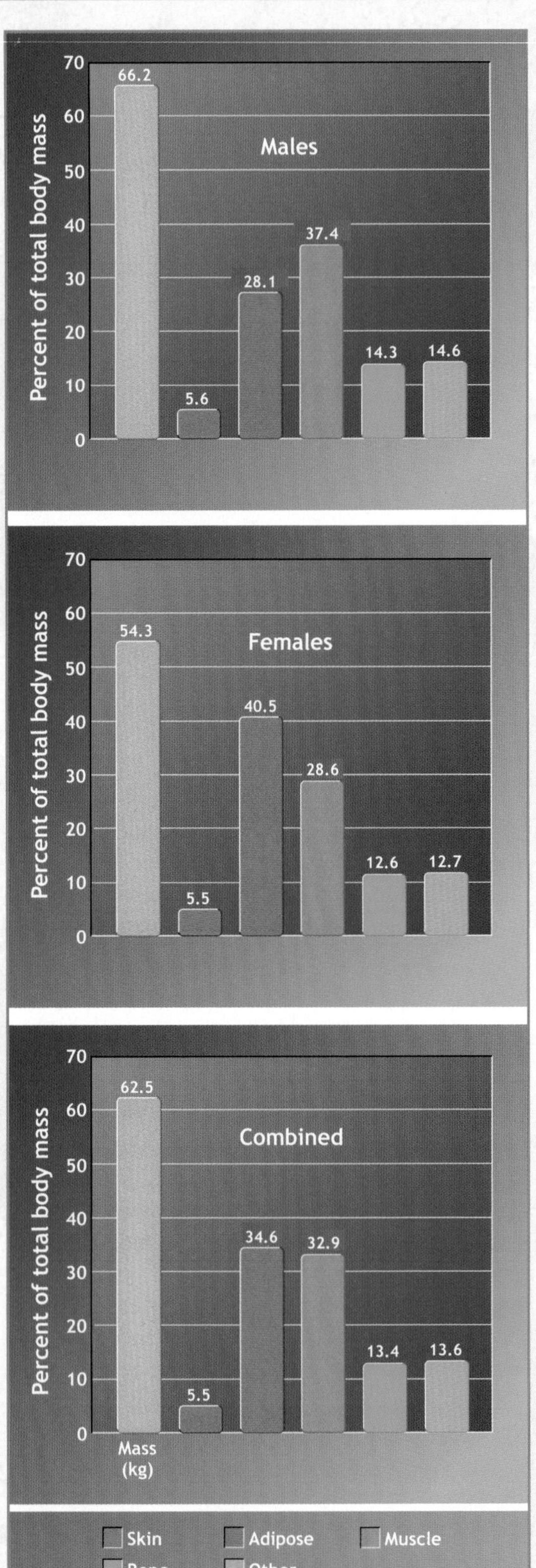

Various tissues in the adult human body expressed as a percentage of total body mass. Body mass in kg.

TABLE 29.8 ➤ BODY COMPOSITIONS OF COLLEGIATE AND PROFESSIONAL FOOTBALL PLAYERS GROUPED BY POSITION

POSITION[a]	LEVEL	N	STATURE (CM)	MASS (KG)	BODY FAT (%)	FFM (KG)
Defensive backs	St. Cloud[b]	15	178.3	77.3	11.5	68.4
	U Mass[c]	12	179.9	83.1	8.8	76.8
	USC[d]	15	183.0	83.7	9.6	75.7
	Gettysburg[e]	16	175.9	79.8	13.6	68.9
	Pro, modern[f]	26	182.5	84.8	9.6	76.7
	Pro, older[f]	25	183.0	91.2	10.7	81.4
Offensive backs and receivers	St. Cloud	15	179.7	79.8	12.4	69.6
	U Mass	29	181.8	84.1	9.5	76.4
	USC	18	185.6	86.1	9.9	77.6
	Gettysburg	18	176.0	78.3	12.9	68.2
	Pro, modern	40	183.8	90.7	9.4	81.9
	Pro, older	25	183.0	91.7	10.0	87.5
Linebackers	St. Cloud	7	180.1	87.2	13.4	75.4
	U Mass	17	186.1	97.1	13.1	84.2
	USC	17	185.6	98.8	13.2	85.8
	Gettysburg	—	—	—	—	—
	Pro, modern	28	188.6	102.2	14.0	87.6
Offensive linemen and tight ends	St. Cloud	13	186.0	99.2	19.1	79.8
	U Mass	23	187.5	107.6	19.5	86.6
	Gettysburg	15	182.6	110.4	26.2	81.0
	USC	25	191.1	106.5	15.3	90.3
	Pro, modern	38	193.0	112.6	15.6	94.7
Defensive linemen	St. Cloud	15	186.6	97.8	18.5	79.3
	U Mass	8	188.8	114.3	19.5	91.9
	USC	13	191.1	109.3	14.7	93.2
	Gettysburg	11	178.0	99.4	21.9	77.6
	Pro, modern	32	192.4	117.1	18.2	95.8
	Pro, older	25	185.7	97.1	14.0	83.5
All positions	St. Cloud	65	182.5	88.0	15.0	74.2
	U Mass	91	184.9	97.3	13.9	83.2
	USC	88	186.6	96.6	11.4	84.6
	Gettysburg	60	178.0	90.6	18.1	73.3
	Pro, modern	164	188.1	101.5	13.4	87.3
	Pro, older	25	183.1	91.2	10.4	81.3
	Dallas-Jets[h]	107	188.2	100.4	12.6	87.7

[a]Grouping according to Wilmore JH, Haskel WL. Body composition and endurance capacity of professional football players. J Appl Physiol 1972;33:564.
[b]Data from Wickkiser JD, Kelly JM. The body composition of a college football team. Med Sci Sports 1975;7:199.
[c]UMass data from Coach Robert Stull and F Katch, University of Massachusetts. Data collected during spring practice, 1985; %fat by densitometry.
[d]USC data from Dr. Robert Girandola, University of Southern California, Los Angeles, 1978, 1993.
[e]Data courtesy of Dr. Kristin Steumple, Department of Exercise and Sport Science, Gettysburg College, Gettysburg, PA, 2000.
[f]Data from Wilmore JH, et al. Football pros' strengths—and CV weakness—charted. Phys Sportsmed 1976;4:45.
[g]Data from Dr. A. R. Behnke.
[h]Data from Katch FI, Katch, VL. Body composition of the Dallas Cowboys and New York Jets football teams, unpublished, 1978.

81.3 kg. Certainly these men were heavy but not fat. The heaviest lineman weighed 118 kg (17.4% body fat; 97.7 kg FFM), whereas the lineman with the most body fat (23.2%) weighed 115.4 kg. Body mass of a defensive back with the least fat (3.3%) was 82.3 kg with an FFM of 79.6 kg.

Table 29.8 presents a clearer picture of average values for body mass, stature, percentage body fat, and FFM of college and professional football players grouped by position.[58,60] The *Pro, older* group consists of 25 players from the 1942 Washington Redskins, the first professional players measured for body composition by hydrostatic weighing. The *Pro, modern* group consists of 164 players from 14 teams in the National Football League (NFL; 69% veterans, 31% rookies). Some 107 members of the 1976 to 1978 Dallas Cowboys and New York Jets make up the third group. Four groups of collegiate players include candidates for spring practice at St. Cloud State College in Minnesota, the University of Massachusetts (UMass), and division III Gettysburg College and teams from the University of Southern California (USC), 1973 to 1977, national champions and participants in two Rose Bowls. Body composition measurements for this data set included hydrostatic weighing with correction for measured residual lung volume.

One would generally expect modern-day professional players to have a larger body size at each position than a representative collegiate group. Although this occurred for comparisons with St. Cloud and UMass players, the USC players gen-

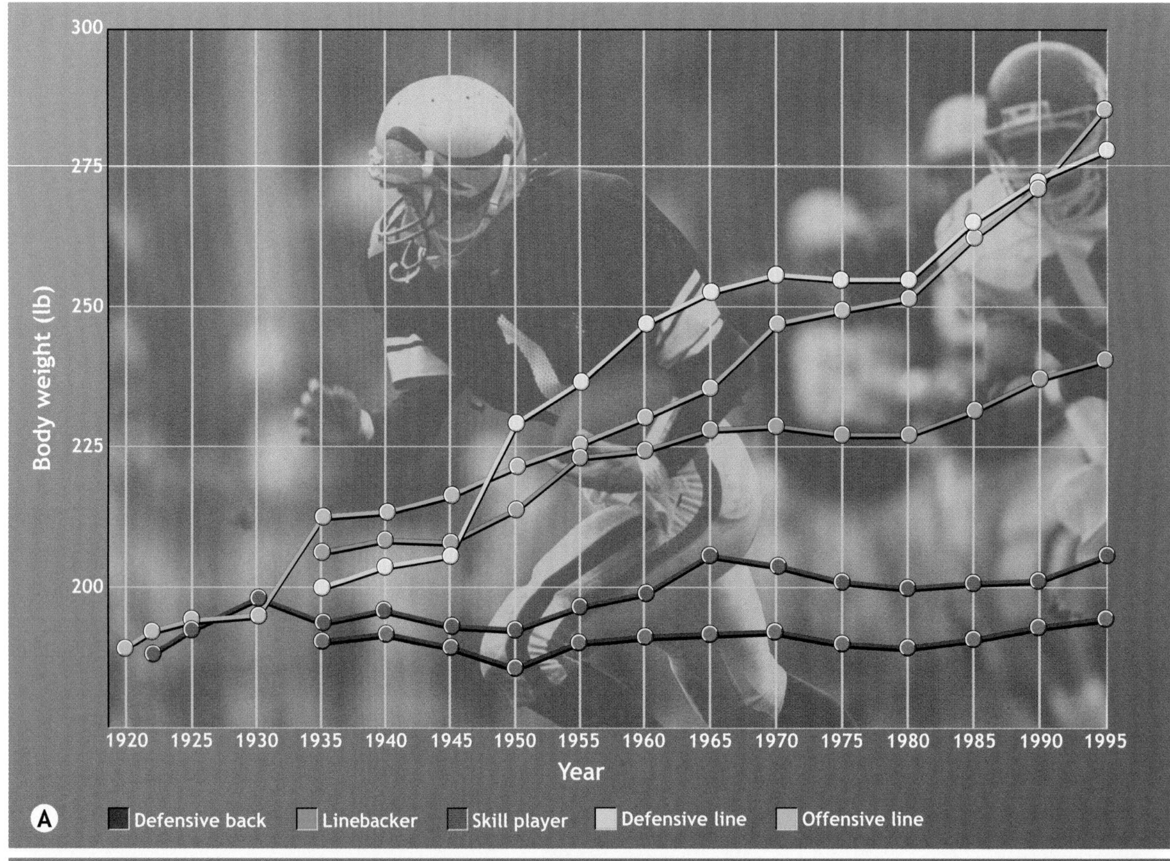

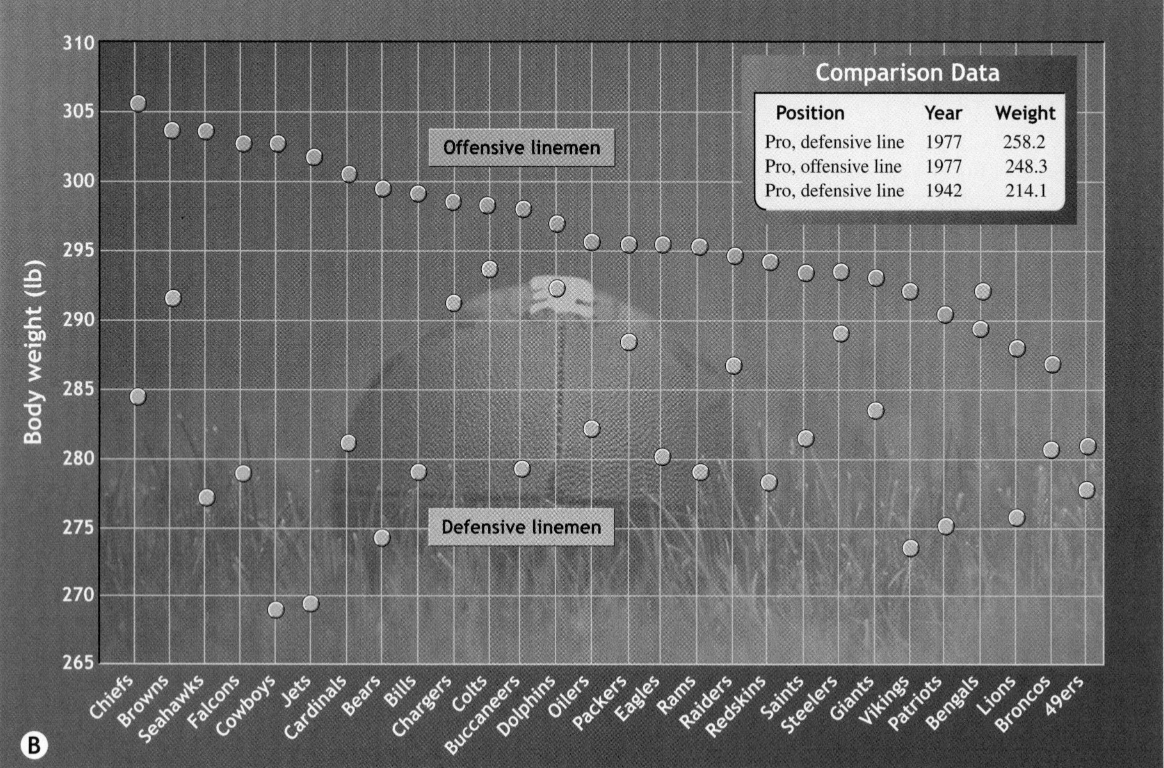

FIGURE 29.8 • **A**. Average body weight by position for all roster players in the NFL between 1920 and 1995. **B**. Average body weight of all roster offensive and defensive linemen in the NFL in 1994. Team rankings progress from the heaviest to lightest body weight for the team's offensive linemen. (From active team rosters for 28 NFL teams as of the first regular-season weekend, September 4–5, 1994). The comparison body weight data for the pro offensive and defensive line (1977) shown in the *inset box* are combined data for the New York Jets and Dallas Cowboys football teams (collected by textbook's authors FK and VK). The 1942 data were provided by Dr. Albert Behnke from his studies of the Washington Redskins. (Data courtesy of the National Football League public relations department.)

erally maintained a physique similar to modern professionals. With the exception of defensive linemen, the USC players at each position showed nearly the same body fat content as current professionals, although they weighed less. For FFM, the USC players weighed no more than 4.4 kg less than professionals at each position. The average defensive lineman in the NFL outweighed his USC counterpart in FFM by only 1.8 kg. Total body mass of the professional linemen, however, significantly exceeded that of USC counterparts, primarily because the professionals possessed 18.2% body fat versus the collegians' 14.7%. These data suggest that elite college and professional players maintain similar body size and body composition.

As a group, professional players 60 years ago were lower in body fat (10.4%), were shorter, and had lower total body mass and FFM than modern professionals. The exceptions, defensive and offensive backs and receivers, were almost identical to more-current players in body size and composition. The biggest differences in physique emerged for the defensive linemen; modern players were 6.7 cm taller, 20 kg heavier, 4.2 percentage points of body fat fatter, and had 12.3 kg more FFM. Obviously, "bigness" was not an important factor in line play during the 1940s. To illustrate this point, the *top* of Figure 29.8 shows the average body mass for all roster players in the NFL (N = 51,333) over a 76-year period.[31] From 1920 to 1985, offensive linemen were the heaviest players; this changed beginning with the 1990 season, when defensive linemen achieved the same body mass as offensive linemen and then surpassed them. While the body mass for offensive linemen appeared to have leveled off at nearly 280 pounds, defensive linemen continued to increase in weight, particularly from 1990 to 1996, when they weighed an average of 16 pounds more (double the weight gain for offensive linemen for the comparable period). On average, offensive linemen were 1.3 pounds per year heavier from 1920 to 1995. At this rate of increase, they should attain 320 pounds by the year 2007 (at an average height of 6 ft 8 in)! At this size, their BMI would be 35.2 kg · m^{-2}, classifying them as high for disease risk (see Fig. 28.1). Even more eye-opening is the BMI for the 2001 Super Bowl football champion's offensive and defensive linemen. Their BMI averaged 38.4 kg · m^{-2} (body mass, 142.4 kg; stature, 192.5 cm), the largest yet reported, and far in excess of the projected 2007 value. Subsequent research must determine if such relatively homogenous groups of elite, physically active, overweight men do in fact experience greater morbidity and mortality than normal-weight peers.

The body weight of offensive and defensive linemen for each of the NFL teams during the 1994 season *(bottom of figure)* ranged from heaviest (Kansas City Chiefs; Super Bowl 1970) to lightest (San Francisco 49ers; Super Bowls 1990 and 1995). For the 1994 season, the average body weight of the winning Super Bowl offensive line (Dallas Cowboys) ranked fifth highest of 28 teams.

A WORRISOME TREND EVEN AMONG LESS-SKILLED AND YOUNGER PLAYERS. Exceptionally high BMIs also occur at less elite levels of collegiate competition. The average BMI of 33.1 kg · m^{-2} for the division III 1999 Gettysburg offensive line (n = 15) and the BMI of 31.7 kg · m^{-2} for other NCAA division III American football linemen (n = 26; 1994–1995) raises similar concern about potential health risks for such large young men (stature, 1.84 m; body mass, 107.2 kg).[47] At the high school level, the BMI of *Parade Magazine*'s All-American football teams increased dramatically beginning in the early 1970s through 1989, and then further increased in rate of gain to the year 2000.[56] The plot in Figure 29.9 shows a clear shift at 1972 in the slope of the regression line (yellow line) relating BMI to

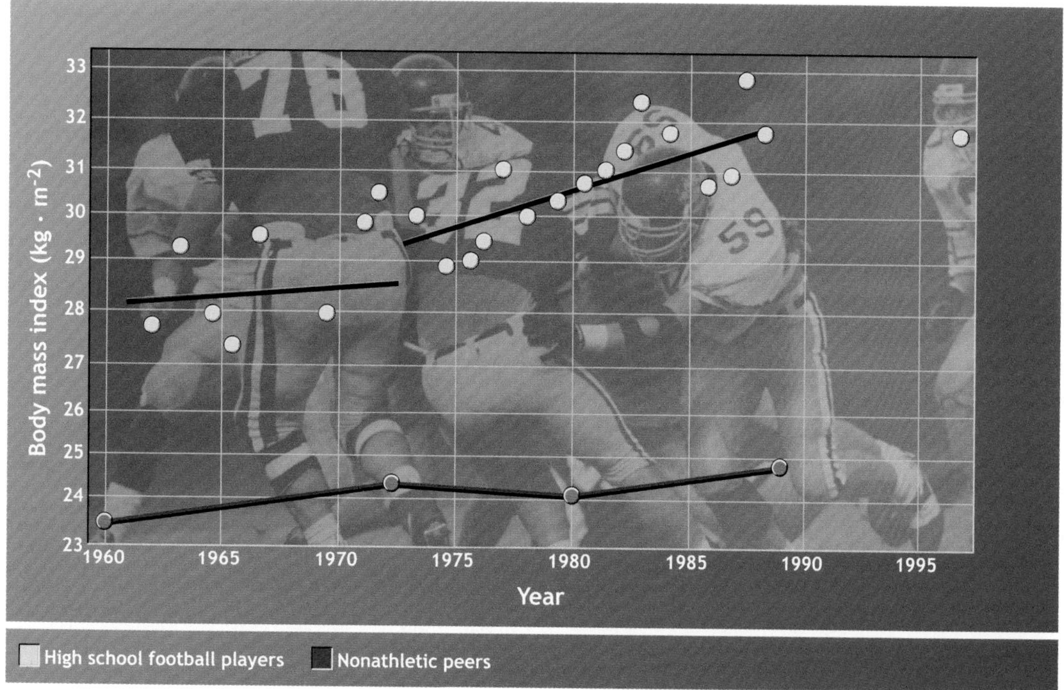

FIGURE 29.9 • BMIs of high school football players over time compared to nonathlete counterparts.

➤➤ PREDICTING BODY FAT FROM SKINFOLDS, GIRTHS, AND BIA MEASUREMENTS FOR DIFFERENT ATHLETIC GROUPS

Appropriate assessment of body composition allows determination of optimal body weight for competition, comparisons between athletes within the same sport, and monitoring changes in the body's lean and fat components resulting from dietary modification and/or exercise training. A valid appraisal of body composition also is an important first step in identifying potential eating disorders and formulating nutritional counseling. In the absence of body fat appraisal by hydrostatic weighing, predictions using skinfolds and/or girth measurements and bioelectric impedence analysis (BIA) have been used for diverse athletic groups.

Because the body's fat-free component can vary, multicomponent models most effectively convert whole body density to percentage body fat. The accompanying table presents population-specific skinfold, anthropometric (girth), and BIA equations for body composition assessment of athletes in general and for those in specific sport categories.

Method	Sport	Gender	Equation	Reference
Skinfolds	All	Women (18-29 y)	Db $(g \cdot cm^{-3})^a$ = 1.096095 - 0.0006952 (Σ4SKF) + 0.0000011 $(\Sigma 4SKF)^2$ - 0.0000714 (age)	28
	All	Boys (14-19 y)	Db $(g \cdot cm^{-3})^a$ = 1.10647 - 0.00162 (subscapular SKF) - 0.00144 (abdomen SKF) - 0.00077 (triceps SKF) + 0.00071 (midaxillary SKF)	17
	All	Men (18-29 y)	Db $(g \cdot cm^{-3})^a$ = 1.112 - 0.00043499 (Σ7SKF) + 0.00000055 (Σ7SKF) - 0.00028826 (age)	27
	Wrestling	Boys (HS)	Db $(g \cdot cm^{-3})^a$ = 1.0982 - 0.000815 (Σ3SKF) - 0.00000084 $(\Sigma 3SKF)^2$	52
BIA	All	Women (NR)	FFM (kg) = 0.73 (HT^2/R) + 0.23 (X_c) + 0.16 (BW) + 2.0	25
	All	Women (college)	FFM (kg) = 0.73 (HT^2/R) + 0.116 (BW) + 0.096 (X_c) - 4.03	39
	All	Men (college)	FFM (kg) = 0.734 (HT^2/R) + 0.116 (BW) +0.096 (X_c) - 3.152	39
	All	Men (19-40 y)	FFM (kg) = 1.949 + 0.701 (BW) + 0.186 (HT^2/R)	41
Anthropometry (girths)	All	Women (18-23 y)	FFM (kg) = 0.757 (BW) + 0.981 (neck C) - 0.516 (thigh C) + 0.79	40
	Ballet	Females (11-25 y)	FFM (kg) = 0.73 (BW) + 3.0	20
	Wrestling	Boys (13-18 y)	Db $(g \cdot cm^{-3})^a$ = 1.12691 - 0.00357 (arm C) - 0.00127 (AB C) + 0.00524 (forearm C)	30
	Football	White men (18-23 y)	%BF = 55.2 + 0.481 (BW) - 0.468 (HT)	23

From Heyward VH, Stolarczyk LM. Applied body composition assessment. Champaign, Il: Human Kinetics, 1996.

4SKF (mm) = sum of four skinfolds: triceps + anterior suprailiac + abdomen + thigh; 7SKF (mm) = sum of seven skinfolds: chest + midaxillary + triceps + subscapular + abdomen + anterior suprailiac + thigh; HT = height (cm); R = resistance (Ω); Xc = reactance (Ω); BW = body weight (kg); C= circumference (cm); thigh (cm) at the gluteal fold; AB (cm): average abdominal circumference = $[(AB_1 + AB_2)/2]$, where AB_1 (cm) = abdominal circumference anteriorly midway between the xyphoid process of the sternum and umbilicus, and laterally between the lower end of the rib cage and iliac crests, and AB_2 (cm) = abdominal circumference at the umbilicus level; NR = age not reported.

[a] Use the following formulas to convert body density (Db) to % body fat (BF): Men %BF = [(4.95/Db) - 4.50] X 100; Women %BF = [(5.01/Db) - 4.57] X 100; Boys (7-12y) %BF = [(5.30/Db) - 4.89] X 100; Boys (13-16y) %BF = [(5.07/Db) - 4.64] X 100; Boys (17-19y) %BF = [(4.99/Db) - 4.55] X 100.

Example Calculations

BOY ATHLETE (18 Y)

Data: Subscapular (SS) skinfold, 10 mm; abdominal (AB) skinfold, 18 mm; triceps (TRI) skinfold, 10 mm; midaxillary (MA) skinfold, 8 mm.

$$\begin{aligned}
Db &= 1.10647 - [0.00162 \times SS_{SKF}] - [0.00144 \times AB_{SKF}] - [0.00077 \times TRI_{SKF}] + [0.00071 \times MA_{SKF}] \\
&= 1.10647 - [0.00162 \times 10] - [0.00144 \times 18] - [0.00077 \times 10] + [0.00071 \times 8] \\
&= 1.10647 - 0.0162 - 0.02592 - 0.0077 + 0.00568 \\
&= 1.06233 \\
\%BF &= [(499 \div Db) - 455] \times 100 \\
&= [(499 \div 1.06233) - 455] \times 100 \\
&= 14.7\%
\end{aligned}$$

FEMALE BALLET DANCER (20 Y)

Data: Body weight, 55.0 kg.

$$\begin{aligned}
FFM (kg) &= [0.73 \times BW] + 3.0 \\
&= 43.15 \text{ kg} \\
\%BF &= [(BW - FFM) \div BW] \times 100 \\
&= [(55 - 43.15) \div 55] \times 100 \\
&= 21.5\%
\end{aligned}$$

MALE FOOTBALL PLAYER (20 Y)

Data: Body weight, 105.0 kg; stature, 188 cm.

$$\begin{aligned}
\%BF &= 55.2 + [0.481 \times BW] - [0.468 \times HT] \\
&= 55.2 + [0.481 \times 105] - [0.468 \times 188] \\
&= 55.2 + 50.51 - 87.98 \\
&= 17.7\%
\end{aligned}$$

year of competition compared to age-matched individuals from large-scale epidemiologic normative data (red line). The investigators suggested that this shift toward a higher BMI coincided with either improved nutrition and training and/or the emerging prevalence among high school athletes of performance-enhancing drugs (chiefly anabolic steroids),[55] a finding confirmed in a subsequent report.[4] Particularly disturbing are the most recent data for high school offensive and defensive linemen, for which the average BMI ranged between 31.8 and 33.5 kg · m^{-2}. The implications for such huge body mass in terms of the students' current health risk (e.g., insulin resistance and type-2 diabetes) and long-term outlook remain to be determined.

OTHER LONGITUDINAL TRENDS IN BODY SIZE. To expand upon longitudinal trends in elite athletes' body size, we determined stature and body mass for two groups of professional athletes: (1) all National Basketball Association (NBA) players from 1970 to 1993 (n ranged from 156 to 400) and (2) professional major league baseball players from 28 teams during the 1986, 1988, 1990, 1992, and 1995 seasons (n = 5031 roster players).

For the NBA players (Fig.29.10A), average body mass increased by 3.8 pounds (1.7 kg) or 1.8% during the 23-year interval. Stature increased more slowly; it changed by only 1 inch, or less than 1%, over the same interval. The NBA players' BMI during this time remained within a narrow range of 0.8 BMI units, from 23.6 to 24.4 kg · m^{-2}. The major league baseball players (shown in *red* in the same figure) show slightly higher mean values than the basketball players. Compared with American professional and collegiate football players, baseball and basketball athletes have maintained BMIs within guidelines considered relatively healthful for minimizing mortality and disease risk.

One might question whether gross body size as reflected by the BMI relates to sports performance variables. For example, Figure 29.10B plots the BMI of National and American League Cy Young award winners and their earned run average (ERA) over the 5-year comparison period. This comparison, while of interest, fails to delineate a clear relation between BMI and performance among the best pitchers in baseball.

MAXIMAL RUNNING PERFORMANCE AND BODY COMPOSITION. Figure 29.11 illustrates maximal acceleration and velocity at 5-yd intervals during a 50-yd run by members of a Super Bowl team during the last week of spring practice prior to the competitive season. Players started the sprint from a bent-forward position similar to a football stance. Ten timing lights placed at 5-yd intervals evaluated speed and acceleration. Each player ran the distance twice, and the fastest time represented the criterion performance. The offensive backs rated fastest; the offensive line had the slowest times. No relationship emerged between any time interval in the 50-yd linear run (commonly used to assess football "speed") and either body mass, fat mass, percentage body fat, or FFM. Stated somewhat differently, the speed a professional player achieves in the 50-yard dash has little relation to selected body composition variables. A fast or slow player is just as likely to have a "desirable" (or "undesirable") body composition as any other player.

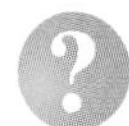

INTEGRATIVE QUESTION

Why doesn't a singular prototype for body composition (%fat, FFM) consistently emerge when one analyzes the body composition of elite athletes in different sports?

High School Wrestlers

Wrestlers represent a unique athletic group who train intensely and undergo repeated bouts of rapid weight loss and regain, and possible chronic undernutrition.[5,13,61] For example, adolescent wrestlers maintain long-term dietary restriction for both energy and protein during the wrestling season.[45] This significantly reduces lean tissue mass, fat stores, and muscular strength and power. Despite warnings from medical and professional groups about rapid weight loss,[1,2] most high school and college wrestlers (except heavyweights) reduce weight a few days before or on competition day. They lose 2 to 6 kg, hoping to gain a competitive advantage by wrestling in a lower weight category.[62] A wrestler who makes weight usually combines food restriction and dehydration, either through fluid and food deprivation or by exercising in a hot environment while wearing plastic or rubber garments. Diuretics, laxatives, extended time in a sauna or steam room, and vomiting also induce weight loss. In one study, 2% of intercollegiate wrestlers also exhibited bulimic behaviors.[54] Unfortunately, the source of information for these athletes about how best to lose weight comes from other wrestlers, not the coach, athletic trainer, or informed parents.[53] A typical wrestler experiences weight loss–weight gain from 7 to 15 times each year and repeats the cycle more than 100 times during a career.[54]

The pattern of weight loss and gain during NCAA division I, II, and III wrestling championships remained consistent among wrestling weight categories but not levels of competition.[48] Twenty hours following the official weigh-in, wrestlers were reweighed before the first round of competition; on average, they gained 4.9% of body mass in 20 hours. The lightest-weight wrestlers gained the most relative weight (4.5 kg or 7.8% of body mass), while heavyweights gained the least weight (0.7% of body mass). Wrestlers who advanced to the second tournament round all regained lost weight, often 7 kg (15.4 lb) in a 12-hour period. To discourage rapid weight loss, the American College of Sports Medicine (ACSM) recommends establishing minimal wrestling weight standards and holding weigh-ins immediately before competition.[1] Current NCAA rules conflict with recommended ACSM guidelines.

PROPOSED LOWEST ACCEPTABLE LEVEL FOR SAFE COMPETITION. Concern about rapid fluid loss before competition relates to the potential for significant reductions in plasma volume, central blood volume, and blood flow to active tissues. As little as 2% weight loss can alter cardiovascular response to submaximal exercise and can increase core temperature and produce undesirable shifts in electrolyte concentrations (see Chapter 25). Monitoring body weight and relative leanness may also benefit pre–high school competitors, because prepubescent wrestlers

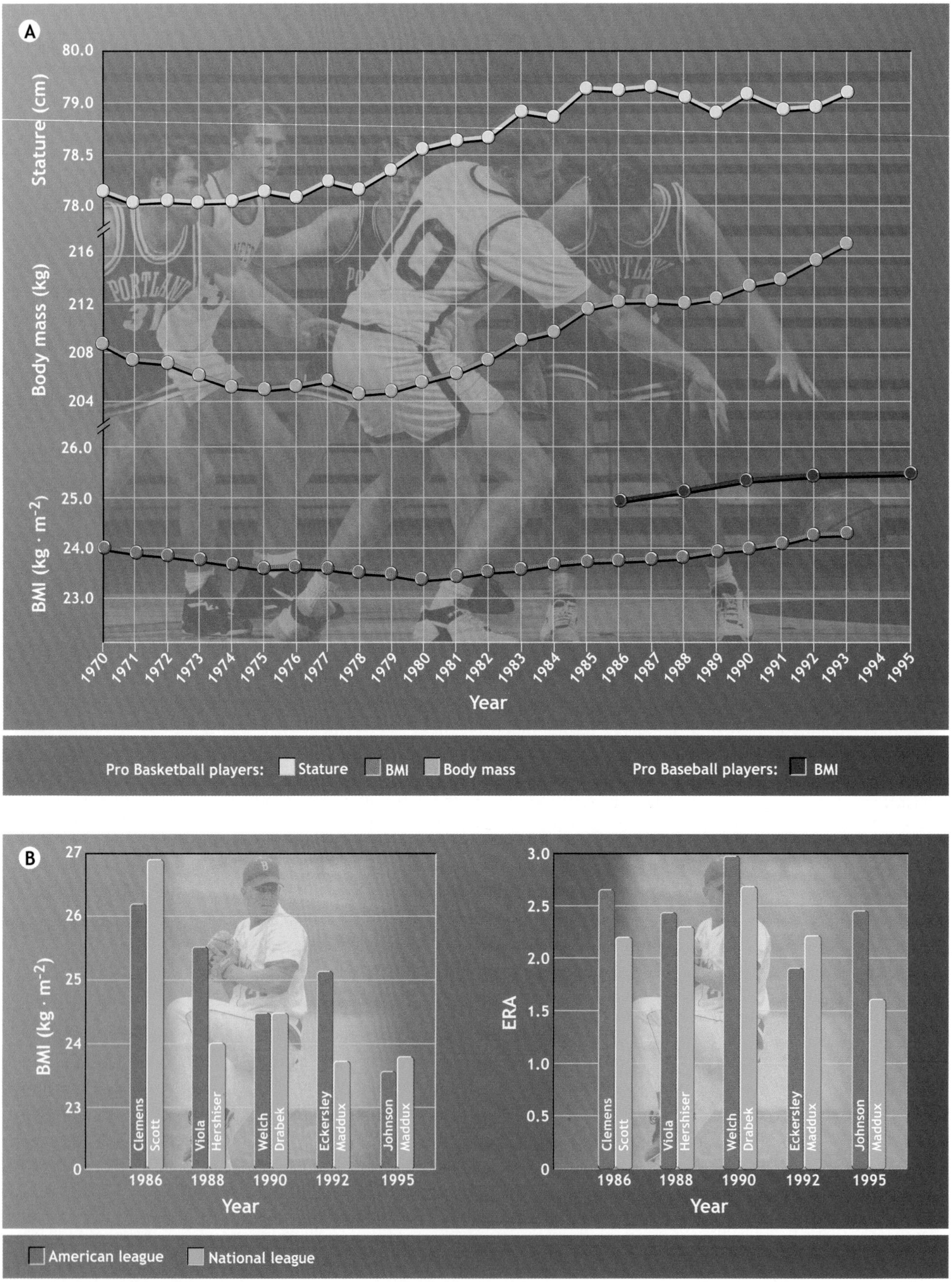

A

Stature (cm)

80.0
79.0
78.5
78.0

Body mass (kg)

216
212
208
204

BMI (kg · m⁻²)

26.0
25.0
24.0
23.0

1970 1971 1972 1973 1974 1975 1976 1977 1978 1979 1980 1981 1982 1983 1984 1985 1986 1987 1988 1989 1990 1991 1992 1993 1994 1995

Year

Pro Basketball players: Stature BMI Body mass

Pro Baseball players: BMI

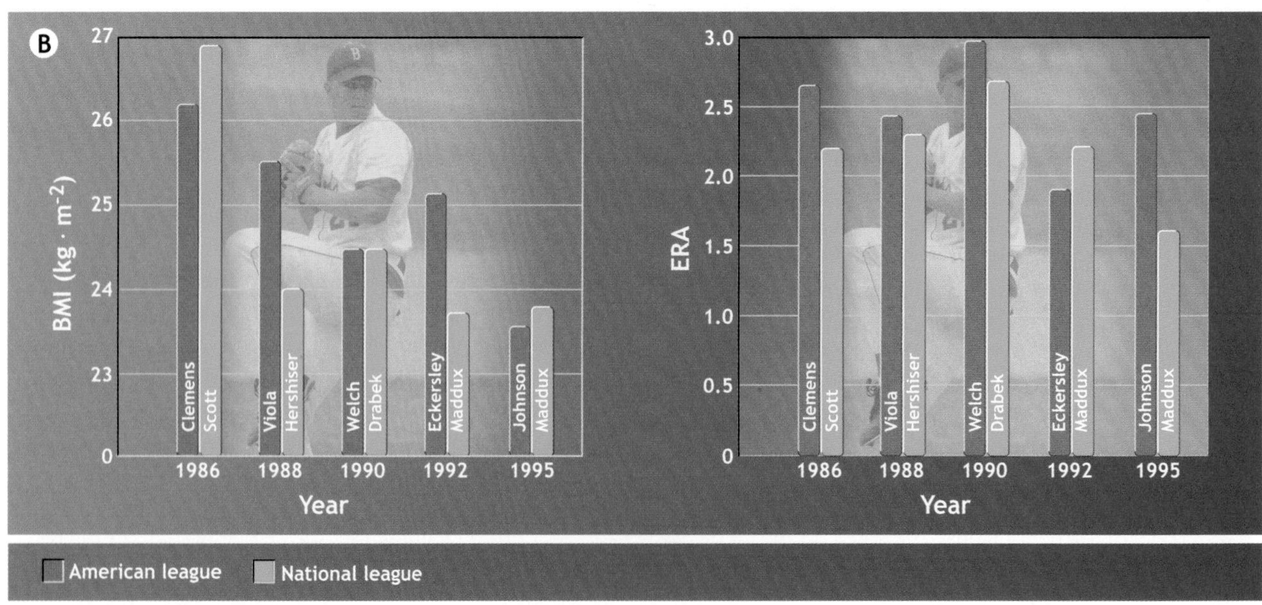

FIGURE 29.10 • **A**. BMI, body mass, and stature of professional NBA players (1970–1993) and BMI of major league baseball players (1986–1995). **B**. BMI for American League and National League Cy Young award winners (best baseball pitcher) along with their corresponding earned run average (ERA). (Data for NBA players from team rosters, compiled by F. Katch; major league baseball data from team rosters courtesy of Major League Baseball.)

Accumulated Run time (s)

Postition	Distance (yd)									
	5	10	15	20	25	30	35	40	45	50
Offensive line	1.30	2.03	2.68	3.26	3.84	4.40	4.95	5.51	6.05	6.61
Defensive line	1.31	1.98	2.62	3.19	3.72	4.28	4.81	5.34	5.87	6.41
Offensive backs	1.22	1.88	2.48	3.00	3.52	4.02	4.51	5.00	5.48	5.97
Wide receivers	1.25	1.91	2.50	3.03	3.54	4.02	4.50	4.98	5.45	5.94
Linebackers	1.24	1.93	2.54	3.10	3.60	4.15	4.66	5.18	5.70	6.19
Defensive backs	1.22	1.89	2.48	3.01	3.52	4.02	4.51	5.00	5.50	5.97

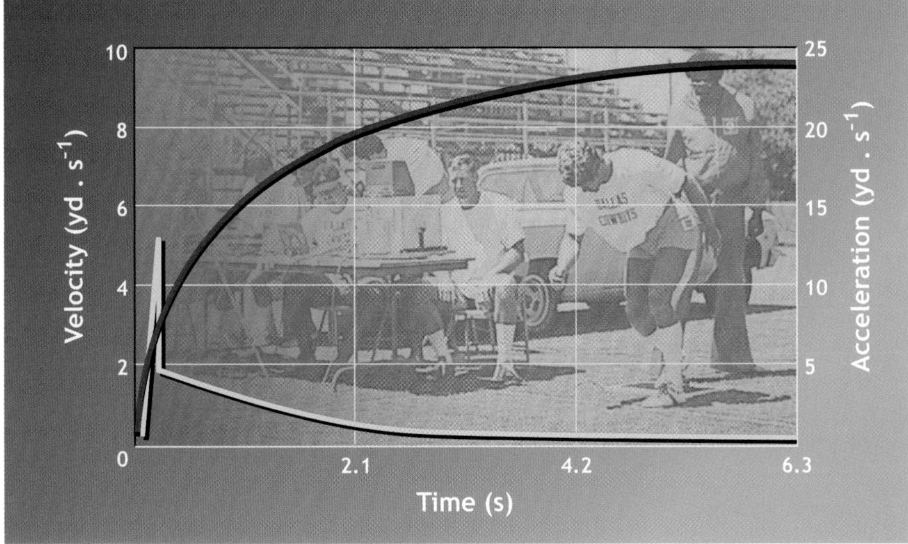

FIGURE 29.11 • Maximal acceleration (*yellow line*) and velocity (*red line*) during a 50-yd running performance by 39 professional football players (Super Bowl champion Dallas Cowboys). *Inset table* displays accumulated run times (s; 5-yd intervals) by position. Timing lights in series recorded sequential run times. (Data courtesy of Dr. Paul Ward.)

possess significantly less body fat than normally active peers.[46] Chapter 30 discusses how to determine minimal weight for wrestlers and presents a prudent approach to reduce body fat.

PHYSICAL CHARACTERISTICS OF HIGH SCHOOL WRESTLERS. Table 29.9 presents the physical characteristics of three groups of high school wrestlers.[11,24] The "certified" Iowa and Minnesota wrestlers competed at one of 12 different weight categories; the "champion" wrestlers competed in state or conference finals. Except for age and skinfolds, little difference exists in physical characteristics of Iowa and Minnesota certified and champion wrestlers. Skinfold measures indicated that the champions were

TABLE 29.9 ➤ ANTHROPOMETRIC COMPARISONS OF CERTIFIED AND CHAMPION IOWA AND MINNESOTA HIGH SCHOOL WRESTLERS AND NEBRASKA WRESTLERS

	CERTIFIED WRESTLERS[a]		CHAMPION WRESTLERS[a]		NEBRASKA WRESTLERS[b]
MEASUREMENT	IOWA (N = 484)	MINN (N = 245)	IOWA (N = 382)	MINN (N = 164)	(N = 409)
Age (y)	15.9	16.8	17.8	17.4	16.4
Stature (cm)	169.9	172.0	171.7	172.5	171.0
Body mass (kg)	64.3	65.3	64.6	64.7	63.2
Chest diameter (cm)	26.8	26.5	27.7	26.6	27.9
Chest depth (cm)	19.0	16.8	19.2	17.3	18.9
Bitrochanteric diameter (cm)	31.0	31.4	31.1	31.5	31.0
Ankles diameter (cm)	14.3	14.3	14.0	14.3	13.8
Skinfolds (mm)					
Scapular	8.4	7.9	6.4	6.8	8.8
Triceps	8.6	9.1	6.0	5.6	8.9
Suprailiac	13.3	12.3	9.1	7.5	11.8
Abdominal	13.1	12.2	8.6	8.3	11.6
Thigh	10.8	13.6	7.7	8.3	9.4
Sum of 5 skinfolds	54.2	55.1	37.8	36.5	50.5

[a]From Clarke KS. Predicting certified weight of young wrestlers; a field study of the Tcheng-Tipton method. Med Sci Sports 1974;6:52.
[b]From Housh TJ, et al. Validity of anthropometric estimations of body compositions in high school wrestlers. Res Q Exerc Sport 1989;60:239.

leaner than less-successful teammates. Because of small body mass differences among the groups, the elite wrestlers competed at a heavier FFM, which may have contributed to success in their weight class. The last column in Table 29.9 presents additional data for 409 Nebraska high school wrestlers. They possessed anthropometric characteristics most similar to the Iowa and Minnesota certified wrestlers. Percentage body fat of the Nebraska wrestlers, determined by hydrostatic weighing, averaged 11.0% (range, 1.5 to 26.0%); minimal wrestling weight at 5% body fat averaged 59.1 kg.

INTEGRATIVE QUESTION

A football coach wishes to field a team whose players are not overly fat. He selects the frequently used BMI to screen out players with excessive body fat. What are the possible outcomes of his decision in terms of football performance?

Male Weight Lifters and Bodybuilders

Resistance-trained athletes, particularly bodybuilders, Olympic weight lifters, and power weight lifters, exhibit remarkable muscular development and FFM, combined with a relatively lean physique.[33] Percentage body fat from underwater weighing averaged 9.3% in bodybuilders, 9.1% in power weight lifters, and 10.8% in Olympic weight lifters. Considerable leanness exists for each group of athletes, even though height–weight tables classify up to 19% of these men as overweight. Groups did not differ in skeletal frame size, FFM, skinfolds, and bone diameters. The only differences occurred for shoulders, chest, biceps (relaxed and flexed), and forearm girths; bodybuilders were larger at each site. The bodybuilders exhibited nearly 16 kg more muscle than predicted for their size; power weight lifters, 15 kg; and Olympic weight lifters, 13 kg.

Female Weight Lifters and Bodybuilders

Bodybuilding gained widespread popularity among women in the United States during the late 1970s. As women aggressively undertook the vigorous demands of resistance training, competition became more intense, and achievement level increased significantly. Bodybuilding success depends upon a slim and lean appearance, complemented by a well-defined yet enlarged musculature, raising interesting questions about the women's body composition. How lean do the competitors become, and does a relatively large muscle mass accompany their low body-fat levels?

Body composition assessment of 10 competitive female bodybuilders revealed an average of 13.2% body fat (range, 8.0 to 18.3%) and 46.6 kg FFM.[18] Except for champion gymnasts, who also average about 13% body fat, bodybuilders were 3 to 4% shorter, 4 to 5% lighter, and had 7 to 10% lower total body fat mass than other top female athletes. The bodybuilders' most striking compositional characteristic, a dramatically large FFM:FM ratio of 7:1, is nearly double the 4.3:1 ratio for other female athletic groups. This difference presumably occurred without steroid use (assessed by questionnaire). Interestingly, 8 of the 10 bodybuilders reported normal menstrual function despite relatively low body fat.

MEN VERSUS WOMEN. Table 29.10 compares body composition, girths, and excess body mass of male and female bodybuilders. Excess mass represents the difference between actual body

TABLE 29.10 ➤ BODY COMPOSITION AND ANTHROPOMETRIC GIRTHS OF MALE AND FEMALE BODYBUILDERS

Sex	Age (y)	Mass (kg)	Stature (cm)	Fat (%)	FFM (kg)	Excess Mass[a] (kg)
Male[b] ($n = 18$)	27.0	82.4	177.1	9.3	74.6	14.8
Female[c] ($n = 10$)	27.0	53.8	160.8	13.2	46.6	1.2

	Males		Females		% Difference (Males vs. Females)	
Body Part (cm)	Raw	Adjusted[d]	Raw	Adjusted[d]	Raw	Adjusted[d]
Shoulders	123.1	37.1	101.7	36.7	17.4	1.1
Chest	106.4	32.1	90.6	32.7	14.9	−1.9
Waist	82.0	24.7	64.5	23.3	21.3	5.7
Abdomen	82.3	24.8	67.7	25.1	15.3	−1.2
Hips	95.6	28.8	87.0	31.4	9.0	−9.0
Biceps relaxed	35.9	10.8	25.8	9.3	28.1	13.9
Biceps flexed	40.4	12.2	28.9	10.4	28.5	14.8
Forearm	30.7	9.2	24.0	8.7	21.8	5.4
Wrist	17.4	5.2	15.1	5.4	13.2	−3.8
Thigh	59.6	17.9	53.0	19.1	11.1	−6.7
Calf	37.3	11.2	32.4	11.7	13.1	−4.5
Ankle	22.8	6.9	26.3	7.3	11.0	−5.8

[a]Body mass minus body mass estimated from height–weight tables.
[b]Reference 33.
[c]Reference 18.
[d]Calculated as $G_i/\sqrt{\text{mass, kg/stature, dm}^{0.7}}$, where G_i equals any one of the girths. The term (mass/stature$^{0.7}$) is a frame structure estimate of perimetric (girth) size. The adjusted values are the perimetric equivalent adjusted girths due to sex differences, because they are corrected for whatever differences may exist as a result of differences in body size.

mass and body mass-for-stature from the Metropolitan Life Insurance tables. Overweight for the men corresponded to a 14.8-kg (18%) excess; and for the women, a 1.2-kg (12%) excess. Obviously, excess body mass in these lean athletes allow primarily reflected FFM as increased skeletal muscle.

Contrasts of the girth data allow comparison of individuals (or groups) who differ in body size. The analysis shows that gender differences in girths, when scaled to body size (referred to as "adjusted" in the table) do not differ as much as the uncorrected absolute girth values. Relative to body size, females exceed the male bodybuilders in 7 of 12 body areas. *This suggests that women can alter muscle size to almost the same relative extent as men, at least when scaled to body size.* The larger hip size in women probably relates to greater fat stores in this location.

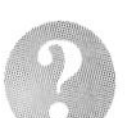

INTEGRATIVE QUESTION

Do established gender differences in body composition justify using sex-specific normative standards when evaluating different components of physical fitness and motor performance?

COMPARATIVE DATA: ANALYSIS OF MUSCULAR AND NONMUSCULAR COMPONENTS

The body profile technique introduced in Chapter 28 provides a distinctive way to partition the anthropometric aspects of body size and shape into muscular and nonmuscular components to consider heterogeneity in body dimensions among individuals and groups. The technique also can track changes in various body components with different training modes, weight loss and gain, growth, and aging. Table 29.11 presents the percentage deviations for the muscular and nonmuscular components for 12 different groups. One can directly compare the percentage deviation scores because the data analysis uses the Behnke reference man and reference woman as standards for comparison, with adjustments among groups to equalize body dimensions for stature.

Professional Ballet Dancers

Ten prima ballerinas from the San Francisco Ballet Company made up the subjects for group 1. Not unexpectedly, 6 of the 11 percentage deviations were negative; those for shoulders, chest, thigh, calf, and ankles were positive.

Champion Bodybuilders

The six muscular sites indicate excessive muscular development for the champion group of 11 Mr. Universe bodybuilders (group 2), particularly biceps, with the largest deviation (+77.9%) of any site among the groups. Expressed as the ponderal (body mass) equivalent for the biceps, the 77.9% deviation equals 127.9 kg. This means that this bodybuilder who weighs 84.2 kg possesses the biceps girth of a 127.9-kg untrained person. The ratio of muscular to nonmuscular girths was 1.396, which confirms the presence of excess muscle.

In contrast to the men, the muscular:nonmuscular ratio for the 10 female champion bodybuilders (group 3) averaged a

TABLE 29.11 ➤ PERCENTAGE DEVIATIONS FOR THE MUSCULAR AND NONMUSCULAR COMPONENTS AMONG INDIVIDUALS AND GROUPS THAT DIFFER SIGNIFICANTLY IN BODY SIZE AND SHAPE

	Group[a]											
Reference Data Group	**1**	**2**	**3**	**4**	**5**	**6**	**7**	**8**	**9**	**10**	**11**	**12**
Age (y)	21.8	32.1	27.1	24.3	18–22	19.5	17.2	17.2	17.0	17.4	17.2	21.2
Body mass (kg)	51.4	84.2	53.4	103.9	78.5	66.2	69.3	58.2	43.4	141.8	59.1	64.6
Stature (cm)	166.4	170.6	160.6	200.3	180.3	167.8	178.1	165.0	161.2	189.7	171.0	172.9
Muscular girths						**Percentage Deviation**						
Shoulders	10.6	28.2	12.9	2.6	1.7	10.7	2.7	−1.0	0.7	−6.4	—	—
Chest	8.6	49.2	19.4	5.8	6.4	14.9	2.2	1.4	3.8	4.1	−1.2	2.0
Biceps	−9.2	77.9	14.9	18.9	2.3	20.2	−2.4	−2.9	5.4	3.1	−10.4	17.3
Forearm	−1.8	43.7	9.1	9.5	3.3	−2.3	1.6	−0.8	2.0	−15.3	2.6	4.0
Thigh	0.0	17.9	−1.6	9.6	6.3	2.5	2.5	−2.2	−20.2	26.1	−4.1	−2.4
Calf	9.8	20.9	3.4	2.6	4.7	1.2	4.4	2.0	1.4	11.0	2.1	2.0
Nonmuscular girths												
Abdomen	−1.2	−28.7	−7.0	−7.1	−2.6	−7.5	−4.5	0.2	−7.8	31.9	−5.9	−7.6
Hips	−3.7	−30.1	−11.0	−9.2	−3.1	−8.0	−0.4	−2.0	−1.4	3.2	2.4	−2.5
Wrist	−5.8	−26.4	−8.3	−20.6	−7.8	−4.2	−4.7	−3.9	16.4	−36.4	3.4	−7.0
Knee	−4.9	−29.0	−12.1	−5.7	−3.8	−10.3	−1.0	4.3	7.6	−12.2	8.7	−0.6
Ankle	0.6	−27.7	−6.1	4.9	−5.9	−6.4	2.6	5.8	11.1	−4.7	—	—

[a]The numbers for the groups refer to the following: 1, professional ballet dancers; 2, champion male body builders; 3, champion female body builders; 4, pro basketball players; 5, male college students; 6, male collegiate gymnasts; 7, senior high school males; 8, senior high school females; 9, smallest boy in a 12th-grade class; 10, largest boy in a 12th-grade class; 11, entering class of Amherst College in 1882; 12, graduating class of Amherst College in 1886. More detailed anthropometric information about groups 1–3, 5, 7–12, including original references, appears in Katch FI, et al. The ponderal somatogram: evaluation of body size and shape from anthropometric girths and stature. Hum Biol 1987;59:439. Data for group 4 pro basketball players represented 17 first-round NBA draft choices measured by authors FK and VK at the 1998 NBA draft (Chicago). Data for group 6 represent 15 Division I male gymnasts from U Mass, Amherst, 1998.

much lower 1.097. Visual assessment of a female bodybuilder suggests that muscular girths predominate, yet the body profile analysis indicates that such appraisal lacks objectivity in differentiating between excess muscle and more-general refinement and shaping of diverse body parts. Specifically, female bodybuilders achieve more-balanced proportions between muscular and nonmuscular components.

Professional Basketball Players

The professional basketball players in group 4 ($n = 17$) are first- and second-round NBA rookie selections in the 1998 draft. The tallest player, at 211.3 cm (83.2 in), weighed 122 kg (269 lb), with a combined 11-girth sum of 729.4 cm. His abdomen (93.5 cm)-to-hips (110.6 cm) ratio was 0.845, his calf (42.2 cm) to thigh (68.5 cm) ratio was 0.616, and his forearm (35.2 cm)-to-biceps flexed (43.8 cm) ratio was 0.804. This player, one of the tallest centers currently in the NBA, had a relatively low 68.6-mm sum of six skinfolds (triceps, 13.2 mm; subscapular, 12.0 mm; abdomen, 17.0 mm; upper thigh, 12.8 mm; calf, 9.8 mm). His upper-body development, particularly the biceps and forearms, represented a much heavier body weight equivalent for someone of the same stature. He had a biceps girth expected of someone who weighed 161.4 kg (39.4-kg, or 87-lb, heavier than his 122-kg body mass) and a forearm girth of a man who weighed 144.7 kg (319 lb) His ponderal equivalent for the shoulders (125.1 kg) and chest (125.8 kg) were in line with his body mass, signifying that his arms were more muscularly developed than his upper trunk. With extensive physical training of the upper trunk (primarily heavy resistance exercise), how much additional muscle will this already large player gain as his body weight increases, probably in excess of 136 kg (300 lb) over a 5- to 10-year playing career? Longitudinal studies of changes in physique status of exceptional athletes would provide answers to such questions.

College-Age Males

Group 5 contains 100 nonathletic men from Eastern Oregon College.

Male Collegiate Gymnasts

The 15 NCAA division I men's gymnasts (group 6) averaged 7.2% body fat (61.4 kg FFM; 12.9 lean:fat ratio). Three men had low body fat, determined by hydrodensitometry (3.1, 3.5, 3.6%), with much larger than expected lean:fat ratios (30.7, 27.6, 17.1). The heaviest gymnast (77.1 kg) also had a relatively large lean:fat ratio (13.2) because of his 5.5% body fat at 72.8-kg FFM. As a group, the gymnasts were heavily muscled in the upper arm and trunk regions. The size of their biceps girth (33.2 cm) would be expected for a group of the same stature who weighed 73.6 kg—the 7.4 kg difference between scale weight (66.2 kg) and the ponderal equivalent weight represents excess muscle. The ponderal equivalent chest weight (70.4 kg) represents 4.2 kg excess muscle, based on this body region (70.4 kg−66.2 kg).

Twelfth-Grade Caucasian Males and Females

Groups 7 and 8 comprise participants in a large-scale multiracial nutritional and anthropometric survey of ninth- through twelfth-grade students at Berkeley High School, Berkeley, California.[26] Despite substantial differences in body mass and stature at identical ages, surprisingly similar percentage deviations emerged for the muscular and nonmuscular components. The absolute dimensions for the various body parts, however, were larger for the boys than for the girls by an amount similar to the gender difference in body mass.

Smallest and Largest Boy in the Twelfth Grade

Groups 9 and 10 are the smallest and largest boy, respectively, of the same age in the 450-member twelfth-grade class at Berkeley High School. The boys differ rather dramatically in body mass (98.4 kg, or 217 lb) and stature (28.5 cm, or nearly 1 ft).

Table 29.12 compares the ponderal equivalents for the muscular and nonmuscular body components of these two boys. The listed **ponderal equivalent** (P-E) value represents body mass equivalents for a person with a specific girth. For example, the P-E of 44.7 kg for the smallest boy represents his body mass projected on the basis of his shoulder girth. Note that this boy weighs 43.4 kg, so his shoulder measurement certainly reflects "normal" development. P-E based on the shoulder measurement of the largest boy is 128.5 kg, yet he weighs 13.3 kg more, 141.8 kg. Expressed somewhat differently, the largest boy in the class possesses a shoulder P-E of someone weighing 128.5 kg. Despite the boy's size, his shoulders remain relatively underdeveloped; this also holds

TABLE 29.12 ➤ PONDERAL EQUIVALENT (P-E) MUSCULAR AND NONMUSCULAR COMPONENTS FOR THE SMALLEST AND LARGEST BOYS IN A TWELFTH-GRADE CLASS[a]

	Smallest Boy Mass = 43.4 kg Stature = 161.2 cm		Largest Boy Mass = 141.8 kg Stature = 189.7 cm	
Variable	Girth (cm)	P-E (kg)	Girth (cm)	P-E (kg)
Muscular				
Shoulders	92.3	44.7	144.2	128.5
Chest	74.7	42.7	126.0	142.9
Biceps	25.6	42.0	43.3	141.6
Forearm	22.1	43.5	33.3	116.3
Thigh	40.6	35.4	82.8	173.2
Calf	29.9	45.0	50.7	152.4
Nonmuscular				
Abdomen	60.9	38.9	123.4	188.0
Hips	75.0	41.6	130.0	147.0
Wrist	15.1	49.1	18.9	90.6
Knee	30.7	45.4	47.0	125.1
Ankle	19.2	46.9	30.1	135.8

[a]Data are for groups 9 and 10 in Table 29.11.
Data courtesy of Dr. AR Behnke.

true for the P-Es projected from his forearms (116.3 kg), wrists (90.6 kg), knees (125.1 kg), and ankles (135.8 kg).

The nonmuscular abdominal component projected a small P-E (38.9 kg) for the smallest boy for his actual weight of 43.4 kg. For the largest boy, an excessively large abdominal component projected a body mass of someone weighing 46.2 kg more or 188.0 kg (415 lb)! The possibility exists that in relatively small children or large adolescents, a large positive deviation for the abdomen P-E signals early obesity onset. If this proves true, then assessment of abdominal P-E with subsequent follow-up may prove useful in detecting and treating childhood obesity.

Entering and Graduating Classes of Amherst College (1882–1886)

We retrieved the remarkable data set for groups 11 (entering class) and 12 (graduating class) from the archival Amherst College records of the pioneer exercise scientist–anthropometrist, Dr. Edward Hitchcock, Jr. Note the dramatic increase in biceps girth and decreases in the nonmuscular abdomen and hip regions over the 4-year period: these changes coincided with the start of daily resistance training using weighted bowling pins.

UPPER LIMIT FOR FAT-FREE BODY MASS

The FFM for Japanese elite sumo wrestlers *(seki-tori)* averages 109 kg.[37] These athletes share the distinction of probably being the world's largest with some American professional football players who weigh 159 kg (350 lb). Because it seems unlikely that athletes in this weight range would possess less than 15% body fat, their FFMs at 15% body fat, theoretically correspond to 135 kg. In reality, however, a football player with a body mass of 159 kg would more likely have 20 to 25% body fat. At 20% body fat, the FFM would be about 127 kg, certainly the highest value ever attained using hydrostatic weighing. But this value remains hypothetical in the absence of reliable data. Even for an exceptionally large professional basketball player (body mass, 138.3 kg [305 lb]; stature, 210.8 cm [83 in]), his percentage body fat is not likely to be less than 10% of body mass, or a fat weight of 13.8 kg and FFM of 114.2 kg. This amount of FFM seems more likely for an upper limit value of 114 kg for an athlete of such dimensions.

To gain additional insight into the question of an upper limit in FFM among athletes, we reviewed more than 30 years of body composition data from our laboratories to determine the largest FFM values determined densitometrically. Thirty-five athletes exceeded an FFM of 100 kg; the top five values were 114.3, 109.7, 108.4, 107.6, and 105.6. The three top values were larger than the two values of 106.5 kg reported for defensive football linemen from 1969–1971 data[3] and for other resistance-trained athletes.[15]

Figure 29.12 presents two analyses of the 35 athletes from our database whose FFMs exceeded 100 kg. Eight of the athletes were former U.S. Olympic shot put and discus performers. The other athletes included 7 offensive NFL linemen and 20 NFL defensive linemen. The *inset tables* provide anthropometric and body composition data. Body fat was determined by repeated trials of underwater weighing with correction for residual lung volume measured by oxygen dilution. Skinfolds were measured in triplicate at each site in rotational order and the average listed. Girths were measured with a cloth anthropometric tape at the same 11 anatomic sites used for Behnke's reference man. The main portion of the figure shows the ponderal body profile analysis for the athletes, separated into muscular and nonmuscular components.

The results for the ponderal body profile show unequivocally (and not unexpectedly) that this group of male athletes scored to the right of the zero reference line for each of the muscular components and negatively for the five nonmuscular components. The calculated P-E of 141.8 kg for the biceps means that for this group of exceptional athletes, their biceps development equals that of individuals expected to weigh about 25 kg more. The P-E weights for forearms (125.9 kg), chest (123.3 kg), and thighs (122.6 kg) confirm that the large muscular components mirror their large FFMs. The lean:fat ratio of 7.3 for these men also supports the data about their unusually large FFMs. For the reference man with a lean body mass (which includes essential fat) of 61.7 kg (15% body fat and 70 kg body mass), the lean:fat ratio of 5.667 remains about 23% less than the ratio for lean athletic groups. In Behnke's system, the male and female reference standards for the P-Es for the 11 body sites approximate body mass—70 kg for the reference man and 56.7 kg for the reference woman. For the muscular components, a large discrepancy between a P-E and scale body mass certainly indicates excess muscularity in that region. For the nonmuscular abdominal site, a positive discrepancy would confirm accretion of excess fat. For the bony regions (knees, wrists, ankles), a negative plot indicates relative smallness in that region, compared with the larger positive deviations for muscular components.

The body composition of an exceptionally large professional football player (NFL Oakland Raiders; unpublished data, Dr. Robert Girandola, Department of Kinesiology, University of Southern California) determined by repeated trials of underwater weighing with correction for residual lung volume exceeded values for FFM presented in Figure 29.12. The player, with a body fat content of 11.3%. (body mass, 141.4 kg; stature, 193 cm; BMI, 38.4 kg · m^{-2}), had a FFM of 125.4 kg, the uppermost value ever reported. With the continuing increase in the body size of pro football offensive and defensive players, this player's large FFM determined in 1997 before he turned professional, will probably not remain the peak value for FFM as body composition data on other large players become available.

Until more data become accessible on the body composition of extremely large and relatively lean athletes (determined by hydrostatic weighing or other acceptable criterion methods), the FFM of 125.4 kg reported for one pro defensive lineman remains the largest ever reported. In the absence of additional data, we assume that 125.4 kg represents the current upper limit of FFM in elite athletes.

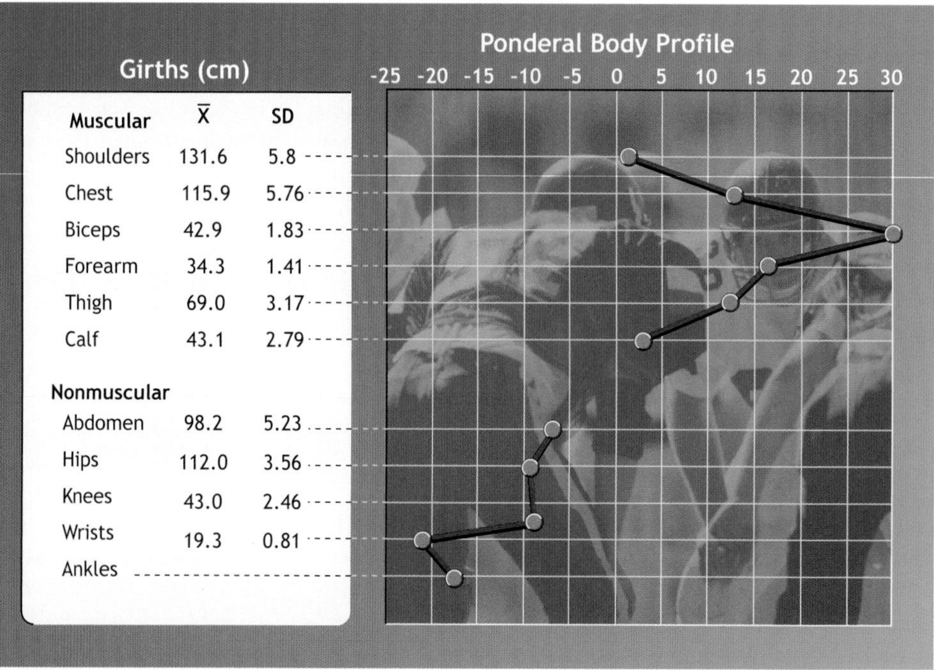

Body Composition

Variable	X̄	SD
Body mass, kg	116.6	5.05
Stature, cm	193.9	3.21
Body fat, %*	11.9	4.06
Body fat, kg	14 . 0	5.31
FFM, kg	102.7	2.45

*Densitometry with correction for residual lung volume by oxygen dilution. Percent fat from the Siri equation (%Fat = [495/Density] - 450)

FIGURE 29.12 • Ponderal body profile and body composition analysis for 35 world-class athletes with FFMs above 100 kg. Description of ponderal body profile described in: Katch FI, Katch VL. The body composition profile: techniques of measurement and applications. Clin Sports Med 1984;2:31.

Summary

1. Body composition assessment reveals that athletes generally have physique characteristics unique to their specific sport. For example, field-event athletes have a relatively large FFM and high percentage body fat, whereas distance runners possess the least amount of lean tissue and fat mass.
2. Champion performance blends unique physique characteristics and highly developed physiologic support systems.
3. Male and female triathletes possess a body composition and aerobic capacity most similar to elite bicyclists.
4. Body composition analysis of American football players reveals that they are among the heaviest of all athletes, yet they maintain a relatively lean body composition. At the highest levels of competition, Division I collegiate and professional football players show remarkable similarity in body size and composition.
5. Competitive male and female swimmers generally have higher body fat levels than distance runners. The difference probably results from self-selection related to economically exercising in the different environments rather than real metabolic effects caused by the environments.
6. Wrestlers undergo both severe training and repeated cycles of sudden weight loss and regain. Most high school and college wrestlers lose 2 to 6 kg, hoping to gain a competitive advantage by wrestling in a lower weight category.
7. Female bodybuilders can probably alter muscle size to the same relative extent as males.
8. The FFM:FM ratio of competitive female bodybuilders significantly exceeds the FFM:FM ratio of other elite female athletes.
9. The body profile analysis, which partitions the body into muscular and nonmuscular components, compares body size and shape among individuals and groups who display extremes in body composition.
10. A value of 125.4 kg represents the current upper limit of FFM of elite athletes, regardless of sport.

References

1. American College of Sports Medicine. Weight loss in wrestlers. Med Sci Sports 1976;8:11.
2. American Medical Association Committee on the Medical Aspects of Sports. Wrestling and weight control. JAMA 1967;201:541.
3. Behnke AR, Wilmore JH. Evaluation and regulation of body build and composition. Englewood Cliffs, NJ: Prentice-Hall, 1974.
4. Buckley WE, et al. Estimated prevalence of anabolic steroid use among high school seniors. JAMA 1988;12:24.
5. Carey D. The validity of anthropometric regression equations in predicting percent body fat in collegiate wrestlers. J Sports Med Phys Fitness 2000;40:254.
6. Carter JEL, Ackland TR. Kinanthropometry in aquatic sports. A study of world class athletes. In: Carter JE, Ackland TR, eds. Human Kinetics Sport Science Monograph Series, vol 5. Champaign, IL: Human Kinetics, 1994.
7. Carter LE, Lucio FD. Body size, skinfolds, and somatotypes of high school and Olympic wrestlers. Perspectives in kinanthropometry. Day JAP, ed. The 1984 Olympic Scientific Congress proceedings, vol 1. Champaign, IL: Human Kinetics, 1986.
8. Carter LE, et al. Advances in somatotype methodology and analysis. Yearbook Phys Anthropol 1983;26:193.
9. Changalur SN, et al. An analysis of male and female Olympic swimmers in the 200-meter events. Can J Sport Sci 1992;17:104.
10. Chollet D, et al. The effects of drafting on stroking variations during swimming in elite male triathletes. Eur J Appl Physiol 2000;82:413.
11. Clarke KC. Predicting certified weight of young wrestlers: a field study of the Tcheng-Tipton Method. Med Sci Sports 1974;6:52.
12. Cureton TK. Physical fitness of champion athletes. Urbana, IL: University of Illinois Press, 1951.
13. Dale KS, Landers DM. Weight control in wrestling: eating disorders or disordered eating? Med Sci Sports Exerc 1999;31:1382.
14. DeGaray AL, et al. Genetic and anthropological studies of Olympic athletes. New York: Academic Press, 1974.
15. Fahey T, et al. Body composition and $\dot{V}O_{2max}$ of exceptional weight-trained athletes. J Appl Physiol 1975;39:559.
16. Flynn ML, et al. Fat storage in athletes: metabolic and hormonal responses to swimming and running. Int J Sports Med 1990;11:433.
17. Forsyth HL, Sinning WE, The anthropometric estimation of body density and leand body weight in male athletes. Med Sci Sports Exerc 1973;5:174.
18. Freedson PS, et al. Physique, body composition, and psychological characteristics of competitive female bodybuilders. Phys Sportsmed 1983;11:85.
19. Grimston SK, Hay JG. Relationships among anthropometric and stroking characteristics of college swimmers. Med Sci Sports Exerc 1986;18:60.
20. Hergenroeder AC, et al. Anthropometric measurements and estimation body composition in ballet dancers. Med Sci Sports Exerc 1993;25:145.
21. Hirata K. Physique and age of Tokyo Olympic champions. J Sports Med Phys Fitness 1966;6:207.
22. Holly RG, et al. Triathlete characterization and response to prolonged strenuous competition. Med Sci Sports Exerc 1986;18:123.
23. Hortobagyi T, et al. Comparison of four methods to assess body composition in black and white athletes. Int J Sports Nutr 1992;2:60.
24. Housh TJ, et al. Validity of anthropometric estimations of body composition in high school wrestlers. Res Q Exerc Sport 1989;60:239.
25. Houtkooper LB, et al. Prediction of fat-free body corrected for bone mass from impedance and anthropometry in adult females. Med Sci Sports Exerc 1989;21:S39.
26. Huenemann RL, et al. Teenage nutrition and physique. Springfield, IL: Charles C Thomas, 1974.
27. Jackson AS, Pollock ML. Generalized equations for predicting body density of men. Brit J Nutr 1978;40:497.
28. Jackson AS, et al. Generalized equations for predicting body density of women. Med Sci Sports 1980;12:175.
29. Jang KT, et al. Energy balance in competitive swimmers and runners. J Swim Res 1987;3:19.
30. Katch FI, McArdle WD. Prediction of body density from simple anthropometric measurements in college-age men and women. Hum Biol 1973;45:445.
31. Katch FI, Monahan KD. Changes in body size of offensive players in the National football League: a 76-year review of 27,744 players. Med Sci Sports Exerc 1998;30:S239.
32. Katch FI, et al. Effects of physical training on the body composition and diet of females. Res Q 1969;40:99.
33. Katch VL, et al. Muscular development and lean body weight in bodybuilders and weight lifters. Med Sci Sports 1980;12:340.
34. Katzmarzyk PT, et al. Familial resemblance for physique: heritabilities for somatotype components. Ann Hum Biol 2000;27:467.
35. Kohlraush W. Zusammenhang von Korperform und Leistung. Ergebnisse der anthropometrischen Messungen an der Athletern der Amsterdamer Olympiade. Int Z Angrew Physiol 1970;2:187.
36. Kohrt WM, et al. Longitudinal assessment of responses by triathletes to swimming, cycling, and running. Med Sci Sports Exerc 1989;21:569.
37. Kondo M, et al. Upper limit of fat-free mass in humans: A study of Japanese sumo wrestlers. Am J Hum Biol 1994;6:613.
38. Leake CN, Carter JE. Comparison of body composition and somatotype of trained female triathletes. J Sports Sci 1991;9:125.
39. Lukaski HC, Bolonchuk WW. Theory and validation of the tetrapolar bioelectrical impedance method to assess human body composition. In Vivo body Composition Studies. Ellis KJ, et al., eds. London:The Institute of Physical Sciences in Medicine, 1987.
40. Mayhew JL, et al. Prediction of body composition in female athletes.
41. Opplinger RA, et al. Bioelectrical impedance prediction of fat-free mass for high school wrestlers validated. Med Sci Sports Exerc 1991;23:573.
42. O'Toole ML. Training for ultraendurance triathletes. Med Sci Sports Exerc 1989;21:209.
43. O'Toole ML. The ultraendurance triathlete: a physiological profile. Med Sci Sports Exerc 1987;19:45.
44. Rebato E, et al. Analysis of sibling resemblance in anthropometric somatotype components. Ann Hum Biol. 2000;27:149.
45. Roemmich JN, Sinning WE. Weight loss and wrestling training: effects of nutrition, growth, maturation, body composition, and strength. J Appl Physiol 1997;82:1751.
46. Sady SP, et al. Physiological characteristics of high-ability prepubescent wrestlers. Med Sci Sports Exerc 1984;16:72.
47. Schmidt WD. Strength and physiological characteristics of NCAA division III American football players. J Strength Cond Res 1999;13:210.
48. Scott JR. et al. Acute weight gain in collegiate wrestlers following a tournament weigh-in. Med Sci Sports Exerc 1994;26:1181.
49. Sinning WE. Body composition, cardiorespiratory function, and rule changes in women's basketball. Res Q 1973;44:313.
50. Sinning WE, Lindberg GD. Physical characteristics of college age women gymnasts. Res Q 1972;43:226.
51. Tanner JM. The physique of the Olympic athlete. London: Allen and Unwin, 1964.
52. Thorland, WG, et al. Midwest wrestling study: Prediction of minimal weight for high school wrestlers. Med Sci Sports Exerc 1991;23:1102.
53. Tipton CM. Making and maintaining weight for interscholastic wrestling. Gatorade Sports Science Exchange 1990;2:1.
54. Tipton CM, Oppliger RA. Nutritional and fitness considerations for competitive wrestlers. World Rev Nutr Diet 1993;71:84.
55. Toohey JV, Cox BA. Steroids and the athlete. Ariz J Health Phys Educ Rec Dance 1971;14:15.
56. Wang MQ, et al. Changes in body size of elite high school football players: 1963–1989. Percept Mot Skills 1993;76:379.
57. Welham WC, Behnke AR. The specific gravity of healthy men. JAMA 1942;118:498.
58. Wickkiser JD, Kelly JM. The body composition of a college football team. Med Sci Sports 1975;7:199.
59. Wilmore JH, Brown CH. Physiological profiles of women distance runners. Med Sci Sports 1974;6:178.
60. Wilmore JH, Haskell WL. Body composition and endurance capacity of professional football players. J Appl Physiol 1972;33:564.
61. Wroble RR, Moxley DP. Acute weight gain and its relationship to success in high school wrestlers. Med Sci Sports Exerc. 1998;30:949.
62. Wroble RR, Moxley DP. Weight loss patterns and success rates in high school wrestlers. Med Sci Sports Exerc 1998;30:625.

CHAPTER 30

Overweight, Obesity, and Weight Control

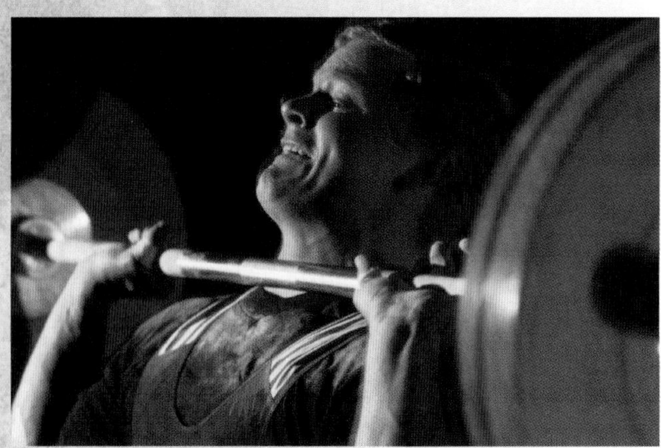

Chapter Objectives

- Discuss the worldwide scope of overfatness and obesity
- Distinguish differences between overweight, overfat, and obesity
- Evaluate the contribution of inherited factors to the development of excess body fat
- List 10 significant health risks of excessive body fat
- Describe the relationship between excess body weight in childhood and adolescence and risk for obesity and poor health in adulthood
- Discuss each of the following criteria for excessive body fat: (1) percentage body fat, (2) regional fat distribution, and (3) fat cell size and number
- Compare fat cell size and number for individuals with average body fat and those classified as massively obese
- Describe general effects of weight gain and weight loss on fat cell size and number in adults
- Outline three approaches to "unbalance" the energy balance equation to induce weight loss
- Describe characteristics of individuals who successfully maintain prolonged weight loss
- Summarize the proposed advantages and disadvantages of ketogenic, high-protein, and very–low-calorie diets for reducing body fat
- Present the rationale for including regular physical activity in a prudent weight-loss program
- Review how moderate increases in physical activity for a previously sedentary, overly fat person affect (1) daily food intake and (2) energy expenditure on a short- and long-term basis
- Outline why combining regular physical activity with moderate food restriction can achieve successful weight loss
- Summarize research about how different exercise modes affect body composition during weight loss
- Explain whether specific (target) exercises induce localized fat loss
- Give diet and exercise advice for gaining body weight to improve appearance or enhance sports performance

➤ **PART 1 • Obesity**

Unfortunately, in our modern scientific era, in which astronauts routinely explore the weightless environment, bioengineers develop surgical procedures to prolong and enhance life's quality, and molecular geneticists unravel basic secrets of subcellular function, no clear answer exists to a seemingly simple question: "Why have so many people become too fat, and what can be done to ameliorate the problem?" A random-digit telephone survey of nearly 110,000 adults in the United States found that nearly 70% struggle to lose weight (29% of men and 40% of women) or just maintain body weight.[189] Only one-fifth of the 45 to 50 million Americans trying to lose weight use the recommended combination of eating fewer calories and engaging in at least 150 minutes of weekly leisure-time physical activity. Those attempting to lose weight spend nearly $40 billion annually on weight-reduction products and services, often using potentially harmful dietary practices and drugs while ignoring sensible weight-loss programs.[30,179] Approximately 2 million Americans pay more than $125 million on appetite-suppressing, over-the-counter diet pills that line drugstore, health food and fitness center, and supermarket shelves, not to mention TV and radio direct marketing and mail order and Internet sales. Despite the upswing in attempts to lose weight, Americans are considerably more overweight than a generation ago, with obesity increasing in all regions of the United States.[142]

WORLDWIDE EPIDEMIC

Figure 30.1 shows the results of a national survey on the prevalence of overweight (defined at the time of this 1994 publication as BMI ≥27) among adults in the United States, compared with the government's objective of the year 2000.[120] Between 1988 and 1991, one-third of adults aged 20 to 74 years classified as overweight. This represents a dramatic increase over previous surveys, with overweight occurrence particularly high among women (Hispanic, African American, Pacific Islanders) and minority groups (*inset table*).

New classifications established on June 18, 1998, by the 24-member expert panel convened by the National Heart Lung and Blood Institute, now define overweight as a BMI of 25 to 29.9 and obesity as a BMI ≥30. As a result of these new standards, the prevalence of overweight and obesity in adults has increased to about 100 million Americans (55% of adults age 20 or older including 35% of college students[128]), with the major increase from a near-doubling of the obesity component (*top inset figure*, Fig. 30.1) to one in four Americans over the past two decades.[121,220] During this time, the average body weight of adult Americans has increased by about 8 pounds. As of January 2000, 25% of the adult population classifies as obese, compared with only 14.5% in 1980. Similar increases in obesity around the world[122,165,214,230]—contributing to the rising tide of diabetes and cardiovascular disease—has led the World Health Organization and the International Obesity Task Force to declare a global obesity epidemic.[202] Obesity is now the second leading cause of preventable deaths in the United States (300,000 deaths yearly, with cardiovascular diseased ranked #1), with a total upper annual cost estimated at $140 billion (www.obesity.org). These results fall short of the Healthy People 2000 goal of reducing overweight prevalence among adults to no more than 20% by the year 2000.[167]

Obesity among youth has more than doubled in the last 15 years with an ever-widening gap between the weights of those deemed overfat and thin. Disturbingly, overweight now claims 15 to 20% of American children and 12% of adolescents (up from 7.6% in 1976–1980). Obesity represents their most common chronic disorder, particularly prevalent among poor and minority children.[28,206] Excessive fatness in youth is even more of an adult health risk than obesity begun in adulthood. Overweight children and adolescents, regardless of their final body weight as adults, exhibit a significantly higher risk of a broad range of illnesses as adults than adolescents of normal weight.[73,210]

REASONS FOR CLASSIFYING OVERWEIGHT AND OBESITY

- Provides meaningful comparisons of body weight status within and between populations
- Identifies individuals and groups at increased risk of morbidity and mortality
- Identifies priorities for intervention at individual and community levels
- Establishes a firm basis for evaluating diverse intervention strategies

Source: World Health Organization

Substantial alterations in the population's gene pool (which require millions of years) cannot explain the dramatic nationwide obesity increase since 1980. Researchers maintain that if the progression of obesity continues, the entire population will be overweight within a few generations. By 2025, 75% of the American population will classify as overweight, with about one-third of these individuals rated obese. More than likely, a sedentary lifestyle and the ready availability of tasty, lipid- and calorie-rich foods served in increasingly larger portions are prime culprits in inducing the expression of unhealthy patterns of pre-existing susceptible genes in the fattening of Western civilization.[13]

Overweight, Overfat, and Obesity: No Unanimity for Terminology

A great deal of confusion surrounds the precise meaning of the terms overweight, overfat, and obesity as applied to body composition and related health risks of excessive body fat. Indeed, each term often takes on a different meaning depending upon the situation and context of use. In most medical literature, the term overweight is meant to describe an overfat condition, even in the absence of accompanying body fat measures. Within this context, obesity then refers to individuals at

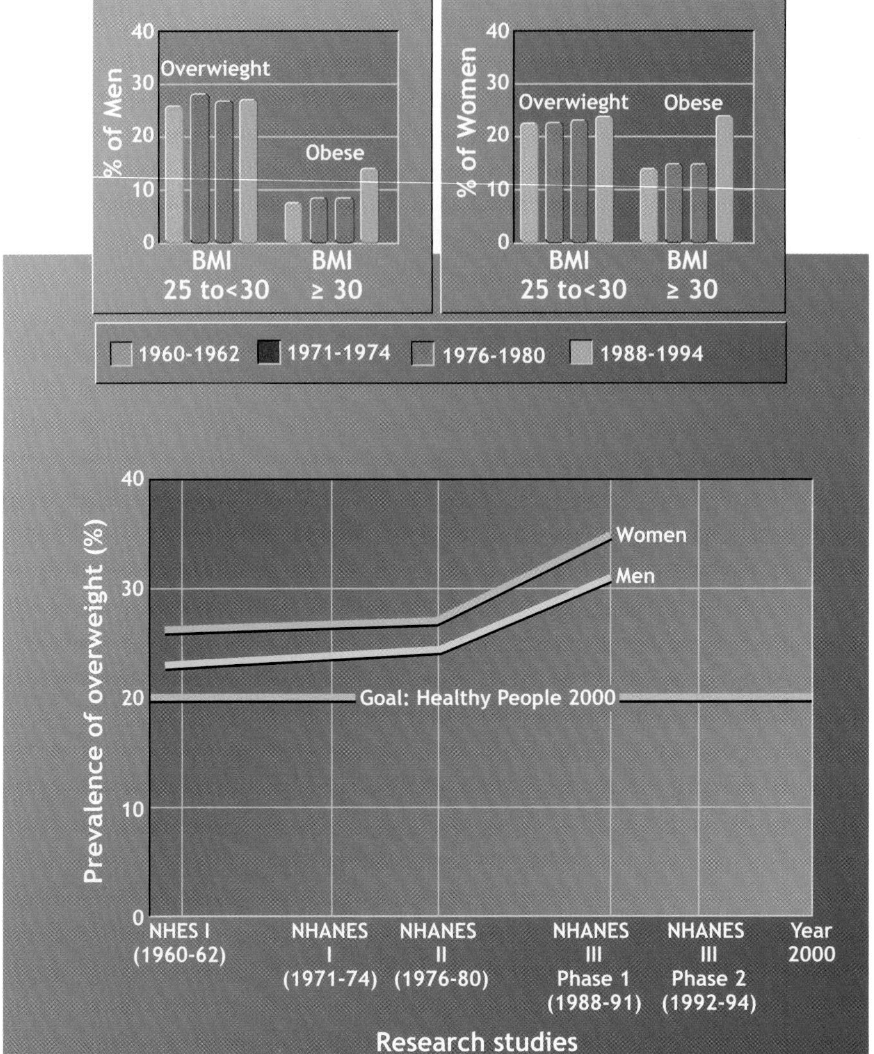

Group	Men (%)*		Women (%)*	
	Overweight	Severely overweight	Overweight	Severely overweight
White	24.4	7.8	24.6	9.6
Black	26.3	10.4	45.1	19.7
Mexican	31.2	10.8	41.5	16.7
Cuban	28.5	10.3	31.9	6.9
Puerto Rican	25.7	7.9	39.8	15.2

*Age-adjusted percentages of overweight and severely overweight persons aged 20-74 y living in the U.S.

FIGURE 30.1 • The fattening of America. Trends in age-adjusted prevalence of overweight in the U.S. population aged 20 through 74 years, compared with the Healthy People 2000 objective for overweight. The *inset table* presents the age-adjusted percentages of overweight and severely overweight persons aged 20 to 74 years from NHANES II (1976-1980) and NHANES I (1971-1974), categorized by ethnicity and gender. NHES, National Health Examination Survey; NHANES, National Health and Nutrition Examination Survey. (From Kuczmarski RJ, et al. Increasing prevalence of overweight among US adults. JAMA 1994;272:205; *inset table* from Kuczmarski RJ, et al. Prevalence of overweight and weight gain in the United States. Am J Clin Nutr 1992;55:495S.) The *inset figure* shows change in the age-adjusted prevalence of overweight and obesity in men and women aged 20 to 74 years from 1960 to 1994. (From National Task Force on the Prevention and Treatment of Obesity. Overweight, obesity, and health risk. Arch Intern Med 2000;160:898.)

the extreme of the overweight continuum. This is precisely the frame of reference currently used to delineate the body fat continuum by means of the BMI (see Chapter 28).

Research and contemporary discussion among diverse disciplines points up the need to distinguish between overweight, overfat, and obesity to insure consistency in use and interpretation. In general, weight-for-height at a given age has provided the most convenient (and easily obtained) index to infer body fat and accompanying health risks. In proper context, however, the overweight condition simply refers to a body weight exceeding some average for stature, and perhaps age, usually by some standard deviation unit or percentage. As discussed in Chapter 28, the overweight condition frequently accompanies an increase in body fat, but not always (e.g., male power athletes), and may or may not coincide with comorbidities like glucose intolerance, insulin resistance, dyslipidemia, and hypertension (e.g., physically fit overfat men and women).

When body fat measures are available (hydrostatic weighing, skinfolds, girths, BIA, DXA), it becomes possible to more accurately place an individual's body fat level on a continuum from low to high, independent of body weight. Overfatness then would refer to a condition where body fat exceeds an age- and/or gender-appropriate average by a predetermined amount. In most situations, "overfatness" represents the correct term when assessing individual and group body fat levels.

The term **obesity** refers to the overfat condition that accompanies a constellation of comorbidities including one or all of the following components of the "**obese syndrome**": glucose intolerance, insulin resistance, dyslipidemia, type 2 diabetes, hypertension, elevated plasma leptin concentrations, increased visceral adipose tissue, and increased risk of coronary heart disease and cancer. Limited research suggests that it is excess body fat, not excess body weight per se that explains the relationship between above average body weight and disease risk.[188] Such findings emphasize the importance of distinguishing the composition of excess body weight in determining an overweight person's disease risk.

Because many men and women may be overweight or overfat but do not exhibit components of the "obese syndrome," we urge caution in using the term obesity (instead of overfatness) in all cases of excessive body weight. However, we acknowledge that these terms are often used interchangeably (as we at times do in this text) to refer to the same condition.

A PROGRESSIVE LONG-TERM PROCESS

Obesity (more precisely, overfatness), defined as an excess accumulation of body fat, is a heterogeneous disorder with a final common pathway in which energy intake chronically exceeds energy expenditure. Disruption in energy balance often begins in childhood, and if this occurs (particularly among older children at the upper decile for body fat), the chance for adult obesity is significantly higher than in children with normal body fat levels.[74,210] For example, obese children at ages 6 to 9 have a 55% chance of being obese as adults—a risk 10 times that of children of normal weight. Simply stated, a child generally does not "outgrow" the overly fat condition. If parental obesity also exists, the child's risk of obesity in adulthood is two to three times that of normal-weight children without obese parents.[219] The child–parent association also results from the family's poor dietary and exercise habits.

Ages 25 to 44 years are the dangerous time for development of excessive fatness by adults.[34] Middle-aged men and women invariably weigh more than college-aged counterparts of the same stature. In the Western world, the average 35-year-old male gains between 0.2 and 0.8 kg of fat each year until the sixth decade of life, despite a progressive *decrease* in food intake. Women tend to gain the most weight; about 14% add more than 30 pounds between ages 25 and 34. Whether "creeping obesity" in adulthood reflects a normal biologic pattern remains unclear.

EXCESSIVE BODY FAT DOES NOT NECESSARILY RELATE TO OVEREATING

If obesity truly represents a unitary disorder, and gluttony and overindulgence singularly cause body fat accretion, then cutting back on food intake should provide permanent weight reduction and improved health. Unfortunately, human obesity results from a complex interaction of factors, including genetic, environmental, metabolic, physiologic, behavioral, social, and perhaps racial influences.[27,72,127,179,229]

Individual differences in specific factors that predispose humans to excessive weight gain include eating patterns and eating environment; food packaging, body image, and variations related to resting metabolic rate; diet-induced thermogenesis; level of spontaneous activity or "fidgeting" (nonexercise activity thermogenesis)[101]; basal body temperature; susceptibility to specific viral infections, levels of cellular adenosine triphosphatase, lipoprotein lipase, and other enzymes; and metabolically active brown adipose tissue.[16,172] Interestingly, while the cause of obesity seldom relates to hormonal aberrations, obesity often triggers a cascade of abnormal hormone responses.[160]

GENETICS INFLUENCES BODY FAT ACCUMULATION

The significant interaction between genetics and environment makes it difficult to quantify the role of each in the development of obesity. One's genetic makeup does not necessarily *cause* obesity, but it does lower the *threshold* for its development (susceptibility genes). Researchers are only now beginning to identify key genes and specific DNA sequence variances that relate to the molecular causes of appetite and satiety and predispose a person to obesity. A more-complete understanding of the genetic role in body fat accretion requires identification of all the genes and their mutations (including the relevant proteins) that contribute to chronic energy imbalance, events that should occur in the not-too-distant future.

Inherited factors contribute to variability in weight gain among individuals fed an identical daily caloric excess and can contribute to the tendency to regain lost weight (see Focus on Research).[15,59] Studies of a relatively large number of individuals representing 9 different kinds of relatives indicate that genetic factors that affect metabolism and appetite determine about 25% of the variation among people in percentage body fat and total fat mass; a larger percentage variation relates to a transmissible (cultural) effect (unhealthy expression patterns of preexisting genes; Fig. 30.2). *In an obesity-producing environment—sedentary and stressful, with ready access to inexpensive, large-portion, high-calorie, good-tasting food—the genetically susceptible (obesity-prone) individual gains weight and possibly lots of it.*[17,51]

Focus on Research

Genetic Tendency to Gain Weight

Bouchard C, et al. The response to long term feeding in identical twins. N Engl J Med 1990;322:1477.

➤ Bouchard and colleagues studied differences in body fat acquisition and its distribution from overfeeding (86,000 "extra" kcal) in 12 pairs of male monozygotic twins for 100 days. Their results provide some of the most persuasive support for an inherited tendency toward obesity.

The twin pairs (average age, 21 y; range, 19 to 27 y) lived in a dormitory under 24-hour supervision for 120 consecutive days. This period included 14 days of baseline testing, 3 days of testing before overfeeding, 100 days of overfeeding, and 3 days of posttesting. Subjects ate normally during baseline testing, with each meal analyzed for nutrient composition and energy content. Body mass remained stable during this time. Subjects were tested during the pre- and postoverfeeding periods for resting metabolic rate; body fat, by hydrostatic weighing; adipose tissue fat composition, by analysis of needle biopsy specimens from the abdominal (umbilicus-level) and femoral (midthigh-level) areas; trunk-fat mass by computed tomographic (CT) scans of abdominal and abdominal visceral areas; and anthropometric assessment that included five trunk and five limb skinfolds and waist and hip circumferences.

After baseline testing, the twins consumed a diet for 6 days a week containing 1000 kcal per day in excess of their baseline energy requirement. Daily meal composition was 50% carbohydrate, 35% lipid, and 15% protein. On day 7, subjects consumed their baseline number of calories. The men ate three meals plus an evening snack, and daily activities included reading, playing cards and video games, watching television, and walking outdoors for 30 minutes. Measurements during overfeeding included body mass (daily), skinfolds (every 5 d), and waist and hip girths (every 25 d).

The *top* figure displays average percentage changes from before to after overfeeding. Body mass increased significantly (average 8.1-kg gain), as did fat mass and FFM. However, the 111% average gain in adipose cell mass dramatically exceeded the 5% FFM increase. The sum of skinfold thickness (used to reflect change in subcutaneous fat) increased 70%, from 76 to 129 mm. Skinfold thickness increased more on the trunk (87%) than on the limbs (50%). Waist and hip girth also increased significantly. The ratio of waist girth-to-hip girth increased, indicating greater fat accretion at the waist than at the hip. Overfeeding increased adipose tissue fat mass in all subcutaneous and visceral sections estimated from CT scans.

Importantly, considerable individual differences existed for changes in body mass and body composition with overfeeding, with greater variation between twin pairs than within pairs. The *bottom* figure displays within-pair differences for the changes in body mass with equivalent excess energy intake. Each colored point represents one twin pair (*A* and *B*). The closer the points fall to the diagonal line, the more similar the twins are. The large differences between twin pairs for changes in body mass exceeded the differences within twin pairs.

A threefold difference emerged for changes in body mass, body composition, trunk fat, and visceral fat between the high and low weight gainers. This clearly indicated that surplus energy intake (with other factors controlled) did not produce similar changes in the outcome variables among twin pairs. Also, neither body mass nor body fat increases predicted visceral fat accumulation. Of clinical significance was the observation that some persons store fat more readily than others on the trunk, in the abdominal cavity, or at both areas—a fat deposition pattern with increased health risk. Bouchard hypothesized that a person's genotype determines adaptations to a sustained energy surplus. More than likely, a yet-undetermined genetic characteristic produces large individual differences in the tendency toward obesity in general and the patterning of fat on the body in particular.

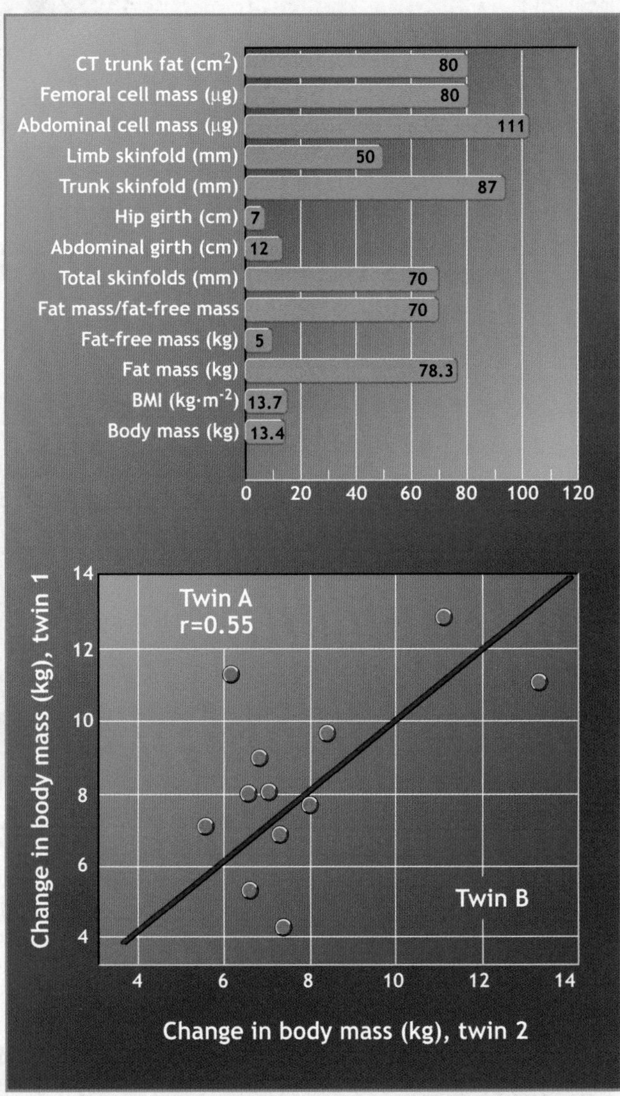

Top. Effects of 100 days of 84,000-kcal overfeeding in 12 pairs of male monozygotic twins. Values are percentage change from before to after overfeeding. *Bottom.* Similarity within twin pairs of changes in body mass in response to overfeeding.

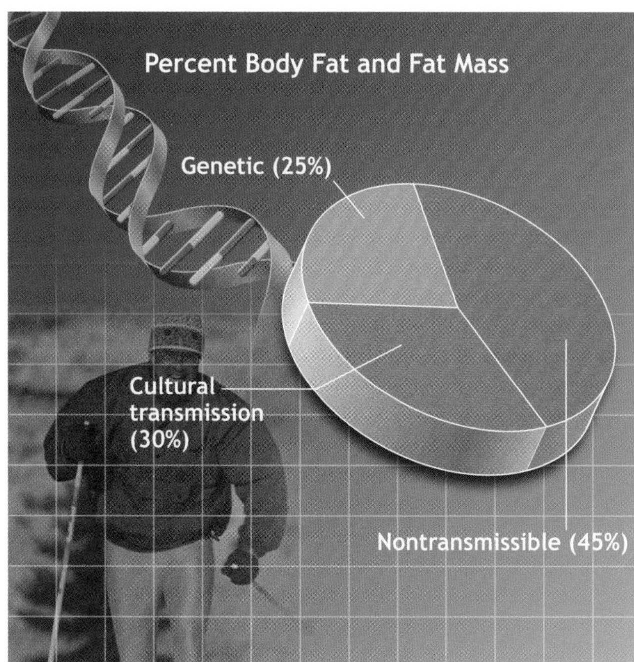

FIGURE 30.2 • Total transmissible variance for body fat. Total body fat and percentage body fat were determined by hydrostatic weighing. (From Bouchard C, et al. Inheritance of the amount and distribution of human body fat. Int J Obes 1988;12:205.)

Mutant Gene?

Studies of twins, adopted children, and specific segments of the population link genetic factors to up to 80% of the risk of becoming obese. Little risk exists for an overweight toddler to grow into an obese adult if both parents are of normal weight. But if a child under age 10, regardless of current body weight, has one or both obese parents (BMI ≥30), the child's risk of becoming an obese adult is more than twice that of the general population, and the risk increases with the severity of obesity in the biologic family members. If a first-degree relative's BMI exceeds 35, the child's obesity risk increases to three times normal; a BMI of 40 corresponds to five times the risk.

Until recently, research had not directly linked human obesity to a mutant gene.[14,174,197] Researchers at the University of Cambridge in England identified a specific defect in two genes that control body weight.[92,144] Two cousins from a Pakistani family in England inherited a defect in the gene that makes leptin (derived from the Greek root *leptos*, meaning thin), a crucial hormone in body weight regulation. Congenital absence of leptin produces continual hunger and marked obesity in these children. The second genetic defect, observed in an English patient, affected the body's response to the "signal" leptin provided. The signal largely determines how much one eats, how much energy one expends, and, ultimately, one's body weight.

Leptin

Studies with animals provide fundamental information about the genetic link to obesity and associated diseases.[53] For example, research with a strain of hybrid mice that balloon up to five times the girth of normal mice supports research that some individuals appear genetically "predestined" to become overly fat. The mutation of a gene called *obese,* or simply *ob*, may disrupt hormonal signals that regulate metabolism, fat storage, and appetite, which tips the energy balance toward body fat accumulation.[229]

The model in Figure 30.3 proposes that the *ob* gene normally becomes activated in adipose tissue (and perhaps muscle tissue), where it encodes and stimulates production of a body fat–signaling, hormonelike protein (***ob* protein**, or **leptin**), which then enters the bloodstream.[158] This satiety signal molecule travels to the ventromedial nucleus, the hypothalamic area that controls appetite and metabolism. Normally, leptin blunts

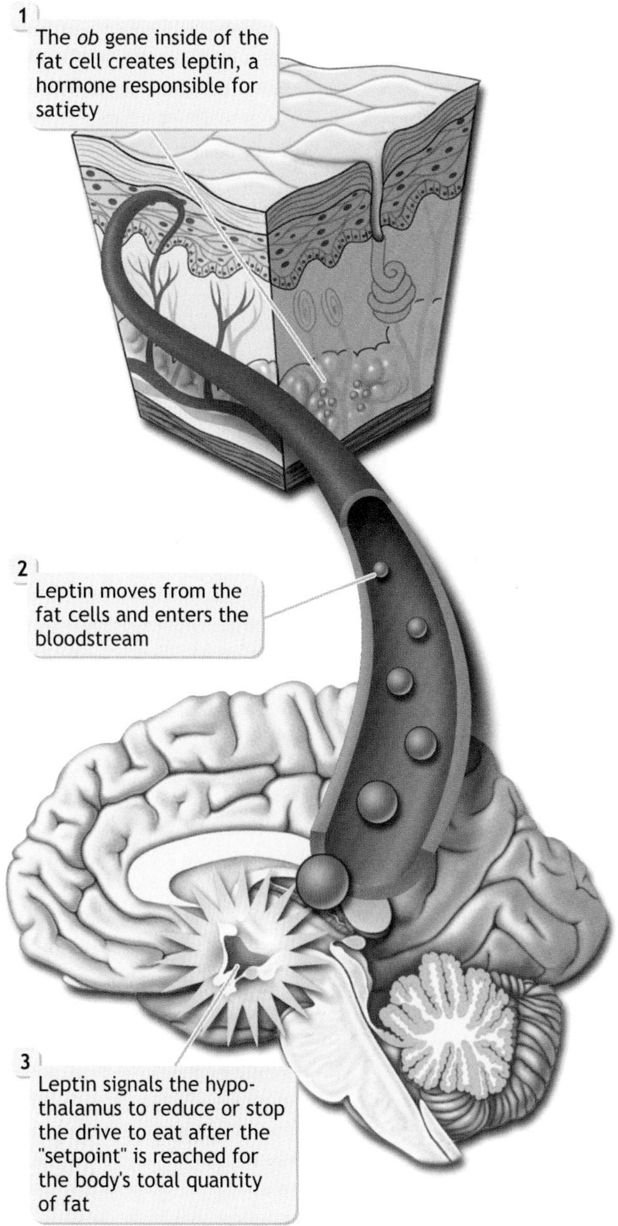

FIGURE 30.3 • A genetic model for obesity. A malfunction of the satiety gene markedly affects production of the satiety hormone leptin. This disrupts events that occur in the hypothalamus, the center responsible for adjusting the body's fat level.

the urge to eat when caloric intake maintains ideal fat stores. Leptin may affect certain neurons in the hypothalamus in a way to (1) stimulate production of chemicals that suppress appetite and/or (2) reduce the levels of brain chemicals that stimulate appetite.[117] These mechanisms would explain how body fat could remain intimately "connected" via a physiologic pathway to the brain for energy balance regulation. In a way, the adipocyte serves an endocrine-like function. With a gene defective for either adipocyte leptin production and/or hypothalamic leptin sensitivity (as probably exists in humans), the brain cannot adequately assess the body's adipose tissue status. Thus, the urge to eat remains constant.

The hormone–hypothalamic biologic control mechanism fits nicely with the set-point theory (see page 842) to explain abnormal body fat accumulation. It also helps explain the extreme difficulty the obese have in sustaining significant fat loss. In children and adults, plasma leptin circulates in direct proportion to adipose tissue mass when energy balance remains in steady state, best described by a single exponential model with four times more leptin in obese than lean subjects. Consequently, human obesity resembles a relative state of leptin resistance similar to obesity-related insulin resistance.[75,129] In fact, high blood leptin concentrations associate strongly with the combination of upper-body obesity, glucose intolerance, hypertriglyceridemia, and hypertension—core metabolic disturbances in the insulin-resistant or metabolic syndrome (see Chapter 20). This unique metabolic disturbance ultimately leads to heart disease, stroke, and type 2 diabetes.[126]

Weight loss reduces serum leptin concentration, and weight gain increases serum leptin.[109,216] Gender, hormones, pharmacologic agents, and the body's current energy requirements also affect leptin production.[31] Even without significant weight loss, a prolonged, moderate energy deficit decreases circulating leptin concentrations, which coincide inversely with hunger sensations.[102] Neither short- nor long-term exercise meaningfully affects leptin, independent of the effects of exercise on total adipose tissue mass.[45,80,155] Subcutaneous recombinant leptin injections produced dose–response relationships with body weight and body fat loss in lean and obese men and women with elevated endogenous serum leptin concentrations.[79] This suggests a potential role for leptin and related hormones in treating obesity.

The linkage of genetic and molecular abnormalities to obesity allows researchers to view overfatness as a disease instead of a psychologic flaw. Early identification of one's genetic predisposition toward obesity makes it possible to begin diet and exercise intervention before obesity sets in and fat loss becomes exceedingly difficult. Pharmaceutical companies may eventually synthesize compounds that produce satiety or affect the resting rate of fat catabolism. These chemicals would produce weight control with a smaller caloric intake and fewer feelings of hunger and deprivation that often accompany conventional diet plans. For example, daily injections of recombinant human leptin accompanied by food restriction produced significantly greater weight loss (7.1 kg) after 6 months in obese patients than dieting plus placebo treatment (1.7 lb).

The following drugs and hormonelike substances combat obesity in persons with a BMI ≥30 (or 27 for persons with comorbid conditions):

- *Present:* **Sibutramine** (brand name, Meridia) is currently approved for use by obese patients who have other risk factors as hypertension, type 2 diabetes, or dyslipidemia. It acts as a pure neurotransmitter reuptake inhibitor of norepinephrine and serotonin, thus prolonging the action of these brain chemicals that inhibit appetite, heightening the sensation of feeling full after a meal. However, it can elevate blood pressure and heart rate. Patients who took Meridia lost an average of 7 to 11 pounds more than those who dieted without the drug over a similar time period. It is used with a behavior-modification program that includes a reduced-calorie diet and increased physical activity. **Orlistat** (brand name, Xenical) blocks intestinal absorption of about 30% of ingested lipids by inhibiting fat-digesting enzymes.[36] It also reduces absorption of vitamin D and other important nutrients, so users should take controlled doses of vitamin supplements. Current drug therapy with either sibutramine or orlistat produces weight loss of about 8 to 10% of initial body weight.
- *Removed from the market:* **Fenfluramine** (sold as Pondimin) and **dexfenfluramine** (a more-effective form of fenfluramine; brand name, Redux) are appetite depressants that promote release of the neurotransmitter hormone serotonin and prevent its uptake by the hypothalamus. **Phentermine** (brand name, Ionamin) is an amphetamine-like drug that stimulates neurotransmitter norepinephrine release in the hypothalamus and interferes with breakdown of serotonin. Combinations of these drugs were marketed as **fen-phen**, a pharmacologic treatment for obesity that produced two different actions on the hypothalamus to depress appetite. On September 15, 1997, their makers withdrew fenfluramine and dexfenfluramine from the market, in response to a request by the Food and Drug Administration. Dangers included increased risk of heart valve defects (in about one-third of users) and rare but lethal primary pulmonary hypertension.[98,217] The combination appears to destroy the body's ability to control levels of serotonin in the bloodstream. Excessive serotonin damages pulmonary blood vessels and possibly the coronary vasculature.
- *In developmental stages:* **β_3-adrenergic agonists** augment daily caloric output by elevating resting metabolism and stimulating release of fatty acids from adipose tissue. **CCK-A promoter** enhances the effect of CCK-A, an intestinal hormone that may inhibit appetite.
- *In several years:* ***Ob*-protein**, a natural body protein, may reduce appetite and accelerate fat metabolism; ***ob*-receptor stimulator**, a drug that mimics appetite-suppressing effects when the *ob* protein binds to its

receptor in the brain, causing leptin receptors to work more effectively. **Neuropeptide-Y blockers** block the effect of and/or synthesis of the hypothalamic brain chemical neuropeptide-Y, which appears to stimulate appetite, control feeding behavior, and depress energy expenditure.

Leptin alone does not determine obesity or explain why some people eat whatever they want and gain little weight, while others become overfat with the same caloric intake. Besides defective leptin production, defective receptor action can increase resistance to endogenous satiety chemicals.[32] A specific gene, the uncoupling protein-2 gene *(UCP2)*, active in all human tissue adds another piece to the obesity puzzle. High activity of the *UCP2* gene activates a protein that burns excess calories as heat energy without coupling to other energy-consuming processes.[58] This **futile metabolism** blunts excess fat storage. Individual differences in gene activation and alterations in metabolic activity lend credence to the common claim "Every little bit of excess I eat turns to fat." Finding a drug that turns on the *UCP2* gene to synthesize more of the heat-generating protein could be a pharmacologic windfall for shedding excess body fat. Other newly discovered molecules that control eating include AGRP (for agouti related protein), a small protein controlled by leptin that may affect hypothalamic cells to increase caloric intake. The brain also synthesizes melanin concentrating hormone when leptin levels increase. An excess of this hypothalamic protein molecule increases an animal's appetite causing it to eat and gain weight. Drugs that inhibit the action of the brain chemicals that control eating may ultimately provide the long-term "cure" for the overfat condition.

LEPTIN, BODY COMPOSITION, AND ANOREXIA NERVOSA. Anorexia nervosa, a condition of disturbed body weight regulation at the extreme low end of the body weight spectrum, triggers a host of metabolic maladaptations, including low leptin levels that accompany reduced fat mass and undernutrition.[2,52,71] If leptin serves as a peripheral signal that regulates energy balance, then a close association should emerge between leptin (lower levels), body composition (low fat mass), and altered metabolic state (depressed BMR) in anorexia nervosa with a reversal toward normal leptin, fat mass, and BMR in rehabilitated anorectics.

Table 30.1 compares body composition, leptin levels, and different expressions of BMR in 16 anorectics (AN), 14 rehabilitated AN patients (recovery >1 y post-AN), and 22 controls.[162] Even after statistical adjustments for differences in fat mass and fat-free body mass (FFM) among groups, marked intra group differences remained in certain variables. For example, the AN subjects had significantly lower leptin concentrations (–76%) and BMRs (–21%) than control subjects. The differences persisted even after adjustment for body fat, suggesting that fat mass might not entirely govern leptin secretion. The return of leptin levels to normal in rehabilitated AN subjects suggests a reversal of energy imbalance from altered metabolism, perhaps from readaptation of previously abnormal neuroendocrine functioning. Thus, physiologic control signals operative in undernutrition probably affect the dysregulation of energy balance and neuroendocrine pathways dif-

TABLE 30.1 ➤ **BODY COMPOSITION, LEPTIN, AND BMR IN ANOREXIA NERVOSA (AN) PATIENTS, REHABILITATED AN PATIENTS, AND CONTROLS**

VARIABLE	PATIENTS WITH AN (n = 16)	REHABILITATED AN PATIENTS (n = 14)	CONTROLS (n = 22)
Age (y)	25 ±5	24 ±5	26 ±6
Weight (kg)	41.6 ±4.9	51.5 ±5.5	56.9 ±5.1
Stature (cm)	163.7 ±5.9	160.5 ±4.7	164.6 ±6.2
BMI	15.5 ±1.2	20.0 ±1.6	21.0 ±1.5
Fat mass			
Absolute (kg)	6.8 ±3.3	13.6 ±4.8	15.7 ±3.7
Relative (%)	16.1 ±6.7	26.0 ±7.3	27.4 ±4.8
Fat-free body mass			
Absolute (kg)	34.7 ±3.5	37.9 ±3.8	41.2 ±3.2
Relative (%)	83.9 ±6.7	74.0 ±7.3	72.6 ±4.8
Leptin, $\mu g \cdot L^{-1}$	1.9 ±1.5	8.4 ±10.5	7.8 ±3.0
Log leptin	0.15 ±0.35	0.75 ±0.40	0.87 ±0.14
Log leptin adjusted for body fat	0.34 ±0.34	0.71 ±0.32	0.75 ±0.32
BMR			
$kJ \cdot min^{-1}$	2.7281 ±0.3691	3.2254 ±0.4082	3.4516 ±0.3405
$kJ \cdot kg$ body $wt^{-1} \cdot min^{-1}$	0.0658 ±0.0067	0.0629 ±0.0071	0.0608 ±0.0052
$kJ \cdot kg$ $FFM^{-1} \cdot min^{-1}$	0.0789 ±0.100	0.0855 ±0.0111	0.0839 ±0.0065
Respiratory quotient	0.80 ±0.06	0.81 ±0.05	0.82 ±0.04

Values are means ± standard deviation.
Modified from Polito A, et al. Basal metabolic rate in anorexia nervosa: relation to body composition and leptin concentrations. Am J Clin Nutr 2000;71:1495.

ferently than in obesity. Poor energy balance regulation also may apply to female athletes, in whom leptin may serve as the metabolic "signal link" between energy availability, adipose tissue, and endocrine control of the reproductive axis.[203]

Influence of Racial Factors

Racial differences in food and exercise habits and cultural attitudes toward body weight help to explain the significantly greater prevalence of obesity among black women (nearly 50%) than among white women (33%). In addition, research with obese women shows that small differences in resting energy expenditure (REE) contribute to the racial differences in obesity.[61,93] On average, black women burned nearly 100 fewer calories each day during rest than their white counterparts, and the slower rate of caloric expenditure persisted even after adjusting for differences in body mass and body composition. A 100-kcal reduction in daily metabolism translates to nearly 1 pound of body fat gained each month. African-American women had a 10% lower total daily energy expenditure than whites owing to a 5% lower REE and 19% lower physical activity energy expenditure.[27] Additionally, obese African-American women had significantly greater decreases in REE than white women following energy restriction and weight loss.[62] The combination of (1) a lower initial REE and (2) more-profound blunting of REE with weight loss suggests that black women (including athletes) may experience greater difficulty achieving a goal body weight than overweight white women.

A Word of Caution

When evaluating purported racial differences in body composition characteristics and their implications, one must carefully evaluate the technologic methods to explore such differences.[212] In addition, interethnic and interracial differences in body size, structure, and fat distribution can mask true differences in body fat at a given BMI. A single, generalized BMI–health risk model would obscure the potential to document chronic disease risks among different population groups.[196] Furthermore, the nature and magnitude of the relationship between body mass or BMI and health risk may vary among racial and ethnic groups. Documenting such body composition components as FFM may also prove important, particularly when scaling racial comparisons by metabolic size.[66]

PHYSICAL INACTIVITY: A CRUCIAL COMPONENT IN EXCESSIVE FAT ACCUMULATION

Physically active lifestyles lessen the "normal" pattern of fat gain in adulthood. For young and middle-aged men who exercise regularly, the time spent in physical activity relates inversely to body fat level.[138] Middle-aged male long-distance runners remain leaner than sedentary counterparts.[224] Surprisingly, no relationship emerged between the runners' body fat level and caloric intake. Perhaps the relatively greater body fat among the middle-aged runners compared to younger runners resulted from less-vigorous training, *not* greater food intake.

From age 3 months to 1 year, the total energy expenditure of infants who later became overweight averaged 21% less than infants with normal weight gain.[176] Native Americans with low daily energy expenditure were at four times greater risk of gaining more than 7.5 kg over a 2-year period than tribal members with higher energy expenditure.[172]

Age-Related Changes in Body Composition of Adult Men and Women

Figure 30.4 shows changes in body composition in a cross section of Japanese men and women from ages 20 to 70 years. Significant declines occurred in stature and lean body mass, while all measures of adiposity increased, the most pronounced being percentage body fat in females between ages 30 and 40 and above age 50. For males, the largest body fat increase occurred from ages 20 to 40. Interestingly, abdominal girth correlated the highest with body fat percentage versus age ($r = 0.75$ for males and females), presumably because of the strong relationships among abdominal girth and intra-abdominal fat discussed in Chapter 28. Coincidentally, thigh girth decreased significantly in males (3.6 cm, 6.6%) and females (2.0 cm, 3.8%) from ages 20 to 70. The loss in thigh girth (and hence upper-leg volume) corresponds to a loss in thigh lean volume due to the diminution in muscle mass (16.1% decline in lean body mass for males and 13.9% for females) with aging. For example, the body mass of females remained essentially unchanged over a 40-year span, yet they accumulated an additional 6.2 kg of body fat (similar loss in lean tissue), a value similar to the 5.2 kg of additional fat gained by males. Males steadily declined in body mass from 66 kg during ages 20 to 29 to 62 kg from ages 60 to 70. The *bottom* of Figure 30.4 illustrates the salient features of the body size changes from loss of stature and changes in posture and girth dimensions.

Benefits of Increased Energy Output with Aging

A study of nearly 7000 male runners 18 years of age and older suggests that maintaining a lifestyle that includes a regular and constant level of endurance exercise does not fully forstall the tendency to add weight through middle age.[224] Figure 30.5 shows the strong inverse association among distance run and BMI and waist circumference in all age categories. Active men typically remained leaner than their sedentary counterparts for each age group, and the men who ran longer distances each week weighed less than those who ran shorter distances. The typical man who maintained a constant weekly running distance through middle age gained 3.3 pounds, and waist size (presumably from intra-abdominal fat) increased about three-fourths of an inch, regardless of distance run. Such findings suggest that by age 50, a physically active man can expect to weigh about 10 pounds more (with a 2-in larger waist) than he weighed at age 20, despite maintaining a constant level of increased physical activity. The

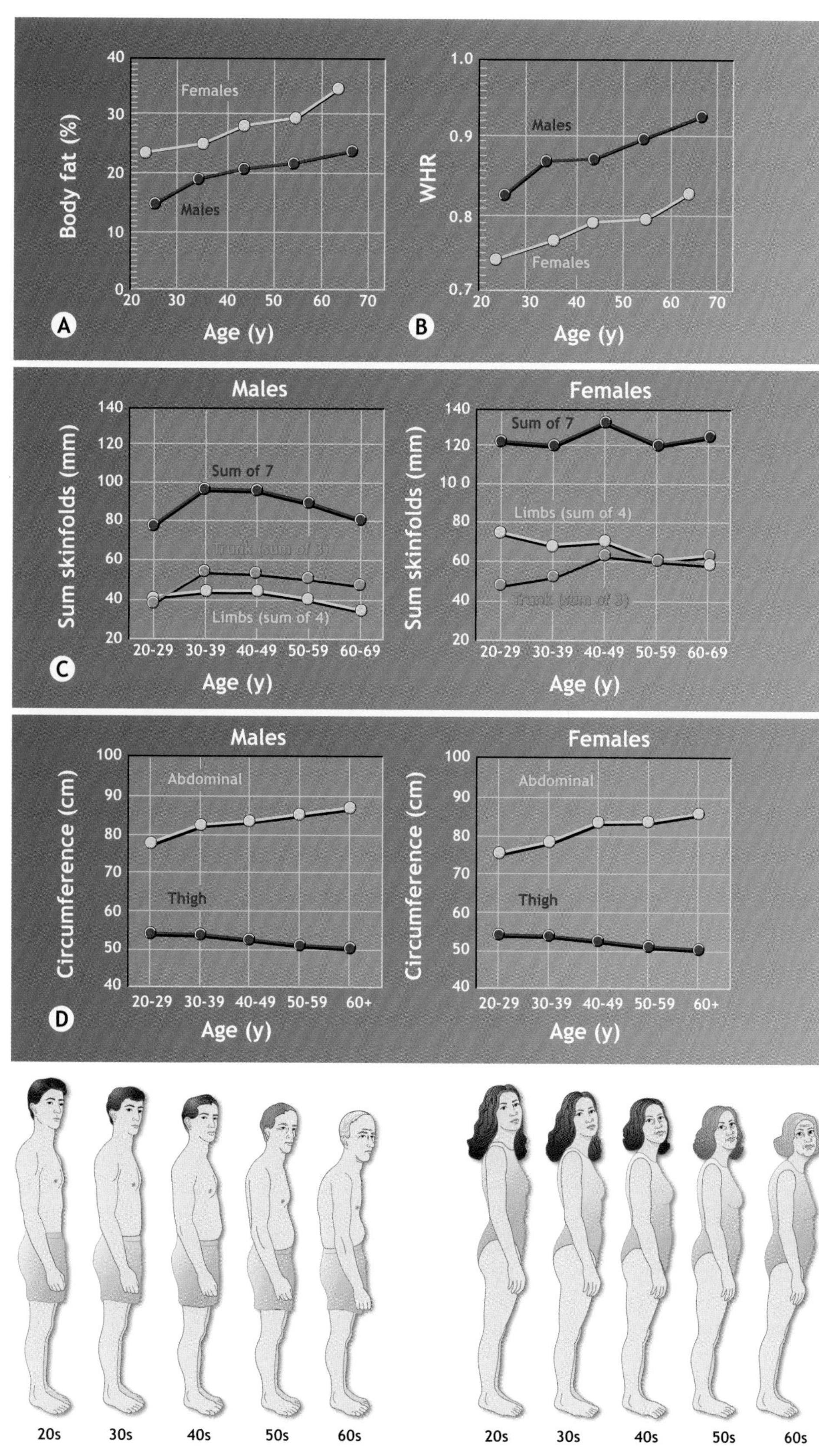

FIGURE 30.4 • Age-related changes in (**A**) percentage body fat, (**B**) waist:hip ratio (WHR), (**C**) sum of skinfolds (subscapular, midaxillary, abdominal, thigh [front and back], and (**D**) abdominal and thigh circumferences) in Japanese men and women. (Detailed data courtesy of Kayo Sakurai, Laboratory for Exercise Physiology and Biomechanics, Chukyo University, Japan. Modified from Sakurai K, et al. Age-related changes in body composition for 643 Japanese aged 20 to 75 years. Med Sci Sports Exerc 1998;30:S238.)

reasons for this proclivity to gain weight and girth remain unknown. Perhaps, reduced levels of testosterone and growth hormone induce age-related change in physique and increase abdominal and visceral fat. For women, increased testosterone levels usually link to visceral fat accumulation. To counter weight gain in middle age, the researchers advise gradually increasing the amount of weekly exercise (1.4 mi. $\cdot$ y^{-1}) starting at about age 30.

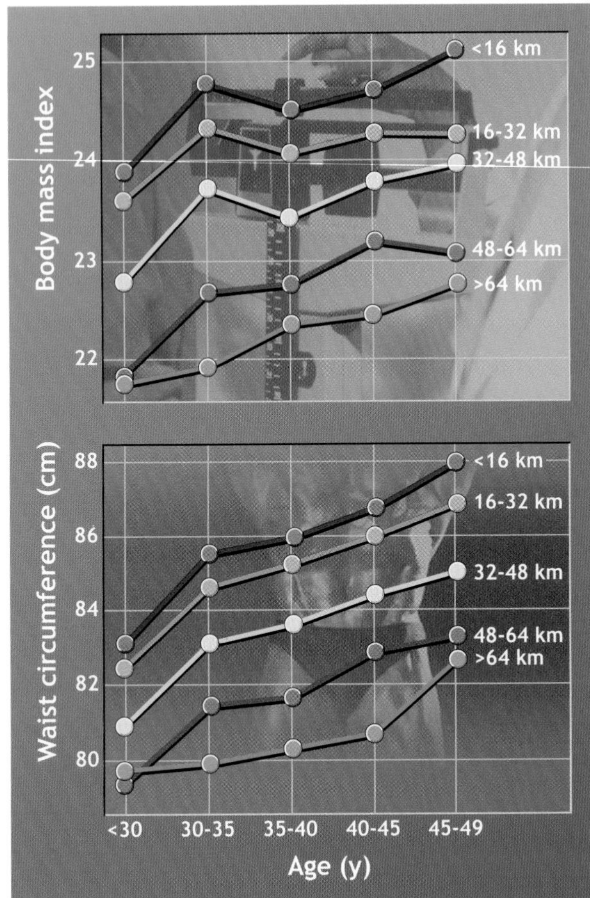

FIGURE 30.5 • Relationship among average body mass index (kg · m^{-2}) (*top*) and waist circumference (*bottom*) and age for men who maintained constant weekly running for varying distances (<16 to >64 km · wk^{-1}). Men who annually increase their running distance by 1.39 miles (2.24 km) per week compensate for the anticipated weight gain during middle age. (From Williams PT. Evidence for the incompatibility of age-neutral overweight and age-neutral physical activity standards from runners. Am J Clin Nutr 1997;65:1391.)

INTEGRATIVE QUESTION

What evidence documents that body fat accumulation among children and adults does not necessarily result from excessive food intake?

HEALTH RISKS OF EXCESSIVE BODY FAT

The June, 1998 guidelines from the National Heart, Lung and Blood Institute and the National Institute of Diabetes, Digestive and Kidney Diseases label obesity a significant societal burden owing to the association between high levels of body weight and body fat with increased risk for adverse health consequences. Obesity is the second leading cause of preventable death in America (cigarette smoking is first). The estimated number of annual deaths attributed to obesity ranges between 280,000 and 325,000, with the higher estimate of premature death for current nonsmokers and never-smokers.[4,24] Hypertension, elevated blood sugar, postmenopausal breast cancer, and elevated total cholesterol and low high-density lipoprotein (HDL)-cholesterol levels heighten an overweight (BMI = 25.0 to 29.9) individual's risks of poor health at any given level of excess weight. In fact, an increasing prevalence of obesity appears to have blunted the previous decline over previous years in coronary disease incidence among middle-aged women.[87] Obese people (BMI ≥30.0) and overweight individuals with two or more heart disease risk factors should reduce weight, while overweight persons without any other risk factors should at least maintain current body weight.

Improved physical fitness interacts with the overfat condition to lower disease risk. For example, nearly 20,000 men age 30 to 83 years who were overweight but physically fit suffered fewer deaths from all causes than unfit but normal weight men.[124] Furthermore, unfit, lean men show a higher risk of all-cause mortality than overfat, fit men.[123] *Such findings support emphasizing increasing physical activity to improve cardiovascular fitness of overweight men and women rather than relying solely on diet to improve the health risk profile.*

Despite the current obesity epidemic, weight control remains low on the list of national public health priorities; it receives far less funding from the National Institutes of Health (NIH) than other widely prevalent diseases.[81,91] Figure 30.6 shows that the economic cost of obesity-related medical problems in the United States was $51.6 billion in 1995—about 7.2% of the $715 billion cost of total illness. Estimated current total health-care costs have risen to nearly $100 billion, or about 10% of the more than $1 trillion dollar cost of remaining ill! Use of health-care resources also increases proportionately with excess body fat.[168] Clearly, maintaining a lean body composition throughout life reduces risk for multiple diseases. Whether weight loss by an already overweight or obese adult reduces health risk to the level of individuals who never gained weight in the first place remains unclear.[99,228] Research must also determine if increased death risk with obesity declines at all levels of obesity as individuals age.[12,24,145]

An Economic Burden for Mature Women

The economic cost to women of obesity is high and that cost continues to increase as a person ages. Researchers at the Institute for Social Research at the University of Michigan (University of Michigan Health & Retirement Study, Ann Arbor, MI) studied the wealth consequences for obese and non-obese women and men between 1992 and 1998. Individual net worth of a moderate to severely obese woman was about 40% less than that of her normal-weight counterpart, even after controlling for health, marital status, and other demographic factors. By 1998, however, an obese woman between ages 57 and 67 reported an individual net worth of about 60% less ($135,670) than her non-obese peer. No significant differences emerged in comparisons among men. Speculation maintains that women are impacted to a greater extent than men by cultural norms of attractiveness, which stigmatize obese women in diverse ways.

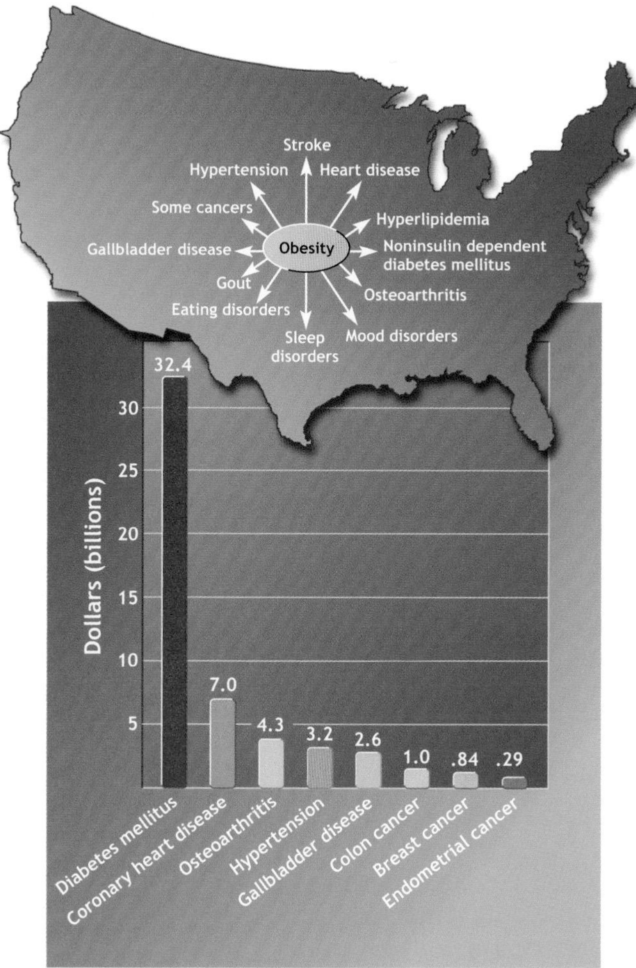

FIGURE 30.6 • Economic cost of major obesity-related illnesses in the United States. (Modified from data in Wolf AM, Colditz GA. Current estimates of the economic costs of obesity. Obes Res 1998;6:97.)

Excessive Fatness in Childhood and Adolescence Predicts Adverse Health Effects in Adulthood

The origin of adult obesity and its adverse health consequences often begins in childhood.[43] Children who gain more weight than peers tend to become overweight adults with increased risk for hypertension, elevated insulin, hypercholesterolemia, and heart disease.[192] Being overweight during adolescence links to adverse health effects 55 years later. The Harvard Growth Study from 1922 to 1935 evaluated 3000 school children annually on a variety of health variables, including triplicate measures of body stature and mass at the same time each year until they left or graduated high school.[37] Of the initial group, the researchers studied 1857 subjects for an additional 8 years. Subjects received designations as either lean (in the 25th to 50th percentile for BMI) or overweight (exceeding 75th percentile for BMI). Compared with leaner subjects, the overweight children as adults showed an overall greater risk of mortality from all causes and a twofold higher coronary heart disease risk. Women overweight in adolescence were eight times more likely to report problems with personal care and routine living tasks (walking, stair climbing, lifting, and a 1.6-fold increase in arthritis) than women rated lean in adolescence.

The alarming rise in obesity during childhood and adolescence requires immediate interventions to prevent subsequent increase in risk for diseases and death as these children become adults. Figure 30.7 shows the percentile cutoffs for a two-level procedure recommended by the American Academy of Pediatrics. BMI classifies young patients as either overweight (BMI >95th percentile; requires in-depth medical assessment) or at risk of becoming overweight (BMI 85th to 95th percentile; requires second-level screening, including family history and risk factor assessment).

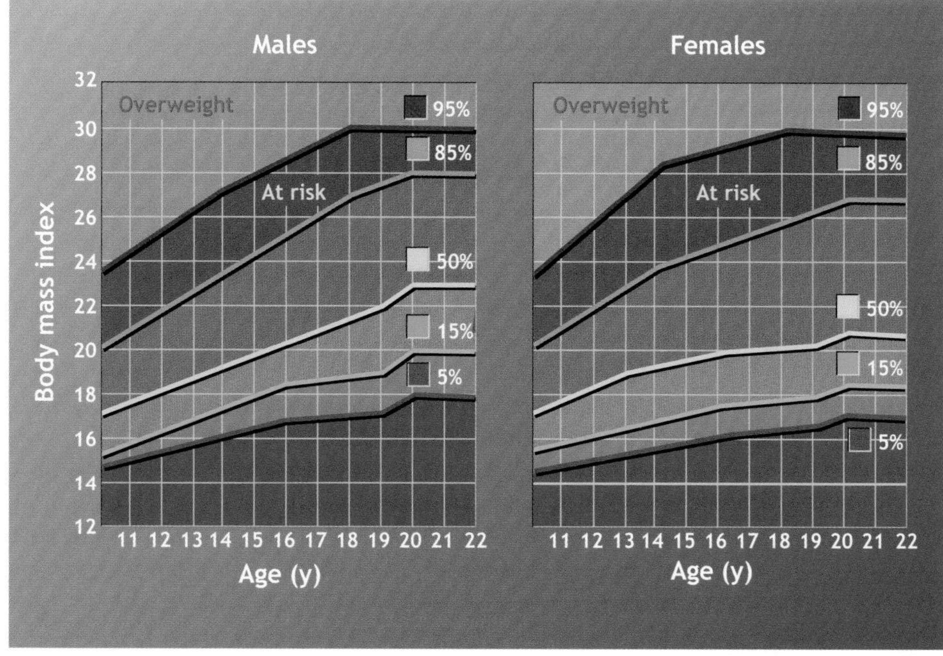

FIGURE 30.7 • Two-level procedure using BMI to identify overweight adolescents and adolescents at risk of becoming overweight. (From Green M, ed. Bright futures: guidelines for health supervision of infants, children and adolescents. Arlington, VA: National Center for Education in Maternal and Child Health, 1994.)

Specific Risks

Considerable information exists regarding increasing levels of body fat and specific health risks in children, adolescents, and adults. Excessive body fat relates closely to the alarming increase in type 2 diabetes among children. For adult diabetics, 70% classify as overweight, and nearly 35% are obese. An NIH report concludes that obesity represents a chronic, degenerative disease, because of multiple biologic hazards for premature illness and death at surprisingly low levels of excess fat.[146] A moderate 4 to 10% increase in body weight after age 20 associates with 1.5 greater risk of death from coronary artery disease and nonfatal myocardial infarction.[180] Even maintaining body weight at the high end of the normal range significantly increases heart disease and cancer risk.[132,222] An 8-year study of nearly 116,000 female nurses observed that all but the thinnest women showed increased risk for heart attack and chest pains.[131] Nurses of average weight experienced 30% more heart attacks than their thinnest counterparts, while the risk for a moderately overweight nurse averaged 80% higher. This means that a woman who gains 9 kg from her late teens to middle age doubles her heart attack risk. A convincing argument maintains that obesity represents an independent and powerful heart disease risk, equal to cigarette smoking, elevated blood lipids, and hypertension. Preliminary findings also indicate that obesity increases risk for low-grade inflammation of the inner lining of arterial vessels. In apparently healthy individuals, arterial wall inflammation can progress unnoticed for years, increasing the individual's risk for heart attack and stroke.

A 16-year follow-up study of the nurses shows that even moderate weight gain after age 18 can prove deadly.[132] One-half of cardiovascular deaths and one-third of colon, endometrial, and breast cancer deaths linked to the overweight condition. Women 30% or more above their desirable body weight showed a fourfold greater chance of dying from heart disease and a twofold greater cancer death risk than age-matched women of below-average body weight. *Such statistics indicate that obesity will soon surpass cigarette smoking as the leading cause of death in the United States.*

Researchers followed a cohort of 82,000 female nurses ages 30 to 55 years every 2 years from 1976 to determine if initial BMI modifies the relation between long-term weight gain or weight loss and hypertension risk.[88] Figure 30.8 depicts the relative risk for hypertension, adjusted for multiple factors linked to hypertension, in three groups stratified for BMI at age 18. For women in the first and second BMI tertiles at age 18 (BMI <22.0), weight loss in later years did not reduce risk for hypertension. Weight gain after age 18 markedly increased hypertension risk compared with women who maintained a stable body weight. In contrast, for women whose BMI exceeded 22.0, subsequent weight loss dramatically decreased risk (relative risk of 0.72 for weight loss of 5.0 to 9.9 kg and 0.57 for loss of 10 kg or more). Weight gain significantly increased hypertension risk in a manner similar to the lighter group of women.

A 5 to 10% weight loss often normalizes an obese person's serum cholesterol and triglyceride levels and reduces blood pressure and overall heart disease risk, including risk of congestive heart failure. The tendency to gain weight with age partially explains the relationship between age and blood pressure. After accounting for cigarette smoking and current disease status, the 27-year study of Harvard alumni showed that men with a body weight 20% or more above "desirable weight" experienced a 2.5 times greater death rate than the leanest men.[123] At all ages, the leanest men showed the least likelihood of dying. In June 1998, the American Heart Association upgraded obesity—on a par with high cholesterol, hypertension, cigarette smoking, and a sedentary lifestyle—to a *major* heart attack risk factor from its former status as a *contributing* risk factor.

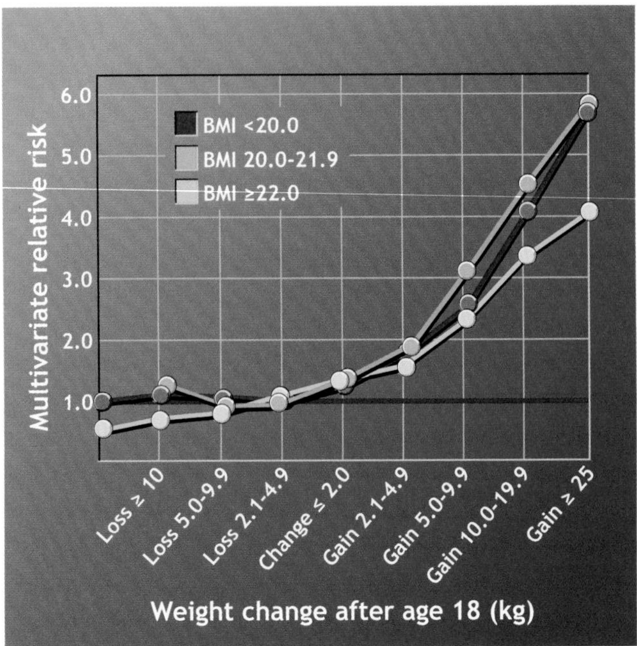

FIGURE 30.8 • Multivariate relative risk for hypertension according to weight change after age 18 years within strata of BMI at age 18. Risk adjusted for: age, BMI at age 18, stature, family history of myocardial infarction, parity, oral contraceptive use, menopausal status, postmenopausal use of hormones, and smoking status. Horizontal red line indicates normal risk. (From Huang Z, et al. Body weight, weight change, and risk for hypertension in women. Ann Intern Med 1998;128:81.)

SPECIFIC HEALTH RISKS OF EXCESSIVE BODY FAT

- Impaired cardiac function from increased mechanical work and autonomic and left ventricular dysfunction
- Hypertension, stroke, and deep-vein thrombosis
- Increased insulin resistance in children and adults and type 2 diabetes (80% of these patients are overweight)
- Renal disease
- Sleep apnea, mechanical ventilatory constraints (particularly in exercise), and pulmonary disease from impaired function because of added effort to move the chest wall
- Problems receiving anesthetics during surgery
- Osteoarthritis, degenerative joint disease, and gout
- Endometrial, breast, prostate, and colon cancers
- Abnormal plasma lipid and lipoprotein levels
- Menstrual irregularities
- Gallbladder disease
- Enormous psychologic burden and social stigmatization and discrimination

CRITERIA FOR EXCESSIVE BODY FAT: HOW FAT IS TOO FAT?

In Chapter 28, we discussed limitations of the height–weight tables and BMI to assess body composition. Three more-appropriate approaches measure a person's fat content:

- Percentage of body mass composed of fat (%body fat)
- Distribution or patterning of fat at different anatomic regions
- Size and number of individual fat cells

Percentage Body Fat

What determines the demarcation between a normal level of body fat and excess? In Chapter 28, we suggested a "normal" body fat range for adult men and women—the "average" percentage body fat value plus or minus one standard deviation. For men and women ages 17 to 50 years, this variation equals 5% body fat units. Using this statistical boundary, overfatness then corresponds to a body fat level that exceeds the average value plus 5% body fat. For example, in young men whose body fat averages 15% of body mass, the borderline for obesity becomes 20% body fat. For older men whose fat averages 25%, obesity is body fat in excess of 30%. For young women, obesity corresponds to body fat content above 30%; for older women, borderline obesity corresponds to about 37% body fat. We emphasize, however, that just because the average value for percentage body fat increases with age, this does *not* dictate that people get fatter as they age. In our opinion, one criterion for determining "too fat" emerges from data for younger men and women—above 20% for men and above 30% for women. With this single gender-specific standard, average age-related population values do not become the reference standard and thus acceptable. We also recognize that this proposed classification standard based on an average for young adults becomes extremely rigorous when applied to the entire population. It probably places 50% of adults in the overly fat category. Interestingly, this comes remarkably close to the data for overweight Americans presented in Figure 30.1, based on the currently recommended overweight classification (i.e., BMI ≥25). It also closely corresponds to preliminary proposed gender-based body fat standards recently computed for young adults from the relationship between BMI and four component estimates of percentage body fat for African Americans and whites.[65]

STANDARDS FOR OVERFATNESS

Men—above 20%; Women—above 30%

We consider that obesity exists along a continuum from the upper limit of normal (20% body fat for men and 30% for women) to as high as 50% and a theoretical maximum of nearly 70% of body mass in the massively obese. This latter group's weight ranges from 170 to 250 kg or higher. In this situation, body fat often exceeds lean body mass, creating a life-threatening situation.

TABLE 30.2 ➤ PERCENTILE RANKINGS FOR TRICEPS SKINFOLDS IN BOYS AND GIRLS AGES 6 TO 18 YEARS

	Percentile			
Age	15th	50th	85th	95th
Boys				
6	6.2	8.4	11.1	14.1
8	6.1	8.8	13.7	17.2
10	6.0	9.1	16.0	20.7
12	5.8	9.4	17.3	23.3
14	5.6	8.9	16.4	23.5
16	5.5	8.5	15.8	21.5
18	5.6	8.5	16.6	21.8
Girls				
6	6.8	10.1	13.4	15.6
8	7.6	11.4	16.4	20.2
10	8.4	12.7	19.0	24.4
12	9.3	14.1	21.3	28.0
14	10.4	15.5	23.3	30.9
16	11.3	26.6	25.1	33.2
18	11.7	17.0	25.8	33.8

From Must J, et al. Reference data for obesity: 85th and 95th percentiles of body mass index (wt/ht^2) and triceps skinfolds. Am J Clin Nutr 1991;53:89.

Criterion for Children

Skinfold measures can broadly assess a child's excess fat in light of the limitations of whole body density for growing children and adolescents discussed in Chapter 28. Table 30.2 presents percentile rankings for triceps skinfolds for boys and girls ages 6 to 18. Generally, a skinfold at or above the 85th percentile raises concern about the child's energy balance and excessive body fatness.

Regional Fat Distribution

The patterning of the body's adipose tissue, independent of total body fat, alters health risks from obesity in children, adolescents, and adults.[56,63,152] Figure 30.9 shows two types of regional fat distribution. The increased health risk from fat deposition in the abdominal area (**central** or **android-type obesity**), particularly internal visceral deposits, may result from this tissue's lively lipolysis with catecholamine stimulation. Fat stored in this area shows greater metabolic responsiveness than fat in the gluteal and femoral regions (**peripheral** or **gynoid-type obesity**). Such increases in central fat more readily support processes that cause heart disease.[194] For men, the percentage of visceral fat increases progressively with age, whereas women begin increasing this fat deposition at the onset of menopause.[111]

Central fat deposition, independent of fat storage in other anatomic areas, reflects an altered metabolic profile. It increases risk for hyperinsulinemia (insulin resistance) and glucose intolerance, type 2 diabetes, endometrial cancer, hypertriglyceridemia, hypercholesterolemia and a negatively altered lipoprotein profile, hypertension, and atherosclerosis.[89] More specifically, ratios of waist:hip girth that exceed 0.80 for women and 0.95 for men relate to increased risk of death, even after adjusting for BMI.[41,60,173,223] Excess weight distri-

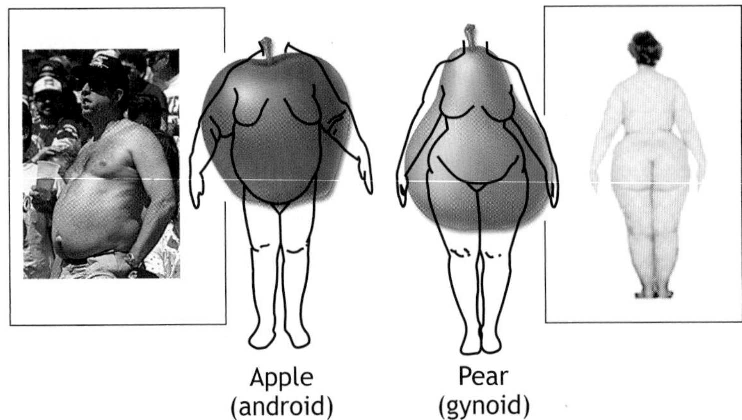

The Waist-to-Hip Ratio

- Waist at navel while standing relaxed, not pulling in stomach
- Hips, over the buttocks where girth is largest
- Divide waist girth by hip girth measure

Ratio for significant health risk
Males: >0.95
Females: >0.80

FIGURE 30.9 • Male (android-pattern) and female (gynoid-pattern) fat patterning, including the waist-to-hip girth ratio threshold for significant health risk.

bution in the abdominal area (and accompanying high blood insulin levels) also increases colorectal cancer risk. For example, when waist girth exceeded 91 cm (36 in) in men and 82 cm (32 in) women, risk was nearly twice that of smaller-girth individuals of similar age and gender.[186]

For children and adolescents, central body fat distribution associates with higher blood cholesterol, triglyceride, and insulin levels and lower HDL-cholesterol in addition to higher blood pressure and increased left ventricular wall thickness.[35,63]

Many clinicians measure waist girth before and during weight loss as a simple gauge of abdominal obesity and to complement information on body fat for individuals in the normal-weight range.[55] *In fact, waist girth alone relates more strongly to direct measures of abdominal visceral adipose tissue accumulation and other heart disease risks than waist:hip ratio.* Women whose waist measurement exceeds 76.2 cm (30 in) have twice the coronary heart disease risk of slimmer counterparts. Table 30.3 presents classification guidelines and associated disease

TABLE 30.3 ➤ CLASSIFICATION OF OVERWEIGHT AND OBESITY BY BMI, WAIST CIRCUMFERENCE, AND ASSOCIATED DISEASE RISK

		Disease Risk[a] Relative to Normal Weight and Normal Waist Circumference	
	BMI, kg · m^{-2}	Men: ≤ 102 cm Women: ≤ 88 cm	Men: > 102 cm Women: > 88 cm
Underweight	<18.5	NR	NR
Normal[b]	18.5–24.9	NR	NR
Overweight	25.0–29.9	Increased	High
Obesity, class			
I	30.0–34.9	High	Very high
II	35.0–39.9	Very high	Very high
III (extreme obesity)	≥40	Extremely high	Extremely high

[a]Disease risk for type 2 diabetes, hypertension, and cardiovascular disease. NR indicates no risk assigned at these BMI levels.
[b]Increased waist circumference can indicate increased risk even in persons of normal weight.
From Executive summary of the clinical guidelines on the identification, evaluation, and treatment of overweight and obesity in adults. Arch Intern Med 1998;158:1855.

risk for overweight and obesity based on BMI or waist girth. *Men with a 102 cm (40-in) or larger waist and women with waist girth larger than 86 cm (35 in) maintain a high risk for various diseases.*

Lipoprotein Lipase Affects Body Fat Distribution

To some extent, genetic characteristics determine one's fat distribution pattern, governed by the regional activity of **lipoprotein lipase (LPL)**.[157] This rate-limiting enzyme facilitates triglyceride uptake and storage by fat cells (**adipocytes**). Variations in LPL activity contribute not only to interindividual differences in fat distribution, but likely affect changes in fat distribution in pregnancy and middle age and may cause less visceral adipose tissue accumulation in blacks than in whites.[33] The significant gender difference in total body fat and pattern of fat distribution also relates to LPL variations; adipocytes in the hip, thigh, and breast regions produce considerable LPL in females, while in males, abdominal adipocytes show greater LPL activity.

Varieties of Human Obesity

Despite current obesity standards, distinguishing the gradations and variations in human obesity extremes remains difficult. Some approaches describe obesity types on the basis of the amount, distribution, and texture of adipose tissue. A classification schema permits quantification of the phenotype; it also appraises different hormonal and biochemical correlates of each obesity type. Unfortunately, many of the terms for describing different levels of obesity—massive, morbid, severe, extreme, gross, super, highly, excessive—do not clearly delineate the magnitude of the condition. To reduce confusion, we use the term **clinically severe obesity** to denote the condition in which total body fat exceeds 3 standard deviations above the average value for percentage body fat. This body fat level (30% men, 40% women) corresponds to a BMI of about 40 ("very high" category in Fig. 28.1).

Figure 30.10 presents six phenotypic patterns observed in female obesity (comparable data are unavailable for males). In addition, the photographic insets complement several of the outline patterns and show examples of clinically

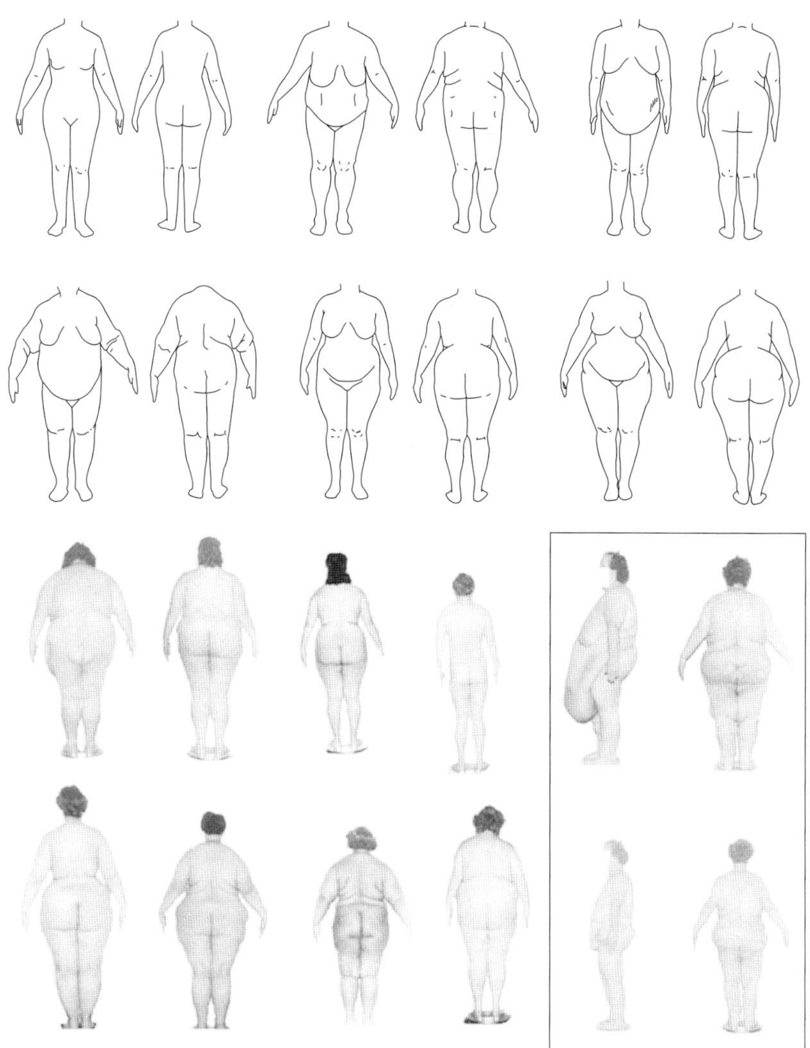

FIGURE 30.10. • Variations in human obesity. Patterns of female body form illustrate the varieties of human obesity. The photographs show examples of body patterns, including intractable obesity in which the abdominal panniculus weighed more than 35 kg before weight loss (*framed lower-right panel*). (Photographs and outline patterns courtesy of Leela S. Craig, M.D.)

severe obesity. The framed panel at *bottom right* shows the effects of a 35-kg weight loss over 15 months by a 49-year-old woman. Most of the weight lost came from the large abdominal panniculus that surgeons partially removed. Interestingly, even with a relatively large decrease in overall body mass, the phenotypic pattern remains relatively invariant.

Adipocyte Size and Number: Hypertrophy Versus Hyperplasia

Adipocyte size and number provide another means to assess and classify obesity. Adipose tissue mass increases in two ways:

1. Existing adipocytes enlarge or fill with fat (**fat cell hypertrophy**)
2. Total adipocyte number increases (**fat cell hyperplasia**)

One technique for studying adipose cellularity involves sucking small fragments of subcutaneous tissue (usually from the triceps, subscapular, buttocks, and/or lower abdomen) into a syringe through a needle inserted directly into the fat depot. Chemical treatment of the tissue sample isolates the individual adipocytes for counting. Dividing fat mass in the sample by adipocyte number determines the average quantity of fat per cell. One can estimate total adipocyte number by determining total body fat by a criterion method such as hydrostatic weighing. For example, an individual who weighs 88 kg with 13% body fat has a total fat mass of 11.4 kg (0.13 × 88 kg). Dividing 11.4 kg by the average fat content per cell estimates total adipocyte number. If the average adipocyte contains 0.60 μg of fat, then this person's body contains 19 billion adipocytes (11.4 kg ÷ 0.60 μg).

Total adipocyte number = Mass of body fat ÷ Fat content per cell

In one of our laboratories, needle biopsy and photomicrographic techniques extracted fat and measured the average fat content of adipocytes at three anatomic sites. Figure 30.11 shows adipocytes from the upper buttocks of one of this textbook's authors whose total fat mass at the time equaled 17.02 kg (body mass, 89.1 kg; 19.1% body fat) with 0.73 μg of fat per cell; the estimated total adipocyte number was 23.3 billion (17.02 kg ÷ 0.73 μg).

Cellularity Differences Between Nonobese and Obese Persons

Figure 30.12 compares body mass, total fat, and adipose tissue cellularity in 25 subjects, 20 of whom classified as clinically obese. The body mass of the obese averaged more than twice that of the nonobese, and they had nearly three times more body fat. For cellularity, adipocytes in the obese averaged 50% larger, with nearly three times more cells (75 vs. 27 billion). *These data illustrate that cell number represents the major structural difference in adipose tissue mass between the clinically severe obese and nonobese.*

Relating total body fat content to both cell size and cell number further demonstrates the contribution of adipocyte number to obesity. As body fat increases, adipocytes eventually reach some biologic upper limit. Once this occurs, cell number becomes the key factor determining any further obesity. Even a doubling of adipocyte size does not explain the large difference in total fat mass between the obese and average person. For comparison, an average-sized person has between 25 and 30 billion adipocytes, whereas the clinically severe obese may have more than three to five times this number when obesity occurs in childhood or adolescence.

Effects of Weight Loss

Figure 30.13 shows results of a classic study of weight loss effects on adipose tissue characteristics of 19 obese adults during two stages of weight loss. During the first stage they

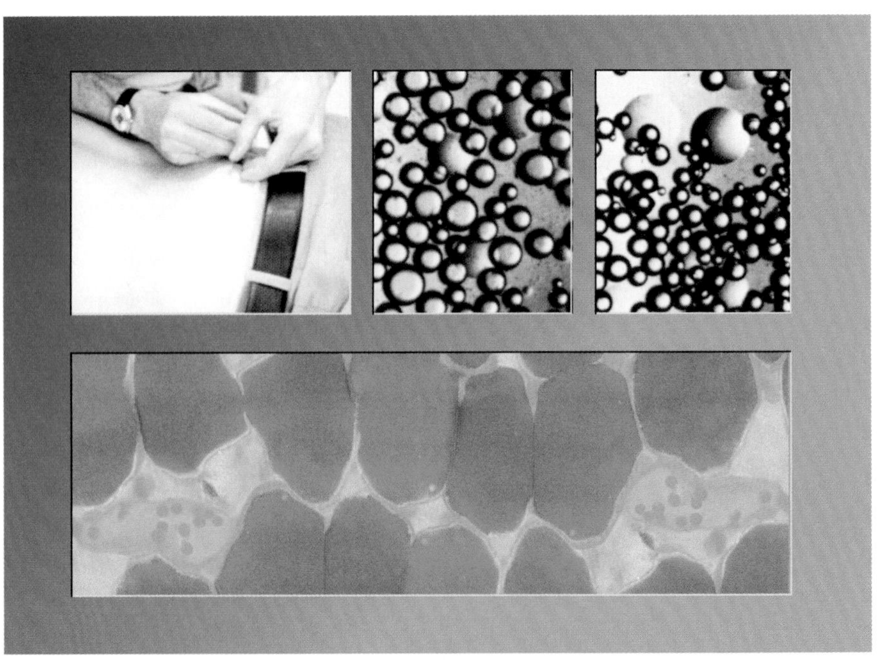

FIGURE 30.11 • (*Upper panel*) Needle biopsy to extract adipocytes from the upper buttocks. The area is sterilized and anesthetized, and the biopsy needle is placed beneath the skin surface. Photomicrographs of the adipocytes from the buttocks of a physically active professor before (*center*) and after (*right*) 6 months of marathon training. Adipocyte diameter averaged 8.6% smaller after training. The average volume of fat in each cell decreased by 18.2%. The large spherical structures in the background are lipid droplets. *Bottom panel.* Cross section of human adipocytes × 440. (From Geneser F. Color atlas of histology. Philadelphia: Lea & Febiger, 1985. Top panel photomicrographs courtesy of P. M. Clarkson, Muscle Biochemistry Laboratory, Exercise Science Department, University of Massachusetts, Amherst, MA.)

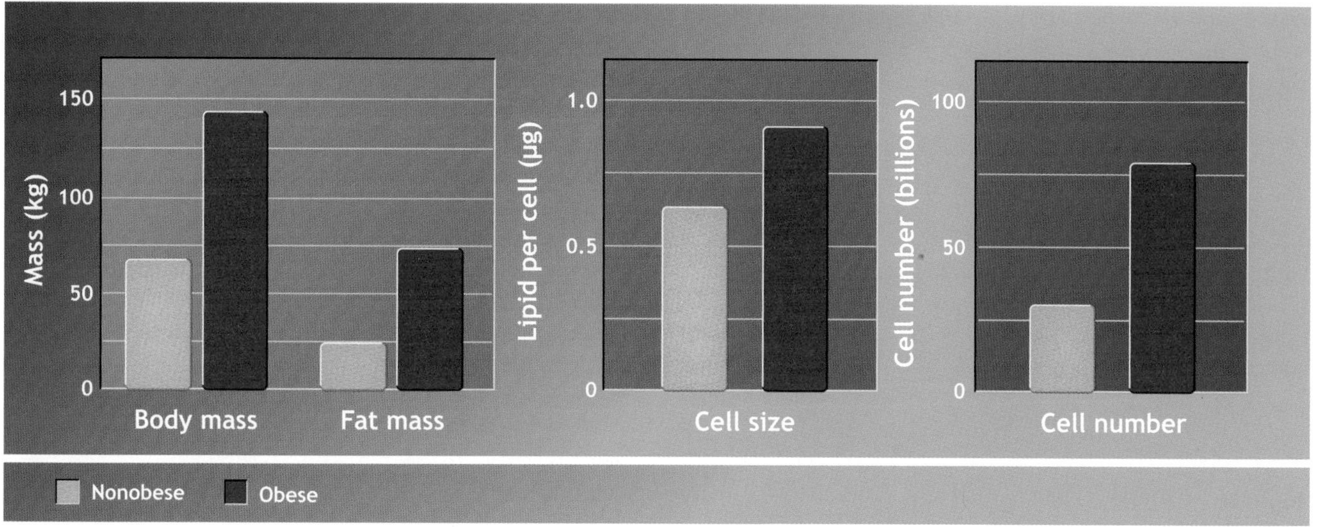

FIGURE 30.12 • Comparison of body mass, total fat mass, and adipocyte size and number in obese and nonobese subjects. (Modified from Hirsch J, Knittle J. Cellularity of obese and non-obese human adipose tissue. Fed Proc 1970;29:1518.)

reduced body mass by 46 kg (149 to 103 kg). Adipocyte number before weight reduction averaged 75 billion; this remained unchanged, even after the 46-kg reduction. Adipocyte size, on the other hand, decreased by 33% from 0.9 to 0.6 μg of lipid per cell. When subjects attained normal body mass of 75 kg by losing an additional 28 kg, cell number still remained unchanged, but cell size continued to shrink to about one-third that in a nonobese comparison group. When the patients achieved a "normal" body mass and body fat level, their adipocytes had become considerably smaller than those of the nonobese. *In adults, the major change in adipose cellularity following weight loss is shrinkage of adipocytes with no*

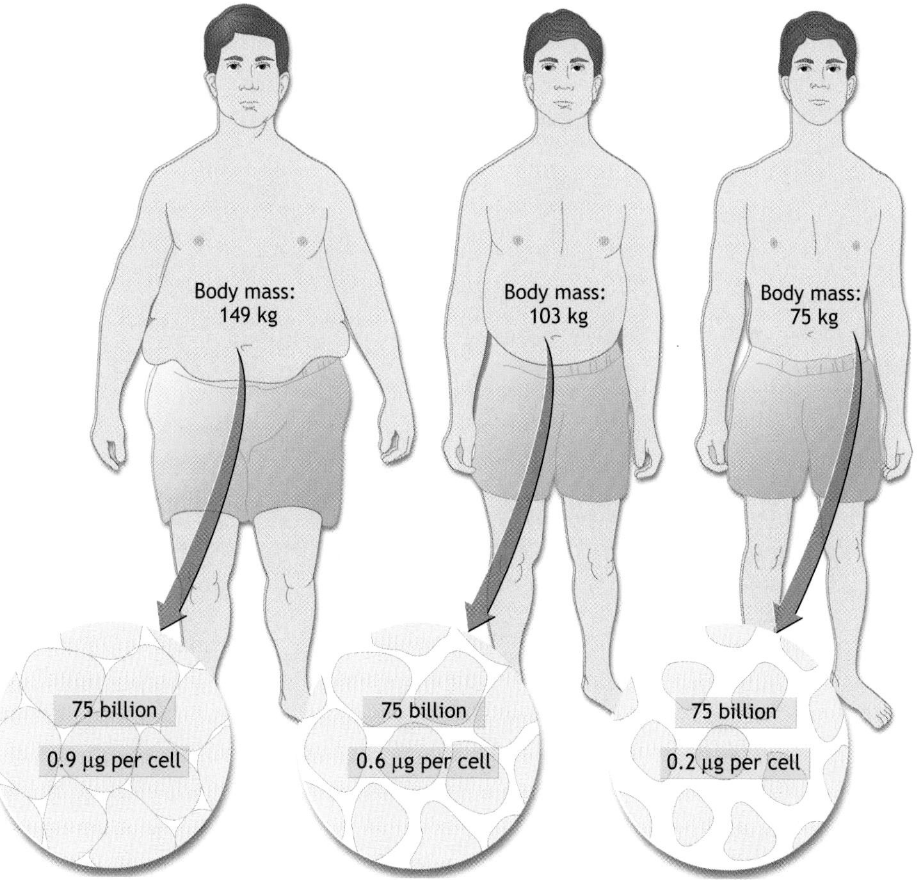

FIGURE 30.13 • Changes in adipose cellularity with weight reduction in obese subjects. (Data from Hirsch J. Adipose cellularity in relation to human obesity. In: Stollerman GH, ed. Advances in internal medicine, vol 17. Chicago: Year-Book, 1971.)

change in cell number. These findings suggest that significant weight loss in obese persons does not really "cure" their obesity, at least in terms of total adipocyte number.

Effects of Weight Gain

An interesting series of studies in the late 1960s and early 1970s evaluated the dynamics of weight gain. In one study, adult male volunteers with an initial average body fat content of 15% deliberately increased daily caloric intake by three times normal to about 7000 kcal for 40 weeks.[193] For a typical subject, body mass increased 25% and percentage body fat nearly doubled from 14.6 to 28.2%. Fat deposition represented 10.5 kg of the 12.7 kg of weight gained during the overfeeding period. In a similar experiment with subjects with no personal or family history of obesity, voluntary overeating increased body mass by 16.4 kg.[183] Comparing cell size and number before and after both of these experiments, the average adipocyte increased substantially in size with *no change* in cell number. When caloric intake decreased and subjects attained normal weight, total body fat declined, and the adipocytes reverted to their original size. *In general, moderate weight gain from overeating in adults causes existing adipocytes to enlarge rather than new adipocytes to develop.*

POSSIBILITY THAT NEW ADIPOCYTES FORM. Extreme accumulation of body fat in adults may stimulate increases in adipose cellularity because adipocyte size may reach an upper limit (probably about 1.0 μg fat), beyond which no further hypertrophy occurs. At extremes of obesity (70% body fat; 170% or more above normal weight), almost all adipocytes attain their hypertrophic limit. In this situation, the preadipocyte pool provides additional adipocytes to increase cell number. *In maturity-onset severe obesity, in which the already obese adult gains even more body fat, hypercellularity may accompany the greatly increasing size of existing adipocytes.*[83] The increased number of cells at this point constitutes a failure of adipocyte regulation that unfortunately leads to further body fat accumulation.

Adipocyte Development

Animal and human research provides important information on adipose tissue growth and development.

Animal Studies

Extensive studies exist on adipose cellularity in rats because these mammals live a relatively short time, enabling researchers to study diet and exercise regimens during important stages of the growth cycle. Figure 30.14 illustrates the general upward trend for body mass, fat mass, and adipocyte size and number in rats during the first 5 months of life. Note that cell number and cell size increase during weeks 6 through

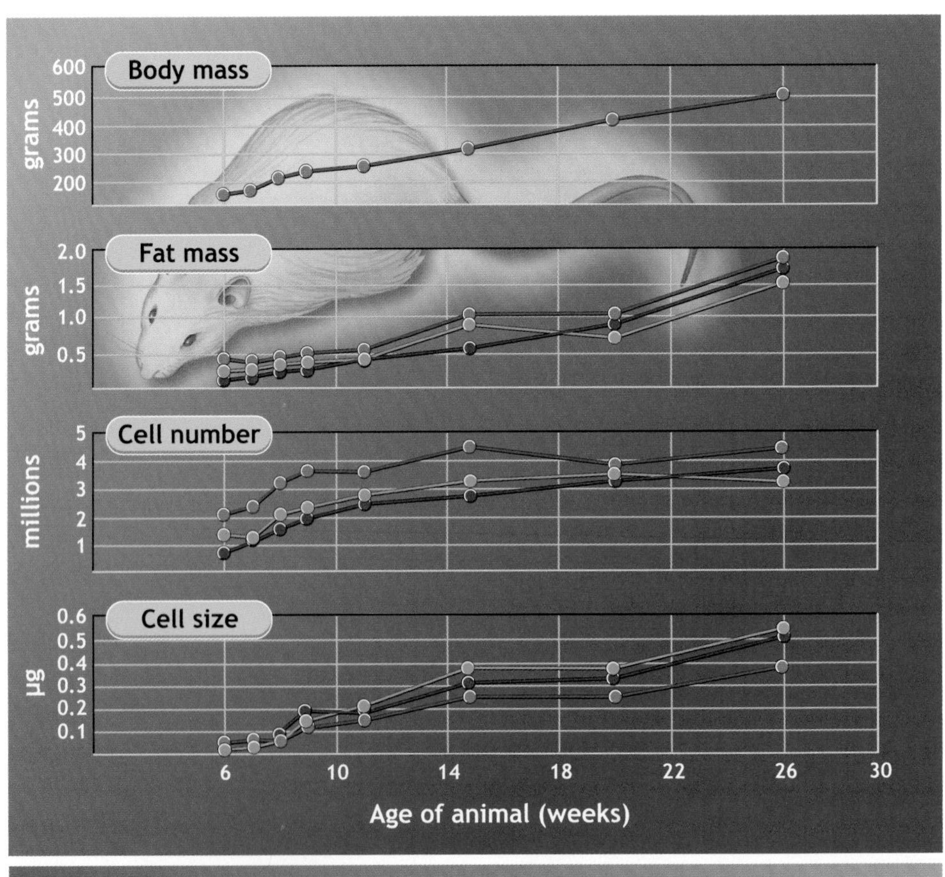

FIGURE 30.14 • Changes in total body mass, and fat mass, adipocyte number, and adipocyte size in three fat pads during the first 5 months of growth in rats. (From Hirsch J, Han PW. Cellularity of rat adipose tissue: effects of growth, starvation, and obesity. J Lipid Res 1969;10:77.)

15, after which further increases in total body fat occur primarily from increased adipocyte size, not because new cells develop.

Human Studies

Cell Size. Cross-sectional studies established adipose cellularity for 34 infants and children who ranged in age from a few days to 13 years.[84] Adipocyte size in newborn infants and children up to age 1 year averaged one-fourth the size in adults; cell size then tripled during the next 6 years, with little further increase to age 13. Data remain scarce concerning changes in adipocyte size between adolescence and adulthood. Adipocyte size probably increases during this growth period because adults possess significantly larger adipocytes than adolescents.

Cell Number. Adipocyte number increases rapidly during the first year of life to reach three times the number at birth. Most of the adipocytes before birth form during the last trimester of pregnancy. Beyond the age of 1 year, cell number increases gradually to about age 10. As with increases in cell size, significant hyperplasia takes place during the adolescent growth spurt; thereafter, cell number remains fairly stable. Percentage body fat increases from 16% at birth to about 25% over the first year.[38] By age 6, body fat decreases to 14% of body mass for girls and 11% for boys. Thereafter, percentage fat progressively increases to average 16% at age 11 years in boys and 27% in girls.

Can Body Fat Be Modified Early in Life?

Certain behaviors may modify body fatness early in life. In humans, for example, maternal nutrition during pregnancy affects body composition of the developing fetus. A mother who gains more than 18 kg generally gives birth to a baby with larger skinfold thickness than a woman who follows the recommended weight gain during pregnancy.[207] Bottle-feeding and early introduction of solid food also associate with childhood obesity. Conversely, breast-feeding, which allows the infant's natural appetite to set limits on food intake, and delayed introduction of solid food may prevent overfeeding, development of poor eating habits, and subsequent obesity.[112]

Prudent caloric intake and regular physical activity during the growth stage may modify the filling of existing adipocytes and proliferation of new ones. Exercise and caloric restriction begun later in life certainly can reduce body fat. As far as we know, only cell size and not cell number decreases. *Early prevention of obesity through proper exercise and diet, rather than correction of existing obesity, offers the greatest potential for curbing the overfat condition so common worldwide among children, teenagers, and adults.*

Summary

1. Obesity (an excess accumulation of body fat), is a heterogeneous disorder with a final common pathway where energy intake chronically exceeds energy expenditure.
2. Over the past 15 to 20 years, the average body weight of adult Americans has increased by about 8 pounds. Currently, 25% of adults classify as obese (BMI $\geq$30), and nearly 55% (100 million adults) are either overweight or obese (BMI $\geq$25).
3. Fifteen to 20% of American children and 12% of adolescents (up from 7.6% in 1976–80) classify as overweight. Excessive body fatness, their most common chronic disorder, is particularly prevalent among poor and minority children.
4. Genetic factors probably account for 25 to 30% of excessive body fat accumulation. Genetic predisposition does not necessarily cause obesity, but given the right environment, the genetically susceptible individual gains body fat. However, substantial alterations in the population's gene pool (which requires millions of years) cannot explain the dramatic worldwide obesity epidemic.
5. A defective gene for adipocyte leptin production and/or hypothalamic leptin insensitivity (plus defects in production and/or sensitivity to other chemicals) causes the brain to assess adipose tissue status improperly. Thus, excessive food intake creates a chronic state of positive energy balance.
6. Excessive body fat is the second leading cause of preventable death in the United States. Comorbid hypertension, elevated blood sugar level, postmenopausal breast cancer, and elevated total cholesterol and low HDL-cholesterol levels increase an overweight person's risk of poor health at any given level of excess weight. Weight loss significantly improves the health risk profile.
7. Standards for overfatness for adult men and women should reflect percentage body fat levels of younger adults more closely (men above 20%; women above 30%).
8. Body fat patterning affects health risks independent of total body fat. Fat distributed in the abdominal region (android-type obesity) poses a greater risk than fat deposited at the thighs and buttocks (gynoid-type obesity).
9. Body fat increases in two ways before adulthood: (1) enlargement of individual adipocytes, termed fat cell hypertrophy, and (2) increase in total cell number, termed fat cell hyperplasia. In extreme cases in adults, adipocyte number increases once cell size reaches the hypertrophic limit.
10. Increases in adipocyte number involve three general time periods: last trimester of pregnancy, first year of life, and adolescent growth spurt prior to adulthood.

➤ Part 2 • Principles of Weight Control: Diet and Exercise

For many adults, body weight fluctuates only slightly during the year, even though annual food intake averages close to 900 kg. This represents an impressive constancy considering that slight increases in daily food intake cause substantial weight gain over time if unaccompanied by compensatory increases in energy expenditure. *The human body functions in accord with the laws of thermodynamics. If total food calories exceed daily energy expenditure, excess calories accumulate and store as fat in adipose tissue.*

ENERGY BALANCE: INPUT VERSUS OUTPUT

In accord with the first law of thermodynamics, the energy balance equation dictates that body mass remains constant when caloric intake equals caloric expenditure. Figure 30.15 shows that any chronic imbalance on the energy output or input side of the equation changes body mass.

Three ways can unbalance the energy balance equation to produce weight loss:

1. Reduce caloric intake below daily energy requirements
2. Maintain normal caloric intake and increase energy expenditure through additional physical activity above daily energy requirements
3. Decrease daily caloric intake and increase daily energy expenditure

When considering the sensitivity of the energy balance equation, note that an energy imbalance of only 1% in daily energy input (positive) and/or output (negative) would increase body weight by 40 to 50 pounds during adulthood. If caloric intake exceeds output by only 100 kcal per day, the surplus calories consumed in a year equals 36,500 kcal (365 days × 100 kcal). Because 0.45 kg (1.0 lb) of body fat contains 3500 kcal (each 1 lb [454 g] of adipose tissue contains about 86% fat, or 390 g × 9 kcal · g^{-1} = 3514 kcal per lb), this caloric excess causes a yearly gain of about 4.7 kg (10.3 lb) of body fat. In contrast, if daily food intake decreases by just 100 kcal, and energy expenditure increases by 100 kcal (e.g., by jogging one extra mile each day), then the yearly deficit equals the energy in 9.5 kg (21 lb) of body fat.

The previous arithmetic represents an overly simplistic accounting for fat accumulation because the diet's composition affects the body's efficiency in converting and storing excess calories as fat. Only about 3% of calories in ingested lipid are lost when the body converts these excess calories to stored fat. In contrast, 25% of carbohydrate calories "burn" during the conversion. Simply stated, the body synthesizes fat more efficiently from dietary lipid than from an equivalent caloric excess of carbohydrate. Whether shifting dietary composition toward higher carbohydrate content actually produces less body fat gain with a caloric excess remains unresolved.[18,85,221]

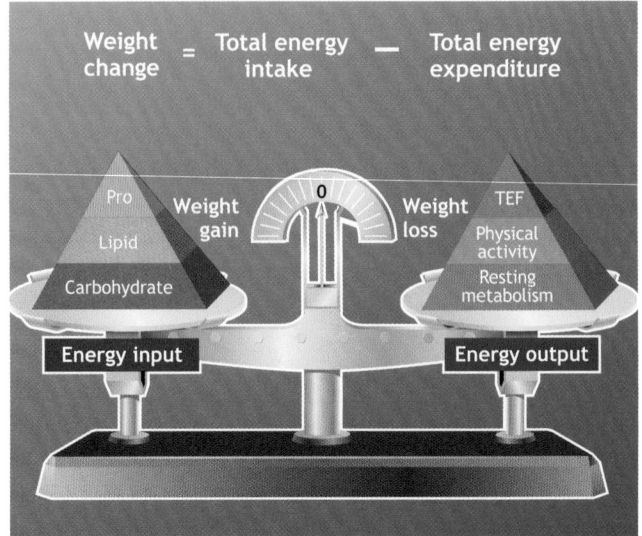

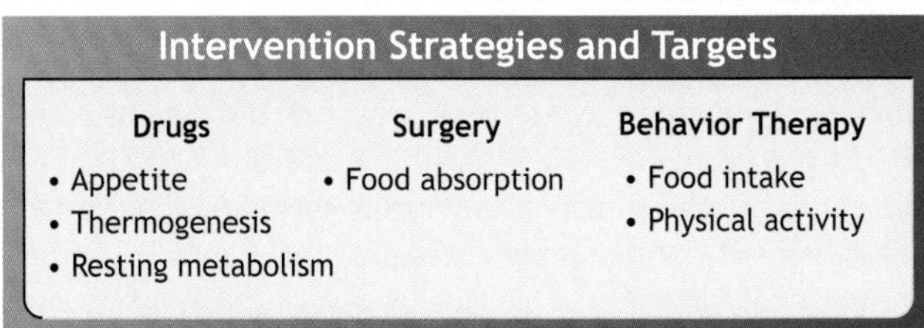

Figure 30.15 • The energy balance equation plus intervention strategies and specific targets to alter energy balance in the direction of weight loss. Pro, protein; TEF, thermic effect of food.

Over the past 10 years, the objective of obesity therapy has changed dramatically. The previous approach assigned a goal body weight that coincided with an "ideal" weight based on body stature and mass. Achieving this body weight heralded the weight-loss program's success. Currently, the World Health Organization, the Institute of Medicine of the National Academy of Sciences, and the National Heart, Lung and Blood Institute recommend that a person with excessive body fat reduce initial body weight by 5 to 15%.[140] This more realistic amount of weight loss generally reduces weight-related comorbidities and complications from hypertension, type 2 diabetes, and dyslipidemia and often exerts a positive effect on the social–psychologic complications related to the obese condition. Setting weight-loss goals beyond the 5 to 15% recommendation often gives patients an unrealistic and potentially unattainable goal in light of current treatment methods.

DIETING FOR WEIGHT CONTROL

Weight loss occurs whenever energy output exceeds energy intake regardless of the diet's macronutrient mixture, reaffirming the first law of thermodynamics. Advantages of relatively high percentages of unrefined complex carbohydrates in the reduced-calorie diet lie in their moderate-to-low glycemic index; high vitamin, mineral, and phytochemical content; low energy density; and low saturated fatty acid levels. A prudent dietary approach to weight loss unbalances the energy balance equation by reducing energy intake by 500 to 1000 kcal below daily energy expenditure. Moderately reduced food intake produces greater fat loss in relation to the energy deficit than more-severe energy restriction.[201] Individuals who create larger daily deficits to lose weight more rapidly tend to regain the weight, in contrast to those who lose weight at a slower rate.[86]

Suppose an overfat woman who normally consumes 2800 kcal daily and maintains a body mass of 79.4 kg wishes to lose weight by dieting. She maintains regular physical activity but reduces food intake to 1800 kcal to create a 1000-kcal daily deficit. In 7 days, the accumulated deficit equals 7000 kcal, or the energy equivalent of 0.9 kg of body fat. Actually, she would lose considerably more than 0.9 kg during the first week, because initially the body's glycogen stores make up a large portion of the energy deficit. Stored glycogen contains fewer calories per gram and considerably more water than stored fat. For this reason, short periods of caloric restriction often encourage the dieter but produce a large percentage of water and carbohydrate loss per unit weight loss, with only a small decrease in body fat. As weight loss continues, a larger proportion of body fat supports the energy deficit created by food restriction (see Fig. 30.21). To reduce body fat by an additional 1.4 kg, the dieter must maintain the reduced caloric intake of 1800 kcal for another 10.5 days; at this point, body fat theoretically decreases at a rate of 0.45 kg every 3.5 days.

Long-Term Success

The potential for successful long-term weight loss maintenance is generally an inverse function of the initial degree of obesity (Fig. 30.16). However, for most individuals, initial success in weight loss relates poorly to long-term success. Participants in supervised weight-loss programs (pharmacologic or behavioral interventions) generally lose about 8 to 10% of their original body mass. Unfortunately, typically one- to two-thirds of the lost weight returns within a year, and almost all of it within 5 years.[96,140,149] Between 90 and 95% of people who lose weight subsequently regain it. Figure 30.17 illustrates clearly that over a 7.3-year follow-up of 121 patients, the tendency to regain weight remained independent of length of the fast (up to 2 mo), amount of weight lost (up to 41.4 kg), or age at obesity onset. Return to original weight occurred in 50% of the dieters within 2 to 3 years, and only seven patients remained at their reduced weights. These discouraging statistics highlight the extreme difficulty of long-term maintenance of a low-calorie diet; it becomes particularly difficult in the relaxed atmosphere of one's home, with ready access to food and often little emotional support.

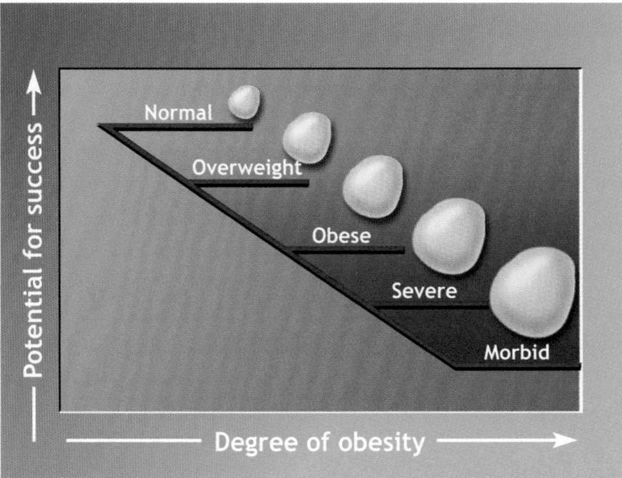

FIGURE 30.16 • Likelihood of success in long-term maintenance of weight loss depends on level of obesity at the start of the intervention.

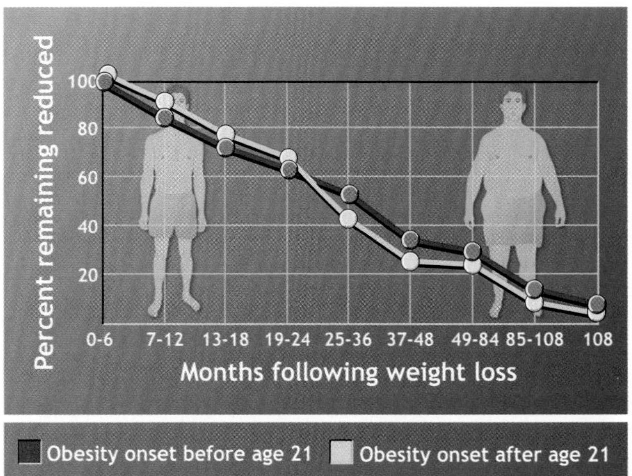

FIGURE 30.17 • Percentage of patients remaining at reduced weights at various time intervals following accomplished weight loss. *Red line,* 60 subjects with obesity onset before age 21; *yellow line,* 42 subjects with obesity onset after age 21. (From Johnson D, Drenick EJ. Therapeutic fasting in morbid obesity. Arch Intern Med 1977;137:1381.)

National Weight Control Registry: Clues to Success

Many success stories exist despite the difficulties usually encountered with losing weight. Among lifetime members of a commercial weight-loss organization that promotes prudent caloric restriction, behavior modification, group support, and moderate physical activity, more than one-half maintained their original weight loss goal after 2 years, and more than one-third had done so after 5 years.[141] Behavior modification, a common intervention in weight loss programs, provides a set of principles and techniques to alter exercise and eating habits. The therapy attempts to increase skills for replacing existing habits with new habits associated with more-healthful behaviors. Behavioral approaches to food intake include (1) pausing before eating to record food about to be eaten, (2) keeping a journal to describe one's mood just before eating, and (3) eating before going to the grocery store. Behavior therapy characteristics include eating well-balanced meals with reduced portion size, restricting daily caloric intake to 500 to 700 kcal, keeping meticulous records of food intake and physical activity, and increasing daily physical activity by 200 to 300 kcal.

A recent project recruited 784 individuals (629 women; 155 men) in the National Weight Control Registry (NWCR), the largest database of individuals who successfully achieved prolonged weight loss. Criteria for NWCR membership included (1) age 18 years or older and (2) maintained weight loss of at least 30 pounds (13.6 kg) for 1 year or longer. Participants averaged 66 pounds (30 kg) of weight loss, and 14% lost more than 100 pounds (45.4 kg). Members maintained the required minimum 30-pound weight loss for a 5.5-year average, and 16% maintained the loss for 10 years or longer. Most participants had been overweight since childhood; nearly one-half had one overweight parent, and more than 25% had both parents overweight. *Genetic background may have predisposed these people to obesity, but an impressive weight loss and its maintenance proves that heredity alone need not predestine a person to the obese condition.*

About 55% of the NWCR members used either a formal program or professional assistance to lose weight; the rest succeeded on their own. Regarding weight-loss methods, 89% modified food intake and maintained relatively high levels of physical activity (2800 kcal weekly on average) to achieve goal weight loss. Only 10% relied solely on diet, and 1% used exercise exclusively. The diet strategy of nearly 90% of participants restricted intake of certain types and/or amounts of foods—44% counted calories, 33% limited lipid intake, and 25% restricted grams of lipid. Forty-four percent ate the same foods they normally ate but in reduced amounts (Table 30.4).

The registry members' belief in the importance of physical activity for weight maintenance is a significant finding; nearly all of them exercised as part of their strategy. Many walked briskly for at least 1 hour daily. About 92% exercised at home, and one-third exercised regularly with friends. Women primarily walked and did aerobic dancing while men chose competitive sports and resistance training. The data in Table 30.4 also show that successful weight loss had far-reaching, positive effects on their lives. At least 85% improved general quality of life, level of energy, physical mobility, general mood, self-confidence, and physical health. Only 13 (1.6%) worsened in any of these areas. Such observations reaffirm that weight loss through diet and exercise can thwart a genetic predisposition to obesity.

TABLE 30.4 ➤ *TOP.* **DIETARY STRATEGIES TO ACHIEVE WEIGHT LOSS OF PARTICIPANTS OF THE NWCR.** *BOTTOM.* **EFFECTS OF WEIGHT LOSS ON VARIOUS DIMENSIONS OF LIFE AS REPORTED BY PARTICIPANTS**

	Percentage		
Strategy	**Women**	**Men**	**Total**
Restricted intake of certain types or classes of foods	87.8	86.7	87.6
Ate all foods but limited quantity	47.2	32.0	44.2
Counted calories	44.8	39.3	43.7
Limited % lipid intake	31.1	36.7	33.1
Counted lipid grams	25.7	21.3	25.2
Followed exchange diet	25.2	11.3	22.5
Used liquid formula	19.1	26.0	20.4
Ate only 1 or 2 food types	5.1	6.7	5.5

Area of Life	**Improved**	**No Difference**	**Worsened**
Quality of life	95.3	4.3	0.4
Level of energy	92.4	6.7	0.9
Mobility	92.3	7.1	0.6
General mood	91.4	6.9	1.6
Self-confidence	90.9	9.0	0.1
Physical health	85.8	12.9	1.3
Interactions with			
Opposite sex	65.2	32.9	0.9
Same sex	5.0	46.8	0.4
Strangers	69.5	30.4	0.1
Job performance	54.5	45.0	0.6
Hobbies	49.1	36.7	0.4
Spouse interactions	56.3	37.3	5.9

From Klem MI, et al. A descriptive study of individuals successful at long-term maintenance of substantial weight loss. Am J Clin Nutr 1997;66:239.

Weight Loss Improves Disease Risk Biomarkers

Weight loss by the obese often exerts a profound effect on biologic factors related to disease risk.[46,139] Figure 30.18 shows the percentage changes from initial body weight and the change in biomarkers of disease risk in obese patients over a 27-month period using two energy-restricting meal plans. In phase 1 during the first 3 months, group A (n = 50) attempted to consume an energy-restricted diet (5.2–6.3 mJ, or 1200–1500 kcal daily) composed of conventional, self-selected meals prepared by the subjects; group B (n = 50), assigned the same caloric intake, substituted two meals and two snack-replacement shakes, soups, hot chocolate, and snack bars (Slim·Fast) for self-selected foods. In phase 2 (mo 4 to 27), all subjects consumed self-selected diets of equal caloric value with one meal and one shake replacement. Unequivocal results emerged from both study phases. Group B's greater weight loss during the 3-month phase 1 period was attributed to a greater actual caloric deficit created with this eating plan. Thereafter, both groups lost on average an additional 0.07% of initial body weight each month (4.2 kg for group A and 3.0 kg for group B). The *bottom figure* shows absolute changes in eight disease biomarkers during phases 1 and 2. Both groups achieved reductions in systolic blood pressure and plasma insulin, glucose, and triglyceride concentrations over the 27-month weight-loss period. These findings support the notion that a modest but sustained weight loss can produce long-term health benefits as reflected by significant improvement in documented risk factors.

Setpoint Theory: A Case Against Dieting

One can crash off large amounts of weight in a relatively short time by simply not eating, but success is short-lived, and eventually the urge to eat wins out and the lost weight returns.

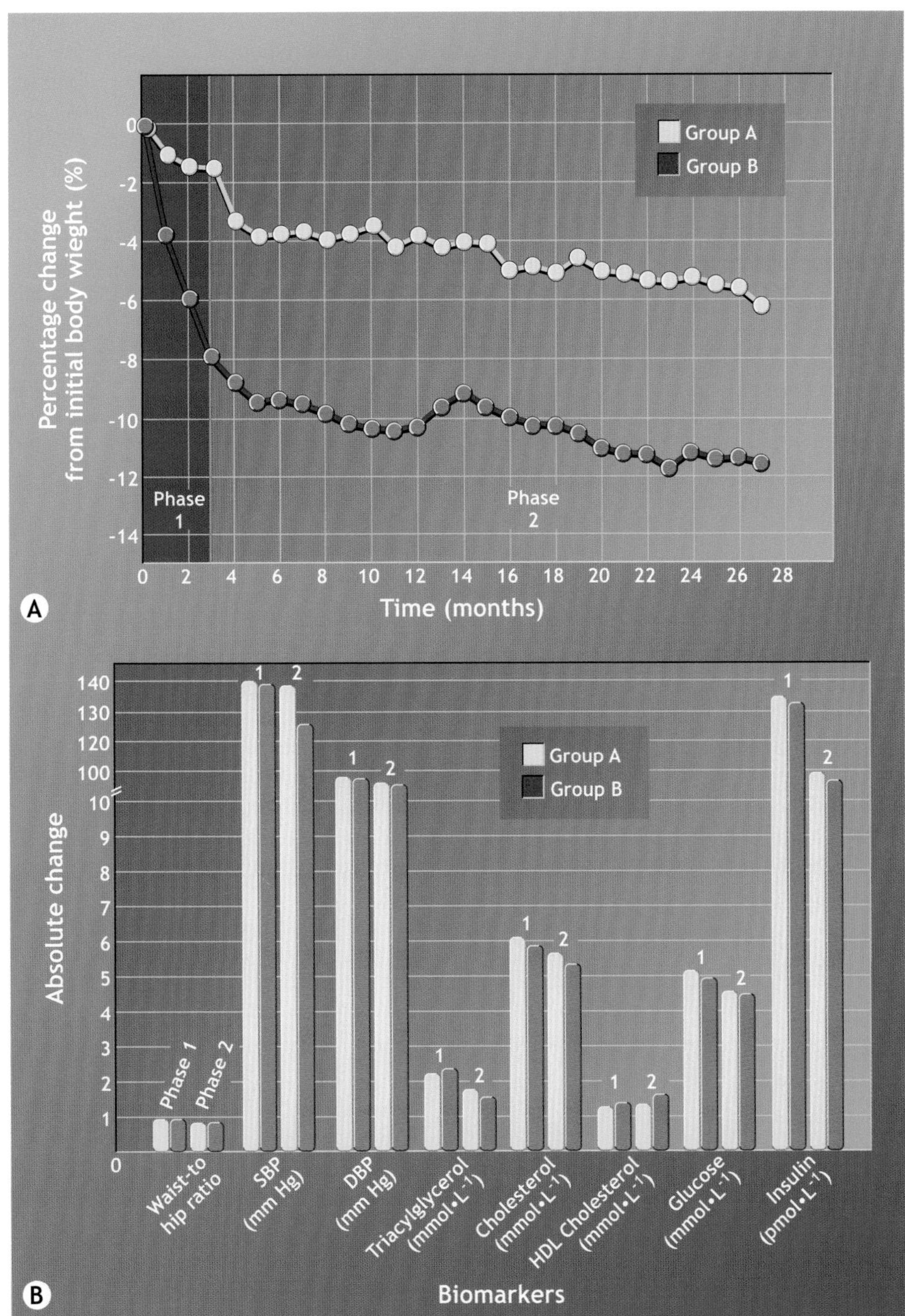

Figure 30.18 • **A**. Average percentage change from initial body weight of obese patients during 27 months of treatment with an energy-restricted diet containing 5.3 to 6.3 kJ (1200 to 1500 kcal). **B**. Absolute changes in biomarkers for groups A (energy-restricted, self-selected, self-prepared meals) and B (Slim-Fast replacement meals) from baseline to 27 months of energy restriction. *SBP*, systolic blood pressure; *DBP*, diastolic blood pressure. (Modified from Detschuneit HH, et al. Metabolic and weight-loss effects of a long-term dietary intervention in obese patients. Am J Clin Nutr 1999;69:198.)

Some argue that the reason for this failure lies in a genetically determined "set point" for body weight (or body fat) that differs from what the dieter would like. The proponents of a **set-point theory** maintain that all persons (fat or thin) have a well-regulated internal control mechanism located deep within the lateral hypothalamus that maintains with relative ease a preset level of body weight and/or body fat within a tight range (±10% from midpoint). In a practical sense, this represents a person's body weight when not counting calories. Exercise and drugs (e.g., fenfluramine, amphetamine, and nicotine) may lower a person's set point, whereas dieting exerts no effect. Each time body weight decreases below one's preestablished set point (losses in body weight and FFM[48]), internal adjustments that affect food intake and regulatory thermogenesis resist the change and conserve and/or replenish body fat. For example, resting metabolism slows and the individual becomes obsessed with food, unable to control the urge to eat. Even when persons overeat and gain body fat above their normal level, the body resists this change by increasing resting metabolism and causing the person to lose interest in food.[85]

Resting Metabolism Decreases

A sustained reduction in resting metabolism represents a well-documented, autoregulatory feedback response to weight loss through dieting.[48,143] Resting metabolism decreases by more than is attributable to loss of either body mass or FFM; severe caloric restrictions can decrease resting metabolism by 45%. This calorie-sparing response takes place independent of the person's weight status or past dieting history. A depressed metabolism conserves energy, causing the diet to progressively become less effective despite a restricted caloric intake. This produces a weight-loss plateau. Further weight loss occurs at a slower pace than the mathematics of the restricted energy intake predict.

Figure 30.19A shows the close coupling between daily total energy expenditure (TEE) required to maintain a constant FFM in obese and nonobese subjects at their usual body weights. When body weight declined by 10% below the usual weight (Fig. 30.19B), TEE declined more than explained by the normal relation between energy expenditure and FFM. Both obese and normal-weight subjects became more energy efficient, requiring disproportionately lower energy intake to maintain the lower body weight. Conversely, increasing body weight by 10% above usual weight (Fig. 30.19C) produced a 15 to 20% unanticipated *increase* in energy expenditure that countered the gain in body fat. These data support the set-point concept, or "command signal" that modulates metabolism to defend a specific level of body fat; unfortunately, regulation occurs at a higher body fat level in the obese.

Figure 30.20 shows further evidence of the body's "defense" against deviations in body weight. The research carefully monitored body mass, resting oxygen consumption (minimal energy requirement), and caloric intake of six obese men for 31 days. During the prediet period, body mass and resting oxygen consumption stabilized with a daily food intake of 3500 kcal. Thereafter, daily caloric intake decreased significantly to 450 kcal. When the subjects switched to the low-calorie diet, body mass and resting metabolism decreased, but the percentage decline in metabolism exceeded the body mass decrease. The *dashed line* (upper figure) represents the expected weight loss for the 450-calorie diet. The decline in resting metabolism (middle figure) conserved energy to make the diet progressively less effective. More than one-half of the total weight loss occurred over the first 8 days of dieting; the remaining weight loss occurred during the final 16 days. A plateau in the theoretical weight-loss curve often frustrates and discourages dieters causing them to abandon the program.

Biologic Feedback Mechanism

Further disconcerting news awaits those who desire permanent fat loss. When overfat people lose weight, adipocytes increase their level of the fat-storing enzyme LPL.[103] Unfortunately, this adaptation facilitates body fat synthesis, and the fatter the person before weight loss, the greater the LPL production with weight loss. In essence, the fatter one is at the start, the more vigorously one's body attempts to regain the lost weight. This observation supports the existence of a biologic feedback mechanism between the brain and body fat levels and helps to explain the difficulty the overfat have maintaining weight loss.

Although the set-point theory delivers unwelcome news for those with a set point "tuned" too high, regular ex-

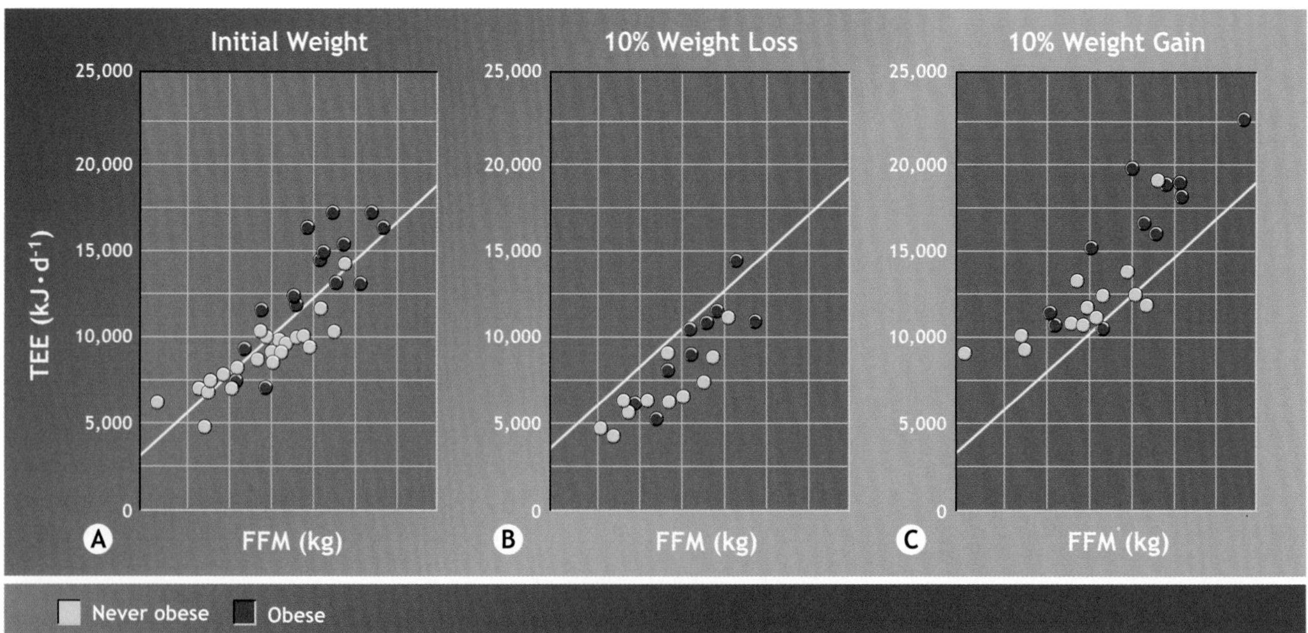

FIGURE 30.19 • Relationship between daily total energy expenditure (TEE) and fat-free body mass (FFM) in obese and normal subjects (**A**) at their usual body weights, (**B**) after 10% weight reduction, and (**C**) after 10% weight gain. (From Leibel RL, et al. Changes in energy expenditure resulting from altered body weight. N Engl J Med 1995;332:621.)

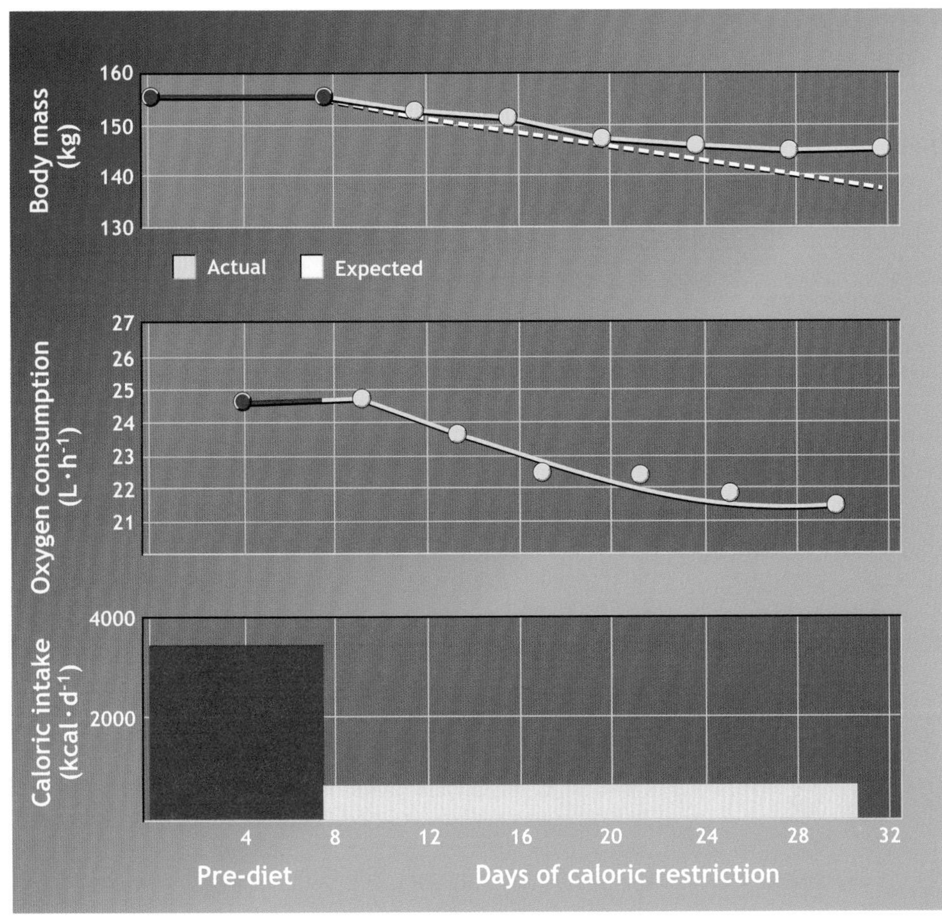

FIGURE 30.20 • Effects of two levels of caloric intake on body mass and resting oxygen consumption. Failure of the actual weight loss to keep pace with that predicted on the basis of food restriction (dashed line) often leaves the dieter frustrated and discouraged. (Adapted from Bray G. Effect of caloric restriction on energy expenditure in obese subjects. Lancet 1969;2:397.)

ercise may lower the set point level. Concurrently, regular exercise conserves and even increases FFM, raises resting metabolism (if FFM increases), and induces metabolic changes that facilitate fat catabolism. These healthful adaptations all augment the weight-loss effort. On page 851 we discuss how food intake tends to decline initially, despite the increase in energy output, for overly fat men and women who exercise regularly. Eventually, as an active lifestyle continues and body fat reserves decrease, caloric intake balances daily energy requirements, and body mass stabilizes at a new, lower level.

Weight Cycling: Going No Place Fast?

The futility of repeated cycles of weight loss and weight gain (**yo-yo effect**) emerged from studies of food efficiency (weight loss–weight gain related to ingested calories) studies of animals. Weight gain often occurs more readily with repeated weight-loss cycles. For example, animals required twice the time to lose the same weight during a second period of caloric restriction and only one-third the time to regain it.[20] Significant controversy exists about extrapolating this response to humans. Additional debate concerns whether the failure to keep off weight raises heart disease risk. Initial reports indicated repeated bouts of weight loss and regain increased the likelihood of death from heart attack. The risk averaged nearly 70% higher for regainers than for those who maintained body weight.[95] In contrast, data from 6500 originally healthy Japanese American men who never smoked showed no ill effects from a repeated cycle of weight loss and regain.[90] Furthermore, periods of rapid weight loss and regain common in dieters do not increase hypertension risk any more than the increased risk from being overweight or gaining weight.[23] Cycles of dieting do not induce adverse psychologic effects of stress level, anxiety, anger, and depression for overweight and normal-weight individuals.[191]

If weight cycling should pose an additional health risk, one can only speculate on the potential for long-term negative effects of repeated weight cycling common among high school and collegiate wrestlers.[200] From a public health perspective, the risks from overweight and obesity far exceed those for weight cycling. *The obese should not use concern for the potential hazards of yo-yo dieting as an excuse to abandon efforts to reduce excess body fat.*

Dieting Extremes

Professional organizations have voiced strong opposition to some dietary practices, particularly extremes of fasting and low-carbohydrate, high-fat, and high-protein diets. Dietary extremes raise concern about athletes and other adolescents and young adults who routinely engage in bizarre and often pathogenic weight-control behaviors (see "In a Practical Sense").

In a Practical Sense

Recognizing Warning Signs of Disordered Eating

Disordered eating refers to a broad spectrum of complex behaviors, core attitudes, coping strategies, and conditions that share an emotionally based, inordinate, and often pathologic focus on body shape and weight.

Anorexia Athletica

There exists a cluster of personality traits among some athletes that often shares a commonality with patients with clinical eating disorders. The same traits that help an athlete excel in sports—compulsive, driven, dichotomous thinker, perfectionist, competitive, compliant and eager to please ("coachable"), and self-motivated—increase the risks for developing disordered eating patterns. This risk grows for individuals whose normal, genetically determined body size and shape deviate from the "ideal" imposed by the sport. The term **anorexia athletica** describes the continuum of subclinical eating behaviors of athletes who fail to meet the criteria for a true eating disorder but who exhibit at least one unhealthy method of weight control, including fasting, vomiting, or use of diet pills, laxatives, or diuretics ("water pills"). Clinical observations indicate a prevalence of disordered eating behaviors of 15 to 60%, depending on the sport.

For many athletes, patterns of disordered eating coincide with the competitive season and abate when the season ends. For them, the preoccupation with body weight may not reflect a true underlying pathology but rather a desire to achieve optimum physiologic function and competitive performance. For a small number of athletes, the season never ends, and they develop a full-blown eating disorder. Anorexia nervosa and bulimia nervosa are the two most common eating disorders. A third category, binge-eating disorder, does not include purging behavior.

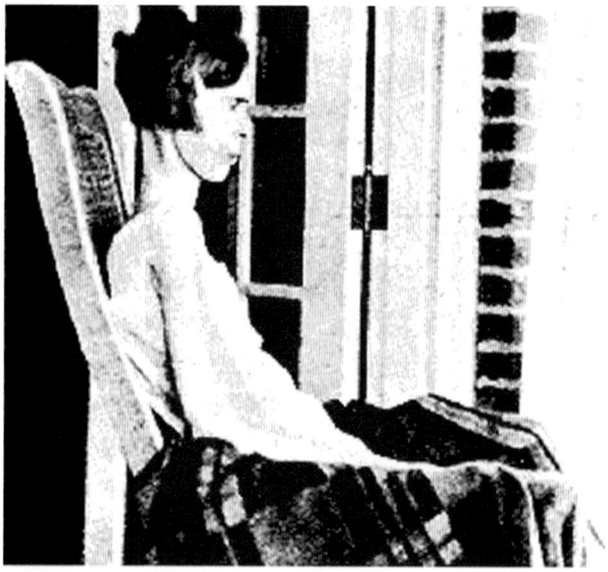

The "first published photo of an anorectic in an American medical journal. By the 1930s there were three essential techniques in the management of anorexia nervosa: change of environment, forced feeding, and psychotherapy. Severe cases were generally treated in private psychiatric hospitals." (From Fasting girls. N Engl J Med 1932;207(5):Oct.)

Anorexia Nervosa

Originally described in ancient writings, **anorexia nervosa** is an unhealthy physical and mental state characterized by a crippling obsession with body size. A "nervous loss of appetite" reflects preoccupation with dieting and thinness and refusal to eat enough food to maintain a normal body weight, which becomes below normal for age and stature. The relentless pursuit of thinness (present in about 1 to 2% of the general population) includes an intense fear of weight gain and fatness (despite a low body weight) and failure to menstruate regularly (amenorrhea). Anorectics have a distorted body image; they actually perceive themselves as fat despite their emaciation.

Anorexia nervosa usually begins with a normal attempt to lose weight through dieting (Table 1). With continued dieting, the individual continues to eat less until practically no food is consumed. Eventually, food restriction becomes an obsession, and the anorectic achieves no sense of satisfaction despite weight loss. As weight loss continues, the anorectic person exhibits denial of the accompanying extreme emaciation.

Bulimia Nervosa

The term *bulimia,* literally meaning "ox hunger," refers to "gorging" or "insatiable appetite." **Bulimia nervosa**, far more common than anorexia nervosa, is characterized by

Low Carbohydrate-Ketogenic Diets

Ketogenic diets emphasize carbohydrate restriction while generally ignoring total calories and the diet's cholesterol and saturated fat content. Advocates maintain that restricting dietary carbohydrate causes the body to mobilize significant fat for energy. This generates excess plasma ketone bodies—by-products of incomplete fat breakdown from inadequate carbohydrate catabolism—which supposedly suppress appetite. Theoretically, the ketones lost in the urine represent unused energy that should further facilitate weight loss. Some extremists claim that urinary energy loss becomes so great that dieters can eat all they want provided they restrict carbohydrates.

At best, the calories lost by urinary ketone excretion probably equal only 100 to 150 kcal per day.[5] This would account for a small weight loss of approximately 0.45 kg per month—not appealing when the major food source is a lipid intake as

IN A PRACTICAL SENSE

➤➤ RECOGNIZING WARNING SIGNS OF DISORDERED EATING—CONT'D

TABLE 1. WARNING SIGNS OF ANOREXIA NERVOSA

- Preoccupation with being too fat despite maintenance of normal body weight
- Loss of menstrual cycle (amenorrhea)
- Frequently commenting about body weight or shape
- Significant loss of body weight
- Weight too low for athletic performance
- Ritualistic concern and preoccupation with dieting, counting calories, cooking, and eating meals
- Excessive concern about body weight, size, and shape, even after weight loss
- Feeling of helplessness in the presence of food
- Severe shifts in mood
- Guilt about eating
- Compulsive need for continuous, vigorous physical activity that exceeds training requirements for a specific sport
- Maintenance of a skinny look (body weight less than 85% of expected weight)
- Prefers to eat in isolation
- Wears baggy clothes to disguise thin-looking appearance
- Episodes of bingeing and purging

frequent episodes of binge eating, almost always followed by purging and intense feelings of guilt and shame (Table 2). Approximately 2 to 4% of all adolescents and adults in the general population (almost exclusively female, including 5% of college women) have bulimia nervosa. Unlike the continual semistarvation of anorexia nervosa, binge eating characterizes bulimia nervosa. The bulimic consumes calorically dense food within several hours, often at night, usually containing between 1000 and 10,000 calories, followed by fasting, self-induced vomiting, taking laxatives or diuretics, or compulsive exercising solely to avoid gaining weight.

Binge-Eating Disorder

Episodes of bingeing, often without the subsequent purging behavior common to bulimia nervosa, characterize **binge-eating disorder**. Individuals eat more rapidly than normal until they can consume no additional food. Food intake greatly exceeds that determined by the physiologic hunger drive. Binge eating, done in private, occurs with feelings of guilt, depression, or self-disgust. These individuals suffer greater self-anger, shame, lack of control, and frustration than non-bingeing overfat individuals. The diagnosis of binge-eating disorder requires that the individual experiences a lack of control over eating and marked psychologic distress when it occurs. The person must binge at least an average of 2 days a week for 6 months. Binge eating differs from the overfat condition in that the same level of self-anger, shame, lack of control, and frustration about binge eating does not necessarily accompany obesity. Little factual information exists about the prevalence of binge-eating disorder; however, it is estimated to occur in approximately 2% of the U.S. population.

References

Dale KS, Landers DM. Weight control in wrestling: eating disorders or disordered eating? Med Sci Sports Exerc 1999;31,1382.

Kinoy BP. Eating disorders: new directions in treatment and recovery. New York: Columbia University Press, 1994.

O'Connor PJ, et al. Eating disorder symptoms in former female college gymnasts: relations with body composition. Am J Clin Nutr 1996;64:840.

Orphanidou CI, et al. Changes in body composition and fat distribution after short-term weight gain in patients with anorexia nervosa. Am J Clin Nutr 1997;65:1034.

Striegel-Moore RH. Risk factors for eating disorders. Ann NY Acad Sci 1997;817:98.

Tanofsky MB, et al. Comparison of men and women with binge eating disorder. Int J Eating Disord 1997;21:49.

Wiederman MW, Pryor T. Substance abuse among women with eating disorders. Int J Eating Disord 1996;20:163.

TABLE 2. WARNING SIGNS OF BULIMIA NERVOSA

- Excessive concern about body weight, body size, and body composition
- Frequent gains and losses in body weight
- Visits to the bathroom following meals
- Fear of not being able to stop eating
- Eating when depressed
- Compulsive dieting after binge-eating episodes
- Severe shifts in mood (depression, loneliness)
- Secretive binge eating but never overeating in front of others
- More frequent criticism of own body size and shape
- Personal or family problems with alcohol or drugs
- Irregular menstrual cycle (oligomenorrhea)

high as 70% of calories consumed. The singular focus of the diet may eventually reduce caloric intake, despite claims that dieters need not consider calorie intake as long as lipid represents the excess. Initial weight loss may also result largely from dehydration caused by an extra solute load on the kidneys that increases water excretion. Water loss does *not* reduce body fat. Low-carbohydrate intake also sets the stage for a significant loss of lean tissue as the body recruits amino acids from muscle to maintain blood glucose via gluconeogenesis—an undesirable side effect for a diet designed to induce body fat loss.

Compared with a well-balanced, low-calorie diet, the ketogenic diet shows no advantage in facilitating fat loss. The diet poses potential hazards for several reasons. It can raise serum uric acid levels, alter electrolyte concentrations to initiate undesirable cardiac arrhythmias, cause acidosis, aggravate kidney problems from the extra solute burden in the renal filtrate, elevate blood lipids, deplete glycogen reserves to contribute to a fatigued state, and cause dehydration. Excessive saturated fatty acid intake profoundly elevates LDL-cholesterol, thus increasing heart disease risk. The diet, definitely contraindicated during pregnancy, can retard fetal development from inadequate dietary carbohydrate.

High-Protein Diets

A modification of a low carbohydrate-ketogenic diet emphasizes a large protein consumption. These low carbohydrate-high protein diets have been extolled to the obese as "last-chance diets." Earlier versions consisted of protein in liquid form advertised as "miracle liquid." Unknown to the consumer, the liquid protein mixture often contained a blend of ground-up animal hooves and horns, with pigskin mixed in a broth with enzymes and tenderizers to "predigest" it. Collagen-based blends produced from gelatin hydrolysis (supplemented with small amounts of essential amino acids) often did not contain the highest quality amino acid mixture and lacked required vitamins and minerals (particularly copper). A negative copper balance often coincides with electrocardiographic abnormalities and rapid heart rate.[57] The diet's safety improves if it contains high-quality protein with ample carbohydrate, essential fatty acids, and micronutrients.[148]

Some argue that extremely high protein intake suppresses appetite through reliance on fat mobilization and subsequent ketone formation. The elevated thermic effect of dietary protein, with its relatively low coefficient of digestibility (particularly for plant protein), ultimately reduces the net calories available from ingested protein compared with a well-balanced meal of equivalent caloric value. This point has some validity, but one must consider other factors when formulating a sound weight-loss program, particularly for the physically active individual. Important considerations include a high-protein diet's potential for (1) strain on liver and kidney function and accompanying dehydration, (2) electrolyte imbalance, (3) glycogen depletion, and (4) lean-tissue loss.

Semistarvation Diets

A therapeutic fast, or **very low calorie diet (VLCD)** may benefit severe clinical obesity where body fat exceeds 40 to 50% of body mass.[3] The diet provides between 400 and 800 kcal daily as high-quality protein foods or liquid meal replacements. Dietary prescriptions usually last for up to 3 months but only as a "last resort" before undertaking more-extreme medical approaches for morbid obesity (≥100 lb above ideal weight) that include various surgical treatments (collectively called bariatric surgery). In laparoscopic surgery, a slender, tubular instrument inserted into the abdominal cavity bands the stomach to reduce its proximal volume.[68] Concurrently, the small intestine is often rearranged to reduce the surface for food absorption.

Dieting with VLCD requires close supervision, usually in a hospital setting. Proponents maintain that severe food restriction breaks established dietary habits, which in turn improves the long-term prospects for success. These diets also may depress appetite to help compliance. Daily medications that accompany a VLCD include calcium carbonate for nausea, bicarbonate of soda and potassium chloride to maintain consistency of body fluids, mouthwash and sugar-free chewing gum for bad breath (from a high level of ketones from fatty acid catabolism), and bath oils for dry skin. *For most individuals, semistarvation does not compose an "ultimate diet" or the proper approach to weight control.* Because a VLCD provides inadequate carbohydrate, the glycogen-storage depots in the liver and muscles deplete rapidly. This impairs physical tasks requiring either high-intensity aerobic effort or shorter-duration anaerobic power output. The continuous nitrogen loss with fasting and weight loss may reflect an exacerbated lean tissue loss. This may occur disproportionately from critical organs like the heart.[153] Finally, the success rate remains poor for prolonged fasting.

Table 30.5 summarizes the principles and main advantages and disadvantages of some of the popular dietary approaches to weight loss. Most diets produce weight loss during the first several weeks, although body water makes up much of the lost weight. In addition, significant lean tissue loss occurs with dieting alone, particularly in the early phase of a VLCD.[119] While one can certainly reduce weight through dieting alone, few people achieve long-term success in altering body size and composition.

FACTORS THAT AFFECT WEIGHT LOSS

Hydration level and duration of the energy deficit affect the amount and composition of weight lost.

Early Weight Loss Is Largely Water

Figure 30.21 shows the general trend for the percentage composition of daily weight loss during 4 weeks of dieting. Water makes up about 70% of the weight lost over the first week of energy deficit. Thereafter, water loss progressively lessens, representing only about 20% of the weight lost during the second and third weeks; concurrently, body fat loss accelerates from 25 to 70%. During the fourth week of dieting, reductions in body fat produce about 85% of the weight loss without further increase in water loss. Protein's contribution to weight loss increases from 5% initially to about 15% by the end of the fourth week.

Hydration Level

Restricting water during the first several days of a caloric deficit significantly increases the *proportion* of body water lost and decreases the *proportion* of fat lost. Although more total weight loss occurs with restricted daily water intake, the additional weight lost comes solely from water as dehydration progresses. Dieters lose the same quantity of body fat regardless of fluid intake level.

TABLE 30.5 ➤ PRINCIPLES, ADVANTAGES, AND DISADVANTAGES OF SOME POPULAR WEIGHT LOSS METHODS

METHOD	PRINCIPLE	ADVANTAGES	DISADVANTAGES	COMMENTS
Surgical procedures	Alteration of gastrointestinal tract changes capacity or amount of absorptive surface	Caloric restriction less necessary	Risks of surgery and postsurgical complications include death	Radical procedures include stomach stapling and removal of section of small intestine (jejunoileal bypass)
Fasting	No energy input ensures negative energy balance	Rapid weight loss (may be a disadvantage) Reduced exposure to temptation	Ketogenic Large portion of weight lost from lean body mass Nutrients lacking	Medical supervision mandatory and hospitalization recommended
Protein-sparing modified fast	Same as fasting except protein or protein with carbohydrate intake assumed to help preserve lean body mass	Same as fasting	Ketogenic Nutrients lacking Some unconfirmed deaths reported, possibly from electrolyte depletion	Medical supervision mandatory Example: *The Last Chance Diet*
One-food–centered diets	Low-caloric intake favors negative energy balance	Easy to follow (initial psychologic appeal)	Too restrictive; nutrients lacking Repetitious nature causes boredom	No food or food combination "burns off" fat Examples: grapefruit diet and egg diet
Low-carbohydrate/high-fat diets	Increased ketone excretion removes energy from the body Fat intake often voluntarily decreased; results in low caloric intake	Inclusion of rich foods has psychologic appeal Initial rapid water loss an incentive	Ketogenic High-fat intake contraindicated for heart and diabetes patients Nutrients lacking	Examples include Taller and Atkins diet; and the "Mayo," "Drinking Man's," and "Air Force" diets
Low-carbohydrate/high-protein diets	Low caloric intake favors negative energy balance	Initial rapid water loss an incentive Increased thermic effect of protein	Expense and repetitious; difficult to sustain	If meat emphasized, the diet becomes high in fat
High-carbohydrate/low-fat diets	Low caloric intake favors negative energy balance	Wise food selections can make the diet nutritionally sound	Initial water retention (from glycogen storage) may be discouraging	Examples include the Pennington diet and the Pritikin diet

Modified and reprinted by permission from Reed PB. Nutrition: an applied science.

Longer-Term Deficit Promotes Fat Loss

Figure 30.22 illustrates the important concept that the caloric equivalent of the weight lost increases as duration of caloric restriction progresses. More specifically, after 2 months on a diet the caloric equivalent of weight loss is more than twice that in the first week. *This points up the importance of maintaining a caloric deficit for an extended duration. Shorter periods of caloric restriction cause a larger percentage of water and carbohydrate loss per unit weight reduction and only a minimal decrease in body fat.*

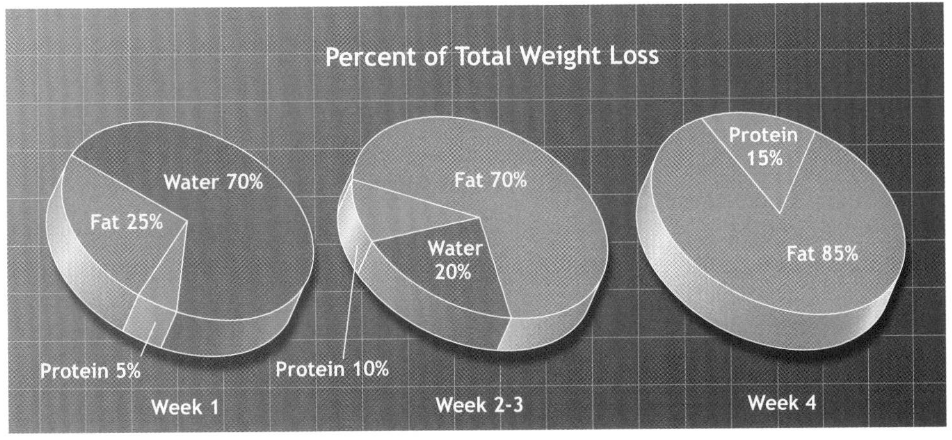

FIGURE 30.21 • Generalized trend for the percentage composition of the weight lost during 4 weeks of caloric restriction.

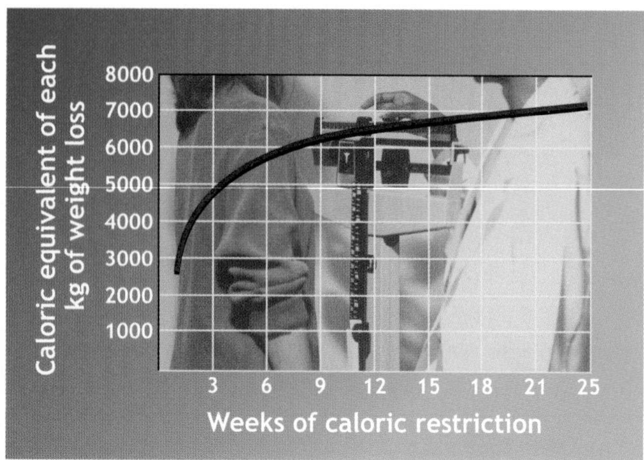

FIGURE 30.22 • General trend for the energy (caloric) equivalent of the weight lost in relation to the duration of caloric restriction. As caloric restriction progresses, the energy equivalent per unit of weight lost increases to about 7000 kcal per kilogram after 20 weeks. This occurs because of the large initial body water loss (no calorie value) early in weight loss.

EXERCISE FOR WEIGHT CONTROL

Despite debate about the precise contributions of physical inactivity and excessive caloric intake to body fat accretion, a sedentary lifestyle consistently emerges as an important factor in weight gain by children, adolescents, and adults.[9,54,137,171,181]

Not Simply Gluttony

Many people view excessive food intake as the sole cause of the overfat condition. Clearly then, some form of caloric restriction by dieting becomes the recommended approach to weight loss. This overly simplistic strategy partly accounts for the dismal success in maintaining weight loss over the long term. *Excess weight gain often parallels reduced physical activity rather than increased caloric intake.* Physically active individuals who eat the most often weigh the least and maintain the highest fitness levels. Per capita caloric intake in the United States has continually decreased over the past 100 years (currently about 400 kcal less each day), yet body mass and body fat have increased steadily. For example, between 1977 and 1987, the average caloric intake of American men and women decreased by 4% (lipid calories by 11%), yet the number of overweight people increased by 8% (BMI increase of 4%).[77] The same period witnessed a 4% decline in energy intake by children and adolescents, yet their average body weight continued to escalate.[221] If energy intake were the *sole* culprit in fat accumulation, then reduced caloric intake (and percentage kcal from lipid) should bring the national body weight to a lower, not higher, level.

Obese infants do not characteristically ingest more calories than recommended dietary standards. For children ages 4 to 6 years, daily energy expenditure averaged 25% below the current recommendation for energy intake at this age. A low level of daily physical activity primarily caused the blunted energy output.[26] More specifically, 50% of boys and 75% of girls in the United States fail to engage in even moderate physical activity three or more times weekly.[1] Time-in-motion photography to document activity patterns of elementary-school children showed that overweight children remained considerably less active than normal-weight peers; excess body weight did not relate to food intake. Caloric intake of overfat high-school girls and boys averaged below that of normal-weight peers.[97,178] Excessive fatness relates directly to the number of hours spent watching television (a consistent marker of inactivity) among children, adolescents, and adults.[6,69] Excessive television watching, playing video games, and otherwise remaining inactive particularly characterizes minority teens. Minimizing time devoted to such behaviors can help combat childhood fat gain.[67,177]

The observation that overfat children often eat the same or even less than peers of average body weight also pertains to less physically active adults as they slowly, progressively gain weight.[198] *Overweight individuals do not eat more on average than persons of normal weight.* Consequently, it remains neither prudent nor justifiable to emphasize dieting alone to effectively induce long-term weight loss.

Increasing Energy Output

Physically active men and women generally maintain a desirable body composition. An increased level of regular physical activity combined with dietary restraint maintains weight loss more effectively than long-term caloric restriction alone[21,106] and may help ex-smokers maintain weight.[64] Even without caloric restriction, a negative energy balance induced by increased caloric expenditure, through either lifestyle activities or formal exercise programs, provides a significant option to unbalance the energy balance equation for weight loss, improved physical fitness, and favorable alterations in body composition and body fat distribution.[114,159,181] Regular exercise possibly produces less accumulation of central adipose tissue associated with aging.[11,108,182] In fact, overweight adult women exhibit a dose-response relationship between exercise, behavior modification, and long-term weight loss.[94] Additional spinoff from regular exercise includes possible prevention of adult-onset obesity, improvement in obesity-related comorbidities, decreased mortality, and beneficial effects on existing chronic diseases.[208,215]

Misconceptions About Exercise

Two arguments attempt to counter the exercise approach to weight loss. One maintains that exercise inevitably increases appetite so that a proportionate increase in food intake negates the caloric deficit exercise produces. The second argument claims that the relatively small calorie-burning effect of a normal exercise workout does not "dent" the body's fat reserves compared with food restriction.

Misconception 1: Exercise and Food Intake

Sedentary people often do not maintain a delicate balance between energy intake and energy expenditure.[134,185] Failure to accurately regulate energy balance at the lower end of the physical activity spectrum contributes to the "creeping obesity" observed in highly mechanized and technically advanced societies. On the other hand, regular exercisers maintain appetite control within a reactive zone in which food intake more readily matches daily energy expenditure.

In considering the effects of exercise on appetite and food intake, one must distinguish exercise type and duration and the participant's body fat status. Lumberjacks, farm laborers, and endurance athletes consume about twice as many daily calories as sedentary individuals. More specifically, marathon runners, cross-country skiers, and cyclists consume about 4000 to 5000 kcal daily, yet they are the leanest people in the population. Obviously, their large caloric intake meets the energy requirements of training while maintaining a relatively lean body composition.

For the overweight person, any small compensatory appetite-stimulating effect of moderate physical activity is more than offset by the extra energy required for exercise. To some extent, the large energy reserve of the overfat person makes it easier to tolerate weight loss and exercise without the obligatory increase in caloric intake typically observed for leaner counterparts.[105,187] *In essence, a weak coupling exists between the short-term energy deficit induced by exercise and energy intake. Increased physical activity by overweight, sedentary individuals does not necessarily alter physiologic needs and automatically produce compensatory increases in food intake to balance additional energy expenditure.*

INTEGRATIVE QUESTION

Respond to the person who claims: "The only way to lose weight is to stop eating. It's that simple!"

Misconception 2: Caloric Stress of Physical Activity

A common misconception concerns the contribution to weight loss of the calories burned in typical exercise. Some argue correctly that it requires an inordinate amount of short-term exercise to lose just 0.45 kg of body fat: for example, chopping wood for 10 hours, playing golf for 20 hours, performing mild calisthenics for 22 hours, or playing ping pong for 28 hours or volleyball for 32 hours. Consequently, a 2- or 3-month exercise regimen produces only a small fat loss in an overfat person. From a different perspective, however, if one played golf (no cart) for 2 hours daily (350 kcal) 2 days per week (700 kcal), it would take about 5 weeks to lose 0.45 kg of body fat. Assuming the person plays year-round, golfing 2 days a week produces a 4.5-kg yearly fat loss, provided food intake remains constant. Even an activity as innocuous as chewing gum burns an extra 11 kcal each hour, a 20% increase over normal resting metabolism. *Simply stated, the calorie-expending effects of exercise add up. A caloric deficit of 3500 kcal equals a 0.45-kg body fat loss, whether the deficit occurs rapidly or systematically over time.*

In estimating the energy cost of performing various physical activities, one assumes that exercise energy expenditure remains constant among people of a particular body size. In Chapter 8, we noted that the energy cost data for most physical activities represent averages, often based on only a few observations. A wide range of values exists because of individual differences in performance style and technique, such environmental factors as terrain, temperature, and wind resistance, and the intensity of participation. Consequently, energy expenditure values for the physical activities presented in Appendix C do not represent constants. Rather, they reflect "average" values applicable under "average" conditions when applied to the "average" person of a given body mass. The data provide approximations for establishing the caloric cost of diverse physical activities.

THE RECOVERY "AFTERGLOW." Controversy exists about the quantitative contribution of excess postexercise oxygen consumption to the total energy expended in physical activity. With low-to-moderate exercise, as performed by most people who exercise for weight control, the contribution of recovery metabolism—the so-called afterglow—to total energy expenditure remains small in relation to exercise energy expediture, ranging up to 75 kcal for exercise durations up to 80 minutes.[161,169] In addition, exercise training causes faster adjustments in postexercise energetics that reduce the magnitude of the total recovery oxygen consumption.[190]

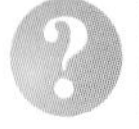

INTEGRATIVE QUESTION

Among physically active men and women, how can those who consume the most calories weigh less than those who consume fewer calories?

EFFECTIVENESS OF REGULAR EXERCISE

The effectiveness of regular exercise for weight loss relates closely to the degree of excess body fat. In general, obese persons lose weight and fat more readily with exercise than normal-weight persons.[181] In addition, aerobic exercise and resistance training, even without dietary restriction, provide significant positive spinoff to the weight loss effort. They alter body composition favorably (reduced body fat and small increase in FFM) for the otherwise healthy overweight person, cardiac patient, and physically challenged individual.[113,209] Overfat children who had 4 months of 40-minute aerobic exercise sessions 5 days a week without dietary restriction accumulated significantly less visceral adipose tissue than nonexercising controls.[154] The active children also gained significantly more FFM and lost significantly more total fat mass and percentage body fat. Adolescent males who participated regularly in vigorous activities showed less abdominal fat than their sedentary counterparts.[44] This indicates that regular exercise and improved aerobic fitness may target fat accumulation in the

TABLE 30.6 ➤ CHANGES IN BODY COMPOSITION AFTER 12 WEEKS OF EITHER RESISTANCE TRAINING OR ENDURANCE TRAINING

	Controls		Resistance Trained		Endurance Trained	
Variable	Pretreatment	Posttreatment	Pretreatment	Posttreatment	Pretreatment	Posttreatment
Relative body fat (%)	20.1 ± 8.5	20.2 ± 8.5	21.8 ± 6.2	18.7 ± 6.6[a]	18.4 ± 7.9	16.5 ± 6.4[a]
Fat mass (kg)	16.2 ± 10.8	16.3 ± 10.5	17.2 ± 7.6	14.8 ± 6.2[a]	14.4 ± 7.9	12.8 ± 7.1[a]
Fat-free body mass (kg)	64.3 ± 5.4	64.4 ± 6.6	61.9 ± 8.3	64.4 ± 9.0[a]	64.1 ± 8.2	64.7 ± 8.6
Total body mass (kg)	80.5 ± 8.1	80.7 ± 8.5	79.1 ± 8.3	79.2 ± 7.6	78.5 ± 8.2	77.5 ± 7.9

[a]Significant difference between pre- to posttest measurements ($P < .05$).
All values means ± SD.
From Broeder CE, et al. Assessing body composition before and after resistance or endurance training. Med Sci Sports Exerc 1997;29:705.

abdominal–visceral area to a greater extent than peripheral fat deposits. Even when an exercise program produces no loss in body weight, substantial reductions occur in both abdominal subcutaneous and visceral fat.[182] This response would certainly blunt a tendency toward insulin resistance and resulting predisposition to type 2 diabetes.

Adding exercise to a weight-loss program favorably modifies the composition of the weight lost in the direction of greater fat loss.[8,110,113,136] In a pioneering study on this topic, each of three groups of adult women maintained a daily caloric deficit of 500 kcal for 16 weeks.[231] The diet group reduced daily food intake by 500 kcal, while the exercise group increased energy output by 500 kcal with a supervised walking and exercise program 5 days a week. The women using diet plus exercise created a daily 500-kcal deficit by reducing food intake by 250 kcal and increasing energy output by 250 kcal through exercise. No significant difference emerged among the three groups for weight loss; each group lost approximately 5 kg. This finding shows that a caloric deficit produces body weight loss regardless of the method used to create the energy imbalance. *For body fat reduction, combining diet and exercise proved most effective.* FFM *increased* by 0.9 kg (exercise group) and 0.5 kg (combination group) with exercise, while dieters *lost* 1.1 kg of lean tissue.

Comparisons of conventional resistance training with endurance training indicate unique resistance-training benefits on body composition.[19,209] Table 30.6 summarizes the effects of 12 weeks of either endurance exercise or resistance training on nondieting, untrained young men. Endurance training significantly reduced percentage body fat (hydrostatic weighing) from reduced fat mass (−1.6 kg; no change in FFM), while resistance training significantly decreased body fat mass (−2.4 kg) and increased the FFM (+2.4 kg). Because FFM remains metabolically more active than body fat, conserving or increasing this tissue depot with exercise training helps maintain a higher level of resting metabolism,[40,47,205] average daily metabolic rate,[195,209] and possibly fat oxidation during rest, all counteracting the age-related increase in adiposity.[25]

Table 30.7 shows the effects of regular exercise for weight loss by six sedentary, obese young men who exercised 5 days a week for 16 weeks by walking 90 minutes each session. The men lost nearly 6 kg of body fat, a decrease in percentage body fat from 23.5 to 18.6%. Exercise capacity also improved, as did HDL-cholesterol (15.6%) and the HDL:LDL cholesterol ratio (25.9%).

Figure 30.23 shows body composition changes for 40 obese women placed into one of four groups: (1) control, no exercise, and no diet; (2) diet only, no exercise (DO); (3) diet plus resistance exercise (D + E), and (4) resistance exercise only, no diet (EO). The women trained 3 days a week for 8 weeks. They performed 10 repetitions each of three sets of eight strength exercises. Body mass decreased significantly for DO (−4.5 kg) and D + E (−3.9 kg), compared with EO (+0.5 kg) and controls (−0.4 kg). Importantly, FFM increased significantly for EO (+1.1 kg), whereas the DO group lost 0.9 kg of FFM. The authors concluded that augmenting a calorie-restriction program with resistance exercise training preserves FFM, compared with dietary restriction alone.

TABLE 30.7 ➤ EFFECTIVENESS OF REGULAR EXERCISE ON BODY COMPOSITION AND BLOOD LIPID CHANGES IN SIX OBESE, YOUNG MEN WITH A 16-WEEK WALKING PROGRAM

Variable	Pretraining[a]	Posttraining[a]	Difference
Body mass (kg)	99.1	93.4	−5.7[b]
Body density, $g \cdot mL^{-1}$	1.044	1.056	+0.012[b]
Body fat (%)	23.5	18.6	−4.9[b]
Fat mass (kg)	23.3	17.4	−5.9[b]
Fat-free body mass (kg)	75.8	76.0	+0.2
Sum of skinfolds (mm)	142.9	104.8	−38.1[b]
HDL cholesterol $mg \cdot dL^{-1}$	32	37	+5.0[b]
HDL/LDL cholesterol	0.27	0.34	+0.07[b]

[a]Values are means.
[b]Statistically significant.
From Leon AS, et al. Effects of a vigorous walking program on body composition, and carbohydrate and lipid metabolism of obese young men. Am J Clin Nutr 1979;33:1776.

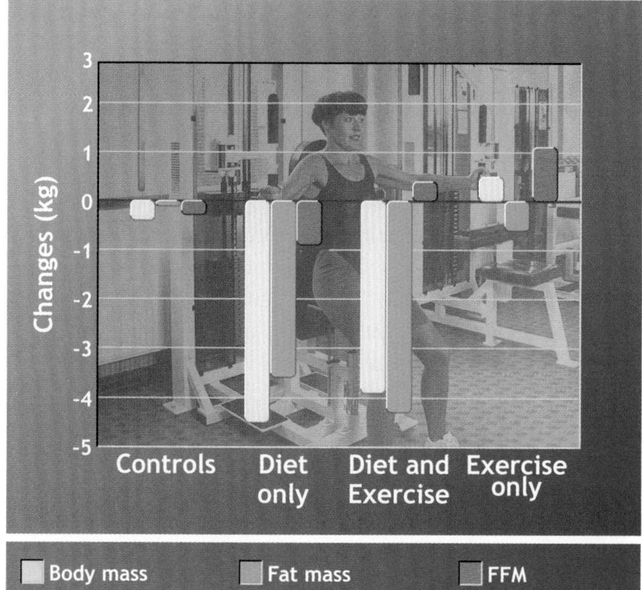

FIGURE 30.23 • Changes in body composition with combinations of resistance exercise and/or diet in obese females. (From Ballor DL, et al. Resistance weight training during caloric restriction enhances lean body weight maintenance. Am J Clin Nutr 1988;47:19.)

Most of the health-related metabolic improvements in the obese with regular exercise relate to total exercise volume and quantity of fat loss rather than to enhanced cardiorespiratory fitness.[41,42,159] Ideal exercise consists of continuous, large-muscle activities with moderate-to-high caloric cost, such as walking, running, rope skipping, stair stepping, cycling, and swimming. Many recreational sports and games are also effective in weight control, although precise quantification and regulation of energy expenditure in these activities becomes difficult. Aerobic exercise also stimulates fat catabolism, establishes favorable blood pressure responses, and generally promotes cardiovascular fitness. Interestingly, aerobic exercise training may elevate resting metabolism independent of any FFM change.[227] No selective effect exists for running, walking, or bicycling; each promotes fat loss with equal effectiveness.[163] Expenditure of an extra 300 kcal daily (e.g., moderate jogging for 30 minutes) should produce a 0.45-kg fat loss in about 12 days. This represents a yearly caloric deficit equivalent to the energy in 13.6 kg of body fat.

Dose-Response Relationship

The total energy expended in physical activity has a dose-response relation to the effectiveness of exercise for weight loss.[8,94] To combat the obesity epidemic, the public health perspective must promote the population's need to increase *total* daily energy expenditure substantially and regularly rather than increase exercise intensity to induce a training response. An overly fat person who starts out with light exercise such as slow walking accrues considerable caloric expenditure simply by extending exercise duration. The focus on exercise duration offsets the inability (and inadvisability) of having the previously sedentary, obese person start a program with more-strenuous exercise. Also, the energy cost of weight-bearing exercise relates directly to body mass; thus, the overweight person expends considerably more calories than someone of average weight.

Walking–Running for Different Durations

The duration of exercise significantly affects fat loss. Table 30.8 lists changes in body fat (predicted from skinfolds) for three groups of men who exercised for 20 weeks by walking and running for either 15, 30, or 45 minutes per workout. Data also include distance run and total duration of weekly workouts, training heart rate, body mass, sum of skinfolds (chest, axilla, triceps, abdomen, suprailiac, and anterior thigh), and waist girth.

The three exercise groups significantly decreased body fat, skinfolds, and waist girth compared with a sedentary control group. Body mass also decreased with exercise, except for the 15-minute group, whose weight remained stable. Comparing the three exercise groups, the 45-minute group lost more body fat than either the 30- or 15-minute groups. The researchers attributed this difference to the greater caloric expenditure with longer exercise (i.e., a dose–response relationship). Individuals who rely on walking as the sole exercise mode for training and weight loss, can use hand, wrist, and ankle weights to increase exercise intensity and calorie output.[25]

Exercise Frequency

To determine the optimal exercise frequency for weight loss, subjects exercised for 30 to 47 minutes for 20 weeks by either running or walking, with exercise intensity maintained between 80 and 95% of maximum heart rate.[164] Training twice weekly produced no significant changes in body mass, skinfolds, or percentage body fat, but training 3 and 4 days weekly did. Furthermore, subjects who trained 4 days a week reduced body mass and skinfolds more than subjects who trained 3 days a week. Percentage body fat decreased similarly in both groups. These findings support a recommendation to exercise *a minimum of* 3 days per week to favorably alter body composition; the additional caloric expenditure with more frequent exercise produces even greater results. The threshold exercise energy expenditure for weight loss probably remains highly individualized. However, the calorie-burning effect of each exercise session should eventually reach *at least* 300 kcal whenever possible. This generally occurs with 30 minutes of moderate-to-vigorous running, swimming, bicycling, or circuit-resistance training or 60 minutes of brisk walking.

INTEGRATIVE QUESTION

Why should one limit weight loss to no more than 2 pounds of body weight weekly?

Start Slowly and Progress Gradually

The initial stage of an exercise–weight-loss program for a previously sedentary, overly fat person should be developmental with moderate energy demands. The individual should adopt long-term goals and personal discipline and restructure eating and exercise behaviors.[135] Unduly rapid training progressions often prove counterproductive because most overfat individuals initially resist increasing their physical activity. During the first few months, intervals of faster-paced walking can replace slow walking. Meaningful changes in body weight and body composition require at least 12 weeks. Most overfat people can realistically expect to reduce body weight by 5 to 15% with programs that focus on modifying eating and exercise behaviors. Behavioral approaches to exercise should bring about lifestyle changes in daily physical activity.[204] For example, walking or bicycling can replace the auto, stair climbing can replace the elevator, and manual tools can replace power tools.[7,49] Eating less and exercising more may prove more effective in a group situation than going it alone. People who joined a weight-loss program with several friends or family members lost more weight than individuals who participated alone.[226]

Self-Selected Energy Expenditures: Mode of Exercise

No selective weight-loss effect exists among diverse modes of big-muscle aerobic exercise to favorably reduce body mass, body fat, skinfold thickness, and girths, although other differences may emerge. For example, Figure 30.24A shows that men and women generally self-select a higher energy expenditure level (with accompanying higher heart rates) at similar ratings of perceived exertion when running for 20 minutes on a treadmill than simulated cross-country skiing (NordicTrack), cycle ergometry, or aerobic riding (HealthRider).[115] Men selected a higher absolute level of exercise intensity and oxygen consumption than women in each exercise mode (Fig. 30.24B), yet treadmill running generated the greatest total oxygen consumed (energy expended) for both groups. These data suggest that for individuals without physical activity limitations, running usually provides the most suitable exercise mode for maximizing energy expenditure during self-selected intensities of continuous exercise. Whether this exercise mode proves more effective in longer-duration programs that use self-selected exercise modes for weight loss awaits verification.

DIET PLUS EXERCISE: THE IDEAL COMBINATION

Combining regular exercise and a reduced-calorie diet provides considerably more flexibility to achieve a negative caloric balance, body fat loss, and metabolic benefits than either exercise alone or diet alone.[50,147,170,211,225] Dietary restraint plus increased physical activity through lifestyle changes offers health and weight-loss benefits similar to those from combining dietary restraint and vigorous structured exercise.[7] Adding exercise to a weight-control program facilitates

TABLE 30.8 ➤ EFFECTS OF THREE TRAINING DURATIONS OF WALKING AND RUNNING ON BODY COMPOSITION CHANGES[a]

	Control (n = 16)		Training Group: 15 Minute (n = 14)		30 Minute (n = 17)		45 Minute (n = 12)	
Variable	Pre	Post	Pre	Post	Pre	Post	Pre	Post
Body mass (kg)	72.1	73.2	76.9	76.3	80.6	78.9	70.9	69.9
Body fat (%)	12.5	13.0	13.7	13.2	14.2	13.6	13.2	12.0
Sum skinfolds (mm)	73.8	79.6	83.0	77.0	90.0	83.8	77.5	67.0
Waist girth (cm)	82.7	84.9	84.3	82.8	88.2	86.1	83.6	81.8

Variable	Week	15 Minute	30 Minute	45 Minute
Distance run per workout (mi)	4	1.56	2.89	4.13
	8	1.54	2.95	4.46
	13	1.79	3.19	4.82
	17	1.75	3.24	5.06
Total time of exercise (min:s)	4	14:58	30:25	41:18
	8	14:11	28:40	42:48
	13	15:51	29:43	43:19
	17	14:53	30:12	42:27
Training heart rate (b · min^{-1})	4	179	175	174
	8	179	174	169
	13	182	175	177
	17	180	175	175
Intensity (%max HR)	4	89.4	83.8	84.5
	8	89.8	73.4	81.0
	13	94.0	90.1	89.5
	17	92.5	90.2	88.1

From Milesis CA, et al. Effects of different durations of physical training on cardiorespiratory function, body composition, and serum lipids. Res Q 1976;47:716.

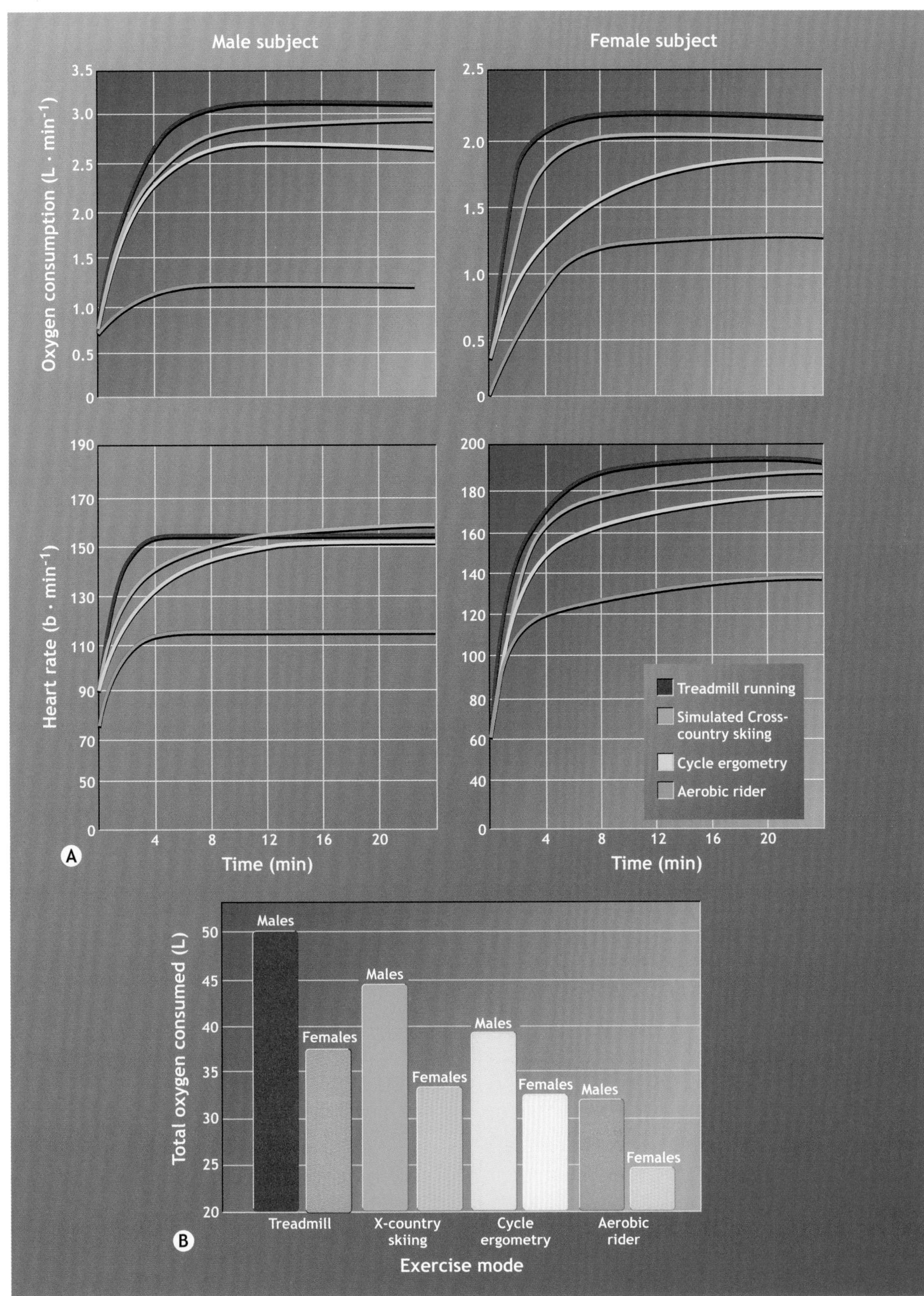

FIGURE 30.24 • A. Oxygen consumption and heart rate for a representative male and female subject during 20 minutes of self-selected exercise consisting of treadmill running, leg-cycle ergometry, simulated cross-country skiing, and aerobic riding. **B**. Total oxygen consumed by males and females during 20 minutes of each form of exercise at the same rating of perceived exertion. (From Kravitz L, et al. Exercise mode and gender comparisons of energy expenditure at self-selected intensities. Med Sci Sports Exerc 1997;29:1028.)

longer-term maintenance of fat loss than total reliance on food restriction.[106,107,156,166] Moderate regular exercise also offsets the decrement in immunoprotective natural killer cell activity associated with weight loss.[184] Table 30.9 summarizes the benefits of exercise to a weight-loss program.

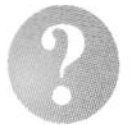

INTEGRATIVE QUESTION

Why might large-scale studies comparing diet only and exercise plus diet often show only a small added weight loss benefit for the exercise-plus-diet group?

How can an overfat person using exercise and dietary restraint to maintain a weight loss of about 1 pound (0.45 kg) a week reduce body mass by 20 pounds (9.1 kg)? A prudent 1-pound per week fat loss requires 20 weeks. The weekly energy deficit to achieve this goal must average 3500 kcal with a daily deficit of 500 kcal. One half-hour of moderate exercise (about 350 "extra" kcal) performed 3 days weekly adds 1050 kcal to the weekly deficit. Consequently, the weekly caloric intake need only decrease by 2400 kcal (about 350 kcal a day) instead of 3500 kcal to lose the desired pound of body fat each week. If the number of exercise days increases from 3 to 5, daily food intake need only decrease by 250 kcal. Extending the duration of the 5-day-per-week workouts from 30 minutes to 1 hour produces the desired weight loss without any reduction in food intake. In this case, the extra physical activity creates the entire 3500 kcal deficit.

If the intensity of the one-hour exercise performed 5 days a week increases by only 10% (cycling at 22 mph instead of 20 mph; running at 6.6 mph instead of 6.0 mph), the number of calories burned each week through exercise increases by an additional 350 kcal (3500 kcal × 0.10). This new weekly deficit of 3850 kcal (550 kcal per day) allows the dieter to *increase* daily food intake by 50 kcal and still maintain a 1-pound weekly fat loss.

Clearly, physical activity combined with mild dietary restriction effectively *unbalances* the energy balance equation for weight loss. This approach produces less-intense feelings of hunger and less psychologic stress than one that relies exclusively on caloric restriction. Furthermore, both aerobic and resistance exercises protect against FFM loss that occurs with weight loss by diet alone.[40,182] This results partly from the favorable effect of regular exercise on mobilization and use of fatty acids from adipose tissue depots.[133,175] Exercise also facilitates protein retention in skeletal muscle and retards its rate of breakdown. *The fat-burning, protein-sparing benefits of regular exercise contribute to facilitated fat loss in a weight-loss program.*

TABLE 30.9 ➤ BENEFITS OF ADDING EXERCISE TO DIETARY RESTRICTION FOR WEIGHT LOSS

- Increases overall size of the energy deficit
- Facilitates lipid mobilization and oxidation, especially from visceral adipose tissue depots
- Increases relative body fat loss by preserving fat-free body mass
- By conserving and even increasing fat-free body mass, blunts the drop in resting metabolism that accompanies weight loss
- Requires less reliance on caloric restriction to create an energy deficit
- Contributes to long-term success of the weight-loss effort
- Provides unique and significant health-related benefits

REALITY CHECK. Regardless of the approach to weight loss, a statement from the National Task Force on the Prevention and Treatment of Obesity best sums up the difficulty in solving the overly fat condition on a long-term basis: *"Obese individuals who undertake weight loss efforts should be ready to commit to lifelong changes in their behavioral patterns, diet, and physical activity."*[148]

The benefits of regular physical activity in weight loss and weight maintenance outlined in Table 30.9 come primarily from highly structured experimental research on relatively small numbers of subjects who significantly increased physical activity with high compliance. On the other hand, large-scale intervention studies (randomized clinical trials) that compare diet only with a combination of diet and regular exercise produce generally less-remarkable results. In some cases, adding exercise did not augment weight loss; when a benefit did occur, the extra weight loss remained small. Clearly, the relatively modest amount of extra physical activity in the exercise group combined with high noncompliance to the exercise regimen in large-scale studies accounts for some blunting of an exercise effect. The key to unlocking the benefits of regular exercise for weight control in the general population lies in effective implementation of psychologic–behavioral factors that favor increased *regular* physical activity.

INTEGRATIVE QUESTION

Outline a prudent, effective plan for a middle-aged woman who wants to shed 10 kg of excess weight. Provide the rationale for each recommendation.

SPOT REDUCTION DOES NOT WORK

The notion of spot reduction emanates from the belief that an increase in a muscle's metabolic activity stimulates relatively greater fat mobilization from the adipose tissue in proximity to the active muscle. Therefore, exercising a specific body area should selectively reduce more fat from that area than having a different muscle group perform exercise of the same caloric intensity. Advocates of spot reduction recommend large numbers of sit-ups or side-bends to reduce excessive abdominal and hip fat. The promise of spot reduction with exercise seems attractive from an aesthetic and health risk standpoint, but unfortunately, critical evaluation of the research evidence does not support its use.[118,151]

INTEGRATIVE QUESTION

How can small adjustments in daily energy expenditure and daily food intake alter body fat content over time? Use specific examples.

To examine claims for spot reduction, researchers compared the girths and subcutaneous fat stores of the right and left forearms of high-caliber tennis players.[76] As expected, the girth of the dominant, or playing, arm exceeded that of the nondominant arm because of a modest muscular hypertrophy from the exercise overload of tennis. Measurements of skinfold thickness, however, clearly showed that regular and prolonged tennis exercise did not reduce subcutaneous fat deposits in the playing arm. Another study evaluated fat biopsy specimens from abdominal, subscapular, and buttock sites before and after 27 days of sit-up exercise training.[100] The number of sit-ups increased from 140 at the end of the first week to 336 on day 27. Despite the significant amount of localized exercise, adipocytes in the abdominal region were no smaller than those in unexercised buttocks or subscapular control regions.

Undoubtedly, the negative energy balance created through regular exercise contributes to reducing total body fat. Exercise stimulates the mobilization of fatty acids via hormones that act on fat depots throughout the body. Body areas of greatest fat concentration and/or lipid-mobilizing enzyme activity supply the greatest amount of this energy. *Exercise does not cause significantly more fatty acid release from the fat pads directly over the active muscle.*

Areas of Fat Loss

Where on the body does fat loss occur when weight is lost? Changes in body composition and body fat distribution in 26 obese women at successive 2.3-kg increments of weight loss over a 14-week period addressed this frequently asked question.[104] Caloric restriction and a 45-minute, 3-day-a-week exercise program (15 min of general calisthenics and 30 min of walking and jogging) affected weight loss. Figure 30.25 displays changes in body composition, skinfolds, and girths for the three subgroups that reduced body mass by 2.3, 4.5, and 9.1 kg. A 4.5-kg weight loss produced nearly twice as much change in overall body composition as a loss of 2.3 kg (top graph). The corresponding change in body composition almost tripled when weight loss doubled from 4.5 to 9.1 kg. Skinfolds (middle graph) and girths (bottom graph) in the trunk region decreased about twice as much as the extremities. *Decreases in body fat with exercise training and/or caloric restriction generally preferentially mobilize and reduce upper-body subcutaneous and deep abdominal fat rather than the more "resistant" fat depots in gluteal and femoral regions.*[39,108]

Possible Gender Difference

An interesting question concerns the possibility of a gender difference in the responsiveness of weight loss to regular exercise. A meta-analysis of 53 research studies on this topic concluded that men generally respond more favorably than women to the effects of exercise on weight loss.[8] One possible explanation involves the gender difference in body fat distribution. As discussed previously, fat distributed in the upper body and abdominal regions (central fat) shows active lipolysis to sympathetic nervous system stimulation and becomes preferentially mobilized for energy during exercise.[199,213] Consequently, the greater upper-body fat distribution in men than in women may contribute to a greater sensitivity to lose fat in the abdominal region with regular exercise. Women also may more effectively preserve energy balance with increased physical activity.[218] Men often reduce energy intake with exercise training, whereas the blunting of food intake may be lower for women. The final answer to this intriguing question awaits further research.

GAINING WEIGHT: THE COMPETITIVE ATHLETE'S DILEMMA

Gaining weight to enhance body composition and exercise performance in activities requiring muscular strength and power or aesthetic appearance poses a unique problem not easily resolved. Most people focus on weight loss to reduce excess body fat and improve overall health and appearance. Weight (fat) gain per se occurs all too readily by tilting the body's energy balance to favor greater caloric intake. Weight gain for athletes should represent muscle mass and accompanying connective tissue. Generally, this form of weight gain occurs if increased caloric intake—carbohydrate for adequate energy and protein sparing, plus the amino acid building blocks of protein for tissue synthesis—accompanies a balanced, progressive resistance exercise program.

Unsupported Hype

Athletes attempting to increase muscle mass often fall easy prey to health food and diet supplement manufacturers who market "high-potency, tissue-building" substances—chromium, boron, vanadyl sulfate, β-hydroxy-β-methyl butyrate, and various protein and amino acid mixtures—none of which reliably increases muscle mass. Concerning protein supplementation, no evidence indicates that commercially prepared mixtures of powdered protein, predigested amino acids, or special high-protein "cocktails" promote muscle growth any more effectively than protein consumed in a well-balanced diet (see Chapter 23).[29,116]

Increase the Lean, Not the Fat

Endurance exercise training usually increases FFM only slightly,[164] but the overall effect reduces body weight because of fat loss from the calorie-burning and possible appetite-depressing effects of this form of exercise. In contrast, heavy muscular overload through resistance training, supported by adequate energy and protein intake (with sufficient recovery), significantly increases muscle mass and strength. Adequate energy intake ensures that no catabolism of protein available for muscle growth occurs from an energy deficit. *Thus, intense aerobic training should not coincide with resistance training to increase muscle mass.*[78,113] More than likely, the added energy (and perhaps protein) demands of concurrent resistance and aerobic exercise training impose a limit on muscle growth and responsiveness to resistance training. A safe (although not proven effective) recommendation increases daily protein intake to about 1.5 g per kg body mass

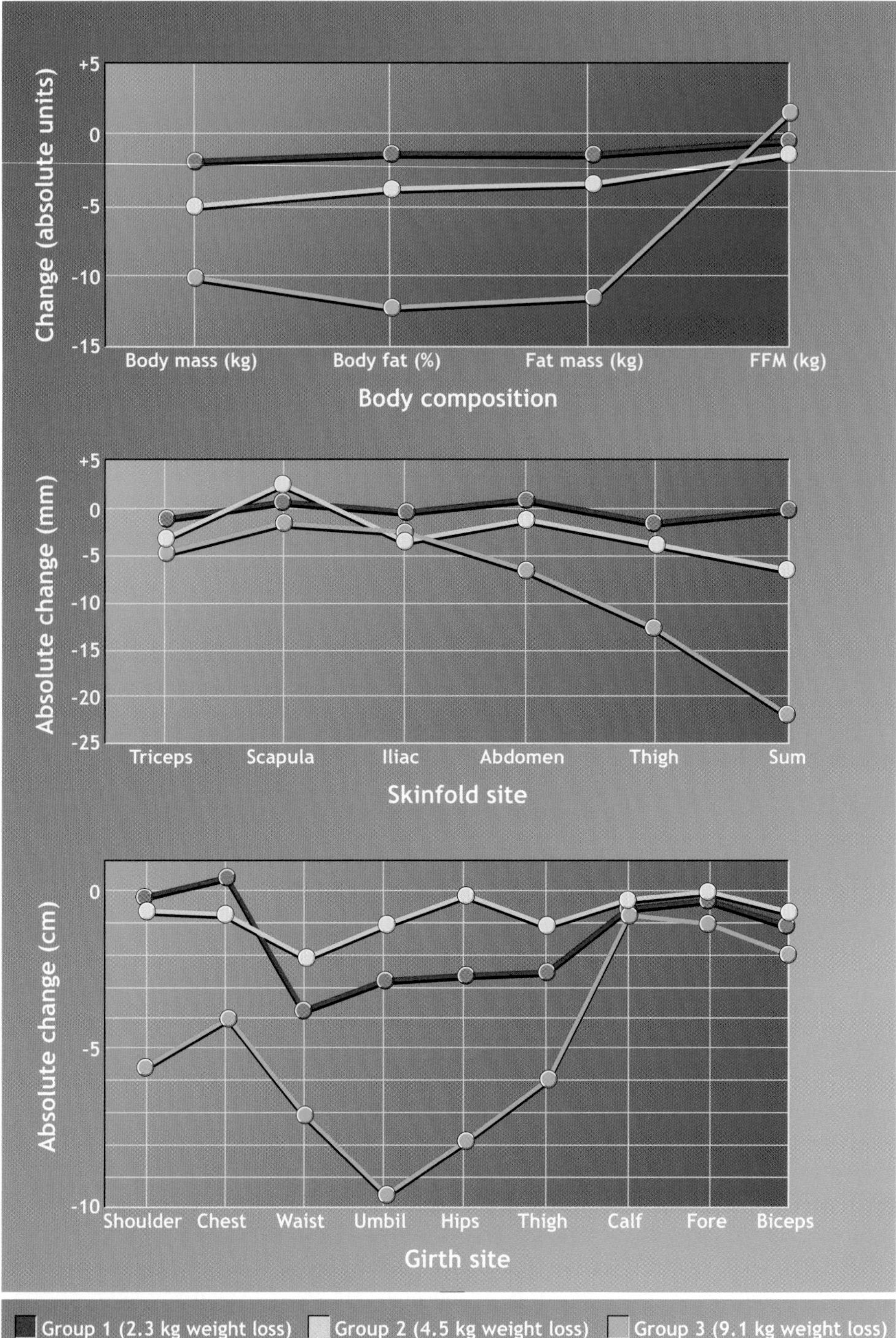

FIGURE 30.25 • Changes in body composition (*top*), skinfolds (*middle*), and girths (*bottom*) with specified weight loss. *Shoulder,* shoulders; *Umbil,* umbilicus abdomen; *Fore,* forearm. (Data from King AC, Katch FI. Changes in body density, fatfolds and girths at 2.3 kg increments of weight loss. Hum Biol 1986;58:708.)

during the resistance-training period.[125] The individual should consume a variety of plant and animal proteins; relying solely on animal protein (high in saturated fatty acids and cholesterol) potentially increases heart disease risk.

If all calories consumed in excess of the energy requirement during resistance training sustained muscle growth, then 2000 to 2500 extra kcal could supply each 0.5-kg increase in lean tissue. In practical terms, 700 to 1000 kcal added to the well-balanced daily meal plan supports a weekly 0.5- to 1.0-kg gain in lean tissue and additional energy needs for training. This ideal situation presupposes that all extra calories synthesize lean tissue.

How Much Gain to Expect

A 1-year program of heavy resistance training for young, athletic men increases body mass by about 20%, the major portion consisting of lean tissue. The rate of lean tissue gain

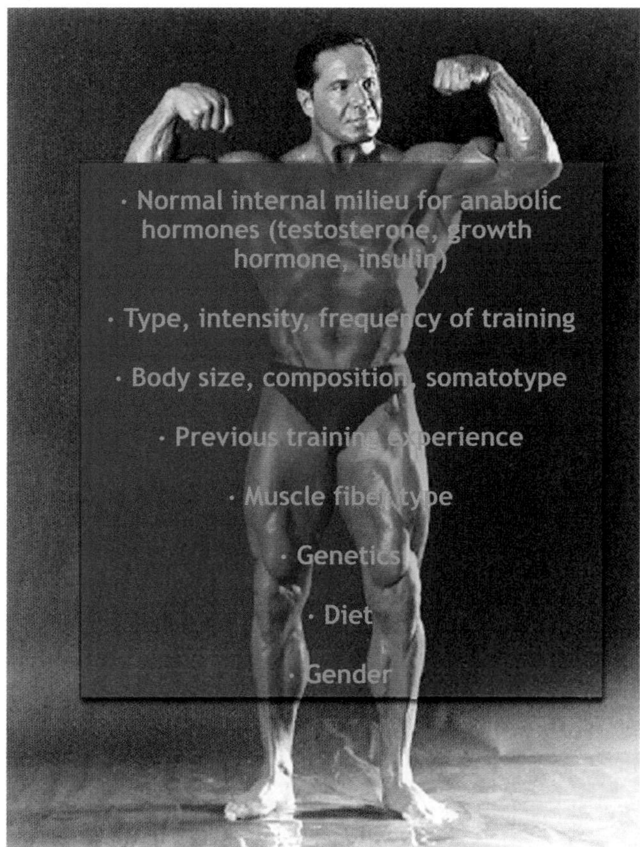

FIGURE 30.26 • Specific factors affecting the magnitude of lean tissue synthesis with resistance training. (Photo courtesy of Bill Pearl.)

rapidly plateaus as training progresses beyond the first year. For athletic women, first year gains in lean tissue mass average 50 to 75% of the absolute values for men, probably owing to women's smaller initial lean body mass. Individual differences in the daily quantity of nitrogen incorporated into body protein (and protein incorporated into muscle) also limit and explain differences among people in muscle mass increases with resistance training. Figure 30.26 presents specific factors affecting the responsiveness of lean tissue synthesis to resistance training.

Athletes with relatively high androgen:estrogen ratios and greater percentages of fast-twitch muscle fibers probably increase lean tissue to the greatest extent. Muscle mass increases most readily at the start of training in individuals with the largest relative FFM (FFM corrected for stature and body fat).[209] Regularly monitoring body mass and body fat verifies whether the combination of training and additional food intake increases lean tissue and not body fat.

INTEGRATIVE QUESTION

Outline recommendations to a high school student who wishes to add body weight to improve appearance and sports performance.

Summary

1. Three ways unbalance the energy-balance equation to produce weight loss: (1) reduce energy intake below daily energy expenditure, (2) maintain normal energy intake and increase energy output, and (3) decrease energy intake and increase energy expenditure.
2. Long-term maintenance of weight loss through dietary restriction has a success rate less than 20%. Typically, one- to two-thirds of the lost weight returns within a year and almost all of it within 5 years.
3. A caloric deficit of 3500 kcal, created through either diet or exercise, represents the equivalent of the calories in 0.45 kg of adipose tissue.
4. Prudent dieting effectively promotes weight loss. Disadvantages of extremes of semistarvation include loss of FFM, lethargy, possible malnutrition, and a depressed resting metabolism. Some of these factors conserve energy and reduce the diet's effectiveness.
5. A sustained reduction in resting metabolism represents a well-documented response to weight loss through dieting.
6. Controversy exists as to whether repeated cycles of weight loss–weight gain (yo-yo effect) increase the body's ability to conserve energy, thus making weight loss with subsequent dieting more difficult. From a public health perspective, the risks from obesity far exceed those from weight cycling.
7. Rapid weight loss during the first few days of caloric deficit mainly reflects loss of body water and stored glycogen; greater fat loss occurs per unit of weight lost as caloric restriction continues.
8. The calories burned in exercise accumulate. Over time, regular extra physical activity creates a considerable energy deficit.
9. The precise role of exercise in appetite suppression or stimulation remains unclear, although moderate increases in physical activity may blunt appetite and depress energy intake of a previously sedentary, overweight person. Most athletes eventually consume enough calories to counterbalance training's added caloric expenditure.
10. Combining exercise with caloric restriction offers a flexible and effective means of weight loss. Exercise enhances fat mobilization and catabolism, accelerating body fat loss. Regular aerobic exercise retards lean tissue loss, while resistance training increases FFM.
11. Selective exercise of specific body areas by spot exercise proves no more effective for localized fat loss than more-general physical activity.
12. Differences in body fat distribution partially explain gender difference in responsiveness to

exercise-induced weight loss. Fat deposited in the upper body and abdominal regions (male-pattern obesity) responds readily to neurohumoral stimulation and becomes preferentially mobilized in exercise compared with fat deposited in gluteal and femoral regions (female-pattern obesity).

13. Athletes should gain weight as lean body tissue (muscle mass and connective tissue). This occurs most readily with a modest increase in caloric intake plus systematic resistance training.
14. Ideally, 700 to 1000 extra kcal per day supports a weekly 0.5- to 1.0-kg gain in lean tissue and resistance training energy requirements. Realistically, individual physiologic variations and training factors also affect weight gain. For this reason, monitor changes in body mass and body fat on a regular basis.

References

1. Aaron DJ, et al. The epidemiology of leisure physical activity in an adolescent population. Med Sci Sports Exerc 1993;25:847.
2. Ahima RS, et al. Role of leptin in the neuroendocrine response to fasting. Nature 1996;382:250.
3. Alban HJ, et al. Metabolic response to low- and very-low-calorie diets. Am J Clin Nutr 1989;49:745.
4. Allison DB, et al. Annual deaths attributable to obesity in the United States. JAMA 1999;282:1530.
5. American Medical Association. A critique of low-carbohydrate ketogenic weight and reduction regimens (a review of Dr. Atkins' diet revolution). JAMA 1973;224:1418.
6. Anderson RE, et al. Relationship of physical activity and television watching with body weight and level of fatness among children. JAMA 1998;279:938.
7. Anderson RE. Effects of lifestyle activity vs structured aerobic exercise in obese women. JAMA 1999;281:335.
8. Ballor DL, Keesey RE. A meta-analysis of the factors affecting changes in body mass, fat mass and fat-free mass in males and females. Int J Obes 1991;15:717.
9. Bar-Or O, et al. Physical activity, genetic, and nutritional considerations in childhood weight management. Med Sci Sports Exerc 1998;30:2.
10. Behnke AR, Wilmore JH. Evaluation and regulation of body build and composition. Englewood Cliffs, NJ: Prentice Hall, 1974.
11. Bemben MG, et al. Age-related patterns in body composition for men aged 20-79 yr. Med Sci Sports Exerc 1995;27:264.
12. Bender R, et al. Effect of age on excess mortality in obesity. JAMA 1999;281:1498.
13. Booth FW, et al. Waging war on modern chronic diseases; primary prevention through exercise biology. J Appl Physiol 88;774:2000.
14. Bouchard C. Genetics of obesity: overview and research directions. In: Bouchard C, ed. The genetics of obesity. Boca Raton, FL: CRC Press, 1994.
15. Bouchard C, et al. The response to long term feeding in identical twins. N Engl J Med 1990;322:1477.
16. Bouchard C, et al. The response to exercise with constant energy intake in identical twins. Obes Res 1994;2:400.
17. Bouchard C. Human variation in body mass: evidence for a role of the genes. Nutr Rev 1997;55:S21.
18. Bray GA, Popkin BM. Dietary fat intake does affect obesity! Am J Clin Nutr 1998;68:1157.
19. Broeder CE, et al. Assessing body composition before and after resistance or endurance training. Med Sci Sports Exerc 1997;29:705.
20. Brownell KD, et al. The effects of repeated cycles of weight loss and regain in rats. Physiol Behav 1986;38:459.
21. Bungard LB, et al. Energy requirements of middle-aged men are modifiable by physical activity. Am J Clin Nutr 1998;69:1136.
22. Buono MJ, et al. Effects of a diet and exercise program on blood lipids, cardiorespiratory function, and body composition in obese women. Med Sci Sports Exerc 1985;17:189.
23. Byers T, et al. Weight cycling, weight gain, and risk of hypertension in women. Am J Epidemiol 1999;150:573.
24. Calle EE, et al. Body-mass index and mortality in a prospective cohort of U.S. adults. N Engl J Med 1999;341:1097.
25. Calles-Escrndón J et al. Basal fat oxidation decreases with aging in women. J Appl Physiol 1995;78:266.
26. Carpenter WH, et al. Total energy expenditure in 4 to 6 year old children. Am J Physiol 1993;27:E706.
27. Carpenter WH, et al. Total daily energy expenditure in free-living older African-Americans and Caucasians. Am J Physiol (Endocrinol Metab) 1998; 274:E96–101.
28. Centers for Disease Control and Prevention. Update: prevalence of overweight among children, adolescents, and adults: United States, 1988–1994. MMWR 1997;46:199.
29. Clarkson PM. Dietary supplements and pharmaceutical agents for weight loss and gain. In: Lamb DR, Murray R, eds. Perspectives in exercise science and sports medicine, vol 10: Exercise, nutrition, and weight control. Carmel, IN: Cooper Publishing, 1998.
30. Cleland R, et al. Commercial weight loss products and programs: what consumers stand to gain and lose. Washington, DC: Federal Trade Commission, Bureau of Consumer Protection, 1998.
31. Considine RV, Caro JF. Leptin: genes, concepts, and clinical perspective. Horm Res 1996;46:249.
32. Considine RV, et al. Serum immunoreactive-leptin concentrations in normal-weight and obese humans. N Engl J Med 1996;334:292.
33. Conway JM, et al. Visceral adipose tissue differences in black and white women. Am J Clin Nutr 1995;61:765.
34. Crawford D, et al. Can anyone successfully control their weight? Findings of a three year community-based study of men and women. Int J Obes Relat Metab Disord 2000;9:1107.
35. Daniels SR, et al. Body fat distribution and cardiovascular risk factors in children. Circulation 1999;99:541.
36. Davidson MH, et al. Weight control and risk factor reduction in obese subjects treated for 2 years with orlistat. JAMA 1999;281:235.
37. Dearborn WF, et al. Data on the growth of public school children (from the materials of the Harvard Growth Study). Monogr Soc Res Child Dev no. 1, 1938.
38. deBruin NC, et al. Quantitative assessment of infant body fat by anthropometry and total-body electrical conductivity. Am J Clin Nutr 1995;61:279.
39. Dengel DR, et al. Comparable effects of diet and exercise on body composition and lipoproteins in older men. Med Sci Sports Exerc 1994;26:1307.
40. Després J-P. Physical activity and adipose tissue. In: Bouchard C, et al., eds. Physical activity, fitness, and health. Champaign, IL: Human Kinetics, 1994.
41. Després J-P. Visceral obesity, insulin resistance, and dyslipidemia: contribution of endurance exercise training to the treatment of the plurimetabolic syndrome. Exerc Sport Sci Rev 1997;25:271.
42. Després J-P, Lamarche B. Low-intensity endurance exercise training, plasma lipoproteins and the risk of coronary heart disease. J Intern Med 1994;236:7.
43. Dietz WH. Health consequences of obesity in youth: childhood predictors of adult disease. Pediatrics 1998;101:518.
44. Dionne I, et al. The association between vigorous physical activities and fat deposition in male adolescents. Med Sci Sports Exerc 2000;32:392.
45. Dirlewanger M, et al. Effect of moderate physical activity on plasma leptin concentrations in humans. Eur J Appl Physiol 1999;79:331.
46. Ditschuneit HH, et al. Metabolic and weight-loss effects of a long-term dietary intervention in obese patients. Am J Clin Nutr 1999;69:198.
47. Dolezal BA, Potteiger JA. Concurrent resistance and endurance training influence basal metabolic rate in nondieting individuals. J Appl Physiol 1998;85:695.
48. Dulloo AG, Jacquet J. Adaptive reduction in basal metabolic rate in response to food deprivation in humans: a role for feedback signals from fat stores. Am J Clin Nutr 1998;68:599.
49. Dunn AL, et al. Comparison of lifestyle and structured interventions to increase physical activity and cardiorespiratory fitness. JAMA 1999;281:327.
50. Ebbeling CB, Rodriguez NR. Effect of exercise combined with diet therapy on protein utilization in obese children. Med Sci Sports Exerc 1999;31:378.
51. Eck Clemens LH, et al. The effect of eating out on quality of diet in premenopausal women. J Am Diet Assoc 1999;99:4421.

52. Eckert ED, et al. Leptin in anorexia nervosa. J Clin Endocrinol Metab 1998;83:791.
53. Elchebly M, et al. Increased insulin sensitivity and obesity resistance in mice lacking the tyrosine phophatase-1B gene. Science 1999;283:1544.
54. Epstein LH, et al. Exercise in treating obesity in children and adolescents. Med Sci Sports Exerc 1996;28:428.
55. Executive summary of the clinical guidelines on the identification, evaluation, and treatment of overweight and obesity in adults. Arch Intern Med 1998;158:1855.
56. Ferguson MA, et al. Fat distribution and hemostatic measures in obese children. Am J Clin Nutr 1998;67:1136–1140.
57. Fisler JS. Cardiac effects of starvation and semi-starvation diets: safety and mechanisms of action. Am J Clin Nutr 1992;56:230S.
58. Fleury C, et al. Uncoupling protein-2: a novel gene linked to obesity and hyperinsulinemia. Nat Genet 1997;15:269.
59. Fogelholm M, et al. Additive effects of mutations in the β_3-adrenergic receptor and uncoupling protein-1 genes on weight loss and weight maintenance of Finnish women. J Clin Endocrinol Metabol 1998;8:4246.
60. Folsom R, et al. Body fat distribution and 5-year risk of death in older women. JAMA 1993;269:483.
61. Foster GD, et al. Resting energy expenditure in obese African American and Caucasian women. Obes Res 1997;5:1.
62. Foster GD, et al. changes in resting energy expenditure after weight loss in obese African American women and white women. Am J Clin Nutr 1999;69:13.
63. Freedman DS, et al. Relation of circumferences and skinfold thicknesses to lipid and insulin concentrations in children and adolescents: the Bogalusa Heart Study. Am J Clin Nutr 1999;69:308.
64. Froom P, et al. Smoking cessation and body mass index of occupationally active men: The Israeli CORDIS Study. Am J Public Health 1999;89:718.
65. Gallagher D, et al. Healthy percentage body fat ranges: an approach for developing guidelines based on body mass index. Am J Clin Nutr, 2000;72:694.
66. Gannon B, et al. Do African Americans have lower-energy expenditure than Caucasians? Int J Obes 2000;24:4.
67. Gordon-Larsen P, et al. Adolescent physical activity and inactivity vary by ethnicity: the National Longitudinal Study of Adolescent Health. J Pediatr 1999;135:301.
68. Gleysteen LJ. Facilitated vertical gastric pouch construction for gastric bypass. Obes Surg 2000;10:174.
69. Gortmaker SL, et al. Television viewing as a cause of increasing obesity among children in the United States. 1986–1990. Arch Pediatr Adolesc Med 1996;150:136.
70. Gower BA, et al. Fat distribution and insulin response in prepubertal African American and white children. Am J Clin Nutr 1998;67:821.
71. Grinspoon S, et al. Serum leptin levels in women with anorexia nervosa. J Clin Endocrinol Metab 1996;81:3861.
72. Grundy SM. Multifactorial causation of obesity: implications for prevention. Am J Clin Nutr 1998;67(suppl):563S.
73. Gunnell DJ, et al. Childhood obesity and adult cardiovascular mortality: a 57-y follow-up study based on the Boyd Orr cohort. Am J Clin Nutr 1998;67:1111.
74. Guo SS, et al. The predictive value of childhood body mass index values for overweight at age 35 yr. Am J Clin Nutr 1994;59:810.
75. Gutin B, et al. Plasma leptin concentrations in obese children: changes during 4-mo periods with and without physical training. Am J Clin Nutr 1999;69:388.
76. Gwinup G, et al. Thickness of subcutaneous fat and activity of underlying muscles. Ann Intern Med 1971;74:408.
77. Heini AF, Weinsier RL. Divergent trends in obesity and fat intake patterns: the American paradox. Am J Med 1997;102:259.
78. Hennessy LC, Watson AWS. The interference effects of training for strength and endurance simultaneously. J Strength Cond Res 1994;8:12.
79. Heymsfield SB, et al. Recombinant leptin for weight loss in obese and lean adults: a randomized, controlled, dose-escalation trial. JAMA 1999;282:1568.
80. Hickey MS, et al. Gender-dependent effects of exercise training on serum leptin levels in humans. Am J Physiol (Endocrinol Metab 35) 1997; 274:E562.
81. Hill JO, Peters JC. Environmental contributions to the obesity epidemic. Science 1998;280:1371.
82. Hill JO, et al. Racial differences in amounts of visceral adipose tissue in young adults: the CARDIA (Coronary Artery Risk Development in Young Adults) Study. Am J Clin Nutr 1999;69:381.
83. Hirsch J, Batchelor BR. Adipose tissue cellularity in human obesity. Clin Endocrinol Metab 1976;5:299.
84. Hirsch J, Knittle J. Cellularity of obese and non-obese human adipose tissue. Fed Proc 1970;29:1518.
85. Hirsch J, et al. Diet composition and energy balance in humans. Am J Clin Nutr 1998;67(suppl):551S.
86. Hovell MF, et al. Long term weight loss maintenance: assessment of behavioral and supplemental fasting regimen. Am J Public Health 1988;78:663.
87. Hu FB, et al. Trends in the incidence of coronary heart disease and changes in diet and lifestyle in women. N Engl J Med 2000;343:530.
88. Huang Z, et al. Body weight, weight change, and risk for hypertension in women. Ann Intern Med 1998;128:81.
89. Hunter GR, et al. Fat distribution, physical activity, and cardiovascular risk factors. Med Sci Sports Exerc 1997;29:362.
90. Iribarren CN, et al. Association of weight loss and weight fluctuation with mortality among Japanese American men. N Engl J Med 1995;333:686.
91. Istook E Jr. Research funding on major disease is not proportionate to taxpayers' needs. J NIH Res 1997;9:26.
92. Jackson RS, et al. Obesity and impaired prohormone processing associated with mutations in the human prohormone convertose 1 gene. Nat Genet 1997;16:303.
93. Jakicic JM, Wing RR. Differences in resting energy expenditure in African American versus Caucasian overweight females. Int J Obes 1998;22:236.
94. Jakicic JM, et al. Effects of intermittent exercise and use of home exercise equipment on adherence, weight loss, and fitness in overweight women. JAMA 1999;282:1554.
95. Jeffrey R, et al. Weight cycling and cardiovascular risk factors in obese men and women. Am J Clin Nutr 1992;55:641.
96. Jeffrey RW, et al. Long-term maintenance of weight loss: current status. Health Psychol 2000;19 (1 suppl):5.
97. Johnson ML, et al. Relative importance of inactivity and overeating in energy balance in obese high school girls. Am J Clin Nutr 1986;44:779.
98. Kahn MA, et al. The prevalence of cardiac valvular insufficiency assessed by transthoracic echocardiography in obese patients treated with appetite-suppressant drugs. N Engl J Med 1998;399:713.
99. Kassirer JP, Angell M. Losing weight—an ill-fated New Year's resolution. N Engl J Med 1998;338:52.
100. Katch FI, et al. Effects of situp exercise training on adipose cell size and adiposity. Res Q Exerc Sport 1984;55:242.
101. Katch FI, et al. The fidget factor. Kansas City: McMeel Publishing, 2000.
102. Keim NL, et al. Relation between circulating leptin concentrations and appetite during a prolonged, moderate energy deficit in women. Am J Clin Nutr 1998;68:794.
103. Kern PA, et al. The effects of weight loss on the activity and expression of adipose-tissue lipoprotein lipase in very obese humans. N Engl J Med 1990;322:1053.
104. King AC, Katch FI. Changes in body density, fatfolds and girths at 2.3 kg increments of weight loss. Hum Biol 1986;58:708.
105. King NA, et al. Effects of exercise on appetite control: implications for energy balance. Med Sci Sports Exerc 1997;29:1070.
106. Klem ML, et al. A descriptive study of individuals successful at long-term maintenance of substantial weight loss. Am J Clin Nutr 1997;66:239.
107. Kohrt WM, et al. Body composition of healthy sedentary and trained, young and older men and women. Med Sci Sports Exerc 1992;24:832.
108. Kohrt WM, et al. Exercise training improves fat distribution patterns in 60- to 70-year-old men and women. J Gerontol 1992;47:M99.
109 Kolaczynski JW, et al. Response of leptin to short term and prolonged overfeeding in humans. J Clin Endocrinol Metab 1996;82:561.
110. Konstantin NP, et al. Effects of dieting and exercise on fat-free body mass, oxygen uptake, and strength. Med Sci Sports Exerc 1985;17:446.
111. Kotani KK, et al. Sexual dimorphism of age-related changes in whole-body fat distribution in the obese. Int J Obes Metab Disord 1994;18:207.
112. Kramer MS. Do breast feeding and delayed introduction to solid food protect against subsequent obesity? J Pediatr 1981;98:883.
113. Kraemer WJ, et al. Compatibility of high-intensity strength and endurance training on hormonal and skeletal muscle adaptations. J Appl Physiol 1995;78:976.
114. Kraemer WJ, et al. Influence of exercise training on physiological and performance changes with weight loss in men. Med Sci Sports Exerc 1999;31:1320.

115. Kravitz L, et al. Exercise mode and gender comparisons of energy expenditure at self-selected intensities. Med Sci Sports Exerc 1997;29:1028.
116. Kreider RB. Dietary supplements and the promotion of muscle growth with resistance exercise. Sports Med 1999;27:97.
117. Kristensen P, et al. Hypothalamic CART is a new anorectic peptide regulated by leptin. Nature 1998;393:72.
118. Krotkiewski M, et al. The effect of unilateral isokinetic strength training on local adipose and muscle tissue morphology, thickness and enzymes. Eur J Appl Physiol 1979;22:221.
119. Krotkiewski M, et al. Increased muscle dynamic endurance associated with weight reduction on a very-low-calorie diet. Am J Clin Nutr 1990;51:321.
120. Kuczmarski RJ, et al. Increasing prevalence of overweight among US adults. JAMA 1994;272:205.
121. Kuczmarski RJ, et al. Varying body mass index cutoff points to describe overweight prevalence among US adults: NHANES III (1988–1994). Obes Res 1997;5:542.
122. Lappalainen R, et al. Recent body-weight changes and weigh loss practices in the European Union. Public Health Nutr 1999;2(1A):135.
123. Lee CD, et al. Cardiorespiratory fitness, body composition, and all-cause and cardiovascular disease mortality in men. Am J Clin Nutr 1999;69:373.
124. Lee I-M, et al. U.S. weight guidelines: is it also important to consider cardiorespiratory fitness? Int J Obes 1998;22:S2.
125. Lemon PWR. Do athletes need more dietary protein and amino acids? Int J Sports Nutr 1995;5:S39.
126. Leyva F, et al. Factors of the metabolic syndrome: Baseline interrelationships in the first follow-up cohort of the HDDRISC Study (HDDRISC-1). Arterioscl Thromb Vasc Biol 1998;18:1198.
127. Lindroos AK, et al. Familial predisposition for obesity may modify the predictive value of serum leptin concentrations for long-term weight change in obese women. Am J Clin Nutr 1998;67:1119.
128. Lowry R, et al. Physical activity, food choice, and weight management goals and practices among US college students. Am J Prev Med 2000;18:27.
129. Luke AH, et al. Leptin and body composition of Nigerians, Jamaicans, and US blacks. Am J Clin Nutr 1998;19:391.
130. Lynch NA, et al. Reductions in visceral fat during weight loss and waking are associated with improvements in $\dot{V}O_{2max}$. J Appl Physiol 2001;90:99.
131. Manson JE, et al. A prospective study of obesity and risk of coronary heart disease in women. N Engl J Med 1990;322:822.
132. Manson JE, et al. Body weight and mortality among women. N Engl J Med 1995;333:677.
133. Martin WA. Effect of acute and chronic exercise on fat metabolism. Exerc Sport Sci Rev 1996;24:203.
134. Mayer J, et al. Relation between calorie intake, body weight and physical work: studies in an industrial male population in West Bengal. Am J Clin Nutr 1956;4:169.
135. McArdle WD, Toner MM. Application of exercise for weight control: the exercise prescription. In: Frankle RT, Yang M-U, eds. Obesity and weight control. Rockville, MD: Aspen, 1988.
136. McMurray RG, et al. Responses of endurance trained subjects to caloric deficits induced by diet or exercise. Med Sci Sports Exerc 1985;17:574.
137. Melby CL, et al. Exercise, macronutrient balance, and weight regulation. In: Lamb DR, Murray R, eds. Perspectives in exercise science and sports medicine, vol. II: Exercise, nutrition, and weight control. Carmel, IN: Cooper Publishing, 1998.
138. Meredith CN, et al. Body composition and aerobic capacity in young and middle-aged endurance-trained men. Med Sci Sports Exerc 1987;19:557.
139. Metz JA, et al. A randomized trial of improved weight loss with a prepared meal plan in overweight and obese patients. Arch Intern Med 2000;160:2150.
140. Miller WC. How effective are traditional dietary and exercise interventions for weight loss? Med Sci Sports Exerc 1999;31:1129.
141. Miller-Kovach K, et al. Weight maintenance among Weight Watchers lifetime members. FASEB J 1998;12:A863.
142. Mokdad AH, et al. The spread of the obesity epidemic in the United States, 1991–1998. JAMA 1999;282:1519.
143. Molé PA, et al. Exercise reverses depressed metabolic rate produced by severe caloric restriction. Med Sci Sports Exerc 1989;21:29.
144. Montague CT, et al. Congenital leptin deficiency is associated with severe early-onset obesity in humans. Nature 1997;387:903.
145. Must A, et al. The disease burden associated with overweight and obesity. JAMA 1999;282:1523.
146. National Institutes of Health. Health implications of obesity, NIH consensus development conference statement, vol 5, no. 9. Washington, DC: U.S. Government Printing Office, 1985.
147. National Institutes of Health, National Heart, Lung, and blood Institute. Obesity evaluation initiative, Clinical guidelines and the identification, evaluation, and treatment of overweight and obesity in adults. Bethesda, MD: National Institutes of Health, June, 1998.
148. National Task Force on the Prevention and Treatment of Obesity. Very-low-calorie diets. JAMA 1993;270:976.
149. National Task Force on the Prevention and Treatment of Obesity. Long-term pharmacotherapy in the management of obesity. JAMA 1996;276:1907.
150. National Task Force on the Prevention and Treatment of Obesity. Obesity, overweight and health risk. Arch Intern Med 2000;160:898.
151. Noland M, Kearney JT. Anthropometric and densitometric responses of women to specific and general exercise. Res Q 1978;49:322.
152. Ostlund RE, et al. The ratio of waist-to-hip circumference, plasma insulin level, and glucose intolerance as independent predictors of the HDL2 cholesterol level in older adults. N Engl J Med 1990;332:229.
153. Owen OE, et al. Protein, fat, and carbohydrate requirements during starvation: anaplerosis and cataplerosis. Am J Clin Nutr 1988;68:12.
154. Owens S, et al. Effect of physical training on total and visceral fat in obese children. Med Sci Sports Exerc 1999;31:143.
155. Pasman WJ, et al. The effect of exercise training on leptin levels in obese males. Am J Physiol (Endocrinol Metab 37) 1998:274:E280.
156. Pavlov KN, et al. Exercise as an adjunct to weight loss and maintenance in moderately obese subjects. Am J Clin Nutr 1989;49:1115.
157. Pérusse L, et al. Familial aggregation of abdominal visceral fat level: results from the Quebec family. Metabolism 1996;45:378.
158. Pérusse L, et al. Acute and chronic effects of exercise on leptin levels in humans. J Appl Physiol 1997;83:5.
159. Pescatello LS, Murphy D. Lower intensity physical activity is advantageous for fat distribution and blood glucose among viscerally obese older adults. Med Sci Sports Exerc 1998;30:1408.
160. Pi-Sunyer FX. Obesity. In: Shils ME, et al. eds. Modern nutrition in health and disease. Philadelphia: Lea & Febiger, 1994.
161. Poehlman ET, et al. The impact of exercise and diet restriction on daily energy expenditure. Sports Med 1991;11:78.
162. Polito A, et al. Basal metabolic rate in anorexia nervosa: relation to body composition and leptin concentrations. Am J Clin Nutr 2000;71:1495.
163. Pollock ML, et al. Effects of mode of training on cardiovascular function and body composition of adult men. Med Sci Sports 1975;7:139.
164. Pollock ML, et al. Frequency of training as a determinant for improvement in cardiovascular function and body composition of middle-aged men. Arch Phys Med Rehabil 1975;56:141.
165. Popkin BM, Doak CM. the obesity epidemic is a worldwide phenomenon. Nutr Rev 1998;56:106.
166. Pronk NP, Wing RR. Physical activity and long-term maintenance of weight loss. Obes Res 1994;2:587.
167. Public Health Service. Healthy people 2000: national health promotion and disease prevention objectives. US Dept. of Health and Human Services publ PHS 90-50212. Washington DC: US Dept. of Health and Human Services; 1990.
168. Quesenberry CP, et al. Obesity, health services use, and health care costs among members of a health maintenance organization. Arch Intern Med 1998;158:466.
169. Quinn TJ, et al. Postexercise oxygen consumption in trained females: effect of exercise duration. Med Sci Sports Exerc 1994;26:908.
170. Racette SB, et al. Effects of aerobic exercise and dietary carbohydrate on energy expenditure and body composition during weight reduction in obese women. Am J Clin Nutr 1995;61:486.
171. Raitakari OT, et al. Associations between physical activity and risk factors for coronary heart disease: the Cardiovascular Risk in Young Finns Study. Med Sci Sports Exerc 1997;29:1055.
172. Ravussin E, et al. Reduced rate of energy expenditure as a risk factor for body-weight gain. N Engl J Med 1988;318:467.
173. Rexrode KM, et al. Abdominal adiposity and coronary heart disease in women. JAMA 1998;280:1843.
174. Ristow M, et al. Obesity associated with a mutation in a genetic regulator of adipocyte differentiation. N Engl J Med 1998;339:953.
175. Riviére D, et al. Lipolytic response of fat cells to catecholamines in sedentary and exercise trained women. J Appl Physiol 1989;66:330.
176. Roberts SB, et al. Energy expenditure and intake in infants born to lean and overweight mothers. N Engl J Med 1988;318:461.

177. Robinson TN. Reducing children's television viewing to prevent obesity: a randomized clinical trial. JAMA 1999;282:1562.
178. Rolland-Cachera MF, Bellisle F. No correlation between adiposity and food intake: why are working class children fatter? Am J Clin Nutr 1986;44:779.
179. Rosenbaum M, et al. Obesity. N Engl J Med 1997;337:396.
180. Rosengren A, et al. Body weight and weight gain during adult life in men in relation to coronary heart disease and mortality. Eur Heart J 1999;20:269.
181. Ross R, et al. Exercise alone is an effective strategy for reducing obesity and related comorbidities. Exer Sport Sci Rev 2000;28:165.
182. Ross R, et al. Reduction in obesity and related comorbid conditions after diet-induced weight loss or exercise-induced weigh loss in men: A randomized controlled trial. Ann Intern Med 2000;133:92.
183. Salans LB, et al. Experimental obesity in man: cellular character of the adipose tissue. J Clin Invest 1971;50:1005.
184. Scanga CB, et al. Effects of weight loss and exercise training on natural killer cell activity in obese women. Med Sci Sports Exerc 1998;30:1668.
185. Schoeller DA. Balancing energy expenditure and body weight. Am J Clin Nutr 1998;68(suppl):956S.
186. Schoen RE, et al. Increased blood glucose and insulin, body size, and incidence of colorectal cancer. J Natl Cancer Inst 1999;91:1147.
187. Schutz Y, et al. Role of fat oxidation in the long-term stabilization of body weight in obese women. Am J Clin Nutr 1992;55:670.
188. Segal KR, et al. Body composition, not body weight, is related to cardiovascular disease risk factors and sex hormone levels in man. J Clin Invest 1987;80:1050.
189. Serdula MK, et al. Prevalence of attempting weight loss and strategies for controlling weight. JAMA 1999;282:1359.
190. Short KR, Sedlock DA. Excess postexercise oxygen consumption and recovery rate in trained and untrained subjects. J Appl Physiol 1997;83:153.
191. Simkin-Silverman L, et al. Lifetime weight cycling and psychological health in normal-weight and overweight women. Int J Eating Disord 1998;24:175.
192. Sinaiko AR, et al. Relation of weight and rate of increase in weight during childhood and adolescence to body size, blood pressure, fasting insulin, and lipids in young adults: the Minneapolis Children's Blood Pressure Study. Circulation 1999;99:1471.
193. Sims EAH, Horton ES. Endocrine and metabolic adaptation to obesity and starvation. Am J Clin Nutr 1968;21:1455.
194. Slyper AH, et al. Low-density lipoprotein and atherosclerosis. JAMA 1994;272:305.
195. Smith DA, et al. Relationship between maximum aerobic power and resting metabolic rate in young adult women. J Appl Physiol 1997;82:156.
196. Solomons NW, Kumanyika S. Implications of racial distinctions for body composition and its diagnostic assessment. Am J Clin Nutr 2000;71:1387.
197. Spiegelman BM, Flier JS. Adipogenesis and obesity: round out the big picture. Cell 1996;87:377.
198. Spitzer L, Rodin J. Human eating behavior: a critical review of studies in normal weight and overweight individuals. Appetite 1981;2:293.
199. Staten MA. The effect of exercise on food intake in men and women. Am J Clin Nutr 1991;53:27.
200. Steen SN, Brownell KD. Patterns of weight loss and regain in wrestlers: has the tradition changed? Med Sci Sports Exerc 1990;22:762.
201. Sweeney ME, et al. Severe vs moderate energy restriction with and without exercise in the treatment of obesity: efficiency of weight loss. Am J Clin Nutr 1993;57:127.
202. Taubes G. As obesity rates rise, experts struggle to explain why. Science 1998;280:1367.
203. Thong FS, et al. Plasma leptin in female athletes: relationship with body fat, reproductive, nutritional, and endocrine factors. J Appl Physiol 2000;88:203.
204. Timperio A, et al. Physical activity beliefs and behaviours among adults attempting weight control. Int J Obes Relat Metab Disord 2000;1:81.
205. Trembly A, et al. Exercise training with constant energy intake. 2: Effect on glucose metabolism and resting energy expenditure. Int J Obes 1990;14:75.
206. Troiano RP, Flegal KM. Overweight children and adolescents: description, epidemiology, and demographics. Pediatrics 1998;101:497.
207. Udall JG, et al. Interaction of maternal and neonatal obesity. Pediatrics 1978;62:17.
208. US Department of Health and Human Services. Physical activity and health: a report of the surgeon general. Atlanta, GA: Centers for Disease Control and Prevention, 1996.
209. VanEtten LMLA, et al. Effect of body build on weight-training induced adaptations in body composition and muscular strength. Med Sci Sports Exerc 1994;26:515.
210. VanHorn L, Greenland P. Prevention of coronary artery disease is a pediatric problem. JAMA 1997;278:1779.
211. Waddem TA. Characteristics of successful weight loss maintenance. In: Pi-Sunyer FX, Allison DB, eds. Obesity treatment: establishing goals, improving outcomes, and establishing the research agenda. New York: Plenum, 1995.
212. Wagner DR, Heyward VH. Measures of body composition in blacks and whites: a comparative review. Am J Clin Nutr 2000;71:1392.
213. Wahrenberg H, et al. Adrenergic regulation of lipolysis in human fat cells during exercise. Eur J Clin Invest 1991;21:534.
214. Wardle J, Griffith J. Socioeconomic status and weight control practices in British adults. J Epidemiol Community Health 2001;55:195.
215. Wei M, et al. Relationship between low cardiorespiratory fitness and mortality in normal-weight, overweight, and obese men. JAMA 1999;282,1547.
216. Weigle DS, et al. Effect of fasting, refeeding, and dietary fat restriction on plasma leptin levels. J Clin Endocrinol Metabol 1997;82:561.
217. Weissman NJ, et al. An assessment of heart-valve abnormalities in obese patients taking dexfenfluramine, sustained-release dexfenfluramine, or placebo. N Engl J Med 1998;339:725.
218. Westerterp KR. Alterations in energy balance with exercise. Am J Clin Nutr 1998;970S.
219. Whitaker RC, et al. Predicting obesity in young adulthood from childhood and parental obesity. N Engl J Med 1997;337:869.
220. Wickelgren I. Obesity: how big a problem? Science 1998;280:1364.
221. Willett WC. Is dietary fat a major determinant of body fat? Am J Clin Nutr 1998;67(suppl):556S.
222. Willett WC, et al. Weight, weight change, and coronary heart disease in women: risk within the "normal" weight range. JAMA 1995;273:461.
223. Williams MJ, et al. Regional fat distribution in women and risk of cardiovascular disease. Am J Clin Nutr 1997;65:855.
224. Williams PT. Relationship of distance run per week to coronary heart disease risk factors in 8283 male runners. The National Runners' Health Study. Arch Intern Med 1997;157:191.
225. Wilmore JH. Increasing physical activity: alterations in body mass and composition. Am J Clin Nutr 1996;63(suppl):456S.
226. Wing RR, et al. Benefits of recruiting participants with friends and increasing social support for weight loss and maintenance. J Consult Clin Psychol 1999;67:132.
227. Withers RT, et al. Energy metabolism in sedentary and active 49- to 70-yr-old women. J Appl Physiol 1998;84:1333.
228. Yanovski SZ, et al. Report of a National Institutes of Health–Centers for Disease Control and Prevention workshop on the feasibility of conducting a randomized clinical trial to estimate the long-term health effects of intentional weight loss in obese persons. Am J Clin Nutr 1999;69:366.
229. Zhang Y, et al. Positional cloning of the mouse *obese* gene and its human homologue. Nature 1994;372:425.
230. Zimmerman MB, et al. A national study of the prevalence of overweight and obesity in 6-12 y-old Swiss children: body mass index, body-weight perceptions and goals. Eur J Clin Nutr 2000;54:568.
231. Zuti WB, Golding LA. Comparing diet and exercise as weight reduction tools. Phys Sportsmed 1976;4:49.

SECTION 7

Exercise, Successful Aging, and Disease Prevention

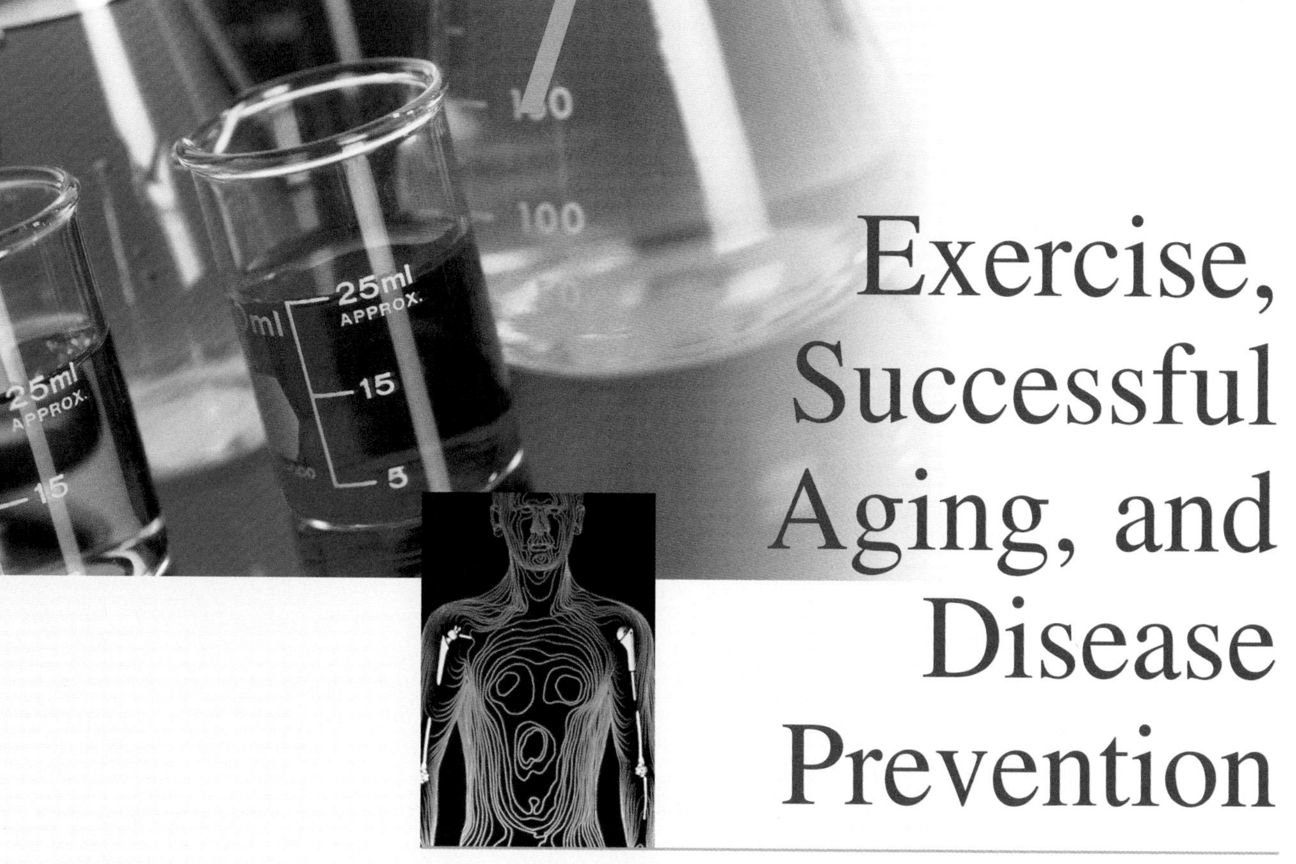

Overview

The physiologic and exercise capacities of older people usually rate below those of younger peers. It remains uncertain whether these differences reflect true biologic aging or the effect of disuse from alterations in lifestyle and reduced physical activity as people age. Encouraging news reveals that older men and women no longer conform to a sedentary stereotype with little or no initiative for active pursuits. There currently exists a meaningful upswing in participation of senior citizens in a broad range of physical activities and exercise programs. Research clearly demonstrates that maintenance of an active lifestyle into later years helps men and women retain a relatively high level of functional capacity. In addition, regular exercise offers significant protection against *and* rehabilitation from a variety of disabilities, diseases, and risk factors, particularly those related to cardiovascular health. Within this framework, the exercise physiologist provides significant skills and contributions through the prudent use of regular exercise in the clinical setting.

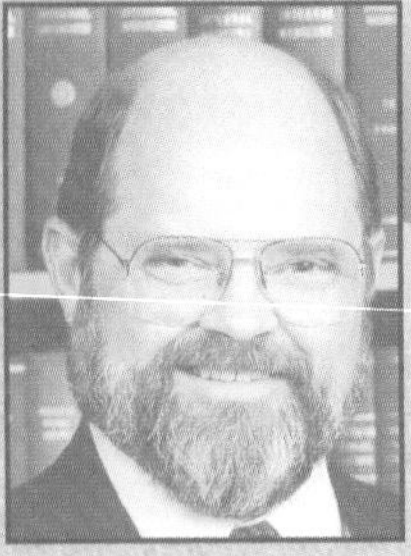

Interview with Dr. Steven N. Blair

Education: BA (Kansas Wesleyan University, Salina, KS); MS and PED (Indiana University, Bloomington, IN); Postgraduate Training (Scholar in Preventive Cardiology, Stanford University School of Medicine, Palo Alto, CA).

Current Affiliation: Director of Epidemiology and Clinical Applications, and Director of Research, The Cooper Institute for Aerobics Research, Dallas, TX.

Honors and Awards: See Appendix E.

Research Focus: My research has two major foci: (1) The Aerobics Center Longitudinal Study, an investigation of the relation of physical activity, cardiorespiratory fitness, and health outcomes and (2) randomized clinical trials of physical activity interventions and their health-related outcomes.

Memorable Publication: Blair SN, et al. Physical fitness and all-cause mortality: a prospective study of healthy men and women. JAMA 1989;262:2395.

Statement of Contributions: ACSM Citation Award
In recognition of his outstanding contributions to the body of knowledge concerning the health implications of a physically active lifestyle.

Dr. Blair is recognized for his insightful, skillful, and persistent application of epidemiological research techniques in the exploration of the health effects of physical activity and physical fitness. His studies of the Cooper Clinic population have markedly advanced our knowledge of the association between physical activity and risk of chronic disease morbidity and mortality. These studies, by demonstrating that moderate levels of physical activity and fitness provide important health benefits, have had a critical impact on public health policy.

Through his research, through his extensive service to the American College of Sports Medicine, and through his highly effective communication with health professionals and with the public, Dr. Blair has made an enormous contribution to exercise science.

➤ What first inspired you to enter the exercise science field? What made you decide to pursue your advanced degree and/or line of research?

I participated in sports in high school and college, and decided during my college career that I wanted to be a physical education teacher and athletic coach.

➤ What influence did your undergraduate education have on your final career choice?

My physical education teachers and coaches encouraged and influenced me to continue my education with graduate school. I had conducted a small, independent research project as an undergraduate and found that I liked defining a problem, collecting data, and trying to make sense of the results. In graduate school, I developed an interest in an academic research career, but I think it was the solid foundation in the liberal arts and specific areas of physical education that influenced my career direction.

➤ Who were the most influential people in your career, and why?

Gene Bissell was a strong early mentor. He is a man of uncompromising principles, dedication, and genuine concern for his students. He once forfeited a win in football when, after the game was over, he realized that an official had missed a call. When Coach Bissell pointed out the infraction, the league office replied that, sometimes calls are missed and that is just one of the breaks of the game. Coach Bissell refused to accept that ruling and insisted that his team he declared the loser.

I had several influential mentors at Indiana University. Karl and Carolyn Bookwalter gave me a research assistantship, helped me with my first publication, and generally introduced me to the world of scientific writing. Arthur Slater-Hammel introduced me to the scientific process, taught me about experimental design, and was the director of my doctoral dissertation. George Cousins was inquisitive and skeptical—two traits I consider essential for a scientist.

My first academic job was at the University of South Carolina. My interests soon turned to preventive cardiology, with a specific interest in exercise as a preventive and therapeutic modality. In the early 1970s I wrote an application for the Multiple Risk Factor Intervention Trial (MRFIT), and we received a grant to serve as one of the 20 MRFIT clinical centers. I learned much from leaders of the MRFIT, including Professors Jerry Stamler, Henry Taylor, Ogelsby Paul, Henry Blackburn, Steve Hulley, Mark Kjelsburg, Lew Kuller, and many others.

In 1978, I had an opportunity to work with Bill Haskell and Peter Wood at the Stanford University Heart Disease Prevention Program. I have had literally hundreds of hours of discussion with them over the years about various issues in exercise science and public health, and I continue to learn from their work and examples.

I also had the great opportunity to develop a relationship with Dr. Ralph S. Paffenbarger, who has considerably influenced my research over the past 20 years. "Paff" has made enormous contributions to the epidemiology of physical activity and health. His work is a model of rigorous methodology, clear thinking, poetic writing, and carefully drawn conclusions. He continues to be a good friend, research collaborator, mentor, and inspiration.

Last, I will mention colleagues at the Cooper Institute. I feel very fortunate that Dr. Cooper had the vision to establish the database for the Aerobics Center Longitudinal Study. My many colleagues at the Cooper Institute have been instrumental in our work over the past 20 years. I have learned much from them, and any success we have had is due in large part to their hard work, dedication, and scientific expertise.

➤ What has been the most interesting/enjoyable aspect of your involvement in science? What was the least interesting/enjoyable aspect?

The most interesting/enjoyable aspect of science for me is the discovery that accompanies research. Nothing is more exciting than seeing the results of an analysis that yield something new and perhaps unexpected.

The least desirable aspects of my scientific life are the constant scrambling for funds to support our research activities and the routine administrative tasks that are inherent in managing an enterprise of 25 to 30 people.

➤ What is your most meaningful contribution to the field of exercise science, and why is it so important?

I think that our work on low cardiorespiratory fitness as a predictor of morbidity and mortality in middle-aged and older women and men is a meaningful contribution to exercise science. Our report on fitness and mortality that was published in the Journal of the American Medical Association *in 1989 seemed to come at the right time and struck a responsive chord in both the scientific and lay communities. This research helped influence several statements on the significance of physical inactivity on public health, which have had a substantial effect on exercise science, public health, and clinical medicine.*

I also am proud of our research on lifestyle physical activity interventions. Our epidemiological studies revealed a curvilinear, dose-response relation between cardiorespiratory fitness and mortality, with the steepest part of the curve at the low end of the fitness continuum. Moderate levels of fitness are associated with reduced risk, and moderate amounts and intensities of physical activity can produce these moderate levels of fitness. We designed a randomized clinical trial to test the hypothesis that behaviorally-based lifestyle physical activity intervention would be as effective as a traditional, structured exercise program in increasing physical activity, improving cardiorespiratory fitness, and improving other health parameters. I am pleased that this work is leading to greater flexibility and more options for exercise programming to achieve health benefits.

➤ What advice would you give to students who express an interest in pursuing a career in exercise science research?

Obtain a strong foundation in science as an undergraduate. Read widely in your area of interest and become familiar with the leading researchers in this area of investigation. Talk to your professors about your plans and seek their advice. Do not be afraid to approach well-known researchers and ask for their advice in making your career choices. Most of them are very nice people and will be flattered if you come well prepared with good questions. As you begin to narrow your choice of institutions for graduate school, make up a visitation schedule and try to visit at least three or four programs that you think match your needs. Go to the very best program that will accept you.

➤ What interests have you pursued outside your professional career?

I like to garden, and my wife and I are proud of our landscaping and flowers. We have season tickets to the symphony, opera, summer musicals, and one of the Dallas theaters. We both use running as our main form of exercise, and we run nearly every day and have over the past 30 years. We like to travel and feel fortunate that my work has afforded us many opportunities to travel in the United States and abroad.

➤ Where do you see the exercise science field (particularly your area of greatest interest) heading in the next 30 years?

Genetic epidemiology will make important contributions to our understanding of which individuals are at greatest risk of a sedentary way of life. We will work out in much greater detail the specific types, amounts, and intensities of activity that prevent or delay specific diseases or conditions. We will finally establish appropriate public health surveillance systems to monitor accurately patterns and trends of physical activity and physical fitness in people of all ages. Physical inactivity will be recognized as the major and most expensive public health problem in the U.S.

We will learn much more about how to help sedentary individuals adopt and maintain physical activity. These advances, however, may not be sufficient to overcome the ever more toxic environment in which we live, as indicated by our continuing to engineer physical activity out of daily life. The threat posed to our public health and well being by an increase in the prevalence of sedentary habits may finally cause us to seriously consider, develop, and implement policy and legislative solutions to encourage more physical activity.

➤ You have the opportunity to give a "last lecture." Describe its primary focus.

I would describe the joys of scientific discovery and the pleasure of collaborating with colleagues to address important public health issues. I would illustrate how hazardous it is to be sedentary and unfit, and how a fit and active way of life can bring benefits to virtually all demographic groups. I would outline the seriousness of the public health problem of inactivity and try to issue a rousing call to action to encourage all to help address this problem. After accepting sustained applause, and even standing ovations and shouts of "Bravo," I would exit the stage and leave the work to the younger generation.

CHAPTER 31

Physical Activity, Health, and Aging

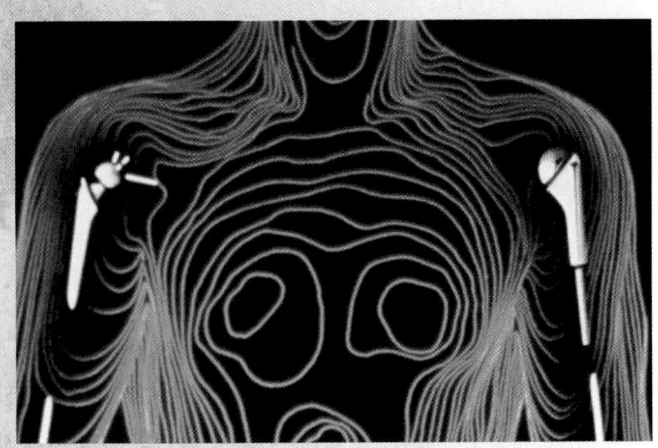

Chapter Objectives

- Summarize aging trends of the American population
- Describe the physical activity level of typical adult American men and women
- Outline the major findings of the Surgeon General's report on the population's physical activity participation
- Answer the question: "How safe is exercising?" List factors that increase the likelihood of experiencing an exercise catastrophe
- Contrast physiologic responses to exercise of children and adults and their implications for evaluating physiologic function and exercise performance
- List important age-related changes in (1) muscular function, (2) nervous system function, (3) cardiovascular function, (4) pulmonary function, and (5) body composition components
- Summarize research findings and potential benefits of moderate resistance training for the elderly
- Discuss the following statement: "A sedentary lifestyle causes losses in functional capacity at least as great as the effects of aging itself"
- Describe research about the role that regular physical activity plays in coronary heart disease prevention and life extension
- Indicate the types and levels of regular physical activity that induce the greatest improvement in risk-factor profile and overall health
- Describe vulnerable plaque and its proposed role in sudden death
- List the major modifiable heart disease risk factors and how regular physical activity affects each
- Outline the normal dynamics of homocysteine, its proposed role in coronary heart disease, and factors that affect its plasma levels
- Discuss the prevalence of heart disease risk factors in children

THE GRAYING OF AMERICA

Elderly persons make up the fastest growing segment of American society. Thirty years ago, age 65 represented the onset of old age. Now gerontologists consider 85 the demarcation of "oldest-old" and age 75, "young-old." Currently, nearly 12% or approximately 35 million Americans exceed age 65, and by the year 2030, 70 million Americans will exceed age 85. Some demographers project that one-half of the girls and one-third of the boys born in developed countries near the end of the 20th century will live in three centuries. In the short term, disease prevention, health care, and more-effective treatment of such age-related diseases as heart disease and osteoporosis help people live longer. Far fewer people now die from infectious childhood diseases, so those with the genetic potential actualize their proclivity for longevity.[66] On a different but parallel front, anticipated breakthroughs in genetic therapies may slow the aging of individual cells. Cellular damage results from (1) accumulated mutations in mitochondrial DNA, perhaps produced by injury and deterioration from oxidative stress and/or (2) gene alterations that blunt synthesis of telomerase, the enzyme that protects telomers at the ends of chromosomes so the cell continues to divide properly. Gene therapies could boost human life spans to a much greater extent than improved medical treatment or even the eradication of certain diseases.

Figure 31.1A shows that, proportionately, centenarians are currently the fastest growing age group in the United States. Numbers range from 30,000 to 50,000, up from the estimate of 15,000 in 1980 and almost none at the beginning of the 20th century. No longer viewed as a quirk of nature, 1 in

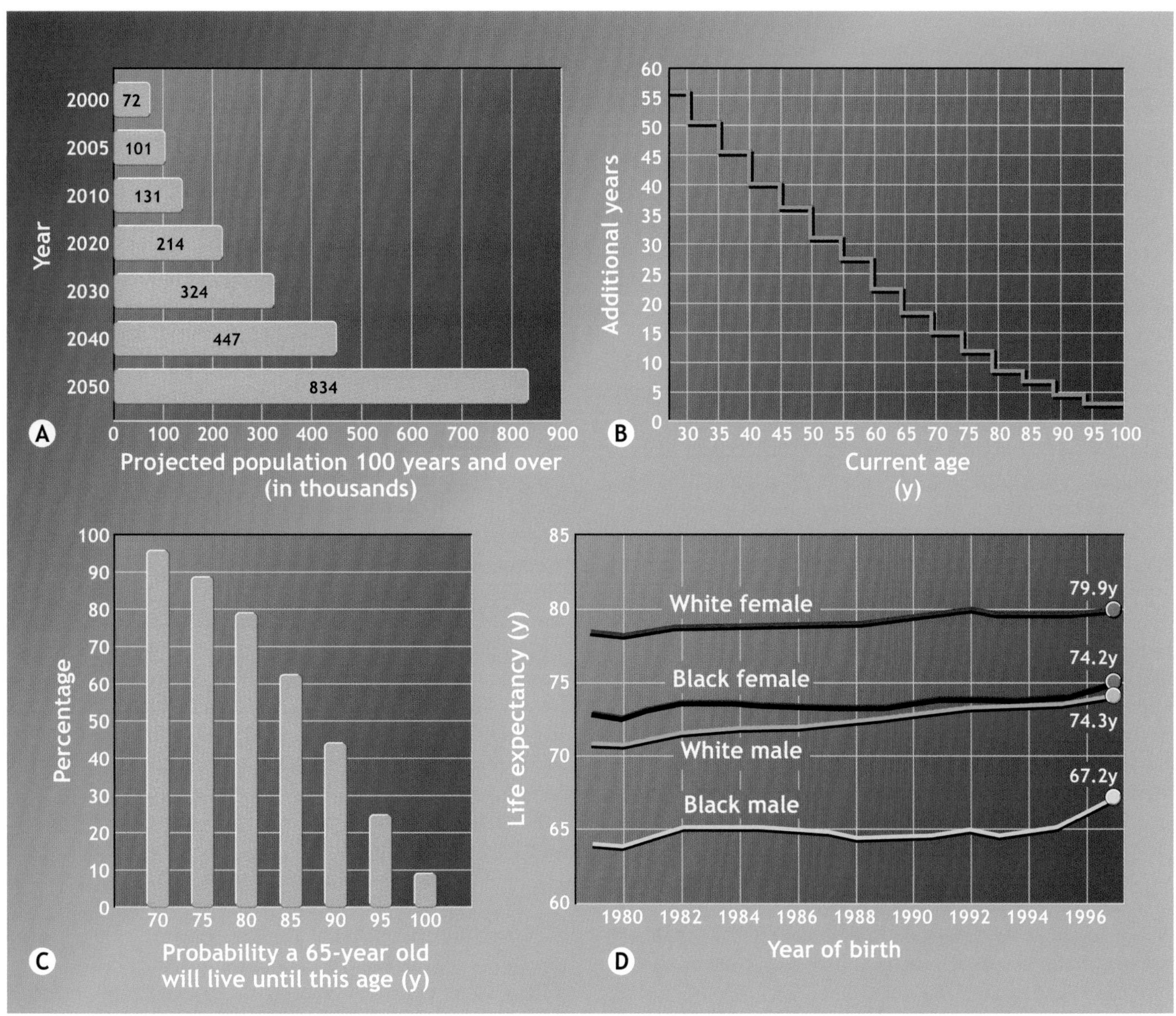

FIGURE 31.1 • The graying of America. **A**. Growth in number of centenarians in the United States. **B**. Additional life expectancy in years for individuals currently at a specific age. **C**. Probability a current 65-year-old will live to a certain age. **D**. Life expectancy trends by year of birth, race, and gender. (Data from U.S. Bureau of the Census, National Center for Health Statistics, Centers for Disease Control and Prevention: Washington, DC, and actuarial tables from insurance companies.)

10,000 Americans now lives to the age of 100. Demographers project that, by the middle of this century, more than 800,000 Americans will exceed age 100, with many maintaining relatively good health. Old-age mortality appears to be on the decline because death rate (number of people per 100 in a specific age group) levels off in the 90-year-old age category (approximately 11 per 100) and decreases to 8 per 100 after age 100. Figures 31.1B and C depict longevity statistics that retirement-pension organizations use to calculate the payout of annuity dividends. For example, a 55-year-old person today can expect to live on average an additional 31.4 years, for a life span of 86 years (Fig. 31.1B). But if this 55-year-old lives an additional 15 years to age 70, life expectancy extends to almost 89 years. Figure 31.1C indicates the proportion of individuals aged 65 years who survive to specified ages. Among current 65-year-olds, 95.5% will live to age 70, 63.3% to age 85, and nearly 10% will achieve 100 years. A child born in 1996 should survive to age 95 or 100 years.

Despite the graying of America, evolution has not kept pace with automation, and humans have failed to adapt effectively to their sedentary lifestyles. Cigarette smoking, elevated body mass index, body fatness, and reduced exercise in midlife and late adulthood provide potent predictors of subsequent disability.[233,234] Inadequate physical activity causes nearly 30% of all deaths from heart disease, colon cancer, and diabetes.[142] Changing to a more physically active lifestyle could significantly reduce mortality from these ailments in older adults and greatly improve cardiovascular and muscular functional capacities, quality of life, and independent living.[29,90,111] The greatest health benefits would derive from strategies that get the population's most sedentary adults into only light-to-moderate patterns of regular physical activity.[2,4,196,240] At any age, behavioral changes such as becoming more physically active, quitting cigarette smoking, and controlling body weight and blood pressure, act independently to delay all-cause mortality and extend life.[165,205] Not only do persons with more-healthful lifestyles survive longer, but the risk of disability is postponed and compressed into fewer years at the end of life.[173] Statistics indicating that the number of 65-and-over competitors in the 1999 New York City Marathon has nearly doubled (404 men and 57 women) since 1990 aptly illustrate the exercise capacities of active older individuals. The winner in the 65- to 69-year-old age group achieved 3:16:13 for the 1998 run, while a 93-year-old man racewalked the distance in 8 hours and 26 minutes.

The New Gerontology

Many gerontologists maintain that research on aging should focus not simply on increasing life span but rather on improving "**healthspan**," the total number of years a person remains in excellent health. The "**new gerontology**" addresses areas beyond age-related diseases and their prevention to recognize that *successful aging* requires maintenance of enhanced physiologic function and physical fitness. Researchers now view much of the physiologic deterioration previously considered "normal aging" as dependent on lifestyle and environmental influences subject to significant modification with proper diet and exercise.[61,117,205] For those achieving older age, low muscular strength, diminished cardiovascular function, and poor joint range of motion, as well as sleep disturbances, relate directly to functional limitations, regardless of disease status.[28,90,150,151,197]

Healthy Life Expectancy: A New Concept

Life expectancy estimates determine the overall length of life based on mortality data, without considering the quality of life as aging progresses. At some point during the life span, some level of disability detracts from longevity. For example, the Centers for Disease Control and Prevention reports that nearly 1 in 10 Americans over age 70 needs help with daily activities such as bathing, and 4 in 10 use assistive devices such as walkers or hearing aids. In addition, approximately one-half of men and two-thirds of women above age 70 have arthritis; one-third of all Americans in this age group also have high blood pressure and 11% have diabetes. Of all seniors, women over age 85 are the most likely to need everyday help; 23% require assistance with at least one basic activity (e.g., dressing or going to the toilet).

To estimate healthful longevity, the World Health Organization (WHO [www.who.int/whr/]) has introduced the concept of **healthy life expectancy**—the expected number of years a person might live in the equivalent of full health. This involves computation of **disability-adjusted life expectancy (DALE)**, which considers the years of ill health, weighted according to severity, and subtracted from expected overall life expectancy to compute the equivalent years of healthy life. The WHO rankings by country show substantially more years lost to disability in poorer countries from the impact of injury, blindness, and paralysis and because the debilitating effects of tropical diseases such as malaria strike children and young adults more frequently. Figure 31.2 shows the DALE for a sample of 14 countries ranked by the WHO. Of the 191 countries evaluated, DALE estimates reached 70 years in 24 countries and 60 years in more than half. Thirty-two countries fell at the lower extreme, at which DALE estimates were less than 40 years. Many of these countries experience major epidemics of HIV/AIDS in addition to other causes of death and disability.

Citizens of Japan experience the longest healthy life expectancy, 74.5 years. Surprisingly, the United States rates 24th, with 70.0 years of healthy life for babies born in 1999 (72.6 y for females and 67.5 y for males). Some groups, such as Native Americans, rural African Americans, and the innercity poor, experience the poor health characteristics of underdeveloped countries. The HIV/AIDS epidemic, tobacco-related diseases, violent deaths, and prevalence of CHD all contribute to the United States' low ranking compared with those of other industrialized nations.

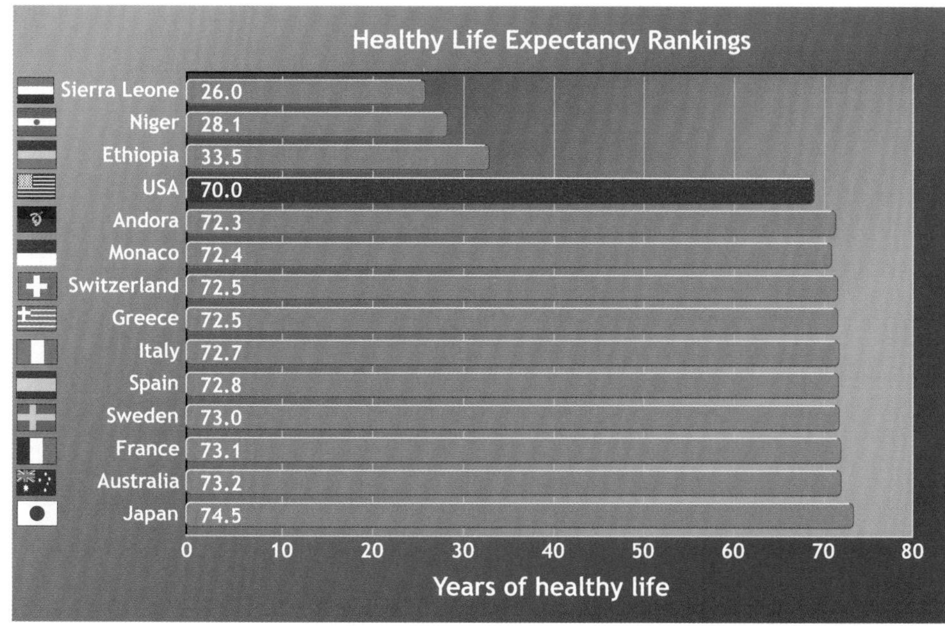

FIGURE 31.2 • Disability-adjusted life expectancy rankings (an estimate of healthy life expectancy) of populations of selected countries as assessed by the World Health Organization. Of all countries surveyed, the US ranked 24th with Japan ranked at the top.

PART 1 • Physical Activity in the Population

PHYSICAL ACTIVITY EPIDEMIOLOGY

Epidemiology involves quantifying factors that influence the occurrence of illness to better understand, modify, and/or control a disease pattern in the general population. The specific field of **physical activity epidemiology** applies the general research strategies of epidemiology to study physical activity as a health-related behavior linked to disease and other outcomes.

Terminology

Physical activity epidemiology applies specific definitions to characterize behavioral patterns and outcomes of the groups under investigation. Relevant terminology includes the following:

- **Physical activity**: Body movement produced by muscle action that increases energy expenditure
- **Exercise**: Planned, structured, repetitive, and purposeful physical activity
- **Physical fitness**: Attributes related to how well one performs physical activity
- **Health**: Physical, mental, and social well-being, not simply absence of disease
- **Health-related physical fitness**: Components of physical fitness associated with some aspect of good health and/or disease prevention (Fig. 31.3)
- **Longevity**: Length of life

Within this framework, physical activity becomes a generic term, with exercise its major component. Similarly, the definition of health focuses on the broad spectrum of well-being that ranges from complete absence of health (near death) to the highest levels of physiologic function. Such definitions often challenge our ability to measure and quantify health and physical activity objectively. However, they do provide a broad perspective to study the role of physical activity in health and disease.

The trend in physical fitness assessment during the past 25 years deemphasizes tests that stress motor performance and athletic fitness (i.e., speed, power, balance, and agility). Instead, current assessment focuses on functional capacities, related to overall good health and disease prevention. The four most common components of **health-related physical fitness** are aerobic and/or cardiovascular fitness, body composition, abdominal muscular strength and endurance, and lower back and hamstring flexibility (see "In a Practical Sense").

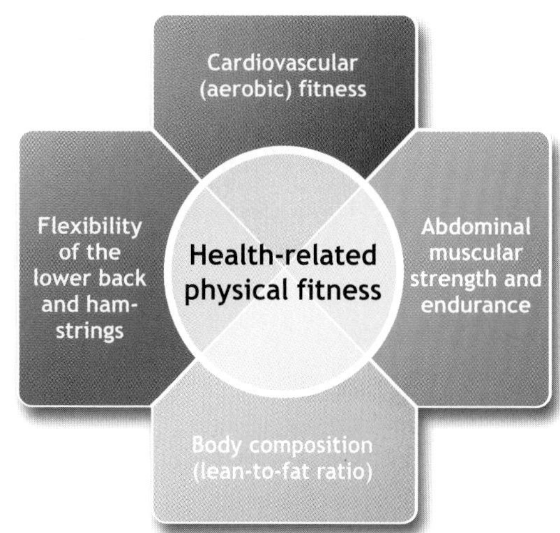

FIGURE 31.3 • Health-related physical fitness components.

IN A PRACTICAL SENSE

ASSESSING LOWER BACK, HAMSTRING, AND SHOULDER–WRIST FLEXIBILITY

Two types of flexibility are: (1) **static flexibility**, full range of motion (ROM) of a specific joint and (2) **dynamic flexibility**, torque or resistance encountered as the joint moves through its ROM. Field tests commonly assess static flexibility indirectly through linear measurement of ROM.

Field Tests of Hip-and-Trunk and Shoulder–Wrist Static Flexibility

Administer a minimum of three trials following a warm-up.

TEST 1: HIP-AND-TRUNK FLEXIBILITY (MODIFIED SIT-AND-REACH TEST)

Starting Position

Sit on the floor with the back and head against a wall, legs fully extended, with the bottoms of the feet against the sit-and-reach box. Place hands on top of each other, stretching arms forward while keeping head and back against the wall. Measure the distance from the fingertips to the box edge with a yardstick. This represents the zero, or starting, point (Fig. A).

Movement

Slowly bend and reach forward as far as possible (move head and back away from the wall), sliding the fingers along the yardstick; hold the final position for 2 seconds (Fig. B).

Score

Total distance reached to the nearest 1/4 inch represents the final score.

MODIFIED SIT-AND-REACH RATINGS

AGE RANGE (Y)	MEN <35	MEN 36–49	RATING	WOMEN <35	WOMEN 36–49
	>17.9	>16.1	**Excellent**	>17.9	>17.4
	17.0–17.9	14.6–16.1	**Good**	16.7–17.9	16.2–17.4
	15.8–17.0	13.9–14.6	**Average**	16.2–16.7	15.2–16.2
	15.0–15.8	13.4–13.9	**Fair**	15.8–16.2	14.5–15.2
	<15.0	<13.4	**Poor**	<15.4	<14.5

TEST 2: SHOULDER–WRIST FLEXIBILITY (SHOULDER AND WRIST ELEVATION TEST)

Starting Position

Lie prone on the floor with the arms fully extended overhead; grasp a yardstick with the hands shoulder-width apart.

Movement

Raise the stick as high as possible.

- Measure the vertical distance (nearest 0.5 in) the yardstick rises from the floor.
- Measure arm length from the acromial process to the tip of longest finger.
- Subtract the average vertical score from arm length.

Score

Arm length − average vertical score (nearest 0.25 in)

SHOULDER-AND-WRIST ELEVATION RATINGS

MEN	RATING	WOMEN
6.00 or less	**Excellent**	5.50 or less
8.25–6.25	**Good**	7.50–5.75
11.50–8.50	**Average**	10.75–7.75
12.50–11.75	**Fair**	11.75–11.00
12.75 or more	**Poor**	12.00 or more

Reference

Modified from Johnson BL, Nelson JK. Practical measurements for evaluation in physical education. 4th ed. New York: Macmillan, 1986.

Test 1: Hip-and-trunk flexibility (modified sit-and-reach test)

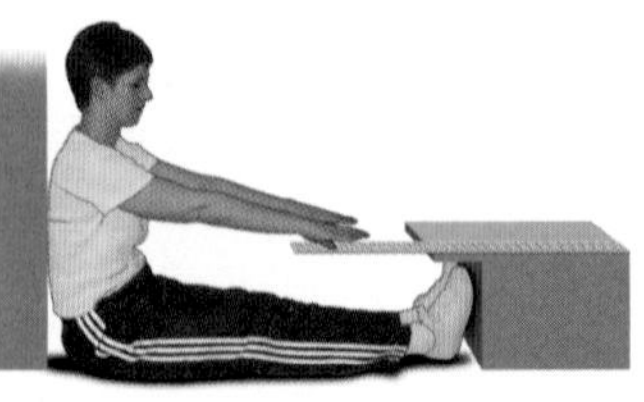

A

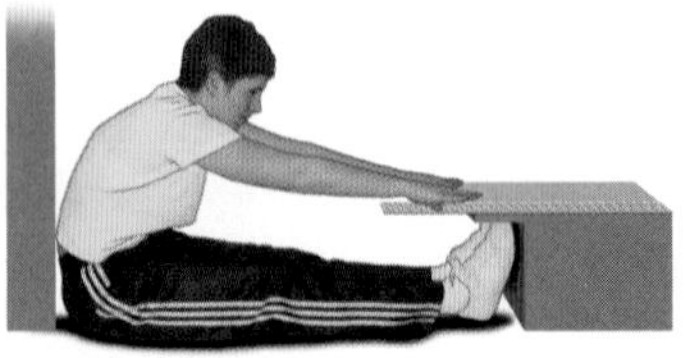

B

Test 2: Shoulder-wrist flexibility (shoulder and wrist elevation test)

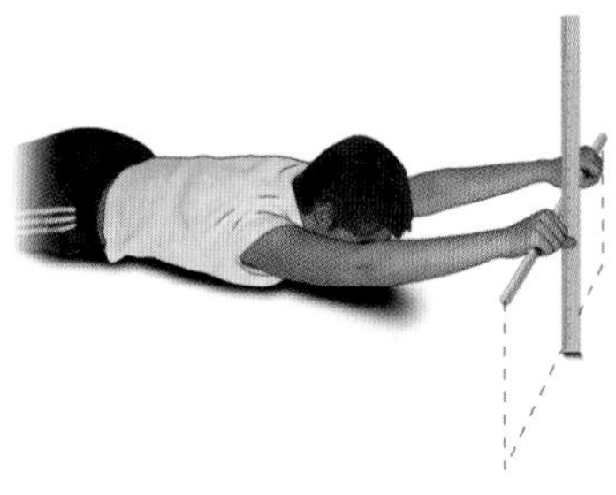

Physical Activity Participation

More than 30 different methods assess physical activity, including direct and indirect calorimetry, self-reports and questionnaires, job classifications, physiologic markers, behavioral observations, mechanical or electronic monitors, and activity surveys. Each approach offers unique advantages but also has disadvantages, depending on the situation and population studied. Obtaining valid estimates of physical activity of large groups is difficult, because such studies, by necessity, apply self-reports of daily activity and exercise participation rather than using direct monitoring or objective measurement. Despite limitations in assessment, a discouraging picture of physical activity participation worldwide emerges consistently, as emphasized for United States citizens in the Surgeon General's report on physical activity as well as data provided by others:[169,225]

Adults

- Only about 15% engage in regular, vigorous physical activity during leisure time, 3 times a week for at least 30 minutes
- More than 60% do not engage in physical activity regularly
- 25% lead sedentary lives (i.e., do not exercise at all)
- Walking, gardening, and yard work are the most popular leisure-time activities
- 22% engage in light-to-moderate physical activity regularly during leisure time (5 times/wk for at least 30 min)
- Physical inactivity occurs more among women than men, blacks and Hispanics than whites, older than younger adults, and less-affluent than wealthier persons
- Participation in fitness activities declines with age; a large number of older citizens have such poor functional capacity that they cannot rise from a chair or bed, walk to the bathroom, or climb a single stair without assistance

Children and Teenagers

- Nearly one-half of those between ages 12 and 21 do not exercise vigorously on a regular basis; a sharp decline in physical activity occurs during adolescence
- 14% report no recent physical activity—more prevalent among females, particularly black females
- 25% engage in light-to-moderate physical activity (e.g., walk or bicycle) nearly every day
- Participation in all types of physical activity declines strikingly as age and school grade increase
- More males participate in vigorous physical activity, strengthening activities, and walking or bicycling than females
- Daily attendance in school physical education programs declined from 42% in early 1990 to less than 25% in 1999

ACTIVITIES OF THOSE AMERICANS WHO REPORT EXERCISING REGULARLY

Activity	Percentage	
	Male	Female
Walking	39	48
Resistance training	20	9
Cycling	16	15
Running	12	6
Stair climbing	10	12
Aerobics	3	10

Healthy People 2000

At best, no more than 20% and possibly less than 10% of adults in the United States, Australia, Canada, and England obtain sufficient regular physical activity at an intensity that imparts discernible health and fitness benefits. Among Americans, a widespread erosion of physical activity patterns becomes particularly apparent with increasing age among adolescents and adults—with the decline in the rate of "regular physical activity" and strengthening patterns greater for adolescent and adult females than males.[35] Current debate suggests that the age-related decline in physical activity among humans has a biologic basis related to altered neurotransmission involving the central dopamine system, the system that regulates motivation for locomotion.[95] Regardless of the cause for progressive inactivity as adults age, *increased* levels of physical activity predict *decreased* levels of morbidity and mortality.[25] Clearly, a need exists to improve the physical activity profile of the population. With this in mind, the Public Health Service established Healthy People 2000 objectives, designed to improve Americans' health status by reducing preventable death, disability, and disease. One important objective focused on upgrading exercise participation by the large number of sedentary men and women, with extra emphasis on developing muscular strength and joint flexibility.

On July 11, 1996, the Surgeon General of the United States acknowledged the importance of physical activity to the nation with release of the first *Surgeon General's Report on Physical Activity and Health.* This wide-ranging report summarized the benefits of regular physical activity in disease prevention. The Surgeon General proposed a national agenda, a call to action that urged the nation to adopt and maintain a physically active lifestyle to combat ailments associated with the country's generally low level of energy expenditure. The following represent major conclusions of the report:

- Men and women of all ages benefit from regular physical activity.
- Significant health benefits accrue from including moderate physical activity (e.g., 30 min of brisk walking or raking leaves, 15 min of running, or 45 min of playing volleyball) on most, if not all days of the week. Achieving this goal improves most American's health and quality of life.[11,51]

The *"Physical Activity Pyramid"* illustrated below summarizes major goals for increasing the level of regular physical activity in the general population, emphasizing diverse forms of behavioral and lifestyle options.

Healthy People 2010

The **Healthy People 2010** initiative, launched on January 25, 2000, builds on the initiatives of the previous two decades as an instrument to improve national health for the first decade of the 21st century. Healthy People 2010 outlines a comprehensive, nationwide health promotion and disease prevention agenda as a roadmap for promoting health and preventing illness, disability, and premature death among all people in the United States.[201] Table 31.1 lists 28 objectives and goals concerning the nation's health.

Healthy People 2010 is designed to achieve two primary goals:

1. Increase quality and years of healthy life
2. Eliminate health disparities among the nation's citizens

Progress will be monitored through achievements within 467 objectives in the 28 focus areas. Many goals and objectives—several of which either directly or indirectly involve upgrading the national level of regular physical activity—converge on interventions designed to reduce or eliminate illness, disability, and premature death among individuals and communities. Others focus on broader issues, such as improving access to quality health care, strengthening public health services, and improving availability and dissemination of health-related information. Each objective has a target for specific improvements and explicit guidelines on how to achieve the stated goal by year 2010. Aside from the United States, the World Health Organization in their World Health Report 2000 aims to stimulate debate about better ways of assessing health system performance to improve the daily lives of people worldwide.

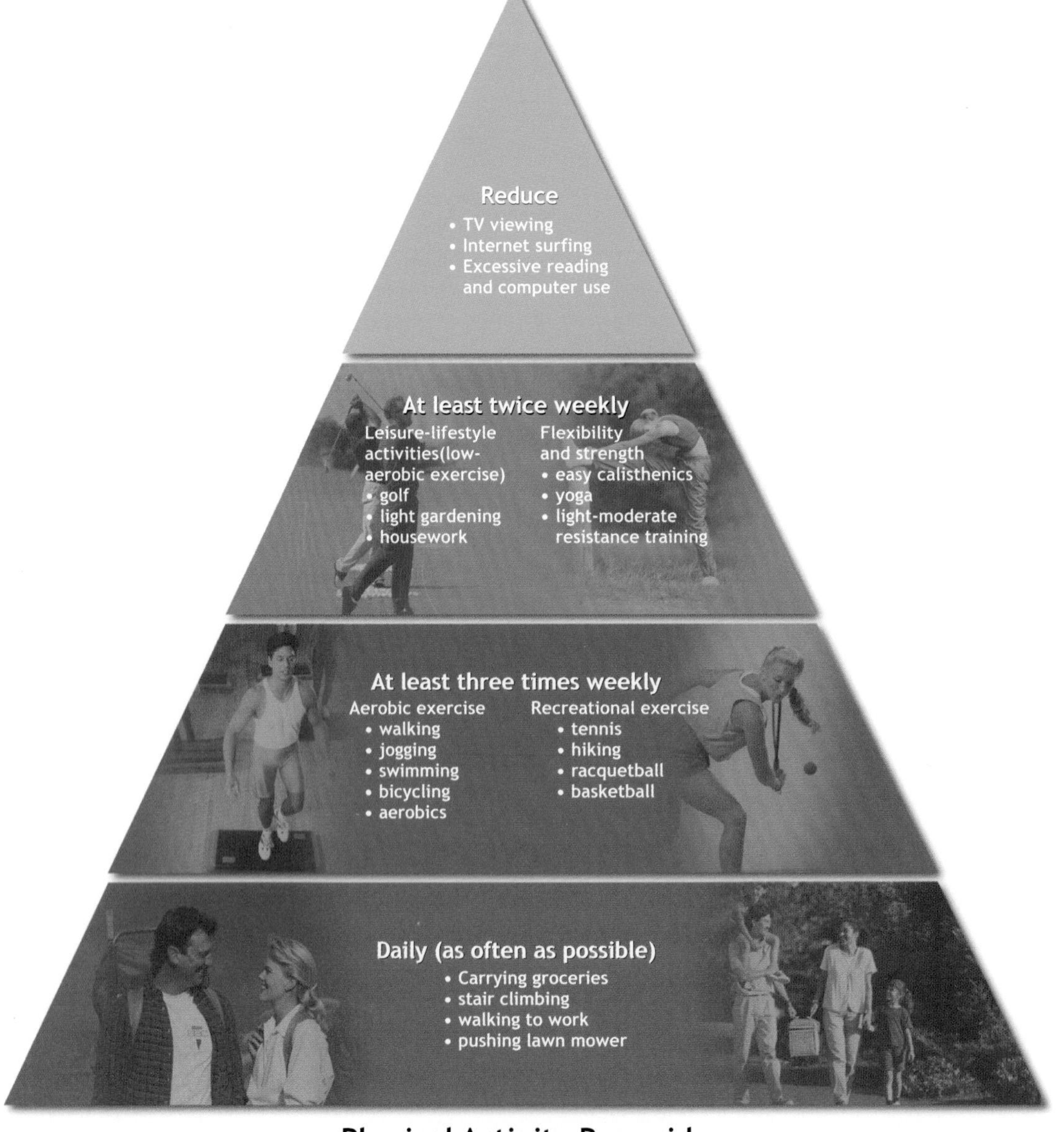

Physical Activity Pyramid

TABLE 31.1 ➤ HEALTHY PEOPLE 2010 OBJECTIVES AND GOALS

1. **Access to Quality Health Services**
   Improve access to comprehensive, high-quality health care services.
2. **Arthritis, Osteoporosis, and Chronic Back Conditions**
   Prevent illness and disability related to arthritis and other rheumatic conditions, osteoporosis, and chronic back conditions.
3. **Cancer**
   Reduce the number of new cancer cases as well as the illness, disability, and death caused by cancer.
4. **Chronic Kidney Disease**
   Reduce new cases of chronic kidney disease and its complications, disability, death, and economic costs.
5. **Diabetes**
   Through prevention programs, reduce the disease and economic burden of diabetes, and improve the quality of life for all persons who have or are at risk for diabetes.
6. **Disability and Secondary Conditions**
   Promote the health of people with disabilities, prevent secondary conditions, and eliminate disparities between people with and without disabilities in the U.S. population.
7. **Educational and Community-Based Programs**
   Increase the quality, availability, and effectiveness of educational and community-based programs designed to prevent disease and improve health and quality of life.
8. **Environmental Health**
   Promote health for all through a healthy environment.
9. **Family Planning**
   Improve pregnancy planning and spacing and prevent unintended pregnancy.
10. **Food Safety**
    Reduce foodborne illnesses.
11. **Health Communication**
    Use communication strategically to improve health.
12. **Heart Disease and Stroke**
    Improve cardiovascular health and quality of life through the prevention, detection, and treatment of risk factors; early identification and treatment of heart attacks and strokes; and prevention of recurrent cardiovascular events.
13. **HIV**
    Prevent HIV infection and its related illness and death.
14. **Immunization and Infectious Diseases**
    Prevent disease, disability, and death from infectious diseases, including vaccine-preventable diseases.
15. **Injury and Violence Prevention**
    Reduce disabilities, injuries, and deaths due to unintentional injuries and violence.
16. **Maternal, Infant, and Child Health**
    Improve the health and well-being of women, infants, children, and families.
17. **Medical Product Safety**
    Ensure the safe and effective use of medical products.
18. **Mental Health and Mental Disorders**
    Improve mental health and ensure access to appropriate, quality mental health services.
19. **Nutrition and Overweight**
    Promote health and reduce chronic disease associated with diet and weight.
20. **Occupational Safety and Health**
    Promote the health and safety of people at work through prevention and early intervention.
21. **Oral Health**
    Prevent and control oral and craniofacial diseases, conditions, and injuries and improve access to related services.
22. **Physical Activity and Fitness**
    Improve health, fitness, and quality of life through daily physical activity.
23. **Public Health Infrastructure**
    Ensure that Federal, Tribal, State, and local health agencies have the infrastructure to provide essential public health services effectively.
24. **Respiratory Diseases**
    Promote respiratory health through better prevention, detection, treatment, and education.
25. **Sexually Transmitted Diseases**
    Promote responsible sexual behaviors, strengthen community capacity, and increase access to quality services to prevent sexually transmitted diseases (STDs) and their complications.
26. **Substance Abuse**
    Reduce substance abuse to protect the health, safety, and quality of life for all, especially children.
27. **Tobacco Use**
    Reduce illness, disability, and death related to tobacco use and exposure to secondhand smoke.
28. **Vision and Hearing**
    Improve the visual and hearing health of the Nation through prevention, early detection, treatment, and rehabilitation.

U.S. Department of Health and Human Services, Healthy People 2010 (Conference edition, two vol), Washington, DC: January 2000.

Safety of Exercising

Several well-publicized reports of sudden death during exercise raised the question of exercise safety.[114,199] Actually, the death rate during exercise has declined over the past 25 years despite an overall increase in exercise participation. In one report of cardiovascular episodes over a 65-month period, 2935 exercisers recorded 374,798 hours of exercise that included 2,726,272 km of running and walking. No deaths occurred during this time, and only two nonfatal cardiovascular complications. This amounted to two complications per 100,000 hours of exercise for women and three complications for men.

Heavy physical exertion does raise a small risk of sudden death (e.g., 1 sudden death per 1.51 million episodes of extertion) during the activity (compared with resting an equivalent time[6]), particularly for sedentary people with a genetic predisposition to sudden death. Nonetheless, the longer-term reduction in overall death risk from regular exercise far outweighs any small potential for acute cardiovascular complications.[125,195] Furthermore, considerably less risk of death exists during physical activity in regular exercisers.[199] For example, a twelve-year follow-up of more than 21,000 male physicians showed that men who exercised at least five times a week had a much lower sudden death risk during vigorous exertion—about sevenfold less—than those who only exercised once a week.[6] The likelihood of an exercise catastrophe—cerebrovascular accident, aortic dissection and rupture, lethal arrhythmias, myocardial infarction—increases under the following conditions:

- Genetic predisposition (family history of sudden death at a young age)
- History of fainting or chest pain with exercise
- Unaccustomed vigorous exercise
- Exercise performed with accompanying psychologic stress
- Extremes of environmental temperature
- Straining-type exercise requiring a significant static muscle-action component (e.g., shoveling wet snow)
- Exercise during viral infection or when not feeling well
- Comingling of some prescription drugs or dietary supplements (e.g., ephedra)

Perhaps not surprisingly, musculoskeletal injuries represent the most prevalent exercise complications. A longitudinal study of aerobic dance injuries in 351 participants and 60 instructors, during nearly 30,000 hours of activity, reported 327 medical complaints.[70] Just 84 of the injuries caused disability (2.8 per 1000 person-hours of participation), and only 2.1% required medical attention. National estimates from self-reported frequency and severity of injuries in five common physical activities—walking, gardening, weight lifting, outdoor bicycling, and aerobics—report relatively low injury rates.[175] Most injuries required no treatment or physical activity reduction. Age does not appear to affect incidence of orthopedic problems for exercise of moderate intensity and duration.[135] For activities involving running, the greatest orthopedic injury risk exists in individuals who exercise for protracted periods.[8]

Prospective epidemiologic research evaluated clinically significant medical incidents and emergencies for 7725 low-risk, apparently healthy corporate fitness enrollees in a supervised facility at a major medical center.[152] Two and one-half years of surveillance reported 15 medically significant events (0.048 per 1000 participant-hours) and two medical emergencies (both recovered) equaling a rate of 0.0063 per 1000 participant-hours. Such an extremely low rate of medical incidents in a supervised health-fitness facility shows that the health-related fitness benefits far outweigh any small risk of participation. A recurring theme in physical activity epidemiology stresses how aging and regular exercise interact to impact physical fitness, health risk, and diseases progression. We explore these interrelationships in the sections that follow.

Sedentary Death Syndrome (SEDS)

A review of the world literature over the last 50 years has led to the conclusion that inactivity alone results in a constellation of problems and conditions eventually leading to premature death. The term **sedentary death syndrome (SEDS)** identifies this condition.[25] Research evidence reveals that:

- SEDS will cause 2.5 million Americans to die prematurely in the next decade.
- SEDS will cost $2–3 trillion in health care expenses in the U.S. in the next decade.
- Chronic diseases have increased because of physical inactivity. In the United States, type 2 diabetes has increased 9-fold since 1958, obesity has doubled since 1980, and heart disease remains the number 1 cause of death.
- Our children are now getting SEDS-related diseases. American children are increasingly overweight, showing fatty streaks in their arteries, and developing type 2 diabetes (a disease formerly restricted to adults).
- SEDS relates to 23 conditions: high blood triglyceride; high blood cholesterol; high blood glucose; type 2 diabetes; hypertension, myorcardial ischemia; arrhythmias; congestive heart failure; obesity; breast depression; chronic back pain; spinal cord injury; stroke; disease cachexia; debilitating illnesses; fall resulting in broken hips; vertebral/femoral fractures.

Increased research efforts are being directed at understanding the biological link between physical inactivity and disease by exploring the molecular and genetic basis of this link. This biological research is being coupled with new research into the behavioral and epidemiological components of SEDS. More medical-based evidence is needed to convince American citizens that physical inactivity promotes unhealthy gene expression and there is an increased need to include regular physical activity in their lives.

Summary

1. Physical activity epidemiology evaluates the nature, extent, and demographics of exercise participation in a large population. Such data often reflect disease occurrence and other health-related outcomes.
2. Researchers paint a discouraging picture of physical activity participation by adult Americans. Only 10 to 15% of adults in the United States obtain enough regular physical activity of adequate intensity to impart significant health and fitness benefits.
3. Health benefits accrue from including a moderate amount of physical activity on most, if not all, days of the week.
4. Intense physical effort raises a small risk of sudden death during the activity compared with resting for an equivalent time, particularly for sedentary people. The longer-term health benefits of regular exercise outweigh the risk of acute cardiovascular complications.
5. The current Healthy People 2010 goals and objectives include 226 targeted health objectives in 28 focus areas for the nation. Several of these either directly or indirectly focus on increasing regular physical activity among all citizens.
6. For activities that involve running, the greatest orthopedic injury potential exists among individuals who exercise for extended durations.

AGE TRENDS

Figure 31.4 shows that physiologic and performance measures improve rapidly during childhood and reach a maximum between late adolescence and approximately age 30. Functional capacity declines thereafter, with deterioration varying at any age, depending on lifestyle characteristics. All physiologic measures typically decline with age, but not all decline at the same rate. Nerve conduction velocity, for example, declines only 10 to 15% from 30 to 80 years, whereas maximum breathing capacity at age 80 averages 40% that at age 30. Some functions that show little if any aging effect at rest (e.g., heart rate), display an appreciable decrement in maximal exercise. Despite decreases in functional capacity and exercise performance, even among active individuals, regular exercise can counter typical aging effects.[75,171,194] For example, aerobic capacity among the physically active averages 25% higher than that of the sedentary in each age category, so that an active 50-year-old person often maintains the functional level of a 20-year-old. The limited number of long-term exercise studies of the same subjects precludes pinpointing how regular exercise overrides the deterioration in function with aging. Many gerontologists believe that the view of aging will change dramatically as people live longer, more physically active lives. Instead of preoccupation with disease and frailty, focus will shift to successful aging.

Differences in Exercise Physiology Between Children and Adults

One must consider the interaction between physical activity and aging when evaluating physiologic responses and exercise performance across a broad age span. The distinct differences between children and adults can be summarized as follows:

- During weight-bearing walking and running, oxygen consumption ($mL \cdot kg^{-1} \cdot min^{-1}$) of children averages 10 to 30% higher than that of adults at a designated submaximal pace.[236] This lower exercise economy, perhaps owing to children's lower ventilatory efficiency, greater body surface area:mass ratio, shorter stride length, and greater stride frequency, makes a standard walking or running pace physiologically more stressful (and performance scores poorer). The exercise disadvantage exists even though children typically maintain equal or somewhat higher aerobic capacities than adults. Also, walking and running economy and the percentage $\dot{V}O_{2peak}$ sustainable during exercise at the lactate threshold continually improve as children age, independent of aerobic capacity changes. This limits the usefulness of a single walking or running performance test to predict $\dot{V}O_{2max}$ throughout childhood and adolescence.[44]
- Children exhibit lower absolute aerobic capacity values ($L \cdot min^{-1}$) than adults because of a smaller fat-free body mass (FFM; Fig. 31.5). Consequently, children are disadvantaged when exercising against a standard external resistance (unadjusted for body size) as in stationary cycling and arm cranking. The fixed oxygen cost ($L \cdot min^{-1}$) of such exercise represents a greater percentage of a child's smaller absolute aerobic capacity. During weight-bearing exercise, in contrast, energy cost relates directly to body mass, so children are not disadvantaged by their smaller body size.
- Children do less well than adults on sprint tests of anaerobic power capacity, most likely because of their inability to generate a high level of blood lactate during maximal exercise. Significantly lower intramuscular levels of the glycolytic enzyme phosphofructokinase may contribute to children's poorer anaerobic exercise performance.

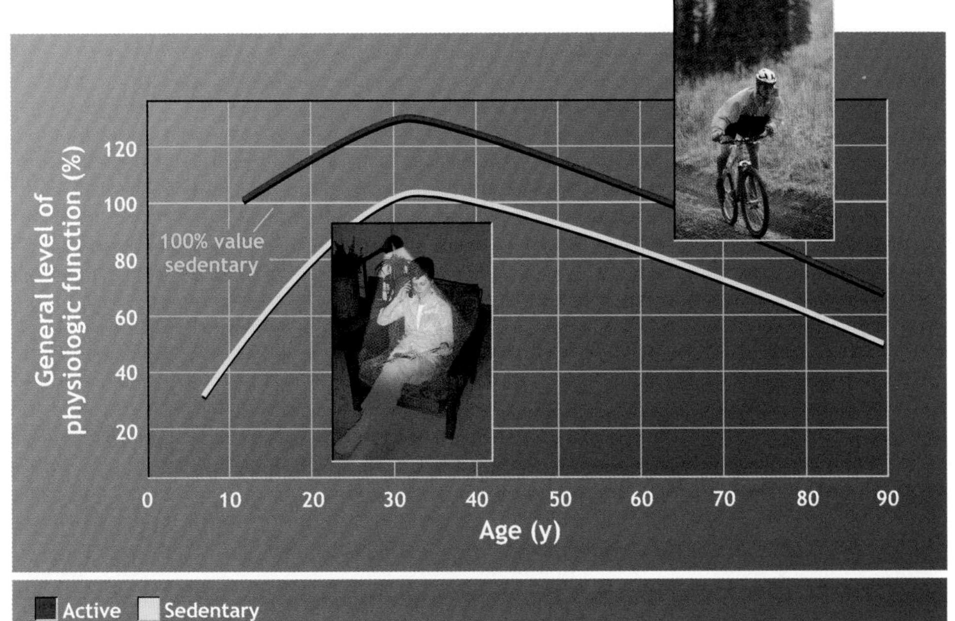

FIGURE 31.4 • Generalized curve for changes in physiologic function with age. Levels expressed as percentage of the 100% value achieved by the typical 20- to 30-year-old sedentary person (*horizontal yellow line*).

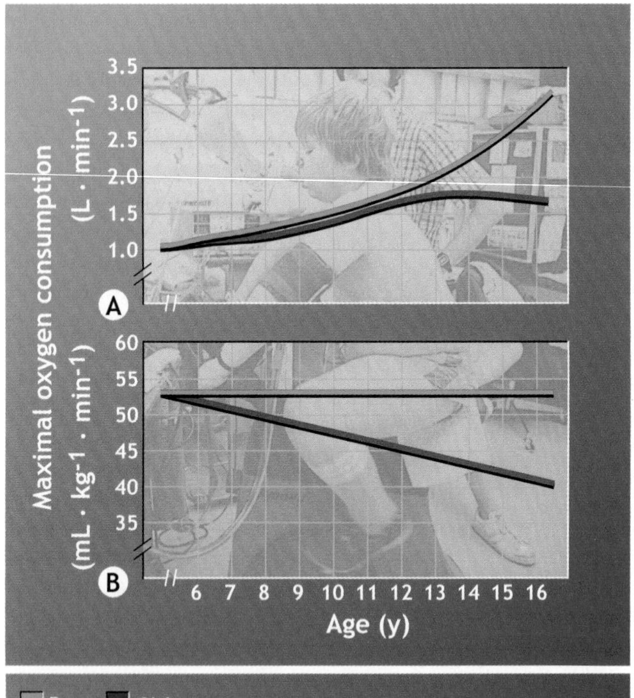

FIGURE 31.5 • **A**. $\dot{V}O_{2max}$ (L · min^{-1}) for boys and girls remains similar until approximately 12 years of age; $\dot{V}O_{2max}$ at age 14 averages 25% higher in boys, and by age 16 the difference exceeds 50%. The differences largely reflect greater muscle mass development in boys and gender differences in daily physical activity. **B**. For boys, $\dot{V}O_{2max}$ (mL · kg^{-1} · min^{-1}) averages about 52 mL · kg^{-1} · min^{-1} from age 6 to 16; for females, the line slopes downward with age, reaching approximately 40 mL · kg^{-1} · min^{-1} at age 16, a value 32% below male counterparts. This difference closely parallels the greater accumulation of body fat in females; extra fat increases the energy cost of exercise but does not increase capacity for aerobic metabolism. (From Krahenbuhl GS, et al. Developmental aspects of maximal aerobic power in children. Exerc Sport Sci Rev 1985;13:503.

- Children breathe relatively larger air volumes (greater ventilatory equivalent) than adults at any level of submaximal exercise oxygen consumption.
- Children and adults significantly increase muscle strength with resistance training. However, prepubescent children, unlike pubescent children and adults, have difficulty increasing muscle mass. This probably results from their relatively low androgen levels.

INTEGRATIVE QUESTION

What factors would explain the relatively poor performances of children compared with adults of equal aerobic capacity in a 10-K run?

Muscular Strength

Age and gender affect muscular strength and muscular power, with the magnitude of each effect influenced by the muscle group studied and the type of muscle action. Some general trends in muscular strength and power of adults with increasing age can be summarized as follows:

- Men and women usually attain their highest strength levels between ages 20 and 40, the time when muscle cross-sectional area is largest. Thereafter, concentric strength of most muscle groups declines, slowly at first and then more rapidly after middle age.
- The accelerated strength loss coincides with weight loss and the increase in chronic diseases such as stroke, diabetes, arthritis, and CHD.[181]
- The capacity for power generation declines faster than for maximal strength.[96]
- Declines in eccentric strength begin at a later age and progress more slowly than those in concentric strength. Strength loss begins at a later age for women than for men.[130]
- Arm strength (e.g., peak torque per unit muscle mass) deteriorates more slowly than leg strength for men and women.[134]
- Strength loss among the elderly directly relates to their limited mobility and fitness status and to the potential for increased incidence of accidents from muscle weakness, fatigue, and poor balance.[101]

Muscle Mass Decrease

Motor unit remodeling is a normal, continual process involving motor end-plate repair and reconstruction. Remodeling progresses by selective denervation of muscle fibers, followed by terminal sprouting of axons from adjacent motor units. Motor unit remodeling gradually deteriorates in old age, leading to **denervation muscle atrophy**, an irreversible degeneration of muscle fibers (particularly type II fibers) and end-plate structures.[31,48,73] This progressively reduces muscle cross section and mass (a condition termed **sarcopenia**), even after adjustment for changes in body mass and stature, particularly in lower-body skeletal muscle mass after the fifth decade.[69,98] Muscle fibers also tend to "type group," in that fast- and slow-twitch fibers lose their typical chessboard distribution and tend to cluster in groups of similar type—perhaps the result of denervation and subsequent fiber death. In addition, older adults have more than twice as much noncontractile content in locomotor muscles as younger adults.[107] The decline in muscle strength with age does not result from an impaired neural drive, because older adults achieve full muscle activation during a maximal voluntary muscle action.[45]

A 40 to 50% reduction in muscle mass from muscle fiber atrophy and actual loss of motor units between ages 25 and 80 is the primary cause of reduced strength, even among healthy, physically active men and women. Figure 31.6A shows that muscle fiber loss appears near age 60. The reduction in total muscle area (Fig. 31.6B) usually parallels reduced fiber size, particularly fast-twitch fibers in the lower extremities. This proportionately increases in the area occupied by the slow-twitch (type I) muscle fibers.

In a longitudinal study of age-related declines in muscular strength, 9 of 12 men initially evaluated for muscular strength and muscle fiber composition 12 years earlier were remeasured.[67] Knee and elbow extensor and flexor strengths, tested at

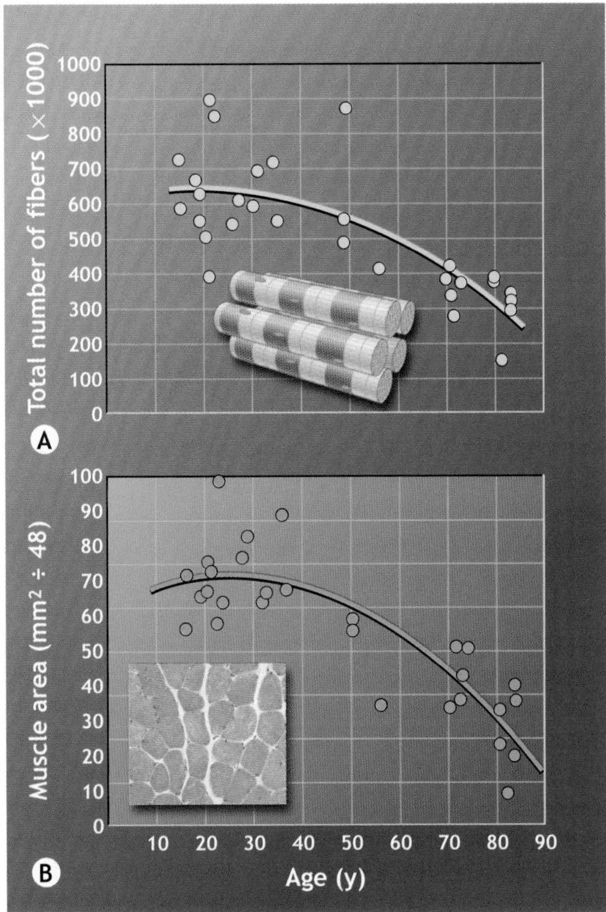

FIGURE 31.6 • Relationship between age and (**A**) total number of muscle fibers and (**B**) muscle cross-sectional area. Muscle size begins to decrease at approximately age 30, decreasing 10% by age 50. Thereafter, muscle area declines more precipitously, largely from decreased total number of muscle fibers. (From Lexell J, et al. What is the cause of the ageing atrophy? Total number, size, and proportion of different fiber types studied in whole vastus lateralis muscle from 15- to 83-year-old men. J Neurol Sci 1988;84:275.)

slow and fast angular velocities, decreased by 20 to 30%. Muscle cross-sectional area for the same muscle groups evaluated by CT scans decreased between 13 and 16%. Muscle biopsies from the vastus lateralis muscle showed a significant 42% reduction in type I fibers without changes in mean fiber type area. Also, the capillary:fiber ratio decreased with aging (0.31 units lower after 12 y). The researchers concluded that changes in muscle cross-sectional area contributed in a major way to the strength decline over a decade from age 65 to 77.

Resistance Training Among the Elderly

Sarcopenia and strength loss with aging reflect the combined effects of progressive neuromotor deterioration and chronic decrease in regular muscle loading. Moderate resistance training provides a remarkably safe way to augment protein synthesis and retention and slow the "normal" and somewhat inevitable loss of muscle mass and strength with aging.[2,144,172] Older men typically demonstrate greater absolute gains in muscle size and strength than female counterparts, but the percentage improvement in hypertrophic and neuromuscular adaptations is similar.[220] Healthy men between ages 60 and 72 years who trained for 12 weeks with standard-resistance exercise at loads equivalent to 80% of their dynamic muscle strength capacity (1-RM) demonstrate how well the elderly respond to resistance training. Figure 31.7 shows that muscle strength increased progressively throughout training. At week 12, knee flexion strength (orange bars) increased by 107%, and knee extension strength by 227%. The improvement rate of 5% per training session matched similar increases reported for young adults. Significant fast- and slow-twitch muscle fiber hypertrophy accompanied the dramatic strength improvements. In other research, muscle cross-sectional area and strength in 70-year-olds who had resistance trained since age 50 equaled values for a group of 28-year-old students.[109] *Older individuals possess impressive plasticity in physiologic,*

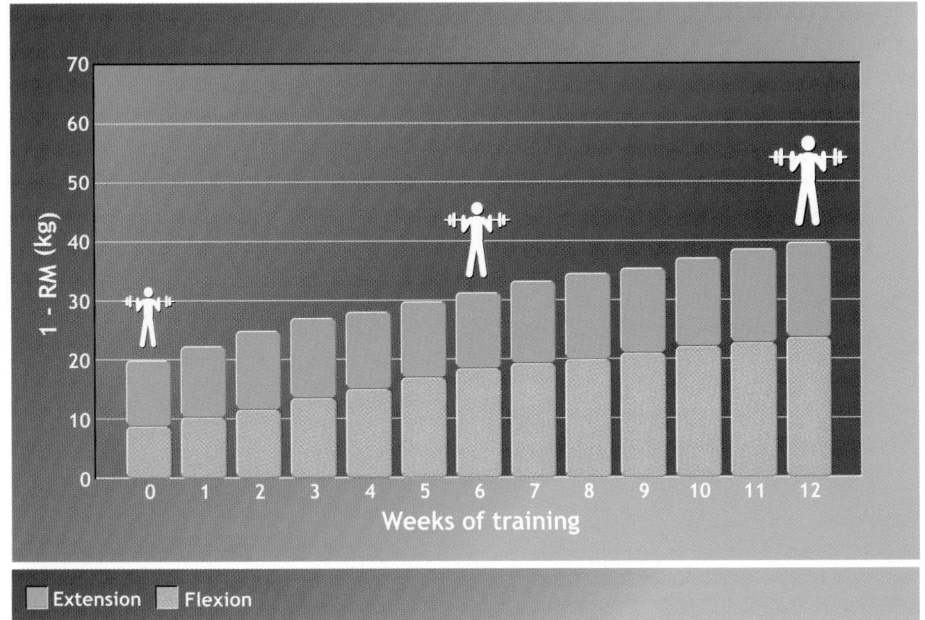

FIGURE 31.7 • Weekly measurements of dynamic muscle strength (1-RM) in left knee extension (*green*) and flexion (*orange*) during resistance training in older men. (From Frontera WR, et al. Strength conditioning in older men: skeletal muscle hypertrophy and improved function. J Appl Physiol 1988;64:1038.)

TABLE 31.2 ➤ STUDIES OF RESISTANCE TRAINING IN OLDER INDIVIDUALS

STUDY	AGE (Y)	GENDER	TRAINING TYPE	STRENGTH GAIN (%)	HYPERTROPHY (%)
1	62–84	M + F	RT	57	NM
2	18–26	M	RT	30	9
	67–72	M	RT	22	NC
3	69–74	M	CT	9–22	NC
4	22–65	M	CT	3–8	19–20
5	63–84	F	RT	7–13	10
6	60–72	M	RT	9–19	9–12
1	62–84	M + F	Iso	45.8	NM
7	41–80	M	Iso	12–24	NM
8	20–26	F	Iso	95	NM
	65–73	F	Iso	72	NM
9	55–78	M + F	CV	1.9–13.4	NM
10	51–87	M	CV (6 wk)	6.4	NC
		M	CV (42 wk)	11.9	1.0
11	65	M + F	CV	5–13	NM
12	65	M	Hdr	15–132	NC

RT, resistance training; CT, circuit training; Iso, isometric training; CV, cardiovascular endurance training; Hdr, hydraulic resistance training; NC, no change; NM, not measured.
1. Perkins LC, Kaiser H. Phys Ther Rev 1961;41:633; 2. Moritaini T, deVries HA. J Gerontol 1980;35:672; 3. Aniansson A, Gustafsson E. Clin Physiol 1981;1:87; 4. Larsson L. Med Sci Sports Exerc 1982;19:203; 5. Aniansson A, et al. Arch Gerontol Geriat 1984;3:229; 6. Frontera WF, et al. J Appl Physiol 1988;64:1038; 7. Liemohm WP. Int J Aging Hum Dev 1975;6:347; 8. Kauffman TL. Arch Phys Med Rehab 1985;66:223; 9. Barry AJ, et al. J Gerontol 1966;21:192; 10. deVries HA, J Gerontol 1970;25:325; 11. Sidney LH, et al. Am J Clin Nutr 1977;30:326; 12. Becque MD. PhD dissertation, University of Michigan, 1989.

structural, and performance characteristics. Muscle responds to vigorous training with marked and rapid improvement into the ninth decade of life.[60] Improved muscle strength, bone density, dynamic balance, and overall functional status with regular exercise may minimize or even reverse the syndrome of physical frailty. Regular exercise also provides the most effective way to reduce orthopedic injury (e.g., high prevalence of falls) in older men and women.[27,119,179] Even for older persons disabled with osteoarthritis of the knee, regular aerobic or resistance exercises induce beneficial effects on measures of disability, pain, and physical performance.[56]

Table 31.2 summarizes relevant literature on changes in muscle strength and size in older adults who participated in resistance training programs. Most programs produced positive responses, with strength improvements ranging between 1.9 and 132% in individuals older than age 60. Mechanisms that explain how the middle aged and elderly respond to resistance training include enhanced motor unit recruitment and innervation patterns and muscular hypertrophy, discussed previously in Chapter 22. As with younger adults, the number of sets and repetitions and the intensity, duration, and frequency of training determine the magnitude of strength adaptations in the elderly.

Neural Function

A nearly 40% decline in the number of spinal cord axons and a 10% decline in nerve conduction velocity reflect the cumulative effects of aging on central nervous system function. These changes likely contribute to the age-related decrement in neuromuscular performance assessed by simple and complex reaction and movement times. Partitioning reaction time into central processing time and muscle action time, aging most adversely affects the time required to detect a stimulus and process the information to produce the response. Because reflexes such as the knee-jerk do not involve processing in the brain, aging affects them less than voluntary responses involving both reaction and movement.[39] Figure 31.8 shows significantly slower movement times for simple and complex tasks by older subjects than for younger subjects of similar physical activity levels. *In all instances, however, the young or old active groups moved considerably faster than the corresponding less-active age group.* These observations suggest that a physically active lifestyle affects neuromuscular functions positively at any age to slow the age-related decline in cognitive performance associated with speed of information processing.[229] As with many other measures of physiologic function, older individuals who remain physically active for 20 years or longer show reaction speeds that equal or exceed those of inactive individuals in their 20s.[204] These findings reinforce the position that regular physical activity slows the biologic aging of select neuromuscular func-

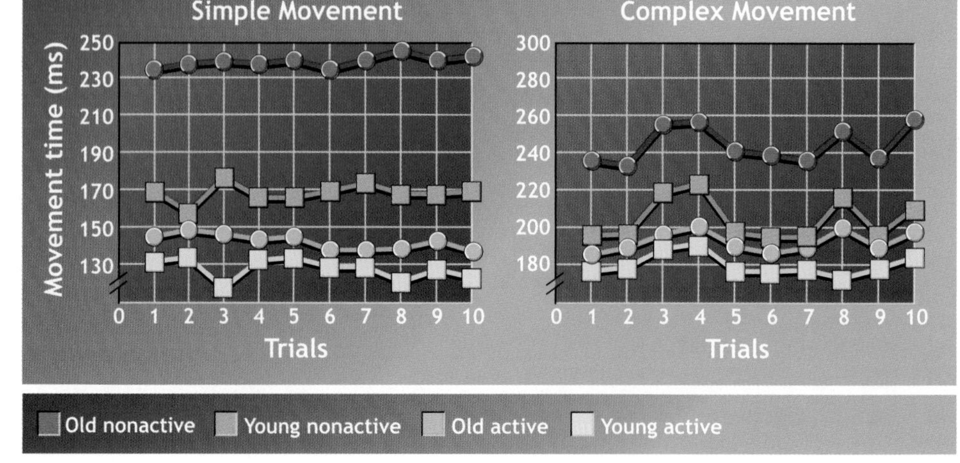

FIGURE 31.8 • Simple and complex movement time in subjects classified as young active, old active, young nonactive, and old nonactive. Note the slower movement times (higher scores) in simple and complex tasks by the old and young nonactive subjects than by their active counterparts. (From Spirduso WW. Reaction and movement time as a function of age and physical activity level. J Gerontol 1975;30:435.)

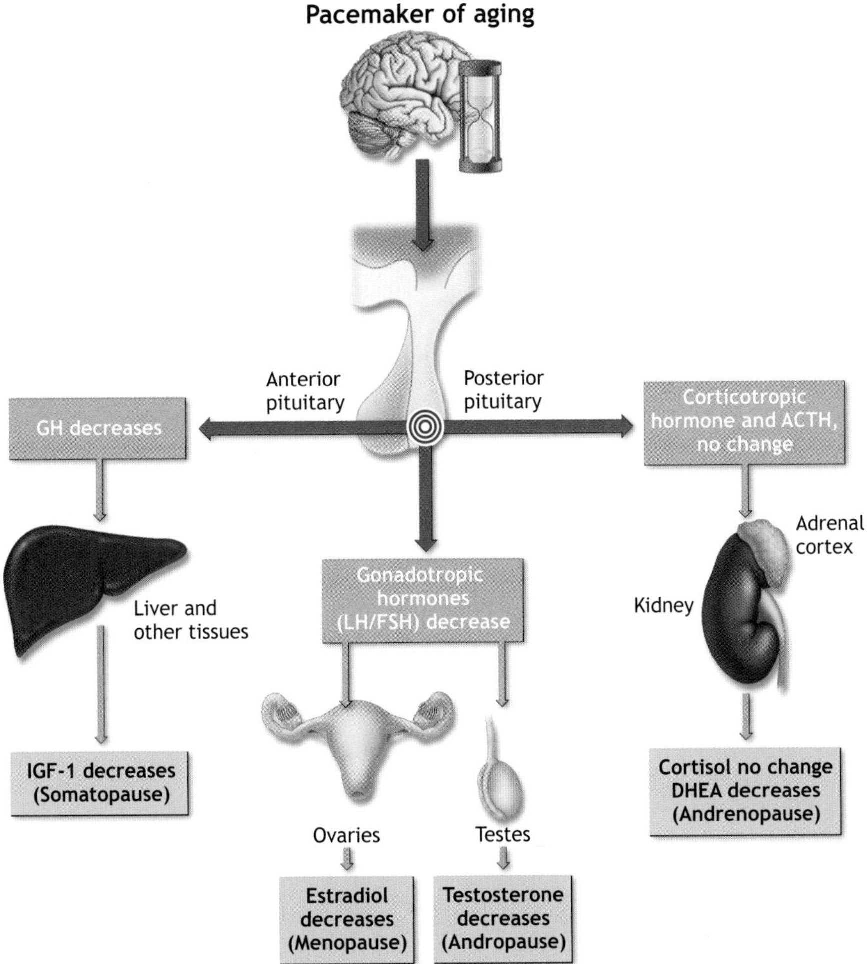

FIGURE 31.9 • Age-related decline in three hormone systems that profoundly affect the rate of biologic aging. *Left,* Decreased growth hormone (GH) release by the anterior pituitary depresses production of IGF-1 by the liver and other tissues, which inhibits cellular growth (a condition of aging termed *somatopause*). *Middle,* Decreased output of gonadotropic luteinizing hormone (LH) and follicle-stimulating hormone (FSH), by the anterior pituitary, coupled with reduced estradiol secretion from the ovaries and testosterone from the testes, causes *menopause* (females) and *andropause* (males). *Right,* Adrenocortical cells responsible for DHEA production decrease their activity (termed *adrenopause*) without clinically evident changes in this gland's corticotropin (ACTH) and cortisol secretion. A central pacemaker in the hypothalamus and/or higher brain areas probably mediates these processes to produce aging-related changes in peripheral organs (ovaries, testicles, and adrenal cortex).

tions. The potential magnitude of these changes and the quantity of physical activity required to induce meaningful responses remain controversial.[198]

Endocrine Changes with Aging

Endocrine function, particularly of the pituitary, pancreas, adrenal, and thyroid glands, changes with age.[117] Approximately 40% of individuals ages 65 and 75 years and 50% of those older than age 80 have impaired glucose tolerance leading to type 2 diabetes. This is the most common form of the disease, and it afflicts 1 in 17 Americans; nearly one-half of these cases remain undiagnosed. Impaired glucose metabolism leading to high blood glucose levels in type 2 diabetes results from:

- Decreased effect of insulin on peripheral tissue (**insulin resistance**)
- Inadequate insulin production by the pancreas to control blood sugar (**relative insulin deficiency**)
- Combined effect of insulin resistance and relative insulin deficiency

With the exception of genetic predisposition and possible effects of aging itself, increased disease prevalence among the elderly largely relates to controllable factors such as poor diet quality, inadequate physical activity, and increased body fat, particularly in the visceral-abdominal region.[3]

Thyroid dysfunction, primarily from lowered pituitary gland release of the thyroid-stimulating hormone thyrotropin (and reduced output of thyroxine), is common among the elderly. This directly affects metabolic function, including decreased glucose metabolism and protein synthesis.

Figure 31.9 depicts changes in three other hormonal systems associated with aging: (1) hypothalamic–pituitary–gonadal axis, (2) adrenal cortex, and (3) growth hormone (GH)/insulin-like growth factor (IGF) axis.

Hypothalamic–Pituitary–Gonadal Axis

Alteration in the interaction between stimulating hormones from the hypothalamus and anterior pituitary gland and gonads decreases estradiol output from the ovaries, which probably initiates the permanent cessation of menses (**menopause**) in the aging female. Changes in hypothalamic–pituitary–gonadal axis activity in males occur more slowly and subtly. For example, serum total and free testosterone gradually decline with aging in males. Age-related decreases in gonadotropic secretions from the anterior pituitary gland characterize male **andropause**.

Adrenal Cortex

Adrenopause refers to the reduced adrenal cortex output of dehydroepiandrosterone (DHEA) and its sulfated ester (DHEAS). In contrast to the glucocorticoid and mineralocorticoid adrenal steroids whose plasma levels remain relatively high with aging, DHEA exhibits a long, progressive decline after age 30. By age 75, the plasma level is only 20 to 30% of that in young adults. This has evoked speculation that plasma DHEA levels might serve as a biochemical marker of biologic aging and disease susceptibility. Research with animals suggests that exogenous DHEA protects against cancer, atherosclerosis, viral infections, obesity, and diabetes; enhances immune function; and even extends life. Despite its quantitative significance as a hormone in humans, researchers know little about DHEA's (1) role in relation to health and aging, (b) cellular or molecular mechanism(s) of action, (c) possible receptor sites, or (d) potential for adverse effects from supplemental use, particularly among young adults with normal DHEA levels. Chapter 23 discusses the case for ergogenic effects of DHEA supplements (and potential risks) on adult men and women.

Growth Hormone/Insulin-Like Growth Factor Axis

Mean pulse amplitude, duration, and fraction of secreted GH gradually decrease with aging, a condition termed **somatopause**. A parallel decrease in circulating IGF-1 levels also occurs. This compound, produced by the liver and other cells, stimulates tissue growth and protein synthesis. The trigger for the age-related GH decrease probably lies in the interaction between the hypothalamus and anterior pituitary gland.

The extent to which changes in gonadal function (menopause and andropause) contribute to adrenopause and somatopause (present in both sexes) remains unknown. A growing body of evidence indicates that functional correlates such as muscle size and strength, body composition and bone mass alterations, and progression of atherosclerosis relate directly to hormonal changes with aging. Hormonal replacement therapy, nutritional supplementation, and regular physical activity may successfully delay or even prevent aspects of hormone-related aging dysfunction.

Pulmonary Function

Mechanical constraints on the pulmonary system progress with age to cause deterioration in static and dynamic lung function measures.[13] Also, pulmonary ventilation and gas exchange kinetics during the transition from rest to submaximal exercise slow substantially.[43] Whether exercise regularly performed throughout life can fully override the "aging" of pulmonary dynamics or tissue oxygen consumption capacity requires further research. In elderly men, however, aerobic training increases the kinetics of gas exchange to a level that approaches values for fit young adults.[14] Likewise, older endurance-trained athletes demonstrate greater pulmonary functional capacity than their sedentary peers. Values for vital capacity, total lung capacity, residual lung volume, maximum voluntary ventilation, $FEV_{1.0}$ and $FEV_{1.0}/FVC$ in athletes above age 60 remain higher than predicted from body size and higher than values for sedentary, healthy individuals.[74] Such findings indicate that regular exercise retards the pulmonary function decline associated with aging.

Cardiovascular Function

Cardiovascular function and aerobic capacity do not escape age-related effects.

Aerobic Capacity

The precise effect of regular aerobic training throughout life on the age-related rate of decline in aerobic capacity remains unresolved. Cross-sectional data reveal that $\dot{V}O_{2max}$ declines between 0.4 and 0.5 mL · kg^{-1} each year (approximately 1%) in adult men and women (Fig. 31.10).[97,241] Extrapolating this average rate of decline reduces aerobic capacity by age 100 to a level that equals the resting oxygen consumption. This represents a somewhat severe estimate because differences probably exist in the age-related rate of decline in $\dot{V}O_{2max}$ in sedentary and active individuals.[75,97,186] Some research indicates that the rate of decline in $\dot{V}O_{2max}$ with advancing age is nearly twice as fast in sedentary men and women as in individuals who maintain relatively intense training programs throughout life. A study of a large cohort of men who varied considerably in age, aerobic capacity, body composition, and lifestyle revealed that maintaining relatively stable physical activity and body composition levels over time produces an average yearly decline in $\dot{V}O_{2max}$ of 0.25 mL · kg^{-1} · min^{-1}. Several longitudinal studies showed no decline in aerobic capacity in individuals who maintained constant training during a 10-year period.[104,170] In contrast, becoming overly fat and sedentary accelerates the rate of $\dot{V}O_{2max}$ decline.

For most individuals, regular aerobic exercise cannot stop the decline in aerobic capacity with aging.[62,214,222] For ex-

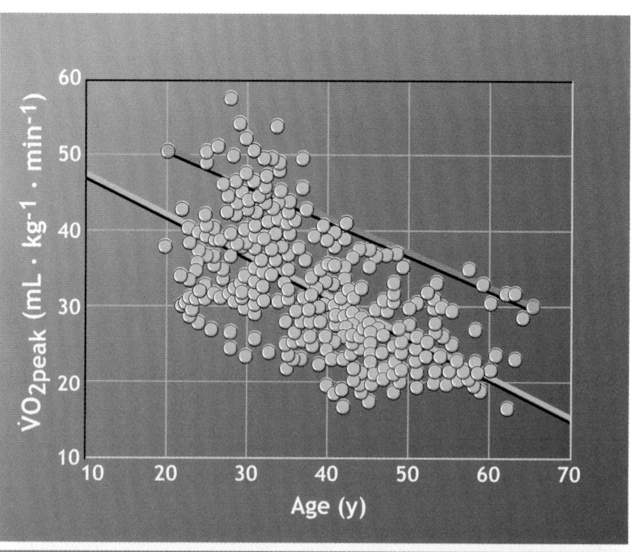

FIGURE 31.10 • Linear regression lines from a cross-sectional assessment of the decline in $\dot{V}O_{2max}$ with age for a large group of female (individual green data points) and male (purple regression line only) employees at the National Aeronautics and Space Administration (NASA)/Johnson Space Center (JSC). (Modified from Jackson AS, et al. Changes in aerobic power of women, ages 20–64 yr. Med Sci Sports Exerc 1996;28:884.)

ample, aerobic capacity of 50-year-old endurance athletes decreased between 8 and 15% per decade despite continued exercise over a 20-year period.[171] Changes in the volume and intensity of exercise training over time likely account for discrepancies in the $\dot{V}O_{2max}$ decline among physically active individuals. *Despite this disparity, research consistently shows that physically active older men and women maintain a higher aerobic capacity than their sedentary counterparts.*

Factors other than physical activity level influence the age-related decline in $\dot{V}O_{2max}$. Heredity undoubtedly plays a crucial role, as does the well-documented increase in body fat and decrease in skeletal muscle mass.[186] In addition, a recent analysis of aerobic capacity of young and older endurance-trained men and women (Fig. 31.11) indicates an average 0.5 L · min^{-1} lower $\dot{V}O_{2max}$ per kg of limb (appendicular) muscle mass for the older athletes, independent of age-associated decreases in muscle and increases in fat.[176] How much the lower aerobic capacity per kg of limb muscle mass in the older subjects reflects reduced oxygen extraction by the active muscles and/or reduced oxygen delivery via decreased cardiac output and/or active muscle blood flow remains undetermined. However, leg blood flow and vascular conductance during cycle ergometer exercise averaged 20 to 30% lower in older endurance-trained men than in younger peers at similar submaximal oxygen consumptions.[178] Consequently, older athletes achieve an equivalent submaximal oxygen consumption at reduced leg blood flows because of increased local oxygen extraction (a-v O_2 difference) from the available blood supply.

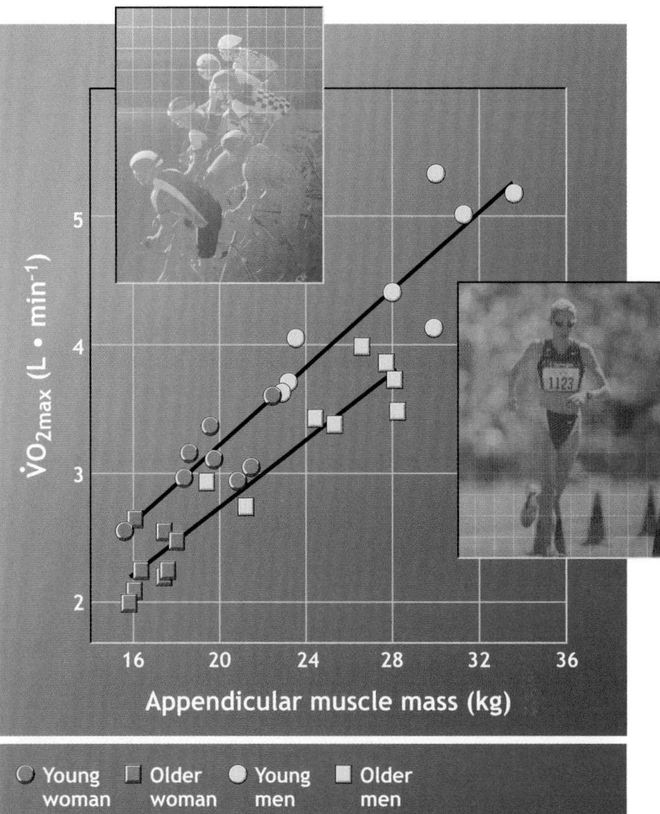

FIGURE 31.11 • Individual maximal oxygen consumption values ($\dot{V}O_{2max}$) related to appendicular muscle mass in young (top line) and older (bottom line) endurance-trained women and men. For an equivalent appendicular muscle mass, $\dot{V}O_{2max}$ averaged 0.5 L · min^{-1} less for older subjects. These data suggest that aerobic capacity per kilogram of appendicular muscle mass decreases with age in highly trained men and women. (From Procter DN, Joyner MJ. Skeletal muscle mass and the reduction of $\dot{V}O_{2max}$ in trained older subjects. J Appl Physiol 1997;82:1411.)

Central and Peripheral Functions

Decrements in central and peripheral functions linked to oxygen transport and use influence the age-related decline in aerobic capacity.

HEART RATE. *A decline in maximum exercise heart rate represents one well-documented change in cardiovascular function with age.* It typically decreases in accord with the following equation, although this provides only a rough approximation:

$$HR_{max} = 220 - \text{age (y)}$$

This age effect reflects reduced medullary outflow of sympathetic activity (depressed β-adrenergic stimulation), which occurs similarly in men and women.[192] Several longitudinal studies of elite athletes show that the decrease in maximum heart rate over a 20-year period (from age 50 to 70 y) is smaller than predicted from the equation typically used to predict maximum heart rate in nonathletes.[171] For untrained older persons, on the other hand, maximum heart rate may be higher than that predicted by 200 age (y), and more accurately predicted by the formula: $HR_{max} = 208 - 0.7 \times \text{age (y)}$.[215] Age exerts no meaningful effect on resting heart rate.

CARDIAC OUTPUT. *Because of a lower maximum heart rate, maximum cardiac output typically decreases with age in trained and untrained men and women.* Reduction in the heart's stroke volume also contributes up to 50% of the age-related reduced capacity for blood flow and oxygen consumption. The decline in stroke volume reflects the combined effects of reduced left ventricular systolic and diastolic myocardial performance, although some physically active individuals maintain contractile function.[116] Healthy elderly individuals often compensate for a diminished maximum heart rate response with an increased cardiac filling (end-diastolic volume), which subsequently increases stroke volume by the Frank-Starling mechanism.[63,241]

PERIPHERAL FACTORS. Reduced peripheral blood flow capacity accompanies age-related decreases in muscle mass. Lower blood flow to active muscle results from a decrease in capillary:muscle fiber ratio and a reduction in arterial cross-sectional area.[202] Scientists must yet determine how aging and regular exercise interact to affect a muscle's oxidative enzymes.[87,177]

Lifestyle or Aging?

Sedentary living produces losses in functional capacity at least as great as the effects of aging. In addition, a high degree of trainability exists among older men and women; positive adaptations in skeletal muscle, substrate metabolism, and cardiovascular function often equal those for younger inidividuals.[32,212] Both low- and higher-intensity exercise enable older individuals to retain cardiovascular functions at a higher level than age-paired sedentary subjects.[148] Active middle-aged men who endurance trained over a 10-year period forestalled the usual 9 to 15% decline in aerobic capacity.[103] At age 55, the men maintained the same values for blood pressure, body mass, and $\dot{V}O_{2max}$ as 10 years earlier.

Endurance Performance

Comparing the endurance performance of athletes of different ages provides further evidence for the impressive effects of regular exercise on preservation of cardiovascular function throughout life. Figure 31.12A shows age-group, world-record times for 50-, 100-, and 200-km runs for men and women of different ages. The world record at each ultradistance (always recorded by the youngest age group) corresponds to an average running pace of approximately 5 minutes 38 seconds per mile for the 50-km run; 6 minutes 33 seconds per mile for the 100-km run, and 7 minutes 28 seconds per mile for the 200-km run. Figure 31.12B presents world-record marathon times, starting at age 4 for males and at age 5 for females and up to age 86 years for men and age 80 years for women. The world record of 2 hours, 7 minutes, 11 seconds by Carlos Lopes (age 37) of Portugal (April 1985) corresponds to a running speed of 4 minutes 51 seconds per mile (20 km · h^{-1} or 12.4 mph).

Endurance performance (marathon) is poorer in children and adolescents and older adults. Considerable performance

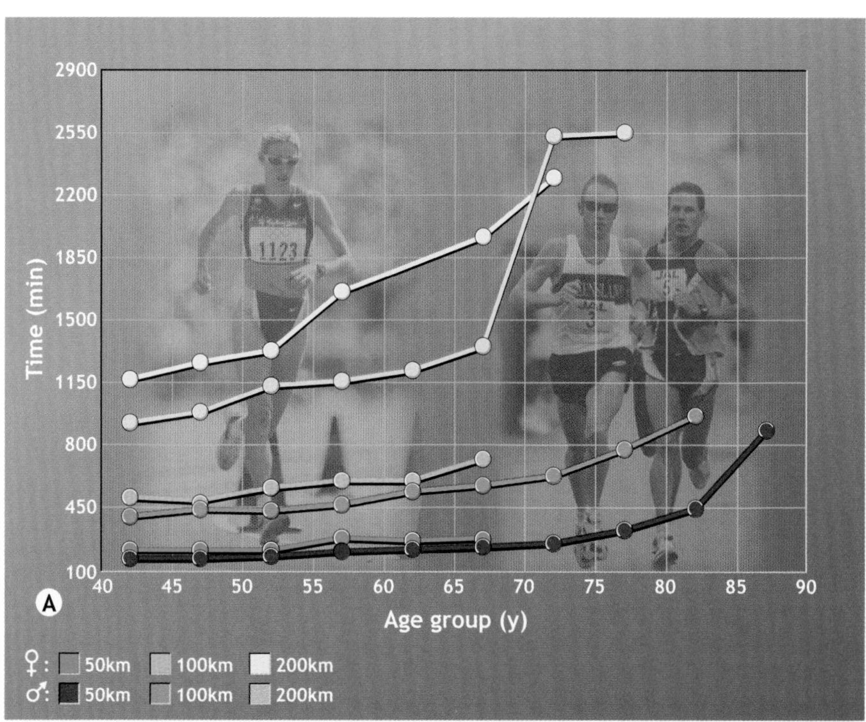

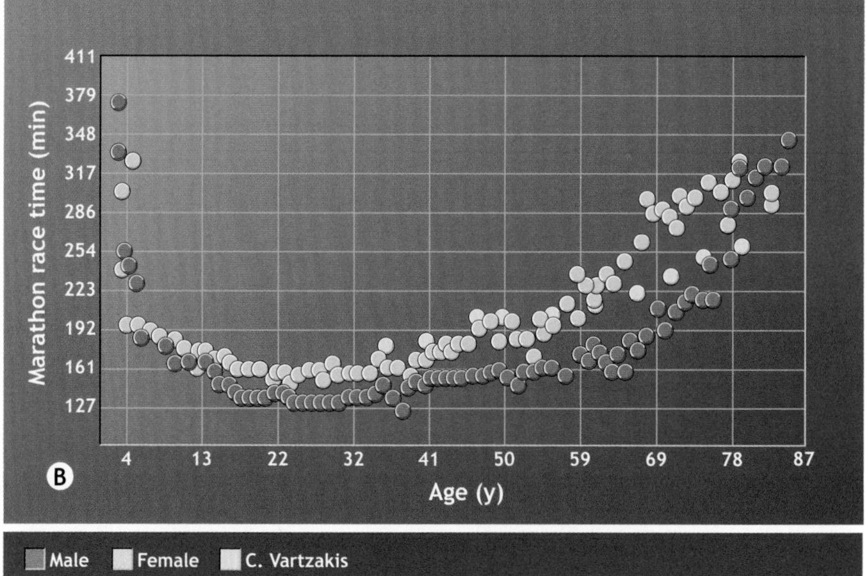

FIGURE 31.12 • **A**. Ultradistance world records by age for men and women. **B**. Plot of world record marathon run times for men and women of different ages. The *yellow data points* represent the remarkable marathon achievements of the Greek runner Christos Vartzakis from age 36 to 79 years. Over a 43-year span, his average speed decreased by 30% from 13.9 km · h^{-1} at age 36 to 9.73 km · h^{-1} at 79 years of age. Interestingly, his marathon time of 3 hours 56 minutes at age 72 bettered the average speed of master's runners 40 years younger competing in the Basa Marathon Race. (Data for ultradistance records courtesy of *Runners World Magazine,* 2000; data on Vartzakis courtesy of Dr. George Rontoyannis, Hellenic Sports Research Institute, Athens, Greece. Data originally published in Rontoyannis G. Sixty-three years of competitive sport activity. Case study. J Sports Med Phys Fitness 1992;32:331.)

decrements occur between age 30 and 86 years; the best marathon time of 340.2 minutes for the 86-year-old men corresponds to a pace of 12.9 minutes per mile, and the record for 80-year-old women of 328.6 minutes equals a pace of 12.5 minutes per mile. The remarkable endurance performances for individuals up to their ninth decade of life affirms the tremendous cardiovascular potential of older men and women who continue vigorous training as they grow older. The similarity in ultraendurance performance times of older men and women (particularly for the 50- and 100-km distances) suggests similar cardiovascular fitness levels between genders among elite athletes with aging.

Aerobic Trainability Among the Elderly: Perhaps a Gender Difference

Exercise training for healthy elderly men enhances the heart's systolic and diastolic properties and increases aerobic capacity to the same relative extent (15 to 30%) as in younger adults.[27,53,128,191] Research has evaluated the contribution of training-induced increases in stroke volume and a-$\bar{v}$ O_2 difference to aerobic fitness improvements in healthy older men and women. Nine to 12 months of endurance training increased $\dot{V}O_{2max}$ by 19% in men and 22% in women (Table 31.3). These values represent the high end of improvement typically observed for younger adults.

However, gender differences emerged in certain aspects of the training response. For men, improved aerobic capacity associated with a 15% larger maximum stroke volume (corresponding cardiac output increase represented two-thirds of the $\dot{V}O_{2max}$ increase) and a 7% greater maximum a-$\bar{v}$ O_2 difference (representing one-third of the $\dot{V}O_{2max}$ increase). For the women, the a-$\bar{v}$ O_2 difference explained the total $\dot{V}O_{2max}$ increase, with no change in left ventricular performance at maximal exercise. This indicates that training-induced increase in aerobic capacity for older women depends on peripheral adaptations in trained muscle and suggests that sex hormones influence gender-related adaptations to endurance training. The lack of a stroke volume increase among older women with training may result from (1) blunting of the normal increase in plasma volume, (2) depression of cardiopulmonary baroreflex sensitivity, and (3) an estrogen-deficiency–related decrease in vascular compliance (i.e., increased vascular stiffness).[202,206] These apparent gender differences in physiology, however, do not impair endurance performance in older women as reflected by male-female similarities in ultradistance running performance (Fig. 31.12A). Research must determine whether a lack of central circulatory adaptation to endurance training in postmenopausal women is a consistent finding and whether the response results from hormonal deficiencies in menopause.[203]

TABLE 31.3 ➤ EFFECTS OF 9 MONTHS OF ENDURANCE TRAINING ON MAXIMAL OXYGEN CONSUMPTION AND CARDIOVASCULAR FUNCTION IN 15 MEN (AGE, 63 ± 3 Y) AND 16 WOMEN (64 ± 3 Y)

	$\dot{V}O_{2MAX}$ L · MIN^{-1}	$\dot{Q}_{MAX}$ L · MIN^{-1}	HR_{MAX} B · MIN^{-1}	SV_{MAX} ML	A-$\bar{V}$ O_2DIFF ML · DL^{-1}
MEN					
Before	2.35	17	170	101	13.8
After	2.8[a]	19[a]	164[a]	116[a]	14.8[a]
WOMEN					
Before	1.36	11.2	161	70	12.2
After	1.66[a]	11.5	164	70	14.4[a]

Values are means; $\dot{V}O_{2max}$, maximal O_2 consumption; $\dot{Q}_{max}$, maximal cardiac output; HR_{max}, maximal heart rate; SV_{max}, stroke volume at maximal exercise; a-$\bar{v}O_2$diff, arteriovenous O_2 content difference at maximal exercise.
[a]$P < .01$ vs. before training.
From Spina RJ, et al. Differences in cardiovascular adaptations to endurance exercise training between older men and women. *J Appl Physiol* 1993; 75:849.

Body Composition

The cross-sectional data in Figure 31.13 show that after age 18, men and women progressively gain body fat until their fifth or sixth decade. After age 60, total body mass decreases

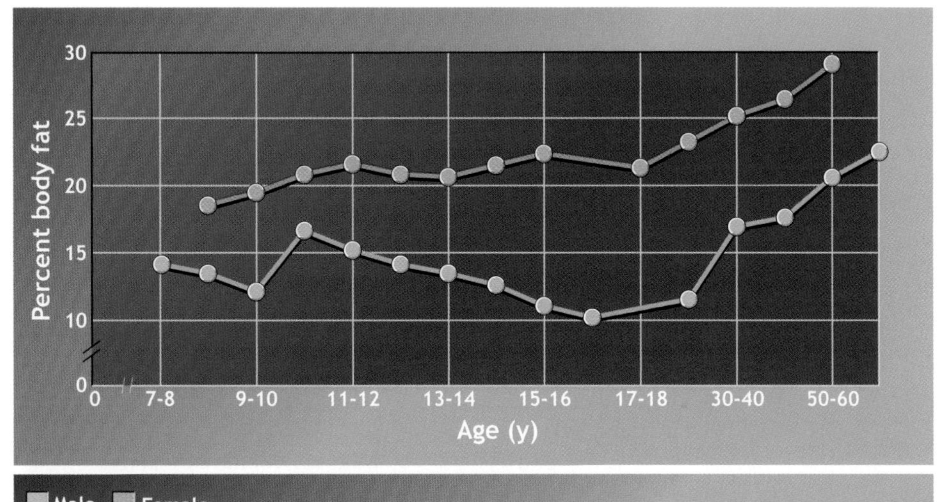

FIGURE 31.13 • Generalized changes in percentage body fat with age.

despite increasing body fat. This results partly from a disproportionately greater death rate among the obese in the upper age group, leaving fewer of these individuals to measure.

Most age-trend studies do not track the same subjects over time; instead, they evaluate different subjects in different age categories at the same time. From such **cross-sectional data**, one attempts to generalize about an individual's expected age-related changes, but sometimes these generalizations are misleading. For example, today's 70- and 80-year-olds typically are shorter than 20-year-old college students. This observation does not necessarily mean that individuals become shorter with age (although this does happen to some extent). Instead, the young adults of this generation receive better nourishment than the 80-year-olds did at age 20.

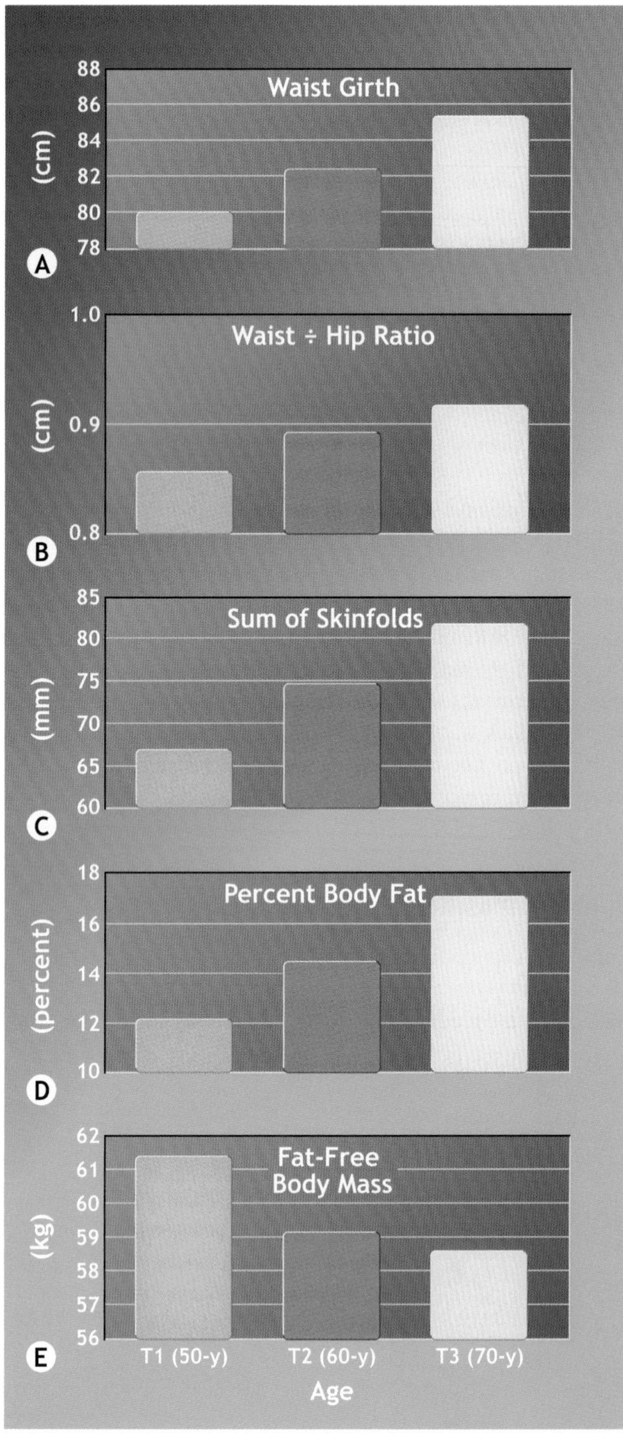

FIGURE 31.14 • Changes in (**A**) waist girth, (**B**) waist:hip girth ratio, (**C**) sum of skinfolds, (**D**) percentage body fat, and (**E**) FFM for 21 endurance athletes who continued to train over a 20-year period, starting at age 50. (From Pollock ML, et al. Twenty-year follow-up of aerobic power and body composition of older track athletes. J Appl Physiol 1997;82:1508.)

The limited **longitudinal data** (data collected on the same subjects over time) show trends in body fat changes similar to those noted in cross-sectional studies.[38] Scientists do not know if the body fat increases during adulthood represent a normal biologic pattern or simply reflect sedentary lifestyle choices. Longitudinal observations of individuals who maintain a physically active lifestyle support a biologic tendency to gain fat as one ages. Figure 31.14 shows body composition changes for 21 endurance athletes who continued to train over a 20-year period, starting at age 50. Despite maintaining a relatively constant body mass during the prolonged period of exercise training, gains occurred in measures of body fat and indicators of abdominal obesity, while FFM declined. The roughly 3% body fat unit increase per decade paralleled similar increases in waist girth. The magnitude of increase in body fat and decrease in FFM, while discouraging to some, average at least 20% less than reported for nonathletes. These data suggest that habitual endurance exercise confers at least some "protection" from the effects of aging on body composition.

Those who train regularly with resistance exercise for many years often demonstrate increased FFM and decreased body fat. Figure 31.15 shows an older resistance-trained athlete; these photos illustrate the impressive potential to increase and then maintain a large muscle mass into late middle-age. Indeed, individuals who begin resistance training in late adolescence seem to defy certain aspects of typical aging. This sport certainly exemplifies the axiom, "Use it-or-lose it!"

Bone Mass

Osteoporosis poses a major problem with aging, particularly among postmenopausal women. This condition produces loss of bone mass as the aging skeleton demineralizes and becomes porous. Bone mass can decrease by 30 to 50% in persons older than age 60. As emphasized in Chapter 2, regular weight-bearing exercise and resistance exercise not only retard bone loss but often increase bone mass in elderly men and women.[119] In postmenopausal women, regular exercise augments hormone replacement therapy to increase total bone mineral density and preserve these gains.[110]

TRAINABILITY AND AGE

Exercise training improves physiologic responses at any age. Several factors affect the magnitude of change, including initial fitness status, genetics, and the specific type of

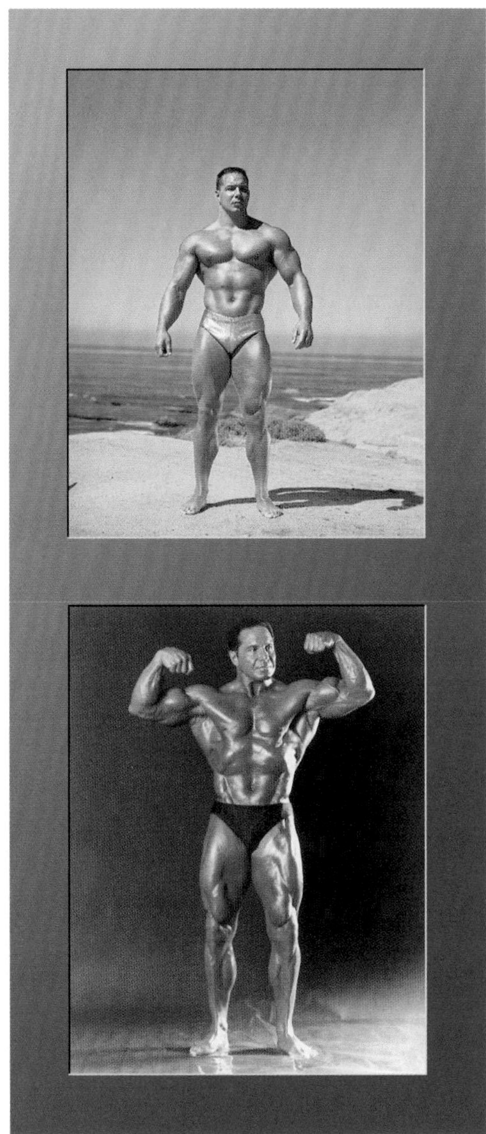

FIGURE 31.15 • Fifty-three consecutive years of resistance training. *Top.* Bill Pearl, one of the greatest bodybuilding champions of all time. Holder of four Mr. Universe titles (1956, 1961, 1967, 1971), he still trains 2.5 hours daily, beginning at 4:30 AM. *Top,* 1967 Mr. Universe, age 37. *Bottom.* Formal pose at age 59. (Photos courtesy of Bill Pearl.)

training. Some researchers believed that aging hindered ability to improve muscular strength and aerobic capacity. They argued that declines in neuromuscular function and impaired cellular capability for protein synthesis and chemical regulation generally diminished trainability with aging.

Research over the past 20 years has modified this classic view of the expected improvements from physical conditioning for people of different ages (Fig. 31.16). Over a broad age range, improvements in physiologic function result from an appropriate training stimulus, often at a rate and magnitude *independent* of the person's age.[31,41] For example, adaptation of muscle fiber size, capillarization, and glycolytic and respiratory enzymes to specific endurance or resistance-training exercise is similar in older men and women and

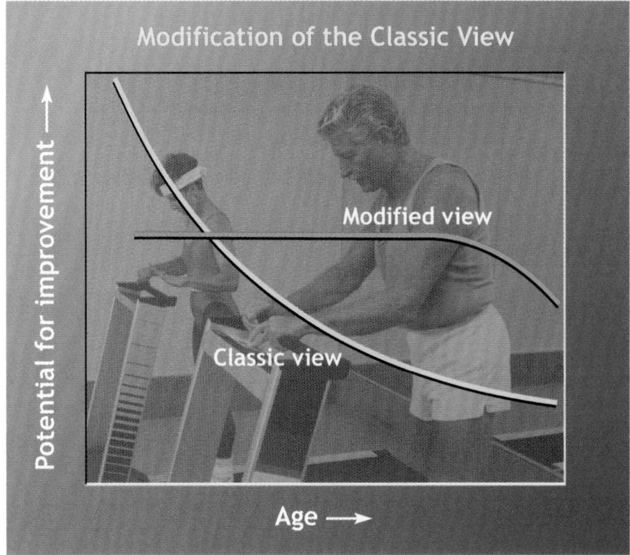

FIGURE 31.16 • New view of old beliefs. Traditional versus the more current view of the expected improvements from physical training with aging.

younger adults. These adaptations emerge most readily with relatively intense exercise that continuously adjusts to training improvements.

Summary

1. Physiologic and performance capabilities usually decline after age 30. Many factors, including diminished physical activity level, affect the rate of decline in physiologic functions.
2. Regular physical activity and exercise training enable older persons to retain higher levels of functional capacity, notably cardiovascular and muscular function.
3. Biologic aging relates to changes in three hormonal systems: hypothalamic–pituitary–gonadal axis, adrenal cortex, and growth hormone/insulin-like growth factor axis.
4. One must consider differences between children and adults in exercise economy, FFM, anaerobic power capacity, and anabolic hormone levels when evaluating their physiologic response and exercise performance.
5. A 40 to 50% reduction in muscle mass from a loss of motor units and muscle fiber atrophy between ages 25 and 80 is the primary cause of the age-associated reduction in muscle strength.
6. Considerable plasticity exists in physiologic, structural, and performance characteristics among older individuals that enable marked and rapid strength improvement with vigorous training into the ninth decade of life.
7. A physically active lifestyle affects neuromuscular functions positively at any age and possibly slows

the age-related decline in cognitive performance associated with speed of information processing.

8. Cross-sectional data indicate that $\dot{V}O_{2max}$ declines approximately 1% each year in adult men and women. Physically active older men and women maintain a higher aerobic capacity than their sedentary peers at any age.
9. Sedentary living causes losses in functional capacity at least as great as aging itself. Regular physical activity improves physiologic function at any age; initial fitness, genetics, and type and amount of training control the magnitude of change.
10. Increased body fat and decreased FFM in aging, active athletes average at least 20% less than nonathletes, which suggests that habitual physical activity confers some protection from the effects of aging on body composition.

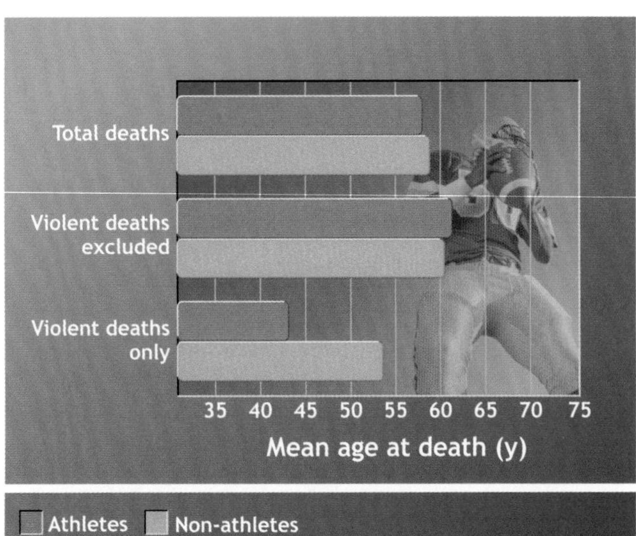

FIGURE 31.17 • Age at death of athletes and nonathletes. No statistically significant differences emerged in comparisons between groups. (From Montoye HJ, et al. The longevity and morbidity of college athletes. Indianapolis, IN: Phi Epsilon Kappa, 1957.)

➤ PART 3 • Physical Activity, Health, and Longevity

Because older fit individuals possess many characteristics of younger people, one might argue that improved physical fitness retards aging and offers health protection and possible longevity.

EXERCISE, HEALTH, AND LONGEVITY

In one of the first studies of the possibility that sport and regular exercise prolongs life, former Harvard oarsmen exceeded their predicted longevity by 5.1 years per man.[83] Other early studies showed similar but more modest life span extension.[9] Methodologic problems that plagued this research included inadequate record keeping, small sample size, improper statistical procedures to estimate expected longevity, and no accounting for socioeconomic status, body type, tobacco use, and family background.

One group of researchers attempted to overcome many of these limitations by studying disease and longevity in former college athletes. No difference emerged in the longevities of ex-athletes and nonathletes (Fig. 31.17). Some equality in genetic background existed between the comparison groups because of the similar average age at death for the grandparents, parents, and siblings of the ex-athletes and nonathletes. These and more-recent findings show that athletic participation as a young adult does *not* ensure good health and longevity later in life.[180] However, maintaining increased physical activity and fitness *throughout life* provides significant health and longevity benefits.[20,57,82,189] A continuing longitudinal study of the health consequences of different fitness levels in 25,341 men and 7080 women shows low aerobic fitness to be a more important precursor of mortality than any of the other significant coronary heart disease (CHD) risk factors (Fig. 31.18).[21] In addition, inverse risk gradients emerged across categories of low, moderate, and high fitness, with a lower death rate among moderately fit individuals than those in the low fitness group. The least fit men and women were nearly twice as likely to die from all causes as their most fit counterparts during an 8-year follow-up period. Increased physical fitness actually countered the negative effects of other important risk factors. Moderately fit smokers with hypertension and high cholesterol lived longer than healthy but sedentary nonsmokers. *Low physical fitness was a more powerful risk factor than high blood pressure, high cholesterol, obesity, and family history.*

Enhanced Quality to a Longer Life: The Harvard Alumni Study

The lifestyles and exercise habits of 17,000 Harvard alumni who entered college between 1916 and 1950 provide evidence that *moderate* aerobic exercise equivalent to jogging approximately 3 miles per day promotes good health and adds several years to life.[164] The results of these long-term studies were as follows:

- Regular exercise countered the life-shortening effects of cigarette smoking and excess body weight.
- Individuals with hypertension who exercised regularly reduced death rate by one-half.
- Regular exercise countered genetic tendencies toward early death. Individuals with one or both parents who died before age 65 (a significant health risk), reduced death risk by 25% with a lifestyle of regular exercise.
- Mortality rate decreased by 50% for active men whose parents lived beyond 65 years.

Figure 31.19 shows that people who exercised more reduced their risk of dying. For example, men who walked 9 or more miles each week showed a 21% lower mortality rate than men who walked 3 miles or less. Life expectancy was higher for men who exercised at the equivalent of light sport

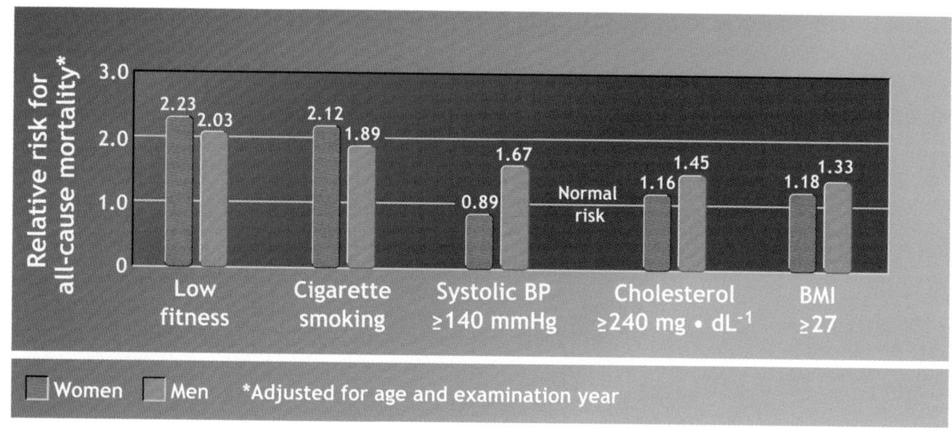

FIGURE 31.18 • Comparative influence of low physical fitness as a precursor of all-cause mortality in men and women. (From Blair S, et al. Influences of cardiorespiratory fitness and other precursors on cardiovascular disease and all-cause mortality in men and women. JAMA 1996;276:205.)

activity than for sedentary men. Life expectancy of Harvard alumni increased steadily from a weekly exercise energy expenditure of 500 kcal up to 3500 kcal, a value equivalent to 6 to 8 hours of strenuous exercise. In addition, the active men lived an average of 1 to 2 years longer than their sedentary classmates. Weekly exercise beyond 3500 kcal offered no additional health or longevity benefits. Exercise carried to extremes associated with *higher* death rates than more moderate activity.

Vigorous Exercise and Longevity

The previously discussed research with Harvard alumni examined only the total amount of weekly physical activity, not its intensity, in relation to heart disease and mortality. Ensuing research with the same group indicates that vigorous regular exercise exerts the greatest effect on extending life.[121] Men who expended at least 1500 kcal weekly in vigorous exercise—equivalent to 6 METs or more, such as jogging or walking briskly, lap swimming, singles tennis, fast cycling, or heavy yard chores for an hour, three or four times a week—during the 20-year study had a 25% lower death rate than the most sedentary men. The most active men showed the greatest life expectancies, largely due to reduced deaths from cardiovascular disease. The benefits of vigorous exercise also extended to overweight smokers. Risk associated with a sedentary lifestyle equaled the risk of smoking one pack of cigarettes per day or being 20% overweight. Subsequent research with these men (and others[5]) showed that the exercise equivalent of a 1-hour brisk walk 5 days weekly or a vigorous workout at least once weekly cut stroke risk almost in half, while brisk walking for 30 minutes 5 days weekly reduced stroke risk by 24%.[122,123] Other stroke-protective activities included stair climbing or participating in such moderate activities as gardening, dancing, and bicycling. An intensive poststroke exercise program also facilitates the stroke survivor's recovery of motor skills.[50]

Epidemiologic Evidence

A critique of 43 studies of the relationship between physical inactivity and CHD concluded that lack of regular exercise contributes to heart disease in a *cause-and-effect* manner; the sedentary person runs almost twice the risk of developing heart disease as the most active individual.[174] *The strength of the association between lack of exercise and heart disease risk equals that observed for hypertension, cigarette smoking, and high serum cholesterol. This makes physical inactivity the greater heart disease risk, since more people lead sedentary lifestyles than possess one or more other primary risks.* The life-protecting benefits of exercise

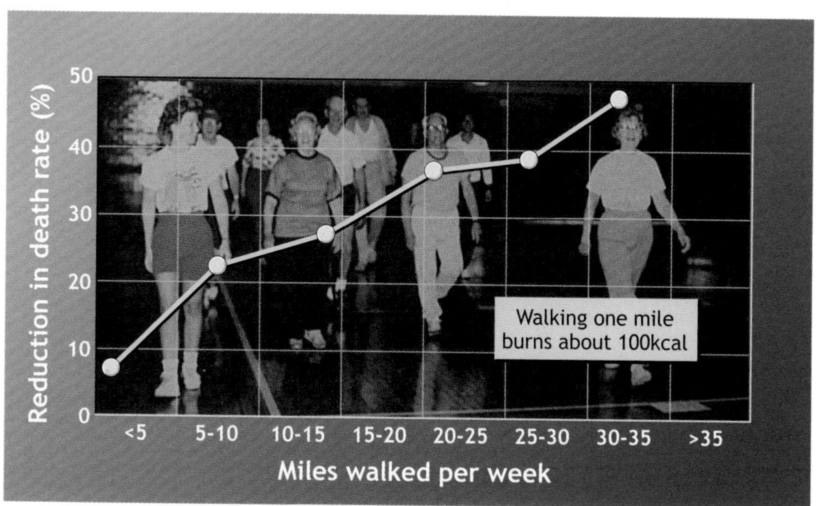

FIGURE 31.19 • Reduced death risk for individuals who participate in regular exercise. (Adapted from Paffenbarger RS Jr, et al. Physical activity, all-cause mortality, and longevity of college alumni. N Engl J Med 1986;314:605.)

link more with preventing early mortality than with extending life span. Surprisingly, only light-to-moderate regular activity such as walking, gardening, stair climbing, and household chores produces health benefits for previously sedentary middle-aged and older men and women. These sedentary citizens represent the largest percentage of the population at greatest risk for chronic disease.[22,76]

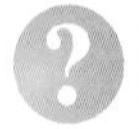

INTEGRATIVE QUESTION

Does physical activity benefit a person even if exercise intensity does not stimulate a training effect?

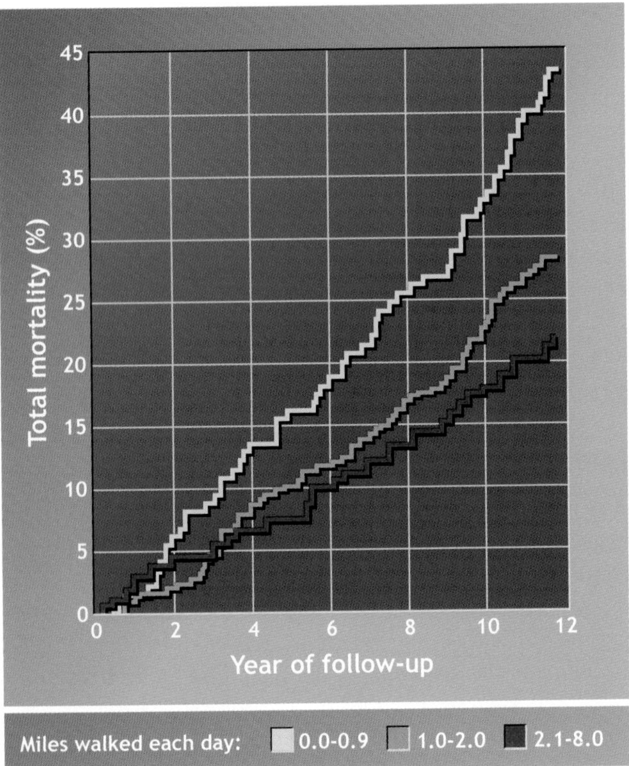

FIGURE 31.20 • Cumulative mortality by year of follow-up and distance walked per day. (To convert distances to kilometers, multiply by 1.609.) (From Hakim AA, et al. Effects of walking on mortality among nonsmoking retired men. N Engl J Med 1998;338:94.)

REGULAR MODERATE EXERCISE PROVIDES SIGNIFICANT BENEFITS

A sedentary lifestyle represents an independent and powerful predictor of CHD risk and mortality.[57,147] Encouraging the most sedentary 25% of the American adult population to become only moderately active yields substantial public health benefits.[11,19,51,115] Figure 31.20 further illustrates the health-related benefits of regular physical activity. The analysis assessed the effect of miles walked each day on overall mortality rate in 707 nonsmoking, physically capable men ages 61 to 81 years. An inverse relationship between distance walked and mortality emerged after adjusting for overall physical activity and other risk factors. For example, men who walked less than 1 mile each day reached a cumulative incidence of death in 7 years that required 12 years for the most active men, who walked at least 2 miles daily. Over 7 years, 43.1% of the less active men died, compared with 21.5% of the most active walkers.

Table 31.4 presents corroborative research findings for leisure-time physical activity of 333 patients between ages 25 to 74 years who suffered a first heart attack and 503 control subjects, selected randomly and matched for age and gender, who had not had a heart attack. After adjustments for heart disease risks (e.g., age, smoking, diabetes, hypertension), regular walkers reduced their risk of a first heart attack by 73%, and those who gardened regularly reduced risk by 66% compared with sedentary peers (risk ratio set at 1.00). Walking exercise or gardening for more than 60 minutes weekly reduced risk similarly to high-intensity leisure-time physical activity. The benefits of walking also applied to women who regularly walked 3 mph or faster for at least 3 hours per week; heart attack risk decreased up to 40% below the risk for sedentary women. For women who walked briskly (≥3.0 mph) for 5 hours per week, the risk decreased by one-half.[139] These findings complement and further support current exercise recommendations from the Centers for Disease Control and Prevention and the American College of Sports Medicine to accumulate 30 minutes or more of moderate-intensity physical activity on most days.

TABLE 31.4 ➤ MODERATE- AND HIGH-INTENSITY LEISURE-TIME PHYSICAL ACTIVITY (LTPA) AND RISK OF PRIMARY CARDIAC ARREST

			Odds Ratio Cardiac Arrest Risk	
Type of LTPA	Case Patients, No. (%)	Controls, No. (%)	Unadjusted	Adjusted[a]
No activity	45 (14)	18 (4)	1.0 (Reference)	1.0 (Reference)
Moderate-intensity	160 (48)	192 (38)	0.36	0.36
High-intensity	128 (38)	293 (58)	0.19	0.36

[a]Adjusted for age, smoking, education, diabetes, hypertension, and health status.
From Lemaitre RN, et al. Leisure-time physical activity and the risk of primary cardiac arrest. Arch Intern Med 1999; 159:686.

Influence of Physical Fitness

A low-level of cardiorespiratory fitness is a strong independent predictor of increased risk for both cardiovascular disease and all-cause mortality.[245] The predictive effect equals that of diabetes mellitus and other heart disease risks.[52,238] One study directly examined aerobic fitness (rather than verbal or written reports of physical activity habits) and heart disease risk of more than 13,000 men and women observed for an average of 8 years. To isolate the effect of physical fitness, the study accounted for cigarette smoking, high cholesterol and blood sugar levels, hypertension, and family history of heart disease. Based on age-adjusted death rates per 10,000 person-years, the least fit group averaged more than three times the death rate of the most fit individuals (Fig. 31.21). Importantly, the greatest health benefits emerged for the group rated just above the most sedentary category. For men, the decrease in death rate from the least fit category to the next category exceeded 38 (64.0 vs. 25.5 deaths per 10,000 person-years), whereas the drop in mortality between the second group and most fit group was only 7. Enhanced aerobic fitness benefited women to a similar extent. To move from the most sedentary category to the next highest group—the change that produced the greatest health benefits—requires only such moderate-intensity exercise as walking briskly for 30 minutes several times weekly.

Studies of Finnish men complement the above findings. Aerobic capacity and leisure-time physical activity showed an inverse, graded, independent association with risk for acute myocardial infarction.[102] Even after adjusting for genetic effects and other familial factors that predict mortality, current aerobic fitness and physical activity level offered significant protection from death.[113] Physical fitness also counters the negative impact of existing disease. For example, an inverse and independent relationship emerged between $\dot{V}O_{2peak}$ and incidence of fatal and nonfatal cardiovascular events and all-cause mortality in male and female hypertensives followed over 16.5 years.[166]

Table 31.5 summarizes 30 years of research relating physical activity level or physical fitness to chronic disease or medical conditions. *Clearly, a strong inverse association exists between regular exercise and level of aerobic fitness and all causes of death, with the greatest impact on diseases of the cardiovascular system. Moderate-intensity regular exercise substantially reduces the risk of dying from heart disease, cancer, and other causes.*[33,105,237]

Structured Exercise Not Necessary

Researchers monitored two groups of 116 sedentary men and 119 women, ages 35 to 60 years during a 2-year randomized clinical trial.[51] One group spent 20 to 60 minutes exercising vigorously (e.g., swimming, stair stepping, walking, or biking) up to 5 days a week at a fitness center. The other group incorporated 30 minutes a day of "lifestyle" exercises (e.g., extra walking, raking leaves, stair climbing, walking around the airport while waiting for a plane, participating in a walking club) most days of the week. The lifestyle participants also learned cognitive and behavioral strategies for increasing daily physical activity.[140] The intervention consisted of 6 months of intensive exercise followed by 18 months of maintenance for each of the programs. At the end of 24 months, *both* groups showed similar and significant improvements in physical activity, cardiorespiratory fitness, systolic and diastolic blood pressure, and body fat percentage. These findings show that the health-derived benefits from regular exercise do not require structured or vigorous exercise.

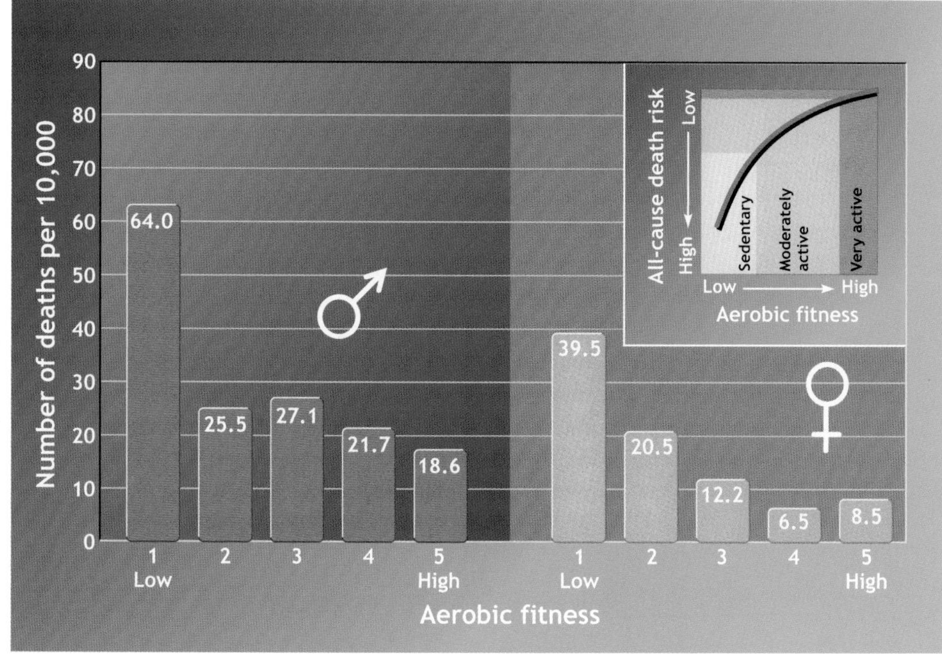

FIGURE 31.21 • Aerobic fitness and longevity. Going from the low fitness category to a moderate level produces the greatest reduction in death risk, with only a small added benefit from further fitness improvements. *Inset figure* shows a generalized curve depicting health benefits from increased daily physical activity and aerobic fitness. (Modified from Blair SN, et al. Physical fitness and all-cause mortality: a prospective study of healthy men and women. JAMA 1989;262:2395.)

TABLE 31.5 ➤ **PHYSICAL ACTIVITY AND/OR PHYSICAL FITNESS AND SELECTED CHRONIC DISEASES OR CONDITIONS, 1963–1993**

Disease or Condition	Number of Studies	Trends Across Activity or Fitness Categories and Strength of Evidence[a]
All-cause mortality	>10	↓↓↓
Coronary artery disease	>10	↓↓↓
Hypertension	5–10	↓↓
Obesity	>10	↓↓
Stroke	5–10	↓
Peripheral vascular disease	<5	→
Cancer		
Colon	>10	↓↓
Rectum	>10	→
Stomach	<5	→
Breast	<5	↓
Prostate	5–10	↓
Lung	<5	↓
Pancreas	<5	→
Type 2 diabetes	<5	↓↓
Osteoarthritis	<5	→
Osteoporosis	5–10	↓↓
Functional capability	5–10	↓↓

[a]→, No apparent difference in disease rates across activity or fitness categories; ↓, *some* evidence of reduced disease rates across activity or fitness categories; ↓↓, *good* evidence of reduced disease rates across activity or fitness categories, control of potential confounders, good methods, some evidence of biological mechanisms; ↓↓↓, *excellent* evidence of reduced disease rates across activity or fitness categories, good control of potential confounders, excellent methods, extensive evidence of biological mechanisms, relationship is considered causal.
From Blair SN. Physical activity, physical fitness, and health. Res Q Exerc Sports 1993;64:365.

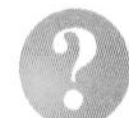

INTEGRATIVE QUESTION

Respond to the statement: "The fact that overwhelming epidemiologic evidence links on-the-job or leisure-time physical activity to reduced CHD risk does not necessarily prove that exercise *causes* improved cardiovascular health."

CAN CHANGING ACTIVITY LEVEL IMPROVE HEALTH?

Although one's current level of physical activity and physical fitness relate to health risk, an important question concerns whether a sustained increase in regular activity can reduce disease risk. To answer this question, previously sedentary, apparently healthy male Harvard alumni reported whether they changed their typical physical activity and other lifestyle habits over an 11- to 15-year period. Figure 31.22 relates changes in health-related lifestyle characteristics to changes in mortality risk. Regardless of age, sedentary men who adopted a more moderate to vigorous level of regular activity had a 51% lower risk of dying than men who remained sedentary. For lifestyle change and heart disease mortality risk, becoming more physically active on a regular basis provided risk reduction benefits equivalent to those from quitting cigarette smoking, reducing body weight, or controlling blood pressure.

Summary

1. Vigorous physical activity early in life contributes little to increased longevity or health in later life. However, a physically active lifestyle throughout life confers significant health benefits.

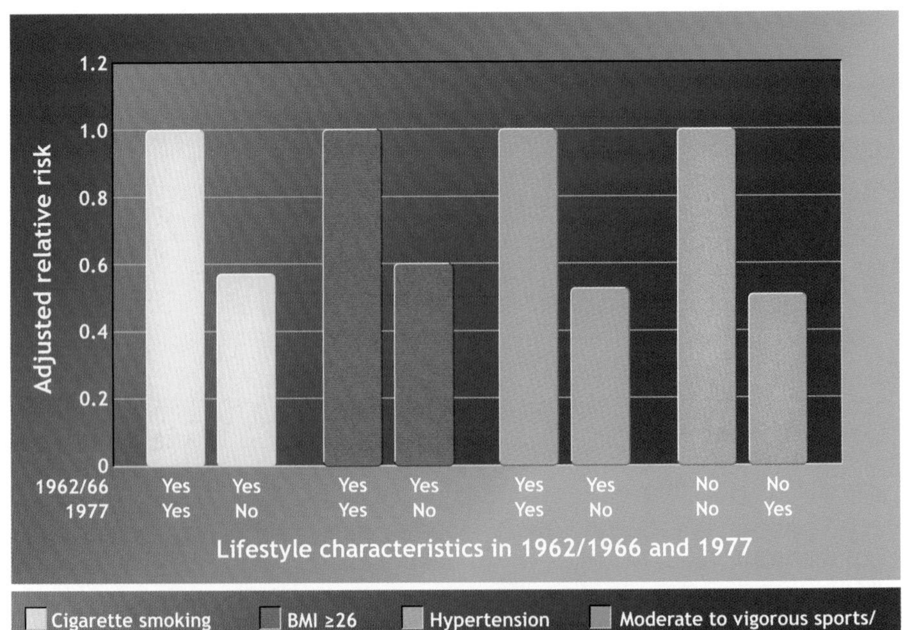

FIGURE 31.22 • Adjusted relative risks for CHD mortality from changes in lifestyle characteristics. Each relative risk is adjusted for age and all other variables in the figure. First bar of each pair represents men with initial unfavorable characteristics (in 1962 or 1966) and at follow-up in 1977. The second bar of the pair shows adjusted relative risks for men achieving favorable changes in the variable of interest between baseline and follow-up. *BMI,* body mass index; *Yes* and *No* refer to presence or absence of trait at date indicated. (Modified from Blair SN. Physical activity, physical fitness, and health. Res Q Exerc Sport 1993;64:365. Data from Paffenbarger RS Jr, et al. The association between changes in physical-activity level and other lifestyle characteristics with mortality among men. N Engl J Med 1993;328:538.)

2. Regular, moderate exercise counters the life-shortening effects of CHD risks including cigarette smoking and excess body weight. A sedentary person runs almost twice the risk of developing heart disease as the most active individuals. More vigorous exercise may extend life by several years.
3. The risk of CHD from sedentary living equals that for hypertension, cigarette smoking, and high serum cholesterol. The life-protecting benefits of exercise relate more to preventing early mortality than to extending overall life span.
4. A moderate amount of regular exercise substantially reduces the risk of dying from heart disease, cancer, and other medically-related maladies. Importantly, the greatest health benefits emerge when a person alters a sedentary lifestyle and becomes just moderately physically active.
5. Strategies that modify lifestyle toward increased daily physical activity beneficially alter factors associated with CHD risk.

➤ PART 4 • Coronary Heart Disease

CHD involves degenerative changes in the intima or inner lining of the larger arteries that supply the myocardium.

CHANGES ON THE CELLULAR LEVEL

Damage to arterial walls begins as a multifactorial response to injury, perhaps from hypertension, cigarette smoking, infection, homocysteine, elevated cholesterol, free radicals, or immunologically mediated factors. One response triggers the chemical modification of various compounds, including the oxidation of low-density lipoprotein cholesterol (LDL-C). This initiates a complex series of changes that produce lesions that sometimes bulge into the vessel lumen or protrude outward into the arterial wall. Lesions initially take the form of fatty streaks, the first signs of atherosclerosis. With further inflammatory damage from continued lipid deposition and proliferation of smooth muscle and connective tissue, the vessel becomes congested with lipid-filled plaques, fibrous scar tissue, or both. Progressive occlusion gradually reduces blood flow capacity, causing the myocardium to become ischemic, or poorly supplied with oxygen.

Vulnerable Plaque: Difficult to Detect Yet Lethal

Vulnerable plaque, a soft type of metabolically active, unstable plaque, does not necessarily produce significant coronary artery narrowing but tends to fissure and burst. The rupture of unstable plaque—the sudden breakdown of fatty plaques in the lining of the coronary arteries—exposes the blood to thrombogenic compounds. This triggers a cascade of chemical events that often culminate in clot formation (thrombus) that leads to myocardial infarction and possible death. The sudden, complete obstruction of a coronary artery frequently occurs in blood vessels with only mild-to-moderate obstructions (<70% blockage). Arterial blockage often occurs before the coronary vessel has narrowed enough to produce angina symptoms or electrocardiographic (ECG) abnormalities or to indicate the need for revascularization procedures (e.g., coronary bypass surgery or balloon angioplasty).[131] Acute disruption and rupture of arterial plaque provides a plausible explanation for sudden death from acute physical and emotional exertion in middle-aged men with coronary artery disease, compared with sudden death under resting conditions.[30] The beneficial effects of cholesterol-lowering strategies on heart disease risk do not always improve coronary blood flow. However, stability of vulnerable plaque may improve with reduction in overall blood cholesterol.[126] This stabilizing effect would reduce the likelihood of rupture of existing coronary artery plaque.

Vascular Degeneration Begins Early in Life

Landmark studies of atherosclerosis in young American soldiers killed in Korea showed advanced lesions in men whose age averaged 22 years.[55] These findings surprised the medical community and focused attention on the possible childhood origins of atherosclerosis. We now know that fatty streaks and clinically significant fibrous plaques develop rapidly during adolescence through the third decade of life.[213] Autopsies of 93 young persons aged 2 to 39 years, most of whom died from trauma, revealed that fatty streaks and fibrous plaques in the aorta and coronary arteries appear early and progress in severity as a young person ages.[16]

Body mass index, systolic and diastolic blood pressure, and total serum cholesterol, triglycerides, and LDL-C strongly and positively related (high-density lipoprotein cholesterol [HDL-C] related negatively) to the extent of vascular lesions in the deceased young people. History of cigarette smoking magnified the vascular damage, a disconcerting fact in light of recent data indicating tobacco use common and on the increase among college students.[184] As the number of risk factors increased, so also did the severity of atherosclerosis in these asymptomatic individuals. Recent analyses of microscopic qualities of coronary atherosclerosis in 760 teenagers and young adults who died as a result of accidents, suicide, and murder indicated that many had arteries so clogged that they could suffer a myocardial infarction.[146] Two percent of those ages 15 to 19 and 20% of those 30 to 34 had advanced plaque formation, the blockages considered most likely to break off and cause a heart attack or stroke. Collectively, the autopsy findings support the wisdom of primary prevention of atherosclerosis through risk factor identification *and* intervention early in childhood or adolescence.

Figure 31.23 shows the progressive occlusion of an artery from a buildup of calcified fatty substances in atherosclerosis. The first overt sign of atherosclerotic change occurs when lipid-laden macrophage cells cluster under the endothelial lining to form a bulge (fatty streak) in the

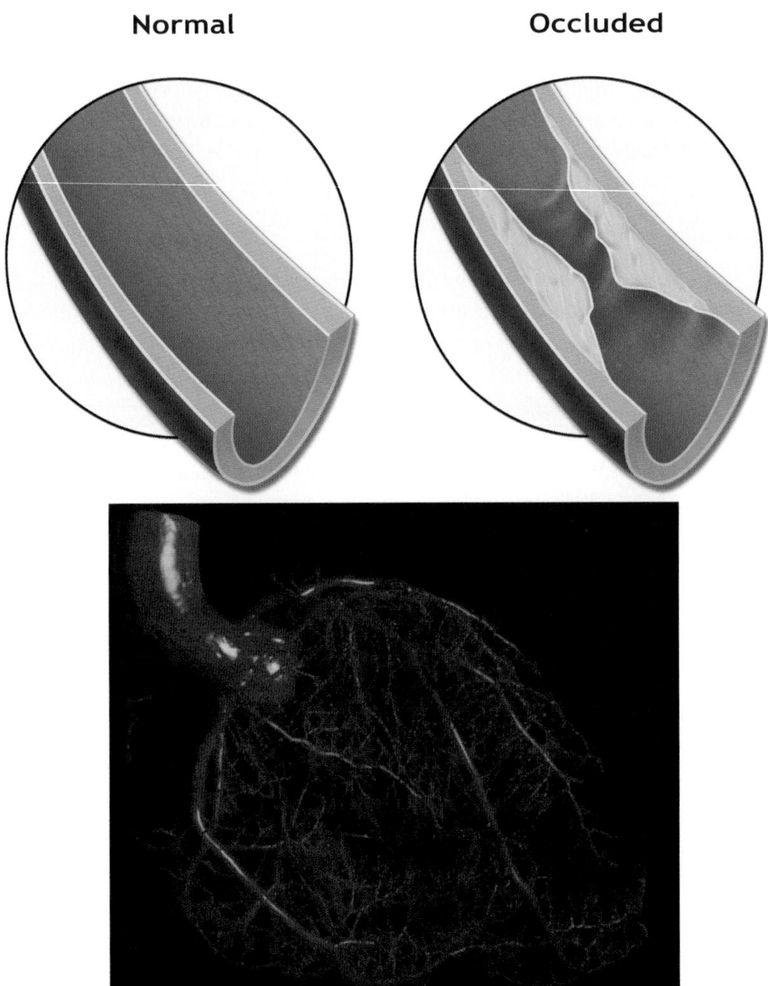

FIGURE 31.23 • *Top left,* Illustration of a cross section of a normal coronary artery. *Top right,* Deterioration of a coronary artery from deposits of fatty substances that roughen the vessel's center. Coronary artery occlusion evokes a myocardial infarction or heart attack. Inset shows cast of coronary artery vasculature.

artery. Over time, proliferating smooth muscle cells accumulate to narrow the lumen (center) of the artery. Typically, a clot (**thrombus**) forms and plugs the artery, depriving the myocardium of normal blood flow (oxygen supply). When the thrombus blocks one of the smaller coronary vessels, a portion of the heart muscle dies (necrosis) and the person suffers a heart attack or **myocardial infarction** (**MI**). MIs are caused by (1) blockage in one or more arteries supplying the heart, thus cutting off myocardial blood supply or (2) sudden spasms (constrictions) of a coronary vessel, causing tissue necrosis from lack of oxygen. MI contrasts with **cardiac arrest** caused by irregular neural–electrical transmission within the myocardium. Cardiac arrest results from chaotic, unregulated beating of the heart's upper chambers (atrial fibrillation) or lower chambers (ventricular fibrillation).

If coronary artery narrowing progresses to cause brief periods of inadequate myocardial perfusion, the person may experience temporary chest pains termed **angina pectoris** (see Chapter 32). These pains usually emerge during exertion because increased physical activity creates a great demand for myocardial blood flow. Anginal attacks provide painful, dramatic evidence of the importance of adequate myocardial oxygen supply.

INTEGRATIVE QUESTION

Design an experiment to evaluate the effects of (1) aerobic exercise training and (2) standard resistance exercise training on cardiovascular risk factors in middle-aged women. Indicate controls, measurement variables, and tests to show a training effect.

Cardiovascular Disease Epidemic

Each year, cardiovascular diseases top the list of the country's most serious health problems. Coronary heart disease is the leading health problem and the primary cause of death. It is also the most expensive condition to treat and resource-intensive chronic conditon. Consider these statistics released by the American Heart Association (AHA) in 2000:

- At least 58.8 million people (one person in four) in the United States suffer from some form of cardiovascular disease. This includes:
  - Hypertension—50,000,000
  - Coronary heart disease—12,000,000
  - Angina pectoris—6,200,000
  - Myocardial infarction—7,000,000
  - Stroke—4,400,000
  - Rheumatic heart disease/rheumatic fever—1,800,000
  - Congenital cardiovascular defects—1,000,000
  - Congestive heart failure—4,600,000
- Cardiovascular disease accounts for almost 1 of every 2.4 deaths.
- Since 1900, cardiovascular disease was the leading cause of death in every year but 1918, and it caused more deaths than the next seven causes combined.
- Every 29 seconds an American suffers a coronary event; each minute someone dies from one.
- A myth prevails that heart disease afflicts predominantly men. Cardiovascular diseases are also the number one killer of women, claiming the lives of more than half a million every year—more than the next 16 causes of death combined.
- No previous symptoms of the disease existed in 57% of men and 64% of women who died suddenly from cardiovascular disease.
- In 1999, cardiovascular disease cost an estimated $286.5 billion, an increase of approximately $12 billion over 1998.
- Stroke killed 159,942 people in 1996. On average, someone in the United States suffers a stroke every 53 seconds, and someone dies every 3.3 minutes.
- Stroke is a leading cause of serious, long-term disability that accounts for more than one-half of all patients hospitalized for a neurologic disease.

Despite these rather discouraging statistics, age-adjusted death rate from cardiovascular disease has decreased by approximately 60% since 1950—307.4 versus 134.6 per 100,000 people for heart disease and 88.8 versus 26.5 per 100,000 for stroke. Still, heart diseases account for approximately 32% of the total mortality in the United States.[36,37,226] Figure 31.24A shows the percentage distribution of the leading causes of death in the United States. Cardiovascular disease accounts for more than 1.5 million MIs and 90,000 strokes annually. Figure 31.24B illustrates the trend in cardiovascular disease (heart diseases and strokes) from 1900 to 1996, including heart disease death rate for men by age category from 1970 to 1996 (Fig. 31.24C). When a heart attack does strike, its severity has decreased over the past decade. A large portion of the decline in incidence and severity relates to risk factor reduction (e.g., 25% of adults smoking now vs. 42% 30 years ago, better pharmacologic control of blood pressure and cholesterol levels, improved exercise behaviors), more effective pharmacologic therapies, and more-intense treatment immediately after a heart attack. Survival rates can reach 96% for those who receive immediate hospital treatment.[72,94,185]

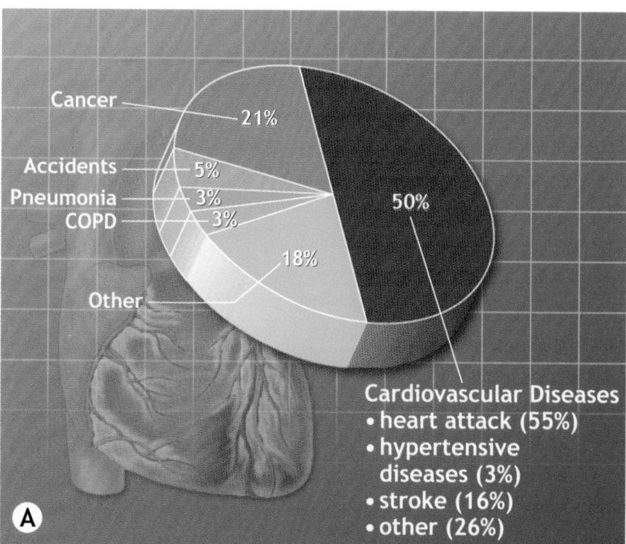

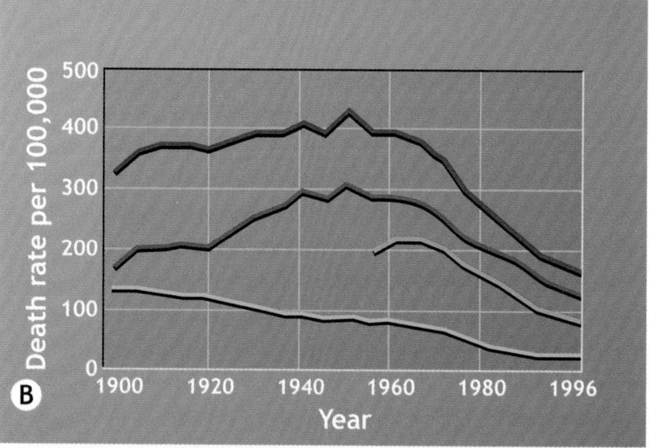

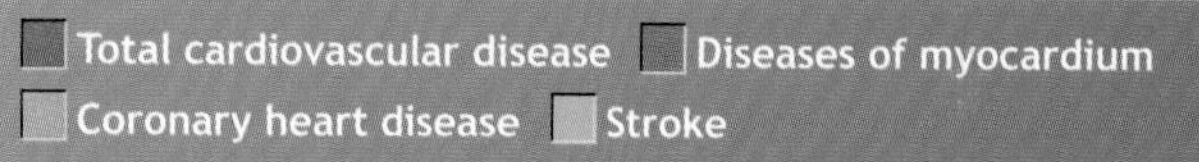

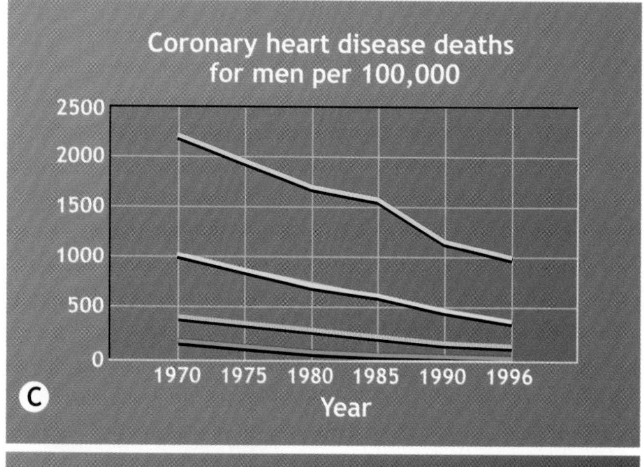

FIGURE 31.24 • **A**. Leading causes of death in the United States. **B**. Declining death rates from heart attacks and stroke per 100,000 between 1900 and 1990. **C**. Coronary heart disease deaths for men per 100,000 by age group between 1970 and 1996. (Data from National Center for Health Statistics and the American Heart Association.)

CORONARY HEART DISEASE RISK FACTORS

Research over the past 40 years has identified various personal characteristics, behaviors, and environmental factors linked to increased CHD susceptibility. Although many of these factors relate strongly to CHD risk, the associations do not necessarily imply a causal relationship (e.g., male-pattern baldness[132]). In some instances, it remains unclear whether risk-factor modification offers effective disease protection.

Until definite proof emerges, it seems prudent to assume that elimination or reduction of one or more of the modifiable risk factors reduces the likelihood of CHD and cumulative disability in later years. For example, a radical heart–risk-reduction program requiring a vegetarian diet that limits fat intake to no more than 10% of total calories and includes regular exercise, stress-management training, and support meetings significantly reduced subsequent heart attack rate and other adverse heart events (e.g., bypass operations and angioplasty procedures).[162] In contrast, patients in conventional care steadily worsened over the same 5-year period. The following lists contain the most frequently implicated **CHD risk factors**:[65,154,205]

Modifiable risk factors

- Diet
- Elevated blood lipid levels
- Hypertension
- Personality and behavior patterns
- Cigarette smoking
- High serum uric acid levels
- Sedentary lifestyle
- Pulmonary function abnormalities
- Excessive body fat
- Diabetes mellitus
- ECG abnormalities
- Tension and stress
- Poor education
- Elevated homocysteine levels

Nonmodifiable risk factors

- Age
- Gender
- Ethnic background
- Male-pattern baldness, particularly lack of hair on the crown of the head; possibly from raised androgen levels
- Family history

Determining the quantitative importance of any single CHD risk factor remains difficult because of the interrelationships among factors, such as blood lipid abnormalities, type 2 diabetes, heredity (gene polymorphism), and obesity.[24,232] For example, early risk factor studies showed that men living in Ireland consumed more saturated fatty acids than blood brothers in the United States, yet the former had a lower incidence of CHD.[224] The higher physical activity level of those living in Ireland was a major difference between groups and explained their lower CHD incidence. High physical activity also explained the low CHD incidence rates for Masai tribesmen of East Africa and farm laborers in Georgia, despite high dietary cholesterol and saturated fatty acid intakes.[145]

Age, Gender, and Heredity

Age represents a CHD risk factor largely because of its association with other risk factors like hypertension, elevated blood lipid levels, and glucose intolerance. Figure 31.25 shows that after age 35 in men and age 45 in women, the chances of dying from CHD increase progressively and dramatically.

At most ages, women show lower risk of death from heart disease than men. For example, a middle-aged man has

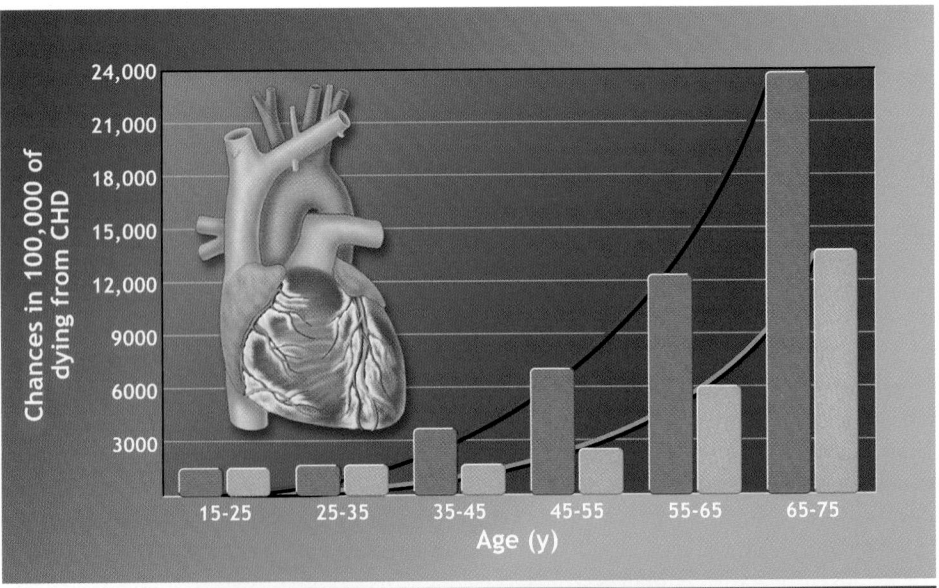

FIGURE 31.25 • Chances of a single individual dying from coronary heart disease (CHD).

a sixfold greater chance of dying from a heart attack than his female counterpart. Perhaps gender-related hormonal differences, including the greater ebb and flow of estrogen levels in women, provide CHD protection.[26,40,81] Despite their gender advantage, heart disease occurs more frequently in American women than in women of other countries. Women also have more lethal and severe first-time heart attacks and suffer a 70 to 100% greater risk of dying within months of a first heart attack than men, particularly women under age 50 (approximately 6% of all heart attacks in women).[85,141,227] Specifically, 17% of women who suffer heart attacks die while still in the hospital, compared with 12% of men. Gender differences in quality of care received may play a role in the poorer survival rate of women who do suffer an MI. The good news is that current trends in smoking reduction, diet improvement, and an increase in postmenopausal hormone use largely account for the current decline in coronary disease in middle-aged women.[89]

Heart attacks that strike at an early age tend to run in families. Familial predisposition probably relates to a genetic role in determining risk of heart disease. In the following sections we examine blood lipid abnormalities, obesity, cigarette smoking, and physical inactivity in relation to CHD (Chapters 15 and 32 discuss hypertension). These modifiable factors represent the "big five" heart disease risks proposed by the American Heart Association. Each exists as a potent, independent CHD risk that can change considerably with lifestyle modification.

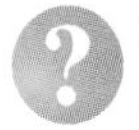

INTEGRATIVE QUESTION

Why doesn't risk factor modification always change disease risk?

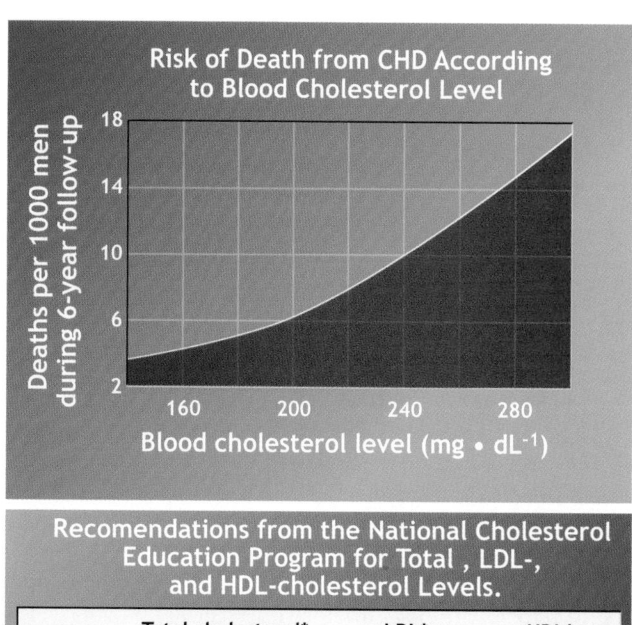

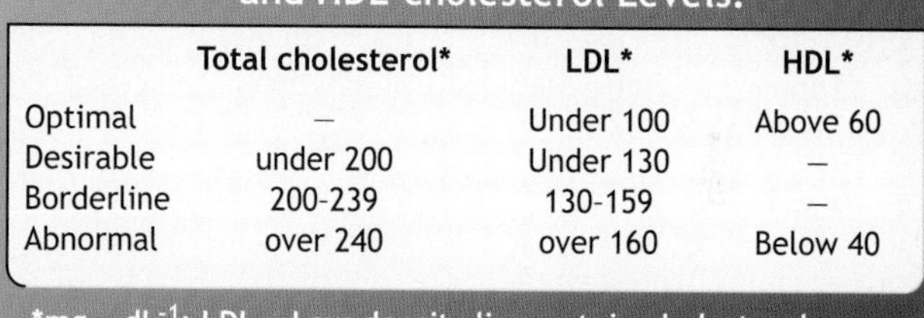

Recomendations from the National Cholesterol Education Program for Total , LDL-, and HDL-cholesterol Levels.

	Total cholesterol*	LDL*	HDL*
Optimal	–	Under 100	Above 60
Desirable	under 200	Under 130	–
Borderline	200-239	130-159	–
Abnormal	over 240	over 160	Below 40

*mg • dL^{-1}; LDL = Low-density lipoprotein cholesterol HDL = High-density lipoprotein cholesterol

FIGURE 31.26 • Death risk from coronary heart disease (CHD) in relation to total serum cholesterol level in 361,662 men ages 35 to 57 years. The *inset table* presents serum cholesterol and lipoprotein level classifications for adults. (Figure adapted from Martin MJ, et al. Serum cholesterol, blood pressure and mortality: implications from a cohort of 361,662 men. Lancet 1986;2:933; Table modified from Lauer MS, Fontanrosa PB. Updated guidelines of cholesterol management. JAMA 2001;285:2508.)

Blood Lipid Abnormalities

Serum cholesterol levels in adults have declined substantially in the United States over the past 35 years, a decline that coincides with a decreased national incidence of CHD. Despite this support for the effectiveness of public health programs geared to lowering heart disease risks, approximately 30% of adults still require intervention for high cholesterol levels.[100]

An abnormal blood lipid level or **hyperlipidemia** is a crucial component in the genesis of atherosclerosis. Figure 31.26 shows the rate of increase in death risk from CHD related to total serum cholesterol. The *inset table* presents serum cholesterol and lipoprotein level classifications for adults. Current guidelines focus less on total cholesterol and more on its lipoprotein components. Adherence to the guidelines will nearly triple the number of adults taking cholesterol-lowering drugs to 36 million Americans and raise by 25% the number who should be on a cholesterol-lowering diet.[118] Early treatment becomes crucial because of a strong association between high serum cholesterol as a young adult and cardiovascular disease in middle age. A cholesterol level of 200 mg · dL^{-1} or lower is usually desirable, although risk for a fatal heart attack begins to rise at 150 mg · dL^{-1}. A cholesterol level of 230 mg · dL^{-1} increases heart attack risk to about twice that of 180 mg · dL^{-1}, and 300 mg · dL^{-1} increases the risk fourfold. For triglycerides, the National Cholesterol Education Program considers 200 mg · dL^{-1} an upper-limit normal triglyceride level, with 200 to 400 mg considered borderline, requiring changes in exercise, diet, and possibly drug treatment if accompanied by other CHD risk factors. *More than likely, triglyceride levels above 100 mg · dL^{-1} pose a cardiac risk.* Individuals with triglyceride levels above 100 mg · dL^{-1} (after 12-h fast) show a 50% greater CHD risk than those with triglycerides below 100 mg · dL^{-1}, even after controlling for HDL-C.[149]

Major clinical drug trials have shown conclusively that reducing cholesterol lowers death rates and prevents heart attacks. Medications that affect blood lipids include (1) bile acid sequestrants (e.g., cholestyramine resin and colestipol hydrochloride), which bind bile acids and stimulate conversion of cholesterol to bile acids and facilitate removal of cholesterol from serum; (2) fibric acid derivatives (e.g., gemfibrozil, probucol, clofibrate), which lower triglycerides and LDL-C (5–20%) and elevate HDL-C (average 6% per year); and (3) the remarkably effective statins (e.g., lovastatin, pravastatin, simvastatin, atorvastatin), which inhibit an enzyme that controls cholesterol synthesis by the cell, increase LDL-C receptors in the liver, and facilitate LDL-C removal from serum (18–55% reduction).

TABLE 31.6 ➤ APPROXIMATE COMPOSITION OF SERUM LIPOPROTEINS

	CHYLOMICRONS	VERY-LOW-DENSITY LIPOPROTEINS (VLDL: PREBETA)	LOW-DENSITY LIPOPROTEINS (LDL: BETA)	HIGH-DENSITY LIPOPROTEINS (HDL: ALPHA)
Density (g · cm^{-3})	0.95	0.95–1.006	1.006–1.019	1.063–1.210
Protein (%)	0.5–1.0	5–15	25	45–55
Lipid (%)	99	95	75	50
Cholesterol (%)	2–5	10–20	40–45	18
Triglyceride (%)	85	50–70	5–10	2
Phospholipid (%)	3–6	10–20	20–25	30

Raising HDL-C by ≥34 mg · dL^{-1} via a 5-year gemfibrozil therapy trial reduced heart attacks, strokes, and death by 24% in patients with initially low HDL-C levels.[23]

Lipids do not circulate freely in blood plasma; they combine with a carrier protein to form lipoproteins composed of a hydrophobic cholesterol core and a coat of free cholesterol, phospholipid, and a regulatory protein (**apolipoprotein** [**Apo**]). Table 31.6 lists the four different lipoproteins, their approximate gravitational densities, and percentage composition in the blood. *Serum cholesterol is a composite of the total cholesterol contained in each of the different lipoproteins.* Although discussions commonly refer to hyperlipidemia, the more meaningful focus addresses the different types of **hyperlipoproteinemia**.

Cholesterol distribution among the various lipoproteins is a more powerful predictor of heart disease risk than total blood cholesterol (Fig. 31.27). Specifically, elevated HDL-C levels relate causally with a lower heart disease risk, even among individuals with total cholesterol below 200 mg · dL^{-1}. Overwhelming evidence links high LDL-C and apolipoprotein (B) levels with increased CHD risk.[116] A more effective evaluation of heart disease risk than either total cholesterol or LDL-C levels divides total cholesterol by HDL-C. *A ratio greater than 4.5 indicates high heart-disease risk; a ratio of 3.5 or lower represents a more desirable risk level.*

LDL-C (synthesized in the liver) and very-low-density lipoprotein cholesterol (VLDL-C) provide the means to transport fats to cells, including the smooth muscle walls of arteries. Upon oxidation, LDL-C participates in artery-clogging, plaque-forming atherosclerosis by stimulating monocyte–macrophage infiltration and lipoprotein deposition.[209] LDL-C's surface coat contains the specific apolipoprotein (Apo B) that facilitates cholesterol removal from the LDL-C molecule by binding to LDL-C receptors of specific cells. Prevention of LDL-C oxidation, on the other hand, slows the progression of CHD. In this regard, the potential benefit of dietary antioxidants such as vitamins C and E and β-carotene on heart-disease risk may lie in their ability to blunt the oxidation of LDL-C (see Chapter 2).[47,79,112,129]

Whereas LDL-C becomes targeted for peripheral tissue and contributes to arterial damage, HDL-C (also produced in the liver and whose levels significantly relate to genetic factors[99]) facilitates **reverse cholesterol transport**. HDL-C promotes surplus cholesterol removal from peripheral tissues (including arterial walls) for transport to the liver for bile synthesis and subsequent excretion via the digestive tract. The apolipoprotein A-1 (Apo A-1) in HDL-C activates the

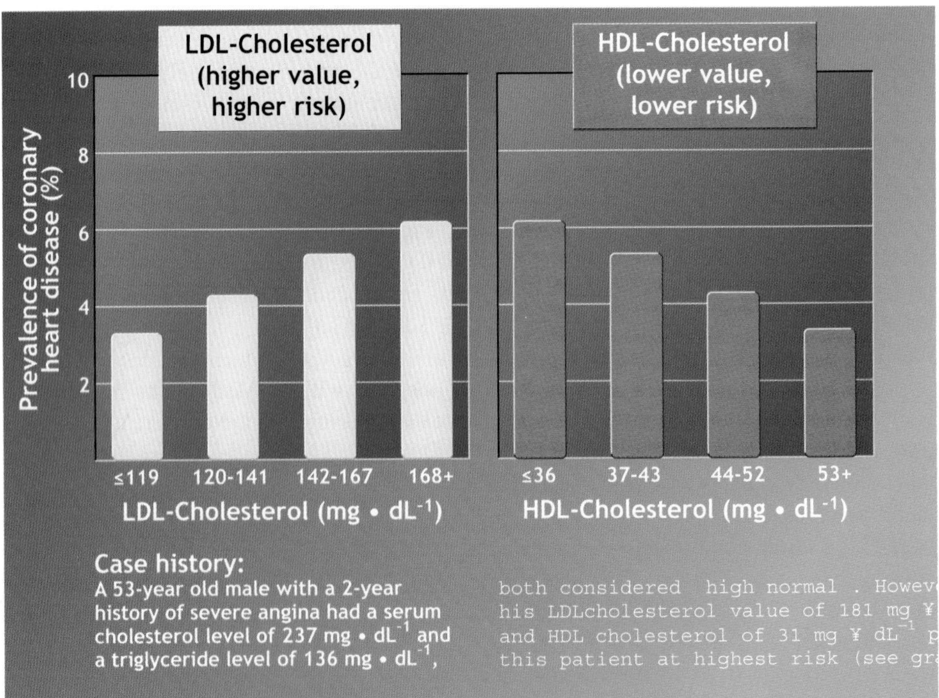

FIGURE 31.27 • Coronary heart disease (CHD) prevalence in relation to levels of low-density lipoprotein cholesterol (LDL-C) and high-density lipoprotein cholesterol (HDL-C). Risk increases directly with increases in LDL-C; conversely, a lower CHD risk accompanies a rise in HDL-C.

enzyme **lecithin acetyl transferase (LCAT)**, which converts free cholesterol into cholesterol esters, thus facilitating removal of cholesterol from lipoproteins and diverse tissues.[163]

Exercise Effects

SHORT-TERM EFFECTS. Reaching the threshold that changes blood lipid and lipoprotein levels in a single exercise session requires considerable physical activity. For example, healthy trained men needed to expend 1100 kcal in one bout of exercise to elevate HDL-C, 1300 kcal of exercise to lower LDL-C, and 800 kcal of exercise to decrease triglyceride levels.[58]

LONG-TERM EFFECTS. A single exercise session produces only transient favorable changes in lipid and apolipoprotein concentrations, yet the change persists with exercising at least every other day.[42]

LDL-C. Exercising regularly usually produces only small reductions in LDL-C level when controlling for serum cholesterol-related factors such as body fat and dietary lipid and cholesterol intake. However, regular exercise may improve the quality of this circulating lipoprotein by promoting a less-oxidized form of LDL-C, thus reducing atherosclerosis risk.[231] In addition, regular aerobic exercise increases the success of dietary efforts to favorably alter high-risk lipoprotein profiles.[207]

HDL-C. Endurance athletes usually maintain relatively high HDL-C levels, and favorable alterations occur for sedentary men and women of all ages who engage in regular moderate-to-vigorous aerobic exercise.[49,51,243] To some extent, exercise intensity and duration exert independent effects in modifying specific CHD risk factors. In general, exercise duration exerts the greatest effect on HDL-C, while exercise intensity most favorably modifies blood pressure and waist girth.[244] In most cases, a favorable change in lipoprotein profile does not require the exercise intensity needed to improve cardiovascular fitness. With perhaps the exception of triglycerides, exercise-induced lipid alterations usually progress independent of body weight changes.[120] For overweight individuals, however, the typical increase in HDL-C with exercise training is diminished without concomitant weight loss.[157,216] Favorable exercise-related lipoprotein changes probably result from enhanced triglyceride clearance from plasma in response to exercise.[190,221]

Protection from Gallstones. The benefits of regular aerobic exercise on modifying cholesterol and lipoprotein profiles extend to protect against painful gallstones and accompanying gallbladder removal, the usual treatment for 500,000 Americans yearly, of whom two-thirds are women. The National Institutes of Health reports that gallstone formation and its consequences are the most common and costly (yearly cost >$5 billion) digestive disease requiring hospitalization and surgery. Overall, women who exercised 30 minutes daily reduced their need for gallbladder surgery by 31%.[124] Physical activity increases the movement of the large intestine and improves blood glucose and insulin regulation; both factors can reduce gallstone risk. Regular exercise may also reduce the cholesterol content of bile, the digestive juice stored in the gallbladder. Eight percent of gallstones are solid cholesterol.

Other Influences

Even trained endurance athletes exhibit considerable variability in HDL-C levels, with some elite runners' values approaching the median value for the general population. Moreover, no single factor—nutrition, body composition, or training status—distinguishes runners with high HDL-C values from those with lower values. This suggests that genetic factors exert a strong influence on the blood lipid profile. In fact, a specific gene produces endothelial lipase (EL), an enzyme that may affect HDL-C production.[99] Excessive activity (turning on) of this gene increases EL synthesis, which might lower HDL-C and increase cardiovascular risk.

Standard resistance training exerts little or no effect on serum levels of triglyceride, cholesterol, or lipoproteins. From a dietary perspective, substituting soy-derived protein for protein from animal sources improves the cholesterol and lipoprotein profile, particularly in persons with high blood cholesterol.[10] A moderate daily alcohol intake—2 oz or 30 mL of 90-proof alcohol, three 6-oz glasses of wine, or slightly less than three 12-oz beers—reduces an otherwise healthy person's risk of heart attack and stroke, independent of physical activity level.[188,243] The heart-protective benefit of alcohol consumption also applies to individuals with type 2 diabetes.[228] Although the mechanism for benefit remains elusive, a moderate alcohol intake increases HDL-C and its subfractions, particularly HDL_2 and HDL_3.[71] In addition, certain components of red wine (e.g., polyphenols) may inhibit LDL-C oxidation, thus blunting a critical step in plaque formation.[158,183] Moderate wine intake also tends to associate with more heart-healthy dietary choices with a positive impact on plasma lipids.[218] Excessive alcohol consumption offers no lipoprotein benefit and increases liver disease and cancer risk.[68]

LIPOPROTEIN(A). **Lipoprotein(a) [Lp(a)]** represents a diverse class of protein particles formed in the liver when two distinct apolipoproteins unite. Lp(a) structurally resembles LDL-C but contains an additional unique apolipoprotein(a) coat. Heredity determines elevated Lp(a) levels, which occur in approximately 20% of the population. When elevated above 25 to 30 mg · dL^{-1} and in conjunction with raised LDL-C levels, the independent risk for atherosclerosis, thrombosis, and acute MI increases significantly.[17,193] Dietary changes and either short- or long-term exercise exert little or no effect on serum Lp(a) concentrations.[78,92,93,136]

Dietary Fiber, Insulin, and CHD Risk. Insulin resistance and associated hyperinsulinemia relate to CHD risk factors of age, obesity, central body fat distribution, smoking, physical inactivity, hypertension, dyslipidemia, and abnormalities in blood-clotting factors. Consequently, many researchers and clinicians now consider insulin resistance and consequent hyperinsulinemia to be independent CHD risk factors.[187]

The combined effects of established CHD risk factors account for approximately 50% of the observed variability in insulin resistance and hyperinsulinemia within the population. The question then is what other factors might contribute to excessive insulin output and, by implication, increased CHD risk. Perhaps total lipid or saturated fatty acid intake and dietary carbohydrates are possible causal factors. In addition, dietary fiber may play a key role in optimizing insulin response.[133] For example, dietary fiber reduces insulin secretion by slowing the rate of nutrient digestion and glucose absorption following a meal. Moreover, because of its inherently high glycemic index, a low-fiber meal tends to stimulate relatively more insulin secretion than a high-fiber meal of equivalent carbohydrate content. Thus, dietary fiber can serve a dual role in heart-disease prevention: (1) attenuating the insulin response to a meal containing carbohydrate and (2) reducing the tendency to accumulate body fat, because of insulin's facilitatory role in fat synthesis. Excessive body fat increases insulin resistance, which ultimately leads to hyperinsulinemia. High circulating insulin levels, in turn, may also cause hypertension, dyslipidemia, abnormalities in blood clotting factors, and perhaps direct vascular injury.

IMMUNOLOGIC FACTORS. An immune response may trigger plaque development within arterial walls. During this process, mononuclear immune cells produce proteins called *cytokines,* some of which stimulate plaque buildup while others inhibit plaque formation. Within this framework, regular exercise may stimulate the immune system to inhibit agents that facilitate arterial disease. For example, 2.5 hours of weekly exercise for 6 months produced a 58% decrease in the production of cytokines that aid in plaque development, while cytokines that inhibit plaque formation increased by nearly 36%.[200] A fruitful line of research should pursue whether regular exercise stimulates the immune system in a way that inhibits infectious agents from initiating arterial disease.

Beyond Cholesterol: Homocysteine and Coronary Heart Disease

In 1969 an autopsy of an 8-year-old boy who died of a stroke revealed that his arteries had the sclerotic look of blood vessels of an elderly man with CHD. His blood also contained excess levels of the amino acid **homocysteine**. This rare genetic error of metabolism, homocystinuria, causes homocysteine levels to increase to hundreds of micromoles (μmol) and produce premature hardening of the arteries and early death from heart attack or stroke. In subsequent years, numerous studies have shown a nearly lockstep association between plasma homocysteine levels and heart attack and mortality in men and women.[54,182,235] In the presence of other conventional CHD risks (e.g., smoking and hypertension) synergistic effects magnify the negative impact of homocysteine on cardiovascular health.[137,247]

All individuals produce homocysteine, a sulfur-containing intermediary product in the metabolism of the essential amino acid methionine. Normally, excess methionine converts to homocysteine, which then converts to cysteine and eventually degrades and voids in the urine. Homocysteine can also recycle back to methionine. Three B vitamins—folic acid, B_6, and B_{12}— facilitate enzymes that affect these interconversions. If the conversion slows because of a genetic defect or vitamin insufficiency, homocysteine levels increase and promote cholesterol's damaging effects on the arterial lumen. Mild-to-moderately elevated plasma homocysteine levels possibly produce damaging effects in the following manner:[155,156,239]

- Injuring vascular endothelium and stimulating growth of smooth muscle cells
- Initiating platelet activation and thrombus formation and possibly coronary artery spasm
- Modifying adhesive properties of the endothelium
- Impairing the vascular responsiveness to L-arginine, the natural precursor of nitric oxide

Figure 31.28 proposes a mechanism for homocysteine's negative impact on cardiovascular health. The homocysteine model helps explain why some people with low-to-normal cholesterol levels contract heart disease.

Hyperhomocysteinemia is a metabolic abnormality present in nearly 30% of CHD patients and 40% of patients with cerebrovascular disease. Excessive homocysteine causes blood platelets to clump, fostering blood clots and deterioration of smooth muscle cells that line the arterial wall. Chronic homocysteine exposure eventually scars and thickens arteries and provides a fertile medium for circulating LDL-C to initiate cell damage. Figure 31.28C gives the relative risk for vascular disease in groups defined by the presence or absence of classic risk factors and elevated plasma homocysteine levels adjusted for age, gender, and research center. Nineteen centers in nine European countries evaluated vascular disease risk associated with increased homocysteine levels. The researchers also quantified the interactive effects among elevated homocysteine and conventional CHD risk factors in women and men younger than age 60, representing 750 cases of atherosclerotic vascular disease and 800 healthy controls. Resting homocysteine levels exerted a significant independent increased risk (on a continuum) for vascular disease similar to that of smoking and hyperlipidemia. A powerful multiplicative interaction effect also emerged in the presence of other risks, particularly cigarette smoking and hypertension. In general, people in the highest quartile for homocysteine levels have nearly twice the risk of heart attack or stroke compared with those in the lowest quartile. Why some people accumulate homocysteine is uncertain, but the evidence points to a deficiency of B vitamins (B_6, B_{12}, and particularly folic acid); lifestyle factors such as cigarette smoking and coffee and high meat intake also associate with elevated homocysteine concentrations.[138,160,161,211]

DISEASES AND DISORDERS LINKED TO ELEVATED PLASMA HOMOCYSTEINE LEVELS

- Heart attack
- Stroke
- Dementia from Alzheimer's disease
- Blood clots in veins (venous thrombosis)
- Osteoporosis
- Recurrent early miscarriage
- Birth defects
- Premature delivery and abnormally low birth weight

No clear standard currently exists for normal or desirable homocysteine levels, although most evidence indicates that the current "normal range" of 8 to 20 μmol per liter of plasma is too high. In fact, evidence suggests as little as 12 μmol can double heart disease risk. Research must also determine whether normalizing homocysteine actually reduces risk of arterial occlusive disease precipitating heart attack and stroke. Otherwise, the debate will continue regarding whether an elevated homocysteine level is simply a CHD risk factor or is an actual cause (not an effect) of CHD.[64,143,159] Nevertheless, sufficient data currently support consuming adequate B vitamins.[29] The dietary intake of folic acid required to lower homocysteine levels remains controversial; some estimates are as high as 400 μg daily as an effective yet safe dosage.[138,208] Even small amounts of this vitamin—plentiful in enriched whole-grain cereals; nuts and seeds; dark green, leafy vegetables; beans and peas; and orange juice—lower homocysteine levels. In 1999, folic acid fortified all white flour, breads,

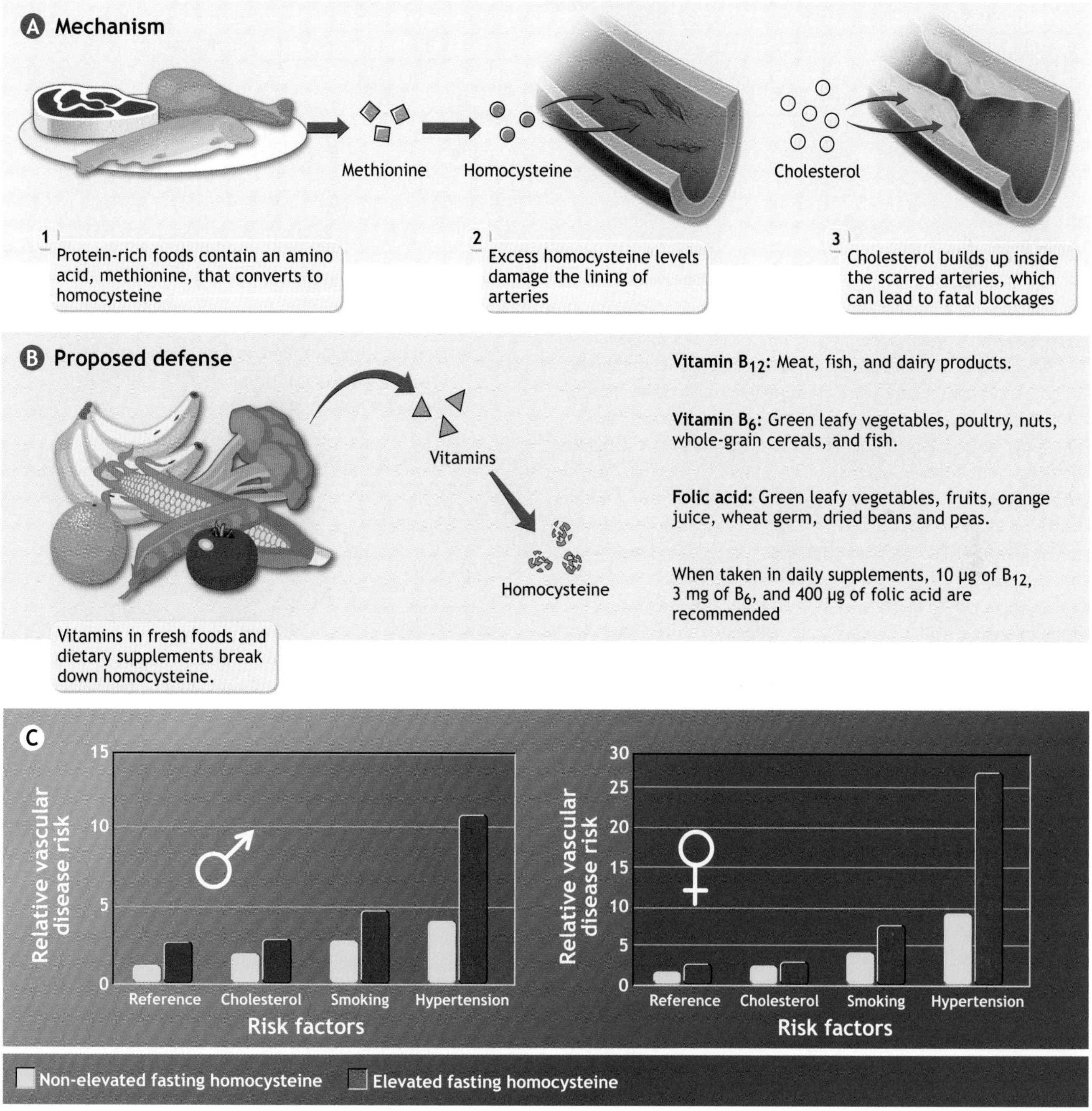

A Mechanism

Methionine

Homocysteine

Cholesterol

1 Protein-rich foods contain an amino acid, methionine, that converts to homocysteine

2 Excess homocysteine levels damage the lining of arteries

3 Cholesterol builds up inside the scarred arteries, which can lead to fatal blockages

B Proposed defense

Vitamins

Homocysteine

Vitamins in fresh foods and dietary supplements break down homocysteine.

Vitamin B_{12}: Meat, fish, and dairy products.

Vitamin B_6: Green leafy vegetables, poultry, nuts, whole-grain cereals, and fish.

Folic acid: Green leafy vegetables, fruits, orange juice, wheat germ, dried beans and peas.

When taken in daily supplements, 10 µg of B_{12}, 3 mg of B_6, and 400 µg of folic acid are recommended

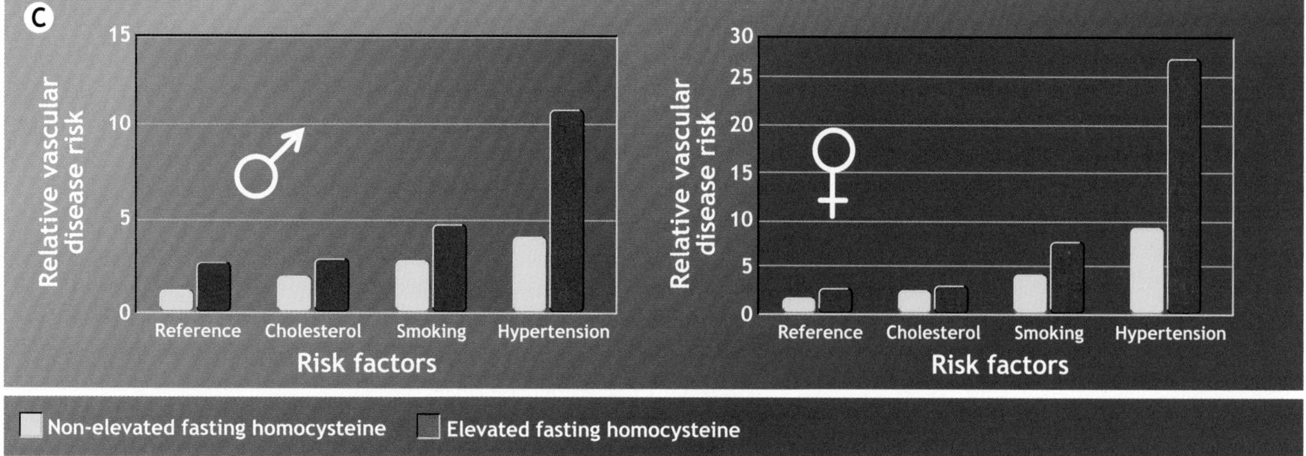

FIGURE 31.28 • **A**. Proposed mechanism for how the amino acid homocysteine damages the lining of arteries and sets the stage for cholesterol infiltration into a vessel. **B**. Proposed defense against the possible harmful effects of elevated homocysteine levels. **C**. Relative risk of all vascular diseases for men and women defined by the presence of classic risk factors with and without elevated plasma total homocysteine levels adjusted for age, gender, and research center. (Graphs from Graham IM, et al. Plasma homocysteine as a risk factor for vascular disease: The European Concerted Action Project. JAMA 1997;277:1775.)

pasta, grits, white rice, and cornmeal. Between 180 and 200 μg is the current RDA for folic acid; 400 μg is probably a better dietary target. *Researchers know little about the effects of regular exercise on homocysteine regulation.*

Excessive Body Fat

Excess body fat has received great notoriety as a CHD risk factor, but its relationship is often codependent with such other risks as hypertension, elevated cholesterol level, type 2 diabetes, and cigarette smoking. The number of annual deaths attributable to overfatness in the U.S. adult population ranges between 262,541 and 383,410.[7] Weight loss and accompanying body fat reduction, whether through diet or exercise, usually normalize cholesterol and triglyceride levels and exert beneficial effects on blood pressure and type 2 diabetes.[91,248] Chapter 30 presents evidence that justifies including excessive body fat as a primary heart disease risk factor contributing to various other diseases.

Cigarette Smoking

Cigarette smoking, either active or passive through environmental exposure, provides one of the strongest indicators of CHD risk; the magnitude of risk directly relates to the number of cigarettes smoked daily. Smokers experience twice the risk of death from heart disease as nonsmokers.[127] The risk increases further for smokers with diabetes and hypertension.[88] The Centers for Disease Control and Prevention estimates that every cigarette smoked steals 7 minutes from a smoker's life. This adds up to 5 million years of potential life Americans lose to cigarettes each year. CHD risk increases the more one smokes (or receives passive exposure[80]), the deeper one inhales, and the stronger the cigarette in terms of tars and noxious by-products. The increasing death rate from heart disease among women in the United States almost parallels their increased cigarette use.[242] British researchers estimate that smokers in their 30s and 40s suffer five times as many heart attacks as nonsmokers in the same age range.[167] When these relatively young smokers suffer a heart attack, an 80% chance exists that smoking caused it; this percentage averages nearly 70% for those in their 50s, and 50% for smokers in their 60s and 70s. Also, smokers run a five times greater risk for stroke than nonsmokers—and those who smoke one pack or more each day are 11 times more likely to suffer a specific type of sudden, deadly stroke most common in younger men and women. Surprisingly, the CHD risk from smoking associates with more deaths than the excess mortality of cigarette smokers from lung cancer; and more bad news, the risk of erectile dysfunction is significantly higher among smokers than among nonsmokers.

Smoking risk usually remains independent of other risk factors. If additional risk factors exist, then smoking accentuates their influence. Cigarette smoking facilitates heart disease through its potentiating effect on serum lipoproteins; individuals who smoke have lower levels of HDL-C than nonsmokers. However, when smoking stops, the HDL-C and heart disease risk return to levels of nonsmokers. *A frightening statistic indicates that within 25 years, smoking will become the world's single leading cause of death and disability.*

Physical Activity

Prospective research studies show clearly that regular physical activity protects against heart disease.[18,153,168,217] Sedentary men and women are approximately twice as likely to suffer a fatal heart attack as their more physically active counterparts. Maintenance of aerobic fitness (independent of actual activity level) throughout life also provides significant protection against CHD risk factors and disease occurrence.[1,82] One could argue that genetic factors contribute significantly more to fitness level than to daily exercise patterns. However, because fitness level relates closely to individual differences in physical activity level among most individuals, regular exercise may assume greater importance than genetics in determining physical fitness and related health benefits. Table 31.7 summarizes possible biologic mechanisms for how regular aerobic exercise protects against CHD.

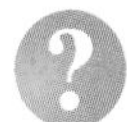

INTEGRATIVE QUESTION

If regular physical activity contributes little to extending life span, what other reasons make sense for maintaining a physically active lifestyle throughout middle and older age?

TABLE 31.7 ➤ POSSIBLE MECHANISMS FOR BENEFICIAL EFFECTS OF REGULAR AEROBIC EXERCISE ON RISK OF CORONARY HEART DISEASE AND MORTALITY

- Improves myocardial circulation and metabolism to protect the heart from hypoxic stress. Improvements include enhanced vascularization and increased coronary blood flow capacity via altered control of coronary vascular smooth muscle, and increased reactivity of coronary resistance vessels. Modest increases in cardiac glycogen stores and glycolytic capacity also prove beneficial if the heart's oxygen supply suddenly becomes compromised.
- Enhances the mechanical properties of the myocardium to enable the exercise-trained heart to maintain or increase contractility during a specific challenge.
- Establishes more-favorable blood-clotting characteristics and other hemostatic mechanisms, including increased fibrinolysis and production of endothelial prostacyclin.
- Normalizes the blood lipid profile to slow or even reverse atherosclerosis.
- Favorably alters heart rate and blood pressure so myocardial work significantly decreases during rest and exercise.
- Suppresses age-related body weight gain and promotes a more desirable body composition and body fat distribution, particularly a reduced level of intra-abdominal adipose tissue.
- Establishes a more favorable neural–hormonal balance to conserve oxygen for the myocardium; improves the mixture of carbohydrate and fat metabolized by the body.
- Provides a favorable outlet for psychologic stress and tension.

Focus on Research

Physical Inactivity: A Significant Coronary Heart Disease Risk

Morris JN, et al. Coronary heart disease and physical activity of work. Lancet 1953;265:1053.

➤ Epidemiologists of the1940s and 1950s did not consider regular exercise a means of protecting against early development of coronary heart disease (CHD). Morris and colleagues demonstrated an impressive link between physical activity in specialized occupations and reduced CHD risk. The researchers compiled statistics on CHD incidence for two groups of workers. One group consisted of 31,000 men aged 35 to 64 years employed by the London Transport Authority. Job classifications included *drivers* and *conductors* of trams and trolley buses and *motormen* and *guards* on the underground railway system. Drivers and motormen classified as sedentary, while a conductor represented a more physically demanding occupation (e.g., walking through a double-decker bus collecting tickets). The second work group consisted of 110,000 *postal workers* and *civil servants*. Physical activity level composed the basic differences between these workers in job requirements: postmen maintained a moderate physical activity level walking delivering mail, while civil servants (postal and telegraph officers, telephone operators, clerks) remained sedentary in office jobs.

The figure shows the CHD incidence (rate per 1000 per age group, determined from medical records) for the first clinical episode of CHD—angina pectoris, myocardial infarction, or death directly attributable to CHD. The London Transport workers exhibited 119 total CHD episodes (3.8% per 1000). In one-quarter of these episodes death occurred within 3 days (34 of 119 cases); in 40%, death ensued within 3 months (49 of 119 cases). Nonetheless, the pattern of CHD incidence differed between conductors and drivers. Drivers contracted the disease at a younger age and had a higher incidence (2.7 vs. 1.9) than conductors; also, drivers showed a rate of immediate mortality twice that of conductors. In contrast, angina occurred twice as frequently in the conductors (0.8 vs. 0.4 per 1000). Overall, conductors exhibited less CHD than drivers, and the disease appeared at a later age. Like the transport workers, the physically active postmen averaged a substantially lower total incidence of CHD and mortality than the sedentary clerks. The physically active group experienced significantly less CHD; when disease did occur, it remained less severe.

Morris offered three possible explanations for the findings:

1. Differences in constitution (e.g., CHD susceptibility) affected existing health status, causing the men to self-select a job category based on its physical requirements.
2. Differences in mental strains from a specific job affected the progression of CHD.
3. Differences in job-related physical activity *caused* group differences in CHD incidence.

While all three explanations seemed plausible, the researchers suggested that differences in on-the-job physical effort provided protection against CHD. Nearly 50 years of subsequent cross-sectional and longitudinal research confirms that increased physical activity confers a protective effect against CHD.

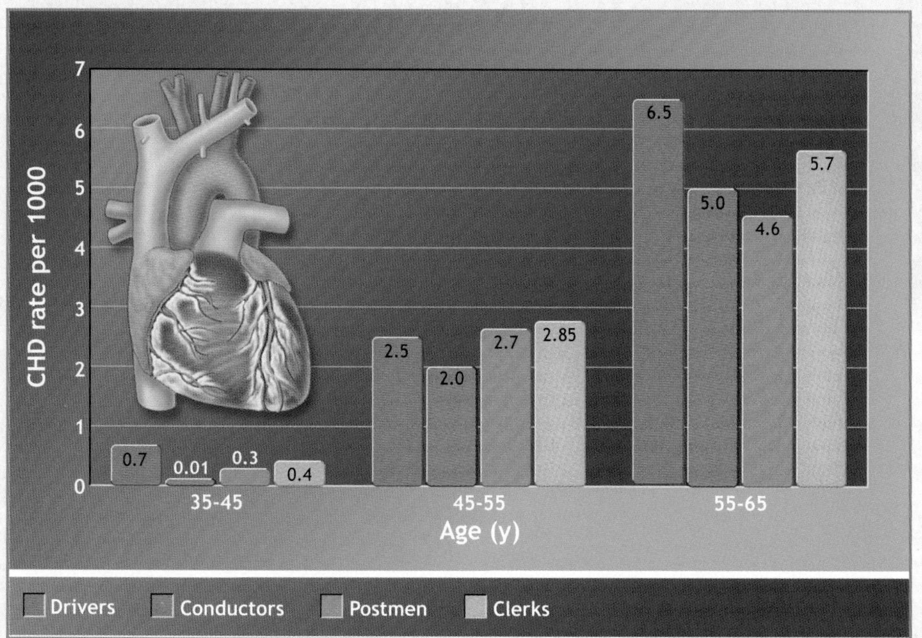

Coronary heart disease (CHD) incidence per 1000 persons for drivers, conductors, postmen, and clerks. Note that within each age and job classification, the most-active workers (conductors and postmen) exhibit the lowest CHD incidence.

CHD Risk Factor Interactions

Many risk factors interact with each other and with CHD.[106] Figure 31.29 shows that the presence of three primary CHD risk factors in the same person magnifies their individual effects. With one risk factor, a 45-year-old man's chance of CHD during the year averages twice the risk for a man without risk factors. With three risk factors present, this man's chance for angina, heart attack, or sudden death increases to five times the level for those with no risk factors.

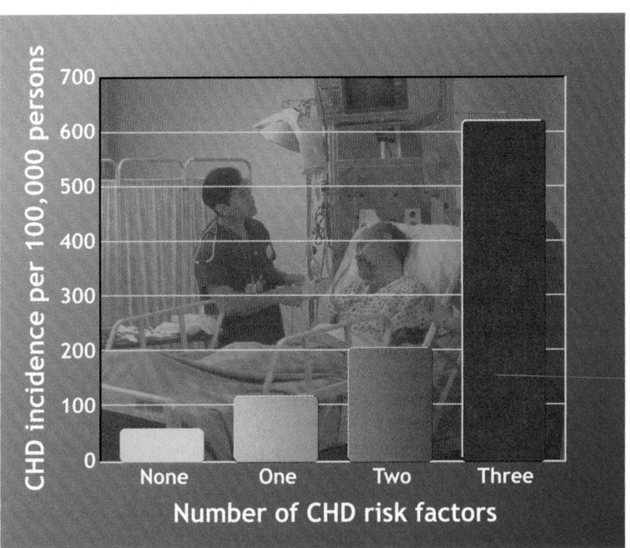

FIGURE 31.29 • General relation between a combination of abnormal risk factors (cholesterol ≥250 mg · dL^{-1}; systolic blood pressure ≥160 mm Hg; smoking ≥1 pack of cigarettes per day) and incidence of coronary heart disease (CHD).

Many CHD risks link in common to behavioral patterns; they become influenced by similar and, in some cases, identical interventions. For example, regular exercise participation exerts a positive influence on obesity, hypertension, type 2 diabetes, stress, and an elevated blood lipid profile. Surprisingly, no other modifiable behavior exerts such a potent positive effect for the greatest number of people, causing many to argue that regular physical activity constitutes the most important behavioral intervention to reduce CHD.

Risk Factors in Children

The frequent occurrence of multiple CHD risk factors in young children emphasizes the need for early CHD initiatives to reduce risk of atherosclerosis later in life.[46,245] Table 31.8 shows that obesity and a family history of heart disease are the two most common risk factors in physically active and apparently healthy boys and girls. A relatively large percentage of these children also showed abnormally high blood lipid concentrations. Of the total group, 65% had one or two risk factors, and 31% had three or more.

As with adults, the association between body fat and serum lipid levels becomes readily apparent in overfat children; the fattest children usually have the highest levels of serum cholesterol and triglycerides. For these children, both general adiposity and visceral adipose tissue also relate to unfavorable hemostatic factors that increase CHD morbidity and mortality in adulthood.[59] Of 62 overfat children aged 10 to 15 years, only one child had just one CHD risk factor.[15] Of the remaining children, 14% had two risk factors, 30% three, 29% four, 18% had five, and the remaining five children (8%) had six. A subsample of these children then enrolled in a 20-week program to evaluate the effects on the risk profile of ei-

TABLE 31.8 ➤ **PREVALENCE OF CHD RISK FACTORS IN BOYS AND GIRLS AGED 7 TO 12 YEARS**

	Prevalence				
Risk Factor	Male	Female	Total	N	Percentage in Total Sample
Obesity (>20% body fat)	10	4	14	47	30
Low $\dot{V}O_{2peak}$ (<31 mL · kg^{-1} · min^{-1})	3	1	4	34	12
Elevated blood lipids					
Cholesterol (>200 mg · dL^{-1})	1	3	4	38	10
Triglycerides (>100 mg · dL^{-1})	4	3	7	38	18
Lipoprotein classification					
Type II	1	1	2	38	5
Type IV	4	3	7	38	18
Family history of CHD	7	5	12	47	26

From Gilliam T, et al. Prevalence of coronary heart disease risk factors in active children, 7 to 12 years of age. Med Sci Sports 1977;9:21.

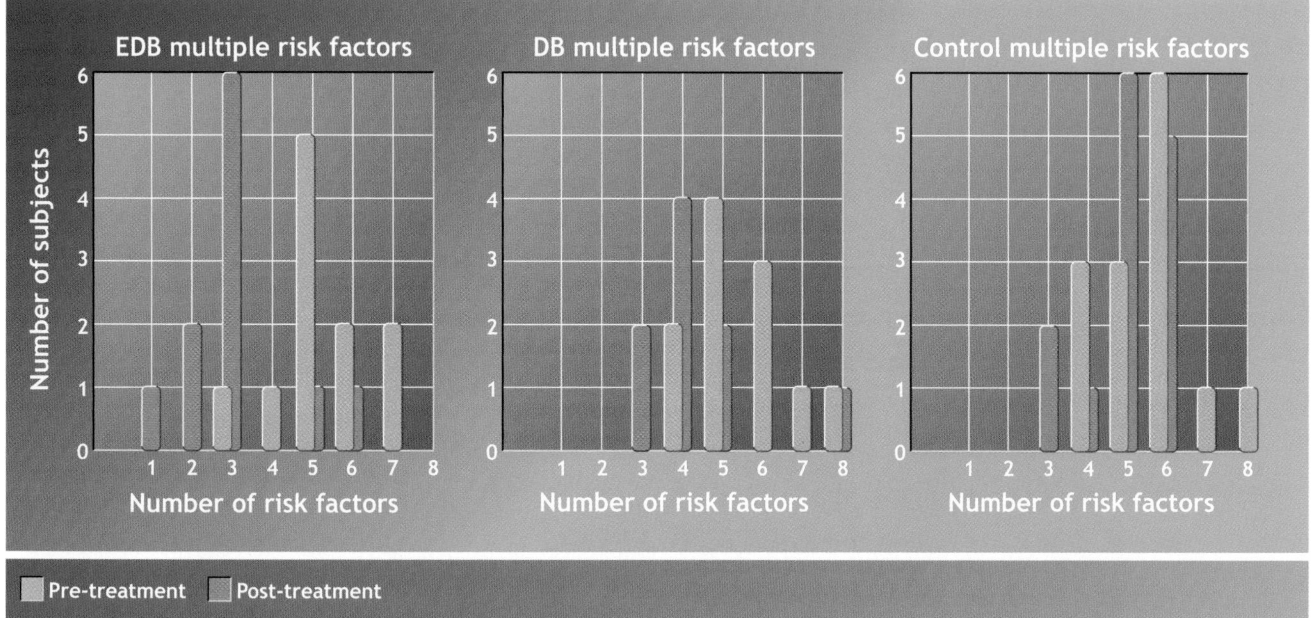

FIGURE 31.30 • Multiple coronary heart disease risk factors for obese adolescents before and after treatment. *DB*, diet + behavior change group; *EDB*, exercise + diet + behavior change group. (From Becque MD, et al. Coronary risk incidence of obese adolescents: reduction by exercise plus diet intervention. Pediatrics 1988;81:605.)

ther (1) diet plus behavior therapy or (2) regular exercise plus diet plus behavior therapy. No changes resulted in multiple-risk reduction in either the control group or those receiving diet plus behavior treatment. In contrast, children undergoing exercise plus diet plus behavior therapy dramatically reduced multiple risks (Fig. 31.30). These encouraging findings demonstrate that a supervised program of moderate food restriction and exercise with behavior modification reduces CHD risk factors in obese adolescents. Adding regular exercise augmented the effectiveness of risk-factor intervention.

Autopsy evidence and the prevalence of CHD risk factors among preadolescents and adolescents indicate that heart disease begins in childhood (see page 893). Usually, the most sedentary children (e.g., those who watch the most TV) have more body fat and a higher BMI than physically active peers.[12] School-based programs aimed at increasing the level of daily physical activity and/or reducing risk factors in children and adolescents increase students' knowledge about risk factors and the benefits of physical activity without impairing academic performance.[108] Such programs may also produce a long-term positive effect on exercise habits and overall health.[223] Future studies must determine if risk intervention improves childhood and subsequent adult behaviors and positively impacts future health. Certainly, if regular physical activity upgrades or at least stabilizes a poor risk factor profile, then school curricula at all grade levels, but especially the kindergarten and elementary grades, should strongly encourage more physically active lifestyles. In this regard, not implementing required daily physical education seems counterproductive from a public health policy standpoint.

Calculating CHD Risk

Risk inventories attempt to assess an individual's susceptibility to CHD. Many of these assessments assign point values to different aspects of lifestyle. In most instances, these scores do not quantify mortality or morbidity risk. Despite this limitation, such qualitative risk assignment provides a valuable tool for assessing general lifestyle behaviors and current heart disease risk.

Figure 31.31 presents a popular risk inventory developed by the American Heart Association. To determine risk profile, review each risk factor and accompanying numerical value that best describes a person's status. Find the box applicable and circle the number in it. For example, a 19-year-old person circles the number 1 in the box labeled 10 to 20 years. After checking all the rows, add the circled numbers. The total number of points represents risk score; see the table in the footnote for relative risk category.

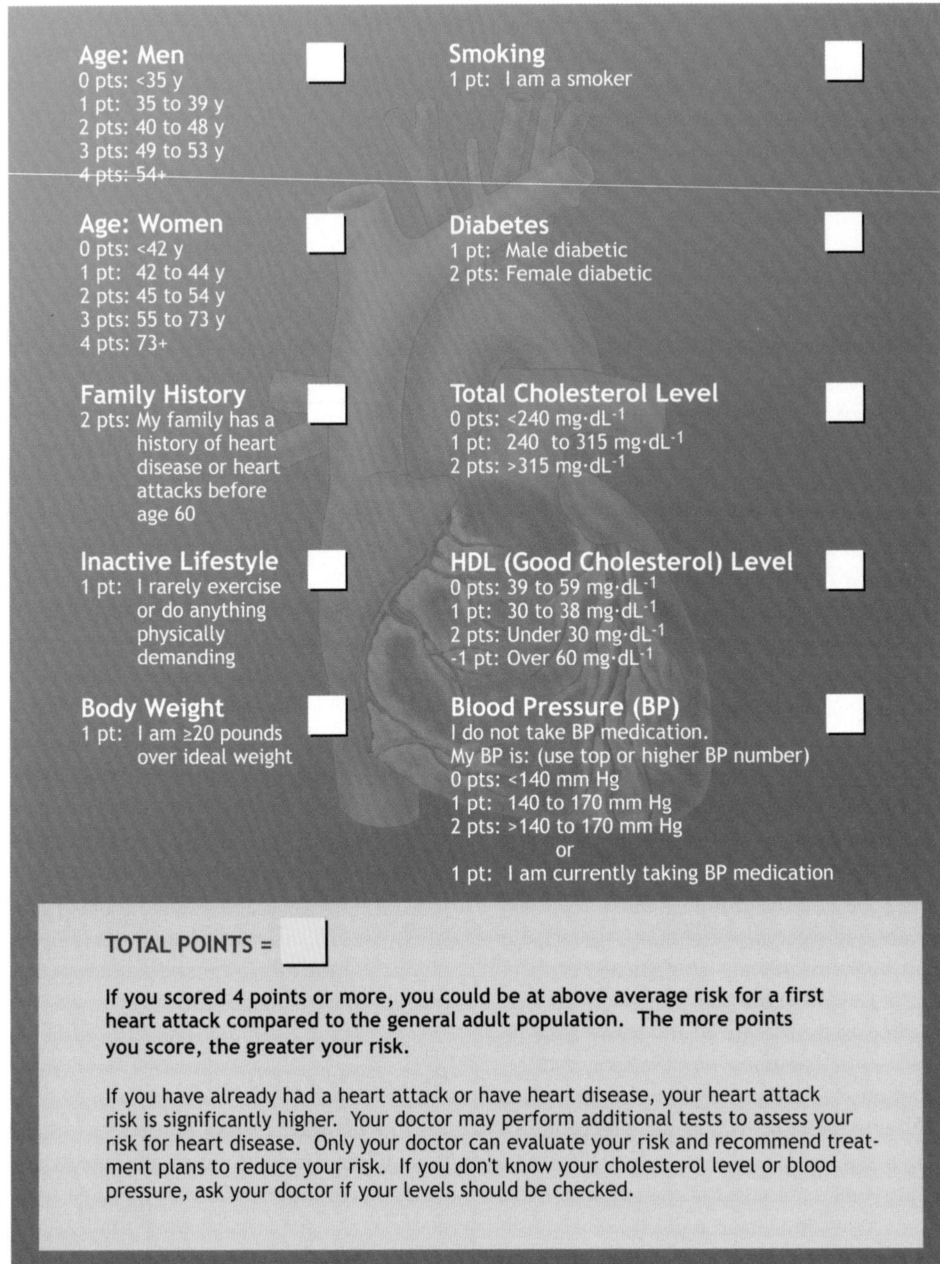

Age: Men
0 pts: <35 y
1 pt: 35 to 39 y
2 pts: 40 to 48 y
3 pts: 49 to 53 y
4 pts: 54+

Smoking
1 pt: I am a smoker

Age: Women
0 pts: <42 y
1 pt: 42 to 44 y
2 pts: 45 to 54 y
3 pts: 55 to 73 y
4 pts: 73+

Diabetes
1 pt: Male diabetic
2 pts: Female diabetic

Family History
2 pts: My family has a history of heart disease or heart attacks before age 60

Total Cholesterol Level
0 pts: <240 mg·dL^{-1}
1 pt: 240 to 315 mg·dL^{-1}
2 pts: >315 mg·dL^{-1}

Inactive Lifestyle
1 pt: I rarely exercise or do anything physically demanding

HDL (Good Cholesterol) Level
0 pts: 39 to 59 mg·dL^{-1}
1 pt: 30 to 38 mg·dL^{-1}
2 pts: Under 30 mg·dL^{-1}
-1 pt: Over 60 mg·dL^{-1}

Body Weight
1 pt: I am ≥20 pounds over ideal weight

Blood Pressure (BP)
I do not take BP medication.
My BP is: (use top or higher BP number)
0 pts: <140 mm Hg
1 pt: 140 to 170 mm Hg
2 pts: >140 to 170 mm Hg
or
1 pt: I am currently taking BP medication

TOTAL POINTS =

If you scored 4 points or more, you could be at above average risk for a first heart attack compared to the general adult population. The more points you score, the greater your risk.

If you have already had a heart attack or have heart disease, your heart attack risk is significantly higher. Your doctor may perform additional tests to assess your risk for heart disease. Only your doctor can evaluate your risk and recommend treatment plans to reduce your risk. If you don't know your cholesterol level or blood pressure, ask your doctor if your levels should be checked.

FIGURE 31.31 • American Heart Association's checklist to evaluate coronary heart disease risk.

Summary

1. CHD represents the single greatest cause of death in the Western world. Its pathogenesis involves degenerative changes in the inner lining of the arterial wall that progressively occlude the blood vessel.
2. Numerous factors increase an individual's susceptibility to CHD. Major risk factors include age and gender, blood lipid abnormalities, hypertension, cigarette smoking, obesity, physical inactivity, diet, family history, and ECG abnormalities during rest and exercise. Prudent treatment attempts to eliminate or reduce "modifiable" CHD risk factors.
3. A serum cholesterol level of 200 mg · dL^{-1} or lower is usually desirable, although many experts recommend lower values for the lowest CHD risk.
4. Treatment of elevated cholesterol should begin early because of a strong association between serum cholesterol level as a young adult and cardiovascular disease in middle age.
5. The distribution of the various lipoproteins, particularly HDL-C and LDL-C, provides a more powerful predictor of heart disease risk than total serum cholesterol concentration alone.
6. LDL-C upon oxidation participates in the artery-clogging, plaque-forming process of atherosclerosis

by stimulating monocyte–macrophage infiltration and lipoprotein deposition.

7. HDL-C facilitates reverse cholesterol transport by removing surplus cholesterol from peripheral tissues (including arterial walls) for transport to the liver for bile synthesis and subsequent excretion via the small intestine.
8. Favorable alterations in HDL-C occur in sedentary men and women of all ages who regularly participate in moderate aerobic exercise.
9. A high level of homocysteine, a metabolic intermediate of the essential amino acid methionine, exerts a powerful independent risk for vascular disease. B-vitamin deficiency, particularly of folic acid, promotes homocysteine buildup.
10. Dietary fiber may exert a dual role in preventing hyperinsulinemia by decreasing circulating insulin levels directly and by thwarting obesity with its associated insulin resistance.
11. Cigarette smokers experience almost twice the risk of death from heart disease as nonsmokers. One mechanism for risk involves the adverse effects of smoking on lipoprotein levels.
12. Sedentary men and women face approximately twice the risk of a fatal heart attack than more physically active counterparts. Maintenance of physical fitness and a physically active lifestyle throughout life significantly lower CHD risk factors and occurrence of disease.
13. The interaction of CHD risk factors magnifies their individual effects on overall disease risk.
14. Programs of nutrition, exercise, and weight control favorably modify many CHD risk factors and usually improve an individual's health outlook. Research must determine if risk intervention in children improves their overall health and ultimately adult health-related behaviors.

References

1. Abbott RF, et al. Cardiovascular risk factors and graded treadmill exercise endurance in healthy adults: the Framingham Offspring Study. Am J Cardiol 1989;63:342.
2. ACSM position stand on exercise and physical activity for older adults. Med Sci Sports Exerc 1998;30:992.
3. ACSM position stand on exercise and type 2 diabetes. Med Sci Sports Exerc 2000;32:1345.
4. ADA/ACSM diabetes mellitus and exercise joint position paper. Med Sci Sports Exerc 1997;29:I.
5. Agnarsson U, et al. Effects of leisure-time physical activity and ventilatory function on risk of stroke in men: the Reykjavík Study. Ann Intern Med 1999;130:987.
6. Albert CM, et al. Triggering of sudden death from cardiac causes by vigorous exertion. N Engl J Med 2000;9:343.
7. Allison DB, et al. Annual deaths attributable to obesity in the United States. JAMA 1999;282:1530.
8. Almeida SA, et al. Epidemiological patterns of musculoskeletal injuries and physical training. Med Sci Sports Exerc 1999;31:1176.
9. Andersen WG. Further studies on the longevity of Yale athletes. Med Times 1916;44:75.
10. Anderson JW, et al. Meta-analysis of the effects of soy protein intake on serum lipids. N Engl J Med 1995;333:276.
11. Anderson RE. Effects of lifestyle activity vs structured aerobic exercise in obese women. JAMA 1999;281:335.
12. Anderson RE, et al. Relationship of physical activity and television watching with body weight and level of fatness among children. JAMA 1998;279:938.
13. Babb TG. Mechanical ventilatory constraints in aging, lung disease and obesity: perspectives and brief review. Med Sci Sports Exerc 1999;31 (1 suppl):S12.
14. Babcock MA, et al. Effects of aerobic endurance training on gas exchange kinetics of older men. Med Sci Sports Exerc 1994;26:447.
15. Becque MD, et al. Coronary risk incidence of obese adolescents: reduction by exercise plus diet intervention. Pediatrics 1988;81:605.
16. Berenson GS, et al. Association between multiple cardiovascular risk factors and atherosclerosis in children and young adults. N Engl J Med 1998;338:1650.
17. Berg K. Lp(a) lipoprotein: an overview. Chem Phys Lipids 1994;67/68:9.
18. Blair SN. Physical activity, physical fitness, and health. Res Q Exerc Sport 1993;64:365.
19. Blair SN, Connelly JC. How much physical activity should we do? The case for moderate amounts and intensities of physical activity. Res Q Exerc Sport 1996;67:193.
20. Blair SN, et al. Changes in physical fitness and all cause mortality: a prospective study of healthy and unhealthy men. JAMA 1995;273:1093.
21. Blair SN, et al. Influences of cardiorespiratory fitness and other precursors on cardiovascular disease and all-cause mortality in men and women. JAMA 1996;276:205.
22. Blair SN, et al. Physical activity, nutrition, and chronic disease. Med Sci Sports Exerc 1997;28:335.
23. Bloomfield-Rubins H, et al. Gemfibrozil for the secondary prevention of coronary heart disease in men with low levels of high-density lipoprotein cholesterol. N Engl J Med 1999;341:410.
24. Boer JM, et al. Parental history of myocardial infarction: lipid traits, gene polymorphisms and lifestyle. Artherosclerosis 2001;155:149.
25. Booth FW, et al. Waging war on modern chronic diseases: primary prevention through exercise biology. J Appl Physiol 2000;88:774.
26. Bousser M-G. Stroke in women. Circulation 1999;99:463.
27. Bouvier F, et al. Left ventricular function and perfusion in elderly endurance athletes. Med Sci Sports Exerc 2001;33:735.
28. Brill PA, et al. Muscular strength and physical function. Med Sci Sports Exerc 2000;32:412.
29. Brönstrup A, et al. Effects of folic acid and combinations of folic acid and vitamin B-12 on plasma homocysteine concentrations in healthy young women. Am J Clin Nutr 1998;68:1104.
30. Burke AP, et al. Plaque rupture and sudden death related to exertion in men with coronary artery disease. JAMA 1999;281:921.
31. Cartee GD. Aging skeletal muscle: response to exercise. Exerc Sport Sci Rev 1994;22:91.
32. Cartee GD. Influence of age on skeletal muscle glucose transport and glycogen metabolism. Med Sci Sports Exerc 1994;26:577.
33. Casazza GA, et al. Exercise training and reduction in some coronary risk factors in female cigarette smokers. Am J Cardiol 1995;75:85.
34. Caspersen CJ. Physical activity epidemiology: concepts, methods, and applications to exercise science. Exerc Sport Sci Rev 1989;17:.
35. Caspersen CJ, et al. Changes in physical activity patterns in the United States, by sex and cross-sectional age. Med Sci Sports Exerc 2000;32:1601.
36. Centers for Disease Control and Prevention. Prevalence of sedentary lifestyle. MMWR 1997;46:941.
37. Centers for Disease Control and Prevention. Decline in deaths from heart disease and stroke— United States, 1900–1999. MMWR 1999;40:649.
38. Chien S, et al. Longitudinal measurements of blood volume and essential body mass in human subjects. J Appl Physiol 1975;39:818.
39. Clarkson PM. The relationship of age and level of physical activity with the fractionated components of patellar reflex time. J Gerontol 1978;3:650.
40. Col NF, et al. Patient-specific decisions about hormone replacement therapy in postmenopausal women. JAMA 1997;277:1140.
41. Coggan AR, et al. Skeletal muscle adaptations to endurance training in 60- to 70-yr-old men and women. J Appl Physiol 1992;72:1780.
42. Crouse SF, et al. Effects of training and a single session of exercise on lipids and apolipoproteins in hypercholesterolemic men. J Appl Physiol 1997;83:2019.
43. Cunningham DA, et al. Gas exchange dynamics with sinusoidal work in young and elderly women. Respir Physiol 1993;91:43.

44. Cureton KJ, et al. Metabolic determinants of the age-related improvement in one-mile run/walk performance in youth. Med Sci Sports Exerc 1997;29:259.
45. DeSerres SJ, Enoka RM. Older adults can maximally activate the biceps brachi muscle by voluntary command. J Appl Physiol 1998;84:284.
46. Després J-P, et al. Physical activity and coronary heart disease risk factors during childhood and adolescence. Exerc Sport Sci Rev 1990;18.
47. Diaz MN, et al. Antioxidants and atherosclerotic heart disease. N Engl J Med 1997;337:408.
48. Doherty TJ, et al. Effects of motor unit losses on strength in older men and women. J Appl Physiol 1993;74:868.
49. Duncan JJ, et al. Women walking for health and fitness: how much is enough? JAMA 1992;266:3295.
50. Duncan P, et al. Randomized-controlled pilot study of a home-based exercise program with individuals with mild and moderate stroke. Stroke 1998;29:2055.
51. Dunn AL, et al. Comparison of lifestyle and structured interventions to increase physical activity and cardiorespiratory fitness. JAMA 1999;281:327.
52. Dvorak RV, et al. Respiratory fitness, free living physical activity, and cardiovascular disease risk in older individuals: a doubly labeled water study. J Clin Endocrinol Metab 2000;85:957.
53. Ehsani AA, et al. Exercise training improves left ventricular systolic function in older men. Circulation 1991;83:96.
54. Eikelboom JW, et al. Homocyst(e)ine and cardiovascular disease: a critical review of epidemiologic evidence. Ann Intern Med 1999;131:362.
55. Enos WF, et al. Coronary disease among United States soldiers killed in action in Korea. JAMA 1953;152:1090.
56. Ettinger WH, et al. A randomized trial comparing aerobic exercise and resistance exercise with a health education program in older adults with knee osteoarthritis: The Fitness Arthritis and Seniors Trial—(FAST). JAMA 1997;277:25.
57. Farrell SW, et al. Influence of cardiorespiratory fitness levels and other predictors on cardiovascular disease mortality in men. Med Sci Sports Exerc 1998;30:899.
58. Ferguson MA, et al. Effects of four different single exercise sessions on lipids, lipoproteins, and lipoprotein lipase. J Appl Physiol 1998;85:1169.
59. Ferguson MA, et al. Fat distribution and hemostatic measures in obese children. Am J Clin Nutr 1998;67:1136.
60. Fiatarone MA, et al. Exercise training and nutritional supplementation for physical frailty in very elderly people. N Engl J Med 1994;330:1769.
61. Finch EE, Tanzi RE. Genetics of aging. Science 1997;278:407.
62. Figzgerald MD, et al. Age-related decline in maximal aerobic capacity in regularly exercising vs. sedentary females: a meta-analysis. J Appl Physiol 1997;83:160.
63. Fleg SL, et al. Impact of age on the cardiovascular response to dynamic upright exercise in healthy men and women. J Appl Physiol 1995;78:890.
64. Folson A, et al. Prospective study of coronary heart disease incidence in relation to fasting total homocysteine, related genetic polymorphisms, and B vitamins. The Atherosclerotic Risk in Communities (ARIC) Study. Circulation 98:204, 1998.
65. Fried LP, et al. Risk factors and 5-year mortality in older adults: the Cardiovascular Health Study, JAMA 1998;279:585.
66. Frisoni GB, et al. Longevity and the epsilon2 allele of apolipoprotein E: the Finnish Centenarians Study. J Gerontol A Biol Sci Med Sci 2001;56:M75.
67. Frontera WR, et al. Aging of skeletal muscle: a 12-yr longitudinal study. J Appl Physiol 2000;88:1321.
68. Fuchs GS, et al. Alcohol consumption and mortality among women. N Engl J Med 1995;332:1245.
69. Gallager D, et al. Appendicular skeletal muscle mass: effects of age, gender, and ethnicity. J Appl Physiol 1997;83:229.
70. Garrick JG, et al. The epidemiology of aerobic dance injuries. Am J Sports Med 1986;14:67.
71. Gaziano JM, et al. Moderate alcohol intake, increased levels of high-density lipoprotein and its subfractions, and decreased risk of myocardial infarction. N Engl J Med 1993;329:1829.
72. Goldberg RJ, et al. A two decades (1975 to 1995) long experience in the incidence, in-hospital and long-term—fatality rates of acute myocardial infarction: a community wide perspective. J Am Coll Cardiol 1999;33:1533.
73. Grabner MD, Enoka RA. Changes in movement capabilities with aging. Exerc Sport Sci Rev 1995;23:65.
74. Hagberg JM, et al. Pulmonary function in young and older athletes and untrained men. J Appl Physiol 1988;65:101.
75. Hagerman FC, et al. A 20-yr longitudinal study of Olympic oarsmen. Med Sci Sports Exerc 1996;28:1150.
76. Hakim AA, et al. Effects of walking on mortality among nonsmoking retired men. N Engl J Med 1998;338:94.
77. Hakim AA, et al. Effects of walking on coronary heart disease in elderly men: The Honolulu Heart Program. Circulation 1999;100:9.
78. Halle M, et al. Lipoprotein (a) in endurance athletes, power athletes, and sedentary controls. Med Sci Sports Exerc 1996;28:962.
79. Harats D, et al. Citrus fruit supplementation reduces lipoprotein oxidation in young men ingesting a diet high in saturated fat: presumptive evidence for an interaction between vitamins C and E in vivo. Am J Clin Nutr 1998;67:240.
80. He J, et al. Passive smoking and the risk of coronary heart disease—a meta-analysis of epidemiologic studies. N Engl J Med 1999;340:920.
81. Heckbert SR, et al. Duration of estrogen replacement therapy in relation to risk of incident of myocardial infarction in postmenopausal women. Arch Intern Med 1997;157:1330.
82. Heim DL, et al. Exercise mitigates the association of abdominal obesity with high-density lipoprotein cholesterol in premenopausal women: results from the third National Health and Nutrition Examination survey. J Am Diet Assoc 2000;100:1347.
83. Hill AB. Cricket and its relation to the duration of life. Lancet 1927;2:949.
84. Hines LM, et al. Genetic variation in alcohol dehydrogenase and the beneficial effect of a moderate alcohol consumption on myocardial infarction. N Engl J Med 2001;344:549.
85. Hochman JS, et al. Sex, clinical presentation, and outcome in patients with acute coronary syndromes. N Engl J Med 1999;341:266.
86. Hofmann AF. Recreational physical activity and the risk of cholecystectomy in women. N Engl J Med 2000;342:213.
87. Houmard JA, et al. Fiber type and citrate synthase activity in human gastrocnemius and vastus lateralis with aging. J Appl Physiol 1998;85:1337.
88. Howard G, et al. Cigarette smoking and progression of atherosclerosis: the Atherosclerosis Risk in Communities (ARIC) Study. JAMA 1998;279:119.
89. Hu FB, et al. Trends in the incidence of coronary heart disease and changes in diet and lifestyle in women. N Engl J Med 2000;343:530.
90. Huang Y, et al. Physical fitness, physical activity, and functional limitation in adults aged 40 and older. Med Sci Sports Exerc 1998;30:1430.
91. Huang Z, et al. Body weight, weight change, and risk for hypertension in women. Ann Intern Med 1998;128:81.
92. Hubinger LM, Mackinnon LT. The effect of endurance training on lipoprotein (a) (Lp(a)) levels in middle-aged males. Med Sci Sports Exerc 1996;28:757.
93. Hubinger LM, et al. Acute effects of treadmill running on lipoprotein(a) levels in males and females. Med Sci Sports Exerc 1997;29:436.
94. Hunink MGM, et al. The recent decline in mortality from coronary heart disease, 1980–1990: the effect of secular trends in risk factors and treatment. JAMA 1997;277:535.
95. Ingram DK. Age-related decline in physical activity: generalization to nonhumans. Med Sci Sports Exerc 2000;32:1623.
96. Izquierdo M, et al. Maximal and explosive force production capacity and balance performance in men of different ages. Eur J Appl Physiol 1999;79:260.
97. Jackson AS, et al. Changes in aerobic power of women, ages 20–64 yr. Med Sci Sports Exerc 1996;28:884.
98. Janssen RJ, et al. Skeletal muscle mass and distribution in 468 men and women aged 18–88 yr. J Appl Physiol 2000;89:81.
99. Jaye M, et al. A novel endothelial-derived lipase that modulates HDL metabolism. Nat Genet 1999;21:424.
100. Johnson CL, et al. Declining serum total cholesterol levels among US adults. JAMA 1993;269:3002.
101. Johnston RB, et al. Effect of lower extremity muscular fatigue on motor control performance. Med Sci Sports Exerc 1998;30:1703.
102. Kakka TA, et al. Relation of leisure-time physical activity and cardiorespiratory fitness to the risk of acute myocardial infarction in men. N Engl J Med 1994;330:1549.
103. Kasch FW. The effects of exercise on the aging process. Phys Sportsmed 1976;4:64.
104. Kasch FW, et al. The effect of physical activity and inactivity on aerobic power in older men (a longitudinal study). Phys Sportsmed 1990;18:73.
105. Kavanagh TT. Exercise in the primary prevention of coronary artery disease. Can J Cardiol 2001;17(2):155.

106. Keil U. Coronary artery disease: the role of lipids, hypertension and smoking. Basic Res Cardiol 2000;95(suppl):I52.
107. Kent-Braun JA, et al. Skeletal muscle contractile and noncontractile components in young and older women and men. J Appl Physiol 2000;88:662.
108. Killen JD, et al. Cardiovascular disease risk reduction for tenth graders. A multiple-factor school-based program. JAMA 1988;260:1728.
109. Klitgaard H, et al. Function, morphology and protein expression of aging skeletal muscle: a cross-sectional study of elderly men with different training backgrounds. Acta Physiol Scand 1990;457(suppl):1.
110. Kohrt WM, et al. HRT preserves increases in bone mineral density and reductions in body fat after a supervised exercise program. J Appl Physiol 1998;84:1506.
111. Kosta T, et al. Habitual physical activity and peak anaerobic power in elderly women. Eur J Appl Physiol 1997;76:81.
112. Kritchevsky SB, et al. Provitamin A carotenoid intake and carotid artery plaques: the Atherosclerosis Risk in Communities Study. Am J Clin Nutr 1998;68:726.
113. Kujala VM, et al. Relationship of leisure-time physical activity and mortality: the Finnish Twin Cohort. JAMA 1998;279:440.
114. Kuller LH, et al. Sudden death and the decline in coronary heart disease mortality. J Chron Dis 1986;39:1001.
115. Kushi LH, et al. Physical activity and mortality in postmenopausal women. JAMA 1997;277:1287.
116. Lamarche B, et al. Fasting insulin and apolipoprotein B levels and low-density lipoprotein particle size as risk factors for ischemic heart disease. JAMA 1998;279:1955.
117. Lamberts SWJ, et al. The endocrinology of aging. Science 1997;278:419.
118. Lauer MS, Fontanarosa PB. Updated guidelines for cholesterol management. JAMA 2001;285:2508.
119. Layne JE, Nelson ME. The effects of progressive resistance training on bone density: a review. Med Sci Sports Exerc 1999;31:25.
120. Leaf DA, et al. Changes in $\dot{V}O_{2max}$, physical activity, and body fat with chronic exercise: effects on plasma lipids. Med Sci Sports Exerc 1997;29:1152.
121. Lee I-M, Paffenbarger RS. Exercise intensity and longevity in men: the Harvard Alumni Study. JAMA 1995;273:1179.
122. Lee I-M, Paffenbarger RS. Physical activity and stroke incidence: The Harvard Alumni Health Study. Stroke 1998;29:2049.
123. Lee I-M, et al. Exercise and risk of stroke in male physicians. Stroke 1999;30:1.
124. Leitzmann MF, et al. Recreational physical activity and risk of cholecystectomy in women. N Engl J Med 1999;341:777.
125. Lemaitre RN, et al. Leisure-time physical activity and the risk of primary cardiac arrest. Arch Intern Med 1999;159:686.
126. Levine GN, et al. Cholesterol reduction in cardiovascular disease: clinical benefits and possible mechanisms. N Engl J Med 1995;332:512.
127. Levy D, et al. Stratifying the patient at risk from coronary disease: new insights from the Framingham Heart Study. Am Heart J 1990;119:712.
128. Levy WC, et al. Endurance exercise training augments diastolic filling at rest and during exercise in healthy young and older men. Circulation 1993;88:116.
129. Lin Y, et al. Estimating the concentration of β-carotene required for maximal protection of low-density lipoproteins in women. Am J Clin Nutr 1998;67:837.
130. Lindle RS, et al. Age and gender comparisons of muscle strength in 654 women and men aged 20–93 yr. J Appl Physiol 1997;83:1581.
131. Little WC, et al. Cause of acute myocardial infarction late after successful coronary artery bypass grafting. Am J Cardiol 1990;65:808.
132. Lotufo PA, et al. Male pattern baldness and coronary heart disease: the Physician's Health Study. Arch Intern Med 2000;160:165.
133. Ludwig DS, et al. Dietary fiber, weight gain, and cardiovascular disease risk factors in young adults. JAMA 1999;282:1539.
134. Lynch NA, et al. Muscle quality. I. Age-associated differences between arm and leg muscle groups. J Appl Physiol 1999;86:188.
135. Macera CA, et al. Age, physical activity, physical fitness, body composition, and incidence of orthopedic problems. Res Q Exerc Sport 1989;60:225.
136. Mackinnon LT, et al. Effects of physical activity and diet on lipoprotein (a). Med Sci Sports Exerc 1997;29:1429.
137. Malinow MR, et al. Plasma homocysteine levels and graded risk for myocardial infarction: findings in two populations at contrasting risk for coronary heart disease. Atherosclerosis 1996;126:27.
138. Malinow MR, et al. Reduction of plasma homocysteine levels by breakfast cereals fortified with folic acid in patients with coronary heart disease. N Engl J Med 1998;15:1009.
139. Manson JE, et al. A prospective study of walking as compared with vigorous exercise in the prevention of coronary heart disease in women. N Engl J Med 1999;341:650.
140. Marcus BH, et al. Evaluation of motivationally tailored vs standard self-help physical activity interventions at the workplace. Am J Health Promotion 1998;6:424.
141. Marrugat J, et al. Mortality differences between men and women following first myocardial infarction. JAMA 1999;280:1405.
142. Martinez ME, et al. Physical activity, body mass index, and prostaglandin E_2 levels in rectal mucosa. J Natl Cancer Inst 1999;91:950.
143. Mayer EL, et al. Homocysteine and coronary atherosclerosis. J Am Coll Cardiol 1996;27:517.
144. McCartney N. Acute responses to resistance training and safety. Med Sci Sports Exerc 1999;31:31.
145. McDonough JR, et al. Coronary heart disease among Negroes and whites in Evans County, Georgia. J Chron Dis 1965;18:443.
146. McGill HC, et al. Association of coronary heart disease risk factors with microscopic qualities of coronary atherosclerosis in youth. Circulation 2000;102:374.
147. McMurray RG, et al. Is physical activity or aerobic power more influential on reducing cardiovascular disease risk factors? Med Sci Sports Exerc 1998;30:1521.
148. Meredith CN, et al. Peripheral effects of endurance training in young and old subjects. J Appl Physiol 1989;66:2844.
149. Miller M, et al. Normal triglyceride levels and coronary artery disease events: the Baltimore Coronary Observational Long-Term Study. J Am Coll Cardiol 1998;May.
150. Morey MC, et al. Is there a threshold between peak oxygen uptake and self-reported physical functioning in older adults? Med Sci Sports Exerc 1998;30:1223.
151. Morey MC, et al. Physical fitness and functional limitations in community-dwelling older adults. Med Sci Sports Exerc 1998;30:715.
152. Morrey MA, Hensrud DD. Risk of medical events in a supervised health and fitness facility. Med Sci Sports Exerc 1999;31:1233.
153. Morris JN. Exercise in the prevention of coronary heart disease: today's best bet in public health. Med Sci Sports Exerc 1994;26:807.
154. NIH Consensus Conference. Triglyceride, high-density lipoprotein, and coronary heart disease. JAMA 1993;269:505.
155. Nakayama MM, et al. T^{-786} mutation in the 5′-flanking of the region of the endothelial nitric oxide synthase gene is associated with coronary spasm. Circulation 1999;99:2855.
156. Nappo F, et al. Impairment of endothelial functions by acute hyperhomocysteinemia and reversal by antioxidant vitamins. JAMA 1999;281:2113.
157. Nicklas BJ, et al. Increases in high-density lipoprotein cholesterol with endurance exercise training are blunted in obese compared with lean men. Metabolism 1997;46:556.
158. Nigdikar SV, et al. Consumption of red wine polyphenols reduces susceptibility of low-density lipoproteins to oxidation in volunteers. Am J Clin Nutr 1998;68:258.
159. Nygård O, et al. Plasma homocysteine levels and mortality in patients with coronary artery disease. N Engl J Med 1997;337:230.
160. Nygård O, et al. Major lifestyle determinants of plasma total homocysteine distribution: the Horland Homocysteine Study. Am J Clin Nutr 1998;67:263.
161. Omenn GS, et al. Preventing coronary heart disease: B vitamins and homocysteine. Circulation 1998;97:421.
162. Ornish D, et al. Intensive lifestyle changes for reversal of coronary heart disease. JAMA 1998;280:2001.
163. Orth-Gomer K, et al. Lipoprotein (a) as a determinant of coronary heart disease in young women. Circulation 1997;95:329.
164. Paffenbarger RS Jr, et al. Physical activity, all-cause mortality, and longevity of college alumni. N Engl J Med 1986;314:605.
165. Paffenbarger RS Jr, et al. Changes in physical activity and other lifeway patterns influencing longevity. Med Sci Sports Exerc 1994;26:857.
166. Pardaens K, et al. Prognostic significance of peak oxygen uptake in hypertension. Med Sci Sports Exerc 1996;28:794.
167. Parish S, et al. Cigarette smoking, tar yields, and non-fatal myocardial infarction: 14000 cases and 32000 controls. Br Med J 1995;311:471.
168. Pate RR, et al. Physical activity and public health: a recommendation from the Centers for Disease Control and Prevention and American College of Sports Medicine. JAMA 1995;273:402.

169. Physical activity trends—United States, 1990–1998. MMWR 2001; March 9: 166..
170. Pollock ML, et al. Effect of age and training on aerobic capacity and body composition of master athletes. J Appl Physiol 1987;62:625.
171. Pollock ML, et al. Twenty-year follow-up of aerobic power and body composition of older track athletes. J Appl Physiol 1997;82:1508.
172. Pollock ML, et al. The recommended quantity and quality of exercise for developing and maintaining cardiorespiratory fitness, strength, and flexibility in healthy adults. Med Sci Sports Exerc 1998;30:975.
173. Powell KE, Blair SN. The public health burdens of sedentary living habits: theoretical but realistic estimates. Med Sci Sports Exerc 1994;26:851.
174. Powell KE, et al. Physical activity and the incidence of coronary heart disease. Annu Rev Public Health 1987;8:253.
175. Powell KE, et al. Injury rates from walking, gardening, weightlifting, outdoor bicycling, and aerobics. Med Sci Sports Exerc 1998;30:1246.
176. Procter DN, Joyner MJ. Skeletal muscle mass and the reduction of $\dot{V}O_{2max}$ in trained older subjects. J Appl Physiol 1997;82:1411.
177. Proctor DN, et al. Oxidative capacity of human muscle fiber types; effects of age and training status. J Appl Physiol 1995;78:2033.
178. Proctor DN, et al. Reduced leg blood flow during dynamic exercise in older endurance-trained men. J Appl Physiol 1998;85:68.
179. Province MA, et al. The effects of exercise on falls in elderly patients: a preplanned meta-analysis of the FICSIT trials. JAMA 1995;273:1341.
180. Quinn TJ, et al. Caloric expenditure, life status, and disease in former male athletes and non-athletes. Med Sci Sports Exerc 1990;22:742.
181. Rantanken T, et al. Grip strength changes over 27 yr in Japanese-American men. J Appl Physiol 1998;85:2047.
182. Ridker PM, et al. Homocysteine and risk of cardiovascular disease among postmenopausal women. JAMA 1999;281:1817.
183. Rifici VA, et al. Red wine inhibits the cell-mediated oxidation of LDL and HDL. J Am Coll Nutr 1999;18:137.
184. Rigotti NA, et al. US college students' use of tobacco products. Results of a national survey. JAMA 2000;284:699.
185. Rosamond WD, et al. Trends in the incidence of myocardial infarction and in mortality due to coronary heart disease, 1987 to 1994. N Engl J Med 1998;339:861.
186. Rosen MJ, et al. Predictors of age-associated decline in maximal aerobic capacity: a comparison of four statistical models. J Appl Physiol 1998;84:2163.
187. Rulge JB, et al. Insulin and risk of cardiovascular disease. Circulation 1998;97:996.
188. Sacco RL, et al. The protective effect of moderate alcohol consumption on ischemic stroke. JAMA 1999;28:913.
189. Sandvik L, et al. Physical fitness as a predictor of mortality among healthy, middle-aged Norwegian men. N Engl J Med 1993;328:533.
190. Schwartz RS, et al. Effects of intensive endurance training on lipoprotein profiles in young and older men. Metabolism 1992;41:644.
191. Seals DR, et al. Enhanced left ventricular performance in endurance trained older men. Circulation 1994;89:198.
192. Seals DR, et al. Exercise and aging: autonomic control of the circulation. Med Sci Sports Exerc 1994;26:568.
193. Seed M, et al. Relationship of serum lipoprotein (a) phenotype to coronary heart disease in patients with familial hypercholesterolemia. N Engl J Med 1990;322:1494.
194. Seiler KS, et al. Gender differences in rowing performance and power with aging. Med Sci Sports Exerc 1998;30:121.
195. Shepard RJ. Exercise and sudden death: an overview. Sport Sci Rev 1995;4:1.
196. Shephard RJ, Baldy GJ. Exercise as cardiovascular therapy. Circulation 1999;99:963.
197. Sherrill DL, et al. Association of physical activity and human sleep disorders. Arch Intern Med 1998;158:1894.
198. Simonen RL, et al. The effect of lifelong exercise on psychomotor reaction time: a study of 38 pairs of male monozygotic twins. Med Sci Sports Exerc 1998;30:1445.
199. Siscovick DS, et al. The incidence of primary cardiac arrest during vigorous exercise. N Engl J Med 1984;311:874.
200. Smith JK. Exercise and atherogenesis. Exerc Sport Sci Rev 2001;29:49.
201. Spain CG, Franks BD. Healthy People 2010: Physical Activity and Fitness. Research Digest (President's Council on Physical Fitness and Sports) 2001; Series 3, No. 13.
202. Spina RJ. Cardiovascular adaptations to endurance exercise training in older men and women. Exerc Sport Sci Rev 1999;27:317.
203. Spina RJ, et al. Effect of exercise training on left ventricular performance in older women free of cardiopulmonary disease. Am J Cardiol 1993;71:99.
204. Spirduso WW, Clifford, P. Replication of age and physical activity effects on reaction and movement time. J Gerontol 1978;33:26.
205. Stampfer MJ, et al. Primary prevention of coronary heart disease in women through diet and lifestyle. N Engl J Med 2000;343:16.
206. Stanchfeld SS, et al. Regulation of blood volume during training in post-menopausal women. Med Sci Sports Exerc 1998;30:92.
207. Stefanick ML, et al. Effects of diet and exercise in men and post-menopausal women with low levels of HDL cholesterol and high levels of LDL cholesterol. N Engl J Med 1998;339:12.
208. Stein JH, McBride PE. Hyperhomocysteinemia and atherosclerotic vascular disease. Arch Intern Med 1998;158:1301.
209. Steinberg D. Low density lipoprotein oxidation and its pathobiological significance. J Biol Chem 1997;272:20963.
210. Stewart JM, et al. Exercise reduces epicardial coronary artery wall stiffness: roles of cGMP and cAMP. Med Sci Sports Exerc 1998;30:215.
211. Stolzenberg-Solomon RZ, et al. Association of dietary protein intake and coffee consumption on serum homocysteine concentrations in an older population. Am J Clin Nutr 1999;69:467.
212. Straton JR, et al. Cardiovascular responses to exercise: effects of aging. Circulation 1994;89:1648.
213. Strong JP, et al. Prevalence and extent of atherosclerosis in adolescents and young adults. JAMA 1999;281:727.
214. Tanaka H, et al. Greater rate of decline in maximal aerobic capacity with age in physically active vs. sedentary healthy women. J Appl Physiol 1997;83:1947.
215. Tanaka H, et al. Age-predicted maximal heart rate revisited. J Am Coll Cardiol 2001;37:153.
216. Thompson PD, et al. Effects of prolonged exercise training without weight loss on high-density lipoprotein metabolism in overweight men. Metabolism 1997;46:217.
217. Thune I, et al. Physical activity improves the metabolic risk profile in men and women. Arch Intern Med 1998;158:1633.
218. Tjønneland A, et al. Wine intake and diet in a random sample of 48,763 Danish men and women. Am J Clin Nutr 1999;69:49.
219. Tolfrey K, et al. Exercise training induced alterations in prepubertal children's lipid-lipoprotein profile. Med Sci Sports Exerc 1998;30:1684.
220. Tracy BL, et al. Muscle quality. II. Effects of strength training in 65 to 75-year-old men and women. J Appl Physiol 1999;86:195.
221. Tran ZV, Weltman A. Differential effects of exercise on serum lipids and lipoprotein levels seen with changes in body weight: a meta analysis. JAMA 1985;254:919.
222. Trappe SW, et al. Aging among elite distance runners: a 22-year longitudinal study. J Appl Physiol 1996;80:285.
223. Trudeau F, et al. Daily primary school physical education: effects on physical activity during adult life. Med Sci Sports Exerc 1999;31:111.
224. Trulson MF, et al. Comparisons of siblings in Boston and Ireland. J Am Diet Assoc 1964;45:225.
225. U.S. Department of Health and Human Services. Healthy People 2000 midcourse review and 1995 revisions. Washington, DC: U.S. Government Printing Office, 1996.
226. U.S. Department of Health and Human Services. Mortality, part B. In: Vital statistics of the United States: various years through 1991. Hyattsville, MD: National Center for Health Statistics, 1995.
227. Vaccarino V, et al. Sex-based differences in early mortality after myocardial infarction. N Engl J Med 1999;341:217.
228. Valmadrid CT, et al. Alcohol intake and risk of coronary heart disease mortality in persons with older-onset diabetes mellitus. JAMA 1999;282:239.
229. Van Boxtel MPJ, et al. Aerobic capacity and cognitive performance in a cross-sectional aging study. Med Sci Sports Exerc 1997;29:1357.
230. Van den Hoogen PC, et al. Blood pressure and long-term coronary heart disease mortality in the Seven Countries study: implications for clinical practice and public health. Eur Heart J 2000;21:1639.
231. Vasankari TJ, et al. Reduced oxidized LDL levels after a 10-month exercise program. Med Sci Sports Exerc 1998;30:1496.
232. Visscher TL, et al. Underweight and overweight in relation to mortality among men aged 40-59 and 50-69 years: the Seven Countries Study. Am J Epidemiol 2000:1;151:660.
233. Visser M, et al. High body fatness, but not low fat-free mass, predicts disability in older men and women: the Cardiovascular Health Study. Am J Clin Nutr 1998;68:584.

234. Vita AJ, et al. Aging, health risks, and cumulative disability. N Engl J Med 1998;338:1035.
235. Wald NJ, et al. Homocysteine and ischemic heart disease: results of a prospective study with implications regarding prevention. Arch Intern Med 1998;158:862.
236. Walker JL, et al. The energy cost of horizontal walking and running in adolescents. Med Sci Sports Exerc 1999;31:311.
237. Wannamethee SG, et al. Changes in physical activity, mortality, and incidence of coronary heart disease in older men. Lancet 1998:351.
238. Wei M, et al. Relationship between low cardiorespiratory fitness and mortality in normal-weight, overweight, and obese men. JAMA 1999;282:1547.
239. Welch GN, Loscalzo J. Homocysteine and atherothrombosis. N Engl J Med 1999;338:1042.
240. Wescott WL, Baechle TR. Strength training past 50. Champaign, IL: Human Kinetics, 1998.
241. Wiebe CG, et al. Exercise cardiac function in young through elderly endurance trained women. Med Sci Sports Exerc 1999;31:684.
242. Willett WC, et al. Relative and absolute excess risks of coronary heart disease among women who smoke cigarettes. N Engl J Med 1987;317:1303.
243. Williams PJ. Interactive effects of exercise, alcohol, and vegetarian diet on coronary artery disease risk factors in 9242 runners: the National Runners' Health Study. Am J Clin Nutr 1997;66:1197.
244. Williams PT. Relationship of heart disease risk factors to exercise quantity and intensity. Arch Intern Med 1998;158:237.
245. Williams PT. Physical fitness and activity as separate heart disease risk factors: a meta-analysis. Exer Sport Sci Rev 2001;33:754.
246. Winkleby MA, et al. Ethnic variation in cardiovascular disease risk factors among children and young adults: findings from the Third National Health and Nutrition Examination survey, 1998–1994. JAMA 1999;281:1006.
247. Wood D. Established and emerging cardiovascular risk factors. Am Heart J 2001;141(2 Pt 2).
248. Xiao-ren P, et al. Effects of diet and exercise in preventing NIDDM in people with impaired glucose tolerance. Diabetes Care 1997;20:537.

CHAPTER 32

Clinical Exercise Physiology for Cancer, Cardiovascular, and Pulmonary Rehabilitation

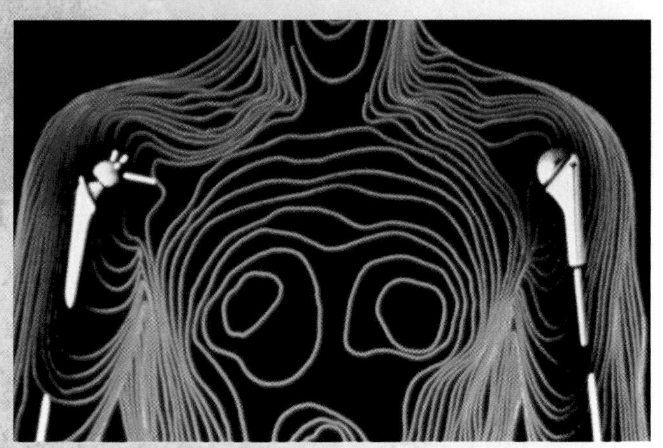

Chapter Objectives

- Discuss the role of the exercise physiologist/health-fitness professional in the clinical setting
- Summarize the exercise benefits for cancer prevention and rehabilitation and make exercise recommendations for persons with cancer
- Review the potential benefits of aerobic exercise for moderate hypertension
- Discuss the role of regular exercise in congestive heart failure
- Discuss the general components in the clinical assessment for cardiac disease
- Summarize noninvasive and invasive procedures to identify specific cardiac dysfunctions
- Describe the three phases of cardiac rehabilitation, including objectives, required levels of supervision, and prudent physical activities
- Give important reasons for including graded exercise stress testing for coronary heart disease screening
- Describe objective indicators of coronary heart disease during an exercise stress test
- List 10 reasons for stopping a stress test
- Define the following terms for stress test results: *true positive, false positive, true negative,* and *false negative*
- Outline an approach for individualizing an exercise prescription
- Discuss the heart transplant patient's responses and adaptations to regular aerobic exercise and resistance training
- Categorize and describe five diseases that affect the pulmonary system
- Outline two proposed mechanisms for exercise-induced bronchospasm and factors that modify its severity
- Describe the benefits to the participant and company of corporate worksite wellness and fitness programs

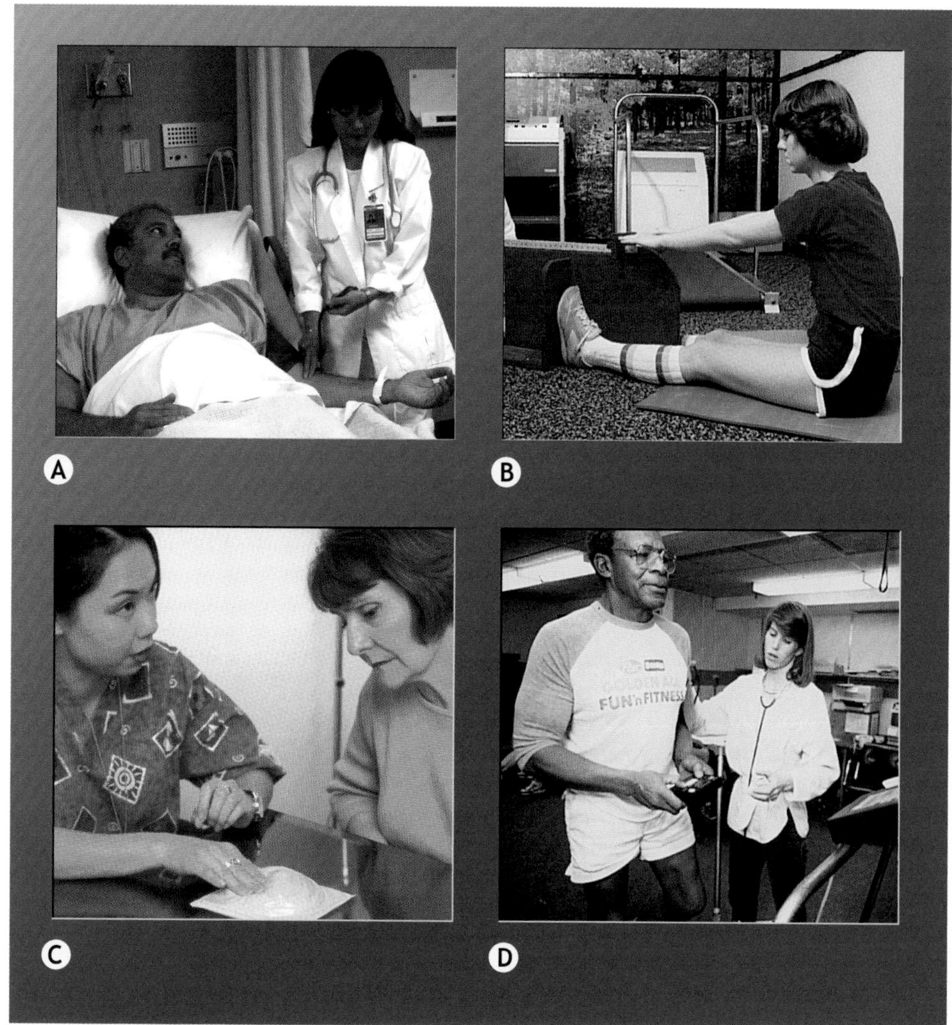

FIGURE 32.1 • The team approach in rehabilitation. Health-care professionals work cooperatively to improve a patient's functional capacity. **A**. Physican/nurse: helps to attain and maintain good health so functional capacity can be improved. **B**. Occupational therapist: helps with ability to function in daily life and safely perform occupational tasks. **C**. Social worker: helps the individual to function within the social system. **D**. Clinical exercise physiologist/physical therapist: helps to improve functional capacity and overall mobility.

THE EXERCISE PHYSIOLOGIST IN THE CLINICAL SETTING

The **clinical exercise physiologist** plays an important part in a team approach to health care and total patient care (Fig. 32.1). In the clinical setting, the exercise physiologist focuses primarily on restoring patient mobility and functional capacity, while working closely with physical therapists, occupational therapists, and the physician. The exercise physiologist has an expanded role in clinical practice because of fundamental relationships among measures of functional capacity, physical fitness, and overall good health. The World Health Organization (WHO) defines health as *"a state of complete physical, mental and social well-being, not merely the absence of disease and infirmity."* This definition considers good health the ability to complete physical tasks successfully and maintain functional independence. Functional capacity measurement provides an objective assessment of a patient's health status and quantifies changes from diverse strategies to improve health and well-being.

Figure 32.2 illustrates a continuum of possible outcomes from disease. Within this context, **disability** refers to

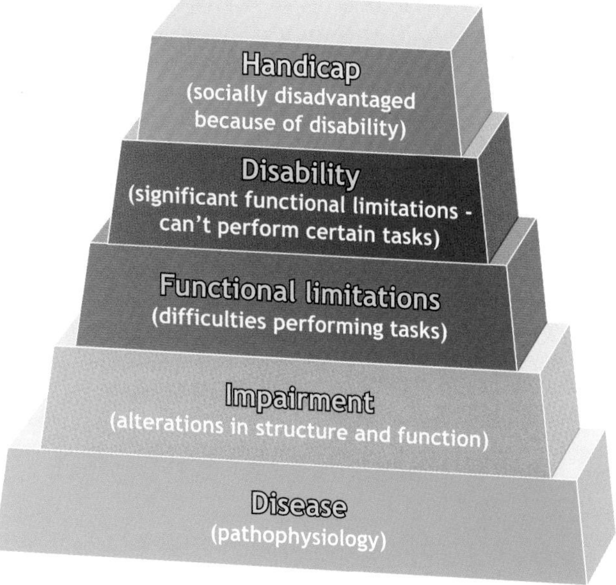

FIGURE 32.2 • Hierarchy of possible outcomes from disease.

an individual's diminished functional capacity, often compounded by an inactive lifestyle,[25,89] whereas **handicap** denotes a physical performance frame of reference defined by society.[165] Handicapped individuals can no longer perform tasks expected by society; having a functional limitation, on the other hand, does not necessarily lead to either disability or handicap.

Vital Link Between Sports Medicine and Exercise Physiology

One traditional view of sports medicine concerns rehabilitating athletes from sports-related injuries. In its broader context, **sports medicine** relates to scientific and medical aspects of physical activity, physical fitness, health, and sports perfor-

TABLE 32.1 ➤ HEALTH BENEFITS OF REGULAR PHYSICAL ACTIVITY[a]

Physical Activity Benefit	Surety Rating	Physical Activity Benefit	Surety Rating
Fitness of body		**Cigarette smoking**	
Improves heart and lung function	****	Improves success in quitting	**
Improves muscular strength/size	****	**Diabetes**	
Cardiovascular disease		Prevention of type 2	****
Coronary heart disease prevention	****	Treatment of type 2	***
Regression of atherosclerosis	**	Treatment of type 1	*
Treatment of heart disease	***	Improvement in diabetic's life quality	***
Prevention of stroke	**	**Infection and immunity**	
Cancer		Prevention of the common cold	**
Prevention of colon cancer	****	Improves overall immunity	**
Prevention of breast cancer	**	Slows progression of HIV to AIDS	*
Prevention of uterine cancer	**	Improves life quality of HIV-infected persons	****
Prevention of prostate cancer	**	**Arthritis**	
Prevention of other cancers	*	Prevention of arthritis	*
Treatment of cancer	*	Treatment/cure of arthritis	*
Osteoporosis		Improvement life quality/fitness	****
Helps increase bone mass and density	****	**High blood pressure**	
Prevention of osteoporosis	***	Prevention of high blood pressure	****
Treatment of osteoporosis	**	Treatment of high blood pressure	****
Blood cholesterol/lipoproteins		**Asthma**	
Lowers blood total cholesterol	*	Prevention/treatment of asthma	*
Lowers LDL-cholesterol	*	Improvement in asthmatic's life quality	***
Lowers triglycerides	***	**Sleep**	
Raises HDL-cholesterol	***	Improvement in sleep quality	***
Low back pain		**Psychologic well-being**	
Prevention of low back pain	**	Elevation in mood	****
Treatment of low back pain	**	Buffers effects of mental stress	***
Nutrition and diet quality		Alleviates/prevents depression	****
Improvement in diet quality	**	Anxiety reduction	****
Increase in total energy intake	***	Improves self-esteem	****
Weight management		**Special issues for women**	
Prevention of weight gain	****	Improves total body fitness	****
Treatment of obesity	**	Improves fitness while pregnant	****
Helps maintain weight loss	***	Improves birthing experience	**
Children and youth		Improves health of fetus	**
Prevention of obesity	***	Improves health during menopause	***
Controls disease risk factors	***		
Reduction of unhealthy habits	**		
Improves odds of adult activity	**		
Elderly and the aging process			
Improvement in physical fitness	****		
Counters loss in heart/lung fitness	**		
Counters loss of muscle	***		
Counters gain in fat	***		
Improvement in life expectancy	****		
Improvement in life quality	****		

****	Strong consensus, with little or no conflicting data
***	Most data supportive, but more research needed for clarification
**	Some supportive data, but much more research needed
*	Little or no data to support

[a]Based on a total physical fitness program that includes physical activity designed to improve both aerobic and musculoskeletal fitness.
From Newman CC. The human body. ACSM's Health Fitness J 1998;2(3):30.

mance. Indeed, the WHO defines physical fitness and sports as the ability to perform muscular work satisfactorily. This definition encompasses one's capacity to perform physical activity at work, at home, or on the athletic field. Sports medicine thus becomes closely linked to clinical exercise physiology, because the sports medicine profession encompasses a broad spectrum of individuals. Patients with low functional capacity recovering from injury, disease, and medical interventions compose one end of the continuum, while the other extreme encompasses healthy, able-bodied and disabled athletes with inordinate levels of physical fitness. Carefully prescribed physical activity contributes to overall good health and quality of life (Table 32.1).[22,89] To this end, exercise physiologists assume an important clinical role in sports medicine by evaluating and reconditioning individuals with diseases and physical disabilities.

PREVALENCE AND TYPES OF DISABILITIES

A variety of medical conditions adversely affect functional capacity and physical performance. Some disabilities occur at birth (e.g., deformed limbs, deafness, blindness, mental retardation, and acquired diseases), whereas others emerge during youth or young adulthood (e.g., injury-related disabilities, diabetes, and general diseases) or later in life (e.g., cardiovascular and pulmonary pathologies).[211]

Figure 32.3 shows data on disability rate by age and gender. In the U.S. population of 275 million in year 2000, an estimated 60 million (22%) individuals were classified as disabled. The remarkable increase in disability with increasing age is of concern because persons older than age 65 represent the population's fastest growing segment (approximately 16% in 2001). For many clinical conditions associated with disability, a continuum ranges from mild to severe pathology. In some cases, the degree of disability does not parallel clinical severity, and many individuals suffer multiple disabilities. Thus, the overall number of individuals in the population with complete or partial disabilities is probably much larger than currently estimated.

Another way to discern the magnitude and impact of disabilities considers the increase in the number of health care professionals. Figure 32.4 shows the number of physical therapy programs in the United States between 1975 and 2000. The enrollment trend has not leveled off during the last 25 years. From

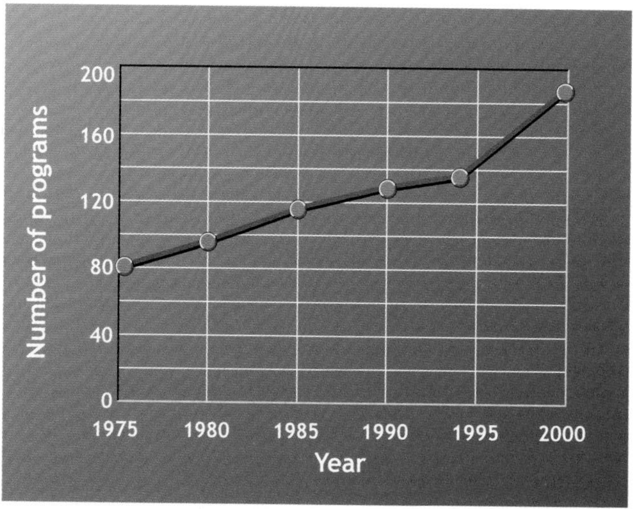

FIGURE 32.4 • Increase in physical therapy programs in United States educational institutions from 1975 to 2000. (Source: Physical Therapy Association. Alexandria, VA.)

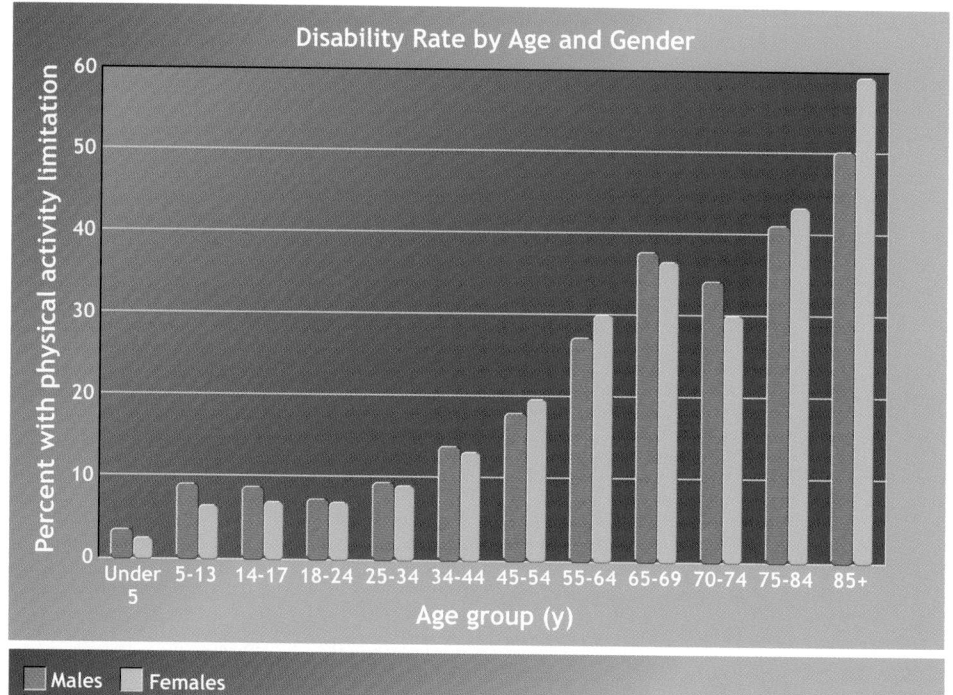

FIGURE 32.3 • Prevalence of disabilities by age and gender. (National Health Interview Survey. U.S. Bureau of the Census, Americans with Disabilities: 1994–95; 1999 update shown [personal communication].)

1975 to 2000, the 290% increase in physical therapy programs in the United States and Canada included 187 accredited programs, with 15 new programs awaiting accreditation in 2001. The number of postgraduate programs has also increased in the last 5 years. As of December 2000, 62 masters and 35 doctoral physical therapy programs existed in the United States.[172]

TRAINING AND CERTIFICATION PROGRAMS FOR EXERCISE PHYSIOLOGISTS

During the past 25 years, exercise has gained widespread acceptance as an integral part of rehabilitative programs of care and health maintenance for a growing list of chronic diseases and disabling conditions. Likewise, expanding public interest in exercise for health promotion has stimulated a parallel need to certify qualified professionals to provide sound advice and supervision regarding physical activities for preventive and rehabilitative purposes. In 1975, the American College of Sports Medicine (ACSM; www.acsm.org) initiated the first ACSM Clinical Track certification program, with a Health/Fitness Track begun in the early 1980s. More than 20,000 certificates have been awarded since 1975; the ACSM continues to be the preeminent organization offering certification programs, newsletters, and continuing education credits (CUEs) to support the professional growth of health–fitness professionals.

The ACSM certifications consist of two different tracks: (1) *Health/Fitness Track* for those who want to provide leadership in fitness assessment and exercise programing of a preventive nature for apparently healthy individuals and for controlling diseases in corporate, commercial, and community settings and (2) *Clinical Track* for professionals who work with groups at high risk or with existing disease in addition to apparently healthy individuals. The accompanying inset table below shows the different levels of certification within each track.

LEVELS OF CERTIFICATION WITHIN ACSM's CLINICAL AND HEALTH/FITNESS TRACKS

CLINICAL TRACK
- Program Director (PD)
- Exercise Specialist (ES)

HEALTH/FITNESS TRACK
- Health/Fitness Director (HFD)
- Health/Fitness Instructor (HFI)
- Exercise Leader (EL)

TABLE 32.2 ➤ ORGANIZATIONS THAT OFFER TRAINING/CERTIFICATION PROGRAMS RELATED TO PHYSICAL ACTIVITY

ORGANIZATION	AREAS OF SPECIALIZATION AND CERTIFICATION
Aerobics and Fitness Association of America (AFAA) www.afaa.com/	Aerobics Fitness Practitioner, Primary Aerobics Instructor, Personal Trainer & Fitness Counselor, Step Reebok Certification, Weight Room/Resistance Training Certification, Emergency Response Certification
American College of Sports Medicine (ACSM) www.acsm.org	Exercise Leader, Health/Fitness Instructor, Exercise Test Technologist, Health/Fitness Director, Exercise Specialist, Program Director
American Council on Exercise (ACE) www.acefitness.com/	Group Fitness Instructor, Personal Trainer, Lifestyle & Weight Management Consultant
Canadian Personal Trainers Network (CPTN) www.cptn.com/	CPTN/OFC Certified Personal Trainer, CPTN Certified Specialty Personal Trainer, CPTN/OFC Assessor of Personal Trainers, CPTN/OFC Course Conductor for Personal Trainers
Canadian Society for Exercise Physiology www.csep.ca/	CFC-Certified Fitness Consultant, PFLC-Professional Fitness and Lifestyle Consultant, AFAC-Accredited Fitness Appraisal Center
Cooper Institute for Aerobics Research www.cooperinst.org/	Certifications in Physical Fitness Specialist, Master Fitness Specialist, Biomechanics of Resistance Training Specialty, Providing Dietary Guidance: Nutrition Specialty, Fitness Specialist for Older Adults Specialty, Special Populations Specialty, Martial Arts Specialist, Group Exercise Leadership, Indoor Cycling Specialty, Aquatics Speciality, Health Promotion Director, Developing Lifestyle Physical Activity Programs, Physical Fitness Specialist, Master Fitness Specialist
International Sports Sciences Association (ISSA) www.issa-usa.com/	Certified Fitness Trainer, Golf Fitness Trainer, Fitness Therapist, Youth Fitness Trainer, Water Fitness Trainer, Aerobic Fitness Trainer; Specialist certificates in Performance Nutrition, Senior Fitness, Sports Conditioning, Martial Arts Conditioning, Fitness for the Physically Limited
Jazzercise www.jazzercise.com/	Certified Jazzercise Instructor
National Strength & Conditioning Association (NSCA) www.ncsa.com/	Certified Strength and Conditioning Specialist (CSCS), Certified Personal Trainer (NSCA-CPT)

Certification at a given level requires a knowledge and skill base commensurate with that specific certification. Additionally, each level has a minimum requirement for experience, level of education, or other ACSM certifications. Certification programs continually undergo review and revision to ensure the highest level of professionalism. Table 32.2 lists examples of other organizations that offer related training and/or certification programs.

CLINICAL APPLICATIONS OF EXERCISE PHYSIOLOGY TO ONCOLOGY, CARDIOVASCULAR DISEASE, AND PULMONARY DISABILITIES

The following sections present clinical applications of exercise physiology for the major areas of oncology, cardiovascular disease, and pulmonary system disabilities. We focus on these disabilities because they are currently the areas of greatest involvement for the exercise physiologist. We also present information regarding the effects of worksite wellness/fitness programs on individual participants and their corporations.

ONCOLOGY

Cancer is a group of diseases collectively characterized by uncontrolled growth and unchecked spread of abnormal cells that form larger-than-normal cell clusters that become tumors (see "On the Horizon"). More than 100 different types of cancers exist, most of which occur in adults.

Cancer Statistics

Cancer is the second leading cause of death in the United States, and approximately one-third of the population has cancer of some type (www.cancernet.nci.nih.gov/). In 2000, approximately 552,200 Americans died from cancer (1500 people per day), with approximately 1.25 million new cancer diagnoses. These estimates exclude noninvasive cancers (except noninvasive urinary bladder cancer), including basal cell and squamous cell cancers. In fact, skin cancers are more prevalent than any others, with 1.35 million basal cell and squamous cell skin cancer diagnoses expected in 2001 (www.skincancer.org). The overall age-adjusted cancer rate is 126 deaths per 1000 individuals.

For *mortality*, lung cancer represents the most prevalent cancer killer of all Americans, followed by cancers of the colon, rectum, breast, and prostate. Even considering men and women separately, lung cancer retains its number one rank as a killer, although mortality rate remains higher for men. Smoking accounts for more than 85% of all lung cancer deaths, and smoking tobacco, chewing smokeless tobacco, and regular exposure to environmental tobacco are blamed for one-third of all cancer deaths in the United States annually. After lung cancer, prostate cancer and colorectal cancer kill men the most often.

Among men, prostate cancer still strikes *most frequently*, and lung cancer moves into second place, followed by colon, rectal, and then bladder cancer. Cancer represents the leading cause of death in young women ages 25 to 44 years.[92] Breast cancer, by far the most prevalent form, exceeds lung, colorectal, and uterine cancers. Surprisingly, minorities (with their different cultural backgrounds and health and nutrition beliefs) consistently exhibit higher rates of cancer than whites.

Figure 32.5 shows estimated new cancer cases (**A**) and estimated deaths (**B**) combined and for male and females separately for 1999 for five different cancers. Figure 32.6 shows estimated new cancer cases by state. In 1999, there were 1,221,800 new cancer cases in the United States. A recent report on cancer incidence reveals a surprising statistic: the number of new cases of all cancers combined per 100,000 persons per year declined 0.8% per year between 1990 and 1997.[183] By far, the greatest decline occurred for men. Cancer death rates also declined 0.8% during the same period, perhaps the result of early diagnosis and aggressive treatment modalities. Public awareness and education programs aimed at early prostate screening for men, breast examinations for women, and colorectal examinations for both have had a positive impact on cancer detection and early treatment. The current population of more than 8 million cancer survivors (many of whom were diagnosed in the 1970s and 1980s) emphasizes the ongoing need for rehabilitative and maintenance options in this important area of medicine.

Cancer Rehabilitation Through Exercise

Regular physical activity helps the cancer patient to recuperate and return to a normal lifestyle with greater independence and functional capacity. For most cancer patients and survivors, loss of body mass and decreased energy level and functional status are the most serious outcomes, particularly following surgery and during chemotherapy and radiation therapy.[35,52,192] Loss of functional status includes difficulty walking more than one block and chronic fatigue that limits completion of routine household chores. Approximately 75% of cancer survivors report extreme fatigue during radiation therapy or chemotherapy, probably from weight loss and decreased muscular strength and cardiovascular endurance,[211] but a home-based regular exercise regimen can reduce feelings of fatigue[194,195] and enhance quality of life (and other biosocial outcomes) following cancer diagnosis.[47] Maintaining and restoring function present challenges to the cancer survivor, even patients considered "cured." Evidence justifies exercise intervention for breast cancer survivors.[92,177,196,224] In addition, nutritional intervention with regular exercise reduces the risk of contracting several forms of cancer.[42,168,185,210,217]

Table 32.3 lists general preventive and intervention goals for a cancer patient who faces sustained periods of inactivity, disuse, and bed rest. *Rehabilitating the patient to a level of function that allows return to work and pursuit of normal recreational activities is the overall goal of the health-*

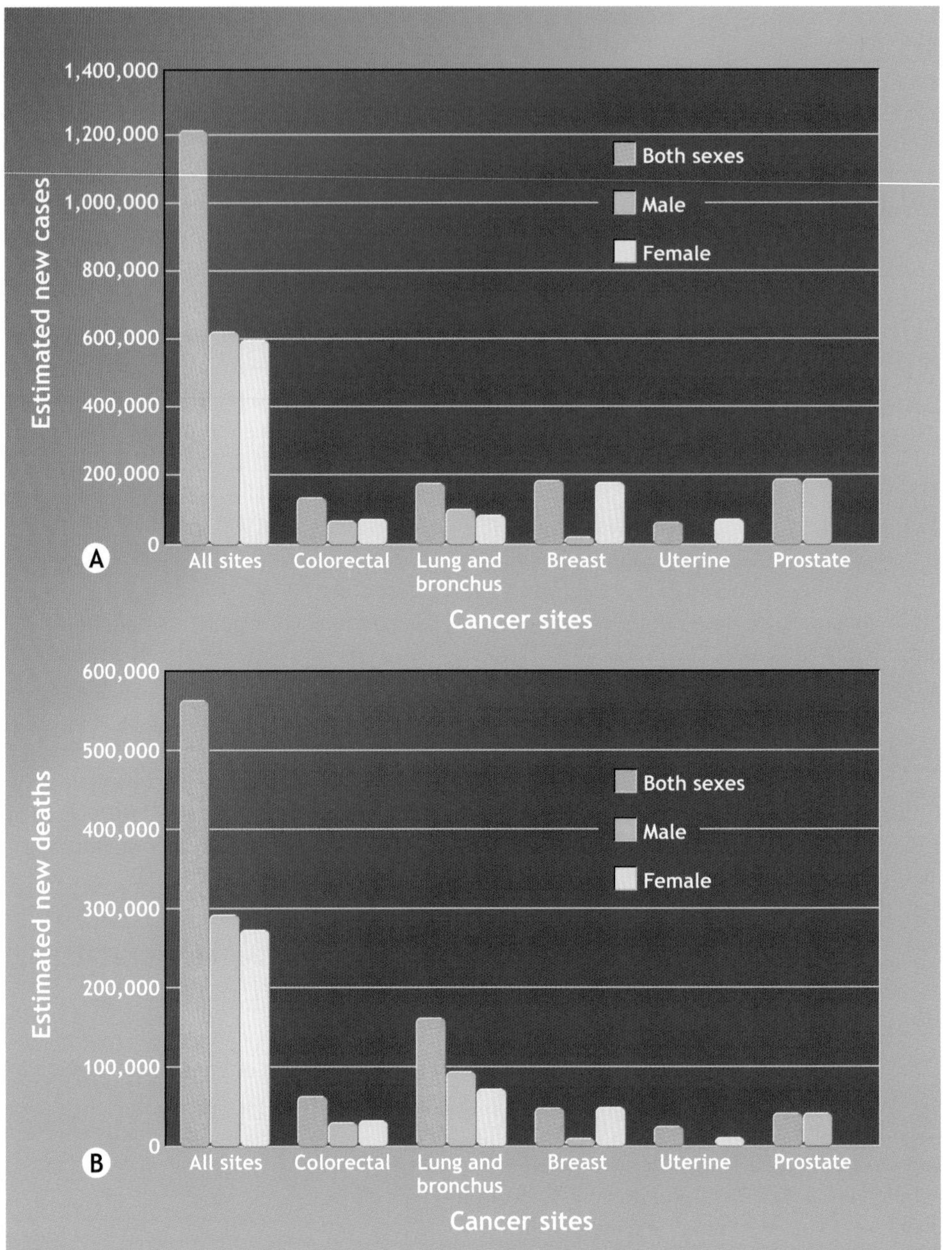

FIGURE 32.5 • A. Estimated number of new cancer cases. **B**. Cancer deaths during 1999. (Source: American Cancer Society, Surveillance Research, 1999.)

care team. Figure 32.7 shows the effects of a 6-week exercise rehabilitation program of treadmill walking weekdays at 80% (138 b · min^{-1}) of peak heart rate during a stress test for five cancer patients suffering severe fatigue.[52] During the first 3 weeks, each patient walked five intervals of 3 minutes, with 3 minutes of active recovery. Exercise duration increased weekly, with the number of exercise intervals reduced until the patient could complete one continuous 30- to 35-minute bout during week 6. Submaximal exercise heart rate and blood lactate concentration decreased significantly during exercise (Fig. 32.7A), while walking speed and distance and maximal performance on the stress test increased (Fig. 32.7B). All subjects increased daily physical activity level without substantial limitations, and they reported improved energy level. This clinical investigation did not meet the rigors of experimental research design (e.g., it lacked nonexercise control patients); nevertheless, the results highlight the positive potential of regular exercise for the physical and emotional rehabilitation of cancer patients.

Protective Effects of Exercise on Cancer

Firm epidemiologic evidence shows a significant inverse relation between amount of occupational or leisure time physical activity and reduction in all-cause cancer risk. For example, one review concludes that the magnitude of the protective effect of physical activity on estrogen-dependent cancer warrants including low-to-moderate exercise as a prudent preventive strategy.[119,217] Other large-scale, community-based studies of colorectal and prostatic hyperplasia indicate that in-

Alaska
0.228 %
New
Hampshire
0.456 %
Washington
0.484 %
Montana
0.466 %
Maine
0.563 %
Oregon
0.418 %
North Dakota
0.486 %
Minnesota
0.411 %
Vermont
0.440 %
Idaho
0.374 %
MA
0.499 %
Wisconsin
0.454 %
South Dakota
0.461 %
Wyoming
0.416 %
New York
0.457 %
Michigan
0.450 %
RI 0.526 %
Nevada
0.464 %
Nebraska
0.445 %
Iowa
0.500 %
CT
0.461 %
Pennsylvania
0.555 %
Utah
0.248 %
New Jersey
0.493 %
California
0.344 %
Illinois
0.472%
Indiana
0.473%
Ohio
0.504 %
Colorado
0.335 %
Delaware 0.511 %
Kansas
0.456 %
Missouri
0.513 %
Virginia
0.427 %
Maryland 0.440 %
Kentucky
0.521 %
West Virginia
0.585 %
Arizona
0.344 %
South Carolina
0.467 %
Oklahoma
0.472 %
New Mexico
0.374 %
Tennessee
0.493 %
Arkansas
0.544 %
North
Carolina
0.470 %
Alabama
0.485 %
Georgia
0.381 %
Texas
0.392 %
Louisiana
0.465 %
Mississippi
0.472 %
Florida
0.590 %
Hawaii
0.360 %

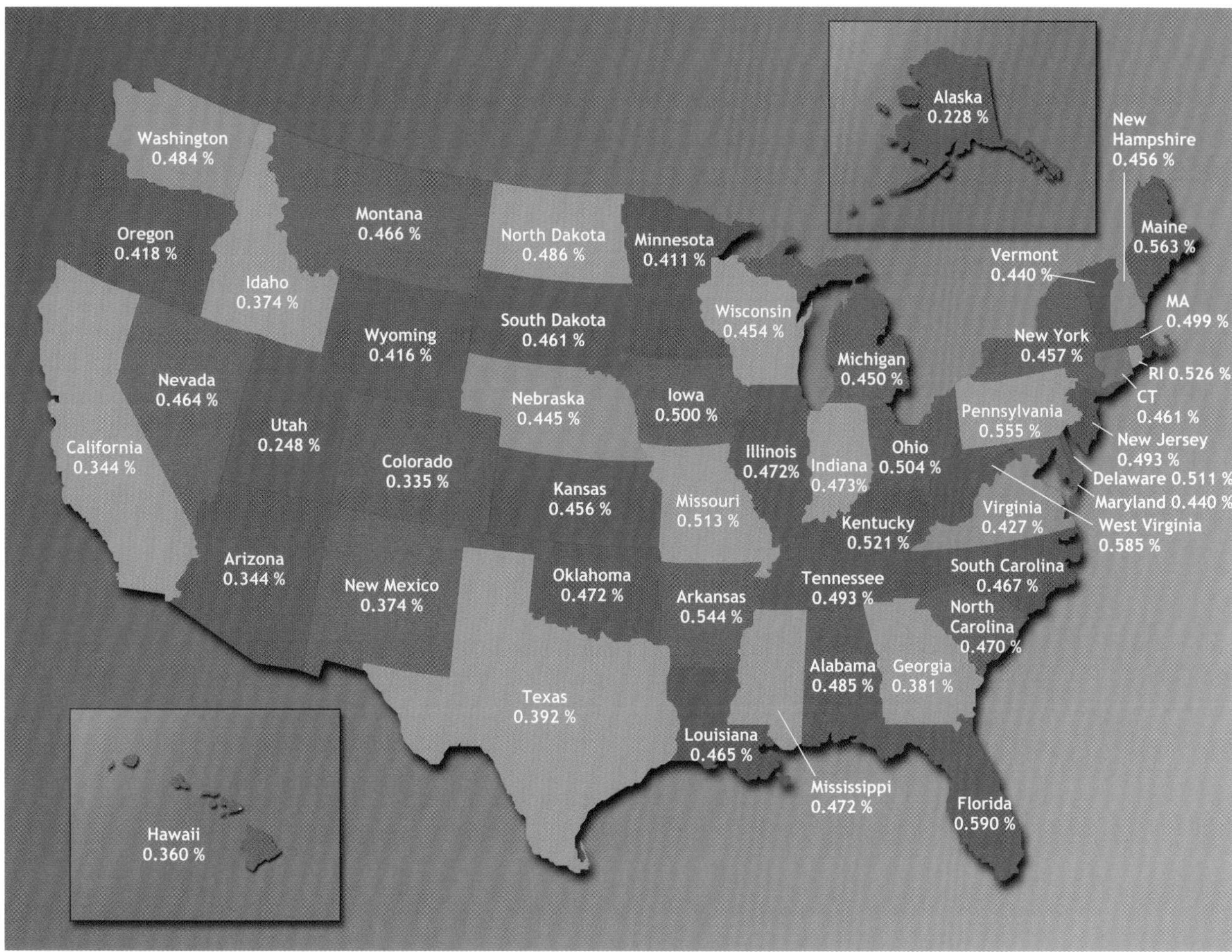

FIGURE 32.6 • Estimates of percentage of each state's total population with *new cases* of cancer in 1999. Excludes basal and squamous cell skin cancers and *in situ* carcinomas except urinary bladder. (Data for cancer estimates from American Cancer Society, Surveillance Research, 1999; data on population by state from U.S. Census.)

creased physical activity significantly reduces cancer risk and mortality.[97,127,137,138,174] For example, a study of nearly 122,000 women found that exercising at least 1 hour daily reduced breast cancer risk by 20%.[185] Furthermore, the proportion of men at high risk for colon cancer would decrease significantly if the men could eliminate the modifiable risk factors including physical inactivity and excessive red meat consumption, obesity, alcohol consumption, cigarette smoking, and low folic acid intake.[175]

Several hypotheses explain how exercise reduces cancer risk. For example, the mechanism for breast cancer risk reduction may involve the lowering effect of exercise on estrogen, a hormone that stimulates breast cell growth. Regular physical activity also lowers circulating levels of blood glucose and insulin and increases corticosteroid hormones. Exercise increases anti-inflammatory cytokine levels and augments insulin-receptor expression in cancer-fighting T cells. In addition, physical activity promotes interferon production, stimulates glycogen synthetase, enhances leukocyte function, improves ascorbic acid metabolism, and exerts beneficial effects on provirus or oncogene activation—all of which could thwart cancerous tumor formation. Physical activity also ap-

TABLE 32.3 ➤ TEN GENERAL TREATMENT GOALS OF THE CLINICAL EXERCISE PHYSIOLOGIST FOR PATIENTS WITH DECONDITIONING, IMMOBILITY, OR DISUSE SYNDROMES

1. Improve patient's overall functional status
2. Improve active motion for nonrestrictive segments and joints
3. Prevent loss of flexibility by active motion and passive movements
4. Stimulate peripheral and central circulation through active motion exercise based on current functional level
5. Increase ventilatory function with systematic breathing exercises
6. Prevent thrombosis through physical activities
7. Prevent loss of motor control and muscle strength and endurance with resistance exercises
8. Reduce the rate of bone loss through weight-bearing aerobic and muscle-strengthening exercises
9. Through active aerobic and resistance exercise, slow the loss of fat-free body mass and subsequent reduction of BMR that accompanies deconditioning
10. Monitor signs of increased fatigue or weakness, lethargy, dyspnea, pallor, dizziness, claudication, or cramping during or following exercise

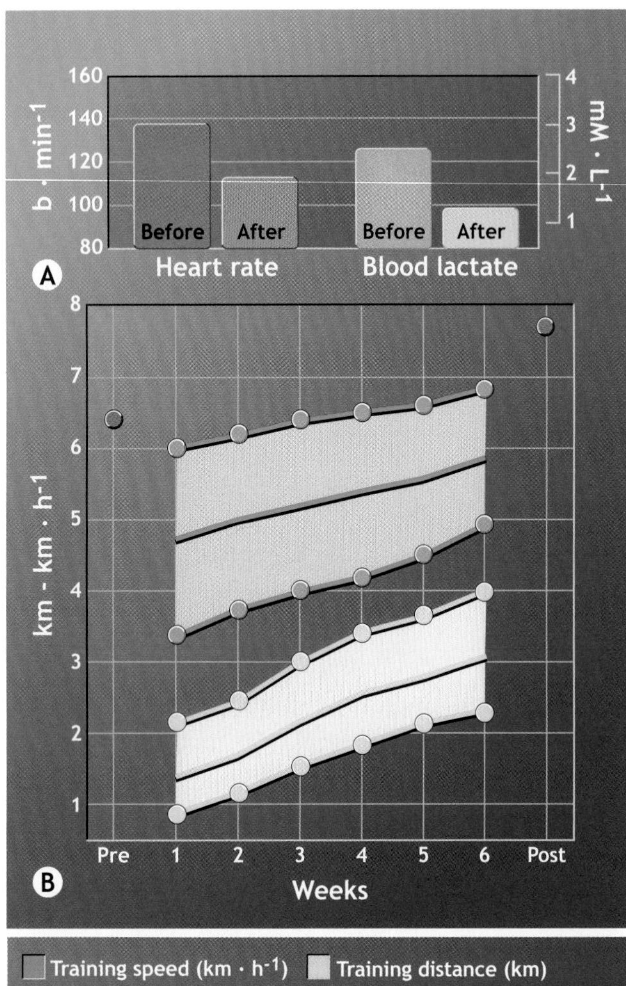

FIGURE 32.7 • **A**. Reduction in heart rate and blood lactate concentration during submaximal walking at 5 km · h^{-1} following six weeks of exercise rehabilitation in five cancer patients suffering severe fatigue. **B**. Weekly changes in training speed (km · h^{-1}) and daily distance walked (km) and pre- and posttraining maximal exercise performance. (From Dimeo F, et al. Aerobic exercise as therapy for cancer fatigue. Med Sci Sports Exerc 1998;30:475.)

pears to reduce the volume and, to a lesser degree, the number of metastatic foci in the lungs of certain rodents fed high-lipid diets.[42] Although few human studies causally link increased physical activity to cancer prevention, the cross-sectional data in Table 32.4 support this link.

Exercise Prescription and Cancer

Research evidence from exercising animals, former athletes, people in active occupations, and those with active recreational lifestyles justifies an important role for physical activity in cancer rehabilitation. Less certainty exists regarding the proper exercise prescription for cancer patients, and little research has addressed the timing of exercise relative to the various phases of cancer treatment. Thus, determining the best time to initiate exercise intervention in the recovery process remains problematic, but results have been encouraging.[147,151] Thirty-five stomach cancer patients were placed in an exercise or control group immediately following curative surgery. From postoperative day 2, patients performed arm and leg ergometer exercise twice daily, 5 days per week for 14 days at 60% of maximal heart rate. The early exercise intervention significantly increased natural killer cell cytotoxic activity in the exercise group compared to the control group. Furthermore, no information exists regarding the proper dose of exercise or the corresponding response of specific cancers to exercise intervention among patients of different ages. In light of limited information, exercise prescription recommendations for cancer rehabilitation generally include symptom-limited, progressive, and individualized physical activities. Ambulation of any kind as soon as practical becomes important for the most sedentary and deconditioned patients. *Emphasis should focus on intervals of low-to-moderate aerobic activity performed several times daily rather than one relatively strenuous bout of continuous exercise.* A dose–response relationship seems to emerge between increased physical activity and improved health and functional capacity among cancer patients.[92] Most sedentary patients derive clinically significant benefits by accumulating up to 30 minutes of daily walking (or equivalent energy expenditure in other activities). Health benefits accrue whether activity takes the form of structured exercise, home-based programs, or sport, household, occupational, or recreational activities.

Cancer patients initially receive a symptom-limited, graded exercise test (GXT) on a treadmill or cycle ergome-

TABLE 32.4 ➤ **PHYSICAL ACTIVITY AND CANCER DEVELOPMENT**[a]

Subjects	Type of Activity	Cancer Type	Protection
Human (M + F)	Normal	Large bowel	Yes
Human (F)	Sports	Breast	Yes
Human (M)	Job	Colon	Yes
Human (M + F)	Job	Colon	Yes
Human (M + F)	Recreation	Left colon	Yes
Human (M)	Sports	Colon	Yes
Human (M)	Recreation	All cause	Yes
Human (M + F)	Sports	All cause	Yes
Animal	Voluntary	Mammary	Yes
Animal	Voluntary	Flank	Yes
Animal	Voluntary	Pancreas	Yes
Animal	Forced	Flank	No
Animal	Forced	Mammary	Yes

[a]Review of 13 studies reporting a relationship between physical activity and cancer protection. All of the human studies surveyed individuals in different settings such as occupational, recreational, sports, and randomly from all settings (normal). Subjects were classified based on levels of physical activity, ranging from sedentary to physically active. M, male; F, female. The recreation and sports studies included estimates of caloric expenditure during the day. Cancer protection was defined as relative risk or percentage increase in the development of the disease. In 12 of the 13 studies, increased protection differed significantly from a chance occurrence.

ter as the basis for their exercise prescription. Testing procedures remain the same as those for healthy individuals, except the patient receives greater attention about their sensations of fatigue. Generally, patients should not exercise to maximum. The exercise prescription initially aims to produce ambulation if the patient has no specific contraindications. The prescription also provides for range-of-motion movements and other exercises to improve muscular strength, augment fat-free body mass (FFM), and improve overall mobility (e.g., submaximal static exercises of the antigravity muscles, deep breathing exercises, and dynamic trunk rotation movements). Exercise progression and intensity are individualized, with initial work:rest ratios of 1:1 increasing to 2:1. Eventually, continuous exercise for up to 15 minutes can replace intermittent exercise bouts.

Breast Cancer Rehabilitation and Exercise

Carcinoma of the breast is the most common form of cancer in white females aged 40 years and older; it causes the greatest number of deaths in women between the ages of 40 and 55 years. In 2000, 183,000 new invasive breast cancer cases were diagnosed and almost 25% of those died (1 every 13 min). This means that one of every nine females contracts breast cancer at some time during her life, with a high rate of reoccurrence.[3] By age 30, the chances of being diagnosed with breast cancer is 1 out of 2000; by age 40, the chances increase tremendously to 1 and 233, and 1 in 22 by age 60. However, the disease is not limited to females: a greater percentage of men than women died from breast cancer in the year 2000 (29% of almost 1400 cases). *Risk factors for breast cancer include family history, personal history of cancer, first menstrual period at an early age, menopause at a late age, first child born after age 30 or no childbirth, and a high-fat diet.*

Improved functional capacity from regular aerobic exercise and circuit-resistance training in breast cancer rehabilitation also produces important "psychologic" benefits. In a study from one of our laboratories, 28 patients recovering from breast cancer surgery enrolled in a 10-week circuit-resistance training program to evaluate the effects of exercise on depression, self-esteem, and anxiety.[197] Patients performed hydraulic resistance exercises in a 14-station aerobic exercise circuit 4 days per week, with the self-paced, individualized program adjusted to meet patient needs and fitness levels. Figure 32.8 shows the changes for depression, trait anxiety, and state anxiety. Exercisers exhibited a 38% decrease in depression, compared with a 13% increase for nonexercising counterparts recovering from breast cancer surgery. The exercisers also showed a 16% decrease in trait anxiety and a 20% reduction in state anxiety, compared with significant increases in both variables for the nonexercising patients. These results demonstrate a potent effect of regular exercise on psychosocial variables during breast cancer rehabilitation. Such findings certainly support structured, moderate exercise in a comprehensive breast cancer rehabilitation program.

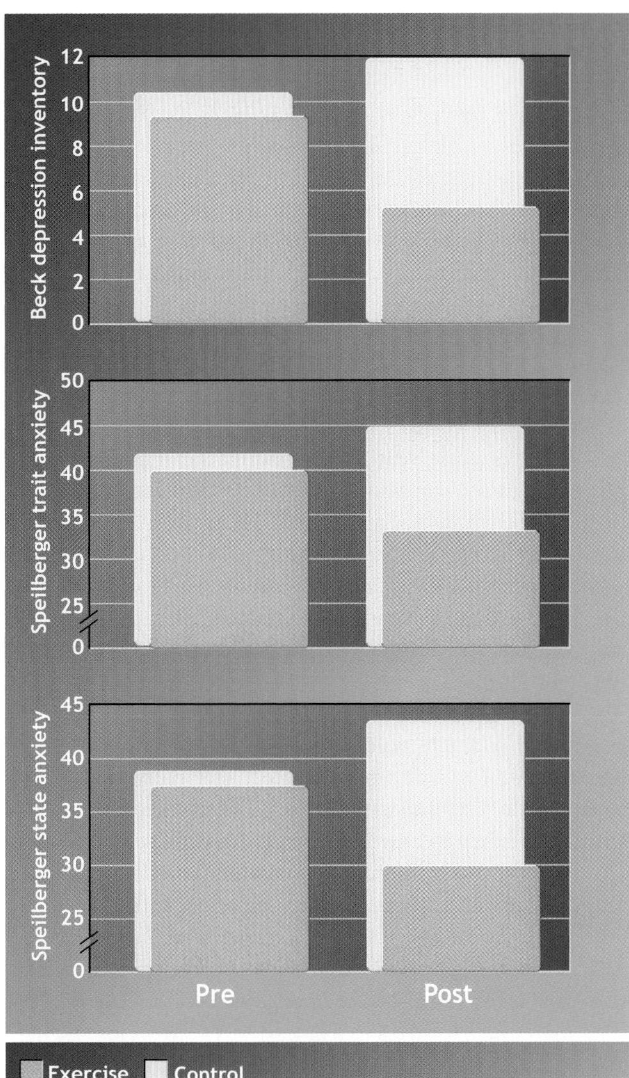

FIGURE 32.8 • Effects of 10 weeks of moderate aerobic exercise on depression (*top*), and trait (*middle*) and state (*bottom*) anxiety in 28 women recovering from breast cancer surgery. (From Segar ML, et al. The effect of aerobic exercise on self-esteem and depressive and anxiety symptoms among breast cancer survivors. Oncol Nurs Forum 1998;25:107.)

Nutrition and Cancer

Diet relates to approximately one-third of the cancer deaths in the United States each year, with another one-third linked to smoking. Many dietary factors affect cancer risk, including type of food, its preparation, portion sizes, diversity, and overall energy balance. Diets with a high proportion of fruits, vegetables, grains, and beans and limited amounts of meat, dairy products, and other high-fat foods may reduce cancer risk, most recently reported for colon cancer.[203]

Based on a review of scientific evidence, the American Cancer Society (www.cancer.org) revised its nutritional guidelines in 1996 (previously updated in 1991). The society's new recommendations agree in principle with the 1992 USDA Food Guide Pyramid, the 1995 Dietary Guidelines for Americans, and the dietary recommendations of other agencies that promote healthful behaviors to prevent coronary heart disease, type 2 diabetes, and other diet-related chronic conditions.

CARDIOVASCULAR DISEASES

Chapter 21 examines the effects of regular exercise on cardiovascular function, aerobic capacity, and exercise performance. In this section, we examine the specific application of exercise in rehabilitating patients with cardiovascular disease.

Overview and Scope of Cardiovascular Disease

Cardiovascular disease, the leading cause of death in industrialized nations, accounts for nearly 1.1 million deaths in the United States each year (www.americanheart.org/). One in four Americans (60 million) experience some form of cardiovascular disease in their lifetime.[6] Fortunately, disease and death rates have declined during the 1990s—a 60% lower coronary heart disease death rate since its peak in the 1960s—partly due to aggressive efforts to reduce risk factors through early screening and implementation of heart disease prevention and rehabilitation programs.[78,186]

Aerobic exercise programs for cardiac patients consider the specific pathophysiology of the disease, the mechanisms that may limit exercise performance, and individual differences in functional capacity. Table 32.5 lists three general categories of heart disease that cause functional impairment. Diseases of the heart muscle (myocardium) predominate, particularly with advancing age. Any one of the following terms indicates myocardial disease: *degenerative heart disease* (DHD), *atherosclerotic cardiovascular disease, arteriosclerotic cardiovascular disease, coronary artery disease* (CAD), or *coronary heart disease* (CHD). In this text, we use CHD.

Because hypertension represents a primary risk for CHD, we first discuss blood pressure stratification and subsequent treatment recommendations. We then review the role of exercise training in preventing and treating hypertension.

Blood Pressure: Classification and Risk Stratification

Hypertension (www.bloodpressure.com), as Chapter 15 discusses, afflicts between 33 and 57% of men and 25 and 60% of women between ages 45 and 74 years (see Fig. 15.8). Hypertension prevalence increases sharply with age and is higher in men than in women and in blacks than in whites. Table 32.6 presents the standard classification of blood pressure for adults age 18 and older. Recommendations for initial screening and subsequent risk stratification and treatment are found in Table 32.7.

TABLE 32.5 ➤ CARDIAC DISEASES THAT CAUSE FUNCTIONAL IMPAIRMENT

DISEASES AFFECTING THE HEART MUSCLE	DISEASES AFFECTING HEART VALVES	DISEASES AFFECTING THE CARDIAC NERVOUS SYSTEM
CHD	Rheumatic fever	Arrhythmias
Angina	Endocarditis	Tachycardia
Myocardial infarct	Mitral valve prolapse	Bradycardia
Pericarditis	Congenital deformations	
Congestive heart failure		
Aneurysms		

TABLE 32.6 ➤ CLASSIFICATION OF BLOOD PRESSURE FOR ADULTS AGE 18 YEARS AND OLDER

CATEGORY	SYSTOLIC (MM HG)		DIASTOLIC (MM HG)
Optimal	<120	and	<80
Normal	120-129	and	80-84
High normal	130-139	or	85-89
Hypertension			
Stage 1	140-159	or	90-99
Stage 2	160-179	or	100-109
Stage 3	≥180	or	≥110

From Sixth report of the Joint Committee on Prevention, Detection, Evaluation, and Treatment of High Blood Pressure (JNVI), Public Health Service, National Institutes of Health, National Heart, Lung and Blood Institute, NIH Publ. no. 98-4080, Nov 1997. This classification should be used with individuals not taking antihypertensive medication and not acutely ill. When systolic and diastolic blood pressures fall into different categories, the higher category should be used to classify status. For example, 160/92 mm Hg would be stage 2 and 174/120 mm Hg, stage 3.

Chronic hypertension damages arterial vessels; it serves as a primary risk for arteriosclerosis, heart disease, stroke, and kidney failure. In many instances, regular exercise provides a prudent first line of defense to treat mild hypertension (140–159 mm Hg systolic; 90–99 mm Hg diastolic) and moderate hypertension (160–179 mm Hg systolic; 100–109 mm Hg diastolic).

Exercise Training and Hypertension

Systolic and diastolic blood pressures decrease by 6 to 10 mm Hg with aerobic exercise training in previously sedentary men and women regardless of age. However, exercise intensity may be a consideration as even a brisk walking program may not provide a satisfactory stimulus to evoke a hypotensive effect.[44] Beneficial results occur with normotensive and hypertensive subjects during rest and exercise.[12,51,80,118,159,212,222] Regular aerobic exercise as preventive therapy also helps to control the tendency for blood pressure to increase over time in individuals at risk for hypertension.[167]

The effects of exercise training on blood pressure become most apparent in patients with mild hypertension.[4,41,82,117,154] Table 32.8 shows that average resting systolic blood pressure in seven middle-aged male patients decreased from 139 to 133 mm Hg following 4 to 6 weeks of interval training. During submaximal exercise, systolic pressure decreased from 173 to 155 mm Hg, while diastolic pressure decreased from 92 to 79 mm Hg. Consequently, training produced approximately a 14% decrease in mean arterial exercise blood pressure. Similar results occurred for an apparently healthy yet borderline hypertensive group of 37 middle-aged men following 6

TABLE 32.7 ➤ RISK STRATIFICATION AND RECOMMENDED TREATMENT FOR HYPERTENSION

Blood Pressure Stages (mm Hg) (see Table 32.6)	Risk Group A (no risk factors; no TOD[a] or CCD[b])	Risk Group B (one risk factor not including diabetes; no TOD or CCD)	Risk Group C (TOD and/or CCD and/or diabetes, with or without other risk factors)
High-normal 130-139/85-89	Lifestyle modification	Lifestyle modification	Drug therapy
Stage 1 140-159/90-99	Lifestyle modification (up to 12 mo)	Lifestyle modification (up to 6 mo)	Drug therapy
Stages 2 and 3 ≥160/≥100	Drug therapy	Drug therapy	Drug therapy

[a]TOD, target organ disease.
[b]CCD, clinical cardiovascular disease.
For example, a person with diabetes, blood pressure of 142/94 mm Hg, and left ventricular hypertrophy classifies as having stage 1 hypertension with target organ disease (left ventricular hypertrophy) and another major risk factor (diabetes). This patient would be classified as stage 1, risk group C, and recommended for immediate drug therapy.
From: Sixth report of the Joint Committee on Prevention, Detection, Evaluation, and Treatment of High Blood Pressure (JNVI), Public Health Service, National Institutes of Health, National Heart, Lung and Blood Institute, NIH Publication no. 98-4080, Nov 1997.

TABLE 32.8 ➤ BLOOD PRESSURE DURING REST AND SUBMAXIMAL EXERCISE BEFORE AND AFTER 4 TO 6 WEEKS OF TRAINING IN SEVEN MIDDLE-AGED CHD PATIENTS

	Rest			Submaximal Exercise		
	Average Value		Difference (%)	Average Value		Difference (%)
Measure[a]	Before	After		Before	After	
Systolic blood pressure (mm Hg)	139	133	−4.3	173	155	−10.4
Diastolic blood pressure (mm Hg)	78	73	−6.4	92	79	−14.1
Mean blood pressure (mm Hg)	97	92	−5.2	127	109	−14.3

[a]Intra-arterial catheter.
Modified from Clausen JP, et al. Physical training in the management of coronary artery disease. Circulation 1969;40:143.

months of regular aerobic exercise.[38] For hypertensive older men and women, 9 months of low-intensity, aerobic exercise lowered systolic blood pressure by 20 mm Hg and diastolic pressure by 12 mm Hg.[82] Figure 32.9 shows changes in resting blood pressure with aerobic training and 1 month of detraining in elderly hypertensive men and women who trained at the lactate threshold three to six times a week for 9 months.[51] Baseline values 3 months prior to training indicate subjects' blood pressures with normal antihypertensive drug therapy. Regular exercise (with continued medication) produced decreases of 15 mm Hg in systolic blood pressure, 11 mm Hg in mean arterial pressure, and 9 mm Hg in diastolic blood pressure. Blood pressure returned to pretraining levels within 1 month for the five subjects who discontinued training.

The precise mechanism(s) for how regular exercise lowers blood pressure remains unknown. Significant contributing factors may include:

- Reduced sympathetic nervous system activity with training and possible normalization of arteriole morphology decrease peripheral resistance to blood flow and so lowers blood pressure.[2,51,57,164]
- Altered renal function facilitates the kidneys' elimination of sodium, which subsequently reduces fluid volume and hence blood pressure.[212]

The ACSM's "Position Stand on Physical Activity, Physical Fitness, and Hypertension" can be accessed at connection.lww.com/go/mcardle.

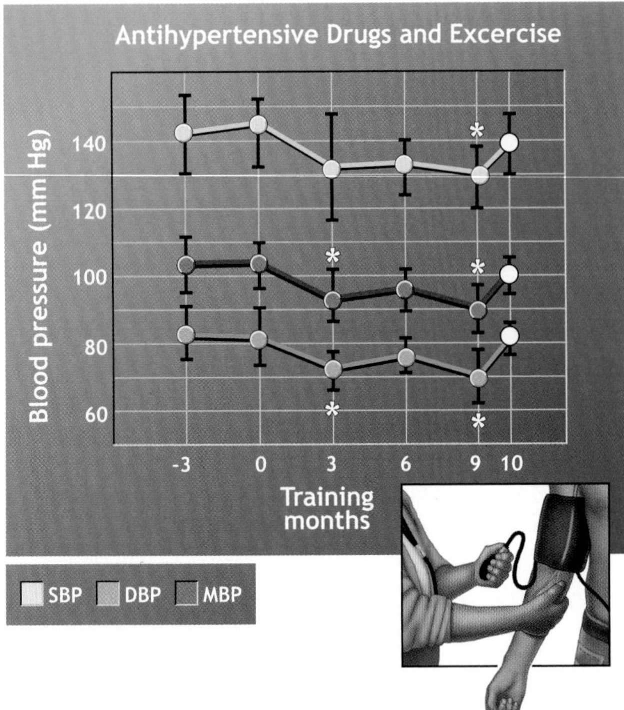

FIGURE 32.9 • Blood pressure changes following 9 months of exercise training at the lactate threshold and after 1 month of detraining (five subjects). Baseline values 3 months before training (−3) indicate subjects' blood pressures with their normal antihypertensive drug therapy only. Statistical analyses compared values during training with the same findings at month 0. *SBP,* systolic blood pressure; *MBP,* mean blood pressure; *DBP,* diastolic blood pressure; *, statistically significant from baseline value. (From Motoyama M, et al. Blood pressure lowering effect of low intensity aerobic training in elderly hypertensive patients. Med Sci Sports Exerc 1998;30:818.)

Not all research supports exercise as a way to treat hypertension. For example, studies with animal models for hypertension have not demonstrated consistent benefit from regular regimens of forced exercise.[69] Even when research shows that regular exercise lowers blood pressure in humans, the studies often have methodological shortcomings and inadequate design. The lack of appropriate control subjects who have their blood pressure measured but do not exercise is usually the most glaring research design weakness. *Despite these limitations, it remains prudent to recommend regular aerobic exercise and proper diet to induce weight loss (where necessary) as a first line of defense in managing borderline hypertension.*[4,80,107,205]

Improved fitness often neutralizes increased mortality associated with elevated blood pressure. Even if exercise does not bring blood pressure to a normal level, aerobic training confers independent health benefits. In one study, aerobically fit individuals with hypertension had a 60% lower mortality rate than their unfit normotensive peers.[21] More-severe elevations in blood pressure require pharmacologic intervention (more than 60 drugs and 30 pill combinations are available for treatment; see Fig. 15.10).

Chronic Resistance Training Effects on Blood Pressure

Despite the relatively large rise in blood pressure during heavy resistance exercise, long-term resistance training does *not* elevate resting blood pressure.[43,60,83,169] In fact, resistance training lessens the typical short-term blood pressure increases during this exercise mode.[60] Trained bodybuilders, for example, show smaller increases in systolic and diastolic blood pressures with resistance exercise than novice bodybuilders and untrained individuals.[60,189] The diminished blood pressure response posttraining becomes most evident when a person exercises at the same absolute load during pretraining and posttraining measurements.[142] Some resistance training protocols lower resting blood pressure,[81,221] but most research finds that aerobic exercise training (not standard resistance training) confers the greater blood pressure–lowering benefits for hypertensives.[108,109,162,167] *As a general guideline, heavy resistance training should not serve as the sole exercise mode to lower blood pressure in hypertensive individuals.*

Diseases of the Myocardium

Recent advances in molecular biology have isolated a possible genetic link to CHD. The gene, termed the **atherosclerosis susceptibility (ATHS) gene** (www.hgmp.mrc.ac.uk), appears on chromosome 19, near the gene that regulates the receptor that removes low-density lipoprotein cholesterol (LDL-C) from the blood.[208] The ATHS gene accounts for nearly 50% of the 13.5 million cases of CHD in the United States.[156] It apparently expresses a set of characteristics—abdominal obesity, low levels of high-density lipoprotein cholesterol (HDL-C), and high levels of LDL-C—that triple a person's risk of myocardial infarction (MI).

Symptoms rarely present in the early stages of CHD. As the disease progresses and coronary arteries narrow, clinical symptoms become evident and advance with increasing severity. The first sign of CHD is often slight angina pain accompanied by decreased functional capacity. This eventually leads to ischemia (reduced blood flow) and possible necrosis of myocardial tissue. In severe cases, the patient usually experiences persistent chest pain, anxiety, nausea, vomiting, and dyspnea. Chronic, untreated angina weakens the myocardium and eventually produces heart failure as cardiac output fails to meet the body's metabolic demands. Often, pulmonary congestion (with a persistent cough) accompanies heart failure, and the patient coughs up blood. At this stage, the patient becomes dyspneic, even when sitting at rest, and can suffer a sudden MI.

The pathogenesis of CHD probably progresses as follows:

- Injury to the endothelial cell wall of the coronary artery
- Fibroblastic proliferation of the inner lining (intima) of the artery
- Further obstruction of blood flow as fat accumulates at the junction of the arterial intima and middle lining
- Cellular degeneration and subsequent formation of hyalin (a clear, homogeneous substance produced in degeneration) within the arterial intima
- Calcium deposition at the edges of hyalinated area

The major disorders caused by reduced myocardial blood supply in CHD include angina pectoris, MI, and congestive heart failure.

Angina Pectoris

Chest-related pain called **angina pectoris** *occurs in approximately 30% of initial manifestations of CHD. This temporary but painful condition indicates that coronary blood flow (and thus oxygen supply) momentarily reaches inadequate levels.* Current theory suggests that metabolites within an ischemic segment of the heart muscle stimulate myocardial pain receptors. The sensation of angina pectoris includes squeezing, burning, and pressing or choking in the chest region, sensations that often mimic the discomforts of benign heartburn (Table 32.9). Anginal pain usually lasts 1 to 3 minutes. Approximately one-third of individuals who experience recurring anginal episodes die suddenly from an MI. Several types of angina exist, including chronic stable angina (often called *walk-through* angina), which occurs at a predictable level of physical exertion. Drugs that promote coronary artery vasodilation and reduce systemic peripheral vascular resistance (e.g., nitroglycerin) commonly treat this condition. Figure 32.10 illustrates the usual pain pattern associated with an acute episode of angina pectoris. Pain generally appears in the left shoulder along the arm to the elbow or occasionally in the midback region, near the left scapula, along the spinal cord.

TABLE 32.9 ➤ COMPARISON OF SYMPTOMS OF ANGINA AND HEARTBURN

ANGINA	HEARTBURN
• Gripping, viselike feelings of pain or pressure behind the breast bone	• Frequent feeling of heartburn
• Pain that radiates to the neck, jaw, back, shoulders, or arms (usually left)	• Frequent use of antacids to relieve pain
• Toothache	• Heartburn wakes person up at night
• Burning indigestion	• Acid or bitter taste in mouth
• Shortness of breath	• Burning chest sensastion
• Nausea	• Discomfort after eating spicy food
• Frequent belching	• Difficulty swallowing

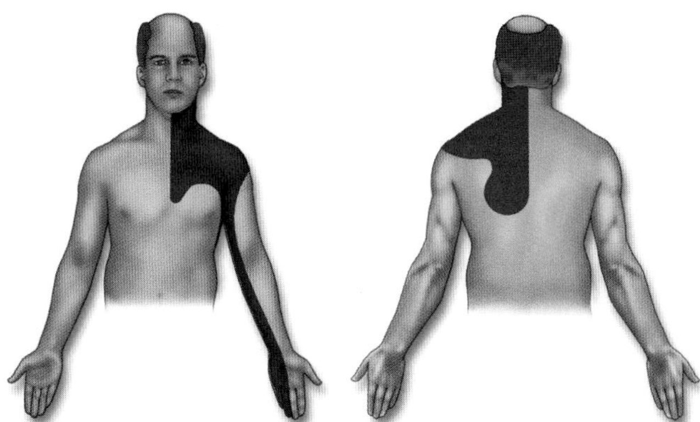

FIGURE 32.10 • Locations for pain generally associated with angina pectoris.

Myocardial Infarction

Each year, 1.5 million **myocardial infarctions** occur with 500,000 fatalities. MI (heart attack, or coronary occlusion) results from a sudden insufficiency in myocardial blood flow, usually from occlusion of a coronary artery. A prior clot (thrombus) formed from plaque accumulation in one or more of the coronary vessels (see Chapter 31) can trigger sudden occlusion. Severe fatigue for several days without specific pain frequently precedes the onset of MI. Figure 32.11 shows the varied locations for pain and discomfort that represent an early warning of an MI. During the infarction, severe, unrelenting chest pain can persist for more than 1 hour.

Congestive Heart Failure

In **congestive heart failure** (**CHF**, chronic decompensation, or simply heart failure), the heart fails to pump enough blood to meet the needs of other organs. CHF results from one or all of the following:

- Narrowed arteries from CHD that limit myocardial blood supply
- Past MI with accompanying scar tissue (necrosis) that diminishes myocardial pumping efficiency
- Chronic hypertension
- Heart valve disease from past rheumatic fever or other pathology
- Primary disease of the myocardium, called *cardiomyopathy*
- Defects present in the heart at birth (congenital heart disease)
- Infection of heart valves and/or myocardium (endocarditis or myocarditis)

A "failing" heart keeps pumping but inefficiently. Heart failure produces shortness of breath and fatigue with minimal exertion. As blood flowing out of the heart slows, blood returning to the heart through the veins backs up, causing fluid to accumulate in the lungs and edema in the legs and ankles. When fluid collects in the lungs, it interferes with breathing, causing shortness of breath, especially when lying down. CHF also affects the kidneys' disposal of sodium and water, further accentuating edema.

CHF, the only form of heart disease on the increase, afflicts approximately 5 million Americans (500,000 new cases diagnosed and 250,000 deaths each year). It is the most common cause for hospitalization of people older than age 65 (responsible for more than 800,000 hospital stays, including many repeat visits). Figure 32.12 shows the consequences of CHF when the heart fails to pump adequately. This figure also shows that nearly one-third (1.4 million) of CHF patients contract the disease before age 60; 20% of patients die within 1 year of diagnosis, and nearly one-half die within 5 years.

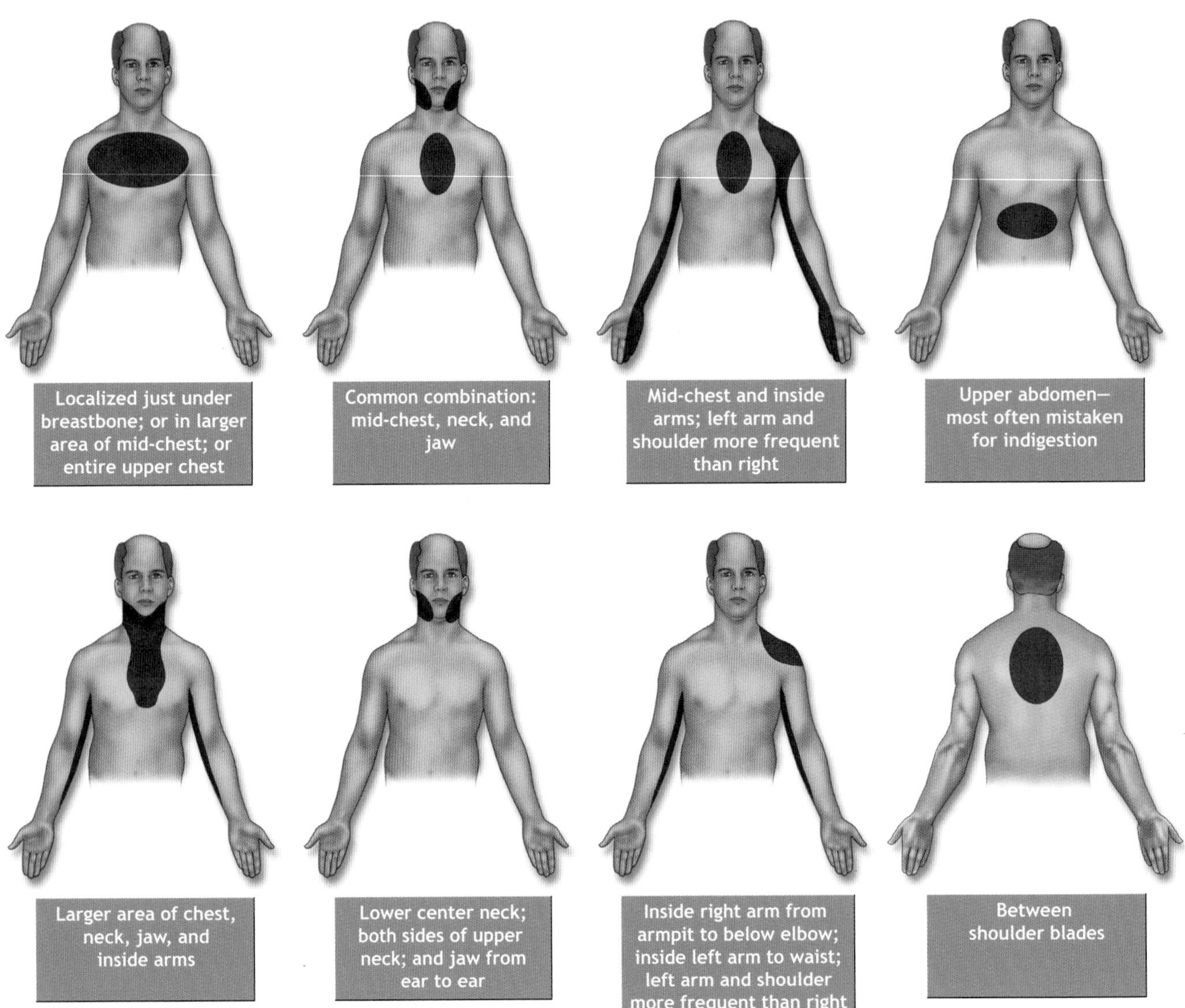

FIGURE 32.11 • Anatomic locations for early warning signs of myocardial infarction. Note the diverse locations for pain.

CHF usually develops slowly as the heart gradually weakens and performs less effectively. Primary causes include (1) chronic hypertension, (2) intrinsic myocardial disease, or (3) structural defects (e.g., diseased heart valves). These conditions produce an oversized, misshapen heart with inadequate pump performance reflected by a low resting left ventricular ejection fraction (LVEF)—a marker of life-threatening heart dysfunction—and failure to increase heart rate with exercise.[64,105] Associated risk factors include diabetes, alcoholism, and chronic lung diseases such as emphysema. CHF symptoms produce extreme disability, but symptom intensity frequently bears little relation to disease severity.[9,166] For example, patients with a low LVEF may not exhibit symptoms, while individuals whose hearts demonstrate essentially normal pump function can experience severe disability. Heart disease and chronic hypertension contribute significantly to disease progression. At the extreme stage, cardiac output from the left and/or right ventricles decreases so much that blood accumulates in the abdomen and lungs and sometimes in the feet and legs. This stage of CHF produces fatigue, shortness of breath, and eventual flooding of the alveoli with blood, a condition termed *pulmonary congestion*. Impaired blood flow may also damage other organs, particularly the kidneys. Nearly 70,000 CHF patients qualify yearly for heart transplantation. Heart failure can affect the right and left heart, although each demonstrates different symptomatologies and progression depending on time of intervention.

CHF TREATMENT AND REHABILITATION. Before the 1980s, treatment for all stages of CHF advocated rest as the first-line defense to reduce stress on the compromised cardiovascular system. Until recently, patients routinely received drugs aimed primarily at easing symptoms (e.g., digitalis to increase the heart's pumping function [inotropic effect]). Current recommendations promote a four-drug regimen with two traditional drugs, digitalis and a diuretic (to increase fluid excretion by kidneys), with newer angiotensin-converting enzyme (ACE) inhibitors and β-blockers. These two latter drugs have

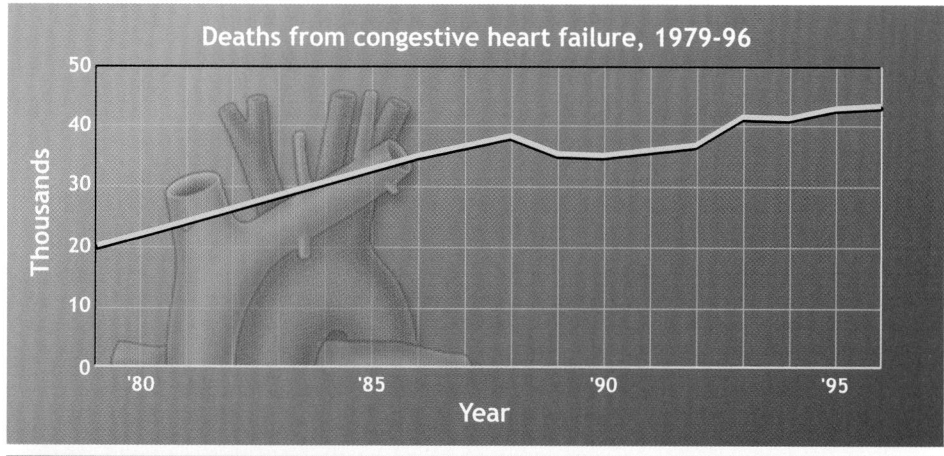

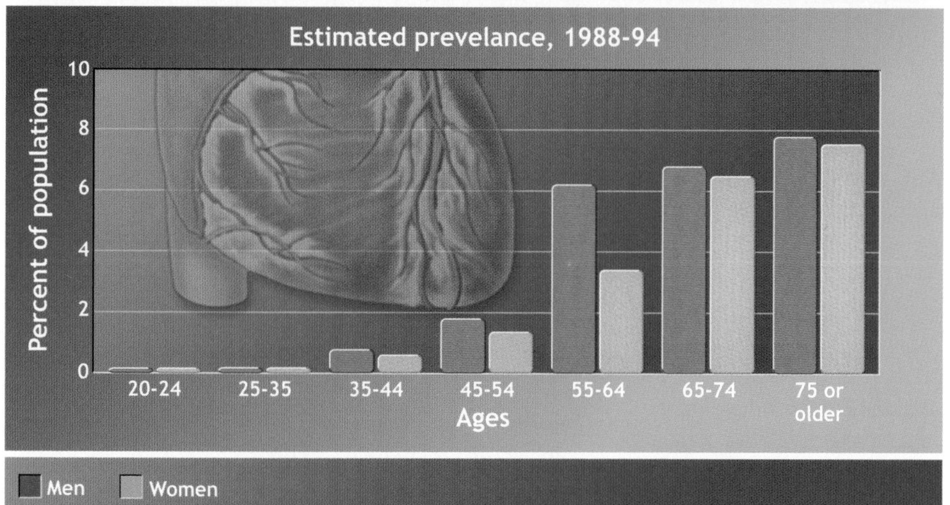

FIGURE 32.12 • Consequences of congestive heart failure (CHF) from impaired pumping ability of either the right or left heart or both. Although the prevalence of and deaths from CHF increase with age, nearly one-third (1.4 million) contract the disease before age 60 years. (Sources: National Center for Health Statistics and American Heart Association, 2000.)

lowered CHF death rates because they block hormones believed to promote disease progression. Recent research also shows dramatic improvement in survival, hospitalization, and symptoms in patients with standard therapy who also received Aldactone (known generically as spironolactone), a relatively inexpensive drug used routinely for heart failure and hypertension, which blocks the fluid-conserving action of aldosterone to a greater extent than ACE inhibitors.[173]

Surgical treatment replaces damaged heart valves or repairs myocardial aneurysms—bulging areas that form on the myocardial wall. Cardiac transplantation represents the extreme treatment of progressive disability from CHF, although the shortage of donor organs remains a serious problem. For patients awaiting a transplant, electrically powered pump implants placed in the abdomen below the heart mechanically assist ventricular function.

Clinicians have reevaluated the role of regular exercise because many of the functional deteriorations in CHF duplicate those that accompany extreme physical deconditioning. Reduced physical fitness and intrinsic changes in skeletal muscle may exacerbate the patient's physical incapacity.[76] Consequently, current therapy advocates regular exercise as an effective adjunct to vasodilator drug therapy in CHF rehabilitation.[84,133]

CHF AND EXERCISE TRAINING. Clinical practice indicates that regular moderate exercise formulated from a symptom-limited GXT and prescribed medications significantly benefit relatively low-risk, stable, compensated patients.[28,31,104,111,113,145,149] These benefits include improvements in functional capacity, exercise tolerance, muscle metabolism, level for dyspnea and the ventilatory response to exercise, risk for arrythmias, quality of life, and shift toward greater dominance of vagal (parasympathetic) tone.

It remains controversial whether the benefits of exercise rehabilitation for CHF link directly to enhanced central circulatory function—either improved myocardial performance per se or disease reversal as reflected by reduced heart size.[16,84] To a large extent, peripheral adaptations with regular exercise contribute to enhanced function and symptomatic improvements.[133,147]

The clinician, after proper classification using risk stratification criteria, supervises an exercise program (commencing with medical supervision) for compensated patients with controlled fluid volume status and absence of unstable or exercise-induced ventricular arrhythmias. The GXT provides the basis for the exercise prescription. For patients with marked exercise intolerance, relatively brief exercise intervals afford benefits (2 to 5 min of light exercise with 1 to 3 min of recovery). The prescription also includes multiple exercise sessions interspersed throughout the day.[147] Because of the usually abnormal heart-rate response in CHF patients, exercising at between 40 and 60% $\dot{V}O_{2peak}$ provides a more objective standard to establish initial exercise intensity. Alternatively, a rating of perceived exertion (RPE) on the Borg scale of "light" to "somewhat hard" (see Fig. 21.20) and/or +2 on the dyspnea scale ("mild, some difficulty;" see Fig. 32.21) generally proves effective. Supervisory personnel should recognize the following warning symptoms of cardiac decompensation:

- Dyspnea
- Hypotension
- Cough
- Angina
- Lightheadedness
- Arrhythmias

After gradually introducing the patient to increased physical activity, exercise duration can increase to 20 to 40 minutes at least three times weekly. After 6 to 12 weeks of supervised exercise, many patients can undertake an unsupervised home exercise program.

Aneurysm

Aneurysm describes an abnormal dilation in the wall of an artery, vein, or cardiac chamber. Vascular aneurysms develop when a vessel wall weakens from trauma, congenital vascular disease, infection, or atherosclerosis. Aneurysms are either arterial or venous and classify according to their specific regions of origin (e.g., thoracic aneurysm). Most aneurysms develop without symptoms and often are discovered during a routine x-ray. The most common symptoms include chest pain with a specific palpable, pulsating mass in the chest, abdomen, or lower back.

Heart Valve Diseases

Medical conditions that relate to heart valve abnormalities include:

- **Stenosis**: Narrowing or constriction that prevents heart valves from opening fully; may result from growths, scars, or abnormal calcified deposits
- **Insufficiency** (also called *regurgitation*): Occurs when a heart valve closes improperly and blood moves back into a heart chamber
- **Prolapse**: Occurs when enlarged valve leaflets in the mitral valve bulge backward into the left atrium during ventricular systole

Valvular abnormalities increase the heart's workload, causing it to pump harder to force blood through a stenosed valve or to maintain cardiac output if blood seeps backward into one of its chambers in diastole. Rheumatic fever, a serious group A streptococcal bacterial infection, causes valvular scarring and heart valve deformity. The most common symptoms are fever and joint pain. Penicillin or other antibiotics are used to treat this inflammatory condition, which usually occurs in children five to 15 years old. In 1997, rheumatic fever and rheumatic heart disease afflicted 1.8 million Americans, and in 1997, killed 5014 individuals.

MITRAL VALVE PROLAPSE. **Mitral valve prolapse (MVP)** occurs in 15 to 20% of the population, predominately in females. Also called *Barlow's syndrome*, MVP diagnoses increased in the 1990s because of its association with endocarditis, atherosclerosis, and muscular dystrophy. MVP probably results from connective tissue abnormalities in the mitral valve leaflets, which deform the valve's shape or structure (enlarged valve leaflets bulge backward into the left atrium during ventricular systole). This valvular "billowing" creates a clicking sound that can be heard with a stethoscope. Regurgitation of blood into the heart's upper chamber occasionally occurs, which can be heard as a murmur. Sixty percent of patients exhibit no symptoms; 40% experience profound fatigue during mild physical activity.

Inflammation Conditions: Endocarditis and Pericarditis

Endocarditis, predominantly of bacterial origin, inflames the cardiac endothelium and damages the tricuspid, aortic, or mitral valves. Patients initially experience musculoskeletal symptoms, including arthritis, low back pain, and general joint weakness. Antibiotic drugs usually treat this disease.

Pericarditis, classified as either acute or chronic (recurring or constrictive pericarditis), presents as inflammation of the heart's outer pericardial lining. Symptoms of acute pericarditis vary; they include chest pain, dyspnea, and increased resting heart rate and body temperature. Over time, the inflammation causes extreme chest pain from fluid accumulation in the pericardial sac that inhibits full myocardial expansion during diastole. The prognosis for acute viral pericarditis remains excellent; chronic pericarditis of bacterial origin represents a more dire condition.

Congenital Malformations

Congenital heart malformations appear in one of every 100 births. They include ventricular or atrial septal defects (hole between the ventricles and atria) and patent ductus arteriosus (shunt caused by an opening between the descending aorta and left pulmonary artery). These defects require surgical repair during childhood.

Cardiac Nervous System Diseases

Cardiac diseases that affect the heart's electrical conduction system include the following: **dysrhythmias (arrhythmias)** that cause the heart to beat too rapidly (**tachycardia**), too slowly (**bradycardia**), or with extra contractions (**ectopic, extrasystole**, or **premature ventricular contractions [PVCs]**) that possibly lead to fibrillation. Dysrhythmias usually produce changes in circulatory dynamics that can cause hypotension (extremely low blood pressure), heart failure, and shock. They often occur after a stroke induced by increased physical exertion or other stressful conditions.

Sinus tachycardia describes a resting heart rate above 100 b · min^{-1}; *bradycardia* indicates a resting heart rate below 60 b · min^{-1}. Sinus bradycardia occurs frequently in endurance athletes and young adults and generally represents a benign dysrhythmia; it actually may benefit cardiac function by producing a longer ventricular filling time during the cardiac cycle.

CARDIAC DISEASE ASSESSMENT

Before initiating an exercise intervention program, the healthcare team decides the extent of health screening, which may include a medical history, physical examination, laboratory assessments, and pertinent physiologic testing.

Purpose of Health Screening and Risk Stratification

Optimizing safety during exercise testing and program participation requires health screening and risk stratification. Assessment of specific risk factors and/or symptoms for chronic cardiovascular, pulmonary, and metabolic diseases optimizes safety during exercise testing and program participation. Proper preparticipation screening accomplishes the following:

- Identifies and excludes persons with medical contraindications to exercise
- Identifies persons requiring in-depth medical evaluation because of age, symptoms, and/or risk factors
- Identifies persons with clinically significant disease who require medical supervision when exercising

Before starting an exercise program, the ACSM recommends using age, health status, symptoms, and risk factor information to classify individuals into one of three risk strata to ensure their safety (see accompanying ACSM Risk Stratification inset). Proper risk stratification provides a basis for recommending further testing, medical assessment, or diagnostic interventions before exercise participation. "In a Practical Sense" provides the **Physical Activity Readiness Questionnaire (Par-Q)** commonly used as a minimal first-pass, preparticipation screening tool.

ACSM RISK STRATIFICATION

LOW RISK

Men <45 years; women <55 years asymptomatic with ≤1 risk factor[a,b]

MODERATE RISK

Men ≥45 years; women ≥55 years, or have ≥2 risk factors[a,b]

HIGH RISK

Individuals with ≥1 sign/symptom of cardiovascular or pulmonary disease[c] or known cardiovascular (cardiac, peripheral vascular, or cerebrovascular), pulmonary (obstructive pulmonary disease, asthma, cystic fibrosis), or metabolic (diabetes, thyroid disorder, renal or liver) disease

[a]Risk factors: family history of heart disease; cigarette smoking; hypertension; hypercholesterolemia; impaired fasting glucose; obesity; sedentary lifestyle

[b]HDL ≥60 mg · dL^{-1} (subtract 1 risk factor from the sum of other risk factors because high HDL decreases CHD risk)

[c]Signs/symptoms of cardiovascular and pulmonary disease: pain, discomfort in chest, neck, jaw, left arm; shortness of breath at rest or with mild exertion; dizziness or syncope; orthopnea or paroxysmal nocturnal dyspnea; ankle edema; tachycardia; intermittent claudication; heart murmur; unusual fatigue or shortness of breath with mild activity

From Franklin BA, et al. ACSM's guidelines for exercise testing and prescription. 6th ed. Baltimore, Lippincott Williams & Wilkins, 2000.

Patient History

A thorough patient history, including past and current medical problems, documents the most common patient complaints and establishes the CHD risk profile. Because most CHD symptoms include chest pain, the differential diagnosis of this pain is a primary focus. Table 32.10 lists symptoms, possible

TABLE 32.10 ➤ DIAGNOSIS OF CHEST PAIN

Pain/Complaint/Findings	Possible Causes	Stimuli	Possible Pathology
Pressure, ache, tightness or burning in midsternum, left shoulder, arm; diaphoresis; nausea; vomiting; S-T segment changes	MI	Exertion; cold; smoking; heavy meal; fluid overload	CHD
Sharp pain worsens with inspiration, improves with sitting	Inflammation	Acute MI	Pericarditis
Chest tightness with breathlessness; low-grade fever	Infection	IV drug use; microbes	Myocarditis; endocarditis
Sharp, stabbing pain; breathlessness; cough; loss of consciousness	Pulmonary	Recent surgery	Pulmonary embolism
Burning pain; indigestion relieved by antacids	Referred pain	Heavy meal, spicy food	Esophageal reflux
Angina pain; breathlessness; wide pulse pressure; ventricular hypertrophy on ECG	Ventricular outflow tract obstruction	Exertion; CHD	Aortic stenosis; mitral valve prolapse

IN A PRACTICAL SENSE

▶▶ PAR-Q FOR ASSESSING READINESS FOR PHYSICAL ACTIVITY

Minimal Preparticipation Screening

Health screening procedures range from self-administered questionnaires to sophisticated diagnostic tests, depending on the target population.

The Physical Activity Readiness Questionnaire (Par-Q) has been recommended as *minimal* screening for entry into moderate-intensity exercise programs. Par-Q was designed to identify the small number of adults for whom physical activity might be inappropriate or those who should receive medical advice concerning the most suitable type of activity.

Original Par-Q

Common sense is your best guide in answering these questions. Please read each question carefully and check *yes* or *no* if it applies to you.

YES ___ NO ___ 1. Has your doctor ever said that you have a heart trouble?
YES ___ NO ___ 2. Do you frequently have pains in your heart and chest?
YES ___ NO ___ 3. Do you often feel faint or have spells of severe dizziness?
YES ___ NO ___ 4. Has a doctor ever said your blood pressure was too high?
YES ___ NO ___ 5. Has your doctor told you that you have a bone or joint problem that has been aggravated by exercise or might be made worse with exercise?
YES ___ NO ___ 6. Is there a good physical reason not mentioned here why you should not follow an activity program even if you wanted to?
YES ___ NO ___ 7. Are you over age 65 and not accustomed to vigorous exercise?

IF YOU ANSWERED *YES* TO ONE OR MORE QUESTIONS:

If you have not recently done so, consult with your personal physician by telephone or in person BEFORE increasing your physical activity and/or taking a fitness test. Show your doctor a copy of this quiz. After medical evaluation, seek advice from your physician as to your suitability for:

- Unrestricted physical activity, probably on a gradually increasing basis
- Restricted or supervised activity to meet your specific needs, at least on an initial basis; check in your community for special programs or services

IF YOU ANSWERED *NO* TO ALL QUESTIONS:

If you answered Par-Q accurately, you have reasonable assurance of your present suitability for:

- *A graduated exercise program*—a gradual increase in proper exercise promotes good fitness development while minimizing or eliminating discomfort
- *An exercise test*—simple tests of fitness (such as the Canadian Home Fitness Test) or more complex types may be undertaken if you so desire
- *Postpone exercising*—if you have a temporary minor illness, such as a common cold, postpone any exercise program

Par-Q was developed by the British Columbia Ministry of Health and conceptualized and critiqued by the Multidisciplinary Advisory Board on Exercise (MABE). Par-Q Validation Report, British Columbia Ministry of Health, May, 1978.

causes, and related pathology of chest pain. A patient history typically includes the following:

- Medical diagnosis of diseases
- Previous physical examination findings to uncover abnormalities
- Recent illnesses, hospitalizations, or surgical procedures
- History of significant symptoms
- Orthopedic problems
- Medications
- Work record
- Family background
- Psychologic record

Physical Examination

The physician usually conducts the physical examination. This includes vital signs (body temperature, heart rate, breathing rate, and blood pressure) and other indications of problems. Assessments encompass auscultation of lungs; palpa-

IN A PRACTICAL SENSE

➤➤ REVISED (R) PAR-Q FOR ASSESSING READINESS FOR PHYSICAL ACTIVITY—CONT'D

rPar-Q (REVISED 1994)

One limitation of the original Par-Q was that about 20% of potential exercisers failed the test—many of these exclusions were unnecessary because subsequent evaluations showed that the individuals were apparently healthy. The revised Par-Q (rPar-Q) was developed to reduce the number of unnecessary exclusions (false positives). The revision can determine the exercise readiness of apparently healthy middle-aged adults with no more than one major risk factor for coronary heart disease.

YES ___ NO ___ 1. Has your doctor ever said that you have a heart condition and recommended only medically supervised activity?

YES ___ NO ___ 2. Do you have chest pain brought on by physical activity?

YES ___ NO ___ 3. Have you developed chest pain in the past month?

YES ___ NO ___ 4. Do you lose your balance because of dizziness, or do you ever lose consciousness?

YES ___ NO ___ 5. Do you have a bone or joint problem that could be worsened by a change in your physical activity?

YES ___ NO ___ 6. Is your doctor currently prescribing drugs (for example, water pills) for high blood pressure or a heart condition?

YES ___ NO ___ 7. Do you know of any other reason why you should not do physical activity?

NOTE: Postpone testing if you have a temporary illness such as a common cold or are not feeling well.

IF YOU ANSWERED *YES* TO ONE OR MORE QUESTIONS:

Talk with your doctor by phone or in person BEFORE you start becoming much more physically active or BEFORE you have a fitness appraisal. Tell your doctor about the Par-Q and which questions you answered YES.

- You may be able to do any activity you want—as long as you start slowly and build up gradually. Or, you may need to restrict your activities to those that are safe for you. Talk with your doctor about the kinds of activities you wish to participate in and follow his or her advice.
- Find out which community programs are safe and helpful for you.

IF YOU ANSWERED *NO* TO ALL QUESTIONS:

If you answered NO honestly to all Par-Q questions you can be reasonably sure that you can:

Start becoming much more physically active—begin slowly and build up gradually; this is the safest and easiest way to go

Take part in a fitness appraisal—this is an excellent way to determine your basic fitness so that you can plan the best way for you to live actively.

DELAY BECOMING MUCH MORE ACTIVE:

If you are not feeling well because of a temporary illness such as a cold or a fever—wait until you feel better, or

If you are or may be pregnant—talk to your doctor before you start becoming more active.

PLEASE NOTE: IF YOUR HEALTH CHANGES SO THAT YOU THEN ANSWER YES TO ANY OF THE ABOVE QUESTIONS, TELL YOUR FITNESS OR HEALTH PROFESSIONAL. ASK WHETHER YOU SHOULD CHANGE YOUR PHYSICAL ACTIVITY PLAN.

Par-Q and you. Gloucester, Ontario: Canadian Society for Exercise Physiology, 1994.

tion and inspection of lower extremities for edema; tests of neurologic function, including reflexes and cognition; and inspection of the skin, especially of the lower extremities in diabetics. Resting cardiorespiratory measures sometimes provide indirect, noninvasive clues to cardiovascular dysfunction. For example, sinus tachycardia or abnormal bradycardia and increased breathing rate and systolic blood pressure can contraindicate exercise without further evaluation.

To prescribe exercise and identify early warning signs, the clinical exercise physiologist must know the patient's heart rate and blood pressure response to graded exercise. For example, a systolic blood pressure increase of 20 mm Hg or more with low-intensity exercise (2 to 4 METs) can reflect abnormal myocardial oxygen demand and signal cardiovascular impairment. Similarly, failure of systolic blood pressure to increase (hypotensive response) may indicate blunted ventricular function; a depressed response with high-intensity exercise (e.g., failure to achieve systolic blood pressures above 140 mm Hg) frequently reflects dormant cardiac disease.

Heart Auscultation

Listening to sounds (**auscultation**) during the cardiac cycle can assess cardiac performance. The exercise physiologist should become familiar with the different abnormal heart sounds and learn how to identify heart murmurs. Auscultation can uncover valvular conditions (e.g., MVP, diagnosed by *click-murmur* sounds) and congenital heart abnormalities (regurgitation sounds in ventricular septal defects).

Laboratory Tests

Laboratory studies using chest x-ray, electrocardiogram (ECG), blood lipid and lipoprotein analyses, and serum enzyme testing contribute to assessing the extent of CHD.

The chest x-ray reveals the size and shape of the heart and lungs, whereas resting and exercise ECGs assess myocardial electrical conductivity and degree of oxygenation. Clinical exercise physiologists need considerable experience reading and interpreting ECGs. Table 32.11 lists six different categories of ECG measurements and interpretations. Chapter 31 discusses various ECG abnormalities and atypical physiologic responses to exercise. Careful ECG monitoring during a GXT provides more-extensive evaluation to target individuals with possible CHD. Table 32.12 presents common ECG changes during exercise and those associated with CHD.

Alterations in serum enzymes often confirm the existence of an acute MI. With myocardial cell death (necrosis) or prolonged ischemia, the following cardiac muscle enzymes leak into the blood because of increased plasma membrane permeability: (1) creatine phosphokinase (CPK), (2) lactate dehydrogenase (LDH), and (3) serum glutamic oxaloacetic transaminase (SGOT). Elevated CPK levels reflect either skeletal or cardiac muscle fiber damage. To pinpoint the source of the enzyme leak, electrophoresis or radioimmunoassay analysis separates CPK into three different isoenzymes: MM-isoenzyme, unique to skeletal muscle; BB-isoenzyme, specific to brain tissue; and MB-isoenzyme, specific for cardiac muscle necrosis. Like CPK, LDH fractionates into different isoenzymes, one of which increases during an MI. An acute MI also raises serum SGOT. Additional blood tests for CHD diagnosis include serum homocysteine (see Chapter 31), lipoprotein (a), fibrinogen, tissue-type plasminogen activator (tPA), and C-reactive protein.

TABLE 32.11 ➤ ECG INTERPRETATION USES ONE OF SIX DIFFERENT CRITERIA

1. Measurements
   - Heart rate (atrial and ventricular)
   - P-R interval (0.12 to 0.20 s)
   - QRS duration (0.06 to 0.10 s)
   - Q-T interval (HR dependent)
   - Frontal plane QRS axis (−30° to +90°)
2. Rhythm diagnosis
3. Conduction diagnosis
4. Wave form description
   - P wave (atrial enlargement)
   - QRS complex (ventricular hypertrophy, infarction)
   - S-T segment (elevated or depressed)
   - T wave (flattened or inverted)
   - U wave (prominent or inverted)
5. ECG diagnosis
   - Within normal limits
   - Borderline abnormal
   - Abnormal
6. Comparison with previous ECG

From Fardy P, Yanowitz FG. Cardiac rehabilitation, adult fitness and exercise testing. Baltimore: Williams & Wilkins, 1996.

TABLE 32.12 ➤ NORMAL AND ABNORMAL ECG CHANGES DURING EXERCISE

Normal ECG Response in Healthy Individuals	Abnormal ECG Response with CHD
1. Slight increase in P wave amplitude	1. Appearance of bundle branch block at a critical HR
2. Shortening of P-R interval	2. Recurrent or multifocal PVCs during exercise and recovery
3. Shift to the right of QRS axis	3. Ventricular tachycardia
4. S-T segment depression <1.0 mm	4. Appearance of bradyarrhythmias, tachyarrhythmias
5. Decreased T wave amplitude	5. S-T segment depression/elevation of >1.0 mm 0.08 s after J point
6. Single or rare PVCs during exercise and recovery	6. Exercise bradycardia
7. Single or rare PVCs or PACs	7. Submaximal exercise tachycardia
	8. Increase in frequency or severity of any known arrhythmia

PVC, premature ventricular contraction; PAC, premature atrial contraction.

Noninvasive Physiologic Tests

Physiologic tests apply either noninvasive or invasive procedures to identify specific cardiac dysfunctions.

ECHOCARDIOGRAPHY. **Echocardiography** uses pulses of reflected ultrasound (echo) to assess the functional and structural characteristics of the myocardium.[61] Ultrasound (high-frequency sound waves) identifies the heart's anatomic components during a cardiac cycle and measures their distances from the echo transducers to accurately estimate heart chamber and vessel size and myocardial wall thickness. Echocardiograms diagnose heart murmurs, evaluate valvular lesions, and quantify congenital defects and myopathies. For this reason, the echocardiogram is preferred to the ECG in recognizing chamber enlargement, inefficient ventricular contractility, myocardial hypertrophy, and other structural abnormalities.

GRADED EXERCISE STRESS TEST. Page 935 of this chapter discusses the rationale for stress testing and outlines four different categories of test protocols for apparently healthy individuals and those with CHD. *The GXT evaluates the ECG under conditions that exceed resting requirements in defined, progressive increments designed to increase myocardial workload.* The GXT also objectifies the functional capacity of patients with known disease and evaluates progress after surgery or other therapeutic interventions.

Table 32.13 lists subjective and objective information obtained during a GXT for designing an exercise prescription. The cardiologist and exercise physiologist supervise the exercise test, interpret the data, and prepare the exercise prescription.

ULTRAFAST CT SCAN. This 10-minute, noninvasive test uses a rapid (ultrafast) electron beam computed tomographic (EBCT) scan to assess calcium deposition within plaque in the linings of the coronary arteries. Test results determine how aggressively to treat blood lipid abnormalities (e.g., diet and exercise vs. drug therapy) and other CHD risk factors. Testing to detect coronary calcium deposition with EBCT is highly sensitive in men and women with significant coronary disease validated by coronary angiography.[79] Exclusion of coronary calcium buildup helps to characterize individuals with a low probability of significant stenosis.

TABLE 32.13 ➤ DATA FROM AN EXERCISE STRESS TEST TO DIAGNOSE AND FORMULATE EXERCISE PRESCRIPTIONS

Subjective data
Angina pain
Dyspnea ratings
Fatigue and weakness
Leg discomfort
Dizziness
Rating of perceived exertion (RPE)
Objective data
• **Physical examination data**
Breathing sounds
Murmurs and gallops
Blood pressure
Pulmonary function tests (before or after exercise)
Heart rate response
Blood gas parameters
• **Physical performance data**
Time on treadmill/cycle ergometer
Maximum work or power output
Rate-pressure product (RPP; HR × systolic blood pressure)
• **Electrocardiogram data**
S-T segment changes
Rate responses
Dysrhythmias
Conduction abnormalities
• **Cardiorespiratory data**
Lactate threshold
Carbon dioxide output
Minute ventilation
Oxygen consumption
Respiratory exchange ratio (R)

Invasive Physiologic Tests

Invasive cardiovascular testing provides information unattainable through noninvasive procedures. This includes the extent, severity, and location of coronary atherosclerosis, degree of ventricular dysfunction, and specific cardiac abnormalities.

RADIONUCLEOTIDE STUDIES. Radionuclide studies require injecting a radioactive isotope (e.g., technetium 99 or comparable substance) into the circulation during rest and exercise. Two examples include:

- **Thallium imaging**: Evaluates areas of myocardial blood flow and tissue perfusion to differentiate between a true-positive and false-positive S-T segment depression obtained by ECG evaluation during a GXT
- **Nuclear ventriculography**: Radiographic imaging procedure that analyzes regional left ventricular contractility following injection of a radioactive isotope contrast material

PHARMACOLOGIC STRESS TESTING. A **pharmacologic stress test** can benefit individuals unable to undergo routine exercise stress testing because of extreme deconditioning, peripheral vascular disease, orthopaedic disabilities, neurologic disease, or other problems. This test involves systematic intravenous drug infusion (e.g., dobutamine, dipyridamole, or adenosine) every 3 minutes until the patient receives the appropriate dosage. Echocardiography and/or thallium scanning then monitor for changes in wall motion abnormalities or coronary perfusion limitations, respectively. Heart rate response, arrhythmias, angina symptoms, S-T segment depression, and blood pressure dynamics also reflect myocardial viability during a pharmacologic stress test.

CARDIAC CATHETERIZATION. **Cardiac catheterization** involves inserting a fine tube (catheter) into a vein or artery that passes into the heart's right or left side. The intracardiac catheter can sample blood, assess pressure differences within the heart's chambers or vessels, and add contrast media to evaluate cardiac function.

CORONARY ANGIOGRAPHY. **Coronary angiography** applies radiography to image the coronary circulation by injecting a contrast medium that flows into the coronary vasculature. The technique is highly effective for evaluating the extent of coronary atherosclerosis; it serves as the gold standard for assessing coronary blood flow and provides the baseline for other test comparisons. Unlike thallium imaging, angiography cannot determine how easily blood flows within portions of the myocardium and cannot be applied during exercise. The accompanying angiogram illustrates angiography to pinpoint impaired blood flow

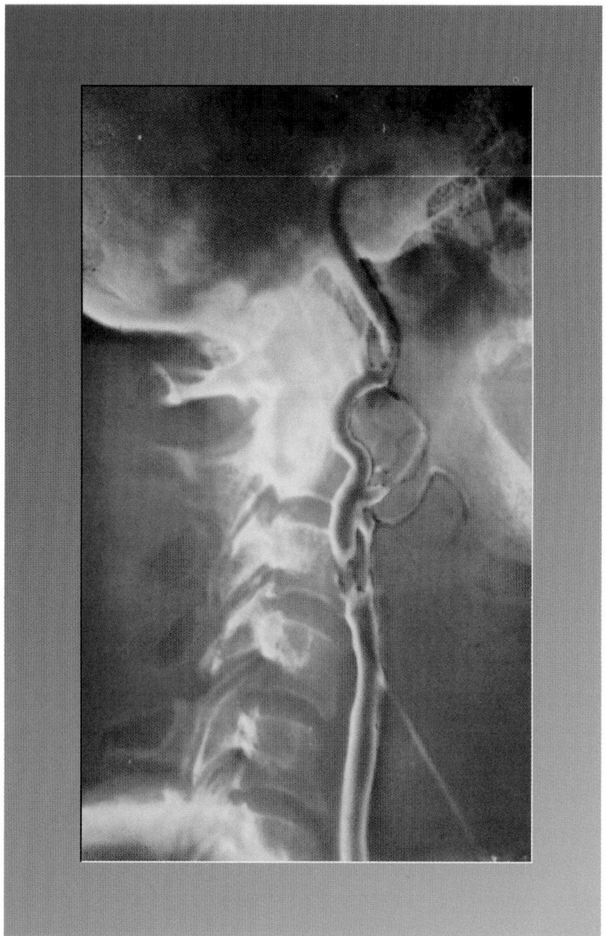

Angiogram showing constriction and absence of blood flow through the right carotid artery. (Courtesy of Dr. Barry Franklin, Beaumont Hospital, Birmingham, MI)

in the carotid artery (shown in *red*). Resectioning a vessel or removing its atherosclerotic plaques can improve blood flow and sometimes reduce the occurrence of a stroke.

CARDIAC REHABILITATION

In addition to the goal of risk factor modification to reduce mortality,[161,202] a comprehensive **cardiac rehabilitation program** focuses on improving a patient's longevity and quality of life.[55] After diagnosis and intervention (e.g., aggressive risk factor reduction, bypass surgery, angioplasty), the exercise physiologist evaluates the cardiac patient for functional capacity and ensuing classification and rehabilitation.[58] Table 32.14 outlines functional and therapeutic classifications of heart disease from the New York Heart Association and guidelines for risk stratification from the American Heart Association (AHA; www.amhrt.org) for categorizing patients for subsequent rehabilitation. Patients differ greatly in symptoms, functional capacities, and rehabilitation strategies. The cardiac rehabilitation program incorporates stringent guidelines to promote low-risk treatment.[59,62,87] CHD patients with mild ischemia tolerate steady-rate exercise at intensities consistent for aerobic training without progressive deterioration in left ventricular function. For patients without ischemia, LVEF in prolonged exercise remains similar to that of healthy controls.[63] Five important aspects of a successful cardiac rehabilitation program include:

1. Appropriate patient selection
2. Concurrent medical, surgical, and pharmacologic therapies
3. Comprehensive patient education
4. Appropriate exercise prescription
5. Careful patient monitoring during rehabilitation

Traditionally, cardiac rehabilitation programs consisted of three distinct phases with different objectives, physical activities, and required supervision. More-contemporary programs have changed on the basis of new theories of risk stratification, recent data on exercise safety, and changes in the health-care industry. Current programs recognize individual differences in rehabilitation when determining program length, degree of supervision, and required ECG monitoring.

Contemporary cardiac rehabilitation includes inpatient and outpatient programs and services, with emphasis on outcome measures. Almost all postsurgery patients benefit from inpatient exercise intervention, risk factor assessment, lifestyle activity counseling, and patient and family education. Patients stay at the hospital an average of 3 to 5 days postsurgery before release.

Inpatient Programs

Inpatient cardiac rehabilitation focuses on the following:

- Medical surveillance
- Identification of patients with significant impairments before discharge
- Rapid patient return to daily activities
- Preparation of patient and family to optimize recovery upon discharge

In-hospital physical activity during the first 48 hours following an MI and/or cardiac surgery is restricted to self-care movements, including arm and leg range of motion and intermittent sitting and standing to maintain cardiovascular reflexes. After several days, patients usually sit and stand without assistance, perform self-care activities, and walk independently up to six times daily, provided none of the following contraindications exist:

- Unstable angina
- Elevated resting blood pressure
- Orthostatic systolic blood pressure above 200 mm Hg with symptoms
- Critical aortic stenosis
- Acute systemic illness or fever
- Uncontrolled atrial or ventricular arrhythmias
- Uncontrolled sinus tachycardia above 120 b · min^{-1}
- Uncompensated CHF
- Active pericarditis or myocarditis
- Recent embolism or thrombophlebitis
- Resting S-T segment displacement of 2 mm or more
- Severe orthopedic conditions

TABLE 32.14 ➤ **A. FUNCTIONAL AND THERAPEUTIC CLASSIFICATIONS OF HEART DISEASE FROM THE NEW YORK HEART ASSOCIATION. B. GUIDELINES FOR RISK STRATIFICATION FROM THE AMERICAN HEART ASSOCIATION WHEN CONSIDERING AN EXERCISE PROGRAM**

A. NEW YORK HEART ASSOCIATION

Functional capacity classification		Therapeutic classification	
Class I:	No limitation of physical activity. Ordinary physical activity does not cause undue fatigue, palpitation, dyspnea, or anginal pain	Class A:	Physical activity need not be restricted
Class II:	Slight limitation of physical activity. Comfortable at rest, but ordinary physical activity results in fatigue, palpitation, dyspnea, or anginal pain	Class B:	Ordinary physical activity need not be restricted, but unusually severe or competitive efforts should be avoided
Class III:	Marked limitation of physical activity. Comfortable at rest, but less than ordinary activity causes fatigue, palpitation, dyspnea, or anginal pain	Class C:	Ordinary physical activity should be moderately restricted, and more strenuous efforts should be discontinued
Class IV:	Unable to carry on any physical activity without discomfort. Symptoms of cardiac insufficiency or of the anginal syndrome may be present even at rest; any physical activity increases discomfort	Class D:	Ordinary physical activity should be markedly restricted
		Class E:	Patient should be at complete rest and confined to bed or chair

B. AMERICAN HEART ASSOCIATION*

AHA CLASSIFICATION	NYHA CLASS	EXERCISE CAPACITY	ANGINA/ISCHEMIA AND CLINICAL CHARACTERISTICS	ECG MONITORING
A. Apparently healthy			Less than 40 years of age; without symptoms, no major risk factors, and normal GXT	No supervision or monitoring required
B. Known stable CHD, low risk for vigorous exercise	I or II	5–6 METs	Free of ischemia or angina at rest or on the GXT; EF = 40 to 60%	Monitored and supervised only during prescribed sessions (6-12 sessions); light resistance training may be included in comprehensive rehabilitation programs
C. Stable CHD with low risk for vigorous exercise but unable to self-regulate activity	I or II	5–6 METs	Same disease states and clinical characteristics as class B but without the ability to self-monitor exercise	Medical supervision and ECG monitoring during prescribed sessions; nonmedical supervision of other exercise sessions
D. Moderate-to-high risk for cardiac complications during exercise	≥III	<6 METs	Ischemia (≥4.0 mm S-T depression) or angina during exercise; two or more previous MIs; EF < 30%	Continuous ECG monitoring during rehabilitation until safety established; medical supervision during all exercise sessions until safety established
E. Unstable disease with activity restriction	≥III	<6 METs	Unstable angina; uncompensated heart failure; uncontrollable arrhythmias	No activity recommended for conditioning purposes; attention directed to restoring patient to class D or higher

*Adapted from American College of Sports Medicine. Guidelines for exercise testing and prescription. 6th ed. Baltimore: Williams & Wilkins, 2000.
NYHA, New York Heart Association; EF, ejection fraction; CHD, coronary heart disease; GXT, graded exercise test.

Outpatient Programs

Upon discharge, the patient should know appropriate and inappropriate physical activities and have a prudent and progressive plan of risk reduction and a specific exercise prescription. Enrollment in an outpatient exercise program is the ideal. Goals for **outpatient cardiac rehabilitation** include:

- Monitoring and supervising patient to detect changes in clinical status
- Returning patient to premorbid vocational/recreational activities
- Assisting patient implement at-home, unsupervised exercise program
- Providing family support and education

Most outpatient program sites encourage multiple physical activities, including resistance exercises, walking, cycling, and swimming. Supervision should include personnel trained in CPR and advanced life support.

PRUDENT PREEXERCISE EVALUATION: EXERCISE STRESS TESTING

Aerobic exercise serves important protective and rehabilitative functions to battle heart disease and improves cardiovascular functional capacity.[202] However, one should view the potential therapeutic benefits of regular exercise in proper perspective. For a sedentary person with undetected significant CHD, a sudden burst of strenuous exercise can inordinately strain cardiovascular function. Medical evaluation before initiating an exercise program reduces this risk considerably. For many people, the **graded exercise stress test (GXT)** provides a crucial component of the medical evaluation.

The GXT generally describes the systematic use of exercise for (1) ECG observations, (2) evaluating patients with exertional discomfort, (3) assessing pharmacologic and therapeutic treatment strategies, and (4) evaluating physiologic adjustments to increasing metabolic demands to objectify physical activity recommendations. Multistage bicycle and treadmill tests are the most common exercise stress testing modes. These tests, graded for exercise intensity, usually include several levels of 3 to 5 minutes of submaximal effort that bring the person to a self-imposed fatigue level or end point. The graded nature of testing allows exercise intensity to increase in small increments to pinpoint ischemic manifestations and rhythm disorders (e.g., anginal pain or ECG abnormalities). If heart disease exists, exercise testing provides a reliable, quantitative index of the person's functional impairment; this objectifies the diagnosis and subsequent exercise prescription.[66,85] Testing generally does not require maximal effort, but the person should exercise to at least 85% of age-predicted maximum heart rate.

A resting ECG precedes the exercise test to provide the important comparative baseline and to certify a person's safety in subsequent graded exercise testing. Unfortunately, exercise stress testing cannot show the extent of CHD or its specific location. Also, 25 to 40% of people with relatively advanced CHD (significant blockage in one or more coronary arteries) achieve a normal GXT evaluation. Interestingly, an abnormal heart rate recovery (i.e., failure of heart rate to decrease by more than 12 $b \cdot min^{-1}$ in the first minute after peak exercise) predicts, independent of ECG assessment, subsequent mortality in patients referred specifically for exercise electrocardiography.[155] This suggests that recovery heart rate provides additional prognostic information to compliment interpretation of the exercise stress test.

Reasons for Stress Testing

Stress testing serves the following six functions in an overall CHD evaluation:

1. *Diagnoses overt heart disease and screens for "silent" coronary disease in seemingly healthy adults.* Approximately 30% of people with confirmed CHD have a normal resting ECG. Graded exercise testing generally uncovers 70% of these abnormalities.
2. *Assesses exercise-related chest symptoms.* In many instances, individuals older than age 40 suffer chest or related pain in the left shoulder or arm during physical exertion. ECG analysis identifies myocardial abnormalities and more precisely diagnoses exercise-induced pain.
3. *Screens candidates for entry into preventive and cardiac rehabilitative exercise programs.* Test results provide an objective framework for designing a program based on a person's current functional capacity and health status. Repeat testing assesses progress and adaptations to regular exercise and provides for program modification.
4. *Uncovers abnormal blood pressure responses.* Individuals with normal resting blood pressure sometimes show greater-than-normal increases in systolic blood pressure during mild-to-moderate exercise, which may signify developing cardiovascular complications.
5. *Monitors effectiveness of therapeutic interventions (drug, surgical, dietary) designed to improve heart disease status and cardiovascular function.* For example, a patient's capacity to achieve a target heart rate without complications often confirms success of coronary bypass surgery.
6. *Quantifies functional aerobic capacity ($\dot{V}O_{2peak}$) and evaluates its deviation from normal standards.*

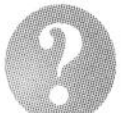

INTEGRATIVE QUESTION

What recommendations should a middle-aged man receive who wants to begin aerobic exercise training because he experiences breathlessness and chest discomfort while walking the golf course?

Who Requires Stress Testing?

Table 32.15 outlines screening and supervisory procedures for exercise testing that conform to policies and practices of the ACSM and the American Medical Association.

Informed Consent

All testing and exercise training must be performed on "informed" volunteers. **Informed consent** should raise the individual's awareness about all potential risks of participation. It must include a written statement that the person had the opportunity to ask questions about the procedures, with sufficient information clearly stated so that consent occurs from a knowledgeable (informed) perspective. A legal guardian or parent must sign the consent form for minors. Individuals need assurance that test results remain confidential and that they can terminate testing or training at any time and for any reason. Table 32.16 presents a sample form for obtaining consent before administering a health-related exercise test.

Stress Testing Contraindications

Absolute contraindications

A stress test should not take place without direct medical supervision if the following contraindications exist:

- Resting ECG suggesting acute cardiac disease
- Recent complicated MI
- Unstable angina pectoris
- Uncontrolled ventricular arrhythmias
- Uncontrolled atrial arrhythmias that compromise cardiac function
- Third-degree AV heart block without pacemaker

TABLE 32.15 ➤ ACSM RECOMMENDATIONS FOR CURRENT MEDICAL EXAMINATION AND EXERCISE STRESS TESTING (GXT) AND PHYSICIAN SUPERVISION OF GXT PRIOR TO PARTICIPATION IN EXERCISE PROGRAM

Risk Category	Medical Examination and GXT	M.D. Supervision
Low risk		
Men <45 years Women <55 years; asymptomatic with ≤1 risk factor[a,b]	Moderate exercise; not necessary Vigorous exercise; not necessary	Moderate exercise; not necessary Vigorous exercise; not necessary
Moderate risk		
Men ≥45 Women ≥55, with ≥2 risk factors[a,b]	Moderate exercise; not necessary Vigorous exercise; recommended	Moderate exercise; not necessary Vigorous exercise; recommended
High risk		
Individuals with ≥1 sign/symptom of cardiovascular or pulmonary disease[c] or known cardiovascular (cardiac, peripheral vascular, or cerebrovascular), pulmonary (obstructive pulmonary disease, asthma, cystic fibrosis), or metabolic (diabetes, thyroid disorder, renal or liver) disease	Moderate exercise; recommended Vigorous exercise; recommended	Moderate exercise; recommended Vigorous exercise; recommended

[a]Risk factors: family history of heart disease; cigarette smoking; hypertension; hypercholesterolemia; impaired fasting glucose; obesity; sedentary lifestyle.
[b]HDL >60 mg · dL^{-1} (subtract 1 risk factor from the sum of other risk factors because high HDL decreases CHD risk).
[c]Signs and symptoms of cardiovascular and pulmonary disease: pain, discomfort in chest, neck, jaw, left arm; shortness of breath at rest or with mild exertion; dizziness or syncope; orthopnea or paroxysmal nocturnal dyspnea; ankle edema; tachycardia; intermittent claudication; heart murmur; unusual fatigue or shortness of breath with mild activity.
Modified from Franklin BA, et al. ACSM's guidelines for exercise testing and prescription. 6th ed. Baltimore: Lippincott Williams & Wilkins, 2000.

- Acute CHF
- Severe aortic stenosis
- Active or suspected myocarditis or pericarditis
- Recent systemic or pulmonary embolism
- Acute infections
- Acute emotional distress

Relative contraindications

A GXT can be administered with caution and with medical personal in the test area under the following conditions:

- Resting diastolic blood pressure ≤115 mm Hg or systolic blood pressure ≤200 mm Hg
- Moderate valvular disease
- Electrolyte abnormalities
- Frequent or complex ventricular ectopy
- Ventricular aneurysm
- Uncontrolled metabolic disease (diabetes, thyrotoxicosis)
- Chronic infectious disease (hepatitis, mononucleosis, AIDS)
- Neuromuscular or musculoskeletal disorders
- Pregnancy (complicated or in the last trimester)
- Psychologic distress and/or apprehension about taking the test

GXT Termination

Graded exercise testing is generally safe when following all guidelines and taking proper precautions. Table 32.17 lists reasons why test termination may be required before the person attains maximum volitional fatigue.

Stress Test Outcomes

The clinical success of the GXT depends on its predictive outcome, that is, how effectively the test correctly diagnoses a person with heart disease.

Four possible GXT outcomes are:

- **True positive** (successful test): The GXT correctly identifies a person with heart disease
- **True negative** (successful test): The GXT correctly identifies a person without heart disease
- **False positive** (unsuccessful test): The GXT incorrectly identifies a normal person as having heart disease
- **False negative** (unsuccessful test): The GXT incorrectly identifies a person with heart disease as normal

A test's **sensitivity** refers to the percentage of persons for whom the test detects an abnormal (positive) response. This represents a true-positive condition that only subsequent follow-up can verify. False-negative (unsuccessful test) results occur 25% of the time and false-positive (unsuccessful test) results approximately 15%. Factors contributing to false-negative results include patient's failure to reach an ischemic threshold, failure to recognize non-ECG signs and symptoms associated with underlying CHD, and technical or observer errors. Various drugs and conditions also increase the probability of false-negative results, particularly if the person takes β-blockers, nitrates, and calcium channel blocking agents.

Test **specificity** refers to the number of true-negative test results—correctly identifying someone without CHD. More false-positive results occur under the influence of the drug digitalis and conditions of hypokalemia, mitral valve prolapse, pericardial disorders, and anemia.

TABLE 32.16 ➤ INFORMED CONSENT FOR A HEALTH-RELATED EXERCISE STRESS TEST

Patient/Subject Name ______________________

1. *Explanation of the exercise test*
   You will perform an exercise test on a cycle ergometer or a motor-driven treadmill. The exercise intensity begins at a level you can easily accomplish and will advance in stages depending on your fitness level. We may stop the test at any time because of signs of fatigue, or you may stop the test when you wish because of feelings of fatigue or discomfort.
2. *Risks and discomforts*
   The possibility exists that certain abnormal changes can occur during the test. These include abnormal blood pressure, fainting, disorder of heart beat, and in rare instances, heart attack, stroke, or death. Every effort will be made to minimize these risks by evaluating preliminary information related to your health and fitness and by observations during testing. Emergency equipment and available trained personnel can deal with unusual situations that may arise.
3. *Responsibilities of the participant*
   Information you possess about your health status or previous experiences of unusual feelings with physical effort may affect the safety and value of your exercise test. Your prompt reporting of how you feel during the exercise test is also important. You are responsible for fully disclosing such information when requested to do so by the testing staff.
4. *Expected benefits from the test*
   The results obtained from the exercise test may assist in diagnosing your illness or evaluating what type of physical activities you might do with low risk of harm.
5. *Questions*
   We encourage you to ask any questions about the procedures used in the exercise test or in the estimation of functional capacity. If you have doubts or questions, please ask us for further explanations.
6. *Freedom of consent*
   Your permission to perform this exercise test is voluntary. You are free to deny consent or stop the test at any point.

I have read this form and all procedures, risks, and potential benefits have been explained. I voluntarily consent to participate in this test.

Date: ______________
Signature of Patient: ____________________
Signature of Witness: ____________________
Questions: ____
____
Responses: ____
Signature of Physician or Authorized Delegate: ____________________ Date: ____________

TABLE 32.17 ➤ CRITERIA FOR TERMINATING A GRADED EXERCISE TEST BY APPARENTLY HEALTHY ADULTS

- Onset of angina or angina-like symptoms
- Significant drop (20 mm Hg) in systolic blood pressure or a failure of the systolic blood pressure to rise with an increase in exercise intensity
- Excessive rise in blood pressure: systolic pressure >260 mm Hg or diastolic pressure >115 mm Hg
- Signs of poor perfusion: light-headedness, confusion, ataxia, pallor, cyanosis, nausea, or cold and clammy skin
- Failure of heart rate to increase with increasing exercise intensity
- Noticeable change in heart rhythm
- Subject requests to stop
- Physical or verbal manifestations of severe fatigue
- Failure of testing equipment
- Early-onset horizontal or downsloping S-T segment depression or elevation (>4 mm)
- Increasing ventricular ectopy, multiform PVCs
- Sustained supraventricular tachycardia

Stress Testing the "Oldest Old"

The stress testing guidelines in Table 32.15 do not apply to individuals 75 years and older, those considered among the "oldest-old."[74] Only a small, highly select subgroup of these men and women participate in vigorous exercise or can successfully complete a stress test. For example, approximately 30% of persons aged 75 to 79 years can achieve a maximal exercise effort, 25% of those aged 80 to 84 years, and 9% of those aged 85 years or older.[93] The oldest-old differ markedly from younger persons in two key areas relative to stress testing: (1) prevalence of asymptomatic CHD and (2) coexistence of other chronic conditions and physical limitations. Elderly, asymptomatic men and women exhibit increased ECG abnormalities, many of which diminish the diagnostic accuracy of the GXT. The prevalence of asymptomatic ischemic episodes uncovered by the exercise ECG increases dramatically among the elderly with no history of MI or ECG abnormalities. Given the large reservoir of asymptomatic CHD among older persons, routine exercise stress testing would likely initiate a cascade of requirements for follow-up invasive cardiac procedures.[219] In the absence of strong evidence supporting aggressive evaluation in the elderly, this practice would place many at unnecessary risk for complications from invasive assessment.[74] For this reason, empirical screening for the elderly prescribes physical activity based on the person's previous exercise experiences and overall sense of well-being. This approach to exercise testing, training, and safety monitoring observes the widely accepted geriatric dictum, "start low and go slow."

Exercise-Induced Indicators of CHD

Physical activity creates the greatest demand for coronary blood flow, thus making exercise testing an effective means of probing for CHD.

Angina Pectoris

Myocardial ischemia—usually from restricted coronary circulation caused by atherosclerosis—stimulates sensory nerves in the walls of the coronary arteries and myocardium. The resulting pain or discomfort generally manifests in the upper chest region, although it frequently feels like increased pressure or constriction in the left shoulder or arm, neck, or jaw (see Fig. 32.10). Impaired cardiac performance—reduced stroke volume and cardiac output and generally diminished left ventricular contractility—also accompanies angina. The pain usually subsides after a few minutes of inactivity without permanent myocardial damage. Although physical activity frequently precipitates an angina episode, angina can also occur at rest (called Prinzmetal's angina or variant angina) with attacks usually occurring in the late evening or nighttime through early morning. In variant angina, caused by a coronary artery spasm, approximately two-thirds of people with it have severe blockage in at least one major coronary vessel.

Electrocardiographic Abnormalities

Alterations in the heart's normal pattern of electrical activity often indicate insufficient myocardial oxygen supply. Such electrical "clues," however, rarely emerge unless myocardial metabolic and blood flow requirements exceed resting conditions.

Figure 32.13A shows a tracing of the dynamic electrical activity of the myocardium throughout the cardiac cycle. Standard ECG paper contains 1-mm and 5-mm squares. Horizontally, each small square represents 0.04 seconds (with normal paper speed of 25 mm · s^{-1}); each large square represents 0.2 seconds. On the vertical axis, a small square indicates a 0.1-mV deflection with a calibration of 10 mm · mV^{-1}. One normal heartbeat (cardiac cycle) consists of five major electrical waves labeled P, Q, R, S, and T. The P wave indicates the electrical impulse (wave of depolarization) before atrial contraction. The Q, R, and S waves, collectively known as the **QRS complex**, represent depolarization of the ventricles immediately before their contraction. Ventricular repolarization generates the T wave. The cause of **S-T segment depression** (Fig. 32.13B) remains unknown, yet this abnormal deviation correlates with other CHD indicators, including coronary artery narrowing. *Individuals with significant S-T segment depression usually have severe, extensive obstruction in one or more coronary arteries.* In addition, the amount of S-T segment depression relates directly to the chances of dying from CHD. Generally, persons with 1- to 2-mm S-T segment depression during exercise exhibit a nearly 5-fold increase in CHD mortality, whereas for those with more than 2-mm depression the death risk increases approximately 20-fold. Current opinion advocates including nonspecific ECG findings in the overall heart disease risk assessment.[49] Even nonspecific minor S-T segment or T-wave abnormalities or both (termed *ST-T abnormalities*) provide a disquieting hint of increased long-term risk of mortality from cardiovascular disease.

During a standard ECG-monitored treadmill test, special electrodes can identify extremely subtle electrical patterns that predict a patient's risk for ventricular fibrillation. The test, termed the **alternans test**, identifies electrical alternation of the heart. Specifically, it uses a device to analyze T-wave alternans, which represent beat-to-beat electrical fluctuations of just one millionth of a volt. T-wave alternans reflect abnormalities in the way myocardial cells recover after transmitting the heart's electrical impulse. Oscillation of the cells' impulse can initiate a chain reaction that ultimately produces arrythmias, fibrillation, and subsequent cardiac arrest in some 350,000 individuals in the United States. Predicting risk for sudden death via T-wave alternans gives high-risk patients medical protection that might include an implanted defibrillator to automatically correct abnormal cardiac electrical activity.

Cardiac Rhythm Abnormalities

Graded exercise testing uncovers abnormalities in the pattern of the heart's electrical activity. A PVC (Fig. 32.13C) during exercise often reflects significant abnormal alteration in cardiac rhythm (**arrhythmia**). In this situation, the normal passage of the depolarization wave through the atrioventricular node does not stimulate the ventricles. Instead, portions of the ventricle spontaneously depolarize. This disorganized electrical activity produces an "extra" ventricular beat (QRS complex) without the P wave (atrial depolarization) that normally precedes it.

PVCs in exercise generally herald the presence of severe ischemic atherosclerotic heart disease, often involving two or more major coronary vessels. This specific myocardial electrical instability with exercise has greater predictive value than S-T segment depression for CHD diagnosis. Patients with exercise-induced PVCs have a 6- to 10-times greater risk of sudden death from abnormal course or fine rapid movements of the ventricles (**ventricular fibrillation**) than patients without this instability. Fibrillation risk becomes more prevalent for individuals with family history of this occurrence. With fibrillation, the ventricles do not contract in a unified manner, and cardiac output falls dramatically. Sudden death ensues unless normal ventricular rhythm returns. One

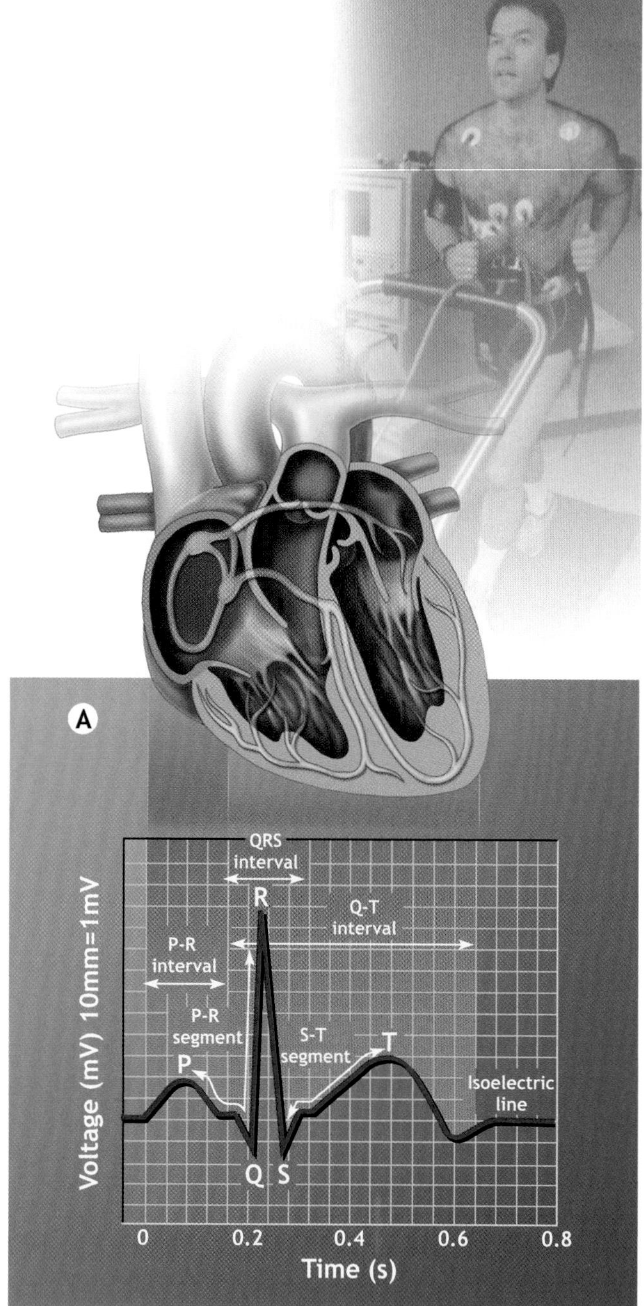

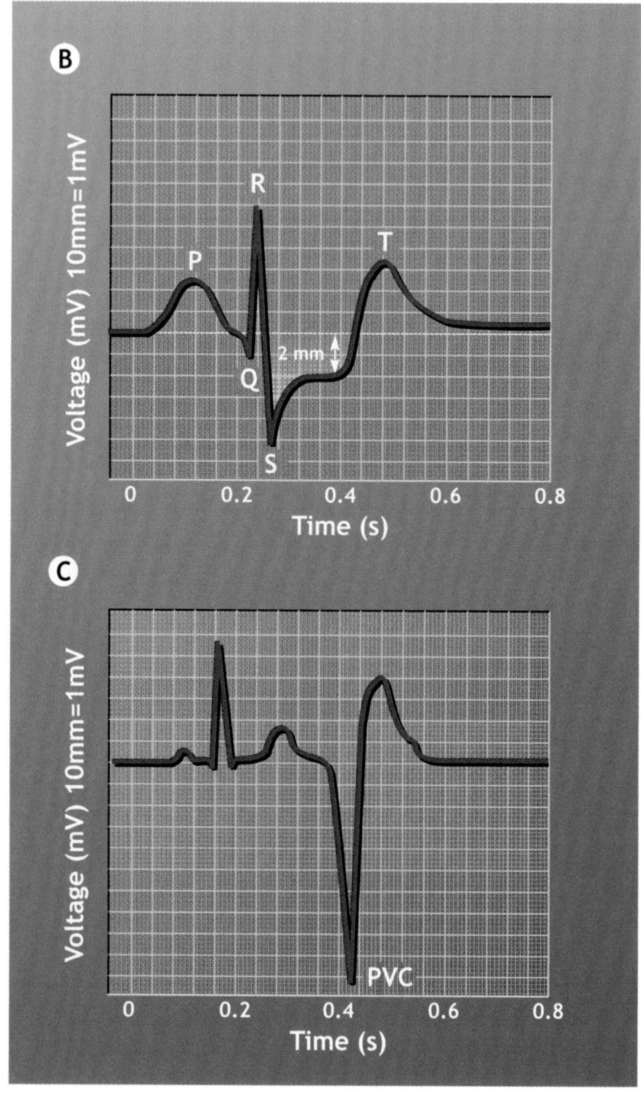

FIGURE 32.13 • A. Normal ECG tracing with an upward-sloping S-T segment. **B**. ECG tracing showing an abnormal horizontal S-T segment depression (*shaded area*) of 2 mm, measured from a stable baseline. **C**. ECG tracing illustrating a premature ventricular contraction (*PVC*).

way to reduce this risk requires implanting an electrical stimulator to correct the abnormal myocardial electrical conductance pattern.

Other CHD Indicators

Blood pressure and heart rate responses to exercise provide two useful non-ECG indices of possible CHD.

- **Hypertensive exercise response:** Normally, systolic blood pressure progressively increases during graded exercise from approximately 120 mm Hg at rest to 160 to 190 mm Hg during peak-intensity exercise. The change in diastolic pressure is generally less than 10 mm Hg. In exercise, systolic blood pressure can rise to well above 200 mm Hg, whereas the diastolic pressure can approach 150 mm Hg. This abnormal hypertensive response provides a significant clue to the presence of cardiovascular disease.
- **Hypotensive exercise response:** Inability for blood pressure to increase during graded exercise reflects cardiovascular malfunction. For example, failure of

systolic blood pressure to increase by at least 20 or 30 mm Hg often results from diminished cardiac reserve.

- **Heart rate response:** A rapid, large increase in heart rate (tachycardia) early in graded exercise often indicates cardiac dysfunction. Likewise, abnormally low exercise heart rates (bradycardia) in non–endurance-trained individuals may reflect unhealthy function of the heart's SA node. Also, inability of heart rate to increase during graded exercise (**chronotropic incompetence**), particularly when accompanied by extreme fatigue, indicates cardiac strain and CHD. An attenuated maximal exercise heart rate in apparently healthy men and women raises cardiovascular disease mortality risk.[116,125] Specifically, failure to achieve at least 85% of age-predicted maximum heart rate during exercise significantly predicts eventual all-cause mortality, independent of any exercise-induced myocardial perfusion defects.[126]

STRESS TEST PROTOCOLS

A 1988 national survey of 1400 exercise stress test centers reported that 71% used a treadmill, 17% a bicycle ergometer, and 12% a step test.[209] Nearly 66% of the treadmill tests used the Bruce protocol; the Balke protocol accounted for 10%. The most recent survey in 2000, based on 75,828 exercise tests performed at Veterans Affairs Medical Centers with cardiology divisions, reported that 78% used the treadmill (82% of those used the Bruce or Modified Bruce protocol). Four major cardiac events occurred (3 MIs and one sustained ventricular tachycardia) representing an event rate of 1.2/10,000.[150]

Bruce and Balke Treadmill Tests

Chapter 11 outlined protocols for the Bruce and Balke GXTs. Each test has distinct advantages and disadvantages. For example, the Bruce test provides more-abrupt increases in exercise intensity between stages. Although this may improve sensitivity to detect ischemic ECG responses, the patient must possess adequate fitness to tolerate increased exercise levels. Both protocols begin at relatively high levels of exercise for cardiac patients and older individuals and thus often require modification. The Bruce protocol incorporates lower initial exercise levels, whereas the Balke test includes a preliminary 2- to 3-minute initial stage at 2 mph, 0% grade.

Choice of a specific exercise test should consider overall health, age, and the person's fitness status. Generally, a stress test starts at a low level with increments in exercise intensity every several minutes. A warm-up, either separately or incorporated within the test protocol, eases the patient into exercise. Total exercise duration should average at least 8 minutes. A test much longer than 15 minutes adds little extra information, because the most-meaningful cardiac and physiologic data emerge within this time interval.

Bicycle Ergometer Tests

Bicycle ergometers have distinct advantages for exercise stress testing. In contrast to the treadmill, power output on the ergometer is readily computed and remains independent of the person's body mass. Most bicycle ergometers are portable, safe, and relatively inexpensive. Generally, two types of ergometers have application for graded exercise testing: (1) electrically braked ergometers and (2) weight-loaded, friction-type ergometers. With electrically braked ergometers, the preselected power output remains fixed within a range of pedaling frequencies. With weight-loaded ergometers, power output, usually expressed in kg-m · min^{-1} or watts (1 W = 6.12 kg-m · min^{-1}), relates directly to frictional resistance and pedaling rate.

The general guidelines for treadmill testing also apply to testing on the bicycle ergometer. Test protocols provide 2- to 4-minute stages of graded exercise with an initial resistance between 0 and 15 or 30 watts; power output generally increases in 15- to 30-watt increments per stage. The subject usually pedals the weight-loaded ergometer at either 50 or 60 revolutions per minute.

Arm-Crank Ergometer Tests

Arm cranking has application for graded exercise testing in special situations (e.g., cardiac assessment during upper-body effort) and for disabled individuals. Chapters 15 and 17 point out that arm exercise lowers $\dot{V}O_{2peak}$ up to 30%, and maximum heart rate generally averages 10 to 15 b · min^{-1} lower than with treadmill or bicycle exercise. Blood pressure is also difficult to measure during arm-crank exercise. Furthermore, *submaximal* arm cranking produces higher blood pressure, heart rate, and oxygen consumption values than the same power output with leg exercise.[170] Nevertheless, graded exercise protocols similar to those developed for leg cycling tests apply to evaluating a patient's response to upper-body exercise. However, the initial frictional resistance remains lower in arm exercise, with smaller increments in power output adjusted accordingly.

INTEGRATIVE QUESTION

What type of exercise prescription would most benefit a patient with CHD who experiences angina during upper-body work in his job as a plasterer or paper hanger?

Stress Testing Safety

The safety of stress testing largely depends on knowing who not to test (prescreening health histories reveal noncandidates for testing), knowing when to terminate a test, and preparing for emergencies. Table 32.18 summarizes the results of 12 reports about exercise stress testing complications (morbidity and mortality during and after the test) involving 2 million exercise tests with different supervision levels.[10,36,67,114,130,193,206,225] Despite differences in testing tech-

TABLE 32-18 ➤ **SUMMARY REPORTS OF INCIDENCE OF MORBIDITY AND/OR MORTALITY DURING OR FOLLOWING A GRADED EXERCISE TEST (1969-1995)**

Study	GXT Tests	Type of Subject	Morbidity Rate (per 10,000)	Mortality Rate (per 10,000)	Total Complications[b] (per 10,000)
1	50,000[a]	Variety	5.2	0.4	5.6
2	18,707	Variety	3.8	0.9	4.7
3					
4	>12,000	Variety	—	2.5	—
5	58,047	Variety	2.1	0.3	2.4
6	71,914[a]	Variety	0.7	0.1	0.8
7	28,133	Variety	3.2	0	3.2
8	4050	Variety	0.3	0	0.3
9	170,000[a]	Variety	2.4	1.0	3.4
10	353,638[a]	Athlete	0	0	0
	712,285[a]	CHD patients	1.4	0.2	1.6
11	518,448[a]	Variety	8.4	0.5	8.9
12	1377[a]	Severe CHD	232	0	232

[a]Direct physician supervision of GXT.
[b]Complications defined as the occurrence of serious arrhythmias during exercise testing (i.e., ventricular fibrillation, ventricular tachycardia, or bradycardia) that mandated immediate medical treatment (cardioversion, use of intravenous drugs, or closed-chest compression).
1. Atterhog JH, et al. Am Heart J 1979;98:572. 2. Cahalin LP, et al. J Cardiopulm Rehabil 1987;7:269. 3. Blessey RL. Exercise Standards and Malpractice Reporter 1989;3:69. 4. DeBrusk RF. Exercise Standards and Malpractice Reporter 1988;2:65. 5. Franklin BA, et al. Chest 1997;111:262. 6. Gibbons L, et al. Circulation 1989;80:846. 7. Knight JA, et al. Am J Cardiol 1995;75:390. 8. Lem V, et al. Heart Lung 1985;14:280. 9. Rochmis P, Blackburn H. JAMA 217:1971;1061. 10. Scherer D, Kaltenbach M. Dtsch Med Wochenschr 1979;33:1161. Stuart RJ Jr, Ellestad MH. Chest 1980;77:94. 12. Young, et al. Circulation 1984;70:184.
(From Franklin BA, et al. ACSM's Guidelines for Exercise Testing and Prescription. 6th Ed. Baltimore: Lippincott Williams & Wilkins, 2000.)

niques, purposes, safety precautions, type and mode of testing, the following conclusions about risk during or immediately following a GXT appear warranted:

- Low risk of death (≤0.01%)
- Low risk of an acute MI (≤0.04%)
- Low risk of complications requiring hospitalization including acute MI or serious arrhythmias (≤0.2%)

Clearly, the risk-benefit ratio favors testing in most situations.

PRESCRIBING EXERCISE

An exercise prescription should improve fitness, promote overall health by reducing risk factors, and ensure a safe and enjoyable exercise experience. *Prescribing exercise involves successful integration of exercise science with behavioral objectives to enhance patient compliance and goal attainment.*[68]

Heart rate and oxygen consumption (or exercise intensity) measured during the stress test provide the basis for the exercise prescription. The prescription individualizes exercise on the basis of current fitness and health status, with emphasis on intensity, frequency, duration, and type of exercise. Starting an exercise program at the proper level takes on added importance for CHD patients, because beginners often do not recognize their limitations.

Practical Illustration

Figure 32.14 illustrates a practical approach that permits functional translation of treadmill or bicycle ergometer exercise test responses to the exercise prescription. The figure depicts data for a male cardiac patient, generated from an algorithm that used exercise test responses from the Bruce treadmill protocol for level-ground ambulation. Heart rate (*A*) was plotted as a function of time, with a mathematical line of best fit (*B*) applied to the data points. A target zone for heart rate *(shaded portion, C)* represented approximately 75% to 85% of the maximum heart rate of 170 b · min^{-1} . The individualized prescription is then detailed for pace (13.8 to 15.4 mi · min^{-1}, *D*) and/or METs (4.1 to 5.9, *E*). The acceptable exercise intensity range in area *C*, based on heart rate response during the exercise test, includes the following recreational activities: touch football, canoeing, and light-to-moderate volleyball, skating, skiing, aerobics, bicycling, tennis and badminton, swimming, skating, and waterskiing. This practical approach to prescribing exercise may improve the prescription's effectiveness (and adherence) for the healthy, previously sedentary individual and CHD patient.

Improvements in CHD Patients

A properly prescribed and monitored exercise program safely improves a cardiac patient's functional capacity. Clinical symptoms (e.g., ECG abnormalities) often improve or disappear.

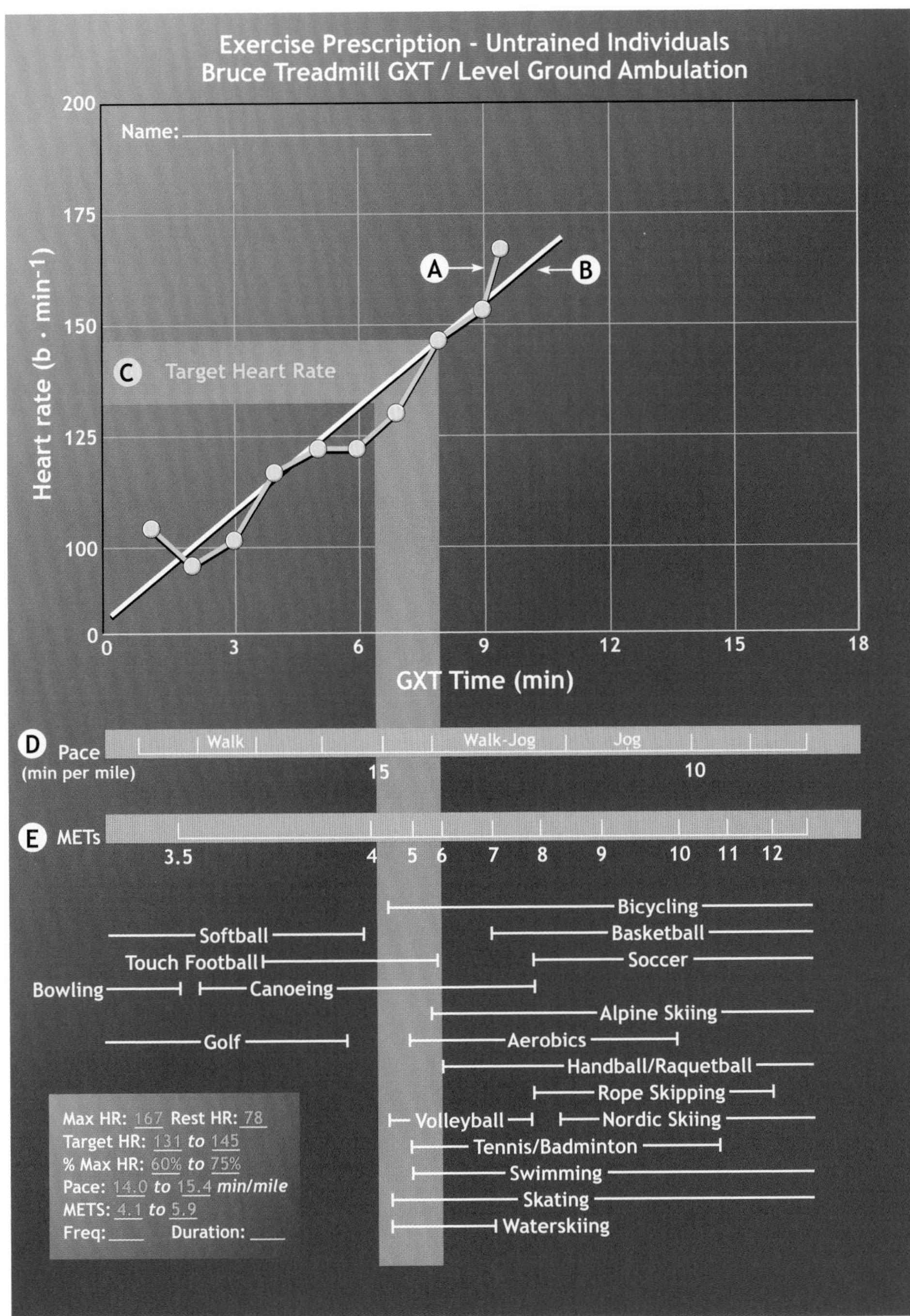

FIGURE 32.14 • Exercise prescription based on functional translation algorithm for level-ground ambulation. Letters in figure identified in text. (Used with permission of Dr. Carl Foster, University of Wisconsin-LaCrosse, LaCrosse, WI.)

This occurs partly because of structural and functional changes in the myocardium. In addition, cardiac patients and normals respond to exercise training with physiologic adjustments that reduce cardiac work at any given external exercise load. For example, reduced exercise heart rate and blood pressure (two major determinants of myocardial workload and oxygen consumption) reduce myocardial effort. This reduction in the rate-pressure product (HR × SBP) delays the onset of anginal pain, allowing exercise of greater intensity and duration. For individuals whose occupations predominantly require arm exercise, training (and testing) should emphasize this musculature, because physical conditioning benefits are highly specific and generally not transferable among muscle groups.[141]

The Program

Joint recommendations of the ACSM and the AHA for cardiovascular screening of children, adolescents, and adults before enrollment or participation in activities at health/fitness facilities can be found on the ancillary website connection.lww.com/go/mcardle.[5] The recommendations also discuss staff qualifications and emergency policies related to cardiovascular safety.

The most effective preventive and rehabilitative exercise programs focus on individual needs. Low- to moderate-intensity exercise regimens evoke greater adherence than intense physical activity.[140] The prescribed exercises usually include rhythmic big-muscle movements that stimulate cardiovascular improvement; examples include walking, jogging, cycling, rope skipping, swimming, stair-climbing and cross-country ski simulation, dynamic calisthenics, and higher-intensity interval training, even among the elderly and patients with chronic heart failure.[1,147,148] On an outpatient basis, less-restricted activities such as mountain biking serve as a recreational adjunct to rehabilitate regularly exercising MI patients with stable CHD.[98]

Chapter 21 discussed guidelines for making decisions concerning training frequency, duration, and intensity. Ideally, the personalized exercise prescription should include a recommendation for weight loss and dietary modification (if necessary), warm-up and cool-down exercises, and a developmental flexibility and strength program. Some heart disease patients exhibit a reduced exercise heart rate response with a correspondingly reduced maximum heart rate. In such cases, target heart rates based on an age-predicted maximum for the general, healthy population grossly overestimate the appropriate training intensity. This supports the wisdom of exercise stress testing each patient to *symptom-limited maximum* and then formulating the exercise prescription from the test's heart rate data.

Supervision Level

The ACSM has categorized several types of exercise programs with specific criteria for entry and supervision (Table 32.19). These programs are either *unsupervised* or *supervised,* with four subdivisions of the supervised category. Unsupervised programs meet the needs of asymptomatic participants of any age with functional capacities of at least 8 METs and no known major risk factors. The supervised exercise programs focus on patients with specific needs. These include asymptomatic physically active or inactive persons of any age with CHD risk factors but no known disease (B4) and symptomatic individuals, including individuals with recent onset of CHD and those with a changed disease status (B1 to B3).

Resistance Exercise Provides Benefits

Resistance exercises added to a cardiac rehabilitation program restore muscular strength, promote preservation of FFM, improve psychologic status and quality of life, and increase glucose tolerance and insulin sensitivity.[68,142,143] Even for patients with advanced heart diease, no adverse effects emerged while performing weightlifting arm exercise at 50, 65, and 85% of 1-RM.[112] In comparisons of resting and exercise responses, no changes occurred in pulmonary wedge pressures, S-T segment of the ECG, or the incidence of dysrhythmias. Contraindications to resistance training for cardiac patients parallel those for aerobic training.[176] The following conditions preclude cardiac patients from participating in resistance training:

- Unstable angina
- Uncontrolled arrhythmias
- Left ventricular outflow obstruction (e.g., hypertrophic cardiomyopathy with obstruction)
- Recent history of CHF without follow-up and treatment
- Severe valvular disease, hypertension (systolic blood pressure >160 mm Hg, and or diastolic blood pressure >105 mm Hg)
- Poor left ventricular function and exercise capacity below 5 METs, with anginal symptoms or ischemic S-T segment depression

RESISTANCE TRAINING PRESCRIPTION. Because of exaggerated blood pressure responses with straining-type exercise, cardiac patients should use only light resistance within the range of 30 to 50% of 1-RM. In the absence of contraindications, elastic bands, light (1 to 5 lb) cuff and hand weights, light free weights, and wall pulleys can be applied initially at entrance to an outpatient program. Low-level resistance training should not be initiated until 2 to 3 weeks post-MI. Barbells and/or weight machines can be used after 4 to 6 weeks of convalescence.

Most cardiac patients begin range-of-motion exercises using relatively light weight for the lower and upper extremities. In accordance with AHA recommendations, they should perform one set of 10 to 15 repetitions to moderate fatigue, using 8 to 10 different exercises (e.g., chest press, shoulder press, triceps extension, biceps curl, lat pull-down, lower back extension, abdominal crunch/curl-up, quadriceps extension or leg press, leg curls, calf raises). Exercises performed 2 to 3 days per week elicit favorable adaptations.[176] The rate-pressure product should not exceed the level prescribed for endurance exercise, and the RPE should range from 11 to 14 on the Borg scale ("fairly light" to "somewhat hard"). To minimize dramatic blood pressure fluctuations during lifting, patients should be warned to avoid straining,

TABLE 32.19 ➤ ACSM CATEGORIES FOR EXERCISE PROGRAMS RELATED TO PATIENT SYMPTOMS

Type	Participants	Entry MET Level	Supervision
A. Unsupervised	Asymptomatic	8+	None
B. Supervised			
1. Inpatient	All symptomatics-post-myocardial infarction, postoperative, pulmonary disease	3	Supervised ambulatory therapy
2. Outpatient	All symptomatics-post-myocardial infarction, postoperative pulmonary disease	3+	Exercise specialist, physician on call
3. In home	Symptomatic + asymptomatic	>3–5	Unsupervised; periodic hospital reevaluation
4. Community	Symptomatic + asymptomatic, 6-8 weeks postinfarct, 4-8 weeks postoperative	>5	Exercise program director + exercise specialist

performing the Valsalva maneuver, and gripping weight handles or bars too tightly.

Cardiac Medications and Exercise Response

Knowledge of the physiologic effects of drug intervention allows the clinical exercise physiologist to properly assess patient response during physical activity. Table 32.20 presents six classifications of common cardiac drugs, along with trade names, side effects, and possible effects on exercise responses.

INTEGRATIVE QUESTION

Why would a weightlifting competition pose a risk to a person with advanced CHD?

TABLE 32.20 ➤ CARDIAC MEDICATIONS: THEIR USE, SIDE EFFECTS, AND EFFECTS ON EXERCISE RESPONSE

TYPE/TRADE NAME	USE	SIDE EFFECTS	EFFECTS ON EXERCISE RESPONSE
I. Antianginal agents			
A. Nitroglycerin compounds [*Amyl nitrate; Isordil; Nitrostat*]	Smooth muscle relaxation; decrease cardiac output	Headache, dizziness, hypotension	Hypotension; increase exercise capacity
B. β-Blockers [*Inderal; Propranolol; Lopressor; Corgard; Biocadren*]	Block β receptors; decrease sympathetic tone; decrease HR, contractility, BP	Bradycardia, heart block, insomnia, nausea, fatigue, weakness, increased cholesterol and blood sugar	Decrease HR; hypotension; decrease cardiac contractility
C. Calcium antagonists [*Verapamil; Nifedipine; Procardia*]	Block influx of calcium; dilate coronary arteries; suppress dysrhythmias	Dizziness, syncope, flushing, hypotension headache, fluid retention	Hypotension
II. Antihypertensive agents			
A. Diuretics [*Thiazides, Lasix, Aldactone*]	Inhibit Na^+ and Cl^- in kidney; increase excretion of sodium and water, and control high BP and fluid retention	Drowsiness, dehydration, electrolyte imbalance; gout, nausea, pain, hearing loss, elevated cholesterol and lipoproteins	Hypotension
B. Vasodilators [*Hydralazine, Captopril, Apresoline, Loniten, Minoxidil*]	Dilate peripheral blood vessels; used in conjunction with diuretics; decrease BP	Increase HR and contractility; headache, drowsiness, nausea, vomiting, diarrhea	
C. Drugs interfering with sympathetic nervous system [*Reserprine, Propranolol, Aldomet, Catapres, Minipress*]	Decrease BP, HR, and cardiac output by dilating blood vessels	Drowsiness, depression, sexual dysfunction, fatigue, dry mouth, stuffy nose, fever, upset stomach, fluid retention, weight gain	Hypotension
III. Digitalis glycosides, derivatives [*Digoxin, Lonoxin, Digitoxin*]	Strengthen heart's pumping force and decrease electrical conduction	Arrhythmias, heart block, altered ECG, fatigue, weakness, headache, nausea, vomiting	Increase exercise capacity; increase myocardial contractility
IV. Anticoagulant agents [*Coumadin, Sodium Heparin, Aspirin, Persantine*]	Prevent blood clot formation	Easy bruising, stomach irritation, joint or abdominal pain, difficulty in swallowing, unexplained swelling, uncontrolled bleeding	
V. Antilipidemic agents [*Cholestyramine, Lopid, Niacin, Atromid-S, Mevacor, Questran Zocor*]	Interfere with lipid metabolism and lowers cholesterol and low-density lipoproteins	Nausea, vomiting, diarrhea, constipation, flatulence, abdominal discomfort, glucose intolerance	
VI. Antiarrhythmic agents [*Cardioquin, Procaine, Quinidine Lidocaine, Dilantin, Propranolol, Bretylium tosylate, Verapamil*]	Alter conduction patterns throughout the myocardium	Nausea, palpitations, vomiting, rash, insomnia, dizziness, shortness of breath, swollen ankles, coughing up blood, fever, psychosis, impotence	Hypotension; decrease HR; decrease cardiac contractility

REHABILITATION FOLLOWING HEART TRANSPLANTATION

Chapter 16 (Fig. 16.11) shows that cardiac transplantation significantly improved peak oxygen consumption, which remained elevated for up to 9 years. Limited data also show that transplant patients respond positively to aerobic exercise training[11,28,110] but not to the same extent as coronary artery bypass surgery patients.[48,163] Generally, heart transplant recipients achieve 55 to 60% of predicted $\dot{V}O_{2max}$ during a GXT.[28] In addition to significant improvements in $\dot{V}O_{2peak}$, training improves blood lactate kinetics. This lowers blood lactate concentration during exercise and recovery, in part from improved lactate removal efficiency.[124] It also appears that graded exercise to fatigue does not pose an oxidative-stress risk (plasma levels of lipid peroxidation) to exercise-trained heart transplant patients, despite their use of immunosuppressive drugs.[102]

Table 32.21 summarizes the results of a randomized, controlled prospective trial of exercise rehabilitation initiated shortly after heart transplantation.[115] Twenty-seven patients discharged within 2 weeks after receiving a heart transplant participated in either a 6-month structured cardiac rehabilitation program or unstructured home therapy. Structured exercise consisted of individualized resistance training and aerobic training (walking) supervised by a physical therapist; the control patients received no formal exercise training. All subjects received graded exercise testing within 1 month of heart transplantation (baseline) and 6 months later. Both groups significantly improved functional capacity from baseline to 6-month follow-up. However, the exercise-trained grouped improved significantly more than controls in $\dot{V}O_{2peak}$ (49 vs. 18%) and total work output (59 vs. 18%). From a practical perspective, transplant patients responded positively to regular exercise training and significantly improved physical activity capacity.

Similar guidelines apply to training the transplant recipient and any postcardiac surgery patient.[106] However, training heart rate guidelines (see Chapter 21) do not apply to the transplant patient because of the sluggish, blunted heart rate responses of the denervated transplanted organ (neural regulation of heart rate absent, hormonal regulation dominant; see Chapter 16). As an alternative, the RPE scale can gauge exercise intensity using ratings between "fairly light" to "somewhat hard" (RPE between 11 and 14). Because of the inordinately slow heart rate response at the onset of exercise, a longer, graded warm-up takes on added importance. Because the transplanted heart does not connect to the afferent nervous system, a patient with advanced CHD in the transplanted heart does not experience the painful warnings of exercise-induced angina pectoris.

TABLE 32.21 ➤ EFFECTS OF A SIX-MONTH STRUCTURED CARDIAC REHABILITATION PROGRAM BEGUN WITHIN ONE MONTH AFTER HEART TRANSPLANTATION (BASELINE) ON CARDIOPULMONARY EXERCISE TEST RESULTS

Variable	Exercise Group (n = 14)			Control Group (n = 13)		
	Baseline	6 Months	Difference (% Change)[a]	Baseline Line	6 Months	Difference (% Change)[a]
Peak oxygen consumption (mL · kg^{-1} · min^{-1})	9.2	13.6	+4.4 (+49)	10.4	12.3	+1.9 (+18)
Workload (W)	59	94	+35 (+59)	66	78	+12 (+18)
Ventilatory equivalent for carbon dioxide ($\dot{V}E/\dot{V}CO_2$)	66	53	−13 (−20)	54	48	−6 (−11)
Ventilatory equivalent for oxygen ($\dot{V}E/\dot{V}O_2$)	79	67	−12 (−15)	64	60	−4 (−6)
Exercise duration (min)	6.9	9.0	+2.1 (+30)	7.2	8.3	+1.1 (+15)
Time to estimated lactate threshold (min)	1.8	3.3	+1.5 (+83)	2.3	2.3	0
Resting heart rate (b · min^{-1})	90	100	+10 (+11)	91	109	+18 (+20)
Peak heart rate (b · min^{-1})	102	125	+23 (+23)	107	134	+27 (+25)
Systolic blood pressure at rest (mm Hg)	126	121	−5 (−4)	130	114	−16 (−12)
Peak systolic blood pressure (mm Hg)	141	148	+7 (+5)	139	148	+9 (+6)
Minute ventilation (L · min^{-1})	38	45	+7 (+18)	46	62	+16 (+35)
Sitting-to-standing rate (# · min^{-1})[b]	10.6	23.9	+13.3 (+125)	12.3	17.9	+5.6 (+46)

[a] Plus signs denote an increase, and minus signs a decrease.

[b] The sitting-to-standing rate is the number of times per minute a patient could rise from a sitting position to a standing position.

From Kobashigawa JA, et al. A controlled trial of exercise rehabilitation after heart transplantation. N Engl J Med 1999;340:272.

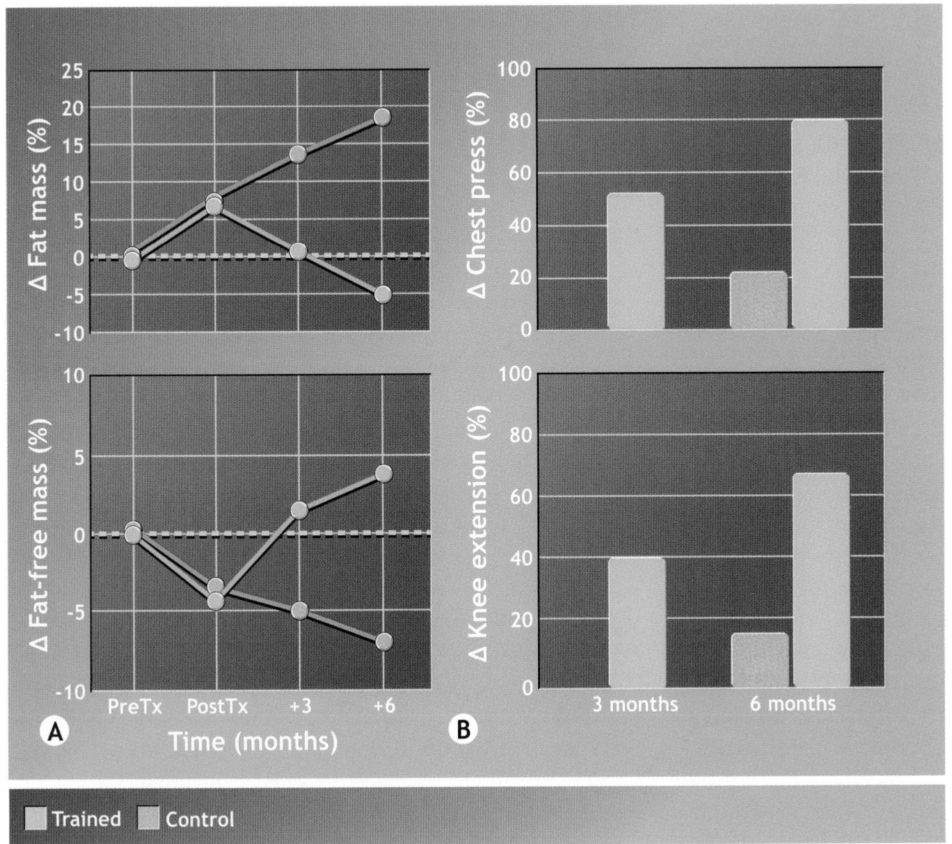

FIGURE 32.15 • A. Changes (Δ) in fat mass and fat-free body mass (FFM) at 2 months posttransplantation and after 3 and 6 months of resistance exercise training or no training. Points represent average values for 14 heart transplant patients randomly assigned before surgery to either a control group or resistance training. **B.** Changes in chest press strength and bilateral knee extension strength after 3 and 6 months of resistance exercise training or no training. The nontraining control group was not tested at 3 months. (From Braith RW, et al. Resistance exercise prevents glucocorticoid-induced myopathy in heart transplant recipients. Med Sci Sports Exerc 1998;30:483.)

Transplant Patients Experience Unique Benefits From Resistance Training

Chronic glucocorticoid therapy to combat tissue rejection causes muscle wasting, strength losses, and reduced bone mineral density and generally hinders a transplant patient's overall recovery and rehabilitation.[29,30] Steroid-induced muscle atrophy and weakness also affect lifestyle negatively, including the patient's recreational pursuits and range of occupational physical tasks. Figure 32.15 shows that a 6-month monitored resistance exercise program for major muscle groups significantly slows the negative alterations in body composition from exogenous glucocorticoid therapy following transplantation.[33] Fourteen heart transplant patients were randomly assigned prior to surgery to either no exercise or resistance training that began 2 months after transplantation and immunosuppressive glucocorticoid therapy. Exercise training consisted of lumbar extensor exercise 1 day a week and upper- and lower-body resistance training 2 days weekly. Initial resistance set at 50% of 1-RM consisted of one set of 10 to 15 repetitions. Resistance increased 5 to 10% with completion of 15 repetitions. Fat mass increased and FFM decreased equally for both groups during glucocorticoid treatment following transplantation (Fig. 32.15A). Six months of resistance training restored FFM to higher levels than before transplantation, while the control group's FFM progressively decreased. Muscular strength increased for both groups during the posttransplant period (Fig. 32.15B), but improvements were four to six times greater for the training group. Additional research indicates that regular resistance exercise training restores bone mineral density toward pretransplant levels, despite continued immunosuppression with glucocorticoids.[32] The following recommendations help to sustain venous return and prevent blood pooling and accompanying hypotension in heart transplant patients during resistance training:[28]

- Alternate between upper- and lower-body exercises during the workout
- Walk for 2 minutes between exercises or perform standing calf raises
- End each training session with a 5-minute, low-intensity cool-down walk

PULMONARY DISEASES

The clinical exercise physiologist's involvement in treating patients with pulmonary disease focuses primarily on improving ventilatory capacity, decreasing the energy cost of breathing, and increasing overall level of physiologic function.[45] The personal history, physical examination, pertinent laboratory data, and imaging studies provide important background information. Cardiovascular system disorders almost always affect pulmonary function, which eventually leads to varying degrees of pulmonary disability. Conversely, pulmonary disease intimately relates to cardiovascular complications. Patients with pulmonary disease and disabilities often benefit from exercise rehabilitation. Pulmonary abnormalities are classified as either obstructive (normal airflow impeded) or restrictive (lung volume dimensions reduced). Despite the convenience of this classification system, pulmonary disorders often reflect both restrictive and obstructive impairment.

Restrictive Lung Dysfunction

Abnormal reduction in pulmonary ventilation, along with diminished lung expansion, decreased tidal volume, and loss of functioning alveolar–capillary units characterize a large and diverse group of pulmonary disorders collectively termed **restrictive lung disease**, or **RLD**.

The genesis of RLD involves pathophysiology of three aspects of pulmonary ventilation: (1) lung compliance, (2) lung volumes and capacities, and (3) work of breathing. **Lung compliance**, a measure of lung and/or chest wall distensibility, refers to the change in lung volume in relation to transpulmonary pressure differentials. In RLD, the chest and lung tissues stiffen and resist expansion under the normal pressure differentials of breathing. The additional resistance to lung expansion requires greater pulmonary force to maintain adequate alveolar ventilation. This greatly increases the energy cost of normal ventilation and accounts for up to 50% of the total oxygen requirement during physical activity.[96] Eventually, the progression of RLD negatively affects all lung volumes and capacities. Figure 32.16 provides examples of typical lung volumes in different conditions associated with RLD. Diminished inspiratory and expiratory reserve volumes occur consistently under all conditions.

Table 32.22 lists major RLD conditions, along with their causes, signs and symptoms, and suggested treatments. Other known causes of RLD include rheumatoid arthritis, immunologic pathology, massive obesity, diabetes mellitus, trauma from injury, penetrating wounds, radiation, burns, other inhalation injuries, poisoning, and complications from drug therapy (including reactions to antibiotics and anti-inflammatory drugs).

Chronic Obstructive Pulmonary Disease

Chronic obstructive pulmonary disease (**COPD**), also termed *chronic airflow limitations* (*CAL*), comprises several respiratory tract diseases that obstruct airflow (e.g., emphysema, asthma, and chronic bronchitis). The disease destroys lung parenchyma, causing a mismatch between regional alveolar air and blood flow. This ultimately affects the lung's mechanical function, compromising gas exchange (ventilation:perfusion ratio) at the alveolar level. *A dramatic decrease in exercise tolerance almost always accompanies COPD.* The disease afflicts 15 to 25 million Americans and ranks as the fifth leading cause of death and second leading cause of morbidity in the United States. The natural history of COPD spans 20 to 50 years and closely parallels a history of chronic cigarette smoking.

Changes in pulmonary function measures, most notably decreased expiratory flow rate and increased residual lung volume, usually form the diagnosis of COPD. The classic disease symptoms include spontaneous spasms of bronchial smooth muscle that produce chronic cough, increased mucus production, inflammation and thickening of the mucosal lining of the bronchi and bronchioles, wheezing, and dyspnea upon exertion. Table 32.23 summarizes differences in anatomic location and pathology among major COPD conditions. Factors predisposing to COPD include chronic cigarette smoking (greater effect in women than men; particularly on the increase among college students[184]), air pollution, occupational exposure to irritating dusts or gases, heredity, infection, allergies, aging, and drugs. *COPD rarely occurs in nonsmokers.* The airways nar-

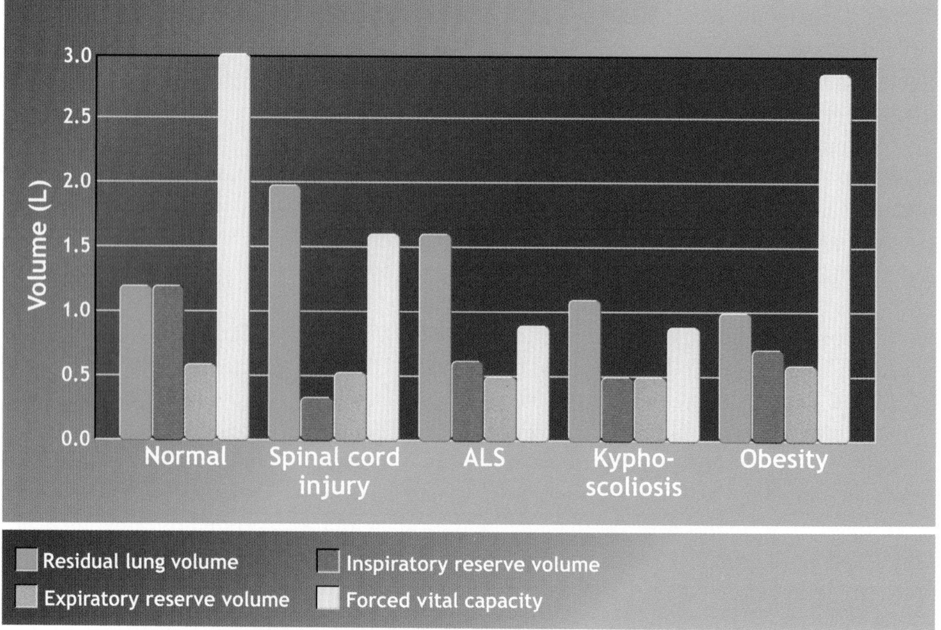

FIGURE 32.16 • Values for lung volumes in different conditions that cause restrictive lung disease. *ALS*, amyotrophic lateral sclerosis.

TABLE 32.22 ➤ **RESTRICTIVE LUNG DISEASES**

Causes/Type	Etiology	Signs and Symptoms	Treatment
I. Maturational			
a. *Abnormal fetal lung development*	Premature birth; (hypoplasia-reduced lung tissue)	Asymptomatic; pulmonary insufficiency	No specific treatment
b. *Respiratory distress syndrome* (hyaline membrane disease)	Insufficient maturation of lungs due to premature birth	↑ respiration rate; ↓ lung volumes; ↓ Pa_{O_2}; acidemia; rapid and labored respiration pressure	Treat mother prior to birth (corticosteroids); hyperalimentation; continuous positive airway
c. *Aging*	Aging and cumulative effects of pollution, noxious gas, inhaled drug use and cigarette smoking	↑ residual volume; ↓ vital capacity; repetitive periodic apnea	No specific treatment; increase physical activity
II. Pulmonary			
a. *Idiopathic pulmonary fibrosis* (IPF)	Unknown origin (perhaps viral or genetic)	↓ lung volumes; pulmonary hypertension; dyspnea; cough; weight loss, fatigue	Corticosteroids; maintain adequate nutrition and ventilation
b. *Coal workers' pneumoconiosis*	Repeated inhalation of coal dust over 10–12 years	↓ TLC, VC, FRC; ↓ lung compliance; dyspnea; ↓ Pa_{O_2}; pulmonary hypertension; cough	Nonreversible, no known cure
c. *Asbestosis*	Chronic exposure to asbestos	↓ lung volumes; abnormal x-ray; ↓ Pa_{O_2}; dyspnea on exertion, shortness of breath	Nonreversible, no known cure
d. *Pneumonia*	Inflammatory process caused by various bacteria, microbes, viruses	↓ lung volumes; abnormal x-ray; tachypneic dyspnea; high fever, chills, cough; pleuritic pain	Drug therapy (antibiotic)
e. *Adult respiratory distress syndrome*	Acute lung injury (fat emboli, drowning, drug induced, shock, blood transfusion, pneumonia)	Abnormal lung function tests; Pa_{O_2} <60 mmHg; extreme dyspnea; cyanotic; headache; anxiety	Intubation and mechanical ventilation
f. *Bronchogenic carcinoma*	Tobacco use	Variable, depending on type and location of growth	Surgery, radiation, chemotherapy; specific drainage
g. *Pleural effusions*	Accumulation of fluid within plueral space; heart failure; cirrhosis	Shortness of breath; pleuritic chest pain; ↓ Pa_{O_2}	
III. Cardiovascular			
a. *Pulmonary edema*	↑ pulmonary capillary hydrostatic pressure secondary to left ventricular failure	↑ respiration rate; ↓ lung volumes; ↓ Pa_{O_2}; arrhythmias; report feeling of suffocation, shortness of breath, cyanotic, cough	Drug therapy, diuretics; supplemental oxygen
b. *Pulmonary emboli*	Complications of venous thrombosis	↓ lung volumes; ↓ Pa_{O_2}; tachycardia; acute dyspnea, shortness of breath; syncope	Heparin therapy; mechanical ventilation
IV. Neuromuscular			
a. *Spinal cord injury*	Trauma paralysis of respiratory muscles	↓ lung volumes; hypoxemia; fatigue; shortness of breath; inability to cough; ↓ voice volume	Active and passive chest wall stretching
b. *Amyotrophic lateral sclerosis*	Degenerative disease of nervous system	↓ lung volumes; ↓ maximum voluntary volume	No treatment except supportive therapy
c. *Poliomyelitis*	Viral infectious disease that attacks motor nerves	Paralysis of diaphragm; shortness of breath	No treatment except supportive therapy
d. *Guillain-Barré syndrome*	Demyelinating disease of motor neurons	Profound muscular weakness; ↓ lung volumes	Passive range-of-motion exercises; active exercise
e. *Neuromuscular diseases (myasthenia gravis, tetanus, muscular dystrophy)*	Diseases of neuromuscular system, genetic or other cause resulting in chronic muscular weakness and wasting	Weakness, fatigue, loss of muscle function and strength, paralysis—affects pulmonary system with eventual loss of function	Drugs; passive and active exercise; supportive therapy
V. Musculoskeletal			
a. *Diaphragmatic paralysis*	Loss or impairment of motor function of diaphragm muscle due to specific lesion	↓ lung volumes; dyspnea, shortness of breath	Not needed
b. *Kyphoscoliosis*	Excessive anteroposterior and lateral curvature of thoracic spine (cause unknown)	↓ lung volumes; exertional dyspnea	Use of orthotic devices; active exercise
c. *Ankylosing spondylitis*	Chronic inflammatory disease of spine (inherited)	Exertional dyspnea	No treatment

TABLE 32.23 ➤ **DIFFERENCES AMONG MAJOR COPD DISEASES**

Name	Area Affected	Result
Bronchitis	Membrane lining bronchial tubes	Inflammation of bronchial lining
Bronchiectasis	Bronchial tubes (bronchi or air passages)	Bronchial dilation with inflammation
Emphysema	Air spaces beyond terminal bronchioles (alveoli)	Breakdown of alveolar walls; air spaces enlarged
Asthma	Bronchioles (small airways)	Bronchioles obstructed by muscle spasm; swelling of mucosa; thick secretions
Cystic fibrosis	Bronchioles	Bronchioles become obstructed and obliterated; plugs of mucus cling to airway walls, leading to bronchitis, atelectasis, pneumonia, or pulmonary abscess

row to obstruct pulmonary airflow in all forms of COPD. Airway narrowing hinders ventilation by trapping air in the bronchioles and alveoli; in essence, the disease increases pulmonary physiologic dead space. The obstruction also increases resistance to airflow (chiefly in expiration), hinders normal gas exchange, and reduces exercise performance by increasing the energy cost of breathing. The latter reduces ventilatory capacity, hindering full arterial oxygen saturation and carbon dioxide elimination. Patients with severe COPD exhibit decreased whole-body mechanical efficiency during exercise.[180] This suggests that factors associated with the respiratory effort also magnify the energy requirements of whole-body exercise to further negatively impact exercise capacity.

Interestingly, poor exercise tolerance and early onset of lactate accumulation in COPD patients do not always link closely to limitations in pulmonary ventilation and gas exchange in exercise. Rather, peripheral skeletal muscle performance deteriorates in COPD as reflected by (1) decreased muscle mass and strength and (2) reduced skeletal muscle oxidative capacity from a marked decrease in type I and increase in type IIb muscle fiber proportions and reduced mitochondrial enzyme activities. Loss of peripheral function possibly results from detraining with a sedentary lifestyle.[134,135] Proper exercise intervention can sometimes reverse peripheral abnormalities associated with COPD.[220]

The following sections focus on the major COPD diseases—chronic bronchitis, emphysema, cystic fibrosis, and exercise-induced bronchospasm.

Chronic Bronchitis

Acute bronchitis, an inflammation of the trachea and bronchi, usually is self-limiting and of short duration. In contrast, **chronic bronchitis** results from prolonged exposure to nonspecific irritants. Over time, the swollen mucous membranes and increased mucus production obstruct the airways, causing wheezing and chronic coughing. Partial or complete airway blockage from mucus secretion causes inadequate arterial oxygen saturation, diminished carbon dioxide elimination, and pulmonary edema. Eventually, the patient develops the characteristic look of a "blue bloater" (Fig. 32.17). Chronic bronchitis develops slowly and worsens over time. Patients

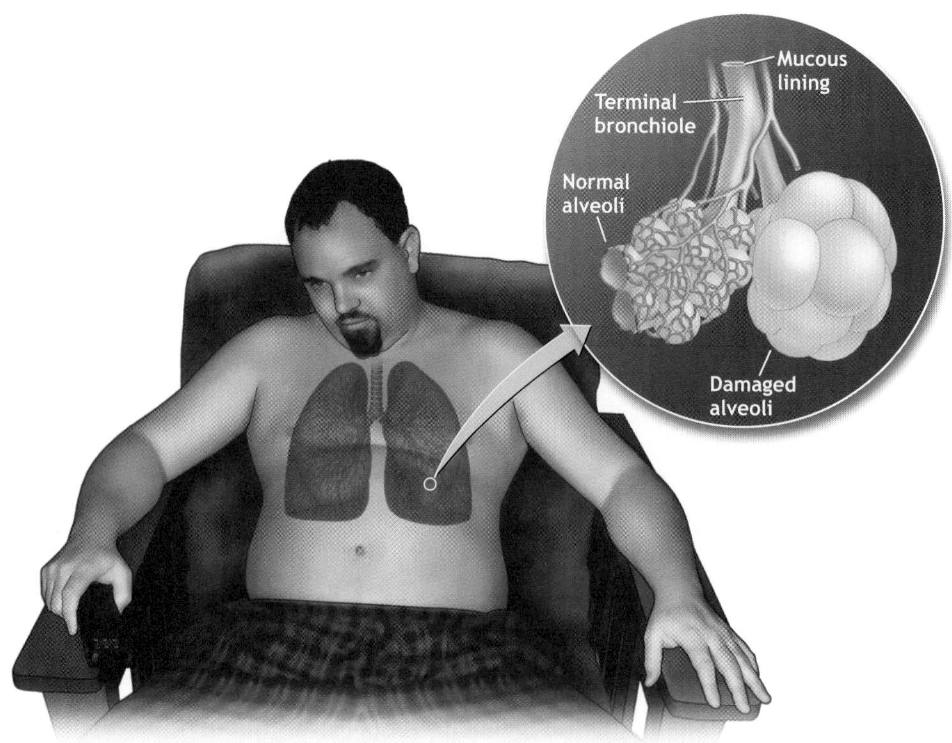

FIGURE 32.17 • A person with chronic bronchitis usually develops cyanosis and pulmonary edema with the characteristic appearance known as the "blue bloater." *Insert.* Effects of chronic bronchitis: misshapen or large alveolar sacs with reduced surface for oxygen and carbon dioxide exchange.

usually have a long history of cigarette smoking. Functional capacity decreases considerably, and fatigue occurs readily with mild exercise. If left untreated, this disease usually leads to premature death.

Emphysema

An abnormal, permanent enlargement of air spaces distal to the terminal bronchioles characterizes **emphysema**. The disease occurs most frequently among chronic cigarette smokers. It develops as a consequence of chronic bronchitis; its symptoms include dyspnea, hypercapnea, persistent cough, cyanosis, and digital clubbing (evidence of chronic hypoxemia; Fig. 32.18). Emphysemic patients consistently demonstrate low exercise capacity and extreme dyspnea with exertion; many patients appear thin-looking and often lean forward with arms braced on the knees to support the shoulders and chest to ease breathing. The chronic effects of trapped air and alveolar distension change the size and shape of the chest, causing the characteristic emphysemic "barrel chest" appearance (Fig. 32.19). Regular exercise does not improve pulmonary function of individuals with emphysema, but it enhances cardiovascular fitness, strengthens both respiratory and nonrespiratory musculature, and improves psychologic status.[17,37] In selected patients with severe emphysema, lung-volume reduction surgery has improved pulmonary function, exercise capacity, and quality of life. Its effects on longevity remain uncertain.[71]

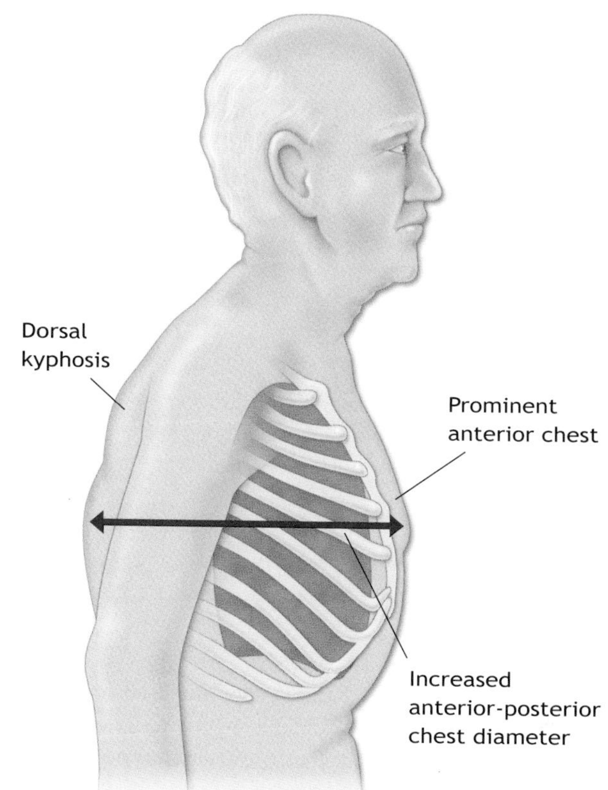

FIGURE 32.19 • Emphysema traps air in the lungs, making exhalation difficult. With time, changes occur in the physical features of the patient, hence the name "pink puffer."

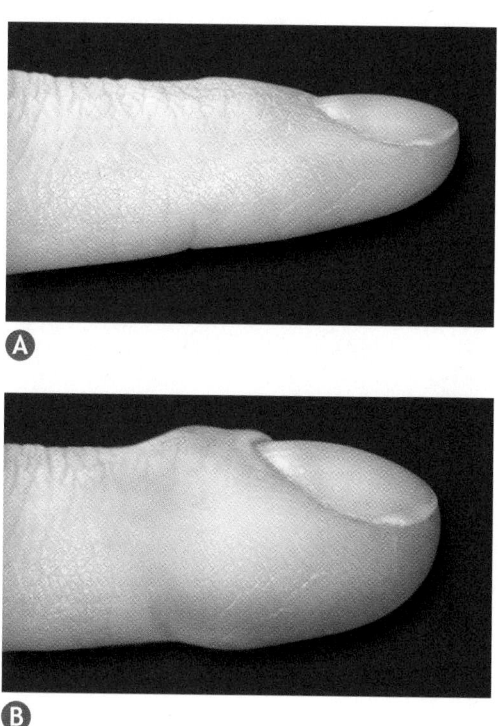

FIGURE 32.18 • Normal digit configuration (**A**) and digital clubbing (**B**). Club fingers and toes indicate chronic tissue hypoxia, a common diagnosis in emphysema.

Cystic Fibrosis

The term **cystic fibrosis** (**CF**; www.cff.org/) originates from the diagnosis of cysts and scar tissue observed on the pancreas during autopsy. Pancreatic cysts and scar tissue often exist but do not reflect the primary characteristics of the disease.[165] Table 32.24 lists clinical signs and symptoms of this inherited and always fatal disease characterized by thickening secretions of all exocrine glands (e.g., pancreatic, pulmonic, and gastrointestinal). Glandular secretions ultimately lead to pulmonary obstruction, mainly in the lung tissue itself. CF, the most common inherited disease (both parents must carry the recessive trait) in whites, afflicts approximately 1 in 2000 white infants in the United States. Approximately 5% (12 million) of Americans carry the gene for CF located on chromosome 7. CF currently afflicts about 30,000 children and adults in the United States.

A positive sweat electrolyte (chloride) test result diagnoses CF. Patients possess a faulty copy of the gene that enables cells to construct a channel through which the chloride ion passes. Consequently, salt accumulates in the cells lining the lungs and digestive tissues, making the surrounding mucus abnormally thick and salty. These mucous secretions, the critical feature of CF, obstruct ducts and passages in the pancreas, liver, and lungs.

Pulmonary impairment is the most common and severe manifestation of CF. Airway obstruction leads to chronic lung

TABLE 32.24 ➤ CLINICAL SIGNS AND SYMPTOMS OF CYSTIC FIBROSIS AND RELATED PULMONARY INVOLVEMENT

Early stage clinical signs and symptoms of cystic fibrosis
- Persistent cough and wheezing
- Recurrent pneumonia
- Excessive appetite but poor weight gain
- Salty skin or sweat
- Bulky, foul-smelling stools (undigested lipids)

Late stage clinical signs and symptoms of cystic fibrosis with pulmonary involvement
- Tachypnea (rapid breathing)
- Sustained chronic cough with mucus production on vomiting
- Barrel chest
- Cyanosis and digital clubbing
- Exertional dyspnea with decreased exercise capacity
- Pneumothorax
- Right heart failure secondary to pulmonary hypertension

hyperinflation. Over time, RLD is superimposed on the obstructive disease, leading to chronic hypoxia, hypercapnea, and acidosis, which increase the risk of arterial desaturation during exercise. The disease progresses to pneumothorax and pulmonary hypertension and eventually death.

Treatment of CF includes antibiotics, the FDA-approved mucos-thinning drug Pulmozyme®, TOBI (tobramycin) solution for inhalation, high dosages of ibuprofen, enzyme supplements, nutritional intervention, and frequent mucous secretion removal. Assessments of physiclal capacity of children with CF suggest a positive role for regular physical activity. For example, aerobic fitness correlates inversely with 8-year mortality.[157] In addition, the anaerobic power of children with CF is significantly lower than healthy counterparts, although they rely more on anaerobic pathways during strenuous exercise.[26,27] Increased minute ventilation with aerobic exercise helps to clear airways of excessive secretions.[190,227] For example, 20 to 30 minutes of aerobic exercise replaces one session of secretion removal for some children. Thus, increasing physical fitness can help delay CF's crippling effects. An abnormally high loss of NaCl in the sweat increases the likelihood of plasma hypoosmolality with concomitant reductions in thirst drive. A flavored drink with relatively high salt content (e.g., 50 mmol · L^{-1}) enhances drinking and reduces exercise dehydration risk in CF patients.[120]

Pulmonary Assessments

Exercise physiologists do not diagnose pulmonary disease, but understanding the different tests and their results assists in planning and implementing exercise interventions. Pulmonary disease diagnosis involves several different objective measures, including chest imaging, flow and volume tests, blood gas analyses, and cytologic and hematologic evaluations.

X-ray

Chest and lung imaging are the most popular pulmonary assessment techniques. These include the conventional x-ray in which roentgen rays (named after German physicist and Nobel laureate Wilhelm Konrad Roentgen [1845–1923]) penetrate the body to provide an image of the chest's anatomy on film (radiograph, or roentgenogram). This standard diagnostic tool screens for abnormalities, provides a baseline for subsequent assessments, and monitors disease progression. A chest radiograph shows body fat, water, tissue, bone, and air space. The low density of air in the lungs allows greater roentgen ray penetration, producing a dark image. Relatively dense bone represents the other extreme; it allows fewer roentgen rays to penetrate its tissue, thus producing a white image. The *top* of Figure 32.20 illustrates a normal chest radiograph taken in the posterioanterior (PA) position.

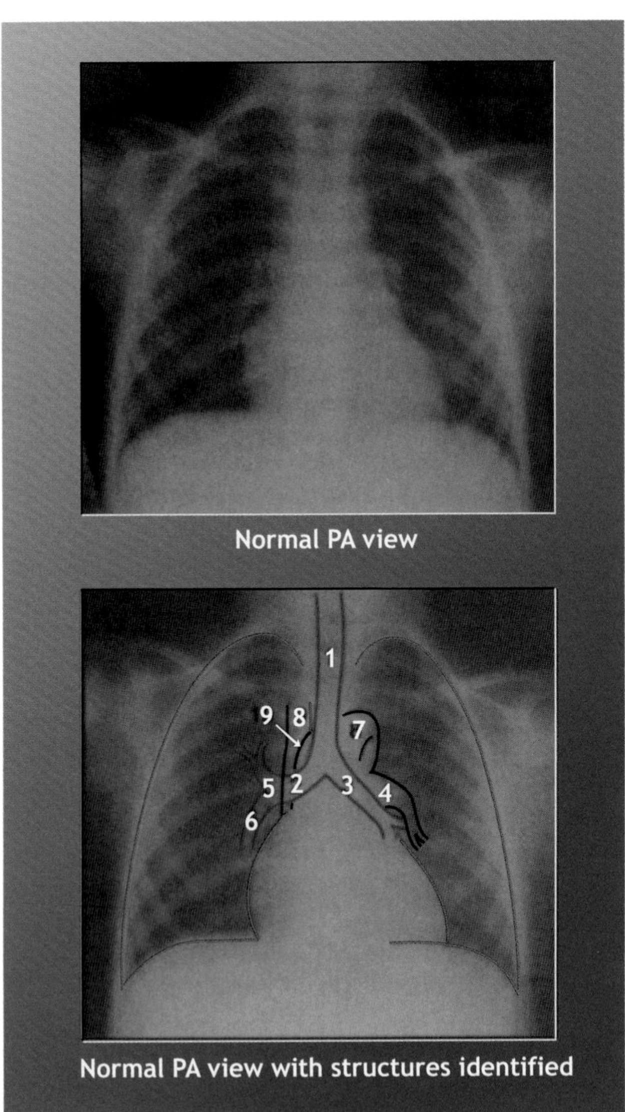

FIGURE 32.20 • Chest x-ray. The *top* radiograph shows a normal chest x-ray in the posterioanterior (PA) view. The *bottom* radiograph shows labeling of the normal anatomic structures. *1,* trachea; *2,* right mainstem bronchus; *3,* left mainstem bronchus; *4,* left pulmonary artery; *5,* pulmonary vein to the right upper lobe; *6,* right interlobular artery; *7,* aortic knob; *8,* superior vena cava; *9,* ascending aorta.

The *bottom* of the figure shows the same radiograph with the normal anatomic structures labeled. Abnormal radiographic densities identify specific lung lesions.

Computed Tomography

Most clinical radiologists consider CT scanning the single greatest advance in radiography of anatomic structures since the discovery of roentgen rays. CT uses a narrow x-ray beam that moves across the body to define adjacent cross-sectional columns of tissue known as a *translation*. Another pass of the beam progresses at a different angle or *rotation*. Repeated translations and rotations in different directions in a given plane with subsequent digitization produces a clear computer-summated image of x-ray transmission data for diagnostic interpretation.

Other Measures

Chapter 12 discussed static and dynamic lung function tests with simple spirometry. Carefully collected spirometric data such as forced vital capacity (FVC), forced expiratory volume in 1 second ($FEV_{1.0}$), maximum voluntary ventilation (MVV), peak expiratory flow (PEF), and lung compliance provide crucial diagnostic information. To measure compliance, the patient swallows a balloon catheter. The technician positions the catheter in the lower third of the esophagus and connects it to a manometer to measure esophageal pressure. The relation of lung volume change to any change in pressure within the catheter then establishes the curve for lung compliance.

Other useful functional tests include pulmonary diffusing capacity (DL or DLCO, expressed in $mL \cdot min^{-1} \cdot mm\ Hg^{-1}$), which measures how much gas enters pulmonary blood per unit time per unit pressure differential across the alveolar–capillary membrane. Flow-volume loops provide graphic representations of events occurring during forced inspiration and expiration. Recording the flow versus volume in an X–Y presentation diagnoses central or peripheral airway obstructions.

Blood gas analyses provide important information for assessing problems related to acid–base balance, alveolar ventilation, and level of arterial oxygen saturation and carbon dioxide elimination. Cytologic and hematologic tests identify microorganisms that cause pulmonary disease.

Pulmonary Rehabilitation and Exercise Prescription

Pulmonary rehabilitation programs have received considerably less attention than programs for cardiovascular and musculoskeletal diseases. The lack of emphasis on pulmonary rehabilitation stems from a failure of rehabilitation to improve pulmonary function significantly or "cure" these potentially deadly diseases. Nevertheless, successful pulmonary rehabilitation places central focus on exercise training because of its positive impact on exercise capacity, respiratory and nonrespiratory muscle functions, ventilatory equivalents for oxygen, psychologic status, quality-of-life variables (e.g., self-esteem and self-efficacy), frequency of hospitalization, and disease progression.[17,40] Much of the disability associated with COPD results from the spiral of progressive physical deconditioning from a sedentary lifestyle (as patients attempt to avoid dyspnea) and is not just the direct effect of the disease.[37,178,199] Frequently, peripheral and respiratory muscle weakness contribute to the COPD patients' poor exercise performance and physiologic incapacity.[88,198] Within this framework, the major goals for pulmonary rehabilitation include:

- Improving health status
- Improving respiratory symptoms (shortness of breath and cough)
- Recognizing early signs that require medical intervention
- Decreasing frequency and severity of respiratory problems
- Maximizing arterial O_2 saturation and CO_2 elimination
- Enhancing daily functional capacity through improved muscular strength, joint flexibility, and cardiorespiratory endurance
- Modifying body composition to enhance functional capacity
- Optimizing nutritional status

The overall pulmonary rehabilitation program emphasizes general patient care, pulmonary respiratory care, exercise and functional training, education about the disease, and psychosocial management. Table 32.25 outlines the important components of an exercise prescription for COPD patients. The training aspects of rehabilitation take on importance for patients with weakness, fatigue, and severe dyspnea that profoundly limit physical activity. Physiologic monitoring during exercise rehabilitation includes measurement of heart rate, blood pressure, respiratory rate, arterial oxygen saturation by pulse oximetry, and dyspnea. Dyspnea monitoring as a target for exercise training involves a perceived **dyspnea scale** (Fig. 32.21), similar to the scale for rating perceived exertion.[65,95] The dyspnea scale emphasizes symptoms of breathing difficulty rather than perceptions of whole-body physical distress that the RPE measures. Self-monitoring exercise intensity in this manner has inherent advantages because (1) respiratory disease usually impairs exercise pulmonary function rather than cardiovascular response and (2) target heart rate for training healthy individuals usually exceeds the peak heart rate achieved when stress testing pulmonary patients. Extreme shortness of breath, fatigue, palpitations, chest discomfort, or a 3 to 5% decrease on pulse oximetry are the most common reasons for stopping exercise.

The pretraining GXT and spirometric analyses form the basis for the exercise prescription.[50] Interpretation of the exercise stress test includes determining (1) whether the test terminated because of cardiovascular or ventilatory end points, (2) the difference between pre- and postexercise pulmonary function (e.g., a decrease of 10% in $FEV_{1.0}$ indicates the need for bronchodilator therapy before exercise), and (3) need for

TABLE 32.25 ➤ COMPONENTS OF THE COPD EXERCISE PRESCRIPTION

Evaluation
- Assess cardiac risk
- Assess exercise capacity with Naughton-type protocol (see Fig. 11.10) using a treadmill or stationary cycle, starting at a low workload and increasing extremely slowly and monitoring desaturation with pulse oximeter
- Determine appropriate exercise levels to prevent arrhythmias or hypoxia in cardiac-impaired patients
- Determine amount of supplemental oxygen needed during exercise
- Determine need for bronchodilators during exercise
- Assess side effects of β-agonist inhalers or aminophylline derivatives during exercise

Supervised exercise
- Direct patient to supervised rehabilitation program if disease is significant
- Set goal of eventually graduating to independent exercise (many patients can do this in about 6 wk)

Independent exercise
- Suggest appropriate training mode: stationary cycling, bicycling, treadmill walking, outdoor walking, stair climbing, or arm ergometry
- Set goal of 60 to 80% of HR_{max} for 20 to 30 minutes, 3 days per week (but build on individual ability)
- Expect 70 to 80% increase over initial work capacity within 6 weeks
- Provide active encouragement and reassurance (especially at first) to overcome anxiety associated with dyspnea

Exercise aids
- Supplemental oxygen
- Bronchodilators (adrenergic agonists and/or aminophylline derivatives)
- Mucolytics
- Corticosteroids (inhaled or oral)
- Monitoring

From Mink BD. Exercise and chronic obstructive pulmonary disease: modest fitness gains pay big dividends. Phys Sportsmed 1997;25(11):43.

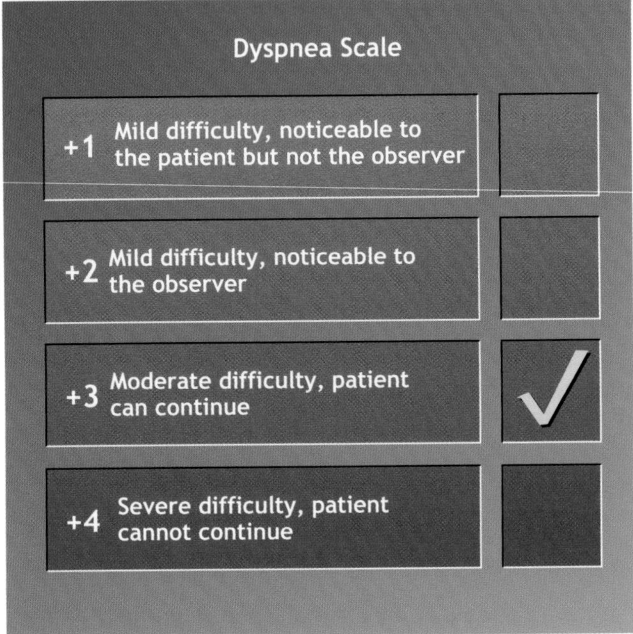

FIGURE 32.21 • Dyspnea scale. Subjective ratings of dyspnea on a scale of 1 to 4 during graded exercise testing. Dyspnea usually accompanies poor exercise capacity and impaired systolic blood pressure response.

supplemental oxygen during exercise (e.g., a pre- to posttest decrease in Pa_{O_2} of more than 20 mm Hg or a Pa_{O_2} below 55 mm Hg).

Exercise prescription (cycling, walking, treadmill exercise, and stair climbing) for patients with **mild lung disease**—shortness of breath with heavy exercise—remains similar to exercise for healthy subjects. Exercise for patients with **moderate lung disease**—shortness of breath with normal daily activities or clinical symptoms of RLD or COPD—usually reaches an intensity no greater than 75% of the ventilatory reserve or the point where the patient becomes noticeably dyspneic. For most patients, this exercise intensity usually falls in the middle of the calculated training heart rate range (50 to 70% of age-predicted maximum with a goal of 60 to 80% of maximum) and corresponds to 40 to 85% of maximum MET level on the GXT. In this case, exercise duration usually averages approximately 20 minutes, 3 times per week. If the patient can exercise only for a shorter duration (e.g., 5 to 15 min per session), exercise frequency can increase to 5 to 7 days weekly.

Patients with **severe lung disease**—shortness of breath during most daily activities and FVC and $FEV_{1.0}$ below 55% of predicted values—require a modified approach to exercise testing and prescription. Usually low-level, discontinuous testing begins at 2 to 3 METs, with increments every 2 to 3 minutes. Exercise prescription uses symptom-limited walking speeds and distances. Brief bouts of interval exercise also provide an option. The low level of the initial training prescription means that patients should exercise a minimum of once daily. Even minimal gains in exercise tolerance add significantly to improving daily function and quality of life.

General exercise and specific expiratory muscle training effectively improve respiratory muscle function and reduce sensations of respiratory effort during exercise in nearly all patients with pulmonary disease.[39,122,207] Two approaches achieve this goal:

1. Resistance training of the ventilatory musculature with a continuous positive airway pressure (CPAP) device; this specifically overloads the respiratory muscles similarly to progressive resistance exercise for nonrespiratory skeletal muscles
2. Increasing respiratory muscle force and endurance capacity through regular aerobic exercise training

INTEGRATIVE QUESTION

Why might exercise prove more effective for coronary heart disease patients than patients with pulmonary disease?

TABLE 32.26 ➤ MAJOR PULMONARY BRONCHODILATOR DRUGS: THEIR USES AND SIDE EFFECTS

DRUG/NAME	ACTION AND CLINICAL USES	SIDE EFFECTS
Sympathomimetics Isoproterenol, ephedrine, Bronkosol, Alupent, Brethine, Proventil, Ventolin	Decrease intracellular calcium; smooth muscle relaxation; bronchodilation	Tachycardia, palpitations, GI distress, nervousness, headache, dizziness
Methylxanthines Amnodur, Elixophyllin, Theodur, Choladril	Increase cAMP; block cAMP decrease	Agitation, hypotension, chest pain, nausea, tachycardia, palpitations, GI distress, nervousness, headache, dizziness
α-Sympatholytics	Block cAMP decrease; bronchodilation	Agitation, hypotension, chest pain, nausea, tachycardia, palpitations, GI distress, nervousness, headache, dizziness
Parasympatholytics Atrovent, atropine sulfate	Block parasympathetic stimulation and prevents increases in cGMP; prevents bronchoconstriction	Central nervous system stimulation with low doses and depression with high doses; delirium, hallucinations, decreased GI activity
Glucocorticoids Prednisone, Cortisol, Azmacort, Vanceril	Decrease inflammatory response; bronchodilation	Obesity, growth suppression, hyperglycemia and diabetes, mood changes, irritability, or depression, thinning of skin, muscle wasting
Cromolyn sodium Intal, Fivent	Prevents influx of calcium ions, thus blocking mast cell release of mediators responsible for bronchoconstriction; bronchodilation	Throat irritation, hoarseness, dry mouth, cough, chest tightness, bronchospasm

Pulmonary Medications

Pulmonary medications include bronchodilators, anti-inflammatory agents, decongestants, antihistamines, mucokinetic agents, respiratory stimulants, depressants, and paralyzing and antimicrobial agents. The drugs promote bronchodilation, facilitate removal of lung secretions, improve alveolar ventilation and arterial oxygenation, and optimize breathing patterns. Table 32.26 lists the most common pulmonary drugs.

EXERCISE AND ASTHMA

Asthma, the most common chronic disease in the industrialized world (www.aafa.org/), afflicts about 17 million Americans, predominantly children and adolescents (notably African American children from inner-city neighborhoods). Asthma, the only chronic disease besides tuberculosis and AIDS, has an increasing death rate. Each day in the United States, 14 people die from asthma, and asthma accounts for almost 2 million emergency room visits (500,000 hospitalizations) and 10 million doctor office visits yearly. Hyperirritability of the pulmonary airways followed by bronchial spasm, edema, and mucus secretion characterize this obstructive pulmonary disease (Fig. 32.22). Common asthma symptoms include chest tightness, coughing, wheezing, and/or shortness of breath.

The annual medical costs for treating asthma in 1998 averaged nearly $7.5 billion. Unfortunately, a high level of physical fitness does not confer immunity from asthma[158]—67 (11%) of the 597 U.S. athletes in the 1984 Olympic games suffered from asthma.[215] (U.S. swimmer Nancy Hogshead, an asthma sufferer, won three gold and one silver medal in these games.) Studies of Finnish elite track and field athletes report physician-diagnosed asthma in 17% of long-distance runners, 8% of power athletes, and 3% of nonathletic controls,[90] while 35% of figure skaters showed a significant increase in airway resistance following skating routines.[136] Bronchospasm following strenuous exercise—a sign of potential "hidden" asthma—occurred in 9% of Philadelphia's high school athletes. Some 13% of black athletes showed bronchospasm compared with only 2% of white athletes.

For nearly 90% of persons with asthma, and 30 to 50% of those suffering from allergic rhinitis and hayfever, exercise provides a potent stimulus for bronchoconstriction, a response termed **exercise-induced bronchospasm**. Reduced vagal tone and increased catecholamine release from the sympathetic nervous system during exercise normally relax pulmonary airway smooth muscle.[15,132,204] Figure 32.22A shows that initial bronchodilation with exercise occurs in healthy persons and asthmatics. For the asthmatic, however, bronchospasm accompanied by excessive mucus secretion follows initial bronchodilation. An acute episode of airway obstruction often occurs within 5 to 15 minutes postexercise (Fig. 32.22B); recovery usually occurs spontaneously within 30 to 90 minutes. One useful technique to detect an exercise-induced asthmatic response applies progressive exercise increments. A spirometric evaluation of FVC and $FEV_{1.0}$ takes place after each exercise period and during 10 to 20 minutes of recovery. *A 10 to 15% reduction in preexercise $FEV_{1.0}/FVC$ confirms the diagnosis of exercise-induced bronchospasm.*[94,121,144] For elite athletes who perform in cold-weather sports (e.g., biathlon, canoe/kayak, cross-country skiing, ice hockey, Nordic combined, and speed skating), combining pulmonary function testing with near-maximal exercise testing, preferably sport-specific exercise testing, in a cold, dry environment provides

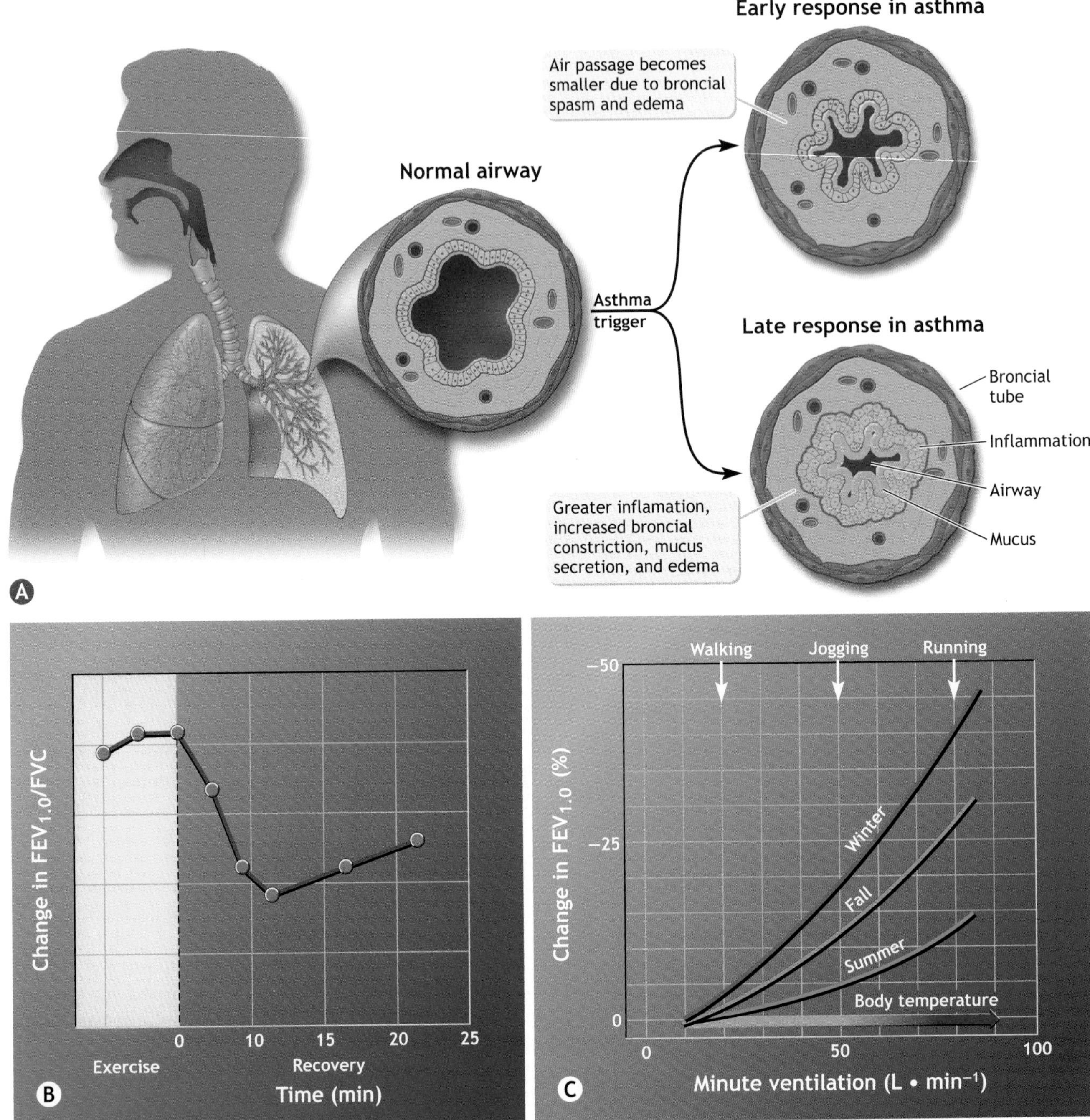

FIGURE 32.22 • **A**. Typical response to an asthma attack. **B**. Pattern of dynamic lung function (*$FEV_{1.0}$/FVC*) during an episode of exercise-induced bronchospasm. **C**. Interaction between exercise intensity (walking, jogging, running) and environmental characteristics. Note that maximal obstruction occurs when inhaling dry air at low temperature (e.g., winter) and minimal obstruction occurs when breathing warm, humid air (e.g., summer). (C modified from McFadden ER Jr, Gilbert IA. Current concepts in exercise-induced asthma. N Engl J Med 1994;330:1362.)

greater sensitivity for screening than laboratory-based (warm air environment) challenges[187] or use of self-reported symptoms for diagnosis.[188]

Sensitivity to Thermal Gradients and Fluid Loss

Several mechanisms help to explain bronchospastic responses to exercise.[8,73,214] One of the more attractive theories relates to alterations in the rate and magnitude of heat and water exchange in the tracheobronchial tree caused by ventilation in exercise and recovery. As the incoming breath of air moves down the respiratory tract, heat and water move away from the airway lining as the air warms and humidifies. The conditioning of inspired air ultimately cools and dries the respiratory mucosa. Drying increases mucosal lining osmolality, with accompanying mast cell degranulation. This in turn releases powerful proinflamatory mediators that trigger bronchoconstriction (e.g., leukotrienes, histamine, and prostaglandins).[128] Rewarming the airways following exercise dilates the bronchial microcirculation, causing hyperemia. Bronchial vasculature engorgement precipitates edema that constricts the airway, independent of any constrictive action of bronchial smooth muscle. Bronchial cooling during exercise and rewarming in recovery also stimulates chemical mediator release that induces bronchoconstriction.

Regardless of the precise mechanism, the large volume of incompletely conditioned inspired air taxes the tracheobronchial tree's smaller airways, causing mucosal temperature to decrease. Heat loss from the airways during exercise relates directly to the degree of bronchoconstriction. In susceptible individuals, the thermal gradient generated by the combination of airway cooling during exercise and subsequent rewarming in recovery intensifies bronchospastic processes.

Environmental Impact

Figure 32.22C shows that a warm-humid (summer) environment suppresses the magnitude of exercise-induced bronchospasm, regardless of air temperature.[14,144] Inhaling ambient air fully saturated with water vapor often abolishes an asthmatic's bronchospastic exercise response. This explains why persons with asthma tolerate walking or jogging on a warm, humid day or swimming in an indoor pool, whereas outdoor winter sports typically trigger an asthmatic attack.[191] The benefit of swimming to the asthma-sensitive individual may not simply relate to the humid environment.[100] Three additional factors contribute to a reduced potential for exercise-induced bronchoconstriction in swimming: (1) interrupted nature of the breathing pattern, (2) lower ventilation volumes, and (3) greater catecholamine response from activation of a relatively small upper-body muscle mass.

Benefits of Warm-Up and Medication

Fifteen to 30 minutes of a light-to-moderate, continuous warm-up or repeat several-minute warm-up intervals initiate a **refractory period** in which subsequent intense exercise does not trigger as severe a bronchoconstrictive response.[15,20,179] The warm-up benefit continues for up to 2 hours, perhaps from prostaglandin release. Prolonging the cool-down period also reduces the severity of postexercise bronchoconstriction; this could occur by slowing airway rewarming and subsequent bronchiole vascular dilation and edema.

Effective preexercise medications limit bronchoconstriction for those desiring to exercise regularly without adversely affecting exercise performance.[99,123,160] Medications include (1) bronchodilators such as theophylline or the leukotriene-receptor antagonist montelukast,[53,128,181] or β_2-agonists (salmeterol)[153] and (2) inhaled heparin therapy or anti-inflammatory agents such as corticosteroids or cromolyn sodium.

Exercise training does not eliminate or cure an asthmatic condition; instead it increases pulmonary airflow reserve and reduces ventilatory work by potentiating exercise bronchodilation. This lets asthmatics maintain higher airflow and sustain relatively intense exercise despite impaired pulmonary function. For asthmatic children, aerobic exercise training (swimming and cycle ergometry) significantly improves $\dot{V}O_{2max}$ and suppresses asthmatic symptoms.[139,152] Research still must determine whether regular aerobic exercise decreases the likelihood of provoking an asthma attack, improves asthmatic control, or decreases medication requirements.

HEALTH/FITNESS PROMOTION AT THE WORK SITE

Since 1980, more than 75 research studies have evaluated comprehensive worksite health/fitness promotion and disease prevention programs. In addition, a pioneering text considered monetary and nonmonetary costs and benefits of enhanced physical fitness related to personal, sociocultural, industrial, environmental, and geriatric sectors of the economy.[200] The primary conclusion drawn from these data indicates positive health outcomes for employees and reduced costs to companies. Areas studied include behavior change, health outcomes, health care costs, worker productivity, absenteeism, and cost benefits.

Behavior Changes/Health Outcomes

Positive health outcomes include reductions in cardiovascular disease risk factors from changes in diet and exercise habits. Much of the research centers on such positive health behaviors as weight loss, reducing fat intake, reducing stress, and using leisure time positively. The following provide examples of positive health outcomes from work site fitness and health promotion programs:

- Two Georgia Pacific Corporation intervention programs helped high-risk employees reduce cholesterol 10% or more using a 1-month educational model with incentives.[46]
- Four years after initiation of an arthritis self-management program, five California counties noted a 20% decline in employee reports of pain and a 40% decrease in physician visits.[131]
- A 2-year work-site intervention program in Minneapolis/St. Paul produced an average weight loss of 4.8 pounds and a 43% increase in smoking cessation.[101]
- An 8-week work-site voluntary program at Coors Brewing Company improved multiple risk factors for cardiovascular disease—decreased systolic blood pressure, total cholesterol, body weight, and risks of ischemia—in participating employees over 8 years at an annual cost below $32 per employee participant per year.[91]

Health Care Costs

The increasing cost of providing employee medical care has eroded profits in all sectors of the economy. A large number of major U.S. corporations that introduced worksite wellness

Focus on Research

Physical Fitness Protects Against Death

Blair S, et al. Physical fitness and all-cause mortality: a prospective study of healthy men and women. JAMA 1989;262:2395.

➤ A report in 1998 by the Centers for Disease Control and Prevention stated that "physical inactivity is one of the major underlying causes of premature mortality in the United States" (Centers for Disease Control and Prevention. Self-reported physical inactivity by degree of urbanization—United States. MMWR 1998;47:1097.) This assertion confirmed that sedentary living causes about one-third of deaths from coronary heart disease, colon cancer, and type 2 diabetes. Increasing the nation's collective level of regular physical activity would therefore reduce the rate of premature deaths from these diseases by two-thirds.

The 1989 study by Blair and associates was the first to reveal the striking relationship between all-cause mortality and physical fitness in a healthy group of 10,224 men and 3120 women. Measurements included maximal treadmill testing for aerobic capacity, including extensive follow-up of a large enough samples of both men *and* women to permit meaningful statistical analyses. The research focused on physical fitness—a biologic attribute as an objective marker for habitual physical activity—rather than physical activity—a behavior, subject to measurement and interpretation difficulties. The dependent variable comprised all-cause and cause-specific mortality followed for up to 110,482 person-years, or an average of more than 8 years. This research and subsequent studies by the same investigators formed the basis for renewed interest and research support about the role of regular physical activity in overall health and disease prevention.

Participants underwent baseline measurements that included personal and family history, physical examination, a questionnaire on demographic characteristics and health habits (including cigarette smoking), anthropometry, resting ECG, blood chemistry, blood pressure, and a maximal treadmill exercise test. Subjects had no known heart problems, hypertension, stroke, diabetes, and resting or exercise ECG abnormalities. Total treadmill test time quantified physical fitness level; treadmill time correlated highly ($r \geq 0.92$) with $\dot{V}O_{2max}$ in men and women. Initial test results placed subjects into one of five aerobic fitness categories (1, low fitness; 5, high fitness), based on gender and age, to assess the link between physical fitness and all-cause and cause-specific mortality.

Figure 1 shows age-specific, all-cause death rates for men *(top)* and women *(bottom)*, categorized by fitness level. For both groups, the decline in death rate with higher fitness became more pronounced with aging. Table 1 shows the age-adjusted all-cause death rates per 10,000 person-years of follow-up (1970–1985), by fitness grouping. Clearly, less-fit women and men experience higher death risk than their more-fit counterparts. Significantly higher relative risk (RR) for all-cause mortality emerged for the least-fit quintile of men and for the two least-fit quintiles of women.

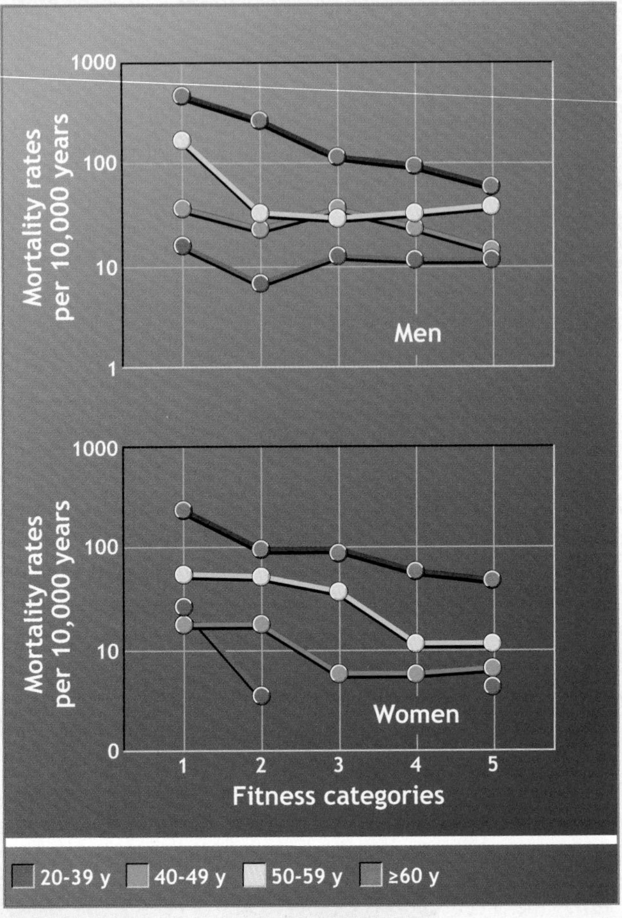

Figure 1. Age-specific, all-cause death rates per 10,000 person-years of follow-up in 10,224 men and 3120 women by physical fitness quintiles as determined by maximal treadmill exercise testing.

Figure 2 shows age-adjusted mortality per 10,000 person-years as a function of metabolic equivalents (METs) and estimated $\dot{V}O_{2max}$ from maximal treadmill testing. The lower limit for mortality risk for men *(orange bars)* and women *(yellow bars)* has an asymptote at about the same point for each age grouping—9 METs ($\dot{V}O_{2max}$ = 31.5 mL · kg^{-1} · min^{-1}) for women and 10 METs ($\dot{V}O_{2max}$ = 35.0 mL · kg^{-1} · min^{-1}) for men. These MET values and corresponding $\dot{V}O_{2max}$ values objectify a lower-limit aerobic fitness cutoff below which health risk increases. Individuals who regularly engage in moderate exercise generally achieve a fitness level above that associated with increased death risk. Brisk walking for 30 to 60 minutes daily provides suf-

Focus on Research

Physical Fitness Protects Against Death

ficient exercise overload to sustain a threshold aerobic fitness standard of 9 METs for women and 10 METs for men.

The data showed a clear, strong, and graded inverse relationship between aerobic fitness and mortality from all causes. The finding remained consistent for men and women, even after adjustment for age, serum cholesterol level, blood pressure, smoking habit, fasting blood glucose level, family history of CHD, and length of follow-up. The strength of the associations and the high prevalence of sedentary habits and low fitness levels produce high attributable risk estimates for the general population.

TABLE 1. AGE-ADJUSTED, ALL-CAUSE DEATH RATES PER 10,000 PERSON-YEARS OF FOLLOW-UP (1970-1985) BY AEROBIC FITNESS CATEGORIES IN WOMEN AND MEN

Fitness Group	Person-Years of Follow-Up	Number of Deaths	Age-Adjusted Rates per 10,000 Person-Years	Relative Risk (RR)
Men				
1 (low)	14,515	75	64.0	3.44
2	16,898	40	25.5	1.37
3	17,287	47	27.1	1.46
4	18,792	43	21.7	1.17
5 (high)	17,557	35	18.6	1.0
Women				
1 (low)	4916	18	39.5	4.65
2	5329	11	20.5	2.42
3	5053	6	12.2	1.43
4	5522	4	6.5	0.76
5 (high)	4613	4	8.5	1.00

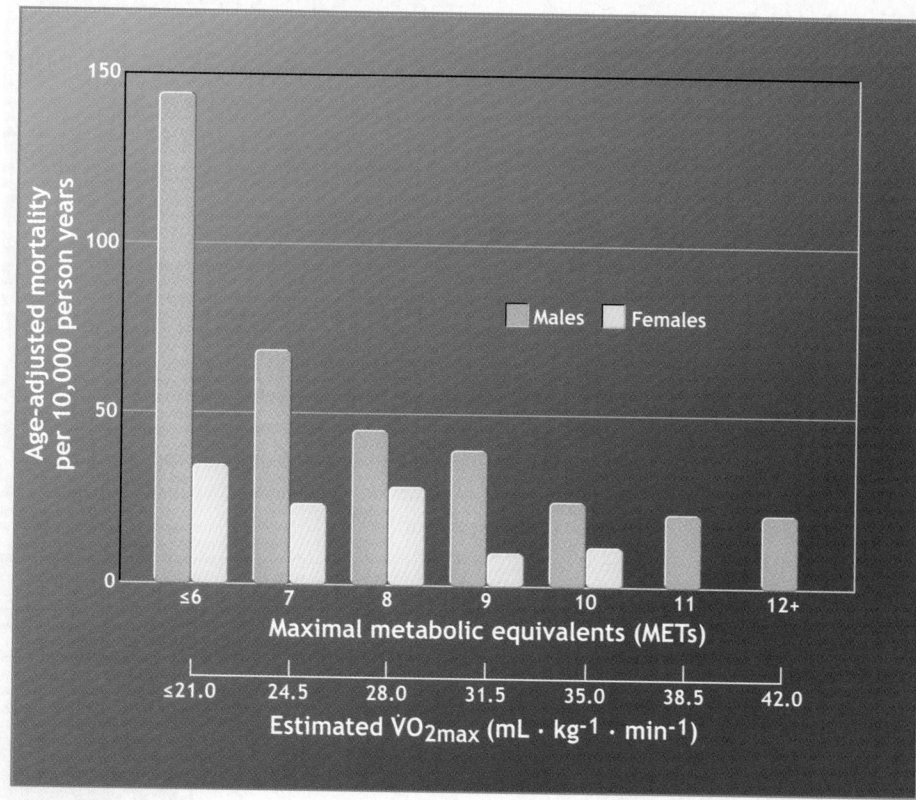

Figure 2. Age-adjusted, all-cause death rates per 10,000 person-years of follow-up by aerobic fitness categories in 3120 women and 10,224 men. Fitness categories expressed as maximal metabolic equivalents (METs) achieved during the maximal treadmill test. Estimated $\dot{V}O_{2max}$ (mL · kg^{-1} · min^{-1}) for each category is presented along the bottom axis.

programs have reduced employee use of health care services. Specific examples are as follows:

- Blue Shield of California demonstrated that a low-cost, mail-delivered health promotion program for 54,902 active and retired public employees saved $8 million in claims during 12 months.[72]
- Bank of America calculated that health promotion geared to retirees saved approximately $4298 per person per year in medical claims.[77,129]
- A 4-year study at General Motors demonstrated the value of counseling and follow-up, compared with screenings only, in a blood pressure–reduction program. At three sites, costs of medical claims for hypertensive individuals declined between $1.89 and $2.72 for every $1.00 spent on the program.[56,77]
- Traveler's Insurance Company saved approximately $1 million on benefit services after starting its employee work-site wellness program.[75]
- Mesa Petroleum reported that wellness/fitness program participants averaged only $173 per year for health care services, compared with $390 for nonparticipants.[182]
- Dupont Corporation credited its fitness program with yearly health care cost savings over a 3-year period of between $1.6 million to $3.0 million.[18]
- General Electric's 18-month study of fitness program members showed a 38% decrease in health care spending versus a 21% increase for nonmembers. The program saved the company an estimated $1 million in medical expenses.[13]
- The Coors' Wellness Center, started in 1981, saved more than $1.4 million in health care costs over 6 years.[91]
- Medical claims for Steelcase Corporation decreased 55% for employees who used company-sponsored and -funded fitness services.[225]

Employee Productivity

Programs that improve employee fitness increase employee productivity.

- The National Aeronautics and Space Administration reported a 12.5% increase in worker productivity for their more fit employees; they also increased stamina, performance, concentration, and decision-making abilities.[46]
- Job performance strongly correlated with exercise adherence in a study of 3231 white-collar employees.[19]
- The Dallas Police Department reported a 39% increase in commendations following the introduction of a physical fitness–lifestyle program.[146]
- Eighty percent of those surveyed about their company-sponsored health and fitness program reported that exercise increased personal work productivity, relieved work-related tension, enhanced concentration, and improved coworker relations. Even nonparticipants responded positively, citing the program as proof of the company's support for employees.

Employee Absenteeism

Work-site fitness and wellness programs reduce employee absenteeism. Healthier, more motivated employees tend to spend more productive hours on the job. For example:

- A 2-year study at Mesa Petroleum reported absenteeism savings of $156 per employee the first year and $303 the second year.[72]
- A comprehensive work-site health-promotion program improved attendance of 2546 participants, saving $149,578 annually.[23]
- Dupont Corporation reduced absenteeism by 47.5% over 6 years when 29,315 blue-collar employees enrolled in fitness programs at four sites, decreasing disability days by 11,726.[18]
- General Mills calculated that reduced absenteeism produced a payback of $3.10 to $3.90 for each dollar spent on its health promotion program during 1985–1986.[216]

Employer Cost Benefits

Corporate "bottom-line" calculations involve return on investment (i.e., the ratio of dollars returned to dollars invested). Wellness and fitness programs often pay an impressive financial dividend. This differentiates them from traditional fringe-benefit offerings, which rarely deliver a tangible investment return.

- Coors Brewing Company reported a $1.24 to $8.33 return for every dollar spent on its full-service wellness program.[218]
- Kennecott Copper Corporation saved $5.78 for each dollar spent on its employee fitness program.[7]
- Johnson & Johnson's wellness program delivered a 30% return on investment during a 12-year period.[34]
- Blue Cross and Blue Shield of Indiana in a 5-year analysis reported a 250% return on investment ($2.50 returned for every $1.00 spent).[200]
- Equitable Life Insurance Company reported a benefit:cost ratio of $5.52 in the first year of its employee fitness program.[103]

Summary

1. The clinical exercise physiologist contributes significantly to total patient care. In the clinical setting, the exercise physiologist focuses on restoring the patient's mobility and functional capacity.
2. *Disability* refers to an individual's diminished functional capacity, often compounded by an inactive lifestyle. *Handicapped* denotes a physical performance frame of reference defined by society.

3. The number of health professionals seeking specialized training has paralleled the increase in disabled persons in the United States.
4. Cancers of the breast, lung, bowel, and uterus are the most prevalent of the more than 100 different types of cancer.
5. Exercise plays an important role in cancer risk reduction, perhaps by increasing levels of anti-inflammatory cytokines, augmenting insulin receptor expression in T cells, or positively affecting provirus and oncogene activation.
6. The exercise prescription for cancer patients is symptom-limited, progressive, and individualized, with improved ambulation the primary goal.
7. A carefully planned, circuit-resistance exercise program decreases depression and state and trait anxieties for women recovering from breast cancer surgery.
8. Cardiovascular disease affects the heart muscle directly, the heart valves, or neural regulation of cardiac function. Each disorder has its specific pathogenesis and intervention strategy.
9. Chronic hypertension damages arterial vessels, significantly increasing risk for arteriosclerosis, heart disease, stroke, and kidney failure. Regular aerobic training usually lowers systolic and diastolic blood pressure.
10. Myocardial pathologies include angina pectoris, myocardial infarction, pericarditis, congestive heart failure (CHF), and aneurysm.
11. Moderate-intensity exercise and prescribed medications provide significant benefits with relatively low risk for stable, compensated CHF patients.
12. Heart valve diseases include stenosis, insufficiency (regurgitation), prolapse, and endocarditis. Congenital malformations include ventricular or atrial septal defects and patent ductus arteriosus. Dysrhythmias (bradycardia, tachycardia, and premature ventricular contractions) are diseases of the heart's nervous system.
13. Cardiac patient assessment includes medical history, physical examination, heart auscultation to uncover murmurs and valvular problems, and laboratory tests (chest x-ray, ECG, blood lipid analyses, serum enzyme testing).
14. Physiologic assessments for CHD include noninvasive tests (echocardiography, exercise stress testing, and ECG analysis). Invasive testing includes radionuclide (thallium) imaging, cardiac catheterization, and coronary angiography.
15. Resistance exercise in cardiac rehabilitation restores and maintains muscular strength, promotes preservation of FFM, improves psychologic status and quality of life, and increases glucose tolerance and insulin sensitivity.
16. Graded exercise stress testing provides a low-risk screening for CHD preventive and rehabilitative exercise programs. Stress-test results provide the objective framework to design an exercise program within a person's current functional capacity and health status.
17. Multistage bicycle and treadmill tests usually include several levels of 3 to 5 minutes of submaximal exercise to a self-imposed fatigue level.
18. Informed consent raises an individual's awareness about potential risks of exercise testing and training. It includes a written statement that the person had an opportunity to ask questions about the procedures, with sufficient information clearly provided so consent occurs from a knowledgeable (informed) perspective.
19. Alterations in the heart's normal electrical activity pattern often indicate insufficient myocardial oxygen supply. Significant S-T segment depression heralds severe, extensive obstruction in one or more coronary arteries.
20. PVCs in exercise generally indicate severe ischemic atherosclerotic heart disease, often involving two or more major coronary vessels. Sudden death from ventricular fibrillation averages 6 to 10 times higher in heart disease patients with frequent PVCs.
21. Significant deviations from normal blood pressure and heart rate responses during graded exercise testing often indicate underlying cardiovascular pathology.
22. Stress tests have four possible outcomes: true positive (test successful); false negative (person with CHD misdiagnosed); true negative (test successful); false positive (healthy person misdiagnosed).
23. With a properly prescribed and monitored exercise program, cardiac patients improve functional capacity to the same extent as healthy people of the same age.
24. Heart transplant patients respond positively to regular exercise training by improving their capacity for physical activity. Adding resistance training diminishes negative effects of immunosuppressive therapy on body composition and muscular strength.
25. RLD and COPD are the two major categories of pulmonary disease. RLD increases chest–lung resistance to inflation. COPD affects expiratory flow capacity and ultimately impedes aeration of alveolar blood.
26. Regular exercise effectively manages various pulmonary diseases, providing that exercise intensity, patient monitoring, and exercise progression receive close attention.
27. Exercise-induced bronchospasm is associated with ambient temperature and humidity and their drying effects on the respiratory mucosa. Drying increases mucosal lining osmolality, stimulating release of powerful mediators that trigger bronchoconstriction. The bronchospastic response lessens when breathing humidified air during exercise.

28. Exercise training does not "cure" asthma: instead, it increases airflow reserve and reduces breathing work during exercise.
29. Employee fitness and wellness programs enhance productivity, reduce absenteeism, and save the company significant medical costs.

References

1. Ahmaidi S, et al. Effects of interval training at the ventilatory threshold on clinical and cardiorespiratory responses in elderly humans. Eur J Appl Physiol 1998;78:170.
2. Amaral SL, et al. Exercise training normalizes wall-to-lumen ratio of the gracilis muscle arterioles and reduces pressure in spontaneously hypertensive rats. J Hypertens 2000;18:1563.
3. American Cancer Society. Cancer facts and figures. Atlanta, GA: American Cancer Society, 1995.
4. American College of Sports Medicine. Position stand. Physical activity, physical fitness, and hypertension. Med Sci Sports Exerc 1993;25:i.
5. American College of Sports Medicine and American Heart Association joint position stand on recommendations for cardiovascular screening, staffing, and emergency policies at health/fitness facilities. Med Sci Sports Exerc 1998;30:1009.
6. American Heart Association. Heart and stroke: statistical update. Dallas: American Heart Association, 2001.
7. American Institute of Preventive Medicine. The cost effectiveness of corporate wellness programs. 1991.
8. Argyros GJ, et al. Water loss without heat flux in exercise-induced bronchospasm. Annu Rev Respir Dis 1993;147:1419.
9. Asakama S, et al. A simple, reliable method of assessing exercise capacity in patients with chronic heart failure. Med Sci Sports Exerc 1999;31:52.
10. Atterhog JH, et al. Exercise testing: a prospective study of complication rates. Am Heart J 1979;98:572.
11. Badenhop DT. The therapeutic role of exercise in patients with orthotopic heart transplant. Med Sci Sports Exerc 1995;27:975.
12. Baglivo HP, et al. Effect of moderate physical training on left ventricular mass in mild hypertensive persons. Hypertension 1990;15(Suppl. I):1.
13. Bailey LC, et al. Preventive program cuts costs of employee back injuries. J Nurs Staff Dev 1989;5:247.
14. Bar-Or O, Inbar O. Swimming and asthma—benefits and deleterious effects. Sports Med 1992;14:397.
15. Beck KC. Control of airway function during and after exercise in asthmatics. Med Sci Sports Exerc 1999;31(suppl):S4.
16. Belardinelli RD, et al. Exercise training improves left ventricular diastolic filling in patients with dilated cardiomyopathy: clinical and prognostic implications. Circulation 1995;91:2775.
17. Belman MJ. Therapeutic exercise in chronic lung disease. In: Pulmonary rehabilitation. Fishman AP, ed. Pulmonary rehabilitation. New York: Marcel Dekker, 1996.
18. Bertera RL. The effects of workplace health promotion on absenteeism and employment costs in a large industrial population. Am J Public Health 1990;80:1101.
19. Bernacki EJ, et al. The relationship of job performance to exercise adherence in a corporate fitness program. J Occup Med 1984;26:529.
20. Bisschop J, et al. Reduction of exercise-induced asthma in children by short, repeated warm ups. Br J Sports Med 1999;33:100.
21. Blair SN, et al. Physical fitness and all-cause mortality: a prospective study of healthy men and women. JAMA 1989;262:2395.
22. Blair SN, et al. Physical activity, nutrition, and chronic disease. Med Sci Sports Exerc 1996;28:335.
23. Blair SN, et al. Health promotion for educators: impact on absenteeism. Prev Med 1986;15:166.
24. Blessey RL. Exercise testing by non-physician health care professionals: complication rates, clinical competencies and future trends. Exerc Stand Malpract Rep 1989;3:69.
25. Blinde EM, McCallister SG. Women, disability, and sport and physical fitness activity: the intersection of gender and disability dynamics. Res Q Exerc Sports 1999;70:303.
26. Boas SR, et al. Factors limiting anaerobic performance in adolescent males with cystic fibrosis. Med Sci Sports Exerc 1996;28:291.
27. Boas SR, et al. Energy metabolism during anaerobic exercise in children with cystic fibrosis and asthma. Med Sci Sports Exerc 1999;31:1242.
28. Braith RW. Exercise training in patients with CHF and heart transplant recipients. Med Sci Sports Exerc 1998;30(suppl):S367.
29. Braith RW, Mitchell MJ. Effect of resistance training on bone metabolism in heart transplant recipients. Congest Heart Failure 1998;4:16.
30. Braith RW, et al. Skeletal muscle strength in heart transplant recipients. J Heart Lung Transplant 1993;12:1018.
31. Braith RW, et al. Neuroendocrine hyperactivity in heart failure is buffered by endurance exercise. Circulation 1996;94:1.
32. Braith RW, et al. Resistance exercise training restores BMD in heart transplant recipients. J Am Coll Cardiol 1997;28:1471.
33. Braith RW, et al. Resistance exercise prevents glucocorticoid-induced myopathy in heart transplant recipients. Med Sci Sports Exerc 1998;30:483.
34. Breslow L, et al. Work site health promotion: its evolution and the J & J experience. Prev Med 1990;19:13.
35. Brown JK. Gender, age, usual weight loss, and tobacco use as predictors of weight loss in patients with lung cancer. Oncol Nurs Forum 1993;20:466.
36. Cahalin LP, et al. The safety of exercise testing performed independently by physical therapists. J Cardiopulm Rehabil 1987;7:269.
37. Casaburi R. Exercise training in chronic obstructive lung disease. In: Casaburi R, Petty TL, eds. Principles and practice of pulmonary rehabilitation. Philadelphia: WB Saunders, 1993.
38. Choquette G, Ferguson RJ. Blood pressure reduction in "borderline" hypertensives following physical training. Can Med Assoc J 1973;108:699.
39. Clark CJ. Pulmonary rehabilitation in chronic respiratory insufficiency: setting up a pulmonary rehabilitation programme. Thorax 1994;49:270.
40. Clark CJ, et al. Low intensity peripheral muscle conditioning improves exercise tolerance and breathlessness in COPD. Eur J Respir J 1996;9:2590.
41. Coconie CC, et al. Effect of exercise training on blood pressure in 70- to 79-yr-old men and women. Med Sci Sports Exerc 1991;23:505.
42. Cohn LA, et al. Voluntary exercise and experimental cancer. Adv Exp Med Biol 1992;322:41.
43. Collander EB, et al. Blood pressure in resistance-trained athletes. Can J Appl Sports Sci 1988;13:31.
44. Cooper AR, et al. What is the magnitude of blood pressure response to a programme of moderate intensity exercise? Randomised controlled trial among sedentary adults with unmedicated hypertension. Br J Gen Pract 2000 ec;50:958.
45. Cooper CB. Determining the role of exercise in patients with chronic pulmonary disease. Med Sci Sports Exerc 1995;27:147.
46. Corporate Health. The newsletter. Association for Fitness in Business, 1991.
47. Courneya KS. Exercise interventions during cancer treatment. Exer Sports Sci Rev 2001;29:60.
48. Daida H, et al. Sequential assessment of exercise tolerance in heart transplantation compared with coronary artery bypass surgery after phase II cardiac rehabilitation. Am J Cardiol 1996;77:696.
49. Daviglus ML, et al. Association of nonspecific minor ST-T abnormalities with cardiovascular mortality: the Chicago Western Electric Study. JAMA 1999;281:524.
50. Debigaré R, et al. Influence of work rate incremental rate on the exercise responses in patients with COPD. Med Sci Sports Exerc 2000;32:1365.
51. Dengel DR, et al. Improvements in blood pressure, glucose metabolism, and lipoprotein lipids after aerobic exercise plus weight loss in obese, hypertensive middle-aged men. Metabolism 1998;47:1075.
52. Dimeo F, et al. Aerobic exercise as therapy for cancer fatigue. Med Sci Sports Exerc 1998;30:475.
53. Drazen JM, et al. Drug therapy: treatment of asthma with drugs modifying the leukotriene pathway. N Engl J Med 1999;340:197.
54. Dubach P, et al. Effect of exercise training on myocardial remodeling in patients with reduced left ventricular function after myocardial infarction. Circulation 1997;95:2060.
55. Engebretson TO, et al. Quality of life and anxiety in a phase II cardiac rehabilitation program. Med Sci Sports Exerc 1999;31:216.
56. Erfurt JC, et al. Worksite wellness programs: incremental comparison of screening and referral alone, health education, follow-up counseling, and plant organization. Am J Health Promot 1991;5:438.

57. Fagard RH, Tipton CM. Physical activity, fitness, and hypertension. In: Bouchard C, et al., eds. Physical activity, fitness, and health. Champaign, IL: Human Kinetics, 1994.
58. Fardy PS, Yanowitz FG. Cardiac rehabilitation, adult fitness, and exercise testing. Baltimore: Williams & Wilkins, 1996.
59. Fletcher GA, et al. Exercise standards: a statement for health care professionals from the American Heart Association. Circulation 1995;91:580.
60. Fleck SJ. Cardiovascular adaptations to resistance training. Med Sci Sports Exerc 1988;20:S146.
61. Fleischmann KE, et al. Exercise echocardiography or exercise SPECT imaging? A meta-analysis of diagnostic test performance. JAMA 1998;280:913.
62. Foster C, et al. Time course of recovery during cardiac rehabilitation. J Cardiopulm Rehabil 1995;15:209.
63. Foster C, et al. Left ventricular function during exercise testing and training. Med Sci Sports Exerc 1997;29:297.
64. Foster C, et al. Physiological and pathological aspects of exercise left ventricular function. Med Sci Sports Exerc 1998;30(suppl):S379.
65. Franco MJ, et al. Comparison of dyspnea ratings during submaximal constant work exercise with incremental testing. Med Sci Sports Exerc 1998;30:479.
66. Franklin BA. Abnormal cardiorespiratory responses to acute aerobic exercise. In: Roitman JL, et al., eds. ACSM's resource manual for guidelines for exercise testing and prescription. 3rd ed. Baltimore: Williams & Wilkins, 1998.
67. Franklin BA, et al. Is direct physician supervision of exercise stress testing routinely necessary? Chest 1997;111:262.
68. Franklin BA, et al. ACSM's guidelines for exercise testing and prescription. 6th ed. Baltimore: Lippincott Williams & Wilkins, 2000.
69. Fregly MJ. Effect of an exercise regimen on development of hypertension in rats. J Appl Physiol 1984;56:381.
70. Fries JF. How may quality of life for rheumatoid arthritis patients be enhanced by current and future treatments? Rheumatology (Oxford) 1999;38(suppl 2):35.
71. Geddes D, et al. Effect of lung-volume-reduction surgery in patients with severe emphysema. N Engl J Med 2000;343:239.
72. Gettman LR. Economic fitness. Fitness Bus 1986;1:11.
73. Gilbert I, et al. Heat and water flux in the intrathoracic airways and exercised induced asthma. J Appl Physiol 1987;63:1681.
74. Gill RM, et al. Role of exercise stress testing and safety monitoring for older persons starting an exercise program. JAMA 2000;284:342.
75. Golaszewski T, et al. A benefit-to-cost analysis of a work-site health promotion program. J Occup Med 1992;34:1164.
76. Green HJ, et al. Normal skeletal muscle Na(+)-K(+) pump concentration in patients with chronic heart failure. Muscle Nerve 2001;24:69.
77. Gregg W, et al. Worksite follow-up and engagement strategies for initiating health risk behavior changes. Health Educ Q 1990;17:455.
78. Goldberg RJ, et al. A two decades (1975 to 1995) long experience in the incidence, in-hospital and long-term—fatality rates of acute myocardial infarction: a community wide perspective. J Am Coll Cardiol 1999;33:1533.
79. Haberl R, et al. Correlation of coronary calcification and angiographically documented stenoses in patients with suspected coronary artery disease: results of 1,764 patients. J Am Coll Cardiol 2001;37:451.
80. Hagberg JM. Physical activity, physical fitness, and blood pressure. In: Leon A, ed. Physical activity and cardiovascular health. Champaign, IL: Human Kinetics, 1997.
81. Hagberg JM, et al. Effect of weight training on blood pressure and hemodynamics in hypertensive adolescents. J Pediatr 104:147, 1984.
82. Hagberg JM, et al. Effects of exercise training on 60- to 69 yr old persons with essential hypertension. Am J Cardiol 1989;64:348.
83. Hagerman FC, et al. Effects of high-intensity resistance training on untrained older men. I. Strength, cardiovascular, and metabolic responses. J Gerontol A Biol Sci Med Sci 2000;55:B336.
84. Hambrecht R, et al. Effects of exercise training on left ventricular function and peripheral resistance in patients with chronic heart failure: A randomized trial. JAMA 2000;283:3095.
85. Hanson P. Exercise testing and training in patients with chronic heart failure. Med Sci Sports Exerc 1994;26:527.
86. Harms CA, Dempsey JA. Cardiovascular consequences of exercise hyperpnea. Exerc Sport Sci Rev 1999;27:37.
87. Haskell WL, et al. Effects of intensive multiple risk factor reduction on coronary atherosclerosis and clinical cardiac events in men and women with coronary artery disease. Circulation 1994;89:975.
88. Hayot M, et al. Relationship between inspiratory muscle function and maximal exercise in patients with chronic obstructive lung disease and patients with chronic heart failure. Am J Respir Crit Care Med 1997;155(suppl):A912.
89. Heath GW, Fentem PH. Physical activity among persons with disabilities—a public health perspective. Exerc Sport Sci Rev 1997;25:195.
90. Helenius IJ, et al. Association between training and risk of asthma in elite athletes. Thorax 1997;51:157.
91. Henritze J, Brammell H. Cost savings at Coors resulting from a health/wellness program. Am J Health Promot 1989;4:25.
92. Hicks JE. Exercise for cancer patients. In: Basmajian JV, Wolf SL, eds. Therapeutic exercise. 5th ed. Baltimore: Williams & Wilkins, 1990.
93. Hollenberg M, et al. Treadmill exercise testing in an epidemiologic study of elderly subjects. J Gerontol A. Biol Sci Med Sci 1998;53A:B259.
94. Hough DO, Dec KL. Exercise-induced asthma and anaphylaxis. Sports Med 1994;18:162.
95. Horowitz MB, et al. Dyspnea ratings for prescribing exercise intensity in patients with COPD. Chest 1996;109:1169.
96. Hsia CC. Cardiopulmonary limitations to exercise in restrictive lung disease. Med Sci Sports Exerc 1999;31(suppl):S28.
97. Hsing AW, et al. Risk factor for colorectal cancer in a prospective study among US white men. Int J Cancer 1998;77:549.
98. Huonker M, et al. Highland mountain hiking and coronary artery disease: exercise tolerance and effects on left ventricular function. Med Sci Sports Exerc 1997;29:1554.
99. Ienna TM, McKenzie CD. The asthmatic athlete: metabolic and ventilatory to exercise with and without pre-exercise medication. Int J Sports Med 1997;18:142.
100. Inbar O, et al. The effect of prone immersion on bronchial responsiveness in children with asthma. Med Sci Sports Exerc 1993;25:1098.
101. Jeffrey RW, et al. An empirical evaluation of the effectiveness of tangible incentives in increasing participation and behavior change in a worksite health promotion program. Am J Health Promot 1993;8:98.
102. Jimenez L, et al. Exercise does not induce oxidative stress in trained heart transplant recipients. Med Sci Sports Exerc 2000;32:2018.
103. Kaman R. The cost of fitness. Fitness Business 1987;2:39.
104. Kao W, Jessup M. Exercise testing and exercise training in patients with congestive heart failure. J Heart Lung Transplant 1994;13:S117.
105. Katz AM. Heart failure: pathophysiology, molecular biology and clinical management. Baltimore: Lippincott Williams & Wilkins, 2000.
106. Kavanagh T. Physical training in heart transplant recipients. J Cardiovasc Risk 1996;3:154.
107. Kelemen MH. Exercise training combined with antihypertensive drug therapy: effects on lipids, blood pressure, and left ventricular mass. JAMA 1990;263:2766.
108. Kelly G. Dynamic resistance exercise and resting blood pressure in adults: A meta analysis. J Appl Physiol 1997;82:1559.
109. Kelley GA, Kelley KS. Progressive resistance exercise and resting blood pressure: A meta-analysis of randomized controlled trials. Hypertension 2000;35:838.
110. Keteyian S, et al. Cardiovascular response of heart transplant patients to exercise training. J Appl Physiol 1991;70:2627.
111. Keteyian SJ, et al. Exercise testing and training of patients with heart failure due to left ventricular systolic dysfunction. J Cardiopulm Rehabil 1997;17:19.
112. King ML, et al. The hemodynamic effects of isotonic exercise using hand-held weights in patients with heart failure. J Heart Lung Transplant 2000;19:1209.
113. Kluess HA, et al. Accelerated skeletal muscle metabolic recovery following exercise training in heart failure. Circulation 1996;94:1.
114. Knight JA, et al. Supervision of clinical exercise testing by exercise physiologists. Am J Cardiol 1995;75:390.
115. Kobashigawa JA, et al. A controlled trial of exercise rehabilitation after heart transplantation. N Engl J Med 1999;340:272.
116. Kohl HW, et al. Maximal exercise hemodynamics and risk of mortality in apparently healthy men and women. Med Sci Sports Exerc 1998;28:601.
117. Kohno K, et al. Depressor effect by exercise training is associated with amelioration of hyperinsulinemia and sympathetic overactivity. Intern Med 2000;39:1013.
118. Kraemer WJ, et al. Resistance training combined with bench-step aerobics enhances women's health profile. Med Sci Sports Exerc 2001;33:259.

119. Kramer MM, Wells CL. Does physical activity reduce risk of estrogen-dependent cancer in women? Med Sci Sports Exerc 1996;28:322.
120. Kriemler S, et al. Preventing dehydration in children with cystic fibrosis who exercise in the heat. Med Sci Sports Exerc 1999;31:774.
121. Kufafka DS, et al. Exercise-induced bronchospasm in high school athletes via a free running test. Chest 1998;114:1613.
122. Lacasse Y, et al. Meta-analysis of respiratory rehabilitation in chronic obstructive pulmonary disease. Lancet 1996;348:1115.
123. LacroixVJ. Exercise-induced asthma. Phys Sportsmed 1999;27(12):75.
124. Lampert E, et al. Short endurance training improves lactate removal ability in patients with heart transplants. Med Sci Sports Exerc 1996;28:801.
125. Lauer MS, et al. Impaired heart rate response to graded exercise prognostic implications of chronotropic incompetence in the Framingham Heart Study. Circulation 1996;93:1520.
126. Lauer MS, et al. Impaired chronotropic response to exercise stress testing as a predictor of mortality. JAMA 1999;281:524.
127. Lee IM, et al. Physical activity and the risk of cancer. Int J Epidemiol 1999;28:286.
128. Leff JA, et al. Montelukast, a leukotriene-receptor antagonist, for the treatment of mild asthma and exercise-induced bronchoconstriction. N Engl J Med 1998;339:147.
129. Leigh JP, Fries JF. Health habits, health care use and costs in a sample of retirees. Inquiry 1992;29:44.
130. Lem V, et al. A nurse-supervised exercise stress testing laboratory. Heart Lung 1985;14:280.
131. Lorig KR, et al. Evidence suggesting that health education for self-management in patients with chronic arthritis has sustained health benefits while reducing health care costs. Arthritis Rheum 1993;36:439.
132. Mahler D. Exercise-induced asthma. Med Sci Sports Exerc 1993;25:554.
133. Maiorana A, et al. Effect of aerobic and resistance exercise training on vascular function in heart failure. Am J Physiol Heart Circ Physiol 2000;279:H1999-.
134. Maltais F, et al. Oxidative capacity of skeletal muscle and lactic acid kinetics during exercise in normal subjects and in patients with COPD. Am J Respir Crit Care Med 1996;153:288.
135. Maltais F, et al. Metabolic and hemodynamic responses of lower limb during exercise in patients with COPD. J Appl Physiol 1998;84:1573.
136. Mannix ET, et al. Exercise-induced asthma in figure skaters. Chest 1996;109:312.
137. Martinez ME, et al. Leisure-time physical activity, body size and colon cancer in women. Nurses' Health Study Research Group. J Natl Cancer Inst 1997;89:948.
138. Martinez ME, et al. Physical activity, body mass index and prostaglandin E2 levels in rectal mucosa. J Natl Cancer Inst 1999;91:950.
139. Matsumoto I, et al. Effects of swimming training on aerobic capacity of exercise induced bronchoconstriction in children with bronchial asthma. Thorax 1999;54:196.
140. Matsusaki M, et al. Influence of workload on the antihypertensive effect of exercise. Clin Exp Pharmacol Physiol 1992;19:471.
141. McArdle WD, et al. Specificity of run training on $\dot{V}O_{2max}$ and heart rate changes during running and swimming. Med Sci Sports 1978;10:16.
142. McCartney N. Role of resistance training in heart disease. Med Sci Sports Exerc 1998;30 (suppl):S396.
143. McCartney N. Acute responses to resistance training and safety. Med Sci Sports Exerc 1999;31:31.
144. McFadden ER Jr, Gilbert IA. Current concepts in exercise-induced asthma. N Engl J Med 1994;330:1362.
145. McKelvie RS, et al. Effects of exercise training in patients with congestive heart failure: a critical review. J Am Coll Cardiol 1995;25:789.
146. Mealey. New fitness for police and firefighters. Phys Sportsmed 1979;7:96.
147. Meyer K. Exercise training in heart failure: recommendations based on current research. Med Sci Sports Exerc 2001;33:525.
148. Meyer K, et al. Interval training in patients with severe chronic heart failure: analysis and recommendations for exrcise procedures. Med Sci Sports Exerc 1997;29:306.
149. Myers J, et al. Influence of high-intensity exercise training on the ventilatory response to exercise in patients with reduced ventricular function. Med Sci Sports Exerc 1999;31:929.
150. Myers J, et al. A survey of exercise testing: methods, utilization, interpretation, and safety in the VAHCS. J Cardiopulm Rehabil 2000;20:251.
151. Na YM, et al. Exercise therapy effect on natural killer cell cytotoxic activity in stomach cancer patients after curative surgery. Arch Phys Med Rehabil 2000;81:777.
152. Neder JA, et al. Short term effects of aerobic training in the clinical management of moderate to severe asthma in children. Thorax 1999;54:202.
153. Nelson JA, et al. Effect of long-term salmeterol treatment on exercise-induced asthma. N Engl J Med 1998;339:141.
154. Nho H, et al. Exercise training in female patients with a family history of hypertension. Eur J Appl Physiol 1998;78:1.
155. Nishima EI, et al. Heart rate recovery and treadmill exercise score as predictors of mortality in patients referred for exercise ECG. JAMA 2000;284:1392.
156. Nishina PM, et al. Linkage of atherogenic lipoprotein phenotype to the low density lipoprotein receptor locus on the short arm of chromosome 19. Proc Natl Acad Sci USA 1992;89:708.
157. Nixon PA, et al. The prognostic value of exercise testing in patients with cystic fibrosis. N Engl J Med 1992;327:1785.
158. Nystad W, et al. Asthma and wheezing among Norwegian elite athletes. Med Sci Sports Exerc 2000;32:266.
159. O'Conner PJ, et al. State anxiety and ambulatory blood pressure following resistance exercise in females. Med Sci Sports Exerc 1993;25:516.
160. O'Kane JW, Woodford GA. Allergen-mediated disease: keeping patients active. Phys Sportsmed 1999;27(9):49.
161. Oldridge NB, et al. Cardiac rehabilitation after myocardial infarction: combined experience of randomized clinical trials. JAMA 1998;260:945.
162. Orbach P, Lowenthal DT. Evaluation and treatment of hypertension in active individuals. Med Sci Sports Exerc 1998;30(suppl):S354.
163. Osada N, et al. Long-term cardiopulmonary exercise performance after heart transplantation. Am J Cardiol 1997;79:451.
164. O'Sullivan SE, Bell C. The effects of exercise and training on human cardiovascular reflex control. J Auton Nerv Syst 2000 3;81:16.
165. O'Toole M. Miller-Keane encyclopedia and dictionary of medicine, nursing and allied health. 5th ed. Philadelphia: WB Saunders, 1992.
166. Packer M, Cohn JN, eds. Consensus recommendations for the management of chronic heart failure. Am J Cardiol 1999;83(2A):1A.
167. Paffenbarger RS Jr, et al. Physical activity and hypertension: an epidemiological view. Ann Med 1991;23:19.
168. Paffenbarger RS Jr, et al. The influence of physical activity on the incidence of site-specific cancers in college alumni. Adv Exp Med Biol 1992;322:7.
169. Pearson AC, et al. Left ventricular diastolic function in weight lifters. Am J Cardiol 1986;58:1254.
170. Pendergast DR. Cardiovascular, respiratory, and metabolic responses to upper body exercise. Med Sci Sports Exerc 1989;21:S121.
171. Peters HP, et al. Potential benefits and hazards of physical activity and exercise on the gastrointestinal tract. Gut 2001;48:435.
172. Physical Therapy Association. Personal communication. July 2000.
173. Pitt B, et al. The effect of spironolactone on morbidity and mortality in patients with severe heart failure. N Engl J Med 1999;341:709.
174. Platz EA, et al. Physical activity and benign prostatic hyperplasia. Arch Int Med 1998;158:2349.
175. Platz EA, et al. Proportion of colon cancer risk that might be preventable in a cohort of middle-aged US men. Cancer Causes Control 2000;11:579.
176. Pollock ML, et al. Resistance exercise in individuals with and without cardiovascular disease. Circulation 2000;101:828.
177. Porock D, et al. An exercise intervention for advanced cancer patients experiencing fatigue: a pilot study. J Palliat Care 2000;16:30.
178. Préfaut C, et al. Pathological basis of exercise training patients with chronic obstructive lung disease. Eur Respir Rev 1995;5:27.
179. Reiff DB, et al. The effect of prolonged submaximal warm-up exercise on exercise-induced asthma. Am Rev Respir Dis 1989;139:479.
180. Reiss TF, et al. Mechanical efficiency in clinically stable patients with COPD. Thorax 1997;52:981.
181. Reiss TF, et al. Montelukast, a once-daily leukotriene receptor antagonist, in the treatment of chronic asthma. Arch Intern Med 1998;158:1213.
182. Report on Mesa Corporate Health and Fitness. Proven Cost Benefits, Mesa, Inc., Texas, 1993.
183. Ries LA, et al. The annual report to the nation on the status of cancer, 1973–1997, with a special section on colorectal cancer. Cancer 2000;88:2398.
184. Rigotti NA, et al. US college students' use of tobacco products. Results of a national survey. JAMA 2000;284:699.
185. Rockhill B, et al. A prospective study of recreational physical activity and breast cancer risk. Arch Intern Med 1999;159:2290.

186. Rosamond WD, et al. Trends in the incidence of myocardial infarction and in mortality due to coronary heart disease, 1987 to 1994. N Engl J Med 1998;339:861.
187. Rundell KW, et al. Exercise-induced asthma screening of elite athletes: field versus laboratory exercise challenge. Med Sci Sports Exerc 2000;32:309.
188. Rundell KW, et al. Self-reported symptoms and exercise-induced asthma in the elite athlete. Med Sci Sports Exerc 2001;33:208.
189. Sale DG, et al. Effect of training on the blood pressure response to weight lifting. Can J Appl Physiol 1994;19:60.
190. Salh W, et al. Effect of exercise and physiotherapy in aiding sputum expectoration. Thorax 1989;44:1006.
191. Sandsund M, et al. Effects of breathing cold and warm air on lung function and physical performance in asthmatic and nonasthmatic athletes during exercise in the cold. Ann NY Acad Sci 1997;813:751.
192. Sarna L. Functional status in women with cancer. Cancer Nurs 1994;17:87.
193. Schere D, Kaltenbach M. Frequency of life-threatening complications associated with exercise testing. Dtsch Med Wochenschr 1979;33:1161.
194. Schwartz AL. Daily fatigue patterns and effect of exercise in women with breast cancer. Cancer Pract 2000;8:16.
195. Schwartz AL, et al. Exercise reduces daily fatigue in women with breast cancer receiving chemotherapy. Med Sci Sports Exerc 2001;33:718.
196. Segal R, et al. Structured Exercise Improves Physical Functioning in Women With Stages I and II Breast Cancer: Results of a Randomized Controlled Trial. J Clin Oncol 2001;19:657.
197. Segar ML, et al. The effect of aerobic exercise on self-esteem and depressive and anxiety symptoms among breast cancer survivors. Oncol Nurs Forum 1998;25:107.
198. Serres I, et al. Impaired skeletal muscle endurance related to physical inactivity and altered lung function in COPD patients. Chest 1998;113:900.
199. Serres I, et al. Skeletal muscle abnormalities in patients with COPD: contribution to exercise intolerance. Med Sci Sports Exerc 1998;30:1019.
200. Shephard RJ. Economic benefits of enhanced fitness. Champaign, IL.: Human Kinetics, 1986.
201. Shephard RJ. Curricular physical activity and academic performance. Pediatr Exerc Sci 1997;9:113.
202. Shephard RJ, Baldy GJ. Exercise as cardiovascular therapy. Circulation 1999;99:963.
203. Slattery ML, et al. A molecular variant of the APC gene at codon 1822: its association with diet, lifestyle, and risk of colon cancer. Cancer Res 2001 1;61:1000.
204. Spector SL. Update on exercise-induced asthma. Ann Allergy 1993;71:571.
205. Stevens VJ, et al. Long-term weight loss and changes in blood pressure: results of the Trials of Hypertension Prevention, phase II. Ann Intern Med 2001 2;134:1.
206. Stuart RJ, Ellestad MH. National survey of exercise stress testing facilities. Chest 1980;77:94.
207. Suzuki S, et al. Expiratory muscle training and sensation of respiratory effort during exercise in normal subjects. Thorax 1995;50:366.
208. Tas J. Genetic predisposition to coronary heart disease and gene for apolipoprotein CIII. Lancet 1991;337:113.
209. Thacker SB, Berkelman RL. Public health surveillance in the United States. Epidemiol Rev 1988;10:164.
210. Uhlenbrock G, Oder U. Can endurance sports stimulate immune mechanisms against cancer and metastasis. Int J Sports Med 1991;12(suppl 1):S63.
211. United States Department of Health and Human Services. Healthy People 2000: national health promotion and disease prevention objectives. DHHS Publ. no. (PHS) 91-50212. Washington, DC: U.S. Government Printing Office, 1990.
212. Urata H, et al. Antihypertensive and volume-depleting effects of mild exercise on essential hypertension. Hypertension 1987;9:245.
213. Vanhees L, et al. Exercise performance and training in cardiac patients with atrial fibrillation. J Cardiopulm Rehabil 2000;20:346.
214. Virant FS. Exercise-induced bronchospasm: epidemiology, pathophysiology, and therapy. Med Sci Sports Exerc 1992;24:851.
215. Voy RO. The U.S. Olympic committee experience with exercise induced bronchospasm, 1984. Med Sci Sports Exerc 1986;18:328.
216. Wagner EH, Guild PA. Choosing an evaluation strategy. Am J Health Promot 1989;4:134.
217. Wells CL. Physical activity and cancer prevention. Focus on breast cancer. ACSM's Health Fitness J 1999;3 (1):13.
218. Wellness Councils of America. This is corporate wellness—and its bottom-line impact. Omaha, NE: Wellness Councils of America, June 1991.
219. Wennberg DE, et al. The association between local diagnostic testing intensity and invasive cardiac procedures. JAMA 1996;275:1161.
220. Whittom F, et al. Histochemical and morphological characteristics of the vastus lateralis muscle in patients with chronic obstructive pulmonary disease. Med Sci Sports Exerc 1998;30:1467.
221. Wiley RL, et al. Isometric exercise training lowers resting blood pressure. Med Sci Sports Exerc 1992;24:749.
222. Wilmore JH, et al. Heart rate and blood pressure changes with endurance training: The Heritage Family Study. Med Sci Sports Exerc 2001;33:107.
223. Willich SN, et al. Cardiac risk factors, medication, and recurrent clinical events after acute cornonary disease. A prospective cohort study. Eur Heart J 2001 15;22:307.
224. Winningham ML, et al. Effects of aerobic exercise on body weight and composition in patients with breast cancer on adjuvant chemotherapy. Oncol Nurs Forum 1989;16:683.
225. Yen LT, et al. Associations between health risk appraisal scores and employee medical claims costs in a manufacturing company. Am J Health Promot 1991;6:46.
226. Young DZ, et al. Safety of maximal exercise testing in patients at high risk for ventricular arrhythmia. Circulation 1984;70:184.
227. Zach M, et al. Cystic fibrosis: physical exercise versus chest physiotherapy. Arch Dis Child 1982;57:587.

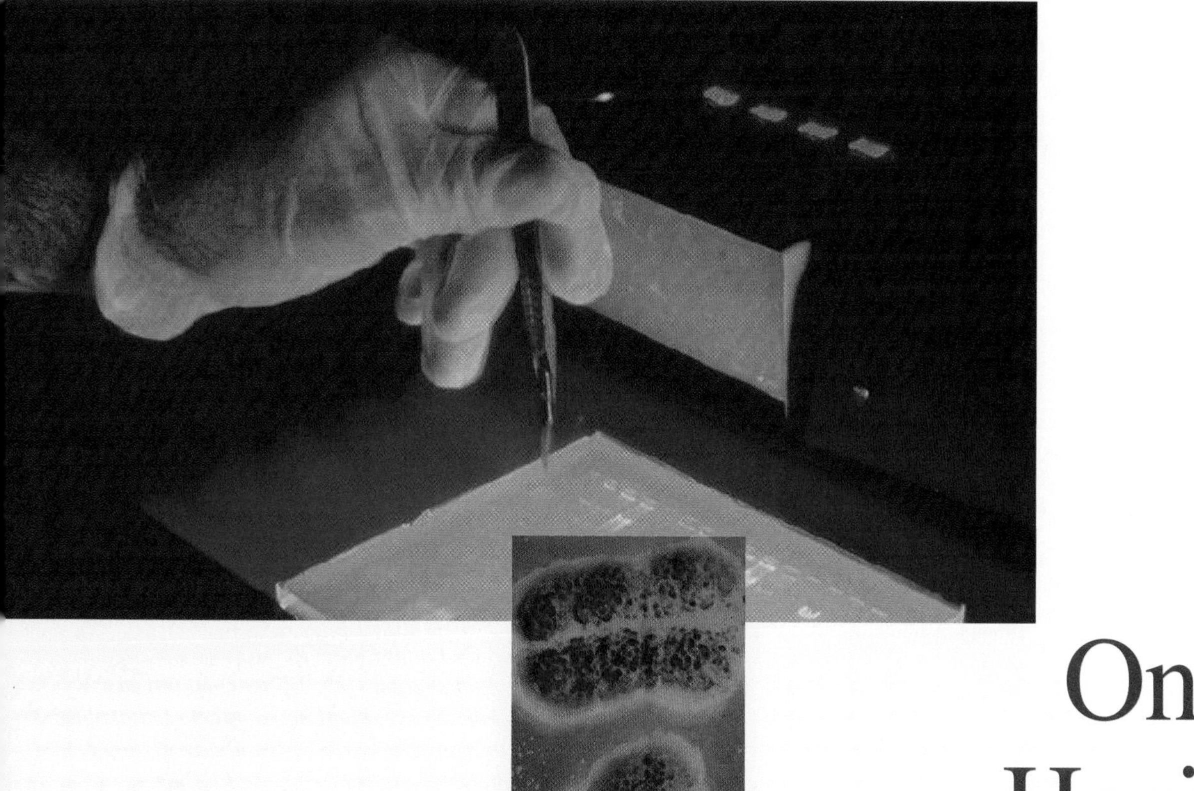

On the Horizon

MOLECULAR BIOLOGY—A NEW VISTA FOR EXERCISE PHYSIOLOGY

The most sensible way to prepare for the challenges and opportunities arising from progress in the identification of the genetic and molecular basis of health and disease is to become familiar with this field and to learn its tools.

Claude Bouchard, Robert Malina, and Louis Pérusse. Genetics of fitness and physical performance. Champaign, IL: Human Kinetics, 1997.

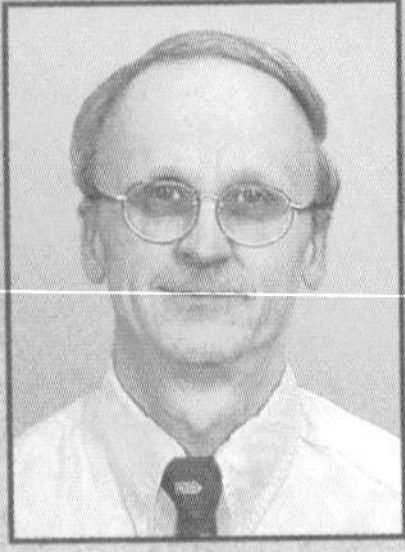

Interview with Frank Booth

Education: BS (Denison University, Granville, OH); PhD (Exercise Physiology, University of Iowa, Ames, IA); Postgraduate Studies; School of Aerospace Medicine, Brooks Air Force Base, San Antonio, TX. Department of Preventive Medicine, Washington University School of Medicine, St. Louis, MO.

Current Affiliation: Professor, Department of Veterinary Biomedical Sciences, College of Veterinary Medicine; Department of Physiology, and Dalton Cardiovascular Research Institute, University of Missouri, Columbia, MO.

Honors and Awards: See Appendix E.

Research Focus: Molecular basis of how physical inactivity increases the risk of unhealthy syndromes and diseases in humans and companion animals.

Memorable Publication: Booth FW. Perspectives on molecular and cellular exercise physiology. J Appl Physiol 1988;65:1461.

Statement of Contributions: ACSM Citation Award
In recognition of outstanding contributions in the basic and applied sciences related to exercise physiology and biochemistry.

Dr. Booth is recognized for his innovation, quantitative, and integrative investigations on the cellular and molecular mechanisms in skeletal muscles associated with the conditions of immobilization, simulated microgravity, acute exercise and training. His findings have given a new meaning and interpretation for the adaptive response of muscle.

Dr. Booth is also deserving of citation for his dedicated leadership and his outstanding example in bringing the discipline of exercise physiology into the realm of molecular biology.

➤ What first inspired you to enter the exercise science field? What made you decide to pursue your advanced degree and/or line of research?

My biology advisor at Denison University, Dr. Robert Haubrich, also was the assistant swim coach. Because I was on the swim team, he and I had many talks together, not only about swimming but science in general, including discussions about exercise and training methods. Dr. Haubrich knew of my interest in biology and sports, and one day after practice gave me a flyer advertising a new graduate program in exercise physiology at the University of Iowa. As soon as I finished reading it, I knew graduate school was what I wanted to pursue, so I applied to the program.

➤ What influence did your undergraduate education have on your final career choice?

The courses I took as part of my biology program, along with Dr. Haubrich's encouragement, were the two primary influences. I loved my comparative anatomy class, where we did animal dissections. This caused me to think about how things worked in humans. My favorite course was philosophy of religion, a course that really made me think.

➤ Who were the most influential people in your career, and why?

Four individuals exerted a profound effect on my thinking about my career. First, Dr. Haubrich made me think critically about the science of exercise, although I didn't think of it as a "real" science back then. On team bus trips, or when I would speak with him in his office, we would discuss science in general. I always wondered what was happening to my body during all those hours in the pool. I recall writing a paper for one of my classes about "metabolic pathways" that really turned me on about the topic.

Second, Dr. Charles Tipton (see "Interview" in the front matter) at the University of Iowa taught me to explore mechanisms of exercise adaptations. He stressed honesty, as he was a real "straight shooter." Dr. Tipton encouraged me to convey what was on my mind and not simply to tell people what they wanted to hear. He was instrumental in getting me to communicate precisely what I thought and to be human yet honest in doing so. From a physiological-metabolic perspective, Dr. Tipton consistently tried to uncover why something occurred. I've never lost that burning desire to seek out basic explanations.

The third person was Dr. James Barnard, a fellow graduate student and now a professor at UCLA. Jim was an exemplary student (perhaps the smartest I've met), always getting "A"s in the hardest courses. His ability and enthusiasm for knowledge motivated me to push myself intellectually, both in coursework and in the laboratory. Jim was a great role model for me.

The fourth person, Dr. John Holloszy (see "Interview" in Section 2), mentored my postdoctoral work and taught me to think more critically. As I was continually around other "postdocs" and scientists who were trying to devise creative ways to explain biologic phenomena, there was no way to "hide" from contributing. More than any person I know, Dr. Holloszy possessed the most amazing intuitive "feel" for which experimental procedures would work and which would not. He taught me the basic tenets about how to do science. My interactions with Dr. Holloszy and the other postdoctoral students in conducting various experiments and writing up the results of our work were invaluable in shaping my career in science.

➤ What has been the most interesting/enjoyable aspect of your involvement in science? What was the least interesting/enjoyable aspect?

I cherish the camaraderie of exercise science colleagues, particularly those with whom I have in-depth discussions about various science topics. The individuals who open up and share the truth about their research are the ones I truly enjoy knowing and relating to. The ideal and most enjoyable environment enables one to speak freely, to really express truthful opinions about a topic. I do not enjoy people who tell you what they want you to hear or know for purposes of personal gain (i.e., to build their own ego or self-promote) instead of communicating with respect for the purity of scientific discovery.

➤ What is your most meaningful contribution to the field of exercise science, and why is it so important?

This is a very difficult question, for which I have no answer. I suspect that the answer will emanate from the judgments of others. However, I do love applying cutting-edge technology to try to answer mechanistic questions concerning exercise. It is important to try to get to the bottom of things, and using new techniques often provides the key to unlocking the required information. Sometimes, it takes months to perfect the procedure you need for an experiment, and then months more to finally get it to work properly.

➤ What advice would you give to students who express an interest in pursuing a career in exercise science research?

It is important for the student to be excited by a course or topic in a course. Sometimes, undergraduate students have difficulty making a decision about their future. I encourage students with an interest in discovering new insights about any exercise-related topic to become involved with a professor's research projects. Even in graduate school, there is a wide range of "true" desire to continue to pursue research interests. However, those students who experience joyous feelings when searching for the unknown will know deep down they have found a suitable path to follow. If a student can find a mentor, then by all means take advantage of the situation, and do whatever it takes to become deeply involved in the intellectual pursuit.

➤ What interests have you pursued outside your professional career?

I am basically a big-time workaholic. Except for evening runs with my dog Swim, I pretty much start in the lab early and end late. I love vigorous exercise and try to do as much as I can when time permits.

➤ Where do you see the exercise science field (particularly your area of greatest interest) heading in the next 20 years?

Our field needs to produce the very best science to counter the cultural trends that have created a sedentary society with all of its ailments and diseases. Discovering the benefits of exercise and conveying those benefits to the public, from the broadest possible topic areas to the molecular basis of disease, remains our best chance to prevent many diseases and upgrade the nation's health. The field needs to cooperate with multiple partners in a major public health effort to convince the world about the long-term health benefits of regular exercise. We as scientists must systematically provide the medical evidence and cross-disciplinary connections to show that exercise, not drugs, exerts the greatest impact on disease to improve health. All of us must become strong advocates, using education and laboratory-based research to convince people everywhere to pursue a healthy lifestyle.

➤ You have the opportunity to give a "last lecture." Describe its primary focus.

The basis of my talk would involve how regular exercise affects daily living. I would focus not just on the physiologic function and performance aspects, but on exercise's effects on chronic ills like diabetes, pulmonary and kidney diseases, heart disease, and cancer. For the ever-increasing number of American citizens living in nursing homes, I would discuss the profound effect of sedentary living on muscular atrophy and reduced strength, two factors that limit these individual's ability to carry out even the simplest tasks of daily living. I would emphasize that relying on pills to tackle disease contributes relatively little to a happy and healthy life. I would also hope to convince the audience that the exercise biologists' role is not simply to study the effects of physical activity or enhance sport performance. The "new" exercise physiologist must reintroduce regular physical activity into an unhealthy, overweight, and sedentary population that is genetically programmed to expect physical activity. I refer to this unhealthy state as SeDS, an abbreviation for sedentary death syndrome.

Achievement of a future, healthy world must involve cooperative effort among diverse public and private organizations that invest enough money in fundamental research to make a real difference. Talking a good game simply will not do it; putting sufficient resources to work will create newer and better opportunities for success through proper research.

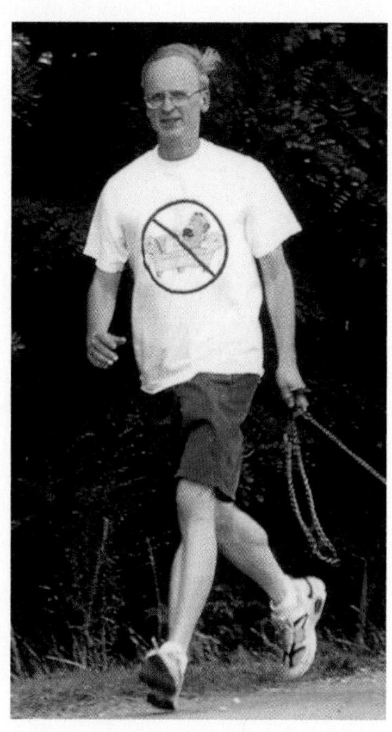

INTRODUCTION

Gene: segment of DNA with an ordered nucleotide sequence for encoding a specific functional substance (i.e., a protein or RNA molecule)

Molecular biology: study of the molecular basis of life

Molecular genetics: study of the structure and sequence of molecules that carry genetic information

Pharmacogenetics: genetic engineering to design specific drugs to target specific disease conditions of an individual's genetic code; this field investigates how genetic diversity affects the efficacy and side effects of targeted drugs

Pharmacogenomics: application of genomic methods and perspectives to study drug-responsive genes

Bioinformatics: understanding the underlying chemical codes of organisms by interpreting gene sequences, converting primary linear code into complex three-dimensional structures, managing automated screens, and running combinatorial chemistry syntheses

Protein: large molecule composed of one or more chains of amino acids in a specific order (determined by the base sequence of nucleotides in the gene coding for the protein). Proteins (perhaps up to 140,000 different structures in the body) provide for unique structure, function, and regulation of cells, tissues, and organs. Examples include hormones, enzymes, and antibodies

Gene expression: converting a gene's coded information by transcription and translation into cellular structures. Expressed genes include those transcribed (copied) from DNA nucleotide sequences into mRNA and then translated by ribosomes into specific nucleotide sequences to form protein

Transcription: RNA polymerase assembles an mRNA molecule complementary to the gene's nucleotide (making an RNA copy of a gene)

The early 1950s ushered in the dawn of the modern age of molecular biology, and the past 10 years of exercise physiology research has, albeit slowly, embraced this field. And so it should. Techniques now available to study how genetic characteristics shape human behavior will soon revolutionize almost every facet of human physical activity and sports medicine. The new generation of exercise physiologists has a wonderful opportunity to study the molecular world of **genes** and their role in human exercise performance and health and disease. Today's exercise physiology students often cooperate in research projects from basic science, clinical and environmental medicine, chemistry, **molecular biology** and **molecular genetics**, **pharmacogenetics**, **pharmacogenomics**, **bioinformatics**, and other newly emerging disciplines in the physical and life sciences.

Many exercise physiology laboratories have begun research programs to study the genetic basis of increased physical activity (and inactivity) related to a multitude of diseases and dysfunctions. This spans the gamut from the role of genetics in training and exercise performance to skeletal muscle adaptations to prolonged microgravity exposure. Occupational, physical, and rehabilitation medicine anticipate the use of gene therapy as a way to transfer genetic material to enhance the patient's production of growth factors. These small **protein** molecules stimulate cell proliferation, migration, and differentiation; promote matrix synthesis to facilitate healing of injured or surgically repaired tissues with limited blood supply; and slow cell growth and/or a finite ability to regenerate (e.g., bone, cartilage, ligaments, tendons).[85] In addition to delivering therapeutic proteins to injured tissues, molecular biology provides a way to potentially engineer new tissues. These biologic substitutes—exogenous structures and/or tissue scaffolding—may eventually link with gene therapy procedures to support tissue regeneration and healing from athletic trauma. Current interest in molecular biology also focuses on how short-term and chronic physical activity act and interact to induce structural and functional adaptations that enhance exercise performance and produce desirable health outcomes.

Booth and colleagues[22,23] assert that future exercise physiology research should emphasize primary disease prevention, with focus on uncovering environmental roots of modern chronic diseases. These maladies annually cause 250,000 premature deaths and play a role in $1 trillion dollars in health care costs for conditions associated with sedentary living, not to mention the toll on human suffering. Dr. Frank Booth, whose contributions we chronicle on pages 968 to 969 and in Appendix E, coined the term S_EDS [sedentary death syndrome] to characterize the effects of a sedentary lifestyle on unhealthy outcomes.

The related fields of molecular biology offer novel ways to study disease mechanisms and strategies that best combat them. Research challenges also emerge in the exercise biology sciences. More specifically, six questions have been posed concerning molecular biology's role in prospective exercise physiology research:[20]

1. How does endurance training coregulate **gene expression** of most mitochondrial proteins in trained skeletal muscle?
2. Which enzymes trigger the shift in the metabolic fuel mixture that occurs with endurance training?
3. What chemical signal(s) induced by resistance training cause skeletal muscle hypertrophy?
4. What DNA regulatory sequences alter **transcription** of a **messenger RNA (mRNA)**?
5. What proteins regulate skeletal muscle function?
6. What important factors affect differential gene expression that occurs in response to changes in a muscle's contractile activity?

A 1999 editorial by Baldwin[9] makes a compelling case that the membership of the American College of Sports Medicine should exploit new fields and technologies involved with "molecular exercise sciences." The views of Booth and Baldwin, not unlike our own, maintain that exercise physiology and sports medicine have progressed over the past decade from an organismal focus, to exercise biochemistry at the organ level, to a current emphasis on molecular dynamics. These scientists posit that our field has already shifted to the molecular age, as evidenced by research emphasis in integrative biology and **proteomics**.

A literature search on PubMed (www.ncbi.nlm.nih.gov:80/entrez) reinforces their point. For the 3-month period between January 1, 2001 and April 1, 2001, almost one-fourth of the citations to the term "muscle" were linked to the term gene (502 citations), and 72 articles concerned genes and human muscle. Not surprisingly, a search for the term "**genome**" yielded 64,112 entries through March, 2001, most occurring within the last 3 years. Funding for research in the genomics area has also increased dramatically. In 1988, the Department of Energy and NIH spent a combined $27.9 million for their genomic programs; in 2000, that amount increased nearly 13-fold to $360.6 million, and hopefully funding will continue to improve in the many disciplines related to molecular medicine.

In this chapter, we introduce molecular biology in general, with specific emphasis on gene expression and **protein synthesis**. Where possible, we link applications to human performance, exercise testing, and sports medicine. Our tour begins with background information on the road to Watson and Crick's pioneering 1953 achievement in deciphering the three-dimensional molecular structure of the **deoxyribose nucleic acid (DNA)** molecule.[134] Their seminal publication, reproduced at the back of this chapter (see page 1050), immediately thrust research in molecular biology to the forefront of scientific exploration worldwide. Their solving the puzzle of the DNA structure led to new techniques and models of how organisms transmit genetic information from parent to offspring and ultimately to successive generations. The spectacular growth of molecular biology affects almost every facet of biomedical research and has forever changed the face of hereditary science. Research in molecular biology will surely fundamentally impact human exercise performance.

In all likelihood, future limits to athletic performance will be determined less by an athlete's innate physiology and anatomy (and commitment to training) and more by surgical enhancement (e.g., more-flexible tendons) and genetic interventions engineered for faster-acting, more-powerful muscles, greater oxygen transport, and more-rapid circulation. The continuing use of banned substances made public at the 2000 Sydney Olympic Games highlights challenges facing the new, independent drug-testing agency to confront the consequences of illegal drug use in the 27th Athens Olympiad in 2004. It would not surprise us if breakthroughs in gene therapy techniques in the coming years infiltrate the athlete's arsenal of "tricks" in time for this Olympiad. This will cause both students and an educated general public to confront specialists in exercise physiology concerning the implications of the molecular biology of gene therapy and "genetic ergogenics," as increasing numbers of athletes cheat with these techniques to gain a competitive edge.

At the end of the chapter, we include lists of (1) references, (2) readings related to molecular biology and **genetics**, twins, and human performance, (3) excellent texts that devote hundreds of pages to the intricacies of the molecular biology of gene transcription and protein synthesis, (4) articles from *Scientific American* concerning molecular biology, (5) useful molecular biology internet sites, and (6) a reprint of Watson and Crick's one-page classic paper in *Nature* about their discovery of DNA's structure that 50 years later unraveled the pieces to the primordial jigsaw puzzle of the **Human Genome Project**.

Messenger RNA (mRNA): molecule that carries genetic information (complementary copy of one of the two DNA strands) between a gene and the ribosomes that translates the genetic information into proteins

Proteomics: systematic analysis of the protein expression of healthy and unhealthy genomes at the molecular level by identifying, characterizing, and quantifying proteins

Protein synthesis: process of creating a protein from amino acid subunits

Deoxyribose nucleic acid (DNA): double-helix molecule (two complementary chains of nucleotides) containing an organism's total hereditary information

Genetics: branch of science that studies patterns of inheritance of specific traits in successive generations

Human Genome Project: government sponsored project led by the Department of Energy and National Institutes of Health to (1) create an ordered set of DNA segments from known chromosomal locations, (2) develop new computational methods to analyze genetic maps and DNA sequence data, and (3) develop new techniques and instruments for detecting and analyzing DNA (i.e., deciphering the complete sequence of genetic instructions in humans). Hundreds of robotic sequencing machines work around the clock to analyze nucleotide sequences using the Sanger-Coulson Dideoxy DNA sequencing method to map different genomes

HISTORY TOUR OF MOLECULAR BIOLOGY

The road to uncovering DNA's three-dimensional structure began with an innocent discovery by Swiss physiologist Friedrich Miescher (1844–1895), Professor of Physiology at the University of Basel, Switzerland and charter member of the 1889 First International Congress of Physiologists. In 1869, Miescher identified what he considered a new biologic substance. Cells from fish sperm and human tissue cells obtained from pus in discarded surgical bandages contained unusual proportions of nitrogen and phosphorus in their **nucleus**. Miescher called the substance *nuclein*, which one of his students, Richard Altman, in 1899 termed nucleic acid because of its slightly acidic properties.

Nucleus: structure that contains the cell's genetic material (chromosomal DNA)

As late as the second half of the nineteenth century, chemists and biologists did not know what role if any genes played in transmitting hereditary information in plants or animals. But this would change when English naturalist, geologist, and biologist, Charles Robert Darwin (1809–1882) (www.bbc.co.uk/education/darwin/biblio/links.htm) proposed a theory of evolution based on **natural selection** of random variation. Darwin developed his theory gradually after many years of geologic and biologic observations on native lands, particularly along the western coast of South America, which included the Galapagos Islands. Darwin's

Natural selection: Darwin's basic idea that species survive because more-favorable phenotypic traits pass down through successive generations

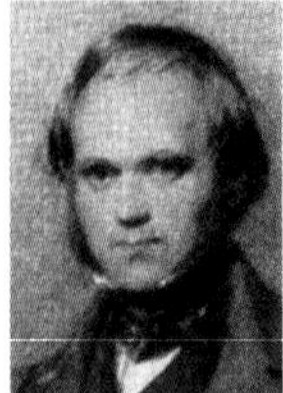

Charles Darwin

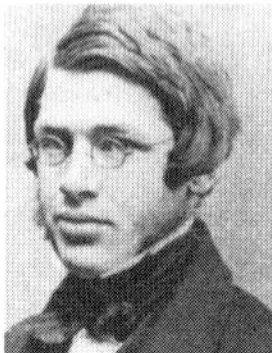

Alfred Wallace

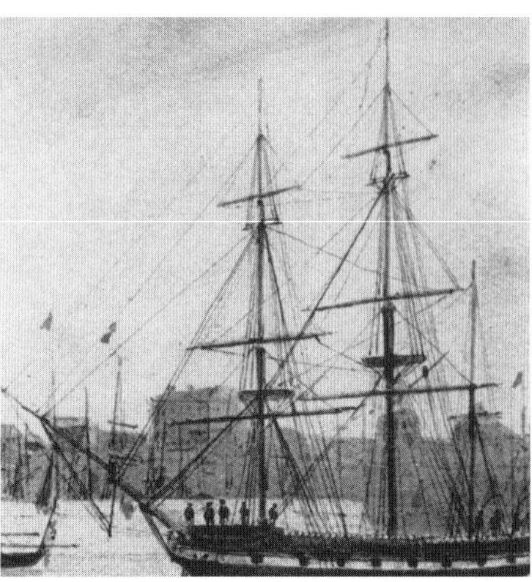

HMS Beagle

insightful observations about the distribution and continuation of animal and plant phenotypic traits were first published on November 26, 1859, 10 years before Miescher discovered nuclein.

Researchers at Brandeis University, Boston have used Darwin's basic ideas about natural selection to create the GOLEM project [Genetically Organized Lifelike Electro Mechanics; (golem03.cs-i.brandeis.edu/index.html)]. They successfully created artificial locomoting machines that mimicked biologic life forms. The simulations demonstrated the feasibility of creating successively more-complex entities from proceeding generations to solve more-difficult simulation tasks. The implications of such "biologic" simulations may have a bearing on the role of natural selection on intelligence and memory.

Another English naturalist, Alfred Russel Wallace (1823–1913), had independently formed his own views regarding natural selection at about the same time Darwin completed his work dealing with evolution theory. Except for sharing his thoughts with selected colleagues in various disciplines, Darwin had not yet made them widely known in formal publications. Darwin's reading of Wallace's 1855 paper about natural selection, *On the Tendency of Varieties to Depart Indefinitely From the Original Type* (reprinted in reference 128) no doubt accelerated his pace to publish the single-volume discourse on evolutionary theory that remains an enduring legacy, forever changing our view about human evolutionary progression through the ages.

Darwin's carefully crafted, thought-provoking treatise, *On the Origin of Species by Means of Natural Selection, or The Preservation of Favoured Races in the Struggle for Life*,[35] indirectly provided empirical "data" on how environmental pressures selected for the survival of a species' observable characteristics (traits) from one generation to the next. His ideas about evolution emerged mainly from insightful observations of subtle differences among plant and animal species during his 4-year, 9- month, and 2-day voyage around the world, begun in 1831 aboard the survey ship HMS *Beagle*.[36] Darwin's theory explained how adaptive modifications to environmental stressors impacted the common descent of current animal and plant species and how natural selection preserved a species' survival.

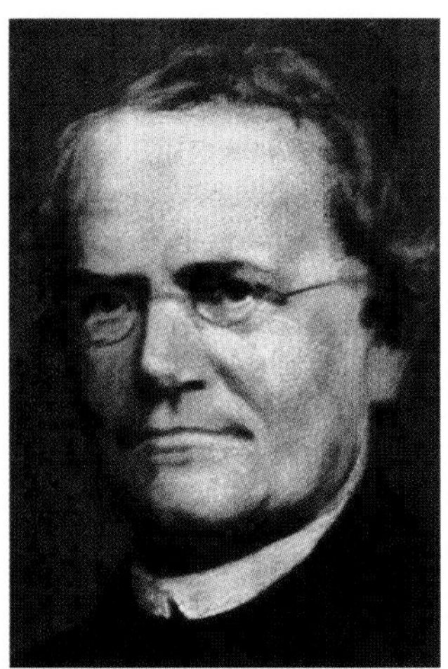

Gregor Johann Mendel

Interestingly, Miescher's discovery of nuclein came 4 years after Austrian monk Gregor Johann Mendel's (1822–1884) elegant 25-year breeding experiments with 10,000 varieties of edible pea plants *Pisum sativum*. Mendel vigilantly tracked the pea's inherited characteristics and submitted his findings in 1865, "Versuche über Pflanzen-Hybriden," to an obscure natural history society journal. The work appeared in 1866 and was later translated into English by William Bateson (1861–1926).[14] Darwin's unifying evolution theory and Mendel's experiments on heredity formed "scientific pillars" of insights embraced by a relatively new field of study—molecular biology—that would subsequently dominate fundamental discoveries in fields such as biology, chemistry, genetics, and medicine.

Mendel's meticulous scientific insights remained relatively obscure for nearly three decades until three scientists (Correns, De Vries, van Tschermak-Seysenegg) rediscovered his research in about 1900. It would take nearly 65 years after Mendel's initial publication (and enormous progress in biochemical techniques) to unravel further secrets highlighting the mysteries of hereditary transmission in human cells. In 1929, Phoebus A. T. Levene (1869–1940) discovered that the essential components of the nucleic acids DNA and **ribonucleic acid (RNA)** were long chains of the repeating **nucleotides**. It remained unclear to Levene and others how these molecules assembled. If the genes indeed contained the hereditary information, scientists needed to know the process involved. Twenty-five years later, a major breakthrough occurred (discussed on the next page) that delivered the biggest biologic thunderbolt since Darwin and stirred a revolution concerning evolutionary theory. This led to at least six other scientific milestones:

Ribonucleic acid: nucleic acid that contains the sugar ribose; usually single stranded

Nucleotide: segment of a nucleic acid containing a 5-carbon sugar, phosphate group, and nitrogen-containing base

1. 1966—cracking the DNA genetic code
2. 1972–1973—start of tremendous advances in biotechnology by splicing pieces of DNA together to form genes (called recombinant molecules) that were inserted into bacteria to produce human proteins

3. 1977—elucidating the complete genetic information of a microorganism, paving the way for the Human Genome Project
4. 1981—creating the first **transgenic** animal by inserting a viral gene into the DNA of a mouse, permitting such animals to serve as models for the study of human diseases
5. 1984—devising the **polymerase chain reaction (PCR)**, an ingenious method of sequencing DNA from minute samples of DNA
6. 1997—cloning the first mammal, the lamb Dolly, from an adult cell

Transgenic: transforming genes from one species into another

Polymerase chain reaction (PCR): technique for artificially amplifying the number of copies of a target DNA sequence, usually by 10^6 to 10^9 times, during repeated cycles of denaturation, annealing with primer, and extension with DNA polymerase

REVOLUTION IN THE BIOLOGIC SCIENCES

In 1953, James D. Watson (1928–) an American postdoctoral student who had earned a Ph.D. in genetics from Indiana University at age 22, teamed with English physicist Francis H. C. Crick (1916–) who was pursuing a Ph.D. in x-ray studies of protein in the Cavendish Laboratory, Cambridge, England. Watson and Crick's breakthrough, deduced from other scientists' research, published and unpublished, posited that the DNA molecule consisted of two polynucleotide linear strands coiled around each other to form a **double helix**.[134]

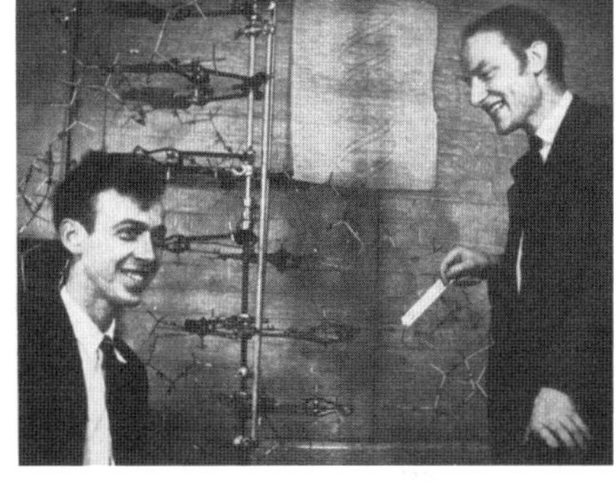

James D. Watson (left) and Francis H.C. Crick (right) at the Cavendish Laboratory next to their DNA ball and wire model. May, 1953.

Nobel laureate James D. Watson said, "We used to think our fate was in our stars. Now we know our fate, in large measure, is in our genes. Never will a more important set of instruction manuals be made available."

The young researchers constructed a ball-and-wire model of DNA, proposing that the two helical strands connected like the steps of a spiral staircase by nucleotide **base pairs** held together by **hydrogen bonds**. Their eventual Nobel Prize rewarded their contribution about DNA's architecture and the three-dimensional fit of its molecular components (fueled in part by substantial theoretical contributions about DNA's helical structure from Kings College, London, colleague Rosalind Franklin [1920–1957; see Introduction, p. lvi]).

In their 1953 landmark publication in *Nature* that described DNA's molecular structure, Watson and Crick state that their research efforts were stimulated by "a knowledge of the general nature of the unpublished experimental results and ideas of Drs. M. H. F. Wilkins and R. E. Franklin and coworkers at King's College, London." This statement, interpreted with the hindsight of many years of investigative efforts by historians and researchers, paints quite a different picture of Rosalind E. Franklin's prior discoveries about DNA's structure, which eventually led Watson and Crick to deduce DNA's final configuration correctly. Franklin's sophisticated x-ray diffraction photo reflecting her expertise with x-ray crystallography (shown to Watson and Crick surreptitiously without Franklin's knowledge; see top of next page) provided the missing pieces about DNA's double helix that empowered Watson and Crick to decipher the puzzle quickly. For historic perspective,

Double helix: two DNA strands twisted in a spiral around each other

Base pairs: two complementary nucleotide bases (G-C or A-T) in a double-stranded DNA molecule held together by hydrogen bonds

Hydrogen bonds: weak, interactive bonding from simultaneous attraction of a positive hydrogen atom to other atoms with negative charges

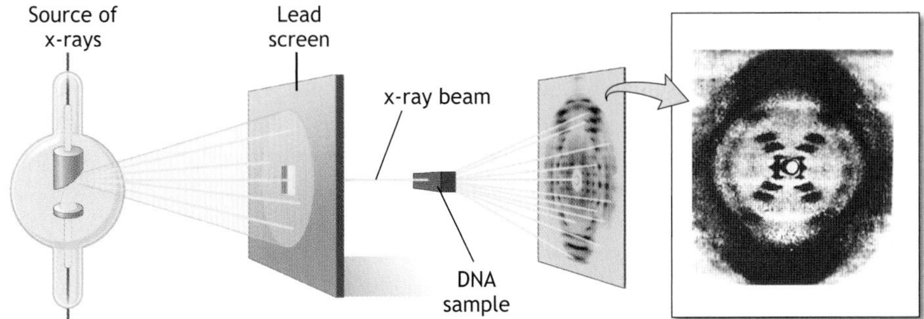

The technique of x-ray crystallography bombards crystals with thin x-ray beams of single (monochromatic) wavelength to determine a substance's three-dimensional crystal structure. The right photo above shows Franklin's x-ray photograph of DNA; she focused the x-ray beam on extra-wet DNA B fibers for a longer than usual time, with a 62-hour exposure time to obtain the vivid photo of DNA's cruciform pattern. Without her knowledge or permission, this recent x-ray photograph was shown and along with knowledge about base-pairing—correctly deduced that DNA must have originated from a helix-shaped molecule.

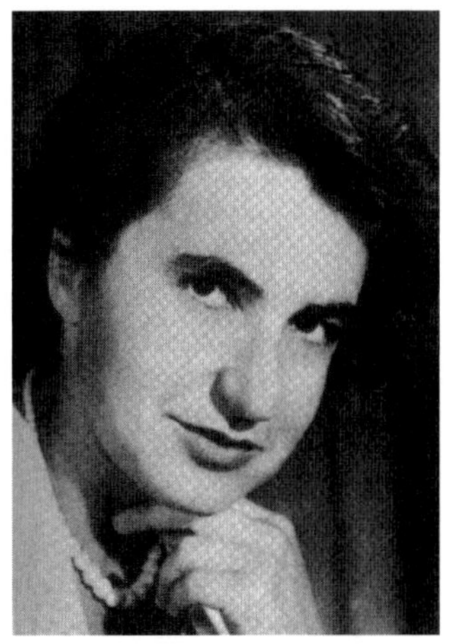

Dr. Rosalind Franklin

we recommend two books with different views about how the DNA puzzle was solved. First, read Watson's colorful personal interpretation of one of the most important discoveries in all of science by one of the scientists who made the discovery.[132] Then read Sayre's compelling and insightful first full account of Rosalind Franklin's previously unacknowledged contribution to discovering DNA's structure.[109]

Template: copy, replica, or pattern; sequence of nucleotides from which a complementary DNA or RNA strand forms

Template strand: original DNA strand that guides the synthesis of a new DNA strand by complementary base pairing

Since Watson and Crick's decisive discovery, we know that DNA's helical structure carries the biologic blueprint for specifying the *order* in which the body's twenty amino acids assemble. Each protein has its own unique amino acid sequence; this sequence ultimately dictates the protein molecule's final shape and distinctive chemical and functional characteristics. We also know that each double-helix strand provides a **template** for synthesizing a new strand, something Watson and Crick had hinted at in their seminal *Nature* paper. A **template strand** represents an original DNA strand. Once faithfully copied, each newly created double-helix strand is a duplicate of its predecessor, with its genetic code sequence preserved. This mechanism of self-replication preserves the genetic flow of information to ensure that successive generations receive the same coded DNA "messages." In fact, all living things on Earth share a common molecular plan. Each of a human's trillions of cells relies on four basic molecular building blocks—nucleic acid, protein, lipid, and polysaccharide—along with other nano-sized biomolecules, to perform their functions efficiently. In addition, all living cells shuttle the flow of information from DNA to RNA to protein. We cannot overstate the full impact of what Watson and Crick deduced about DNA's structural configuration. Their contribution and subsequent years of investigation have affected every facet of biomedical science, from how primordial DNA formed and survived to the nature of deadly diseases and the all-out search for their eventual cure. Their unraveling of DNA's structure also profoundly affected all of science, but particularly subsequent discoveries about the human genome (see next section).

The field of molecular biology has shown explosive growth during the past 40 years. Discoveries have been so startling that almost every year since 1958 a Nobel Prize has been awarded for research related to molecular biology. Table 1 lists the Nobel Prize winners in the fields of chemistry and physiology or medicine. Note that since its 1901 inception, four of the only ten women awarded a Nobel Prize in science won for molecular biology-related research.[87] Marie Curie won in both physics (1903) and chemistry (1911). Table A at the end of this chapter (page 1046) presents a timeline for "genetics" from before Mendel to salient discoveries in genetics and molecular biology, culminating with elucidation of the genetic sequence of the fruit fly *Drosophila melanogaster* in September 1999, the first human genome in June 2000, more than 95% of the genetic code of the laboratory mouse 4 months later in October 2000, and the complete genome sequence of the dimorphic bacterium *Caulobacter crescentus* in April, 2001.[94]

Human genome: the full complement of genetic material in a human cell; contains about 80,000 to 140,000 genes and from 3.12 (Celera Genomics estimate) to 3.15 (National Human Genome Research Institute estimate) billion nucleotide base pairs

X chromosome: sex chromosome present in two copies in female animals

Y chromosome: sex chromosome present in one copy in male animals

Genotype: the individual's genetic makeup at the molecular level comprising the entire set of genes

Phenotype: observable characteristics or attributes resulting from the expression of genes

Escherichia coli (E. coli): rod-like anaerobic bacterium with 4.6 million base pairs, found in the colon of humans and other mammals; studied in many disciplines for its genetic characteristics

HUMAN GENOME

The **human genome** represents the full complement of genetic material in a human cell. A private company, Celera Genomics (www.celera.com/), and the publically funded National Human Genome Research Institute (www.nhgri.nih.gov/) announced on June 26, 2000, their completion of the first assembly draft of the human genome. The organizations disagree about the genome's full size and the number of human genes. However, scientists know for sure that the total number of base pairs determines **genome** size. The genome, distributed among 23 pairs of **chromosomes**, each repeated over and over like a genetic stutter without interruption, imparts our individual uniqueness. At conception, one complete chromosome set from the father (22 plus an **X or Y sex chromosome**) joins with one complete set from the mother (22 plus an X sex chromosome) to give each human offspring 46 chromosomes. The helical DNA structures (**genotype**) contain the genetic blueprint or "roadmap" of the instructions for almost every aspect of our being (**phenotype**). The phenotype reflects the expression of our gene pool from the physical dimensions, texture, color, composition, and shape of every internal and external body part to our personalities with all their idiosyncrasies. The human genome greatly exceeds the genome size of other organisms. For example, the bacterium ***Escherichia coli*** (*E. coli*; primary member of the large bacterial family *Enterobacteriaceae*) contains 4.6 million base pairs, while yeast contains

TABLE 1 ➤ NOBEL PRIZES AWARDED IN RESEARCH RELATED TO CELL AND MOLECULAR BIOLOGY FROM 1958 TO 2000

YEAR	SCIENTIST	PRIZE[a]	RESEARCH
2000	Arvid Carlsson Paul Greengard Eric Kandel	P or M	Slow synaptic neural transmission among neural cells, biology of memory, and development of selective serotonin reuptake inhibitors
1999	Günter Blobel	P or M	Proteins' intrinsic signals govern cell transport and localization
1998	Robert F. Furchgott Louis J. Ignarro Ferid Murad	P or M	Nitric acid as a signaling molecule in cardiovascular regulation
1997	Rolf M. Zinkernagel Peter C. Doherty	P or M	Immune system recognition of virus-infected cells
1996	Jens C. Skou	Chemistry	Na^+/K^+-ATPase
	Paul Boyer John Walker		Mechanism of ATP synthesis
	Stanley B. Prusiner	P or M	Protein structure of prions
1995	Edward B. Lewis **Christiane Nüsslein-Volhard** Eric Wieschaus	P or M	Genetic control of embryonic development
1994	Alfred Gilman Martin Rodbell	P or M	Structure and function of GTP-binding (G) proteins
1993	Richard Roberts Phillip Sharp	P or M	Split genes and RNA processing
	Kary Mullis	Chemistry	Polymerase chain reaction (PCR)
	Michael Smith		Site-directed mutagenesis (SDM)
1992	Edmond Fischer Edwin Krebs	P or M	Alteration of enzyme activity by phosphorylation/dephosphorylation
1991	Erwin Neher Bert Sakmann	P or M	Measurement of ion flux by patch-clamp recording
1989	J. Michael Bishop Harold Varmus	P or M	Cellular genes capable of causing malignant transformation
	Thomas R. Cech Sidney Altman	Chemistry	Ability of RNA to catalyze reactions
1988	Johann Deisenhofer Robert Huber Hartmut Michel	Chemistry	Bacterial photosynthetic reaction center
1987	Susumu Tonegawa	P or M	DNA rearrangements responsible for antibody diversity
1986	**Rita Levi-Montalcini** Stanley Cohen	P or M	Factors that affect nerve outgrowth
1985	Michael S. Brown Joseph L. Goldstein	P or M	Regulation of cholesterol metabolism and endocytosis
1984	Georges Köhler César Milstein	P or M	Monoclonal antibodies
	Niels K. Jerne		Antibody formation
1983	**Barbara McClintock**	P or M	Mobile elements in the genome
1982	Aaron Klug	Chemistry	Structure of nucleic acid–protein complexes
1980	Paul Berg	Chemistry	Recombinant DNA technology
	Walter Gilbert Frederick Sanger		DNA sequencing technology
	Baruj Benacerraf Jean Dausset George D. Snell	P or M	Major histocompatibility complex
1978	Werner Arber Daniel Nathans Hamilton Smith	P or M	Restriction endonuclease technology
	Peter Mitchell	Chemistry	Chemiosmotic mechanism of oxidative phosphorylation
1976	D. Carleton Gajdusek	P or M	Prion-based diseases
1975	David Baltimore Renato Dulbecco Howard M. Temin	P or M	Reverse transcriptase and tumor virus activity
1974	Albert Claude Christian de Duve George E. Palade	P or M	Structure and function of internal components of cells
1972	Gerald Edelman Rodney R. Porter	P or M	Immunoglobulin structure
	Christian B. Anfinsen	Chemistry	Relationship between primary and tertiary structure of proteins
1971	Earl W. Sutherland Jr.	P or M	Mechanism of hormone action and cyclic AMP
1970	Bernard Katz Ulf S. von Euler	P or M	Nerve impulse propagation and transmission
	Luis F. Leloir	Chemistry	Role of sugar nucleotides in carbohydrate synthesis
1969	Max Delbrück Alfred D. Hershey Salvador E. Luria	P or M	Genetic structure of viruses
1968	H. Gobind Khorana Marshall W. Nirenberg	P or M	Genetic code
	Robert W. Holley		Transfer RNA structure
1966	Peyton Rous	P or M	Tumor viruses
1965	F. Francois Jacob Andres M. Lwoff Jacques L. Monod	P or M	Bacterial operons and messenger RNA
1964	**Dorothy C. Hodgkin**	Chemistry	Structure of complex organic molecules
1963	John C. Eccles Alan L. Hodgkin Andrew F. Huxley	P or M	Ionic basis of nerve membrane potentials
1962	Francis H. C. Crick James D. Watson Maurice H. F. Wilkins	P or M	Three-dimensional structure of DNA
	John C. Kendrew Max F. Perutz	Chemistry	Three-dimensional structure of globular proteins
1961	Melvin Calvin	Chemistry	Biochemistry of CO_2 assimilation during photosynthesis
1960	F. MacFarlane Burnet Peter B. Medawar	P or M	Clonal selection theory of antibody formation
1959	Arthur Kornberg Severo Ochoa	P or M	Synthesis of DNA and RNA
1958	George W. Beadle Joshua Lederberg Edward L. Tatum	P or M	Gene expression
	Frederick Sanger	Chemistry	Primary structure of proteins

[a]P or M, physiology or medicine. *Note:* corecipients for some awards were excluded if their primary research did not involve molecular and cell biology. Frederick Sanger won two Nobels (1958, 1980); his important contributions helped to pave the way for future human genome research.
Bold type identifies females.

Escherichia coli (E. coli)

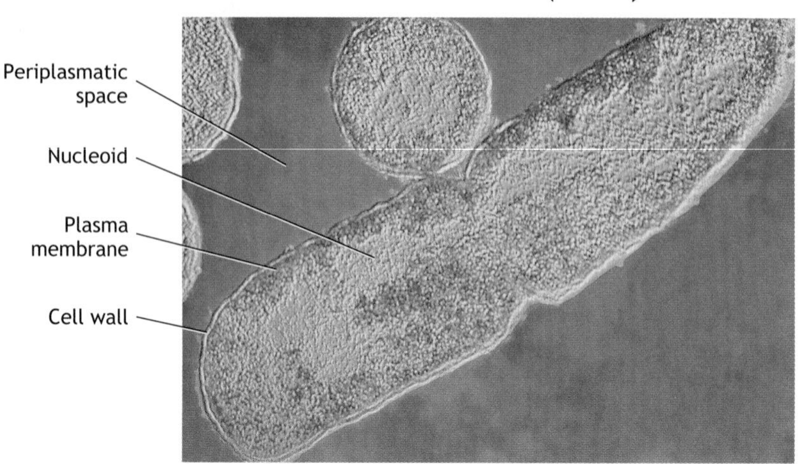

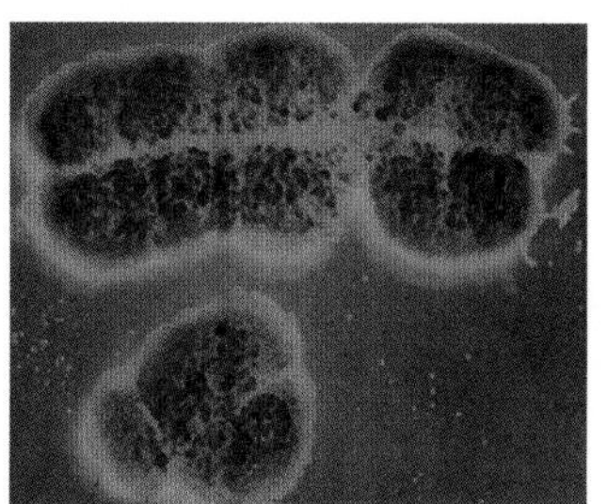
Human males have X (larger; top) and Y (smaller; bottom) chromosomes

Diploid: having two representatives of every chromosome (e.g., two copies of each gene)

Neurofibromatosis: hereditary disorder characterized clinically by the combination of patches of hyperpigmentation in both cutaneous and subcutaneous tumors over the entire body

Pseudogene: stretch of DNA similar in nucleotide sequence to normal DNA but containing defective (mutated) genes, rendering it nonfunctional for transcription and translation

Megabase: one billion base pairs

15 million base pairs. In contrast, the smallest human chromosome (the so-called male or Y chromosome) consists of 50 million base pairs, and the largest human chromosome contains 250 million base pairs. For some idea of the enormity of the genetic structures, consider the following analogy:

> A double-spaced 8.5 × 11–inch page of text using normal margins contains about 3000 letters or roughly 250 words. Porting the human genome to pages would equal the number of letters in 1000 copies of the Sunday *New York Times* or 1200 copies of the 4th edition of our 900-page *Exercise Physiology* text. Stated another way, reading one letter of code every second would require about 100 years without a break to peruse the entire genome! A single DNA strand in one **diploid** human cell with 23 pairs of chromosomes, if unwound and stacked end to end, would stretch to the height of a person 60 inches tall, yet it occupies a width of only 50 trillionths of an inch; and it's not only DNA's remarkably large size but also its relative molecular weight. For example, the chromosome of *E. coli* has a molecular weight of 2500×10^6, contrasted with a molecular weight of only 180 for the monosaccharide glucose.

To unravel the submicroscopic secrets of genetic material, sophisticated detection techniques help scientists "decode" the human genome. Most of the DNA sequences never become part of the final transcript that ultimately directs protein synthesis. By the year 2003, the Human Genome Project (www.ornl.gov/TechResources/Human_Genome/home.html) hopes to achieve its major objective of sequencing the total DNA of the human genome. As of November 2000, more than one-half of the genome had been identified, sequenced, and recorded in public databases (e.g., www.sanger.ac.us/HGP/Chr22/; http://www.gdb.org/). The December 1999 issue of *Nature* featured a milestone scientific achievement—the sequence or "genetic map" for 12 contiguous segments of human chromosome 22, the second smallest of the 23 chromosomes (chromosome 22 contains about 1.6 to 1.8% of the total genomic DNA).[43] At least 27 human disorders link to chromosome 22 genes, including ovarian, colon, and breast cancers; cataracts; schizophrenia; **neurofibromatosis**; mental retardation; and disorders of the nervous system and fetal development.

Scientists view this monumental genomic accomplishment as somewhat like completing an intricately detailed inaugural chapter in the human genetic instruction book composed of many complex chapters. An international collaboration from eight laboratories in the United Kingdom, Japan, the United States, Canada, and Sweden disclosed that chromosome 22 contained at least 545 genes (and 134 **pseudogenes**) in its 33.4-**megabase** structure. Through July 2001, sequencing of chromosone 1 to 22 is nearly complete (100%); for chromosone Y, it is 62.4% and 85.2% for chromosone X. Five large science centers currently work on about 85% of the Human Genome Project: the Whitehead Institute in Cambridge, MA; Washington University School of Medicine in St. Louis, MO; Baylor College of Medicine in Houston, TX; the Joint Genome Institute in Walnut Creek, CA; and the Sanger Center in Cambridge, England. Government-supported laboratories in France, Germany, Japan, and China also support genome research. The companies involved in the Human Genome Project must still resolve important questions before conquering the final structure of the human genome:

1. Correcting any sequencing errors in the base pairs to solidify the validity of the genome
2. Determining the missing "gaps" in the many short sequences of bases
3. Locating 100% of the genes, even if prior analysis predicted some stretches of DNA did not contain any genes (which turned out not to be the case when new genes were located on fruit fly heterochromatin)—making it likely such genes would be located in human heterochromatin

4. Locating the non–protein-coding genes (some genes code for RNA, not protein)
5. Identifying the functions of genes—crucial milestones that will ultimately lead to understanding the mechanisms responsible for preserving health and controlling disease

In a material sense, a relatively few discrete genetic instructions ultimately determine all of the subtlety of our species, including the thousands of years of accomplishment in fields of study from architecture to poetry and medicine to computer science and zoology. Anatomic and psychologic differences between any two unrelated individuals really reflect relatively few differences in their genomic blueprint—perhaps one or two gene sequences out of thousands. For example, the person next door, the basketball great Michael Jordan, and the brilliant Austrian physicist Lise Meitner (1878–1968[112]; deprived of a Nobel Prize for contributing to the discovery of nuclear fission because of her religion and professional animosities) are far more alike than different, yet the variety among individuals approaches infinity!

Dr. Lise Meitner

NUCLEIC ACIDS

Figure 1 shows the central configurational differences between the two nucleic acids, DNA and RNA; the three *yellow text boxes* highlight the important differences. Both structures carry and then transmit the hereditary information among the same type of cells when they divide (i.e., liver cells produce liver cells) and from generation to generation through reproductive cells. Within all living cells, genes encode the hereditary set of instructions that determine an organism's unique characteristics, from a simple bacterium such as *Streptococcus pneumoniae* to the complex multicellular organism *Homo sapiens*. As organisms within a species increase in complexity, the total information stored within the genome also increases tremendously. In subsequent sections, we describe just how much encoded information must be transcribed and translated to ultimately create proteins, which characterize thousands of unique cells, tissues, and organs that define the organism. Think of DNA as the raw material or building blocks of genes, and RNA as the link or intermediary to protein synthesis.

DNA and RNA

The **nucleic acids** DNA and RNA consist of polarized **polymers** of repeating subunits or nucleotides. A nucleotide consists of a nitrogen-containing organic base having 6 carbon atoms, a 5-carbon sugar, and a phosphate molecule (Fig. 2). A nucleotide's main support structure (backbone) consists of the sugar and phosphate molecules. The sugar phosphate backbone lies on the outside of the helix, with the amine bases on the inside. In this configuration, a base on one strand

Nucleic acid: large molecule containing nucleotide subunits

Polymer: high-molecular-weight substance linked together by repeating similar or identical subunits (e.g., glucose polymer starch); long-chain molecule linkage forms a two- and three-dimensional network

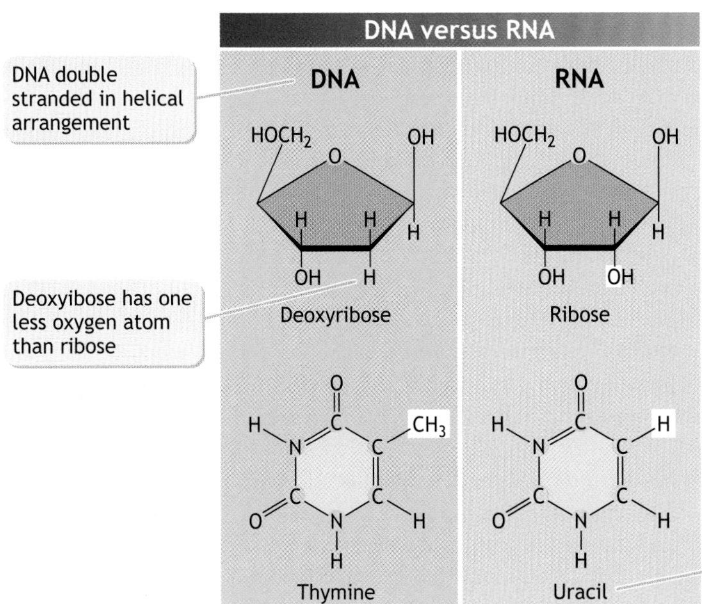

FIGURE 1 • Differences in molecular configuration between DNA and RNA.

FIGURE 2 • The components of a nucleotide, nucleotide-numbering nomenclature, and how nucleotides join together by phosphodiester bonding.

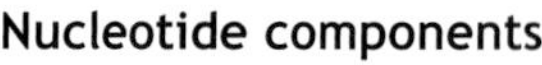

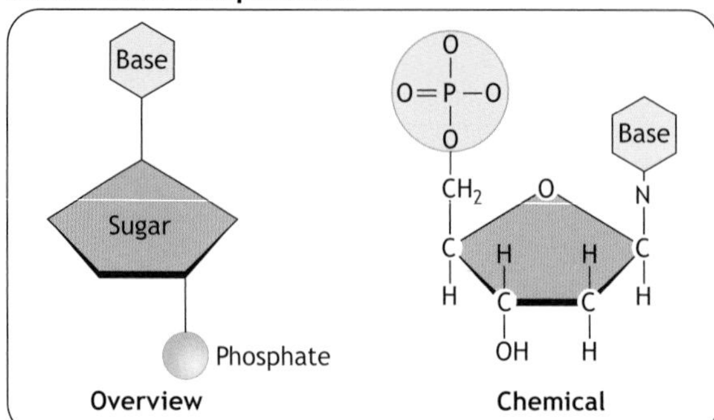

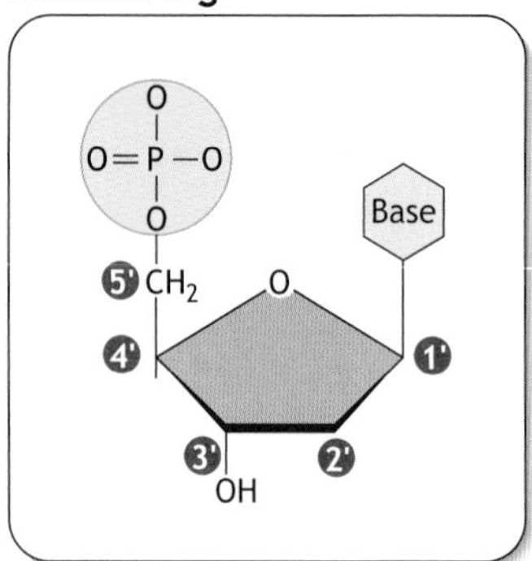

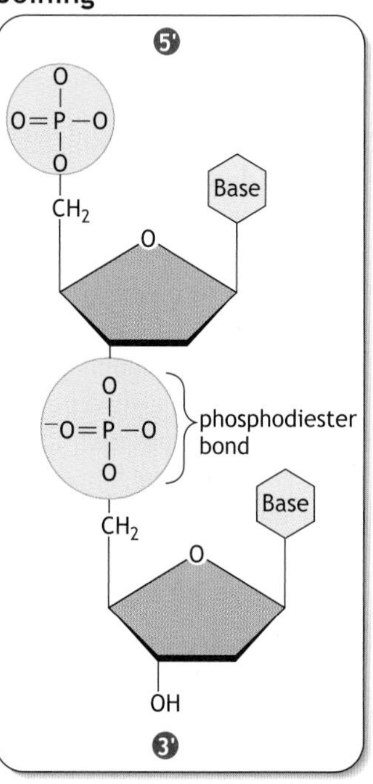

Polynucleotide: two or more nucleotides joined together; the phosphate at carbon 5′ of one sugar combines at the 3′ position of another sugar

Deoxyribose: sugar with five carbon atoms

Metaphase: step in mitosis (or meiosis) where microtubules organize into a spindle, and chromosomes move to the cell's equator to align in pairs, but have not yet migrated to the poles

Histone: positively charged small nuclear protein molecule cluster that binds to DNA (DNA winds around it) before it uncoils at the replication site; histones neutralize negatively charged DNA

Nucleosome: DNA coiled around a cluster of histone proteins; linked nucleosomes form chromatin

Electron microscope: Electron beams with wavelengths thousands of times shorter than visible light replace light, allowing significantly greater resolution and magnification. The electrons pass through an ultra-thin, specially prepared stained section of an embedded and dehydrated specimen maintained in a vacuum

points at a base on the second strand When nucleotides join to form **polynucleotides**, they link at specific carbon locations on the sugar molecule. These locations, numbered, in the red circles from 1′ to 5′, begin with 1′ to the right of the oxygen (O) atom in the ring. The "prime" symbol (′) distinguishes the carbons in the sugar from carbons in the base. Note from Figure 1 that RNA has one additional O atom in its sugar. Thus, the ribose sugar in RNA differs from the **deoxyribose** sugar in DNA. Nucleotides link when the phosphate at carbon 5′ of one sugar combines at the carbon 3′ position of another sugar. The phosphate group attaches to the 5′ carbon; the base attaches to the 1′ carbon. DNA and RNA synthesis always proceeds in the 5′ to 3′ direction.

The *top* of Figure 3 shows the successive levels (stages) of DNA packaging in a chromosome, proceeding from condensed **metaphase** (upper left) to supercoiled (middle right), loosely condensed, and uncondensed chromatin fiber stages. The negatively charged DNA molecule encircles and binds to a cluster of positively charged eight **histone** proteins. The histone (purple ball-like structure) clamps the DNA to the core of the molecule. The term **nucleosome** describes DNA wrapped around the puck-shaped histone proteins. Examining this region by **electron microscopy** reveals that one beadlike nucleosome contains 146 nucleotide base pairs wound twice like a rope around one cluster of the eight histones. The cluster contains two each of four different protein subunits (H2A, H2B, H3, H4), with each specific subunit having a different molecular mass. A DNA strand with about 60 base pairs and a ninth histone molecule links each cluster to the next one. During replication, the DNA uncoils from the histone core. The DNA molecule shown at the *bottom* of the figure eventually packs into the single metaphase chromosome displayed at the top left of the figure.

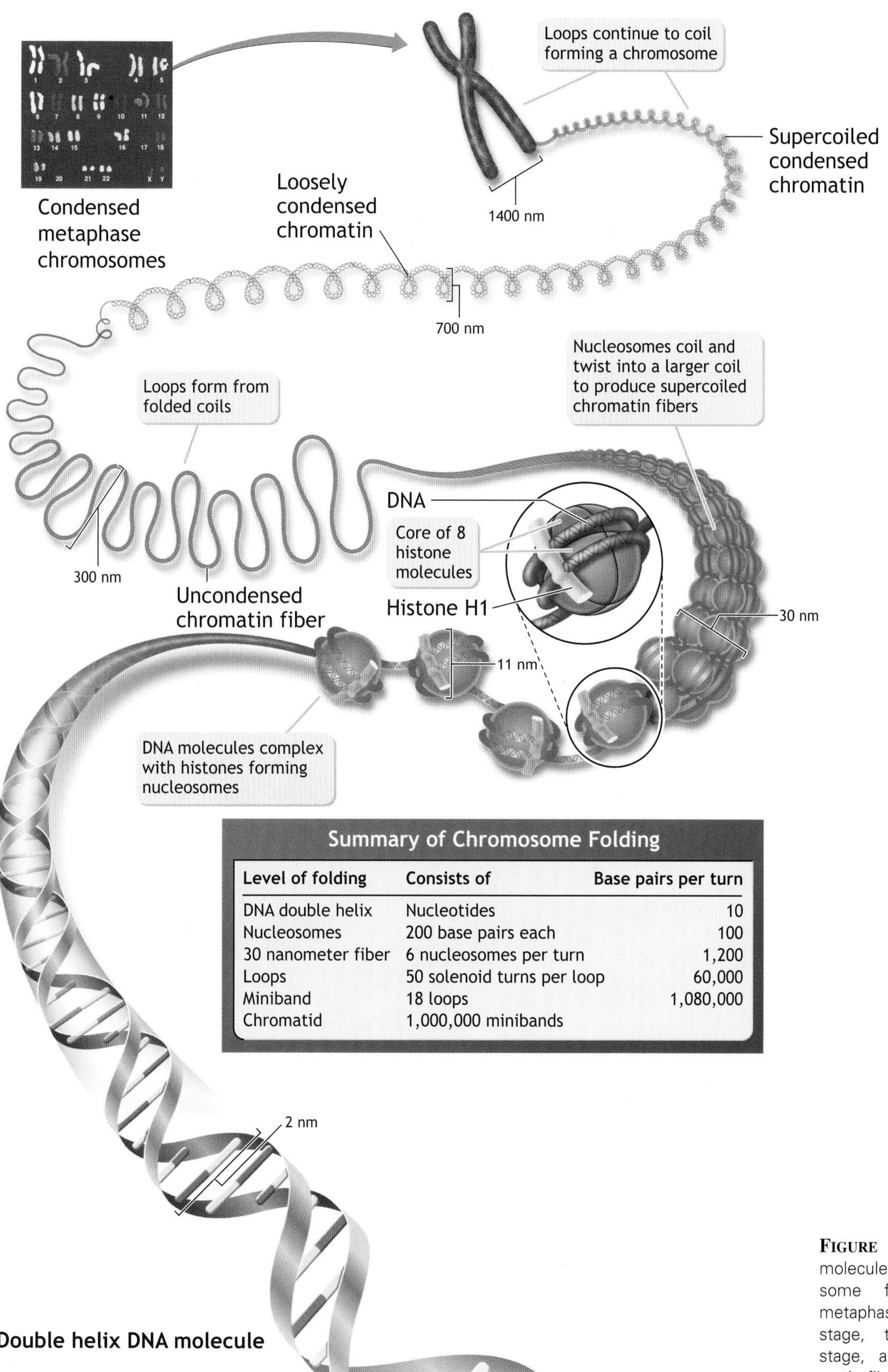

Summary of Chromosome Folding

Level of folding	Consists of	Base pairs per turn
DNA double helix	Nucleotides	10
Nucleosomes	200 base pairs each	100
30 nanometer fiber	6 nucleosomes per turn	1,200
Loops	50 solenoid turns per loop	60,000
Miniband	18 loops	1,080,000
Chromatid	1,000,000 minibands	

FIGURE 3 • Double-helix DNA molecule packaged in a chromosome from the condensed metaphase stage, to supercoiled stage, to loosely condensed stage, and uncondensed chromatin fiber stage. The *inset table* provides details about chromosome folding from the DNA double helix to the chromatid. nm (nanometer) = one-millionth mm.

Chromatid: one of the two double-stranded DNA daughter molecules of a duplicated, mitotic chromosome joined by a centromere

Mitosis: separation of duplicated chromosomes to create identical daughter cells with mirror-image (genetically identical) chromosomes; prophase, metaphase, anaphase, and telophase compose the four phases of mitosis

Centromere: region of a mitotic chromosome (indentation) before replication where two daughter chromatids join

Daughter chromosome: descendent chromosome following replication from the original (mother) chromosome

Dehydration synthesis: removal of the equivalent of a water molecule from two subunit molecules that forms a new, larger molecule

Phosphodiester bond: strong covalent bond formed when two nucleotides link together eliminating a water molecule; bonding involves the phosphate molecule from one nucleotide and the hydroxyl (OH) molecule of another nucleotide

Covalent bond: sharing one or more pairs of electrons between two atoms

The *inset table* of Fig. 3 provides relevant information about chromosome folding in the DNA double helix, nucleosomes, 30-nm fiber, loops, minibands, and **chromatids**.

The packaging of DNA within cells reflects a remarkable architectural accomplishment. The *inset table* summarizes DNA folding and how compacting the molecule enhances the efficiency of replication. In the compacted configuration as chromosomes, no transcription takes place to ensure that DNA remains intact to survive **mitosis**. The chromatids (listed in the *last line of the table*) with 1 million minibands represent duplicate strands of DNA held together by a **centromere** just before the DNA separates into two **daughter chromosomes**. The unnumbered figure below on page 987 shows the details for chromosome 2 and the general nomenclature for identifying specfic genes on the short p and long q arms of a chromosome. The architectural details of a condensed metaphase chromosome are shown on the right of the figure.

Linking Nucleotides: Phosphodiester Bonding

The chemical reaction when two nucleotides link together eliminates a water molecule, a process termed **dehydration synthesis**, which involves the phosphate molecule from one nucleotide and the hydroxyl (OH) molecule of another nucleotide. The resultant **phosphodiester bond** (Fig. 4) shown for RNA and DNA creates a relatively strong **covalent bond**. The new polymer, now two units long, still has free phosphate and OH

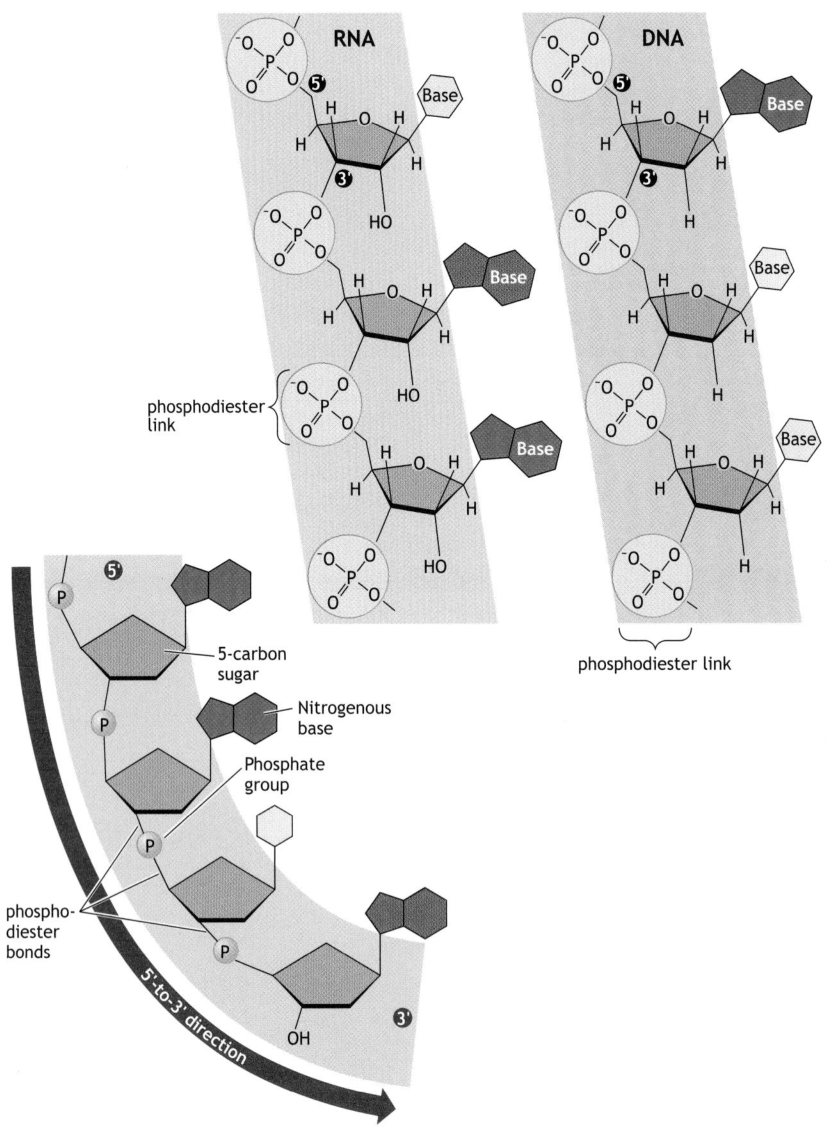

FIGURE 4 • Linking of nucleotides by phosphodiester bonding in RNA and DNA. The general schema shown at the bottom left illustrates the relative position of the sugar, base, and phosphate groups within a nucleotide along the 5′-to-3′ direction, including phosphodiester bonding.

groups for linking to other nucleotides. This linkage forms an incredibly long chain with thousands of nucleotides, although the example shows only a few. In DNA measurement, the term **kilobase (kb)** represents a unit of DNA fragment length equal to 1000 nucleotides. Another nucleic acid, adenosine triphosphate (or ATP) contains a 5-carbon sugar base **(adenine)** and three phosphate groups. Unlike DNA and RNA that transfer genetic information, ATP continually transfers *chemical energy* throughout life to power the body's cells until death.

Kilobase (kb): a unit of length for DNA fragments equal to 1000 nucleotides

Adenine: one of the four bases in DNA; always pairs with thymine

Complementary strand: when one DNA strand runs in the 5′ to 3′ direction, the complementary strand runs oppositely from 3′ to 5′

Antiparallel: arranged in parallel but with opposite orientation as in DNA

Structure of DNA

Figure 5 shows the DNA molecule composed of a sequence of sugar phosphate chains with hydrogen bonding between the nitrogenous bases. In the double-strand DNA molecule the strands are not identical. They lie parallel but line up in opposite directions. One strand runs in the 5′ to 3′ direction, and its **complementary strand** runs from 3′ to 5′. The *top left* of the figure illustrates the **antiparallel** arrangement of the DNA strands, including a close-up view of the hy-

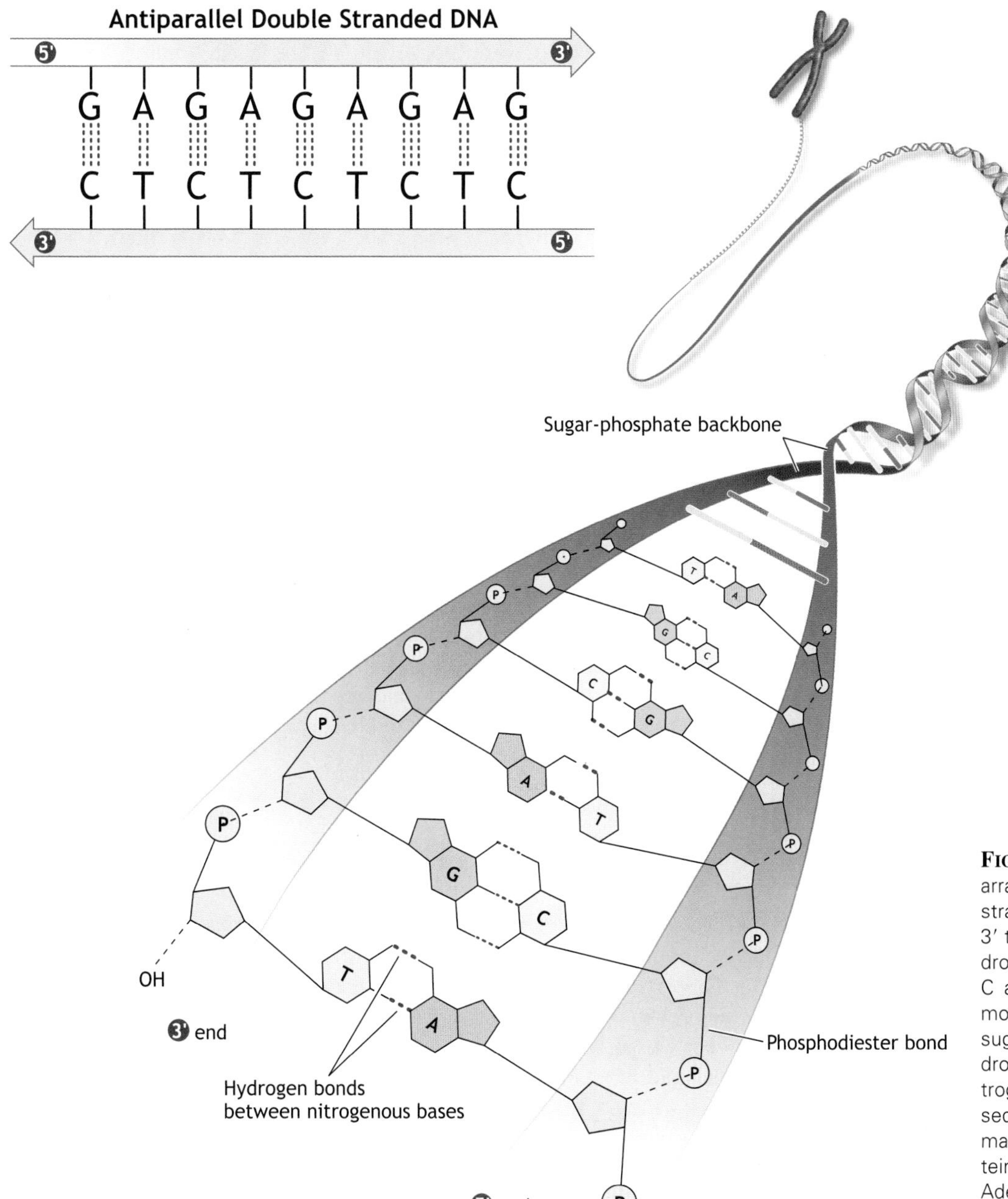

Figure 5 • *Top.* Antiparallel arrangement of a DNA double strand from the 5′ to 3′ and 3′ to 5′ directions. Note the hydrogen bonding between G and C and A and T. *Bottom.* DNA molecule with its sequence of sugar-phosphate chains and hydrogen bonding between nitrogenous bases. The specific sequence of base pairs ultimately determines every protein's specific characteristics. Adenine always binds with thymine.

Guanine: one of the four bases in DNA; always pairs with cytosine

Cytosine: one of the four bases in DNA; always pairs with guanine

Thymine: one of the four bases in DNA; always pairs with adenine

Chargaff's rule: pyrimidine content (T + C) equals purine content (A + G), where ([T] = [A]; [G] = [C]); (A + T)/(G + C) remains variable between different organisms but constant within an organism

Complementary: pairing in DNA between bases A-T or T-A, and C-G or G-C

Purine: nitrogen-containing, double-ring basic compound in nucleic acids; purines in DNA and RNA include adenine and guanine

Pyrimidine: nitrogen-containing, single-ring basic compound in nucleic acids; pyrimidines in DNA include cytosine and thymine and cytosine and uracil in RNA

Uracil: base that replaces thymine in RNA that pairs with the adenine base

Transfer RNA (tRNA): RNA molecules that transport a specific amino acid to ribosomes; translates information in the mRNA nucleotide into the amino acid sequence of a polypeptide

Ribosomal RNA (rRNA): structural part of a ribosome that contains RNA molecules

Polymerase (DNA or RNA): enzyme that catalyzes nucleic acid synthesis on preexisting nucleic acid templates; assembles RNA from ribonucleotides or DNA from deoxyribonucleotides

Primer: a short nucleotide segment that pairs with a single DNA strand at a free 3′-OH end (template strand) so DNA polymerase can synthesize a DNA chain; cells use RNA primers, while the PCR method uses DNA primers

Primase: enzyme that synthesizes the RNA primer to initiate DNA synthesis

drogen bonding between the base pairs that holds the parallel spiral ribbons together. The deduction by Watson and Crick of the antiparallel nature of the DNA strand resolved one of the remaining mysteries about DNA's structure, and ultimately how replication proceeds.

Base Pairing

One of the "golden rules" of DNA's molecular arrangement displayed in Figure 6 relates to the pairing of the four bases, the letters of the DNA alphabet. **Guanine** (G) always links with **cytosine** (C) and adenine (A) always links with **thymine** (T) in the same proportions within all DNA molecules. Stated somewhat differently, whenever a G base occurs in one of the strands, a C base occurs opposite it in the opposing strand. Likewise, when an A base occurs in one strand, a T base occurs in the other strand. The proportionality of the four bases was confirmed in 1950 by Erwin Chargaff (1905–) at Columbia University who determined the relative amounts of each base in DNA. **Chargaff's rule** determined that the molar amount of thymine always equaled the molar amount of adenine, and similarly, molar amounts of guanine always equaled cytosine on one DNA strand ([T] = [A]; [G] = [C]). Watson and Crick relied on this information to piece together DNA' s structure. In their model, each rung of the DNA ladder consists of a purine connected to a pyrimidine. The term *base pairing* refers to the joining of **complementary** bases (G with C or A with T). The G and A nitrogenous bases consist of two rings (called a **purine**), while the two other base pairs C and T have a single ring (called a **pyrimidine**). Thus, each base pair consists of one larger purine base mated to a smaller pyrimidine base. Adenine and thymine form two strong hydrogen bonds between the base pairs, but not with G or C. Similarly, G and C form three strong hydrogen bonds to keep the C–G base pair intact, but not with A or T. The additive effect of millions of relatively weak hydrogen bonds within the DNA molecule keeps the helix from separating. Applying Chargaff's rule within an organism, the pyrimidine content (T + C) equals the purine content (A + G); however, the relative amounts of pyrimidines and purines differ among organisms.

The *top* of Figure 6 illustrates the DNA double-helix molecule, with the base pairing and hydrogen bonding for A–T and G–C. Precise x-ray measurements have determined that the DNA double helix has a width of 2.0 nm (nanometers; 10^{-9} m, or 10 Å = one-millionth mm, or 1000 nm = 1 μm), with exactly 10 base pairs in each full turn and that the height of each turn equals 3.4 nm. The *bottom* of the figure shows the five bases classified as either a purine or pyrimidine. Note the pyrimidine base **uracil**. In RNA (next section), uracil replaces thymine, so that adenine pairs with uracil as A–U. The inclusion of uracil helps to distinguish RNA from DNA—besides RNA's extra oxygen atom in the ribose sugar and usually single-strand configuration. The simple mnemonic "cut the pie" helps to associate the pyrimidine or purine bases: **CUT** represents **c**ytosine, **u**racil, and **t**hymine, with the **py**rimidines represented by **pie**.

The heat required to dissociate the H bonds between two strands of DNA determines the DNA molecule's melting temperature. A proportionality exists between the number of bonds in the base pair and the energy required to break the bonds. Thus, the three hydrogen bonds holding C and G together require more heat to break (higher melting point) than the two hydrogen bonds between A and T.

Forms of RNA

The three forms of RNA include:

1. Messenger RNA (mRNA) molecules, which serve as a template for protein synthesis based on the molecular sequence from a small section of the DNA molecule
2. **Transfer RNA (tRNA)** molecules, which, as their name implies, transfer amino acids to the growing peptide chain on the ribosome
3. **Ribosomal RNA (rRNA)** molecules, which account for about 50% of the mass of ribosomes; the structures aid in assembling amino acids into polypeptides

Each of the three RNA forms has its own **polymerase** or complex enzyme: polymerase I is associated with rRNA, polymerase II with mRNA, and polymerase III with tRNA. RNA polymerases, unlike their DNA counterparts, do not require a **primer** to initiate RNA chain synthesis. The term **primase** refers to the RNA polymerase that produces the primer for DNA syn-

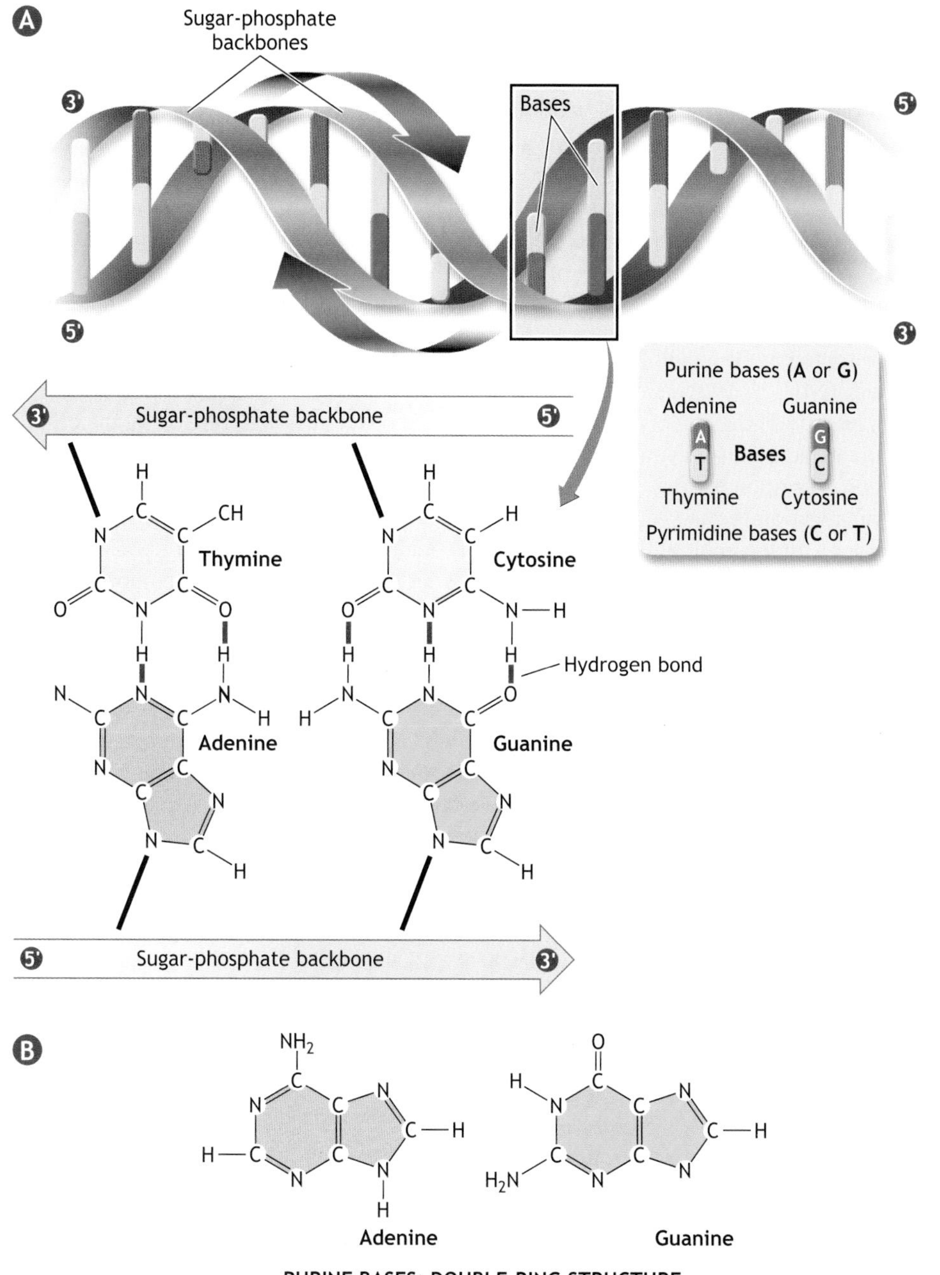

FIGURE 6 • A. Configuration details of the DNA double-helix molecule with base pairing and hydrogen bonding for adenine (A)–thymine (T) and guanine (G)–cytosine (C). The two spiral ribbons represent the sugar (deoxyribose)-phosphate backbone of DNA. Note that two hydrogen bonds shown in dark red form between A and T and three form between G and C. This happens because the two polynucleotide chains that contain them lay antiparallel to each other. **B**. The five bases classified as purines (A and G) or pyrimidines (C, uracil, T).

thesis. The three RNA polymerases have between 6 and 10 protein subunits that differ in molecular structure and regulatory function. About 97% of cellular RNA exists as rRNA; mRNA accounts for about 2%, and tRNA less than 1%. Compared with the DNA in a single chromosome that contains up to 250 million base pairs, RNA contains no more than a few thousand, which makes an RNA molecule considerably shorter. This makes sense because RNA carries only part of the information from one segment of the DNA molecule that it copied. In a subsequent section on protein synthesis beginning on page 988, we discuss how mRNA duplicates DNA's genetic information, and the roles of rRNA and tRNA in protein synthesis.

Codons and Nature's Genetic Code

First presented by Marshall Nirenberg and Johann Matthaei of the National of Institutes of Health (NIH) in 1961 at the International Congress of Biochemistry in Moscow (and 3 years later by Philip Leder and M. Nirenberg), the coded message carried by the mRNA molecule exists as a series of three bases or **codons**. Each three-letter codon block of information corresponds to one of the body's 20 amino acids. A codon codes for one amino acid, but most amino acids are represented by more than one codon. If only one base coded for an amino acid, only four amino acids could be coded instead of 20. Even if two adjacent bases coded for an amino acid, there would still not be enough combinations to make 20 amino acids. Fortunately, scientists deduced that three bases coding for an amino acid ($4^3 = 64$ combinations) met the requirement to include all the amino acids. For example, the triplet sequence A-U-G on mRNA displayed in Figure 7 (green box within yellow panel) refers to a specific code for the amino acid **methionine**. The A (adenine) is called the first letter, U (uracil) the second letter, and G (guanine) the third letter. With only 20 amino acids and 64 codons, several codons code for more than one amino acid. In fact, as mentioned, most amino acids have more than one codon or sequence of letters with no intervening code disrupting the sequence.

Codon: sequence of three DNA or RNA bases (nucleotides) that encode (specify) a single amino acid

Methionine: nutritionally essential amino acid; most natural source of active methyl groups in the body. The triplet sequence A-U-G on mRNA codes this amino acid

Sequencing of Codons

The amino acid serine exemplifies a four-codon sequence that differs only in the base occupying the third nucleotide or letter. The sequence is U-C-U, U-C-C, U-C-A, and U-C-G, with identical first two letters. The first two bases are the defining letters of the codon sequence. Reading from the 5′ end of each codon, the first and second letters remain generally constant for each amino acid, while the base in the third position wobbles. Thus, for example, the codon for phenylalanine contains a U or C as the third letter. Because both U-U-U and U-U-C code for phenylalanine, phenylalanine is inserted into a newly synthesized polypeptide if U-U-U or U-U-C were "read" during **translation** or protein synthesis.

Codon Table. Similar to the English alphabet with its 26 letters, the *codon table* in Figure 7 provides the genetic code "alphabet," but with only four distinct letters—the code words in the analogy. When we exclude the three **stop codons** (red boxes) that signal termination of linkages in polypeptide chains, the remaining 61 codons represent the useful information for protein synthesis. The stop codons, U-A-A, U-A-G, and U-G-A, signal the end of a genetic message (i.e., termination of protein synthesis), like periods at the end of a sentence. When the translation machinery encounters one of these chain terminators, translation halts, releasing the polypeptide from the translation complex. Recall that the start codon for methionine (A-U-G) initiates polypeptide formation; it also can code for methionine within peptide chains.

Translation: polypeptide formation (protein synthesis) on a ribosome using the amino acid sequence specified by an mRNA's nucleotide sequence

Stop codon: 3 of the 64 codon combinations that terminate a polypeptide assembly

HOW DNA REPLICATES

A **DNA replication fork** refers to the Y-shaped region of replicating DNA molecules. As the double helix unwinds, nucleotide duplication occurs on both strands at a rate of about 50 nucleotide additions per second. Each strand serves as the template to create two new daughter strands by complementary base pairing. This mechanism provides each daughter helix with one intact strand from the parent (original strand) and one newly synthesized strand. Each strand, a complementary mirror image of the other, can serve as a template to reconstruct the other strand. Figure 8 presents a schematic overview of DNA replication.

DNA replication fork: Y-shaped region of replicating DNA molecules where the enzymes replicating a DNA molecule bind to an untwisted, single DNA strand

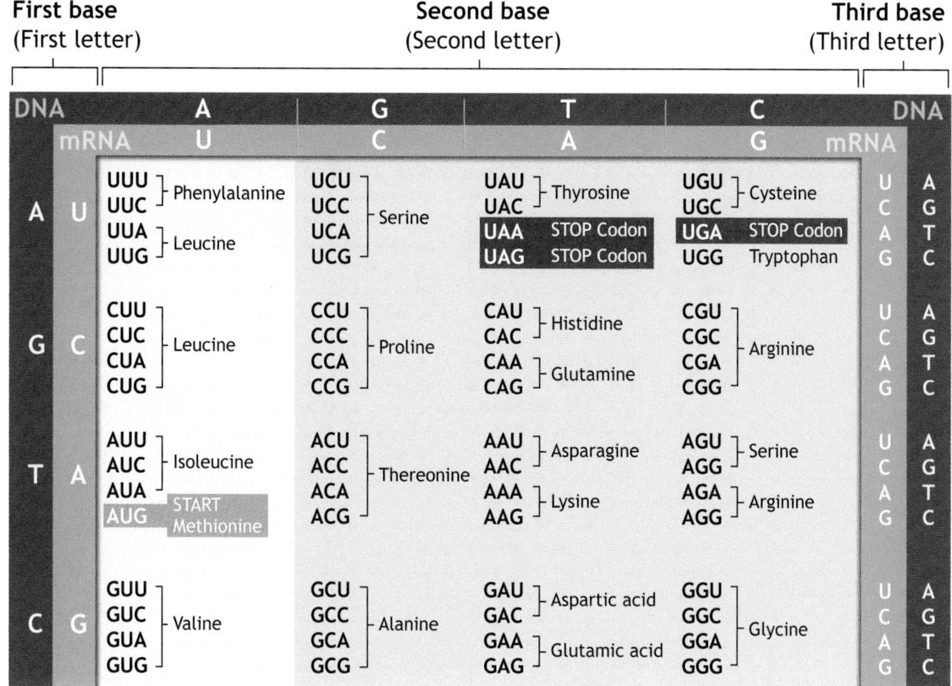

FIGURE 7 • The codon table—the alphabet of the universal genetic code. From the time that Watson and Crick correctly deduced DNA's helical structure in 1953, different coding schemes attempted to explain DNA's alphabetic configuration (including imaginative proposals by physicists George Gamow, Richard Feynman, and Edward Teller[58]); in 1964, Paul Leder and Marshall Nirenberg established the final code-breaking sequences for RNA synthesis.[79] The three-letter codon "word" in mRNA is complementary to the corresponding three-letter codon within DNA from which it had been transcribed.

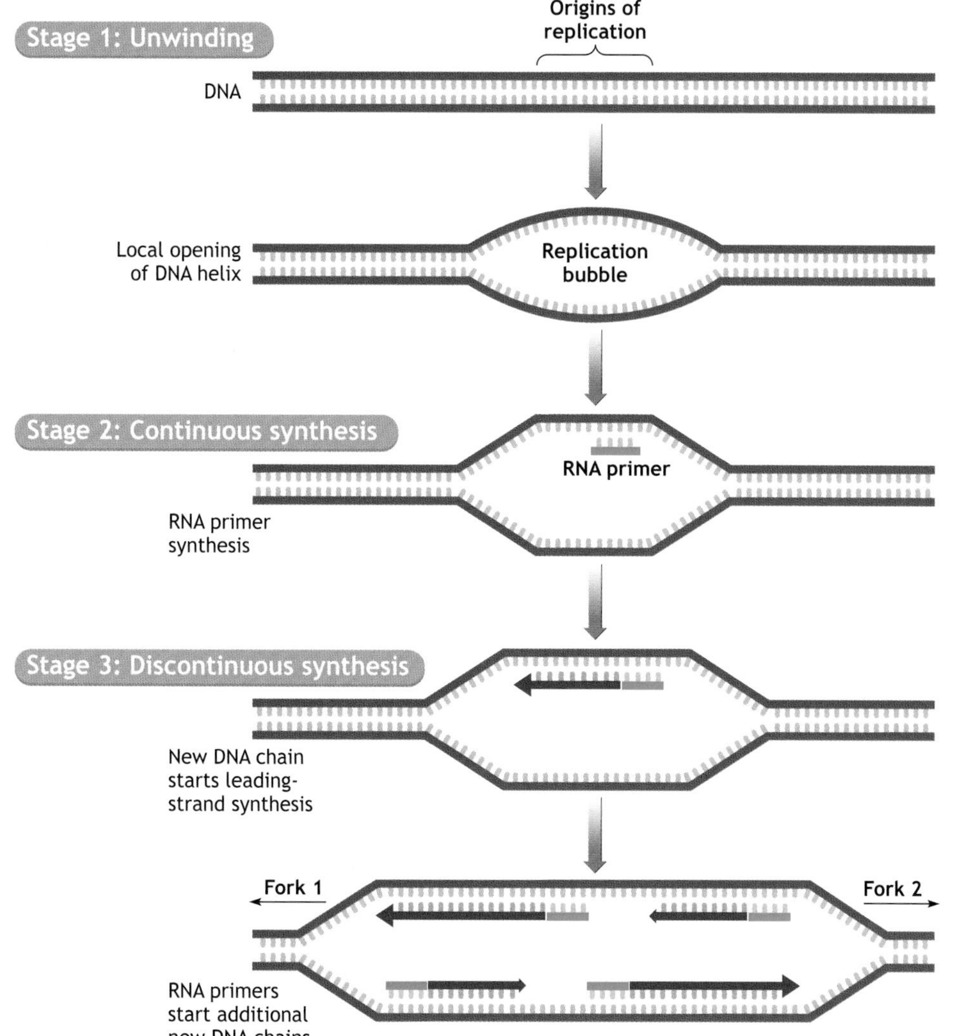

FIGURE 8 • Replication bubble and DNA replication. Note the straight (not helical) double strands of DNA in stage 1 after untwisting by DNA gyrase and unwinding by helicase. The DNA resembles an elongated bubble as the double strand opens and DNA begins to divide (stage 2, continuous synthesis). In stage 3 (discontinuous synthesis), replication proceeds in opposite directions along each end of the Y-shaped replication forks.

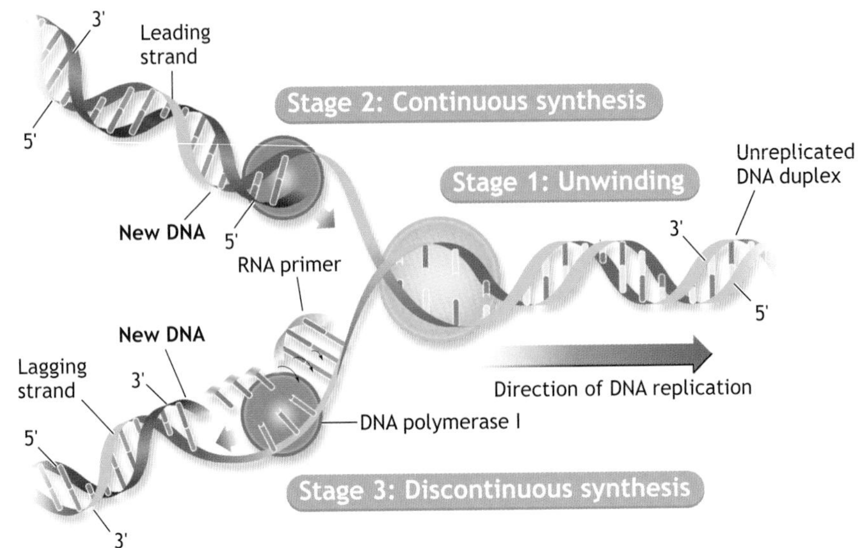

Figure 9 • Three stages of DNA replication. Stage 1, unwinding; stage 2, continuous synthesis; stage 3, discontinuous synthesis.

Origins of replication: sites on DNA where replication begins

RNA primer: small segment of 10 RNA nucleotides complementary to the parent DNA template that adds DNA nucleotides to it to synthesize a new DNA strand

Single-strand binding protein (SSB): protein that keeps separated strands of DNA from rejoining

DNA polymerase: enzymes responsible for creating new DNA strands during replication or repair

Leading strand: new DNA daughter strand formed during continuous synthesis of DNA

Continuous synthesis: process of creating a DNA strand

Lagging strand: new shorter DNA strand formed during discontinuous synthesis; joined end to end by DNA ligase away from the replication fork

Discontinuous synthesis: RNA primer 10 nucleotides long under the influence of DNA polymerase I that adds 1000 nucleotides ahead of the lagging strand's 5′ end until its gap fills

DNA polymerase I: enzyme that makes small bits of DNA to fill in gaps between Okazaki fragments during stage 3 discontinuous synthesis

DNA ligase: enzyme that binds short Okazaki fragments of the lagging strand into a continuous strand in DNA replication during stage 3 discontinuous synthesis

Okazaki segments: short DNA segments 100–200 nucleotides long assembled by discontinuous replication in the 5′ to 3′ direction away from the replication fork; forms the lagging strand

Replication begins with the untwisted, unzipped appearance of two DNA strands on the *top left,* where replication starts at specific zones called **origins of replication** and ends where **RNA primers** (green) start new DNA chains on the leading strand. Several origins of replication exist along a chromosome, replicating simultaneously in *opposite* directions. Multiple replications reduce the time to propagate DNA by an order of magnitude, since complete duplication of one strand of human DNA takes approximately 6 hours. The number of base pairs along the chromosome's replication region ranges from 10,000 up to 1 million, with the average at about 100,000 base pairs.

Stages of DNA Replication

Figure 9 amplifies the three stages of DNA replication illustrated in Figure 8. In stage 1, helicase enzymes *(orange)* unwind the molecule's double helix. This stabilizes the strands, while **single-strand binding protein (SSB)** maintains separation between the two DNA strands. In stage 2, **DNA polymerase** *(purple sphere)* immediately acts on DNA's **leading strand** to add nucleotides *toward* the strand's 3′ end *(red).* The process of creating the strand, called **continuous synthesis**, proceeds uninterrupted. The other DNA strand, known as a **lagging strand**, is created in shorter segments, with gaps in its structure *away* from the replication fork, compared with the leading strand. In stage 3 **discontinuous synthesis**, a 10-nucleotide RNA primer, under the influence of **DNA polymerase I**, adds 1000 nucleotides ahead of the lagging strand's 5′ end until its gap fills. Thus, new DNA nucleotides replace the existing RNA nucleotides. **DNA ligase** then affixes the newly created, smaller **Okazaki fragments** 100–200 nucleotides long to the lagging strand in the 5′ to 3′ direction to make a complete DNA strand.

Pivotal Role for DNA Polymerase

DNA polymerase plays the central role in life's processes because this enzyme consistently duplicates the genetic information from generation to generation. The rich instructional bank of DNA information has been modified and improved over more than 3 billion years to build proteins and other molecules atom by atom according to selective molecular directions. For every cell that divides, DNA polymerase duplicates all of its DNA so cells transfer one copy to each daughter cell. DNA polymerase can be considered the most accurate of the thousands of enzymes because it creates an exact DNA copy, transmitting less than one "error" in a billion bases. Stated another way, one might find only one mistake in a thousand novels. The excellent match of C to G and A to T provides much of the specificity needed for this high accuracy, but DNA polymerase adds an extra step. After it copies each base, it "proofreads" it and deletes any wrong base sequence from its grasp. Polymerases can vary in structure from relatively "simple" to complex. In humans, polymerases are complex structures that unwind the helix, build an RNA primer, and construct a new strand. Some even have a ring-shaped structure that clamps the polymerase to the DNA strand. Polymerase function varies from day-to-day DNA repair and maintenance to the complex task of DNA replication when the cell divides. Herein, we discuss the important role of DNA polymerase in forensic medicine in building a large quantity of identical DNA strands from only a miniscule amount of DNA from a crime scene or paternity case.

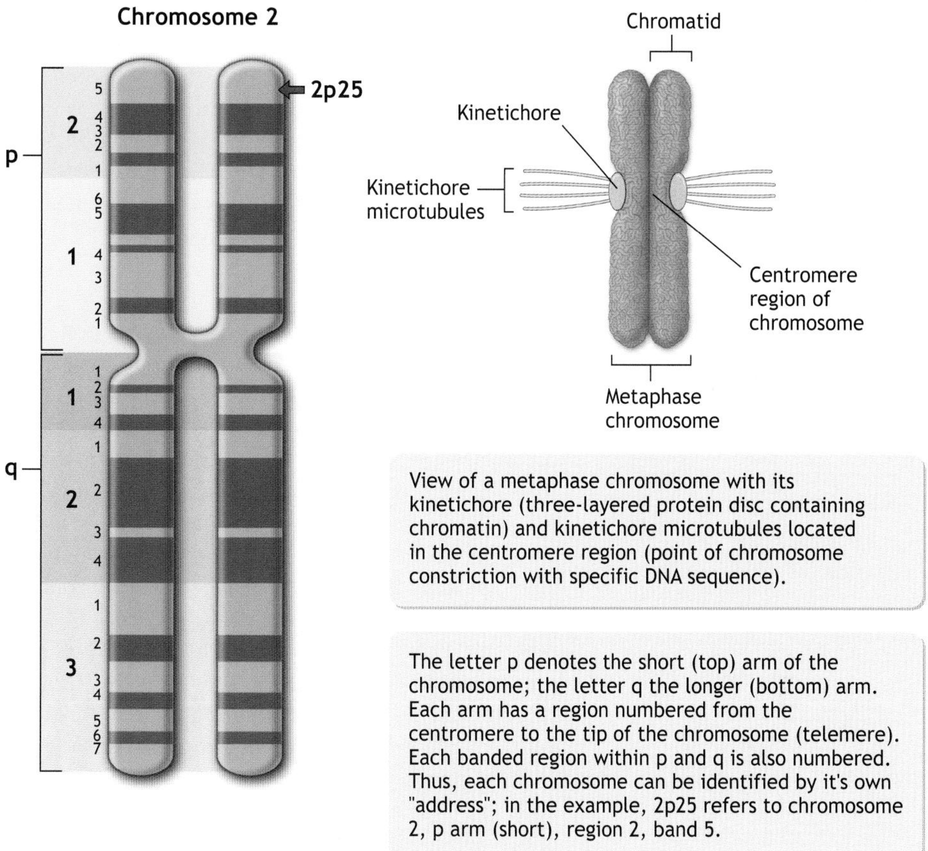

Left. Identification of gene 2p25 on chromosome 2. *Right.* Metaphase chromosome.

What Controls DNA Synthesis?

Several molecular control mechanisms trigger DNA synthesis in cells. The **cell cycle** illustrated in Figure 10 depicts the four phases of a cell's life. Like a clock or thermostat, each phase has defined "on" and "off" periods regulated by enzymes that start and terminate a particular stage. DNA replication (synthesis) occurs in the S phase, which lasts approximately 6 hours. The three checkpoints identified by the stars serve as the thermostat's sensors, each with specific regulator enzymes called **cyclins** governing a specific

Cell cycle: four stages of a cell's life cycle

Cyclins: specific cell-regulator enzymes that activate and deactivate protein kinases in the cell cycle and help to control progression from one stage in the cycle to the next. They are destroyed after their function by a ubiquitin-signaled process

Figure 10 • Four stages of the cell cycle and its molecular control mechanisms. Note the three checkpoints and the question(s) posed prior to DNA synthesis during the S phase.

G_1: period within the cell cycle preceding DNA synthesis

G_2: period within the cell cycle from the end of DNA synthesis and start of the M phase

Telophase: final stage in mitosis (or meiosis); the spindle disappears and daughter sets of separated chromosomes decondense, the cytoplasm splits, a nuclear envelope resurrounds the chromosomes, and nucleoli appear

Kinase: enzyme that shuttles a phosphate group (PO_4) from ATP or another nucleoside triphosphate to a different molecule

Protein kinase: enzyme that transfers phosphate groups to other proteins, changing their activity

function. Toward the end of the G_1 (growth) stage, cyclin enzymes achieve a critical activity level that triggers a response when the cell achieves adequate size within a favorable environment. If cell size and environment prove satisfactory, the cell proceeds to S phase for DNA synthesis. Following DNA synthesis, the G_1 cyclins degrade as the cell prepares to enter mitosis (M phase). The next checkpoint occurs between the G_2 and M phases, a crucial time in the cell cycle. When the DNA has been replicated without error, the cell enters mitosis and then progresses to complete **telophase**. Mitosis produces two cells genetically identical to the original parent cell.

Cell Life Cycle Controllers

Figure 10 provides details of the workings of cell life cycle controllers. Cyclin-dependent **kinases** (cdk_1 and cdk_2) activate specific cyclins. Once this occurs, the complex of the two **protein kinases** regulates how the cell proceeds through its cycle. After each stage, cyclin degradation temporarily halts cdk activity. With mitosis complete, the process begins again, accumulating cyclins for the next initial G_1 growth stage.

The cdk_2 protein "turns on" in the transition between the G_1 and S stages; cdk_1 drives the cell cycle from stage G_2 to M stage. In other words, the cyclin-dependent protein kinases phosphorylate their target cyclin proteins through the different stages of the cell cycle. Signaling proteins called growth factors operate in concert during the cycle. For example, mitosis-promoting factor (MPF) governs the sequence of events between the G_1 and M phases of the cell cycle. Other growth factors also exert their effect. For example, the hormone **erythropoietin** produced by the kidneys (see Chapters 20, 23, 24) initiates proliferation of red blood cell precursors and their maturation to erythrocytes. Nerve growth factor (NGF) modulates neuronal cell growth during development of the nervous system, interleukin-2 participates in immune cell proliferation, and **insulin-like growth factor** (**IGF**) facilitates many metabolic events related to cellular growth and development. A unique feature of growth factors relates to how they control the transition stages during cellular growth and differentiation. Failure to work in concert with cyclins and kinases during cellular proliferation terminates control of cellular proliferation, causing cells to continue to divide unchecked. This can serve both positive and negative functions. The latter produce lethal effects because DNA synthesis would progress to the M stage by successfully reproducing a mutant **cancer** gene. If highly specialized genes called tumor suppressors (e.g., the *p53* gene) cannot halt the cell cycle long enough for DNA repair enzymes to function, then cell growth proceeds rapidly and unchecked to produce tumors. Also, deleterious mutations can pass to progeny cells; the successive buildup of mutations in all likelihood ultimately develops cancer.

Insulin-like growth factor (IGF): small protein hormone with the potent effect of increasing aspects of cellular growth and development. IGF-1 (also known as somatomedin C) controls the general effects of growth hormone on growth

Cancer: accelerated, unplanned growth and division of mutant cells that form larger-than-normal cell clusters that become tumors

PROTEIN SYNTHESIS: TRANSCRIPTION AND TRANSLATION

Protein synthesis involves two prominent events:

1. Transcription in the cell nucleus that creates a single-strand RNA copy of the genetic information stored in the double-stranded DNA molecule
2. Translation in the cell cytoplasm of RNA to form proteins

In essence, the DNA molecule's nucleotide base sequence defines the protein's ultimate three-dimensional shape. Our tour of protein synthesis begins by considering a "roadmap" of the prominent events in assembling proteins from precursor biomolecules. The story originates in the cell's ribosomes and ends with creation of a fully **functional protein**—a unique molecule whose structure dictates its operation and specific mode of action.

Functional protein: protein with its own set of genetically determined information to carry out specific function(s)

Generalized Overview

DNA gyrase: enzyme that relaxes supercoiled DNA

Supercoiled DNA: configuration of twisted DNA packed into a cell prior to replication

Figure 11 provides a generalized overview of six stages in protein synthesis. Prior to stage 1, the DNA under enzyme control "untwists" to expose its code. Before DNA's hydrogen bonds break, DNA topoisomerase enzymes (e.g., **DNA gyrase**) "relaxes" the **supercoiled DNA** by literally cutting the DNA to create a double-stranded break, but maintains hold of both ends of the DNA. The two halves of the molecule then rotate relative to each other (they untwist) before rejoining. Once the strand untwists,

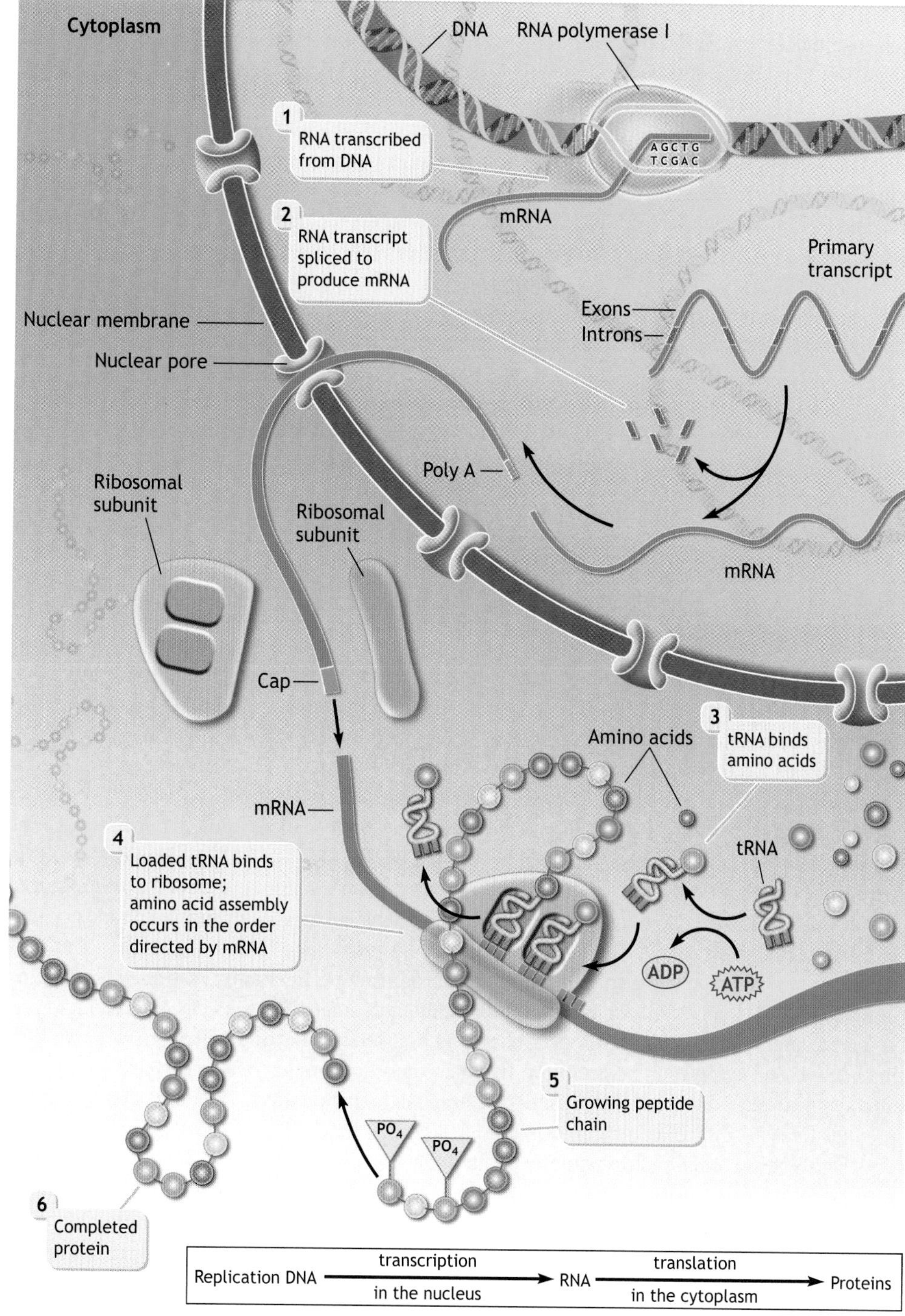

FIGURE 11 • Generalized overview of six stages (*numbered yellow boxes*) in protein synthesis. Notable features include the schematic depiction of events during *transcription* (stages labeled *1* and *2* within the cell's nucleus) and *translation* (stages labeled *3* to *6* in the cell's cytoplasm). The *bottom inset* summarizes the two principle aspects of protein synthesis (transcription and translation) following replication of the DNA molecule.

DNA helicase unwinds the helical DNA molecule by separating the hydrogen bonds between the base pairs. The single-strand binding protein (SSB) binds to one of the unpaired DNA strands to inhibit its remerging with its neighbor (complementary) strand. This prevents the strands from recoiling and reforming the double helix. **DNA polymerase III (Pol III)** serves as a "verifier" to ensure that the bases pair correctly. If they do, the enzyme joins the nucleotides together. If not, the mismatched base pair is rejected. A previous section (How DNA Replicates) provides further details about the DNA **replication bubble** and three stages of DNA replication.

Stage 1 signifies the start of transcription. This involves copying a discrete section of the genetic sequence directly from the DNA template to the growing RNA strand. The enzyme **RNA polymerase I** in Figure 11 (labeled 1 because it was discovered before the other polymerases) binds to the specific **promoter** (initiator) region at the beginning of a gene. Linking to a specific

DNA helicase: enzyme that catalyzes the unwinding of double-helical DNA by using energy released from ATP hydrolysis

DNA polymerase III (Pol III): enzyme involved in making DNA when chromosomes replicate

Replication bubble: site where DNA divides

RNA polymerase: enzyme that synthesizes RNA from a DNA template

Promoter: site on DNA where RNA polymerase binds and initiates transcription (promotes gene expression); required for expression and regulation of gene transcription

nitrogenous base sequence, it "alerts" transcription to initiate formation of the complementary RNA strand. When RNA polymerase arrives at the end of the gene, it receives a "stop" signal from one of three nucleotide sequences (U-A-A, U-A-G, U-G-A; see Fig. 7) and disengages from the DNA. The newly assembled RNA strand, called the **primary RNA transcript** of the gene (stage 2), is processed and eventually exits the nucleus to the cytoplasm through the octagon disk-shaped **nuclear pore complex**. This complex selectively transports proteins across the nuclear envelope after specific protein receptors dock with the protein, allowing it to enter its channel and pass to the cytoplasm. Note that once mRNA leaves the nucleus in stage 2, it links to the ribosome's poly A-site and waits to bind to the appropriately coded amino acid floating freely in the cytoplasm. A specific orientation of mRNA on the ribosome exposes only one codon at a time to match and bind with its anticodon contained on a tRNA.

Primary RNA transcript: mRNA molecule transcribed as an exact complement to a gene

Nuclear pore complex: octagon, disk-shaped structure that allows proteins to cross the nuclear envelope into the cytoplasm after protein receptors dock with the protein

Within the cytoplasm, translation proceeds through stage 3 (tRNA binds amino acids), stage 4 (tRNA binds to a ribosome, signifying the start of amino acid assembly), and stage 5 (the peptide chain increases in length), until stage 6, when a fully functional protein forms. The *inset at the bottom* of Figure 11 summarizes the two key aspects of protein synthesis following DNA molecule **replication:**

Replication: duplication of DNA prior to cell division

1. Transcription of information in the genetic code from DNA molecules to RNA molecules in the nucleus (RNA synthesis) for decoding
2. Translation of genetic information in the cytoplasm to synthesize proteins

Transcription of the Genetic Code: RNA Synthesis and Gene Expression

A **gene**, located along a specific chromosome at a specific site, contains the sequence (code or "plan") required to synthesize a protein. The gene within the DNA molecule ranges from several thousand to millions of bases. Unlocking the regulation of a particular gene provides the driving force for many molecular biologists' passion for the field.

The *left side* of Figure 12 highlights the five stages of gene expression in human cells. The same two basic sequences of molecular events occur whether in the simplest **bacteria** (**prokaryotes**) that dominated the Earth during its first 2 billion or so years of evolution or in **eukaryotes** that evolved about 1.5 billion years ago. The eukaryotes include thousands of uni- and multicellular organisms (including humans) with membrane-bound **organelles**. The cells of these organisms include a true nucleus with chromosomes. In contrast, prokaryotes have no defined nucleus, generally have no membrane-bound organelles, the DNA remains single stranded, and the main events—transcription and translation—occur coupled, not separately in the nucleus and cytoplasm, respectively. In eukaryotes, in contrast, translating the code for protein synthesis does not occur until the RNA strand exits the nucleus. The *right side* of the figure illustrates the flow of genetic information that Francis Crick in 1956 termed **central dogma**.

Bacteria: primitive, single-celled organisms used to study genetic characteristics and to clone mammalian genes

Prokaryote: cell or organism lacking a structurally discrete nucleus or nuclear membrane; contains a single circular chromosome

Eukaryotes: multicellular organisms with membrane-bound organelles and a true nucleus containing multiple linear chromosomes (Greek; from *eu-karyon* or true nucleus)

Organelle: intracellular structure within a cell that carries out specialized functions (e.g., mitochondrion)

Central dogma: Crick's belief, more powerful than a hypothesis, that the genetic information flow creates proteins from DNA (transcription in the nucleus) and RNA (translation in the cytoplasm) to protein

The Watson and Crick hypothesis posited that chromosomal DNA functions as the template for RNA molecules. These molecules then move to the cytoplasm to dictate a protein's amino acid *arrangement*. The *down arrow* from DNA emphasizes the proposition that DNA provides the template for self-replication. The *next* phase emphasizes that all cellular RNA molecules were made on (transcribed from) DNA templates. Concomitantly, RNA templates determined (translated) the proteins. The unidirectionality of the *two arrows* between Stages 3 and 4 and 4 and 5 indicates that protein templates would never determine RNA sequences, nor would RNA templates create DNA. With few exceptions, the central dogma has stood the test of time and remains essentially valid. Except in some instances in which the reproductive cycle of **retroviruses** adds a step using a reverse transcriptase enzyme, proteins almost never serve as templates for RNA. If they did, the arrows would go bidirectionally between DNA and RNA. Interestingly, at the time Crick proposed the central dogma, little direct experimental support existed for this mechanistic concept that RNA served as the template for DNA.

Retrovirus: RNA virus that can enter a cell using reverse transcriptase to reproduce a copy of itself into the genome. A retrovirus carrying an oncogene can transform a host cell into a cancerous cell

Examples of Gene Expression

Beginning with conception, gene expression lays the eventual groundwork for each person's diverse cells, tissues, organs, and systems. Gene expression explains why no two people match exactly in any outer or even inner physical traits. No two hearts, livers, kid-

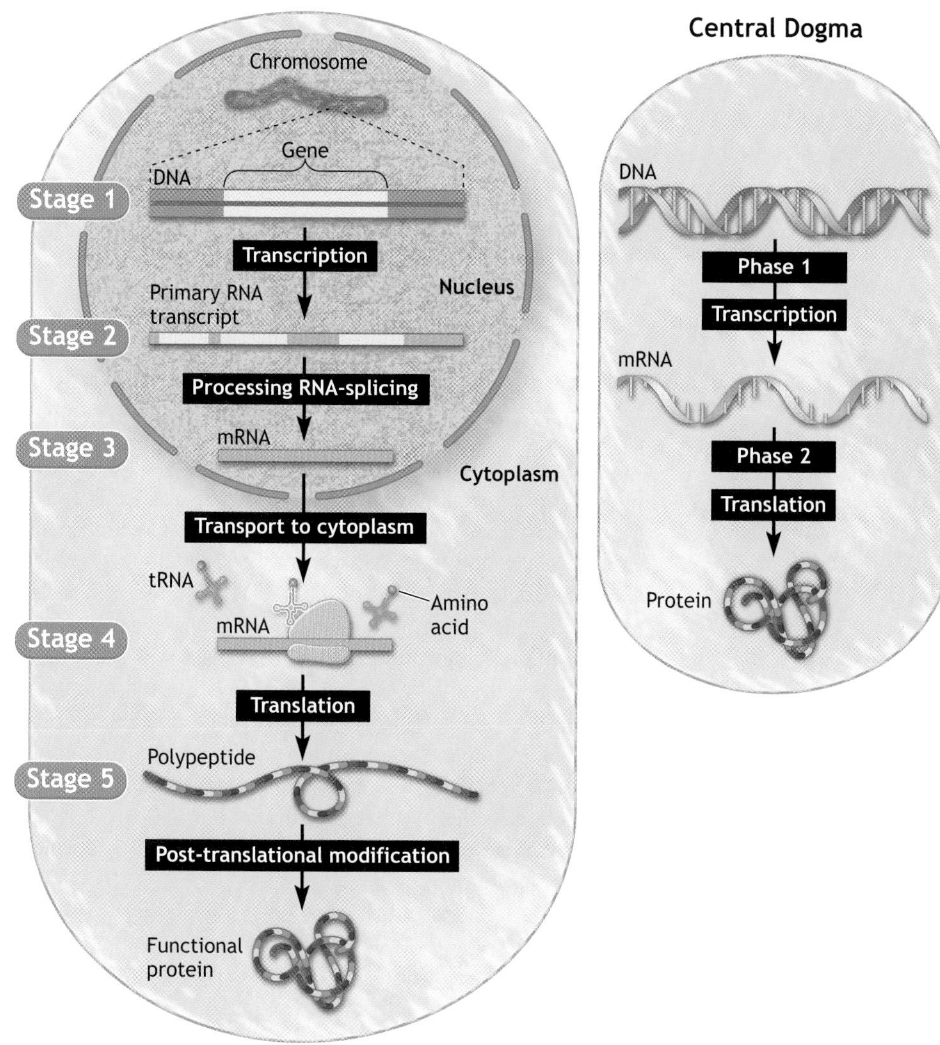

Figure 12 • *Left.* Five stages of gene expression in eukaryotes. Transcription (stage 1) produces an mRNA copy of the gene. In translation (stage 4), the information in mRNA molecules "directs" which amino acid to produce and where to position the amino acids when the ribosomes synthesize polypeptides. Translation refers to the creation (assembly) of a protein on the ribosome; mRNA copies the specific coded information from the DNA strand. Post-translational modifications can alter polypeptides in their transition to a functional protein (stage 5). *Right.* Crick's 1956 working hypothesis (central dogma) posits that two distinct phases play the defining role in expressing the genetic information encoded in DNA molecules. In phase 1 (transcription), RNA polymerase enzyme assembles a mRNA molecule with its nucleotide sequence complementary to the gene's nucleotide sequence. In phase 2 (translation), a ribosome assembles a polypeptide (protein) where mRNA's nucleotide sequence specifies the final amino acid configuration.

neys, brains, vertebrae, adrenal glands, intra-abdominal fat distributions, teeth, nostrils, ears, or fingerprints match precisely. Even identical twins with the same starting genetic machinery have unique and subtle outward physical characteristics and often not-so-subtle distinctive personalities. At times, some aspect of gene expression remains repressed or "off," no longer needing to remain active or "on." Most of the time, gene expression "fits" or modulates to the body's current metabolic state, persisting throughout the individual's life span. The biologic catalysts—the enzymes containing a minimum of 100 amino acid residues—effectively control the genetic machinery and subsequent transformation and control of different energy forms. Six potential regions within the nucleus and cytoplasm shown in Figure 13 regulate gene expression. When the mRNA travels to the cytoplasm from the nucleus, protein regulation via translation in the cytoplasm at sites 3 to 6 can begin, as can further modifications once a protein forms as indicated at site 6.

Protein Enzymes

Acting as biomolecular switches, enzymes selectively regulate thousands of cellular activities, coupling some and uncoupling others, all orchestrated in fractions of a second throughout an organism's life. To categorize different kinds of enzymes, the Enzyme Commission (EC) of the International Union of Biochemistry and Molecular Biology (ICBMB) devised

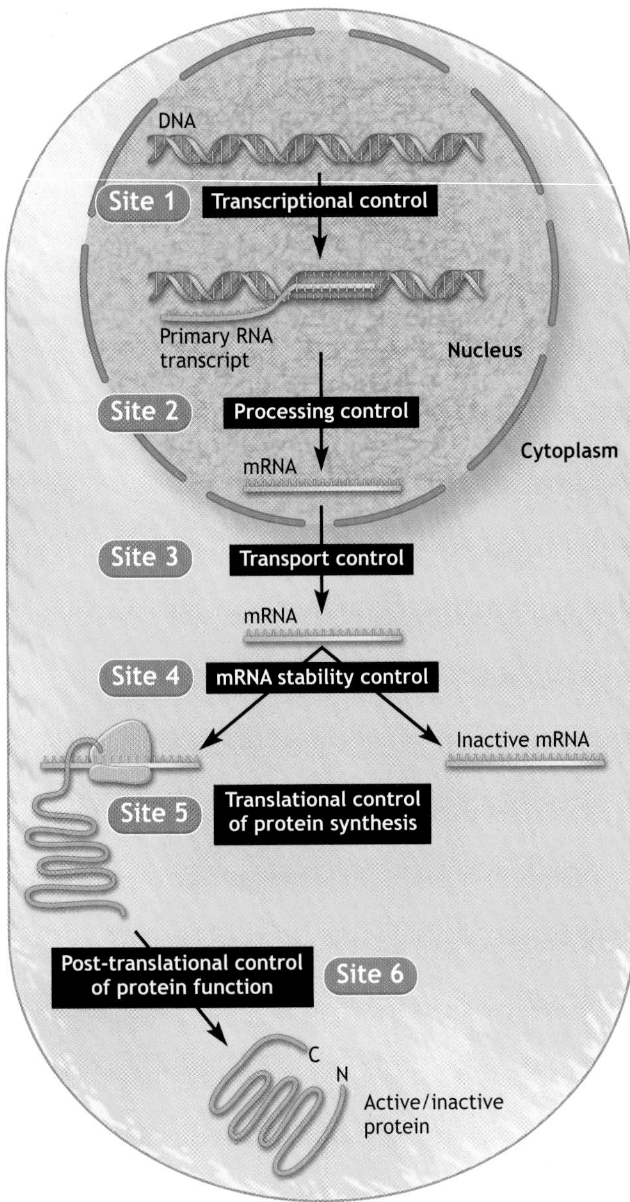

FIGURE 13 • Six potential sites regulate gene expression.

a nomenclature and numbering system for enzymes. The following six major classes of enzymes exist, each with subgroups and sub-subgroups:

1. *Oxidoreductases:* catalyze oxidation–reduction reactions
2. *Transferases:* catalyze transfer of functional groups between molecules
3. *Hydrolases:* catalyze hydrolytic cleavage
4. *Lyases:* catalyze removal of a group from or addition of a group to a double bond, or other changes involving electron rearrangement
5. *Isomerases:* catalyze intramolecular rearrangement
6. *Ligases:* catalyze reactions that join two molecules

The EC assigns a number with four parts to each enzyme. For example, hexokinase has the designation EC2.7.1.2. This means hexokinase belongs to transferases, the second major enzyme class, and the next two numbers denote the subclass and sub-subclass specified in the ICBMB reference. The last numbered entry, a serial number, refers to the order in which the enzyme was added to the list (hexokinase was second). In exercise physiology, we encounter many different enzymes, particularly in the complex reactions of the citric acid (Krebs) cycle. For example, the ligase enzyme pyruvate carboxylase (EC 6.4.1.1) catalyzes the conversion reaction of pyruvate to oxaloacetate, while pyruvate decarboxylase (EC 4.1.1.1) catalyzes pyruvate to acetaldehyde. What main classes do these two enzymes belong to?

Control of Transcription

Factors that affect gene expression during transcription include diverse "switches" or regulator enzyme **activator proteins** and **repressor proteins**. These operate at the site of the active gene and also at sites thousands of nucleotides away from the starting site. This geography of operation provides great regulatory freedom in how genes initially switch on and off prior to and during transcription. For example, some enzymes accelerate the capture of RNA polymerase to enhance transcription, while others repress transcription by delaying different sequences of events. In essence, activator and repressor proteins control transcription rate in the following two ways:

Activator protein: binds to DNA at enhancer sites to position RNA polymerase correctly on the gene

Repressor protein: blocks action of RNA polymerase on DNA that turns genes "off"

Enhancer site: where gene expression increases from contact with the transcription complex

Coactivator protein: transmits signals from activator proteins to basal factors

Coding region: location on the DNA strand where transcription occurs

1. Activator proteins bind to DNA at sites called enhancer sites. Figure 14 shows the transcription complex (proteins involved in transcription) correctly positioning RNA polymerase at the proper gene location. The folding of the DNA strand brings the **enhancer site** into close proximity to the transcription complex. This increases communication between the activator proteins and transcription complex. Another group of proteins, termed **coactivator proteins**, transmits signals from activator proteins to other factors (called basal factors) close to the DNA strand, helping to position RNA polymerase correctly at the precise location in DNA's **coding region**.
2. Repressor proteins bind to "silencer" protein binding sites along the DNA strand. The silencer sequence, adjacent to or overlapping the enhancer region, can prevent an activator protein from binding to a neighboring enhancer site. This delays or cancels transcription from initiating a discrete mRNA coding sequence.

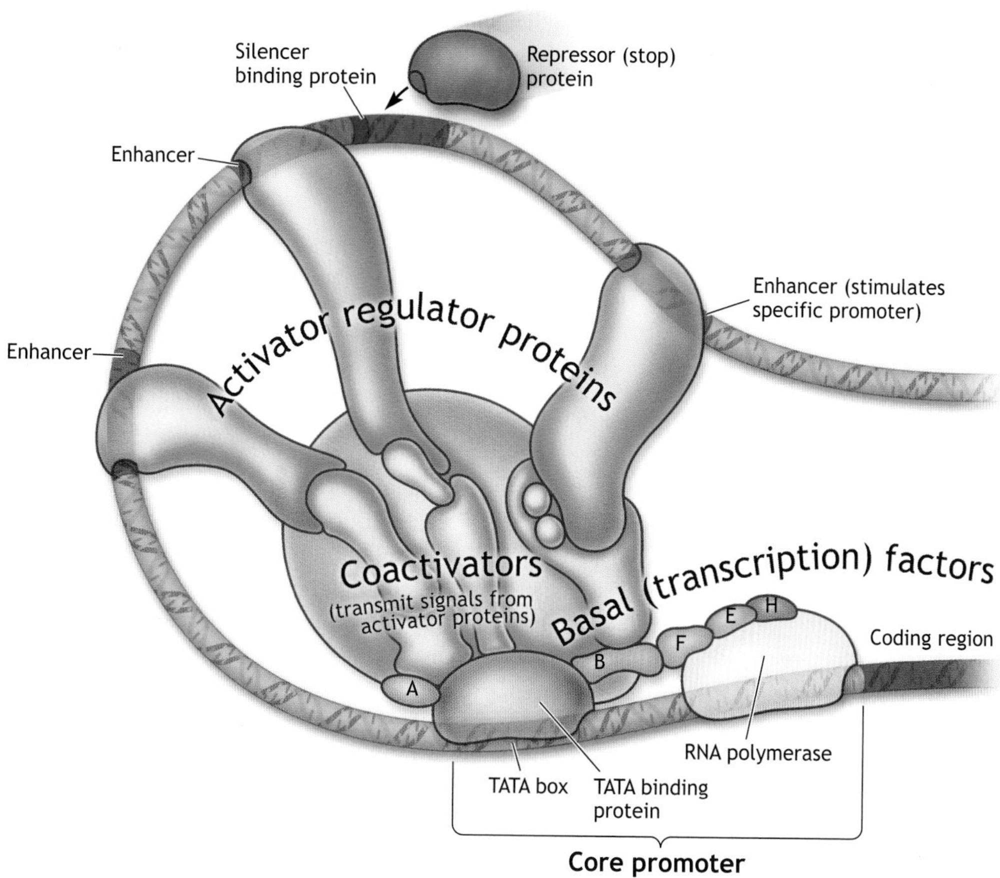

FIGURE 14 • Structure of transcription complex involved in transcriptional control. At the start of the coding sequence along DNA's double helix (purple rope-like structure), the basal (transcription) factors labeled (from *left to right*) A, TATA binding protein, B, F, E, and H correctly position RNA polymerase and then release it to transcribe mRNA.

Enzyme Turnover Number

Some enzymes fulfill their functions more quickly than others. An important way to measure an enzyme's performance relates to how quickly it binds to and releases from its substrate(s) during biomolecular reactions; that is, its turnover rate or number. To encourage a reaction, an enzyme must correctly position or orient itself with its substrate. The electrical properties of a substrate change, depending in part on its correct spatial arrangement with the substrate. In essence, the enzyme's positive and negative charges align with the substrate's positive and negative charges to favorably continue a chemical reaction.

The *top of the unnumbered figure on page 994* shows an enzyme arranging to link up with its intended substrate to create an enzyme–substrate complex. Once the enzyme fulfills its function, the complex breaks down, releasing its product. The enzyme then almost instantaneously catalyzes another reaction. The rate of end-product formation depends on two factors: (1) the concentration of substrate and (2) the nature of the enzyme–substrate complex. Note that as the concentration of substrate increases, the reaction rate moves toward its maximum. At this point, all of the enzymes' active sites fully engage the substrate's active sites. Continued new product formation now depends only on the rapidity of substrate processing, referred to as **turnover number**. This can vary tremendously, from 1 to 10,000 molecules per second, but a turnover number of 1000 substrate molecules per second characterizes many enzymes. A high turnover ensures that enzymes remain "turned on" at their optimal concentration during gene expression.

Turnover number: the units of enzyme activity per mole of enzyme (μmol · min^{-1} · mol^{-1} of enzyme). The turnover number (also called catalytic constant) allows relative catalytic comparisons among enzymes. For example, catalase (5×10^4) is about 2500 times more active than amylase (1.9×10^4)

The enzyme's binding sites, while they remain in the "on" position with their substrate for extremely brief periods, may do so more dynamically than previously believed. Instead of remaining coupled for the entire period, other similar binding sites may switch places with the originally bound site (analogous to "hit-join-and-run"), suggesting that enzyme molecules maintain more mobility than previously thought. Future research will determine whether changes in binding site cycling will allow other proteins in the signaling chain to participate in still other gene-regulating pathways. If so, then the elaborate nature of enzyme

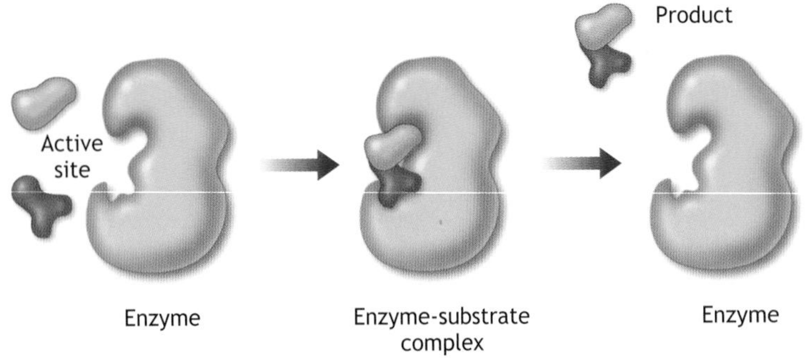

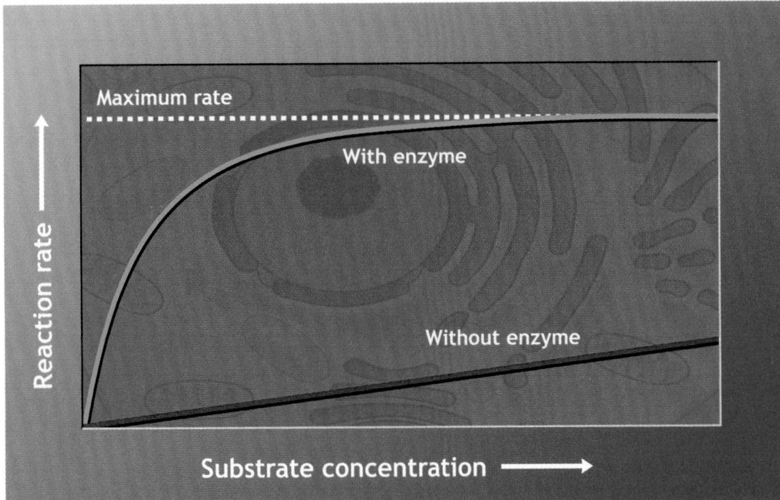

Top. Enzyme-substrate interaction. *Bottom.* Reaction rate versus substrate concentraton with and without enzyme action.

Housekeeping genes: genes automatically switched "on" all the time to maintain essential cell functions

Genetic code: sequence of nucleotides, coded in triplets (codons) along the mRNA that determine the amino acid sequence in protein synthesis. The gene's DNA sequence can predict the mRNA sequence; the genetic code in turn predicts the amino acid sequence

Ribosome: small cellular component (organelle) composed of specialized ribosomal RNA; site of polypeptide (protein) synthesis

Exon: protein-coding DNA sequence of a gene

Intron: DNA base noncoding sequence that interrupts a gene's protein-coding sequence; the sequence transcribes into RNA, but gets excised from the "message" before it translates into protein

turnover rates and unique protein–receptor interactions take on even greater complexity than previously believed.

Gene Expression and Human Exercise Performance

The next decades in exercise physiology research will build upon the rapidly developing knowledge base about gene expression and the human gene map for performance and health-related phenotypes (See Med Sci Sports Exerc 2001;33:885; with annual updates). In the not-too-distant future, sport scientists will routinely incorporate simplified molecular biologic techniques to assess an individual's potential for strength, speed, endurance, and other traits important to exercise performance. While it might seem far-fetched now, choosing astronauts for extended-duration missions to other planets may rely on molecular biology to "select" candidates with more-resistant genes to protect against bone loss or spatial disorientation with prolonged microgravity. Coaches and trainers in future decades will undoubtedly apply technologies from molecular medicine to genetically screen young children for gene clusters that indicate potential for desirable athletic traits (and traits related to training responsiveness), such as predominance of a specific fiber type, abundance of targeted aerobic enzymes, muscle capillaries, or left ventricular cavity size. Today, sports scientists use laboratory and field testing to screen athletes for performance and physiologic capacities. Similar application and acceptance of molecular genetics, however, will require mastery of the new technologies with ethical issues considered.

Gene expression is tightly controlled. When muscle tissue rebuilds, gene expression for actin and myosin protein filament enlargement remains "on" while gene expression for generating new muscle cells remains "off," because cellular hypertrophy not hyperplasia usually prevails. These "on–off" genes are referred to as "**housekeeping genes.**" In bodily processes such as coding for the proteins involved in aerobic metabolism, gene expression does not shut down but remains continually on until death. The same applies to all cell and tissue metabolic activities controlled by enzymes that dominate cellular and subcellular events. Organisms from bacteria to humans use the same two basic principles of gene expression. First, an RNA duplicate is made of a particular gene with its unique coding sequence on a DNA template that represents some combination in succession of G, C, T, A. Second, the RNA copy containing the sequence of the **genetic code** on the **ribosome** (located outside the nucleus) orchestrates the sequential construction of amino acids into a protein possessing unique biomolecular characteristics.

Exons and Introns

The RNA primary transcript molecule contains all of the information needed from the gene to create a protein. The RNA primary transcript structure discovered by Crick,[133] called a coding region or **exon**, shown in the green primary transcript within the purple nucleus in Figure 11, also contains additional, unwanted stretches of nucleotide "spacers," or noncoding regions termed **introns** (five introns also shown in *pink* within the primary transcript of Fig. 11). In fact, 97% of DNA consists of introns. An example of just three exons and two introns in Figure 15 shows the individual numbering for the base pair sequences within each exon and intron. For example, the numbers 1–30 designate the base pairs for the first exon along the RNA strand, while 105–146 signify the base pairs for the last exon. The two introns with their base pairs have the numbers 30–31 and 104–105. During transcription, note the removal of intron links 30–31 and 104–105, leaving the remaining three exons that splice together (their base pairs now numbered 1–146) to create the final mRNA transcript. This must occur before the mRNA strand leaves the nucleus and enters the cytoplasmic space (cytosol).

The cytoplasm cannot receive partially processed transcripts. Intron removal likely occurs because these structures provide no known usable code for any part of the polypeptide initially specified by the gene. These clusters of repeated, apparently nonfunctional and random DNA sequences scattered throughout the genome exist as either short interspersed elements of 500 or fewer base pairs (called SINEs) or long interspersed elements of more than 1000 base pairs (LINEs) in length. The mature mRNA transcript displayed at the *bottom* of Figure 14 contains the correct sequence of codes to create proteins. The example shows the specified order for seven amino acids inserted into the elongating polypeptide chain, determined originally during translation based on codon sequence.

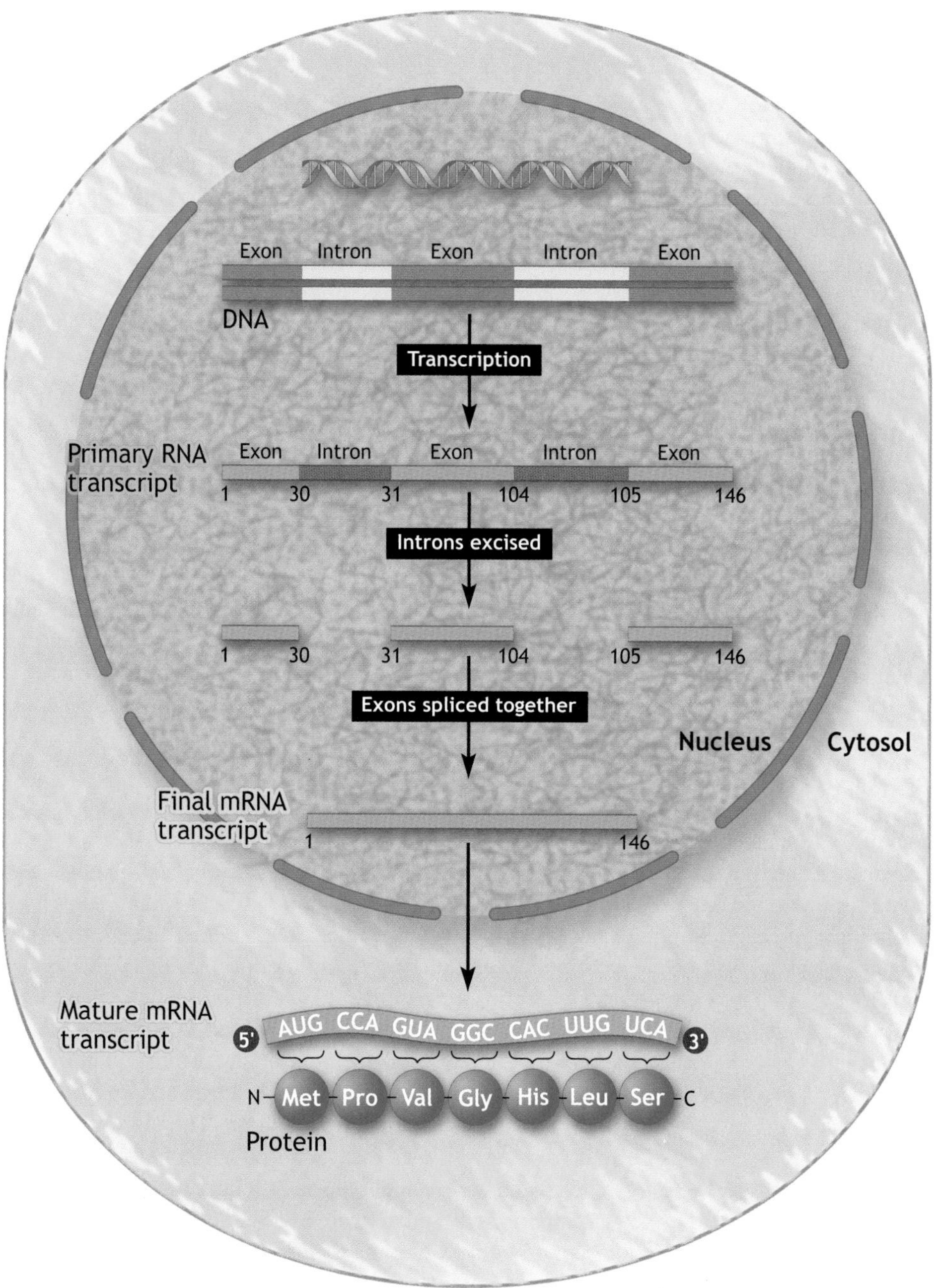

FIGURE 15 • Example of exons and introns, individual numbering for the base pair sequences, and intron excision and exon splicing to form the final (mature) mRNA transcript. For this structure, note the three-letter codons shown in white lettering along the green mRNA, and the corresponding amino acids listed in the blue circles below. The codon table in Figure 7 (page 985) lists the full names for these amino acids.

RNA Splicing

RNA splicing: excision of unwanted sequence of introns from the primary transcript so the exons fuse together

Polypeptide: unbranched string of amino acids linked by peptide bonds formed during gene translation

RNA splicing removes unwanted intron sequences from the primary transcript, which enables translation to avoid those sequences. Introns usually occupy an area 10 to 30 times greater than exons. The final, mature mRNA strand is shorter than the primary transcript owing to the excision of about 90% of the introns in the primary transcript prior to translation. Consider exon splicing a unique phase of protein construction at the start of protein assembly. Splicing manipulates intron sequencing in many ways to form **polypeptides**. The hemoglobin (Hb) molecule, for example, requires 432 nucleotides to encode its 144 amino acids, yet before intron excision, 1356 nucleotides exist in the primary mRNA transcript of the Hb gene. Regulation of gene expression occurs by changes in how splicing takes place during different stages of a cell's development and the type of cell involved.

mRNA Packaging: Polyadenylic Acid and Guanosine Triphosphate—Tails and Caps

Polyadenylic acid [Poly (A)] tail: chain 100–200 adenine nucleotides long; joins one end at the 3′ region of the final transcripted mRNA before the RNA transcript migrates through the nuclear pore

Guanosine triphosphate (GTP): Initiates translation when it binds mRNA at the 5′ end of the molecule to the smaller of the ribosome's two subunits; referred to as the "cap" on the final transcripted mRNA

Before the RNA transcript migrates through the nuclear pore as the final transcripted mRNA, a **polyadenylic acid (Poly[A]) tail**, 100–200 adenine nucleotides long joins one end at the 3′ region via the action of the enzyme poly(A) polymerase, and a terminal portion or "cap" (methylated **guanosine triphosphate** or **GTP**) joins near the 5′ other end. Much as a college student wears a cap and gown during the graduation ceremony before entering the "real" world, so mRNA must be "capped and tailed" to prepare the transcripted molecule for translation before it exits the nucleus to take part in subsequent protein synthesis. The newly formed cap performs the important function of initiating translation when it binds the mRNA to the smaller of the ribosome's two subunits.

The *top* of Figure 16 shows how the GTP cap and poly(A) tail join to RNA. Note that the capping enzyme *(*symbolized by the shorter curved purple arrow*)* cleaves two phosphates *(*circles enclosed in red*)* from GTP and one phosphate from the mRNA strand. In forming the cap, the GTP now attaches near the end of the first base of the mRNA. The *bottom* of Figure 16 illustrates the addition of the poly(A) tail when a specific endonuclease enzyme (depicted in orange) recognizes the sequence A-A-U-A-A-A on the mRNA and snips the strand near that point. This permits a tail of 100–200 adenine residues to affix to the 3′ end of the mRNA strand. The addition of poly(A) promotes mRNA stability. It permits the mRNA molecule to maintain translation for up to several weeks, sometimes producing 100,000 protein molecules. Recall that transcription using DNA occurs inside the cell's nucleus, whereas ribosomal assembly takes place in the cytoplasm. The capping and tailing function enables the mRNA to exit the nucleus to begin the next phase of protein synthesis.

Exiting the Nucleus

The mRNA now contains a copy of the specific nucleotide sequence from the DNA gene. The mRNA then shuttles the "coded message," after the transcription stage, through the nuclear membrane into the cytoplasm where protein synthesis (translation) begins. Translation includes three main stages: (1) initiation, (2) elongation, and (3) termination. Using high resolution x-ray crystallography, researchers have determined that a tunnel-like groove runs through the middle of the larger size 50S subunit, providing the location that links amino acids together.[95] Thirty-one separate proteins affix to the outside of the subunit where they also reach inside the ribosome. Because a protein needs to be within a 3–Å distance to induce any effect, and because the proteins on the surface and those that reach around remain within 18 Å, the source of any protein interaction must be RNA. In this case, adenosine 2486 is the nucleotide in question with an associated nitrogen atom. Therefore, the RNA gives the catalytic power to protein synthesis—in essence, ribosomes serve as ribozymes. This finding helps to explain why some bacteria remain resistant to antibiotics. A mutation on one of the ribosomal proteins within the ribosomal groove locks up with part of the antibiotic molecule, preventing the peptide from exiting the region and thus preventing further antibiotic binding and subsequent damage to the bacteria.

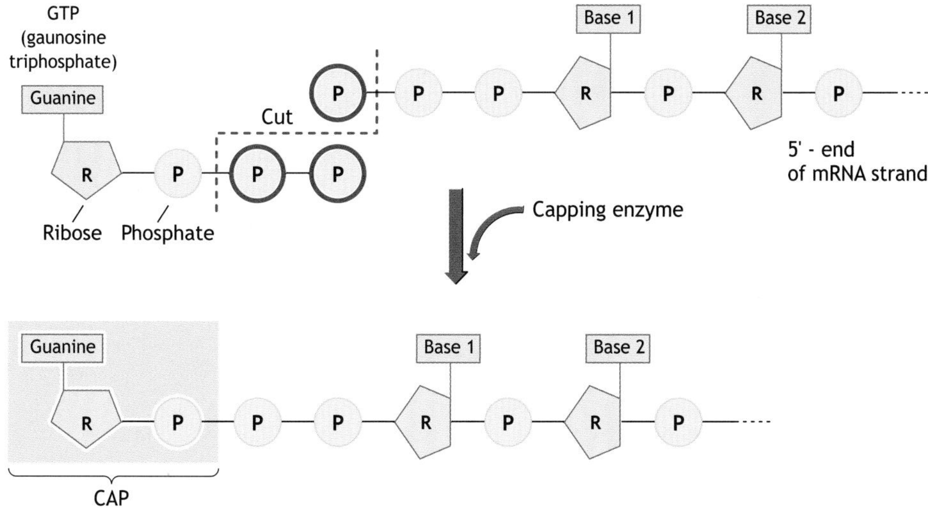

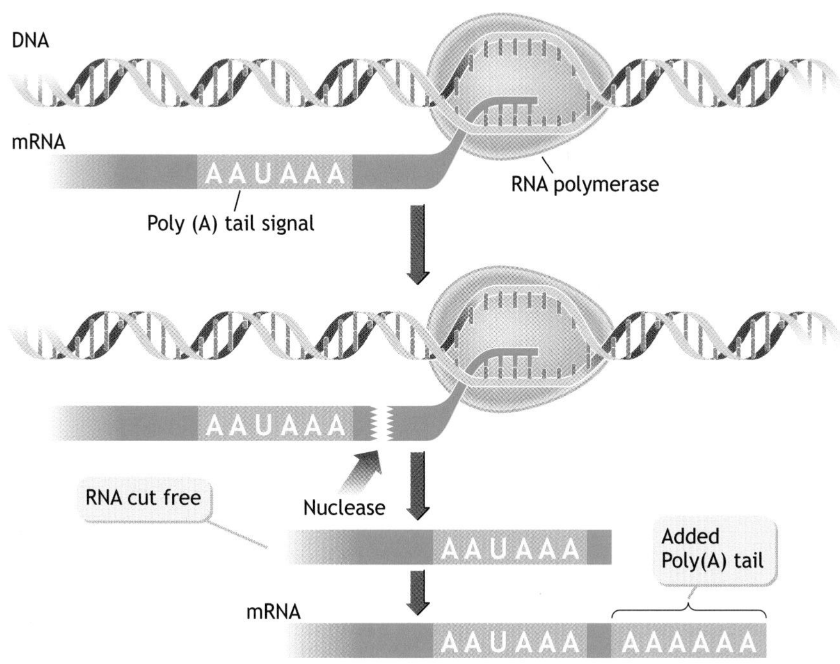

FIGURE 15 • *Top.* Addition of a guanosine triphosphate (GTP) cap to mRNA. The red dashes indicate where the "cut" occurs by the action of the capping enzyme. *Bottom.* Addition of a poly (A) tail to mRNA. The mRNA molecule exits the nucleus once capping and tailing occurs, carrying the "coded message" for the upcoming translation phase in protein synthesis.

Translation of the Genetic Code: Ribosomal Assembly of Polypeptides

Translation initiates protein construction. Once the mRNA enters the cytoplasm through the nuclear pore, it seeks out a ribosome with which to bind. The millions of ribosomes in the cell's cytoplasm originated in the nucleus. A ribosome consists of a large and a small subunit, the latter fitting into a depression on the ribosome's larger surface. A ribosome has three sites that associate with mRNA: (1) **A-site** (A for attachment), (2) **P-site** (P for polypeptide), and (3) **E-site** (E for exit).

Ribosomes and Polypeptide Synthesis: Initiation of Protein Construction

The cell's ribosomes provide the catalysts for initiating protein synthesis and serve as submicroscopic factories to produce polypeptides. Figure 17 illustrates a four-step sequence of a ribosome binding to one end of an mRNA molecule and the subsequent three nucleotide

FIGURE 17 • Ribosomes, the initiators for protein synthesis. Polypeptide synthesis proceeds from the top in step 1 with the anticodon of tRNA complementary to the mRNA codon. The tRNA occupies the ribosome's A-site, with an anticodon complementary to the mRNA's codon at the opposite A-site. The ribosome translocates down the mRNA one codon at a time. Step 2. The lengthening polypeptide chain *fMet* is transferred to Leu, the incoming amino acid. The ribosome ejects the original tRNA (step 3) with its amino acid, exposing the next codon on the mRNA chain. When the tRNA molecule recognizes the next exposed codon, it binds to that codon, thus lengthening the growing peptide chain (step 4). *fMet* represents an addition to the lengthening polypeptide chain already occupied by Leu (Met, the amino acid methionine; Leu, leucine).

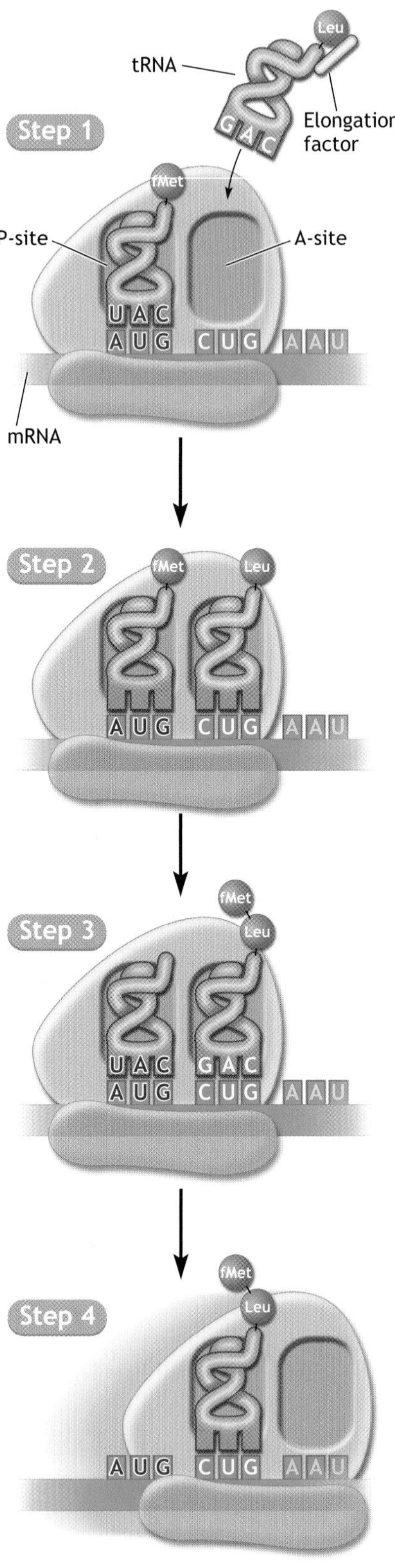

Polypeptide chain: repeated polypeptide units

Peptide bonding: chemical linking that binds amino acids in a protein; formed when the carboxyl group of one amino acid reacts with a second amino acid's amino group

increments down the mRNA molecule. Decoding of genetic information occurs when the ribosomes bound to mRNA translate a genetic code sequence. The tRNA then interacts with a specific amino acid, adding one at a time to the end of the progressively elongating **polypeptide chain**. Sequential linking of amino acids by **peptide bonding** ultimately forms the specific protein with its unique genetically determined information to achieve its function(s).

Role of tRNA

The tRNA molecule has a three-dimensional structure resembling a cloverleaf, with an amino acid at one end and three nitrogenous bases that match the mRNA's codon (called an **anticodon**) at the other end. The tRNA with matching codon serves as a relay or go-between in protein synthesis. In effect, the tRNA acts as a "personal shuttle" to deliver a specific free-floating amino acid to the ribosome's A-site. For example, the triplet U-A-C represents the codon for the amino acid methionine. When the tRNA with the matching U-A-C anticodon (it carries no other amino acid) interacts with the free-floating U-A-C amino acid, it binds to it by action of the activating enzyme **aminoacyl-tRNA synthetase.** Each amino acid's specific activating enzyme serves two purposes: (1) it deciphers and then binds (couples) to a specific amino acid and (2) it identifies the anticodon on the tRNA molecule. Some activating enzymes decipher the sequence of one anticodon and thus only one tRNA, while others recognize multiple tRNA molecules. Thus, the activating enzyme "reads" the genetic code on both the particular amino acid, such as tryptophan, and its tRNA tryptophan anticodon sequence A-C-C. Figure 18 shows three views of tRNA: (1) a computer-generated model, (2) a three-dimensional representation that highlights internal base pairing with hydrogen bonding, and (3) a two-dimensional cloverleaf model with the tRNA anticodon shown in blue. This example represents the complementary three-nucleotide sequence C-A-U matching mRNA's codon G-U-A.

Anticodon: three complementary bases at the end of a tRNA molecule that recognize and bind to an mRNA codon

Aminoacyl-tRNA synthetase: activating enzyme that covalently links amino acids to the 3′ ends of their cognate tRNA

Polypeptide Elongation and Termination

The polypeptide chain increases in length when an amino acid from tRNA **translocates** to it. The A-U-G codon shown in Figure 17 within the mRNA message initiates the "start" signal for peptide elongation. The same A-U-G sequence that encodes tryptophan also encodes

Translocation: movement along the ribosome by an mRNA molecule a distance of three nucleotide blocks (one codon) at a time

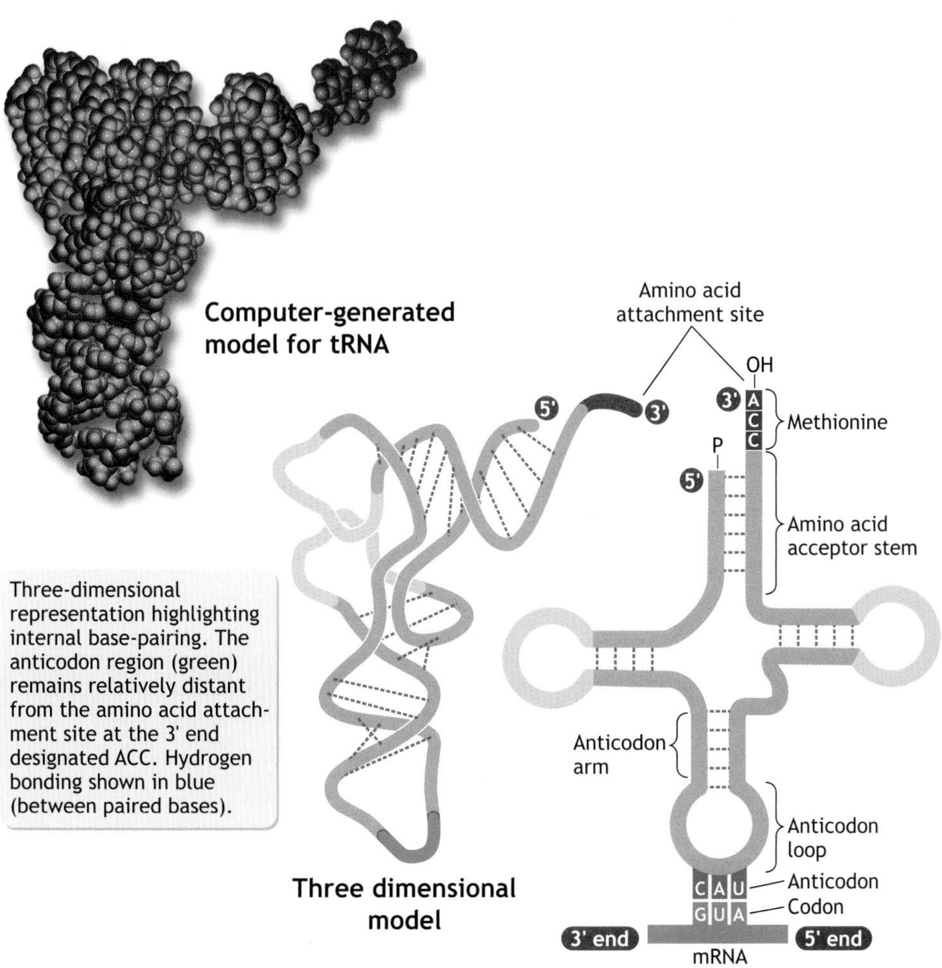

FIGURE 18 • Three views of tRNA: computer-generated model, three-dimensional model, and cloverleaf model. Note that the anticodon displayed in the cloverleaf model (complementary three-nucleotide sequence) matches up with the mRNA codon using complementary (antiparallel) binding between the anticodon (blue) and codon (green).

methionine. The first A-U-G message "sensed" in the mRNA molecule initiates translation. The ribosome translocates down the mRNA a distance of three nucleotide blocks (one codon) at a time. After each third nucleotide, the ribosome ejects the original tRNA with its amino acid, exposing the next codon on the mRNA chain. When the tRNA molecule recognizes the next exposed codon, it binds to it, thus lengthening the growing peptide chain. The elongation procedure for building the polypeptide continues repeatedly until a stop codon terminates the process.

Figure 19 schematically illustrates the three stages in polypeptide termination. The three "stop" codons, or base sequences, include U-A-A, U-A-G, and U-G-A. These codons "turn off" the signal in the mRNA message, preventing addition of another amino acid sequence to the chain. Stage 1 shows the stop codon U-A-A on the mRNA strand within the A-site of the ribosome, where one of three kinds of releasing factors—eRF1, eRF2, or eRF3—locks into position to split apart the linking covalent bond. In stage 2, the polypeptide chain releases from tRNA at the ribosome's P-site, to effectively end protein synthesis. Once the polypeptide and tRNA uncouple from the termination complex, the small and large ribosomal units recycle along with mRNA in stage 3 for further mRNA translation.

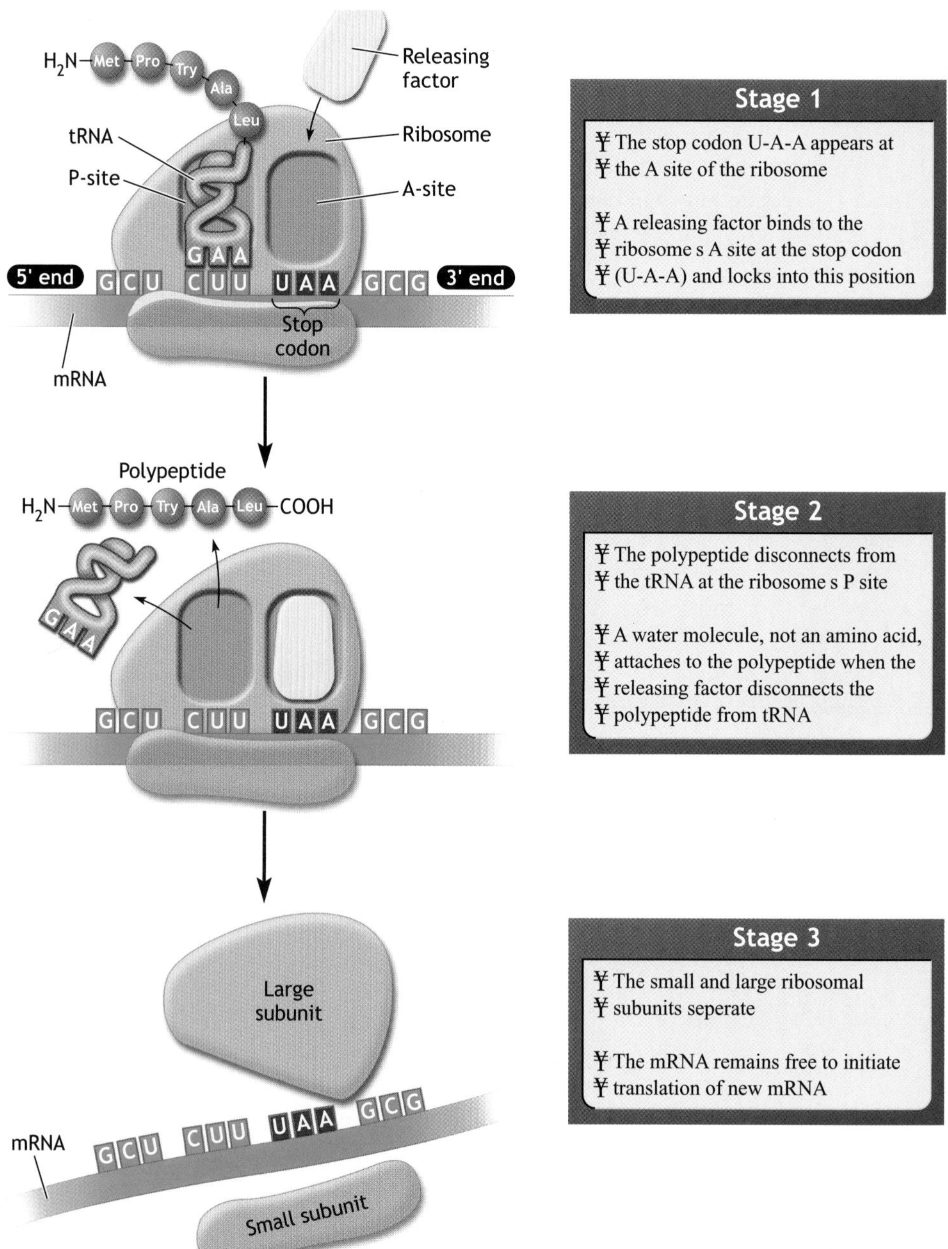

FIGURE 19 • Three stages in polypeptide termination.

Protein Delivery System: The Golgi Complex

Once the ribosome produces its polypeptide, newly formed strands can exit a cell through its outer membrane into the external interstitial fluid environment. The highly membranous **Golgi complex** structures within the cell provide the transfer mechanism for moving materials from the cell to its external environment. Italian physiologist and microscopist Camillo Golgi (1843–1926), who shared the 1906 Nobel Prize in physiology or medicine for his work on nervous system anatomy, first called attention in 1898 to these minute intracellular structures using the light microscope. Many biologists of his time doubted the existence of such structures; 60 years later, the electron microscope confirmed their existence in exquisite detail.

The Golgi complex receives a polypeptide from the cell's **endoplasmic reticulum**. Figure 20 shows polypeptide transport into the Golgi complex where the molecule may become a **glycoprotein**. When a polysaccharide binds to a lipid, it forms a **glycolipid**. Glycoproteins or glycolipids then collect within the flattened, membranous sacs called the cisternae region of the Golgi complex, where specialized enzymes modify the protein component. The transport vesicles that hold proteins that pass from the endoplasmic reticulum pinch off and break away from the roughened endoplasmic surfaces. The tiny vesicles, attached to the cell's outer membrane, expel their contents to the extracellular spaces via secretory vesicles. In essence (but not always), the Golgi complex takes up the polypeptide on one of its surfaces and then modifies and repackages it into molecules that leave the Golgi complex via a transport vesicle at its other membrane.

Golgi complex: stack of membrane-bound vesicles between the endoplasmic reticulum and plasma membrane involved in posttranslational modification of proteins, and sorting and delivering them to different intracellular compartments

Endoplasmic reticulum: tubules, vesicles, and flattened sac structures of the cell's endomembrane system; ribosomes cover its outer rough, granular surface

Glycoprotein: protein complexed with a polysaccharide

Glycolipid: polysaccharide bound to a lipid

Termination of Protein Synthesis

The end-point of protein synthesis creates one of thousands of completed or functional proteins, each with a specific function and mode of action depending in part on its structure. The inset table below shows eight categories of proteins and their biologic functions:

Protein Category	Function	Example
1. Contractile	Form muscles	Actin, myosin
2. Enzyme	Catalyze biological processes	Protease
3. Hormone	Regulate body functions	Cortisol
4. Protective	Fight infection	Antibodies
5. Storage	Store nutrients	Calcium within bone
6. Structural	Form structures	Endoplasmic reticulum
7. Transport	Deliver substances among cells, tissues, organs	Hemoglobin
8. Toxic	Defense mechanism	Snake venom (disintegrins)

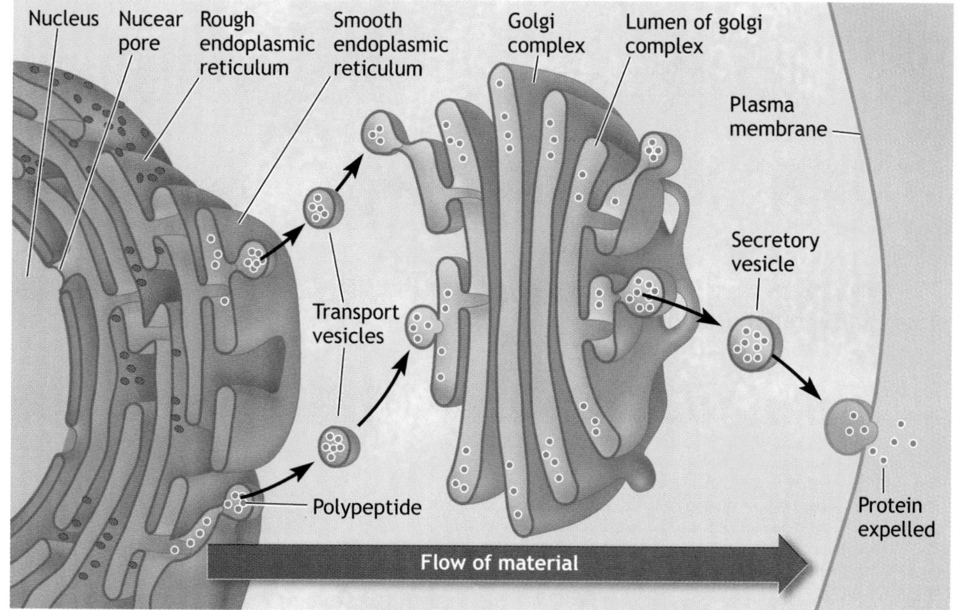

FIGURE 20 • Polypeptide transport into the Golgi complex. The Golgi complex accepts polypeptides on one of its surfaces after the ribosomes release them, repackaging them as glycoproteins, and expels them contained in secretory vesicles for final expulsion through the plasma membrane or delivery to another cell area. The Golgi structures modify proteins within their lumen for use within cells or outside of cells once they pass through the plasma membrane.

Primary structure: specific linear sequence of amino acids determined by the nucleotide sequence of the gene that encodes the protein

Secondary structure: coiled protein similar to the pairing of strands in DNA or folded back onto itself to give a flat look; formed from regular repeating interactions among closely linked residues in the primary sequence using hydrogen bonding

α Helix: one possible secondary structure of polypeptides; right-handed peptide chain maintained by hydrogen (H) bonds between carbon (C) and oxygen (O) atoms of every fifth amino acid along the chain. The degree of rotation remains regular for bonds on either side of the α carbon (with nitrogen, C, H, and amino side chain attached to it) along the polypeptide chain

Tertiary structure: final 3-dimensional folding of a polymer chain; interactions between residues remain farther apart

Quaternary structure: a highly complex, 3-dimensional structure or functional protein formed by joining two or more polypeptides

It usually takes between 20 seconds and 2 minutes to synthesize most proteins depending on the protein's complexity. The Hb molecule and its amino acid sequence serves as an excellent example of the four levels of protein structure (Fig. 20). This generalized example begins with the linear sequence of amino acids from the amino acid at the amino-terminal end through to the carboxyl-terminal residue. The polypeptide strand formed when peptide linkages join amino acid monomers represents protein's **primary structure**. In a **secondary structure**, the protein can twist into a three-dimensional form known as an ***α* helix**. It can also fold back onto itself to give a flat look (*β*-pleated sheets), with regular repeating interactions using hydrogen bonding among closely linked residues in the primary sequence. Interactions among residues farther apart in the primary structure determine a **tertiary structure**, such as disulfide bond formation between two cysteine residues. In this conformation, the protein literally folds up on itself, much like a roll of pretzel dough twisting into a pretzel. The topology of the *α* helices and *β*-pleated sheets play important roles in determining the final shape assumed by a protein.[32] The complex Hb molecule consists of two *α* subunits and two *β* subunits (tetramer). The term **quaternary structure** refers to protein's subunit structure; Hb contains multiple subunits.

Hemoglobin and the Evolutionary Tree

Figure 21 shows that the Hb molecule contains two *α* and two *β* chains; the heme group is associated with each chain. The central iron atom (shown in *red*) binds with one oxygen molecule and acts as a magnet to attract and hold it. Interestingly, our closest blood relative, the chimpanzee, has an identical *α* chain. The Hb amino acid sequence in cows and pigs diverges from that of humans by about 12%, while for chickens the divergence increases to 25%. Molecular biologists have constructed an evolutionary tree for many proteins (e.g., the iron-containing mitochondrial cytochromes) as a way of tracking evolutionary history.

Some proteins change relatively slowly, taking hundreds of millions of years to evolve. Histones change at a rate of 0.25 mutations per 100 amino acids per 100 million years. In contrast, other proteins like neurotoxins and immunoglobulins mutate more quickly (rates of 110 to 140). Variation in the resistance to change makes "sense" because crucial cellular functions like energy generation in the citric acid cycle or correct folding of DNA requires that gene sequences remain almost invariant. Proteins sensitive to relatively large variations in their operational properties sustain faster evolutionary changes.

Proteolysis: The Ultimate Fate of Proteins

Proteolysis: protein degradation

Proteosome: proteolytic enzyme that degrades unwanted proteins in the cytoplasm of eukaryotic cells

Ubiquitin: small protein that attaches by covalent bonding to a protein "marked" for destruction by proteosomes

Protein synthesis from amino acids and degradation into amino acid constituents progress unabated throughout life. The rates of protein synthesis and degradation, a process called **proteolysis**, regulate the organism's total protein content at any given time, independent of the proteins' structural configurations (bone or muscle) or functions (metabolic and intracellular enzymes). For example, the structural proteins* in bone may not decay significantly for months or years, while enzyme proteins in intermediary metabolism or those that regulate cell growth may survive for only minutes or fractions of a second. The enzymes that control proteolysis, known as proteases, hydrolyze the amino acids' peptide bonds, breaking them into their constituent molecules. A relatively large trash can–shaped **proteosome**, formed from protease enzymes, degrades the unwanted proteins in the cell's cytoplasm (Fig. 22). These cylindrical structures capture proteins destined for destruction by recognizing a small marker or tag protein (**ubiquitin**) that attaches by covalent bonding to an active site on the protein.

*Collagen, the most plentiful structural protein, accounts for about one-fourth of the body's protein. In essence, it forms molecular cables that strengthen the tendons and plentiful, resilient sheets that support the skin and internal organs. This simple protein, composed of three chains wound together in a tight triple helix, contains more than 1400 amino acids in each chain. Collagen forms from a repeated sequence of three amino acids; every third amino acid is glycine, a small amino acid that fits perfectly inside the helix. Many of the remaining positions in the chain are filled by two amino acids, proline and hydroxyproline, the latter a modified version of proline. Hydroxyproline formation involves modifying normal proline amino acids after building the collagen. The reaction requires vitamin C to assist in the addition of oxygen. Unfortunately, vitamin C deficiency slows hydroxyproline production and stops new collagen construction, ultimately causing scurvy. When heated, collagen's triple helix unwinds and the chains separate. When the denatured mass of tangled chains cools down, it soaks up the surrounding water like a sponge, forming gelatin, used commonly in cooking.

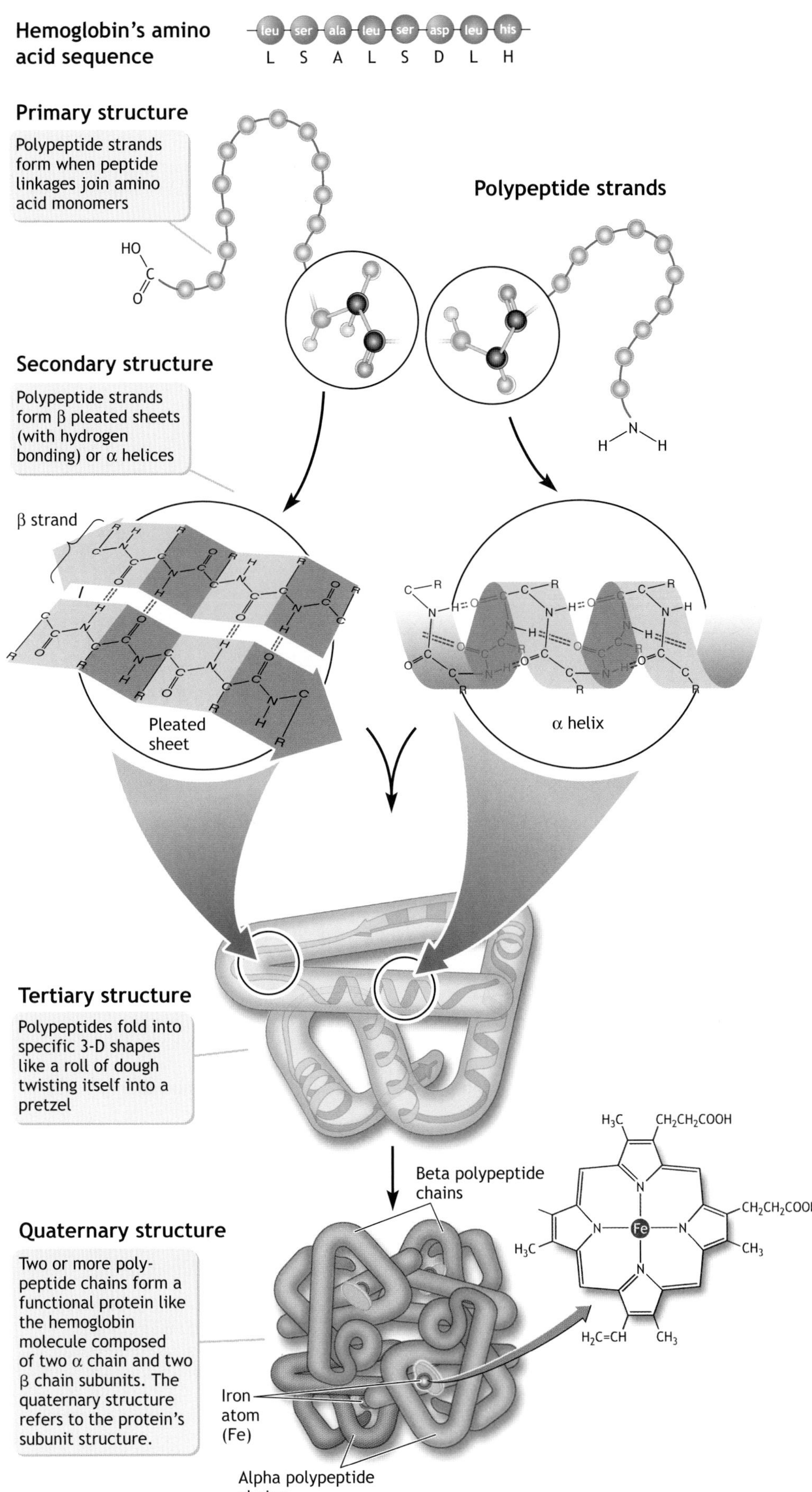

FIGURE 21 • Four protein structures (primary, secondary, tertiary, quaternary) in the synthesis of the complex hemoglobin molecule first deciphered by Max Perutz in 1960 and published in *Nature* (1960; 185: 416). The purified molecule's precise arrangement was calculated from the way its crystals diffracted a beam of x-rays. Hemoglobin's tertiary structure contains eight α-helical regions; the quaternary structure contains four polypeptide chains (two α and two β). Knowledge of the configuration of new protein structures has increased exponentially since Perutz first worked out the details of hemoglobin's structure; as of July 9, 2001, the Protein Data Bank (www.rcsb.org/pdb/) contained 15,531 unique structures into which proteins can fold. Of these, x-ray diffraction identified 12,817 unique structures and 2384 by NMR.

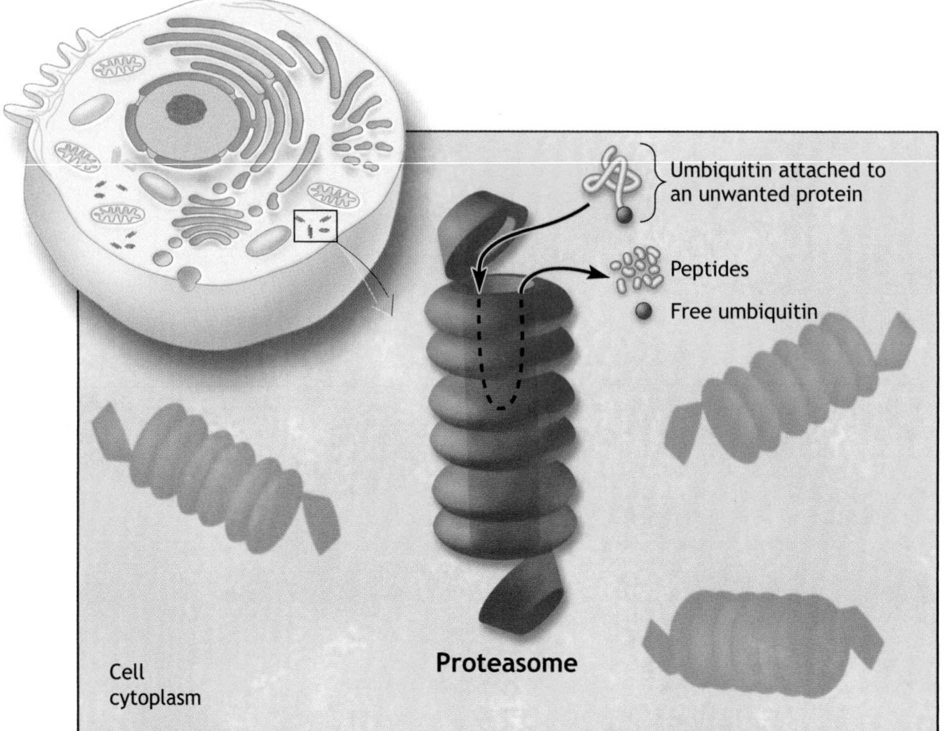

Figure 21 • Proteosomes in the cell cytoplasm maintain a balance between protein synthesis and protein degradation. The free ubiquitin tag (displayed in *red*) attaches to an active site on the designated protein, identifying it for degradation to its peptide components within the proteosome's cylindrical structure. Once ejected, the ubiquitin recycles to another unwanted protein.

Once tagged, the ubiquinated protein enters the proteosome, which degrades it to smaller peptide units before expelling it along with the ubiquitin tag. Proteosomes degrade many types of proteins, from denatured or misfolded ones to misformed or oxidized amino acids.

Summary of Main Sequence of Events in Protein Synthesis

Table 3 charts the sequence of key events in the flow of genetic information in living cells from DNA⟶RNA⟶protein.

Table 3 ➤ ESSENTIAL CONCEPTS AND SEQUENCE OF EVENTS IN PROTEIN SYNTHESIS

- A nucleotide sequence from DNA provides the genetic information required to begin the transcription into RNA
- The enzyme RNA polymerase binds to the specific promoter region of a gene; nucleotide sequences in the DNA indicate where to begin and end transcription
- RNA polymerase manufactures messenger RNA (mRNA) molecules to mirror the base sequence of DNA; transcription copies a sequence of the genetic code direction from DNA to an mRNA strand; this includes both coding and noncoding segments of genetic information
- The RNA transcript contains the information it needs to create a protein; RNA splicing removes random, intervening sequences of unwanted "junk" nucleotides (introns) from mRNA
- The mRNA strand (linked entrons) carrying a duplicate copy of the genetic code shuttles the "coded message" (sequence of codons), exiting the nucleus and entering the cytoplasm to begin protein synthesis
- Translation initiates protein construction; the A-U-G codon acts as the "start" signal
- In the cytoplasm, the mRNA molecule searches to bind with a ribosome (ribonucleoprotein, a "protein-manufacturing machine"
- The anticodon of transfer RNA (tRNA) positions itself to matchup with a three-nucleotide sequence of codons, each codon corresponding to one amino acid; the codon contains a copy or transcription of the DNA code
- For the four RNA nucleotides, 64 different codons in the genetic code exist, with each amino acid having at least one (and usually more than one) codon
- Binding takes place at the ribosome's attachment site between the tRNA molecule (carrying the same genetic sequence on its anticodon) and the complementary base sequence of the mRNA codon (e.g., G-A-C with C-U-G)
- The ribosome, coupled to one end of the mRNA molecule, shifts (translocates) over one codon (three nucleotide blocks) to the polypeptide site, allowing exposure of a new codon; a new incoming tRNA (with its amino acid) links to the ribosome's attachment site; the amino acid at the ribosome's polypeptide region releases and binds to a new amino acid on tRNA at the ribosome's attachment site; thus, the tRNA with one amino acid now gains another amino acid, then another one, and so on; successively adding new amino acids elongates the peptide chain
- Protein synthesis terminates when a chain-terminating nonsense "stop" codon (UAA, UAG, UGA) turns off the signal for adding more amino acids to the peptide chain
- A complete (fully assembled) protein exists in one of four geometric configurations (primary, secondary, tertiary, quaternary) shown in Figure 21

MUTATIONS

The slightest aberration in the sequence of the 3 billion letters of the genome can produce catastrophic effects on health and well-being. Fortunately, an exquisite array of internal repair mechanisms (specialized protein complexes) correct mismatches along the double helix, thus avoiding a phalanx of dreadful, life-altering genetic disorders. Still, on a daily basis, factors in the external environment continually threaten the body's DNA from cosmic and ultraviolet radiation bombardment to radioactive decay and gamma waves, including dangerously reactive free radical species (see page 1009). A **mutation** results from a minor alteration or "misspelling" in DNA sequence that cripples the corresponding RNA or protein. **Sickle-cell anemia** provides a salient example when an abnormality occurs in the hemoglobin molecule as illustrated in the second row of the inset table below:

Normal hemoglobin β-chain amino acids						
Valine	Histidine	Leucine	Threonine	Proline	Glutamic acid	Glutamic acid
					↓	
Sickle-cell anemia hemoglobin β-chain amino acids						
Valine	Histidine	Leucine	Threonine	Proline	**Valine**	Glutamic acid

In the sickle cell condition, the amino acid valine shown in *red* substitutes for glutamic acid and alters hemoglobin's β chain because of a codon change from G-A-A to G-U-A. Many human diseases generally form from protein abnormalities caused by a change in the sequence of only one of the 3×10^9 or more DNA nucleotide pairs in the human genome. Not all of the coding sequences in amino acids make "sense." The term **junk DNA** describes such DNA sequences. These inherited sequences perform no currently known "genetically useful" purpose,[16,127] yet they remain part of the chromosomes. Junk DNA replicates inside a cell the same way any other DNA molecule replicates, but without an ability for gene expression. In this sense it too is considered defective.

Mutation: gene with permanently altered or defective genetic information that causes heritable changes

Sickle-cell anemia: usually fatal hereditary disease affecting hemoglobin; develops when the amino acid valine substitutes for glutamic acid, thus changing its codon nucleotide sequence from G-A-A to G-U-A. The disease afflicts 2 of every 1000 African Americans. Erythrocyte-shape becomes irregular, thin, elongated, and crescent-shaped, severely affecting oxygen-transport capacity

Junk DNA: DNA sequences that perform no currently known useful purpose but still remain part of chromosomes

Varieties of Mutations

The guiding principle of central dogma, discussed previously on pages 990 and 991, implicitly states that any change in the inherited genetic material produces a ripple effect on replication, transcription, and translation. This ultimately means that a mutation in the original daughter chromosomes passes on sets of characteristics to the next generation so the offspring inherits the mutation. One can do little short of a temporary, stop-gap measure using **genetic engineering** to replace the defective sequences or arrest their development a distance far removed from the gene. For example, small deletions hundreds of thousands of bases away from a particular gene (called *PAX6*) can alter the gene's expression and actually cause a mutation in which a typical characteristic (e.g., iris in the eye) fails to develop, producing a developmental syndrome called aniridia. Poorly understood processes can somehow *silence* genes up to 90 million bases down the chromosome. However, once the DNA template is used during transcription to make an RNA copy of the inherited mutated sequences, the altered RNA translates the defective code during protein synthesis. Because all of the body's vital processes depend on proteins for their intended functions, mutated genes pose a very real health hazard.

The doggerel below provides eight examples of different types of mutations and what can happen to disrupt the orderly sequence in the genetic code:

MUTATION TYPE	EXAMPLE OF DISRUPTION IN THE CODING SEQUENCE
Wild type	The cat sat on the mat
Substitution	The **r**at sat on the mat
Insertion (single)	The cat s**p**at on the mat
Insertion (multiple)	The cat**tle** sat on the mat
Deletion (single)	The c-t sat on the mat
Deletion (multiple)	The cat --- -- the mat
Inversion (small)	The **tac** sat on the mat
Inversion (large)	**Tam echt no tas tac echt**

A graphic example points up the probability for "errors" to creep into the DNA sequence. If the total DNA compacted in the body's 10 trillion cells was laid end to end like a long link of sausages, it would stretch from the Earth to the sun 667 times—not a trivial length because of the 93-million mile one-way distance to the sun! Thus, a single ge-

Genetic engineering: laboratory-altered DNA that changes its characteristics, usually in four stages that involve: (1) cleaving the source DNA, (2) creating recombinants, (3) cloning copies of recombinants, and (4) locating cloned copies for the desired gene. Screening makes the desired clones resistant to antibiotics and gives them different properties for easy identification

Single nucleotide polymorphism (SNP): polymorphism due to variation at a single nucleotide

Allele: abbreviation for "allelomorph"; refers to a gene's different DNA forms or sequences

Locus: location of a specific gene on a chromosome

Polymorphism: a locus where two or more alleles have gene frequencies that exceed 0.01 in a population

Photolithography: optimal technology for etching (transferring) electrical circuits on suitable media (silicon wafer with silicon dioxide)

Mutagen: ionizing radiation, ultraviolet radiation, or a chemical agent that disrupts the genetic machinery (sequence of DNA code) and causes mutations

Teratogen: agent that causes extreme mutations

Carcinogen: any agent that causes cancer; for example, smoke from cigarettes contains known carcinogenic agents (e.g., carbon monoxide, formaldehyde, and the metals aluminum, copper, lead, mercury, zinc)

Benign tumor: tumor that remains in one location; it no longer responds to normal growth control and lacks capacity to invade distant sites

Malignant tumor: tumor that invades other tissues and forms secondary or tertiary cancers

Sarcoma: cancers forming from connective, muscle, or bone tissues

Carcinoma: cancers formed from epithelial tissue

Metastasize: spread of cancerous cells from the original tumor mass to form secondary cancers (metastases) elsewhere in the body

Oncogene: mutant gene that promotes the loss of cellular growth control, transforming a cell to a malignant state. Many oncogenes directly or indirectly control a cell's growth rate

netic code mismatch can wreak havoc on the "normal" sequence of DNA nucleotides and, hence, genes. A defect in code sequence often remains quiescent for nearly a lifetime before it emerges. For example, it may take 60 years before a seemingly minor misalignment in a receptor gene devastates heart function, causing congestive heart failure within a few months. When researchers identify this human gene variant years before its expression, as discussed below, they will prescribe highly specific drugs to combat the defect. Within the next decade, new classes of drugs will target specific mutated cells, instead of the current "shot-gun" approach that attempts to cripple just about all cells with a massive pharmacologic overdose. A case in point concerns a stretch of genes along chromosome 21, where mutations give rise to Alzheimer's disease, amyotrophic lateral sclerosis (Lou Gehrig's disease), epilepsy, deafness, autoimmune disease, birth defects, and manic depression. For Down syndrome (named after English physician John Langdon Down [1828–1896] who observed individuals in a British asylum in 1866 and published "Observations on an Ethnic Classification of Idiots"), researchers have been on a quest to develop animal models of this genetic form of mental insufficiency and other genetic abnormalities in hopes of developing genetically engineered strategies to eradicate them.

Single Nucleotide Polymorphisms

Pharmaceutical and computer chip manufacturers have partnered to develop techniques to identify specific molecular markers called **single nucleotide polymorphisms**, or **SNPs** (pronounced *snips*), thousands of which reside within each person's genetic code. Most of these tiny nucleotide genetic code "snippets" are normally configured, with no deviant code. Some, however, have a single "mismatch" in the nucleotide sequence that predisposes an individual to a particular disease or injury (e.g., ligament tear in football or gymnastics) or renders their immune system resistant to drug treatment. Identifying a specific gene variant allows appropriate lifestyle changes (e.g., nutrition, weight loss, exercise training) to prevent emergence of the disease or disability or delay its onset. Thirteen major multi-national companies have formed a nonprofit alliance (SNP Consortium LTD: snp.cshl.org) to identify 300,000 variants on human chromosomes by the year 2002 and develop drugs that target the disease by its genetic profile.

SNP assessment (Fig. 23) uses microarrays of chips (biochips) and a "library" of artificial DNA to compare the individual's DNA sample with the chips' existing gene sequences. This makes it imperative to achieve 100% accuracy, because even a small error (incorrect identification) could prove disastrous from a worldwide health standpoint. For example, 99.9% accuracy in matching the 300,000 biochip SNPs for only 1000 people would create 300,000 errors! As of April 1, 2001, researchers had identified and published on the Internet the code for 856,666 mapped SNPs. Once SNP biochips become widely available, the next step requires development of technologies that follow the trail from where the gene gives its instructions to create a specific protein to where the proteins reside in the body. The technique of **photolithography** for etching microcircuits on a silicon chip could also encode a single biochip containing the entire human genome. Within this decade, disposable, microfabricated "lab-on-a-chip" technologies will enable widespread, less expensive assay techniques than those currently available.[51] Figure 23 illustrates the four-step procedure to identify SNPs and their specific genetic sequences or anomalies.

A new generation of technologies for DNA sequencing permits assays for high-throughput SNP genotyping on a microfabricated capillary array electrophoresis (CAE) microchip with 96 channels.[88] The new approaches allow for complex, sensitive, specific, and high-speed analysis.[75,78] The latest CAE sequencers can analyze as little as 0.3 μL of sample in less than 90 seconds, using a four-color fluorescence scanner, allowing more sequencing of genotyping reactions at lower cost. The challenge to molecular biologists is to map as many SNP-genotypes as possible (hence the need for faster sequencers) for purposes of analyzying an individual's genome, since the latter is linked to the predisposition/susceptibility to many diseases.[29,30,50,101]

Cancer

The body's defense mechanisms include "error-correcting" proteins that literally "erase" an apparent aberration in DNA sequencing. Unfortunately, the external effects of ionizing and ultraviolet radiation and chemical and pharmacologic **mutagens** exert catastrophic effects on genetic machinery, specifically the code sequence in DNA. In extreme cases of mutations, structural defects in embryos produce gross deformities such as missing limbs and multiple organs. In these cases, the extreme form of chemical mutagen, known as a **teratogen** (*teras* in Greek means monster), produces the effect.

The term **carcinogen** refers to any agent that causes cancer. In cancer, cell growth proceeds unchecked, forming larger-than-normal cell clusters that become tumors. A **benign tumor** remains in one location; cells from a **malignant tumor** migrate to invade other tissues and form secondary cancers. Cancers that form from connective tissue, muscle, or bone are called **sarcomas**; the most prevalent cancers (breast, lung), called **carcinomas**, originate from epithelial tissue. Malignant tumors tend to **metastasize**, or spawn cells that invade healthy tissue, when they travel via the lymphatic or vascular circulation to form new secondary cancers termed metastases. Mutation of a gene into an **oncogene** (cancer-causing gene) often produces numerous cancers, many of which cannot be eradicated by surgery and/or drugs that target specific cells. Cancer occurs from a failure to "turn on" specific genes that code nucleotide sequences to repress uncontrolled cell division. A tumor cell can develop from a mutation in any of the stages that regulate cell growth and differentiation. In colon cancer, for example, loss of the *APC* gene (adenomatous polyposis coli) on chromosome 5q alters the gut's normal epithelial tissue lining. This leads to

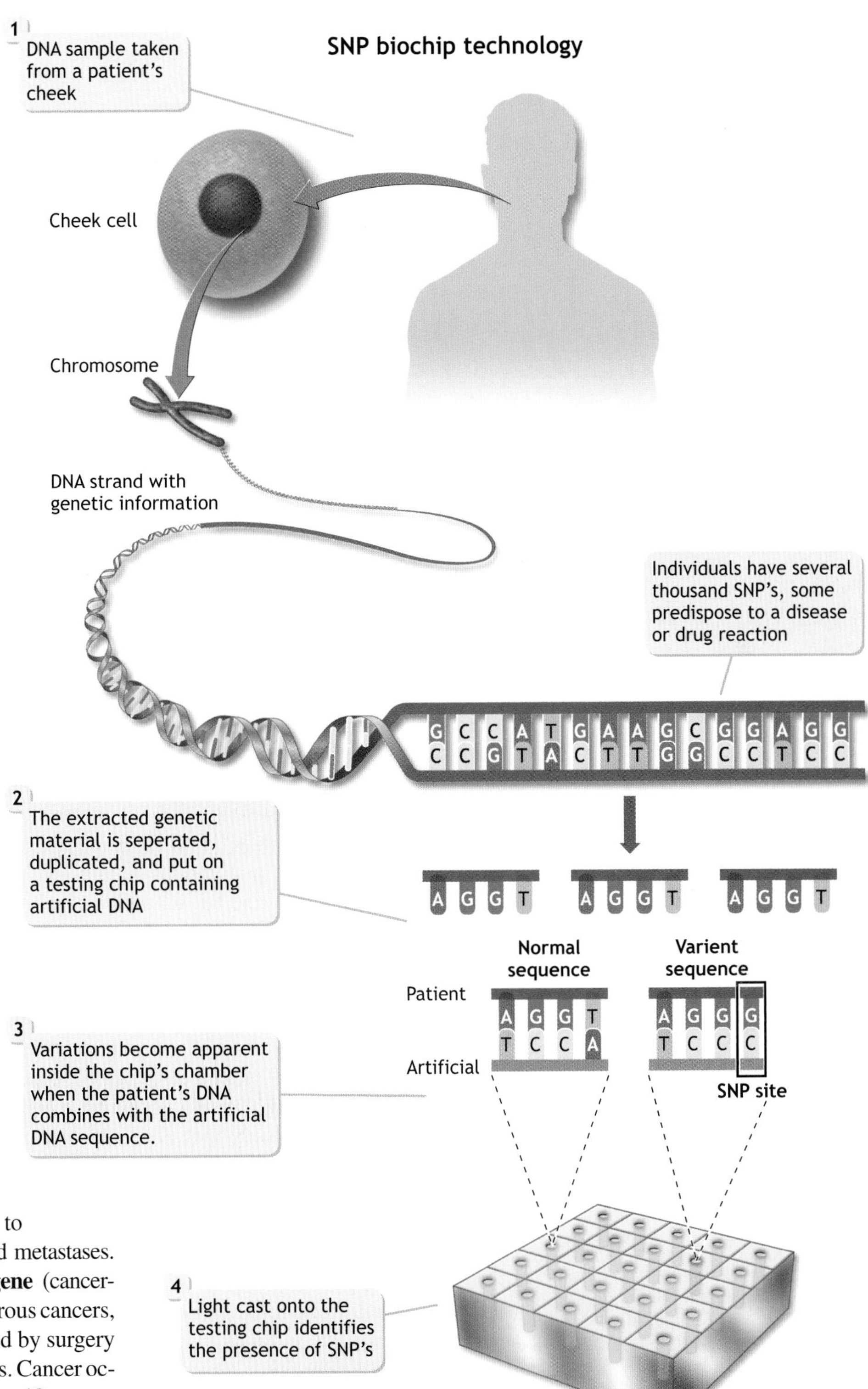

FIGURE 23 • Four main stages in SNP biochip technology that looks at many genes at once to determine which are expressed in a particular cell type. Thousands of individual genes can be spotted on a single square inch slide. Note the relative size of the SNP biochip made possible by barcode scanning the microarrays on the biochip. Rapidly identifying the microarrays allows them to link to genes, probe samples, reagents, and experimental protocols. Consult www.lab-on-a-chip.com for research links about microarry technology.

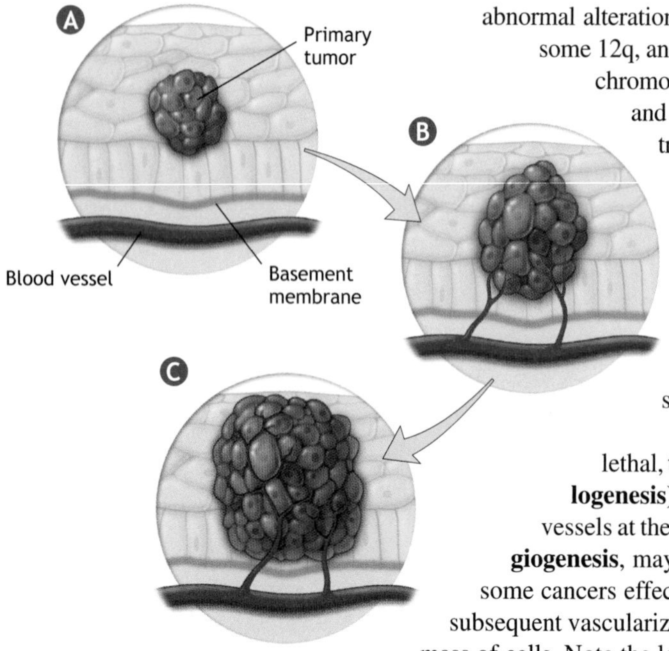

A Primary tumor

Blood vessel Basement membrane

B

C

Progressive vascularization of a tumor.

Proto-oncogene: gene that produces a protein that regulates cell growth; altering a proto-oncogene can transform it to a cancer-causing oncogene

Vasculogenesis: in vivo formation of blood vessels by differentiation of vascular precursor cells. In implanted bioartificial organs, molecular biology techniques can stimulate the growth of new blood vessels or treat peripheral vascular diseases, wounds, and ulcers from compromised microvasculature

Angiogenesis: new blood vessel formation, usually during embryo development but can also occur abnormally around malignant tumors

Gene therapy: introducing genes into cells (genetic surgery) to alter phenotype (i.e., cure diseases like cystic fibrosis using engineered adenovirus carrying a "good" gene to replace the crippled cystic fibrosis gene). Gene therapy cures symptoms but cannot correct the genetic defect in next-generation germ cells

Apoptosis: death of a cell following preprogrammed "instructions"; the dead cell is eventually removed by phagocytosis. A small family of proteases called caspases transmit the apoptotic death signal.

abnormal alterations in DNA, activation of the *k-ras* **proto-oncogene** on chromosome 12q, and loss of two other genes (*DCC* on chromosome 18q and *p53* on chromosome 17p). These alterations induce malignant colon carcinoma and metastasis. A new cell imaging technology (imaging mass spectrometry) can pinpoint the exact location in tissues that produce high levels of the protein thyosin beta-4 believed to trigger tumor growth.[115] Digital computer images that identify the location of specific tissue proteins allow researchers to determine when new proteins invade tumor cells or when normally-produced proteins disappear. Protein imaging opens a new vista in cancer screening for searching out specific molecules for comparison between normal and disease states, and developing strategies to arrest existing cancers.

Researchers know that as some cancerous cells become more lethal, they form into primitive channels to create blood vessels (**vasculogenesis**). The new blood vessels eventually connect with preexisting vessels at the edge of the tumor. This process, completely independent of **angiogenesis**, may explain why therapies that attack angiogenesis may not treat some cancers effectively. The above left *inset figure* shows angiogenesis and the subsequent vascularization of tumors. First, the tumor proliferates as it forms a small mass of cells. Note the lack of blood vessels in *A*. Without blood vessels, the tumor remains small. Second, protein factors in *B* stimulate the endothelial cells of nearby blood vessels to grow toward the tumor cells. Third, blood vessels in *C* proliferate, creating almost unlimited tumor growth. Note the approximate quadrupling of tumor cells.

Researchers hope to develop **gene therapy** strategies to attack tumor growth. This approach uses a peptide that targets tumor blood vessels, invades cells, and literally "tricks" cancer cells into killing themselves. The peptide contains two domains: (1) one that seeks out tumor blood vessels and (2) one that triggers cell suicide or programmed cell death (**apoptosis**;[74] *apopt,* falling off, *osis,* process). This normally-occurring process in both invertebrate and vertebrate biology should be considered one of nature's defensive mechanisms to purge the organism of cells damaged by mutation, viral invasion, external radiation, malignancy, and other deleterious cellular events (not always abnormalities). In fact, a recent review[104] discusses possible mechanisms of apoptotic cell death in diverse tissues induced by various exercise modes, including eccentric muscle activity in humans and wheel running in rodents[105] and skeletal muscle inactivity due to chronic heart failure.[1] The authors recommend additional research to investigate (1) shifts in pro- and anti-apoptotic proteins during chronic exercise training and (2) cell's molecular signals that might enhance apoptotic events in skeletal muscle activity. Additional research needs to closely investigate how hormonal changes affect different signaling proteins, oxidant production by the electron transport chain, and how mitochondria regulate apoptotic rate.

Other more tangible examples of apoptosis include the continual shedding of the outer protective skin layer. Also, before birth, up to 85% of neural cells in the brain and spinal cord literally "disappear" (or die) before regeneration occurs again. Apoptosis-inducing factor (AIF), released from mitochondria, translocates into the nucleus and triggers programmed cell death. AIF plays an essential role in cell death during cavitation of embryoid bodies during morphogenesis.[69] Researchers are studying four main areas of apoptosis: (1) molecular mechanisms involved in the induction of apoptosis, (2) control of the intracellular protease pathways responsible for induction, (3) biochemical events during apoptosis, particularly events that mediate cell death, and (4) role of mechanisms in normal development and disease. An intriguing question remains to be answered: what are the consequences of failure to initiate apoptosis in response to DNA damage?[108]

In the not-too-distant future, anticancer drugs will eradicate specific cancers once SNPs or a related technology identify them. A subsequent section discusses the fight against mutation-caused diseases, using a new generation of genetically engineered vaccines.

Mitochondrial DNA Mutations and Diseases

Normally, we view the chromosomes as the sole repository for DNA. However, DNA also exists in mitochondria. The complete human mitochondrial genome consists of 16,569 base pairs,[4] with the genetic blueprint for 37 molecules that produce about 90 % of the body's energy needs.[130] In Chapters 5 and 6, we describe energy release during cellular respiration when electron transfer ultimately produces water by uniting oxygen and hydrogen in the synthesis of significant quantities of energy-rich ATP. Researchers have determined the mitochondrial DNA (mtDNA) codes for 13 proteins that regulate respiratory chain oxidation and for 24 RNA molecules (2 tRNA, 22 rRNA) that manufacture subunits of respiratory chain proteins.[129–131] Thus, a defect (mutation) in mtDNA can induce devastating and unpredictable effects on basic cellular metabolic processes, particularly in neural, muscular, renal, and endocrine tissues. Figure 24 lists 12 diseases from mutations in mtDNA. The ring of DNA displayed in the schematic view shows different base pairs of mtDNA, numbered counterclockwise from the top center position labelled O_H in white. Mitochondrial DNA mutations also may be implicated in aging, affecting the impact of **free radicals** on tissues of the cardiovascular system.[64,128] In addition to studying serious human diseases caused by deleterious mutations, other uses of mtDNA fall into two additional categories: (1) forensic medicine, and (2) molecular anthropology. In forensic medicine, mtDNA analysis proves particularly useful because the high number of nucleotide polymorphisms (sequence variants) allow discrimination among individuals and/or biological samples. Even when degraded by environmental insult or time, minute samples of body fluids or fragments of hair, skin, muscle, bone, and blood may yield enough material for typing the mtDNA locus.[7,68,81,116] The likelihood of recovering mtDNA in small or degraded biological samples exceeds that for nuclear DNA. Mitochondrial DNA molecules exist in hundreds to thousands of copies per cell compared to only two nuclear copies per cell. Also, because mtDNA is inherited only from the mother, any maternally related individual can provide a reference sample in situations where an individual's DNA cannot be directly compared with a biologic sample. In molecular anthropology, mtDNA analysis examines the extent of genetic variation in humans and the relatedness of world populations.[28,102,106] Because of its unique mode of maternal inheritance, mtDNA can reveal ancient population histories, which might show migration patterns, expansion dates, and geographic homelands. Mitochondrial DNA has been extracted and sequenced from a Neanderthal skeleton, providing evidence that modern humans do not share a close relationship with Neanderthals in the human evolutionary tree.[100]

Free radical: highly reactive ionized atom or molecule with a single unpaired electron in the outer orbit; can cause a mutation by reacting violently with DNA

NEW HORIZONS IN MOLECULAR BIOLOGY

Watson and Crick's pioneering achievements in deciphering the molecular structure of DNA ushered in a new era. Currently, various microscopic and genetic engineering techniques affect not only medically related research but also strategies involving human exercise performance. The successful sequencing of the human genome, announced on June 26, 2000, was one of the most remarkable scientific feats in the history of medical science. Understanding the genetic blueprint of human life will speed the discovery of innovative new drugs to battle existing diseases. A year before this monumental achievement, the scientists who first mapped human chromosome 22 poignantly stated the following in their quest to decipher a section of the code:[43]

> Knowledge of the complete genomic DNA sequence of an organism allows a systematic approach to defining its genetic components. The genomic sequence provides access to the complete structures of all genes, including those without known function, their control elements, and, by inference, the proteins they encode, as well as all other biologically important sequences. Furthermore, the sequence is a rich and permanent source of information for the design of further biological studies of the organism and for the study of evolution through cross-species sequence comparison. The power of this approach has been amply demonstrated by the determination of the sequences of a number of microbial and model organisms. The next step is to obtain the complete sequence of the entire human genome.

Disease	Features
Alzheimer's disease	Progressive loss of cognitive capacity
CPEO (chronic progressive external ophthalmoplegia)	Paralysis of eye muscles and mitochondrial myopathy
Diabetes mellitus	High blood glucose levels; numerous complications
Dystonia	Abnormal movements involving muscular rigidity; degeneration of brain's basal ganglia
KSS (Kearns-Sayre syndrome)	CPEO combined with retinal degeneration, heart disease, hearing loss, diabetes, kidney failure
Leigh's syndrome	Progressive motor and verbal skill loss and degeneration of basal ganglia (potentially lethal childhood disease)
LHON (Leber's hereditary optic neuropathy)	Permanent or temporary blindness stemming from optic nerve damage
MELAS (mitochondrial encephalomyopathy, lactic acidosis and strokelike episodes)	Dysfunction of brain tissue (often causing seizures, transient regional paralysis and dementia) with mitochondrial myopathy and toxic blood acidity
MERRF (myoclonic epilepsy and ragged red fibers)	Seizures combined with mitochondrial myopathy, hearing loss, and dementia
Mitochondrial myopathy	Deterioration of muscle; poor exercise tolerance; muscle often displays ragged red fibers filled with abdormal mitochondria
NARP (neurogenic muscle weakness, ataxia and retinitis pigmentosa)	Muscle strength and coordination loss; regional brain degeneration and retinal deterioration
Pearson's syndrome	Childhood bone marrow dysfunction (leading to loss of blood cells) and pancreatic failure; survivors often progress to KSS

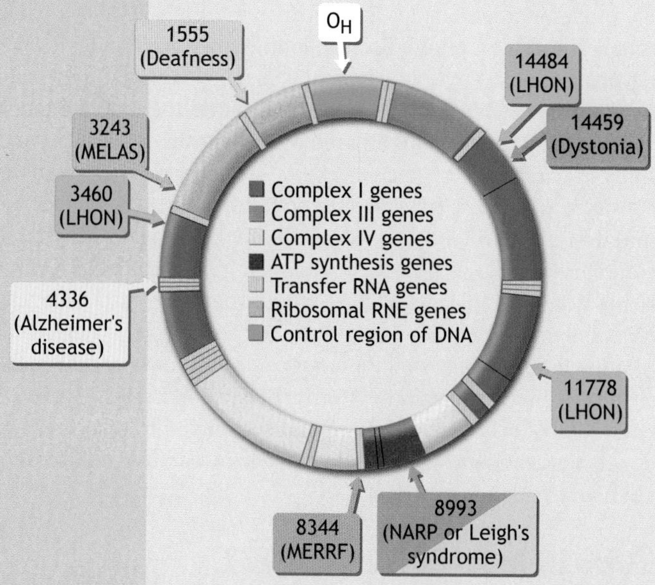

FIGURE 24 • Mitochondrial DNA diseases. The ring of DNA displayed in the *central schematic view* shows the genes associated with a particular disorder. Many of the mitochondrial DNA diseases are inherited, but they also can occur spontaneously in the developing embryo and become widespread during fetal development. The mutations also can form in different tissues (at different times during the life span), often taking years to become fully expressed and often potentially lethal or severely debilitating. (Adapted from Wallace DC, et al. Report of the committee on human mitochondrial DNA. In: Cuticchia AJ, ed. Human gene mapping: a compendium. Baltimore: Johns Hopkins University Press, 1995: 910–954. Also available at (www.gen.emory.edu/mitomap.html).

Microscope Technologies

To provide some idea of the capabilities of microscopic technologies germane to molecular biology, we compare four procedures, three of which have helped to unravel the secrets locked within the chemical configuration of structures that house the genetic code. Before detailing the different technologies, consider units of measurement and how they relate to what the human eye can observe and what the most powerful microscopes can reveal. Figure 25 displays nine different sublevels of organization, ranging from the minimum resolvable minute cellular structures revealed by electron microscopy of 0.2 nm to what the unaided eye observes by just looking at a small piece of skin at the outer region of the biceps.

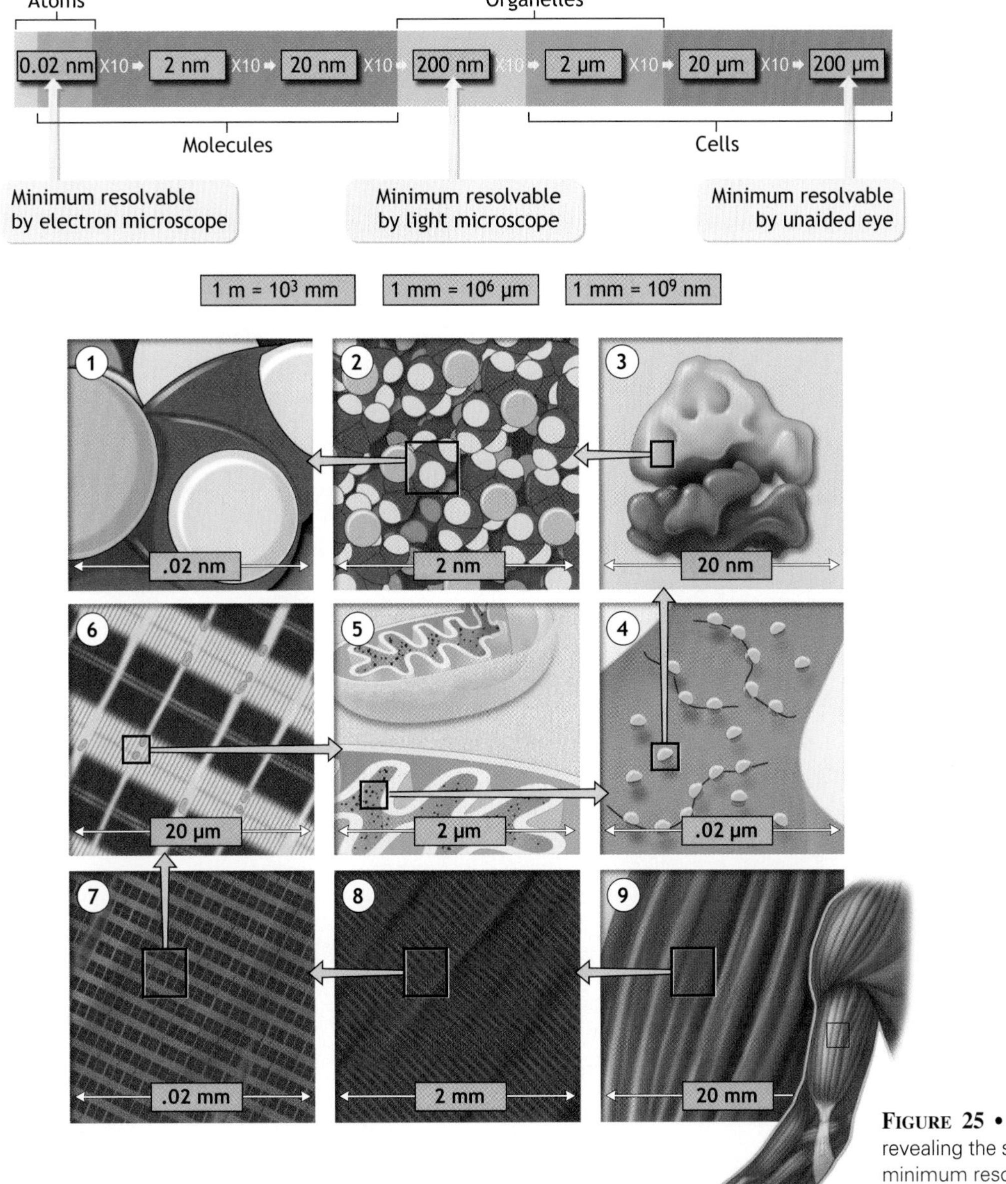

FIGURE 25 • *Top.* Units of measurement for revealing the size of cellular structures from the minimum resolvable distance viewing an object directly (0.2 mm) or through the light (200 nm) and electron (0.2 nm; 200 μm) microscopes. *Bottom.* Nine different sublevels of organization from the macro level at the biceps to the atomic level.

The examples show each succeeding sublevel of detail using a multiplier of 10. Even with the most powerful electron microscopes, individual atoms cannot yet be seen. However, single molecules of labeled ATP (and other molecules) have been imaged using total internal reflection **fluorescence microscopy** (TIRFM). The technique of assessing single molecules has broad application in studies of the mechanism of molecular motors (motility.york.ac.uk85/).[33,73,124]

Fluorescence microscope: microscope shown in Figure 26B that illuminates fluorescent-stained objects

Light Microscope

The **light microscope** shown Figure 24A magnifies the interior of cells one thousand times. This represents a quantum leap in technology from the primitive microscope first used in 1655 by British experimental physicist Robert Hooke (1635–1703) to describe what he termed "cells" in sections of cork, and Dutch microscopist Anton van Leeuwenhoek's (1632–1723) 1674 discovery of the single-celled protozoa and later observations of bacte-

Light microscope: microscope shown in Figure 26A that uses light, fixation of an object, and suitable lens that magnifies objects up to 1000 times with a resolution of 0.2 μm

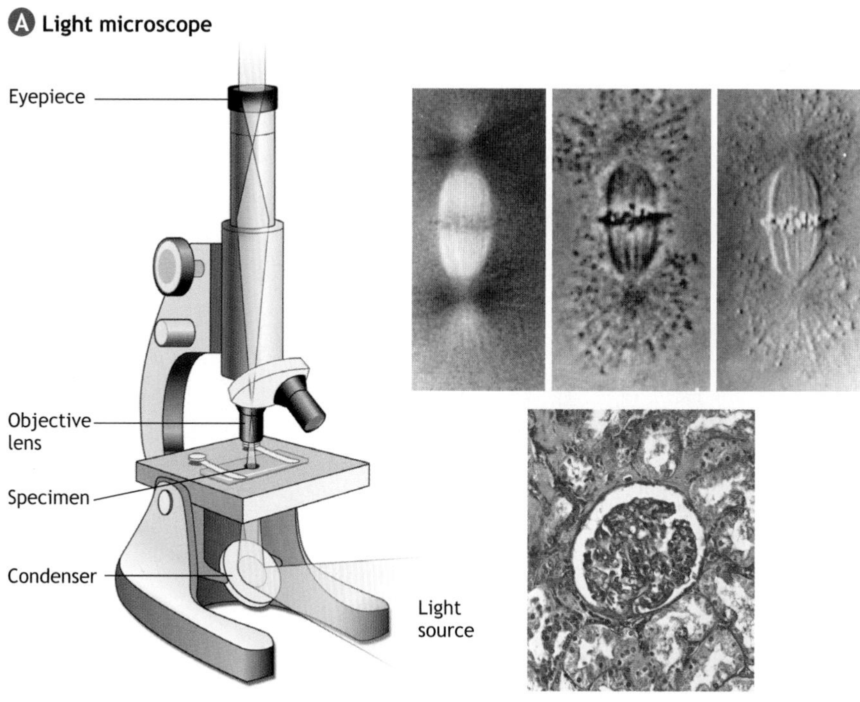

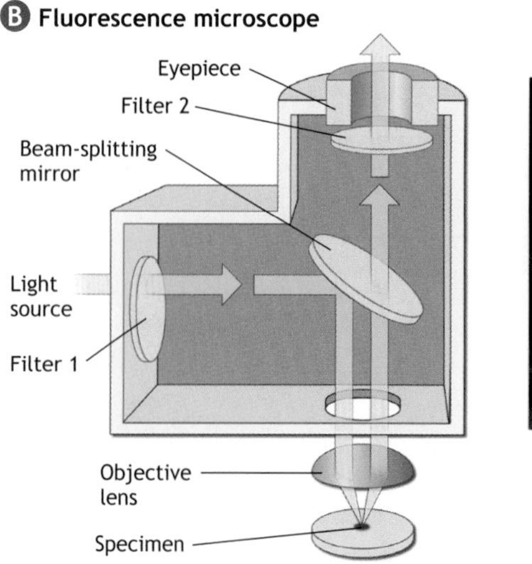

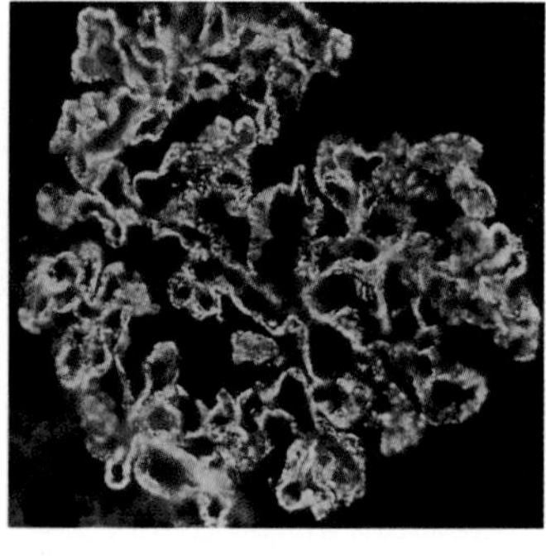

FIGURE 26 • Four different microscopes evaluate cell structures. **A**. Light microscope. **B**. Fluorescence microscope. **C**. Scanning electron microscope (SEM). **D**. Transmission electron microscope (TEM).

ria. The images at the right of the microscope represent the same structure viewed by three different light microscopes, each with a more complex lens system. Each microscope uses a different system of interchangeable lenses to exploit how light travels when it passes through the cell's interior to give a different portrayal of the image. A standard light microscope, in which a bright light focuses on the specimen through lenses in the condenser provided the three images involved in cell division, including a more detailed view shown in color. The **phase-contrast light microscope** uses a different optical system than that shown in *panel A,* as does the **interference-contrast light microscope** that obtained close-up image in *panel C.* In the fluorescence microscope shown in Figure 26B, light passes through two filters labeled *1* and *2* in the illustration. The first filters any light within the specimen except wavelengths that "excite" a previously applied fluorescent dye. The second blocks the wavelength of the excited **fluorescent** dye but allows only those wavelengths emitted from the fluorescent dye to pass. Fluorescent dyes absorb light at one wavelength and emit light at longer wavelengths. In staining for DNA in the mitotic spin-

Phase-contrast light microscope: category of light microscope

Interference-contrast light microscope: category of light microscope

Fluorescence: a molecule absorbs light of one wavelength and then emits light of another longer, lower energy wavelength

C Scanning electron microscope

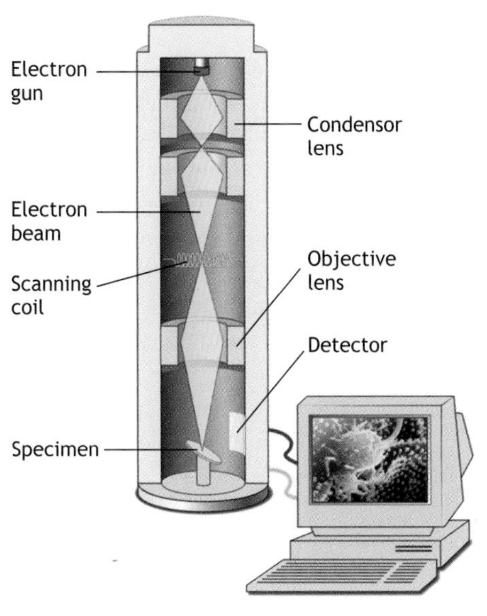

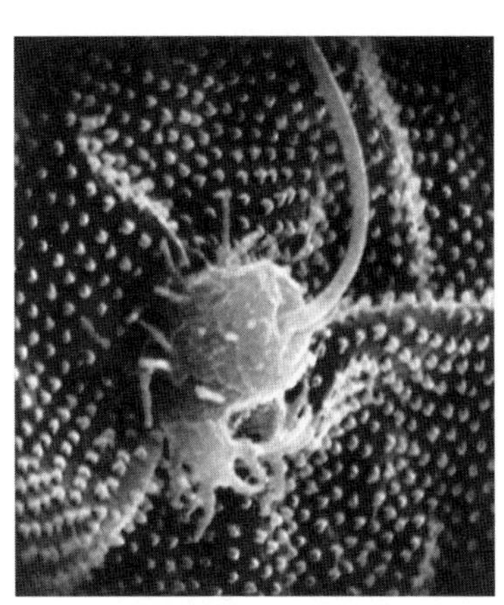

D Transmission electron microscope

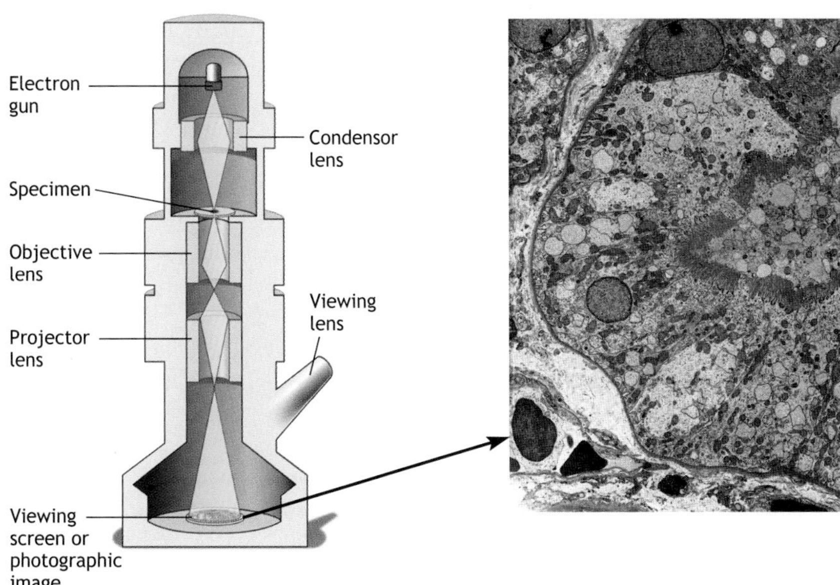

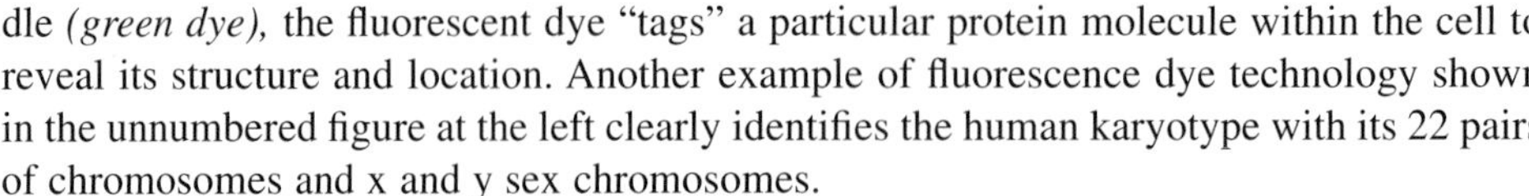

dle *(green dye),* the fluorescent dye "tags" a particular protein molecule within the cell to reveal its structure and location. Another example of fluorescence dye technology shown in the unnumbered figure at the left clearly identifies the human karyotype with its 22 pairs of chromosomes and x and y sex chromosomes.

The development of precise technologies (i.e., molecular combing) enables researchers to analyze individual DNA molecules for in-depth genetic abnormalities and patterns. This makes pinpointing disease-related genes an easier task, and consequently, development of new drugs to eradicate inborn or environmentally-induced errors within the genetic alphabet.

The human karyotype prepared by 24-color FISH (fluorescent in situ hybridization) uniquely identifies each of the 22 pairs of chromosomes and one sex chromosome (total of 46 chromosomes at conception). Recent advances in fluorescence in situ imaging technology has improved the resolution from 1 million to 10 million bases.

Electron Microscopes

The electron microscope, invented in the 1950s, represented a technologic advance for unraveling the innermost secrets about cell structures and functions. Many pioneers in muscle contraction theory relied on data from electron microscopy to elucidate structural components of a muscle's intricate protein filament structures during contraction and relaxation.[17] In 1964, H. E. Huxley proposed his sliding-filament mechanism of muscle contraction from studies using the electron microscope.[66]

SCANNING ELECTRON MICROSCOPE. The **scanning electron microscope (SEM)** shown in Figure 26C uses electron beams with wavelengths thousands of times shorter than those of visible light. These waves replace light, allowing significantly greater resolution and magnification. Electromagnetic coils focus the beam on the specimen, similar to the lens of a light microscope. The electrons pass through an ultrathin, stained specimen coated with a thin film of a heavy metal. The detector measures the electrons scattered or emitted by the beam as it passes through the dehydrated specimen and provides a highly detailed image magnified 1 million times (resolution of 2 nm). To prepare the sample, the tissue goes into a fixing solution and then is washed and dehydrated in successively higher acetone or alcohol concentrations. The tissue then is placed into a dilute solution of plastic embedding medium, then into a specimen vial, and a final embedding mixture for polymerization in an oven. The hard, plastic-containing specimen is then set in an **ultramicrotome** (figure at left) for slicing with a glass or diamond knife. The ultrathin sections are lifted from the surface with a copper grid, dried, and stained with the electron-dense, heavy metal solution (salts of uranium and lead) in preparation for viewing. The scanned images have a resolution between 3 and 20 nm and provide exquisite, detailed three-dimensional images.

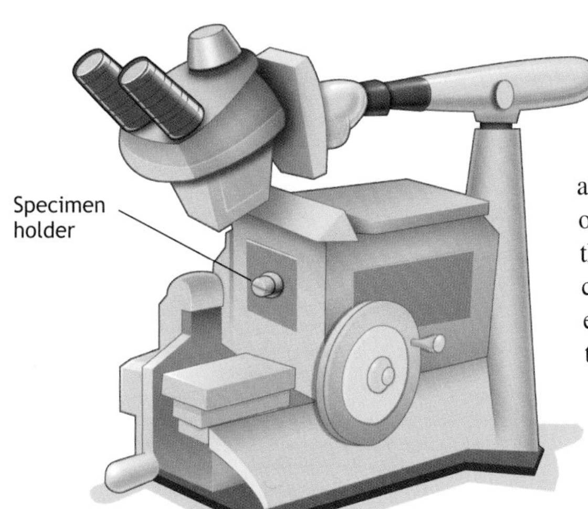

Ultramicrotome

TRANSMISSION ELECTRON MICROSCOPE. Figure 26D shows an extremely thin slice of a prepared substance (biopsy of lung tissue) within the vacuum of the transmission electron microscope (TEM). Multiple stains reveal different parts of a structure, because each stain clings to a different structural part.

LASER SCANNING CONFOCAL MICROSCOPY. In **Laser scanning confocal microscopy** (LSCM; also known as confocal scanning laser microscopy or CSLM; see unnumbered figure on top of next page), an expanded laser light beam creates high-resolution images and three-dimensional reconstructions of biologic specimens (www.loci.wisc.edu/confocal/confocal.html). The projected beam becomes a scanning beam with an objective lens that focuses a small spot onto a fluorescent specimen. After conversion into a static beam, the reflected and emitted fluorescent light mixture focuses onto a photodetector (photomultiplier) via a dichroic mirror (beam splitter). The dichroic mirror splits the reflected light, while emitted fluorescent light passes through to the photomultiplier. A confocal aperture (pinhole) placed in front of the photodetector selectively allows fluorescent light to pass from points on the specimen not within the focal plane. This greatly reduces out-of-focus information (both above and below the focal plane). The spot focused on the pinhole center is known as the "confocal spot." Most confocal microscopes are

Scanning electron microscope (SEM): uses electron beams with wavelengths thousands of times shorter than visible light to produce significantly greater resolution and magnification

Ultramicrotome: microtome that cuts specimen sections 0.01 μm thick or less for electron microscopy

Laser scanning confocal microscopy (LSCM): laser light beam creates high resolution images and 3-D reconstructions of biologic specimens

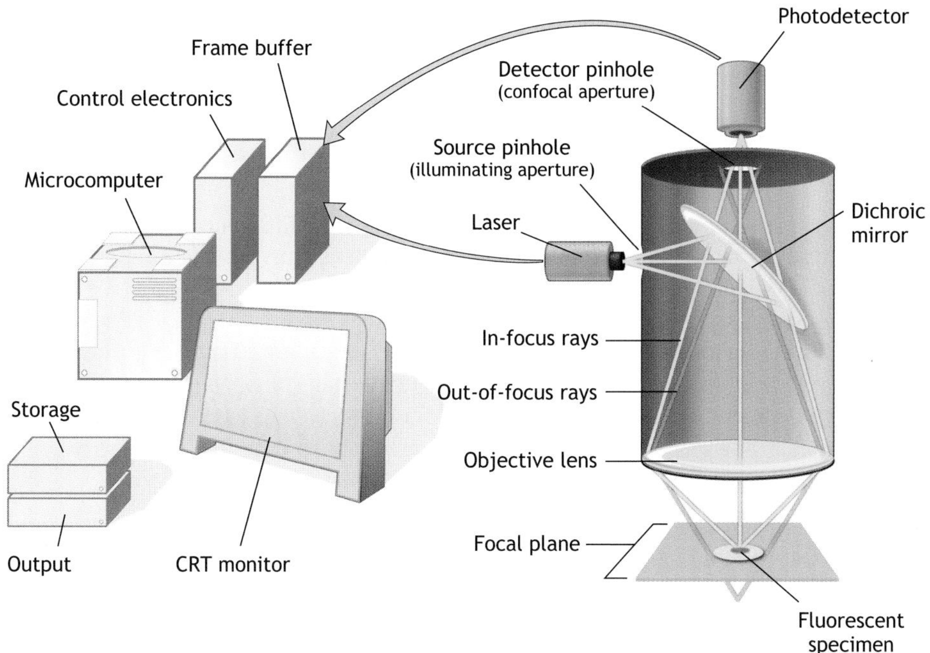

Laser scanning confocal microscopy. The image shown on the CRT monitor, a virus infected cell structure, was the fluorescent specimen scanned by the microscope.

PET scanner: provides detailed images of biochemical activity in the body without surgery. Patients are injected with a low dose of a short-lived radioactive sugar that concentrates in tissues for easy visualization

Pathogens: any virus, microorganism, or other substance that causes disease; *Streptococcus* bacteria cause scarlet fever, rheumatic fever, and pneumonia in humans. In plants, destructive diseases caused by bacteria (mostly pseudomonads) include blights, soft rots, and wilts. Viruses cannot replicate independently; they exist only within the cells of other organisms. Viruses usually contain a protein coating (capsid) and lipid-rich protein envelope around the capsid ("a piece of bad news wrapped up in a protein") and reproduce using the metabolic apparatus of their host

coupled to a conventional microscope. Advanced software now permits four-dimensional microscopy to study three-dimensional specimens as they grow or change over time (www.loci.wisc.edu/); additional techniques include multiple-photon excitation fluorescence (www.its.caltech.edu/~pinelab/2photon.html) and computational optical scanning, and a variety of optimal techniques for experimental intervention into living specimens.

Positron Emission Tomography (PET). The **PET scanner** provides detailed images of biochemical activity in the body without surgery for diagnosing heart disease, stroke, epilepsy, Parkinson's disease, and cancer. Patients are injected with a low dose of a short-lived radioactive sugar. Detectors assess release of gamma rays from the sugar, which concentrates in the tissues under study. The unnumbered tomographic images of the brain on the right taken with a 32-ring PET scanner clearly show areas of interest detected by different colored radiopharmaceuticals. In this example, the image shows glucose (bright yellow) used in excess of normal requirements, as in a growing tumor. Unlike magnetic resonance imaging (MRI), which primarily examines *anatomy* in detail, the PET scan can visualize body *functions* during the course of a disease like cancer and accurately show its extent (i.e., whether it is malignant or benign and treatment effects). In Alzheimer's disease, for example, a PET scan can recognize abnormal brain patterns years before a physician can confirm the disease. In Parkinson's disease, the presence of a labeled amino acid (F-DOPA) quantifies a deficiency in dopamine synthesis. Early confirmation of the deficiency leads to a different treatment modality than is used if the deficiency cannot be established. Several web sites provide excellent information about PET scanning (www.muc.ucla.edu/; www.laxm.nuc.ucla.edu:8000/lpp/).

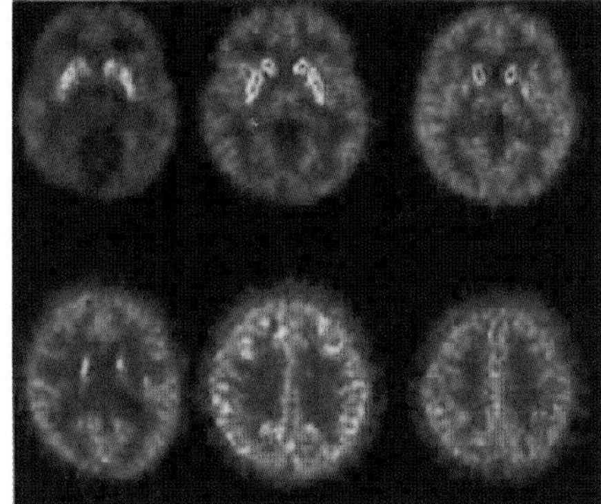

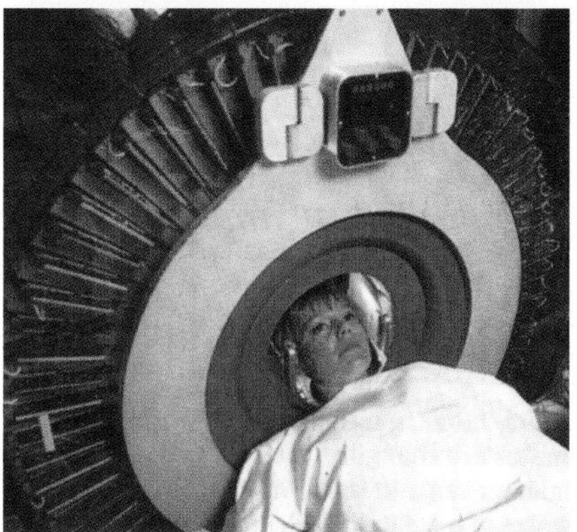

Top. Excess glucose shows as yellow colored regions in the brain PET scan. *Bottom.* Patient undergoing brain scan with the 32-ring PET scanner.

Medically Related Research

Almost every aspect of medicine now benefits from molecular biology/molecular genetics research. Within the past 10 years, researchers have developed new techniques to fight many diseases, including cancer, AIDS, asthma, diabetes, influenza, rheumatic fever, and malaria. The new disease-fighters use genetic engineering to improve the immunologic antigen defense machinery against viral, bacterial, fungal, or parasitic **pathogens**. Because all pathogens contain antigens in their structure, a new generation of genetically engineered vaccines will severely blunt their destructive effects. Figure 27 provides a capsule view of four disease-fighting approaches with vaccine techniques that manipulate the genetic code.

Vector: plasmid, retrovirus, or bacterial or yeast artificial chromosome used to transfer a segment of foreign DNA among cells or species to produce more end product. The vector represents the genome that transports alien DNA into a host cell

Virus: small structure that grows by infecting other cells; adenovirus, retrovirus, adeno-associated viruses represent the most commonly used viral gene vectors

Immune response: immediate defensive reaction of the immune system upon encountering an invasion by a foreign substance like a pathogen

1. *Live **vector** vaccines.* Genes from a dangerous virus such as HIV are inserted into a **virus** that is harmless to humans. When injected, the altered virus prompts a strong **immune response** to combat the pathogen.
2. *Reassortment virus vaccines.* Combining genes from different pathogenic strains creates a decoy virus that looks dangerous to the pathogen but remains harmless while triggering an appropriate immune response.
3. *Naked DNA vaccines.* A pathogen's DNA is injected directly into the body. The cells incorporate the DNA, using the preprogrammed specific genetic "instructions" to create antigens to fight offending pathogens or existing tumors.
4. *Recombinant subunit vaccines.* Culturing a pathogen's genetic code (genes) produces massive quantities of a specific antigen. The disease-fighting vaccine is made from the cultured antigens rather than from the whole pathogen.

Some genetically engineered vaccines trick the immune system into creating antibodies to seek out and destroy undesirable molecules before they cross the blood–brain barrier. For example, small cocaine molecules escape the body's protein antibody defenses without mechanisms to stop it. Engineered vaccines can create a larger cocaine derivative, which the immune system can then recognize and disarm. This aspect of genetic design, although currently more expensive than cloning to make drug therapies, offers new hope in battling addictive diseases.

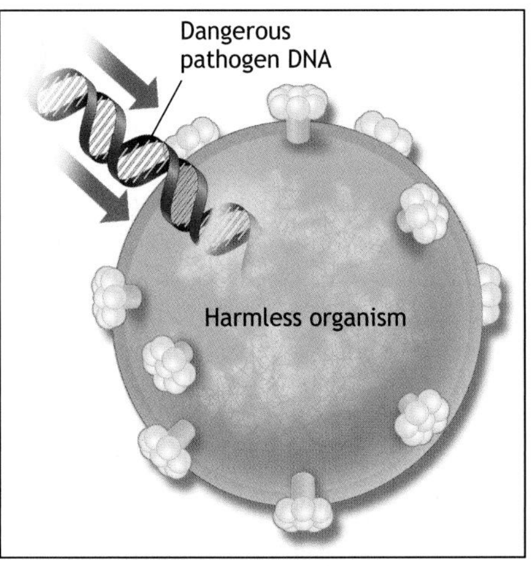

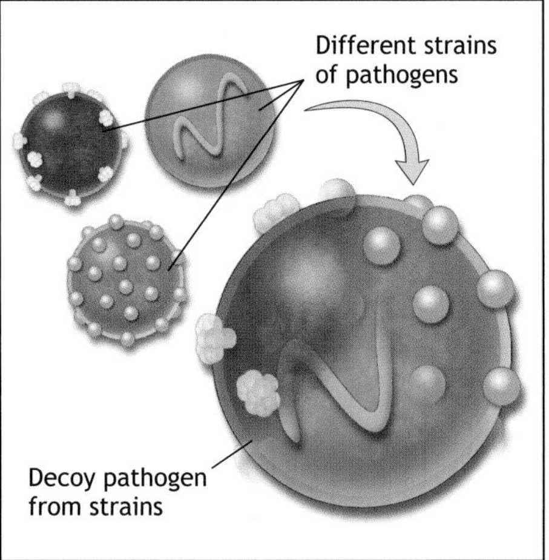

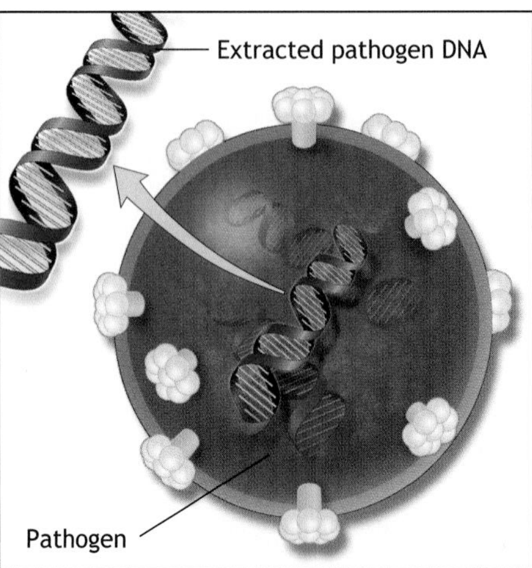

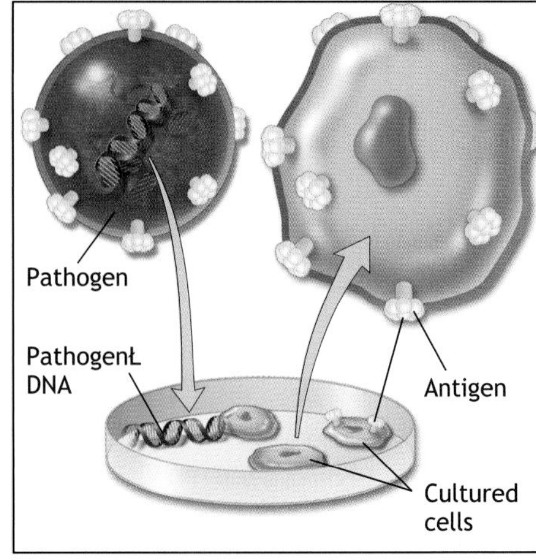

FIGURE 27 • Genetic engineering a new generation of four vaccine types to fight human diseases.

Figure 28 lists the body's 22 numbered chromosomes, including X and Y chromosomes, and specific genes on each chromosone linked to cancers and metabolic/endocrine, neurologic/psychiatric, and cardiovascular disorders. The *right side of the figure on page 1018* profiles chromosome 17, for which seven deadly cancers have already been identified. The *bottom* of the figure on page 1019 shows the mechanism of action of different chemical carcinogens on this particular nucleotide sequence of the tumor suppressor gene *p53*. About 50% of human cancers occur from inactivating this gene. Each carcinogen produces a distinctive nucleotide substitution. Note the C or G substitution that displaces six T nucleotides.

Many areas of medicine other than cancer benefit from new findings in molecular biology. For example, people with advanced sleep-phase syndrome (ASPS) cannot resist the urge either to sleep or to wake up early. Research indicates that ASPS does not reflect a learned behavior or some other factor, but follows a specific inherited pattern. Eventually, researchers may tie disorders to a single gene, opening new vistas to the genetics of the biologic clock in humans,[72,119,121] with potential applications to many aspects of human performance. Some of the same medical research techniques have found their way into the arsenal of technologies to probe secrets about topics of interest to exercise physiologists. These include blood pressure control, endurance and strength training adaptations, maturational shifts related to caloric input and output, hormonal balance with exercise, and pulmonary, cardiovascular, and body weight regulation (including anorexia nervosa[53]).

Gene splicing: attaching a fragment of DNA from one species (e.g., mammal) to another species (e.g., bacterium) to clone mammalian DNA

Recombinant DNA: forming a hybrid DNA molecule by fusing DNA fragments from different species; attaching a segment of DNA from one species to a second species, followed by inserting the hybrid molecule into a host organism such as a bacterium

Reverse transcriptase: enzyme that allows a single-stranded RNA template to synthesize a double-stranded DNA copy for insertion elsewhere in the genome

cDNA: single-stranded DNA complementary to an RNA and synthesized from it using reverse transcriptase. This kind of DNA only codes exons

Bacteriophage: any virus that infects bacteria

Restriction endonuclease: enzyme that cleaves a specific short DNA nucleotide sequence whenever it occurs at a target site

DNA Technologies

By isolating a small fragment of DNA from a chromosome in an animal species (including humans), scientists can "remake" an exact copy of the DNA segment in a test tube, preserving the precise sequence of its nucleotide base pairs. Researchers use several terms to describe this process of eventual gene reconfiguration or manipulation on chromosomes—genetic engineering, **gene splicing**, or **recombinant DNA**.

A crucial step along the path to genetic engineering occurred in 1967 when Dr. Arthur Kornberg synthesized biologically active DNA. This was followed in 1970 in classic experiments by Drs. David Baltimore, Renato Dulbecco, and Howard Temin who won the 1975 Nobel Prize in physiology or medicine for discoveries concerning the interaction between tumor viruses and a cell's genetic material. They discovered that a specific enzyme tumor virus (**reverse transcriptase**) made a DNA copy from RNA. The researchers used purified mRNA from muscle or liver tissue to show that this enzyme interacts with the mRNA. Reverse transcriptase duplicates the mRNA to the specific sequence of complementary DNA (**cDNA**). DNA polymerase can then convert the single-stranded DNA to a double strand for eventual cloning into a **bacteriophage** or other vector. These experiments proved transfer of the content stored in the genetic material to DNA; subsequent experiments also proved that purified DNA from one cell introduced into other cells produce new particles of RNA tumor virus.

In 1973, two American researchers, Stanley Cohen, cofounder of Genentech, one of the first biotechnology corporations, at Stanford University and Herbert Boyer (1986 Nobel Prize in physiology or medicine with Rita Levi-Montalcini for discovering cell growth factors) at the University of California, San Francisco, building upon the research described above, introduced the recombinant DNA technique shown schematically in unnumbered figure at right. They successfully cut DNA from an amphibian gene (primitive frog *Xenopus*) into segments, using a **restriction endonuclease** enzyme (*Eco*RI) to cut the plasmid (figure at right). They then

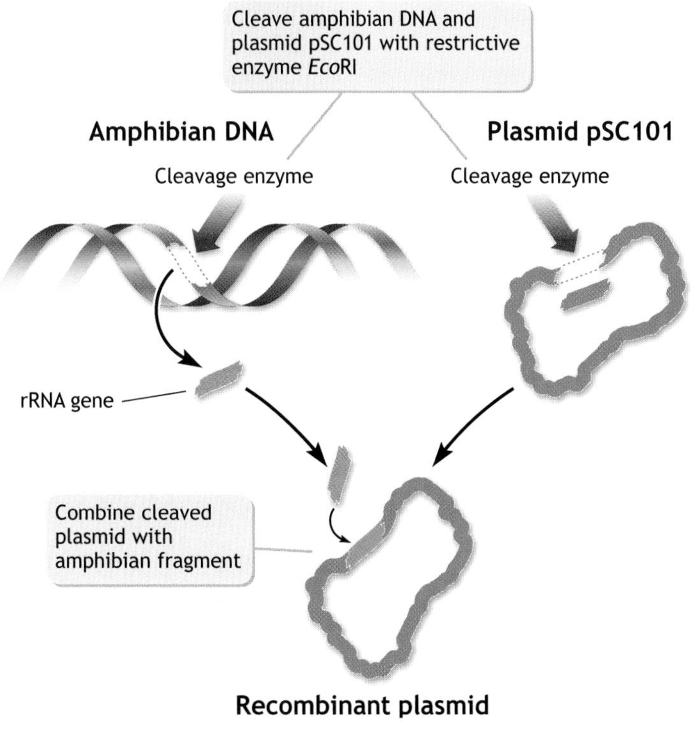

Drs. Stanley Cohen and Herbert Boyer produce the first recombinant DNA organism in 1973. They combined the cleaved plasmid (pSC101 shown at the right) with a fragment of amphibian DNA (shown on the left) using restriction endonuclease enzyme (*Eco*R1) to produce the recombinant plasmid shown at the bottom.

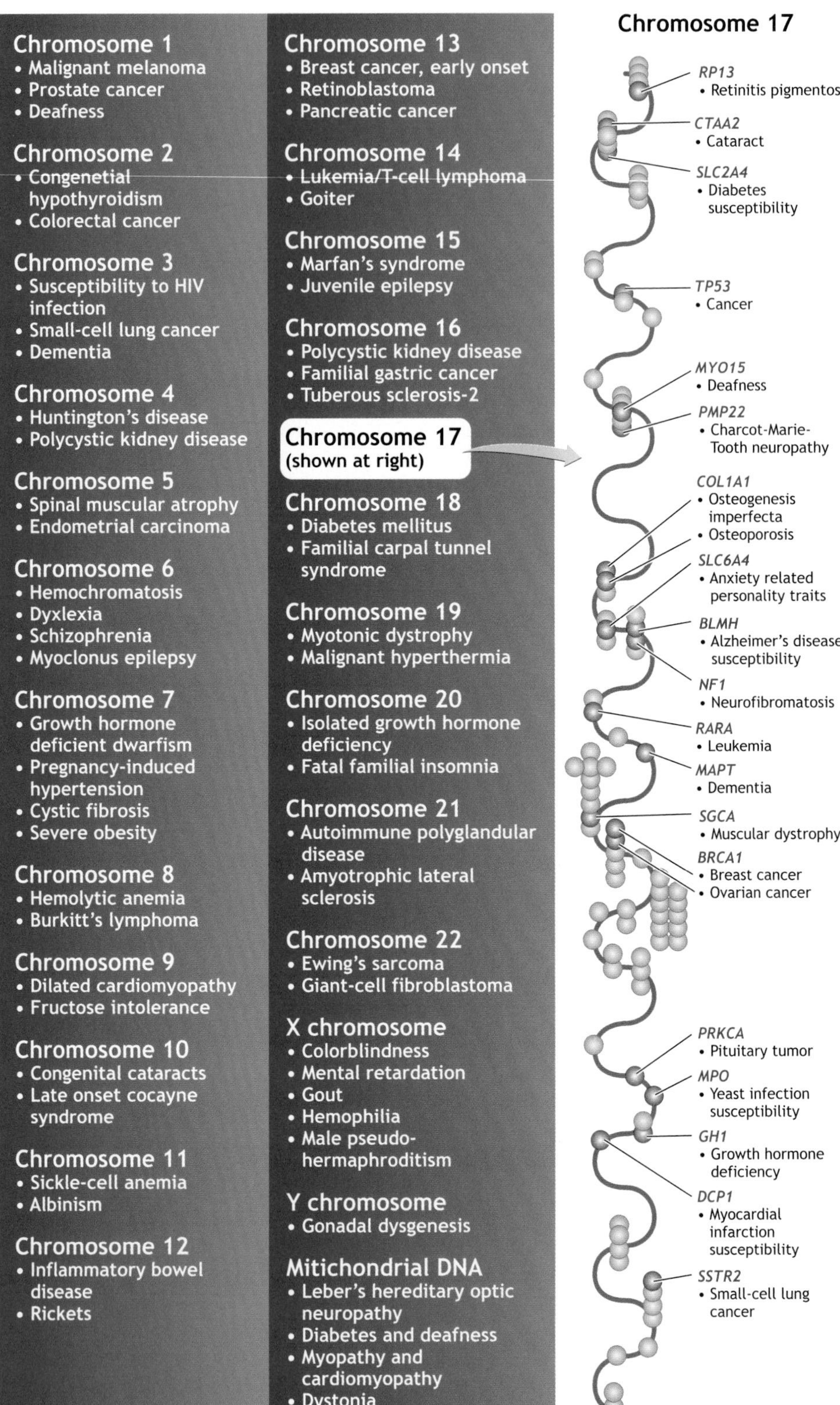

FIGURE 28 • Links on the body's chromosomes to specific cancer, metabolic/endocrine, neurologic/psychiatric, and cardiovascular disorders. *Right.* Close-up of disorders found on chromosome 17. On this chromosome, red designates the specific gene name and its location.

rejoined the 9000-nucleotide segment to form a circular plasmid called pSC101, so-named by Cohen because it was the 101st plasmid he isolated.

Their experimental procedure (explained further in the section on RNA cloning), produced the first plasmid to clone a vertebrate gene. In essence, the frog–bacterial molecule represented recombinant DNA using gene splicing to rejoin the two ends of the

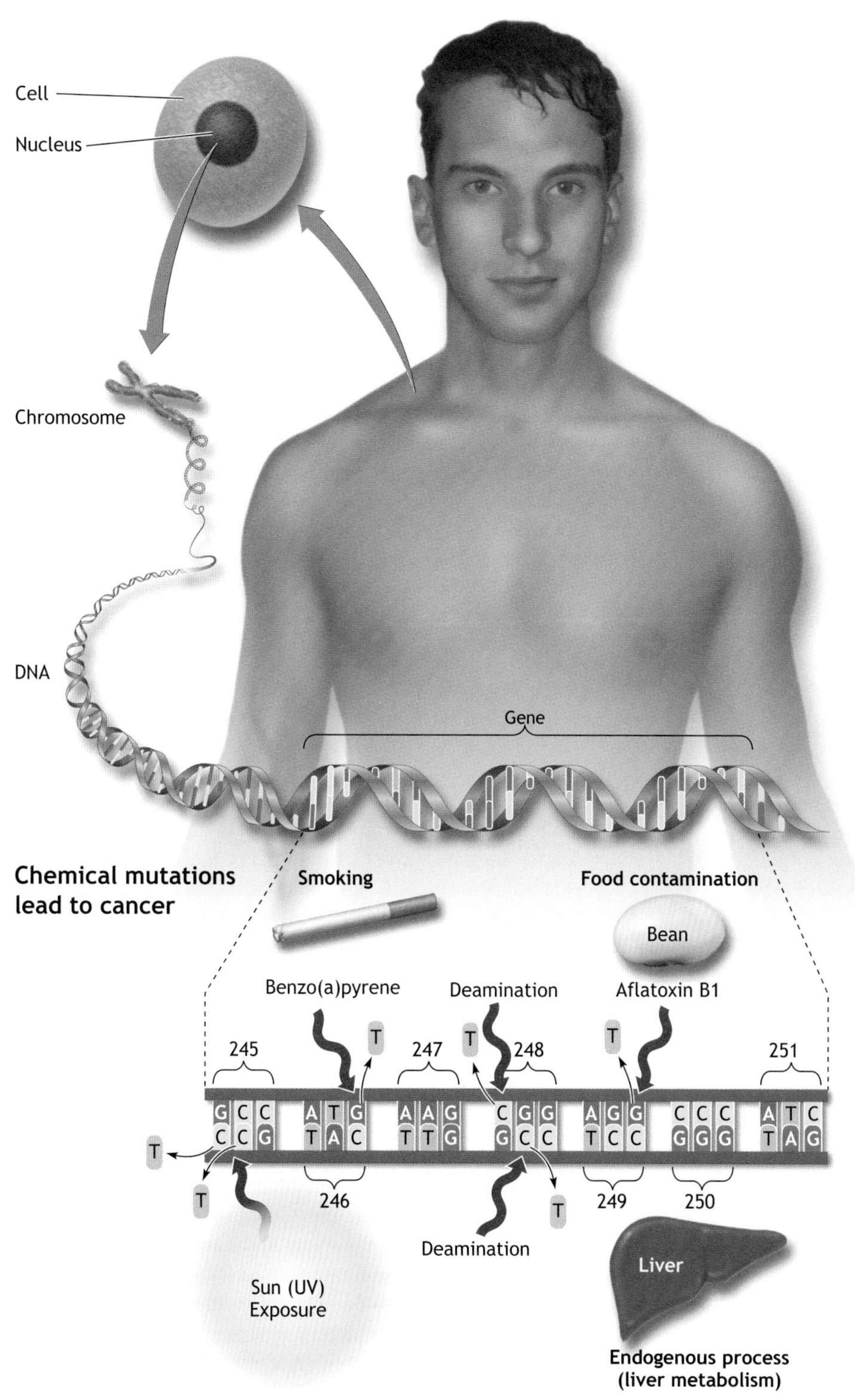

Figure 28 *(cont'd)* • Graphic illustrating how different carcinogens (chemical and other) affect the nucleotide sequence of the *p53* gene responsible for about 50% of human cancers. The *p53* gene's name comes from the product it encodes, a polypeptide with a molecular mass of 53,000 daltons (1 dalton equals one-twelfth the mass of carbon 12; for comparison, a water molecule weighs 18 daltons, and hemoglobin weighs 64,500 daltons).

pSC101 plasmid. This technique can be likened to "cutting" and "pasting" text or images from one section of a document to another in a computer software program. The endonuclease first cleaves the amphibian DNA setting it free. The two ends of the rRNA gene now join the pSC101 plasmid cleaved by *Eco*R1. Fundamentally, gene splicing creates a new genetic blueprint in a test tube that leapfrogs nature's own genetic engineering methods based on natural selection—a process that normally comingles genes within the Earth's plant and animal species over tens of millions of years of evolution.

With the opening of trade routes and exploration in the ancient world, different sizes, shapes, and characteristics of plant and animal species from one location gained options to "share" their genetic code with similar species in other more distant locations thousands of miles away. Thus, unknowingly, humans helped to selectively breed (genetically engineer) plants and animals, in effect revising and updating the original gene pool that now forms the great variety of flowers, vegetables, and animals around us. What took nature millions of years to accomplish, scientists can now duplicate in a day and produce thousands of copies of DNA's exact nucleotide sequence from a particular gene in a given genome. By manipulating DNA's configuration, a newly created gene can be inserted into cells of plants and animals, creating new cells or species with unique characteristics expressed by the new genetic instructions.

Cloning: creating a cell(s) or molecule(s) from a single ancestral cell or molecule

Genomic library: collection of DNA fragments from an organism's genome. A library includes noncoding DNA and cDNA

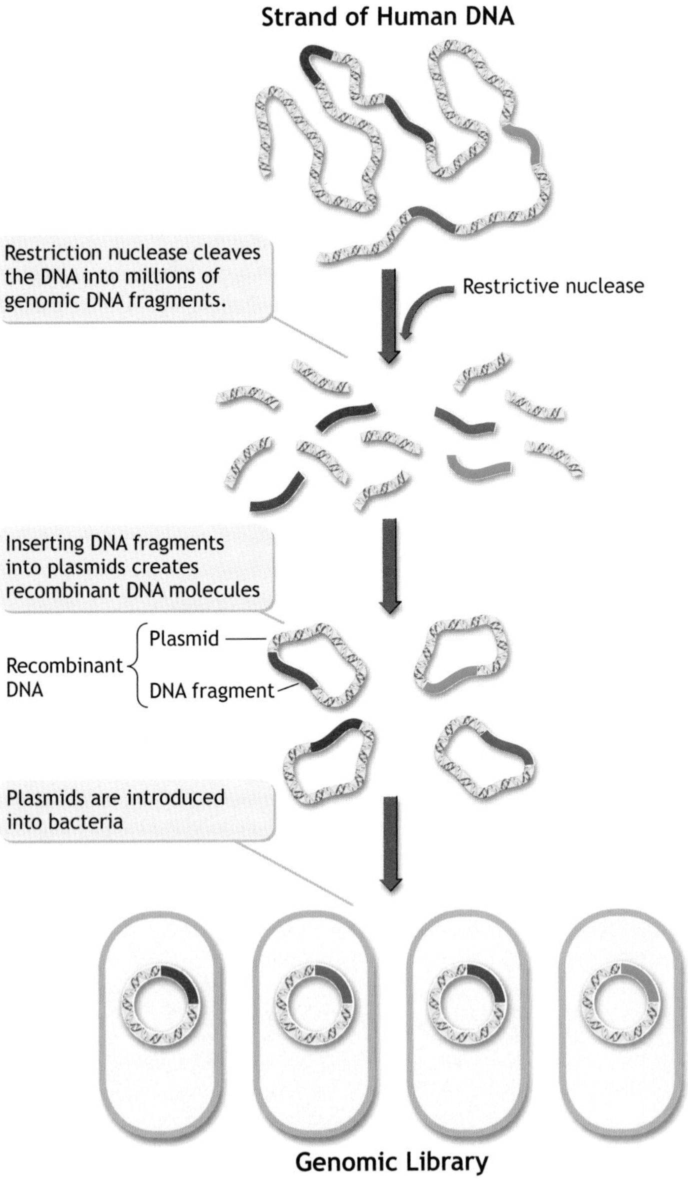

DNA Cloning Isolates Human Genes

DNA **cloning** progresses in several stages. The first involves mechanically breaking the genetic material within a DNA sample or, alternatively, using restriction endonucleases that precisely cut the nucleotide sequence along DNA's double helix into smaller segments to facilitate manipulation. The collection of DNA pieces formed by endonuclease cleavage represents single, random segments of all of the organism's DNA, which includes all of the genetic material. The term **genomic library** describes the collection of cloned fragments. Many genomic libraries exist in the public domain (e.g., www.gdb.org), so researchers can use them without having to reduplicate the particular DNA sequences of interest. Figure 29 shows formation of a genomic library.

A restriction endonuclease cleaves a short strand of human double-helix chromosomal DNA, usually four to six base pairs in length, into millions of fragments. One of the most widely used chemical techniques, **gel electrophoresis** (Greek *phoresis*, "to be carried"), perfected by 1948 Chemistry Nobel laureate Arne Wilhelm Tiselius (1902–1971), separates DNA fragments within an electric field. The DNA strands, inserted into a circular plasmid carrier molecule, recombine the DNA (hence the term *recombinant DNA*). This occurs when the enzyme DNA ligase with addition of ATP covalently links the DNA fragment to the previously opened **plasmid** composed of several thousand nucleotide pairs. Once inserted, the ligase rejoins the ends of the plasmid to produce the new recombinant plasmid molecule known as a vector. Recombinant plasmids are then inserted into bacteria (e.g., *E. coli*) to ensure that only one bacterium receives one plasmid. At this stage, the total culture of bacteria represents the genomic library illustrated in Figure 29.

The next stage of DNA cloning grows the bacterium in a nutrient-rich broth, which sustains cell multiplication that doubles its number every hour. This also therefore doubles the number of recombinant DNA copies. By simple multiplication, doubling the number of DNA copies each hour over 24 hours produces almost

Strand of Human DNA
Restriction nuclease cleaves the DNA into millions of genomic DNA fragments.
Restrictive nuclease
Inserting DNA fragments into plasmids creates recombinant DNA molecules
Recombinant DNA
Plasmid
DNA fragment
Plasmids are introduced into bacteria
Genomic Library

FIGURE 29 • Creating a genomic library from human DNA. The library consists of bacteria with specific DNA fragments contained in carrier substances such as plasmids. Note in the example how four different-colored DNA segments (red, blue, purple, green) from the original human DNA shown at the top end up within the bacterial host. The rest of the DNA fragments also can make clones.

17 million new copies from a single bacterium! The bacteria are then broken apart (lysed), and the millions of DNA copies culled from the larger bacterial chromosome and other cellular contents to provide pure replicas of the original DNA segment. Recovering this segment occurs after the specific **restriction enzyme** isolates it from plasma DNA for separation by gel electrophoresis (refer to Figure 30).

Gel electrophoresis: separation of electrically charged substances (like proteins) through a gel mesh according to size. Smaller substances migrate faster than larger substances when they pass through the electric field from the top (negative) to bottom (positive) electrode through a slab of agarose gel, a polysaccharide extracted from seaweed

Plasmid: small circular molecule in bacteria without chromosomal DNA; serves as a vector for transferring genes among cells

Practical Application in Bioremediation

Implementation of bacterial cloning has practical applications in the field of bioremediation that uses bacteria to degrade dangerous compounds. For example, the pink-colored, rotten cabbage smelling-like bacteria Deinococcus *radiodurans* (D. *radi*) shown in the unnumbered figures below have been genetically cloned from strains of E. *coli* previously made resistant to toxic wastes. D. *radi* was isolated in 1956 from a can of ground beef that had been "sterilized" by gamma radiation but still spoiled. Researchers determined that D. *radi* survived approximately 17kGy (1.7 million rads), a value equal to 3000 times the lethal dose of radiation for humans. The economic value of D. *radi* is straightforward; easily producing trillions of copies of the new bacterium will save hundreds of billions of dollars in biohazard cleanup. For example, because D. *radi* consumes heavy metals and radioactive wastes, it can scavange toxic wastes buried at 1000 sites throughout the United States and other sites worldwide, a legacy from nuclear weapons production between 1945 and 1986. Researchers have also fused a gene that encodes toluene dioxygenase (the enzyme that decomposes toluene) to a D. *radi* promoter (site that activates the gene), and then inserted it into one of the bacterium's chromonsomes. The resulting recombinant bacterium "upgraded" D. *radi* for degrading toluene and other organic compounds at levels exceeding those at radioactive waste sites. D. *radi* not only survives high radiation doses, but also long periods of dehydration and ultraviolet irradiation. D. *radi* apparently repairs its radiation damaged DNA base pairs by use of redundant genetic "signals." The two billion year-old microbe has from four to ten DNA molecules. The protein, RecA, matches the damaged DNA base pairs and splices them together. During the repair process, cell-building activities shut down and the broken DNA pieces maintained in place. The complete genome of D. *radi* has been decoded (see Timeline, 1999; Table 3) and can be accessed from the TIGR web site, www.tigr.org/. The DNA of D. *radi* consists of 3.3 million chemical base units. The genome contains two circular chromosomes, one about 2.6 million and the other 400,000 base pairs in length, and two smaller circular molecules (megaplasmid of 177,000 base pairs and plasmid of 45,000 base pairs). Despite its high tolerance for radioactivity, D. *radi* decomposes at 45°C.

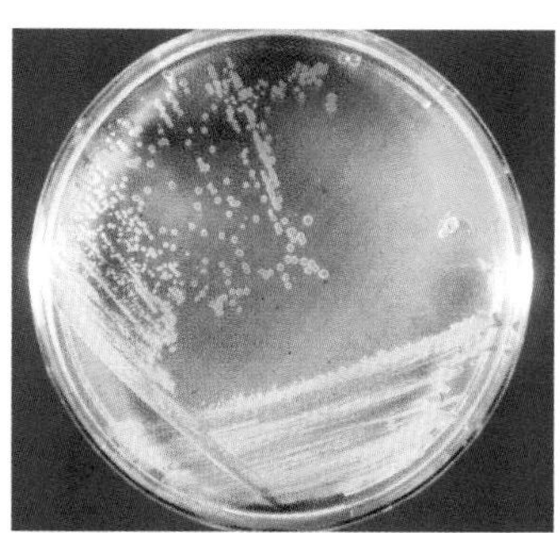

Left. Electron photomicrograph of D. *radi* (sequenced in the DOE Microbial Genome Program as a cluster of four cells or tetrad). D. *radi* and related species have been identified worldwide, including in Antarctic granite and in tanks of powerful ^{60}Cobalt irradiators in Denmark. *Right.* D. *radi* growing on a nutrient agar plate; the orange color is from carotenoid pigment. (Images from the Uniformed Services University of the Health Sciences, Bethesda, MD; www.usuhs.mil/).

Restriction enzyme: cuts DNA at precise locations, and with DNA ligase, reassembles the pieces into a desired order. Cutting between G and A leaves overhanging "sticky end" chains because base pairs formed between the two overhanging portions "glue" the two strands together where the sticky ends match, assembling them into customized genomes (e.g., designer bacteria that make insulin or growth hormone, or genes for disease resistance added to agricultural plants)

Locating Specific Genes with Plasmids

Creating cloned DNA involves locating a specific gene within the plasmid or viral culture. Consider the analogy of entering a five-story department store without signs or a computer database to search for a single unmarked item. One could begin searching on the first floor, proceeding to every shelf and cupboard of every floor until finding the item, but the inefficiency of this strategy seems obvious. To facilitate locating a specific gene, a specific **DNA probe** of known nucleotide sequence, labeled with colored fluorescent markers or radioisotopes, searches the pool of millions of copies of DNA fragments. The probes, used in **hybridization** reactions, capture a single DNA or RNA strand to form another nucleic acid with a complementary nucleotide sequence. The probe searches the genomic library until it locates a matching code on a specific chromosomal gene or a specific RNA sequence in cells or tissues.

Searching for a single gene remains complicated, because the gene can contain both coding exons and noncoding introns. If the clone with its isolated sequences contains only exons (i.e., only the uninterrupted coding sequences), then the new genomic library is called

DNA probe: radioactive or fluorescent-labeled nucleotide that identifies, isolates (targets), or binds to a gene or gene product

Hybridization: selective binding of two complementary nucleic acid strands (DNA or RNA) to detect specific nucleotide sequences

cDNA library: contains the genes' coding regions, including leading and trailing mRNA sequences

a **cDNA library** (the *c* refers to a copy or complementary DNA). Different cDNA libraries reflect different tissues because the libraries contain the specifically transcribed mRNA from the original source tissue. A cDNA library contains the gene's coding regions, often including the leading and trailing sequences of the mRNA. The absence of chromosomal DNA serves as a cDNA clone's most distinguishing feature. The enzyme reverse transcriptase uses the source cell or tissue mRNA to construct DNA. Cloning cDNA molecules is similar to cloning genomic DNA fragments. Each different type of tissue (e.g., heart, liver, kidney) has a different cDNA library associated with it. Cloned DNA makes it possible to manufacture exact copies of "pure" genetic material relatively quickly from among millions of nucleotide sequences. The uninterrupted coding sequence for a particular gene gives the cDNA clone a clear advantage for duplicating the gene in bulk or deducing a protein's amino acid sequence. Like genomic libraries, cDNA libraries exist in the public domain for sharing among researchers; commercial vendors also make them available for purchase. Many Internet sites provide valuable links to databases (e.g.,www.ddbj.nig.ac.jp/links-e/html) for mammals and other vertebrates, fungi, plants, eukaryotes, prokaryotes, viruses, specific gene groups, and large-scale genome sequencing centers. The unnumbered figure below illustrates the basic difference in creating genomic DNA and cDNA libraries. In both cases, fragments of digested DNA (shown as *purple* fragments) are inserted into cloning vectors such as phage.

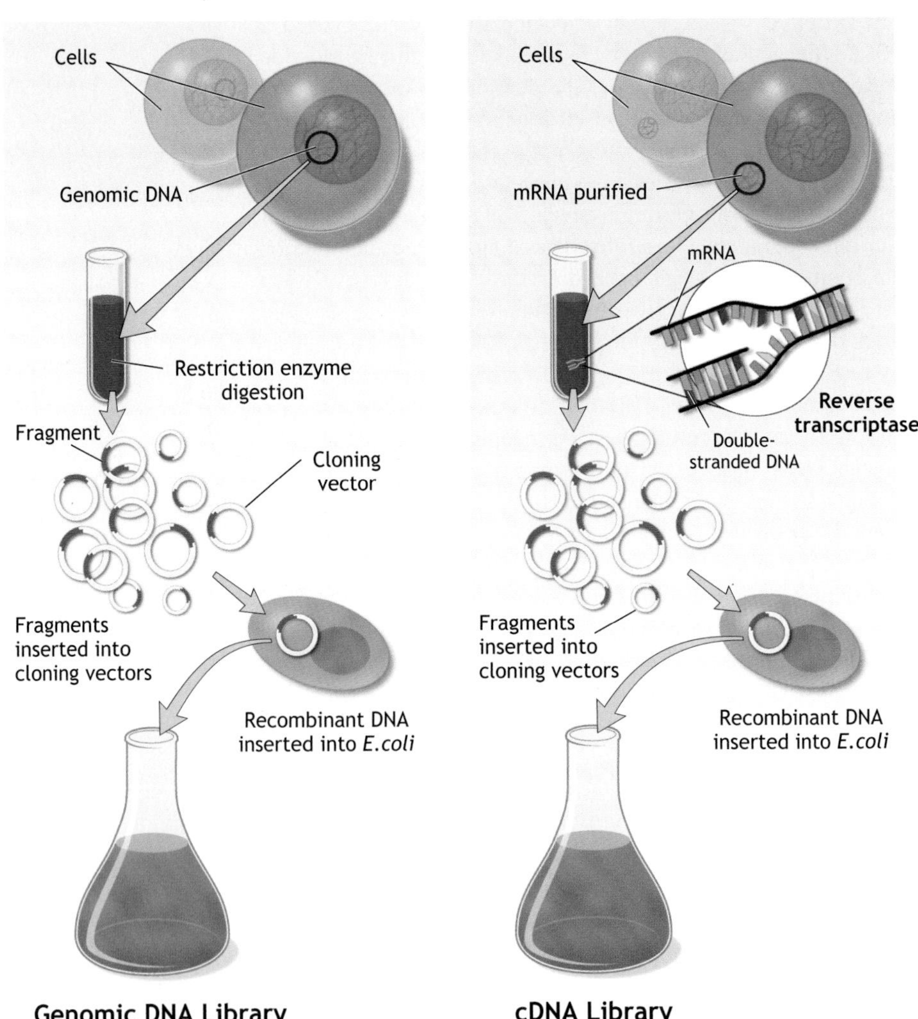

Electrophoresis and Gel Transfer Methods

The electrophoresis technique moves charged particles such as proteins through an electrically charged supporting medium. The negatively charged phosphate groups of DNA molecules migrate to the positive (anode) pole of the apparatus. Figure 30 shows two ways of

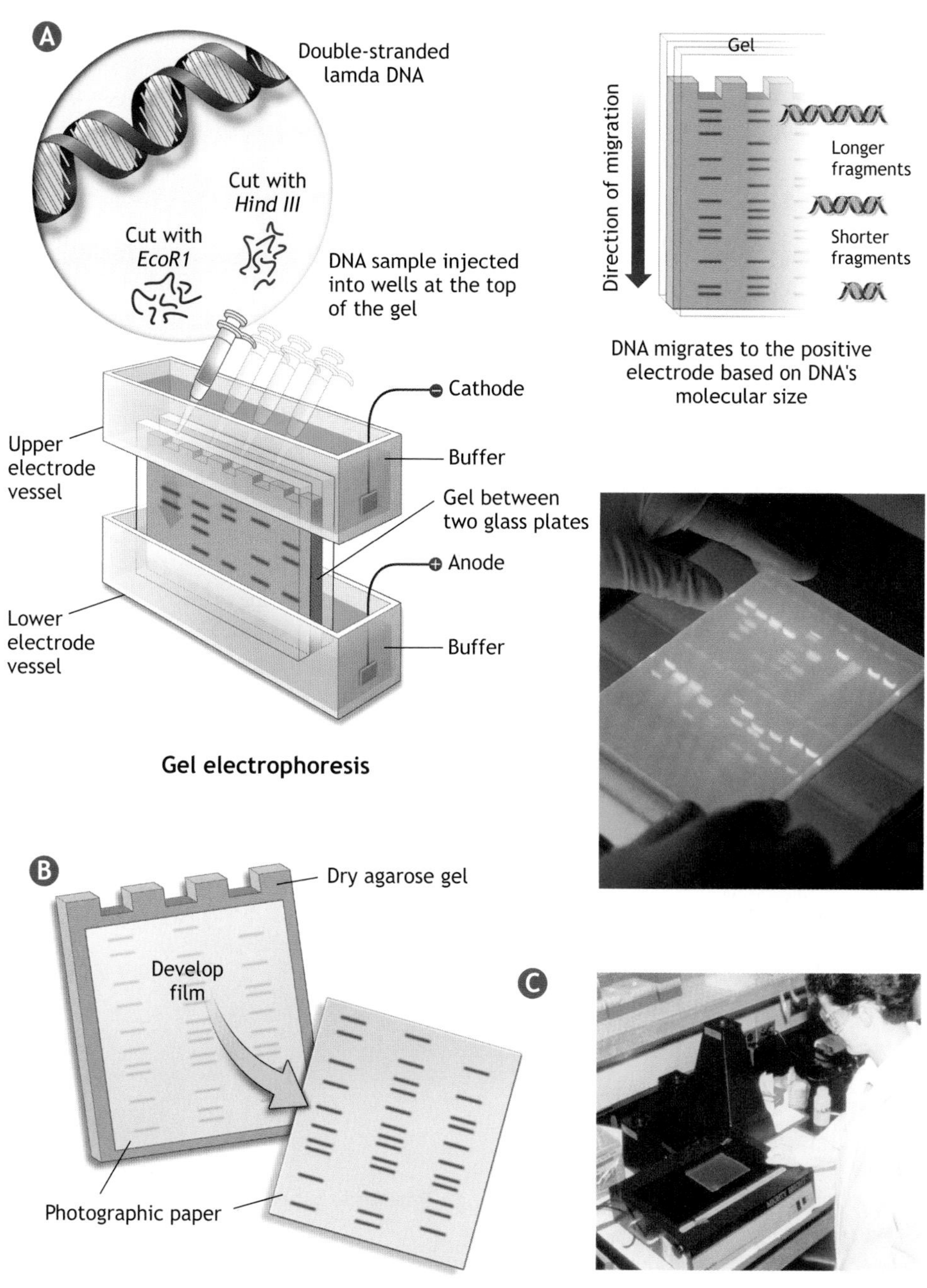

FIGURE 30 • Gel electrophoresis: separating DNA fragments by molecular size. **A**. Two restriction endonucleases cleave DNA into two segments for placement at the top of a thin agarose gel slab supported in a vertical position. An electric current separates the DNA fragments as they pass through the hydrated gel according to their mobility; small fragments move more quickly through the electric current and fixate at the bottom of the gel at the positive electrode. Larger fragments settle nearer to the top. The top right photo reveals the DNA bands fluoresced under ultraviolet light. Note: The restriction enzyme takes the initials of the bacterial type and strain from its source; *Eco*R1 refers to *E. coli* strain RY13, and the 1 means this restriction enzyme was found first in the strain. The cleavage site is 5′–GAATTC–3′ and 3′–CTTAAG–5′; the *HindIII* source is *Haemophilus influenzae* R_d. The cleavage site is 5′–AAGCTT–3′ and 3′–TTCGAA–5′. **B**. Autoradiography technique displays radioisotope ^{32}P-labeled DNA bands on exposed photographic paper placed over the agarose gel. **C**. Dr. Kristin Stuempfle, Department of Health and Exercise Sciences, Gettysburg College, reviewing the film of a sequencing gel on a light box.

separating DNA fragments. The top example (*A*) shows cutting the same DNA molecule from the λ (bacteriophage) genome with two different restriction endonucleases, *EcoR1* and *HindIII* (hundreds of other enzymes with distinct specificities have been isolated). Small fragments migrate faster than large fragments when they pass through the electric field from top (negative) to bottom (positive) through a slab of agarose gel. Heating the gel causes its protein fibers to congeal and form a grid through which DNA fragments pass. Separating DNA fragments by size in an electric field makes it relatively easy to distinguish among DNA segments. Note the bands at the *lower right panel* of the gel. These represent smaller DNA fragments than the upper longer fragments. The DNA shows up clearly in the bottom right photo because soaking the medium with a DNA- or RNA-specific dye (ethidium bromide) stains DNA orange (pink-like in photo), which becomes clearly visible under **ultraviolet light**. Extraction of DNA provides samples of pure DNA fragments. Purified DNA can be used in cloning experiments or for matching in size to other DNA fragments.

Ultraviolet light: electromagnetic rays at higher frequencies than the violet end of the visible spectrum

Radioisotope: isotope that becomes more stable by emitting radiation

Southern blotting: technique that detects single-stranded DNA from transferring DNA fragments to nylon paper with a DNA-binding probe

Northern blotting: hybridization technique that binds a DNA probe to a target RNA molecule; the technique detects a specific RNA sequence in a cell

Western blotting: technique for separating genetic fragments using a probe (usually an antibody) that binds to a target protein

In vitro: in an artificial environment such as a test tube or culture medium

Anneal: rejoin separated single complementary strands of DNA to form a double helix

Figure 30B shows an alternative technique using the labeled **radioisotope** ^{32}P to expose DNA bands when photographic paper placed over the gel reveals β particles emitted from the isotope. Figure 31 illustrates three gel transfer methods to separate fragments of genetic material and proteins: **Southern blotting**, **Northern blotting**, and **Western blotting**.

DNA Amplification with the Polymerase Chain Reaction

The polymerase chain reaction (PCR) method developed in 1987 by Dr. Kerry Mullis (1993 Nobel Prize in chemistry) represents a milestone in molecular biology.[91] The PCR method, carried out **in vitro** without prior transfer in living cells, artificially amplifies an extremely small amount of DNA and rapidly creates billions of copies of a specific region of a single DNA molecule. Figure 32A illustrates the basic concept of the PCR where purified DNA polymerase copies a DNA template in cycles of replication. In the first step of the initial cycle, a minute amount of double-stranded DNA is heated to about 94°C for several minutes to denature (separate) the strands. Each strand has a known sequence of nucleotides on either side of the target nucleotides. Next, two short, specifically designed synthetic primers of known DNA sequence (shown in *green* and *red*) hybridize or **anneal** to one of the two separated strands at the exact beginning and ending position of the target DNA nucleotide sequence. In other words, only the target sequence, bracketed by the primers, duplicates because no primers attach elsewhere along the DNA fragment.

The annealing process cannot withstand the initial high temperature required to separate the double helix so it occurs at a lower 54°C. At this temperature, the single-stranded DNA fragments match complementary nucleotide sequences at the ends of the target DNA

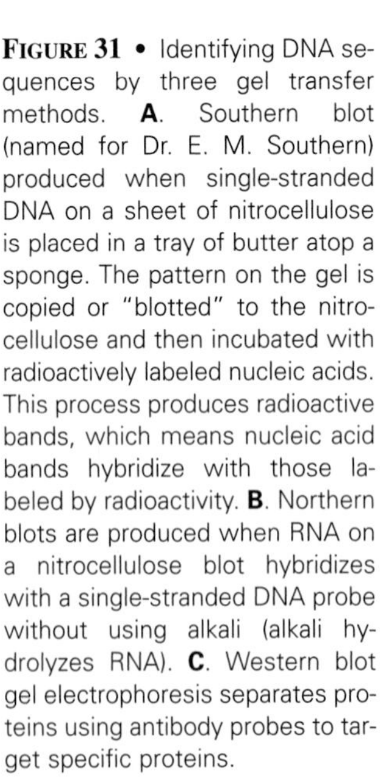

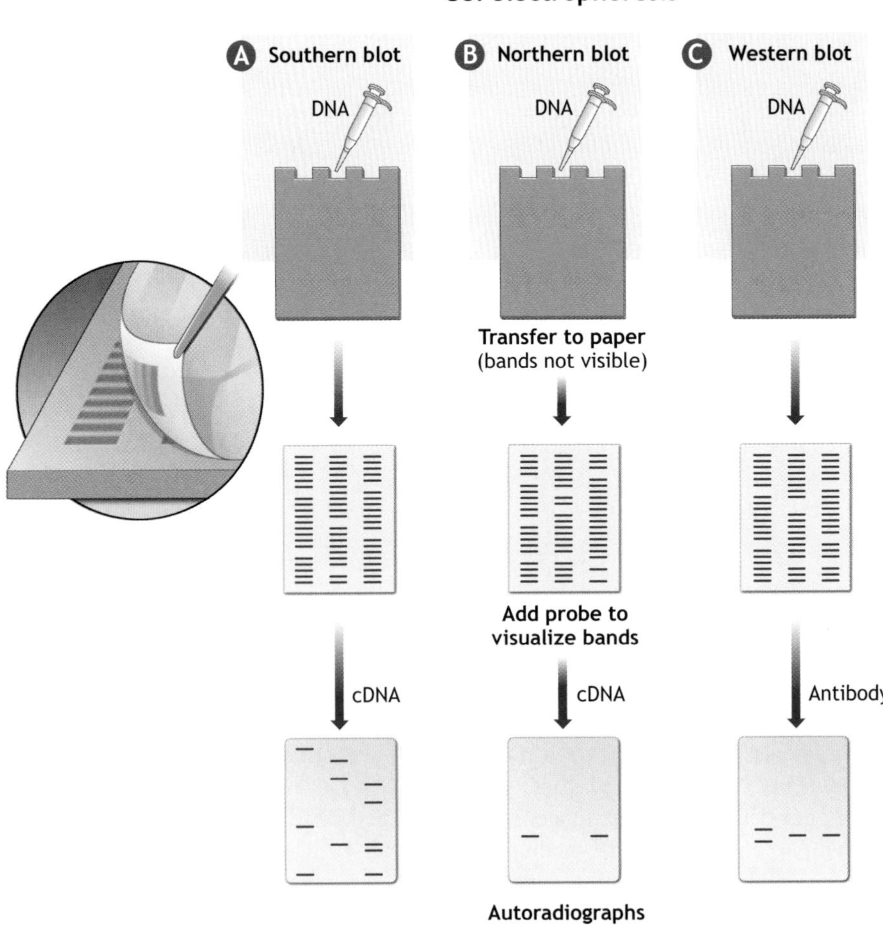

FIGURE 31 • Identifying DNA sequences by three gel transfer methods. **A**. Southern blot (named for Dr. E. M. Southern) produced when single-stranded DNA on a sheet of nitrocellulose is placed in a tray of butter atop a sponge. The pattern on the gel is copied or "blotted" to the nitrocellulose and then incubated with radioactively labeled nucleic acids. This process produces radioactive bands, which means nucleic acid bands hybridize with those labeled by radioactivity. **B**. Northern blots are produced when RNA on a nitrocellulose blot hybridizes with a single-stranded DNA probe without using alkali (alkali hydrolyzes RNA). **C**. Western blot gel electrophoresis separates proteins using antibody probes to target specific proteins.

sequence. DNA synthesis would not proceed without appropriate primers. Adding a heat-resistant DNA polymerase to the reaction in step 3 synthesizes a new DNA strand, now creating two strands. The most widely used polymerase (Taq) is isolated from the heat-resistant bacterium ***Thermus aquaticus***. The temperature, now increased to 70°C for another minute or two, lets the polymerase elongate new DNA strands that begin at the primers.

***Thermus aquaticus*:** thermally stable bacterium that survives at very high temperatures found in hot springs and geysers. The bacterium provides the important *Taq* DNA-replicating polymerase; voted 1989 "Molecule of the Year" by the prestigious journal *Science*

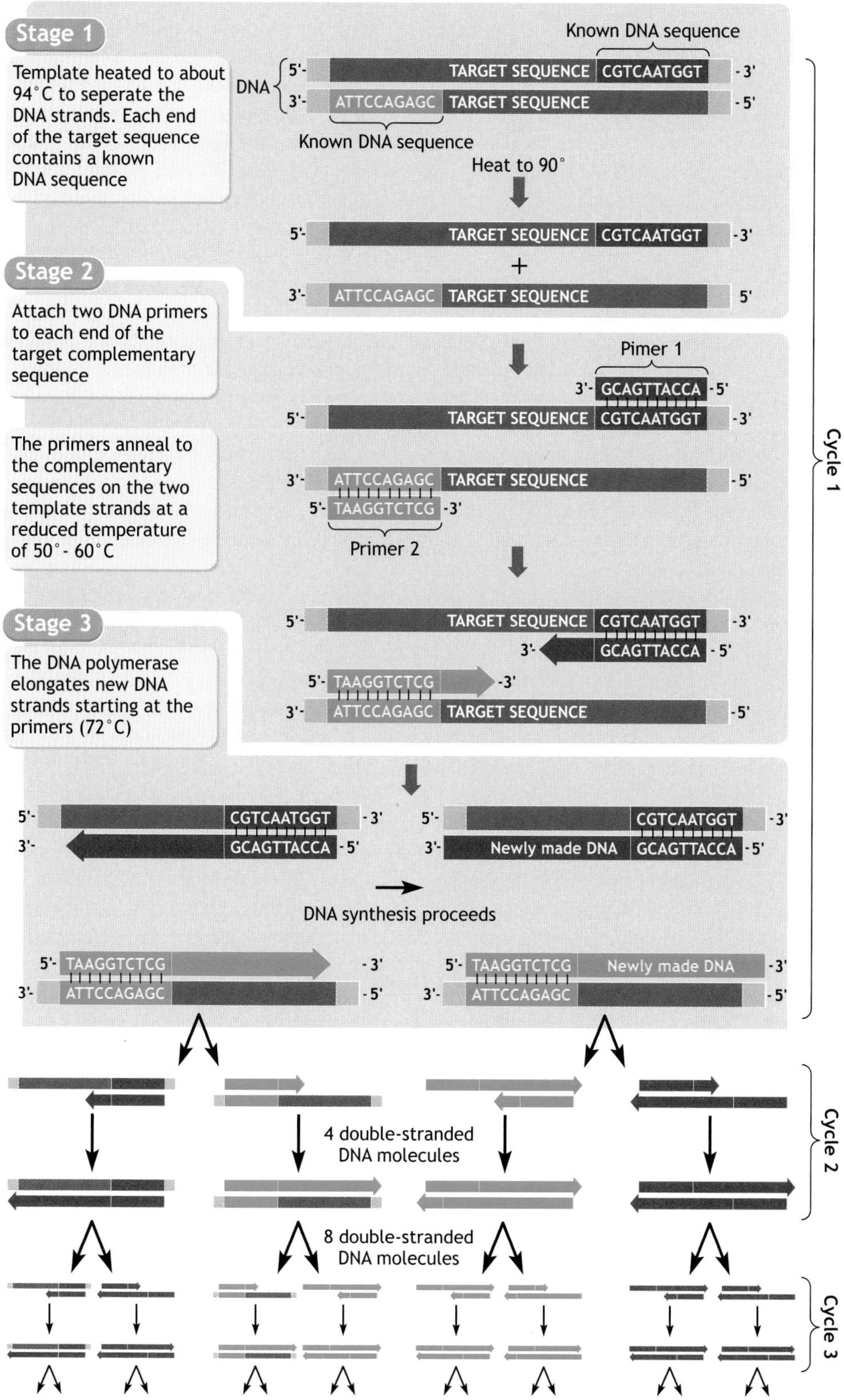

FIGURE 32 • Artificial DNA amplification using the PCR method. *Cycle 1.* Three stages during the first PCR cycle. *Cycle 2.* Second PCR cycle produces four double strands of DNA. *Cycle 3.* Third cycle produces eight double-stranded DNA molecules. Each succeeding cycle produces twice as much DNA as was produced in the previous cycle. Thirty cycles produce more than 1 billion DNA fragments. Several hours of production creates hundreds of billions of copies. The thermocycler PCR apparatus controls reaction temperature to ensure that repeated replication cycles and separation occur systematically on a preset schedule. The Internet site (info.med.yale.edu/genetics/ward/tavi/Guide.html) provides a step-by-step protocol guide for standard PCR and a variant termed multiplex PCR (for downloading as a PDF document).

Because the PCR technique requires that reactants cycle through a varied temperature profile during incubation, the PCR apparatus (thermocycler) automatically progresses through a preset thermal sequence. This first cycle, repeated 20 to 40 times, doubles the amount of DNA synthesized in each succeeding cycle.

The PCR method only clones DNA fragments with known beginning and ending sequences. With prior knowledge of the code, it takes only 20 repeat cycles to duplicate enough target DNA to produce 1,048,536 copies (2^{20}) of the original sequence. The second and third cycles displayed in Figure 30 show how the PCR method eventually copies millions (or billions) of the original DNA sequence. The second cycle repeats the first cycle. It progresses through each temperature change, first to separate strands at about 94°C, then to anneal the primers at a cooler 54°C, and finally through polymerase action to make two additional DNA strands at 72°C. Note that the third cycle produces eight double-stranded DNA molecules; after seven cycles, the newly created DNA consists of double strands with flush ends (same length) uniquely identical to the original target sequence. The next 17 cycles produce the additional 1,048,528 copies, and just 10 more cycles produce one-thousand million more target molecules!

Applications of PCR

The PCR technique affects numerous fields besides molecular biology, including biotechnology, entomology and the environmental sciences, molecular epidemiology, forensic science, genetic engineering, most medical specialties, microbiology, proteomics, the food industry, and even apparel manufacturing. For the 2000 Sydney Olympic Games, a special ink containing a small DNA snippet from a saliva swab from two Australian athletes was affixed to labels, tags, pins, and stickers of official Olympic merchandise to thwart counterfeiters. An electronic scanner could check the invisible ink to verify an item's authenticity. The same DNA-marking strategy, impossible to reverse-engineer, can verify rare and one-of-a-kind objects from premium grade oil to fine wine. PCR also can identify diverse viruses and bacteria or any DNA extracted from a current or ancient plant or animal organism. It identifies the unique sequence of a miniscule amount of DNA nucleotide material, even in substances millions of years old.

The amplification potential for PCR remains truly awesome. It requires only one-tenth of one-millionth of a liter (0.1 μL) of a substance such as saliva or another body fluid or tissue to prove that the genetic sample's sequence originated from a specific person or species. The PCR method can easily produce 1 μg of substance (about 500 base pairs long), equal to one-millionth of a gram (10^{-6}), enough to completely sequence or clone DNA. In fact, beginning with less than a picogram (0.000 000 000 001 or 10^{-12}) of DNA with a chain length of 10,000 nucleotides (about 100,000 molecules), in several hours PCR can produce several micrograms of DNA (10^{11} molecules). Interestingly, scientists have identified the genetic blueprint of insects trapped within 80 million–year-old amber (fossilized pine resin) from a miniscule amount of DNA, using present-day insects to "match" the DNA sequences. In a controversial report published in *Nature*, (October 2000), scientists reported reviving a bacterium (spore) from a drop of fluid trapped for 250 million years in a crystal of rock salt excavated 1850 feet below the Earth's surface. In extinct fossils, on the other hand, not enough DNA sequences exist for cloning because the DNA decomposes significantly every 5000 years. Thus, while some gene fragments may survive, cloning a "Jurassic Park" prehistoric monster falls outside the realm of possibility with today's available molecular archeology technologies.

In forensic medicine, a single hair salvaged from a crime scene can be matched for its DNA sequence to hair samples from a suspect or victim. When a PCR-generated DNA sequence matches the original DNA template strand sequence, chances of misidentifying the true suspect become almost infinitesimal against a coincidental DNA match. In fact, if an individual's known DNA profile matches the DNA profile from the crime scene, the probability is 82 billion to 1 that the DNA comes from that person!

Paternity: fatherhood

Autoradiography: process that produces an image (autoradiograph) on a photographic film placed flat on an electrophoresis gel; shows the position of radioactive molecules "transferred" to the gel

Paternity cases routinely involve DNA analysis using PCR techniques such as DNA fingerprinting **autoradiography** to identify parental offspring correctly (see Fig. 33). In the

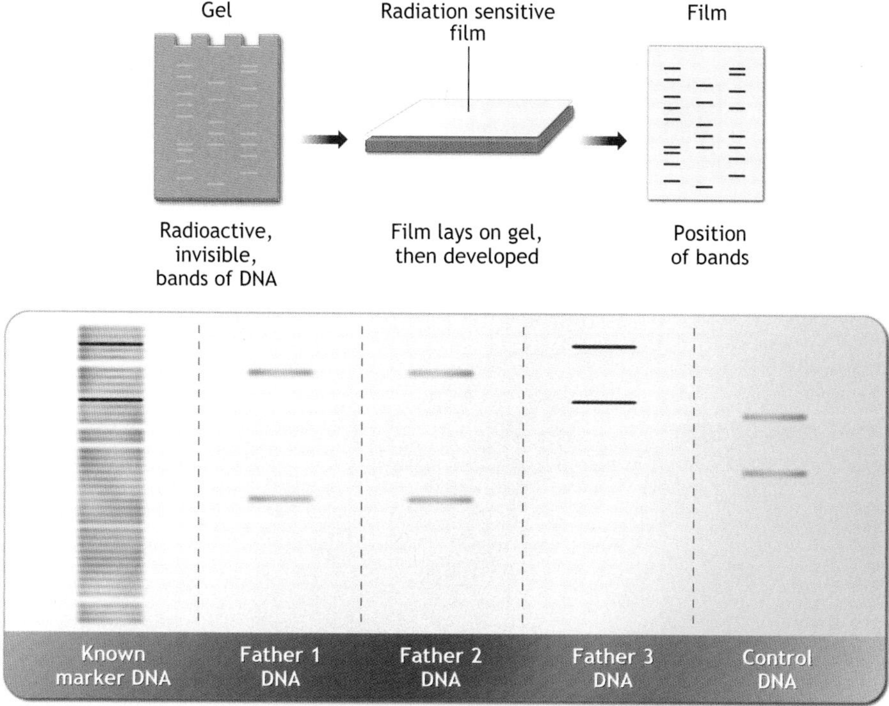

Figure 33 • DNA fingerprinting autoradiography compares DNA fragments after their separation by gel electrophoresis to identify the child's father. Matched patterns of DNA banding from different tissues or body fluids confirm the original DNA source. Specific restriction enzymes sever the DNA fragments at precise sites in the chain. Thus, snippets of DNA, known as RFLPs (**r**estriction **f**ragment **l**ength **p**olymorphisms), have different lengths and hence different molecular weights. A match between the known marker DNA and the sample (e.g., father 3) provides prima facia, direct evidence that father 3 is the biologic father. By the end of the year 2000, 43 previously convicted criminals were exonerated on the basis of DNA analysis of forensic evidence, often years following incarceration. Several hundred more criminal cases based on DNA analysis are currently pending. We recommend the following book for its riveting (but disturbing), frank discussion about criminal justice system and the important role DNA fingerprinting should play to ensure that the accused have the opportunity to present objective evidence (data) about criminal wrongdoing:

figure's example, the DNA from suspected fathers 1 and 2 did not match the known marker DNA from the child; thus father 3, with an exact banding match, was deemed the biologic father. The control DNA from a known source verifies the validity of the test procedures. The many variations of the PCR method allow researchers to produce hybrid genes with desirable (or undesirable) traits. Fusing DNA segments from different biologic specimens opens a tremendous avenue to study genetic variation in cells and tissues. It also elucidates how "errors" in specific gene sequences relate to diseases, and how genetic engineering can combat them.

Injection Experiments

Injection **transfection**, performed in cultured cells, refers to a microtechnique for introducing an outside (exogenous) DNA donor source into a recipient host. Injection of purified DNA with a known sequence of nucleotides for a particular gene presents a potentially desirable strategy for expressing an outcome trait in the host. Injection strategies have been useful in exercise physiology-related animal research. By injecting a gene with a particular trait into the egg of a mother, the new trait can be "turned on" in the offspring. This allows researchers to observe the effects of "knocking out" a section of one gene and replacing it with another segment to glean insight into the functional role of that gene product.

Consider the example in Figure 32 that illustrates the basic principle of microinjection applied to a rodent (mouse) model. Immediately after the **gametes** join (one egg and one sperm), a microinjection technique using a thin glass needle inserts a target gene (**transgene**) into the larger male **pronucleus** just before the cells fuse into a single egg. The egg(s) is then surgically harvested and implanted into the womb of a female rodent who serves as the "foster" mother. When the mother produces progeny, the newborns, referred to as **founder mice**, should carry a copy of the transgene on a single chromosome (i.e., be **heterozygous** for the transgene). When two founder mice breed, 25% of the progeny receive two copies of the transgene (i.e., are **homozygous** for the transgene), 50% have one transgene, and 25% have no transgenes. These percentages follow basic laws of inheritance discovered by geneticist Gregor Mendel (see page 972). Researchers have used hundreds of

Transfection: introduction of an external donor source of DNA into a recipient host

Gamete: egg or sperm

Transgene: genetic engineering technique that places a foreign gene in the cells of a different species

Pronucleus: fertilized egg containing the haploid egg or sperm nucleus

Founder mice: original engineered mice (with one copy of a transgene) bred together to create transgenic animals

Heterozygous: two different copies (alleles) of the same gene

Homozygous: two identical copies (alleles) of the same gene

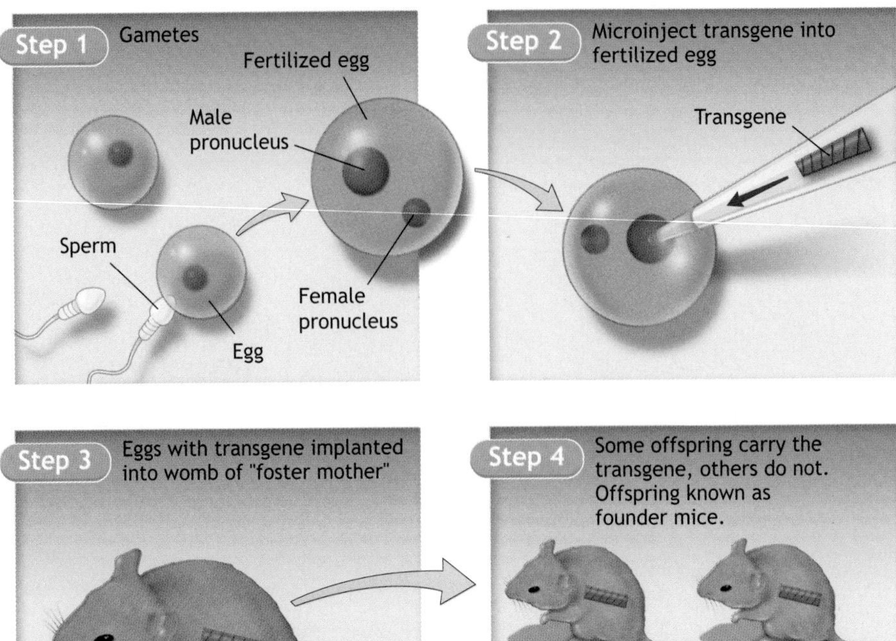

Figure 34 • Generalized procedure for creating transgenic offspring by injecting a target gene (transgene) into a fertilized egg. Some of the progeny, called founder mice, carry the transgene in their chromosomes, but the process may fail in others.

strains of transgenic organisms created with the above procedures to study the metabolic and developmental characteristic of many diseases.

Working with transgenic organisms has proved beneficial for experimenting with different genetic manipulations (including mutated genes) to shed light on possible mechanisms for disease conditions. Consider four ways researchers carry out such experiments:

Knockin animal model: harbors a specific mutation in a predetermined gene created and subsequently analyzed for altered drug responses

Knockout animal model: specific gene(s) inactivated (disabled) by inserting a gene cassette that disrupts the coding sequence (or operation) linked to a specific target gene

1. Replacing a normal gene with a mutant gene ("trading places") and observing effects on the offspring (a **knockin animal model**)
2. Inactivating or interrupting a normal gene's function and observing effects on the offspring (a **knockout animal model**)
3. Adding a mutant gene and observing the combined effects of the mutant gene *and* normal gene on the offspring
4. Increasing the expression of a given protein by increasing the number of copies of a gene

Because of its relevance to exercise physiology, we take a closer look on page 1030 at strategies for disabling genes related to obesity using the knockout technique elegantly described in 1994 by University of Utah researchers.

Cloning a Mammal

Totipotent: the cell possesses the required genetic information or "blueprint" to form an intact organism

Nuclear transfer: DNA removed from an unfertilized egg and introduced into the nucleus of a specially prepared cell by an electrical pulse or chemical to fuse the two substances together to initiate their development

Scientists at the Roslin Institute, Scotland, in 1997 tapped the complete genetic library contained within the zygote (i.e., cell **totipotent** potentiality) to clone the Dorset sheep "Dolly." This milestone represented the first such viable intact donor derived from adult mammalian cells.[138] The researchers removed an unfertilized oocyte (egg cell) from an adult ewe and replaced its nucleus with the nucleus from a mammary gland cell of an adult sheep. They then implanted this egg in another ewe, producing the healthy offspring sheep. The idea behind the **nuclear transfer** experiment was to produce genetically engineered transgenic mammals inexpensively that could reliably produce large quantities of pharmaceuticals in their milk. A likely benefit would be large quantities of human proteins for drug synthesis to treat diseases such as cystic fibrosis, hemophilia, and emphysema, with potential benefits toward aging and cancer research. Milk produced from transgenic sheep, goats, and cattle can yield up to 40 g of protein per liter at relatively low cost, circumventing the need to use purified, expensive blood to harvest protein with risk of contamination from AIDS or hepatitis C. Proteins produced in human cell cultures have high cost and relatively low yields. Transgenetically produced proteins have application in the **nutriceutical** industry, **xenotransplantation**, animal models of disease, and cell therapy.

The first Dolly experiments represented a milestone in cloning technology, but not before unleashing a firestorm of criticism concerning ethical and scientific issues related to the possibilities of eventual experiments with human cloning. Figure 35 shows that Dolly possesses the same genes as the cells from the ewe's udder. The reproductive cell cycle developed normally following intermediate stages (keeping donor cells "**quiescent**" so their DNA did not replicate or divide) until the early embryo developed. The researchers then transplanted the embryo into a receptive ewe (Scottish blackface sheep). Following several hundred unsuccessful implants, Dolly was born from the implanted ewe and survived. Dolly subsequently gave birth through normal mating to produce three additional, healthy lambs.

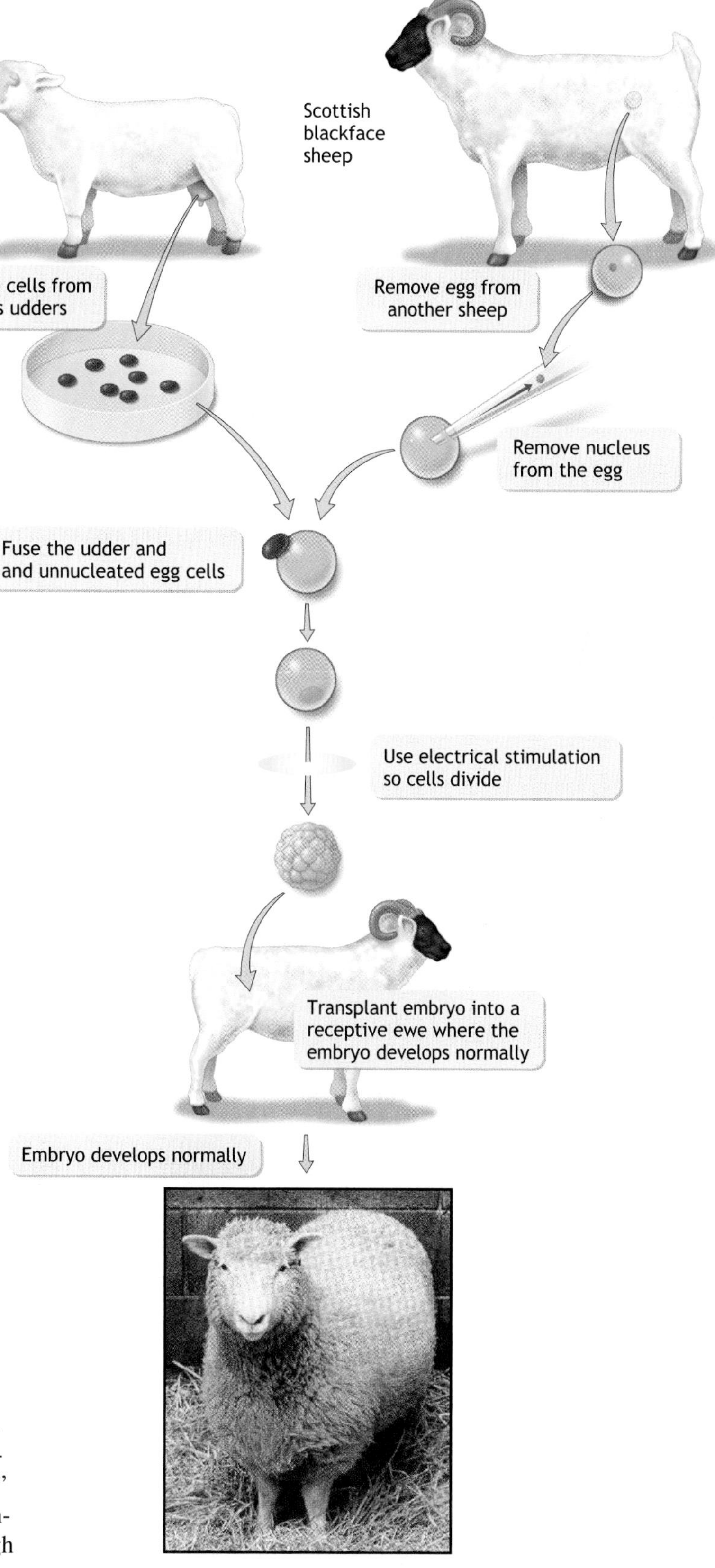

FIGURE 35 • Steps in cloning a mammal. Dorset sheep Dolly (bottom photo) has identical genes as the ewe that donated the original genes (Dorset sheep, upper left).

Subsequent research with a technique called "gene-targeting" offers new hope for correcting genetic defects caused by "faulty" genes.[86] Scottish researchers inserted a human DNA sequence (the human gene for α-1 antitrypsin, a malfunctioning enzyme in familial emphysema) into a specific chromosome region of an adult sheep cell. These modified cells were then fused with sheep eggs from each nucleus into a fertilized sheep egg stripped of its original nucleus. The eggs were grown into embryos and then implanted in ewes. The nuclear transfer technique produced two cloned lambs, Cupid and Diana, whose modified cells contained specific targeted changes in their genetic machinery. In addition to implanting a therapeutic transgene, the researchers included a targeting sequence that ensured the gene "turned on" only in the mammary glands to produce high concentrations of α-1 antitrypsin in milk. This breakthrough technology allows researchers to "turn off" genes at precise locations, thereby controlling subsequent protein function. For example, altered genetic sequences in pigs or other animals could neuter xenoreactive transplantation antigens involved in tissue rejection, thereby enhancing organ transplants from animals to humans. In this way, animals could serve as organ banks for humans. Enhancing favorable genetic

Nutriceutical: genetically engineered product that alters or modifies characteristics of a product or its by-product

Xenotransplantation: transfer of organs or tissues from a donor of one species to a recipient of another. Successful transplants require that the immune system of the recipient accept the donor organ successfully

Quiescent: having all but the most fundamental functions of a cell or group of cells stopped; in essence, with switched-off genes that define the special functions of the cell (i.e., restricting food supply or creating an unfavorable internal cellular environment)

Gene cassette: artificially constructed DNA segment containing a genetic marker with restriction sites at both ends of the nucleotide segment

Pseudopregnant: ovulation induced by sterile copulation

Germ line: cell lineage consists of mature reproductive germ cells (sperm, egg)

Pro-opiomelanocortin (POMC): precursor of neurotransmitters (β-endorphin) and hormones (melanocortin peptides), whose roles include pigmentation, adrenocortical function, food intake and fat storage, and immune and neural functions

Neurohormone: hormone formed by neurosecretory cells and liberated by nerve impulses (e.g., norepinephrine)

traits (and deleting undesirable ones explained in the next section on knockout genes) could improve animal milk and meat quality by making products tastier and more nutritious. Likewise, inactivating genes responsible for neuropathogenic disease offers substantial medical benefits, including diminished worldwide health-care costs when the newer technologies become more cost-effective.

Gene Knockout Technique

Mice provide a useful model for studying genetic manipulations because of great control afforded the experimental subjects, environment, and shorter life span. For example, researchers can study a strain of normal-sized mice with black fur, obese mice with black fur, obese mice with white fur, and so on. Genetic "tampering" could verify whether the gene actually modulated the specific effect, independent of its influence on fur color. Deactivating a gene(s) within the DNA known to produce an obese strain of mice should produce litters of normal-weight mice.

Figure 36 shows the experimental strategy for creating a transgenic mouse with a knocked-out gene.

- A DNA fragment receives a genetically modified gene (**gene cassette** shown in *purple*), thus altering the target gene's usual nucleotide sequence.
- Growth of the cell culture produces one or more cell colonies containing the altered gene. Finding such a colony means the mutant gene altered the DNA fragment.
- Inject the genetically altered cells into the developing embryo of a previously mated female mouse.
- Place the developing embryo into a normal **pseudopregnant** mouse who gives birth to a litter where most progeny possess cells with the altered gene.
- Mating two offspring with the mutant gene can produce an offspring with the mutant gene on each of two chromosomes. The grafted transgene can also be incorporated into the mice from another strain of mouse into a totally different organism.

If the original gene alteration inactivated the function of one of the genes, then the transgenic mouse inherits the mutant gene that replaced or "knocked out" the primary target gene. This strain of mice can be reliably bred to produce progeny with the foreign gene now permanently part of their **germ line** DNA. In studying the etiology of cancer, for example, two transplanted oncogenes (*ras* and *myc*) remain dominant in the host and always produce a mouse with cancer. The same strategy can apply to study mechanisms of obesity described below.

Knockout Mice to Study Mechanisms of Obesity

Researchers have developed transgenic mice lacking the gene that encodes for the complex molecule **pro-opiomelanocortin (POMC)**, produced mainly in the brain and skin.[142] POMC, a precursor of melanocortin peptides, possess a wide range of physiologic properties, including roles in food intake and body fat accumulation. The researchers originally intended to study POMC-deficient mice to evaluate **neurohormone** signaling and CNS functioning. Their strain of transgenic mutant mice overate and became obese, with altered pigmentation that produced yellowish fur on their abdomen instead of typical brownish-black fur. They also showed significantly less adrenal tissue than litter mates of normal size and color. Figure 37A shows that after 1 month of age, the body weight of the mutant mice steadily increased to twice the weight of normal litter mates.

These findings coincided with a previous report describing a rare genetic disease in two children caused by a mutant *Pomc* gene.[76] These red-haired children had no melanocortins, and they developed severe obesity soon after birth and suffered adrenal insufficiency. *Panel D* in Figure 37 shows the rapid weight gain of this young girl and boy whose weight far exceeded typical age standards. The connection between the mice and children was striking; functional characteristics caused by the *Pomc* gene mutation in humans paralleled those in the transgenic mice with yellow pigmentation and obesity.

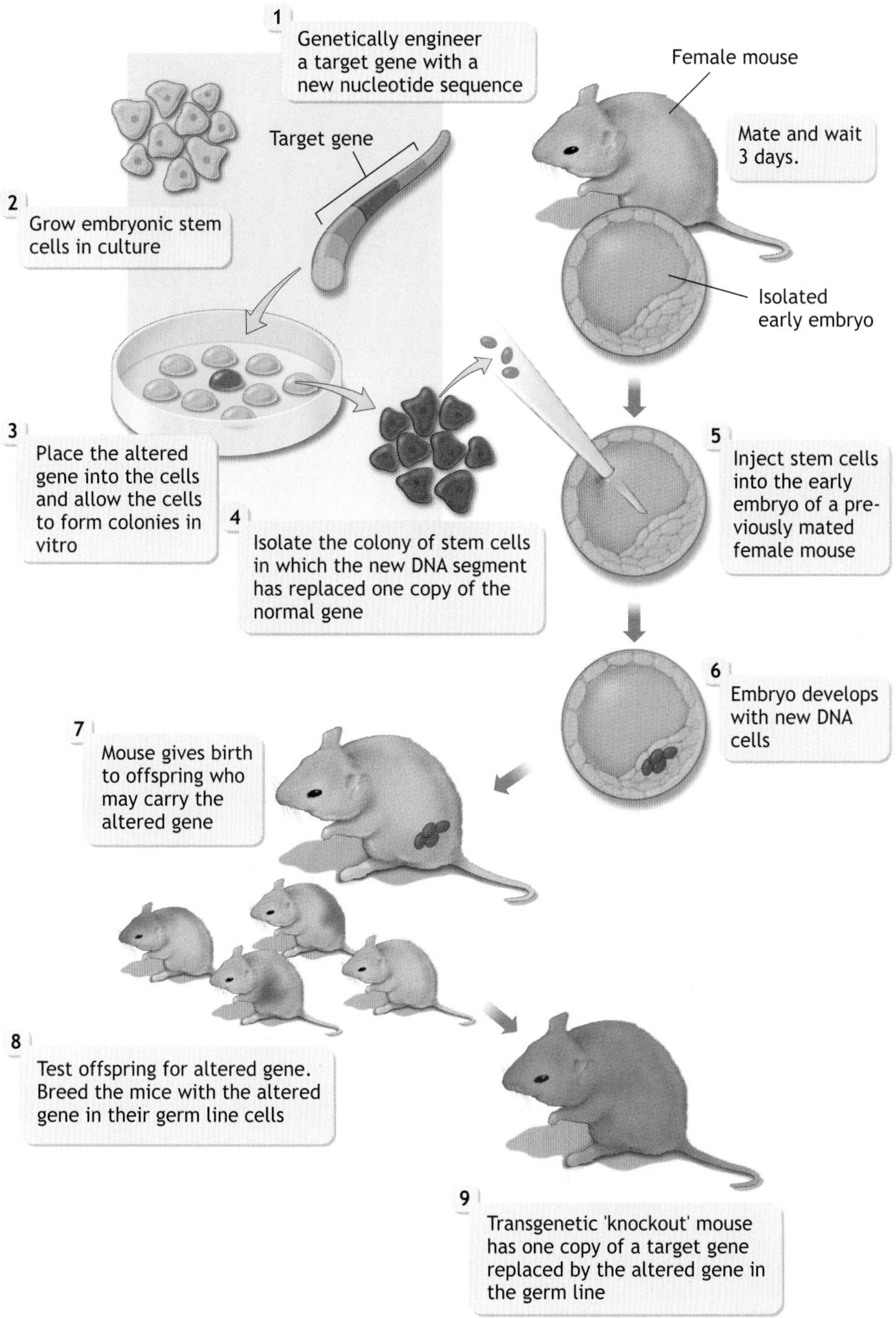

FIGURE 36 • Creating a transgenic mouse with a knocked-out gene.

Injecting the obese, POMC-deficient mice with the melanocortin peptide, α-melanocyte-stimulating-hormone agonist (α-MSH) produced a significant body weight loss within 1 day; within 1 week, body weight decreased by about 38% and declined further to 48% after the second week (Figure 37B). A reversal also occurred in the pigmentation of the mice, and their fur lost its yellowish tinge. Within 10 days of terminating α-MSH "therapy," the mice began to regain lost weight, reaching preinjection weight in another 14 days. Their yellow fur color in the ventral and dorsal sites also reappeared. In contrast, α-MSH injections and subsequent cessation of treatment produced no effect on body mass or fur pigmentation in normal control litter mates. The researchers explained that weight loss during treatment exceeded expectations from the energy-balance equation. This occurred although the mutant mice ate significantly more food daily than the control mice (35.7 g vs. 24.2 g;

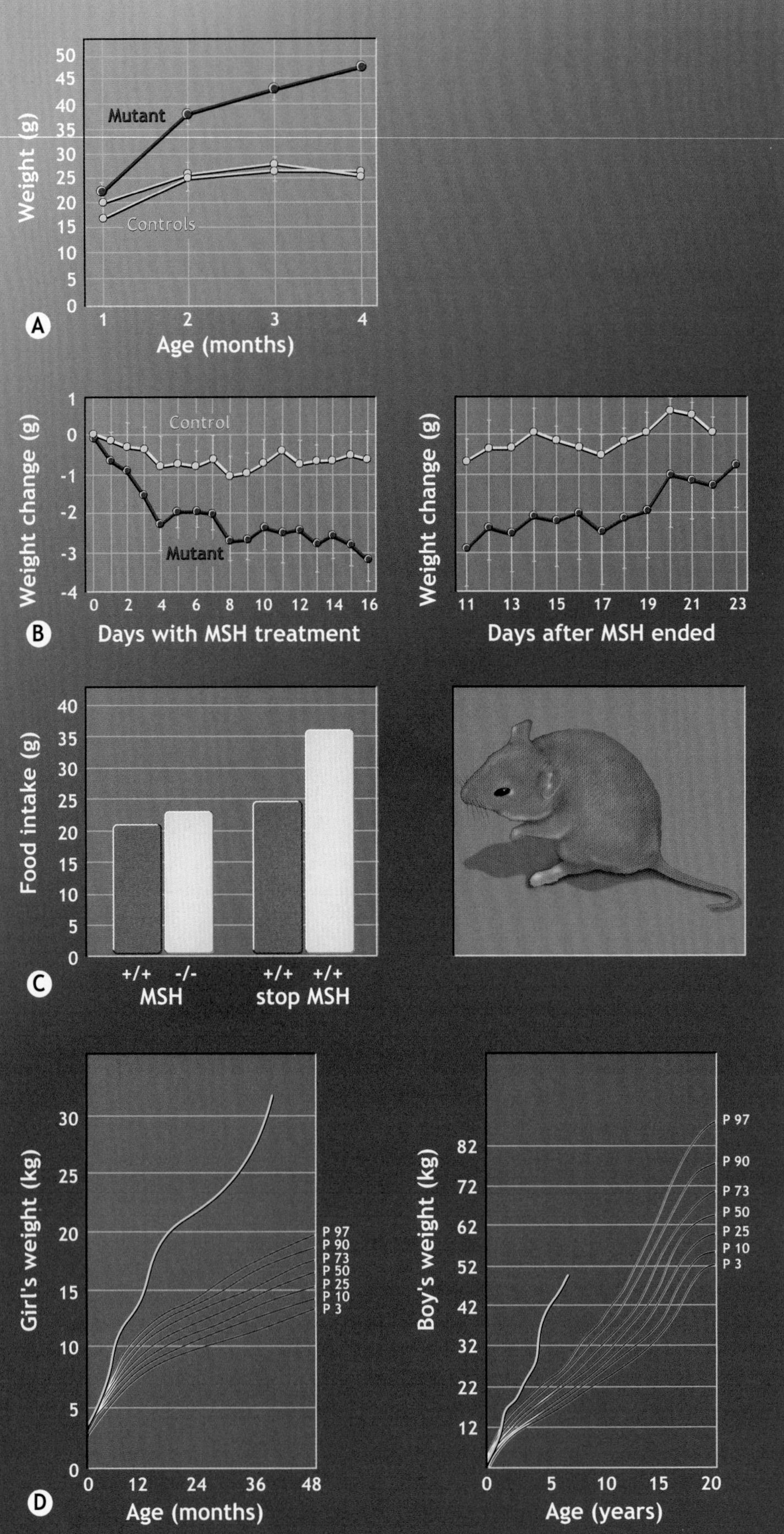

FIGURE 37 • POMC-deficient transgenic mice provide new clues to obesity. **A**. Body weight gain in mutant and control mice. **B**. Change in body weight with and without treatment. **C**. Differences in food intake with and without treatment. **D**. Extreme weight gain in a young boy and girl with the POMC mutation. The white lines represent growth curves for children representing the 3rd through 97th percentile (p). (Data from A, B, and C modified from Yaswen L, et al. Obesity in the mouse model of pro-opiomelanocortin deficiency responds to peripheral melanocortin. Nat Med 1999;5:1066. Data in D from Krude H, et al. Severe early-onset obesity, adrenal insufficiency and red hair pigmentation caused by POMC mutations in humans. Nat Genet 1998;19:155.)

Fig. 34C). Because fat cells contain melanocortin receptors, and these receptors induce **lipolysis**, melanocortin-based drugs may eventually prove helpful as therapeutic agents to combat obesity. Interestingly, injections of MSH analogs also reduced excess body fat in another strain of obese transgenic mice, deficient in the hormone **leptin**.[60] In studies of 87 unrelated Italian obese children and adolescents, three new mutations were identified within the POMC signal peptide (substitution of Ser with Thr at codon 7; Ser with Leu at codon 9; Arg with Gly at codon 236).[38] The researchers believe the mutations in codons 7 and 9 of the signal peptide alter the translocation of pre-POMC into the endoplasmic reticulum, and therefore, explain the linkage between POMC and the genetic predisposition to obesity, a view shared by others studying this association. Further studies of genetic variations in the POMC coding region should provide new insights concerning the etiology of obesity.[39,45,77] On-going experiments with transgenic animal and human models will help researchers understand the etiology of obesity and its treatment.[96] Extremes in obesity have been linked to DNA polymorphisms in the translated portion of the leptin (LEP) gene.[83] Leptin-regulated endocannabinoids (marijuana-like substances naturally produced in the brain) stimulate appetite and play a role in food regulation as a component in the leptin signaling cascades.[41] In the not-too-distant future, excess body fat may provide a ready source of stem cells from which to create replacement tissues (e.g., bone, muscle, cartilage) for diseased or damaged ones.[145] Incorporating a person's own stem cells would avoid rejection of transplanted tissue and circumvent moral objections concerning the use of human embryonic stem cells.

Lipolysis: splitting up (hydrolysis) or chemical decomposition of triglyceride

Leptin: protein hormone involved with appetite and fat storage

Newer approaches also apply genetic techniques using **antisense RNA** to suppress expression of a target gene as a way to assess gene function. By incompletely blocking the function of knockout genes, researchers should be able to uncover unexpected roles for sequenced genes.[42] The field of proteomics (using sophisticated imaging software and molecular scanners integrated with protein chemistry techniques) also offers a new approach to study how proteins expressed in a genome act in complex, biologic processes.[62] For example, scientists have developed an ion channel "nanopore" technique that discriminates among almost identical DNA molecules that differ by only one base pair or one nucleotide.[125] This level of differentiation permits highly accurate molecular identification to unscramble intricacies of gene expression, and ultimately to develop strategies that target mutagens.

Antisense RNA: RNA complementary in sequence to mRNA, thus capable of base pairing with it by using the nontemplate strand of DNA to transcribe RNA from it. Analogous to two original strands in DNA base-pairing with each other. In practice, synthesis of an oligonucleotide hybridizes a mutant mRNA sequence, stopping its translation into protein

HUMAN PERFORMANCE RESEARCH

Molecular biologists studying physical activity and exercise training seek to decipher signaling pathways by which genes transcribe the effects of a mechanical stressor and resultant phenotypic expression. For example, resistance training applies muscular overload of the biceps as a mechanical stressor,[97,126] while increasing upper-arm strength and size represent expression of a phenotype characteristic. Crucial, unanswered questions concern "where" and "how" skeletal overload translates into newly acquired "strength" and muscular hypertrophy. The answers likely reside within signal transduction pathways leading from cell surface receptors to the nucleus, resulting in transcription of genes and subsequent protein synthesis.[13,59] Little doubt remains that scientists will progressively uncover the secrets of the genome as they learn more about the intricacies of how different signaling processes interact, integrate, and differentiate to produce function and consequences, and possibly even share common intermediates.[15,59]

Consider a seemingly simple series of movements such as releasing the bowstring when shooting an arrow and the highly complex maneuvers of a triple back summersault from a 10-m diving platform. The movement patterns of both activities require precise coordination and integration of neural stimulation and muscular action. In turn, each component of the movement demands specific timing and force requirements to achieve a desired outcome. At the molecular level, thousands of enzymes govern such precision requirements, each turning on and off at precisely the right time and in the correct sequence to make the movement successful (or unsuccessful). A better understanding of signaling processes governing enzyme activity between stressors and genes may someday explain the how and why of individual differences in human movement capacities. For example, why does one identical twin perform better than their twin in a particular activity? Identical twins come from the same genetic pool, so one would expect few differences in performance between them, but this is not the case. Even if twins had identical experiences in mastering the mechanics of an activity, from practice time to coaching, their performance levels would differ. Fractions of a second or tenths of a centimeter often mean the difference between victory and second place—whether the performers are twins or Olympic-caliber athletes. A combination of biochemical individuality and known allelic variations should enable researchers to determine optimal nutritional profiles (i.e., targeted doses of vitamins, minerals, and other nutrients) to create personalized comprehensive lifestyle prescriptions tailored to the needs of each person.[46] A tremendous challenge also exists among the disciplines to determine the molecular basis of disease expression, as for example, for type 2 diabetes that has increased 39% in the United States from 1990 to 1999.[3,89]

When reduced to the most fundamental level, all physical activities, or aspects of all life, ultimately depend on the multiplicity of molecular events that turn genes on and off. The new generation of molecular exercise scientists must expand research to uncover how different signaling mechanisms regulate transcriptional, translational, and posttranslational events. Elucidation of these mechanisms will enable scientists to manipulate experimental variables to answer questions related to our field. For example, how does long-term exercise intensity and duration alter levels of a specific mRNA or an upstream signaling molecule such as Ca^{+2}, an intermediary involved in multiple signal transduction cascades?[47] A simple muscle contraction corresponds to a 100-fold increase in intramuscular Ca^{+2} concentration (from 10^{-7} M to 10^{-5} M). Some researchers believe the huge Ca^{+2} influx, which coincides with myofilament cross-bridge cycling (see Chapter 18), serves as an important signaling messenger that links a muscle's function to transcriptional dynamics.[6] Other exercise-related physiologic regulators of transcription include hypoxia and cellular oxidative stress (or redox). The hypoxic state affects production of erythropoietin (EPO gene) and **glucose transporter-1 (GLUT-1)**.[44] Understanding the functional characteristics of how genes operate under hypoxic conditions will provide key information about oxygen delivery to cells and ultimately its use via citric-acid–cycle reactions, electron transport, and ATP synthesis associated with oxidative energy transformations.[63,144]

Glucose transporter-1 (GLUT-1): facilitates glucose transport across the plasma membrane independently of the hormone insulin

Reactive oxygen species (ROS): oxygen free radical formed from imprecise coupling during oxygen's reduction to water in the final stage of electron transport–oxidative phosphorylation

Thioredoxin: protein involved in oxidation-reduction reactions to balance the cell's redox state

Oxygen free radicals and reducing agents (i.e., antioxidants) also modulate transcription.[114] In Chapter 6, we discuss how the mitochondrion's reduction of oxygen to form water serves as the final common step in ATP synthesis. Imprecise coupling of this pathway forms free radicals of oxygen. Diverse antioxidants within skeletal muscle then scavenge and quench most of these **reactive oxygen species (ROS)**.[111] However, during high-intensity endurance exercise when aerobic metabolism increases 15- to 20-fold, ROS form in greater numbers and possibly produce damaging effects similar to lipid peroxidation.[37,90,139,140] The protein **thioredoxin**, which reduces oxidized proteins, helps to balance a cell's redox state during energy metabolism and also appears to affect transcriptional activity.[61,65] Determining how ROS influence transcription will pave the way for improved understanding of long-term health effects (or potential risks) of aerobic-type activities. Researchers have discovered that endurance training nearly doubles mitochondrial protein and mitochondrial mass.[64,92] This means that having a robust experimental model (endurance exercise/training) from which to study gene expression will surely lead to important discoveries about the essence of endurance exercise effects and adaptations per se. In fact, experiments have already described alterations in mRNA gene expression with long-term electrical stimulation,[143] including exercise effects related to muscle mitochondrial and overall cellular activity[21,49,56,67,70,93,98,120,122,130,141] and molecular-related alterations in skeletal muscle and muscle fiber type.[15,18,19,48,110,118] Microgravity's effects on gene expression in skeletal muscle provide a fruitful area for further study.[2,8,10,11,12,25-27,37,40,54,55,57,99,117,135,144] Studies of identical twins attempt to explain why one individual tends to participate regularly in sports and physical activities while the other twin shows little inclination to remain physically active. As part of the Heritage Family Study,[31,71,103,107,113,136,137] a search for genes related to body composition changes following 20 weeks of exercise training from 364 sib-pairs from 99 Caucasian families provided evidence of linkage of fat-free mass and insulin-like growth factor 1 genes, including gene sites for BMI and fat mass, and plasma leptin levels with the low-density lipoprotein receptor gene.[31] Further study of the genomic basis of training-induced changes in body composition with systematic endurance-type training will help to enlighten mechanisms in body weight regulation.

Another viable area for application of molecular biology research to the sport sciences involves various gene therapy techniques (viral and nonviral delivery strategies) (1) to treat acute and chronic musculoskeletal injuries such as muscle tears, cartilage defects, and tendon ruptures; (2) to reconstruct ligaments, osseous nonunions, and meniscus tears; and (3) to transplant tissue or genetic material. One hopes that inserting relevant genes directly into target tissues, or systemically via vectors into the bloodstream, will increase the probability of successful therapy and accelerated recuperation.[85] Researchers in the molecular biology sciences are just now beginning to track down the flaws in human DNA that cause debilitating muscoskeletal disease, as for example, those involved with lumbar disks.[5,80,84,123] One must temper such expectations by perhaps justifiable concerns that genetic engineering's potential benefits could also result in "tinkering" with issues related to doping and drug testing.

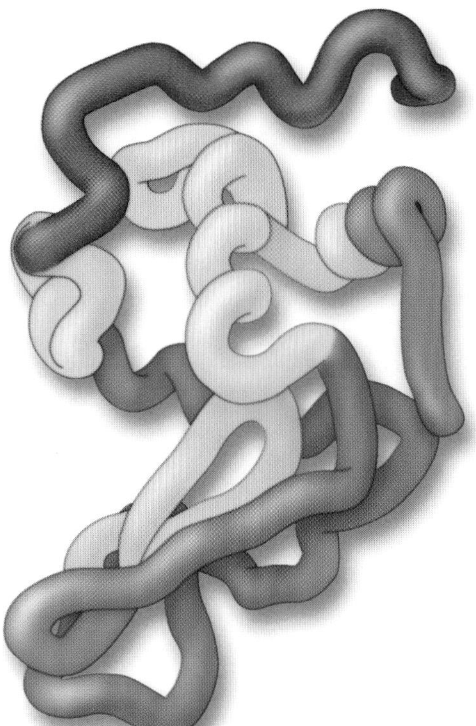

FIGURE 38 • Computer-generated model of hen egg white **lysozyme** (HEWL) color coded to show regions of high *(red)* and lower *(blue and yellow)* stability constants when binding to monoclonal antibody D1.3 (along the *red* area). Lysozyme, discovered by Sir Alexander Fleming (1881–1955) 5 years before he discovered penicillin, protects against bacterial infection. This small enzyme, the first ever to have its structure solved, attacks the bacterial protective cell wall. Some bacteria build a protective outer layer of carbohydrate chains interlocked by short peptide strands, which brace their delicate plasma membranes against their high intracellular osmotic pressure. Lysozyme breaks these carbohydrate chains, destroying the cell membrane's structural integrity, and the bacteria burst under their own internal pressure. The lysozyme from hen egg whites protects proteins and fats that nourish the developing chick. (Figure constructed using program GRASP [trantor.bioc.columbia.edu/grasp/]. Dr. Ernesto Freire. Professor of Biology and Biophysics. Director of the Biocalorimetry Center. The Johns Hopkins University, Baltimore.)

Lysozyme: enzyme that destroys the structural layer of some bacterial cell walls

New techniques of molecular and cell biology such as nuclear magnetic resonance–detected carbon-14, nitrogen-15, and hydrogen exchange now make it possible to study aspects of protein structure and functions.[52] For example, the computer-generated structural model of a protein in Figure 38 shows color-coded regions of high- and low-stability constants when binding to another molecule such as **monoclonal antibody** D1.3. The *red region* that interacts directly with D1.3 shows the highest stability; the *yellow* and *blue regions* remain unaffected by D1.3 binding. Thus, high and low regions of stability within a protein molecule may relate differently to its functional associations with other molecules. The important implication for protein synthesis is that sites within the conformational structure of a molecule may serve dual functions, depending on the molecule's configuration and structural residues.

Monoclonal antibody: pure antibody of a single type that only recognizes a single antigen; produced in cell culture as a fusion product from a cancer cell and an antibody-producing cell

As far as we know, no research in exercise molecular biology has studied whether exercise training might induce changes in a protein's structure. Will these changes alter the regions(s) within the molecule for cooperative binding or interactions among binding pathways with other molecules?

Crucial questions concern what "signals" control cooperation among different molecules, and whether changes occur selectively in some proteins (in certain regions within the molecule) and not others? A question such as the following, for example, requires an answer: "What contribution do both genetics and environmental factors affect the complex etiology of many common and debilitating diseases?"[24] The model describing gene-exercise interaction (Fig. 39) affects health status indirectly by altering gene expression that itself impacts intermediate phenotypes and disease outcome. In addition, increased physical activity (exercise) and training influence health. A crucial challenge remains: scientists must identify the function and interaction of the genes in this schema.

We hope that during the first decade of the third millennium, researchers from varied disciplines will cross boundaries to solve unanswered questions in exercise physiology. Working together, exercise physiologists trained in molecular biology (or molecular biologists with training in exercise physiology) can profit from the insights of biologists, geneti-

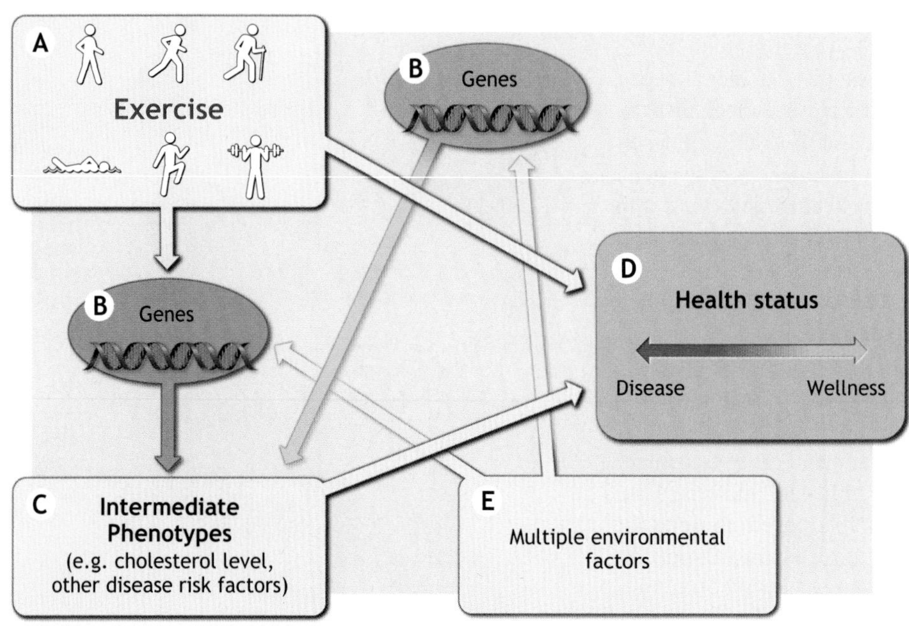

FIGURE 39 • Model of gene-exercise interaction, intermediate phenotype and multiple environmental factor interactions in determining health status along the disease–wellness continuum. (Adapted from Bray MS. Genomics, genes, and environmental interaction: the role of exercise. J Appl Physiol 2000;88:788.) Note: The journal Medicine & Science in Sports & Exercise announced plans to publish an annual update of the human gene map for performance and health-related fitness phenotypes. The inaugural issue (Rankinen T, et al. Med Sci Sports Exerc 2001; 33:855) contains specific reference to genes and their location published through December 2000. The initial work was a collaboration among scientists at five laboratories who have worked in the area pertaining to the genetics of fitness and performance.

cists, pharmacologists, and chemists who study human physical activity at the molecular level. Then shared explorations will benefit all humanity.

> . . . there can be no doubt that this treasure of genetic information will irrevocably change our view of our place in the world. Our children will be diagnosed for diseases they have not even developed and treated with drugs that match their body chemistry. Our grandchildren may be plucked from a pool of cells bathing in a petri dish after being screened for hidden flaws in their DNA. And our great-grandchildren will have dominion over the generations to come, with the capability to engineer traits into the genetic material as easily as sewing a button on a shirt.
>
> Kevin Davies. Cracking the genome. New York: The Free Press, 2001.

References

1. Adams V, et al. Apoptosis in skeletal myocytes of patients with chronic heart failure is associated with exercise intolerance. J Am Coll Cardiol 1999;33:959.
2. Allen DL, et al. Myonuclear number and myosin heavy chain expression in rat soleus single muscle fibers after spaceflight. J Appl Physiol 1996;81:145.
3. Almind K, et al. Putting the genes for type II diabetes on the map. Nat Med 2001;7:277.
4. Anderson S, et al. Sequence and organization of the human mitochondrial genome. Nature 1981;290:457.
5. Annunen S, et al. An allele of COL9A2 associated with intervertebral disc disease. Science 1999;285:409.
6. Baar K, et al. Transcriptional regulation in response to exercise. Exerc Sport Sci Rev 1999;27:333.
7. Baker LE, et al. A silica-based mitochondrial DNA extraction method applied to forensic hair shafts and teeth. J Forensic Sci 2001;46:126.
8. Baldwin KM. Effect of spaceflight on the functional, biochemical, and metabolic properties of skeletal muscle. Med Sci Sports Exerc 1996;28:983.
9. Baldwin KM. Research in sports medicine and exercise sciences in the 21st Century. Sports Med Bull 1999;34:9.
10. Baldwin KM, et al. Interactive effects of loading and thyroid states on skeletal isomyosins. Int J Sports Med 1997;18(Suppl 4):S296.
11. Balon TW, Yerneni KK. Redox regulation of skeletal muscle glucose transport. Med Sci Sports Exerc 2001;33:382.
12. Bamman MM, et al. Impact of resistance exercise during bed rest on skeletal muscle sarcopenia and myosin isoform distribution. J Appl Physiol 1998;84:157.
13. Barr K, Esser K. Phosphorylation of p70S6k correlates with increased skeletal muscle mass following resistance exercise. Am J Physiol 1999;276(Cell Physiol 45):C120.
14. Bateson W. Experiments in plant hybridization. Cambridge, MA: Harvard University Press, 1950.
15. Baumann H, et al. Exercise training induces transitions of myosin isoform subunits within histochemically typed human muscle fibres. Pflugers Arch 1987;409:349.
16. Beckers M, et al. Active genes in junk DNA? Characterization of DUX genes embedded with 3.3 kb repeated elements. Gene 2001;264:51.
17. Bennet HS. The structure of striated muscle as seen by the electron microscope. In: Bourne, GH, ed. Structure and function of muscle, vol 1. New York: Academic Press, 1960.
18. Bigard XA, et al. Endurance training affects myosin heavy chain phenotype in regenerating fast-twitch muscle. J Appl Physiol 1996;81:2658.
19. Bigard AX, et al. Changes in myosin heavy chain profile of mature regenerated muscle with endurance training in rat. Acta Physiol Scand 1999;165:185.
20. Booth FW. Application of molecular biology in exercise physiology. Exerc Sport Sci Rev 1988;16:1.
21. Booth FW. Cytochrome c protein synthesis rate in rat skeletal muscle. J Appl Physiol 1991;71(4):1225.
22. Booth F, Gordon S. Advocacy is needed to promote research into diseases of physical inactivity. Exerc Sport Sci Rev 2000;28:145.
23. Booth FW, et al. Waging war on modern chronic diseases: primary prevention through exercise biology. J Appl Physiol 2000;88:774.
24. Bray MS. Genomics, genes, and environmental interaction: the role of exercise. J Appl Physiol 2000;88:788.

25. Caiozzo VJ, et al. Effect of spaceflight on skeletal muscle: mechanical properties and myosin isoform content of a slow muscle. J Appl Physiol 1994;76:1764.
26. Caiozzo VJ, et al. Microgravity-induced transformations of myosin isoforms and contractile properties of skeletal muscle. J Appl Physiol 1996;81:123.
27. Campbell WG, et al. Differential global gene expression in red and white skeletal muscle. Am J Physiol Cell Physiol 2001;280:C763.
28. Cann RL. Genetic clues to dispersal in human populations: retracing the past from the present. Science 2001;291:1742.
29. Cargill M, Daley GQ. Mining for SNPs: putting the common variants—common disease hypothesis to the test. Pharmacogenomics 2000;1:27.
30. Cargill M, et al. Characterization of single-nucleotide polymorphisms in coding regions of human genes. Nat Genet 1999;22:231.
31. Chagnon YC, et al. Genomic scan for genes affecting body composition before and after training in Caucasians from HERITAGE. J Appl Physiol 2001;90:1777.
32. Chiti F, et al. Mutational analysis of acylphosphatase suggests the importance of topology and contact order in protein folding. Nat Struct Biol 1999;6:1005.
33. Cross RA. Molecular motors: kinesin's dynamically dockable neck. Curr Biol 2000;10: R124.
34. Daly MJ. Engineering radiation-resistant bacteria for environmental biotechnology. Curr Opin Biotechnol 2000;11(3):280.
35. Darwin CR. On the origin of species by means of natural selection, or the preservation of favoured races in the struggle for life. London, 1859; reprinted Cambridge, MA: Harvard University Press, 1964.
36. Darwin CR. Charles Darwins's diary of the voyage of HMS Beagle. Barlow N, ed. 1933; reprinted New York: Krause Reprints, 1969.
37. Davies KJ, et al. Free radicals and tissue damage produced by exercise. Biochem Biophys Res Commun 1982;107:1198.
38. del Giudice EM, et al. Molecular screening of the proopiomelanocortin (POMC) gene in Italian obese children: report of three new mutations. Int J Obes Relat Metab Disord 2001;25:61.
39. Delplanque J, et al. Linkage and association studies between the proopiomelanocortin (POMC) gene and obesity in caucasian families. Diabetologia 2000;43:1554.
40. Diffee GM, et al. Activity-induced regulation of myosin isoform distribution: comparison of two contractile activity programs. J Appl Physiol 1993;74:2509.
41. DiMarzo V, et al. Leptin-regulated endocannabinoids are involved in maintaining food intake. Nature 2001;410:822.
42. Driver S, et al. Oligonucleotide-based inhibition of embryonic gene expression. Nat Biotech 1999;17:1184.
43. Dunham I, et al. The DNA sequence of human chromosome 22. Nature 1999;402:489.
44. Ebert BL, et al. Hypoxia and mitochondrial inhibitors regulate expression of glucose transporter-1 via distinct cis-acting sequences. J Biol Chem 1995;270:29083.
45. Echwald SM, et al. Mutational analysis of the proopiomelanocortin gene in Caucasians with early onset obesity. Int J Obes Relat Metab Disord 1999;23:293.
46. Eckhardt RB. Genetic research and nutritional individuality. J Nutr 2001;131:336S.
47. Evans MJ, Scarpulla RC. Interaction of nuclear factors with multiple sites in the somatic cytochrome c promoter: characterization of upstream NRF-1, ATF, and intron Sp1 recognition sequences. J Biol Chem 1999;264:14361.
48. Fluck M, et al. Skeletal muscle CaMKII enriches in nuclei and phosphorylates myogenic factor SRF at multiple sites. Biochem Biophys Res Commun 2000 13;270:488.
49. Freire E. The propagation of binding interactions to remote sites in proteins: analysis of the binding of the monoclonal antibody D1.3 to lysozyme. Proc Natl Acad Sci USA 1999;96:10118.
50. Friddle C, et al. Full-genome scan for linkage in 50 families segregating the bipolar affective disease phenotype. Am J Hum Genet 2000;66:205
51. Fu A, et al. A microfabricated fluorescence-activated cell sorter. Nat Biotech 1999;17(11):1109.
52. Fujikawa-Adachi K, et al. Human mitochondrial carbonic anhydrase VB. cDNA cloning, mRNA expression, subcellular localization, and mapping to chromosome X. J Biol Chem 1999;23:274:21228.
53. Fumeron F, et al. Association of a functional 5-HT transporter gene polymorphism with anorexia nervosa and food intake. Mol Psychiatry 2001;6:9.
54. Gordon SE, et al. ANG II is required for optimal overload-induced skeletal muscle hypertrophy. Am J Physiol Endocrinol Metab 2001;280:E150.
55. Gordon SE, et al. Selected Contribution: Skeletal muscle focal adhesion kinase, paxillin, and serum response factor are loading dependent. J Appl Physiol 2001;90:1174.
56. Haddad F, et al. Myosin heavy chain expression in rodent skeletal muscle: effects of exposure to zero gravity. J Appl Physiol 1993;75:2471.
57. Hardingham GE, et al. Distinct functions of nuclear and cytoplasmic calcium in the control of gene expression. Nature 1997;385:260.
58. Hayes B. The invention of the genetic code. Am Sci 1998;86:8.
59. Heft MA, et al. Signaling pathways in cardiac myocyte hypertrophy. J Mol Cell Cardiol 1997;29:2873.
60. Heymsfield SB, et al. Recombinant leptin for weight loss in obese and lean adults. A randomized, controlled dose-escalation trial. JAMA 1999;282:1568.
61. Hochachka PW, et al. Unifying theory of hypoxia tolerance: molecular/metabolic defense and rescue mechanisms for surviving oxygen lack. Proc Natl Acad Sci USA 1996;93:9493.
62. Hochstrasser DF. Proteome in perspective. Clin Chem Lab Med 1998;36(11):825.
63. Holloszy JO. Biochemical adaptations in muscle: effects of exercise on mitochondrial oxygen uptake and respiratory enzyme activity in skeletal muscle. J Biol Chem 1967;242:2278.
64. Holmgren A. Thioredoxin and glutaredoxin systems. J Biol Chem 1989;264:13963.
65. Hosoda K, et al. New members of uncoupling protein family implicated in energy metabolism. Clin Exp Pharmacol Physiol 1999;26:561.
66. Huxley HE. The mechanism of muscular contraction. Science 1969;164:1356.
67. Jackson MJ, et al. Electron spin resonance studies of intact mammalian skeletal muscle. Biochim Biophys Acta 1985;847:185.
68. Jamieson A. Forensic biology: its past, present, and future. Biologist (London) 2000;47:69.
69. Joza N, et al. Essential role of the mitochondrial apoptosis-inducing factor in programmed cell death. Nature 2001;410, 549.
70. Jubrias SA, et al. Large energetic adaptations of elderly muscle to resistance and endurance training. J Appl Physiol 2001;90:1663.
71. Katzmarzyk PT, et al. Fitness, fatness, and estimated coronary heart disease risk: the HERITAGE Family Study. Med Sci Sports Exerc 2001;33:585.
72. Kayumov L, et al. A randomized, double-blind, placebo-controlled crossover study of the effect of exogenous melatonin on delayed sleep phase syndrome. Psychosom Med 2001;63:40.
73. Keller D, Bustamante C. The mechanochemistry of molecular motors. Biophys J 2000;78:541.
74. Kerr JF, et al. Apoptosis: a basic biological phenomenon with wide-ranging implications in tissue kinetics. Br J Cancer 1972;26:239.
75. Kheterpal I, Mathies RA. Capillary array electrophoresis DNA sequencing. Anal Chem 1999;71:31.
76. Krude H, et al. Severe early-onset obesity, adrenal insufficiency and red hair pigmentation caused by POMC mutations in humans. Nat Genet 1998;19:155.
77. Krude I, Gruters I. Implications of proopiomelanocortin (POMC) mutations in humans; the POMC deficiency syndrome. Trends Endocrinol Metab 2000;11:15.
78. Lagally ET, et al. Single-molecule DNA amplification and analysis in an integrated microfluidic device. Anal Chem 2001;73:565.
79. Leder P, Nirenberg M. RNA code-words and protein synthesis, II. Nucleotide sequence of a valine RNA codeword. Proc Natl Acad Sci USA 1964;52:420.
80. Lohiniva J, et al. Splicing mutations in the COL3 domain of collagen IX cause multiple epiphyseal dysplasia. Am J Med Genet 2000;90:216.
81. Lorente JA, et al. Missing person identification: genetics at work for society. Science 2000;290:2257.
82. Makarova KS, et al. Genome of the extremely radiation-resistant bacterium deinococcus radiodurans viewed from the perspective of comparative genomics. Microbiol Mol Biol Rev 2001;65:44.
83. Mammes O, et al. Association of the G-2548A polymorphism in the 5′ region of the LEP with overweight. Ann Hum Genet 2000;64:391.
84. Marini JC. Genetic risk factors for lumbar disk disease. JAMA 2001;1843.
85. Martinek V, et al. Gene therapy and tissue engineering in sports medicine. Phys Sportsmed 2000;28:34.
86. McCreath J, et al. Production of gene-targeted sheep by nuclear transfer from cultured somatic cells. Nature 2000;405:1066.

87. McGrayne SB. Nobel Prize women in science: their lives, struggles, and momentous discoveries. 2nd ed. Secaucus, NJ: Citadel Press Book, Carol Publishing, 1998.
88. Medintz I, et al. High-performance multiplex snp analysis of three hemochromatosis-related mutations with capillary array electrophoresis microplates. Genome Res 2001;11:413.
89. Mokdad AH, et al. The continuing increase of diabetes in the US. Diabetes Care 2001;Feb;24(2):412.
90. Moyes CD, et al. Regulation of muscle mitochondrial design. J Exp Biol 1998;201:299.
91. Mullis KB. The unusual origin of the polymerase chain reaction. Sci Am 1990;262:36.
92. Murakami T, et al. Induction of nuclear respiratory factor-1 expression by an acute bout of exercise in rat muscle. Biochim Biophys Acta 1998;1381:113.
93. Nader GA, Esser KA. Intracellular signaling specificity in skeletal muscle in response to different modes of exercise. J Appl Physiol 2001;90:1936.
94. Nierman WC, et al. Complete genome sequence of Caulobacter crescentus. Proc Natl Acad Sci 2001;98:4136.
95. Nissen P, et al. RNA tertiary interactions in the large ribosomal subunit: The A-minor motif. Proc Natl Acad Sci USA 2001;98:2087.
96. North MA. Advances in the molecular genetics of obesity. Curr Opin Genetics Develop 1999;9:283.
97. Oishi Y. Relationship between myosin heavy chain IId isoform and fibre types in soleus muscle of the rat after hindlimb suspension. Eur J Appl Physiol 1993;66:451.
98. Oishi Y, et al. Changes in fibre-type composition and myosin heavy-chain IId isoform in rat soleus muscle during recovery period after hindlimb suspension. Eur J Appl Physiol 1994;68:102.
99. Okumoto T, et al. Severe endurance training fails to change myosin heavy-chain distribution of diaphragm. Respir Physiol 1996;104:39.
100. Ovchinnikov IV, et al. Molecular analysis of Neanderthal DNA from the northern Caucasus. Nature 2000;404:490.
101. Pajunkanta P, et al. Two loci on chromosomes 2 and X for premature coronary heart disease identified in early- and late-settlement populations of Finland. Am J Hum Genet 2000;67:1481.
102. Pennisi E. Tracking the sexes by their genes. Science 2001;291:1733.
103. Perusse L, et al. Familial aggregation of submaximal aerobic performance in the HERITAGE Family study. Med Sci Sports Exerc 2001;33:597.
104. Phaneuf S, Leeuwenburgh C. Apoptosis and exercise. Med Sci Sports Exerc. 2001;33:393.
105. Podhorska-Okolov M, et al. Apoptosis of myofibres and satellite cells: exercise-induced damage in skeletal muscle of the mouse. Neuropath Appl Neurobiol 1998;24:518.
106. Rew DA. Mitochondrial DNA, human evolution and the cancer genotype. Eur J Surg Oncol 2001;27:209.
107. Rivera MA, et al. Angiogenin gene-race interaction for resting and exercise BP phenotypes: the HERITAGE Family Study. J Appl Physiol 2001;90:1232.
108. Rich T, et al. Defying death after DNA damage. Nature. 2000 12;407:777.
109. Sayre A. Rosalind Franklin & DNA. New York: WW Norton, 1975.
110. Sen CK. Oxidants and antioxidants in exercise. J Appl Physiol 1995;79:675.
111. Sen CK, Roy S. Antioxidant regulation of cell adhesion. Med Sci Sports Exerc 2001;33:377.
112. Sime RL. Lise Meitner: a life in physics. Berkeley: University of California Press, 1996.
113. Skinner JS, et al. Age, sex, race, initial fitness, and response to training: the HERITAGE Family Study. J Appl Physiol 2001;90:1770.
114. Staron RS, et al. Comparison of soleus muscles from rats exposed to microgravity for 10 versus 14 days. Histochem Cell Biol 1998;110:73.
115. Stoecki M, Chaurand P, Hallahan DE, Caprioli RM. Imaging mass spectrometry: A new technology for the analysis of protein expression in mammalian tissues. Nat Med 2001;7:493.
116. Stone AC, et al. Mitochondrial DNA analysis of the presumptive remains of Jesse James. J Forensic Sci 2001;46:173.
117. Sullivan VK, et al. Myosin heavy chain composition in young and old rat skeletal muscle: effects of endurance exercise. J Appl Physiol 1995;78:2115.
118. Swoap SJ. In vivo analysis of the myosin heavy chain IIB promoter region. Am J Physiol 1998;266:C681.
119. Takahashi Y, et al. Predisposing factors in delayed sleep phase syndrome. Psychiatry Clin Neurosci 2000;54:356.
120. Tikunov BA, et al. Quantitative electrophoretic analysis of myosin heavy chains in single muscle fibers. J Appl Physiol 2001;90:1927.
121. Toh KL, et al. An hPer2 phosphorylation site mutation in familial advanced sleep phase syndrome. Science 2001;9;291:1040.
122. Tsika RW, et al. Interaction of compensatory overload and hindlimb suspension on myosin isoform expression. J Appl Physiol 1987;62:2180.
123. Unger SL, et al. Multiple epiphyseal dysplasia: radiographic abnormalities correlated with genotype. Pediatr Radiol 2001;31:10.
124 Veigel C, et al. The motor protein myosin-I reduces its working stroke in two steps. Nature 1999;395:530.
125. Vercoutere W, et al. Rapid discrimination among individual DNA hairpin molecules at single-nucleotide resolution using an ion channel. Nat Biotechnol 2001;19:248.
126. Virbasius GL, Scarpulla RC. Activation of the human mitochondrial transcription factor A gene by nuclear respiratory factors: a potential regulatory link between nuclear and mitochondrial gene expression in organelle biogenesis. Proc Natl Acad Sci USA 1994;91:1309.
127. Vogel G. The human genome. Objection #2: why sequence the junk? Science 2001;291:1184.
128. Wallace AR. Contributions of the theory of natural selection. London: Macmillan, 1870.
129. Wallace DC. Mitochondrial genetics: a paradigm for aging and degenerative diseases. Science 1992;256:628.
130. Wallace DC, et al. 1995. Report of the Committee on Human Mitochondrial DNA. In: Cuticchia AJ, ed. Human gene mapping: a compendium. Baltimore: Johns Hopkins University Press, 1995.
131. Wallace DC. Mitochondrial DNA in aging and disease. Sci Am 1997;277:40.
132. Watson JD. The double helix. New York: Atheneum, 1968.
133. Watson JD. Molecular biology of the gene. 4th ed. Boston: Addison-Wesley,1988.
134. Watson JD, Crick FHC. Molecular structure of nucleic acids. A structure for deoxyribose nucleic acid. Nature 1953;171:737.
135. Widrick JJ, et al. Effect of a 17 day spaceflight on contractile properties of human soleus muscle fibres. J Physiol (Lond) 1999;516:915.
136. Wilmore JH, et al. Cardiac output and stroke volume changes with endurance training: the HERITAGE Family Study. Med Sci Sports Exerc 2001;33:99.
137. Wilmore JH, et al. Heart rate and blood pressure changes with endurance training: the HERITAGE Family Study. Med Sci Sports Exerc 2001;33:107.
138. Wilmut I, et al. Viable offspring derived from fetal and adult mammalian cells. Nature 1997;385:810.
139. Witt EH, et al. Exercise, oxidative damage and effects of antioxidant manipulation. J Nutr 1992;122:766.
140. Wu P, et al. Mechanism responsible for inactivation of skeletal muscle pyruvate dehydrogenase complex in starvation and diabetes. Diabetes 1999;48:1593.
141. Xia Y, et al. Electrical stimulation of neonatal cardiomyocytes results in the sequential activation of nuclear genes governing mitochondrial proliferation and differentiation. Proc Natl Acad Sci USA 1997;94:11399.
142. Yaswen L, et al. Obesity in the knockout mice model of pro-opiomelanocortin deficiency responds to peripheral melanocortin. Nat Med 1999;5:1066.
143. Zelzer E, et al. Insulin induces transcription of target genes through the hypoxia-inducible factor HIF-1 alpha/ARNT. EMBO J 1998;17:508.
144. Zhou MY, et al. Myosin heavy chain isoforms of human muscle after short-term spaceflight. J Appl Physiol 1995;78:1740.
145. Zuk PA, et al. Multilineage cells from human adipose tissue: implications for cell-based therapies. Tissue Engineering. 2001;7, 211.

Suggested Readings: Books

Alberts B, et al. Molecular biology of the cell. 3rd ed. New York: Garland Publishing, 1994.

Alberts B, et al. Essential cell biology. An introduction to the molecular biology of the cell. Garland Publishing. New York, 1998.

Apps DK, et al. Biochemistry. A concise text for medical students. 5th ed. Baillière London: Tindall, 1992.

Bishop J, Waldholz M. Genome. New York: Simon & Shuster, 1990.

Bouchard C, et al. Genetics of fitness and physical performance. Champaign, IL: Human Kinetics, 1997.

Bowler PJ. Charles Darwin. The man and his influence. New York: Cambridge University Press, 1990.

Box JF, Fisher R.A. The life of a scientist. New York: John Wiley & Sons, 1978.

Brandon C, Tooze J. Introduction to protein structure. New York and London: Garland Publishing, 1991.

Clarke DP. Molecular biology made simple and fun. 2nd ed. Vienna, IL: Cache River Press, 2000.

Cook-Deegan R. The gene wars. New York: Norton, 1994.

Crick FHC. What mad pursuit. New York: Basic Books, 1988.

Davies K. Cracking the genome: inside the race to unlock human DNA. New York: Free Press, 2001.

DeRobertis EDP, DeRobertis EMF Jr. Cell and molecular biology. 8th ed. Philadelphia: Lea & Febiger, 1987.

Dudek RW. High-yield cell and molecular biology. Baltimore: Lippincott Williams & Wilkins, 1999.

Dwyer J, et al. Actual innocence. New York: Doubleday, 2000.

Freifelder D, Malacinski GM. Essentials of molecular biology. Boston: Jones & Bartlett Publishers, 1993.

Hamer DH, Copeland P. Living with our genes. New York: Doubleday, 1998.

Hartl DL, Jones EW. Genetics. Principles and analysis. 4th ed. Sudbury, MA: Jones & Bartlett, 1998.

Houdebine LM. ed. Treansgenic animals: generation and use. New York: Gordon and Breach, 1997.

Jorde LB, et al. Medical genetics. 2nd ed. St. Louis: Mosby, 1999.

Judson HF. The eight day of creation. Cold Spring Harbor, NY: Cold Spring Harbor Laboratory Press, 1996.

Karp G. Cell and molecular biology. 2nd ed. New York: John Wiley & Sons, 1999.

Kolata G. Clone. New York: William Morrow, 1999.

Lewin B, et al. Genes VI. 6th ed. New York: Oxford University Press, 1997.

Lodish H. Molecular cell biology. 4th ed. New York: WH Freeman, 1999.

Lodish H, Darnell JE. A student's companion in molecular cell biology. 3rd ed. New York: WH Freeman, 2000.

Malina RM, Bouchard C. Sport and human genetics. Champaign, IL: Human Kinetics, 1986.

Mange EJ, Mange AP. Basic human genetics. 2nd ed. Sunderland, MA: Sinauer Associates, 1999.

Marks DB, et al. Basic medical biochemistry. A clinical approach. Baltimore: Williams & Wilkins, 1996.

Mathews CK. Biochemistry. 3rd ed. Old Tappan, NJ: Pearson Education, 2000.

McConkey EH. Human genetics: the molecular revolution. Boston: Jones & Bartlett, 1993.

Miesfeld RL, ed. Applied molecular genetics. New York: John Wiley & Sons, 1999.

Paolella P. Introduction to molecular biology. Boston: WCB/McGraw-Hill, 1998.

Purves WK, et al. Life. The science of biology. 5th ed. Sunderland, MA: Sinauer Associates, 1998.

Raven PH, Johnson GB. Biology. 4th ed. Dubuque, IA: Wm C Brown, 1996.

Ridley M. Genome: The autobiography of a species in 23 chapters. New York: HarperCollins Publishers, 1999.

Rothwekk NV. Understanding genetics: a molecular approach. New York: Wiley-Liss, 1993.

Russel PJ. Fundamentals of genetics. 2nd ed. Old Tappan, NJ: Pearson Education, 2000.

Russel PJ. Genetics. 5th ed. Old Tappan, NJ: Pearson Education, 2000.

Schlief R. Genetics and molecular biology. Baltimore: Johns Hopkins University Press, 1993.

Schumm DE. Core concepts in clinical molecular biology. Baltimore: Lippincott Williams & Wilkins, 1997.

Stracham T, Read AP. Human molecular genetics. 2nd ed. New York: John Wiley & Sons, 1999.

Stryer L. Biochemistry. 4th ed. New York: WH Freeman, 1995.

Voit D, Voit JG. Biochemistry. 2nd ed. New York: John Wiley & Sons, 1995.

Watson JD. Molecular biology of the gene. 5th ed. Old Tappan, NJ: Pearson Education, 2000.

Watson J.D. Recombinant DNA. 2nd ed. New York: Freeman, 1995.

Wilmut I, Campbell K, Tudge C. The second creation. New York: Farrar Straus & Giroux, 2000.

Suggested Readings: Additional

Abbott A. Structures by numbers. Nature 2000;408:130.

Adam SA. Transport pathways of macromolecules between the nucleus and the cytoplasm. Curr Opinion Genet Dev 1999;11:402.

Adams MD, et al. The genome sequence of Drosophila melanogaster. Science 2000;287:2185.

Adwalla P, et al. Linkage disequilibrium and recombination in hominid mitochondrial DNA. Science 1999;286:2524.

Allan VJ, Schroer TA. Membrane motors. Curr Opin Genet Dev 1999;11:476.

Altshuler D, et al. An SNP map of the human genome generated by reduced representation shotgun sequencing. Nature 2000;407:513.

Ames BW. Identifying environmental chemical causing mutations and cancer. Science 1979; 204:587.

An P, et al. Familial aggregation of resting blood pressure and heart rate in a sedentary population: the HERITAGE Family Study. Health, risk factors, exercise training, and genetics. Am J Hyperten 1999;12:264.

Anerson WF. Uses and abuses of human gene transfer. Hum Gene Ther 1992;3:1.

Ashburner M, et al. Gene ontology: tool for the unification of biology. The Gene Ontology Consortium. Nat Genet 2000;25:25.

Avery OT, et al. Studies on the chemical nature of the substance inducing transformation of pneumococcal types. J Exp Med 1944;79:137.

Beadle GW, Tatum EL. Genetic control of biochemical reactions in Neurospora. Proc Nat Acad Sci USA 1941; 27:499.

Benzer S. Fine structure of a genetic region in bacteriophage. Proc Nat Acad Sci USA;41:344.

Bishop AC, et al. A chemical switch for inhibitor-sensitive alleles of any protein kinase. Nature 2000;407:395.

Blackburn EH. Telomers and their synthesis. Science 1990; 249:489.

Boluyt MO, et al. Regional variation in cardiac myosin isoforms of female F344 rats during aging. 1999;54A:B313.

Borecki IB, et al. Evidence for at least two major loci influencing human fatness. Am J Hum Genet 1998;63:831.

Botstein D, et al. Yeast as a model organism. Science 1997; 277:1259.

Bouchard C. Genetics of obesity: overview and research directions. In: Bouchard C, ed. The genetics of obesity. Boca Raton, FL: CRC Press, 1994.

Bouchard C, et al. Control of cell proliferation by Myc. Trends Cell Biol 1998;8:202.

Bouchard C. Genetics of overweight and obesity. Arch Pediatr 1999;6(suppl 2):158s.

Brenner S, et al. An unstable intermediate carrying information from genes to ribosomes for protein synthesis. Nature 1961; 190:576.

Broder S, Venter JC. et al. Whole genomes: the foundation of new biology and medicine. Curr Opin Biotechnol 2000;11:581.

Broder S, Venter JC. Sequencing the entire genomes of free-living organisms: the foundation of pharmacology in the new millennium. Annu Rev Pharmacol Toxicol 2000;40:97.

Burke DT, et al. Cloning of large segments of exogenous DNA into yeast by means of artificial chromosome vectors. Science 1987;236:806.

Caetano AR, et al. A comparative gene map of the horse (Equus caballus). Genome Res 1999:1239.

Caskey CT. Molecular medicine: a spin-off from the helix. JAMA 1993;269:1986.

Cavazzana-Calvo M, et al. Gene therapy of human severe combined immunodeficiency (SCID)-X1 diseaase. Science 2000;287:2396.

Chagnon YC, et al. Linkages and associations between the leptin receptor (LEPR) gene and human body composition in the Quebec Family Study. Int J Obes Relat Metab Disord 1999;23:278.

Clasey JL, et al. The use of anthropometric and dual-energy X-ray absorptiometry (DXA) measures to estimate total abdominal and abdominal visceral fat in men and women. Obes Res 1999;7:256.

Collins FS, McKusick VA. Implications of the Human Genome Project for medical science. JAMA 2001;285:540.

Collins FS, Mansoura MK. The human genome project. Cancer 2001;91:221.

Collins FS, Haseltine WA. Of genes and genomes: what lies between the base pairs. J Investig Med 2000;48:295.

Crick FHC, et al. General nature of the genetic code for proteins. Nature 1961;192:1227.

Crick FHC. Split genes and RNA splicing. Science 1979; 204:264.

Crow, JF. Francis Galton: Count and measure, measure and count. Genetics 1993;135:1.

De Souza SJ, et al. The correlation between introns and the three-dimensional structure of proteins. Gene 1997;205:141.

Despres JP, et al. Plasma post-heparin lipase activities in the HERITAGE Family Study: the reproducibility, gender differences, and associations with lipoprotein levels. Health, risk factors, exercise training and genetics. Clin Biochem 1999;32:157.

Despres JP, et al. Race, visceral adipose tissue, plasma lipids, and lipoprotein lipase activity in men and women: the Health, Risk Factors, Exercise Training, and Genetics (HERITAGE) family study. Arterioscler Thromb Vasc Biol 2000;20:1932.

Dickson D, Macilwain C. It's a G: the one-billionth nucleotide. Nature 1999;402:331.

Dionne I, et al. Gender difference in the effect of body composition on energy metabolism. Int J Obes Relat Metab Disord 1999;23:312.

Doucet E, et al. Fasting insulin levels influence plasma leptin levels independently from the contribution of adiposity: evidence from both a cross-sectional and an intervention study. J Clin Endocrinol Metab 2000;85:423.

Drake JW. Spontaneous mutation. Ann Rev Genetics 1991; 25:125.

Driver S, et al. Oligonucleotide-based inhibition of embryonic gene expression. Nat Biotech 1999;17:1184.

Dujon B. The yeast genome project: What did we learn? Trends Genetics 1996; 12:263.

Durfy SJ. Ethics and the human genome project. Arch Pathol Lab Med 1993;117:466.

Ellerby HM, et al. Anti-cancer activity of targeted pro-apoptotic peptides. Nat Med 1999;5:1032.

Fanning AS, Anderson JM. Protein modules as organizers of membrane structure. Curr Opinion Genet Dev 1999;11:432.

Fatina C, et al. RAS genes influence exercise-induced left ventricular hypertrophy: an elite athletes study. Med Sci Sports Exerc 2000;32:1868.

Fisher RA. Has Mendel's work been rediscovered? Ann Science 1936; 1:115.

Fraser AG. et al. Functional genomic analysis of C. elegans chromosome 1 by systematic RNA interference. Nature 2000;408:325.

Fu A, et al. A microfabricated activated-activated cell sorter. Nat Biotech 1999;17:1109.

Fu Y, et al. Mutagenesis analysis of human SM22: characterization of actin binding. J Appl Physiol 2000;89:1985.

Garenc C, et al. Linkage and association studies of the lipoprotein lipase gene with postheparin plasma lipase activities, body fat, and plasma lipid and lipoprotein concentrations: the HERITAGE Family Study. Metabolism 2000;49:432.

Gayagay G, et al. Elite endurance athletes and the ACE I allele: the role of genes in athletic performance. Hum Genet 1998;103:48.

Gehring WJ, Ikeo K. Pax6: mastering eye morphogenesis and eye evolution. Trends Genet 1999;15:371.

Goodsell DS. Biomolecules and nanotechnology. Am Sci 2000;88:230.

Goodsell DS, Olson AJ. Structural symmetry and protein function. Annu Rev Biophys Biomol Struct 2000;29:105.

Gilbert W, et al. Origin of genes. Proc Natl Acad Sci USA 1997;94:7698.

Gilbert W, et al. Origin of life: the RNA world. Nature 1986;319:618.

Gilbert W, et al. The correlation between introns and the three-dimensional structure of proteins. Gene 1997;205:141.

Grant SF, et al. Long PCR detection of the C4A null allele in B8-C4AQ0-C4B1-DR3. J Immunol Methods 2000;244:41.

Grant SF, et al. Long PCR detection of the C4A null allele in B8-C4AQ0-C4B1-DR3. J Immunol Methods 2000;244:41.

Greider CW, Blackburn EH. The telomer terminal transferase of Tetrahymena is a ribonucleoprotein enzyme with two kinds of a primer specificity. Cell 1987; 51:887.

Gudmundsson H, et al. Inheritance of human longevity in Iceland. Eur J Hum Genet 2000;8:743.

Gudmundsson H, et al. Inheritance of human longevity in Iceland. Eur J Hum Genet 2000;8:743.

Gulcher J, et al. Genetic homogeneity of Icelanders. Nat Genet 2000;26:395.

Gulcher J, et al. Genetic homogeneity of Icelanders. Nat Genet 2000;26:395.

Gulcher J, et al. The genealogic approach to human genetics of disease. Cancer J 2001 Jan-Feb;7(1):61.

Gulcher JR, et al. Protection of privacy by third-party encryption in genetic research in Iceland. Eur J Hum Genet 2000;8:739.

Gulcher JR, et al. Protection of privacy by third-party encryption in genetic research in Iceland. Eur J Hum Genet 2000;8:739.

Gulcher JR, Stefansson K. The Icelandic Healthcare Database and informed consent. N Engl J Med 2000;342:1827.

Hamer DH, et al. A linkage between DNA markers on the X chromosome and male sexual orientation. Science 1993; 261:321.

Hardy GH. Mendelian proportions in a mixed population. Science 1908; 28:49.

Helgason A, et al. Estimating Scandinavian and Gaelic ancestry in the male settlers of Iceland. Am J Hum Genet 2000;67:697.

Helgason A, et al. mtDna and the islands of the North Atlantic: estimating the proportions of Norse and Gaelic ancestry. Am J Hum Genet 2000;68:723.

Helgason A, et al. mtDNA and the origin of the Icelanders: deciphering signals of recent population history. Am J Hum Genet 2000;66:999.

Helgason A, et al. mtDNA and the origin of the Icelanders: deciphering signals of recent population history. Am J Hum Genet 2000;66:999.

Hershey AD, Chase M. Independent functions of viral protein and nucleic acid in growth of bacteriophage. J Gen Physiol 1952; 36;39.

Hershey AD, Rotman, R. Genetic recombination between host-range and placque-type mutants of bacteriophage in single bacterial cell. Genetics 1948;34:44.

Hershey AD. Genes and hereditary characteristics. Nature 1970; 23;226.

Hershey AD. Idiosyncrasies of DNA structure. Science 1970; 19;168:1425.

Hinney A, et al. Candidate gene polymorphisms in eating disorders. Eur J Pharmacol 2000;410:147.

Hong Y, et al. Familial clustering of insulin and abdominal visceral fat: the HERITAGE Family Study. J Clin Endocrinol Metab 1998;83:4239.

Hong Y, et al. Evidence of a major locus for lipoprotein lipase (LPL) activity in addition to a pleiotropic locus for both LPL and fasting insulin: results from the HERITAGE Family Study. Atherosclerosis 1999;144:393.

Hong Y, et al. Evidence of pleiotropic loci for fasting insulin, total fat mass, and abdominal visceral fat in a sedentary population: the HERITAGE Family Study. Obes Res 2000;8:151.

Huey KA, et al. Temporal effects of inactivty on myosin heavy chain gene expression in rat slow muscle. Muscle Nerve 2001;24:517.

Ingvarsson T, et al. The inheritance of hip osteoarthritis in Iceland. Arthritis Rheum 2000;43:2785.

Jones CR, et al. Familial advanced sleep-phase syndrome: a short-period circadian rhythm variant in humans. Nat Med 1999;5:1062.

Kadonaga JT, Grunstein M. Chromosomes and expression mechanisms. Chromatin: the packaging is the message. Curr Opin Genet Dev 1999;9:129.

Karjalainen J, et al. Angiotensinogen gene M235T polymorphism predicts left ventricular hypertrophy in endurance athletes. J Am Coll Cardiol 1999;34:494.

Katzmarzyk PT, et al. Familial resemblance for physique: heritabilities for somatotype components. Ann Hum Biol 2000; 27:467.

Katzmarzyk PT, et al. Familial risk of obesity and central adipose tissue distribution in the general Canadian population. Am J Epidemiol 1999;149:933.

Katzmarzyk PT, et al. Linkage and association of the sodium potassium-adenosine triphosphatase alpha2 and beta1 genes with respiratory quotient and resting metabolic rate in the Quebec Family Study. J Clin Endocrinol Metab 1999;84:2093.

Katzmarzyk PT, et al. Physique, subcutaneous fat, adipose tissue distribution, and risk factors in the Quebec Family Study. Int J Obes Relat Metab Disord 1999;23:476.

Katzmarzyk PT, et al. Seven-year stability of indicators of obesity and adipose tissue distribution in the Canadian population. Am J Clin Nutr 1999;69(6):1123.

Katzmarzyk PT, et al. Stability of indicators of the metabolic syndrome from childhood and adolescence to young adulthood: the Quebec Family Study. J Clin Epidemiol 2001;54:190.

Katzmarzyk PT, et al. Television viewing, physical activity, and health-related fitness of youth in the Quebec Family Study. J Adol Health 1998;23:318.
Kawai, J, et al. Functional annotation of a full-length mouse cDNA collection. Nature 2001;409: 685.
Kim JJ, et al. Protection from immunodeficiency virus challenges in thesus macaques by multicomponent DNA immunization. Virology 2001;285:204.
Knoppers BM, Chadwick R. The Human Genome Project: under an international ethical microscope. Science 1994;265:2035.
Lahn BT, Page DC. Four evolutionary strata on the human X chromosome. Science 1999; 286:964.
Lander ES, et al. Initial sequencing and analysis of the human genome. Nature 2001;409:860.
Lander ES, Weinberg RA. Genomics: journey to the center of biology. Science 2000;287:1777.
Laitinen T, et al. A susceptibility locus for asthma-related traits on chromosome 7 revealed by genome-wide scan in a founder population. Nat Genet 2001;28:87
Larose M, et al. A new gene related to obesity identified by suppression subtractive hybridization. Int J Obes Relat Metab Disord 2001;25:770.
Leathes JB. Function and design. Science 1926;64:187.
Lemieux I, et al. The small, dense LDL phenotype as a correlate of postprandial lipemia in men. Atherosclerosis 2000;153:423.
Lichtenstein P, et al. Environmental and heritable factors in the causation of cancer—analysis of cohorts of twins from Sweden, Denmark, and Finland. N Engl J Med 2000:343:78.
Lovel-Badge R, Boncinelli E. Genetics of disease. Sampling a witch's brew: the genetics of complex systems. Curr Opin Genet Dev 1999;9:263.
Lueking A, *et al.* Protein microarrays for gene expression and antibody screening. Anal Biochem 1999;270:103.
Lyon M. Gene action in the X chromosome of the mouse (Mus musculus L.) Nature 1961;190:372.
Marintchev A, et al. Solution structure of the single-strand break repair protein XRCC1 N-terminal domain. Nat Struct Biol 1999;6:884.
McClintock B. The origin and behavior of mutable loci in maize. Proc Nat Acad Sci USA 1950;36:344.
McClintock B. Control of gene action in maize. Brookhaven Symposium Quant Biol 1965;18:162.
McKinsey TA, Olson EN. Cardiac hypertrophy: sorting out the circuitry. Curr Opin Genet Dev 1999;9:267.
Meselson M, Stahl, FW. The replication of DNA in Escherichia coli. Proc Nat Acad Sci USA 1958;44: 671.
Mewes HW, et al. MIPS: a database for genomes and protein sequences. Nucleic Acid Res 2000;28:37.
Montgomery HE, et al. Human gene for physical performance. Nature 1998;393:221.
Morgan TH. Sex limited inheritance in Drosophila. Science 1910;32:120.
Muller HJ. Artifical transmutation of the gene. Science 1927;66:84.
Murry JC, et al. A comprehensive human linkage map with centimorgan density. Science 1994;265:2049.
Myers et al. A whole-genome assembly of Drosophila. Science 2000 24;2872196.
Nüsslein-Volhard C, Wieschaus E. Mutations affecting segment number and polarity in Drosophila. Nature 1980; 287: 795.
O'Brien SJ, et al. Genomics. On choosing mammalian genomes for sequencing. Science 2001;292:2264.
O'Brien SJ, Stanyon R. Phylogenomics. Ancestral primate viewed. Nature 1999;402:365.
Pascot A, et al. Age-related increase in visceral adipose tissue and body fat and the metabolic risk profile of premenopausal women. Diabetes Care 1999;22:1471.
Perusse L, Bouchard C. Gene-diet interactions in obesity. Am J Clin Nutr 2000;72:1285S.
Perusse L, et al. Etiology of massive obesity: role of genetic factors. World J Surg 1998;22:907.
Perusse L, et al. Familial aggregation of amount and distribution of subcutaneous fat and their responses to exercise training in the HERITAGE Family Study. Obes Res 2000;8:140.
Perusse L, et al. A genome-wide scan for abdominal fat assessed by computed tomography in the Quebec Family Study. Diabetes 2001;50:614.
Perusse L, et al. Genotype-environment interaction in human obesity. Nutr Rev 1999;57:S3.
Perusse L, et al. The human obesity gene map: the 1998 update. Obes Res 1999;7:111.
Perusse L, et al. Role of genetic factors in childhood obesity and in susceptibility to dietary variations. Ann Med 1999;31(Suppl 1):19.
Pizza M, et al. Identification of vaccine candidates against serogroup B meningococcus by whole-genome sequencing. Science 2000;10;287.
Prescott JC, et al. Telomerase: Dr. Jekyll or Mr, Hyde? Curr Opin Genet Dev 1999;9:368.
Polejaeva IA, et al. Cloned pigs produced by nuclear transfer from adult somatic cells. Nature 2000;407:86.
Raju TN. The Nobel chronicles. 1995: Edward B Lewis (b 1918), Christiane Nusslein-Volhard (b 1942), and Eric Francis Wieschaus (b 1947). Lancet 2000;356:81.
Rankinen T, et al. AGT M235T and ACE ID polymorphisms and exercise blood pressure in the HERITAGE Family Study. Am J Physiol Heart Circ Physiol 2000;279(1):H368.
Rankinen T, et al. Linkage of the Na,K-ATPase alpha 2 and beta 1 genes with resting and exercise heart rate and blood pressure: cross-sectional and longitudinal observations from the Quebec Family Study. J Hyperten 1999;17:339.
Rankinen T, et al. No association between the angiotensin-converting enzyme ID polymorphism and elite endurance athlete status. J Appl Physiol 2000;88:1571.
Rankinen T, et al. NOS3 Glu298Asp genotype and blood pressure response to endurance training: the HERITAGE family study. Hypertension 2000;36:885.
Rauramaa R, et al. The RsaI polymorphism in the alpha-fibrinogen gene and response of plasma fibrinogen to physical training—a controlled randomised clinical trial in men. Thromb Haemost 2000;83:803.
Ravussin E, Bouchard C. Human genomics and obesity: finding appropriate drug targets. Eur J Pharmacol 2000 27;410:131.
Reeves RH. Recounting a genetic story. Nature 2000;405:283.
Rice T, et al. Familial aggregation of body mass index and subcutaneous fat measures in the longitudinal Quebec family study. Gen Epidemiol 1999;16:316.
Rice T, et al. Segregation analysis of body mass index in a large sample selected for obesity: the Swedish Obese Subjects Study. Obes Res 1999;7:246.
Rivera MA, et al. A mitochondrial DNA D-loop polymorphism and obesity in three cohorts of women. Int J Obes Relat Metab Disord 1999;23:666.
Rivera MA, et al. Linkage between a muscle-specific CK gene marker and VO_{2max} in the HERITAGE Family Study. Med Sci Sports Exerc 1999;31:698.
Rivera MA, et al. Three mitochondrial DNA restriction polymorphisms in elite endurance athletes and sedentary controls. Med Sci Sports Exerc 1998;30:687.
Ronnemaa T, et al. Serum lipids, lipoproteins, and lipid metabolizing enzymes in identical twins discordant for obesity. J Clin Endocrinol Metab 1998;83:2792.
Rosmond R, et al. A polymorphism of the 5'-flanking region of the glucocorticoid receptor gene locus is associated with basal cortisol secretion in men. Metabolism 2000;49:1197.
Rosmond R, et al. Hypertension in obesity and the leptin receptor gene locus. J Clin Endocrinol Metab 2000;85:3126.
Rosmond R, et al. Tsp509I polymorphism in exon 2 of the glucocorticoid receptor gene in relation to obesity and cortisol secretion: cohort study. Brit Med J 2001 17;322:652.
Rubin GM. The draft sequences. Comparing species. Nature 2001;409:820.
Rubin GM, et al. A brief history of Drosophila's contributions to genome research. Science 2000;287:2216.
Rubin GM, et al. Comparative genomics of the eukaryotes. Science 2000;287:2204.
Rubin GM, et al. A Drosophila complementary DNA resource. Science 2000;287:2222.
Sachidanandam R, et al. A map of human genome sequence variation containing 1.42 million single nucleotide polymorphisms. Nature 2001;409:928.
Sager R, Ramanis Z. Recombination of nonchromosomal genes in Chlamydomonas. Proc Nat Acad Sci USA 1965;53:1053.
Salanoubat M, et al. Sequence and analysis of chromosome 3 of the plant Arabidopsis thaliana. Nature 2000;408:820.
Seidell JC, et al. Abdominal adiposity and risk of heart disease. JAMA 1999;281:2284.
Selmer, et al. Crystal structure of Thermotoga maritima ribosome recycling factor: a tRNA mimic. Science 1999;286:2349.
Sigurgardottir S, et al. The mutation rate in the human mtDNA control region. Am J Hum Genet 2000;66:1599.

Skalka A, et al. Segmental distribution of nucleotides in the DNA of bacteriophage lambda. J Mol Biol 1968;28;34:1.

St-Amand J, et al. Apolipoprotein E polymorphism and the relationships of physical fitness to plasma lipoprotein-lipid levels in men and women. Med Sci Sports Exerc 1999;31:692.

Stanforth PR, et al. Accuracy of prediction equations to estimate submaximal $\dot{V}O_2$ during cycle ergometry: the HERITAGE Family Study. Med Sci Sports Exerc 1999;31:183.

Sveinbjornsdottir S, et al. Familial aggregation of Parkinson's disease in Iceland. N Engl J Med 2000;343:1765.

Tavazoie S, et al. Systematic determination of genetic network architecture. Nat Genet 1999;22:28.

Tremblay A, et al. Fat balance and ageing: results from the Quebec Family Study. Br J Nutr 1998;79:413.

Ukkola O, et al. Interactions among the glucocorticoid receptor, lipoprotein lipase, and adrenergic receptor genes and plasma insulin and lipid levels in the Quebec Family Study. Metabolism 2001;50:246.

Venter JC, et al. The sequence of the human genome. Science 2000;291:1304.

Wallace DC. Mitochondrial diseases: genotype versus phenotype. Trends Genetics 1993;9:128.

Watson JD, Crick, FHC. Genetical implications of the structure of deoxyribonucleic acid. Nature. 1953;171:964.

Wiemann S, et al. Toward a catalog of human genes and proteins: sequencing and analysis of 500 novel complete protein coding human cDNAs. Genome Res 2001;11:422.

Weisnagel SJ, et al. Decreased fasting and oral glucose stimulated C-peptide in nondiabetic subjects with sequence variants in the sulfonylurea receptor 1 gene. Diabetes 2001;50:697.

Wieschaus E. Embryonic transcription and the control of developmental pathways. Genetics 1996; 142:5.

Wilson J, et al. Successful ex vivo gene therapy directed to liver in a patient with familial hypercholesterolaemia. Nature Genetics 1994;6:335.

Wolfarth B, et al. A polymorphism in the $\text{alpha}_{2a\text{–adenoreceptor}}$ gene and endurance athlete status. Med Sci Sports Exerc 2000;32:1709.

Wong FS, et al. Identification of an MHC class I-restricted autoantigen in type 1 diabetes by screening an organ-specific cDNA library. Nat Med 1999;5:1026.

Wright CE, et al. In vivo regulation of the beta-myosin heavy chain gene in hypertensive rodent heart. Am J Physiol Cell Physiol 2001;280:C1262.

York D, Bouchard C. How obesity develops: insights from the new biology. Endocrine 2000;13:143.

Ziauddin J, Sabatini M. Microarrays of cells expressing defined cDNAs. Nature 2001;411:107.

Suggested Readings: Twins

Arden NK, et al. Genetic influences on muscle strength, lean body mass, and bone mineral density: a twin study. J Bone Miner Res 1997;12:2076.

Beunen G. Thomis M. Genetic determinants of sports participation and daily physical activity. Int J Obes 1999;23(Suppl 3):S55.

Bonora E. Relationship between regional fat distribution and insulin resistance. Int J Obes Relat Metab Disord 2000;2:S32.

Boomsma DI, et al. Resemblances of parents and twins in sports participation and heart rate. Behav Genet 1989;19:123.

Bouchard C, et al. Genetic effect in resting and exercise metabolic rates. Metabolism 1989;38:364.

Bouchard C, et al. Genetics of aerobic and anaerobic performances. Exerc Sport Sci Rev 1992;20:27.

Bouchard C, et al. Submaximal power output in adopted and biological siblings. Ann Hum Biol 1984;11:303.

Bouchard C, et al. Using MZ twins in experimental research to test for the presence of a genotype-environment interaction effect. Acta Gen Med Gemell 1990;39:85.

Carmelli D, Reed T. Stability and change in genetic and environmental influences on hand-grip strength in older male twins. J Appl Physiol 2000;89:1879.

Cesari M, et al. Are fasting plasma homocyst(e)ine levels heritable? A study of normotensive twins. J Invest Med 2000;48:351.

Chatterjee S, et al. Physical and motor fitness in twins. Jpn J Physiol 1995;45(3):519.

Chen WJ, et al. Diagnosis of zygosity by questionnaire and polymarker polymerase chain reaction in young twins. Behav Genet 1999;29(2):115.

Christensen K, et al. Genetic and environmental influences on functional abilities in Danish twins aged 75 years and older. J Gerontol A Biol Sci Med Sci 2000;55:M446.

Ener S. Coronary artery disease in identical twins. Ann Thorac Surg 2000;70:692.

Faith MS, et al. Evidence for independent genetic influences on fat mass and body mass index in a pediatric twin sample. Pediatrics 1999;104:61.

Ferrari S, et al. Genetic aspects of osteoporosis. Curr Opin Rheumatol 1999;11:294.

Finkel D, et al. Genetic and environmental influences on functional age: a twin study. J Gerontol B. Psychol Sci Soc Sci 1995;50:104.

Fontaine E, et al. Resting metabolic rate in monozygotic and dizygotic twins. Acta Genet Med Gemell 1985;34:41.

Friedlander Y, et al. Sib-air linkage analysis of longitudinal changes in lipoprotein risk factors and lipase genes in women twins. J Lipid Res 2000;41:1302.

Gabler S, et al. Fitness of twinning. Hum Biol 1994;66:699.

Gagnon J, et al. The Trp64 Arg mutation of the $\beta3$ adrenergic receptor gene has no effect on obesity phenotypes in the Québec Family Study and Swedish Obese Subjects Cohorts. J Clin Invest 1996;98:2086.

Gibbons LE, et al. Determinants of isokinetic and psychophysical lifting strength and static back muscle endurance: a study of male monozygotic twins. Spine 1997;22:2983.

Heitmann BL, et al. Are genetic determinants of weight gain modified by leisure-time physical activity? A prospective study of Finnish twins. Am J Clin Nutr 1997;66:672.

Kaminer Y, et al. Bulimia in a pair of monozygotic twins. J Nerv Ment Dis 1988;176:246.

Karlsson J, et al. Muscle strength and muscle characteristics in monozygous and dizygous twins. Acta Physiol Scand 1979;106:319.

Komi PV, Karlsson J. Physical performance, skeletal muscle enzyme activities, and fibre types in monozygous and dizygous twins of both sexes. Acta Physiol Scand 1979;105:1.

Lauderdale DS, et al. Familial determinants of moderate and intense physical activity: a twin study. Med Sci Sports Exerc 1997;29:1062.

Lo SS, et al. Effects of acute hyperglycaemia on cardiac function: an echocardiographic study of monozygotic twins. Int J Cardiol 2000;74:139.

Loos R, et al. Gender-specific regional changes in genetic structure of muscularity in early adolescence. J Appl Physiol 1997;82:1802.

Maes HHM, et al. Inheritance of physical fitness in 10-yr-old twins and their parents. Med Sci Sports Exerc 1996;28:1479.

McCreath KJ, et al. Production of gene-targeted sheep by nuclear transfer from cultured somatic cells. Nature 2000;405:1066.

Neale MC, Cardon LR. Methodology for genetic studies of twins and families. Dordrecht: Kluwer, 1992.

Nelson TL, et al. Genetic and environmental influences on waist-to-hip ratio and waist circumference in an older Swedish twin population. Int J Obes Relate Metab Disord 1999;23:449.

Pelling AL, et al. A human genomic library enriched in transcriptionally active sequences (aDNA Library). Genome Res 2000;10:874.

Pérusse L, et al. Inter-generation transmission of physical fitness in the Canadian population. Can J Sport Sci 1988;13:8.

Prud'Homme D, et al. Sensitivity of maximal aerobic power to training is genotype-dependent. Med Sci Sports Exerc 1984;16:489.

Reed T, et al. Genetic influences and grip strength norms in the NHLBI twin study males aged 59–69. Ann Hum Biol 1991;18:425.

Reed T, et al. Ten-year follow-up for male twins divided into high- or low-risk groups for ischemic heart disease based on risk factors measured 25 years previously. Ann Epidemiol 2000;10:278.

Segal NL. Behavioral aspects of intergenerational human cloning: twin-based perspective. Twin Res 1999;2:53.

Simoneau J-A, Bouchard C. Genetic determinism of fibre type proportion in human skeletal muscle. FASEB J 1992;9:77.

Simoneau JA, et al. Inheritance of human skeletal muscle and anaerobic capacity adaptation to high-intensity intermittent training. Int J Sports Med 1986;7:167.

Sklad M, et al. Development of general strength in mono and dizygotic twins. Biol Sport 1992;9:1091.

Sullivan PF, et al. Genetic epidemiology of binging and vomiting. Br J Psychiatry 1998;173:75.

Thomis MA, et al. Multivariate genetic analysis of maximal isometric muscle force at different elbow angles. J Appl Physiol 1997;82:959.

Thomis MAI, et al. Inheritance of static and dynamic arm strength and some of its determinants. Acta Physiol Scand 1998;163:59.

Thomis MAI, et al. Strength training: importance of genetic factors. Med Sci Sports Exerc 1998;30:724.
Treloar SA, et al. Age at menarche as a fitness trait: nonadditive genetic variance detected in a large twin sample. Am J Hum Genet 1990;47:137.
Wade T, et al. A genetic analysis of the eating and attitudes associated with bulimia nervosa: dealing with the problem of ascertainment in twin studies. Behav Genet 1999;29:1.

References: Scientific American

Adleman LM. Computing with DNA. Sci Am 1998:279(2):54–61.
Allen RD. The microtubule as an intracellular engine. Sci Am 1987;256(2):26–33.
Andersen JL, et al. Muscle, genes and athletic performance. Sci Am 2000;283(3):48–55.
Axel R. The molecular logic of smell. Sci Am 1995;273(4):154–159.
Baer E. Advanced polymers. Sci Am 1986;255(4):157–165.
Baltimore D, Heilman C. HIV vaccines: prospects and challenges. Sci Am 1998;279(1):98–103.
Bayley H. Building doors into cells. Sci Am 1997;277(3):62–69.
Beardsley T. Evolution evolving. New findings suggest mutation is more complicated than anyone thought. Sci Am 1997;277(3):15,18.
Beardsley T. Getting wired. New observations may show how neurons form connections. Sci Am 1999;280(6):24,26.
Beardsley T. Mutations galore. Sci Am 1999;280(4):32,36.
Beardsley T. The start of something big? Dolly has become a new icon for science. Sci Am 1997;276(5):15–16.
Beardsley T. Stem cells come of age. Sci Am 1999;281(1):30–31.
Beardsley T. Trends in human genetics: vital data. Sci Am 1996;27(3):100–105.
Beck G, Habicht G. Immunity and the invertebrates. Sci Am 1996;275(5): 60–66.
Berns MW. Laser scissors and tweezers. Sci Am 1998;278(4):62–67.
Berridge MJ. The molecular basis of communication within the cell. Sci Am 1985;253(4):124–135.
Birge RR. Protein based computers. Sci Am 1995;272(3):90–95.
Blaese RM. Gene therapy for cancer. Sci Am 1997;276(6):111–115.
Blaser MJ. The bacteria behind ulcers. Sci Am 1996;274(2):104–109.
Boon T. Teaching the immune system to fight cancer. Sci Am 1993;266(3):122–132.
Brown K. The human genome business today. Sci Am 2000;283(1):50–57.
Brown, K. Seeds of concern. Sci Am 2001;284(4):52.
Campbell, A. How viruses insert their DNA into the DNA of the host cell. Sci Am 1976; 235(6):102.
Capecci MR. Targeted gene replacement. Sci Am 1994;270(3):52–59.
Cavenee WK, White RL. The genetic basis of cancer. Sci Am 1995;272(3): 72–81.
Cech TR. RNA as an enzyme. Sci Am 1986;255(5):76–84.
Cerman A, et al. Glucose and aging. Sci Am 1987;256(5):82–88.
Chambon. P. Split genes. Sci Am 1981;244(5):60.
Changeus J-P. Chemical signaling in the brain. Sci Am 1993;269(5): 58–62.
Chilton, M.-D. A vector for introducing new genes into plants. Sci Am 1983;248(6):50.
Close FE, Page PR. Glueballs. Sci Am 1998;279(5):80–93.
Cohen JS, Hogan ME. The genetic medicines. Sci Am 1994;271(6):76–82.
Cohen, SN. The manipulation of genes. Sci Am 1975; 233(1):24.
Collins S, Jegalian KG. Deciphering the code of life. Sci Am 1999;279:86–91.
Collins FS, Jegalian, KG. Deciphering the code of life. Sci Am 1999;281(6):87.
Crick FC. The genetic code III. Sci Am 1966;215:55–62.
DeDuvc C. Microbodies in the living cell. Sci Am 1983;248:74.
De Roberts, EM et al. Homeobox genes and the vertebrate body plan. Sci. Am 1990;263(1):46.
Doolittle RF. Proteins. Sci Am 1985;253(4):74–85.
Doolittle WF. Uprooting the tree of life. Sci Am 2000;282(2):90–95.
Dugatkin LA, Godin J-GJ. How females choose their mates. Sci Am 1998; 278(4):56–61.
Duke RC, et al. Cell suicide in health and disease. Sci Am 1996;275(6): 80–87.
Englehard VH. How cells present antigens. Sci Am 1994;271(2):.
Ezzell C. Beyond the human genome. Sci Am 2000;283(1):.
Feldman M, Eisenbach L. What makes a cell metastatic? Sci Am 1988; 259(5):40–47.
Felgner PL. Nonviral strategies for gene therapy. Sci Am 1997;276(6):102–106.
Friedman T. Overcoming the obstacles to gene therapy. Sci Am 1997; 276(6):96–101.
Friend CM. Catalysis on surfaces. Sci Am 1993;268(4):74–85.
Gasser, CS, Fraley, RT. Transgenic crops. Sci Am 1992;266(6):62.
Gershenfeld N, Chuang IL. Quantum computing with molecules. Sci Am 1998;278(6):66–73.
Gerstein M, Levitt M. Simulating water and the molecules of life. Sci Am 1998;279(5):100–105.
Gibb WW. Gaining on fat. Sci Am 1996;275(2):88–94.
Gibbs WW. Trailing a virus. Sci Am 1999;281(2):80–87.
Glover DM, et al. The centrosome. Sci Am 1993;268(6):62–69.
Godson GN. Molecular approaches to malaria vaccines. Sci Am 1985; 252(5):32–39.
Golde DW, Gasson JC. Hormones that stimulate the growth of blood cells. Sci Am 1988;258(1):34–42.
Goldstein GW, Betz AL. The blood–brain barrier. Sci Am 1986;255(3): 70–79.
Gottlieb DI. BABAergic neurons. Sci Am 1988;258(2):38–45.
Greenspan RJ. Understanding the genetic construction of behavior. Sci Am 1995;272(4):72–78.
Greider CW, Blackburn EH. Telomers, telomerase, and cancer. Sci Am 1996;274(2):92–97.
Grimaldi, DA. Captured in amber. Sci Am 1996;274(4):84.
Grivell, LA. Mitochondrial DNA. Sci Am 1983;248(3):78.
Groce CM, Klein G. Chromosome translocation and human cancer. Sci Am 1985;252(3):44–61.
Grunstein, M. Histones as regulators of genes. Sci Am 1992;267(4):68.
Haseltine WA. Discovering genes for new medicines. Sci Am 1997;276(3): 92–97.
Ho DY, Saplosky RM. Gene therapy for the nervous system. Sci Am 1997; 276(6):116–120.
Hoberman JM, Yesalis CE. The history of synthetic testosterone. Sci Am 1995;272(2):76–81.
Hogle JM, et al. The structure of poliovirus. Sci Am 1987;256():28–35.
Holliday, R. A different kind of inheritance. Sci Am 1989; 60(60):60.
Horwitz AF. Integrins and health. Sci Am 1997;276(5):68–75.
Howard K. The bioinformatics gold rush. Sci Am 2000;283(1):58–63.
Hunter T. The proteins of oncogenes. Sci Am 1984;252(2):70.
Hynes RO. Fibronectins. Sci Am 1986;254(6):32–41.
Ingber DE. The architecture of life. Sci Am 1998;278(1):48–57.
Jain RK. Barriers to drug delivery in solid tumors. Sci Am 1994;271(1):58–65.
Jegalian, K, Lahn, BT. Why the Y is so wired. Sci Am 2001;284(2):56.
Johnson HM, et al. How interferons fight disease. Sci Am 1994;270(5): 68–75.
Jordan VC. Designer estrogens. Sci Am 1998;279(4):60–69.
Joyce GF. Directed molecular evolution. Sci Am 1992;267(6):90–97.
Karplus M, McCammon JA. The dynamics of proteins. Sci Am 1986; 254(4):30–39.
Kempermann G, Gage FH. New nerve cells for the adult brain. Sci Am 1999;280(5):48–67.
Kornberg, A. The nucleosome. Sci Am 1981;244(2):52.
Lacy PE. Treating diabetes with transplanted cell. Sci Am 1995;273(1):50–59.
Landry DW. Immunotherapy for cocaine addiction. Sci Am 1997;276(2):2–45.
Langridge WHR. Edible vaccines. Sci Am 2000;283(3):66–71.
Lanza RP, et al. Xenotransplantation. Sci Am 1997;277(1):54–59.
Laver G, et al. Disarming flu viruses. Sci Am 1999;280(1):78–87.
Lawn RM, Vehar GA. The molecular genetics of haemophilia. Sci Am 1986;254:48.
Lerner RA, Tramantono A. Catalytic antibodies. Sci Am 1988;258(3):58–70.
Losick, R, Kaiser, D. Why and how bacteria communicate. Sci Am 1997;276(2):68.
Maniatis, T, Ptashne, M. A DNA operator-repressor system. Sci Am 1976;234(1):64.
Marrack P, Kappler JW. How the immune system recognizes the body. Sci Am 1993;269(3):81–89.
McGinnis W, Kuziora M. The molecular architects of body design. Sci Am 1994;270(2):58–66.
Miller RV. Bacterial gene swapping in nature. Sci Am 1998;278(1):66–73.
Mirsky S. What cloning means for gene therapy. Sci Am 1997;276(6): 122–123.
Moxon RE, Wills C. DNA microsatellites: agents of evolution? Sci Am 1999;280(1):94–99.

Mullis KB. The unusual origin of the polymerase chain reaction. Sci Am 1990;262(4):36–43.
Murray AW, Szastak JW. Artificial chromosomes. Sci Am 1987;257(5): 60–70.
Myerowitz EM. The genetics of flower development. Sci Am 1994; 271(5):6–65.
Nemeroff CB. The neurobiology of depression. Sci Am 1998;278(6):42–57.
Nesse RM, Williams GC. Evolution and origins of disease. Sci Am 1998; 279(5):86–93.
Neufeld PJ, Colman N. When science takes the witness stand. Sci Am 1990;262(5):46–53.
Nirenberg MW. The genetic code II. Sci Am 1963;208:80–94.
Nossal GJV. Life, death, and the immune system. Sci Am 1993;269(3): 72–79.
Novick, RP. Plasmids. Sci Am 1980;243(6):103.
O'Brien SJ, Dean M. In search of AIDS-resistance genes. Sci Am 19; sept 97
Oldstone MJS. Vital alteration of cell function. Sci Am 1989;261(2):34–41.
Orgel LE. The origin of life on the earth. Sci Am 1994;271(4):76–83.
Ostro MJ. Liposomes. Sci Am 1987;256(1):90–95.
Pääbo S. Ancient DNA. Sci Am 1993;269(5):86–92.
Perutz MF. The hemoglobin molecule. Sci Am 1964;19;211:64.
Plomin R, DeFries JC. the genetics of cognitive abilities and disabilities. Sci Am 1998;278(5):62–83.
Ptashne M. How gene activators work. Sci Am 1989;260(1):24–31.
Radman M, Wagner R. The high fidelity of DNA duplications. Sci Am 1988;259(2):24–30.
Rasmussen H. The cycling of calcium as an intracellular messenger. Sci Am 1989;260(4):44–51.
Rebek J Jr. Synthetic self-replicating tumors. Sci Am 1994;271(1):48–55.
Reed MA, Tour JM. Computing with molecules. Sci Am 2000;282(6): 86–93.
Rennie J. The body against itself. Sci Am 1990;263(6):76–85.
Rennie J. DNA's new twists. Sci Am 1993;266(3):122–132.
Rennie, J. Gading the gene tests. Sci Am 1994;270(6):88.
Rhodes D, Klug A. Zinc fingers. Sci Am 1993;268(2):56–65.
Riddle RD, Tabin CJ. How limbs develop. Sci Am 1999;280(2):74–79.
Rodier PM. The early origins of autism. Sci Am 2000;282(2):56–63.
Rose MR. Can human aging be postponed? Sci Am 1999;279:106–111.
Ross J. The turnover of messenger RNA. Sci Am 1989;260(4):28–35.
Rothman JE, Lelio O. Budding vesicles in cells. Sci Am 1996;274(3): 70–77.
Ruoslahti E. How cancer spreads. Sci Am 1996;275(5):72–77.
Schwartz RH. T cell anergy. Sci Am 1993;269(3):62–71.
Scott JD, Pawson T. Cell communication: the inside story. Sci Am 2000; 282(6):72–79.
Smith, DVS, Magolskee, RF. Making sense of taste. Sci Am 2001;284(3):32.
Smith KA. Interleukin 2. Sci Am 1990;262(3):26–33.
Snyder SH. The molecular basis of communication between cells. Sci Am 1985;253(4):114–123.
Stahl FW. Genetic recombination. Sci Am 1987;256(2):90–101.
Stossel TP. The machinery of cell crawling. Sci Am 1994;271(3):54–63.
Strauss, E. Counting the lives of a cell. Sci Am Presents 2000;11(2):51.
Streit W, Kincaid-Colton CA. The brain's immune system. Sci Am 1995;273(5):54–61.
Stroud RM. A family of protein cutting enzymes. Sci Am 1974;231:74–88.
Stryer L. The molecules of visual excitation. Sci Am 1987;257(1):32–41.
Tattersall, I. Out of Africa again . . . and again. Sci Am 1997;276(6):88.
Thompson EOP. The insulin molecule. Sci Am 1955;192:36–41.
Tjian R. Molecular machines that control genes. Sci Am 1995;272(2):54–61.
Todorov IN. How cells maintain stability. Sci Am 1990;262(6):32–39.
Tomalia DA. Dendrimer molecules. Sci Am 1995;272(5):62–69.
Trichopoulos, D. et al. What causes cancer? Sci Am 1996;275(3):80.
Tsien, JZ. Building a brainier mouse. Sci Am 2000;282(4):62.
Urry DW. Elastic biomolecular molecules. Sci Am 1995;272(1):64–69.
Velander VH, et al. Transgenic livestock as drug factories. Sci Am 1997; 276(1):70–75.
Wallace DC. Mitochondrial DNA in aging and disease. Sci Am 1997; 277(2):40–47.
Weber K, Osborn M. The molecules of the cell matrix. Sci Am 1985; 253(4):92–103.
Weinberg R. Finding the anti-oncogene. Sci Am 1988;259(3):44.
Weinberg, RA. How cancer arises. Sci Am 1996;275(3):62.
Weindruch R. Caloric restriction and aging. Sci Am 1996;274(1):46–53.
Weiner DB, Kennedy RC. Genetic vaccines. Sci Am 1999;281(1):50–57.
Weissman IL, Cooper MD. How the immune system develops. Sci Am 1993;269(3):72–79.
Welch WJ. How cells respond to stress. Sci Am 1993;268(5):56–64.
White, R, Lalouel, J.-M. Chromosome mapping with DNA markers. Sci Am 1988; 58(2):40.
Wilmut I. Cloning for medicine. Sci Am 1998;279(6):58–65.
Young JD-E, Cohn ZA. How killer cells kill. Sci Am 1988;258(1):28–34.
Young MW. The tick-tock of the biological clock. Sci Am 2000;282(3):64–71.

Molecular Biology on the Internet

Access Excellence (www.accessexcellence.com/)
Alliance for Cellular Signaling (afcs.swmed.edu/)
American Society of Gene Therapy (www.asgt.org/)
Art in the Genetic Age (www.geneart.org/)
Bacterial Artificial Chromosomes (www.ornl.gov/meetings/bacpac/index.html)
Beginner's Guide to Molecular Biology (www.iacr.bbsrc.ac.uk/notebook/courses/guide/)
Biobase (biobase.dk/)
Biocompare (www.biocompare.com)
Biological Structure Resource (ndbserver.rutgers.edu:80/)
Biology Links: Biochemistry and Molecular Biology (mcb.harvard.edu/BioLinks/biochem.html)
Biomolecular Engineering Research Center (bmerc-www.bu.edu/)
BioOnline (www.bio.com/)
BIOSCI (www.bio.net/)
BioSpace Site Search (www.biospace.com/b2/navigate/site_search.cfm)
Biotech Chronicles (www.accessexcellence.org/AB/BC/index.html#Anchor-33869)
Biotech Life Science Dictionary (biotech.icmb.utexas.edu/pages/dictionary.html)
Brown Lab (cmgm.stanford.edu/pbrown/)
Brutlag Bioinformatics Group (motif.stanford.edu/)
Build-Your-Own DNA Kit (dna2z.com/kits/whatsdna.html)
Cells Alive! (cellsalive.com/)
Cancer Genome Anatomy Project (www.ncbi.nlm.nih.gov/ncicgap/)
CMS Molecular Biology Resource (www.unl.edu/stc-95/ResTools/cmshp.html)
Cold Spring Harbor Laboratory (www.cshl.org/)
Computational Biology at ORNL (compbio.ornl.gov/)

Computational Molecular Biology at NIH (molbio.info.nih.gov/molbio/)
Coriell Institute for Medical Research (locus.umdnj.edu/nigms/)
Cytogenetics Gallery (genscope.concord.org/)
Dennis Kunkel's Microscopy (www.pbrc.hawaii.edu/~kunkel/)
Department of Energy Microbial Cell Project (microbialcellproject.org/)
DNA from A to Z (dna2z.com/a2z/index.html)
DNA Learning Center (vector.cshl.org/)
DNA-o-Gram Generator (dna2z.com/DNA-o-gram/)
DNA Vaccine Web (www.genweb.com/Dnavax/dnavax.html)
Doubletwist (www.doubletwist.com)
EcoCyc: Encyclopedia of *E. coli* Genes and Metabolism (ecocyc.PangeaSystems.com/ecocyc/ecocyc.html)
Electronic Scholarly Publishing (www.esp.org/)
Endoplasmic Reticulum: Structure and Function (cellbio.utmb.edu/cellbio/rer1.htm#Menu)
Environmental Molecular Sciences Laboratory (www.emsl.pnl.gov:2080/)
ExPASy Molecular Biology Server (www.expasy.ch/)
Flybase (flybase.bio.indiana.edu:82/)
Gene Map of the Human Genome (www.ncbi.nlm.nih.gov/SCIENCE96/)
Genentech (www.genentech.com/)
Genes and Disease (www.ncbi.nlm.nih.gov/disease/)
Genesolutions.com (www.genesolutions.com/)
Gene Therapy Clinical Trials (www.wiley.co.uk/genetherapy/clinical/)
Genetic Enginering News (www.genengnews.com/)
Genetics Computer Group (www.gcg.com/)
Genetics Education Center (www.kumc.edu/gec/)
Genetics Glossary. U.S. Department of Energy (www.bis.med.jhmi.edu/Dan/DOE/prim6.html)
Genome Database (www.gdb.org/)
Genomes to Life (www.DOEGenomesToLife.org/)
Genomics News Wire (www.genomicsnews.com/)
Genscope (genscope.concord.org/)
Glycolysis (colossus.chem.indiana.edu/topics/glycolysis.html)
Harvard University Dept of Molecular & Cellular Biology (www.ncbi.nlm.nih.gov/UniGene/Mm.Home.html)
History of Life (www.ucmp.berkeley.edu/historyoflife/histoflife.html)
HotMolecBase (bioinformatics.weizmann.ac.il/hotmolecbase/)
Howard Hughes Medical Institute (http:www.hhmi.org/)
Human Chromosome 16 Project (informa.bio.caltech.edu/idx_www_tree.html)
Human Gene Therapy (www.humangenetherapy.com/index.html)
Human Genome Project Information (www.ornl.gov/hgmis/)
Human Genome Sequencing Center (www.hgsc.bcm.tmc.edu/index.html)
Human Genome Sequencing Department (www-hgc.lbl.gov/)
Hypertextbook Cell Biology Chapter Directory (esg-www.mit.edu:8001/esgbio/cb/cbdir.html)
Image Library of Biological Macromolecules (www.imb-jena.de/IMAGE.html)
Institute for Human Gene Therapy (www.med.upenn.edu/ihgt/info/links2.html)
Introduction to Amino Acids (www.cryst.bbk.ac.uk/education/AminoAcid/overview.html)
ISREC Bioinformatics Group (www.isrec.isb-sib.ch/)
Jackson Laboratory (www.jax.org/)
Joint Genome Institute (www.jgi.doe.gov/tempweb/JGI_microbial/html/index.html)
Laboratory for Optimcal and computational Instrumentation (www.loci.wisc.edu/)
Links to BioWeb Servers (www.bis.med.jhmi.edu/biolinks.html)
List of Chemistry Servers (www.chem.ucla.edu/chempointers.html)
Mary Ann Liebert, Publishers (www.liebertpub.com/)
Metabolic Database (cgsc.biology.yale.edu/metab.html)
Microbial Genome Program (www.science.doe.gov/ober/microbial.html)
MITOMAP (www.gen.emory.edu/mitomap.html)
Molecular Art/Molecular Science (www.scripps.edu/pub/goodsell/)
Molecular Biologist Toolkit (www.hslib.washington.edu/basic_sciences/molbio/)
Molecular Biology Desk Reference (molbio.info.nih.gov/molbio/desk.html)
Molecular Genetics Jump Station (www.horizonpress.com/gateway/molbiol.html)
Molecular Physiology of CNS Development (rsb.info.nih.gov/mol-physiol/homepage.html)
Molecules R Us (molbio.info.nih.gov/cgi-bin/pdb)
National Biotechnology Facility (www.nbif.org/)
National Center for Biotechnology Information (NCBI) (www.ncbi.nlm.nih.gov/)
National Gene Vector Laboratory (www-ngvl.med.umich.edu/)
National Human Genome Research Institute (www.nhgri.nih.gov/)
Natural and Accelerated Bioremediation Research (NABIR) Program (www.lbl.gov/NABIR)
Nature (www.nature.com/nature/)
Neurosciences on the Internet (www.nEuroguide.com/)
NIH Office of Recombinant DNA Activities (www.nih.gov/od/orda/)
NOVA (www.pbs.org/wgbh/nova/genome/)
Office of Science (www.science.doe.gov/)
Pedro's BioMolecular Research Tools (www.public.iastate.edu/~pedro/research_tools.html)
Primer on Molecular Genetics: Glossary (www.bis.med.jhmi.edu/Dan/DOE/prim6.html)
Protein Crystallography on the Web (px.cryst.bbk.ac.uk/)
Protein Data Bank (www.rcsb.org/pdb/)
Rasmol & Chime: Molecular Visualization Freeware (www.umass.edu/microbio/rasmol/)
Recombinant Capital (www.recap.com/mainweb.nsf)
Research Genetics (www.resgen.com/)
Reverse Transcription Homepage (staffa.wi.mit.edu/sabatini_public/reverse_transfection/frame.htm)
RNA World (www.imb-jena.de/RNA.html)
Rotavirus Online (rotavirus.com/home/index.htm)
The Sanger Center (www.sanger.ac.uk/)
Society for Developmental Biology (sdb.bio.purdue.edu/)
Stanford Genomic Resources (genome-www.stanford.edu/)
TIGR. The Institute for Genomic Research (www.tigr.org/)
Timeline of Biotechnology (www.biospace.com/articles/timeline.cfm)
UniGene-Mus Musculus (www.ncbi.nlm.nih.gov/UniGene/Mm.Home.html)
Urbanowicz on Darwin (www.csuchico.edu/~curban/Darwin/DarwinSem-S95.htm)
Virtual Cell (ampere.scale.uiuc.edu/%7Em-lexa/cell/cell.html)
Voyage of the Beagle (www.literature.org/authors/darwin-charles/the-voyage-of-the-beagle/)
Web Gene Server (www.itba.mi.cnr.it/webgene/)
Whitehead Institute for Biomedical Research (www.genome.wi.mit.edu/)
WWW Sites for Biologists (golgi.harvard.edu/BioLinks/Huge.html)

TABLE A ➤ TIMELINE OF EVENTS ABOUT "GENETICS" BEFORE MENDEL, FOLLOWED BY NOTABLE EVENTS IN GENETICS AND MOLECULAR BIOLOGY TO THE PRESENT

DATE	EVENT
BEFORE MENDEL	
420 BC	Socrates speculated about why children and parents seemed to differ in so many physical and psychologic characteristics
400 BC	Hippocrates believed that semen contributed to a child's physical and mental characteristics and that a woman passed on physical and mental traits via an analogous fluid
320 BC	Aristotle denounced Hippocrates's ideas believing a father's semen contributes a child's inherited characteristics; he taught that mothers provided the raw materials to create the child and that a "force" in mother's blood creates female babies
1000 AD	Hindu philosophers teach that parents pass on all their characteristics to offspring—"A man of base descent can never escape his origins"
1100–1700	Spontaneous generation remains the governing theory that organisms arise from nonliving matter, and how traits pass to new generation
1630	William Harvey deduces that males contribute sperm or pollen and females contribute eggs to reproduce their kind by sexual means
1655	Englishman Robert Hooke designs a microscope to examine thin slices of cork, observing honeycomb compartments he calls *cellulae* (Latin for "small rooms," known now as cells)
1657	Dutch naturalist Antonie van Leeuwenhoek observed the first living cells; he called them *animalcules* (little animals; protozoa and bacteria) and believed they played a role in fermentation
1724	Cross-fertilization of corn discovered
1838	Mathias Schleiden studied plants, observing that all plants "are aggregates of fully individualized, independent, separate beings, namely the cells themselves"
1839	Theodor Schwann developed the cell theory—cells serve as the basic building units of all animal tissues
1858	Naturalists Charles Darwin and Alfred Wallace independently propose their ideas about natural section—animal populations that survive adapt their hereditary characteristics and variations (see pages 971–972)
1859	Charles Darwin publishes *On the Origin of Species by Means of Natural Selection, or The Preservation of Favoured Races in the Struggle for Life*
1865	Gregor Mendel, Austrian botanist and monk, presents his "Laws of Heredity" to the Natural Science Society, based on his 25-year cross-breeding experiments with 10,000 varieties of edible pea plants
AFTER MENDEL	
1868	Swiss biologist Friedrich Miescher isolates "nuclein" (now called DNA) from cells of open wounds and fish sperm
1882	German embryologist Walther Fleming discovers thin threads in nuclei (known now as chromosomes) that divide lengthwise in salamander larvae; he names mitosis; Robert Koch discovers the cause (bacterium) of a human microbial disease
1883	German physiologist August Weismann proposes the germ plasm theory that both parents contribute chromosomes equally to transmit hereditary characteristics to offspring
1900	Hugo De Vries, Carl Correns, and Erich van Tschermak-Seysenegg independently rediscover Mendel's research.
1902	American geneticist Walter Sutton develops chromosomal theory of heredity (similar chromosomes pair with one another during meiosis, each going to a different cell); he called Mendel's "factors" *genes*
1907	Thomas Hunt Morgan proves with fruit flies that chromosomes play a role in heredity
1908	British physician Archibald Garrod describes inborn errors of metabolism, recognizing that inherited diseases might reflect genetic enzyme deficiencies
1910	T. H. Morgan proves that chromosomes carry genes, and "crossing-over" experiments determine gene location (Principle of Linkage)
1911	T. H. Morgan maps gene location on fruit fly chromosomes
1912	Lawrence Bragg discovers that x-rays elucidate the molecular structure of crystalline substances, leading to x-ray crystallography and Rosalind Franklin's discovery of DNA's helical structure in the early 1950s
1915–1917	J. Frederick Twort (1915) first isolates viruses that infect bacteria; K. Felix d'Herelle (1917) establishes the existence of viruses that infect bacteria and invents a method to culture them; he also demonstrates that a virus (which he named *bacteriophage* or devourer of bacteria) reproduces only in live bacteria
1916	Publication of journal *Genetics*
1917–1918	Sewell Wright shows that enzymes mediate discrete biochemical steps determining coat colors in guinea pigs, mice, rats, rabbits, and large mammals
1926	T. H. Morgan publishes the influential *The Theory of the Gene*; Hermann Muller discovers that x-rays produce mutations in fruit flies, paving the way for future discoveries in genetics
1927	Herman Muller (1946 Nobel Prize for production of mutations by x-ray irradiation) treats sperm with heavy doses of x-rays and induces true "gene mutations" in germ cells (mutagenesis)
1928	British microbiologist Frederick Griffith proposes that an unknown "factor" transformed the harmless R strain of diplococcus to the virulent or pathogenic S strain *(Streptococcus pneumoniae)*; mice injected with R lived; mice injected with S died; adding both S and R killed the mice, proving that one strain passed to the other strain
1929	Phoebus Levine discovers the sugar deoxyribose
1931	Curt Stern proves that genetic exchanges of traits such as eye color involve the physical exchange of parts of chromosomes called "crossing over"

TABLE A ➤ TIMELINE OF EVENTS ABOUT "GENETICS" BEFORE MENDEL, FOLLOWED BY NOTABLE EVENTS IN GENETICS AND MOLECULAR BIOLOGY TO THE PRESENT—cont'd

DATE	EVENT
AFTER MENDEL—cont'd	
1935	Wendell Stanley crystallizes tobacco mosaic virus; Andrie Belozersky isolates pure DNA
1937	Frederick Bawden discovers that tobacco mosaic virus contains RNA
1938	The term "molecular biology" comes into use
1941	George Beadle and Edward Tatum use the bread mold *Neurospora* to confirm the "one gene–one enzyme" hypothesis (one gene–one polypeptide)—each gene determined a specific enzyme that performs a specific metabolic task
1944	Oswald Avery, Colin MacLeod, Maclyn McCarty at Rockerfeller Institute confirm that DNA, not proteins, serve as the hereditary material in bacteria ("transforming principle"); if proteins were involved, proteases would block transformation, but they did not; Frederick Sanger uses chromatography to determine the amino acid sequence of insulin
1945	Salvador Luria and Max Delbrück develop a phage model to study how genetic information transfers to host bacterial cells
1946	Edward Tatum and Joshua Lederberg discover that bacteria can exchange genetic material directly by plasma conjugation
1947	Barbara McClintock first reports on "transposable elements" (known today as jumping genes or transposons)
1950	Erwin Chargaff discovers that in DNA the number of thymines always equaled the number of adenines, and the number of guanines always equaled the number of cytosines ([T] = [A]; [G] = [C]) (known as "Chargaff's rule")
1952	Joshua Lederberg discovers bacterial structures (plasmids) that contain extrachromosomal genetic material; Lederberg and Norton Zinder prove that bacterial genes can infiltrate more than one cell (transduction)—a virus takes DNA from one bacterial cell and transports the genes to another cell it infects; Alfred Hershey (early 1960s Director of the Cold Spring Harbor Genetics Research Unit with members Nobel laureate Barbara McClintock and John Cairns [1969 Nobel Prize laureate for the genetic structure of viruses]) and assistant Martha Chase "tag" the DNA (^{32}P) and protein (^{35}S) in bacteriophage T2 (which attacks bacteria) to determine their roles during replication—that phage DNA, not its protein component, contains the phage genes; only the viral DNA (not viral protein) entered the cell in significant amounts to produce new viruses, which verified its role as the genetic carrier; electron microscopy verifies the structure of ribosomes; William Hayes discovers conjugation; Jean Brachet shows that protein synthesis involves RNA
1953	James Watson and Francis Crick publish their landmark paper in *Nature* (see page 1050) concerning their deduction about the 3-D, helical, complementary, antiparallel configuration of DNA; W. Hayes discovers that plasmids can transfer genetic markers among bacteria
1956	Francis Fraenkel-Conrat demonstrates genetic "self-assembly" by reassembling the tobacco mosaic virus from its constituent elements; Francis Crick and George Gamow (physicist) propose the "central dogma"—genetic information flows unidirectionally from DNA to mRNA to protein
1958	Arthur Kornberg purifies the enzyme DNA polymerase I from *E. coli* and uses it to create DNA in a test tube Jérôme Lejeune discovers that children with Down syndrome contained a forty-seventh chromosome (trisomy)
1959	Francois Jacob and Jacques Monod discover repressors and operons—clusters of controlling genes in DNA that regulate "on" and "off" transcriptional control functions
1961	Marshall Nirenberg and Johann Matthaei use the base uracil to create mRNA (poly-U), the UUU codon for phenylalanine, a step toward cracking the DNA code Syndney Brenner, François Jacob, and Matthew Meselson provide biochemical proof using density-gradient centrifugation that genes code for proteins through messenger RNA
1964	Paul Leder and M. Nirenberg crack the genetic code, interpreting the triplet mRNA codons that specify each of the 20 amino acids Geneticist Charles Yanofsky and colleagues at Stanford, studying the mold *Neurospora crassa*, discover that suppressor mutations restored a mutant's active enzyme that previously produced an inactive protein.
1965	Alfred Hershey and Elizabeth Burgi demonstrate that bacteriophage lamba DNA has 20 base-long, single-stranded tails at each end. The tails' base sequences were complementary, allowing their "sticky ends" to find each other and form circular DNA molecules; Ruth Sager and Zenta Ramanis discover intragenic recombination in nonchromosomal genes due to DNA in the cellular organelles.
1967	Mary Weiss and Howard Green join human and mouse cells together (somatic cell fusion) to add the gene for thymidine kinase to chromosome 17 (forming a hybrid cell); this powerful technique assists in gene mapping and other human genetic analyses
1970	Peter Duesberg and Peter Vogt discover the first oncogene from experiments with retroviruses and map the genetic structure of these viruses; David Baltimore and Howard Temin independently purify reverse transcriptase restriction enzyme that cuts DNA at specific locations; Swedish scientists stain mammalian chromosomes that show a banding pattern
1972	Hugh McDevitt observes that specific genes control immune responses, suggesting heritability of acquired diseases
1973	Stanley Cohen, Ann Chang, and Herbert Boyer produce the first recombinant DNA organism (created DNA using *E. coli* restriction enzyme to splice genomes into a novel combination); Paul Berg suggests that the NIH establish guidelines about DNA splicing techniques; Bruce Ames develops a test to identify DNA damaged by unwanted chemicals; improved method developed for DNA electrophoresis using agarose gel and ethidium bromide staining

TABLE A ➤ **TIMELINE OF EVENTS ABOUT "GENETICS" BEFORE MENDEL, FOLLOWED BY NOTABLE DISCOVERIES IN GENETICS AND MOLECULAR BIOLOGY TO THE PRESENT—cont'd**

DATE	EVENT
AFTER MENDEL—cont'd	
1975	At an international conference, scientists call for establishing guidelines for recombinant-DNA research
1976	Venture capitalist Robert Swanson with biochemist H. Boyer form Genentech, Inc. whose mission is to develop, manufacture, and market pharmaceuticals
1977	Genentech scientists first use *E. coli* to produce a human protein—somatostatin (growth hormone–releasing factor); this milestone, using a recombinant gene to clone a protein, unleashed a biotechnologic revolution that continues today; Bill Rutter and Howard Goodman isolate the rat gene for insulin
1978	Genentech scientists with the City of Hope National Medical Center use recombinant DNA technology to produce human insulin; Stanford scientists transplant a mammalian gene; David Botstein and colleagues discover restriction fragment length polymorphisms (RFLPs—genetic variation in the length of mutant regions of DNA fragments produced by interaction with restriction enzymes; used in "genetic fingerprinting"); Steen Willadsen performs the first successful embryo splitting, dividing sheep embryos in two
1979	John Baxter clones the human growth hormone gene
	Arnold Levine and David Lane discover the p53 gene
1980	U.S. Supreme Court (Diamond *v.* Chakrabarty, 447 U.S. 303, 1980) upholds a patent for inventing a human-made, genetically created bacterium capable of breaking down crude oil, opening up commercialization of genetic engineering
	Researchers, using a bacterium, insert a gene that codes for the protein interferon; Martin Cline and colleagues create a transgenic mouse; Christiane Nüsslein-Volhard and Eric Wieschaus first report mutations in each of three major classes of genes in *Drosophilia* concerned with early embryonic development (awarded Nobel Prize in 1995 honoring their work)
1981	Mary Harper and colleagues use in situ hybridization to map the insulin gene
1982	FDA approves Genentech's application to market genetically engineered human insulin (licensed to Eli Lilly and Company)
1983	Kery Mullis at Cetus Corporation develops the polymerase chain reaction (PCR) technique, which allows making almost unlimited copies of specific regions of DNA from a tiny sample, amplifying it to a large enough quantity for analysis, revolutionizing molecular biology research (refer to Fig. 32); Jay Levy isolates the AIDS virus almost simultaneously with the Pasteur Institute and NIH.
1984	Chiron Corporation clones and sequences the HIV genome
	Alec Jeffreys discovers genetic "fingerprinting" that revolutionizes forensic medicine (confirmed the skeletal remains of Nazi war criminal Josef Mengele) and validiy of paternity and immigration cases
1985	Axel Ullrich and his team at Genentech sequence the human insulin receptor, leading to diabetes treatment with human insulin; NIH approves guidelines for human gene therapy experiments; Cal Bio clones the gene that encodes human lung surfactant protein; biotechnology companies field test genetically engineered plants resistant to insects, bacteria, and viruses
1986	Peter Schultz combines antibodies and enzymes (catalytic antibodies) to produce pharmaceuticals by cutting, splicing, and modifying biologic molecules at specific points; the Health and Environmental Research Advisory Committee of the Department of Energy prepare an initial report about the possibility of initiating the human genome project
	Yuri Dubrova and colleagues (including Sir Alec Jeffreys) present the first direct evidence that radiation from Chernobyl causes heritable mutations in humans (*Nature.* 1996 25;380:683); FDA approves Hepatitis B, the first genetically engineered human vaccine
1987	Genentech receives FDA approval to market Activase (Alteplase, recombinant), a tissue plasminogen activator (t-PA), to dissolve blood clots in patients with coronary disease; David Burke, Georges Carle, and Maynard Olson develop a high-capacity cloning system using in vitro construction of linear DNA transformed into a yeast plasmid and maintained as artificial chromosome vectors (maintained as yeast artificial chromosomes or YACs)
1988	Philip Leder and Timothy Stewart patent the first genetically altered transgenic mouse ("Harvard Mouse" susceptible to breast cancer); genetic engineering companies begin cross-licensing agreements for products with parallel products (e.g., Hoffman-LaRoche, Inc, and Cetus Corporation cross-license Interleukin-1 and Polyethylene Glycol Modified IL-2); the DOE and the NIH signed a memorandum of understanding to "coordinate research and technical activities related to the human genome." (www.nhgri.nih.gov/HGP/#When); (www.nhgri.nih.gov/HGP_goals/5yrplan.html)
1989	UC Davis scientists develop a recombinant vaccine against the rinderpest virus
	National Center for Human Genome Research founded with James Watson first director (now called The National Human Genome Research Institute [NHGRI: www.nhgri.nih.gov/])
1990	Mary-Claire King at UC Berkeley proves that the BRCA1 breast cancer gene on chromosome 17 has a familial basis, and that the gene can stop (suppress) and reverse several types of cancers; biotechnology companies receive patents for genetically engineered pharmaceuticals; the Human Genome Project to map and sequence the genomes of model organisms officially begins with a multiphase, $200 million budget for 15 years; formal launch of the International Human Genome Project; Calgene Inc., successfully field tests genetically engineered cotton plants; scientists introduce the bioluminescent gene *Agrobacterium tumefaciens* from the firefly into tobacco plant cells, producing a tobacco plant that glows green after receiving the catalyst luciferin

TABLE A ➤ **TIMELINE OF EVENTS ABOUT "GENETICS" BEFORE MENDEL, FOLLOWED BY NOTABLE DISCOVERIES IN GENETICS AND MOLECULAR BIOLOGY TO THE PRESENT—cont'd**

DATE	EVENT
AFTER MENDEL—cont'd	
1990, cont'd	Geneticist W. French Anderson successfully uses gene therapy for the first time in a four-year old girl with the rare autosomal recessive diseases adenosine deaminase (ADA) deficiency; Alan Handyside and Robert Winston at London's Hammersmith Hospital pioneer *in vitro* fertilization
1991	The online *Mendelian Inheritance in Man* database publishes a catalog of genetic diseases and their cytogenetic map locations (www.ncbi.nlm.gov/omim/); scientists begin the full-scale genome sequencing of *E. coli*
1992	U.S. Army institutes program to collect blood and tissue samples from new recruits (genetic "dog tag" surveillance) to better identify soldiers killed in action; British and American researchers discover a technique for vitro testing of embryos for genetic disorders (e.g., hemophilia, cystic fibrosis)
1993	Daniel Cohen and an international team of scientists produce a rough map of the 23 pairs of human chromosomes.
1994	The FDA approves Calgene Inc.'s Flavr-Savr tomato for sale in the U.S., the first genetically engineered food product (designed to stay firm after harvest and remain on the vine longer to ripen to full flavor); the *BRCA1* gene, implicated in familial breast cancer, also plays a role in noninherited breast cancers; scientists worldwide discover many genes linked to inherited and noninherited diseases (hearing loss, sudden infant death syndrome, cerulean cataracts, melanoma, dyslexia, thyroid cancer, dwarfism, prostate cancer, bipolar disorder); first nonvirus genome reported in *Science* (1994;265:) for the bacterium *Haemophilus influenzae*
1995	Duke researchers transplant hearts from genetically altered pigs into baboons, proving the feasibility of cross-species transplants; leptin, a protein product of the obesity (*ob*) gene triggers weight loss in experimental animals; scientists develop the STS gene mapping technique; scientists develop a transgenic mouse carrying a gene for a form of inherited Alzheimer's disease characterized by more brain amyloid protein (APP)
1996	The FDA approves Biogen's recombinant interferon drug Avonex for treating multiple sclerosis; scientific collaboration sequences the entire genome of the most complex organism yet studied, *Saccharomyces cerevisiae* (baker's yeast), with 12 million base pairs; scientists sequence the genome of the ancient organism archaea, neither a eukaryote or prokaryote; researchers determine the 3-D structure of T cells; the FDA develops an inexpensive diagnostic biosensor test for the toxic strain of *E. coli;* scientists discover a gene involved with Parkinson's disease
1997	Charles Roberts, Gary Silberstein, and Charles Daniel discover the WT1 tumor suppressor gene implicated in breast cancer; Ian Wilmut and Keith Campbell (Roslin Institute, Edinburgh) clone "Dolly" the sheep, the first mammal successfully cloned from an adult cell; scientists develop the first artificial human chromosome; Japanese researchers configure bits of DNA as "logic" elements (instructions) for a computer; scientists sequence the genomes of *E. coli, H. pylori,* and *B. burgdorferi* (Lyme disease pathogen); Azim Surani merged mouse thymocytes (type of white blood cells) with mouse embryonic germ cells—stem cells that develop into sperm or egg cells. The reprogrammed cells wouldn't form embryos, but instead develop directly into needed cells or tissues (*EMBO* 1997;16:6510)
1998	Scientists successfully grow embryonic stem cells; Japanese scientists clone eight calves using cells from a single adult cow; John Sulston (Sanger Center, Cambridge, England) and Robert Waterston (Washington University, St. Louis, MO) sequence the complete genome for the worm *C. elegans* (*Science* 1998;282:2012); Rod MacKinnon and associates of Rockerfeller University determine the first crystal structure of a membrane channel (Cell 1998;95:649)
	Scientists develop a new cloning technique with a mouse model that creates three generations of cloned clones; John Sulston (Sanger Center, Cambridge, England) and Robert Waterston (Washington University, St. Louis, MO)
1999	An international collaboration of scientists determines the DNA sequence of human chromosome 22 (*Nature* 1999;402:489)
2000	FDA approves the drug Taxol for treating early stage breast cancer; researchers discover that existing AIDS patients can become infected with a stronger form of the virus; Gerald Schatten and colleagues subdivide the embryos of primates, producing a live offspring (107 rhesus monkey embryos divided into two to nine pieces to form 368 embryos; one survived, producing a baby monkey); CuraGen Corporation announces the first functional genomics map of an entire genome (yeast); Celera Corporation and the Human Genome Project announce the deciphering of the human genome (June 26, 2000)
	Celera's estimates 3.12 billion bases for the human genome, 30 million fewer that the public consortium estimate. The Celera estimate includes 26.4 million DNA segments of about 500 letters (14.5 billion letters). This requires more than 500 million trillion DNA comparisons using 20,000 hours on Celera's super-computer (800 Alpha EV6 and EV67 processors with 64-bit architecture and 80 terabytes of memory, equivalent to about 5 to 6 times the Library of Congress). Craig Venter and Gerald Rubin sequence the genome of the fruit fly *Drosophilia melanogaster*
2001	William Nierman and colleagues complete the genomic sequence of *Caulobacter crescentus*; Richard Peek and associates at Vanderbilt University use whole-genome microarrays to determine how genetic differences between strains of *Helicobacter pylori* influence gastric cancer type and the severity; American and Japanese researchers characterize gene expression in 49 embryonic and adult mouse tissues using DNA microarrays with 13,600 genes; University of Buffalo researchers demonstrate horizontal gene transfer between different families of mouth bacteria; Arnold Levine receives the first Albany Medical Center Prize in Medicine and Biomedical Research for discovering the p53 gene that normally protects against cancer but causes cancer when it mutates (single mutation in the 135th position of the gene's 393 amino acids)

FIRST PUBLISHED REPORT OF THE DNA STRUCTURE*

Molecular Structure of Nucleic Acids

A Structure for Deoxyribose Nucleic Acid

We wish to suggest a structure for the salt of deoxyribose nucleic acid (D.N.A.). This structure has novel features which are of considerable biological interest.

A structure for nucleic acid has already been proposed by Pauling and Corey[1]. They kindly made their manuscript available to us in advance of publication. Their model consists of three intertwined chains, with the phosphates near the fibre axis, and the bases on the outside. In our opinion, this structure is unsatisfactory for two reasons: (1) We believe that the material which gives the X-ray diagrams is the salt, not the free acid. Without the acidic hydrogen atoms it is not clear what forces would hold the structure together, especially as the negatively charged phosphates near the axis will repel each other. (2) Some of the van der Waals distances appear to be too small.

Another three-chain structure has also been suggested by Fraser (in the press). In his model the phosphates are on the outside and the bases on the inside, linked together by hydrogen bonds. This structure as described is rather ill-defined, and for this reason we shall not comment on it.

We wish to put forward a radically different structure for the salt of deoxyribose nucleic acid. This structure has two helical chains each coiled round the same axis (see diagram). We have made the usual chemical assumptions, namely, that each chain consists of phosphate diester groups joining β-D-deoxyribofuranose residues with 3′,5′ linkages. The two chains (but not their bases) are related by a dyad perpendicular to the fibre axis. Both chains follow right-handed helices, but owing to the dyad the sequences of the atoms in the two chains run in opposite directions. Each chain loosely resembles Furberg's[2] model No. 1; that is, the bases are on the inside of the helix and the phosphates on the outside. The configuration of the sugar and the atoms near it is close to Furberg's 'standard configuration', the sugar being roughly perpendicular to the attached base. There is a residue on each chain every 3 · 4 A. In the z-direction. We have assumed an angle of 36° between adjacent residues in the same chain, so that the structure repeats after 10 residues on each chain, that is, after 34 A. The distance of a phosphorus atom from the fibre axis is 10 A. As the phosphates are on the outside, cations have easy access to them.

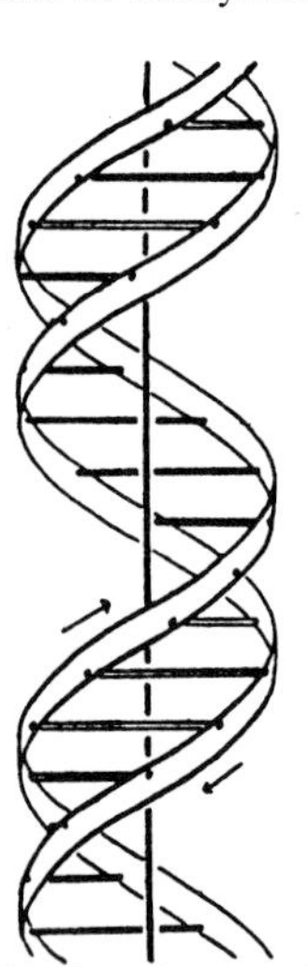

This figure is purely diagrammatic. The two ribbons symbolize the two phosphate–sugar chains, and the horizontal rods the pairs of bases holding the chains together. The vertical line marks the fibre axis

The structure is an open one, and its water content is rather high. At lower water contents we would expect the bases to tilt so that the structure could become more compact.

The novel feature of the structure is the manner in which the two chains are held together by the purine and pyrimidine bases. The planes of the bases are perpendicular to the fibre axis. They are joined together in pairs, a single base from one chain being hydrogen-bonded to a single base from the other chain, so that the two lie side by side with identical z-co-ordinates. One of the pair must be a purine and the other a pyrimidine for bonding to occur. The hydrogen bonds are made as follows: purine position 1 to pyrimidine position 1; purine position 6 to pyrimidine position 6.

If it is assumed that the bases only occur in the structure in the most plausible tautomeric forms (that is, with the keto rather than the enol configurations) it is found that only specific pairs of bases can bond together. These pairs are: adenine (purine) with thymine (pyrimidine), and guanine (purine) with cytosine (pyrimidine).

In other words, if an adenine forms one member of a pair, on either chain, then on these assumptions the other member must be thymine; similarly for guanine and cytosine. The sequence of bases on a single chain does not appear to be restricted in any way. However, if only specific pairs of bases can be formed, it follows that if the sequence of bases on one chain is given, then the sequence on the other chain is automatically determined.

It has been found experimentally[3,4] that the ratio of the amounts of adenine to thymine, and the ratio of guanine to cytosine, are always very close to unity for deoxyribose nucleic acid.

It is probably impossible to build this structure with a ribose sugar in place of the deoxyribose, as the extra oxygen atom would make too close a van der Waals contact.

The previously published X-ray data[5,6] on deoxyribose nucleic acid are insufficient for a rigorous test of our structure. So far as we can tell, it is roughly compatible with the experimental data, but it must be regarded as unproved until it has been checked against more exact results. Some of these are given in the following communications. We were not aware of the details of the results presented there when we devised our structure, which rests mainly though not entirely on published experimental data and stereochemical arguments.

It has not escaped our notice that the specific pairing we have postulated immediately suggests a possible copying mechanism for the genetic material.

Full details of the structure, including the conditions assumed in building it, together with a set of co-ordinates for the atoms, will be published elsewhere.

We are much indebted to Dr. Jerry Donohue for constant advice and criticism, especially on interatomic distances. We have also been stimulated by a knowledge of the general nature of the unpublished experimental results and ideas of Dr. M. H. F. Wilkins, Dr. R. E. Franklin and their co-workers at King's College, London. One of us (J. D. W.) has been aided by a fellowship from the National Foundation for Infantile Paralysis.

J. D. Watson
F. H. C. Crick

Medical Research Council Unit for the
Study of the Molecular Structure of
Biological Systems,
Cavendish Laboratory, Cambridge.
April 2.

[1]Pauling, L., and Corey, R. B., *Nature,* **171,** 346 (1953); *Proc. U.S. Nat. Acad. Sci.,* **39,** 84 (1953).
[2]Furberg, S., *Acta Chem. Scand.,* **6,** 634 (1952).
[3]Chargaff, E., for references see Zamenhof, S., Brawerman, G. and Chargaff, E., *Biochim. et Biophys. Acta,* **9,** 402 (1952).
[4]Wyatt, G. R., *J. Gen. Physiol.,* **36,** 201 (1952).
[5]Astbury, W. T., Symp. Soc. Exp. Biol. 1, Nucleic Acid, 66 (Camb. Univ. Press, 1947).
[6]Wilkins, M. H. F., and Randall, J. T., *Biochim. et Biophys. Acta,* **10,** 192 (1953).

*Reprinted by permission from *Nature,* April 25, 1953, p. 737.

Appendix A

The Metric System and Conversion Constants in Exercise Physiology

Appendix A has three parts. Part 1 deals with the metric system, Part 2 discusses the Système International d'Unités (SI units), and Part 3 presents conversion factors for clinical hematology and clinical chemistry.

➤ Part 1 • The Metric System

Most measurements in science are expressed in terms of the **metric system**. This system uses units that are related to one another by a power of 10. The prefix *centi-* means one-hundredth, *milli-* means one-thousandth, and *kilo-* is derived from a word that means one thousand. In the following sections, we show the relationship between metric units and English units of measurement that are relevant to the material presented in this book.

➤ UNITS OF LENGTH

Metric Unit	Equivalent Metric Units	Equivalent English Units
meter (m)	100 cm; 1000 mm	39.37 in; 3.28 ft; 1.09 yd
centimeter (cm)	0.01 m; 10 mm	0.3937 in
millimeter (mm)	0.001 m; 0.1 cm	0.03937 in

UNITS OF MASS (WEIGHT)

Use the following conversions for common units of mass (weight) and volume. For example, 1 ounce = 0.06 pound. Two ounces would therefore equal 2 × 0.06 = 0.12 pound, and 16 ounces = 0.96 pound (16 × 0.06).

➤ UNITS OF MASS (WEIGHT)

Metric Unit	Equivalent Metric Units	Equivalent English Units
kilogram (kg)	1000 g 1,000,000 mg	35.3 oz; 2.2046 lb
gram (g)	0.001 kg 1000 mg	0.353 oz
milligram (mg)	0.000001 kg 0.001	0.0000353 oz

➤ UNITS OF VOLUME

Metric Unit	Equivalent Metric Units	Equivalent English Units
liter (L)	1000 mL	1.057 qt
milliliter (mL) or cubic centimeter (cc)	0.001 L	0.001057 qt

➤ TEMPERATURE

To convert Fahrenheit to Celsius: °C = (°F − 32) ÷ 1.8
To convert Celsius to Fahrenheit: °F = (1.8 × °C) + 32
On the Fahrenheit scale, water freezes at 32°F and boils at 212°F.
On the Celsius scale, water freezes at 0°C and boils at 100°C.

➤ UNITS OF SPEED

MPH	KM · HR^{-1}	M · S^{-1}	MPH	KM · HR^{-1}	M · S^{-1}
1	1.6	0.47	11	17.7	5.17
2	3.2	0.94	12	19.3	5.64
3	4.8	1.41	13	20.9	6.11
4	6.4	1.88	14	22.5	6.58
5	8.0	2.35	15	24.1	7.05
6	9.6	2.82	16	25.8	7.52
7	11.2	3.29	17	27.4	7.99
8	12.8	3.76	18	29.0	8.46
9	14.4	4.23	19	30.6	8.93
10	16.0	4.70	20	32.2	9.40

COMMON EXPRESSIONS OF WORK, ENERGY, AND POWER

Watts	Kilocalories (kcal)	Foot-Pounds (ft-lb)
1 watt = 0.73756 ft-lb · s^{-1}	1 kcal = 3086 ft-lb	1 ft · lb = 3.2389 × 10^{-3} kcal
1 watt = 0.01433 kcal · min^{-1}	1 kcal = 426.8 kg-m	1 ft · lb = 0.13825 kg-m
1 watt = 1.341 × 10^{-3} hp or 0.0013 hp	1 kcal = 3087.4 ft-lb	1 ft · lb = 5.050 × 10^{-3} hp · h^{-1}
1 watt = 6.12 kg-m · min^{-1}	1 kcal = 1.5593 × 10^{-3} hp · h^{-1}	

Terminology and Units of Measurement

The American College of Sports Medicine suggests that the following terminology and units of measurement be used in scientific endeavors to promote consistency and clarity of communication, and to avoid ambiguity. The terms defined below utilize the units of measurement of the Système International d'Unités (SI units).

Exercise: Any and all activity involving generation of force by the activated muscle(s) that results in disruption of a homeostatic state. In dynamic exercise, the muscle may perform shortening (concentric) contractions or be overcome by external resistance and perform lengthening (eccentric) contractions. When muscle force results in no movement, the contraction should be termed static or isometric.

Exercise intensity: A specific level of maintenance of muscular activity quantified in terms of power (energy expenditure or work performed per unit of time), isometric force sustained, or velocity of progression.

Endurance: The time limit of a person's ability to maintain either a specific isometric force or a specific power level involving combinations of concentric or eccentric muscular contractions.

Mass: A quantity of matter of an object, a direct measure of the object's inertia (note: mass = weight ÷ acceleration due to gravity; unit: gram or kilogram).

Weight: The force with which a quantity of matter is attracted toward Earth by normal acceleration of gravity (traditional unit: kilogram).

Energy: The capability of producing force, performing work, or generating heat (unit: joule or kilojoule).

Force: That which changes or tends to change the state of rest or motion in matter (unit: newton).

Speed: Total distance traveled per unit of time (unit: meters per second).

Velocity: Displacement per unit of time. A vector quantity requiring that direction be stated or strongly implied (unit: meters per second or kilometers per hour).

Work: Force expressed through a distance but with no limitation on time (unit: joule or kilojoule). Quantities of energy and heat expressed independently of time should also be presented in joules. The term "work" should *not* be employed synonymously with muscular exercise.

Power: The rate of performing work; the derivative of work with respect to time; the product of force and velocity (unit: watt). Other related processes such as energy release and heat transfer should, when expressed per unit of time, be quantified and presented in watts.

Torque: Effectiveness of a force to produce axial rotation (unit: newton · meter).

Volume: A space occupied, for example, by a quantity of fluid gas (unit: liter or milliliter). Gas volumes should be indicated as ATPS, BTPS, or STPD.

Amount of a substance: The amount of a substance is frequently expressed in moles. A mole is the quantity of a chemical substance that has a weight in mass units (e.g., grams) numerically equal to the molecular weight, or that in the case of a gas has a volume occupied by such a weight under specified conditions. One mole of a respiratory gas is equal to 22.4 liters at STPD.

➤ PART 2 • SI Units

The uniform numerical value system is known as the Système International d'Unités, or its abbreviation, SI. SI was developed through international cooperation to create a universally acceptable system of measurement. SI ensures that units of measurement are uniform in concept and style. The SI system permits quantities in common use to be more easily compared. Many scientific organizations endorse the concept of the SI, and leading journals in nutrition, health, and exercise science now require that laboratory data be presented in SI units. The information in this appendix has been summarized from a detailed description about the SI published in the following article:

Young DS. Implementation of SI units for clinical laboratory data. Style specifications and conversion tables. Ann Intern Med 1987;106:114.

➤ DEFINITIONS OF COMMON SI UNITS

Degree Celsius (°C)	The degree Celsius (centigrade) is equivalent to K − 273.16.
Radian (rad)	The radian is the plane angle between two radii of a circle which subtend on the circumference of an arc equal in length to the radius.
Joule (J)	The joule is the work done when the point of application of a force of one newton is displaced through a distance of one meter in the direction of the force. 1 J = 1 N · m.
Kelvin (K)	The kelvin is the fraction 1/273.16 of the thermodynamic temperature of the triple point of water.
Kilogram (kg)	The kilogram is a unit of mass equal to the mass of the international prototype of the kilogram.
Meter (m)	The meter is the length equal to 1,650,763.73 wavelengths in vacuum of the radiation that corresponds to the transition between the levels $2p_{10}$ and $5d_5$ of the krypton 86 atom.
Newton (N)	The newton is that force which, when applied to a mass of 1 kilogram, gives it an acceleration of 1 meter per second squared. 1 N = 1 kg · m/s^2.
Pascal (Pa)	The pascal is the pressure produced by a force of 1 newton applied, with uniform distribution, over an area of 1 square meter. 1 Pa = 1 N/m^2.
Second (s)	The second is the duration of 9,192,631,770 periods of the radiation that corresponds to the transition between the two hyperfine levels of the ground state of the cesium 133 atom.
Watt (W)	The watt is the power that in 1 second gives rise to the energy of 1 joule. 1 W = 1 J/s.

➤ BASE UNITS OF SI NOMENCLATURE

Physical Quantity	Base Unit	SI Symbol
Length	meter	m
Mass	kilogram	kg
Time	second	s
Amount of substance	mole	mol
Thermodynamic temperature	kelvin	K
Electric current	ampere	A
Luminous intensity	candela	cd

➤ GENERAL SI STYLE GUIDELINES

Guidelines	Example	Incorrect Style	Correct Style
Lowercase letters are used for symbols or abbreviations	kilogram	Kg	kg
Exceptions:			
	kelvin	k	K
	ampere	a	A
	liter	l	L
Symbols are not followed by a period	meter	m.	m
Exception: end of sentence	mole	mol.	mol
Symbols are not to be pluralized	kilograms	kgs	kg
	meters	ms	m
Names and symbols are not to be combined	force	kilogram · meter · s^{-2}	kg · m · s^{-2}
			kg · m/s^2
When numbers are printed, symbols are preferred		100 meters	100 m
		2 moles	2 mol
A space should be placed between number and symbol		50ml	50 mL
The product of units is indicated by a dot above the line		kg × m/s^2	kg · m · s^{-2}
			kg · m/s^2
Only one solidus (/) should be used per expression		mmol/L/s	mmol/(L · s)
A zero should be placed before the decimal		.01	0.01
Decimal numbers are preferable to fractions		¾	0.75
		75%	0.75
Spaces are used to separate long numbers		1,500,000	1 500 000
Exception: optional with four-digit number		1000	1000 or 1 000

➤ COMMON PREFIXES USED WITH SI UNITS OF MEASUREMENT

Prefix	Abbreviation	Multiplication factor
tera	T	1,000,000,000,000 = 10^{12}
giga	G	1,000,000,000 = 10^{9}
mega	M	1,000,000 = 10^{6}
kilo	k	1,000 = 10^{3}
hecto	h	100 = 10^{2}
deci	d	0.1 = 10^{-1}
centi	c	0.01 = 10^{-2}
milli	m	0.001 = 10^{-3}
micro	μ	0.000,001 = 10^{-6}
nano	n	0.000,000,001 = 10^{-9}
pico	p	0.000,000,000,001 = 10^{-12}

For SI units in exercise physiology, the term *body weight* is properly referred to as mass (kg), height should be referred to as stature (m), second is s, minute is min, hour is h, week is wk, month is mo, year is y, day is d, gram is g, liter is L, hertz is Hz, joule is J, kilocalorie is kcal, ohm is Ω, pascal is Pa, revolutions per minute is rpm, volt is V, and watt is W. These abbreviations or symbols are used for the singular or plural form.

➤ CONVERSION FACTORS FOR USE IN THE EXERCISE SCIENCES

To Convert	Into	Multiply By
A		
ampere-hours	coulombs	3,600.0
ampere-hours	faradays	0.03731
angstrom units	inches	3.937×10^{-9}
angstrom units	meters	1×10^{-10}
angstrom units	micrometers	1×10^{-4}
B		
BTU	ergs	1.0550×10^{-10}
BTU	foot-pounds	778.3
BTU	gram-calories	252.0
BTU	horsepower-hours	3.931×10^{-4}
BTU	joules	1,054.8
BTU	kilogram-calories	0.2520
BTU	kilogram-meters	107.5
BTU	kilowatt-hours	2.928×10^{-4}
BTU/hour	foot-pounds/second	0.2162
BTU/hour	gram-calorie/second	0.0700
BTU/hour	horsepower-hours	3.929×10^{-4}
BTU/hour	watts	0.2931
BTU/minute	foot-pounds/second	12.96
BTU/minute	horsepower	0.02356
BTU/minute	kilowatts	0.01757
BTU/minute	watts	17.57
BTU/square foot/minute	watts/square inch	0.1221
C		
calories, gram (mean)	BTU (mean)	3.9685×10^{-3}
centigrade (celsius)	Fahrenheit	(C° × 9/5) + 32
centigrams	grams	0.01
centiliters	fluid ounces (U.S.)	0.3382
centiliters	cubic inches	0.6103
centiliters	drams	2.705
centiliters	liters	0.01
centimeters	feet	3.281×10^{-2}
centimeters	inches	0.3937
centimeters	kilometers	1×10^{-5}
centimeters	meters	0.01
centimeters	miles	6.214×10^{-6}
centimeters	millimeters	10.0
centimeters	mils	393.7
centimeters	yards	1.094×10^{-2}
centimeter-dynes	centimeter-grams	1.020×10^{-3}
centimeter-dynes	meter-kilograms	1.020×10^{-8}
centimeter-dynes	pound-feet	7.376×10^{-8}
centimeter-grams	centimeter-dynes	980.7
centimeter-grams	meter-kilograms	1×10^{-5}
centimeter-grams	pound-feet	7.233×10^{-6}
centimeters of mercury	atmospheres	0.01316
centimeters of mercury	feet of water	0.4461
centimeters of mercury	kilograms/square meter	136.0
centimeters of mercury	pounds/square foot	27.85
centimeters of mercury	pounds/square inch	0.1934
centimeters/second	feet/minute	1.1969
centimeters/second	feet/second	0.03281
centimeters/second	kilometers/hour	0.036
centimeters/second	knots	0.1943
centimeters/second	meters/minute	0.6
centimeters/second	miles/hour	0.02237
centimeters/second	miles/minute	3.728×10^{-4}
centimeters/second/second	feet/second/second	0.03281
centimeters/second/second	km/hour/second	0.036
centimeters/second/second	meters/second/second	0.01
centimeters/second/second	miles/hour/second	0.02237
cubic centimeters	cubic feet	3.531×10^{-5}
cubic centimeters	cubic inches	0.06102
cubic centimeters	cubic meters	1×10^{-6}
cubic centimeters	cubic yards	1.308×10^{-6}
cubic centimeters	gallons (U.S. liq.)	2.642×10^{-4}
cubic centimeters	liters	0.001
cubic centimeters	pints (U.S. liq.)	2.113×10^{-3}
cubic centimeters	quarts (U.S. liq.)	1.057×10^{-3}
cubic feet	bushels (dry)	0.8036
cubic feet	cubic centimeters	28,320.0
cubic feet	cubic inches	1,728.0
cubic feet	cubic meters	0.02832
cubic feet	cubic yards	0.03704
cubic feet	gallons (U.S. liq.)	7.48052
cubic feet	liters	28.32
cu feet	pints (U.S. liq.)	59.84
cubic feet	quarts (U.S. liq.)	29.92
cubic feet/minute	cubic centimeters/second	472.0
cubic feet/minute	gallons/second	0.1247
cubic feet/minute	liters/second	0.4720
cubic feet/minute	pounds of water/minute	62.43
cubic feet/second	million gal/day	0.646317
cubic feet/second	gallons/minute	448.831
cubic inches	cubic centimeters	16.39
cubic inches	cubic feet	5.787×10^{-4}
cubic inches	cubic meters	1.639×10^{-4}
cubic inches	cubic yards	2.143×10^{-5}
cubic inches	gallons	4.329×10^{-3}
cubic inches	liters	0.01639
cubic inches	pints (U.S. liq.)	0.03463
cubic inches	quarts (U.S. liq.)	0.01732
cubic meters	bushels (dry)	28.38
cubic meters	cubic centimeters	1×10^{-6}
cubic meters	cubic feet	35.31
cubic meters	cubic inches	61,023.0
cubic meters	cubic yards	1.308
cubic meters	gallons (U.S. liq.)	264.2
cubic meters	liters	1,000.0
cubic meters	pints (U.S. liq.)	2,113.0
cubic meters	quarts (U.S. liq.)	1,057.0
cubic yards	cubic centimeters	7.646×10^{5}
cubic yards	cubic feet	27.0

➤ CONVERSION FACTORS FOR USE IN THE EXERCISE SCIENCES—*continued*

To Convert	Into	Multiply By
cubic yards	cubic inches	46,656.0
cubic yards	cubic meters	0.7646
cubic yards	gallons (U.S. liq.)	202.0
cubic yards	liters	764.6
cubic yards	pints (U.S. liq.)	1,615.9
cubic yards	quarts (U.S. liq.)	807.9
cubic yards/ minute	cubic ft/second	0.45
cubic yards/ minute	gallons/second	3.367
cubic yards/ minute	liters/second	12.74
D		
days	seconds	86,400.0
decigrams	grams	0.1
deciliters	liters	0.1
decimeters	meters	0.1
degrees (angle)	quadrants	0.01111
degrees (angle)	radians	0.01745
degrees (angle)	seconds	3,600.0
degrees/second	radians/second	0.01745
degrees/second	revolutions/ minute	0.1667
degrees/second	revolutions/ second	2.778×10^{-3}
dekagrams	grams	10.0
dekaliters	liters	10.0
dekameters	meters	10.0
drams	grams	1.7718
drams	ounces	0.0625
dynecentimeter	ergs/second	0.01
dynesquare centimeter	atmospheres	9.869×10^{-7}
dynesquare centimeter	inches of mercury at 0°C	2.953×10^{-5}
dynesquare centimeter	inches of water at 4°C	4.015×10^{-4}
dynes	grams	1.020×10^{-3}
dynes	joules/centimeter	1×10^{-7}
dynes	jouls/meter (newtons)	1×10^{-5}
dynes	kilograms	1.020×10^{-6}
dynes	poundals	7.233×10^{-5}
dynes	pounds	2.248×10^{-6}
dynes/square centimeter	bars	1×10^{-6}
E		
ergs	BTU	9.480×10^{-11}
ergs	dyne-centimeters	1.0
ergs	foot-pounds	7.3670×10^{-8}
ergs	gram-calories	0.2389×10^{-7}
ergs	gram-centimeters	1.020×10^{-3}
ergs	horsepower hours	3.7250×10^{-14}
ergs	joules	1×10^{-7}
ergs	kilogram-calories	2.389×10^{-11}
ergs	kilogram-meters	1.020×10^{-8}
ergs	kilowatt-hours	0.2778×10^{-13}
ergs	watt-hours	0.2778×10^{-10}
ergs/second	BTU/minute	$5,688 \times 10^{-9}$
ergs/second	foot-pounds/minute	4.427×10^{-6}
ergs/second	foot-pounds/second	7.3756×10^{-8}
ergs/second	horsepower	1.341×10^{-10}
ergs/second	kilogram-calories/ minute	1.433×10^{-9}
ergs/second	kilowatts	1×10^{-10}
F		
feet	centimeters	30.48
feet	kilometers	3.048×10^{-4}
feet	meters	0.3048
feet	miles (naut.)	1.645×10^{-4}
feet	miles (stat.)	1.894×10^{-4}
feet	millimeters	304.8
feet	mils	1.2×10^{4}
feet of water	atmospheres	0.02950
feet of water	inches of mercury	0.8826
feet of water	kilograms/square centimeter	0.03048
feet of water	kilograms/square meter	304.8
feet of water	pounds/square foot	62.43
feet of water	pounds/square inch	0.4335
feet/minute	centimeters/second	0.5080
feet/minute	feet/second	0.01667
feet/minute	kilometers/hour	0.01829
feet/minute	meters/minute	0.3048
feet/minute	miles/hour	0.01136
feet/second	centimeters/second	30.48
feet/second	kilometers/hour	1.097
feet/second	knots	0.5921
feet/second	meters/minute	18.29
feet/second	miles/hour	0.6818
feet/second	miles/minute	0.01136
feet/second/ second	centimeters/second	30.48
feet/second/ second	kilometers/hour/ second	1.097
feet/second/ second	meters/second/ second	0.3048
feet/second/ second	miles/hour/second	0.6818
feet/100 feet	percent grade	1.0
foot-candles	lumens/square meter	10.764
foot-pounds	BTU	1.286×10^{-3}
foot-pounds	ergs	1.356×10^{7}
foot-pounds	gram-calories	0.3238
foot-pounds	horsepower-hours	5.050×10^{-7}
foot-pounds	joules	1.356
foot-pounds	kilogram-calories	3.24×10^{-4}
foot-pounds	kilogram-meters	0.1383
foot-pounds	kilowatt-hours	3.766×10^{-7}
foot-pounds/ minute	BTU/minute	1.286×10^{-3}
foot-pounds/ minute	foot-pounds/ second	0.01667
foot-pounds/ minute	horsepower	3.030×10^{-5}
foot-pounds/ minute	kilogram-calories/ minute	3.24×10^{-4}
foot-pounds/ second	kilowatts	2.260×10^{-5}
foot-pounds/ second	BTU/hour	4.6263
foot-pounds/ second	BTU/minute	0.07717
foot-pounds/ second	horsepower	0.818×10^{-3}

➤ CONVERSION FACTORS FOR USE IN THE EXERCISE SCIENCES—*continued*

To Convert	Into	Multiply By
foot-pounds/second	kilogram-calories/minute	1.01945
foot-pounds/second	kilowatts	1.356×10^{-3}
G		
gallons	cubic centimeters	3,785.0
gallons	cubic feet	0.1337
gallons	cubic inches	231.0
gallons	cubic meters	3.785×10^{-3}
gallons	cubic yards	4.951×10^{-3}
gallons	liters	3.785
gallons (liq. British imp.)	gallons (U.S. liq.)	1.20095
gallons (U.S.)	gallons (imp.)	0.83267
gallons of water	pounds of water	8.3453
gallons/minute	cu feet/second	2.228×10^{-3}
gallons/minute	liters/second	0.06308
gallons/minute	cubic feet/hour	8.0208
grams	dynes	980.7
grams	grains	15.43
grams	joules/centimeter	9.807×10^{-5}
grams	joules/meter (newtons)	9.807×10^{-3}
grams	kilograms	0.001
grams	kilograms	0.001
grams	milligrams	1,000.0
grams	ounces (avoirdupois)	0.03527
grams	ounces (troy)	0.03215
grams	poundals	0.07093
grams	pounds	2.205×10^{-3}
grams/centimeter	pounds/inch	5.600×10^{-3}
grams/cubic centimeter	pounds/cubic foot	62.43
grams/cubic centimeter	pounds/cubic inch	0.03613
grams/cubic centimeter	pounds/mil-foot	3.405×10^{-7}
grams/liter	grains/gallon	58.417
grams/liter	pounds/1000 gallons	8.345
grams/liter	pounds/cubic foot	0.062427
grams/liter	parts/million	1,000.0
grams/square centimeter	pounds/square foot	2.0481
gram-calories	BTU	3.9683×10^{-3}
gram-calories	ergs	4.1868×10^{7}
gram-calories	foot-pounds	3.0880
gram-calories	horsepower-hours	1.5596×10^{-6}
gram-calories	kilowatt-hours	1.1630×10^{-6}
gram-calories	watt-hours	1.1630×10^{-3}
gram-calories/second	BTU/hour	14.286
gram-centimeters	BTU	9.297×10^{-8}
gram-centimeters	ergs	980.7
gram-centimeters	joules	9.807×10^{-5}
gram-centimeters	kilogram-calories	2.343×10^{-8}
gram-centimeters	kilogram-meters	1×10^{-5}
H		
horsepower	BTU/minute	42.44
horsepower	foot-pounds/minute	33,000.0
horsepower	foot-pounds/second	550.0
horsepower (metric) (542.5 foot-pounds/second)	horsepower (550 foot-pounds/second)	0.9863
horsepower (550 foot-pounds/second)	horsepower (metric) (542.5 foot-pounds/second)	1.014
horsepower	kilogram-calories/minute	10.68
horsepower	kilowatts	0.7457
horsepower	watts	745.7
horsepower (boiler)	BTU/hour	33,479.0
horsepower (boiler)	kilowatts	9.803
horsepower-hours	BTU	2,547.0
horsepower-hours	ergs	2.6845×10^{13}
horsepower-hours	foot-pounds	1.98×10^{6}
horsepower-hours	gram-calories	641,190.0
horsepower-hours	joules	2.684×10^{6}
horsepower-hours	kilogram-calories	641.1
horsepower-hours	kilogram-meters	2.737×10^{5}
horsepower-hours	kilowatt-hours	0.7457
hours	days	4.167×10^{-2}
hours	weeks	5.952×10^{-3}
I		
inches	centimeters	2.540
inches	meters	2.540×10^{-2}
inches	miles	1.578×10^{-5}
inches	millimeters	25.40
inches	mils	1,000.0
inches	yards	2.778×10^{-2}
inches of mercury	atmospheres	0.03342
inches of mercury	feet of water	1.133
inches of mercury	kilograms/square centimeter	0.03453
inches of mercury	kilograms/square meter	345.3
inches of mercury	pounds/square foot	70.73
inches of mercury	pounds/square inch	0.4912
inches of water (at 4°C)	atmospheres	2.458×10^{-3}
inches of water (at 4°C)	inches of mercury	0.07355
inches of water (at 4°C)	kg/square centimeter	2.540×10^{-3}
inches of water (at 4°C)	ounces/square inch	0.5781
inches of water (at 4°C)	pounds/square foot	5.204

➤ CONVERSION FACTORS FOR USE IN THE EXERCISE SCIENCES—*continued*

To Convert	Into	Multiply By
inches of water (at 4°C)	pounds/square inch	0.03613
J		
joules	BTU	9.480×10^{-4}
joules	ergs	1×10^{7}
joules	foot-pounds	0.7376
joules	kg-calories	2.389×10^{-4}
joules	kg-meters	0.1020
joules	watt-hours	2.778×10^{-4}
joules/centimeter	grams	1.020×10^{4}
joules/centimeter	dynes	1×10^{7}
joules/centimeter	joules/meter (newtons)	100.0
joules/centimeter	poundals	723.3
joules/centimeter	pounds	22.48
K		
kilograms	dynes	980,665.0
kilograms	grams	1,000.0
kilograms	joules/centimeter	0.09807
kilograms	joules/meter (newtons)	9.807
kilograms	poundals	70.93
kilograms	pounds	2.205
kilograms	tons (long)	9.842×10^{-4}
kilograms	tons (short)	1.102×10^{-3}
kilograms/cubic meter	grams/cubic centimeter	0.001
kilograms/cubic meter	pounds/cubic foot	0.06243
kilograms/cubic meter	pounds/cubic inch	3.613×10^{-5}
kilograms/cubic meter	pounds/mil-foot	3.405×10^{-10}
kilograms/meter	pounds/foot	0.6720
kilograms/square centimeter	dynes	980,665.0
kilograms/square centimeter	atmospheres	0.9678
kilograms/square centimeter	feet of water	32.81
kilograms/square centimeter	inches of mercury	28.96
kilograms/square centimeter	pounds/square foot	2,048.0
kilograms/square centimeter	pounds/square inch	14.22
kilograms/square meter	atmospheres	9.678×10^{-5}
kilograms/square meter	bars	98.07×10^{-6}
kilograms/square meter	feet of water	3.281×10^{-3}
kilograms/square meter	inches of mercury	2.896×10^{-3}
kilograms/square meter	pounds/square foot	0.2048
kilograms/square meter	pounds/square inch	1.422×10^{-3}
kilograms/square millimeter	kilograms/square meter	1×10^{6}
kilogram-calories	BTU	3.968
kilogram-calories	foot-pounds	3,088.0
kilogram-calories	horsepower-hours	1.560×10^{-3}
kilogram-calories	joules	4,186.0
kilogram-calories	kilogram-meters	426.9
kilogram-calories	kilojoules	4.186
kilogram-calories	kilowatt-hours	1.163×10^{-3}
kilogram-meters	BTU	9.294×10^{-3}
kilogram-meters	ergs	9.804×10^{7}
kilogram-meters	foot-pounds	7.233
kilogram-meters	joules	9.804
kilogram-meters	kilogram-calories	2.342×10^{-3}
kilogram-meters	kilowatt-hours	2.723×10^{-6}
kilolines	maxwells	1,000.0
kiloliters	liters	1,000.0
kilometers	centimeters	1×10^{5}
kilometers	feet	3,281.0
kilometers	inches	3.937×10^{4}
kilometers	meters	1,000.0
kilometers	miles	0.6214
kilometers	millimeters	1×10^{6}
kilometers	yards	1,094.0
kilometers/hour	centimeters/second	27.78
kilometers/hour	feet/minute	54.68
kilometers/hour	feet/second	0.9113
kilometers/hour	knots	0.5396
kilometers/hour	meters/minute	16.67
kilometers/hour	miles/hour	0.6214
kilometers/hour/second	centimeters/second/second	27.78
kilometers/hour/second	feet/second/second	0.9113
kilometers/hour/second	meters/second/second	0.2778
kilometers/hour/second	miles/hour/second	0.6214
kilowatts	BTU/minute	56.92
kilowatts	foot-pounds/minute	4.426×10^{4}
kilowatts	foot-pounds/second	737.6
kilowatts	horsepower	1.341
kilowatts	kilogram-calories/minute	14.34
kilowatts	watts	1,000.0
kilowatt-hours	BTU	3,413.0
kilowatt-hours	ergs	3.600×10^{13}
kilowatt-hours	foot-pounds	2.655×10^{6}
kilowatt-hours	gram-calories	859,850.0
kilowatt-hours	horsepower-hours	1.341
kilowatt-hours	joules	3.6×10^{6}
kilowatt-hours	kilogram-calories	860.5
kilowatt-hours	kilogram-meters	3.671×10^{5}
kilowatt-hours	pounds of water evaporated from and at 212°F	3.53
kilowatt-hours	pounds of water raised from 62° to 212°F	22.75

➤ CONVERSION FACTORS FOR USE IN THE EXERCISE SCIENCES—*continued*

To Convert	Into	Multiply By
L		
liters	bushels (U.S. dry)	0.02838
liters	cubic centimeters	1,000.0
liters	cubic feet	0.03531
liters	cubic inches	61.02
liters	cubic meters	0.001
liters	cubic yards	1.308×10^{-3}
liters	gallons (U.S. liq.)	0.2642
liters	pints (U.S. liq.)	2.113
liters	quarts (U.S. liq.)	1.057
liters/minute	cubic feet/second	5.886×10^{-4}
liters/minute	gallons/second	4.403×10^{-3}
M		
meters	centimeters	100.0
meters	feet	3.281
meters	inches	39.37
meters	kilometers	0.001
meters	miles (nautical)	5.396×10^{-4}
meters	miles (statute)	6.214×10^{-4}
meters	millimeters	1,000.0
meters	yards	1.094
meters/minute	cms/second	1.667
meters/minute	feet/minute	3.281
meters/minute	feet/second	0.05468
meters/minute	kilometers/hour	0.06
meters/minute	knots	0.03238
meters/minute	miles/hour	0.03728
meters/second	feet/minute	196.8
meters/second	feet/second	3.281
meters/second	kilometers/hour	3.6
meters/second	kilometers/minute	0.06
meters/second	miles/hour	2.237
meters/second	miles/minute	0.03728
meters/second/second	centimeters/second/second	100.0
meters/second/second	feet/second/second	3.281
meters/second/second	kilometers/hour/second	3.6
meters/second/second	miles/hour/second	2.237
meter-kilograms	centimeter-dynes	9.807×10^{7}
meter-kilograms	centimeter-grams	1×10^{5}
meter-kilograms	pound-feet	7.233
miles (nautical)	feet	6,080.27
miles (nautical)	kilometers	1.853
miles (nautical)	meters	1,853.0
miles (nautical)	miles (statute)	1.1516
miles (nautical)	yards	2,027.0
miles (statute)	centimeters	1.609×10^{5}
miles (statute)	feet	5,280.0
miles (statute)	inches	6.336×10^{4}
miles (statute)	kilometers	1.609
miles (statute)	meters	1,609.0
miles (statute)	miles (nautical)	0.8684
miles (statute)	yards	1,760.0
miles/hour	centimeters/second	44.70
miles/hour	feet/minute	88.0
miles/hour	feet/second	1.467
miles/hour	kilometers/hour	1.609
miles/hour	kilometers/minute	0.02682
miles/hour	knots	0.8684
miles/hour	meters/minute	26.82
miles/hour	miles/minute	0.1667
miles/hour/second	centimeters/second/second	44.70
miles/hour/second	feet/second/second	1.467
miles/hour/second	kilometers/hour/second	1.609
miles/hour/second	meters/second/second	0.4470
miles/minute	centimeters/second	2,682.0
miles/minute	feet/second	88.0
miles/minute	kilometers/minute	1.609
miles/minute	knots/minute	0.8684
miles/minute	miles/hour	60.0
mil-feet	cubic inches	9.425×10^{-6}
milliliters	kilograms	1,000.0
millimicrons	meters	1×10^{-9}
milligrams	grains	0.01543236
milligrams	grams	0.001
milligrams/liter	parts/million	1.0
millihenries	henries	0.001
milliliters	liters	0.001
millimeters	centimeters	0.1
millimeters	feet	3.281×10^{-3}
millimeters	inches	0.03937
millimeters	kilometers	1×10^{-6}
millimeters	meters	0.001
millimeters	miles	6.214×10^{-7}
millimeters	mils	39.37
millimeters	yards	1.094×10^{-3}
minutes (angles)	degrees	0.01667
minutes (angles)	quadrants	1.852×10^{-4}
minutes (angles)	radians	2.909×10^{-4}
minutes (angles)	seconds	60.0
N		
newtons	dynes	1×10^{5}
O		
ohms (international)	ohms (absolute)	1.005
ohms	megohms	1×10^{-6}
ohms	microhms	1×10^{6}
ounces	drams	16.0
ounces	grains	437.5
ounces	grams	28.349527
ounces	pounds	0.0625
ounces	ounces (troy)	0.9115
ounces	tons (long)	2.790×10^{-5}
ounces	tons (metric)	2.835×10^{-5}
ounces (fluid)	cubic inches	1.805
ounces (fluid)	liters	0.02957
ounces (troy)	grains	480.0
ounces (troy)	grams	31.103481
ounces (troy)	ounces (avoirdupois)	1.09714
ounces (troy)	pennyweights (troy)	20.0
ounces (troy)	pounds (troy)	0.08333
ounces/square inch	dynes/square centimeter	4,309.0
ounces/square inch	pounds/square inch	0.0625
P		
pints (liquid)	cubic centimeters	473.2
pints (liquid)	cubic feet	0.01671

➤ CONVERSION FACTORS FOR USE IN THE EXERCISE SCIENCES—*continued*

To Convert	Into	Multiply By
pints (liquid)	cubic inches	28.87
pints (liquid)	cubic meters	4.732×10^{-4}
pints (liquid)	cubic yards	6.189×10^{-4}
pints (liquid)	gallons	0.125
pints (liquid)	liters	0.4732
pints (liquid)	quarts (liquid)	0.5
pounds (avoirdupois)	ounces (troy)	14.5833
pounds	drams	256.0
pounds	dynes	44.4823×10^{4}
pounds	grains	7,000.0
pounds	grams	453.5924
pounds	joules/centimeter	0.04448
pounds	joules/meter (newtons)	4.448
pounds	kilograms	0.4536
pounds	ounces	16.0
pounds	ounces (troy)	14.5833
pounds	poundals	32.17
pounds	pounds (troy)	1.21528
pounds	tons (short)	0.0005
pounds of water	cubic inches	27.68
pounds of water	gallons	0.1198
Q		
quarts (dry)	cubic inches	67.20
quarts (liquid)	cubic centimeters	946.4
quarts (liquid)	cubic feet	0.03342
quarts (liquid)	cubic inches	57.75
quarts (liquid)	cubic meters	9.464×10^{-4}
quarts (liquid)	cubic yards	1.238×10^{-3}
quarts (liquid)	gallons	0.25
quarts (liquid)	liters	0.9463
R		
radians	degrees	57.30
revolutions	degrees	360.0
revolutions	quadrants	4.0
revolutions	radians	6.283
revolutions/minute	degrees/second	6.0
revolutions/minute	radians/second	0.1047
revolutions/minute	revolutions/second	0.01667
revolutions/minute/minute	radians/second/second	1.745×10^{-3}
revolutions/minute/minute	revolutions/minute/second	0.01667
revolutions/minute/minute	revolutions/second/second	2.778×10^{-4}
revolutions/second	degrees/second	360.0
revolutions/second	radians/second	6.283
revolutions/second	revolutions/minute	60.0
revolutions/second/second	radians/second/second	6.283
revolutions/second/second	revolutions/minute/minute	3,600.0
revolutions/second/second	revolutions/minute/second	60.0
S		
seconds (angle)	degrees	2.778×10^{-4}
seconds (angle)	minutes	0.01667
seconds (angle)	quadrants	3.087×10^{-6}
seconds (angle)	radians	4.848×10^{-6}
square centimeters	circular mils	1.973×10^{5}
square centimeters	square feet	1.076×10^{-3}
square centimeters	square inches	0.1550
square centimeters	square meters	0.0001
square centimeters	square miles	3.861×10^{-11}
square centimeters	square millimeters	100.0
square centimeters	square yards	1.196×10^{-4}
square feet	acres	2.296×10^{-5}
square feet	circular mils	1.833×10^{8}
square feet	square centimeters	929.0
square feet	square inches	144.0
square feet	square meters	0.09290
square feet	square miles	3.587×10^{-8}
square feet	square millimeters	9.290×10^{4}
square feet	square yards	0.1111
square inches	circular mils	1.273×10^{6}
square inches	square centimeters	6.452
square inches	square feet	6.944×10^{-3}
square inches	square millimeters	645.2
square inches	square mils	1×10^{6}
square inches	square yards	7.716×10^{-4}
square kilometers	acres	247.1
square kilometers	square centimeters	1×10^{10}
square kilometers	square feet	10.76×10^{6}
square kilometers	square inches	1.550×10^{9}
square kilometers	square meters	1×10^{6}
square kilometers	square miles	0.3861
square kilometers	square yards	1.196×10^{6}
square meters	acres	2.471×10^{-4}
square meters	square centimeters	1×10^{4}
square meters	square feet	10.76
square meters	square inches	1,550.0
square meters	square miles	3.861×10^{-7}
square meters	square millimeters	1×10^{6}
square meters	square yards	1.196
square miles	acres	640.0
square miles	square feet	27.88×10^{6}
square miles	square kilometers	2.590
square miles	square meters	2.590×10^{6}
square miles	square yards	3.098×10^{6}
square millimeters	circular mils	1,973.0
square millimeters	square centimeters	0.01
square millimeters	square feet	1.076×10^{-5}
square millimeters	square inches	1.550×10^{-3}
square yards	acres	2.066×10^{-4}
square yards	square centimeters	8,361.0
square yards	square feet	9.0
square yards	square inches	1,296.0
square yards	square meters	0.8361
square yards	square miles	3.228×10^{-7}
square yards	square millimeters	8.361×10^{5}
T		
temperature (°F) + 460	absolute temperature (°F)	1.0
temperature (°F) − 32	temperature (°C)	5/9
temperature (°F) + 460	absolute temperature (°F)	1.0
temperature (°F) − 32	temperature (°C)	5.9
tons (metric)	kilograms	1,000.0
tons (metric)	pounds	2,205.0

➤ CONVERSION FACTORS FOR USE IN THE EXERCISE SCIENCES—*continued*

To Convert	Into	Multiply By
W		
watts	BTU/hour	3.4129
watts	BTU/minute	0.05688
watts	ergs/second	107.0
watts	foot-pounds/ minute	44.27
watts	foot-pounds/ second	0.7378
watts	horsepower	1.341×10^{-3}
watts	horsepower (metric)	1.360×10^{-3}
watts	kilogram-calories/ minute	0.01433
watts	kilowatts	0.001
watts (absolute)	BTU (mean)/ minute	0.056884
watts (absolute)	joules/second	1.0
watt-hours	BTU	3.413
watt-hours	ergs	3.60×10^{-10}
watt-hours	foot-pounds	2,656.0
watt-hours	gram-calories	859.85
watt-hours	horsepower-hours	1.341×10^{-3}
watt-hours	kilogram-calories	0.8605
watt-hours	kilogram-meters	367.2
watt-hours	kilowatt-hours	0.001
watts (international)	watts (absolute)	1.0002
Y		
yards	centimeters	91.44
yards	kilometers	9.144×10^{-4}
yards	meters	0.9144
yards	miles (nautical)	4.934×10^{-4}
yards	miles (statute)	5.682×10^{-4}
yards	millimeters	914.4

➤ Part 3 • Clinical Hematology and Clinical Chemistry

➤ SI CONVERSION TABLE FOR COMMON VALUES IN CLINICAL HEMATOLOGY AND CLINICAL CHEMISTRY

Component	Present Reference Intervals (Examples)	Present Unit	Conversion Factor	SI Reference Intervals	SI Unit Symbol	Significant Digits	Suggested Minimum Increment
Hemoglobin (B)							
Mass concentration							
—female	12.0–15.0	g/dL	10	120–150	g/L	XXX	1 g/L
—male	13.6–17.2	g/dL	10	136–172	g/L	XXX	1 g/L
Substance conc. Hb [Fe]							
—female	12.0–15.0	g/dL	0.6206	7.45–9.30	mmol/L	XX.XX	0.05 mmol/L
—male	13.6–17.2	g/dL	0.6206	8.45–10.65	mmol/L	XX.XX	0.05 mmol/L
Alkaline phosphatase (S)	30–120	U/L	0.01667	0.5–2.0	μkat/L	X.X	0.1 μkat/L
Amino acid nitrogen (P)	4.0–6.0	mg/dL	0.7139	2.9–4.3	mmol/L	X.X	0.1 mmol/L
Amino acid nitrogen (U)	50–200	mg/24 h	0.07139	3.6–14.3	mmol/d	X.X	0.1 mmol/d
Androstenedione (S)							
—male >18 y	0.2–3.0	μg/L	3.492	0.5–10.5	mmol/L	XX.X	0.5 nmol/L
—female >18 y	0.8–3.0	μg/L	3.492	3.0–10.5	nmol/L	XX.X	0.5 nmol/L
Bilirubin, total (S)	0.1–1.0	mg/dL	17.10	2–18	μmol/L	XX	2 μmol/L
Calcium (S)							
—male	8.8–10.3	mg/dL	0.2495	2.20–2.50	mmol/L	X.XX	0.02 mmol/L
—female <50 y	8.8–10.0	mg/dL	0.2495	2.20–2.50	mmol/L	X.XX	0.02 mmol/L
—female >50 y	8.8–10.2	mg/dL	0.2495	2.20–2.56	mmol/L	X.XX	0.02 mmol/L
Calcium (U), normal diet	<250	mg/24 h	0.02495	<6.2	mmol/d	X.X	0.1 mmol/d
Cholesterol (P)							
—<29 y	<200	mg/dL	0.02586	<5.20	mmol/L	X.XX	0.05 mmol/L
—30–39 y	<225	mg/dL	0.02586	<5.85	mmol/L	X.XX	0.05 mmol/L
—40–49 y	<245	mg/dL	0.02586	<6.35	mmol/L	X.XX	0.05 mmol/L
—>50 y	<265	mg/dL	0.02586	<6.85	mmol/L	X.XX	0.05 mmol/L
Ferritin (S)	18–300	ng/mL	1.00	18–300	μg/L	XX0	10 μg/L
Glucose (P)—fasting	70–110	mg/dL	0.05551	3.9–6.1	mmol/L	XX.X	0.1 mmol/L
Hemoglobin (B)							
—male	14.0–18.0	g/dL	10.0	140–180	g/L	XXX	1 g/L
—female	11.5–15.5	g/dL	10.0	115–155	g/L	XXX	1 g/L
Insulin (P,S)	5–20	μU/mL	7.175	35–145	pmol/L	XXX	5 pmol/L
	5–20	mU/L	7.175	35–145	pmol/L	XXX	5 pmol/L
	0.20–0.84	μg/mL	172.2	35–145	pmol/L	XXX	5 pmol/L

B, blood; P, plasma; S, serum; U, urine.

➤ SI CONVERSION TABLE FOR COMMON VALUES IN CLINICAL HEMATOLOGY AND CLINICAL CHEMISTRY—*continued*

Component	Present Reference Intervals (Examples)	Present Unit	Conversion Factor	SI Reference Intervals	SI Unit Symbol	Significant Digits	Suggested Minimum Increment
Iron (S)							
—male	80–180	μg/dL	0.1791	14–32	μmol/L	XX	1 μmol/L
—female	60–160	μg/dL	0.1791	11–29	μmol/L	XX	1 μmol/L
Lipoproteins (P)							
Low density [LDL]— as cholesterol	50–190	mg/dL	0.02586	1.30–4.90	mmol/L	X.XX	0.05 mmol/L
High density [HDL]— as cholesterol							
Male	30–70	mg/dL	0.02586	0.80–1.80	mmol/L	X.XX	0.05 mmol/L
Female	30–90	mg/dL	0.02586	0.80–2.35	mmol/L	X.XX	0.05 mmol/L
Testosterone (P)							
—female	0.6	ng/mL	3.467	2.0	nmol/L	XX.X	0.5 nmol/L
—male	4.6–8.0	ng/mL	3.467	14.0–28.0	nmol/L	XX.X	0.5 nmol/L
Thyroid tests:							
Thyroid-stimulating hormone [TSH] (S)	2–11	μU/mL	1.00	2–11	mU/L	XX	1 mU/L
Thyroxine [T_4] (S)	4.0–11.0	μg/dL	12.87	51–142	nmol/L	XXX	1 nmol/L
Thyroxine binding globulin [TBG] (S)—[as thyroxine]	12.0–28.0	μg/dL	12.87	150–360	nmol/L	XX0	1 nmol/L
Thyroxine, free (S)	0.8–2.8	ng/dL	12.87	10–36	pmol/L	XX	1 pmol/L
Triiodothyronine [T_3] (S)	75–220	ng/dL	0.01536	1.2–3.4	nmol/L	X.X	0.1 nmol/L
T_3 uptake (S)	25–35	%	0.01	0.25–0.35	1	0.XX	0.01
Tolbutamide (P)— therapeutic	50–120	mg/L	3.699	180–450	μmol/L	XX0	10 μmol/L
Transferrin (S)	170–370	mg/dL	0.01	1.70–3.70	g/L	X.XX	0.01 g/L
Triglycerides (P) [as triolein]	<160	mg/dL	0.01129	<1.80	mmol/L	X.XX	0.02 mmol/L
Vitamin A [retinol] (P,S)	10–50	μg/dL	0.03491	0.35–1.75	μmol/L	X.XX	0.05 μmol/L
Vitamin B_1 [thiamine hydrochloride] (U)	60–500	μg/24 h	0.002965	0.18–1.48	μmol/d	X.XX	0.01 μmol/d
Vitamin B_2 [riboflavin] (S)	2.6–3.7	μg/dL	26.57	70–100	nmol/L	XXX	5 nmol/L
Vitamin B_6 [pyridoxal] (B)	20–90	ng/mL	5.982	120–540	nmol/L	XXX	5 nmol/L
Vitamin B_{12} [cyano-cobalamin] (P,S)	200–1000	pg/mL	0.7378	150–750	pmol/L	XX0	10 pmol/L
		ng/dL	7.378		pmol/L		
Vitamin C [ascorbic acid]	0.6–2.00	mg/dL	56.78	30–110	μmol/L	X0	10 μmol/L
Vitamin D_3 [cholecalciferol] (P)	24–40	μg/mL	2.599	60–105	nmol/L	XXX	5 nmol/L
25 OH-cholecalciferol	18–36	ng/mL	2.496	45–90	nmol/L	XXX	5 mmol/L
Vitamin E [alpha-tocopherol] (P,S)	0.78–1.25	mg/dL	23.22	18–29	mol/L	XX	1 mol/L

B, blood; P, plasma; S, serum; U, urine.

Appendix B

Nutritive Values for Common Foods, Alcoholic and Nonalcoholic Beverages, and Specialty and Fast-Food Items

This appendix has three parts. Part 1 lists nutritive values for common foods, Part 2 lists nutritive values for alcoholic and nonalcoholic beverages, and Part 3 presents nutritive values for specialty and fast-food items. The nutritive values of foods and alcoholic and nonalcoholic beverages are expressed in 1-ounce (28.4 g) portions so comparisons can readily be made between the different food categories. For example, the protein content of 1.55 g for 1 ounce of banana nut bread can be compared directly to the protein content of 6.28 g for 1 ounce of processed American cheese.

Part 1 • Nutritive Values for Common Foods[a]

The foods are grouped into categories and are listed in alphabetical order within each category. The categories include breads, cakes and pies, cookies, candy bars, chocolate, desserts, cereals, cheese, fish, fruits, meats, eggs, dairy products, vegetables, and typical salad bar entries. An additional section labeled Variety consists of food items such as soups, sandwiches, salad dressings, oils, some condiments, and other "goodies." The nutritive value for each food is expressed per ounce or 28.4 g of that food item. The specific values for each food include the caloric content (kcal) for 1 ounce, protein, total fat, carbohydrate, calcium, iron, vitamin B_1, vitamin B_2, fiber content, and cholesterol.

[a] The information about the nutritive value of the foods was taken from a variety of sources. This includes primarily data from Watt BK, Merrill AL. Composition of foods—raw, processed and prepared. U.S. Department of Agriculture, Washington, DC, 1963; Adams C, Richardson M. Nutritive value of foods. Home and Garden Bulletin No. 72, rev, Washington, DC, U.S. Government Printing Office, 1981; and Pennington JAT, Church HN. Food Values of Portions Commonly Used. 14th ed. New York: Harper & Row, 1985. Other sources include a comprehensive database on the Cyber mainframe computer at the University of Massachusetts, the consumer relations departments of manufacturers, and journal articles that evaluated specific foods items. *NA indicates data not available.*

➤ BREADS

	KCAL	PROTEIN (G)	FAT (G)	CHO (G)	CA (MG)	FE (MG)	B_1 (MG)	B_2 (MG)	FIBER (G)	CHOLESTEROL (MG)
Banana nut	91	1.55	4.00	12.7	10.0	0.470	0.054	0.046	0.66	18.3
Boston brown—canned	60	1.26	0.39	13.2	25.8	0.567	0.038	0.025	1.34	1.9
Cornmeal muffin—recipe	91	1.89	3.15	13.2	41.6	0.567	0.069	0.069	1.00	14.5
Croutons—dry	105	3.69	1.04	20.5	35.0	1.020	0.099	0.099	0.09	0
Cracked wheat	74	2.63	0.99	14.2	18.1	0.755	0.108	0.108	1.50	0
Cracked wheat—toast	88	3.00	1.17	16.9	21.6	0.899	0.100	0.128	1.82	0
French—chunk	81	2.67	1.10	14.3	31.6	0.875	0.130	0.097	0.57	0
Italian	78	2.55	0.25	16.0	4.7	0.756	0.116	0.066	0.47	0
Mixed grain	74	2.27	1.05	13.6	30.6	0.907	0.113	0.113	1.78	0
Mixed grain—toast	80	2.47	1.15	14.8	33.3	0.986	0.099	0.123	1.97	0
Oatmeal	74	2.37	1.25	13.6	17.0	0.794	0.130	0.075	1.10	0
Oatmeal—toast	80	2.47	1.36	14.8	18.5	0.863	0.110	0.081	1.20	0
Pita pocket	78	2.94	0.42	15.6	23.2	0.685	0.129	0.061	0.45	0
Pumpernickel	71	2.60	0.98	13.6	20.4	0.777	0.097	0.147	1.67	0
Pumpernickel—toast	78	2.86	1.08	15.0	22.5	0.857	0.088	0.162	1.87	0
Raisin—	77	2.15	1.12	15.0	28.4	0.879	0.093	0.176	0.68	0
Raisin—toast	92	2.57	1.34	17.6	33.8	1.080	0.081	0.209	0.81	0
Rye—light	74	2.40	1.04	13.6	22.7	0.771	0.116	0.090	1.87	0
Rye—light—toast	84	2.73	1.18	15.5	25.8	0.876	0.107	0.103	2.15	0
Vienna	79	2.72	1.10	14.4	31.2	0.873	0.130	0.100	0.91	0
White	76	2.35	1.10	13.8	35.7	0.806	0.133	0.088	0.54	0
White—toast	84	2.67	1.26	15.7	40.6	0.915	0.121	0.103	0.64	0
Whole wheat	69	2.84	1.22	12.9	20.2	0.964	0.100	0.059	2.10	0
Whole wheat—toast	79	3.42	1.47	14.4	22.5	1.090	0.090	0.066	2.74	0
Bread crumbs—dry grated	111	3.69	1.42	20.7	34.6	1.160	0.099	0.099	1.15	1.4
Bread crumbs—soft	76	2.35	1.10	13.9	35.9	0.806	0.134	0.088	0.54	0
Bread sticks wo/salt	109	3.40	0.82	21.3	7.9	0.255	0.017	0.020	0.43	0
Bread sticks w/salt	86	2.67	0.89	16.4	13.0	0.243	0.016	0.024	0.41	0

➤ CAKES AND PIES

	KCAL	PROTEIN (G)	FAT (G)	CHO (G)	CA (MG)	FE (MG)	B_1 (MG)	B_2 (MG)	FIBER (G)	CHOLESTEROL (MG)
Cakes										
Angel food cake	67	1.71	0.09	15.2	23.5	0.123	0.014	0.057	0	0
Boston cream pie	61	0.59	1.89	10.4	6.1	0.142	0.002	0.043	0	4.7
Carrot cake	103	1.05	5.32	13.2	6.9	0.304	0.030	0.035	0	14.6
Cheesecake	86	1.54	5.45	8.1	15.9	0.136	0.009	0.037	0	52.4
Choc cupcake/choc frosting	97	1.24	3.29	16.5	16.9	0.575	0.029	0.041	0	15.2
Coffee cake	91	1.78	2.70	14.8	17.3	0.480	0.054	0.059	0	18.5
Dark fruitcake	109	1.32	4.62	16.5	27.0	0.791	0.053	0.053	0	13.2
Gingerbread cake	91	1.15	2.86	15.2	12.2	0.706	0.042	0.038	0	7.8
Pound cake	113	1.89	4.72	14.2	18.9	0.472	0.047	0.057	0	30.2
Sheet cake—plain	104	1.32	3.96	15.8	18.1	0.429	0.046	0.049	0	20.1
Sheet cake—white frosting	104	0.94	3.28	18.0	14.3	0.281	0.030	0.037	0	16.4
Sponge cake	83	2.01	1.27	16.0	10.8	0.524	0.043	0.046	0	58.8
White cake/coconut	109	1.30	4.05	17.0	13.7	0.454	0.041	0.053	0	1.2
White cake/white frosting	104	1.20	3.59	16.8	13.2	0.399	0.080	0.052	0	1.2
Yellow cake/chocolate frosting	101	1.03	4.48	15.9	9.5	0.509	0.020	0.058	0	15.6
Pies										
Apple pie	73	0.66	3.14	10.7	5.0	0.300	0.031	0.023	0	0
Apple pie—fried	85	0.73	4.67	10.7	4.0	0.312	0.030	0.020	0	4.7
Banana cream pie	46	0.90	1.85	6.7	21.0	0.156	0.022	0.042	0	2.2
Blueberry pie	68	0.72	3.05	9.9	4.7	0.377	0.031	0.025	0	0
Boston cream pie	61	0.59	1.89	10.4	6.1	0.142	0.002	0.043	0	4.7

➤ CAKES AND PIES—*continued*

	KCAL	PROTEIN (G)	FAT (G)	CHO (G)	CA (MG)	FE (MG)	B_1 (MG)	B_2 (MG)	FIBER (G)	CHOLESTEROL (MG)
Pies—*continued*										
Cherry pie	74	0.77	3.19	10.9	6.6	0.569	0.034	0.025	0	0
Cherry pie—fried	83	0.68	4.74	10.7	3.7	0.233	0.020	0.020	0	4.3
Chocolate cream pie	50	1.20	2.04	6.9	25.9	0.175	0.024	0.049	0	2.4
Coconut cream pie	57	1.03	2.79	7.2	24.0	0.198	0.021	0.042	0	2.5
Coconut custard pie	66	1.69	3.85	6.3	25.0	0.304	0.029	0.055	0	31.4
Cream pie	85	0.56	4.29	11.0	8.6	0.205	0.011	0.028	0	1.5
Custard pie	55	1.43	2.65	6.3	23.1	0.269	0.026	0.050	0	27.6
Lemon meringue pie	72	0.95	2.90	10.7	5.1	0.283	0.020	0.028	0	27.7
Mincemeat pie	70	0.65	2.13	12.8	6.9	0.360	0.028	0.024	0	0
Peach pie	73	0.63	3.14	10.9	4.8	0.340	0.031	0.028	0	0
Pecan pie	120	1.30	4.87	18.9	7.2	0.380	0.045	0.034	0	28.1
Pumpkin pie	52	1.28	2.23	7.3	30.0	0.373	0.019	0.042	0	15.5
Strawberry chiffon pie	65	0.85	3.46	8.0	7.7	0.254	0.022	0.023	0	7.1

➤ COOKIES

	KCAL	PROTEIN (G)	FAT (G)	CHO (G)	CA (MG)	FE (MG)	B_1 (MG)	B_2 (MG)	FIBER (G)	CHOLESTEROL (MG)
Animal cookies	120	1.90	2.89	22.0	3.0	0.918	0.080	0.130	0	0.1
Brownies w/nuts	135	1.84	8.93	15.6	12.8	0.567	0.070	0.070	0	25.5
Butter cookies	130	1.76	4.82	20.2	36.3	0.170	0.011	0.017	0	4.1
Fig bars	106	1.02	1.93	21.4	20.2	0.689	0.039	0.037	0	13.7
Lady fingers	102	2.19	2.19	18.3	11.6	0.515	0.019	0.039	0	101.0
Oatmeal raisin cookies	134	1.64	5.45	19.6	9.8	0.600	0.049	0.044	0	1.1
Peanut butter cookies	145	2.36	8.27	16.5	12.4	0.650	0.041	0.041	0	13.0
Sandwich type cookies	138	1.42	5.67	20.6	8.5	0.992	0.064	0.050	0	0
Shortbread cookies	137	1.77	7.09	17.7	11.5	0.709	0.089	0.080	0	23.9
Sugar cookies	139	1.18	7.09	18.3	29.5	0.532	0.053	0.035	0	17.1
Vanilla wafers	131	1.42	4.96	20.6	11.3	0.567	0.050	0.070	0	17.7

➤ CANDY BARS

	KCAL	PROTEIN (G)	FAT (G)	CHO (G)	CA (MG)	FE (MG)	B_1 (MG)	B_2 (MG)	FIBER (G)	CHOLESTEROL (MG)
Almond Joy	151	1.69	7.82	18.5	2.0	0.778	0	0	0	0
Sugar-coated almonds	146	3.10	9.12	14.6	39.6	0.775	0.042	0.156	0	0
Bittersweet chocolate	141	1.90	9.73	15.7	13.0	1.040	0.015	0.050	0	0
Caramel—plain or chocolate	115	1.00	2.99	22.0	41.9	0.399	0.010	0.050	0	1.0
Chocolate candy kisses	154	2.10	8.98	15.9	52.9	0.499	0.020	0.080	0	0
Chocolate-coated almonds	161	3.92	12.70	8.0	47.8	1.090	0.052	0.186	0	0
Chocolate-covered coconut	133	0.91	7.10	17.5	8.4	0.614	0.008	0.016	0	0
Chocolate-covered mints	116	0.50	2.99	23.0	16.0	0.299	0.010	0.020	0	0
Chocolate-covered peanuts	159	5.00	11.70	9.8	32.9	0.689	0.086	0.043	0	0
Chocolate-covered raisins	111	1.06	2.71	20.6	12.2	0.663	0.034	0.025	0	0
Chocolate fudge	115	0.56	2.78	21.0	22.0	0.299	0.010	0.030	0	1.0
Chocolate fudge with nuts	114	1.06	4.99	18.8	22.0	0.299	0.016	0.030	0	7.4
English toffee	195	0.89	16.90	9.8	0	0.177	0.470	0.044	0	0
Gum drops	98	0	0.20	24.8	2.0	0.100	0	0	0	0
Hard candy	109	0	0	27.6	6.0	0.100	0	0	0	0
Jelly beans	104	0	0.10	26.4	1.0	0.299	0	0	0	0
Kit-Kat	138	1.98	7.25	16.5	42.9	0.369	0.020	0.073	0	0
Krackle	149	2.00	8.09	16.9	50.0	0.400	0.017	0.075	0	0

➤ CANDY BARS—*continued*

	KCAL	PROTEIN (G)	FAT (G)	CHO (G)	CA (MG)	FE (MG)	B_1 (MG)	B_2 (MG)	FIBER (G)	CHOLESTEROL (MG)
Malted milk balls	135	2.30	6.99	17.8	62.9	0	0	0	0	0
M&M's plain chocolate	140	1.95	6.08	19.5	46.7	0.449	0.015	0.073	0	0
M&M's peanut chocolate	144	3.23	7.25	16.5	35.4	0.402	0.016	0.056	0	0
Mars bar	136	2.27	6.24	17.0	48.2	0.312	0.014	0.093	0	0
Milk chocolate—plain	145	2.00	8.98	16.0	49.9	0.399	0.020	0.100	0	6.0
Milk chocolate w/almonds	150	2.90	10.40	15.0	60.9	0.559	0.030	0.130	0	4.5
Milk chocolate w/peanuts	155	4.89	11.70	10.0	31.9	0.679	0.112	0.065	0	3.0
Milk chocolate and rice cereal	140	2.00	6.99	18.0	47.9	0.200	0.010	0.080	0	6.0
Milky Way	123	1.53	4.25	20.3	40.6	0.232	0.013	0.070	0	6.6
Mr. Goodbar	151	3.62	9.05	13.9	39.2	0.567	0.030	0.072	0	4.2
Reese's Peanut Butter Cup	151	3.65	9.07	13.9	21.7	0.430	0.020	0.032	0	1.6
Snickers	134	3.08	6.62	17.0	32.4	0.227	0.013	0.050	0	0
Vanilla fudge	118	0.70	3.15	22.0	29.9	0.030	0.006	0.025	0	10.0
Vanilla fudge with nuts	122	1.00	5.01	18.3	25.0	0.159	0.017	0.026	0	8.5

➤ CHOCOLATE

	KCAL	PROTEIN (G)	FAT (G)	CHO (G)	CA (MG)	FE (MG)	B_1 (MG)	B_2 (MG)	FIBER (G)	CHOLESTEROL (MG)
Baking chocolate	145	3.49	15.00	7.5	22.0	1.900	0.015	0.099	0	0
Bittersweet chocolate	141	1.90	9.73	15.7	13.0	1.040	0.015	0.050	0	0
Milk chocolate—plain	145	2.00	8.98	16.0	49.9	0.399	0.020	0.100	0	6.0
Semisweet chocolate chips	143	1.17	10.20	16.2	8.5	0.967	0.017	0.023	0	0
Dark chocolate—sweet	150	1.00	9.98	16.0	7.0	0.599	0.010	0.040	0	0
Chocolate cupcake/ chocolate frosting	97	1.24	3.29	16.5	16.9	0.575	0.029	0.041	0	15.2
Chocolate candy kisses	154	2.10	8.98	15.9	52.9	0.499	0.020	0.080	0	0
Chocolate chip cookies	122	1.54	5.94	18.9	11.0	0.540	0.068	0.155	0	3.4
Chocolate-coated almonds	161	3.92	12.70	8.0	47.8	1.090	0.052	0.186	0	0
Chocolate-coated peanuts	159	5.00	11.70	9.8	32.9	0.689	0.086	0.043	0	0
Chocolate-covered mints	116	0.50	2.99	23.0	16.0	0.299	0.010	0.020	0	0
Chocolate-covered raisins	111	1.06	2.71	20.6	12.2	0.663	0.034	0.025	0	0
Chocolate cream pie	50	1.20	2.04	6.9	25.9	0.175	0.024	0.049	0	2.4
Chocolate fudge	115	0.56	2.78	21.0	22.0	0.299	0.010	0.030	0	1.0
Chocolate fudge with nuts	114	1.06	4.99	18.8	22.0	0.299	0.016	0.030	0	7.4
Cake flour-baked value	103	2.08	0.28	22.4	4.5	1.250	0.154	0.096	0	0
Reese's Peanut Butter Cup	151	3.65	9.07	13.9	21.7	0.430	0.020	0.032	0	1.6
Chocolate pudding/recipe	42	0.88	1.25	7.3	27.3	0.142	0.005	0.039	0	4.3
Chocolate pudding instant	34	0.85	0.818	5.9	28.4	0.065	0.009	0.039	0	3.1

➤ DESSERTS AND BREAKFAST PASTRIES

	KCAL	PROTEIN (G)	FAT (G)	CHO (G)	CA (MG)	FE (MG)	B_1 (MG)	B_2 (MG)	FIBER (G)	CHOLESTEROL (MG)
Apple brown betty	43	0.30	1.60	7.40	5.4	0.130	0.016	0.012	0	3.8
Apple cobbler	55	0.53	1.74	9.57	8.8	0.206	0.023	0.019	0	0.3
Apple crisp	53	0.33	1.93	9.09	7.4	0.278	0.018	0.013	0	0
Apple dumpling	55	0.32	2.37	8.64	7.1	0.253	0.012	0.013	0	0
Banana nut bread	91	1.60	4.00	12.70	10.0	0.470	0.054	0.046	0	18.3
Bread and raisin pudding	60	1.20	2.47	8.54	27.7	0.304	0.030	0.048	0	24.4
Cheesecake	86	1.50	5.45	8.10	15.9	0.136	0.009	0.037	0	52.4
Cherry cobbler	44	0.53	1.37	7.52	8.5	0.391	0.019	0.021	0	0.3
Cherry and cream cheese torte	79	1.28	3.96	10.00	28.5	0.266	0.015	0.052	0	11.2
Vanilla milkshake	32	0.98	0.841	5.09	34.5	0.026	0.013	0.052	0	3.2
Cream puff w/custard fill	72	1.24	4.54	6.83	16.4	0.276	0.015	0.040	0	58.8

➤ DESSERTS AND BREAKFAST PASTRIES—*continued*

	KCAL	PROTEIN (G)	FAT (G)	CHO (G)	CA (MG)	FE (MG)	B_1 (MG)	B_2 (MG)	FIBER (G)	CHOLESTEROL (MG)
Chocolate eclair w/custard fill	79	1.20	4.43	8.96	18.6	0.258	0.019	0.041	0	50.4
Gelatin salad	17	0.43	0	3.99	0.5	0.024	0.002	0.002	0	0
Peach cobbler	28	0.50	1.35	7.96	7.6	0.197	0.018	0.017	0	0.3
Peach crisp	34	0.31	1.06	6.18	4.8	0.203	0.010	0.010	0	0
Crepe, unfilled	49	2.06	1.32	7.07	25.0	0.475	0.045	0.070	0.21	43.0
Pancakes—plain	63	2.10	2.10	9.45	28.4	0.525	0.063	0.074	0.42	16.8
Croissant	117	2.32	6.02	13.40	10.0	1.040	0.085	0.065	0.54	6.5
Danish pastry—plain	109	1.99	5.97	12.90	29.8	0.547	0.080	0.085	0	24.4
Danish pastry w/fruit	102	1.74	5.67	12.20	7.41	0.567	0.070	0.061	0	24.4
Doughnut—cake-type	119	1.33	6.75	13.90	13.0	0.454	0.068	0.068	0	11.3
Doughnut—jelly-filled	99	1.48	3.84	13.00	12.2	0.349	0.052	0.044	0	0
Doughnut—yeast-raised	111	1.89	6.28	12.30	8.0	0.661	0.132	0.057	0	9.9
Chocolate pudding	42	0.88	1.25	7.28	27.3	0.142	0.005	0.039	0	4.3
Tapioca pudding	38	1.43	1.44	4.85	29.7	0.120	0.012	0.052	0	27.3
Vanilla pudding	32	0.99	1.10	4.50	33.1	0.089	0.009	0.046	0	4.1
Chocolate pudding—instant	34	0.85	0.82	5.89	28.4	0.065	0.009	0.039	0	3.1
Rice pudding	33	0.86	0.86	5.80	28.6	0.107	0.021	0.039	0	3.2
Butterscotch pudding pop	47	1.19	1.29	7.80	37.8	0.020	0.015	0.055	0	0.5
Chocholate pudding pop	49	1.34	1.34	8.20	42.8	0.179	0.015	0.055	0	0.5
Vanilla pudding pop	46	1.19	1.29	7.80	37.8	0.020	0.015	0.055	0	0.5

➤ CEREALS (WITHOUT MILK)

	KCAL	PROTEIN (G)	FAT (G)	CHO (G)	CA (MG)	FE (MG)	B_1 (MG)	B_2 (MG)	FIBER (G)	CHOLESTEROL (MG)
All-Bran	70	3.99	0.50	21.0	23.00	4.49	0.369	0.429	8.490	0
Alpha Bits	111	2.20	0.60	24.6	7.99	1.80	0.399	0.399	0.650	0
Apple Jacks	110	1.50	0.10	25.7	2.99	4.49	0.399	0.399	0.200	0
Bran Buds	73	3.95	0.68	21.6	18.90	4.52	0.371	0.439	7.860	0
Bran Chex	90	2.95	0.81	22.6	16.80	4.51	0.347	0.150	5.200	0
Buc Wheats	110	2.00	1.00	24.0	59.90	8.09	0.674	0.764	2.000	0
C.W. Post—plain	126	2.54	4.44	20.3	13.70	4.50	0.380	0.438	0.643	0
C.W. Post w/raisins	123	2.45	4.05	20.3	14.00	4.51	0.358	0.413	0.660	0
Cap'n Crunch	120	1.46	2.60	22.9	4.60	7.53	0.506	0.544	0.709	0
Cap'n Crunchberries	118	1.46	2.35	23.0	8.91	7.32	0.478	0.543	0.324	0
Cap'n Crunch—Peanut Butter	125	2.03	3.64	21.5	5.67	7.37	0.486	0.567	0.324	0
Cheerios	110	4.24	1.77	19.4	47.30	4.44	0.394	0.394	3.000	0
Cocoa Krispies	109	1.50	0.39	25.2	4.73	1.81	0.394	0.394	0.354	0
Cocoa Pebbles	117	1.35	1.49	24.7	5.40	1.75	0.405	0.405	0.312	0
Corn Bran	98	1.97	1.02	23.9	32.30	9.60	0.299	0.551	5.390	0
Corn Chex	111	2.00	0.10	24.9	2.99	1.80	0.399	0.070	0.499	0
Corn Flakes—Kellogg's	110	2.30	0.09	24.4	1.00	1.80	0.367	0.424	0.594	0
Corn Flakes—Post Toasties	110	2.30	0.09	24.4	1.00	0.70	0.367	0.424	0.594	0
Corn grits—enriched yellow dry	105	2.49	0.33	22.5	0.55	1.10	0.182	0.107	3.270	0
Corn grits—enriched ckd	17	0.41	0.06	3.7	0.12	0.18	0.028	0.018	0.527	0
Cracklin' Oat Bran	108	2.60	4.16	19.4	18.90	1.80	0.378	0.425	4.280	0
Cream of Rice	15	0.24	0.01	3.3	0.93	0.05	0.012	0	0.163	0
Cream of Wheat	16	0.42	0.07	3.4	6.27	1.27	0.028	0.008	0.395	0
Crispy Wheat 'n Raisins	99	2.00	0.46	23.1	46.80	4.48	0.396	0.396	1.320	0
Farina—cooked	14	0.41	0.02	3.0	0.49	0.14	0.023	0.015	0.389	0
Fortified Oat Flakes	105	5.32	0.41	20.5	40.20	8.09	0.354	0.413	0.827	0
40% Bran Flakes—Kellogg's	91	3.60	0.54	22.2	13.80	8.14	0.369	0.430	0.850	0
40% Bran Flakes—Post	92	3.20	0.45	22.3	12.70	4.50	0.374	0.435	3.800	0
Froot Loops	111	1.70	1.00	25.0	2.99	4.49	0.399	0.399	0.299	0
Frosted Mini-Wheats	102	2.93	0.27	23.4	9.15	1.83	0.366	0.457	2.160	0
Frosted Rice Krispies	109	1.30	0.10	25.7	1.00	1.80	0.399	0.399	0.998	0

➤ CEREALS (WITHOUT MILK)—*continued*

	KCAL	PROTEIN (G)	FAT (G)	CHO (G)	CA (MG)	FE (MG)	B_1 (MG)	B_2 (MG)	FIBER (G)	CHOLESTEROL (MG)
Fruit & Fiber w/apples	90	2.99	1.00	22.0	9.98	4.49	0.374	0.424	4.190	0
Fruit & Fiber w/dates	90	2.99	1.00	21.0	9.98	4.49	0.374	0.424	4.190	0
Fruitful Bran	92	2.50	0	22.5	8.34	6.75	0.313	0.354	4.170	0
Fruity Pebbles	115	1.10	1.50	24.4	2.99	1.80	0.399	0.399	0.226	0
Golden Grahams	109	1.60	1.09	24.1	17.40	4.50	0.363	0.436	1.670	0
Granola—homemade	138	3.49	7.69	15.6	17.70	1.12	0.170	0.072	2.970	0
Granola—Nature Valley	126	2.89	4.92	18.9	17.80	0.95	0.098	0.048	2.960	0
Grape Nuts	100	3.28	0.11	23.2	10.90	1.22	0.398	0.398	1.840	0
Grape Nuts Flakes	102	2.99	0.30	23.2	11.00	4.49	0.399	0.399	1.900	0
Honey & Nut Corn Flakes	113	1.80	1.50	23.3	2.99	1.80	0.399	0.399	0.299	0
Honey Bran	96	2.51	0.57	23.2	13.00	4.54	0.405	0.405	3.160	0
Honey Comb	111	1.68	0.52	25.3	5.15	1.80	0.387	0.387	0.387	0
Honey Nut Cheerios	107	3.09	0.69	22.8	19.80	4.47	0.344	0.430	0.790	0
King Vitamin	115	1.49	1.62	24.0	NA	17.10	0.124	1.430	0.135	0
Kix	109	2.49	0.70	23.3	34.80	8.06	0.398	0.398	0.398	0
Life	104	5.22	0.52	20.3	99.20	7.47	0.612	0.644	0.902	0
Lucky Charms	111	2.57	1.06	23.1	31.90	4.52	0.354	0.443	0.624	0
Malt-O-Meal	14	0.43	0.03	3.1	0.59	1.13	0.057	0.028	0.354	0
Maypo—cooked	1	0.02	0.01	0.1	0.52	0.04	0.003	0.003	0.012	0
Nutri-Grain—barley	106	3.11	0.21	23.4	7.60	1.00	0.346	0.415	1.660	0
Nutri-Grain—corn	108	2.30	0.68	24.0	0.68	0.60	0.338	0.405	1.750	0
Nutri-Grain—rye	102	2.48	0.21	24.0	5.67	0.80	0.354	0.425	2.160	0
Nutri-Grain—wheat	102	2.45	0.32	24.0	7.73	0.80	0.387	0.451	1.800	0
Oatmeal—prepared	18	0.73	0.29	3.1	2.42	0.19	0.032	0.006	0.497	0
Rolled Oats	109	4.55	1.78	19.0	14.70	1.19	0.206	0.038	3.090	0
Instant Oatmeal w/apples	26	0.74	0.30	5.0	30.00	1.15	0.091	0.053	0.552	0
Instant Oatmeal w/bran & raisins	23	0.71	0.28	4.4	25.20	1.10	0.081	0.092	0.480	0
Instant Oatmeal w/maple	30	0.84	0.35	5.8	29.60	1.16	0.097	0.059	0.530	0
Instant Oatmeal w/cinnamon & spice	31	0.85	0.34	6.2	30.30	1.17	0.099	0.60	0.510	0
Instant Oatmeal w/raisins & spice	29	0.77	0.32	5.7	29.60	1.18	0.092	0.065	0.556	0
100% Bran	77	3.57	1.42	20.7	19.80	3.49	0.687	0.773	8.380	0
100% Natural	135	3.02	6.02	18.0	48.90	0.83	0.085	0.150	3.390	0
100% Natural—w/apples	130	2.92	5.32	19.0	42.80	0.79	0.090	0.158	1.300	0
100% Natural—w/raisins and dates	128	2.89	5.23	18.7	41.20	0.80	0.077	0.165	1.080	0
Product 19	108	2.75	0.17	23.5	3.44	18.00	1.460	1.720	0.369	0
Puffed Rice	111	1.79	0.20	25.5	2.03	0.30	0.030	0.028	0.227	0
Puffed Wheat	104	4.25	0.24	22.4	7.09	1.35	0.047	0.070	5.430	0
Quisp	117	1.42	2.08	23.6	8.50	5.96	0.510	0.718	0.378	0
Raisin Bran—Kellogg's	91	3.07	0.46	21.4	14.50	13.90	0.293	0.332	3.410	0
Raisin Bran—Post	86	2.68	0.55	21.4	13.70	4.56	0.373	0.430	3.190	0
Raisins, Rice & Rye	96	1.60	0.06	24.2	6.16	3.45	0.308	0.370	0.308	0
Ralston—cooked	15	0.62	0.09	3.2	1.57	0.18	0.022	0.020	0.370	0
Rice Chex	112	1.49	1.00	25.2	3.88	1.79	0.400	0.298	1.840	0
Rice Krispies	109	1.86	0.20	24.2	3.91	1.76	0.391	0.391	0.312	0
Roman Meal—dry	91	4.07	0.60	20.4	18.40	1.31	0.142	0.069	0.905	0
Roman Meal—cooked	17	0.77	0.11	3.9	3.45	0.25	0.028	0.014	0.877	0
Shredded Wheat	102	3.09	0.71	22.5	11.00	1.20	0.070	0.080	3.100	0
Shredded wheat—generic	97	3.06	0.45	16.4	11.20	0.89	0.082	0.075	2.900	0
Special K	111	5.58	0.10	21.3	7.97	4.48	0.399	0.399	0.266	0
Sugar Corn Pops	108	1.40	0.10	25.6	0.10	1.80	0.399	0.399	0.100	0
Sugar Frosted Flakes	108	1.46	0.08	25.7	0.81	1.78	0.405	0.405	0.446	0
Sugar Smacks	106	2.00	0.50	24.7	2.99	1.80	0.369	0.429	0.319	0
Super Golden Crisp	106	1.80	0.26	25.6	6.01	1.80	0.344	0.430	0.430	0
Team	111	1.82	0.48	24.3	4.05	1.73	0.371	0.425	0.270	0
Total	105	2.84	0.60	22.3	172.00	18.00	1.460	1.720	2.060	0
Trix	108	1.50	0.40	24.9	5.99	4.49	0.399	0.399	0.184	0
Wheat & Raisin Chex	97	2.68	0.21	22.6	NA	4.04	0.263	0.315	1.890	0
Wheat Chex	104	2.77	0.68	23.3	11.00	4.50	0.370	0.105	2.100	0

➤ CEREALS (WITHOUT MILK)—*continued*

	KCAL	PROTEIN (G)	FAT (G)	CHO (G)	CA (MG)	FE (MG)	B_1 (MG)	B_2 (MG)	FIBER (G)	CHOLESTEROL (MG)
Wheat germ—toasted	108	8.25	3.09	14.0	12.50	2.19	0.474	0.233	3.910	0
Wheat germ w/brown sugar, honey	107	6.19	2.30	17.2	8.98	1.93	0.349	0.180	3.390	0
Wheatena—cooked	16	0.58	0.13	3.4	1.28	0.16	0.002	0.006	0.385	0
Wheaties	99	2.74	0.51	22.6	43.00	4.50	0.391	0.391	2.540	0
Whole wheat berries	16	0.54	0.11	3.2	1.70	0.17	0.023	0.006	0.680	0
Whole wheat cereal—cooked	18	0.58	0.11	3.9	1.99	0.18	0.020	0.014	0.457	0

➤ CHEESE

	KCAL	PROTEIN (G)	FAT (G)	CHO (G)	CA (MG)	FE (MG)	B_1 (MG)	B_2 (MG)	FIBER (G)	CHOLESTEROL (MG)
American—processed	106	6.28	8.84	0.45	174	0.110	0.008	0.111	0	27.0
American cheese food—cold pack	94	5.23	6.78	2.36	145	0.240	0.009	0.274	0	18.0
American cheese spread	82	5.16	6.00	2.48	159	0.090	0.014	0.380	0	16.0
Blue	100	6.09	8.14	0.66	150	0.090	0.008	0.395	0	21.0
Brick	105	6.40	8.40	0.79	191	0.130	0.004	0.159	0	27.0
Brie	95	5.87	7.84	0.13	52	0.140	0.020	0.147	0	28.0
Camembert	85	5.60	6.86	0.13	110	0.094	0.008	0.138	0	20.0
Caraway	107	7.13	8.27	0.87	191	0.100	0.009	0.196	0	25.0
Cheddar	114	7.05	9.38	0.36	204	0.197	0.008	0.106	0	29.9
Cheshire	110	6.60	8.66	1.36	182	0.060	0.013	0.198	0	28.9
Colby	112	6.73	9.08	0.73	194	0.216	0.004	0.171	0	27.0
Cottage	29	3.54	1.20	0.76	17	0.040	0.006	0.115	0	4.2
Cottage—lowfat 2%	26	3.90	0.55	1.03	20	0.045	0.007	0.052	0	2.4
Cottage—lowfat 1%	21	3.51	0.29	0.77	18	0.040	0.006	0.115	0	1.3
Cottage—dry curd	24	4.89	0.12	0.52	9	0.065	0.007	0.004	0	2.0
Cottage—w/fruit	35	2.80	0.96	3.78	14	0.031	0.005	0.115	0	3.1
Cream	99	2.10	9.87	0.75	23	0.337	0.005	0.056	0	30.9
Edam	101	7.07	7.79	0.40	207	0.125	0.010	0.274	0	25.0
Feta	75	4.49	6.19	1.16	140	0.180	0.040	0.315	0	25.0
Fontina	110	7.25	8.62	0.44	156	0.060	0.006	NA	0	32.9
Gjetost	132	2.74	8.32	12.00	113	0.130	0.009	0.170	0	25.0
Gorgonzola	111	6.99	8.98	0	149	0.120	0.010	0.512	0	25.0
Gouda	101	7.06	7.72	0.63	198	0.070	0.009	0.232	0	31.9
Gruyere	117	8.44	9.05	0.10	286	0.060	0.017	0.095	0	30.9
Liederkranz	87	4.99	7.99	0	110	0.120	0.010	0.389	0	21.0
Limburger	93	5.67	7.59	0.14	141	0.040	0.023	0.227	0	26.0
Monterey jack	106	6.93	8.56	0.19	212	0.200	0.004	0.119	0	26.0
Mozzarella—skim, low moist	80	7.60	4.67	0.89	207	0.076	0.006	0.150	0	15.0
Mozzarella—whole milk, regular	80	5.50	5.75	0.63	147	0.050	0.004	0.106	0	22.0
Mozzarella—whole milk, moist	90	6.10	7.19	0.43	163	0.060	0.005	0.119	0	25.0
Muenster	104	6.40	8.42	0.32	203	0.125	0.004	0.178	0	27.0
Neufchatel	74	2.82	6.70	0.83	21	0.080	0.004	0.113	0	22.0
Parmesan—hard	111	10.00	7.30	0.91	335	0.230	0.010	0.453	0	19.0
Parmesan—grated	129	11.80	8.50	1.06	389	0.270	0.013	0.527	0	22.0
Pimento processed	106	6.26	8.82	0.49	174	0.120	0.008	0.404	0	27.0
Port du salut	100	6.73	7.99	0.16	84	0.140	0.004	0.151	0	34.9
Provolone	100	7.13	7.54	0.61	214	0.146	0.005	0.248	0	20.0
Ricotta—part skim	39	3.23	2.25	1.45	77	0.126	0.006	0.052	0	8.8
Ricotta—whole milk	49	3.19	3.68	0.86	59	0.108	0.004	0.024	0	14.3
Romano	110	9.00	7.63	1.03	301	0.230	0.010	0.339	0	28.9
Romano—grated	128	10.50	8.86	1.20	350	0.270	0.013	0.394	0	32.9
Roquefort	105	6.10	8.93	0.57	188	0.172	0.010	0.512	0	26.0
Swiss	107	8.03	7.79	0.96	272	0.050	0.006	0.074	0	26.0
Swiss processed	95	7.00	6.97	0.60	219	0.170	0.004	0.078	0	24.0

➤ FISH

	KCAL	PROTEIN (G)	FAT (G)	CHO (G)	CA (MG)	FE (MG)	B_1 (MG)	B_2 (MG)	FIBER (G)	CHOLESTEROL (MG)
Bass—freshwater raw	32	5.36	1.05	0	22.7	0.422	0.028	0.009	0	19.3
Bluefish—baked/broiled	45	7.43	1.42	0	2.6	0.174	0.022	0.030	0	17.9
Bluefish—fried in crumbs	58	6.44	2.78	1.33	2.3	0.151	0.017	0.023	0	17
Bluefish—raw	35	5.67	1.20	0	2.0	0.136	0.016	0.023	0	16.7
Carp—raw	36	5.05	1.59	0	11.6	0.352	0.013	0.011	0	18.7
Catfish—channel—raw	33	5.16	1.20	0	11.3	0.275	0.013	0.030	0	16.4
Cod—baked w/butter	37	6.46	0.94	0	5.7	0.139	0.025	0.022	0	17.0
Cod—batter-fried	56	5.56	2.92	2.13	22.7	0.142	0.011	0.011	0	15.6
Cod—baked/broiled	30	6.46	0.24	0	4.0	0.139	0.025	0.022	0	15.6
Cod—poached	29	6.24	0.24	0	4.0	0.139	0.025	0.022	0	15.6
Cod—steamed	29	6.24	0.24	0	4.0	0.139	0.025	0.022	0	15.9
Cod—smoked	22	5.19	0.17	0	4.0	0.113	0.023	0.020	0	14.2
Cod—Atlantic—raw	23	5.05	0.19	0	4.5	0.108	0.022	0.018	0	12.2
Cod liver oil	255	0	28.40	0	0	0	0	0	0	162.0
Eel—smoked	94	5.27	7.88	0.23	26.9	0.198	0.040	0.099	0	19.8
Haddock—breaded/fried	58	5.67	3.00	2.33	11.3	0.384	0.020	0.033	0.01	18.3
Haddock—smoked	33	7.14	0.27	0	13.9	0.397	0.013	0.014	0	21.8
Haddock—raw	22	5.36	0.20	0	9.4	0.298	0.010	0.010	0	16.2
Herring—pickled	74	4.03	5.10	2.73	21.8	0.346	0.010	0.039	0	3.7
Herring—smoked/ kippered	62	6.97	3.52	0	23.8	0.428	0.036	0.090	0	22.7
Herring—canned w/liquid	59	5.64	3.86	0	41.7	0.879	0.007	0.051	0	27.5
Mackerel—fried	49	7.00	2.35	0	4.3	0.445	0.045	0.116	0	19.8
Mackerel—Atlantic— baked/broiled	74	6.78	5.05	0	4.3	0.445	0.045	0.117	0	21.3
Mackerel—Atlantic—raw	58	5.27	3.94	0	3.4	0.462	0.050	0.088	0	19.8
Mackerel—Pacific—raw	45	6.12	2.84	0	2.3	0.567	0.043	0.096	0	22.7
Northern pike—raw	25	5.47	0.20	0	16.2	0.156	0.017	0.018	0	11.0
Ocean perch—breaded/ fried	62	5.34	3.67	2.33	30.7	0.400	0.033	0.037	0.03	15.3
Pollock—baked/broiled	28	6.60	0.31	0	19.3	0.149	0.014	0.057	0	19.8
Pollock—poached	36	6.60	0.31	0	17.0	0.149	0.010	0.050	0	19.8
Salmon—broiled/baked	61	7.74	3.10	0	2.0	0.157	0.061	0.048	0	24.7
Coho salmon—steamed/ poached	52	7.77	2.14	0	8.22	0.252	0.057	0.031	0	13.9
Smoked salmon— Chinook	33	5.17	1.22	0	03.0	0.240	0.007	0.029	0	6.7
Atlantic salmon— small can	36	5.05	1.62	0	3.1	0.204	0.057	0.097	0	17.0
Pink salmon—raw	33	5.64	0.98	0	11.3	0.218	0.040	0.057	0	14.7
Sardines	59	7.00	3.24	0	108.0	0.826	0.023	0.064	0	40.4
Sea trout steelhead—raw	30	4.73	1.02	0	4.8	0.077	0.023	0.057	0	23.5
Sea trout steelhead— cooked	37	6.07	1.42	0	5.7	0.088	0.024	0.064	0	32.3
Shad—baked with bacon	57	6.58	3.20	0	6.8	0.170	0.037	0.074	0	17.0
Smelt—rainbow—raw	28	4.99	0.69	0	17.0	0.255	0.016	0.034	0	19.8
Snapper—baked or broiled	36	7.46	0.49	0	11.3	0.068	0.015	0.021	0	13.3
Snapper—raw	28	5.81	0.38	0	9.1	0.051	0.013	0.017	0	10.5
Sole/flounder—baked w/butter	40	5.34	2.00	0	5.3	0.093	0.023	0.032	0	22.7
Sole/flounder—baked/ broiled	33	6.84	0.43	0	5.3	0.093	0.023	0.032	0	19.3
Sole/flounder— batter-fried	83	4.47	5.10	4.07	16.7	0.239	0.057	0.042	0.01	15.0
Sole/flounder—breaded/ fried	53	4.96	2.55	2.54	11.3	0.128	0.037	0.034	0	15.0
Sole/flounder—steamed	26	5.67	0.33	0	4.5	0.079	0.017	0.027	0	14.7
Sole/flounder—raw	26	5.33	0.34	0	5.1	0.102	0.025	0.022	0	13.6
Lemon sole—raw	23	4.85	0.21	0	4.8	0.088	0.026	0.023	0	17.0
Lemon sole—fried w/crumbs	56	4.56	3.12	2.64	26.9	0.176	0.020	0.023	0	18.4
Lemon sole—steamed	26	5.84	0.26	0	6.0	0.147	0.026	0.026	0	17.0

➤ FISH—*continued*

	KCAL	PROTEIN (G)	FAT (G)	CHO (G)	CA (MG)	FE (MG)	B_1 (MG)	B_2 (MG)	FIBER (G)	CHOLESTEROL (MG)
Swordfish—raw	34	5.61	1.14	0	1.1	0.230	0.010	0.027	0	11.0
Swordfish—broiled/baked	44	7.20	1.46	0	1.7	0.295	0.012	0.033	0	14.2
Trout—baked/broiled	43	7.47	1.22	0	24.3	0.690	0.024	0.064	0	20.7
Tuna—oil pack	56	8.26	2.34	0	3.8	0.395	0.010	0.030	0	5.0
Tuna—water pack	37	8.38	0.14	0	3.4	0.409	0.010	0.033	0	16.0
Tuna—raw	31	6.63	0.27	0	4.5	0.207	0.123	0.013	0	12.8
Whiting—flour/bread-fried	54	5.13	1.56	1.98	11.3	0.198	0.023	0.020	0	18.4

➤ FRUITS

	KCAL	PROTEIN (G)	FAT (G)	CHO (G)	CA (MG)	FE (MG)	B_1 (MG)	B_2 (MG)	FIBER (G)	CHOLESTEROL (MG)
Apple w/peel	16	0.055	0.100	4.31	2.05	0.051	0.005	0.004	0.709	0
Apple slices w/peel—fresh	17	0.054	0.100	4.33	2.06	0.052	0.005	0.004	0.709	0
Apple juice—canned/ bottled	13	0.017	0.032	3.32	1.94	0.105	0.006	0.005	0.034	0
Apple juice—frozen concentrate	47	0.144	0.105	11.60	5.78	0.258	0.003	0.015	0.089	0
Applesauce—sweetened	22	0.052	0.052	5.67	1.11	0.111	0.003	0.008	0.397	0
Apricot—fresh halves	14	0.397	0.110	3.15	4.02	0.154	0.009	0.011	0.538	0
Apricot halves—light syrup	18	0.150	0.013	4.67	3.34	0.110	0.005	0.006	0.319	0
Apricot nectar—canned	16	0.104	0.025	4.08	2.03	0.108	0.003	0.004	0.170	0
Avocado—average	46	0.563	0.340	2.10	3.07	0.284	0.030	0.035	2.720	0
Banana—fresh slices	26	0.293	0.136	6.63	1.74	0.088	0.013	0.028	0.578	0
Blackberries—canned	26	0.370	0.040	6.54	5.98	0.184	0.008	0.011	1.011	0
Blackberries—fresh	15	0.205	0.110	3.62	9.06	0.158	0.008	0.011	1.910	0
Blackberries—frozen	18	0.334	0.122	4.45	8.26	0.173	0.008	0.013	1.460	0
Blueberries—fresh	16	0.190	0.108	4.00	1.76	0.047	0.014	0.014	0.763	0
Blueberries—frozen unsweetened	14	0.119	0.181	3.46	2.19	0.051	0.009	0.010	0.658	0
Boysenberries—frozen	14	0.314	0.075	3.46	7.73	0.240	0.015	0.010	1.100	0
Sour cheeries—frozen	13	0.260	0.124	3.13	3.66	0.150	0.012	0.010	0.384	0
Sweet cherries—fresh	20	0.340	0.272	4.69	4.10	0.110	0.014	0.017	0.430	0
Sweet cherries—frozen	25	0.325	0.037	6.34	3.39	0.099	0.008	0.013	0.224	0
Cranberries—whole—raw	14	0.110	0.057	3.58	2.09	0.057	0.009	0.006	1.190	0
Cranberry/apple juice	19	0.015	0.090	4.82	2.02	0.017	0.001	0.006	0.070	0
Cranberry juice cocktail	16	0.009	0.015	4.03	0.90	0.043	0.002	0.002	0.085	0
Date—whole—each	78	0.557	0.127	20.80	9.22	0.342	0.026	0.028	2.300	0
Figs—medium—fresh	21	0.215	0.085	5.44	10.20	0.102	0.017	0.014	1.050	0
Fig—dried—each	72	0.864	0.330	18.50	40.80	0.634	0.020	0.025	3.140	0
Fruit cocktail—heavy syrup	21	0.111	0.020	5.36	1.78	0.081	0.005	0.005	0.280	0
Fruit cocktail—light syrup	16	0.114	0.020	4.23	1.80	0.082	0.005	0.005	0.284	0
Grapefruit half—pink/red	9	0.157	0.028	2.18	3.00	0.034	0.010	0.006	0.369	0
Grapefruit half—white	10	0.195	0.029	2.38	3.36	0.017	0.010	0.006	0.368	0
Grapefuit sections—fresh	9	0.179	0.028	2.29	3.33	0.025	0.010	0.006	0.370	0
Grapefruit sections— canned	17	0.160	0.028	4.38	4.02	0.114	0.010	0.006	0.313	0
Grapefruit juice—fresh	11	0.142	0.029	2.60	2.53	0.056	0.011	0.006	0.113	0
Grapefruit juice— sweetened	13	0.164	0.026	3.15	2.27	0.102	0.011	0.007	0.076	0
Grapefruit juice— unsweetened	11	0.148	0.028	2.54	1.95	0.057	0.012	0.006	0.077	0
Grapefruit juice— frozen concentrate	41	0.548	0.137	9.86	7.67	0.140	0.041	0.022	0.383	0
Grapes—Thompson	20	0.188	0.163	5.03	3.01	0.073	0.026	0.016	0.333	0
Grape juice—bottled/ canned	17	0.158	0.021	4.25	2.47	0.068	0.007	0.010	0.141	0
Grape juice—frozen concentrate	51	0.184	0.088	12.60	3.68	0.102	0.015	0.026	0.492	0

➤ FRUITS—*continued*

	KCAL	PROTEIN (G)	FAT (G)	CHO (G)	CA (MG)	FE (MG)	B_1 (MG)	B_2 (MG)	FIBER (G)	CHOLESTEROL (MG)
Grape juice—prep frozen	15	0.053	0.026	3.62	1.13	0.029	0.004	0.007	0.142	0
Kiwi fruit	17	0.280	0.127	4.22	7.46	0.112	0.007	0.015	0.962	0
Lemon—fresh wo/peel	8	0.313	0.083	2.64	7.33	0.171	0.011	0.006	0.582	0
Lemon juice—fresh	7	0.107	0.081	2.45	2.09	0.009	0.008	0.003	0.099	0
Lemon juice—bottled	6	0.114	0.081	1.84	3.02	0.036	0.012	0.003	0.085	0
Lime—fresh	9	0.199	0.055	2.99	9.30	0.169	0.008	0.006	0.228	0
Lime juice—fresh	8	0.124	0.029	2.56	2.54	0.009	0.006	0.003	0.113	0
Lime juice—bottled	6	0.115	0.115	1.84	3.46	0.069	0.009	0.001	0.099	0
Loganberries—fresh	20	0.430	0.088	3.69	8.50	0.181	0.014	0.010	1.760	0
Loganberries—frozen	16	0.430	0.089	3.68	7.33	0.181	0.014	0.010	1.760	0
Mango—fresh—slices	19	0.146	0.077	4.83	2.92	0.360	0.016	0.016	0.997	0
Mango—fresh—whole	19	0.145	0.078	4.82	2.88	0.356	0.016	0.016	1.010	0
Cantaloupe—cubes	10	0.250	0.079	2.37	3.19	0.060	0.006	0.006	0.284	0
Casaba melon—cubes	8	0.255	0.028	1.75	1.50	0.113	0.017	0.006	0.284	0
Honeydew melon—cubes	10	0.128	0.028	2.60	1.67	0.020	0.022	0.005	0.307	0
Melon balls—mixed—frozen	9	0.239	0.023	2.25	2.79	0.008	0.005	0.006	0.295	0
Mixed fruit—dried	69	0.697	0.139	18.20	10.60	0.767	0.012	0.045	1.220	0
Mixed fruit—frozen—thawed	28	0.397	0.052	6.87	2.04	0.079	0.005	0.010	0.386	0
Nectarine	14	0.267	0.129	3.34	1.25	0.044	0.005	0.012	0.554	0
Orange	13	0.266	0.035	3.33	11.30	0.029	0.025	0.011	0.680	0
Orange sections—fresh	13	0.266	0.035	3.34	11.30	0.029	0.025	0.011	0.680	0
Mandarin oranges—canned	17	0.113	0.011	4.61	2.03	0.101	0.015	0.012	0.478	0
Orange juice—fresh	13	0.199	0.057	2.95	3.09	0.057	0.025	0.008	0.113	0
Orange juice—frozen concentrate	45	0.679	0.059	10.80	9.05	0.099	0.079	0.018	0.313	0
Orange juice—frozen	13	0.191	0.016	3.05	2.50	0.031	0.023	0.005	0.057	0
Papaya—whole fresh	11	0.173	0.040	2.78	6.71	0.028	0.008	0.009	0.482	0
Papaya—slices fresh	12	0.174	0.040	2.77	6.68	0.060	0.008	0.009	0.482	0
Papaya nectar—canned	16	0.049	0.043	4.12	2.72	0.098	0.002	0.001	0.170	0
Peaches—fresh	12	0.199	0.026	3.14	1.30	0.031	0.005	0.012	0.489	0
Peach slices—frozen/thawed	27	0.177	0.037	6.80	0.91	0.105	0.004	0.010	0.467	0
Peach halves—heavy syrup	21	0.130	0.028	5.67	1.05	0.077	0.003	0.007	0.315	0
Peach halves—light syrup	15	0.126	0.010	4.13	1.05	0.101	0.002	0.007	0.402	0
Peach halves—dried	68	0.020	0.216	17.40	8.07	1.150	0	0.060	2.330	0
Peach nectar—canned	15	0.076	0.006	3.95	1.48	0.054	0	0.004	0.170	0
Pears—Bartlett	17	0.111	0.113	4.29	3.24	0.070	0.006	0.011	0.779	0
Pear halves—heavy syrup	21	0.057	0.036	5.42	1.44	0.061	0.004	0.006	0.395	0
Pear halves—light syrup	16	0.054	0.007	4.30	1.44	0.082	0.003	0.005	0.395	0
Pear nectar—canned	17	0.030	0.003	4.47	1.25	0.073	0	0.004	0.204	0
Pineapple slices—heavy syrup	22	0.098	0.034	5.72	3.91	0.108	0.025	0.007	0.270	0
Pineapple slices—light syrup	15	0.103	0.034	3.81	3.91	0.110	0.026	0.007	0.268	0
Pineapple—frozen sweetened	24	0.113	0.029	6.29	2.55	0.113	0.028	0.009	0.496	0
Pineapple juice—frozen concentrate	51	0.369	0.029	12.60	11.00	0.255	0.065	0.017	0.255	0
Plums	16	0.223	0.176	3.69	1.29	0.030	0.012	0.027	0.550	0
Plums—canned—heavy syrup	25	0.102	0.028	6.59	2.53	0.238	0.005	0.010	0.434	0
Plums—canned—light syrup	18	0.105	0.029	4.61	2.70	0.243	0.005	0.011	0.444	0
Prunes—dried	68	0.739	0.145	17.80	14.50	0.702	0.023	0.046	2.700	0
Prune juice—bottled	20	0.172	0.009	4.95	3.43	0.334	0.005	0.020	0.310	0
Raisins—seedless	85	0.914	0.130	22.50	13.90	0.594	0.044	0.025	1.670	0
Raspberries—fresh	14	0.256	0.157	3.27	6.22	0.162	0.009	0.026	1.770	0
Raspberries—canned w/liquid	26	0.235	0.034	6.62	2.99	0.120	0.006	0.009	1.200	0

➤ FRUITS—*continued*

	KCAL	PROTEIN (G)	FAT (G)	CHO (G)	CA (MG)	FE (MG)	B_1 (MG)	B_2 (MG)	FIBER (G)	CHOLESTEROL (MG)
Raspberries—frozen	29	0.197	0.044	7.42	4.30	0.184	0.005	0.013	1.300	0
Rhubarb—raw—diced	6	0.253	0.056	1.29	39.50	0.062	0.006	0.009	0.737	0
Rhubarb—cooked w/sugar	33	0.111	0.013	8.85	41.10	0.060	0.005	0.006	0.624	0
Strawberries—fresh	9	0.173	0.105	2.00	4.00	0.108	0.006	0.019	0.736	0
Strawberries—frozen	10	0.120	0.030	2.59	4.38	0.213	0.006	0.010	0.736	0
Tangerine—fresh	13	0.179	0.054	3.17	4.05	0.028	0.030	0.006	0.574	0
Tangerines—canned—light syrup	17	0.127	0.028	4.61	2.03	0.105	0.015	0.012	0.453	0
Watermelon	9	0.175	0.121	2.04	2.24	0.048	0.023	0.006	0.114	0

➤ MEATS

	KCAL	PROTEIN (G)	FAT (G)	CHO (G)	CA (MG)	FE (MG)	B_1 (MG)	B_2 (MG)	FIBER (G)	CHOLESTEROL (MG)
Beef chuck—pot-roasted	108	7.20	8.64	0	3.67	0.840	0.020	0.065	0	29.0
Beef chuck—pot-roasted lean	77	8.80	4.34	0	3.67	1.040	0.024	0.080	0	30.0
Beef round—pot-roasted lean and fat	74	8.44	4.20	0	1.67	0.920	0.020	0.069	0	27.0
Beef round—pot-roasted lean	63	8.97	2.74	0	1.33	0.980	0.021	0.074	0	27.0
Ground beef—lean	77	7.00	5.34	0	3.00	0.600	0.013	0.060	0	24.7
Ground beef—regular	82	6.67	5.94	0	3.00	0.700	0.010	0.053	0	25.3
Sirloin steak—lean	57	8.10	2.53	0	2.33	0.700	0.026	0.056	0	21.7
T-bone steak—lean and fat	92	6.80	6.97	0	2.67	0.720	0.026	0.059	0	23.7
Beef lunchmeat—thin-sliced	50	7.96	1.09	1.62	2.99	0.759	0.023	0.054	0	12.0
Beef lunchmeat—loaf/roll	87	4.06	7.42	0.82	2.99	0.659	0.030	0.062	0	18.0
Beef rib—oven-roasted—lean	68	7.70	3.90	0	3.34	0.740	0.023	0.060	0	22.7
Beef round—oven roasted—lean	54	8.14	2.12	0	1.67	0.834	0.028	0.076	0	23.0
Beef rump roast—lean only	51	8.40	1.89	0	1.13	0.567	0.026	0.049	0	19.6
Beef brains—pan-fried	56	3.57	4.50	0	2.67	0.630	0.037	0.074	0	566.0
Beef heart	47	8.17	1.59	0.12	1.67	2.130	0.040	0.436	0	54.7
Beef kidney	41	7.23	0.97	0.27	5.00	2.070	0.054	1.150	0	110.0
Beef liver—fried	61	7.57	2.27	2.23	3.00	1.780	0.060	1.170	0	137.0
Beef tongue—cooked	80	6.27	5.87	0.09	2.00	0.960	0.009	0.009	0	30.4
Beef tripe—raw	28	4.14	1.12	0	36.00	0.553	0.002	0.047	0	26.9
Beef tripe—pickled	17	3.29	0.40	0	25.00	0.389	0	0.028	0	15.0
Corned beef—canned	71	7.67	4.24	0	5.67	0.590	0.006	0.042	0	24.3
Corned beef hash—canned	49	2.35	1.29	2.82	3.74	0.567	0.016	0.052	0.153	17.0
Beef—dried/cured	47	8.24	1.10	0.44	2.00	1.280	0.050	0.230	0	45.9
Beef and vegetable stew	26	1.85	1.27	1.74	3.36	0.336	0.017	0.020	0.393	8.2
Beef stew—canned	22	1.64	0.88	2.06	2.66	0.368	0.008	0.014	0.150	1.7
Burrito—beef and bean	63	3.40	2.84	6.48	26.70	0.437	0.042	0.047	0.810	8.4
Tostada w/beans and beef	49	2.72	3.06	2.98	27.50	0.319	0.012	0.036	0.583	9.1
Beef w/macaroni and tomato	24	1.25	0.73	3.16	3.81	0.300	0.024	0.021	0.291	2.8
Beef enchilada	69	3.09	3.26	3.69	60.20	0.418	0.017	0.039	0.465	8.9
Frankfurter—beef	92	3.20	8.36	0.68	3.48	0.378	0.014	0.029	0	13.4
Frankfurter—beef and pork	91	3.20	8.26	0.73	2.98	0.328	0.056	0.034	0	14.4
Beef pot pie—frozen	52	1.99	2.73	4.77	2.42	0.436	0.022	0.018	0.109	5.0
Beef pie—recipe	70	2.84	4.05	5.27	3.92	0.513	0.039	0.039	0.155	5.7
Beef taco	75	4.94	4.80	3.67	30.90	0.469	0.010	0.049	0.407	16.2
Chicken meat—all-fried	62	8.67	2.59	0.48	4.86	0.383	0.024	0.056	0.002	26.5
Chicken meat—all-roasted	54	8.20	2.10	0	4.25	0.342	0.020	0.050	0	25.3
Chicken meat—all-stewed	50	7.74	1.90	0	4.05	0.330	0.014	0.046	0	23.5

➤ MEATS—*continued*

	KCAL	PROTEIN (G)	FAT (G)	CHO (G)	CA (MG)	FE (MG)	B_1 (MG)	B_2 (MG)	FIBER (G)	CHOLESTEROL (MG)
Boned chicken w/broth	47	6.17	2.26	0	3.99	0.439	0.004	0.037	0	17.6
Chicken—dark meat—fried	68	8.22	3.30	0.74	5.06	0.423	0.026	0.070	0.002	27.3
Chicken—dark meat—roasted	58	7.76	2.75	0	4.25	0.377	0.020	0.064	0	26.3
Chicken—dark meat—stewed	55	7.37	2.55	0	4.05	0.385	0.016	0.057	0	24.9
Chicken—light meat—fried	54	9.31	1.57	0.12	4.45	0.322	0.020	0.036	0	25.3
Chicken—light meat—roasted	49	8.77	1.28	0	4.25	0.302	0.018	0.033	0	23.9
Chicken—light meat—stewed	45	8.18	1.17	0	3.64	0.265	0.012	0.033	0	21.7
Chicken breast—no skin	47	8.80	0.99	0	4.29	0.295	0.020	0.032	0	24.0
Chicken breast meat—stewed	43	8.20	0.86	0	3.58	0.250	0.012	0.034	0	21.8
Chicken drumstick—batter-fried	76	6.22	4.45	2.36	4.73	0.382	0.032	0.061	0.008	24.4
Chicken drumstick—roasted	61	7.69	3.16	0	3.27	0.376	0.020	0.061	0	26.2
Chicken wing—batter-fried	92	5.64	6.19	3.10	5.79	0.365	0.030	0.043	0.012	22.6
Chicken wing—flour-fried	91	7.40	6.28	0.67	4.43	0.354	0.017	0.039	0.009	23.0
Chicken wing—roasted	83	7.48	5.53	0	4.17	0.359	0.012	0.037	0	24.2
Chicken gizzards—simmered	44	7.73	1.04	0.32	2.58	1.180	0.008	0.070	0	54.9
Chicken hearts—simmered	52	7.49	2.23	0.03	5.27	2.560	0.017	0.206	0	68.7
Chicken livers—simmered	44	6.90	1.55	0.25	4.05	2.400	0.043	0.496	0	179.0
Chicken roll—light meat	45	5.52	2.08	0.69	11.90	0.274	0.018	0.037	0	13.9
Chicken frankfurter	73	3.67	5.52	1.93	27.00	0.567	0.019	0.033	0	28.4
Chicken á la king	54	3.12	3.93	1.93	14.70	0.289	0.012	0.049	0.154	25.6
Chicken and noodles	43	2.60	2.13	3.07	3.07	0.278	0.006	0.020	0.142	12.2
Chicken chow mein	29	2.60	1.25	1.13	6.58	0.284	0.009	0.026	0.466	8.5
Chicken curry	26	2.21	1.53	0.64	2.52	0.170	0.009	0.019	0.033	5.3
Chicken frankfurter	72	3.67	5.52	1.93	27.00	0.567	0.019	0.033	0	28.4
Chicken pot pie—frozen	53	1.84	2.84	5.08	3.70	0.382	0.020	0.020	0.210	4.9
Chicken roll—light meat	45	5.52	2.08	0.69	11.90	0.274	0.018	0.037	0	13.9
Chicken salad w/celery	97	3.82	8.90	0.47	5.92	0.239	0.012	0.028	0.109	17.3
Chicken patty sandwich	79	4.48	4.06	6.10	7.95	0.338	0.052	0.047	0.244	12.3
Chicken broth—from dry	2	0.16	0.13	0.17	1.74	0.009	0	0.004	0.001	0.1
Chicken broth—from cube	2	0.11	0.04	0.18	0.04	0.014	0.001	0.003	0	0.1
Chicken noodle soup	9	0.48	0.29	1.10	2.00	0.092	0.006	0.007	0.085	0.8
Tostada w/beans and chicken	45	3.50	2.06	3.38	29.30	0.305	0.013	0.034	0.668	9.6
Chicken taco	63	5.60	3.03	3.67	31.60	0.237	0.014	0.043	0.407	16.5
Chicken enchilada	64	3.38	2.48	3.69	60.50	0.359	0.018	0.036	0.465	9.1
Turkey dark meat—roasted	53	8.10	2.05	0	9.11	0.662	0.018	0.070	0	24.0
Turkey white meat—roasted	44	8.48	0.91	0	5.47	0.380	0.017	0.037	0	19.6
Turkey breast—barbecued	40	6.39	1.40	0	2.00	0.120	0.010	0.030	0	16.0
Turkey gizzards	46	8.34	1.10	0.17	4.32	1.540	0.009	0.093	0	65.6
Turkey hearts	50	7.58	1.73	0.58	3.72	1.950	0.019	0.250	0	64.0
Turkey livers	48	6.80	1.69	0.97	3.02	2.210	0.015	0.404	0	177.0
Turkey loaf	31	6.38	0.45	0	2.00	0.113	0.011	0.030	0	11.6
Turkey roll	41	5.27	2.03	0.15	11.40	0.358	0.025	0.064	0	11.9
Turkey bologna	56	3.86	4.27	0.27	23.40	0.432	0.015	0.047	0	28.0
Turkey frankfurter	64	4.05	5.22	0.42	36.50	0.485	0.023	0.050	0	24.6
Turkey ham	36	5.37	1.49	0.42	2.49	0.776	0.020	0.075	0	15.9
Turkey pastrami	37	5.22	1.75	0.43	2.49	0.403	0.022	0.075	0	14.9
Turkey salami	55	4.62	3.89	0.15	5.47	0.463	0.029	0.075	0	22.9
Turkey pot pie—frozen	51	1.80	2.75	4.65	7.79	0.256	0.020	0.020	0.110	2.4

➤ EGGS

	KCAL	PROTEIN (G)	FAT (G)	CHO (G)	CA (MG)	FE (MG)	B_1 (MG)	B_2 (MG)	FIBER (G)	CHOLESTEROL (MG)
Egg white, cooked	13	2.68	0	0.33	3.20	0.008	0.002	0.072	0	0
Egg yolk, cooked	108	4.76	8.73	0.07	44.40	1.620	0.044	0.121	0	355.0
Egg, fried in butter	56	3.54	3.45	0.38	15.70	0.536	0.018	0.148	0	129.0
Egg, hard cooked	40	3.52	2.79	0.34	13.80	0.474	0.014	0.132	0	113.0
Egg, poached	40	3.50	2.79	0.34	13.80	0.474	0.014	0.132	0	113.0
Egg, scrambled w/ milk and butter	40	2.88	2.57	0.61	23.90	0.412	0.013	0.106	0	93.9
Egg raw—large	40	3.52	2.79	0.34	13.80	0.474	0.017	0.139	0	113.0
Egg white—raw	13	2.68	0	0.33	3.20	0.008	0.002	0.075	0	0
Egg yolk, raw	108	4.76	8.73	0.07	44.40	1.620	0.051	0.126	0	355.0
Egg substitute, frozen	45	3.20	3.15	0.91	20.80	0.562	0.034	0.110	0	0.5
Egg substitute, powder	125	15.60	3.66	6.12	90.70	0.879	0.062	0.493	0	162.0

➤ DAIRY PRODUCTS

	KCAL	PROTEIN (G)	FAT (G)	CHO (G)	CA (MG)	FE (MG)	B_1 (MG)	B_2 (MG)	FIBER (G)	CHOLESTEROL (MG)
Milk—1% lowfat	12	0.93	0.30	1.36	34.9	0.014	0.011	0.047	0	1.16
Milk—2% lowfat	14	0.94	0.56	1.36	34.5	0.012	0.011	0.047	0	2.56
Milk—skim	10	0.97	0.05	1.38	34.9	0.012	0.010	0.040	0	0.46
Milk—whole	17	0.93	0.95	1.32	33.8	0.014	0.010	0.046	0	3.83
Buttermilk	12	0.94	0.25	1.35	33.0	0.014	0.010	0.044	0	1.04
Milk—instant nonfat dry	102	9.96	0.21	14.80	349.0	0.088	0.117	0.496	0	5.00
Canned skim milk—evaporated	22	2.11	0.06	3.22	82.0	0.078	0.013	0.088	0	1.11
Canned whole milk—evaporated	38	1.91	2.20	2.81	73.9	0.054	0.014	0.090	0	8.33
Carob flavor mix—powder	106	0.47	0.05	26.50	0	1.300	0.002	0	4.020	0
Chocolate milk—1%	18	0.92	0.28	2.96	32.5	0.068	0.010	0.047	0.425	0.79
Chocolate milk—2%	20	0.91	0.57	2.95	32.2	0.068	0.010	0.046	0.425	1.93
Chocolate milk—whole	24	0.90	0.96	2.94	31.8	0.068	0.010	0.046	0.425	3.52
Hot cocoa—with whole milk	25	1.03	1.03	2.93	33.8	0.088	0.012	0.049	0.340	3.74
Instant breakfast w/2% milk	25	1.52	0.47	3.50	31.0	0.807	0.040	0.048	0	1.82
Instant breakfast w/1% milk	23	1.51	0.25	3.50	31.3	0.807	0.040	0.048	0	1.00
Instant breakfast w/skim milk	22	1.55	0.04	3.50	31.4	0.804	0.039	0.041	0	0.40
Instant breakfast w/whole milk	28	1.51	0.82	3.47	30.4	0.807	0.040	0.047	0	3.33
Egg nog	38	1.08	2.12	3.84	36.8	0.057	0.010	0.054	0	16.60
Kefir	20	1.13	0.55	1.07	42.6	0.060	0.055	0.054	0	1.22
Malt powder—chocolate-flavored	107	1.49	1.08	24.80	17.6	0.648	0.049	0.057	0.540	1.35
Malted milk powder	117	3.12	2.30	21.50	85.0	0.209	0.143	0.260	0.405	5.40
Malted milk drink—chocolate-flavored	25	1.00	0.95	3.19	32.5	0.064	0.014	0.047	0.043	3.64
Chocolate milkshake	36	0.96	1.05	5.80	32.0	0.088	0.016	0.069	0.035	3.70
Strawberry milkshake	32	0.95	0.80	5.35	32.0	0.030	0.013	0.055	0.024	3.10
Vanilla milkshake	32	0.98	0.84	5.09	34.5	0.026	0.013	0.052	0.019	3.20
Ovaltine powder—chocolate-flavored	102	2.00	0.85	23.70	134.0	6.190	0.719	0.772	0.013	0
Ovaltine powder—malt-flavored	104	2.53	0.24	23.60	106.0	5.820	0.772	1.010	0.040	0
Ovaltine drink—chocolate-flavored	24	1.02	0.94	3.12	41.9	0.510	0.067	0.104	0.001	3.53
Ovaltine drink—malt-flavored	24	1.06	0.89	3.10	39.7	0.480	0.072	0.124	0.003	3.53
Milk—goat	20	1.00	1.17	1.27	37.9	0.014	0.014	0.039	0	3.25

➤ DAIRY PRODUCTS—*continued*

	KCAL	PROTEIN (G)	FAT (G)	CHO (G)	CA (MG)	FE (MG)	B_1 (MG)	B_2 (MG)	FIBER (G)	CHOLESTEROL (MG)
Milk—sheep	31	1.70	1.99	1.52	54.8	0.028	0.018	0.100	0	0
Milk—soybean	9	0.78	0.54	0.51	1.2	0.163	0.046	0.020	0	0
Ice cream—regular-vanilla	57	1.02	3.05	6.76	37.5	0.026	0.011	0.070	0	12.60
Ice cream—rich-vanilla	67	0.79	4.54	6.13	28.9	0.019	0.008	0.054	0	16.90
Ice cream—soft-serve	62	1.15	3.69	6.28	38.7	0.070	0.013	0.073	0	25.00
Creamsicle ice cream bar	44	0.52	1.33	7.56	19.8	0	0.009	0.034	0	0
Drumstick ice cream bar	88	1.23	4.68	10.20	31.7	0.047	0.009	0.043	0	0
Fudgesicle ice cream bar	35	1.48	0.08	7.22	50.0	0.039	0.012	0.070	0	0
Ice milk	40	1.12	1.22	6.28	38.0	0.039	0.016	0.075	0	3.90
Ice milk—soft-serve, 3% fat	36	1.30	0.75	6.22	44.4	0.045	0.019	0.088	0	2.10
Yogurt—coffee-vanilla	24	1.40	0.35	3.90	48.5	0.020	0.012	0.057	0	1.42
Yogurt—lowfat with fruit	29	1.24	0.31	5.37	43.0	0.020	0.010	0.050	0	1.25
Yogurt—lowfat-plain	18	1.49	0.43	2.00	51.8	0.022	0.012	0.060	0	1.75
Yogurt—nonfat milk	16	1.62	0.05	2.17	56.5	0.025	0.014	0.066	0	0.50
Yogurt—whole milk	17	0.98	0.92	1.32	34.3	0.014	0.008	0.040	0	3.68

➤ VEGETABLES

	KCAL	PROTEIN (G)	FAT (G)	CHO (G)	CA (MG)	FE (MG)	B_1 (MG)	B_2 (MG)	FIBER (G)	CHOLESTEROL (MG)
Alfalfa sprouts	9	1.13	0.200	1.07	9.5	0.272	0.021	0.036	1.030	0
Artichoke hearts—marinated	28	0.680	0.250	2.18	6.5	0.270	0.010	0.029	1.780	0
Asparagus—raw spears	6	0.865	0.063	1.05	6.4	0.193	0.032	0.035	0.395	0
Asparagus—canned spears	5	0.606	0.184	0.70	3.9	0.177	0.017	0.025	0.454	0
Bamboo shoots—sliced, raw	8	0.738	0.088	1.47	3.8	0.143	0.043	0.020	0.738	0
Bamboo shoots—sliced, canned	5	0.489	0.113	0.91	2.2	0.090	0.007	0.007	0.706	0
Bean sprouts—fresh, raw	9	0.861	0.050	1.68	3.8	0.258	0.024	0.035	0.736	0
Bean sprouts—boiled	6	0.576	0.025	1.19	3.4	0.185	0.014	0.029	0.572	0
Bean sprouts—stir fried	14	1.220	0.059	3.00	3.7	0.549	0.040	0.050	0.777	0
Black beans—cooked	37	2.500	0.152	6.72	7.8	0.593	0.069	0.017	2.540	0
Green beans—raw, uncooked	9	0.515	0.034	2.02	10.6	0.363	0.024	0.030	0.644	0
Green beans—fresh, cooked	10	0.535	0.082	2.24	13.2	0.363	0.021	0.027	0.737	0
Green beans—frozen, cooked	8	0.386	0.038	1.73	12.8	0.233	0.014	0.021	0.880	0
Green beans—canned/drained	6	0.326	0.028	1.28	7.6	0.256	0.004	0.016	0.378	0
Red kidney beans—dry	94	6.690	0.234	16.90	40.5	2.330	0.150	0.062	6.160	0
Lima beans—dry, large	96	6.080	0.194	18.00	22.9	2.130	0.144	0.057	8.600	0
Lima beans—fresh—cooked	35	1.930	0.090	6.70	9.0	0.695	0.040	0.027	2.670	0
Lima beans—dry, small	98	5.790	0.397	18.20	18.4	2.270	0.136	0.048	8.500	0
Lima beans—canned/drained	27	1.530	0.100	5.20	8.0	0.487	0.010	0.013	2.420	0
Beans w/franks—canned	40	1.900	1.860	4.37	13.6	0.490	0.016	0.016	1.950	1.7
Pork and beans—canned	32	1.500	0.413	5.95	17.4	0.470	0.013	0.017	1.560	1.9
Navy beans—dry, cooked	40	2.460	0.162	7.77	19.9	0.703	0.057	0.017	2.490	0
Pinto beans—dry, cooked	39	2.320	0.148	7.28	13.6	0.741	0.053	0.026	3.230	0
Refried beans—canned	30	1.770	0.303	5.24	13.2	0.500	0.014	0.016	2.470	0
Soybeans—dry	118	10.400	5.650	8.55	78.5	4.450	0.248	0.247	1.570	0
White beans—dry	95	5.990	0.334	17.70	36.0	2.190	0.210	0.059	0.766	0
White beans—dry, cooked	40	2.550	0.182	7.32	20.7	0.808	0.067	0.017	2.230	0
Yellow wax beans—raw	9	0.515	0.034	2.02	10.6	0.294	0.024	0.030	0.644	0
Yellow wax beans—raw	10	0.535	0.082	2.24	13.2	0.363	0.021	0.027	0.726	0
Yellow wax beans—frozen	8	0.386	0.038	1.73	12.8	0.233	0.014	0.021	0.880	0
Beets—cooked	9	0.300	0.014	1.90	3.1	0.176	0.009	0.004	0.539	0

➤ VEGETABLES—*continued*

	KCAL	PROTEIN (G)	FAT (G)	CHO (G)	CA (MG)	FE (MG)	B_1 (MG)	B_2 (MG)	FIBER (G)	CHOLESTEROL (MG)
Beets—pickled slices	18	0.227	0.028	4.63	3.1	0.116	0.006	0.014	0.587	0
Broccoli—raw, chopped	8	0.844	0.097	1.49	13.5	0.251	0.019	0.034	0.934	0
Broccoli—raw spears	8	0.845	0.098	1.49	13.5	0.250	0.018	0.034	0.935	0
Broccoli—frozen, cooked spears	8	0.879	0.034	1.51	14.5	0.173	0.015	0.023	0.826	0
Brussels sprouts—raw	12	0.960	0.084	2.54	11.6	0.396	0.039	0.026	1.260	0
Brussels sprouts—cooked	11	1.090	0.145	2.45	10.2	0.342	0.030	0.023	1.220	0
Brussels sprouts—frozen, cooked	12	1.030	0.112	2.36	7.0	0.210	0.029	0.032	1.230	0
Cabbage—raw, shredded	7	0.340	0.049	1.52	13.0	0.162	0.015	0.009	0.680	0
Cabbage—cooked	6	0.272	0.070	1.35	9.5	0.110	0.016	0.016	0.661	0
Bok choy—raw, shredded	4	0.425	0.057	0.62	30.0	0.227	0.011	0.020	0.486	0
Bok choy—cooked	3	0.442	0.045	0.51	26.3	0.295	0.009	0.018	0.454	0
Red cabbage—raw	8	0.393	0.073	1.74	14.6	0.142	0.018	0.009	0.648	0
Red cabbage—cooked	6	0.299	0.057	1.32	10.6	0.102	0.010	0.006	1.567	0
Carrot—whole, raw	12	0.291	0.055	2.87	7.5	0.142	0.028	0.017	1.906	0
Carrot—grated, raw	12	0.289	0.052	2.88	7.7	0.142	0.027	0.016	0.907	0
Carrots—sliced, cooked	13	0.309	0.050	2.97	8.7	0.176	0.010	0.016	0.992	0
Carrots—frozen, cooked	10	0.338	0.031	2.34	8.2	0.136	0.008	0.010	1.050	0
Carrots—canned, drained	7	0.183	0.054	1.57	7.4	0.181	0.005	0.009	0.435	0
Carrot juice	11	0.267	0.041	2.63	6.7	0.130	0.026	0.015	0.385	0
Cauliflower—raw	7	0.561	0.051	1.39	7.9	0.164	0.022	0.016	0.720	0
Cauliflower—cooked	7	0.530	0.050	1.31	7.8	0.119	0.018	0.018	0.622	0
Cauliflower—frozen, cooked	5	0.457	0.061	1.06	4.9	0.116	0.010	0.015	0.535	0
Celery—raw, chopped	5	0.189	0.033	1.03	10.4	0.137	0.009	0.009	0.472	0
Swiss chard—raw	5	0.510	0.057	1.06	14.5	0.510	0.011	0.025	0.512	0
Swiss chard—cooked	6	0.533	0.023	1.17	16.5	0.642	0.010	0.024	0.616	0
Collards—fresh	5	0.445	0.062	1.07	33.0	0.299	0.009	0.018	0.590	0
Collards—fresh, cooked	4	0.313	0.043	0.75	22.0	0.116	0.005	0.012	0.798	0
Collards—frozen, cooked	10	0.840	0.115	2.02	59.5	0.317	0.013	0.033	0.794	0
Corn—kernels, raw	24	0.913	0.335	5.38	0.6	0.147	0.057	0.017	1.220	0
Corn on the cob—cooked	31	0.943	0.363	7.14	0.6	0.173	0.061	0.020	1.190	0
Corn—cooked from frozen	23	0.857	0.020	5.80	0.6	0.085	0.020	0.020	1.190	0
Corn—canned, drained	23	0.743	0.283	5.26	1.4	0.142	0.009	0.014	0.398	0
Corn—canned cream-style	21	0.494	0.119	5.14	0.9	0.108	0.007	0.015	0.354	0
Cucumber slices w/peel	4	0.153	0.037	0.82	4.0	0.079	0.009	0.006	0.329	0
Eggplant—cooked	8	0.236	0.066	1.88	1.7	0.099	0.022	0.006	1.060	0
Escarole/curly endive—chopped	5	0.354	0.057	0.95	14.7	0.235	0.023	0.022	0.369	0
Garbanzo/chickpeas—dry	103	5.470	1.720	17.20	29.9	1.770	0.135	0.060	5.390	0
Garbanzo/chickpeas—cooked	47	2.500	0.735	7.78	13.8	0.819	0.033	0.018	1.920	0
Jerusalem artichoke—raw	22	0.567	0.004	4.95	4.0	0.964	0.057	0.017	0.369	0
Kale—fresh, chopped	14	0.935	0.198	2.84	38.0	0.482	0.031	0.037	1.650	0
Kohlrabi—raw slices	8	0.482	0.028	1.76	6.9	0.113	0.014	0.006	0.405	0
Kohlrabi—cooked	8	0.510	0.030	1.96	7.0	0.113	0.011	0.006	0.395	0
Leeks—chopped, raw	17	0.425	0.085	4.00	16.7	0.594	0.017	0.008	0.668	0
Leeks—cooked, chopped	9	0.230	0.057	2.16	8.5	0.310	0.007	0.006	0.927	0
Lentils—dry	96	7.960	0.273	16.20	14.6	2.550	0.135	0.069	3.400	0
Lentils—cooked from dry	33	2.560	0.106	5.73	5.3	0.944	0.048	0.020	1.430	0
Lentils—sprouted, raw	30	2.540	0.156	6.30	7.0	0.909	0.065	0.036	1.150	0
Lettuce—butterhead	4	0.367	0.062	0.66	9.5	0.085	0.017	0.017	0.397	0
Lettuce—iceberg	4	0.286	0.054	0.59	5.4	0.142	0.013	0.009	0.347	0
Lettuce—romaine	5	0.459	0.057	0.67	10.2	0.312	0.028	0.028	0.482	0
Mushrooms—raw, sliced	7	0.593	0.119	1.32	1.4	0.352	0.029	0.127	0.508	0
Mushrooms—cooked	8	0.614	0.134	1.46	1.7	0.494	0.020	0.085	0.625	0
Mushrooms—canned, drained	7	0.530	0.082	1.40	3.1	0.224	0.017	0.063	0.596	0
Mustard greens—fresh	7	0.764	0.057	1.39	29.4	0.414	0.023	0.031	0.764	0
Mustard greens—cooked	4	0.640	0.068	0.60	21.0	0.316	0.012	0.018	0.587	0
Okra pods—cooked	9	0.530	0.048	2.04	17.9	0.128	0.037	0.016	0.624	0

➤ **VEGETABLES—*continued***

	KCAL	PROTEIN (G)	FAT (G)	CHO (G)	CA (MG)	FE (MG)	B_1 (MG)	B_2 (MG)	FIBER (G)	CHOLESTEROL (MG)
Okra slices—cooked	11	0.589	0.085	2.32	27.1	0.190	0.028	0.035	0.709	0
Onions—chopped, raw	10	0.335	0.074	2.07	7.1	0.105	0.017	0.003	0.454	0
Onion slices—raw	10	0.335	0.074	2.08	7.2	0.105	0.017	0.003	0.454	0
Onion—dehydrated flakes	91	2.530	0.122	23.70	72.9	0.446	0.022	0.018	2.510	0
Onion rings—frozen, heated	115	1.520	7.570	10.80	8.8	0.482	0.079	0.040	0.240	0
Parsley—freeze-dried	81	8.910	1.420	11.90	40.5	15.200	0.304	0.648	22.000	0
Parsley—fresh, chopped	9	0.624	0.085	1.96	36.9	1.760	0.023	0.031	1.550	0
Parsnips—sliced, raw	21	0.341	0.085	5.09	10.0	0.167	0.026	0.014	1.280	0
Fresh peas—uncooked	23	1.530	0.113	4.10	7.0	0.416	0.075	0.037	1.380	0
Peas—cooked	24	1.520	0.060	4.43	7.8	0.438	0.073	0.042	1.360	0
Peas—frozen, cooked	22	1.460	0.078	4.04	6.7	0.443	0.080	0.050	1.280	0
Peas—edible pods, fresh	12	0.794	0.057	2.15	12.1	0.589	0.043	0.023	0.794	0
Split peas—dry	97	6.970	0.328	17.10	15.5	1.250	0.206	0.061	4.030	0
Peas + carrots—frozen, cooked	14	0.875	0.120	2.87	6.4	0.266	0.064	0.020	1.170	0
Green chili pepper—raw	11	0.557	0.057	2.68	5.0	0.340	0.026	0.026	0.504	0
Red chili peppers—raw/ chopped	11	0.567	0.057	2.68	4.9	0.340	0.026	0.026	0.454	0
Jalapeño peppers—canned, chopped	7	0.225	0.170	1.39	7.5	0.792	0.008	0.014	0.850	0
Baked potato with skin	31	0.653	0.028	7.16	2.8	0.386	0.030	0.009	0.660	0
Baked potato—flesh only	26	0.556	0.029	6.10	1.5	0.100	0.030	0.006	0.436	0
Potato skin—oven-baked	56	1.220	0.029	13.20	9.8	1.080	0.035	0.034	1.130	0
Potato + peel—microwaved	30	0.692	0.028	6.83	3.1	0.350	0.034	0.009	0.660	0
Peeled potato—boiled	24	0.485	0.029	5.67	2.1	0.088	0.028	0.005	0.426	0
French fries—oven-heated	63	0.980	2.480	9.64	2.3	0.380	0.035	0.009	0.567	0
French fries—frozen, w/vegetable oil	90	1.140	4.690	11.20	5.7	0.215	0.050	0.008	0.567	0
Cottage-fried potatoes	62	0.975	2.320	9.64	2.8	0.425	0.034	0.009	0.567	0
Hash-brown potatoes	30	0.343	1.980	3.02	1.1	0.115	0.010	0.003	0.567	0
Mashed potatoes prep and milk	22	0.548	0.166	4.98	7.4	0.077	0.025	0.011	0.405	0.5
Mashed potatoes—milk and margarine	30	0.533	1.200	4.74	7.3	0.074	0.024	0.014	0.405	0.5
Potato pancakes	88	1.730	4.700	9.85	7.8	0.451	0.039	0.035	0.563	34.7
Potatoes au gratin mix	26	0.653	1.170	3.65	23.5	0.090	0.006	0.023	0.487	1.4
Scalloped potatoes—recipe	24	0.813	1.040	3.05	16.2	0.163	0.020	0.026	0.289	3.4
Potato chips	148	1.590	10.000	14.70	7.0	0.339	0.040	0.006	1.360	0
Potato flour	100	2.260	0.226	22.60	9.3	4.880	0.119	0.040	0.317	0
Pumpkin—canned	10	0.311	0.080	2.28	7.4	0.394	0.007	0.015	0.519	0
Red radishes	4	0.170	0.151	1.01	5.7	0.082	0.001	0.013	0.624	0
Rutabaga—cooked cubes	10	0.314	0.053	2.19	12.0	0.133	0.020	0.010	0.434	0
Sauerkraut—canned w/ liquid	5	0.258	0.040	1.21	8.7	0.417	0.006	0.006	0.529	0
Soybeans—mature, raw	37	3.700	1.900	3.17	19.4	0.599	0.096	0.033	0.656	0
Spinach—cooked from fresh	7	0.843	0.074	1.06	38.4	1.010	0.027	0.067	0.702	0
Summer squash—raw slices	6	0.334	0.061	1.23	5.7	0.130	0.018	0.010	0.425	0
Zucchini squash—cooked	5	0.181	0.014	1.11	3.6	0.099	0.012	0.012	0.567	0
Acorn squash—boiled/ mashed	10	0.190	0.023	2.49	7.5	0.159	0.028	0.002	0.680	0
Butternut squash—baked, cube	12	0.256	0.026	2.97	11.6	0.170	0.020	0.005	0.794	0
Spaghetti squash—baked/ boiled	8	0.187	0.073	1.83	6.0	0.095	0.010	0.006	0.794	0
Winter squash—boiled	10	0.319	0.050	2.40	5.2	0.136	0.018	0.006	0.794	0
Sweet potato—baked in skin	29	0.487	0.032	6.89	8.0	0.129	0.020	0.036	0.850	0
Candied sweet potatoes	39	0.246	0.920	7.91	7.3	0.324	0.005	0.012	0.545	0

➤ VEGETABLES—*continued*

	KCAL	PROTEIN (G)	FAT (G)	CHO (G)	CA (MG)	FE (MG)	B_1 (MG)	B_2 (MG)	FIBER (G)	CHOLESTEROL (MG)
Tofu (soybean curd)	22	2.290	1.360	0.53	29.7	1.520	0.023	0.015	0.343	0
Tomato—fresh, whole	6	0.251	0.060	1.23	2.1	0.136	0.017	0.014	0.415	0
Tomatoes—whole, canned	6	0.265	0.070	1.22	7.4	0.171	0.013	0.009	0.298	0
Tomato sauce—canned	9	0.376	0.047	2.04	3.9	0.218	0.019	0.016	0.425	0
Tomato paste—canned	24	1.070	0.249	5.33	9.9	0.848	0.044	0.054	1.210	0
Tomato juice—canned	5	0.215	0.017	1.20	2.6	0.164	0.013	0.009	0.220	0
Turnip cubes—raw	8	0.255	0.028	1.76	8.5	0.085	0.011	0.009	0.587	0
Mixed vegetables—frozen, cooked	17	0.812	0.043	3.70	7.2	0.232	0.020	0.034	1.120	0
Vegetable juice cocktail	6	0.178	0.026	1.29	3.1	0.119	0.012	0.008	0.178	0
Water chestnuts—raw	30	0.398	0.027	6.77	3.2	0.170	0.040	0.057	0.869	0
Watercress—fresh	3	0.650	0.033	0.37	33.4	0.050	0.025	0.033	0.719	0
White yams—raw	34	0.438	0.049	7.90	8.7	0.153	0.032	0.009	0.822	0

➤ SALAD BAR

	KCAL	PROTEIN (G)	FAT (G)	CHO (G)	CA (MG)	FE (MG)	B_1 (MG)	B_2 (MG)	FIBER (G)	CHOLESTEROL (MG)
Alfalfa sprouts	8.59	1.130	0.196	1.070	9.45	0.272	0.021	0.036	1.030	0
Artichoke hearts, marinated	28.00	0.680	2.250	2.180	6.50	0.270	0.010	0.029	1.780	0
Asparagus	6.35	0.867	0.062	1.050	6.35	0.193	0.032	0.035	0.432	0
Avocado	45.70	0.563	4.340	2.100	3.07	0.284	0.030	0.035	2.720	0
Bacon, regular	163.00	8.640	14.000	0.164	2.98	0.482	0.195	0.080	0	23.9
Bean sprouts	8.50	0.861	0.050	1.680	3.82	0.258	0.024	0.035	0.7365	0
Beets	8.67	0.300	0.013	1.900	3.00	0.176	0.009	0.004	0.567	0
Beets, canned, diced	9.00	0.260	0.040	2.040	4.34	0.517	0.003	0.012	0.590	0
Broccoli, raw	7.73	0.844	0.097	1.490	13.50	0.251	0.019	0.034	0.934	0
Cabbage	6.48	0.340	0.049	1.520	13.00	0.162	0.015	0.009	0.680	0
Cabbage, red	7.70	0.393	0.073	1.740	14.60	0.142	0.018	0.009	0.648	0
Carrots, grated	12.40	0.289	0.052	2.880	7.73	0.142	0.027	0.016	0.907	0
Cauliflower	6.80	0.561	0.051	1.390	7.94	0.164	0.022	0.016	0.720	0
Celery	4.54	0.189	0.030	1.030	10.40	0.137	0.009	0.009	0.472	0
Chicken salad	96.70	3.820	8.900	0.469	5.92	0.239	0.012	0.028	0.109	17.3
Crab, cooked	23.90	5.050	0.561	0.140	12.90	0.104	0.012	0.044	0	18.0
Croutons, dry bread cubes	105.00	3.690	1.040	20.500	35.00	1.020	0.099	0.099	0.085	0
Cucumber slices	3.69	0.153	0.037	0.824	3.99	0.079	0.009	0.006	0.329	0
Egg, chopped	40.40	3.520	2.790	0.338	13.80	0.475	0.014	0.133	0	113
Escarole/curly endive	4.82	0.354	0.057	0.953	14.70	0.235	0.023	0.022	0.369	0
Garbanzo/chickpeas, cooked	46.50	2.500	0.735	7.780	13.80	0.819	0.033	0.018	1.920	0
Green pepper, sweet	6.80	0.244	0.130	1.500	1.70	0.357	0.024	0.014	0.454	0
Ham salad	51.50	5.000	3.000	0.880	2.00	0.280	0.244	0.072	0	16
Ham, minced	74.20	4.620	5.860	0.526	2.70	0.216	0.203	0.054	0	20.2
Leeks	17.30	0.425	0.085	4.000	16.70	0.594	0.017	0.008	0.688	0
Lettuce, butterhead	3.69	0.366	0.062	0.658	9.47	0.085	0.017	0.017	0.370	0
Lettuce, iceberg	3.69	0.287	0.054	0.592	5.37	0.142	0.013	0.009	0.370	0
Lettuce, loose leaf	5.11	0.369	0.085	0.992	19.20	0.397	0.014	0.023	0.391	0
Lettuce, romaine	4.54	0.459	0.057	0.673	10.20	0.312	0.028	0.028	0.482	0
Lobster meat	27.80	5.800	0.168	0.364	17.20	0.111	0.020	0.019	0	20.3
Mushrooms, raw	7.09	0.593	0.119	1.320	1.42	0.352	0.029	0.127	0.508	0
Onions	9.57	0.335	0.074	2.070	7.09	0.105	0.017	0.003	0.454	0
Parmesan cheese, grated	129.00	11.800	8.500	1.060	389.00	0.270	0.013	0.109	0	22.0
Peas, cooked	22.30	1.460	0.078	4.040	6.73	0.443	0.080	0.050	1.280	0
Sesame seed kernels, dried	167.00	7.480	15.500	2.660	37.20	2.210	0.204	0.024	1.950	0
Shrimp, boiled	28.00	5.930	0.306	0	11.00	0.876	0.009	0.009	0	55.3
Spinach, fresh	6.23	0.810	0.099	0.992	28.00	0.770	0.022	0.054	0.947	0
Sunflower seeds, dry	162.00	6.460	14.000	5.320	32.90	1.920	0.650	0.070	1.970	0
Tomatoes	5.51	0.252	0.061	1.230	1.89	0.135	0.017	0.014	0.416	0
Tuna salad	53.00	4.550	2.630	2.670	4.84	0.282	0.009	0.019	0.340	3.73
Turkey meat	41.30	5.270	2.030	0.149	11.40	0.358	0.025	0.064	0	11.9

➤ **VARIETY**

	KCAL	PROTEIN (G)	FAT (G)	CHO (G)	CA (MG)	FE (MG)	B_1 (MG)	B_2 (MG)	FIBER (G)	CHOLESTEROL (MG)
Chips and crackers										
Doritos—nacho flavor	139	2.20	6.79	18.00	17.0	0.399	0.040	0.030	1.10	0
Doritos—taco flavor	140	2.60	6.59	17.60	44.9	0.699	0.080	0.090	1.10	0
Potato chips—sour cream and onion	153	2.40	9.48	14.60	21.0	0.474	0.040	0.055	1.35	1.0
Wheat cracker—thin	124	3.19	4.96	17.70	10.6	1.060	0.142	0.106	1.84	0
Whole wheat crackers	124	3.19	5.32	17.70	10.6	1.850	0.070	0.106	2.94	0
Condiments										
Catsup	30	0.52	0.11	7.17	6.2	0.228	0.026	0.020	0.45	0
Mustard	21	1.34	1.25	1.81	23.8	0.567	0.024	0.057	0.11	0
Soy sauce	14	1.46	0.02	2.40	4.7	0.567	0.014	0.036	0	0
Deli meats										
Bologna—beef	89	3.32	8.04	0.56	3.7	0.394	0.016	0.036	0	16.0
Bratwurst	92	4.05	7.90	0.84	13.8	0.292	0.070	0.064	0	17.8
Keilbasa sausage	88	3.76	7.70	0.61	12.0	0.414	0.064	0.061	0	18.5
Knockwurst sausage	87	3.37	7.88	0.05	2.9	0.258	0.097	0.040	0	16.3
Liverwurst	93	4.00	8.10	0.63	7.9	1.810	0.077	0.291	0	44.1
Pepperoni sausage	140	5.94	12.50	0.80	2.8	0.397	0.09	0.07		9.79
Polish sausage	92	3.99	8.13	0.46	3.0	0.409	0.142	0.042	0	20.0
Salami—beef	72	4.17	5.69	0.70	2.47	0.567	0.036	0.073	0	17.3
Salami—pork and beef	72	3.94	5.70	0.64	3.68	0.755	0.068	0.106	0	18.5
Salami—turkey	55	4.62	3.89	0.15	5.47	0.463	0.029	0.075	0	22.9
Salami—dry—beef and pork	120	6.49	9.75	0.74	2.84	0.425	0.170	0.082	0	22.7
Turkey pastrami	37	5.22	1.75	0.43	2.49	0.403	0.022	0.075	0	14.9
Mexican foods										
Beef taco	75.2	4.94	4.80	3.67	30.9	0.469	0.01	0.049	0.407	16.2
Beef enchilada	69.0	3.09	3.26	3.69	60.2	0.418	0.017	0.039	0.465	8.93
Cheese enchilada	78.0	3.12	4.2	3.78	108.0	0.324	0.015	0.050	0.465	10.2
Chicken enchilada	63.6	3.38	2.48	3.69	60.5	0.359	0.018	0.036	0.465	9.10
Corn tortilla, enriched, regular	61.4	1.89	0.964	12.30	39.7	0.567	0.047	0.028	2.27	0
Corn torilla, enriched, thin	61.0	1.64	0.95	12.30	39.8	0.567	0.046	0.028	2.26	0
Corn tortilla, fried	82.2	2.08	2.84	12.30	39.7	0.567	0.047	0.028	2.27	0
Enchirito	60.4	3.15	2.75	3.31	51.5	0.410	0.015	0.037	0.748	9.18
Flour tortilla	84	2.07	2.15	15.50	17.0	0.440	0.102	0.062	0.800	0
Refried beans, canned	30.3	1.77	0.303	5.24	13.2	0.500	0.014	0.016	2.47	0
Nuts and seeds										
Almonds—dried, chopped	167	5.65	14.80	5.78	75.5	1.040	0.060	0.220	3.36	0
Almonds—whole, toasted	167	5.77	14.40	6.48	80.0	1.400	0.037	0.170	3.99	0
Sunflower seeds—dry	162	6.46	14.00	5.32	32.9	1.920	0.650	0.070	1.97	0
Oils and shortening										
Cocoa butter oil	251	0	28.40	0	0	0	0	0	0	0
Corn oil	251	0	28.40	0	0	0.001	0	0	0	0
Cottonseed oil	251	0	28.40	0	0	0	0	0	0	0
Olive oil	251	0	28.40	0	0.1	0.109	0	0	0	0
Palm oil	251	0	28.40	0	0.1	0.003	0	0	0	0
Palm kernel oil	251	0	28.40	0	0	0	0	0	0	0
Peanut oil	251	0	28.40	0	0	0.008	0	0	0	0
Safflower oil	251	0	28.40	0	0	0	0	0	0	0
Sesame oil	250	0	28.40	0	0	0	0	0	0	0
Soybean oil	251	0	28.40	0	0	0.007	0	0	0	0
Sunflower oil	251	0	28.40	0	0	0	0	0	0	0
Walnut oil	251	0	28.40	0	0	0	0	0	0	0
Wheat germ oil	250	0	28.40	0	0	0	0	0	0	0
Vegetable shortening	251	0	28.40	0	0	0	0	0	0	0
Pasta and noodles										
Spaghetti, cooked firm, hot	41	1.42	0.142	8.53	3.1	0.454	0.051	0.028	0.482	0

➤ VARIETY—*continued*

	KCAL	PROTEIN (G)	FAT (G)	CHO (G)	CA (MG)	FE (MG)	B_1 (MG)	B_2 (MG)	FIBER (G)	CHOLESTEROL (MG)
Pasta and noodles—*continued*										
Spaghetti, cooked tender, hot	31	1.01	0.111	6.48	3.0	0.405	0.04	0.022	0.425	0
Whole wheat spaghetti, cooked	35	1.53	0.113	7.49	4.3	0.244	0.048	0.020	1.040	0
Spaghetti w/sauce and cheese, canned	22	0.68	0.227	4.42	4.5	0.318	0.040	0.032	0.284	0.3
Spaghetti w/sauce and cheese, homemade	30	1.02	1.02	4.20	9.07	0.260	0.028	0.020	0.284	0.9
Spaghetti w/sauce and meat, canned	30	1.36	1.13	4.42	6.01	0.374	0.017	0.020	0.312	2.6
Spaghetti w/sauce and meat, homemade	38	2.17	1.37	4.46	14.20	0.423	0.029	0.034	0.314	10.2
Spaghetti sauce, homemade	23	0.77	1.25	2.95	6.70	0.380	0.026	0.017	0.343	0
Spaghetti sauce, canned	31	0.52	1.35	4.52	7.97	0.184	0.016	0.017	0.343	0
Spaghetti meat sauce	30	1.03	1.30	3.72	4.95	0.385	0.028	0.022	0.193	2.3
Spaghetti sauce, dry, packet	79	1.70	0.28	18.20	48.20	0.765	NA	0.162	0.057	0
Spaghetti sauce w/ mushrooms, packet	85	2.84	2.55	13.90	113.00	0.510	NA	0.136	0.085	0
Egg noodles, cooked	35	1.17	0.35	6.60	3.19	0.400	0.039	0.023	0.624	8.9
Chow mein noodles, dry	139	3.72	6.93	16.40	8.82	0.252	0.032	0.019	1.100	3.2
Spinach noodles, dry	108	3.97	1.08	20.20	11.60	1.290	0.278	0.133	1.930	0
Spinach noodles, cooked	32	1.13	0.36	5.97	3.37	0.429	0.043	0.027	0.569	0
Chicken and noodles, recipe	43	2.60	2.13	3.07	3.07	0.278	0.006	0.020	0.142	12.2
Chicken and noodles, frozen	32	2.17	1.30	2.49	15.70	0.393	0.009	0.018	0.022	8.0
Noodles, ramen—beef, cooked	28	0.76	0.94	4.17	NA	NA	NA	NA	0.500	NA
Noodles, ramen, chicken, cooked	25	0.76	0.85	3.63	NA	NA	NA	NA	0.512	NA
Noodles, ramen, oriental	26	0.74	1.07	3.83	NA	NA	NA	NA	0.512	NA
Lasagna, frozen entree	38	2.32	1.71	2.61	34.00	0.343	0.026	0.045	0.194	12.4
Pizza										
Pizza—cheese	69	3.54	2.13	9.21	52.00	0.378	0.080	0.069	0.510	13.2
Pizza—mozzarella	80	7.60	4.67	0.89	207.00	0.076	0.006	0.097	0	15.0
Pizza—Canadian bacon	52	6.82	2.36	0.38	3.00	0.229	0.231	0.055	0	16.3
Pizza—pepperoni	140	5.94	12.50	0.81	2.80	0.397	0.090	0.070	0	9.8
Pizza—onion	10	0.34	0.07	2.07	7.10	1.105	0.017	0.003	0.450	0
Popcorn										
Popcorn—plain, air popped	106	3.50	1.42	21.30	3.50	0.709	0.106	0.035	4.600	0
Popcorn—cooked in oil/salted	142	2.32	7.99	15.50	7.70	0.696	0.026	0.052	3.090	0
Popcorn—syrup-coated	109	1.60	0.81	24.30	1.60	0.405	0.106	0.016	0.810	0
Rice										
Brown—dry	102	2.13	0.54	21.90	9.04	0.510	0.096	0.014	0.965	0
Brown—cooked	34	0.709	0.17	7.23	3.40	0.170	0.026	0.006	0.483	0
White—regular, dry	103	1.90	0.11	22.80	6.74	0.828	0.125	0.009	0.340	0
White—regular, cooked	31	0.567	0.03	6.86	2.84	0.397	0.03	0.003	0.102	0
White—converted, dry	105	2.10	0.15	23.00	17.00	0.828	0.124	0.010	0.624	0
White—converted, cooked	30	0.599	0.02	6.60	5.35	0.227	0.03	0.003	0.180	0

➤ **VARIETY—*continued***

	KCAL	PROTEIN (G)	FAT (G)	CHO (G)	CA (MG)	FE (MG)	B_1 (MG)	B_2 (MG)	FIBER (G)	CHOLESTEROL (MG)
Rice—*continued*										
White—instant, dry	106	2.13	0.06	23.40	1.42	1.300	0.125	0.008	0.737	0
White—instant, prepared	31	0.624	0.03	6.86	0.85	0.227	0.037	0.003	0.216	0
Wild—cooked	26	1.02	0.06	5.39	1.42	0.312	0.031	0.045	0.709	0
Rice bran	78	3.77	5.44	14.40	21.50	5.500	0.64	0.070	6.150	0
Rice polish	75	3.43	3.62	16.40	19.40	4.560	0.521	0.051	0.680	0
Salad dressings										
Blue cheese salad dressing	143	1.37	14.80	2.09	22.90	0.057	0.003	0.028	0.020	7.6
Caesar's salad dressing	126	2.66	12.70	0.67	44.40	0.239	0.007	0.025	0.050	33.9
French dressing	150	0.16	16.00	1.81	3.55	0.113	0	0	0.220	0
Italian dressing—low-calorie	15	0.02	1.18	1.37	0.59	0.059	0	0	0.080	1.7
Mayonnaise	203	0.31	22.60	0.77	5.67	0.168	0.005	0.012	0	16.8
Imitation mayonnaise	66	0	5.67	3.78	0	0	0	0	0	7.6
Ranch salad dressing	104	0.86	10.70	1.31	28.40	0.075	0.010	0.040	0	11.1
Russian salad dressing	140	0.45	14.50	3.00	5.44	0.174	0.014	0.014	0.080	18.4
Thousand Island dressing	107	0.26	10.10	4.30	3.52	0.170	0.006	0.009	0.060	7.3
Thousand Island dressing—low-calorie	45	0.22	3.00	4.58	3.12	1.174	0.006	0.008	0.340	3.4
Vinegar and oil dressing	124	0	14.20	0	0	0	0	0	0	0
Salads, prepared										
Chicken salad w/celery	97	3.82	8.90	0.47	5.92	0.239	0.012	0.028	0.110	17.3
Coleslaw	20	0.36	0.74	3.52	12.80	0.166	0.019	0.017	0.570	2.3
Egg salad	68	2.91	6.01	0.45	14.50	0.525	0.019	0.070	0	97.4
Ham salad spread	62	2.46	4.39	3.01	2.24	0.168	0.123	0.034	0.030	10.4
Macaroni salad—no cheese	75	0.54	6.66	3.52	5.50	0.229	0.020	0.014	0.270	4.9
Potato salad w/mayo and eggs	41	0.76	2.32	3.16	5.44	0.185	0.022	0.017	0.420	19.3
Tuna salad	53	4.55	2.53	2.67	4.84	0.282	0.009	0.019	0.340	3.7
Waldorf salad	85	0.72	8.33	2.62	8.82	0.196	0.020	0.013	0.720	4.3
Sandwiches										
Avocado and cheese—white	64	2.02	4.00	5.39	43.1	0.418	0.057	0.059	0.98	4.4
Avocado and cheese—whole wheat	62	2.14	3.97	5.24	37.8	0.477	0.047	0.05	1.76	4.3
BLT—whole wheat	68	2.49	3.77	6.45	11.4	0.570	0.077	0.043	1.55	4.1
BLT—white	70	2.30	3.77	6.70	18.2	0.489	0.092	0.055	0.43	4.2
Grilled cheese—wheat	91	4.22	5.37	7.10	87.4	0.565	0.057	0.076	1.59	11.8
Grilled cheese—part whole wheat	95	4.39	5.82	6.59	103.0	0.526	0.067	0.093	0.61	13.3
Grilled cheese—white	97	4.22	5.79	6.88	103.0	0.441	0.068	0.092	0.30	13.3
Chicken salad—wheat	80	3.00	4.25	8.13	14.7	0.679	0.066	0.046	1.88	6.2
Chicken salad—white	85	2.83	4.63	8.05	22.7	0.552	0.080	0.060	0.39	7.1
Corn dog	84	2.55	5.10	6.97	8.7	0.495	0.072	0.043	0.03	9.5
Corned beef and swiss on rye	83	5.26	4.59	4.90	63.8	0.768	0.044	0.078	0.97	16.4
English muffin (egg/cheese/bacon)	74	3.70	3.70	6.37	40.5	0.637	0.095	0.103	0.32	43.8
Egg salad—wheat	79	2.60	4.56	7.44	17.0	0.744	0.063	0.059	1.67	48.8
Egg salad—soft white	83	2.41	4.90	7.25	24.5	0.636	0.075	0.074	0.30	41.6
Ham—rye	59	3.84	2.09	6.10	12.0	0.474	0.182	0.073	1.24	7.1
Ham—whole wheat	59	3.79	2.04	6.84	12.4	0.617	0.164	0.060	1.54	6.1
Ham—soft white	61	3.74	2.08	6.60	18.6	0.504	0.186	0.073	0.29	6.7
Ham and swiss—rye	68	4.65	3.23	5.08	63.5	0.389	0.147	0.079	0.99	10.8
Ham and cheese—wheat	67	4.20	3.23	5.72	40.5	0.527	0.136	0.066	1.27	9.7
Ham and cheese—soft white	69	4.20	3.36	5.43	48.0	0.428	0.152	0.078	0.23	10.6
Ham salad—wheat	75	2.45	4.02	7.83	11.5	0.569	0.104	0.045	1.52	5.6

➤ VARIETY—*continued*

	KCAL	PROTEIN (G)	FAT (G)	CHO (G)	CA (MG)	FE (MG)	B_1 (MG)	B_2 (MG)	FIBER (G)	CHOLESTEROL (MG)
Sandwiches—*continued*										
Ham salad—white	78	2.25	4.26	7.71	17.5	0.454	0.119	0.057	0.28	6.2
Hotdog/frankfurter and bun	87	2.80	5.10	7.04	19.6	0.570	0.095	0.062	0.40	7.6
Patty melt—ground beef/rye	91	5.09	6.07	3.96	36.5	0.533	0.040	0.072	0.81	17.1
Peanut butter and jam—whole wheat	92	3.40	3.85	12.30	15.4	0.751	0.070	0.045	2.29	0
Peanut butter and jam—white	98	3.29	4.14	12.80	23.4	0.632	0.085	0.059	0.85	0
Reuben—grilled	58	3.43	3.38	3.53	43.6	0.633	0.030	0.052	0.80	10.4
Roast beef—whole wheat	64	4.00	2.52	6.71	12.3	0.760	0.061	0.054	1.53	6.2
Roast beef—white	67	3.97	2.63	6.46	18.5	0.665	0.072	0.066	0.27	6.9
Tuna salad—wheat	72	3.29	3.29	8.03	13.0	0.667	0.057	0.040	1.74	5.5
Tuna salad—white	76	3.18	3.47	7.92	19.6	0.555	0.068	0.052	0.44	6.2
Turkey—whole wheat	62	4.09	2.33	6.67	11.6	0.554	0.056	0.044	1.53	6.0
Turkey—white	64	4.07	2.42	6.41	17.8	0.435	0.066	0.055	0.27	6.7
Turkey and ham—rye	58	3.74	2.12	6.18	12.3	0.743	0.060	0.079	1.23	8.4
Turkey and ham—whole wheat	59	3.71	2.07	6.90	12.6	0.846	0.060	0.064	1.54	7.2
Turkey and ham—white	60	3.65	2.10	6.67	18.8	0.762	0.071	0.078	0.28	8.0
Turkey and ham w/ cheese—rye	68	4.22	3.46	5.04	44.2	0.616	0.050	0.083	0.99	12.1
Turkey and ham w/ cheese—wheat	67	4.14	3.25	5.77	40.5	0.716	0.051	0.070	1.27	10.6
Turkey and ham w/ cheese—white	69	4.13	3.38	5.48	48.3	0.636	0.059	0.082	0.23	11.6
Sauces										
Bordelaise sauce	24	0.33	1.46	1.10	3.80	0.179	0.008	0.010	0.01	3.8
Hot chili sauce, red pepper	5	0.25	0.17	1.10	2.51	0.137	0.003	0.026	2.29	0
Teriyaki sauce	24	1.69	0.09	4.52	6.30	0.488	0.008	0.020	0	0
Seafood										
Anchovy—raw	37	5.78	1.37	0	41.7	0.921	0.016	0.073	0	19.6
Frog legs—raw meat	21	4.65	0.085	0	5.1	0.539	0.040	0.070	0	14.2
Lobster meat—cooked	28	5.80	0.17	0.36	17.2	0.111	0.020	0.019	0	20.3
Scampi—fried in crumbs	69	6.07	3.49	3.26	19.0	0.357	0.037	0.039	0.04	50.2
Shrimp—boiled	28	5.93	0.31	0	11.0	0.876	0.009	0.009	0	55.3
Squid (calamari)—fried in flour	50	5.10	2.12	2.20	11.0	0.287	0.016	0.130	0	73.7
Soups										
Cream of celery	20	0.38	1.27	2.00	9.04	0.141	0.007	0.011	0.09	3.2
Chicken, chunky	20	1.43	0.75	1.95	2.71	0.195	0.010	0.020	0.03	3.4
Chicken and dumpling	23	1.30	1.28	1.39	3.34	0.144	0.004	0.017	0.10	7.6
Chicken gumbo	13	0.60	0.32	1.89	5.53	0.201	0.006	0.009	0.05	0.9
Chicken-noodle—chunky	14	1.50	0.70	0.24	2.84	0.170	0.009	0.020	0.09	2.1
Chili with beans	32	1.62	1.56	3.38	13.20	0.973	0.014	0.030	0.91	4.8
Clam chowder—New England	19	1.08	0.75	1.90	21.40	0.169	0.008	0.027	0.11	2.5
Minestrone—chunky	15	0.60	0.33	2.45	7.20	0.209	0.006	0.014	0.12	0.6
Cream of mushroom	29	0.46	2.15	2.10	7.23	0.119	0.007	0.019	0.06	0.4
Mushroom—barley	14	0.43	0.51	1.69	2.82	0.113	0.006	0.020	0.17	0
Onion—canned	13	0.87	0.40	1.89	6.10	0.156	0.008	0.006	0.11	0
Oyster stew	14	0.49	0.89	0.94	4.96	0.227	0.005	0.008	0	3.1
Pea—prepared w/milk	27	1.40	0.79	3.59	19.30	0.224	0.017	0.030	0.07	2.0
Cream of potato	17	0.39	0.53	2.59	4.52	0.107	0.008	0.008	0.10	1.5
Split pea and ham	22	1.31	0.47	3.17	3.90	0.253	0.014	0.011	0.19	0.8
Tomato—canned	19	0.47	0.43	3.75	3.05	0.396	0.020	0.011	0.11	0
Tomato-beef-noodle	32	1.00	0.97	4.78	3.95	0.252	0.019	0.020	0.03	0.9

➤ VARIETY—*continued*

	KCAL	PROTEIN (G)	FAT (G)	CHO (G)	CA (MG)	FE (MG)	B_1 (MG)	B_2 (MG)	FIBER (G)	CHOLESTEROL (MG)
Soups—continued										
Tomato bisque prepared w/milk	22	0.71	0.75	3.32	21.00	0.099	0.013	0.030	0.01`	2.5
Turkey—chunky	16	1.23	0.53	1.69	6.00	0.229	0.010	0.029	0.12	1.1
Turkey noodle	16	0.88	0.45	1.95	2.60	0.212	0.017	0.014	0.03	1.1
Cream vegetable—dry mix	126	2.27	6.84	14.80	1.42	0.539	1.470	0.127	0.22	1.2
Vegetable	16	0.49	0.45	2.77	4.96	0.249	0.012	0.010	0.37	0
Miscellanous										
Garlic cloves	42	1.80	0.14	9.38	51.30	0.482	0.057	0.030	0.47	0
Gelatin salad/dessert	17	0.43	0	3.99	0.50	0.024	0.002	0.002	0.02	0
Quiche Lorraine	97	2.09	7.73	4.67	34.00	0.226	0.018	0.052	0.09	45.9
Spinach souffle	45	2.29	3.84	0.59	47.90	0.279	0.019	0.064	0.79	38.4

➤ PART 2 • Nutritive Values for Alcoholic and Nonalcoholic Beverages

The nutritive values for alcoholic and nonalcoholic beverages are expressed in 1-ounce (28.4-g) portions. We have also included the nutritive values for the minerals calcium, iron, magnesium, phosphorus, and potassium and the vitamins thiamine, riboflavin, niacin, and cobalamin. Alcoholic beverages contain no cholesterol or fat.

➤ ALCOHOLIC BEVERAGES (1 OUNCE)

				MINERALS					VITAMINS			
	KCAL	PROTEIN (G)	CHO (G)	CA (MG)	FE (MG)	MG (MG)	P (MG)	K (MG)	B_1 (MG)	B_2 (MG)	NIACIN (MG)	B_{12} (MG)
Beer, regular	12	0.072	1.1	1.4	0.009	1.83	3.50	7.09	0.002	0.007	0.128	0.005
Beer, light	8	0.057	0.4	1.4	0.011	1.42	3.44	5.13	0.003	0.008	0.111	0.002
Brandy	69	0	10.6	2.5	0.012		1.01	1.01	0.002	0.002	0.004	0
Champagne	22	0.043	0.6	1.6	0.093	2.40	1.90	22.60	0	0.003	0.019	0
Dessert wine, dry	36	0.057	1.2	2.3	0.068	2.55	2.55	26.20	0.005	0.005	0.060	0
Dessert wine, sweet	44	0.057	3.3	2.3	0.057	2.55	2.64	26.20	0.005	0.005	0.060	0
Gin, rum, vodka, scotch, whiskey—80 proof	64	0	0	0	0.010	0	0	1.01	0	0	0	0
Gin, rum, vodka, scotch, whiskey—86 proof	71	0	0	0	0.012	0	1.16	0.55	0.002	0.002	0.004	0
Gin, rum, vodka, scotch, whiskey—90 proof	74	0	0	0	0.010	0	0	0.86	0	0	0	0
Sherry, dry	28	0.024	0.3	2.1	0.052	1.96	2.60	17.80	0.002	0.002	0.024	0
Sherry, medium	40	0.066	2.3	2.3	0.071	2.27	1.89	23.60	0.002	0.008	0.035	0
Vermouth, dry	34	0.028	1.6	2.0	0.096	1.42	1.89	11.30	NA	NA	0.011	0
Vermouth, sweet	44	0.014	4.5	1.7	0.099	1.13	1.65	8.50	NA	NA	0.011	0
Wine, dry white	19	0.029	0.2	2.6	0.093	2.62	1.67	17.40	0	0.001	0.019	0
Wine, medium white	19	0.028	0.2	2.5	0.085	3.03	3.84	22.60	0.001	0.001	0.019	0
Wine, red	20	0.055	0.5	2.2	0.122	3.60	3.84	31.50	0.001	0.008	0.023	0.004
Wine, rosé	20	0.055	0.4	2.4	0.108	2.74	4.08	28.10	0.001	0.004	0.020	0.002
Creme de menthe	105	0	11.8	0	0.023	0	0	0	0	0	0.001	0
Bloody Mary	22	0.153	0.9	1.9	0.105	2.10	4.02	41.40	0.010	0.006	0.123	0
Bourbon and soda	26	0	0	1.0	0.244	0.24	0.48	0.48	0	0	0.005	0
Daiquiri	52	0	1.9	0.9	0.043	0.47	1.89	6.14	0.004	0.	0.012	0
Manhattan	64	0	0.9	0.5	0.025	0.01	1.99	7.46	0.003	0.001	0.026	0
Martini	63	0	0.1	0.4	0.024	0.40	0.81	5.26	0	0	0.004	0
Piña colada	53	0.120	8.0	2.2	0.062		2.01	20.10	0.008	0.004	0.033	0
Screwdriver	23	0.160	2.5	2.1	0.023	2.26	3.86	43.30	0.018	0.004	0.046	0
Tequila	31	0.099	2.4	1.7	0.077	1.98	2.80	29.30	0.010	0.005	0.054	0
Tom Collins	16	0.013	0.4	1.3	NA	0.38	0.12	2.30	0	0	0.004	0
Whiskey sour	42	0	3.7	0.3	0.021	0.26	1.60	5.08	0.003	0.002	0.006	0
Coffee and cream liqueur	93	0.784	5.9	4.2	0.036	0.60	13.90	9.05	0	0.016	0.022	0
Coffee liqueur	95	0	13.3	0.5	0.016	0.54	1.64	8.18	0.001	0.003	0.040	0

➤ NONALCOHOLIC BEVERAGES (1 OUNCE)

				Minerals					Vitamins			
	Kcal	Protein (g)	CHO (g)	Ca (mg)	Fe (mg)	Mg (mg)	P (mg)	K (mg)	B_1 (mg)	B_2 (mg)	Niacin (mg)	B_{12} (mg)
Hot cocoa with whole milk	25	1.030	2.9	33.8	0.088	6.350	30.60	54.400	0.012	0.049	0.041	0.099
Cocoa mix + water—diet	7	0.561	1.3	13.3	0.110	4.870	19.80	59.800	0.006	0.030	0.024	0
Coffee—brewed	0.2	0.016	0.1	0.5	0.113	1.590	0.32	15.400	0	0.002	0.063	0
Coffee—instant dry powder	1.4	0.016	0.3	0.8	0.019	1.100	2.05	67.70	0	0	0.061	0
Coffee—cappuccino	9.2	0.059	1.6	1.0	0.022	1.330	3.84	17.600	0	0	0.048	0
Coffee—Swiss mocha	7.7	0.078	1.3	1.1	0.036	1.360	4.37	17.900	0	0	0.039	0
Coffee whitener—												
nondairy,	38.5	0.284	3.2	2.6	0.009	0.060	18.20	54.1	0	0	0	0
liquid powder	155	1.360	15.6	6.3	0.326	1.200	120.00	230.0	0	0.047	0	0
Cola beverage, regular	12	0	3.0	0.7	0.009	0.230	3.52	0.306	0	0	0	0
Diet cola—w/aspartame	0	0	0	1.0	0.009	0.319	2.40	0	0.001	0.007	0	0
Club soda	0	0	0	1.4	0.012	0.319	0	0.479	0	0	0	0
Cream soda	15	0	3.8	1.5	0.015	0.229	0	0.306	0	0	0	0
Diet soda—avg. assorted	0	0	0.0	1.1	0.011	0.200	3.03	0.559	0	0	0	0
Egg nog—commercial	38	1.080	3.8	36.8	0.057	5.250	31.00	46.900	0.010	0.054	0.030	0.127
Five Alive citrus	13	0.135	3.1	1.7	0.021	1.950	2.70	34.000	0.015	0.003	0.060	0
Fruit-flavored soda pop	13	0	3.2	1.1	0.020	0.305	0.15	1.520	0	0	0.002	0
Fruit punch drink—canned	13	0.015	3.4	2.1	0.058	0.610	0.31	7.160	0.006	0.006	0.006	0
Gatorade	5	0	1.3	2.8	NA	NA	0	2.840	NA	NA	NA	0
Ginger ale	10	0.008	2.5	0.9	0.051	0.232	0.08	0.387	0	0	0	0
Grape soda, carbonated	12	0	3.2	0.9	0.024	0.305	0	0.229	0	0	0	0
Kool-Aid w/ NutraSweet	0	0	0	0	0	0.028	0	0	0	0	0	0
Kool-Aid w/sugar added	12	0	3.0	0	0	0	0	0	0	0	0	0
Lemon-lime soda	12	0	3.0	0.7	0.019	0.154	0.08	0.308	0	0	0.004	0
Lemonade drink from dry	11	0	2.9	7.6	0.016	0.322	3.65	3.540	0	0	0.004	0
Lemonade frozen conc	51	0.078	13.3	1.9	0.205	1.420	2.46	19.200	0.007	0.027	0.020	0
Limeade frozen conc	53	0.052	14.0	1.4	0.029	7.800	1.69	16.800	0.003	0.003	0.028	0
Chocolate milkshake	36	0.962	5.8	32.0	0.088	4.700	28.90	56.800	0.016	0.069	0.046	0.097
Strawberry milkshake	32	0.952	5.4	32.0	0.030	3.600	28.40	51.700	0.013	0.055	0.050	0.088
Vanilla milkshake	32	0.982	5.1	34.5	0.026	3.500	29.00	49.300	0.013	0.052	0.052	0.101
Orange drink/carbonated	14	0	3.5	1.5	0.018	0.305	0.31	0.686	0	0	0	0
Pepper-type soda	12	0	2.9	0.9	0.010	0.077	3.16	0.154	0	0	0	0
Root beer	12	0.008	3.0	1.5	0.014	0.306	0.15	0.230	0	0	0	0
Pineapple-grapefruit drink	13	0.068	3.3	2.0	0.087	1.700	1.59	17.500	0.009	0.005	0.076	0
Pineapple-orange drink	14	0.352	3.3	1.5	0.076	1.590	1.13	13.200	0.009	0.005	0.059	0
Tang orange juice crystals	13	0.170	0.06	3.1	4.57	0.002	0.02	0.008	0	0	0	0
Tonic water/Quinine water	10	0	2.5	0.4	0.019	0.077	0	0.077	0	0	0	0
Tea—brewed	0	0.001	0.1	0	0.006	0.796	0.16	10.500	0	0.004	0.012	0
Herbal tea—brewed	0	0	0	0.6	0.022	0.319	0	2.390	0.003	0.001	0	0
Perrier water	0	0	0	3.8	0	0.148	0	0	0	0	0	0
Poland Springs bottled water	0	0	0	0.4	0.001	0.239	0	0	0	0	0	0

Note: Alcoholic beverages contain no fat or cholesterol; light beer contains 0.5 g fiber, and regular beer contains 1.2 g fiber per 8 oz serving. All of the other nonmixed alcoholic beverages have no fiber.

Note: Other nonalcoholic beverages are listed in the sections on fruits and vegetables.

PART 3 • Nutritive Values for Specialty and Fast-Food Items

Nutrient information was kindly provided by the manufacturer or its representative and is reproduced as presented in their literature. Unlike Parts 1 and 2, nutritive values are not given for 1-ounce portions but for the actual amounts of the foods as sold commercially. To make a direct comparison of the kcal values and the various nutrients, we recommend that the weight of the food and its nutrients be expressed relative to 1-ounce (28.4-g) portions.

ARBY'S

Food Item	Serving Size (g)	kcal	Protein (g)	Fat (g)	CHO (g)
Bacon Cheddar Deluxe	225	561	28	34	78
Baked Potato Plain	312	291	8	1	0
Beef 'n Cheddar	190	490	24	21	51
Chicken Breast Sandwich	210	592	28	27	57
Chocolate Shake	300	384	9	11	32
French Fries	71	211	2	8	6
Hot Ham 'n Cheese Sandwich	161	353	26	13	50
Jamocha Shake	305	424	8	10	31
Junior Roast Beef	86	218	12	8	22
King Roast Beef	192	467	27	19	49
Potato Cakes	85	201	2	14	13
Regular Roast Beef	147	353	22	15	32
Super Roast Beef	234	501	25	22	40
Superstuffed Potato Broccoli and Cheddar	340	541	13	22	24
Superstuffed Potato Deluxe	312	648	18	38	72
Superstuffed Potato Mushroom and Cheese	300	506	16	22	21
Superstuffed Potato Taco	425	619	23	27	145
Turkey Deluxe	197	375	24	17	39
Vanilla Shake	250	295	8	10	30

Source: Arby's Inc. Nutritional information provided by Consumer Affairs, Arby's Inc., Atlanta, GA, 1986.

BURGER KING

Food Item	Serving Size (g)	kcal	Protein (g)	Total Carbohydrate (g)	Total Fat (g)	Cholesterol (mg)	Sodium (mg)	Dietary Fiber (g)	Percentage of U.S. RDA* Vit A	Vit C	Ca	Fe
Burgers												
Whopper sandwich	270	640	27	45	39	90	870	3	10	15	8	25
Whopper with cheese sandwich	294	730	33	46	46	115	1300	3	15	15	25	25
Double Whopper sandwich	351	870	46	45	56	170	940	3	10	15	8	40
Double Whopper with cheese sandwich	375	960	52	46	63	195	1360	3	15	15	25	40
Whopper Jr. sandwich	168	420	21	29	24	60	570	2	4	8	6	20

➤ BURGER KING—*continued*

Food Item	Serving Size (g)	kcal	Protein (g)	Total Carbohydrate (g)	Total Fat (g)	Cholesterol (mg)	Sodium (mg)	Dietary Fiber (g)	Percentage of U.S. RDA* Vit A	Vit C	Ca	Fe
Burgers—*continued*												
Whopper Jr. with cheese sandwich	180	460	23	29	28	75	780	2	8	8	15	20
Hamburger	129	330	20	28	15	55	570	1	2	0	4	15
Cheeseburger	142	380	23	28	19	65	780	1	6	0	15	15
Double cheeseburger	213	600	41	29	36	135	1040	1	8	0	20	25
Double cheeseburger with bacon	221	640	44	29	39	145	1220	1	8	0	20	25
Sandwiches/Side Orders												
BK Big Fish sandwich	255	720	25	59	43	60	1090	2	2	2	6	20
BK Broiler Chicken sandwich	248	540	30	41	29	80	480	2	4	10	4	30
Chicken sandwich	229	700	26	54	43	60	1400	2	°	°	10	20
Chicken Tenders (6 piece)	88	250	16	14	12	35	530	2	°	°	°	4
Broiled Chicken salad†	302	200	21	7	10	60	110	3	100	25	15	20
Garden salad†	215	90	6	7	5	15	110	3	110	50	15	6
Side salad†	133	50	3	4	3	5	55	2	50	20	6	2
French fries (medium, salted)	116	400	5	43	20	0	240	3	°	4	°	6
Onion rings	124	310	4	41	14	0	810	5	°	°	°	°
Dutch apple pie	113	310	3	39	15	0	230	2	°	10	°	8
Drinks												
Vanilla shake (medium)	284	310	9	53	7	20	230	1	6	6	30	°
Chocolate shake (medium)	284	310	9	54	7	20	230	3	6	°	20	10
Chocolate shake (medium, syrup added)	341	460	11	87	7	20	300	1	6	6	30	°
Strawberry shake (medium, syrup added)	341	430	9	83	7	20	260	1	6	6	30	°
Coca-Cola Classic (medium)	22 (fl oz)	260	0	70	0	0	@	0	°	°	°	°
Diet Coke (medium)	22 (fl oz)	1	0	<1	0	0	@	0	°	°	°	°
Sprite (medium)	22 (fl oz)	260	0	66	0	0	@	0	°	°	°	°
Tropicana orange juice	311	140	2	33	0	0	0	0	0	100	0	0
Coffee	355	5	0	1	0	0	5	0	°	°	°	°
Milk—2% low fat	244	120	8	12	5	20	120	0	10	4	30	°
Breakfast												
Croissan'wich with bacon, egg and cheese	118	350	15	18	24	225	790	<1	8	°	15	10
Croissan'wich with sausage, egg and cheese	159	530	20	21	41	255	1000	<1	8	°	15	15

➤ BURGER KING—*continued*

Food Item	Serving Size (g)	kcal	Protein (g)	Total Carbohydrate (g)	Total Fat (g)	Cholesterol (mg)	Sodium (mg)	Dietary Fiber (g)	Percentage of U.S. RDA* Vit A	Vit C	Ca	Fe
Breakfast, *continued*												
Croissan'wich with ham, egg and cheese	144	350	18	19	22	230	1390	<1	8	°	15	10
French toast sticks	141	500	4	60	27	0	490	1	°	°	6	15
Hash browns	71	220	2	25	12	0	320	2	10	8	°	2
A.M. Express grape jam	12	30	0	7	0	0	0	0	0	0	0	0
A.M. Express strawberry jam	12	30	0	8	0	0	5	0	0	0	0	0
Condiments/ Toppings												
Processed American cheese	25	90	6	0	8	25	420	0	6	°	15	°
Lettuce	21	0	0	0	0	0	0	0	°	°	°	°
Tomato	28	5	0	1	0	0	0	0	2	8	°	°
Onion	14	5	0	1	0	0	0	0	°	°	°	°
Pickles	14	0	0	0	0	0	140	0	0	0	0	0
Ketchup	14	15	0	4	0	0	180	0	4	°	°	°
Mustard	3	0	0	0	0	0	40	0	0	0	0	0
Mayonnaise	28	210	0	<1	23	20	160	0	°	°	°	°
Tartar sauce	28	180	0	0	19	15	220	0	°	°	°	°
Land O' Lakes whipped classic blend	10	65	0	0	7	0	75	0	8	°	°	°
Bull's Eye barbecue sauce	14	20	0	5	0	0	140	0	°	°	°	2
Bacon bits	3	15	1	0	1	5	0	0	°	°	°	°
Croutons	7	30	<1	4	1	0	75	0	°	°	°	°
Burger King Salad Dressings												
Thousand Island dressing	30	140	0	7	12	15	190	<1	30	°	°	°
French dressing	30	140	0	11	10	0	190	0	15	°	°	°
Ranch dressing	30	180	<1	2	19	10	170	<1	°	°	°	°
Bleu cheese dressing	30	160	2	1	16	30	260	<1	°	°	°	°
Reduced calorie light Italian dressing#	30	15	0	3	0.5	0	50	0	°	°	°	°
Dipping Sauces												
A.M. Express dip	28	80	0	21	0	0	20	0	°	°	°	°
Honey dipping sauce	28	90	0	23	0	0	10	0	°	°	°	°
Ranch dipping sauce	28	170	0	2	17	0	200	0	°	°	°	°
Barbecue dipping sauce	28	35	0	9	0	0	400	0	2	2	°	°
Sweet & sour dipping sauce	28	45	0	11	0	0	50	0	°	°	°	°

Source: Burger King Corporation, Miami, FL, 1996. For additional information, call 1-800-937-1800.
† = Without dressing @ = Depends on the water supply ° = Less than 2% of the U.S. RDA
★ = Values for vitamins A and C and minerals calcium and iron represent percent daily values based on a 2000 kcal diet # = Regular Italian dressing—150 kcal—16 g. fat.
— = Negligible.

➤ DAIRY QUEEN

Food Item	Serving Size (g)	Description	kcal	Protein (g)	Fat (g)	CHO (g)	Ca (mg)	Fe (mg)	Vitamin A (IU)	Vitamin C (mg)	Vitamin B_1 (mg)	Vitamin B_2 (mg)
Banana Split	383		540	9	11	103	—	—	—	—	—	—
Big Brazier	213	deluxe	470	28	24	36	111	5.2	—	<2.5	0.34	0.37
Big Brazier	184	regular	184	27	23	37	113	5.2	—	<2.0	0.37	0.39
Big Brazier	213	w/cheese	553	32	30	38	268	5.2	495	<2.3	0.34	0.53
Blizzard Banana Split	—	regular	763	—	—	—	—	—	—	—	—	—
Blizzard Banana Split	—	large	1333	—	—	—	—	—	—	—	—	—
Blizzard chocolate sandwich cookies	—	regular	600	—	—	—	—	—	—	—	—	—
Blizzard chocolate sandwich cookies	—	large	1050	—	—	—	—	—	—	—	—	—
Blizzard German chocolate	—	regular	794	—	—	—	—	—	—	—	—	—
Blizzard German chocolate	—	large	1460	—	—	—	—	—	—	—	—	—
Blizzard, Heath	—	regular	824	—	—	—	—	—	—	—	—	—
Blizzard, Heath	—	large	1212	—	—	—	—	—	—	—	—	—
Blizzard, M&M	—	regular	766	—	—	—	—	—	—	—	—	—
Blizzard, M&M	—	large	1154	—	—	—	—	—	—	—	—	—
Brazier cheese dog	113		330	15	19	24	168	1.6	—	—	—	0.18
Brazier chili dog	128		330	13	20	25	86	2.0	—	11.0	0.15	0.23
Brazier dog	99		273	11	15	23	75	1.5	—	11.0	0.12	0.15
Brazier French fries	71	regular	200	2	10	25	tr	0.4	tr	3.6	0.06	tr
Brazier French fries	113	large	320	3	16	40	tr	0.4	tr	4.8	0.09	0.03
Brazier onion rings	85		300	6	17	33	20	0.4	tr	2.4	0.09	tr
Brazier regular	106		260	13	9	28	70	3.5	—	<1.0	0.28	0.26
Brazier w/cheese	121		318	18	14	30	163	3.5	—	<1.2	0.29	0.29
Buster Bar	149		460	10	29	41	—	—	—	—	—	—
Chicken sandwich	220		670	29	41	46	—	—	—	—	—	—
Cone	213	large	340	9	10	57	—	—	—	—	—	—
Cone	142	regular	240	6	7	38	—	—	—	—	—	—
Cone	85	small	140	3	4	22	—	—	—	—	—	—
Dairy Queen Parfait	284		460	10	11	81	300	1.8	400	tr	0.12	0.43
Dilly Bar	85		240	4	15	22	100	0.4	100	tr	0.06	0.17
Dilly Bar	85		210	3	13	21	—	—	—	—	—	—
Dipped, cone	234	large	510	9	24	64	—	—	—	—	—	—
Dipped, cone	156	regular	340	6	16	42	—	—	—	—	—	—
Dipped, cone	92	small	190	3	9	25	—	—	—	—	—	—
Double Delight	255		490	9	20	69	—	—	—	—	—	—
Double hamburger	210		530	36	28	33	—	—	—	—	—	—
Double w/cheese	239		650	43	37	34	—	—	—	—	—	—
Chocolate dipped cone	234	large	450	10	20	58	300	0.4	400	tr	0.12	0.51
Chocolate dipped cone	156	medium	300	7	13	40	200	0.4	300	tr	0.09	0.34
Chocolate dipped cone	78	small	150	3	7	20	100	tr	100	tr	0.03	0.17

➤ DAIRY QUEEN—*continued*

Food Item	Serving Size (g)	Description	kcal	Protein (g)	Fat (g)	CHO (g)	Ca (mg)	Fe (mg)	Vitamin A (IU)	Vitamin C (mg)	Vitamin B_1 (mg)	Vitamin B_2 (mg)
Chocolate malt	588	large	840	22	28	125	600	5.4	750	6.0	0.15	0.85
Chocolate malt	418	medium	600	15	20	89	500	3.6	750	3.6	0.12	0.60
Chocolate malt	241	small	340	10	11	51	300	1.8	400	2.4	0.06	0.34
Chocolate sundae	248	large	400	9	9	71	300	1.8	400	tr	0.09	0.43
Chocolate sundae	184	medium	300	6	7	53	200	1.1	300	tr	0.06	0.26
Chocolate sundae	106	small	170	4	4	30	100	0.7	100	tr	0.03	0.17
Cone	213	large	340	10	10	52	300	tr	400	tr	0.15	0.43
Cone	142	medium	230	6	7	35	200	tr	300	tr	0.09	0.26
Cone	71	small	110	3	3	18	100	tr	100	tr	0.03	0.14
Float	397		330	6	8	59	200	tr	100	tr	0.12	0.17
Freeze	397		520	11	13	89	300	tr	200	tr	0.15	0.34
Sandwich	60		140	3	4	24	60	0.4	100	tr	0.03	0.14
Fiesta sundae	269		570	9	22	84	200	tr	200	tr	0.23	0.26
Fish sandwich	170		400	20	17	41	60	1.1	tr	tr	0.15	0.26
Fish sandwich w/cheese	177		440	24	21	39	150	0.4	100	tr	0.15	0.26
Float	397		410	5	7	82	—	—	—	—	—	—
Freeze	397		500	9	12	89	—	—	—	—	—	—
French fries	71	regular	200	2	10	25	—	—	—	—	—	—
French fries	113	large	320	3	16	40	—	—	—	—	—	—
Frozen dessert	113		180	4	6	27	—	—	—	—	—	—
Hot dog	100		280	11	16	21	—	—	—	—	—	—
Hot dog w/cheese	114		330	15	21	21	—	—	—	—	—	—
Hot dog w/chili	128		320	13	20	23	—	—	—	—	—	—
Hot Fudge brownie delight	266		600	9	25	85	—	—	—	—	—	—
Malt	588	large	1060	20	25	187	—	—	—	—	—	—
Malt	418	regular	760	14	18	134	—	—	—	—	—	—
Malt	291	small	520	10	13	91	—	—	—	—	—	—
Mr. Misty	439	large	340	0	0	84	—	—	—	—	—	—
Mr. Misty	330	regular	250	0	0	63	—	—	—	—	—	—
Mr. Misty	248	small	190	0	0	48	—	—	—	—	—	—
Mr. Misty float	404		440	6	8	85	200	tr	120	tr	0.12	0.17
Mr. Misty float	411		390	5	7	74	—	—	—	—	—	—
Mr. Misty freeze	411		500	9	12	91	—	—	—	—	—	—
Mr. Misty Kiss	89		70	0	0	17	—	—	—	—	—	—
Onion rings	85		280	4	16	31	—	—	—	—	—	—
Parfait	283		430	8	8	76	—	—	—	—	—	—
Peanut Buster Parfait	305		740	16	34	94	—	—	—	—	—	—
Shake	588	large	990	19	26	168	—	—	—	—	—	—
Shake	418	regular	710	14	19	120	—	—	—	—	—	—
Shake	291	small	490	10	13	82	—	—	—	—	—	—
Single hamburger	148		360	21	16	33	—	—	—	—	—	—
Single w/cheese	162		410	24	20	33	—	—	—	—	—	—
Strawberry shortcake	312		540	10	11	100	—	—	—	—	—	—
Sundae	248	large	440	8	10	78	—	—	—	—	—	—
Sundae	177	regular	310	5	8	56	—	—	—	—	—	—
Sundae	106	small	190	3	4	33	—	—	—	—	—	—
Super Brazier	298		783	53	48	35	282	7.3	—	<3.2	0.39	0.69
Super Brazier chili dog	210		555	23	33	42	158	4.0	—	18.0	0.42	0.48
Super Brazier dog	182		518	20	30	41	158	4.3	tr	14.0	0.42	0.44

➤ DAIRY QUEEN—*continued*

Food Item	Serving Size (g)	Description	kcal	Protein (g)	Fat (g)	CHO (g)	Ca (mg)	Fe (mg)	Vitamin A (IU)	Vitamin C (mg)	Vitamin B_1 (mg)	Vitamin B_2 (mg)
Super Brazier dog w/cheese	203		593	26	36	43	297	4.4	—	14.0	0.43	0.48
Super hot dog	175		520	17	27	44	—	—	—	—	—	—
Super hot dog w/cheese	196		580	22	34	45	—	—	—	—	—	—
Super hot dog w/chili	218		570	21	32	47	—	—	—	—	—	—
Triple hamburger	272		710	51	45	33	—	—	—	—	—	—
Triple w/cheese	301		820	58	50	34	—	—	—	—	—	—

Source: International Dairy Queen, Inc., Minneapolis, MN, 1982. Nutritional information reviewed and edited by Dr. David J. Aulik in cooperation with Raltech Scientific Services.

➤ JACK IN THE BOX

Menu Item	Serving Size (g)	Calories (per serving)	Protein (g)	Fat (g)	Carbohydrates (g)	Percentage of U.S. RDA: Calcium	Iron	Vitamin A	Vitamin C
Sandwiches									
Beef Gyro	260	620	27	32	55	8	30	4	15
Chicken Fajita Pita	189	290	24	8	29	25	15	10	10
Chicken sandwich	160	400	20	18	38	15	10	4	0
Chicken supreme	245	620	25	36	48	20	15	10	4
Country fried steak sandwich	153	450	14	25	42	6	15	2	8
Fish supreme	245	590	22	32	51	20	20	10	8
Grilled chicken fillet	211	430	29	19	36	15	35	6	10
Smoked chicken cheddar & bacon	223	540	30	30	37	30	15	10	15
Sourdough ranch chicken sandwich	225	490	29	21	45	—	10	—	0
Spicy crispy chicken sandwich	224	560	24	27	55	10	15	4	8
Hamburgers									
Hamburger	97	280	13	11	31	10	15	2	2
Cheeseburger	110	330	16	15	32	20	15	6	2
Double cheeseburger	152	450	24	24	35	25	20	10	0
Jumbo Jack	229	560	26	32	41	10	25	4	10
Jumbo Jack with cheese	242	610	29	36	41	20	30	6	10
Bacon bacon cheeseburger	242	710	35	45	41	25	30	8	15
Grilled sourdough burger	223	670	32	43	39	20	25	15	10
Ultimate cheeseburger	280	830	47	57	33	30	35	15	0
¼ lb burger	172	510	26	27	39	15	20	6	0
The Colossus burger	272	940	52	60	48	30	35	10	6
Teriyaki Bowls									
Chicken Teriyaki bowl	440	580	28	1.5	115	10	10	110	15
Beef Teriyaki bowl	440	580	28	3	124	15	25	100	10
Soy sauce	9	5	**	0	**	0	0	0	0
Breakfast									
Breakfast Jack	121	300	18	12	30	20	15	8	15
Pancake platter	231	610	15	22	87	10	10	8	10
Sausage crescent	156	580	22	43	28	15	15	10	0
Scrambled egg platter	213	560	18	32	50	15	25	15	15
Scrambled egg pocket	183	430	29	21	31	20	20	20	0
Sourdough breakfast sandwich	147	380	21	20	31	25	20	15	15
Supreme crescent	153	530	23	33	34	15	20	15	20
Hash browns	57	160	1	11	14	0	2	0	10
Country Crock Spread	5	25	0	3	0	0	2	4	0
Grape jelly	14	40	0	0	9	0	0	0	0
Pancake syrup	42	120	0	0	30	0	0	0	0

➤ JACK IN THE BOX—*continued*

Menu Item	Serving Size (g)	Calories (per serving)	Protein (g)	Fat (g)	Carbohydrates (g)	Percentage of U.S. RDA: Calcium	Iron	Vitamin A	Vitamin C
Salads									
Chef salad	324	320	19	30	9	35	15	90	35
Taco salad	397	470	23	34	30	40	25	30	15
Side salad	111	50	3	7	**	6	0	60	15
Bleu cheese dressing	70	260	22	**	14	0	0	0	0
Buttermilk house dressing	70	360	36	**	8	0	0	0	0
Low calorie Italian dressing	70	25	2	**	2	0	0	0	0
Thousand Island dressing	70	310	30	**	12	0	0	0	0
Mexican Food									
Taco	78	190	11	7	15	10	6	0	0
Super taco	126	280	17	12	22	15	10	0	4
Guacamole	25	50	4	**	3	*	*	2	70
Salsa	28	10	0	0	2	*	*	2	*
Sides and Desserts									
Seasoned curly fries	109	360	5	20	39	2	8	0	8
Small French fries	68	220	3	11	28	0	4	0	30
Regular French fries	109	350	4	17	45	0	6	0	40
Jumbo fries	123	400	5	19	51	0	8	0	45
Onion rings	103	380	5	23	38	2	10	0	4
Sesame breadsticks	16	70	2	2	12	0	0	0	0
Tortilla chips	28	140	2	6	18	0	0	0	0
Hot apple turnover	110	350	3	19	48	0	10	0	15
Cheesecake	99	310	8	18	29	10	2	0	0
Chocolate chip cookie dough cheesecake	102	360	7	18	44	15	6	6	0
Cinnamon Churritos	75	330	3	21	34	2	30	0	0
Finger Foods									
Egg rolls—3 piece	165	440	3	24	54	8	15	0	6
Egg rolls—5 piece	285	750	5	41	92	15	20	0	10
Chicken strips (breaded)—4 piece	112	290	25	13	18	0	4	0	0
Chicken strips (breaded)—6 piece	177	450	39	20	28	0	6	0	0
Chicken Taquitos—5 piece	136	350	19	15	34	15	10	4	2
Chicken Taquitos—8 piece	218	560	30	25	54	20	15	8	4
Barbecue sauce	28	45	1	0	11	0	0	0	0
Buttermilk house sauce	25	130	**	13	3	0	*	0	2
Hot sauce	13	5	**	0	1	0	0	0	0
Sweet & sour sauce	28	40	**	0	11	0	0	0	0
Drinks									
Orange juice	183	80	1	0	20	2	2	8	160
Lowfat milk (2%)	244	120	8	5	12	30	0	10	4
Vanilla milk shake (regular)	304	350	9	7	62	30	0	0	0
Chocolate milk shake (regular)	322	330	11	7	59	35	4	0	0
Strawberry milk shake (regular)	298	330	9	7	60	30	0	0	0
Iced tea (small)	16	0	0	0	0	0	0	0	0
Coffee (small)	8	5	0	0	1	0	0	0	0

Source: Jack In The Box; nutritional information provided by Foodmaker, Inc., San Diego, CA.

➤ KENTUCKY FRIED CHICKEN

Food Item	Serving Size (g)	kcal	Protein (g)	CHO (g)	Fat (g)	Cholesterol (mg)	Vit A (mg)	Vit C (mg)	Thia (mg)	Ribo (mg)	Nia (mg)	Ca (mg)	Fe (mg)
Original Recipe Chicken													
Wing	55	178	12.2	6.0	11.7	64	<100	<1.0	0.03	0.08	3.7	47.9	1.2
Side breast	90	267	18.8	10.8	16.5	77	<100	<1.0	0.06	0.13	6.9	68.0	1.2
Center breast	115	283	27.5	8.8	15.3	93	<100	<1.0	0.09	0.17	11.5	68.0	1.0
Drumstick	57	146	13.1	4.2	8.5	67	<100	<1.0	0.05	0.12	3.2	21.2	1.1
Thigh	104	294	17.9	11.1	19.7	123	104	<1.0	0.08	0.30	5.5	65.1	1.3
Extra Tasty Crispy Chicken													
Wing	65	254	12.4	9.3	18.6	67	<100	<1.0	0.04	0.06	3.3	17.8	0.6
Side breast	110	343	21.7	14.0	22.3	81	<100	<1.0	0.09	0.10	8.5	30.4	0.8
Center breast	135	342	33.0	11.7	19.7	114	<100	<1.0	0.11	0.13	13.1	33.3	0.8
Drumstick	69	204	13.6	6.1	13.9	71	<100	<1.0	0.06	0.12	3.7	12.9	0.7
Thigh	119	406	20.0	14.4	29.8	129	131	<1.0	0.10	0.21	6.5	49.0	1.2
Kentucky Nuggets	16	46	2.8	2.2	2.9	11.9	<100	<1.0	<0.01	0.03	1.00	2.4	0.1
Barbecue sauce	28.3	35	0.3	7.1	0.6	<1.0	<370	<1.0	<0.01	0.01	0.19	6.1	0.2
Sweet 'n sour	28.3	58	0.1	13.0	0.6	<1.0	<100	<1.0	<0.01	0.02	0.04	4.7	0.2
Honey	14.2	49	0.0	12.1	<0.01	<1.0	<100	<1.0	<0.01	0.00	0.04	0.6	0.1
Mustard	28.3	36	0.9	6.1	0.9	<1.0	<100	<1.0	<0.01	0.01	0.16	10.2	0.3
Chicken Littles	47	169	5.7	13.8	10.1	18	<100	<1.0	0.16	0.12	2.2	22.6	1.7
Buttermilk biscuits	65	235	4.5	28.0	11.7	1	<100	<1.0	0.24	0.19	2.6	95.0	1.6
Mashed potatoes w/gravy	98	71	2.4	11.7	1.6	<1	<100	<1.0	<0.01	0.04	1.2	21.8	0.04
French fries	77	244	3.2	31.1	11.9	2	<100	15.7	0.15	0.05	2.0	12.5	0.06
Corn on the cob	143	176	5.1	31.9	3.1	<1	272	2.3	0.14	0.11	1.8	7.2	0.08
Coleslaw	91	119	1.5	13.2	6.6	5	310	21.5	0.03	0.03	0.2	32.8	0.02
Colonel's Chicken sandwich	166	482	20.8	38.6	27.3	47	<100	<1.0	0.38	0.27	11.1	46.1	1.3

Source: Public Affairs Department, KFC Corporation, Louisville, KY.

➤ LONG JOHN SILVER'S

Food Item	Serving Size (g)	Description	kcal	Protein (g)	Fat (g)	CHO (g)
3 Pc. Nugget dinner		6 chicken nuggets, Fryes, slaw	699	23	45	54
Apple pie	113		280	2	11	43
Barbecue sauce	34		45	0	0	11
Battered shrimp dinner		6 battered shrimp, Fryes, slaw	771	17	45	60
Bleu cheese dressing	45		225	4	23	3
Breaded clams			465	13	25	46
Breaded fish sandwich platter		Fish sandwich, Fryes, slaw	835	30	42	84
Breaded oysters		6 pieces	460	14	19	58
Breaded shrimp platter		Breaded shrimp, Fryes, slaw, 2 hush puppies	962	20	57	93
Cherry pie	113		294	3	11	46
Chicken planks		4 pieces	458	27	23	35
Clam chowder	187		128	7	5	15
Clam dinner		Clams, Fryes, slaw	955	22	58	100
Coleslaw			138	1	8	16
Coleslaw, drained on fork	98		182	1	15	11
Combo salad		4.25 oz seafood salad, 2 oz salad shrimp, 6 oz lettuce, 2.4 oz tomato, 1 pkg crackers	397	27	29	21

➤ LONG JOHN SILVER'S—*continued*

Food Item	Serving Size (g)	Description	kcal	Protein (g)	Fat (g)	CHO (g)
Corn on the cob	150	1 ear	176	5	4	29
Fish & Chicken		1 fish, 2 tender chicken planks, Fryes, slaw	935	36	55	73
Fish & Fryes		3 fish, Fryes	853	43	48	64
Fish & Fryes		2 fish, Fryes	651	30	36	53
Fish & More		2 fish, Fryes, slaw, 2 hush puppies	978	34	58	92
Fish w/batter		2 pieces	319	19	19	19
Fish w/batter		3 pieces	477	28	28	28
Four nuggets and Fryes			427	16	24	39
Fryes	85		247	4	12	31
Fryes			275	4	15	32
Honey-Mustard sauce	35		56	—	—	14
Hush Puppies	47	2 pieces	145	3	7	18
Hush Puppies		3 pieces	158	1	7	20
Kitchen–breaded fish (three piece dinner)		3 kitchen breaded fish, Fryes, slaw, 2 hush puppies	940	35	52	84
Kitchen–breaded fish (two piece dinner)		2 kitchen-breaded fish, Fryes, slaw, 2 hush puppies	818	26	46	76
Lemon Meringue pie	99		200	2	6	37
Ocean chef salad		6 oz lettuce, 1.25 oz shrimp, 2 oz seafood blend, 2 tomato wedges, ¾ oz cheese	229	27	8	13
Ocean scallops		6 pieces	257	10	12	27
One fish and Fryes			449	16	24	42
One fish, two nuggets, and Fryes			539	23	30	46
Oyster dinner		6 oysters, Fryes, slaw	789	17	45	78
Pecan pie	113		446	5	22	59
Peg leg w/batter		5 pieces	514	25	33	30
Pumpkin pie	113		251	4	11	34
Reduced calorie Italian dressing	49		20	0	1	3
Scallop dinner		6 scallops, Fryes,	747	17	45	66
Sea salad dressing	45		220	4	21	5
Seafood platter shrimp, 2 scallops, Fryes, slaw		1 fish, 2 battered	976	29	58	85
Seafood salad		5.6 oz seafood salad, 6 oz lettuce, 2.4 oz tomato	426	19	30	22
Shrimp & Fish dinner		1 fish, 3 battered shrimp, Fryes, slaw, 2 hush puppies	917	27	55	80
Shrimp salad shrimp, 6 oz lettuce, 2.4 oz tomato		4.5 oz salad	203	28	3	16
Shrimp w/batter		5 pieces	269	9	13	31
Sweet-n-sour sauce	30		—	—	—	—
Tartar sauce	30		117	—	11	5
Tender chicken plank dinner		3 chicken planks, Fryes, slaw	885	32	51	72

➤ LONG JOHN SILVER'S—*continued*

Food Item	Serving Size (g)	Description	kcal	Protein (g)	Fat (g)	CHO (g)
Tender chicken plank dinner		4 chicken planks, Fryes, slaw	1037	41	59	82
Thousand Island dressing	48		223	—	22	8
Three piece fish dinner		3 fish, Fryes, slaw, 2 hush puppies	1180	47	70	93
Treasure chest		2 pc fish, 2 peg legs	467	25	29	27
Two planks and Fryes			551	22	28	51

Source: Long John Silver's Seafood Shoppes; sampling and nutrient analysis conducted independently by the Department of Nutrition and Food Science, University of Kentucky, April 10, 1986.

➤ McDONALD'S

Menu Item	Serving Size	Calories	Protein (g)	Carbohydrates (g)	Total Fat (g)	Cholesterol (mg)	Sodium (mg)	Dietary Fiber (g)	Percentage of U.S. RDA: Vitamin A	Vitamin C	Calcium	Iron
Sandwiches												
Hamburger	160 g	270	12	34	10	30	520	2	2	4	15	15
Cheeseburger	120 g	320	15	35	14	45	750	2	6	4	15	15
Quarter Pounder	172 g	420	23	37	21	70	690	2	4	4	15	25
Quarter Pounder with cheese	200 g	530	28	38	30	95	1160	2	10	4	15	25
McLean deluxe	214 g	350	24	38	12	60	800	3	8	15	15	25
McLean deluxe with cheese	228 g	400	27	39	17	70	1040	3	10	15	15	25
Big Mac	216 g	530	25	47	28	80	960	3	6	4	20	25
Filet-O-Fish	143 g	360	14	40	16	35	690	2	2	°	10	10
McGrilled chicken Classic	189 g	260	24	33	4	45	500	2	4	8	10	10
McChicken sandwich	190 g	510	17	44	30	50	820	2	2	2	15	15
French Fries												
Small French fries	68 g	210	3	26	10	0	135	2	°	15	°	2
Large French fries	147 g	450	6	57	22	0	290	5	°	30	2	6
Super Size French fries	176 g	540	8	68	26	0	350	6	°	35	2	8
Chicken McNuggets/Sauce												
Chicken McNuggets (4 piece)	73 g	200	12	10	12	40	350	0	°	°	°	4
Chicken McNuggets (6 piece)	109 g	300	19	16	18	65	530	0	°	°	2	6
Chicken McNuggets (9 piece)	165 g	450	28	24	27	95	800	0	°	°	2	8
Hot Mustard (1 pkg)	28 g	60	1	7	3.5	5	240	<1	°	°	°	4
Barbecue sauce (1 pkg)	28 g	45	0	10	0	0	250	0	°	6	°	°
Sweet 'n sour sauce (1 pkg)	28 g	50	0	11	0	0	140	0	6	°	°	°
Honey (1 pkg)	14 g	45	0	12	0	0	0	0	°	°	°	°
Honey mustard (1 pkg)	14 g	50	0	3	4.5	10	85	0	°	°	°	°
Salads												
Chef salad	313 g	210	19	9	11	180	730	2	90	35	16	10
Fajita chicken salad	285 g	160	20	9	6	65	400	3	160	50	4	10
Garden salad	234 g	80	6	7	4	140	60	2	60	35	6	8
Side salad	139 g	45	3	4	2	70	35	1	50	20	4	4
Croutons (1 pkg)	11 g	50	1	7	1.5	0	125	0	°	°	2	2
Bacon bits (1 pkg)	3 g	15	1	0	1	5	90	0	°	°	°	°

➤ **McDONALD'S—*continued***

Menu Item	Serving Size	Calories	Protein (g)	Carbohydrates (g)	Total Fat (g)	Cholesterol (mg)	Sodium (mg)	Dietary Fiber (g)	Percentage of U.S. RDA: Vitamin A	Vitamin C	Calcium	Iron
Salad Dressings												
Bleu cheese (1 pkg)	60 g	190	2	8	17	30	650	0	2	°	6	2
Ranch (1 pkg)	60 g	230	1	10	21	20	550	0	°	2	4	°
1000 Island	63 g	190	1	16	13	25	510	1	2	2	2	2
Lite Vinaigrette (1 pkg)	62 g	50	0	9	2	0	240	0	6	6	°	°
Red French reduced calorie (1 pkg)	68 g	160	0	23	8	0	490	0	4	6	°	°
Breakfast												
Egg McMuffin	137 g	290	17	27	13	235	730	1	10	2	15	15
Sausage McMuffin	112 g	360	13	26	23	45	750	1	4	°	15	10
Sausage McMuffin with Egg	163 g	440	19	27	29	255	820	1	10	°	15	15
English muffin	55 g	140	4	25	2	0	220	1	°	°	10	8
Sausage biscuit	119 g	430	10	32	29	35	1130	1	°	°	8	15
Sausage biscuit with egg	170 g	520	16	33	35	245	1220	1	6	°	10	15
Bacon, egg and cheese biscuit	152 g	450	17	33	27	240	1340	1	10	°	10	15
Biscuit	76 g	260	4	32	13	0	840	1	°	°	6	10
Sausage	43 g	170	6	0	16	35	290	0	°	°	°	2
Scrambled eggs (2)	102 g	170	13	1	12	425	190	0	10	°	6	6
Hash browns	53 g	130	1	14	8	0	330	1	°	4	°	2
Hotcakes (plain)	150 g	310	9	53	7	15	610	2	°	°	10	15
Hotcakes (margarine 2 pats and syrup)	222 g	580	9	100	16	15	760	2	8	°	10	15
Cheerios (1 pkg)	19 g	70	2	15	1	0	180	2	15	15	2	25
Wheaties (1 pkg)	23 g	80	2	18	0.5	0	160	2	15	15	4	30
Muffins/Danish												
Fat free apple bran muffin	70 g	170	4	38	0	0	200	1	°	°	4	6
Apple danish	105 g	360	5	51	16	40	290	1	10	°	8	6
Cheese danish	105 g	410	7	47	22	70	340	0	15	°	8	6
Cinnamon Raisin danish	105 g	430	5	56	22	50	280	1	10	°	10	8
Raspberry danish	105 g	400	5	58	16	45	300	1	10	°	8	6
Desserts/Shakes												
Vanilla lowfat frozen yogurt cone	90 g	120	4	24	0.5	5	85	0	°	2	15	2
Strawberry lowfat frozen yogurt sundae	178 g	240	6	51	1	5	115	1	°	2	20	2
Hot caramel lowfat frozen yogurt sundae	182 g	310	7	63	3	5	200	1	2	2	25	°
Hot fudge sundae	179 g	290	8	54	5	5	190	2	°	2	25	4
Nuts (sundaes)	7 g	40	2	2	3.5	0	0	0	°	°	°	°
Baked apple pie	77 g	260	3	34	13	0	200	<1	°	40	2	6
McDonaldland cookies (1 pkg)	56 g	260	4	41	9	0	270	1	°	°	°	10
Vanilla shake—small	414 mL	340	11	62	5	25	220	0	4	6	40	2
Chocolate shake—small	414 mL	340	12	64	5	25	300	1	4	6	45	4
Strawberry shake—small	414 mL	340	12	63	5	25	220	0	4	10	40	4
Milk/Juices												
1% lowfat milk (8 fl oz)	1 crtn	100	8	13	2.5	10	115	0	10	4	30	°
Orange juice (6 fl oz)	177 mL	80	1	20	0	0	20	0	2	90	2	2
Apple juice (6 fl oz)	177 mL	80	0	20	0	0	0	0	°	°	°	2

Source: McDonald's Corporation, Oak Brook, IL 60521, (708) 575-3663, 1996.

° = less than 2% of the U.S. RDA

➤ PIZZA HUT

Food Item (1 slice)	kcal	Protein (g)	Fat (g)	CHO (g)	Ca (mg)	Fe (mg)	Vitamin A (IU)	Vitamin C (mg)	Vitamin B_1 (mg)	Vitamin B_2 (mg)
Thick 'n' chewy, beef	620	38	20	73	400	7.2	750	<1.2	0.68	0.60
Thick 'n' chewy, cheese	560	34	14	71	500	5.4	1000	<1.2	0.68	0.68
Thick 'n' chewy, pepperoni	560	31	18	68	400	5.4	1250	3.6	0.68	0.68
Thick 'n' chewy, pork	640	36	23	71	400	7.2	750	1.2	0.90	0.77
Thick 'n' chewy, supreme	640	36	22	74	400	7.2	1000	9.0	0.75	0.85
Thick 'n' crispy, beef	490	29	19	51	350	6.3	750	<1.2	0.30	0.60
Thick 'n' crispy, cheese	450	25	15	54	450	4.5	750	<1.2	0.30	0.51
Thick 'n' crispy, pepperoni	430	23	17	45	300	4.5	1000	<1.2	0.30	0.51
Thick 'n' crispy, pork	520	27	23	51	350	6.3	1000	<1.2	0.38	0.68
Thick 'n' crispy, supreme	510	27	21	51	350	7.2	1250	2.4	0.38	0.68

Source: Research 900 and Pizza Hut, Inc., Wichita, KS.

➤ ROY ROGERS

Food Item	Serving Size (g)	kcal	Protein (g)	Fat (g)	CHO (g)
Apple danish	71	249	4.5	11.6	31.6
Bacon cheeseburger	180	581	32.3	39.2	25.0
Biscuit	63	231	4.4	12.1	26.2
Breakfast crescent sandwich	127	401	13.3	27.3	25.3
Breakfast crescent sandwich w/bacon	133	431	15.4	29.7	25.5
Breakfast crescent sandwich w/ham	165	557	19.8	41.7	25.3
Breakfast crescent sandwich w/sausage	162	449	19.9	29.4	25.9
Breast and wing	196	604	43.5	36.5	25.4
Brownie	64	264	3.3	11.4	37.3
Caramel sundae	145	293	7.0	8.5	51.5
Cheese danish	71	254	4.9	12.2	31.4
Cheeseburger	173	563	29.5	37.3	27.4
Cherry danish	71	271	4.4	14.4	31.7
Chicken breast	144	412	33.0	23.7	16.9
Chocolate shake	319	358	7.9	10.2	61.3
Coleslaw	99	110	1.0	6.9	11.0
Crescent roll	70	287	4.7	17.7	27.2
Egg and biscuit platter	165	394	16.9	26.5	21.9
Egg and biscuit platter w/bacon	173	435	19.7	29.6	22.1
Egg and biscuit platter w/ham	200	442	23.5	28.6	22.5
Egg and biscuit platter w/sausage	203	550	23.4	40.9	21.9
French fries	85	268	3.9	13.5	32.0
Hamburger	143	456	23.8	28.3	65.6
Hot chocolate	8 oz	123	3.0	2.0	22.0
Hot fudge sundae	151	337	6.5	12.5	53.3
Hot topped potato plain	227	211	5.9	0.2	47.9
Hot topped potato w/bacon 'n cheese	248	397	17.1	21.7	33.3
Hot topped potato w/broccoli 'n cheese	312	376	13.7	18.1	39.6
Hot topped potato w/oleo	236	274	5.9	7.3	47.9
Hot topped potato w/sour cream 'n chives	297	408	7.3	20.9	47.6
Hot topped potato w/taco beef 'n cheese	359	463	21.8	21.8	45.0
Large fries	113	357	5.3	18.4	42.7
Large roast beef	182	360	33.9	11.9	29.6
Large roast beef w/cheese	211	467	39.6	20.9	30.3
Leg	53	140	11.5	8.0	5.5
Macaroni	100	186	3.1	10.7	19.4
Milk	8 oz	150	8.0	8.2	11.4
Orange juice	8 oz	99	1.5	0.2	22.8
Orange juice	8 oz	136	2.0	0.3	31.3

➤ ROY ROGERS—*continued*

Food Item	Serving Size (g)	kcal	Protein (g)	Fat (g)	CHO (g)
Pancake platter (w/syrup, butter)	165	452	7.7	15.2	71.8
Pancake platter (w/syrup, butter) w/bacon	173	493	10.4	18.3	72.0
Pancake platter (w/syrup, butter) w/ham	200	506	14.3	17.3	72.4
Pancake platter (w/syrup, butter) w/sausage	203	608	14.2	29.6	71.8
Potato salad	100	107	2.0	6.1	10.9
Roast beef sandwich	154	317	27.2	10.2	29.1
Roast beef sandwich w/cheese	182	424	32.9	19.2	29.9
RR bar burger	208	611	36.1	39.4	28.0
Salad bar Thousand Island	2 T	160	NA	16.0	4.0
Salad bar bacon 'n tomato	2 T	136	NA	12.0	6.0
Salad bar bacon bits	1 T	24	4.0	1.0	38.0
Salad bar blue cheese dressing	2 T	150	2.0	16.0	2.0
Salad bar cheddar cheese	¼ cup cheese	112	5.8	9.0	0.8
Salad bar Chinese noodles	¼ cup noodles	55	1.5	2.8	6.5
Salad bar chopped eggs	2 T	55	4.0	4.0	0.7
Salad bar croutons	2 T	132	5.5	0	31.0
Salad bar cucumbers	5–6 slices	4	NA	0	1.0
Salad bar green peas	¼ cup	7	0.5	0	1.2
Salad bar green peppers	2 T	4	0.3	0	1.0
Salad bar lettuce	1 cup	10	NA	0	4.0
Salad bar low cal Italian	2 T	70	NA	6.0	2.0
Salad bar macaroni salad	2 T	60	1.0	3.6	6.2
Salad bar mushrooms	¼ cup	5	0.5	0	0.7
Salad bar potato salad	2 T	50	1.0	3.0	5.5
Salad bar ranch	2 T	155	NA	14.0	4.0
Salad bar shredded carrots	¼ cup	12	0.6	0	24.0
Salad bar sliced beets	¼ cup	16	0.5	0	3.8
Salad bar sunflower seeds	2 T	101	4.0	9.0	5.0
Salad bar tomatoes	3 slices	20	0.8	0	4.8
Strawberry shake	312	315	7.6	10.2	49.4
Strawberry shortcake	205	447	10.1	19.2	59.3
Strawberry sundae	142	216	5.7	7.1	33.1
Thigh	98	296	18.4	19.5	11.7
Thigh and leg	151	436	29.9	27.5	17.2
Vanilla shake	306	306	8.0	10.7	45.0
Wing	52	192	10.5	12.8	8.5

Source: Roy Rogers Restaurants, Marriott Corporation, Washington, DC. Nutritional data furnished by Lancaster Laboratories, 1985.

➤ TACO BELL

Food Item	kcal	Protein (g)	Fat (g)	Calories from Fat	Saturated Fat	Cholesterol (mg)	Na (mg)	Percent U.S. RDA Ca	Fe
Tacos and Tostadas									
Chicken soft taco	223	14	10	90	4	58	553	6	8
Soft taco	223	12	11	100	5	32	539	5	10
Soft taco supreme	268	13	15	140	8	47	551	8	11
Steak soft taco	217	12	9	80	4	31	569	5	6
Taco	180	10	11	100	5	32	276	8	5
Taco supreme	225	11	15	130	7	47	287	10	6
Tostada	242	9	11	100	4	14	593	17	8
Burritos									
7 layer burrito	485	15	21	190	8	28	1115	25	25
Bean burrito	391	13	12	110	4	5	1138	19	20
Beef burrito	432	22	19	170	8	57	1303	16	22

➤ TACO BELL—*continued*

Food Item	kcal	Protein (g)	Fat (g)	Calories from Fat	Saturated Fat	Cholesterol (mg)	Na (mg)	Percent U.S. RDA Ca	Percent U.S. RDA Fe
Burritos—*continued*									
Big beef burrito supreme	525	25	25	220	11	72	1418	20	25
Burrito supreme	443	18	19	170	9	47	1184	20	21
Chicken burrito	345	17	13	110	5	57	854	14	14
Chicken burrito supreme	520	27	23	200	9	125	1130	15	50
Chili cheese burrito	391	17	18	160	9	47	980	30	17
Combo burrito	412	17	16	140	6	32	1221	17	21
Steak burrito supreme	500	26	23	200	11	75	1350	20	15
Specialty Items									
Beef MexiMelt	262	13	14	130	7	38	711	23	8
Cinnamon twists	139	1	6	50	0	0	189	°	2
Mexican pizza	574	19	38	340	12	50	1003	31	25
Nachos	345	7	18	160	6	9	398	23	4
Nachos BellGrande	633	22	34	300	12	49	952	36	20
Nachos supreme	364	12	18	160	5	17	470	19	15
Pintos 'n cheese	190	9	9	80	4	14	640	15	7
Taco salad	838	31	55	490	16	79	1132	25	34
Side Orders and Condiments									
Green sauce	4	0	0	0	0	0	136	°	°
Guacamole	36	0	3	30	1	0	132	4	°
Hot taco sauce	2	0	0	0	0	0	91	°	°
Mild taco sauce	0	0	0	0	0	0	6	°	°
Nacho cheese sauce	51	2	4	40	2	4	196	6	°
Picante sauce	3	0	0	0	0	0	132	2	0
Pico de Gallo	6	0	0	0	0	0	65	°	°
Ranch dressing	136	1	14	130	3	20	330	2	°
Red sauce	10	0	0	0	0	0	261	°	°
Salsa	27	1	0	0	0	0	709	5	3
Seasoned rice	110	2	3	30	1	5	230	°	8
Sour cream	44	1	4	40	3	15	11	2	°

Source: Taco Bell Corporation, Irvine, CA. 1996.
° = trace

➤ WENDY'S

Food Item	Serving Size (g)	kcal	Protein (g)	CHO (g)	Fat (g)	Cholesterol (mg)	Vit A (mg)	Vit C (mg)	Thia (mg)	Ribo (mg)	Nia (mg)	Ca (mg)	Fe (mg)
Sandwiches													
½ lb hamburger patty	74	180	19	—	12	65	—	—	4	—	20	—	20
Plain single	126	340	24	30	15	65	—	—	25	20	30	10	30
Single with everything	210	420	25	35	21	70	5	15	25	20	30	10	30
Wendy's Big Classic	260	570	27	47	33	90	10	20	30	25	35	15	35
Jr. Hamburger	111	260	15	33	9	34	2	4	25	20	20	10	20
Jr. cheeseburger	125	310	18	33	13	34	2	4	25	50	20	10	20
Jr. bacon cheeseburger	155	430	22	32	25	50	2	15	30	50	20	10	20
Jr. Swiss deluxe	163	360	18	34	18	40	4	10	25	60	25	10	20
Kids' meal hamburger	104	260	15	32	9	35	2	2	25	20	20	20	20
Kids' meal cheeseburger	116	300	18	33	13	35	2	2	25	50	20	10	20

➤ WENDY'S—*continued*

Food Item	Serving Size (g)	kcal	Protein (g)	CHO (g)	Fat (g)	Cholesterol (mg)	Vit A (mg)	Vit C (mg)	Thia (mg)	Ribo (mg)	Nia (mg)	Ca (mg)	Fe (mg)
Sandwiches—*continued*													
Grilled chicken fillet	70	100	18	—	3	55	—	—	4	4	35	—	6
Grilled chicken sandwich	175	340	24	36	13	60	2	8	30	25	50	10	20
Chicken breast fillet	99	220	21	11	10	55	—	—	8	8	60	—	70
Chicken sandwich	219	430	26	41	19	60	2	8	30	25	70	10	80
Chicken club sandwich	205	506	30	42	25	70	2	15	35	30	80	10	80
Fish fillet sandwich	170	460	18	42	25	55	2	2	40	35	20	10	15
Kaiser bun	65	200	6	37	3	10	—	—	25	20	10	10	10
White bun	56	160	5	30	3	tr	—	—	20	20	10	10	10
Sandwich Toppings													
American cheese slice	18	70	4	—	6	15	6	—	—	4	—	12	—
Bacon	6	30	2	—	3	5	—	4	4	—	2	—	—
Ketchup	14	17	—	4	—	NA	4	4	—	—	—	—	—
Lettuce	10	1	—	—	—	0	—	—	—	—	—	—	—
Mayonnaise	13	90	—	—	10	10	—	—	—	—	—	—	—
Mustard	5	4	—	—	—	0	—	—	—	—	—	—	—
Onion	10	4	—	—	—	0	—	—	—	—	—	—	—
Pickles	14	2	—	—	—	0	—	—	—	—	—	—	—
Tomatoes	21	4	—	—	—	0	—	6	—	—	—	—	—
Honey mustard	14	71	—	4	6	5	—	—	—	—	—	—	—
Tartar sauce	21	120	—	—	14	15	—	—	15	10	—	—	—
Superbar—Pasta													
Alfredo sauce	56	35	1	5	1	tr	—	—	—	—	—	6	—
Fettucini	56	190	4	27	3	10	—	—	10	6	6	—	6
Garlic toast	18.3	70	2	9	3	tr	4	—	6	2	2	2	2
Pasta medley	56	60	2	9	2	tr	6	15	6	4	4	—	4
Rotini	56	90	3	15	2	tr	—	—	6	4	6	—	4
Spaghetti sauce	56	28	—	7	0	tr	—	—	—	—	—	—	—
Spaghetti meat sauce	56	60	4	8	2	10	4	4	—	2	4	—	4
Garden Spot Salad Bar													
Alfalfa sprouts	28	8	1	1	0	0	—	4	—	2	—	—	—
Applesauce, chunky	28	22	—	6	—	0	—	—	—	—	—	—	—
Bacon bits	14	40	5	—	14	10	—	2	6	4	6	—	—
Bananas	28	26	—	7	—	0	—	4	—	2	—	—	—
Breadsticks	7.5	30	1	5	1	0	—	—	2	2	2	2	2
Broccoli	43	12	1	2	0	0	6	65	2	2	—	2	2
Cantaloupe	57	20	—	5	0	0	20	30	—	—	—	—	—
Carrots	27	12	—	2	0	0	80	4	2	—	—	—	—
Cauliflower	57	14	1	3	0	0	—	70	4	2	2	2	2
Cheddar chips	28	160	3	12	12	5	—	—	2	—	4	6	2
Cheese, shredded (imitation)	28	90	6	1	6	tr	4	—	—	15	—	20	—
Chicken salad	56	120	7	4	8	tr	—	4	—	4	6	—	2
Chives	28	71	6	18	1	0	195	313	15	25	8	25	30
Chow mein noodles	14	74	1	8	4	0	—	—	6	4	4	—	4
Coleslaw	57	70	—	8	5	5	4	25	—	—	—	2	—
Cottage cheese	105	108	13	3	4	15	6	—	—	10	—	6	—
Croutons	14	60	2	8	3	—	—	—	4	4	4	—	4
Cucumbers	14	2	—	—	0	0	—	—	—	—	—	—	—
Eggs (hard cooked)	20	30	3	—	2	90	4	—	—	6	—	—	—
Garbanzo beans	28	46	3	8	1	0	—	—	2	—	—	—	6
Green peas	28	21	1	4	0	0	4	8	6	2	—	—	2
Green peppers	37	10	—	2	0	0	2	60	2	—	—	—	—
Honeydew melon	57	20	—	5	0	0	—	25	2	—	2	—	—
Jalapeño peppers	14	2	—	—	0	0	—	—	—	—	—	—	—
Lettuce—iceberg	55	8	—	1	0	0	2	4	2	—	—	—	2
Lettuce—romaine	55	9	1	1	0	0	15	20	4	4	—	2	4
Mushrooms	17	4	—	—	0	0	—	—	—	4	4	—	—
Olives, black	28	35	—	2	3	0	—	—	—	—	—	2	4
Oranges	56	26	—	7	0	0	—	50	4	—	—	2	—

➤ **WENDY'S—*continued***

Food Item	Serving Size (g)	kcal	Protein (g)	CHO (g)	Fat (g)	Cholesterol (mg)	Vit A (mg)	Vit C (mg)	Thia (mg)	Ribo (mg)	Nia (mg)	Ca (mg)	Fe (mg)
Garden Spot Salad Bar—*continued*													
Parmesan cheese	28	130	12	1	9	20	6	—	—	6	—	40	—
Parmesan cheese (imitation)	28	80	9	4	3	tr	20	—	—	—	—	50	—
Pasta salad	57	35	2	6	—	0	—	—	—	2	2	—	2
Peaches	57	31	—	8	0	0	2	2	—	—	2	—	—
Pepperoni, sliced	28	140	5	2	12	35	—	—	160	4	10	—	2
Pineapple chunks	100	60	—	16	0	0	—	15	6	—	—	—	2
Potato salad	57	125	—	6	11	10	—	10	2	—	2	—	2
Pudding—butterscotch	57	90	1	11	4	tr	—	—	—	—	—	6	2
Pudding—chocolate	57	90	—	12	4	tr	—	—	2	2	—	15	2
Red onions	9	2	—	—	0	0	—	—	—	—	—	—	—
Red peppers, crushed	28	120	5	15	4	0	200	15	10	15	20	2	15
Seafood salad	56	110	4	7	7	tr	—	2	—	2	—	20	2
Strawberries	56	17	—	4	0	0	—	50	—	2	—	—	—
Sour topping	28	58	—	2	5	0	—	—	—	—	—	—	—
Sunflower seeds and raisins	28	140	5	6	10	0	—	—	30	4	6	2	10
Three-bean salad	57	60	1	13	—	—	4	—	—	—	—	—	2
Tomatoes	28	6	—	1	0	0	2	10	—	—	—	—	—
Tuna salad	56	100	8	4	6	tr	—	4	—	4	25	—	2
Turkey ham	28	35	5	—	1	15	—	—	—	4	6	—	4
Watermelon	57	18	—	4	0	0	2	10	4	—	—	—	—
Salad Dressings													
Blue cheese	15	9	—	—	10	10	—	—	—	—	—	—	—
Celery seed	15	70	—	3	6	5	—	—	—	—	—	—	—
French	15	60	—	4	6	0	—	—	—	—	—	—	—
French, sweet red	15	70	—	5	6	0	—	—	—	—	—	—	—
Hidden Valley ranch	15	50	—	—	6	5	—	—	—	—	—	—	—
Italian Caesar	15	80	—	—	9	5	—	—	—	—	—	—	—
Italian, golden	15	45	—	3	4	0	—	—	—	—	—	—	—
Salad oil	28	250	0	0	28	0	—	—	—	—	—	—	—
Thousand Island	15	70	—	2	7	5	—	—	—	—	—	—	—
Wine, vinegar	15	2	—	—	0	0	—	—	—	—	—	—	—
Reduced calorie bacon and tomato	15	45	—	3	4	—	—	—	—	—	—	—	—
Reduced calorie Italian	15	25	—	2	2	0	—	—	—	—	—	—	—
Prepared Salads													
Chef salad	331	180	15	10	9	120	110	110	15	25	6	25	15
Garden salad	277	102	7	9	5	0	110	110	10	20	6	20	10
Taco salad	791	660	40	46	37	35	80	80	30	45	25	80	35
Superbar—Mexican Fiesta (where available)													
Cheese sauce	56	39	1	5	2	tr	—	—	—	—	—	6	—
Picante sauce	56	18	—	4	—	NA	10	30	2	—	2	—	2
Refried beans	56	70	4	10	3	tr	—	—	4	2	—	2	6
Rice, Spanish	56	70	2	13	1	tr	6	—	45	—	8	4	10
Taco chips	40	260	4	40	10	0	—	—	2	4	—	8	4
Taco meat	56	110	10	4	7	25	—	—	8	6	10	4	10
Taco sauce	28	16	—	3	—	tr	4	2	—	—	—	—	—
Taco shells	11	45	—	6	3	0	—	—	—	—	—	—	—
Tortilla, flour	37	110	3	19	3	NA	—	—	4	2	2	8	2
French fries (small) 3.2 oz**	91	240	3	33	12	0	—	10	10	2	10	—	4
Chili (regular) 9 oz	255	220	21	23	7	45	15	15	8	10	10	8	35
Cheddar cheese, shredded	28	110	7	1	10	30	10	—	—	6	—	20	—
Sour cream	28	60	1	1	6	10	6	—	—	2	—	4	—
Crispy chicken nuggets (6)	93	280	14	12	20	50	—	—	6	6	30	4	4

➤ **WENDY'S—*continued***

FOOD ITEM	SERVING SIZE (G)	KCAL	PROTEIN (G)	CHO (G)	FAT (G)	CHOLESTEROL (MG)	PERCENTAGE OF U.S. RDA VIT A (MG)	VIT C (MG)	THIA (MG)	RIBO (MG)	NIA (MG)	CA (MG)	FE (MG)
Nugget sauces													
Barbecue	28	50	—	11	—	0	6	—	—	—	—	—	4
Honey	14	45	—	12	—	0	—	—	—	—	—	—	—
Sweet and sour	28	45	—	11	—	0	—	—	—	—	—	—	2
Sweet mustard	28	50	—	9	1	0	—	—	—	—	—	—	—
Hot Stuffed Baked Potatoes													
Plain	250	270	6	63	—	0	—	50	20	6	20	2	20
Bacon and cheese	362	520	20	70	18	20	10	60	35	15	35	8	24
Broccoli and cheese	350	400	8	58	16	tr	14	60	20	10	20	10	15
Cheese	318	420	8	66	15	10	10	50	20	100	20	6	20
Chili and cheese	403	500	15	71	18	25	15	60	20	100	25	8	28
Sour cream and chives	323	500	8	67	23	25	50	75	20	10	20	10	20
Beverages													
Frosty, small***	243	400	8	59	14	50	10	—	8	30	2	30	6
Cola, small	8*	100	0	25	0	0	—	—	—	—	—	—	—
Lemon-lime soft drink, small	8*	100	0	24	0	0	—	—	—	—	—	—	—
Diet cola	8*	1	0	—	0	0	—	—	—	—	—	—	—
Coffee	6*	2	0	—	0	0	—	—	—	—	—	—	—
Decaf coffee	6*	2	0	—	0	0	—	—	—	—	—	—	—
Hot chocolate	6*	110	2	22	1	tr	—	—	—	8	—	6	2
Lemonade	8*	90	0	24	0	0	—	15	—	4	—	—	2
Choc milk	8*	160	7	24	5	15	15	4	6	20	—	25	4
Milk, 2%	8*	110	8	11	4	20	10	4	6	20	—	30	—
Tea (hot or iced)	6*	1	0	0	0	0	—	—	—	—	—	—	—
Chocolate chip cookie	64	275	3	40	13	15	2	—	8	8	6	2	8

Source: Consumer Relations, Wendy's International, Dublin, OH.

*Fluid ounces.

**To determine nutritional information for a large order of fries, multiply figures by 1.3; Biggie fries, multiply by 1.87; large chili, multiply by 1.5; 9-piece nuggets, multiply by 1.5; 20-piece nuggets, multiply by 3.3.

***To determine nutritional information for a medium Frosty, multiply figures by 1.3; large Frosty, multiply by 1.7. For a medium soft drink, multiply by 1.5; large soft drink, multiply by 2. For a Biggie soft drink, multiply by 3.5.

Appendix C

Energy Expenditure in Household, Occupational, Recreational, and Sports Activities[a,b]

HOW TO USE APPENDIX C

Refer to the column that comes closest to current body mass. Multiply the number in this column by the number of minutes you spend in an activity. Suppose that an individual weighing 62.3 kg (137 lb) spends 30 minutes playing a casual game of billiards. To determine the energy cost of participation, multiply the caloric value per minute (2.6 kcal) by 30 to obtain the 30-minute gross expenditure of 78 kcal. If the same individual does aerobic dance for 45 minutes, the *gross* (value includes resting energy expenditure) energy expended would be calculated as 6.4 kcal × 45 minutes, or 288 kcal.

[a]All values for energy expenditure are in kilocalories (kcal) per minute.

YOUR BODY WEIGHT KG	47	50	53	56	59	62	65	68
Activity LB	104	110	117	123	130	137	143	150
Archery								
hunting (walking)		3.5	3.9	4.1	4.3	4.6	4.8	5.0
nonhunting, recreational		2.9	3.2	3.4	3.6	3.8	4.0	4.2
Backpacking								
without load	5.7	6.1	6.4	6.8	7.1	7.5	7.9	8.2
with 11-lb load	6.1	6.5	6.8	7.2	7.6	8.0	8.4	8.8
with 22-lb load	6.6	7.0	7.4	7.8	8.3	8.7	9.1	9.5
with 44-lb load	7.0	7.4	7.8	8.2	8.7	9.1	9.6	10.0
Badminton								
leisure	4.6	4.9	5.1	5.4	5.7	6.0	6.3	6.6
tournament	7.0	7.3	7.7	8.1	8.6	9.0	9.4	9.9
Baking, general (F)	1.6	1.8	1.9	2.0	2.1	2.2	2.3	2.4
Baseball								
catcher		4.5	4.8	5.1	5.4	5.6	5.9	6.2
infielder		3.8	4.3	4.5	4.7	5.0	5.2	5.5
outfielder		3.7	4.1	4.3	4.5	4.8	5.0	5.2
pitcher		4.6	5.2	5.5	5.8	6.1	6.4	6.7
playing catch		2.1	2.3	2.5	2.6	2.7	2.8	3.0
Basketball								
game (pickup, playground)		6.6	7.4	7.8	8.3	8.7	9.1	9.5
game (structured, with officials)		7.0	7.9	8.3	8.8	9.2	9.7	10.1
nongame, general shooting around		5.0	5.6	5.9	6.2	6.5	6.8	7.1
officiating		3.7	4.2	4.4	4.6	4.9	5.1	5.4
shooting baskets, practice		5.7	6.5	6.9	7.2	7.6	8.0	8.3
wheelchair		5.4	6.0	6.4	6.7	7.1	7.4	7.7
wheelchair competition, full-court game		5.4	6.0	6.3	6.7	7.0	7.3	7.7
Baton twirling	6.3	6.8	7.3	7.6	8.1	8.5	8.9	9.3
Bench stepping								
30 step-cycles/min 6 in. bench		6.7	7.5	7.9	8.4	8.8	9.2	9.7
30 step-cycles/min 8 in. bench		7.3	8.3	8.8	9.2	9.7	10.2	10.6
30 step-cycles/min 10 in. bench		8.0	9.0	9.5	10.0	10.5	11.0	11.5
30 step-cycles/min 12 in. bench		8.7	9.9	10.4	11.0	11.6	12.1	12.7
Billiards ("pool")	2.0	2.1	2.2	2.4	2.5	2.6	2.7	2.9
Bookbinding	1.8	1.9	2.0	2.1	2.2	2.4	2.5	2.6
Bowling	4.4	4.8	5.2	5.4	5.7	6.0	6.3	6.6
Boxing								
in ring, match	10.4	11.1	11.8	12.4	13.1	13.8	14.4	15.1
sparring, practice	6.5	6.9	7.3	7.7	8.1	8.6	9.0	9.4
Calisthenics, warm-ups	3.4	3.7	4.0	4.2	4.4	4.7	4.9	5.1
Canoeing								
2.0–3.9 mph, light effort		2.4	2.8	2.9	3.1	3.3	3.4	3.6
4.0–5.9 mph, moderate effort		5.7	6.5	6.9	7.2	7.6	8.0	8.3
more than 5.9 mph vigorous effort		9.9	11.1	11.8	12.4	13.0	13.7	14.3
camping trip		3.3	3.7	3.9	4.1	4.3	4.6	4.8

Note: Symbols (M) and (F) denote experiments for males and females, respectively.

71 157	74 163	77 170	80 176	83 183	86 190	89 196	92 203	95 209	98 216
5.2	5.4	5.7	5.9	6.1	6.3	6.5	6.8	7.0	7.2
4.3	4.5	4.7	4.9	5.1	5.3	5.5	5.6	5.8	6.0
8.6	9.0	9.3	9.7	10.0	10.4	10.8	11.1	11.5	11.9
9.2	9.5	9.9	10.3	10.7	11.1	11.5	11.9	12.3	12.6
9.9	10.4	10.8	11.2	11.6	12.0	12.5	12.9	13.3	13.7
10.4	10.9	11.3	11.8	12.2	12.6	13.1	13.5	14.0	14.4
6.9	7.2	7.5	7.8	8.1	8.3	8.6	8.9	9.2	9.5
10.4	10.8	11.2	11.6	12.1	12.5	12.9	13.4	13.8	14.3
2.5	2.6	2.7	2.8	2.9	3.0	3.1	3.2	3.3	3.4
6.5	6.7	7.0	7.3	7.6	7.8	8.1	8.4	8.6	8.9
5.7	6.0	6.2	6.4	6.7	6.9	7.2	7.4	7.6	7.9
5.5	5.7	5.9	6.2	6.4	6.6	6.9	7.1	7.3	7.5
7.0	7.3	7.5	7.8	8.1	8.4	8.7	9.0	9.3	9.6
3.1	3.2	3.4	3.5	3.6	3.8	3.9	4.0	4.2	4.3
9.9	10.4	10.8	11.2	11.6	12.0	12.5	12.9	13.3	13.7
10.6	11.0	11.5	11.9	12.3	12.8	13.2	13.7	14.1	14.6
9.5	9.7	9.9	10.1	10.4	10.6	10.8	11.0	11.2	11.4
7.5	7.8	8.1	8.4	8.7	9.0	9.3	9.7	10.0	10.3
5.6	5.8	6.1	6.3	6.5	6.8	7.0	7.2	7.5	7.7
8.7	9.1	9.4	9.8	10.2	10.5	10.9	11.3	11.6	12.0
8.1	8.4	8.8	9.1	9.4	9.8	10.1	10.5	10.8	11.1
8.0	8.4	8.7	9.0	9.4	9.7	10.1	10.4	10.7	11.1
3.0	3.1	3.2	3.4	3.5	3.6	3.7	3.9	4.0	4.1
10.1	10.5	10.9	11.4	11.8	12.2	12.6	13.1	13.5	13.9
11.1	11.6	12.0	12.5	13.0	13.5	13.9	14.4	14.9	15.3
12.0	12.5	13.0	13.5	14.0	14.5	15.0	15.6	16.1	16.6
13.2	13.8	14.4	14.9	15.5	16.0	16.6	17.2	17.7	18.3
2.7	2.8	2.9	3.0	3.2	3.3	3.4	3.5	3.6	3.7
6.9	7.2	7.5	7.7	8.1	8.4	8.6	8.9	9.2	9.5
15.8	16.4	17.1	17.8	18.4	19.1	19.8	20.4	21.1	21.8
9.8	10.2	10.6	11.0	11.5	11.9	12.3	12.7	13.1	13.5
5.3	5.5	5.8	6.0	6.2	6.5	6.7	6.9	7.1	7.3
3.7	3.9	4.0	4.2	4.4	4.5	4.7	4.8	5.0	5.1
8.7	9.1	9.4	9.8	10.2	10.5	10.9	11.3	11.6	12.0
14.9	15.5	16.2	16.8	17.4	18.1	18.7	19.3	20.0	20.6
5.0	5.2	5.4	5.6	5.8	6.0	6.2	6.4	6.7	6.9

YOUR BODY WEIGHT—*continued*

ACTIVITY	KG 47 LB 104	50 110	53 117	56 123	59 130	62 137	65 143	68 150
Canoeing, continued								
competition, crew or sculling		9.9	11.1	11.8	12.4	13.0	13.7	14.3
pleasure, general		2.9	3.2	3.4	3.6	3.8	4.0	4.2
white water (recreational)		4.1	4.6	4.9	5.2	5.4	5.7	6.0
Car washing	3.3	3.5	3.7	3.9	4.1	4.3	4.5	4.8
Card playing	1.2	1.3	1.3	1.4	1.5	1.6	1.6	1.7
Carpentry, general	2.4	2.6	2.8	2.9	3.1	3.2	3.4	3.5
Carpet sweeping (F)	2.2	2.3	2.4	2.5	2.7	2.8	2.9	3.1
Carpet sweeping (M)	2.3	2.4	2.5	2.7	2.8	3.0	3.1	3.3
Circuit resistance training								
Free weights	4.0	4.3	4.5	4.8	5.0	5.3	5.5	5.8
Hydra-Fitness	6.2	6.6	7.0	7.4	7.8	8.2	8.6	9.0
Nautilus	4.3	4.6	4.9	5.2	5.5	5.8	6.0	6.3
Universal	5.3	5.8	6.2	6.5	6.9	7.2	7.5	7.9
Cleaning (F)	2.9	3.1	3.3	3.5	3.7	3.8	4.0	4.2
Cleaning (M)	2.7	2.9	3.1	3.2	3.4	3.6	3.8	3.9
Coal mining								
drilling coal, rock	4.4	4.7	5.0	5.3	5.5	5.8	6.1	6.4
erecting supports	4.1	4.4	4.7	4.9	5.2	5.5	5.7	6.0
shoveling coal	5.1	5.4	5.7	6.0	6.4	6.7	7.0	7.3
Cooking (F)	2.1	2.3	2.4	2.5	2.7	2.8	2.9	3.1
Cooking (M)	2.3	2.4	2.5	2.7	2.8	3.0	3.1	3.3
Cricket								
batting	3.9	4.2	4.4	4.6	4.9	5.1	5.4	5.6
bowling	4.2	4.5	4.8	5.0	5.3	5.6	5.9	6.1
fielding	3.7	3.9	4.1	4.3	4.8	4.8	5.0	5.3
Croquet	2.8	3.0	3.1	3.3	3.5	3.7	3.8	4.0
Cycling								
leisure, 5.5 mph	3.0	3.2	3.4	3.6	3.8	4.0	4.2	4.4
leisure, 9.4 mph	4.8	5.0	5.3	5.6	5.9	6.2	6.5	6.8
racing, fast	8.0	8.5	9.0	9.5	10.0	10.5	11.0	11.5
Dancing								
aerobic, easy	4.3	4.8	5.2	5.6	5.9	6.2	6.4	6.7
aerobic, medium	4.8	5.2	5.5	5.8	6.1	6.4	6.7	7.0
aerobic, intense	6.3	6.7	7.1	7.5	7.9	8.3	8.7	9.2
ballroom	2.4	2.6	2.7	2.9	3.0	3.2	3.3	3.5
choreographed	5.0	5.2	5.5	5.8	6.1	6.4	6.7	7.0
"twist," "lambada"	8.0	8.4	8.9	9.4	9.9	10.4	10.9	11.4
modern	3.4	3.6	3.8	4.0	4.3	4.5	4.7	4.9
Digging trenches	6.8	7.3	7.7	8.1	8.6	9.0	9.4	9.9
Drawing (standing)	1.7	1.8	1.9	2.0	2.1	2.2	2.3	2.4
Eating (sitting)	1.1	1.2	1.2	1.3	1.4	1.4	1.5	1.6
Electrical work	2.7	2.9	3.1	3.2	3.4	3.6	3.8	3.9
Farming								
barn cleaning	6.3	6.8	7.2	7.6	8.0	8.4	8.8	9.2
driving harvester	1.9	2.0	2.1	2.2	2.4	2.5	2.6	2.7
driving tractor	1.8	1.9	2.0	2.1	2.2	2.3	2.4	2.5
feeding cattle	4.2	4.3	4.5	4.8	5.0	5.3	5.5	5.8
feeding animals	3.1	3.3	3.4	3.6	3.8	4.0	4.2	4.4
forking straw bales	6.7	6.9	7.3	7.7	8.1	8.6	9.0	9.4
milking by hand	2.5	2.7	2.9	3.0	3.2	3.3	3.5	3.7
milking by machine	1.1	1.2	1.2	1.3	1.4	1.4	1.5	1.6
shoveling grain	4.2	4.3	4.5	4.8	5.0	5.3	5.5	5.8
Fencing								
competition	7.2	7.6	8.1	8.5	9.0	9.4	9.9	10.8
practice	3.6	3.9	4.2	4.4	4.6	4.9	5.1	5.3
Field hockey	6.5	6.7	7.1	7.5	7.9	8.3	8.7	9.1
field game (competition, structured)	6.6	7.0	7.4	7.8	8.3	8.7	9.1	9.5
practice	5.6	6.1	6.5	6.9	7.2	7.6	8.0	8.3

71	74	77	80	83	86	89	92	95	98
157	**163**	**170**	**176**	**183**	**190**	**196**	**203**	**209**	**216**
14.9	15.5	16.2	16.8	17.4	18.1	18.7	19.3	20.0	20.6
4.3	4.5	4.7	4.9	5.1	5.3	5.5	5.6	5.8	6.0
6.2	6.5	6.7	7.0	7.3	7.5	7.8	8.1	8.3	8.6
5.0	5.2	5.5	5.7	5.7	5.9	6.1	6.3	6.5	6.9
1.8	1.9	1.9	2.0	2.1	2.2	2.2	2.3	2.4	2.5
3.7	3.8	4.0	4.2	4.3	4.5	4.6	4.8	4.9	5.1
3.2	3.3	3.5	3.6	3.7	3.9	4.0	4.1	4.3	4.4
3.4	3.6	3.7	3.8	4.0	4.1	4.3	4.4	4.6	4.7
6.1	6.3	6.6	6.8	7.1	7.4	7.6	7.9	8.1	8.4
9.4	9.7	10.2	10.5	10.9	11.4	11.7	12.1	12.5	12.9
6.6	6.8	7.1	7.4	7.7	8.0	8.2	8.5	8.8	9.1
8.3	8.6	8.9	9.3	9.6	10.0	10.3	10.7	11.0	11.4
4.4	4.6	4.8	5.0	5.1	5.3	5.5	5.7	5.9	6.1
4.1	4.3	4.5	4.6	4.8	5.0	5.2	5.3	5.5	5.7
6.7	7.0	7.2	7.5	7.8	8.1	8.4	8.6	8.9	9.2
6.2	6.5	6.8	7.0	7.3	7.6	7.8	8.1	8.4	8.6
7.7	8.0	8.3	8.6	9.0	9.3	9.6	9.9	10.3	10.6
3.2	3.3	3.5	3.6	3.7	3.9	4.0	4.1	4.3	4.4
3.4	3.6	3.7	3.8	4.0	4.1	4.3	4.4	4.6	4.7
5.9	6.1	6.4	6.6	6.9	7.1	7.4	7.6	7.9	8.1
6.4	6.7	6.9	7.2	7.5	7.7	8.0	8.3	8.6	8.8
5.6	5.9	6.2	6.5	6.8	7.1	7.4	7.7	8.0	8.3
4.2	4.4	4.5	4.7	4.9	5.1	5.3	5.4	5.6	5.8
4.5	4.7	4.9	5.1	5.3	5.5	5.7	5.9	6.1	6.3
7.1	7.4	7.7	8.0	8.3	8.6	8.9	9.2	9.5	9.8
12.0	12.5	13.0	13.5	14.0	14.5	15.0	15.5	16.1	16.6
6.9	7.2	7.5	7.8	8.1	8.4	8.8	9.1	9.4	9.7
7.3	7.6	7.9	8.2	8.5	8.9	9.2	9.5	9.8	10.1
9.6	10.0	10.4	10.8	11.2	11.6	12.0	12.4	12.8	13.2
3.6	3.8	3.9	4.1	4.2	4.4	4.5	4.7	4.8	5.0
7.3	7.6	7.9	8.2	8.5	8.9	9.2	9.5	9.8	10.1
11.9	12.4	12.9	13.4	13.9	14.4	15.0	15.5	16.0	16.5
5.1	5.3	5.6	5.8	6.0	6.2	6.4	6.7	6.9	7.1
10.3	10.7	11.2	11.6	12.0	12.5	12.9	13.3	13.8	14.2
2.6	2.7	2.8	2.9	3.0	3.1	3.2	3.3	3.4	3.5
1.6	1.7	1.8	1.8	1.9	2.0	2.0	2.1	2.2	2.3
4.1	4.3	4.5	4.6	4.8	5.0	5.2	5.3	5.5	5.7
9.6	10.0	10.4	10.8	11.2	11.6	12.0	12.4	12.8	13.2
2.8	3.0	3.1	3.2	3.3	3.4	3.6	3.7	3.8	3.9
2.6	2.7	2.8	3.0	3.1	3.2	3.3	3.4	3.5	3.6
6.0	6.3	6.5	6.8	7.1	7.3	7.6	7.8	8.1	8.3
4.6	4.8	5.0	5.2	5.4	5.6	5.8	6.0	6.2	6.4
9.8	10.2	10.6	11.0	11.5	11.9	12.3	12.7	13.1	13.5
3.8	4.0	4.2	4.3	4.5	4.6	4.8	5.0	5.1	5.3
1.6	1.7	1.8	1.8	1.9	2.0	2.0	2.1	2.2	2.3
6.0	6.3	6.5	6.8	7.1	7.3	7.6	7.8	8.1	8.3
11.2	11.7	12.1	12.6	13.1	13.5	14.0	14.4	14.9	15.5
5.6	5.8	6.1	6.3	6.5	6.8	7.0	7.2	7.4	7.7
9.5	9.9	10.3	10.7	11.1	11.5	11.9	12.3	12.7	13.1
9.9	10.4	10.8	11.2	11.6	12.0	12.5	12.9	13.3	13.7
8.7	9.1	9.4	9.8	10.2	10.5	10.9	11.3	11.6	12.0

YOUR BODY WEIGHT—*continued*

ACTIVITY	KG 47 LB 104	50 110	53 117	56 123	59 130	62 137	65 143	68 150
Fishing								
boat, sitting	2.1	2.2	2.3	2.5	2.6	2.7	2.8	3.0
general	3.3	3.5	3.7	3.9	4.1	4.3	4.6	4.8
ice, sitting	1.7	1.8	1.9	2.0	2.1	2.2	2.3	2.4
riverbank, walking	4.1	4.4	4.6	4.9	5.2	5.4	5.7	6.0
riverbank, standing	2.9	3.1	3.2	3.4	3.6	3.8	4.0	4.2
stream, in waders	5.0	5.3	5.6	5.9	6.2	6.5	6.8	7.1
Food shopping (F)	3.0	3.1	3.3	3.5	3.7	3.8	4.0	4.2
Football								
competition (structured play)	7.4	7.9	8.3	8.8	9.3	9.8	10.2	10.7
playing catch	2.1	2.2	2.3	2.5	2.6	2.7	2.8	3.0
touch, flag, general	6.6	7.0	7.4	7.8	8.3	8.7	9.1	9.5
Forestry								
ax chopping, fast	14.0	14.9	15.7	16.6	17.5	18.4	19.3	20.2
ax chopping, slow	4.0	4.3	4.5	4.8	5.0	5.3	5.5	5.8
barking trees	5.8	6.2	6.5	6.9	7.3	7.6	8.0	8.4
carrying logs	8.7	9.3	9.9	10.4	11.0	11.5	12.1	12.6
felling trees	6.2	6.6	7.0	7.4	7.8	8.2	8.6	9.0
hoeing	4.2	4.6	4.8	5.1	5.4	5.6	5.9	6.2
planting by hand	5.1	5.5	5.8	6.1	6.4	6.8	7.1	7.4
sawing by hand	5.7	6.1	6.5	6.8	7.2	7.6	7.9	8.3
sawing, power	3.5	3.8	4.0	4.2	4.4	4.7	4.9	5.1
stacking firewood	4.2	4.4	4.7	4.9	5.2	5.5	5.7	6.0
trimming trees	6.1	6.5	6.8	7.2	7.6	8.0	8.4	8.8
weeding	3.4	3.6	3.8	4.0	4.2	4.5	4.7	4.9
Frisbee								
general	2.4	2.6	2.8	2.9	3.1	3.3	3.4	3.6
Ultimate Frisbee (competition)	5.1	5.4	5.8	6.1	6.4	6.7	7.1	7.4
Furriery	3.9	4.2	4.4	4.6	4.9	5.1	5.4	5.6
Gardening								
digging	5.9	6.3	6.7	7.1	7.4	7.8	8.2	8.6
hedging	3.3	3.9	4.1	4.3	4.5	4.8	5.0	5.2
mowing	5.3	5.6	5.9	6.3	6.6	6.9	7.3	7.6
raking	2.5	2.7	2.9	3.0	3.2	3.3	3.5	3.7
Golf								
carrying clubs (caddy)	4.5	4.8	5.1	5.4	5.7	6.0	6.3	6.5
driving range	2.4	2.6	2.8	2.9	3.1	3.3	3.4	3.6
general	3.7	3.9	4.2	4.4	4.6	4.9	5.1	5.4
pulling clubs in cart	4.1	4.4	4.6	4.9	5.2	5.4	5.7	6.0
using power cart	2.9	3.1	3.2	3.4	3.6	3.8	4.0	4.2
Gymnastics	3.0	3.3	3.5	3.7	3.9	4.1	4.3	4.5
Handball	6.9	7.2	7.7	8.1	8.5	9.0	9.4	9.8
Horse-grooming	6.0	6.4	6.8	7.2	7.6	7.9	8.3	8.7
Horseback riding								
galloping	6.4	6.9	7.3	7.7	8.1	8.5	8.9	9.3
trotting	5.2	5.5	5.8	6.2	6.5	6.8	7.2	7.5
walking	1.9	2.1	2.2	2.3	2.4	2.5	2.7	2.8
Horseshoes	3.3	3.4	3.5	3.7	3.9	4.1	4.3	4.5
Housework								
mopping floors	2.8	3.1	3.3	3.5	3.7	3.8	4.0	4.2
dusting	3.0	3.3	3.4	3.6	3.8	4.0	4.2	4.4
laundry	3.1	3.4	3.5	3.7	3.9	4.1	4.3	4.5
washing windows	3.2	3.5	3.6	3.8	4.0	4.2	4.4	4.6
vacuuming	3.0	3.3	3.4	3.6	3.8	4.0	4.2	4.4
Hunting	4.1	4.4	4.7	4.9	5.2	5.5	5.7	6.0
Ice hockey								
game (structured)	6.6	7.0	7.4	7.8	8.3	8.7	9.1	9.5
practice	6.2	6.6	7.0	7.4	7.7	8.1	8.5	8.9
Ironing clothes	1.6	1.7	1.7	1.8	1.9	2.0	2.1	2.2

71	74	77	80	83	86	89	92	95	98
157	**163**	**170**	**176**	**183**	**190**	**196**	**203**	**209**	**216**
3.1	3.2	3.4	3.5	3.6	3.8	3.9	4.0	4.2	4.3
5.0	5.2	5.4	5.6	5.8	6.0	6.2	6.4	6.7	6.9
2.5	2.6	2.7	2.8	2.9	3.0	3.1	3.2	3.3	3.4
6.2	6.5	6.7	7.0	7.3	7.5	7.8	8.1	8.3	8.6
4.3	4.5	4.7	4.9	5.1	5.3	5.5	5.6	5.8	6.0
7.5	7.8	8.1	8.4	8.7	9.0	9.3	9.7	10.0	10.3
4.4	4.6	4.8	5.0	5.1	5.3	5.5	5.7	5.9	6.1
11.2	11.7	12.1	12.6	13.1	13.5	14.0	14.5	15.0	15.4
3.1	3.2	3.4	3.5	3.6	3.8	3.9	4.0	4.2	4.3
9.9	10.4	10.8	11.2	11.6	12.0	12.5	12.9	13.3	13.7
21.1	22.0	22.9	23.8	24.7	25.5	26.4	27.3	28.2	29.1
6.0	6.3	6.5	6.8	7.1	7.3	7.6	7.8	8.1	8.3
8.7	9.1	9.5	9.8	10.2	10.6	10.9	11.3	11.7	12.1
13.2	13.8	14.3	14.9	15.4	16.0	16.6	17.1	17.7	18.2
9.4	9.8	10.2	10.6	11.0	11.4	11.7	12.1	12.5	12.9
6.5	6.7	7.0	7.3	7.6	7.8	8.1	8.4	8.6	8.9
7.7	8.1	8.4	8.7	9.0	9.4	9.7	10.0	10.4	10.7
8.7	9.0	9.4	9.8	10.1	10.5	10.9	11.2	11.6	12.0
5.3	5.6	5.8	6.0	6.2	6.5	6.7	6.9	7.1	7.4
6.2	6.5	6.8	7.0	7.3	7.6	7.8	8.1	8.4	8.6
9.2	9.5	9.9	10.3	10.7	11.1	11.5	11.9	12.3	12.6
5.1	5.3	5.5	5.8	6.0	6.2	6.4	6.6	6.8	7.1
3.7	3.9	4.0	4.2	4.4	4.5	4.7	4.8	5.0	5.1
7.7	8.0	8.4	8.7	9.0	9.3	9.7	10.0	10.3	10.6
5.9	6.1	6.4	6.6	6.9	7.1	7.4	7.6	7.9	8.1
8.9	9.3	9.7	10.1	10.5	10.8	11.2	11.6	12.0	12.3
5.5	5.7	5.9	6.2	6.4	6.6	6.9	7.1	7.3	7.5
8.0	8.3	8.6	9.0	9.3	9.6	10.0	10.3	10.6	11.0
3.8	4.0	4.2	4.3	4.5	4.6	4.8	5.0	5.1	5.3
6.8	7.1	7.4	7.7	8.0	8.3	8.6	8.9	9.1	9.4
3.7	3.9	4.0	4.2	4.4	4.5	4.7	4.8	5.0	5.1
5.6	5.8	6.1	6.3	6.5	6.8	7.0	7.2	7.5	7.7
6.2	6.5	6.7	7.0	7.3	7.5	7.8	8.1	8.3	8.6
4.3	4.5	4.7	4.9	5.1	5.3	5.5	5.6	5.8	6.0
4.7	4.9	5.1	5.3	5.5	5.7	5.9	6.1	6.3	6.5
10.3	10.7	11.2	11.5	12.0	12.5	12.9	13.3	13.7	14.2
9.1	9.5	9.9	10.2	10.6	11.0	11.4	11.8	12.2	12.5
9.7	10.1	10.6	11.0	11.4	11.8	12.2	12.6	13.0	13.4
7.8	8.1	8.5	8.8	9.1	9.5	9.8	10.1	10.5	10.8
2.9	3.0	3.2	3.3	3.4	3.5	3.6	3.8	3.9	4.0
4.7	4.9	5.1	5.3	5.5	5.7	5.9	6.1	6.3	6.5
4.4	4.6	4.8	5.0	5.2	5.4	5.6	5.8	6.0	6.2
4.6	4.7	4.9	5.1	5.3	5.5	5.7	5.9	6.1	6.3
4.7	4.9	5.1	5.3	5.5	5.7	5.9	6.1	6.3	6.5
4.8	5.0	5.2	5.4	5.6	5.8	6.0	6.2	6.4	6.6
4.6	4.8	5.0	5.2	5.4	5.6	5.8	6.0	6.2	6.4
6.2	6.5	6.7	7.0	7.2	7.5	7.8	8.0	8.2	8.5
9.9	10.4	10.8	11.2	11.6	12.0	12.5	12.9	13.3	13.7
9.3	9.7	10.1	10.5	10.9	11.3	11.7	12.1	12.5	12.9
2.3	2.4	2.5	2.6	2.7	2.8	2.9	3.0	3.1	3.2

YOUR BODY WEIGHT—*continued*

ACTIVITY KG / LB	47 / 104	50 / 110	53 / 117	56 / 123	59 / 130	62 / 137	65 / 143	68 / 150
Judo	8.3	8.8	9.3	9.8	10.3	10.9	11.4	11.9
Jumping rope								
70 per min	7.6	8.1	8.6	9.1	9.6	10.0	10.5	11.0
80 per min	7.7	8.2	8.7	9.2	9.7	10.2	10.7	11.2
125 per min	8.3	8.9	9.4	9.9	10.4	11.0	11.5	12.0
145 per min	9.3	9.9	10.4	11.0	11.6	12.2	12.8	13.4
Kendo	9.3	9.7	10.2	10.8	11.4	12.0	12.6	13.2
Knitting, sewing	1.1	1.1	1.2	1.2	1.3	1.4	1.4	1.5
Lacrosse	7.0	7.4	7.9	8.3	8.7	9.2	9.6	10.1
Locksmith	2.8	2.9	3.0	3.2	3.4	3.5	3.7	3.9
Lying at ease	1.0	1.1	1.2	1.2	1.3	1.4	1.4	1.5
Machine-tooling								
machining	2.3	2.4	2.5	2.7	2.8	3.0	3.1	3.3
operating lathe	2.5	2.6	2.8	2.9	3.1	3.2	3.4	3.5
operating punch press	4.2	4.4	4.7	4.9	5.2	5.5	5.7	6.0
tapping and drilling	3.2	3.3	3.4	3.6	3.8	4.0	4.2	4.4
welding	2.4	2.6	2.8	2.9	3.1	3.2	3.4	3.5
working sheet metal	2.3	2.4	2.5	2.7	2.8	3.0	3.1	3.3
Marching, rapid	6.7	7.1	7.5	8.0	8.4	8.8	9.2	9.7
Mountain climbing	7.4	7.9	8.4	8.9	9.4	9.9	10.3	10.8
Motorcycle riding	6.5	6.9	7.3	7.7	8.1	8.5	8.9	9.3
Music playing								
accordion (sitting)	1.5	1.6	1.7	1.8	1.9	2.0	2.1	2.2
cello (sitting)	2.0	2.1	2.2	2.3	2.4	2.5	2.7	2.8
conducting	1.9	2.0	2.1	2.2	2.3	2.4	2.5	2.7
drums (sitting)	3.1	3.3	3.5	3.7	3.9	4.1	4.3	4.5
flute (sitting)	1.7	1.8	1.9	2.0	2.1	2.2	2.3	2.4
horn (sitting)	1.4	1.5	1.5	1.6	1.7	1.8	1.9	2.0
organ (sitting)	2.6	2.7	2.8	3.0	3.1	3.3	3.4	3.6
piano (sitting)	1.9	2.0	2.1	2.2	2.4	2.5	2.6	2.7
trumpet (standing)	1.5	1.6	1.6	1.7	1.8	1.9	2.0	2.1
violin (sitting)	2.2	2.3	2.4	2.5	2.7	2.8	2.9	3.1
woodwind (sitting)	1.5	1.6	1.7	1.8	1.9	2.0	2.1	2.2
Paddleball	8.5	8.9	9.4	10.0	10.5	11.0	11.6	12.1
Paddle tennis	8.4	8.6	9.1	9.6	10.1	10.7	11.1	11.7
Painting								
inside projects	1.6	1.7	1.8	1.9	2.0	2.1	2.2	2.3
outside projects	3.7	3.9	4.1	4.3	4.5	4.8	5.0	5.2
scraping	3.1	3.2	3.3	3.5	3.7	3.9	4.1	4.3
Planting seedings	3.3	3.5	3.7	3.9	4.1	4.3	4.6	4.8
Plastering	3.7	3.9	4.1	4.4	4.6	4.8	5.1	5.3
Printing press work	1.7	1.8	1.9	2.0	2.1	2.2	2.3	2.4
Racquetball	8.4	8.9	9.4	10.0	10.5	11.0	11.6	12.1
Roller skating								
inside, rink	5.4	5.7	6.0	6.4	6.7	7.1	7.4	7.7
outside, pavement	5.8	6.2	6.6	7.0	7.3	7.7	8.1	8.4
Rope jumping								
110 rpm	6.7	7.1	7.5	7.9	8.4	8.8	9.2	9.7
120 rpm	6.4	6.8	7.3	7.7	8.1	8.5	8.9	9.3
130 rpm	6.0	6.4	6.8	7.1	7.5	7.7	8.3	8.7
Rowing								
machine, moderate	5.7	6.0	6.3	6.7	7.0	7.4	7.7	8.1
machine, race pace	8.6	8.9	9.4	10.0	10.5	11.0	11.6	12.1
skull, leisure	4.7	5.0	5.3	5.5	5.9	6.2	6.4	6.8
skull, race pace	8.7	8.9	9.4	10.0	10.5	11.0	11.6	12.1
Running, cross-country	7.8	8.2	8.6	9.1	9.6	10.1	10.6	11.1
Running, on flat surface								
11 min, 30 s per mile	6.3	6.8	7.2	7.6	8.0	8.4	8.8	9.2
9 min per mile	9.1	9.7	10.2	10.8	11.4	12.0	12.5	13.1

71	**74**	**77**	**80**	**83**	**86**	**89**	**92**	**95**	**98**
157	**163**	**170**	**176**	**183**	**190**	**196**	**203**	**209**	**216**
12.4	13.0	13.5	14.0	14.5	15.1	15.6	16.1	16.6	17.2
11.5	12.0	12.5	13.0	13.4	13.9	14.4	14.9	15.4	15.9
11.6	12.1	12.6	13.1	13.6	14.1	14.6	14.6	15.6	16.1
12.6	13.1	13.6	14.2	14.7	15.2	15.8	16.3	16.8	17.3
14.0	14.6	15.2	15.8	16.4	16.9	17.5	18.1	18.7	19.3
13.7	14.3	14.9	15.5	16.1	16.7	17.3	17.8	18.4	19.0
1.6	1.6	1.7	1.8	1.8	1.9	2.0	2.0	2.1	2.2
10.4	10.7	11.0	11.2	11.5	11.8	12.1	12.4	12.7	13.0
4.0	4.2	4.4	4.6	4.7	4.9	5.1	5.2	5.4	5.6
1.6	1.6	1.7	1.8	1.8	1.9	2.0	2.0	2.1	2.2
3.4	3.6	3.7	3.8	4.0	4.1	4.3	4.4	4.6	4.7
3.7	3.8	4.0	4.2	4.3	4.5	4.6	4.8	4.9	5.1
6.2	6.5	6.8	7.0	7.3	7.6	7.8	8.1	8.4	8.6
4.6	4.8	5.0	5.2	5.4	5.6	5.8	6.0	6.2	6.4
3.7	3.8	4.0	4.2	4.3	4.5	4.6	4.8	4.9	5.1
3.4	3.6	3.7	3.8	4.0	4.1	4.3	4.4	4.6	4.7
10.1	10.5	10.9	11.4	11.8	12.2	12.6	13.1	13.5	13.9
11.3	11.7	12.2	12.7	13.2	13.7	14.1	14.6	15.0	15.6
9.7	10.1	10.5	10.9	11.3	11.7	12.1	12.5	12.9	13.3
2.3	2.4	2.5	2.6	2.7	2.8	2.8	2.9	3.0	3.1
2.9	3.0	3.2	3.3	3.4	3.5	3.6	3.8	3.9	4.0
2.8	2.9	3.0	3.1	3.2	3.4	3.5	3.6	3.7	3.8
4.7	4.9	5.1	5.3	5.5	5.7	5.9	6.1	6.3	6.6
2.5	2.6	2.7	2.8	2.9	3.0	3.1	3.2	3.3	3.4
2.1	2.1	2.2	2.3	2.4	2.5	2.6	2.7	2.8	2.8
3.8	3.9	4.1	4.2	4.4	4.6	4.7	4.9	5.0	5.2
2.8	3.0	3.1	3.2	3.3	3.4	3.6	3.7	3.8	3.9
2.2	2.3	2.4	2.5	2.6	2.7	2.8	2.9	2.9	3.0
3.2	3.3	3.5	3.6	3.7	3.9	4.0	4.1	4.3	4.4
2.3	2.4	2.5	2.6	2.7	2.8	2.8	2.9	3.0	3.1
12.6	13.2	13.7	14.2	14.8	15.3	15.8	16.4	16.9	17.4
12.2	12.7	13.2	13.7	14.2	14.2	15.2	15.8	16.3	16.8
2.4	2.5	2.6	2.7	2.8	2.9	3.0	3.1	3.2	3.3
5.5	5.7	5.9	6.2	6.4	6.6	6.9	7.1	7.3	7.5
4.5	4.7	4.9	5.0	5.2	5.4	5.6	5.8	6.0	6.2
5.0	5.2	5.4	5.6	5.8	6.0	6.2	6.4	6.7	6.9
5.5	5.8	6.0	6.2	6.5	6.7	6.9	7.2	7.4	7.6
2.5	2.6	2.7	2.8	2.9	3.0	3.1	3.2	3.3	3.4
12.6	13.2	13.7	14.2	14.8	15.3	15.8	16.4	16.9	17.4
8.1	8.4	8.8	9.1	9.4	9.8	10.1	10.5	10.8	11.1
8.8	9.2	9.6	9.9	10.3	10.7	11.1	11.4	11.8	12.2
10.1	10.5	10.5	11.3	11.8	12.2	12.6	13.1	13.5	13.9
9.8	10.1	10.6	10.9	11.4	11.8	12.2	12.6	13.0	13.4
9.1	9.4	9.8	10.2	10.6	11.0	11.3	11.7	12.1	12.5
8.5	8.9	9.3	9.7	10.1	10.6	11.1	11.6	12.1	12.6
12.6	13.2	13.7	14.2	14.8	15.3	15.8	16.4	16.9	17.4
7.2	7.6	8.0	8.4	8.8	9.2	9.6	10.0	10.4	10.8
12.6	13.2	13.7	14.2	14.8	15.3	15.8	16.4	16.9	17.4
11.6	12.1	12.6	13.0	13.5	14.0	14.5	15.0	15.5	16.0
9.6	10.0	10.5	10.9	11.3	11.7	12.1	12.5	12.9	13.3
13.7	14.3	14.9	15.4	16.0	16.6	17.2	17.8	18.3	18.9

YOUR BODY WEIGHT	KG	47	50	53	56	59	62	65	68
ACTIVITY	LB	104	110	117	123	130	137	143	150
Running, on flat surface, continued									
8 min per mile		9.8	10.8	11.3	11.9	12.5	13.1	13.6	14.2
7 min per mile		10.7	12.2	12.7	13.3	13.9	14.5	15.0	15.6
6 min per mile		11.8	13.9	14.4	15.0	15.6	16.2	16.7	17.3
5 min, 30 s per mile		13.6	14.5	15.3	16.2	17.1	17.9	18.8	19.7
Running—marathon									
5 h. 02 min (11:30 min/mi; 140 m/min)		5.5	5.8	6.2	6.5	6.9	7.2	7.6	7.9
4 h. 42 min (10:45 min/mi; 150 m/min)		5.9	6.3	6.7	7.1	7.5	7.9	8.2	8.6
4 h. 24 min (10:05 min/mi; 160 m/min)		6.5	6.9	7.3	7.7	8.1	8.5	8.9	9.3
4 h. 10 min (9:32 min/mi; 170 m/min)		7.0	7.4	7.8	8.2	8.7	9.1	9.6	10.0
3 h. 55 min (9:00 min/mi; 180 m/min)		7.4	7.9	8.3	8.8	9.3	9.8	10.2	10.7
3 h. 43 min (8:30 min/mi; 190 m/min)		7.9	8.4	8.9	9.4	9.9	10.4	10.9	11.4
3 h. 31 min (8:05 min/mi; 200 m/min)		8.4	8.9	9.4	10.0	10.5	11.0	11.6	12.1
3 h. 21 min (7:40 min/mi; 210 m/min)		8.8	9.4	10.0	10.5	11.1	11.7	12.2	12.8
3 h. 12 min (7:20 min/mi; 220 m/min)		9.3	9.9	10.5	11.1	11.7	12.3	12.9	13.5
3 h. 04 min (7:00 min/mi; 230 m/min)		9.8	10.4	11.0	11.7	12.3	12.9	13.5	14.2
Sailing, leisure		2.1	2.2	2.3	2.5	2.6	2.7	2.9	3.0
Scrubbing floors		5.1	5.5	5.8	6.1	6.4	6.8	7.1	7.4
Scuba diving		10.9	11.2	11.5	11.8	12.1	12.4	12.7	13.0
Shoe repair, general		2.2	2.3	2.4	2.5	2.7	2.8	2.9	3.1
Sitting quietly		1.0	1.1	1.1	1.2	1.2	1.3	1.4	1.4
Skateboarding		4.1	4.4	4.6	4.9	5.2	5.4	5.7	6.0
Skiing, hard snow									
level, moderate speed		5.6	6.0	6.3	6.7	7.0	7.4	7.7	8.1
level, walking speed		6.7	7.2	7.6	8.0	8.4	8.9	9.3	9.7
uphill, "fast" speed		12.9	13.7	14.5	15.3	16.2	17.0	17.8	18.6
Skiing, soft snow									
leisure (F)		4.6	4.9	5.2	5.5	5.8	6.1	6.4	6.7
leisure (M)		5.2	5.6	5.9	6.2	6.5	6.9	7.2	7.5
Skindiving									
considerable motion		13.0	13.8	14.6	15.5	16.3	17.1	17.9	18.8
moderate motion		9.7	10.3	10.9	11.5	12.2	12.8	13.4	14.0
Snorkeling		4.3	4.6	4.9	5.2	5.5	5.8	6.0	6.3
Snowshoeing, soft snow									
hiking, open fields, trails		6.6	7.0	7.4	7.8	8.3	8.7	9.1	9.5
jogging, moving fast with lightweight snowshoes		11.9	12.7	13.4	14.2	15.0	15.7	16.5	17.3
Snowmobiling			3.1	3.2	3.4	3.6	3.8	4.0	4.2
Soccer									
Casual, general		5.7	6.1	6.5	6.9	7.2	7.6	8.0	8.3
Competition		8.3	8.8	9.3	9.8	10.3	10.9	11.4	11.9
Softball									
fast or slow pitch, general		4.1	4.4	4.6	4.9	5.2	5.4	5.7	6.0
infield/outfield		4.7	5.0	5.3	5.6	5.9	6.2	6.5	6.8
officiating		3.3	3.5	3.7	3.9	4.1	4.3	4.6	4.8
pitching		5.0	5.3	5.6	5.9	6.2	6.5	6.8	7.1
Squash		9.9	10.5	11.1	11.8	12.4	13.0	13.7	14.3
Standing quietly (M)		1.3	1.4	1.4	1.5	1.6	1.7	1.8	1.8
Steel mill, working in									
fettling		4.3	4.5	4.7	5.0	5.3	5.5	5.8	6.1
forging		4.7	5.0	5.3	5.6	5.9	6.2	6.5	6.8
hand rolling		6.4	6.9	7.3	7.7	8.1	8.5	8.9	9.3
merchant mill rolling		6.8	7.3	7.7	8.1	8.6	9.0	9.4	9.9
removing slag		8.4	8.9	9.4	10.0	10.5	11.0	11.6	12.1

71 157	**74 163**	**77 170**	**80 176**	**83 183**	**86 190**	**89 196**	**92 203**	**95 209**	**98 216**
14.8	15.4	16.0	16.5	17.1	17.7	18.3	18.9	19.4	20.0
16.2	16.8	17.4	17.9	18.5	19.1	19.7	20.3	20.8	21.4
17.9	18.5	19.1	19.6	20.2	20.8	21.4	22.0	22.5	23.1
20.5	21.4	22.3	23.1	24.0	24.9	25.7	26.6	27.5	28.3
8.3	8.6	9.0	9.3	9.7	10.0	10.4	10.7	11.1	11.4
9.0	9.4	9.8	10.1	10.5	10.9	11.3	11.7	12.1	12.4
9.7	10.1	10.6	11.0	11.4	11.8	12.2	12.6	13.0	13.4
10.5	10.9	11.3	11.8	12.2	12.7	13.1	13.5	14.0	14.4
11.2	11.6	12.1	12.6	13.1	13.5	14.0	14.5	14.9	15.4
11.9	12.4	12.9	13.4	13.9	14.4	14.9	15.4	15.9	16.4
12.6	13.2	13.7	14.2	14.8	15.3	15.8	16.4	16.9	17.4
13.3	13.9	14.5	15.0	15.6	16.2	16.7	17.3	17.9	18.4
14.1	14.7	15.3	15.9	16.5	17.1	17.6	18.2	18.8	19.4
14.8	15.4	16.0	16.7	17.3	17.9	18.5	19.2	19.8	20.4
3.1	3.3	3.4	3.5	3.7	3.8	3.9	4.1	4.2	4.3
7.7	8.1	8.4	8.7	9.0	9.4	9.7	10.0	10.4	10.7
13.3	13.6	13.9	14.2	14.5	14.8	15.1	15.4	15.7	16.0
3.2	3.3	3.5	3.6	3.7	3.9	4.0	4.1	4.3	4.4
1.5	1.6	1.6	1.7	1.7	1.8	1.9	1.9	2.0	2.1
6.2	6.5	6.7	7.0	7.3	7.5	7.8	8.1	8.3	8.6
8.4	8.8	9.2	9.5	9.9	10.2	10.6	10.9	11.3	11.7
10.2	10.6	11.0	11.4	11.9	12.3	12.7	13.2	13.6	14.0
19.5	20.3	21.1	21.9	22.7	23.6	24.4	25.2	26.0	26.9
7.0	7.3	7.5	7.8	8.1	8.4	8.7	9.0	9.3	9.6
7.9	8.2	8.5	8.9	9.2	9.5	9.9	10.2	10.5	10.9
19.6	20.4	21.3	22.1	22.9	23.7	24.6	25.4	26.2	27.0
14.6	15.2	15.9	16.5	17.1	17.7	18.3	19.0	19.6	20.2
6.6	6.8	7.1	7.4	7.7	8.0	8.2	8.5	8.8	9.1
9.9	10.4	10.8	11.2	11.6	12.0	12.5	12.9	13.3	13.7
18.0	18.8	19.5	20.3	21.1	21.8	22.6	23.3	24.1	24.9
4.3	4.5	4.7	4.9	5.1	5.3	5.5	5.6	5.8	6.0
8.7	9.1	9.4	9.8	10.2	10.5	10.9	11.3	11.6	12.0
12.4	13.0	13.5	14.0	14.5	15.1	15.6	16.1	16.6	17.2
6.2	6.5	6.7	7.0	7.3	7.5	7.8	8.1	8.3	8.6
7.1	7.4	7.7	8.0	8.3	8.6	8.9	9.2	9.5	9.8
5.0	5.2	5.4	5.6	5.8	6.0	6.2	6.4	6.7	6.9
7.5	7.8	8.1	8.4	8.7	9.0	9.3	9.7	10.0	10.3
14.9	15.5	16.2	16.8	17.4	18.1	18.7	19.3	20.0	20.6
1.9	2.0	2.1	2.2	2.2	2.3	2.4	2.5	2.6	2.6
6.3	6.6	6.9	7.1	7.4	7.7	7.9	8.2	8.5	8.7
7.1	7.4	7.7	8.0	8.3	8.6	8.9	9.2	9.5	9.8
9.7	10.1	10.6	11.0	11.4	11.8	12.2	12.6	13.0	13.4
10.3	10.7	11.2	11.6	12.0	12.5	12.9	13.3	13.8	14.2
12.6	13.2	13.7	14.2	14.8	15.3	15.8	16.4	16.9	17.4

YOUR BODY WEIGHT

	KG 47	50	53	56	59	62	65	68
Activity	**LB 104**	**110**	**117**	**123**	**130**	**137**	**143**	**150**
Steel mill, working in, continued								
tending furnace	5.9	6.3	6.7	7.1	7.4	7.8	8.2	8.6
tipping molds	4.3	4.6	4.9	5.2	5.4	5.7	6.0	6.3
Surfing	3.9	4.1	4.3	4.5	4.8	5.0	5.3	5.5
Stock clerking	2.5	2.7	2.9	3.0	3.2	3.3	3.5	3.7
Swimming, fitness swims								
back stroke	7.9	8.5	9.0	9.5	10.0	10.5	11.0	11.5
breast stroke	7.6	8.1	8.6	9.1	9.6	10.0	10.5	11.0
butterfly		8.6	9.1	9.6	10.1	10.7	11.1	11.7
crawl, fast	7.3	7.8	8.3	8.7	9.2	9.7	10.1	10.6
crawl, slow	6.0	6.4	6.8	7.2	7.6	7.9	8.3	8.7
side stroke	5.7	6.1	6.5	6.8	7.2	7.6	7.9	8.3
treading, fast	8.0	8.5	9.0	9.5	10.0	10.5	11.1	11.6
treading, normal	2.9	3.1	3.3	3.5	3.7	3.8	4.0	4.2
Table tennis (ping pong)	3.2	3.4	3.6	3.8	4.0	4.2	4.4	4.6
Tailoring								
cutting	2.0	2.1	2.2	2.3	2.4	2.5	2.7	2.8
hand-sewing	1.5	1.6	1.7	1.8	1.9	2.0	2.1	2.2
machine-sewing	2.2	2.3	2.4	2.5	2.7	2.8	2.9	3.1
pressing	2.9	3.1	3.3	3.5	3.7	3.8	4.0	4.2
Tennis								
competition	6.9	7.3	7.8	8.2	8.7	9.1	9.5	9.9
recreational	5.1	5.5	5.8	6.1	6.4	6.8	7.1	7.4
Typing								
electric (computer)	1.3	1.4	1.4	1.5	1.6	1.7	1.8	1.8
manual	1.5	1.6	1.6	1.7	1.8	1.9	2.0	2.1
Volleyball								
beach, competition	7.2	7.7	8.2	8.6	9.1	9.5	10.0	10.5
beach, recreational	5.7	6.1	6.5	6.9	7.2	7.6	8.0	8.3
general ,recreational (6- to 9- member (team)	2.4	2.6	2.8	2.9	3.1	3.3	3.4	3.6
gymnasium, competition	3.3	3.5	3.7	3.9	4.1	4.3	4.6	4.8
no sand, competition (indoors, outdoors)	6.2	6.6	7.0	7.4	7.7	8.1	8.5	8.9
wallyball, general	5.7	6.1	6.5	6.9	7.2	7.6	8.0	8.3
water	2.4	2.6	2.8	2.9	3.1	3.3	3.4	3.6
Walking, leisure outdoors								
asphalt road	3.8	4.0	4.2	4.5	4.7	5.0	5.2	5.4
fields and hillsides	3.9	4.1	4.3	4.6	4.8	5.1	5.3	5.6
grass track	3.8	4.1	4.3	4.5	4.8	5.0	5.3	5.5
plowed field	3.6	3.9	4.1	4.3	4.5	4.8	5.0	5.2
Walking, treadmill level								
2.0 mph	2.4	2.6	2.8	3.0	3.1	3.3	3.4	3.6
2.5 mph	3.0	3.2	3.4	3.6	3.8	4.0	4.2	4.4
3.0 mph	3.6	3.8	4.0	4.2	4.4	4.6	4.8	5.0
3.5 mph	4.0	4.3	4.6	4.8	5.1	5.3	5.6	6.1
4.0 mph	4.6	4.9	5.2	5.4	5.7	6.0	6.3	6.6
Wallpapering	2.3	2.4	2.5	2.7	2.8	3.0	3.1	3.3
Water polo, recreational	7.0	7.4	7.7	8.1	8.5	8.9	9.3	9.7
Water polo, competition	9.4	9.9	10.4	11.0	11.5	12.0	12.5	13.1
Water-skiing	5.6	6.0	6.4	6.7	7.1	7.5	7.8	8.2
Watch repairing	1.2	1.3	1.3	1.4	1.5	1.6	1.6	1.7
Whitewater rafting, recreational	4.1	4.4	4.6	4.9	5.2	5.4	5.7	6.0
Window cleaning	2.9	3.0	3.1	3.3	3.5	3.7	3.8	4.0
Wind surfing	3.3	3.5	3.7	3.9	4.1	4.3	4.6	4.8
Wrestling, competition	9.1	9.7	10.3	10.8	11.4	12.0	12.6	13.2
Writing (sitting)	1.4	1.5	1.5	1.6	1.7	1.8	1.9	2.0
Yoga	2.9	3.1	3.3	3.5	3.7	3.8	4.0	4.2

71	**74**	**77**	**80**	**83**	**86**	**89**	**92**	**95**	**98**
157	**163**	**170**	**176**	**183**	**190**	**196**	**203**	**209**	**216**
8.9	9.3	9.7	10.1	10.5	10.8	11.2	11.6	12.0	12.3
6.5	6.8	7.1	7.4	7.6	7.9	8.2	8.5	8.7	9.0
5.7	6.0	6.3	6.5	6.8	7.0	7.2	7.4	7.6	7.9
3.8	4.0	4.2	4.3	4.5	4.6	4.8	5.0	5.1	5.3
12.0	12.5	13.0	13.5	14.0	14.5	15.0	15.5	16.1	16.6
11.5	12.0	12.5	13.0	13.4	13.9	14.4	14.9	15.4	15.9
12.2	12.7	13.2	13.7	14.2	14.2	15.2	15.8	16.3	16.8
11.1	11.5	12.0	12.5	12.9	13.4	13.9	14.4	14.8	15.3
9.1	9.5	9.9	10.2	10.6	11.0	11.4	11.8	12.2	12.5
8.7	9.0	9.4	9.8	10.1	10.5	10.9	11.2	11.6	12.0
12.1	12.6	13.1	13.6	14.1	14.6	15.1	15.6	16.2	16.7
4.4	4.6	4.8	5.0	5.1	5.3	5.5	5.7	5.9	6.1
4.8	5.0	5.2	5.4	5.6	5.8	6.1	6.3	6.5	6.7
2.9	3.0	3.2	3.3	3.4	3.5	3.6	3.8	3.9	4.0
2.3	2.4	2.5	2.6	2.7	2.8	2.8	2.9	3.0	3.1
3.2	3.3	3.5	3.6	3.7	3.9	4.0	4.1	4.3	4.4
4.4	4.6	4.8	5.0	5.1	5.3	5.5	5.7	5.9	6.1
10.2	10.6	11.1	11.5	11.9	12.4	12.8	13.2	13.7	14.1
7.7	8.1	8.4	8.7	9.0	9.4	9.7	10.0	10.4	10.7
1.9	2.0	2.1	2.2	2.2	2.3	2.4	2.5	2.6	2.6
2.2	2.3	2.4	2.5	2.6	2.7	2.8	2.9	2.9	3.0
10.9	11.4	11.9	12.3	12.8	13.2	13.7	14.2	14.6	15.1
8.7	9.1	9.4	9.8	10.2	10.5	10.9	11.3	11.6	12.0
3.7	3.9	4.0	4.2	4.4	4.5	4.7	4.8	5.0	5.1
5.0	5.2	5.4	5.6	5.8	6.0	6.2	6.4	6.7	6.9
9.3	9.7	10.1	10.5	10.9	11.3	11.7	12.1	12.5	12.9
8.7	9.1	9.4	9.8	10.2	10.5	10.9	11.3	11.6	12.0
3.7	3.9	4.0	4.2	4.4	4.5	4.7	4.8	5.0	5.1
5.7	5.9	6.2	6.4	6.6	6.9	7.1	7.4	7.6	7.8
5.8	6.1	6.3	6.6	6.8	7.1	7.3	7.5	7.8	8.0
5.8	6.0	6.2	6.5	6.7	7.0	7.2	7.5	7.7	7.9
5.5	5.7	5.9	6.2	6.4	6.6	6.9	7.1	7.3	7.5
3.7	3.9	4.1	4.2	4.4	4.5	4.7	4.9	5.0	5.2
4.5	4.7	4.9	5.1	5.3	5.5	5.7	5.9	6.1	6.3
5.3	5.5	5.7	5.9	6.2	6.5	6.7	6.9	7.1	7.3
6.1	6.4	6.6	6.9	7.1	7.4	7.7	7.9	8.2	8.4
6.9	7.2	7.5	7.8	8.1	8.4	8.7	8.9	9.2	9.5
3.4	3.6	3.7	3.8	4.0	4.1	4.3	4.4	4.6	4.7
10.1	10.5	10.9	11.3	11.7	12.1	12.5	12.9	13.3	13.7
13.6	14.1	14.7	15.2	15.7	16.3	16.8	17.3	17.9	18.4
8.7	9.1	9.4	9.8	10.1	10.5	10.9	11.2	11.6	12.0
1.8	1.9	1.9	2.0	2.1	2.2	2.2	2.3	2.4	2.5
6.2	6.5	6.7	7.0	7.3	7.5	7.8	8.1	8.3	8.6
4.2	4.4	4.5	4.7	4.9	5.1	5.3	5.4	5.6	5.8
5.0	5.2	5.4	5.6	5.8	6.0	6.2	6.4	6.7	6.9
13.8	14.3	14.9	15.5	16.1	16.7	17.2	17.8	18.4	19.0
2.1	2.1	2.2	2.3	2.4	2.5	2.6	2.7	2.8	2.8
4.4	4.6	4.8	5.0	5.1	5.3	5.5	5.7	5.9	6.1

Appendix D

Metabolic Computations in Open-Circuit Spirometry

STANDARDIZING GAS VOLUMES: ENVIRONMENTAL FACTORS

Gas volumes obtained during physiologic measurements are usually expressed in one of three ways: *ATPS, STPD,* or *BTPS.*

ATPS refers to the volume of gas at the specific conditions of measurement, at *A*mbient *T*emperature (273°K+ambient temperature, °C), ambient *P*ressure, and *S*aturated with water vapor. Gas volumes collected during open-circuit spirometry and pulmonary function tests are measured initially at ATPS.

A volume of a gas varies, however, depending on its temperature, pressure, and content of water vapor, even though the absolute number of gas molecules remains constant. These environmental influences are summarized as follows:

Temperature:	The volume of a gas varies *directly* with temperature. Increasing temperature causes the molecules to move more rapidly; the gas mixture expands, and the volume increases proportionately *(Charles' law).*
Pressure:	The volume of a gas varies *inversely* with pressure. Increasing pressure on a gas forces the molecules closer together, causing the volume to decrease in proportion to the increase in pressure *(Boyle's law).*
Water vapor:	The volume of a gas varies depending on its water vapor content. The volume of a gas is greater when it is saturated with water vapor than it is when the same gas is dry (i.e., contains no moisture).

These three factors—temperature, pressure, and the relative degree of saturation of the gas with water vapor—must be considered, especially when gas volumes are to be compared under different environmental conditions and used subsequently in metabolic and physiologic calculations. The standards that provide the frame of reference for expressing a volume of gas are either STPD or BTPS.

STPD refers to the volume of a gas expressed under *S*tandard conditions of *T*emperature (273°K or 0°C), *P*ressure (760 mm Hg), and *D*ry (no water vapor). Expressing a gas volume STPD, for example, makes it possible to evaluate and compare the volumes of expired air measured while running in the rain at high altitude, along a beach in the cold of winter, or in a hot desert environment below sea level. *In all metabolic calculations, gas volumes are always expressed at STPD.*

1. To reduce a gas volume to standard temperature (ST), the following formula is applied:

$$\text{Gas volume ST} = V_{ATPS} \times \frac{273°K}{273°K + T°C} \quad (1)$$

where T°C = temperature of the gas in the measuring device and 273°K = absolute temperature Kelvin, which is equivalent to 0°C.

2. The following equation is used to express a gas volume at standard pressure (SP):

$$\text{Gas volume SP} = V_{ATPS} \times \frac{P_B}{760 \text{ mm Hg}} \quad (2)$$

where P_B = ambient barometric pressure in mm Hg and 760 = standard barometric pressure at sea level, mm Hg.

3. To reduce a gas to standard dry (SD) conditions, the effects of water vapor pressure at the particular environmental temperature must be subtracted from the volume of gas. Because expired air is 100% saturated with water vapor, it is not necessary to determine its percent saturation from measures of relative humidity. The vapor pressure in moist or completely humidified air at a particular ambient temperature can be obtained in Table D.1 and is expressed in mm Hg. This vapor pressure (P_{H_2O}) is then subtracted from the ambient

TABLE D.1 ➤ VAPOR PRESSURE (P_{H_2O}) OF WET GAS AT TEMPERATURES NORMALLY ENCOUNTERED IN THE LABORATORY

T (°C)	P_{H_2O} (mm Hg)	T (°C)	P_{H_2O} (mm Hg)
20	17.5	31	33.7
21	18.7	32	35.7
22	19.8	33	37.7
23	21.1	34	39.9
24	22.4	35	42.2
25	23.8	36	44.6
26	25.2	37	47.1
27	26.7	38	49.7
28	28.4	39	52.4
29	30.0	40	55.3
30	31.8		

barometric pressure (PB) to reduce the gas to standard pressure dry (SPD) as follows:

$$\text{Gas volume SPD} = V_{ATPS} \times \frac{P_B - P_{H_2O}}{760} \quad (3)$$

By combining equations (1) and (3), any volume of moist air can be converted to STPD as follows:

$$\text{Gas volume STPD} = V_{ATPS}\left(\frac{273}{273 + T°C}\right)\left(\frac{P_B - P_{H_2O}}{760}\right) \quad (4)$$

Fortunately, these computations need not be carried out, because the appropriate *STPD correction factors* have already been calculated for moist gas in the range of temperatures and pressures ordinarily encountered in most laboratories. These factors are presented in Table D.2. Multiplying any gas volume ATPS by the appropriate correction factor gives the same gas volume STPD that would be obtained if values for the ambient temperature, barometric pressure, and water vapor pressure were substituted in equation (4).

The term *BTPS* refers to a volume of a gas expressed at *B*ody *T*emperature (usually 273°K + 37°C or 310°K), ambient *P*ressure (whatever the barometer reads), and *S*aturated with water vapor with a partial pressure of 47 mm Hg at 37°C. Conventionally, pulmonary physiologists express lung volumes such as vital capacity, inspiratory and expiratory capacity, residual lung volume, and the dynamic measures of lung function such as maximum breathing capacity at body temperature and moist, or BTPS. The following equation converts a gas volume ATPS to BTPS:

TABLE D.2 ➤ FACTORS TO REDUCE MOIST GAS TO A DRY GAS VOLUME AT 0°C AND 760 mm Hg

Barometric	Temperature (°C)																	
Reading	15	16	17	18	19	20	21	22	23	24	25	26	27	28	29	30	31	32
700	0.855	851	847	842	838	834	829	825	821	816	812	807	802	797	793	788	783	778
702	857	853	849	845	840	836	832	827	823	818	814	809	805	800	795	790	785	780
704	860	856	852	847	843	839	834	830	825	821	816	812	807	802	797	792	787	783
706	862	858	854	850	845	841	837	832	828	823	819	814	810	804	800	795	790	785
708	865	861	856	852	848	843	839	834	830	825	821	816	812	807	802	797	792	787
710	867	863	859	855	850	846	842	837	833	828	824	819	814	809	804	799	795	790
712	870	866	861	857	853	848	844	839	836	830	826	821	817	812	807	802	797	792
714	872	868	864	859	855	851	846	842	837	833	828	824	819	814	809	804	799	794
716	875	871	866	862	858	853	849	844	840	835	831	826	822	816	812	807	802	797
718	877	873	869	864	860	856	851	847	842	838	833	828	824	819	814	809	804	799
720	880	876	871	867	863	858	854	849	845	840	836	831	826	821	816	812	807	802
722	882	878	874	869	865	861	856	852	847	843	838	833	829	824	819	814	809	804
724	885	880	876	872	867	863	858	854	849	845	840	835	831	826	821	816	811	806
726	887	883	879	874	870	866	861	856	852	847	843	838	833	829	824	818	813	808
728	890	886	881	877	872	868	863	859	854	850	845	840	836	831	826	821	816	811
730	892	888	884	879	875	871	866	861	857	852	847	843	838	833	828	823	818	813
732	895	890	886	882	877	873	868	864	859	854	850	845	840	836	831	825	820	815
734	897	893	889	884	880	875	871	866	862	857	852	847	843	838	833	828	823	818
736	900	895	891	887	882	878	873	869	864	859	855	850	845	840	835	830	825	820
738	902	898	894	889	885	880	876	871	866	862	857	852	848	843	838	833	828	822
740	905	900	896	892	887	883	878	874	869	864	860	855	850	845	840	835	830	825
742	907	903	898	894	890	885	881	876	871	867	862	857	852	847	842	837	832	827
744	910	906	901	897	892	888	883	878	874	869	864	859	855	850	845	840	834	829
746	912	908	903	899	895	890	886	881	876	872	867	862	857	852	847	842	837	832
748	915	910	906	901	897	892	888	883	879	874	869	864	860	854	850	845	839	834
750	917	913	908	904	900	895	890	886	881	876	872	867	862	857	852	847	842	837
752	920	915	911	906	902	897	893	888	883	879	874	869	864	859	854	849	844	839
754	922	918	913	909	904	900	895	891	886	881	876	872	867	862	857	852	846	841
756	925	920	916	911	907	902	898	893	888	883	879	874	869	864	859	854	849	844
758	927	923	918	914	909	905	900	896	891	886	881	876	872	866	861	856	851	846
760	930	925	921	916	912	907	902	898	893	888	883	879	874	869	864	859	854	848
762	932	928	923	919	914	910	905	900	896	891	886	881	876	871	866	861	856	851
764	936	930	926	921	916	912	907	903	898	893	888	884	879	874	869	864	858	853
766	937	933	928	924	919	915	910	905	900	896	891	886	881	876	871	866	861	855
768	940	935	931	926	922	917	912	908	903	898	893	888	883	878	873	868	863	858
770	942	938	933	928	924	919	915	910	905	901	896	891	886	881	876	871	865	860

TABLE D.3 ➤ **BTPS[a] FACTORS**

T (°C)	BTPS	T (°C)	BTPS
20	1.102	29	1.051
21	1.096	30	1.045
22	1.091	31	1.039
23	1.085	32	1.032
24	1.080	33	1.026
25	1.075	34	1.020
26	1.068	35	1.014
27	1.063	36	1.007
28	1.057	37	1.000

[a]Body temperature, ambient pressure, and saturated with water vapor.

Gas volume BTPS =

$$V_{ATPS}\left(\frac{P_B - P_{H_2O}}{P_B - 47 \text{ mm Hg}}\right)\left(\frac{310}{273 + T°C}\right) \quad (5)$$

As was the case with the correction to STPD, appropriate BTPS *correction factors* are available for converting a moist gas volume at ambient conditions to a volume BTPS. These BTPS factors for a broad range of ambient temperatures are presented in Table D.3. The factors have been computed assuming a barometric pressure of 760 mm Hg, and small deviations (±10 mm Hg) from this pressure introduce only a minimal error.

CALCULATION OF OXYGEN CONSUMPTION

In determining oxygen consumption by open-circuit spirometry, we are interested in knowing how much oxygen has been removed from the *inspired air*. Because the composition of inspired air remains relatively constant (CO_2 = 0.03%, O_2 = 20.93%, N_2 = 79.04%), it is possible to determine the oxygen removed from the inspired air by measuring the amount and composition of the expired air. This measurement indicates that the expired air contains more carbon dioxide (usually 2.5 to 5.0%), less oxygen (usually 15.0 to 18.5%), and more nitrogen (usually 79.04 to 79.60%). However, nitrogen is inert in terms of metabolism; any change in its concentration in expired air reflects the fact that the number of oxygen molecules removed from the inspired air is not replaced by the same number of carbon dioxide molecules produced in metabolism. This results in the volume of expired air (VE, STPD) being unequal to the inspired volume (VI, STPD). For example, if the respiratory quotient is less than 1.00 (i.e., less CO_2 produced in relation to O_2 consumed), and 3 liters of air are inspired, *less* than 3 liters of air will be expired. This produces a higher nitrogen concentration in expired air than in inspired air. This is not to say that nitrogen has been produced, only that nitrogen molecules now represent a larger percentage of VE compared to VI. In fact, VE differs from VI in direct proportion to the change in nitrogen concentration between the inspired and expired volumes. Thus, VI can be determined from VE using the relative change in nitrogen in an equation known as the *Haldane transformation.*

$$V_I, STPD = V_E, STPD \times \frac{\%N_2E}{\%N_2I} \quad (6)$$

where $\%N_2I$ = 79.04 and $\%N_2E$ = percent nitrogen in expired air computed from gas analysis as $[(100 - (\%O_2E + \%CO_2)]$.

The volume of O_2 in the inspired air (VO_2I) can then be determined as follows:

$$VO_2I = V_I \times \%O_2I \quad (7)$$

Substituting equation (6) for VI,

$$VO_2I = V_E \times \frac{\%N_2E}{79.04\%} \times \%O_2I \quad (8)$$

where $\%O_2I = 20.93\%$

The amount or volume of oxygen in the expired air (VO_2E) is computed as

$$VO_2E = V_E \times \%O_2E \quad (9)$$

where $\%O_2E$ is the fractional concentration of oxygen in expired air determined by gas analysis (chemical or electronic methods).

The amount of O_2 removed from the inspired air *each minute* ($\dot{V}O_2$) can then be computed as follows:

$$\dot{V}O_2 = (\dot{V}_I \times \%O_2I) - (\dot{V}_E \times \%O_2E) \quad (10)$$

By substitution

$$\dot{V}O_2 = \left\{\left[\left(\dot{V}_E \times \frac{\%N_2E}{79.04\%}\right) \times 20.93\%\right] - (\dot{V}_E \times \%O_2E)\right\} \quad (11)$$

where $\dot{V}O_2$ = volume of oxygen consumed per minute, expressed in milliliters or liters, and $\dot{V}_E$ = expired air volume per minute expressed in milliliters or liters.
Equation (11) can be simplified to:

$$\dot{V}O_2 = \dot{V}_E\left[\left(\frac{\%N_2E}{79.04\%} \times 20.93\%\right) - \%O_2E\right] \quad (12)$$

The final form of the equation is:

$$\dot{V}O_2 = \dot{V}_E[(\%N_2E \times 0.265) - \%O_2E] \quad (13)$$

The value obtained within the brackets in equations (12) and (13) is referred to as the *true O_2;* this represents the "oxygen extraction" or, more precisely, the percentage of oxygen consumed for any volume of air *expired.*

Although equation (13) is the equation used most widely to compute oxygen consumption from measures of expired air, it is also possible to calculate $\dot{V}O_2$ from direct measurements of both $\dot{V}_I$ and $\dot{V}_E$. In this case, the Haldane transformation is not used, and oxygen consumption is calculated directly as:

$$\dot{V}O_2 = (\dot{V}_I \times 20.93) - (\dot{V}_E \times \%O_2E) \quad (14)$$

In situations in which only $\dot{V}_I$ is measured, the $\dot{V}_E$ can be calculated from the Haldane transformation as:

$$\dot{V}_E = \dot{V}_I \frac{\%N_2I}{\%N_2E}$$

By substitution in equation (14), the computational equation is:

$$\dot{V}O_2 = \dot{V}_I\left[\%O_2I - \left(\frac{\%N_2I}{\%N_2E} \times \%O_2E\right)\right] \quad (15)$$

CALCULATION OF CARBON DIOXIDE PRODUCTION

The carbon dioxide production per minute ($\dot{V}CO_2$) is calculated as follows:

$$\dot{V}CO_2 = \dot{V}_E(\%CO_{2_E} - \%CO_2I) \quad (16)$$

where $\%CO_{2_E}$ = percent carbon dioxide in expired air determined by gas analysis, and $\%CO_2I$ = percent carbon dioxide in inspired air, which is essentially constant at 0.03%.

The final form of the equation is:

$$\dot{V}CO_2 = \dot{V}_E(\%CO_2E - 0.03\%) \quad (17)$$

CALCULATION OF RESPIRATORY QUOTIENT

The respiratory quotient (RQ) is calculated in one of two ways:

1. $RQ = \dot{V}CO_2 / \dot{V}O_2$ (18)

or

2. $RQ = \dfrac{(\%CO_2E - 0.03\%)}{\text{“true” } O_2}$ (19)

SAMPLE METABOLIC CALCULATIONS

The following data were obtained during the last minute of a steady-rate, 10-minute treadmill run performed at 6 miles per hour at a 5% grade.

$\dot{V}_E$: 62.1 liters, ATPS
Barometric pressure: 750 mm Hg
Temperature: 26°C
$\%O_2$ expired: 16.86 (O_2 analyzer)
$\%CO_2$ expired: 3.60 (CO_2 analyzer)
$\%N_2$ expired: [100 − (16.86 + 3.60)] = 79.54

Determine the following:

1. $\dot{V}_E$, STPD
2. $\dot{V}O_2$, STPD
3. $\dot{V}CO_2$ STPD
4. RQ
5. $kcal \cdot min^{-1}$

1. $\dot{V}_E$, STPD (use equation 4 or STPD correction factor in Table D.2).

$$\dot{V}_E, STPD = \dot{V}_E, ATPS\left(\frac{273}{273 + T°C}\right)\left(\frac{P_B - P_{H_2O}}{760}\right)$$

$$= 62.1\left(\frac{273}{299}\right)\left(\frac{750 - 25.2}{760}\right)$$

$$= 62.1\ (0.913 \times 0.954)$$

$$= 54.07\ L \cdot min^{-1}$$

2. $\dot{V}O_2$, STPD (use equation 13)

$$\dot{V}O_2, STPD = \dot{V}_E, STPD\ [(\%N_2E \times 0.265) - \%O_2E]$$

$$= 54.07\ [(0.7954 \times 0.265) - 0.1686]$$

$$= 54.07\ (0.0422)$$

$$= 2.281\ L \cdot min^{-1}$$

3. $\dot{V}CO_2$, STPD (use equation 17)

$$\dot{V}CO_2, STPD = \dot{V}_E, STPD\ (\%CO_2E - 0.03\%)$$

$$= 54.07\ (0.0360 - 0.0003)$$

$$= 54.07\ (0.0357)$$

$$= 1.930\ L \cdot min^{-1}$$

4. RQ (use equation 18 or 19)

$$RQ = \dot{V}CO_2/\dot{V}O_2$$

$$= \frac{1.930\ L\ CO_2 \cdot min^{-1}}{2.281\ L\ O_2 \cdot min^{-1}}$$

$$= 0.846$$

or

$$RQ = \frac{(\%CO_2E - 0.03\%)}{\text{“true” } O_2}$$

$$= \frac{3.60 - .03}{4.22}$$

$$= 0.846$$

Because the exercise was performed in a steady rate of aerobic metabolism, the obtained RQ of 0.846 can be applied in Table 8.1 to obtain the appropriate caloric transformation. In this way, the exercise oxygen consumption can be transposed to kcal of energy expended per minute as follows:

5. Energy expenditure ($kcal \cdot min^{-1}$) = $\dot{V}O_2$ ($L \cdot min^{-1}$) × caloric equivalent per liter O_2 at the given steady-rate RQ

$$\text{Energy expenditure} = 2.281 \times 4.862$$

$$= 11.09\ kcal \cdot min^{-1}$$

Assuming that the RQ value reflects the nonprotein RQ, a reasonable estimate of both the percentage and quantity of lipid and carbohydrate metabolized during each minute of the run can be obtained from Table 8.1.

Percentage kcal derived from lipid = 50.7%
Percentage kcal derived from carbohydrate = 49.3%
Grams of lipid utilized = 0.267 g per liter of oxygen or approximately 0.61 g per minute (0.267 × 2.281 L O_2)
Grams of carbohydrate utilized = 0.580 g per literof oxygen or approximately 1.36 g per minute (0.580 ×2.281 L O_2)

Appendix E

Honors and Awards of Interviewees

STEVEN N. BLAIR

Fellow: American College of Epidemiology, American Epidemiological Society, Council on Epidemiology, American Heart Association, American College of Sports Medicine (ACSM), American Academy of Kinesiology and Physical Education, (AAKPE), The Society of Behavioral Medicine, North American Association for the Study of Obesity, The Advancement of Sound Science Coalition; Health Educator of the Year Award, South Carolina Association for Health Education Honor Award, Association for Research, Administration, Professional Councils, and Societies, American Association Health, Physical Education, Recreation, & Dance (AAHPERD); Scholar Award, Southern District American Association for Health, Physical Education, Recreation, & Dance (AAHPERD); South Carolina AAHPERD Scholar Award; W.W. Patty Distinguished Alumni Award, Indiana University; Wellner Distinguished Scholar, Frostburg State University; Citation Award, ACSM; Doctor Honoris Causa degree, Free University of Brussels; R. Tait McKenzie Recognition Award, AAHPERD; Presidential Citation, AAHPERD; Distinguished Scholar, University of Memphis; Healthy American Fitness Leader; IHRSA Person of the Year; Doctor of Health Science Degree, Lander University; IDEA Lifetime Achievement Award; ICSSPE Gold Medal; Surgeon General's Medallion; Honor Award, Texas Regional Chapter of the ACSM; Award of Meritorious Achievement of the American Heart Association; Landsdowne Scholar, University of Victoria; William G. Anderson Commemorative Award; President, AAKPE; President, ACSM.

FRANK W. BOOTH

Outstanding teaching recognition (Basic Sciences Teaching Award, Best Teacher Award, Outstanding Advisor Award, Best Teacher in Physiology, John H. Freeman Outstanding Teaching Award for best Basic Science teacher, Dean's Teaching List, Graduate School of Biomedical Sciences Dean's Excellence in Teaching Awards, Most approachable lecturer award); Citation Classic in *Current Contents* 31, April 18, 1988; MERIT Award, NIH; Citation Award, American College of Sports Medicine; Board of Trustees, American College of Sports Medicine; Vice President, American College of Sports Medicine; Board of Directors, Texas Space Consortium; Chair, Muscle Biology Peer Review Panel, NASA (2000).

CLAUDE BOUCHARD

Honor Award Canadian Association of Sport Sciences; Honor and Citation Awards, American College of Sports Medicine; Benjamin Delessert Award in Nutrition (French); Willendorf Award, International Association for the Study of Obesity; Sandoz Award, Canadian Atherosclerosis Society; Albert Creff Award in Nutrition, French National Academy of Medicine; American Academy of Kinesiology; TOPS Award, North American Association for the Study of Obesity; W. Henry Sebrell Award, Weight Watchers Foundation; Honoris Causa Doctorate in Science, Katholieke Universiteit Leuven; member, Royal Academy of Medicine of Belgium; Donald B. Brown Research Chair on Obesity, Laval University; and President, International Association for the Study of Obesity.

DAVID L. COSTILL

Ball State University Outstanding Researcher Award; McClintock Award for Research and Writing; Ball State University Alumni Association Study-Abroad Award; Runner's World National Running Award 1976-1977. President, American College of Sports Medicine; Elected to Fellowship, American Academy of Kinesiology, U.S . Olympic Committee on Sports Medicine; James Ashmore Research Award, American Diabetes Association; Nurmi Scientific Achievement Award; Peter V. Karpovich Distinguished Lecturer, Springfield College, MA. Citation Award, American College of Sports Medicine, Senior International Research Fellowship (Fogarty Institute of the National Institutes of Health), Oslo, Norway; Nurmi Scientific Achievement Award; Alliance Scholar. American Alliance for Health, Physical Education, Recreation and Dance; Delbert Oberteuffer Lecture, Ohio State University, Columbus, OH; D. B. Dilland Wolffe Lectures, American College of Sports Medicine, Las Vegas, NV; The Tom Anderson Memorial Lecture, Christchurch, New Zealand; C. H. McCloy Research Lecturer, American Alliance for Health, Physical Education, Recreation and Dance; Senator Dick Lugar's Vitae Bonae Award; Honor Award, American College of Sports Medicine; Appointed John and Janice Fisher Chair in Exercise Science, Ball State University; Thomas K. Cureton Award, National Fitness Leaders Association.

BARBARA L. DRINKWATER

Honor Award and Citation Award, American College of Sports Medicine; President, American College of Sports Medicine; Joseph B. Wolffe Memorial Lecturer, American College of Sports Medicine; Fellow, American College of Sports Medicine; Member, American Physiological Society; Member, American Academy of Kinesiology and Physical Education; Distinguished Alumni Award, University of North Carolina; Distinguished Achievement Award, Douglass College, Rutgers University; DeMontfort University, UK Honorary D. Sc.; Research Award, Council on Aging and Adult Development; Raymond A. Weiss Lecturer, C. H. McCloy Lecturer, R. Tait McKenzie Lecturer, Honor Award, American Association, Physical Education, Health, Recreation, and Dance.

JOHN O. HOLLOSZY

American College of Sports Medicine (ACSM) Citation and Honor Awards; Research Group on Biochemistry of Exercise Honor Award for Scientific Achievements; International Olympic Committee Prize 2000; Elected Member or Fellow of the American Society of Biological Chemists, American Physiological Society, American Society of Clinical Investigation, American Institute of Nutrition and American Society for Clinical Nutrition, the Gerontological Society of America, American Diabetes Association, ACSM, American Heart Association (AHA) and AHA Council on Epidemiology, American Federation for Clinical Research, Sigma XI, and the American Geriatrics Society.

LORING B. ROWELL

Established Investigator of the American Heart Association; Fullbright Scholar; Citation Award (ACSM, 1983); Honor Award (ACSM, 1997); Editorial Boards (*American Journal of Physiology*, *Journal of Applied Physiology*, *Circulation Research*); NIH Study section.

BENGT SALTIN

International Olympic Committee Prize, 2002; Docent in exercise physiology, Karolinska Institute, Stockholm; Member of the Danish Academy of Sciences; American College of Sport Science Citation Award and Honor Award; Doctor Honoris Causa, University of Paris, France, University of Athens, Greece, University of Guelph, Canada, Aristotle University, Thessaloniki, Greece, Norwegian University of Physical Education, Oslo, Norway, University of Tartu, Estonia, University of Jyväskylä, Finland; The Order of the Dannebrog, 1st degree (Royal Danish Order of Chivalry); The Novo Nordisk Award 1999; First 1973 Wolff Lecture, American College of Sports Medicine; First 1989 International Olympic Committee Conference Opening lecture; A.D. Adolph Inauguration Lecture; 1996 Opening Pre-Olympic International Olympic Committee Conference Lecture; 1998 Gollnick Tutorial Lecture, American College of Sports Medicine; First President of the European College of Sport Science; First Editor-in-Chief of the Scandinavian Journal of Medicine and Science in Sports; Member of panels evaluating basic biological and physiological research in Lithuania and Norway; Board member and President of the International Orienteering Federation.

CHARLES M. TIPTON

Honor Award and Citation Award, American College of Sports Medicine; Honor Award, Environmental and Exercise Physiology Section, American Physiological Society; Gatorade Award for Excellence in Teaching; Recognition Award, Southwest Regional Chapter, American College of Sports Medicine; Vice-President for Physiology, American College of Sports Medicine; President, American College of Sports Medicine; Editor-In-Chief, *Medicine and Science in Sports and Exercise*; Associate Editor, *Journal of Applied Physiology*; FASEB Visiting Scholar to Minority Schools; Member, NASA-AIBS-IDI Review Panels for Fluids and Electrolytes, Physiology, Space Medicine, Countermeasures, Cardiopulmonary Physiology, Muscle Function and Atrophy, and Research Facilities. Member and Chair, NIH Applied Physiology and Bioengineering Study Section, Member NIH Physician-Scientists Study Section; Chair, APS Section for Environmental and Exercise Physiology.

Index

Page numbers in *italics* denote figures; those followed by a t denote tables.